W9-BGM-324

The 5-Minute Pediatric Consult

SIXTH EDITION

ASSOCIATE EDITORS

Louis M. Bell, Jr., MD
Professor of Pediatrics at the University of Pennsylvania
Associate Chair of Clinical Activities
Chief, Division of General Pediatrics
The Department of Pediatrics
Children's Hospital of Philadelphia
Philadelphia, Pennsylvania

Peter M. Bingham, MD
Associate Professor
Department of Pediatric Neurology
University of Vermont
Burlington, Vermont

Esther K. Chung, MD, MPH
Professor of Pediatrics
Jefferson Medical College, Thomas Jefferson University
Nemours – Philadelphia
Philadelphia, Pennsylvania
Nemours/A.I. duPont Hospital for Children
Wilmington, Delaware

David F. Friedman, MD
Clinical Assistant Professor of Pediatrics at the University
    of Pennsylvania
Perelman School of Medicine
Division of Pediatric Hematology
Children's Hospital of Philadelphia
Philadelphia, Pennsylvania

Kathleen M. Loomes, MD
Associate Professor of Pediatrics, Perelman School of
    Medicine at the University of Pennsylvania
Division of Gastroenterology, Hepatology and Nutrition
The Children's Hospital of Philadelphia
Philadelphia, Pennsylvania

Petar Mamula, MD
Associate Professor of Pediatrics at the
    University of Pennsylvania
Division of Gastroenterology, Hepatology and Nutrition
Children's Hospital of Philadelphia
Philadelphia, Pennsylvania

Maria R. Mascarenhas, MBBS
Associate Professor of Pediatrics at the
    University of Pennsylvania
Division of Gastroenterology, Hepatology and Nutrition
Children's Hospital of Philadelphia
Philadelphia, Pennsylvania

Ronn E. Tanel, MD
Associate Professor of Pediatrics
UCSF School of Medicine
Director, Pediatric Arrhythmia Center
Division of Pediatric Cardiology
UCSF Children's Hospital
San Francisco, California

ASSISTANT EDITOR

Charles I. Schwartz, MD
Clinical Assistant Professor of Pediatrics
University of Pennsylvania School of Medicine
Philadelphia, Pennsylvania

MANAGING EDITOR

Cheryl Polchenko
General Pediatrics
Children's Hospital of Philadelphia
Philadelphia, Pennsylvania

The 5-Minute Pediatric Consult

SIXTH EDITION

Editor

M. William Schwartz, MD
Emeritus Professor of Pediatrics
Perelman School of Medicine University of Pennsylvania
Formerly, Senior Physician
Children's Hospital of Philadelphia
Philadelphia, Pennsylvania

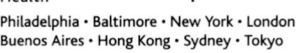. Wolters Kluwer | Lippincott Williams & Wilkins
Health
Philadelphia · Baltimore · New York · London
Buenos Aires · Hong Kong · Sydney · Tokyo

Acquisitions Editor: Rebecca Gaertner
Managing Editor: Nicole Walz
Project Manager: Bridgett Dougherty
Senior Manufacturing Manager: Benjamin Rivera
Marketing Manager: Kimberly Schonberger
Design Coordinator: Teresa Mallon
Production Services: Aptara, Inc.

6th Edition
© 2012 by Lippincott Williams & Wilkins, a Wolters Kluwer business
530 Walnut Street
Philadelphia, PA 19106
LWW.com

5th Edition © 2008 by Lippincott Williams & Wilkins; 4th Edition © 2005 by Lippincott Williams & Wilkins

All rights reserved. This book is protected by copyright. No part of this book may be reproduced in any form or by any means, including photocopying, or utilizing by any information storage and retrieval system without written permission from the copyright owner, except for brief quotations embodied in critical articles and reviews.

The 5-Minute Logo 〔5〕 is a registered trademark of Lippincott Williams & Wilkins. This mark may not be used without written permission from the publisher.

Printed in China

Library of Congress Cataloging-in-Publication Data

The 5-minute pediatric consult / [edited by] M. William Schwartz; associate editors, Louis M. Bell, Jr. ...[et al.]; assistant editor, Charles I. Schwartz. – 6th ed.
       p. ; cm. – (5-minute consult series)
   Five-minute pediatric consult
   Includes bibliographical references and index.
   ISBN 978-1-4511-1656-4 (hardback : alk. paper)
   ISBN 978-1-4511-8338-2
   I. Schwartz, M. William, 1935-   II. Title: Five-minute pediatric consult.   III. Series: 5-minute consult.
   [DNLM: 1. Pediatrics–Handbooks. WS 39]
   618.92–dc23

                                                                      2012012664

Care has been taken to confirm the accuracy of the information presented and to describe generally accepted practices. However, the authors, editors, and publisher are not responsible for errors or omissions or for any consequences from application of the information in this book and make no warranty, expressed or implied, with respect to the currency, completeness, or accuracy of the contents of the publication. Application of this information in a particular situation remains the professional responsibility of the practitioner.

The authors, editors, and publisher have exerted every effort to ensure that drug selection and dosage set forth in this text are in accordance with current recommendations and practice at the time of publication. However, in view of ongoing research, changes in government regulations, and the constant flow of information relating to drug therapy and drug reactions, the reader is urged to check the package insert for each drug for any change in indications and dosage and for added warnings and precautions. This is particularly important when the recommended agent is a new or infrequently employed drug.

Some drugs and medical devices presented in this publication have Food and Drug Administration (FDA) clearance for limited use in restricted research settings. It is the responsibility of health care providers to ascertain the FDA status of each drug or device planned for use in their clinical practice.

The publishers have made every effort to trace copyright holders for borrowed material. If they have inadvertently overlooked any, they will be pleased to make the necessary arrangements at the first opportunity.

To purchase additional copies of this book, call our customer service department at (800) 638-3030 or fax orders to (301) 223-2320. International customers should call (301) 223-2300.

Visit Lippincott Williams & Wilkins on the Internet: at LWW.com. Lippincott Williams & Wilkins customer service representatives are available from 8:30 am to 6 pm, EST.

                                                  10 9 8 7 6 5 4 3 2 1

CCS0512

WS: To Susan, David, Charlie, Brandie, Mitchell, Caroline, and Chloe

LB: To my mom and dad, Deasue and Louis. Thank you for all of the intangibles

PB: For Nishan, at the beginning

EC: In Memory of Dr. Ed Baik Chung and Dr. Okhyung Kang and Dennis, Marissa and Emma Lee

DF: To Marisa, Elias, Henry, and Isabel

KML: To my mother Joan

PM: To my family and patients

MM: To my wonderful family. Thanks for all your support

RT: To Sarah, Meghan, Lauren, and my many teachers and mentors

PREFACE

This sixth edition of *The 5-Minute Pediatric Consult* attests to the continuing value to the readers of the content and innovative format. A sixth edition! Wow! I look back on the history of this text and now website with pride and much pleasure. When the first edition was proposed in 1995, the new format of the 5-Minute series intrigued me. The innovative design, fitting well into the evolving computer technology, first Personal Digital Assistants and then the internet, has led to wide acceptance of this presentation that provides easy access to important information. The popularity of *The 5-Minute Pediatric Consult* is a testimony to the excellent work of the authors and editors who write the chapters, and to the editorial and production staff who transform the pages into the final book and website.

This edition contains many chapters rewritten by a group of new authors as well as refinement of all chapters. There are a number of new topics written by child psychiatrists such as separation anxiety, substance abuse, and obsessive compulsive disorders. My thanks to Pace Ducket for recruiting these authors. We added new topics such as narcolepsy, dental trauma, fragile X syndrome, thoracic insufficiency syndrome, and vaccine reactions.

I have been fortunate to have a team of associate editors, many have been on this project for all six editions, while others joined us later but continued the high level of professionalism and dedication to this book. I appreciate the efforts of Lou Bell, Peter Bingham, Esther Chung, David Friedman, Kathy Loomes, Petar Mamula, Maria Mascarenhas, and Ronn Tanel. My gratitude to all of them for their efforts to continue the reputation of high quality known in *The 5-Minute Pediatric Consult*. One of the principles for working on this project is it should be fun. I know it has been enjoyable for me. As the internet and notebooks become more popular, my old fashioned bias for real books will continue despite the prediction that books will be obsolete in the future. I hope not.

Being involved in many ways with educating medical students at Penn and residents at Children's Hospital of Philadelphia, and visiting many hospitals, I was able to see firsthand how this book was helpful to trainees, primary care pediatricians, and nurses, and thus, justifying the name of *The 5-Minute Pediatric Consult*. The spread of the book to other countries in many translations was gratifying and exceeded my initial expectations.

At a recent medical school reunion, I was struck by the memories of my classmates who all shared similar experience in the 4 years of school but had quite a diverse record of recollections that they entered into the reunion booklet. One of my memories was the experience at grand rounds where the chief of medicine related the story that he asked his mentor and previous chief of medicine to continue to come to grand rounds and participate in the department's activities. The older doctor agreed with the proviso that when he began to repeat himself and show some major memory defects, that he would get a tap on the shoulder as an indicator of it was time to step off the stage. The former chief did not want to be remembered as the old man with a poor memory who stayed too long. One day he got a tap on his shoulder; he knew what that meant. Our memories of him remain positive. On the other hand, our former chief of pediatrics would sleep through grand rounds and when prodded to answer a question, he began to talk about his favorite disease, even though it was not the topic of the session; so much for his reputation. These contrasting observations have helped form some of my professional philosophies. I always made sure that I did not stay too long, mainly to allow for the next generation to have opportunities that I was fortunate to have in my career. Therefore, with this sixth edition, I am retiring from editorship of *The 5-Minute Pediatric Consult* and look to the future of the book under the new team.

Before I go, I do want to express my appreciation and special thanks to Cheryl Polchenko, managing editor and a good pal, who has held all the pieces together and assured the completion of these editions. In every group there is a special person who quietly stands out, Cheryl is that person. *Grazie mille!* Likewise, that staff at Wolters Kluwer Health (that was Lippincott that was Williams & Wilkins). My friends and associates at Wolters Kluwer Health made working on this project a great pleasure. Thanks to Sonya Seigafuse, Rebecca Gaertner, and Nicole Walz who worked on the sixth edition and to Tim Hiscock, Katie Millet, and Joyce Murphy from the past editions. I appreciate them being so helpful. Sandhya Joshi headed the production team that turned the manuscripts into this book. *Molte grazie* to all of them.

At this time of reflection, I also want to acknowledge people, most of whom are no longer with us but their influence on me remains. First my parents who were book lovers and set a great example for the joys of reading and the value of education. Then my teachers, mentors, and colleagues including Willis Hunt, an eccentric but lovable biology teacher, Isaac Starr, my research mentor who showed that one could be a first rate scientist as well a gentleman (I loved his advice that "all the easy things have been done already."), Harold Farmer, a general internist who demonstrated an enthusiasm for teaching and for delving into medical history, and Francis Wood who set the example that excellent medical care has to be combined with compassionate doctor–patient communication. My fond memories of training at Children's Hospital of Philadelphia include my mentors: David Cornfeld, John Hope, Bob Kaye, Alfred Bongiovani, Bill Rashkind, and Henry Cecil as well as colleagues, Mike Genel, Tom Moshang, Bill Sharrar, Fred Burg, and Ed Chaney, all great friends. A special recognition of Bruce Tempest, former roommate, source of many good insights, both medical and cultural and an integral part of helping medical students learn firsthand about Navajo culture. Of course, I value the lessons from patients and families who taught me the most about patient care. Thanks to all.

WILLIAM SCHWARTZ, MD
Philadelphia 2012

CONTRIBUTING AUTHORS

Nicholas S. Abend, MD
Assistant Professor of Neurology and
    Pediatrics
Perelman School of Medicine at the
    University of Pennsylvania
Children's Hospital of
    Philadelphia
Philadelphia, Pennsylvania

Akinyemi Ajayi, MD, FCCP, FAASM
Children's Lung, Asthma and Sleep
    Specialists and the Children's Sleep
    Laboratory
Orlando, Florida

Ali Al-Omari, MD
Pediatric Orthopaedic Fellow
Department of Orthopaedic Surgery
The Children's Hospital of Philadelphia
Philadelphia, Pennsylvania

Lindsey G. Albenberg, DO
Division of Gastroenterology, Hepatology,
    and Nutrition
Children's Hospital of Philadelphia
Philadelphia, Pennsylvania

Craig A. Alter, MD
Division of Endocrinology and Diabetes
The Children's Hospital of Philadelphia
Professor of Clinical Pediatrics
The Perelman School of Medicine
University of Pennsylvania
Philadelphia, Pennsylvania

Timothy Andrews, MD
Private Practice
Allergy and Asthma Associates
Arnold, Maryland

William Anninger, MD
Assistant Professor of Ophthalmology
Children's Hospital of Philadelphia
Perelman School of Medicine at the
    University of Pennsylvania
Philadelphia, Pennsylvania

Garrick A. Applebee, MD
Assistant Professor of Neurology and
    Pediatrics
University of Vermont College of Medicine
Medical Director
Vermont Regional Sleep Center
Fletcher Allen Health Care
Burlington, Vermont

Lee Atkinson-McEvoy, MD
Associate Clinical Professor of Pediatrics
Associate Division Chief, General
    Pediatrics
UCSF Benioff Children's Hospital
San Francisco, California

Edward F. Attiyeh, MD
Assistant Professor of Pediatrics
Children's Hospital of Philadelphia
Perelman School of Medicine at the
    University of Pennsylvania
Philadelphia, Pennsylvania

J. Christopher Austin, MD, FAAP, FACS
Associate Professor
Department of Urology
Pediatric Urology
Oregon Health and Science University
Portland, Oregon

Oluwakemi B. Badaki-Mukan, MD, CM
Instructor of Pediatrics
Department of Pediatrics
Pediatric Emergency Medicine Research
    Fellow
Department of Emergency Medicine

Mark L. Bagarazzi, MD
Chief Medical Officer
Inovio Pharmaceuticals, Inc.
Blue Bell, Pennsylvania

Charles Bailey, MD, PhD
Divisions of Hematology & Oncology
Department of Pediatrics
Children's Hospital of Philadelphia
Philadelphia, Pennsylvania

Naomi Balamuth, MD
Assistant Professor
Department of Pediatrics
The Children's Hospital of Philadelphia
Philadelphia, Pennsylvania

Robert N. Baldassano, MD
Professor
University of Pennsylvania, School of
    Medicine
Director
Center for Pediatric Inflammatory Bowel
    Disease
The Children's Hospital of Philadelphia
Philadelphia, Pennsylvania

Christina Bales, MD
Assistant Professor of Clinical Medicine
Perelman School of Medicine of the
    University of Pennsylvania
Attending Physician
Division of Gastroenterology, Hepatology,
    and Nutrition
Department of Pediatrics
The Children's Hospital of Philadelphia
Philadelphia, Pennsylvania

Diane Barsky, MD
Attending Physician
Division of Gastroenterology, Hepatology
    and Nutrition
Children's Hospital of Philadelphia
Philadelphia, Pennsylvania

Hamid Bassiri, MD, PhD
Clinical Associate and Attending
Division of Infectious Diseases
Children's Hospital of Philadelphia
Philadelphia, Pennsylvania

Suzanne E. Beck, MD
Associate Professor of Clinical Pediatrics
University of Pennsylvania School of
    Medicine
Philadelphia, Pennsylvania

Julia Belkowitz, MD
Assistant Regional Dean for Student
    Affairs
Assistant Professor of Clinical Pediatrics
University of Miami Miller School of
    Medicine
Miami, Florida

Amanda K. Berry, MSN, CRNP
Pediatric Nurse Practitioner
Division of Urology
The Children's Hospital of Philadelphia
Philadelphia, Pennsylvania

Timothy Beukelman, MD, MSCE
Associate Professor
Department of Pediatrics
Division of Rheumatology
University of Alabama at Birmingham
Birmingham, Alabama

Anita Bhandari, MD
Assistant Professor of Pediatrics
Division of Pediatric Pulmonology
Connecticut Children's Medical Center
Hartford, Connecticut

Sumit Bhargava, MD
Clinical Associate Professor
Department of Pediatrics
Stanford School of Medicine
Attending Pulmonologist and Sleep
    Physician
Lucille Packard Childrens Hospital
Palo Alto, California

Diana X. Bharucha-Goebel, MD
Division of Neurology
Children's Hospital of Philadelphia
Philadelphia, Pennsylvania

Gil Binenbaum, MD, MSCE
Attending Surgeon
The Children's Hospital of Philadelphia
Assistant Professor of Ophthalmology
The Perelman School of Medicine at the
    University of Pennsylvania
Philadelphia, Pennsylvania

Mercedes M. Blackstone, MD
Attending Physician
Pediatric Emergency Medicine
Children's Hospital of Philadelphia
Assistant Professor of Clinical Pediatrics
Perelman School of Medicine at the
    University of Pennsylvania
Philadelphia, Pennsylvania

Peter Matthew Kennedy de Blank, MD, MSCE
Neuro-Oncology Fellow
Division of Oncology
Children's Hospital of Philadelphia
Philadelphia, Pennsylvania

Christopher P. Bonafide, MD, MSCE
Assistant Professor of Pediatrics
University of Pennsylvania
Division of General Pediatrics
The Children's Hospital of Philadelphia
Philadelphia, Pennsylvania

James Boyd, MD
Assistant Professor of Neurology
University of Vermont College of Medicine
Burlington, Vermont

Laura K. Brennan MD
Attending Physician
Division of General Pediatrics
The Children's Hospital of Philadelphia
Philadelphia, Pennsylvania

Lee J. Brooks, MD
Clinical Professor of Pediatrics
University of Pennsylvania
Attending Physician
Children's Hospital of Philadelphia
Philadelphia, Pennsylvania

Jeffrey P. Brosco, MD, PhD
Director
Pediatrics Program
Professor of Clinical Pediatrics
Department of Pediatrics
University of Miami Miller School of
    Medicine
Miami, Florida

Kurt Brown, MD
Senior Director
Clinical Research
Group Director
Neuroscience Therapeutic Area
AstraZeneca
Wilmington, Delaware

Valerie I. Brown, MD, PhD
Assistant Professor
Division of Pediatric Hematology/
    Oncology
Department of Pediatrics
Vanderbilt Children's Hospital
Vanderbilt-Ingram Cancer Center
Nashville, Tennessee

Ann B. Bruner, MD
Mountain Manor Treatment Center
Baltimore, Maryland

Leah Burke, MD
Associate Professor
Departments of Pediatrics and Medicine
University of Vermont College of Medicine
Attending Physician
Fletcher Allen Health Care
Burlington, Vermont

Genevieve L. Buser, MD, MSHP
Pediatric Infectious Diseases Fellow
Children's Hospital of Philadelphia
Philadelphia, Pennsylvania

Francesca Byrne, MD
Department of Pediatric Cardiology
University of California, San Francisco
San Francisco, California

Michael D. Cabana, MD, MPH
Professor of Pediatrics
Epidemiology & Biostatistics
University of California, San Francisco
Department of Pediatrics
San Francisco, California

Andrew C. Calabria, MD
Attending Physician
Division of Endocrinology and Diabetes
The Children's Hospital of Philadelphia
Assistant Professor of Pediatrics
Perelman School of Medicine
University of Pennsylvania
Philadelphia, Pennsylvania

Robert M. Campbell, Jr, MD
Director
The Center for Thoracic Insufficiency
    Syndrome
Pediatric Orthopaedist
Division of Orthopaedic Surgery
The Children's Hospital of Philadelphia
Professor of Orthopaedic Surgery
The University of Pennsylvania School of
    Medicine
Philadelphia, Pennsylvania

Douglas A. Canning, MD
Director
Division of Urology
The Children's Hospital of Philadelphia
Professor of Urology in Surgery
Perelman School of Medicine, University
    of Pennsylvania
Philadelphia, Pennsylvania

William B. Carey, MD
Director of Behavioral Pediatrics
Division of General Pediatrics
The Children's Hospital of Philadelphia
Clinical Professor of Pediatrics
University of Pennsylvania School of
    Medicine
Philadelphia, Pennsylvania

Vanessa S. Carlo, MD
Assistant Professor of Pediatrics
Thomas Jefferson University
Philadelphia, Pennsylvania

Michael C. Carr, MD, PhD
Associate Director
Pediatric Urology
Children's Hospital of Philadelphia
Philadelphia, Pennsylvania

Leslie Castelo-Soccio, MD, PhD
Attending Physician, Pediatrics and
    Dermatology
Section of Dermatology
The Children's Hospital of Philadelphia
Philadelphia, Pennsylvania

Elizabeth Candell Chalom, MD
Assistant Professor of Pediatrics
University of Medicine and Dentistry
  of New Jersey
Chief, Pediatric Rheumatology
Saint Barnabas Medical Center
Livingston, New Jersey

Candice Chen, MD, MPH
Assistant Research Professor
Department of Health Policy
School of Public Health and Health
  Services
The George Washington University
Washington, DC

Cindy W. Christian, MD
Chair
Child Abuse and Neglect Prevention
The Children's Hospital of Philadelphia
Professor of Pediatrics
The Perelman School of Medicine at the
  University of Pennsylvania
Philadelphia, Pennsylvania

Matthew S. Christman, MD
Fellow
Pediatric Urology
Division of Urology
The Children's Hospital of
  Philadelphia
Philadelphia, Pennsylvania

Esther K. Chung, MD, MPH, FAAP
Professor of Pediatrics
Jefferson Medical College
Thomas Jefferson University
Nemours - Philadelphia
Philadelphia, Pennsylvania

Meryl S. Cohen, MD
Associate Professor of Pediatrics
Perelman School of Medicine
The Children's Hospital of Philadelphia
University of Pennsylvania
Philadelphia, Pennsylvania

Joy L. Collins, MD, FACS, FAAP
Assistant Professor of Clinical Surgery
University of Pennsylvania
Attending Surgeon
Department of General and Thoracic
  Surgery
The Children's Hospital of Philadelphia
Philadelphia, Pennsylvania

Stephen H. Contompasis, MD
Associate Professor of Pediatrics
University of Vermont College of Medicine
Burlington, Vermont

Lawrence Copelovitch, MD
Assistant Professor of Pediatrics
Division of Nephrology
The Children's Hospital of Philadelphia
Perelman School of Medicine at the
  University of Pennsylvania
Philadelphia, Pennsylvania

Rosalyn Diaz Crescioni, MD
Department of Gastroenterology
Puerto Rico Children's Hospital
Bayamón, Puerto Rico

Randy Q. Cron, MD, PhD
Professor of Pediatrics & Medicine
Director of Pediatric Rheumatology
University of Alabama at Birmingham
Birmingham, Alabama

Kristin E. D'Aco, MD
Fellow
Clinical and Biochemical Genetics
Children's Hospital of Philadelphia
Philadelphia, Pennsylvania

George A. Datto, MD
Department of Pediatrics
Nemours
A. I. duPont Hospital for Children
Wilmington, Delaware

Richard S. Davidson, MD
Professor of Orthopedic Surgery
Department of Orthopedic Surgery
Children's Hospital of Philadelphia
University of Pennsylvania School of
  Medicine
Philadelphia, Pennsylvania

Michelle Denburg, MD
Renal Physician
Children's Hospital of Philadelphia
Philadelphia, Pennsylvania

Mark F. Ditmar, MD
Clinical Associate Professor
Department of Pediatrics
Thomas Jefferson University
Philadelphia, Pennsylvania

Dennis J. Dlugos, MD
Director
Pediatric Regional Epilepsy Program
The Children's Hospital of Philadelphia
Associate Professor of Neurology and
  Pediatrics
Perelman School of Medicine at the
  University of Pennsylvania
Philadelphia, Pennsylvania

John P. Dormans, MD
The Richard M. Armstrong, Jr. Endowed
  Chair
Pediatric Orthopaedic Surgery
Professor of Orthopaedic Surgery at the
  University of Pennsylvania School of
  Medicine
Chief of Orthopaedic Surgery
The Children's Hospital of Philadelphia
Division of Orthopaedic Surgery
Philadelphia, Pennsylvania

Monica Dowling, PhD
Assistant Professor Clinical Pediatrics
Clinical Psychology
University of Miami
Miller School of Medicine
Mailman Center for Child Development
Miami, Florida

Naomi Dreisinger, MD, MS, FAAP
Director
Pediatric Emergency Department
Beth Israel Medical Center
Asst. Professor
Pediatrics
Albert Einstein College of Medicine
New York City, New York

Nancy Drucker, MD
Pediatric Cardiology
Fletcher Allen Health Care
Associate Professor
University of Vermont College of Medicine
Burlington, Vermont

C. Pace Duckett, MD
Adjunct Faculty
Department of Psychiatry
University of Pennsylvania
Philadelphia, Pennsylvania

Michelle Dunn, MD
Clinical Assistant Professor in Pediatrics
University of Pennsylvania Perelman
  School of Medicine
Attending Physician
General Pediatrics
Children's Hospital of Philadelphia
Philadelphia, Pennsylvania

Sadiqa Edmonds, MD
Fellow
Division of Pediatric Emergency Medicine
Children's Hospital of Philadelphia
Philadelphia, Pennsylvania

Alcia Edwards-Richards, MD
Pediatric Nephrology Fellow
University of Miami
Miami, Florida

Deborah B. Ehrenthal, MD, MPH
Director of Health Services Research for
    Women and Children
Department of Medicine and Obstetrics
    and Gynecology
Christiana Care Health System
Newark, Delaware

Gary A. Emmett, MD, FAAP
Professor of Pediatrics
Thomas Jefferson University
Philadelphia, Pennsylvania

Yasemen Eroglu, MD
Department of Gastroenterology
    Physicians and Surgeons
Doernbecher Children's Hospital
Oregon Health and Science University
Portland, Oregon

Stephen J. Falchek, MD
Instructor
Departments of Pediatrics and Neurology
Thomas Jefferson University
Interim Division Chief
Division of Pediatric Neurology
A.I. duPont Hospital for Children
Wilmington, Delaware

Marni J. Falk, MD
Assistant Professor
Division of Human Genetics
Department of Pediatrics
The Children's Hospital of Philadelphia
    and University of Pennsylvania
    Perelman School of Medicine
Philadelphia, Pennsylvania

Kristen A. Feemster, MD, MPH, MSHP
Assistant Professor of Pediatrics
Perelman School of Medicine
University of Pennsylvania
Division of Infectious Diseases
The Children's Hospital of Philadelphia
Philadelphia, Pennsylvania

Ciarán Della Fera
Student
School of Medicine
University of Massachusetts
Worcester, Massachusetts

Douglas Finefrock, MD
Assistant Program Director
Department of Emergency Medicine
Albert Einstein College of Medicine of
    Veshiva University
New York City, New York

Richard S. Finkel, MD
Director, Neuromuscular Program
Division of Neurology
The Children's Hospital of Philadelphia
Clinical Professor in Neurology and
    Pediatrics
Pearlman School of Medicine
University of Pennsylvania
Philadelphia, Pennsylvania

Kristin N. Fiorino, MD
Assistant Professor
Department of Pediatrics
Attending Physician
Division of Gastroenterology, Hepatology,
    and Nutrition
The Children's Hospital of Philadelphia
Philadelphia, Pennsylvania

Brian T. Fisher, DO, MSCE, MPH
Assistant Professor of Pediatrics
The Children's Hospital of Philadelphia
Perelman School of Medicine at the
    University of Pennsylvania
Philadelphia, Pennsylvania

Michael J. Fisher, MD
Associate Professor
Division of Oncology
Department of Pediatrics
Children's Hospital of Philadelphia
Philadelphia, Pennsylvania

Jonathan Fleenor, MD, FACC, FAAP
Pediatric Cardiology
Children's Hospital of the King's
    Daughters
Norfolk, Virginia

John M. Flynn, MD
Professor of Orthopaedic Surgery
The University of Pennsylvania School of
    Medicine
Associate Chief of Orthopaedics
The Children's Hospital of Philadelphia
Philadelphia, Pennsylvania

Matthew Isaac Fogg, MD
Allergy and Asthma Specialists, PC
Attending Allergist
St. Christopher's Hospital for Children
Clinical Assistant Professor of Pediatrics
Drexel University College of Medicine
Philadelphia, Pennsylvania

Brian John Forbes, MD, PhD
Associate Professor
Ophthalmology & Pediatrics
Perelman School of Medicine at the
    University of Pennsylvania
Department of Ophthalmology
The Children's Hospital of Philadelphia
Philadelphia, Pennsylvania

James P. Franciosi, MD, MS
Assistant Professor
Department of Gastroenterology
University of Cincinnati
Cincinnati Children's Hospital
Cincinnati, Ohio

David F. Friedman, MD
Clinical Assistant Professor of Pediatrics
    at the University of Pennsylvania
Perelman School of Medicine
Division of Pediatric Hematology
Children's Hospital of Philadelphia
Philadelphia, Pennsylvania

Joshua R. Friedman, MD, PhD
Assistant Professor
Department of Pediatrics
The Children's Hospital of Philadelphia
The Perelman School of Medicine at the
    University of Pennsylvania
Philadelphia, Pennsylvania

Sarah M. Frioux, MD
Major
U.S. Army
Department of Pediatrics
Tripler Army Medical Center
Tripler AMC, Hawaii

Theodore J. Ganley, MD
Director of Sports Medicine
The Children's Hospital of Philadelphia
Associate Professor of Orthopaedic
    Surgery
The University of Pennsylvania School of
    Medicine
Philadelphia, Pennsylvania

Ana Catarina Garnecho, MD
Developmental-Behavioral Pediatrics
Neurodevelopmental Center
Department of Pediatrics
Memorial Hospital of Rhode Island
Warren Alpert School Medical School of
    Brown University

Jackie P.-D. Garrett, MD
Fellow Physician
Division of Allergy and Immunology
Children's Hospital of Philadelphia
Philadelphia, Pennsylvania

Jeffrey S. Gerber, MD, PhD
Assistant Professor of Pediatrics
University of Pennsylvania School of
  Medicine
Division of Infectious Diseases
The Children's Hospital of Philadelphia
Philadelphia, Pennsylvania

Lynette A. Gillis, MD
Associate Professor
Department of Pediatrics
Divisions of Pediatric Gastroenterology,
  Hepatology, and Nutrition and Medical
  Genetics
Vanderbilt University Medical Center
Nashville, Tennessee

Jenifer A. Glatz, MD
Assistant Professor of Pediatrics
Pediatric Cardiology Children's Hospital at
  Dartmouth
Manchester, New Hampshire

Samuel B. Goldfarb, MD
Division of Pulmonary Medicine
The Children's Hospital of
  Philadelphia
Philadelphia, Pennsylvania

Jeremy Golding, MD
Clinical Professor of Family Medicine and
  OB-GYN
University of Massachusetts Medical
  School
Quality Officer-Department of Family
  Medicine
UMass Memorial Health Care/
  Hahnemann Family Health Center
Boston, Massachusetts

Kelly C. Goldsmith, MD
Attending Physician
Department of Oncology
Children's Hospital of Philadelphia
Philadelphia, Pennsylvania

Scott M. Goldstein, MD
Adjunct Clinical Assistant Professor of
  Ophthalmology
Oculoplastic Service
Wills Eye Institute
Jefferson Medical College
Philadelphia, Pennsylvania

John M. Good, MD
Clinical Faculty
University of New Mexico
General Pediatrics
Lovelace Sandia Health Systems
Albuquerque, New Mexico

Vani Gopalareddy, MD
Associate Professor of Pediatrics
Director of Hepatology and Liver
  Transplantation
Levine Children's Hospital at Carolinas
  Medical Center
Charlotte, North Carolina

Marc Gorelick, MD, MSCE
Sr. Associate Dean for Clinical Affairs
Professor of Pediatrics, and Chief of
  Pediatric Emergency Medicine
Medical College of Wisconsin
Jon E. Vice Chair in Emergency Medicine
Children's Hospital of Wisconsin
Milwaukee, Wisconsin

Neera Goyal, MD, MSc
Assistant Professor of Pediatrics
Division of Neonatology and Pulmonary
  Biology
Division of Hospital Medicine
Cincinnati Children's Hospital Medical
  Center
Cincinnati, Ohio

William R. Graessle, MD
Associate Professor of Pediatrics
Cooper Medical School of Rowan
  University
Camden, New Jersey

Ernie Graham, MD
Department of Gyn/Ob
Johns Hopkins University School of
  Medicine
Baltimore, Maryland

Rose C. Graham, MD, MSCE
Adjunct Assistant Professor of Pediatrics
University of North Carolina School of
  Medicine
Chapel Hill, North Carolina
Attending Physician
Pediatric Gastroenterology
Mission Children's Specialists
Asheville, North Carolina

Abby M. Green, MD
Fellow
Division of Infectious Diseases
The Children's Hospital of Philadelphia
Philadelphia, Pennsylvania

Adda Grimberg, MD
Associate Professor of Pediatrics
Perelman School of Medicine
University of Pennsylvania
Scientific Director
Diagnostic and Research Growth Center
The Children's Hospital of Philadelphia
Philadelphia, Pennsylvania

Andrew B. Grossman, MD
Clinical Assistant Professor of Pediatrics
Perelman School of Medicine at the
  University of Pennsylvania
Attending Physician
Division of Gastroenterology, Hepatology,
  and Nutrition
The Children's Hospital of Philadelphia
Philadelphia, Pennsylvania

Blaze Robert Gusic, MD, FAAP
Las Vegas, Nevada

Chad R. Haldeman-Englert, MD
Assistant Professor
Department of Pediatrics
Wake Forest Baptist Medical Center
Winston-Salem, North Carolina

J. Nina Ham, MD
Assistant Professor of Pediatrics
Pediatric Diabetes and Endocrinology
  Section
Baylor College of Medicine
Houston, Texas

Brian D Hanna, MDCM, PhD
Director
Section of Pulmonary Hypertension
Division of Cardiology
The Children's Hospital of Philadelphia
Clinical Professor of Pediatrics
Perelman School of Medicine
University of Pennsylvania
Philadelphia, Pennsylvania

Jessica K. Hart, MD
Pediatric Hospitalist
Department of General Pediatrics
Children's Hospital of Philadelphia
Philadelphia, Pennsylvania

Sandra G. Hassink, MD
Director Nemours Obesity Initiative
A. I. duPont Hospital for Children
Wilmington, Delaware

Cheryl Hausman, MD
Medical Director
Children's Hospital of Philadelphia Care
  Network
University City
Philadelphia, Pennsylvania

Fiona M. Healy, MD
Department of Pediatric Pulmonology
Philadelphia, Pennsylvania

David Hehir, MD
Assistant Professor of Pediatrics
Divisions of Cardiology and Critical Care
Children's Hospital of Wisconsin
Medical College of Wisconsin
Milwaukee, Wisconsin

Eugene R. Hershorin, MD
Associate Professor of Clinical Pediatrics
Chief – Division of General Pediatrics
Associate Chair – Department of
    Pediatrics
University of Miami Miller School of
    Medicine
Miami, Florida

Robert J. Hoffman, MD, MS
Associate Professor
Department of Emergency Medicine
Albert Einstein College of Medicine
Bronx, New York;
Research Director
Department of Emergency Medicine
Beth Israel Medical Center
New York, New York
Director, Clinical Toxicology
Emergency Services Institute
Sheikh Khalifa Medical City
Abu Dhabi, United Arab Emirates

Jessica Hoseason, MD
Resident
Doernbecher Children's Hospital
Oregon Health and Science University
Portland, Oregon

Arvind Hoskoppal, MD, MHS
Pediatric Cardiology Fellow
UCSF
San Francisco, California

Evelyn K. Hsu, MD
Assistant Professor
Gastroenterology, Hepatology
Seattle Children's Hospital
Seattle, Washington

Marleine F. Ishak, MD
Pediatric Pulmonology
Yale University
New Haven, Connecticut

Sujit Iyer, MD
Pediatric Emergency Medicine
Director of Medical Education – DCMC
    Emergency Department
Dell Children's Medical Center of Central
    Texas
Austin, Texas

Oksana A. Jackson, MD
Assistant Professor of Surgery
Division of Plastic Surgery
Perelman School of Medicine at the
    University of Pennsylvania and the
    Children's Hospital of Philadelphia
Philadelphia, Pennsylvania

Cynthia R. Jacobstein, MD, MSCE
Assistant Professor of Clinical Pediatrics
Department of Pediatrics
Division of Emergency Medicine
Children's Hospital of Philadelphia
Philadelphia, Pennsylvania

Douglas Jacobstein, MD
Attending Physician
Division of Pediatric Gastroenterology and
    Nutrition
Sinai Hospital of Baltimore
Baltimore, Maryland

Irfan Jafree, MD
Electrophysiology Fellow
Department of Neurology
University of Vermont College of Medicine
Burlington, Vermont

**John Lynn Jefferies, MD, MPF, FACC,
FAAP**
Associate Professor
Pediatric Cardiology
Director
Advanced Heart Failure, Cardiomyopathy,
    and Ventricular Assist Device Programs
Co-Director
Cardiovascular Genetics
Associate Director
Heart Institute Research Core
Cincinnati Children's Hospital Medical
    Center
University of Cincinnati
Cincinnati, Ohio

Anne K. Jensen, BA
Medical Student
Division of Ophthalmology
Children's Hospital of Philadelphia
Philadelphia, Pennsylvania

Payal S. Kadia, MD
Fellow
Pediatric Emergency Medicine
Children's Hospital of Philadelphia
Philadelphia, Pennsylvania

Binita M. Kamath, MBBChir, MRCP, MTR
Staff Physician
Division of Gastroenterology, Hepatology
    and Nutrition
The Hospital for Sick Children
Associate Scientist
Research Institute
Assistant Professor
University of Toronto
Toronto, Canada

Robert D. Karch, MD, MPH, FAAP
Director
Pediatric Hospital Medicine
Nemours Children's Hospital
Orlando, Florida

Sara Karjoo, MD
Pediatric Gastroenterology, Hepatology
    and Nutrition
Children's Hospital of Philadelphia
Philadelphia, Pennsylvania

Michael D. Keller, MD
Division of Allergy/Immunology
Children's Hospital of Philadelphia
Philadelphia, Pennsylvania

Andrea Kelly, MD, MSCE
Assistant Professor of Pediatrics
Division of Endocrinology & Diabetes
Children's Hospital of Philadelphia
Perelman School of Medicine at the
    University of Pennsylvania
Philadelphia, Pennsylvania

Janice Anne Kelly, MD
Clinical Associate Professor of Pediatrics
University of Pennsylvania
Division of Gastroenterology and Nutrition
Children's Hospital of Philadelphia
Philadelphia, Pennsylvania

Judith Kelsen, MD
Assistant Professor of Pediatrics
The Children's Hospital of Philadelphia
Division of Gastroenterology
Philadelphia, Pennsylvania

Shellie M. Kendall, MD
Clinical Fellow
Pediatric Cardiology
University of California, San Francisco
San Francisco, California

Melissa Kennedy, MD
Attending Physician
Children's Hospital of Philadelphia
Philadelphia, Pennsylvania

Hans B. Kersten, MD
Associate Professor of Pediatrics
St. Christopher's Hospital for
    Children
Drexel University College of Medicine
Philadelphia, Pennsylvania

Leslie Kersun, MD, MSCE
Inpatient Medical Director
Division of Oncology
The Children's Hospital of
    Philadelphia
Assistant Professor of Pediatrics
Perelman School of Medicine at the
    University of Pennsylvania
Philadelphia, Pennsylvania

Jason Y. Kim, MD, MSCE
Division of Infectious Diseases
The Children's Hospital of
    Philadelphia
Assistant Professor of Clinical
    Pediatrics
Perelman School of Medicine
Philadelphia, Pennsylvania

Terry Kind, MD, MPH
Associate Professor of Pediatrics
Director
Pediatric Medical Student Education
Department of Community Pediatric
    Health
Children's National Medical Center
The George Washington University
Washington, DC

Jeremy King, DO
Pediatric Gastroenterologist
Kapiolani Medical Specialists
Assistant Professor
Pediatrics
John A. Burns School of Medicine
Honolulu, Hawaii

Matthew P. Kirschen, MD
Pediatrics
Stanford, California

Thomas F. Kolon, MD
Associate Professor of Urology
Perelman School of Medicine at the
    University of Pennsylvania
Program Director
Pediatric Urology Fellowship
Children's Hospital of Philadelphia
Philadelphia, Pennsylvania

Sanjeev V. Kothare, MD
Division of Epilepsy & Clinical
    Neurophysiology
Associate Professor
Department of Neurology
Harvard Medical School
Interim Medical Director
Center for Pediatric Sleep Disorders
Fellowship Director
Pediatric Sleep Medicine Training
    Program
Children's Hospital Boston
Boston, Massachusetts

Renee K. Kottenhahn, MD, FAAP
Clinical Associate Professor of Pediatrics
Jefferson Medical College of Thomas
    Jefferson University
Philadelphia, Pennsylvania
Associate Director
Pediatric Practice Program and Attending
    Physician
Department of Pediatrics
Christiana Care Health Services
Wilmington, Delaware

Wendy J. Kowalski, MD
Attending Neonatologist
Department of Neonatology
Lehigh Valley Hospital
Allentown, Pennsylvania

Richard M. Kravitz, MD
Associate Professor of Pediatrics
Medical Director
Pediatric Sleep Laboratory
Department of Pediatrics
Duke University Medical Center
Durham, North Carolina

Matthew P. Kronman, MD, MSCE
Assistant Professor, Division of Infectious
    Diseases
Department of Pediatrics
University of Washington/Seattle
    Children's Hospital
Seattle, Washington

Julie You Kwon, MD
Division of Ophthalmology
Children's Hospital of Philadelphia
Philadelphia, Pennsylvania

Michele P. Lambert, MD, MTR
Assistant Professor of Pediatrics at the
    Children's Hospital of Philadelphia
Division of Hematology
Perelman School of Medicine at the
    University of Pennsylvania
Philadelphia, Pennsylvania

David R. Langdon, MD
Clinical Director
Division of Endocrinology
Children's Hospital of Philadelphia
Clinical Associate Professor
University of Pennsylvania School of
    Medicine
Philadelphia, Pennsylvania

Judith B. Larkin, MD, FAAP
Instructor in Pediatrics
Nemours Pediatrics, Philadelphia
Thomas Jefferson University Hospital
Philadelphia, Pennsylvania
A. I. duPont Hospital for Children
Wilmington, Delaware

Christopher LaRosa, MD
A. I. duPont Hospital for Children
Wilmington, Delaware

Jerry G. Larrabee, MD
Division Chief
Pediatric Primary Care
Department of Pediatrics
University of Vermont
Burlington, Vermont

Dale Young Lee, MD
Fellow
Pediatric Gastroenterology, Hepatology,
    and Nutrition
Children's Hospital of Philadelphia
Philadelphia, Pennsylvania

Rebecca K. Lehman, MD
Assistant Professor
Department of Neurosciences
Division of Pediatric Neurology
Medical University of South Carolina
Charleston, South Carolina

Alycia Leiby, MD
Goryeb Children's Hospital/Atlantic
    Health System
Pediatric Gastroenterology and Nutrition
Morristown, New Jersey

Diva D. De León, MD
Assistant Professor of Pediatrics
Division of Endocrinology/Diabetes
The Children's Hospital of Philadelphia
Perelman School of Medicine at the
    University of Pennsylvania
Philadelphia, Pennsylvania

Daniel H. Leung, MD
Assistant Professor of Pediatrics
Gastroenterology, Hepatology, and
  Nutrition
Texas Children's Hospital
Baylor College of Medicine
Medical Director
Viral Hepatitis Clinic
Houston, Texas

Leonard J. Levine, MD
Assistant Professor of Pediatrics
Department of Pediatrics
Drexel University College of
  Medicine
Attending Physician
Division of Adolescent Medicine
St. Christopher's Hospital for
  Children
Philadelphia, Pennsylvania

Lorraine E. Levitt Katz, MD
Associate Professor
Division of Endocrinology
Children's Hospital of Philadelphia
Philadelphia, Pennsylvania

Norman Lewak, MD
Clinical Professor of Pediatrics
University of California, San Francisco
San Francisco, California

Daniel J. Licht, MD
Assistant Professor of Neurology and
  Pediatrics
Division of Neurology
The Children's Hospital of Philadelphia
Philadelphia, Pennsylvania

Henry Lin, MD
Fellow
Pediatric Gastroenterology, Hepatology,
  and Nutrition
The Children's Hospital of Philadelphia
Philadelphia, Pennsylvania

Rochelle G. Lindemeyer, DMD
Attending Dentist
Director
Pediatric Dentistry Residency
  Program
Department of Dentistry
Children's Hospital of Philadelphia
Philadelphia, Pennsylvania

Steven Liu, MD
Pediatric Gastroenterologist
Children's Center for Digestive
  Healthcare
Atlanta, Georgia

Kathleen M. Loomes, MD
Associate Professor of Pediatrics
Perelman School of Medicine at the
  University of Pennsylvania
Division of Gastroenterology, Hepatology
  and Nutrition
The Children's Hospital of
  Philadelphia
Philadelphia, Pennsylvania

Alexander Lowenthal, MD
Senior Echocardiography Fellow
Lucile Packard Children's Hospital at
  Stanford
Palo Alto, California

Sheela N. Magge, MD, MSCE
Assistant Professor of Pediatrics
University of Pennsylvania Perelman
  School of Medicine
Division of Endocrinology and
  Diabetes
The Children's Hospital of
  Philadelphia
Philadelphia, Pennsylvania

Shannon Manzi, PharmD
Team Leader, Emergency Services
Department of Pharmacy
Children's Hospital Boston
Boston, Massachusetts

Petar Mamula, MD
Associate Professor of Pediatrics
University of Pennsylvania Perelman
  School of Medicine
Division of Gastroenterology, Hepatology
  and Nutrition
The Children's Hospital of
  Philadelphia
Philadelphia, Pennsylvania

Yang Mao-Draayer, MD, PhD
Associate Professor
Department of Neurology
University of Michigan
Ann Arbor, Michigan

Bradley S. Marino, MD, MPP, MSCE
Associate Professor of Pediatrics
University of Cincinnati College of
  Medicine
Director
Heart Institute Research Core
Director
Heart Institute Neurodevelopmental
  Clinic
Attending Physician
Cardiac Intensive Care Unit
Divisions of Cardiology and Critical Care
  Medicine
Cincinnati Children's Hospital Medical
  Center
Cincinnati, Ohio

Jennifer A. Markowitz, MD
Department of Neurology
Children's Hospital of Boston
Boston, Massachusetts

Jonathan Markowitz, MD, MSCE
Director
Children's Center for Digestive Health
Greenville, South Carolina

Maria R. Mascarenhas, MBBS
Associate Professor of Pediatrics at the
  University of Pennsylvania
Division of Gastroenterology, Hepatology
  and Nutrition
Children's Hospital of Philadelphia
Philadelphia, Pennsylvania

Kiran Maski, MD
Instructor
Department of Neurology
Children's Hospital Boston
Boston, Massachusetts

Oscar Henry Mayer, MD
Division of Pulmonology
The Children's Hospital of
  Philadelphia
Assistant Professor of Clinical
  Pediatrics
Perelman School of Medicine of the
  University of Pennsylvania
Philadelphia, Pennsylvania

Erin E. McGintee, MD
Attending Physician
Allergy and Immunology
ENT and Allergy Associates, LLP
East Hampton, New York

Susan McKamy, PharmD, BCPS
Assistant Clinical Professor
Department of Clinical Pharmacy
School of Pharmacy
University of California, San Francisco
San Francisco, California
Clinical Lead Pharmacist
Miller Children's Hospital of Long Beach
Long Beach, California

Heather McKeag, MD
Assistant Professor of Pediatrics
Tufts University School of Medicine
Department of Pediatrics
Floating Hospital for Children at Tufts
   Medical Center
Boston, Massachusetts

Lisa Mcleod, MD
Department of Pediatrics
Children's Hospital of Philadelphia
Philadelphia, Pennsylvania

Maureen McMahon, MD
Instructor
Department of Pediatrics
Jefferson Medical College
Philadelphia, Pennsylvania
Pediatrician
Department of Pediatrics
A.I. duPont Hospital for Children
Wilmington, Delaware

Hugh J McMillan, MD, MSc
Assistant Professor of Pediatrics
Division of Neurology
Children's Hospital of Eastern Ontario
Ottawa, Ontario

Margaret M. McNamara, MD
Associate Professor of Pediatrics
University of California San Francisco
San Francisco, California

William McNett, MD
Associate Professor
Pediatrics
Jefferson Medical College
Philadelphia, Pennsylvania

Avani S. Mehta, MD
Fellow
Pediatric Emergency Medicine
Children's Hospital of Philadelphia
Philadelphia, Pennsylvania

Devendra I. Mehta, MBBS, MSc, MRCP
Assistant Professor
Department of Pediatrics
Thomas Jefferson University
Pediatric Gastroenterologist
Department of Pediatrics
Nemours Children's Clinic
Orlando, Florida

Michelle E. Melicosta, MD, FAAP
U.S. Army Health Center
Wiesbaden, Germany

Heather L. Meluskey, BS, BSN, RN
Pulmonary Hypertension Nurse
   Coordinator
Department of Cardiology
The Children's Hospital of Philadelphia
Philadelphia, Pennsylvania

Calies Menard-Katcher, MD
Division of Gastroenterology, Hepatology
   and Nutrition
Children's Hospital of Philadelphia
Philadelphia, Pennsylvania

Jondavid Menteer, MD
Assistant Professor of Pediatrics
Children's Hospital Los Angeles
Keck School of Medicine
Los Angeles, California

Laura M. Mercer-Rosa, MD, MSCE
Assistant Professor in Pediatrics
Perelman School of Medicine
University of Pennsylvania
Philadelphia, Pennsylvania

Kevin E. C. Meyers, MBBCh
Associate Professor of Pediatrics
Nephrology Division
Department of Pediatrics
The Children's Hospital of Philadelphia
University of Pennsylvania
Philadelphia, Pennsylvania

Edmund A. Milder, MD
Fellow
Pediatric Infectious Diseases
Children's Hospital of Philadelphia
Philadelphia, Pennsylvania
Medical Corps
United States Navy

Carol A. Miller, MD
Clinical Professor
Pediatrics
University of California San Francisco
   School of Medicine
San Francisco, California

Monte D. Mills, MD
Director
Division of Ophthalmology
The Children's Hospital of Philadelphia
Associate Professor
Ophthalmology
Perelman School of Medicine, University
   of Pennsylvania
Philadelphia, Pennsylvania

Jane E. Minturn, MD, PhD
Division of Oncology
The Children's Hospital of Philadelphia
Assistant Professor of Pediatrics
Perelman School of Medicine at the
   University of Pennsylvania
Philadelphia, Pennsylvania

Sabina Mir, MBBS
Pediatric Gastroenterology, Hepatology
   and Nutrition
Texas Children's Hospital
Baylor College of Medicine
Houston, Texas

Rakesh D. Mistry, MD, MS
Assistant Professor of Pediatrics
University of Pennsylvania School of
   Medicine
Attending Physician
Children's Hospital of Philadelphia
Philadelphia, Pennsylvania

Kimberly Molina, MD
Assistant Professor of Pediatrics
Division of Pediatric Cardiology
University of Utah
Salt Lake City, Utah

Divya Moodalbail, MD
Pediatric Nephrology Fellow
The Children's Hospital of Philadelphia
Philadelphia, Pennsylvania

Sogol Mostoufi-Moab, MD, MSCE
Assistant Professor of Pediatrics
Divisions of Oncology and Endocrinology
The Children's Hospital of Philadelphia
Philadelphia, Pennsylvania

Amanda Muir, MD
Fellow
Department of Gastroenterology,
   Hepatology and Nutrition
The Children's Hospital of Philadelphia
Philadelphia, Pennsylvania

Frances M. Nadel, MD, MSCE
Associate Professor, Clinical Pediatrics
Department of Pediatrics
Perelman School of Medicine at the
    University of Pennsylvania
Attending Physician
Division of Emergency Medicine
Children's Hospital of Philadelphia
Philadelphia, Pennsylvania

Luz I. Natal-Hernandez, MD
Pediatric Cardiology
UCSF Medical Center
San Francisco, California

Jane Nathanson, MD
Pediatric Resident
The Children's Hospital of Philadelphia
Philadelphia, Pennsylvania

Seth L. Ness, MD, PhD
Director
Medical Leader
Neuroscience Therapeutic Area
Janssen Research and Development LLC
Janssen Pharmaceutical Companies of
    Johnson & Johnson
Titusville, New Jersey

Jason G. Newland, MD, Med
Associate Professor of Pediatrics
Children's Mercy Hospitals & Clinics
University of Kansas City, Missouri

Jessica Newman, DO
Fellow
Division of Infectious Diseases
Department of Internal Medicine
University of Kansas Medical Center
Kansas City, Kansas

Ross Newman, DO
Assistant Professor of Pediatrics
University of Missouri-Kansas City
Children's Mercy Hospital and Clinics
Kansas City, Missouri

Thomas Nguyen, MD
Assistant Program Director
Residency
Department of Emergency Medicine
Albert Einstein College of Medicine of
    Veshiva University
New York City, New York

Sheila M. Nolan, MD, MSCE
Global Medical Monitor
Vaccine Clinical Research
Pfizer Inc.
Pearl River, New York

Robert Noll, MD, FAAP
Director
Pediatric Hospital Medicine and
    Emergency Care
Department of Pediatrics
Crozer-Chester Medical Center
Chester, Pennsylvania
Clinical Assistant Professor of Pediatrics
Jefferson Medical College of Thomas
    Jefferson University
Philadelphia, Pennsylvania

Cynthia F. Norris, MD
Clinical Associate in Pediatrics
Acute Care Unit
Department of Pediatrics
Medical Director
Division of Hematology
The Children's Hospital of Philadelphia
Philadelphia, Pennsylvania

Bruce A. Ong, MD, MPH
Pediatric Pulmonary Fellow
Division of Pulmonary Medicine and
    Cystic Fibrosis Center
The Children's Hospital of Philadelphia
Philadelphia, Pennsylvania

Kevin C. Osterhoudt, MD, MS, FAAP,
FAACT, FACMT
Medical Director
The Poison Control Center
The Children's Hospital of Philadelphia
Associate Professor of Pediatrics and
    Emergency Medicine
The Perelman School of Medicine at the
    University of Pennsylvania
Philadelphia, Pennsylvania

Erica Pan, MD, MPH, FAAP
Associate Clinical Professor
Department of Pediatrics
Division of Infectious Diseases
University of California, San Francisco
San Francisco, California
Deputy Health Officer
Director
Division of Communicable Disease
    Control & Prevention
Alameda County Public Health Department
Oakland, California

Howard B. Panitch, MD
Professor of Pediatrics
Perelman School of Medicine
University of Pennsylvania
Director of Clinical Programs
Division of Pulmonary Medicine
The Children's Hospital of Philadelphia
Philadelphia, Pennsylvania

Rita Panoscha, MD
Clinical Associate Professor
Department of Pediatrics
The Child Development and Rehabilitation
    Center and Oregon Health and Science
    University
Portland, Oregon

Juliann M. Paolicchi, MA, MD
Director
Pediatric Comprehensive Epilepsy Center
Associate Professor
Weill Cornell Medical Center
New York City, New York

Carolyn Paris, MD
Attending Physician
Department of Emergency Medicine
Seattle Children's Hospital
Assistant Professor
University of Washington School of
    Medicine
Seattle, Washington

Ushama Patel, MD
Albert Einstein Practice Inc.
Philadelphia, Pennsylvania

Elena Elizabeth Perez, MD, PhD
Associate Professor
Division of Allergy, Immunology,
    Rheumatology
Department of Pediatrics
University of South Florida
St. Petersburg, Florida

Nadja G. Peter, MD
Craig-Dalsimer Division of Adolescent
    Medicine
Department of Pediatrics
Children's Hospital of Philadelphia
Philadelphia, Pennsylvania

Christopher J. Petit MD
Assistant Professor
Lillie Frank Abercrombie Section of
    Cardiology
Department of Pediatrics
Texas Children's Hospital
Baylor College of Medicine
Houston, Texas

Virginia M. Pierce MD
Fellow
Division of Infectious Diseases
Department of Pediatrics
Children's Hospital of Philadelphia
Philadelphia, Pennsylvania

Nelangi M. Pinto, MD, MSCI
Assistant Professor
Division of Cardiology
Department of Pediatrics
University of Utah
Salt Lake City, Utah

Jonathan R. Pletcher, MD
Assistant Professor
Department of Pediatrics
University of Pittsburgh School of
    Medicine
Clinical Director
Division of Adolescent Medicine
Children's Hospital of Pittsburgh
Pittsburgh, Pennsylvania

Charles A. Pohl, MD
Professor
Department of Pediatrics
Jefferson Medical College of Thomas
    Jefferson University
Pediatrician
Department of Pediatrics
A. I. duPont Hospital for Children
Wilmington, Delaware

Jill C. Posner, MD, MSCE
Associate Professor of Clinical Pediatrics
Department of Pediatrics
The Children's Hospital of Philadelphia
Perelman School of Medicine
The University of Pennsylvania
Philadelphia, Pennsylvania

Matthew L. Prowler, MD
Department of Psychiatry
Hospital of University of Pennsylvania
Philadelphia, Pennsylvania

Graham E Quinn, MD, MSCE
Division of Ophthalmology
Children's Hospital of Philadelphia
University of Pennsylvania Perelman
    School of Medicine
Philadelphia, Pennsylvania

Christopher P. Raab, MD
Clinical Instructor in Pediatrics
Thomas Jefferson University
Philadelphia, Pennsylvania
Staff Physician
Division of Diagnostic Referral
Nemours/A. I. duPont Hospital for
    Children
Wilmington, Delaware

William V. Raszka, Jr., MD
Department of Pediatrics
University of Vermont College of Medicine
Burlington, Vermont

Jennifer Reid, MD
Assistant Professor of Pediatrics
Department of Pediatrics
University of Washington School of
    Medicine
Seattle Children's Hospital
Seattle, Washington

Anne F. Reilly, MD, MPH
Associate Professor of Clinical Pediatrics
Perelman School of Medicine at the
    University of Pennsylvania
Philadelphia, Pennsylvania

Daniel H. Reirden, MD
University of Colorado School of Medicine
Children's Hospital of Colorado
Sections of Adolescent Medicine and
    Infectious Disease
Aurora, Colorado

Amy E. Renwick, MD
Director of Primary and Consultative
    Pediatrics
Division of General Pediatrics
Alfred I. duPont Hospital for Children
Wilmington, Delaware
Assistant Professor of Pediatrics
Jefferson Medical College
Philadelphia, Pennsylvania

David C. Rettew, MD
Associate Professor of Psychiatry and
    Pediatrics
Program Director
Child & Adolescent Psychiatry Fellowship
Director
Pediatric Psychiatry Clinic
Vermont Center for Children, Youth, and
    Families
Burlington, Vermont

Molly J. Richards, MD
Assistant Professor of Pediatrics
University of Colorado School of Medicine
Department of Adolescent Medicine
Children's Hospital Colorado
Aurora, Colorado

Jeffrey D. Roizen, MD, PhD
Fellow and Instructor
Department of Endocrinology and
    Diabetes
The Children's Hospital of Philadelphia
Philadelphia, Pennsylvania

Michelle T. Rook, MD, MSc
Assistant Professor Division of
    Gastroenterology, Hepatology and
    Nutrition
The Children's Hospital of Philadelphia
University of Pennsylvania
Philadelphia, Pennsylvania

Howard M. Rosenberg, DDS, MSD, Med
Associate Professor
Pediatric Dentistry
Department of Preventive and Restorative
    Sciences
University of Pennsylvania School of
    Dental Medicine
Philadelphia, Pennsylvania

Marianne Ruby, MD
Clinical Instructor
Department of Obstetrics and
    Gynecology
Thomas Jefferson University
Philadelphia, Pennsylvania

Rebecca L. Ruebner, MD
Department of Pediatrics
Division of Nephrology
Children's Hospital of Philadelphia
Philadelphia, Pennsylvania

Richard M. Rutstein, MD
Medical Director
Special Immunology Service
Children's Hospital of Philadelphia
Professor of Pediatrics
Perelman School of Medicine at the
    University of Pennsylvania
Philadelphia, Pennsylvania

Matthew J. Ryan, MD
Assistant Professor of Pediatrics
Perelman School of Medicine at the
    University of Pennsylvania
Attending Physician
Division of Gastroenterology, Hepatology
    and Nutrition
The Children's Hospital of Philadelphia
Philadelphia, Pennsylvania

Nicole Ryan, MD
Assistant Professor
Department of Neurology
Children's Hospital of Philadelphia
Philadelphia, Pennsylvania

Ann E. Salerno, MD
Division Chief, Pediatric Nephrology
UMass Memorial Children's Medical
 Center
Assistant Professor of Pediatrics
University of Massachusetts Medical
 School
Worcester, Massachusetts

Denise A. Salerno, MD, FAAP
Pediatric Clerkship Director
Associate Chair for Undergraduate
 Education
Department of Pediatrics
Temple University School of Medicine
Philadelphia, Pennsylvania

Matthew G. Sampson
U of M Pediatrics Nephrology
C.S. Motts Children's Hospital
Ann Arbor, Michigan

Wudbhav N. Sankar, MD
Assistant Professor of Orthopaedic Surgery
Children's Hospital of Philadelphia
University of Pennsylvania School of
 Medicine
Philadelphia, Pennsylvania

Vered Yehezkely Schildkraut, MD
Consultant
Pediatric Gastroenterology
Department of Gastroenterology and
 Clinical Nutrition
The Royal Children's Hospital
Pediatric Gastroenterology Department
Monash Medical Centre
Melbourne, Australia

Samantha A. Schrier, MD
Fellow
Divisions of Human Genetics and
 Biochemical Genetics
The Children's Hospital of Philadelphia
Philadelphia, Pennsylvania

Charles I. Schwartz, MD, FAAP
Assistant Clinical Professor of Pediatrics
University of Pennsylvania Perelman
 School of Medicine
Chairman of the Department of Pediatrics
Phoenixville Hospital
Phoenixville, Pennsylvania

Teena Sebastian, MD
Department of Pediatrics
Albert Einstein Medical Center
Philadelphia, Pennsylvania

Steven M. Selbst, MD
Pediatric Residency Program Director
Professor and Vice-Chair for Education
Department of Pediatrics
Jefferson Medical College
Thomas Jefferson University
Philadelphia, Pennsylvania
Nemours/Alfred I. duPont Hospital for
 Children
Wilmington, Delaware

Edisio Semeao, MD
Attending Physician
Department of Gastroenterology
Division of Gastroenterology, Hepatology
 and Nutrition
The Children's Hospital of Philadelphia
Philadelphia, Pennsylvania

Deborah Sesok-Pizzini, MD, MBA
Medical Director
Blood Bank and Transfusion Medicine
The Children's Hospital of Philadelphia
Associate Professor of Clinical Pathology
 and Laboratory Medicine
Perelman School of Medicine at the
 University of Pennsylvania
Philadelphia, Pennsylvania

Christine B. Sethna, MD, EdM
Assistant Professor
Hofstra School of Medicine
Interim Divisional Director
Pediatric Nephrology
Cohen Children's Medical Center of
 New York
New Hyde Park, New York

Kara N. Shah, MD, PhD
Director
Division of Dermatology
Cincinnati Children's Hospital
Associate Professor
Departments of Pediatrics and
 Dermatology
University of Cincinnati College of
 Medicine
Cincinnati, Ohio

Samir S. Shah, MD, MSCE
Director
Division of Hospital Medicine
Cincinnati Children's Hospital Medical
 Center
Associate Professor
Department of Pediatrics
University of Cincinnati College of
 Medicine
Cincinnati, Ohio

Julia F. Shaklee, MD
Division of Pediatric Infectious Diseases
The Children's Hospital of Philadelphia
Philadelphia, Pennsylvania

Raanan Shamir, MD
Chairman
Institute of Gastroenterology, Nutrition
 and Liver Diseases
Schneider Children's Medical Center of
 Israel
Professor of Pediatrics
Sackler Faculty of Medicine
Tel-Aviv University
Israel

Andi L. Shane, MD, MPH
Assistant Professor
Division of Infectious Diseases
Emory University School of Medicine
Atlanta, Georgia

David D Sherry, MD
Chief
Rheumatology Section
Professor of Pediatrics
The Children's Hospital of Philadelphia
University of Pennsylvania
Philadelphia, Pennsylvania

Aseem R. Shukla, MD, FAAP
Director
Pediatric Urology
Associate Professor of Urology and
 Pediatrics
University of Minnesota Amplatz
 Children's Hospital
Minneapolis, Minnesota

Daniel Shumer, MD
Pediatric Chief Resident
Vermont Children's Hospital
University of Vermont
Burlington, Vermont

Alyssa Siegel, MD
Clinical Assistant Professor
Division of General Pediatrics
The Children's Hospital of Philadelphia
Philadelphia, Pennsylvania

Hugh Silk, MD, MPH, FAAFP
Clinical Associate Professor
University of Massachusetts Medical
 School
Department of Family Medicine and
 Community Health
Family Medicine Residency – Hahnemann
 Family Health Center
Worcester, Massachusetts

Kim Smith-Whitley, MD
Director
Comprehensive Sickle Cell Center
Clinical Director
Division of Hematology
The Children's Hospital of Philadelphia
Associate Professor
Perelman School of Medicine
University of Pennsylvania
Philadelphia, Pennsylvania

Michael J. Smith, MD, MSCE
Assistant Professor of Pediatrics
University of Louisville School of Medicine
Louisville, Kentucky

Sabrina E. Smith, MD, PhD
Adjunct Assistant Professor of Neurology
University of Pennsylvania School of
    Medicine
Children's Hospital of Philadelphia
Philadelphia, Pennsylvania

Howard M. Snyder, III, MD
Director of Surgical Teaching
Division of Urology
The Children's Hospital of Philadelphia
Professor of Urology
University of Pennsylvania Perelman
    School of Medicine
Philadelphia, Pennsylvania

Patrick Solari, MD
Clinical Assistant Professor
Department of Pediatrics
Seattle Children's Hospital/University of
    Washington School of Medicine
Seattle, Washington

Danielle Soranno, MD
Fellow
Division of Nephrology
Children's Hospital of Philadelphia
Philadelphia, Pennsylvania

**Raman Sreedharan, MD, DCH,
MRCPCH**
Attending Physician
Division of Gastroenterology, Hepatology
    and Nutrition
Children's Hospital of Philadelphia
Clinical Assistant Professor of Pediatrics
Perelman School of Medicine
University of Pennsylvania
Philadelphia, Pennsylvania

**Andrew P. Steenhoff, MBBCh, DCH,
FCPaed(SA)**
Assistant Professor
Department of Pediatrics
Perelman School of Medicine
University of Pennsylvania
Attending Physician
Division of Infectious Diseases
The Children's Hospital of Philadelphia
Philadelphia, Pennsylvania

Julie W. Stern, MD
Clinical Associate Professor
University of Pennsylvania
Division of Oncology
The Children's Hospital of Philadelphia
Philadelphia, Pennsylvania

Sheila Stille, DMD
Program Director
General Practice Residency in Dentistry
University of Massachusetts
Worcester, Massachusetts

Kathleen E. Sullivan, MD, PhD
Chief
Division of Allergy and Immunology
Professor of Pediatrics
Children's Hospital of Philadelphia
Philadelphia, Pennsylvania

John I. Takayama, MD, MPH
Professor of Clinical Pediatrics
Department of Pediatrics
University of California San Francisco
UCSF Benioff Children's Hospital
San Francisco, California

Ronn E. Tanel, MD
Associate Professor of Pediatrics
Department of Pediatrics
UCSF School of Medicine
Director
Pediatric Arrhythmia Center
Division of Pediatric Cardiology
UCSF Benioff Children's Hospital
San Francisco, California

Carl Tapia, MD
Assistant Professor of Pediatrics
Texas Children's Hospital
Houston, Texas

Danna Tauber, MD, MPH
Assistant Professor
Department of Pediatrics
Drexel University College of Medicine
Attending Physician
Section of Pulmonology
St Christopher's Hospital for Children
Philadelphia, Pennsylvania

Jesse A. Taylor, MD
Assistant Professor
Co-Director
CHOP Cleft Team
Plastic, Reconstructive, and Craniofacial
    Surgery
The University of Pennsylvania and
    Children's Hospital of Philadelphia
Philadelphia, Pennsylvania

David T. Teachey, MD
Assistant Professor
Department of Pediatrics
Divisions of Pediatric Hematology and
    Oncology
Blood and Marrow Transplant
Children's Hospital of Philadelphia
University of Pennsylvania, School of
    Medicine
Philadelphia, Pennsylvania

Bruce Tempest, MD
Medical Director (retired) USPHS
Indian Health Service
Gallup Indian Medical Center
Gallup, New Mexico

Alexis Teplick, MD
Pediatrics
Children's Recovery Hospital
Campbell, California

Michelle Terry, MD
Clinical Associate Professor
Department of Pediatrics
University of Washington
Seattle, Washington

Sunil Thummala, MD, MBA
Neurologist
Paris Regional Medical Center
Paris, Texas

Leonel Toledo, MD
Assistant Physician
Department of Pediatrics
The Children's Hospital of Philadelphia
Philadelphia, Pennsylvania

James R. Treat, MD
Assistant Professor of Pediatrics and
    Dermatology
Perelman School of Medicine at the
    University of Pennsylvania
Fellowship Director
Pediatric Dermatology
Children's Hospital of Philadelphia
Philadelphia, Pennsylvania

Vikas Trivedi, MD
Orthopedic Surgeon
Massachusetts General Hospital
Boston, Massachusetts

Nicholas Tsarouhas, MD
Professor of Clinical Pediatrics
University of Pennsylvania School of
  Medicine
Medical Director
Emergency Transport Team
Associate Medical Director
Emergency Department
The Children's Hospital of Philadelphia
Philadelphia, Pennsylvania

Shamir Tuchman, MD, MPH
Assistant Professor of Pediatrics
Division of Pediatric Nephrology
Children's National Medical Center
George Washington University School of
  Medicine
Washington, DC

Judith A. Turow, MD, FAAP
Clinical Associate Professor of Pediatrics
Division of General Pediatrics
Thomas Jefferson University Hospital
Philadelphia, Pennsylvania

John Y. Tung, MBBS, BSc, MRCPH
Attending Physician
Department of Pediatrics
Division of Gastroenterology
A.I. duPont Children's Hospital
Wilmington, Delaware

Charles Vanderpool, MD
Resident Physician
Department of Pediatrics
Vanderbilt University Medical Center
Resident Physician
Department of Pediatrics
Vanderbilt Childrens Hospital
Nashville, Tennessee

Senbagam Virudachalam, MD
Fellow in Academic General Pediatrics
Department of Pediatrics
The Children's Hospital of Philadelphia
Philadelphia, Pennsylvania

Waqar Waheed, MD
Assistant Professor of Neurology
University of Vermont
Burlington, Vermont

Elizabeth M. Wallis, MD
Fellow in Academic General Pediatrics
The Children's Hospital of Philadelphia
Philadelphia, Pennsylvania

Daniel Walmsley, DO, FAAP
Assistant Professor of Pediatrics
Department of Pediatrics
Jefferson Medical College/Nemours
  Pediatrics
Philadelphia, Pennsylvania

Katherine A. Wayman, MD
Chief Resident Neurology
Fletcher Allen Health Care
Burlington, Vermont

Jessica Wen, MD
Assistant Professor of Pediatrics
Division of Gastroenterology, Hepatology
  and Nutrition
The Children's Hospital of Philadelphia
Philadelphia, Pennsylvania

Peter Weiser, MD
Assistant Professor
Division of Pediatric Rheumatology
Department of Pediatrics
Children's Hospital of Alabama
University of Alabama at Birmingham
Birmingham, Alabama

Alexis Weymann
Pediatric Residency Program
The Children's Hospital of Philadelphia
Philadelphia, Pennsylvania

Terri Brown Whitehorn, MD
Assistant Professor of Clinical Pediatrics
Perelman School of Medicine – University
  of Pennsylvania
Philadelphia, Pennsylvania

Sarah E. Winters, MD
Attending Physician
Primary Care
The Children's Hospital of Philadelphia
Philadelphia, Pennsylvania

Char M. Witmer, MD, MSCE
Assistant Professor
Department of Pediatrics
Division of Hematology
The Children's Hospital of Philadelphia
Philadelphia, Pennsylvania

Margaret Wolff, MD
Fellow in Pediatric Emergency Medicine
University of Pennsylvania School of
  Medicine
Division of Emergency Medicine
Children's Hospital of Philadelphia
Philadelphia, Pennsylvania

Tracie Wong, MD
Assistant Professor of Pediatrics
University of Pennsylvania School of
  Medicine
Attending Physician
Division of GI, Hepatology and Nutrition
Children's Hospital of Philadelphia
Philadelphia, Pennsylvania

George A. (Tony) Woodward, MD,
MBA
Chief
Division of Emergency Medicine
Medical Director
Transport Services
Seattle Children's Hospital
Professor of Pediatrics
University of Washington School of
  Medicine
Seattle, Washington

Paige L. Wright, MD
Assistant Professor
Department of Pediatrics
University of Washington School of
  Medicine
Academic Faculty
Emergency Services Department
Children's Hospital and Regional Medical
  Center
Seattle, Washington

Hsi-Yang Wu, MD
Associate Professor of Urology
Stanford University Medical Center
Lucile Packard Children's Hospital
Palo Alto, California

Albert C. Yan, MD
Chief
Section of Pediatric Dermatology
Children's Hospital of Philadelphia
Associate Professor
Pediatrics and Dermatology
Perelman School of Medicine at the
  University of Pennsylvania
Philadelphia, Pennsylvania

Yvette Yatchmink, MD, PhD
Associate Professor of Pediatrics
   (Clinical)
Division of Developmental-Behavioral
   Pediatrics
Warren Alpert Medical School of Brown
   University
Providence, Rhode Island

Stephen A. Zderic, MD
Professor of Surgery in Urology
The Perelman School of Medicine at the
   University of Pennsylvania
The John W. Duckett Endowed Chair
The Children's Hospital of
   Philadelphia
Philadelphia, Pennsylvania

Andrew F. Zigman
Department of Pediatric Surgery
Kaiser Permanente Surgery Department
Portland, Oregon

Karen P. Zimmer, MD, MPH, FAAP
Assistant Professor
Johns Hopkins School of Medicine
Medical Director
ECRI Institute
Baltimore, Maryland

Raezelle Zinman, MDCM
Clinical Professor of Pediatrics
University of Pennsylvania
Division of Pulmonary Medicine
Children's Hospital of Philadelphia
Philadelphia, Pennsylvania

Catherine S. Zorc, MD
Fellow in Academic General
   Pediatrics
Division of General Pediatrics
Children's Hospital of Philadelphia
Philadelphia, Pennsylvania

Kathleen M. Zsolway, DO
Medical Director
General Pediatrics Faculty Practice
The Children's Hospital of
   Philadelphia
Clinical Associate Professor of
   Pediatrics
University of Pennsylvania
Philadelphia, Pennsylvania

CONTENTS

The 5-Minute Pediatric Consult

SIXTH EDITION

ABDOMINAL MASS

Rose C. Graham

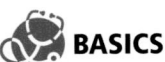 **BASICS**

DEFINITION
An unusually enlarged abdominal or retroperitoneal organ (i.e., hepatomegaly, splenomegaly, or enlarged kidney) or a defined fullness in the abdominal cavity not directly associated with an abdominal organ.

EPIDEMIOLOGY
- 60% of abdominal masses in children are due to organomegaly.
- 40% of abdominal masses in children are due to anomalies of development, neoplasms, or inflammatory conditions.

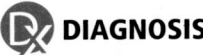 **DIAGNOSIS**

DIFFERENTIAL DIAGNOSIS
- **Stomach**
  - Gastroparesis
  - Duplication
  - Foreign body/bezoar
  - Gastric torsion
  - Gastric tumor (lymphoma, sarcoma)
- **Intestine**
  - Feces (constipation)
  - Meconium ileus
  - Duplication
  - Volvulus
  - Intussusception
  - Intestinal atresia or stenosis
  - Malrotation
  - Inflammatory bowel disease complications (abscess, phlegmon)
  - Appendiceal or Meckel diverticulum abscess
  - Toxic megacolon
  - Lymphoma, adenocarcinoma
  - Carcinoid
  - Foreign body
  - Duodenal hematoma (trauma)
- **Liver**
  - Hepatomegaly due to intrinsic liver disease:
    - Hepatitis (viral, autoimmune)
    - Metabolic disorders (Wilson disease, glycogen storage disease)
    - Congenital hepatic fibrosis
  - Cystic disease (Caroli disease)
  - Tumor (hepatic adenoma, hepatoblastoma, hepatocellular carcinoma or diffuse neoplastic process such as lymphoma)
  - Vascular tumor (hamartoma, hemangioma, hemangioendothelioma)
  - Vascular obstruction/congestion (Budd–Chiari syndrome, congestive heart failure)
  - Focal nodular hyperplasia
- **Spleen**
  - Storage disease (Gaucher, Niemann–Pick)
  - Langerhans cell histiocytosis
  - Leukemia
  - Hematologic (hemolytic disease, sickle cell disease, hereditary spherocytosis/elliptocytosis)
  - Wandering spleen

- **Pancreas**
  - Pseudocyst (trauma)
  - Pancreatoblastoma
- **Gallbladder/biliary tract**
  - Choledochal cyst
  - Hydrops
  - Obstruction (stone, stricture, trauma)
- **Kidney**
  - Multicystic dysplastic kidney
  - Hydronephrosis/ureteropelvic obstruction
  - Polycystic disease
  - Wilms tumor
  - Renal vein thrombosis
  - Cystic nephroma
  - Mesoblastic nephroma
- **Bladder**
  - Posterior urethral valves
  - Neurogenic bladder
- **Adrenal**
  - Adrenal hemorrhage
  - Adrenal abscess
  - Neuroblastoma
  - Pheochromocytoma
- **Uterus**
  - Pregnancy
  - Hematocolpos
  - Hydrometrocolpos
- **Ovary**
  - Cysts (dermoid, follicular)
  - Torsion
  - Germ cell tumor
- **Peritoneal**
  - Ascites
  - Teratoma
- **Abdominal wall**
  - Umbilical/inguinal/ventral hernia
  - Omphalocele/gastroschisis
  - Trauma (rectus hematoma)
  - Tumor (fibroma, lipoma, rhabdomyosarcoma)
- **Omentum/mesentery**
  - Cysts
  - Mesenteric fibromatosis
    - Mesenteric adenitis
  - Tumors (liposarcoma, leiomyosarcoma, fibrosarcoma, mesothelioma)
- **Other**
  - Lymphangioma
  - Fetus in fetu
  - Sacrococcygeal teratoma

APPROACH TO THE PATIENT
When evaluating a pediatric abdominal mass, an organized approach is paramount in determining its etiology.
- **Phase 1:** Determine the location of the abdominal mass and its association with intra-abdominal organs via a thorough and careful abdominal examination.
- **Phase 2:** Perform diagnostic tests:
  - Ultrasound is the most efficient way to start the evaluation.

Hints for Screening Problems
- In neonates, a palpable liver edge can be normal; the total liver span is most important.
- In infants, a full bladder is often mistaken for an abdominal mass.
- In infants, most abdominal masses are of renal origin and nonmalignant.
- Severe constipation in older children and adolescents can present as a large, hard mass extending from the pubis past the umbilicus.
- Gastric distention should be considered in all children who present with a tympanitic epigastric mass.

HISTORY
- **Question:** Weight loss?
- *Significance:* Tumor, inflammatory bowel disease
- **Question:** Fever?
- *Significance:* Abscess, malignancy
- **Question:** Jaundice?
- *Significance:* Liver/biliary disease
- **Question:** Hematuria or dysuria?
- *Significance:* Renal disease
- **Question:** Vomiting?
- *Significance:* Intestinal obstruction
- **Question:** Frequency and quality of bowel movements?
- *Significance:* Constipation, intussusception, compression of bowel by mass
- **Question:** Bleeding or bruising?
- *Significance:* Coagulopathy
- **Question:** History of abdominal trauma?
- *Significance:* Pancreatic pseudocyst, duodenal hematoma
- **Question:** Sexual activity?
- *Significance:* Pregnancy
- **Question:** Age of patient?
- *Significance:*
  - Often a helpful clue in investigating the cause of the abdominal mass
  - In neonates, the most common origin of abdominal masses is the genitourinary system (cystic kidney disease, hydronephrosis).
  - In infants and preschool-aged children, the most common malignant tumors are Wilms tumor and neuroblastoma.
  - In adolescent-aged girls, ovarian disorders, hematocolpos, and pregnancy are more common causes of abdominal masses.

PHYSICAL EXAM
- **Finding:** General appearance?
- *Significance:* Ill-appearance or cachexia point toward infection or malignancy.
- **Finding:** Location of abdominal mass?
- *Significance:*
  - Left lower quadrant: Constipation, ovarian process, ectopic pregnancy
  - Left upper quadrant: Anomaly of the kidney or splenomegaly
  - Right lower quadrant: Abscess (inflammatory bowel disease), intestinal phlegmon, appendicitis, intussusception, ovarian process, ectopic pregnancy
  - Right upper quadrant: Involves liver, gallbladder, biliary tree, or intestine
  - Epigastric: Abnormality of the stomach (bezoar, torsion), pancreas (pseudocyst), or enlarged liver
  - Suprapubic: Pregnancy, hydrometrocolpos, hematocolpos, posterior urethral valves
  - Flank: Renal disease (cystic kidney, hydronephrosis, Wilms tumor)
- **Finding:** Characteristics of abdominal mass?
- *Significance:* Mobility, tenderness, firmness, smoothness, and/or irregularity of the surface of the mass can provide clues to its significance.
- **Finding:** Hard and immobile mass?
- *Significance:* Tumor
- **Finding:** Extension of mass across midline or into pelvis?
- *Significance:* Tumor, hepatomegaly, splenomegaly
- **Finding:** Percussion of mass?
- *Significance:* Dullness indicates a solid mass; tympany indicates a hollow viscus.
- **Finding:** Shifting dullness, fluid wave?
- *Significance:* Ascites
- **Finding:** Skin exam?
- *Significance:* Bruising and petechiae may occur with coagulopathy related to liver disease and malignant infiltration of bone marrow; café au lait spots are associated with neurofibromas.
- **Finding:** Lymphadenopathy or lymphadenitis?
- *Significance:* Systemic process either malignant or infectious

DIAGNOSTIC TESTS & INTERPRETATION
- **Test:** CBC
- *Significance:* Anemia or hemolysis
- **Test:** Chemistry panel
- *Significance:*
  - Renal disease: BUN and creatinine levels
  - Liver disease (bilirubin, ALT, AST, alkaline phosphatase, GGT, albumin, PT/PTT)
  - Gallbladder disease (bilirubin, GGT)
  - Pancreatic disease: Amylase/lipase levels
  - Intestinal disease: Hypoalbuminemia
- **Test:** Uric acid and lactate dehydrogenase levels
- *Significance:* Elevated in the setting of rapid cell turnover of solid tumors

Imaging
- Plain abdominal radiographs:
  - Rule out intestinal obstruction, identify calcifications, fecal impaction.
- Abdominal ultrasound:
  - Can usually identify the origin of the mass and differentiate between solid and cystic tissue; disadvantages are operator variability and a limited exam when bowel gas obscures underlying abdominal tissues.
- CT scan:
  - Can provide more detail when there is overlying gas or bone; if malignancy is suspected should do chest, abdomen, and pelvis CT.
- MRI:
  - Vascular lesions of liver, major vessels, and tumors
- Radioisotope cholescintigraphy (HIDA) scan:
  - Liver, gallbladder
    - Meckel scan can identify gastric mucosa contained within a Meckel diverticulum or intestinal duplication.
- Voiding cystourethrography or intravenous urography:
  - Wilms tumor, cystic kidney disease, posterior urethral valves, hydronephrosis
- Upper GI study and barium enema:
  - May be of benefit when the mass involves the intestine

 TREATMENT

General Measures
- Immediate hospitalization for patients who present with an abdominal mass and signs and/or symptoms of intestinal obstruction
- Initial diagnostic studies should include an abdominal ultrasound and a surgical or oncological consultation as indicated.
- The remaining causes of abdominal masses require urgent care and timely evaluation and referral to appropriate specialists.

ISSUES FOR REFERRAL
Except for the diagnosis of constipation, the presence of an abdominal mass requires immediate attention, and diagnostic studies should be performed expeditiously at a facility capable of diagnosing pediatric disorders.

Admission Criteria
- Immediate hospitalization for patients who present with an abdominal mass and signs and/or symptoms of intestinal obstruction (intussusception, volvulus, gastric torsion, bezoar, foreign body):
  - Toxic megacolon
  - Ovarian torsion
  - Ectopic pregnancy
  - Biliary obstruction (stone, hydrops)
  - Fever
  - Pancreatitis (pseudocyst)
- The remaining causes of abdominal masses require urgent care and timely evaluation and referral to appropriate specialists.

ADDITIONAL READING

- Chandler JC, Gauderer MWL. The neonate with an abdominal mass. *Pediatr Clin North Am.* 2004;51: 979–997.
- Golden CB, Feusner JH. Malignant abdominal masses in children: Quick guide to evaluation and diagnosis. *Pediatr Clin North Am.* 2002;49: 1369–1392.
- Mahaffey SM, Rychman RC, Martin LW. Clinical aspects of abdominal masses in children. *Semin Roentgenol.* 1988;23:161–174.
- Merten DF, Kirks DR. Diagnostic imaging of pediatric abdominal masses. *Pediatr Clin North Am.* 1985;32:1397–1426.

 CODES

ICD9
- 789.1 Hepatomegaly
- 789.2 Splenomegaly
- 789.30 Abdominal or pelvic swelling, mass, or lump, unspecified site

ICD10
- R16.0 Hepatomegaly, not elsewhere classified
- R16.1 Splenomegaly, not elsewhere classified
- R19.00 Intra-abd and pelvic swelling, mass and lump, unsp site

ABDOMINAL MIGRAINE

Matthew P. Kirschen
Joel Friedlander

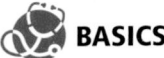

BASICS

DESCRIPTION
Recurrent attacks of periumbilical pain with nausea, vomiting, anorexia, headache, and pallor

EPIDEMIOLOGY
Incidence
- Occurs mostly in children, with a mean onset at age 7 year (3–10 years)
- Peak symptoms 10–12 years of age
- More common in girls (3:2)

Prevalence
- May affect as many as 1–4% of children at some point in their lives
- Declining frequency toward adulthood

RISK FACTORS
Genetics
Parents of affected children often have history of migraine headaches and motion sickness.

ETIOLOGY
- May involve neuronal activity originating in the hypothalamus with involvement of the cortex and autonomic nervous system
- Serotonin is implicated, and blockade of serotonin receptors may prevent abdominal migraine.
- May involve some as yet ill-defined local intestinal vasomotor factors

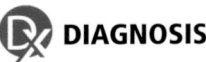

DIAGNOSIS

Rome III criteria—2 episodes within 12 months meeting all of the following criteria:
- Paroxysmal intense periumbilical pain that lasts >1 hour
- Intervening episodes of health between episodes
- Pain that interferes with activity
- Pain associated with ≥2 of the following: Anorexia, nausea, vomiting, headache, photophobia, or pallor
- No evidence of inflammatory, anatomic, metabolic, or neoplastic process

HISTORY
- Pain usually lasts <6 hours.
- Pain can be located anywhere in abdomen, but more often in upper quadrants.
- No abdominal pain between attacks
- Repetition of identical abdominal crises, anywhere from 1 time per week to several times a year
- Migraine in the history of patient or relatives
- Occasionally, other migraine phenomena such as nausea, vomiting, perspiration, body temperature changes, focal paresthesias, radiation of pain to a limb, visual disturbances, or general malaise
- Impaired consciousness (some degree of lethargy may occur)
- Ask about a family history of migraine headache or unexplained bouts of abdominal pain as children.

PHYSICAL EXAM
- Physical exam, including complete neurologic and abdominal exam, is usually unremarkable.
- Complete eye exam including fundoscopic exam should be done to evaluate for papilledema.

DIAGNOSTIC TESTS & INTERPRETATION
- Even if a patient meets most criteria for abdominal migraine, studies as outlined below should be strongly considered to ensure that a more serious disorder does not exist.
- Abdominal migraine is a diagnosis of exclusion.

Lab
- CBC with differential
- ESR and CRP
- Urinalysis
- Pregnancy test
- Amylase and lipase
- Stool hemoccult
- Stool culture
- Lactose breath test for lactose intolerance
- Lead level
- Evaluation for porphyria or familial Mediterranean fever

- Metabolic evaluation (must be performed during a symptomatic period): Urine organic acids, plasma amino acids, ammonia, lactate, blood gas, acylcarnitine profile, imaging

Diagnostic Procedures/Radiologic Imaging
- Obstruction series to assess for intermittent or partial bowel obstruction
- Upper GI to rule out anatomic abnormalities
- US or CT scan to rule out mass lesion or chronic appendicitis
- Renal US to rule out ureteropelvic junction (UPJ) obstruction
- Barium enema (during painful crisis) to rule out intussusception
- EEG may help differentiate between abdominal migraine and epilepsy.
- Visual evoked response (VER) to red and white flashlight: Children with abdominal migraine may display a specific fast-wave activity response.
- Rarely, brain imaging with CT or MRI may be useful for evaluating causes of intermittent hydrocephalus.

DIFFERENTIAL DIAGNOSIS
- Infection:
  - Giardia
- Environmental:
  - Lead intoxication
- Tumors
- Metabolic:
  - Porphyria, lactose intolerance, female carriers of (X-linked) ornithine transcarbamylase (OTC) gene mutation, organic acidemias
- Psychosocial:
  - Functional abdominal pain/irritable bowel syndrome
- Surgical:
  - Appendicitis, intussusception, biliary colic
- Inflammation:
  - Inflammatory bowel disease, peptic ulcer disease, mesenteric adenitis
- GI:
  - Irritable bowel syndrome, gastroesophageal reflux, wandering spleen, cyclical vomiting syndrome, recurrent abdominal pain, functional abdominal pain, constipation, superior mesenteric artery (SMA) syndrome, recurrent pancreatitis

- Anatomic:
  - Meckel diverticulum, UPJ obstruction
- Neurologic:
  - Abdominal epilepsy—but has a shorter duration of pain (minutes), altered consciousness during event, abrupt onset, abnormal discharges in EEG in 80%
  - Temporal lobe epilepsy
  - Intermittent hydrocephalus (possibly secondary to a 3rd ventricle colloid cyst)

ALERT
Because it is usually a diagnosis of exclusion, many patients go through a large workup to rule out other causes of pain, sometimes including laparotomy.

TREATMENT

MEDICATION (DRUGS)
- Medications can be used to abort acute attacks or be taken as daily prophylaxis.
- For most patients, risks of side effects and complications from the use of these medications may outweigh the relief of pain, especially in children who are experiencing infrequent episodes.
- Limited data exist on abortive agents for abdominal migraines; however, several agents have shown benefit in specialty-based clinical practice, including metoclopramide, steroids, intranasal sumatriptan, and NSAIDs (although the latter may be avoided if there are clinical concerns for gastritis or peptic ulcer disease). Consider benzodiazepines (i.e. lorazepam) and antiemetics (i.e. odansetron) for vomiting predominant symptoms.
- Suggested prophylactic treatments are similar to those for migraine headaches and include tricyclic antidepressants (e.g., amitriptyline), topiramate, propranolol, cyproheptadine, and valproic acid. If EEG or other data point to possible epilepsy, empiric treatment with anticonvulsants may be considered.

ADDITIONAL TREATMENT
General Measures
- Trigger avoidance:
  - An event diary should be kept to identify possible migraine triggers.
  - Avoiding triggers is the most optimal strategy for preventing recurrent attacks:
    - Common triggers include caffeine, nitrites, amines, emotional arousal, travel, prolonged fasting, altered sleep, exercise, and/or flickering lights.
- Cognitive therapies:
  - Behavioral therapies and lifestyle modification (regular sleep, hydration, and exercise) may also be of benefit. Biofeedback in conjunction with other cognitive therapies and/or relaxation programs may be helpful. Assistance from a trained pediatric mental health professional might be necessary.

ONGOING CARE

FOLLOW-UP RECOMMENDATIONS
- Most children outgrow abdominal migraine symptoms (~60%) by early adolescence.
- A substantial percentage of patients (~70%) may later develop more typical migraine headaches.
- Although nonspecific EEG changes are seen more commonly among these children, very few go on to develop epilepsy.
- 10% of children who have a diagnosis of migraine headaches have previously suffered from unexplained recurrent abdominal pain.
- Adult migraine headache sufferers experience abdominal pain more frequently than do tension headache sufferers.

PATIENT EDUCATION
- To help child during bouts of pain, allow the child to do whatever makes him or her comfortable—rest, positioning, quiet.
- Whether the patient should be excused from school depends on various factors:
  - Frequency, severity, and duration of pain
  - Age, maturity, and coping skills of the child

ADDITIONAL READING

- Catto-Smith AG, Ranuh R. Abdominal migraine and cyclical vomiting. *Semin Pediatr Surg*. 2003;12(4): 254–258.
- Cuvellier JC, Lépine A. Childhood periodic syndromes. *Pediatr Neurol*. 2010;42(1):1–11.
- Lewis DW. Pediatric migraine. *Neurol Clin*. 2009;27(2):481–501.
- Li BU, Balint JP. Cyclic vomiting syndrome: Evolution in our understanding of a brain-gut disorder. *Adv Pediatr*. 2000;47:117–160.
- Popovich DM, Schentrup DM, McAlhany AL. Recognizing and diagnosing abdominal migraines. *J Pediatr Health Care*. 2010;24(6):372–377.
- Rasquin A, Di Lorenzo C, Forbes D, et al. Childhood functional gastrointestinal disorders: Child/adolescent. *Gastroenterology*. 2006;130: 1527–1537.

- Russell G, Abu-Arafehl, Symon DN. Abdominal migraine: Evidence for existence and treatment options. *Pediatr Drugs*. 2002;4:1–8.
- Tan V, Sahami AR, Peebes R, et al. Abdominal migraine and treatment with intravenous valproic acid. *Psychosomatics*. 2006;47(4):353–355.
- Weydert JA, Ball TM, Davis MF. Systematic review of treatments for recurrent abdominal pain. *Pediatrics*. 2003;111:e1–e11.

CODES

ICD9
346.20 Variants of migraine, not elsewhere classified, without mention of intractable migraine without mention of status migrainosus

ICD10
- G43.101 Migraine with aura, not intractable, with status migrainosus
- G43.109 Migraine with aura, not intractable, without status migrainosus
- G43.111 Migraine with aura, intractable, with status migrainosus

FAQ

- Q: Does this mean my child will develop migraine headaches?
- A: There is no accurate way to predict whether your child will develop migraine headaches.
- Q: I have 2 younger children. What chance do they have of developing abdominal migraines?
- A: Although migraine headaches do tend to run in families, there is no known Mendelian inheritance pattern.
- Q: What can I do to help my child during bouts of pain?
- A: First, allow the child to do whatever makes him or her comfortable. This may mean resting, positioning, or being quiet. Acetaminophen or NSAID based pain relievers may help to a certain degree. Whether the patient should be excused from school depends on various factors such as the frequency, severity, and duration of the pain as well as the age, maturity, and coping skills of the child.

ABDOMINAL PAIN

Kurt A. Brown

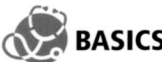 **BASICS**

DEFINITION
A child's complaint of abdominal pain can originate from GI and non-GI causes but also commonly can be the manifestation of referred pain from extra-abdominal sites.

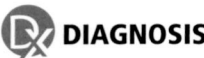 **DIAGNOSIS**

DIFFERENTIAL DIAGNOSIS
- **Congenital/anatomic**
  - Incarcerated hernia
  - Intussusception
  - Malrotation with volvulus
  - Ovarian torsion
  - Testicular torsion
  - Ureteropelvic junction obstruction
- **Infectious**
  - Cystitis and urinary tract infections
  - Fitz-Hugh–Curtis syndrome
  - Gastroenteritis (bacterial, viral or parasitic)
  - Helicobacter pylori gastritis
  - Mononucleosis
  - Pharyngitis
  - Pelvic inflammatory disease
  - Peritonitis
  - Pneumonia
  - Psoas abscess
  - Sepsis
  - Tubo-ovarian abscess
  - Varicella
- **Toxic, environmental drugs**
  - Anticholinergic drugs
  - Intestinal foreign body
  - Heavy-metal (i.e., lead) ingestion
  - Mushroom poisoning
  - Food poisoning
  - Sympathomimetic drugs
- **Trauma**
  - Child abuse
  - Duodenal hematoma
  - Perforated viscus
  - Splenic hematoma/rupture
- **Tumor**
  - Any tumor, benign or malignant, leading to viscus obstruction
  - Leukemia
  - Lymphoma
  - Wilms tumor
- **Genetic/metabolic**
  - Diabetic ketoacidosis
  - Lactase deficiency

- **Allergic/inflammatory**
  - Appendicitis
  - Cholecystitis
  - Eosinophilic gastroenteritis
  - Henoch–Schönlein purpura
  - Hepatitis
  - Inflammatory bowel disease
  - Intestinal adhesions
  - Mesenteric adenitis
  - Necrotizing enterocolitis
  - Pancreatitis
  - Peptic ulcer or gastritis
  - Esophagitis or duodenitis
- **Functional**
  - Depression
  - Functional abdominal pain
  - Malingering
  - Munchausen syndrome (+/− by proxy)
  - Stress
- **Miscellaneous**
  - Abdominal migraine
  - Cholelithiasis
  - Colic
  - Constipation
  - Dysmenorrhea
  - Ectopic pregnancy
  - Endometriosis
  - Ileus
  - Intestinal pseudo-obstruction
  - Irritable bowel syndrome
  - Lactose intolerance
  - Mittelschmerz
  - Nephrolithiasis
  - Ovarian cyst
  - Pregnancy
  - Porphyria
  - Sickle cell disease
  - Typhlitis

APPROACH TO THE PATIENT
- **Phase 1:** Careful and complete history and physical exam to narrow this extensive differential diagnosis:
  - Identify emergencies
  - Separate acute pain conditions from chronic pain
- **Phase 2:** Directed laboratory evaluations should be made to support more likely portions of the differential diagnosis.

HISTORY
- **Question:** Location and duration of pain?
- *Significance:* Acute vs. chronic illness
- **Question:** Onset and progression of symptoms?
- *Significance:* Evolution of painful process
- **Question:** Presence of hematochezia?
- *Significance:* Colonic bleeding or massive upper GI bleeding
- **Question:** Abdominal distention?
- *Significance:* Distention of an abdominal viscus by air, stool, or fluid
- **Question:** Radiation of pain?
- *Significance:* Certain entities characteristically have radiation of pain (i.e., pancreatitis to the back, appendicitis to the right lower quadrant).

- **Question:** Pain relieved by bowel movements?
- *Significance:* Etiology may be related to colonic distension (by air or stool) or inflammation (colitis).
- **Question:** Bowel movement pattern: Decrease in frequency or change in caliber?
- *Significance:* Constipation, tumor, or something else?
- **Question:** Relationship to emesis?
- *Significance:* Usually upper intestinal tract obstruction, liver or gall bladder disorders (pain etiology—see Table 1)
- **Question:** Signs and symptoms of abdominal pain?
- *Significance:* The farther the complaint of pain is away from the periumbilical region, the more likely the pain etiology represents organic disease. True nighttime waking with pain is more often correlated with organic disease than functional pain.

PHYSICAL EXAM
- **Finding:** Location of pain?
- *Significance:* See Table 1
- **Finding:** Re-examination by the same health care provider for changing characteristics?
- *Significance:* Evolution of abdominal process
- **Finding:** Rebound tenderness?
- *Significance:* Peritoneal irritation from peritonitis or appendicitis; potential need for surgical intervention
- **Finding:** Rectal examination?
- *Significance:* Peritoneal irritation, further localization of pain, masses, presence and consistency of stool, and/or occult heme

DIAGNOSTIC TESTS & INTERPRETATION
- **Test:** CBC with differential
- *Significance:* Total WBC count is nonspecific and may be a poor indicator of intestinal inflammation. Anemia is seen in lead poisoning, malignancy, and bleeding. Low platelets are seen in hypersplenism.
- **Test:** ESR
- *Significance:* Nonspecific indicator of systemic inflammation, such as inflammatory bowel disease
- **Test:** Urinalysis
- *Significance:* General screen for urinary tract abnormalities, infection, and collagen disease
- **Test:** Comprehensive metabolic panel
- *Significance:* Sodium, potassium, chloride, carbon dioxide, blood urea nitrogen, creatinine, glucose, total protein, albumin, alanine aminotransferase, uric acid, lactate dehydrogenase

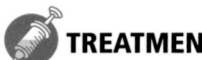 **TREATMENT**

General Measures
- Every effort should be made to ensure that the patient is clinically stable.
- Frequent evaluation of vital signs and physical exam is a means of assessing evolving pain and ensuring that the patient is well enough for potential discharge.

ISSUES FOR REFERRAL
Persistent abdominal pain without clear etiology or chronic GI diseases should be referred to a pediatric gastroenterologist.

Table 1. Classic clinical findings in disorders characterized by abdominal pain

Disorder	Typical clinical picture	Definitive diagnostic test
Peptic ulcer disease	Burning or sharp midepigastric pain that occurs 1–3 hours after meals and is exacerbated by spicy food and relieved by antacids; family history of peptic ulcer disease	Endoscopy
Pancreatitis	Episodic left upper quadrant pain or epigastic that occurs 5–10 minutes after meals, radiates to the back, and is exacerbated by fatty foods	Pancreatic ultrasound or CT scan; Serum amylase and lipasis level (↑)
Urinary tract infection	Suprapubic pain, burning on urination, urinary frequency, urinary urgency	Urine culture; Urinalysis
Renal calculi	Severe periodic cramping pain that occurs in the flank and occasionally radiates to the groin; costovertebral angle tenderness; family history of renal calculi	Urinalysis; Renal ultrasound
Periappendiceal abscess	Right lower quadrant pain; rebound and direct tenderness; anorexia and vomiting; fever	Laparoscopy; WBC count (↑)
Gallbladder disease	Right upper quadrant pain that occurs 5–10 minutes after meals and is exacerbated by fatty foods; family history of gallstones	Gallbladder ultrasound
Menstrual pain	Cramping suprapubic pain that occurs during the menses	Trial with NSAIDs
Pelvic inflammatory disease	Suprapubic pain	Cervical culture
Functional abdominal pain (irritable bowel syndrome)	Cramping periumbilical pain that is exacerbated by eating and relieved by defecation	Trial with Metamucil
Lactose intolerance	Cramping periumbilical pain that increases following ingestion of dairy products and is accompanied by flatulence and bloating	Trial with a milk-free diet; Breath hydrogen study for lactose deficiency
Inflammatory bowel disease	Right lower quadrant cramping and tenderness; anemia; guaiac-positive stool	Colonoscopy; Barium enema; Upper GI series; ESR (↑), platelet count (↑), WBC count (↑)
Esophagitis	Epigastric and substernal pain that is relieved by antacids and exacerbated by lying down; history of iron deficiency; anemia; guaiac-positive stool	Endoscopy
Lead poisoning	Abdominal pain; history of pica; microcytic anemia; basophilic stippling	Serum lead level
Pancreatic pseudocyst	Left upper quadrant pain; recurrent vomiting; history of abdominal pain	Abdominal ultrasound
Sickle cell disease	Periumbilical pain that responds to rest and rehydration	Sickle cell preparation; Hemoglobin electrophoresis
Abdominal epilepsy	Periodic severe abdominal pain that is often associated with seizures	Trial with anticonvulsants
Abdominal migraine	Severe abdominal pain; family history of migraine; recurrent headache, fever, and vomiting; unilateral or occipital headache; somatic complaints	Trial with antimigraine medications
Depression	Social withdrawal; decreased activity; irritability; poor attention span; difficulty sleeping	Trial with antidepressant medications
School avoidance	Nonspecific abdominal pain; severe anxiety reaction; pain that is more severe on weekdays and improves on weekends	

CT, computed tomography; ESR, erythrocyte sedimentation rate; GI, gastrointestinal; NSAIDS, nonsteroidal antiinflammatory drugs; UTI, urinary tract infection; WBC, white blood cell; ↑, increased.

ADDITIONAL READING

- Alfven G. One hundred cases of recurrent abdominal pain in children: Diagnostic procedures and criteria for a psychosomatic diagnosis. *Acta Paediatr.* 2003;92:43–49 [erratum appears in *Acta Paediatr.* 2003;92:641].
- American Academy of Pediatrics Subcommittee on Chronic Abdominal Pain; North American Society for Pediatric Gastroenterology, Hepatology, and Nutrition. Chronic abdominal pain in children. *Pediatrics.* 2005;115(3):e370–e81.
- Apley J. Psychosomatic aspects of gastrointestinal problems in children. *Clin Gastroenterol.* 1977; 6:311–320.
- Berger MY, Gieteling MJ, Benninga MA. Chronic abdominal pain in children. *BMJ.* 2007;334: 997–1002.
- Chitkara DK, Rawat DJ, Talley NJ. The epidemiology of childhood recurrent abdominal pain in Western countries: A systematic review. *Am J Gastroenterol.* 2005;100(8):1868–1875.
- Collins BS, Thomas DW. Chronic abdominal pain. *Pediatr Rev.* 2007;28(9):323–331 [erratum appears in *Pediatr Rev.* 2007;28(12):469].
- Huertas-Ceballos A, Macarthur C, Logan S. Dietary interventions for recurrent abdominal pain (RAP) in childhood. *Cochrane Database Syst Rev.* 2002;2: CD003019.
- Huertas-Ceballos A, Macarthur C, Logan S. Pharmacological interventions for recurrent abdominal pain (RAP) in childhood. *Cochrane Database Syst Rev.* 2002;1:CD003017.
- McCollough M, Sharieff GQ. Abdominal pain in children. *Pediatr Clin North Am.* 2006;53(1): 107–137, vi.
- Weydert JA, Ball TM, Davis MF. Systematic review of treatments for recurrent abdominal pain. *Pediatrics.* 2003;111(1):e1–e11.
- Zeiter DK, Hyams JS. Recurrent abdominal pain in children. *Pediatr Clin North Am.* 2002;49:53–71.

 CODES

ICD9
- 560.0 Intussusception
- 756.70 Anomaly of abdominal wall, unspecified
- 789.00 Abdominal pain, unspecified site

ICD10
- K56.1 Intussusception
- Q79.59 Other congenital malformations of abdominal wall
- R10.9 Unspecified abdominal pain

ABNORMAL BLEEDING

Char Witmer

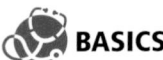 **BASICS**

DEFINITION
Abnormal bleeding may present as:
- Frequent or significant mucocutaneous bleeding (epistaxis, bruising, gum bleeding, or menorrhagia)
- Bleeding in unusual sites such as muscles, joints, or internal organs
- Excessive postsurgical bleeding

ETIOLOGY
Abnormal bleeding can be the result of a coagulation factor deficiency, an acquired or congenital disorder of platelet number or function, or inherited or acquired collagen vascular disorders.

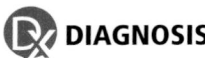 **DIAGNOSIS**

DIFFERENTIAL DIAGNOSIS
Platelet disorders may be quantitative or qualitative, collagen vascular disorders can be acquired or inherited, and disorders of coagulation factors can be congenital or acquired.

- **Thrombocytopenia: Defective production**
  - Congenital/genetic:
    ○ Thrombocytopenia with absent radii syndrome
    ○ Amegakaryocytic thrombocytopenia
    ○ Fanconi anemia
    ○ Metabolic disorders
    ○ Wiskott–Aldrich syndrome
    ○ Bernard–Soulier syndrome
    ○ Other rare familial syndromes (e.g., May–Hegglin anomaly)
  - Acquired:
    ○ Aplastic anemia
    ○ Drug-associated marrow suppression
    ○ Virus-associated marrow suppression (e.g., HIV)
    ○ Chemotherapy
    ○ Radiation injury
    ○ Nutritional deficiencies (e.g., vitamin B12 and folate)
  - Marrow infiltration:
    ○ Neoplasia (e.g., leukemia, neuroblastoma)
    ○ Histiocytosis
    ○ Osteopetrosis
    ○ Myelofibrosis
    ○ Hemophagocytic syndromes
    ○ Storage diseases
- **Thrombocytopenia: Increased destruction**
  - Idiopathic thrombocytopenia
  - Neonatal alloimmune thrombocytopenia
  - Maternal autoimmune thrombocytopenia
  - Drug induced (heparin, sulfonamides, digoxin, chloroquine)
  - Sepsis/disseminated intravascular coagulopathy
  - Infection: Viral, bacterial, fungal, rickettsial
  - Microangiopathic process (e.g., thrombotic thrombocytopenic purpura/hemolytic uremic syndrome)
  - Kasabach–Merritt syndrome
  - Hypersplenism

- **Platelet function disorders**
  - Storage pool disorders (e.g., dense granule deficiency, Hermansky–Pudlak or Chediak–Higashi syndrome)
  - Platelet receptor abnormalities (e.g., Glanzmann thrombasthenia, adenosine 5'-diphosphate receptor defect)
  - Drugs (e.g., aspirin, NSAIDs, guaifenesin, antihistamines, phenothiazines, anticonvulsants)
  - Uremia
  - Paraproteinemia
- **Coagulation disorders**
  - Prolongation of activated partial thromboplastin time (aPTT):
    ○ Deficiency of factor VIII, IX, XI, or XII
    ○ Acquired inhibitor or lupus anticoagulant
    ○ Von Willebrand disease (aPTT may be normal)
  - Prolongation of prothrombin time (PT):
    ○ Mild vitamin K deficiency
    ○ Liver disease, mild to moderate
    ○ Deficiency of factor VII
    ○ Factor VII inhibitor
  - Prolongation of PT and aPTT:
    ○ Liver disease, severe
    ○ Disseminated intravascular coagulopathy
    ○ Severe vitamin K deficiency
    ○ Hemorrhagic disease of the newborn
    ○ Deficiency of factor II, V, or X or fibrinogen
    ○ Dysfibrinogenemia
    ○ Hypoprothrombinemia associated with a lupus anticoagulant
  - Normal screening laboratory tests:
    ○ Von Willebrand disease
    ○ Factor XIII deficiency
    ○ Alpha-2-antiplasmin deficiency
    ○ Plasminogen activator inhibitor-I deficiency
- **Vessel wall disorders**
  - Congenital:
    ○ Hereditary hemorrhagic telangiectasia
    ○ Ehlers–Danlos syndrome
    ○ Osteogenesis imperfecta
    ○ Marfan syndrome
  - Acquired:
    ○ Vasculitis (systemic lupus erythematosus, Henoch–Schönlein purpura, and others)
    ○ Scurvy

APPROACH TO THE PATIENT
- **Phase 1**
  - Includes a thorough history and physical exam
  - Familial history specifically of bleeding or consanguinity is an important component of this phase.
  - Standard screening laboratory tests include PT, aPTT, and platelet count.
- **Phase 2**
  - If a bleeding disorder is suspected but the initial screening tests are negative, testing for von Willebrand disease, factor XIII deficiency, and dysfibrinogenemia is warranted.
  - Consider platelet aggregation studies.
- **Phase 3**
  - Any abnormal screening tests need further evaluation with additional testing to define the specific disorder (e.g., factor assays).

HISTORY
By taking into account the patient's age, sex, clinical presentation, past medical history, and family history, the most likely cause of bleeding can be usually determined.
- **Question:** Sex of patient?
- *Significance:* Hemophilia is X-linked.
- **Question:** Family history of bleeding?
- *Significance:* Suggests an inherited bleeding disorder
- **Question:** Bleeding in unusual places without significant trauma (intracranial, joints)?
- *Significance:* May indicate significant factor deficiency—hemophilia
- **Question:** Several surgeries in the past without bleeding?
- *Significance:* An inherited bleeding disorder is less likely.
- **Question:** Poorly controlled epistaxis?
- *Significance:* Localized trauma (nose-picking) can cause unilateral epistaxis.
- **Question:** Sepsis?
- *Significance:* Suggests disseminated intravascular coagulopathy
- **Question:** Mucocutaneous bleeding (gum bleeding, bruises, epistaxis, menorrhagia)?
- *Significance:* May indicate a platelet disorder or von Willebrand disease
- **Question:** Purpura or petechiae?
- *Significance:* May signify platelet disorders, von Willebrand disease, or vasculitis
- **Question:** Recent medications?
- *Significance:* Aspirin and NSAIDs (e.g., ibuprofen) affect platelet function.
- **Question:** Presence of renal or liver disease?
- *Significance:*
  - Azotemia contributes to bleeding.
  - Liver disease reduces clotting factors.
- **Question:** Severe malnutrition?
- *Significance:* May lead to scurvy, vitamin K deficiency, or decreased hepatic synthesis of coagulation factors
- **Question:** Sudden onset of petechiae?
- *Significance:* May indicate idiopathic thrombocytopenia

PHYSICAL EXAM
- **Finding:** Petechiae in skin and mucous membranes?
- *Significance:* Disorder of platelet number or function, von Willebrand disease, or vasculitis
- **Finding:** Small bruises in unusual places?
- *Significance:* Possible platelet disorder or von Willebrand disease
- **Finding:** Large bruises or palpable bruises?
- *Significance:* Coagulation deficiencies, severe platelet disorders, or von Willebrand disease
- **Finding:** Delayed wound healing?
- *Significance:* Factor XIII deficiency or dysfibrinogenemia
- **Finding:** Purpura localized to lower body (buttocks, legs, ankles)?
- *Significance:* Henoch–Schönlein purpura

DIAGNOSTIC TESTS & INTERPRETATION

- **Test:** Phase 1: Initial laboratory screening
  - Platelet count
  - PT and aPTT
- *Significance:* Screening tests normal, bleeding disorder suspected
- **Test:** Phase 2:
  - Definitive platelet testing includes platelet aggregation and adenosine triphosphate release studies with ristocetin, collagen, thrombin, arachidonic acid, and adenosine 5'-diphosphate.
- *Significance:* Qualitative platelet defect suspected
  - Factor VIII:C
  - Von Willebrand factor antigen (VIIIR:Ag)
  - Von Willebrand factor activity (ristocetin cofactor)
  - Von Willebrand factor multimeric analysis—only send after the diagnosis of von Willebrand disease has been established
  - Thrombin time and fibrinogen assay to screen for afibrinogenemia or dysfibrinogenemia
  - Factor XIII deficiency suspected: Factor XIII assay (urea clot lysis study)
- *Significance:* Von Willebrand disease suspected
- **Test:** Phase 3: Discriminating laboratory studies for abnormal phase 1 tests
- *Significance:*
  - When thrombocytopenia is present:
    - Inspection of blood smear (screening for bone marrow diseases)
  - Mean platelet volume (may be normal or elevated in destructive causes, elevated in congenital macrothrombocytopenias, low in Wiskott–Aldrich syndrome)
  - Bone marrow aspiration (rarely necessary)
  - When disseminated intravascular coagulopathy is suspected (infection, liver disease, massive trauma, PT and aPTT prolonged):
    - Fibrinogen
    - D-dimer or fibrin split products
    - Peripheral smear inspection for RBC fragments
  - Prolonged aPTT (inhibitor screen [50:50 mixing study of patient's and normal plasma]):
  - If aPTT fully corrects with mixing, this is consistent with a factor deficiency:
    - Assess for specific factor deficiencies: Factor VIII, IX, XI, XII
  - If partial or no correction after mixing study:
    - Inhibitor is present.
    - Confirmatory test for the presence of a lupus anticoagulant with a platelet-neutralizing procedure or DRVVT
- **Test:** Prolonged PT
- *Significance:*
  - Inhibitor screen should also be considered for prolonged PT.
  - Specific factor levels (VII)
- **Test:** Prolonged PT and aPTT
- *Significance:*
  - Test for disseminated intravascular coagulopathy, liver disease, and fibrinogen disorders, as described previously
  - Vitamin K deficiency, moderate to severe
  - Factor assays: V, X, II (prothrombin), and fibrinogen

CLINICAL PEARLS

- Children with bleeding disorders are more likely to have large bruises (>5 cm), palpable bruises, and bruises on more than one body part.
- Uncommon sites for bruising for all ages include the back, buttocks, arms, and abdomen.
- The aPTT may be extremely prolonged in patients with deficiencies of the contact factors (prekallikrein, high molecular weight kininogen [HMWK], factor XII). These deficiencies do not result in bleeding.
- Improper specimen collection including heparin contamination or underfilling of the specimen tube can result in artificially prolonged clotting times.
- Do not forget to consider nonaccidental injury as a cause of increased bruising.
- Factor XII deficiency and lupus anticoagulant are not associated with abnormal bleeding.

ALERT

Pitfalls of testing:
- **PFA-100**
  - Low specificity and sensitivity
  - Affected by medications (NSAIDs)
  - Not recommended as a screening test
- **Bleeding time**
  - Prolonged when platelets <100,000/mm^3
  - Affected by medications such as aspirin, NSAIDs, antihistamines
  - Does not correlate well with bleeding risk
  - Accurate result depends on proper technique.
  - Not recommended as a screening test
- **PT and aPTT**
  - Normal ranges are age dependent.
  - Polycythemia (hematocrit 65%) or underfilling of the specimen tube may result in a spuriously prolonged result.
  - Heparin contamination results in a spuriously prolonged result.
- **Von Willebrand disease studies**
  - Values fluctuate over time and may be periodically normal in affected individuals.
  - May require repeated testing to make diagnosis

EMERGENCY CARE

- Pressure, elevation, and ice are generally helpful for most bleeding disorders when active bleeding is present.
- More definitive care is dictated by the nature of the underlying hemostatic defect:
  - Platelet transfusions are useful in disorders of thrombocytopenia owing to decreased production and for intrinsic qualitative platelet disorders, but not for immune platelet disorders.
  - Frozen plasma should be used only in severe cases when the exact diagnosis is not readily available but a defect in coagulation is suspected.
- Head injuries in patients with thrombocytopenia or hemophilia require immediate medical attention.

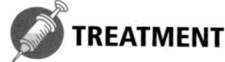 **TREATMENT**

General Measures
- Pressure on wound
- Elevation
- Topical application of thrombin
- Topical application of clot-activating polymers

ADDITIONAL READING

- Buchanan GR. Bleeding signs in children with idiopathic thrombocytopenic purpura. *J Pediatr Hematol Oncol.* 2003;25(Suppl 1):S42–S46.
- Khair K, Liesner R. Bruising and bleeding in infants and children: A practical approach. *Br J Haematol.* 2006;133:221–231.
- Koreth R, Weinert C, Weisdorf DJ, et al. Measurement of bleeding severity: A critical review. *Transfusion.* 2004;44:605–617.
- Lillicrap D, Nair SC, Srivastava A, et al. Laboratory issues in bleeding disorders. *Haemophilia.* 2006;12:68–75.
- Manno CS. Difficult pediatric diagnoses—bruising and bleeding. *Pediatr Clin North Am.* 1991;38:637–655.
- Sarnaik A, Kamat D, Kannikeswaran N. Diagnosis and management of bleeding disorder in a child. *Clin Pediatr.* 2010;49:422–431.

 CODES

ICD9
- 626.2 Excessive or frequent menstruation
- 782.7 Spontaneous ecchymoses
- 784.7 Epistaxis

ICD10
- D69.1 Qualitative platelet defects
- R04.0 Epistaxis
- R23.3 Spontaneous ecchymoses

FAQ

- Q: What are the proper preoperative screening tests for bleeding disorders prior to elective surgery such as tonsillectomy?
- A: A thorough personal history, familial history, and physical exam are by far the most important screening tests. A bleeding time or PFA-100 is not recommended. A CBC, PT, and aPTT are often requested by the surgeon, but normal results do not ensure that a bleeding complication will not occur. Overall, the sensitivity and specificity of these screening tests is poor.
- Q: Bruising is a normal part of childhood. How does one know when bruising is "too much"?
- A: Small bruises on boney prominences on the front of the body are common in children and probably reflect trauma rather than a bleeding disorder. Children with bleeding disorders are more likely to have large bruises (>5 cm), palpable (raised) bruises, and bruises on more than one body part. Uncommon sites for bruising for all ages include the back, buttocks, arms, and abdomen.

ACETAMINOPHEN POISONING

Kevin C. Osterhoudt

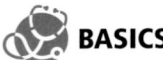 **BASICS**

DESCRIPTION
- Acetaminophen poisoning may occur after acute or chronic overdose.
- After acute overdose, a serum acetaminophen level above the treatment line of the Rumack-Matthew acetaminophen poisoning nomogram should be considered possibly hepatotoxic.
- Acetaminophen is sold under many brand names and is often an ingredient in combination pain reliever preparations.
- Serious hepatotoxicity after a single acute overdose by young children is rare compared with that by adolescents.
- Most toddlers with acetaminophen hepatotoxicity suffer repeated supratherapeutic dosing.

EPIDEMIOLOGY
- Analgesics are the most common drugs implicated in poisoning exposures among children younger than 6 years.
- Acetaminophen preparations make up ~48% of all analgesic poisoning exposures reported to poison control centers.

Incidence
In 2003, acetaminophen poisoning was responsible for 1/2 of all adult cases of acute liver failure.

RISK FACTORS
- Depression
- Pain syndromes
- Glutathione depletion: Prolonged vomiting, alcoholism, etc.
- CYP2E1 induction: Alcoholism, isoniazid therapy

GENERAL PREVENTION
- Acetaminophen should be stored with child-resistant caps, out of sight of young children.
- Proper use of acetaminophen products should be taught to patients with pain or fever.

PATHOPHYSIOLOGY
- Most absorbed acetaminophen is metabolized through formation of hepatic glucuronide and sulfate conjugates.
- Some acetaminophen is metabolized by the CYP450 mixed-function oxidase system, leading to the formation of the toxic *N*-acetyl-p-benzoquinoneimine (NAPQI).

- NAPQI is quickly detoxified by glutathione under usual circumstances.
- After overdose, metabolic detoxification can become saturated:
  - Drug elimination half-life becomes prolonged.
  - Proportionately more NAPQI is produced.
  - Glutathione supply cannot meet detoxification demand.
  - Hepatotoxicity or renal toxicity may ensue.

ETIOLOGY
- Single acute overdose of >150 mg/kg or 10 g
- Repeated overdose of >100 mg/kg/d, or 6 g/d, for >2 days

COMMONLY ASSOCIATED CONDITIONS
- Acetaminophen is often marketed in combination with other pharmaceuticals, which may complicate a drug overdose situation.
- Adolescents frequently overdose on more than 1 drug preparation.

 DIAGNOSIS

HISTORY
- Medical history of pain or fever:
  - Acetaminophen ingestion should be explored in any patient being treated for pain or fever.
- Amount of acetaminophen ingested:
  - A single, acute ingestion of <150 mg/kg (≤10 g in adolescents) is unlikely to cause significant toxicity among otherwise healthy individuals.
- Timing of ingestion:
  - Allows application of the Rumack-Matthew nomogram
- Sustained-release preparation:
  - Acetaminophen is now available in sustained-release form.
- Medication list:
  - Use of isoniazid or other CYP2E1 hepatic enzyme inducers may increase risk for toxicity.
- Signs and symptoms:
  - Initially may be clinically silent
  - Vomiting
  - Anorexia

PHYSICAL EXAM
Right upper quadrant tenderness may suggest acetaminophen-induced hepatitis.

DIAGNOSTIC TESTS & INTERPRETATION
Lab
- Serum acetaminophen level:
  - Allows application of the Rumack-Matthew nomogram after acute overdose
  - Rumack-Matthew nomogram applies only to single, acute acetaminophen overdose scenarios.
- Hepatic transaminases:
  - Aspartate aminotransferase (AST) is the most sensitive of the widely available measures to assess acetaminophen hepatotoxicity and begins to rise 12–24 hours after significant overdose
- Liver and kidney function tests:
  - As the AST rises, it is important to follow liver and kidney function with tests such as serum glucose, prothrombin (PT) and partial thromboplastin (PTT) times, serum creatinine, plasma pH, and serum albumin.
  - The PT and PTT may be slightly elevated owing to direct effect of elevated blood acetaminophen concentrations or *N*-acetylcysteine therapy, without signifying liver injury.
  - The decline of an elevated serum AST may indicate either liver recovery or profound liver failure and must be interpreted in context.
- Salicylate level:
  - May be a coingestant in the setting of analgesic drug overdose

Pathological Findings
Hepatic zone III (centrilobular) necrosis

DIFFERENTIAL DIAGNOSIS
- Infectious hepatitis
- Other drug-induced hepatitis

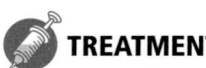 **TREATMENT**

MEDICATION (DRUGS)
First Line
- Single acute overdose:
  - Activated charcoal, 1–2 g/kg (maximum 75 g), may be administered if acetaminophen is judged to be present in the stomach or proximal intestine (usually within 2 hours of ingestion).
  - *N*-acetylcysteine should be administered if a serum acetaminophen level obtained >4 hours after overdose falls above the treatment line of the Rumack-Matthew nomogram.
  - Patients presenting to medical care >7 hours after overdose should be given a loading dose of *N*-acetylcysteine while waiting for the serum acetaminophen level result.

- Oral *N*-acetylcysteine dose: 140 mg/kg loading dose, followed by 70 mg/kg maintenance doses q4h (see "FAQ")
- Intravenous *N*-acetylcysteine dose: 150 mg/kg loading dose over 1 hour, then 12.5 mg/kg/hr for 4 hours, then 6.25 mg/kg/hr (see "FAQ")
- Repeated supratherapeutic ingestion:
  - Consider *N*-acetylcysteine therapy if:
    ○ Ingestion of >100 mg/kg or 6 g/d for consecutive days
    ○ Patient is symptomatic
    ○ AST level is elevated
    ○ Acetaminophen level is higher than would be expected given dosing, and AST level is normal
- Once started, *N*-acetylcysteine therapy should be continued until:
  - The serum acetaminophen level is nondetectable
  - A simultaneous serum AST has not risen, or, if elevated, liver enzymes and liver function are clearly improving

Second Line
- Acetaminophen poisoning and oral *N*-acetylcysteine therapy are emetogenic: Chill and cover the *N*-acetylcysteine. Consider antiemetic therapy with drugs such as metoclopramide and/or ondansetron. Enteral *N*-acetylcysteine may be given slowly via nasogastric or nasoduodenal tube.
- Intravenous *N*-acetylcysteine has been associated with anaphylactoid reactions, which may require cessation or slowing of infusion, antihistamines, corticosteroids, and/or epinephrine.

ADDITIONAL TREATMENT
General Measures
Evaluate for possible polypharmacy overdose.

ISSUES FOR REFERRAL
- Patients with AST approaching 1,000 IU/L should be considered for transfer to a liver transplant center.
- Mental health services should be provided to victims of intentional overdose.

SURGERY/OTHER PROCEDURES
Liver transplant should be considered per transplant center protocols. The King's College Hospital Criteria include:
- pH <7.30 after resuscitation, or
- PT >1.8 times control, plus
- Serum creatinine >3.3 mg/dL, plus
- Encephalopathy

IN-PATIENT CONSIDERATIONS
Admission Criteria
- *N*-acetylcysteine therapy
- Psychiatric evaluation warranted

Discharge Criteria
- *N*-acetylcysteine therapy concluded
- No concern for developing liver injury

ONGOING CARE

FOLLOW-UP RECOMMENDATIONS
Patient Monitoring
- Cardiorespiratory monitoring is warranted during intravenous *N*-acetylcysteine therapy.
- Intensive care monitoring is warranted during fulminant hepatic failure.

PATIENT EDUCATION
- Drug administration education should be offered to victims of chronic overdose.
- Home safety education should be provided after pediatric exploratory ingestions.

PROGNOSIS
- Among previously healthy children, hepatotoxicity is rare with single doses <150–200 mg/kg.
- After single acute acetaminophen overdose, likelihood of hepatotoxicity may be determined by using the Rumack-Matthew nomogram.
- *N*-acetylcysteine therapy prevents hepatic failure in >99% of acetaminophen-poisoned patients if administered within 8 hours of overdose.
- *N*-acetylcysteine therapy is less efficacious when administered >8 hours after overdose, but should still be offered.
- Repetitive dosing of >75 mg/kg/d should be evaluated cautiously, especially in the presence of the following:
  - Febrile illness
  - Vomiting or malnourishment
  - Anticonvulsant or isoniazid therapy

COMPLICATIONS
- Hepatic failure
- Renal insufficiency
- Anaphylactoid shock may complicate intravenous *N*-acetylcysteine therapy.

ADDITIONAL READING

- American Academy of Pediatrics. Committee on Drugs. Acetaminophen toxicity in children. *Pediatrics*. 2001;108:1020–1024.
- Betten DP, Cantrell FL, Thomas SC, et al. A prospective evaluation of shortened course oral N-acetylcysteine for the treatment of acute acetaminophen poisoning. *Ann Emerg Med*. 2007;50:272–279.
- Bronstein AC, Spyker DA, Cantilena LR, et al. 2009 annual report of the American Association of Poison Control Centers' National Poison Data System. *Clin Toxicol*. 2010;48:979–1178.
- Chun LJ, Tong MJ, Busuttil RW, et al. Acetaminophen hepatotoxicity and acute liver failure. *J Clin Gastroenterol*. 2009;43:342–349.
- Dart RC, Erdman AR, Olson KR, et al. Acetaminophen poisoning: An evidence-based consensus guideline for out-of-hospital management. *Clin Toxicol*. 2006;44:1–18.
- Heard KJ. Acetylcysteine for acetaminophen poisoning. *New Engl J Med*. 2008;359:285–292.
- Hendrickson RG. Acetaminophen. In: Nelson LS, Lewin NA, Howland MA, et al., eds. *Goldfrank's toxicologic emergencies*, 9th ed. New York: McGraw-Hill; 2011:483–499.

CODES

ICD9
965.4 Acetaminophen poisoning by aromatic analgesics, not elsewhere classified

ICD10
- T39.1X4A Poisoning by 4-Aminophenol derivatives, undetermined, initial encounter
- T39.1X4D Poisoning by 4-Aminophenol derivatives, undetermined, subsequent encounter
- T39.1X4S Poisoning by 4-Aminophenol derivatives, undetermined, sequela

FAQ
- Q: What is "patient-tailored" *N*-acetylcysteine (**NAC**) therapy?
- A: The duration of *N*-acetylcysteine therapy used to be dependent upon the pharmaceutical form administered, but is now tailored to the patient based on serum acetaminophen level and liver function.
- Q: Should **NAC** be given PO or IV?
- A: Both seem to be similarly efficacious. Oral administration of **NAC** is complicated by taste aversion and vomiting. IV **NAC** may lead to anaphylactoid shock. No cost–benefit studies are available for direct comparison of patient-tailored courses of oral **NAC** and IV **NAC**.

ACNE
Marney Gundlach

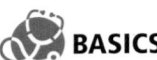

BASICS

DESCRIPTION
Acne vulgaris is a disorder of pilosebaceous follicles (PSFs). PSFs are found on the face, chest, back, and upper arms. Acne lesions include microcomedones, closed comedones (whiteheads or CCs), open comedones (blackheads or OCs), inflammatory lesions (erythematous papules [Pap], pustules [Pus], nodules [Nod], or cysts), scars, and macules. No universally accepted classification system for acne exists. One scheme is:

	OC/CC	Pap/Pus	Nod/Scars
Mild	+	+/−	+/−
Moderate	+	+	+/−
Severe	+	+	+

Other forms of acne:
- Acne conglobata: Large connecting cysts or abscesses causing severe disfigurement
- Acne fulminans: Severe acne associated with fever, arthritis, and systemic symptoms
- Acne rosacea: In adults; no comedones
- Steroid acne: Uniform papules or pustules seen after using topical or systemic steroids
- Neonatal acne: Inflammatory acne in up to 20% of neonates; resolves without treatment

RISK FACTORS
Genetics
Familial patterns exist, but no inheritance pattern has been demonstrated.

PATHOPHYSIOLOGY
Four factors contribute to PSF obstruction:
- Increased sebum production: Adrenarche causes increased androgen production, which enlarges sebaceous glands and increases sebum production. Production peaks in teens and decreases in 20s.
- Hyperkeratinization: Epithelial cells lining the PSF don't shed well. Cells and sebum obstruct the PSF, creating a microcomedone.
- Proliferation of *Propionibacterium acnes*: Anaerobic, gram-positive diphtheroid colonizes PSFs and produces free fatty acids (FFAs).
- Inflammation
  - *P. acnes* attract neutrophils (PMNs) to PSFs, which ingest bacteria-releasing hydrolytic enzymes. Inflammation caused by enzymes and FFAs damaging follicles
  - Acne severity related to interactions of *P. acnes* with immune mediators, not absolute concentrations of *P. acnes*
  - Educate patients that OCs are due to lipid oxidation and melanin, not dirt.

ETIOLOGY
- Environmental factors (work grease exposure, hair grease use) may increase lesion numbers.
- Friction from athletic helmets, shoulder pads, chin straps, or bra straps may worsen acne.

COMMONLY ASSOCIATED CONDITIONS
- Polycystic ovarian syndrome (PCOS)
- SAPHO syndrome: Synovitis, acne, pustulosis, hyperostosis, and osteitis
- Adrenal tumors
- Late-onset congenital adrenal hyperplasia

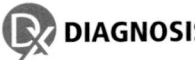

DIAGNOSIS

HISTORY
- Age of onset: early or late onset of acne may indicate androgen excess.
- Medications (including some oral contraceptive pills [OCPs], lithium, progestin implants, depot medroxyprogesterone, isoniazid, nicotine products, and steroids) may worsen acne.
- Menstrual history: Premenstrual flares may occur owing to androgen effects of progesterone.
- Androgen excess (history of or current)
  - Prepubertal: Early-onset acne or body odor, increased growth, adrenarche or pubarche, genital maturation, or clitoromegaly
  - Postpubertal: Alopecia, hirsutism, truncal obesity, acanthosis nigricans, or irregular menses
- Psychological impact: Ask patients about self-esteem, depression, and suicidal ideations.

PHYSICAL EXAM
- Skin: Note distribution of OCs, CCs, and inflammatory lesions on the face, chest, and back. May diagram facial lesions with global assessment of acne severity (number, size, extent, and scarring). Pomade acne may be seen around hairline.
- Note signs of androgen excess (see "History").

DIAGNOSTIC TESTS & INTERPRETATION
Lab
- Consider for patients with early- or late-onset acne, signs of androgen excess, or acne unresponsive to traditional therapy.
- Most boys have normal hormone levels.
- Girls may have increased levels of DHEAS and free testosterone and decreased levels of sex hormone–binding globulin (SHBG). Consider also total testosterone, FSH, and LH for PCOS.
- Lab monitoring while using isotretinoin should include complete blood count, triglycerides, cholesterol, and transaminases.

DIFFERENTIAL DIAGNOSIS
- Adenoma sebaceum
- Gram-negative folliculitis
- Keratosis pilaris

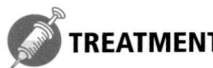

TREATMENT

MEDICATION (DRUGS)
Topical Agents
Patients assume acne should improve with vigorous cleansing of the skin. Instead, this may worsen acne and irritation from topical agents.

- Benzoyl peroxide (BP): Bactericidal, decreases FFAs.
  - Use for mild inflammatory and comedonal acne; or as adjunct with oral or topical antibiotics to prevent antibiotic resistance.
  - Available as lotion, cream, wash, and gel in 2.5–10%; 5% concentration up to twice daily effective for most patients; 10% solution has similar effectiveness as 5% but with increased side effects.
  - Side effects include drying, erythema, burning, peeling, stinging, and rarely contact dermatitis.
  - Counsel patients that BP may bleach clothing and linens.
- Topical antibiotics (erythromycin, clindamycin, sulfacetamide) decrease concentration of *P. acnes* and inflammatory mediators; may decrease FFAs.
  - Use for mild or moderate inflammatory acne; no comedolytic effects; apply once or twice daily. Do not use as monotherapy.
  - Side effects: Well tolerated but may include drying or irritation; patients may complain about the smell of sulfacetamide.
  - Often combined with BP; combination products are more expensive. Can use separate generic prescriptions of BP and topical antibiotics together
  - Combining with topical retinoid in clinical trials yields faster results and greater clearing than topical antibiotics alone.
- Retinoids promote epithelial shedding from the PSF, promote comedone drainage, prevent new comedone formation (by decreasing obstruction), and are anti-inflammatory.
  - Side effects include erythema, dryness, irritation, initial acne flares, hypo- or hyperpigmentation, and photosensitivity (advise use of sunscreen with SPF 15–30).
  - 1st-line therapy for most patients; may increase penetration of other topical agents by improving cell shedding
  - Treatment started with lowest strength, small amount every 3rd night and increased to nightly application over 3 weeks. Increase concentration as tolerated. Applying at night may decrease photosensitivity.
- Tretinoin
  - Available as cream, gel, and liquid (increasing potency, respectively). Apply to dry skin.
  - Approved for children ≥13 years
  - Sporadic reports of congenital malformations have occurred with tretinoin (pregnancy category C); may discuss with women of childbearing age.
- Adapalene
  - Cream, gel, solution, or pledgets
  - Adapalene gel 0.1% is better tolerated than tretinoin gel 0.025%.
  - Approved for children ≥13 years
- Tazarotene
  - Cream and gel. Apply to dry skin.
  - More irritating than other retinoids
  - Approved for children ≥12 years
  - Teratogenicity concerns; contraindicated in pregnancy (Category X)
- Salicylic acid promotes comedolysis with drying and peeling, effective for comedonal acne:
  - 0.5–5% cream, wash, lotion, or gel once or twice daily
  - Less effective than topical retinoids at preventing new lesions, but less irritating
  - Consider for patients with comedonal acne who cannot use retinoids or who have a large surface area to treat (e.g., back).
- Azelaic acid: Anticomedonal and antibacterial; decreases hyperpigmentation:
  - 20% cream applied twice daily
  - Side effects include itching, burning, tingling, stinging, and erythema.
  - Consider for patients with comedonal acne who cannot use retinoids or who have a large surface area to treat (e.g., back).

Oral Agents

- Oral antibiotics (tetracycline, doxycycline, minocycline): Same as topical antibiotics plus inhibit PMN chemotaxis, decrease inflammation:
  - Tetracycline is cheapest but has least efficacy; also 4×/day dosing
  - Minocycline and doxycycline given 1–2× daily, dosed at 1 mg/kg
  - Use for acne that is moderate to severe, widespread, or treatment resistant.
  - Use with retinoids; do not use alone.
  - Antibiotic resistance may be seen in 25% of patients; limit treatment length. After 12 weeks, may switch to retinoid monotherapy with no change in clinical response.
  - More effective than topical antibiotics, but more systemic effects
- Isotretinoin decreases sebum production, is anti-inflammatory, and reduces *P. acnes*:
  - Used for acne that is recalcitrant or with significant scarring only, given side effects.
  - Dose starts at 0.5 mg/kg/d in 2 divided doses for 4 weeks, and is increased as tolerated up to 1 mg/kg/d; total course usually 15–20 weeks; total cumulative dose should not exceed 120–150 mg/kg.
    - For patients with severely inflamed acne, start at lower dose to prevent initial acne flares or pretreat with oral corticosteroids.
  - FDA-mandated registry (iPledge; see https://www.ipledgeprogram.com/) for all patients on isotretinoin; prescribed only by physicians experienced with its use
  - Side effects:
    - Teratogenicity (obtain 2 negative pregnancy tests in women prior to starting)
    - Depression and suicide have been reported in patients on isotretinoin (causality not established, but counsel about this risk).
    - Rare, sporadic reports of serious skin infections including erythema multiforme, Stevens-Johnson syndrome, and toxic epidermal necrolysis
    - Pseudotumor cerebri when combined with tetracycline (contraindicated)
    - Other side effects: Hyperlipidemia, dry skin, headaches, cheilitis, impaired glucose control in diabetics
- OCPs (for women):
  - Combined OCPs work by (1) estrogen increasing SHBG, which decreases free testosterone, decreasing gonadotropin secretion, which decreases ovarian androgen production; and (2) androgen receptor blocking, which prevents dihydrotestosterone (DHT) formation in the PSFs.
  - Suggested as an adjunct for women with moderate to severe acne not responding to topical retinoids
  - Use OCPs with a low-androgen progestin. OCPs shown in RCTs to improve acne:
    - Ethinyl estradiol (35 mcg) and norgestimate
    - Ethinyl estradiol (20 or 30 mcg) and levonorgestrel
    - Ethinyl estradiol (20-30-35 mcg) and norethindrone
    - Ethinyl estradiol (30 mcg) and drospirenone 3 mg
    - Ethinyl estradiol (30 mcg) and chlormadinone 2 mg

- May need 3–6 months to see improvement.
- Side effects include nausea, breast tenderness, weight gain, breakthrough menstrual bleeding, myocardial infarction, ischemic stroke, and DVTs.
- Use caution in girls who smoke tobacco.
- Spironolactone
  - Blocks androgen receptor in sebaceous gland
  - Give 50–150 mg daily.
  - Off-label use, usually in combination with oral antibiotics

ALERT

- *Clostridium difficile* pseudomembranous colitis may occur rarely with topical clindamycin.
- Do not use isotretinoin with tetracycline, minocycline, or doxycycline owing to increased risk of pseudotumor cerebri.
- BP inactivates tretinoin; when used together, apply BP in the morning and tretinoin at night.
- Tetracycline, minocycline, and doxycycline are category D drugs (unsafe in pregnancy).

ADDITIONAL TREATMENT
General Measures
- Goal is to reduce number and severity of lesions and prevent scarring. Treat until no new lesions form.
- Tell patients that 6–8 weeks (time for microcomedone to mature) are required for clinical improvement.
- Scars warrant aggressive treatment targeting inflammation.
- In general, creams and lotions are less drying than solutions or gels. More-drying formulations may be better for patients with oily skin or for quick-drying prior to applying makeup; less-drying formulations may be needed for patients with sensitive skin/eczema.

COMPLEMENTARY & ALTERNATIVE THERAPIES
- Limited empirical studies on CAM and acne. RCTs of the following showed that they were not as effective as 5% BP, but resulted in less skin irritation:
  - Tea tree oil: A mixture of terpenes and alcohols with antibiotic and antifungal properties; 5% solution may be effective at treating comedonal and inflammatory acne; may be associated with male gynecomastia
  - Gluconolactone 14% solution may be effective on comedonal and inflammatory acne.

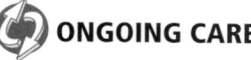 ONGOING CARE

PATIENT EDUCATION
- http://www.skincarephysicians.com/acnenet/index.html
- http://www.aap.org/publiced/BR_Teen_Acne.htm

COMPLICATIONS
- Scarring may be permanent.
- Self-esteem: Acne severity correlated to social variables including embarrassment and lack of enjoyment in social activities among teenagers.
- Patients with mild to moderate acne showed clinical depression and >5% suicidal ideation. Depression scores improve in correlation with response to acne treatment.
- Suicide

ADDITIONAL READING

- Antoniou C, Dessinioti C, Stratigos AJ, et al. Clinical and therapeutic approach to childhood acne: An update. *Ped Dermatol*. 2009;26:373–380.
- Krowchuk DP. Managing adolescent acne: A guide for pediatricians. *Pediatr Rev*. 2005;26:250–261.
- Magin PJ, Adams J, Heading GS, et al. Topical and oral CAM in acne: A review of the empirical evidence and a consideration of its context. *Complement Ther Med*. 2006;14:62–76.
- Strauss J, Krowchuck DP, Leyden JJ, et al. Guidelines of care for acne vulgaris management. *J Am Acad Dermatol*. 2007;56:651–663.
- Zaenglein AL, Thibout DM. Expert committee recommendations for acne management. *Pediatrics*. 2006;188:1188–1199.

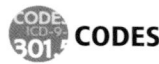 CODES

ICD9
- 706.1 Other acne
- 695.3 Rosacea

ICD10
- L70.0 Acne vulgaris
- L70.1 Acne conglobata
- L70.9 Acne, unspecified

FAQ

- Q: What treatment is recommended for patients with comedonal and inflammatory acne?
- A: Topical retinoid + topical/oral antibiotic + BP
- Web site with patient FAQs: http://www.skincarephysicians.com/acnenet/FAQ.html

ACQUIRED HYPOTHYROIDISM

Adda Grimberg

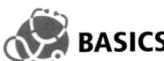 **BASICS**

DESCRIPTION
Hypothyroidism that occurs after the neonatal period

EPIDEMIOLOGY
Incidence
- May develop at any age
- Autoimmune thyroid disorders occur more frequently in children and adolescents with type 1 diabetes mellitus.

Prevalence
Chronic lymphocytic thyroiditis prevalence correlates with iodine intake; countries with the highest dietary iodine also have the highest prevalence.

RISK FACTORS
Genetics
- Family history of thyroid disease or other autoimmune endocrinopathies increases risk.
- Genetic predisposition in patients with chronic lymphocytic thyroiditis; 30–40% of patients have a family history of thyroid disease, and up to 50% of their 1st-degree relatives have thyroid antibodies.
- Weak associations of chronic lymphocytic thyroiditis with certain human leukocyte antigen haplotypes
- Autoimmune thyroid disease may be part of Schmidt syndrome (type II polyglandular autoimmune disease).
- Genetic syndromes associated with higher incidence of autoimmune thyroiditis:
  - Down syndrome
  - Turner syndrome (especially those with isochromosome Xq)

ETIOLOGY
- Myriad causes (see "Differential Diagnosis")
- Can result from thyroid gland dysfunction (primary hypothyroidism) or from pituitary/hypothalamic dysfunction leading to understimulation of the thyroid gland (secondary and tertiary hypothyroidism)

COMMONLY ASSOCIATED CONDITIONS
- Vitiligo
- Other autoimmune endocrinopathies
- Pernicious anemia

DIAGNOSIS

HISTORY
- Linear growth failure can be the 1st sign of thyroid dysfunction.
- Declining school performance is a sensitive marker for lethargy and reduced focusing.
- Radiation exposure, history of diabetes, family history of autoimmune disease
- Signs and symptoms:
  - Early primary hypothyroidism can be asymptomatic.
  - Hypothyroid-related symptoms indicate progression from compensated to uncompensated hypothyroidism.
  - Hypothyroidism may be preceded in some cases by temporary hyperthyroidism (Hashitoxicosis).
  - Goiter may be the presenting sign of acquired hypothyroidism; tenderness suggests an infectious process.

PHYSICAL EXAM
- Bradycardia: Thyroid hormone has cardiac effects.
- Short stature (or fall-off on growth curve) and increased upper/lower segment ratio: Euthyroidism is required to maintain normal growth.
- Goiter: Note consistency, symmetry, nodularity, signs of inflammation:
  - May give a clue regarding cause of hypothyroidism
  - May provide a clinical marker to follow during therapy
- Myxedema (water retention) is not limited to subcutaneous tissue; it may also lead to cardiac failure, pleural effusions, and coma.
- Muscle hypertrophy, yet muscle weakness most obvious in arms, legs, and tongue; hypothyroidism causes disordered muscle function.
- Delayed relaxation phase of deep tendon reflexes due to slowed muscle contraction
- Pale, cool, dry, carotenemic skin due to decreased cell turnover
- Increase in lanugo hair in children; can be reversed with treatment
- Sexual development is an important factor.
- Hypothyroidism can be associated with:
  - Delayed puberty (due to low thyroid hormone level)
  - Precocious puberty and galactorrhea (due to elevated TSH)

DIAGNOSTIC TESTS & INTERPRETATION
Lab
- T_4 (low) and TSH (elevated): Elevated TSH with normal T_4 indicates compensated primary hypothyroidism.
- Free T_4: The most sensitive marker for secondary/tertiary hypothyroidism (TSH elevation lost; total T_4 may still be low normal)
- Antithyroglobulin and antimicrosomal (antiperoxidase) antibodies are markers for chronic lymphocytic thyroiditis.
- The following conditions may test false-positive for acquired hypothyroidism:
  - Thyroid-binding globulin deficiency: Low total T_4, but normal free T_4 and TSH
  - Peripheral resistance to thyroid hormone: Normal/high total T_4
  - "Euthyroid sick" syndrome: low T_4 and T_3; normal/low TSH; increased shunting to reverse T_3
- The following tests may be affected in acquired hypothyroidism:
  - Serum creatinine: Elevated due to reduced glomerular filtration rate
  - LDL cholesterol level: Elevated due to decreased LDL receptor expression
  - Creatine kinase: Increased; hypothyroidism is a rare cause of rhabdomyolysis.

Imaging
Head MRI for suspected secondary/tertiary hypothyroidism or pituitary or hypothalamic lesion

DIFFERENTIAL DIAGNOSIS
- Immunologic:
  - Chronic lymphocytic thyroiditis (Hashimoto thyroiditis)
  - Polyglandular autoimmune syndrome (Schmidt syndrome)
- Infectious:
  - Postviral subacute thyroiditis
  - Associated with congenital infections:
    ○ Rubella
    ○ Toxoplasmosis
- Environmental:
  - Goitrogen ingestion:
    ○ Iodides
    ○ Expectorants
    ○ Thioureas
- Iatrogenic:
  - Following surgical thyroidectomy for thyroid cancer, hyperthyroidism, or extensive neck tumors
  - Following radioiodine ablative therapy for hyperthyroidism or thyroid cancer
  - Following irradiation to the head or neck for cancer treatment
  - Medications: lithium, amiodarone, iodine contrast dyes, tiratricol (an OTC fat-loss supplement)

- Metabolic:
  - Cystinosis
  - Histiocytosis X
- Congenital:
  - Late-onset congenital-large ectopic gland
- Genetic syndromes:
  - Down syndrome
  - Turner syndrome
- Secondary or tertiary hypothyroidism
  - Hypothalamic or pituitary disease
- Consumptive hypothyroidism:
  - Due to increased type 3 iodothyronine deiodinase activity in hemangiomas

 TREATMENT

MEDICATION (DRUGS)
L-Thyroxine (synthetic thyroid hormone) replacement
- Indicated for the treatment of overt or compensated hypothyroidism
- 2–5 mcg/kg/d PO, once daily
- Monitor T_4 and TSH and titrate dose to maintain normalized thyroid function tests.
- Duration of therapy:
  - Lifetime
  - In 30% of the cases, children with chronic lymphocytic thyroiditis will undergo spontaneous remission.
  - Need for treatment can be reassessed after growth is completed.

 ONGOING CARE

FOLLOW-UP RECOMMENDATIONS
Patient Monitoring
- Whenever starting medication or adjusting dose, check T_4 and TSH at 4–6 weeks to assess adequacy of the new dose.
- Monitor response to treatment by measuring T_4 and TSH levels to ensure compliance.

PATIENT EDUCATION
Pharmacies in recent years have been recommending that L-thyroxine be administered on an empty stomach. The Drugs and Therapeutics Committee of the Pediatric Endocrine Society recommended that consistency in administration, coupled with regular dose titration to thyroid function tests, is more important than improving absorption by restricting intake to only times of empty stomach.

PROGNOSIS
- If patients are compliant, prognosis is excellent.
- Treated patients often resume growth at a rate greater than normal (catch-up growth).
- In children in whom treatment has been delayed, catch-up growth may not fully normalize height to predicted values.
- Other signs and symptoms resolve at a variable rate.
- Goiters in chronic lymphocytic thyroiditis may not completely regress with treatment (enlargement due to persistent inflammation does not correct, though TSH-mediated hypertrophy will).

COMPLICATIONS
- Most significant complication is impaired linear growth.
- Puberty can also be affected.
- Myxedema coma may occur.
- Encephalopathy of varied clinical presentation has been associated with high titers of thyroid antibodies, especially antimicrosomal; responds well to corticosteroid treatment.

ADDITIONAL READING

- Ai J, Leonhardt JM, Heymann WR. Autoimmune thyroid diseases: Etiology, pathogenesis, and dermatologic manifestations. *J Am Acad Dermatol.* 2003;48:641–659.
- Ban Y, Tomer Y. Genetic susceptibility in thyroid autoimmunity. *Pediatr Endocrinol Rev.* 2005;3:20–32.
- Barbesino G, Chiovato L. The genetics of Hashimoto's disease. *Endocrinol Metab Clin North Am.* 2000;29:357–374.
- Haugen BR. Drugs that suppress TSH or cause central hypothyroidism. *Best Pract Res Clin Endocrinol Metab.* 2009;23:793–800.
- Hunter I, Greene SA, MacDonald TM, et al. Prevalence and aetiology of hypothyroidism in the young. *Arch Dis Child.* 2000;83:207–210.
- Nabhan ZM, Kreher NC, Eugster EA. Hashitoxicosis in children: Clinical features and natural history. *J Pediatr.* 2005;146:533–536.
- Pearce EN, Farwell AP, Braverman LE. Thyroiditis. *N Engl J Med.* 2003;348:2646–2655.
- Ranke MB. Catch-up growth: New lessons for the clinician. *J Pediatr Endocrinol Metab.* 2002;15(Suppl 5):S1257–S1266.
- Roldan MB, Alonso M, Barrio R. Thyroid autoimmunity in children and adolescents with type 1 diabetes mellitus. *Diabetes Nutr Metab Clin Exp.* 1999;12:27–31.
- Stathatos N, Wartofsky L. Perioperative management of patients with hypothyroidism. *Endocrinol Metab Clin N Am.* 2003;32:503–518.
- Surks MI, Ortiz E, Daniels GH, et al. Subclinical thyroid disease: Scientific review and guidelines for diagnosis and management. *JAMA.* 2004;291:228–238.
- Weber G, Vigone MC, Stroppa L, et al. Thyroid function and puberty. *J Pediatr Endocrinol Metab.* 2003;16(Suppl 2):S253–S257.
- Zeitler P, Solberg P, Drugs and Therapeutics Committee of the Lawson Wilkins Pediatric Endocrine Society. Food and levothyroxine administration in infants and children. *J Pediatr.* 2010;157:13–14.e1.

 CODES

ICD9
244.9 Unspecified acquired hypothyroidism
ICD10
E03.4 Atrophy of thyroid (acquired)

FAQ

- Q: What happens if my child forgets a dose?
- A: Give the dose as soon as you remember. If it is the next day, give 2 doses.
- Q: How long will my child have to take these pills?
- A: Probably for life.
- Q: Are there any side effects from the medication?
- A: No. The medication contains only the hormone that your child's thyroid gland is not making. The hormone is made synthetically, so there is also no infectious risk.
- Q: If my child takes twice the dose, will his or her growth catch up faster?
- A: Your child may grow a little faster but will also have adverse effects from having too much thyroid hormone.
- Q: Does the medication have to be taken at any particular time of day?
- A: No, but consistently choosing the same time of day helps to remember to take it. Do not take simultaneously with soy products or raloxifene (an antiestrogen medication) because they can cause malabsorptions of levothyroxine.
- Q: What if my child needs surgery?
- A: Treatment of hypothyroidism such that the patient is euthyroid (normal thyroid status) prior to surgery is preferable whenever possible (only exception is ischemic heart disease requiring surgery). Euthyroid sick syndrome, which is common in very ill patients, should not be treated.

ACUTE DRUG WITHDRAWAL

Robert J. Hoffman
Naomi Dreisinger

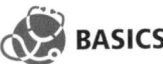 **BASICS**

DESCRIPTION
- Drug withdrawal is a physiologic response to an effectively lowered drug concentration in a patient with tolerance to that drug.
- Withdrawal results in a predictable pattern of symptoms that are reversible if the drug in question or another appropriate substitute is reintroduced.
- Sedative-hypnotic withdrawal is the most common life-threatening withdrawal syndrome in children. This includes withdrawal from barbiturates, benzodiazepines, as well as gamma hydroxybutyrate and similar substances.
- Other substances that are associated with withdrawal syndromes include opioids, selective serotonin reuptake inhibitors, and caffeine.

EPIDEMIOLOGY
- The most common life-threatening withdrawal syndrome, alcohol withdrawal, rarely occurs in children.
- Neonates born to alcohol-dependent mothers are at risk.

RISK FACTORS
Patients receiving sedatives or analgesics capable of causing tolerance are at risk. This is particularly true with infusions or high doses of such substances in previously naïve patients.

GENERAL PREVENTION
- Clinician familiarity with tolerance and withdrawal associated with prescribed medications allows appropriate drug tapering.
- Drug abuse prevention is appropriate for all children.

PATHOPHYSIOLOGY
- Altered CNS neurochemistry is the most important and clinically relevant aspect of withdrawal pathophysiology.
- Under normal conditions, the CNS maintains a balance between excitation and inhibition. While there are several ways to achieve this balance, excitation is constant and actions occur through removal of inhibitory tone.
- Relative to adults and younger children, adolescents are more prone to development of dependence and withdrawal syndromes due to immaturity of their prefrontal cortex.

ETIOLOGY
- Neonates:
  - Maternal alcohol, caffeine, opioid, sedative-hypnotic, or selective serotonin reuptake inhibitor use may result in a neonatal abstinence syndrome.
  - Treatment with caffeine, opioids, or sedative-hypnotics may result in an abstinence syndrome.
- Older children:
  - Subsequent to treatment with caffeine, opioids, or sedative-hypnotics, an abstinence syndrome may result.
  - Substance abuse, particularly opioids, gamma hydroxybutyrate or other sedative-hypnotics may result in an abstinence syndrome.
  - Frequent caffeine or nicotine use may lead to an abstinence syndrome.
- Use of opioid antagonists such as naloxone, naltrexone, and nalmephene are associated with opioid withdrawal.

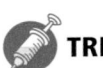 **DIAGNOSIS**

- Drug withdrawal is a clinical diagnosis.
- Patients should be evaluated for associated diagnoses such as traumatic injury, pneumonia, etc.

HISTORY
- Typically, a history of substance exposure, either direct exposure or maternal use, will be elicited.
  - Exposure may be to prescribed medication or abusable substances.
  - Substance use by the mother or child might intentionally be concealed.
- The timing of withdrawal varies depending on the half-life of the substance involved.
  - The shorter the half-life, the sooner the onset of withdrawal and typically the more severe withdrawal symptoms.
- Alcohol or sedative-hypnotics:
  - Withdrawal from these may result in tremulousness, diaphoresis, agitation, insomnia, altered mental status, or withdrawal seizures.
  - Baclofen withdrawal is more frequently severe or life-threatening relative to benzodiazepine withdrawal. History of pump manipulation or malfunction should be sought.
- Caffeine:
  - Withdrawal may result in dysphoria, headache, behavioral changes, or agitation.
- Opioids:
  - Nausea, vomiting, diarrhea, irritability, yawning, sleeplessness, diaphoresis, lacrimation, tremor, and hypertonicity may result.
  - Neonates can also have seizures, a high-pitch cry, skin mottling, and excoriation. These latter signs and symptoms are more typical of opioid withdrawal and rarely occur with neonatal alcohol withdrawal.
- Nicotine:
  - Dysphoria, agitation, behavioral changes, and increased appetite may all occur.
- SSRIs:
  - Neonatal withdrawal from SSRIs may result in jitteriness, agitation, crying, shivering, increased muscle tone, breathing and sucking problems, as well as seizure.
  - Children withdrawing from SSRIs may have jitteriness, agitation, dysphoria, behavioral changes, shivering, increased muscle tone, and seizure.

PHYSICAL EXAM
- Vital signs including temperature should be evaluated regularly. Vital sign changes are tachycardia and hypertension may occur concomitantly with acute drug withdrawal.
- Technology-dependent patients, such as children with an intrathecal baclofen pump, should have evaluation of the machine to determine if it is working properly.
- Most cases of substance withdrawal only result in behavioral changes.
- Opioid withdrawal may be accompanied by diaphoresis, mydriasis, yawning, and lacrimation.
- Sedative-hypnotic withdrawal may result in hypertension, tachycardia, hyperthermia, agitation, hallucinations, and seizure.

DIAGNOSTIC TESTS & INTERPRETATION
Imaging
Neuroimaging to rule out intracranial pathology may rarely be indicated.

Diagnostic Procedures/Other
- No routine lab tests are indicated for patients with substance withdrawal.
- Tests necessary to rule out differential diagnoses should be obtained when appropriate.

DIFFERENTIAL DIAGNOSIS
- Hypoglycemia
- Intoxication with sympathomimetics, anticholinergics, theophylline, caffeine, aspirin, or lithium
- Thyroid storm
- Serotonin syndrome
- Neuroleptic malignant syndrome
- Encephalitis
- Meningitis
- Sepsis

TREATMENT

MEDICATION (DRUGS)
- Symptom-triggered treatment has been demonstrated to be superior to fixed-regimen treatment in terms of patient outcome as well as length of stay.
- Patients experiencing withdrawal from benzodiazepines or barbiturates after treatment in a chronic or intensive care setting may be treated by reinstituting the drug and then tapering.
- Iatrogenic withdrawal induced by use of opioid antagonists should not be treated by opioid administration.
  - Withdrawal induced by naloxone should abate rapidly due to the brief half-life of naloxone.
  - Withdrawal induced by naltrexone or nalmephene will be much longer lasting. Symptomatic treatment may be indicated.

- There is no fixed quantity of drug to use for any withdrawal syndrome. Each patient requires a unique quantity of drug.
  - Repeated dosing should continue until the symptoms are controlled, at which point maintenance and then tapering can occur.
- Sedative-hypnotic withdrawal:
  - Ideally, withdrawal is treated with the same class of substance, such as benzodiazepine or barbiturate, if not the precise same drug.
  - Benzodiazepines are particularly useful due to the rapid onset of effect.
  - Diazepam has active metabolites that assist in tapering the drug.
  - Propofol is an outstanding medication for treatment of severe alcohol or sedative-hypnotic withdrawal in adults.
    - Propofol may be used in pediatric cases refractory to benzodiazepines and barbiturates.
    - Use is associated with respiratory depression.
    - Clinicians must be capable of airway management and expect airway support to be necessary when propofol is used.
    - Propofol use is safe in children, but rare cases of metabolic acidemia have occurred when prolonged infusions are used. Prolonged use of propofol infusion should be accompanied by close observation for acidemia.
- Opioid withdrawal:
  - Heroin (as well as other opioids) withdrawal is best treated with an opioid of similar potency and equal or longer duration of action.
  - Methadone is a preferred treatment for withdrawal in adolescents and adults, but most neonatologists have limited or no experience with this drug.
  - Paregoric and tincture of opium remain the most commonly used therapies for neonatal withdrawal.
  - Patients who experience opioid withdrawal in the setting of chronic or intensive care may be treated by reinstituting infusion or dosing of the drug they were on before withdrawal symptoms and then tapering this, typically by 10% daily.
- Caffeine withdrawal:
  - Caffeine as soft drink or tea taken to treat headache or agitation
  - Neonatal caffeine abstinence symptoms may be treated by reinstituting 75–100% of the caffeine dosage that was discontinued. This amount is then tapered, typically by 10% daily.
- Nicotine withdrawal is not typically treated in children.
- Use of nicotine patch, gum, or other delivery methods is used to increase success rate of abstinence rather than for medical management of the withdrawal syndrome.

ADDITIONAL TREATMENT
General Measures
- Initial Stabilization
  - Initial management is aimed at evaluating and supporting airway, breathing, circulation, serum glucose, and ECG. (A, B, C, D, E)
- Supportive care is the most important general principle.
- The illness is managed with intent of close monitoring and addressing issues as they arise.

ISSUES FOR REFERRAL
- Any patient with substance abuse issues should be referred for appropriate psychiatric or drug counseling.
- Most cases of substance withdrawal are best handled by an addiction specialist, medical toxicologist, intensivist, or other clinician experienced with management of withdrawal.

IN-PATIENT CONSIDERATIONS
Admission Criteria
- In-patient treatment for alcohol or sedative-hypnotic withdrawal is mandatory.
- Although withdrawal from opioids and selective serotonin reuptake inhibitors is not life-threatening, admission with initial management as an inpatient is preferable.

IV Fluids
- Maintenance IV fluid may be required in patients who are unable to take PO.
- Dehydration was once a leading cause of death among patients with alcohol withdrawal.

Discharge Criteria
- Inpatients who have been converted from parenteral to oral medications and are controlled with oral medications may be discharged for home tapering.
- Patients who never require parenteral therapy may be discharged with oral replacement medication after consultation with the appropriate specialist.

 ONGOING CARE

FOLLOW-UP RECOMMENDATIONS
- If disposition will be discharge, it is crucial to ensure that the patient's condition is stable before discharge.
- If there is any question regarding whether the patient can be appropriately managed as an outpatient, initial in-patient management is preferable.

Patient Monitoring
- Sedative-hypnotic withdrawal or any other withdrawal syndrome with severe symptoms is best cared for with initial cardiopulmonary monitoring until vital sign abnormalities are controlled with appropriate replacement therapy.
- Patients should be closely monitored until vital signs are within acceptable limits.
- Vigilance for agitation or delirium with sedative-hypnotic withdrawal is necessary.
- Vigilance to detect oversedation and respiratory depression is necessary.

PATIENT EDUCATION
Patients or parents should be aware of withdrawal symptoms to be vigilant for detecting future events.

PROGNOSIS
- With appropriate therapy, withdrawal is well tolerated.
- Poor prognostic factors are primarily related to comorbidities.

COMPLICATIONS
Complications of hypertension, tachycardia, hyperthermia, and CNS agitation or seizure may occur with sedative-hypnotic withdrawal.

ADDITIONAL READING

- Anon. Neonatal complications after intrauterine exposure to SSRI antidepressants. *Prescrire Int.* 2004;13:103–104.
- Coles CD, Smith IE, Fernhoff PM, et al. Neonatal ethanol withdrawal: Characteristics in clinically normal, nondysmorphic neonates. *J Pediatr.* 1984;105:445–451.
- Dyer JE, Roth B, Hyma BA. Gamma-hydroxybutyrate withdrawal syndrome. *Ann Emerg Med.* 2001;37: 147–153.
- Nordeng H, Lindeman R, Perminov KV, et al. Neonatal withdrawal syndrome after in utero exposure to selective serotonin reuptake inhibitors. *Acta Paediatr.* 2001;90:288–291.
- Robe LB, Gromisch DS, Iosub S. Symptoms of neonatal ethanol withdrawal. *Curr Alcohol.* 1981;8:485–493.
- Scott CS, Decker JL, Edwards ML, et al. Withdrawal after narcotic therapy: A survey of neonatal and pediatric clinicians. *Pharmacotherapy.* 1998: 1308–1312.
- Tobias JD. Tolerance, withdrawal, and physical dependency after long-term sedation and analgesia of children in the pediatric intensive care unit. *Crit Care Med.* 2000;28:2122–2132.

CODES

ICD9
- 291.81 Alcohol withdrawal
- 292.0 Drug withdrawal
- 779.5 Drug withdrawal syndrome in newborn

ICD10
- F13.939 Sedatv/hyp/anxiolytc use, unsp w withdrawal, unsp
- F19.939 Other psychoactive substance use, unsp with withdrawal, unsp
- P96.1 Neonatal w/drawal symp from matern use of drugs of addiction

ACUTE KIDNEY INJURY

Rebecca Ruebner
Lawrence Copelovitch

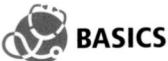 **BASICS**

DESCRIPTION
- Acute kidney injury (AKI), previously referred to as acute renal failure (ARF), is defined as any insult to the kidney, with a sudden decrease of normal kidney function that compromises the normal renal regulation of fluid, electrolyte, and acid–base homeostasis.
- In practical terms, AKI is characterized by a reduction in the glomerular filtration rate (GFR) that results in an abrupt increase in the concentrations of serum creatinine and BUN.
- AKI in the most severe cases may lead to irreversible end-stage renal failure.
- In AKI, the urine output is variable: Anuria, oliguria, and in some cases polyuria can all be observed at presentation.
- Oliguria: Urine output <0.5 mL/kg/h in infants or <500 mL/1.73 m^2/d in older children
- Anuria: Total cessation of urinary output
- Polyuria: Urine output >2 L/m^2/d in infants and children or 3 L/d in adults

EPIDEMIOLOGY
Incidence
- AKI due to acute tubular necrosis (ATN) is commonly seen in hospitalized patients. The combination of ischemia plus nephrotoxic agents (aminoglycosides, amphotericin B, contrast, chemotherapeutic agents) place these patients at increased risk.
- AKI secondary to dehydration, NSAID toxicity, or medication-induced interstitial nephritis is common in the outpatient setting

PATHOPHYSIOLOGY
AKI is commonly precipitated by an ischemic or nephrotoxic event. Initial vasodilatation is followed by intense vasoconstriction, with blood redistributed from the cortex to the juxtamedullary nephrons. Delivery of oxygen to the kidney is impaired, leading to ATN. Intratubular debris and cast formation develop. Tubular fluid leaks backward across the injured tubular membrane, which, in addition to tubular obstruction, causes further hemodynamic changes.

ETIOLOGY
AKI has many causes, which can be subcategorized into 3 groups:
- Prerenal:
  – Decreased perfusion of the kidney secondary either to decreased intravascular volume (e.g., dehydration), decreased effective circulating blood volume (e.g., CHF), or from altered intrarenal hemodynamics (e.g., NSAIDs)
  – Common form of AKI in children
- Postrenal:
  – Obstructive process (either structural or functional)
  – Obstruction can reside in the lower tract or bilaterally in the upper tracts (unless the patient has a single kidney).
  – This form of renal failure is more common in newborns.

- Intrinsic: Disorders that directly affect the kidney. This form can be subcategorized as follows:
  – ATN is the end result of either ischemic- or toxin-mediated damage to the tubules. Ischemic induced ATN is the result of prolonged and severe prerenal AKI, which is no longer immediately reversible with the restoration of appropriate renal perfusion. Toxin-mediated ATN can be caused by many medications (e.g., aminoglycosides), poisons (e.g., mercury), or endogenous toxins (e.g., myoglobinuria).
  – Glomerular disorders include the various forms of acute glomerulonephritis (e.g., postinfectious, rapidly progressive [crescentic]).
  – Vascular lesions compromise glomerular blood flow. Hemolytic-uremic syndrome is the most common disorder that causes intrinsic AKI in children.
  – Interstitial nephritis most often occurs as a result of exposure to medications such as NSAIDs. It may also be associated with infections (e.g., pyelonephritis), systemic diseases, or tumor infiltrates.

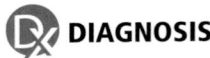 **DIAGNOSIS**

HISTORY
- Previous infection (acute glomerulonephritis), neurogenic bladder, single kidney (obstruction)
- Therapy with nonsteroidal anti-inflammatory agents, β-lactam antibiotics, acyclovir (acute interstitial nephritis), nephrotoxic drugs (e.g., aminoglycosides, amphotericin B, cisplatin [ATN])
- Toxins: Exposure to heavy metals, organic solvents (ATN)
- Gross hematuria: Glomerulonephritis (tea colored), renal calculi (bright red blood)
- Positive family history of hemolytic-uremic syndrome
- Trauma: Crush injury (ATN)
- Review of symptoms: Various systemic symptoms (acute glomerulonephritis)
- Signs and symptoms: Fever, rash (acute interstitial nephritis, acute glomerulonephritis), bloody diarrhea, pallor (hemolytic-uremic syndrome), severe vomiting or diarrhea (prerenal), abdominal pain (obstruction), hemorrhage, shock (ATN), anuria (acute glomerulonephritis, obstruction), polyuria (ATN, acute interstitial nephritis)

PHYSICAL EXAM
- General: Weight and hydration status; shock (i.e., prerenal, ATN), edema (e.g., acute glomerulonephritis), jaundice (i.e., hemolytic-uremic syndrome, ATN)
- Eyes: Uveitis (i.e., acute interstitial nephritis)
- Lungs: Rales (i.e., acute glomerulonephritis)
- Heart: Gallop (i.e., acute glomerulonephritis)
- Abdomen/Pelvis: Mass (i.e., obstruction)
- Skin: Rash (i.e., acute interstitial nephritis, acute glomerulonephritis), petechiae (i.e., hemolytic-uremic syndrome)
- Joints: Arthritis (i.e., acute glomerulonephritis)

DIAGNOSTIC TESTS & INTERPRETATION
Lab
- All patients with AKI should have a urinalysis with microscopic exam, serum chemistries, and a CBC:
  – Urinalysis: Specific gravity (>1.020 suggests prerenal AKI), proteinuria (>3+ intrinsic, glomerular AKI), eosinophiluria (acute interstitial nephritis), pyuria (pyelonephritis), granular casts (prerenal, ATN), pigmenturia (ATN), erythrocyte casts (glomerulonephritis acute interstitial nephritis, ATN)
  – Serum chemistries: Hyponatremia, acidosis, hyperkalemia, hyperphosphatemia, hypocalcemia, BUN/creatinine >20 (i.e., prerenal)
  – CBC: Microangiopathic hemolytic anemia, thrombocytopenia (i.e., hemolytic-uremic syndrome), eosinophilia (i.e., acute interstitial nephritis)
- Selected patients require further studies, including serologies, urine electrolytes, imaging, and renal biopsy:
  – Serologies: Hypocomplementemia (acute glomerulonephritis), antineutrophil cytoplasmic antibodies (acute glomerulonephritis), antinuclear antibodies (acute glomerulonephritis)
  – The fractional excretion of sodium (FENa) is a useful urinary index that determines tubular function. FENa = [(UNa/PNa)/(Ucreat/Pcreat)] × 100. The FENa should not be obtained after diuretics are administered. FENa >2: acute interstitial nephritis, ATN; FENa <1: hemolytic-uremic syndrome, acute glomerulonephritis, prerenal.

Imaging
- Chest radiograph: Cardiomegaly or pulmonary edema (fluid overload)
- Renal US: Hydronephrosis, trabeculated bladder (i.e., obstruction), increased echogenicity (i.e., ATN, acute interstitial nephritis, acute glomerulonephritis, hemolytic-uremic syndrome), abnormal Doppler study (renal venous thrombosis)

Diagnostic Procedures/Other
Renal biopsy: Indicated in patients with prolonged, unexplained AKI or suspicion for crescentic glomerulonephritis

DIFFERENTIAL DIAGNOSIS
- Chronic kidney disease: Insidious, associated with poor growth, polyuria, rickets, delayed growth, and anemia
- Azotemia (elevated BUN): Hypercatabolic states including corticosteroid therapy or upper GI bleeding
- Elevated creatinine: Caused by rhabdomyolysis, drugs (trimethoprim-sulfa, cimetidine)

TREATMENT

MEDICATION (DRUGS)

- Excretion and evacuation of many medications is influenced by AKI. Careful attention to drug dosing and levels can minimize toxicity.
- Preventive: Mannitol or furosemide therapy to prevent AKI remains controversial. They may be used prophylactically (e.g., amphotericin B, cisplatin, contrast media) or in cases of hemoglobinuria or myoglobinuria to increase urine flow. Physicians consider that this may convert renal failure from oliguric to nonoliguric.

ADDITIONAL TREATMENT

Additional Therapies

- Supportive:
  - Establish an effective circulatory volume. If the patient is in shock, administer fluids (e.g., normal saline, lactated Ringer solution) liberally, even if there is no urine output.
  - Maintain a normal intravascular volume. Carefully monitor urine output, and provide appropriate fluids accordingly. Consider fluid restriction and diuretics if the patient suffers volume overload.
  - Monitor serum potassium levels frequently. Avoid drugs, fluids, or foods containing potassium in patients with oliguria or anuria.
  - Avoid nephrotoxic medications when possible.
  - Hyponatremia is usually due to free water excess and should be managed with fluid restriction. Hypertonic saline should be used if only CNS symptoms are present.
  - Hypocalcemia, if mild, may be treated by phosphate restriction. Severe hypocalcemia requires treatment with calcium gluconate (100 mg/kg) given slowly.
  - Severe acidosis (pH <7.2) requires supplementation with bicarbonate. However, this may cause hypernatremia, fluid overload, and symptomatic hypocalcemia.
  - The effect of aggressive nutritional support is controversial, with the exception of use in a significantly malnourished or hypercatabolic child.
  - Hypertension should be treated aggressively if encephalopathy is present.
  - Dialysis or hemofiltration is indicated for refractory acidosis, severe hyperkalemia, volume overload, and uremic symptoms (e.g., pericarditis, lethargy, bleeding diathesis) or for the removal of toxins (e.g., uric acid, salicylate).
- Specific:
  - Each cause of renal failure may necessitate specific treatment, such as fluid resuscitation (i.e., prerenal), urologic intervention (i.e., obstruction), and corticosteroids (i.e., acute interstitial nephritis, some forms of acute glomerulonephritis).

IN-PATIENT CONSIDERATIONS

Initial Stabilization

- If hypovolemic, rapidly establish euvolemia with 0.9% NS boluses.
- If urine output remains low after euvolemia is established, begin fluid restriction (insensibles and urine output).
- In severe hyperkalemia (>6.5 mEq/L), consider:
  - Calcium gluconate (100 mg/kg IV) over 5–10 minutes if severe
  - Glucose (0.5 g/kg) and insulin (0.1 U/kg) IV over 30 minutes
  - Sodium bicarbonate (1–2 mEq/kg) IV over 10–30 minutes if acidotic
  - When administering sodium bicarbonate, monitor serum calcium carefully since the hypocalcemia may worsen.
  - Kayexalate (1 g/kg) PO or PR in sorbitol
  - Furosemide (1–2 mg/kg) if renal function is adequate
  - Hemodialysis or peritoneal dialysis

ONGOING CARE

FOLLOW-UP RECOMMENDATIONS

- Patients usually remain hospitalized until their renal function improves. Long-term follow-up to monitor sequelae is indicated in patients with prolonged anuria.
- The likelihood of recovery from AKI depends on the amount of urine output and the underlying cause.
- Patients with nonoliguric AKI (e.g., toxin-mediated ATN, interstitial nephritis, hemolytic-uremic syndrome) have lower complication rates than those with oliguric AKI.

PROGNOSIS

- Generally, patients with nonoliguric renal failure have a lower mortality rate than patients with oliguria or anuria.
- The mortality rate increases in patients with multisystem organ failure, despite good supportive care.

COMPLICATIONS

- A significant postobstructive diuresis can be seen after treatment for obstructive AKI.
- Fluid overload, resulting in congestive heart failure, hypertension, or hyponatremia
- Hyperkalemia, affecting cardiac function by causing arrhythmias
- Uremia, manifest by mental status changes, increased risk of bleeding, and infection
- Metabolic acidosis
- Hypocalcemia, causing tetany

ADDITIONAL READING

- Andreoli SP. Acute renal failure. *Curr Opin Pediatr.* 2002;14:183–188.
- Malinoski DJ, Slater MS, Mullins RJ. Crush injury and rhabdomyolysis. *Crit Care Clin.* 2004;20: 171–192.
- Singri N, Ahya SN, Levin ML. Acute renal failure. *JAMA.* 2005;289:747–751.

CODES

ICD9

- 584.9 Acute kidney failure, unspecified
- 866.00 Injury to kidney without mention of open wound into cavity, unspecified injury

ICD10

- S37.009A Unspecified injury of unspecified kidney, initial encounter
- S37.009D Unspecified injury of unspecified kidney, subsequent encounter
- S37.009S Unspecified injury of unspecified kidney, sequela

FAQ

- Q: What is the expected recovery time in patients with AKI who present with anuria?
- A: Recovery time depends on the etiology of the AKI. Children with hemolytic-uremic syndrome may recover in days to weeks. Those with ATN recover days after treatment for the cause. Children whose disorder results from obstruction usually recover as soon as the obstruction is removed.
- Q: When should renal function return to normal?
- A: Renal function may never return to normal in patients with long-standing anuria. In other cases, after recovery occurs, serum creatinine levels return to normal within weeks.
- Q: Which indices should be observed after a patient recovers from AKI?
- A: Patients recovering from AKI should have BP and urinalysis for proteinuria monitored regularly. Serum creatinine should be measured if the course of AKI was prolonged.

ACUTE LYMPHOBLASTIC LEUKEMIA

Susan R. Rheingold

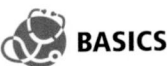 **BASICS**

DESCRIPTION

- Acute lymphoblastic leukemia (ALL) is a malignant proliferation of white blood cells characterized by an excess of lymphoblasts.
- Risk stratification is based on clinical features at diagnosis (age and WBC count), biologic and cytogenetic characteristics of the lymphoblasts, and response to initial therapy.
- Risk stratification determines therapy intensity and prognosis.
  - Low risk: Favorable cytogenetics (trisomy 4, 10, or t(12;21) (TEL/AML1), age 1–10 years, WBC count <50,000 at diagnosis, precursor B phenotype, and no minimal residual disease (MRD) at end-induction.
  - Standard risk: Age 1–10 years; WBC count <50,000, precursor B phenotype, non-contributory cytogenetics, no extramedullary involvement (CNS or teste), and no minimal residual disease (MRD) at end-induction.
  - High risk: Age 1–10 years with WBC count >50,000; age >10 years regardless of WBC count or phenotype; all T-cell phenotype, extramedullary involvement, and no/very low minimal residual disease (MRD) at end-induction.
- Very high risk: Unfavorable cytogenetics (hypodiploid, MLL), positive minimal residual disease at end of induction/induction failure. Traditionally patients with t(9;22) ALL (Philadelphia +) were considered very high risk but outcomes have improved drastically with targeted molecular therapy.
- Infants <1 year of age at diagnosis have poor outcomes and are treated on intensive infant protocols.

EPIDEMIOLOGY

- ALL is the most common cancer of childhood, accounting for 30% of cancer diagnoses in children ≤15 years of age.
- More common in Caucasians and males

Incidence

- Incidence of ALL is 1/1,700 in children <15 years of age.
- Peak incidence is between 2 and 5 years of age.

RISK FACTORS

- Prior cancer therapy—chemotherapy or radiation.
- Early exposure to viruses (i.e., daycare) appears to be protective.
- Twin with ALL.
- Genetic syndrome listed below.

Genetics

Increased risk of leukemia with the following:

- Trisomy 21 (≤15% risk), Neurofibromatosis type 1, Fanconi anemia, Bloom syndrome, Ataxia Telangiectasia, Schwachman–Diamond syndrome
- Li–Fraumeni p53 Syndrome (Familial cancer syndrome).
- Congenital immunodeficiencies (e.g., Wiskott–Aldrich syndrome).
- 5–25% risk of ALL in monozygotic twin (5% in dizygotic) before 5 years of age

PATHOPHYSIOLOGY

Leukemia cells are derived from a lymphoblastic precursor cell that acquires multiple genetic mutations that lead to rapid clonal proliferation; lack of cell maturation; and resistance to normal cell death processes (apoptosis). This lymphoblastic proliferation leads to overgrowth and the crowding out of normal bone marrow precursors causing ineffective hematopoiesis and infiltration of lymphatic tissue and end-organs

ETIOLOGY
ASSOCIATED CONDITIONS

- Trisomy 21 (Down syndrome)
- Li–Fraumeni Syndrome
- Neurofibromatosis type 1
- Ataxia telangiectasia
- Bloom syndrome
- Immunodeficiencies

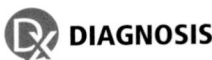 **DIAGNOSIS**

SIGNS AND SYMPTOMS
HISTORY

- Bleeding (cutaneous and mucosal), easy bruising, epistaxis
  - Low platelet count
  - Coagulopathy
- Bone pain, limp, refusal to bear weight:
  - Infiltrative disease of marrow
  - Pathologic fractures
- Fatigue, pallor, headache:
  - Anemia
- Stridor, orthopnea, shortness of breath, wheezing, any respiratory distress:
  - Mediastinal mass, pleural effusion
  - Venous stasis due to hyperleukocytosis
- Oliguria, anuria:
  - Renal failure most likely from tumor lysis syndrome
- Ocular pain, blurred vision, photophobia:
  - Leukemic infiltration of orbit, optic nerve, retina, iris, cornea, or conjunctiva
- Headache, vomiting, seizures, lethargy:
  - Leukemic infiltration CNS
  - Stroke due to hyperleukcytosis

PHYSICAL EXAM

- Pallor
  - Anemia
- Lymphadenopathy (generalized)
  - Infiltration with leukemia
- Hepatosplenomegaly
  - Infiltration with leukemia
- Bone tenderness
  - Bone marrow infiltration, fracture
- Petechiae and purpura, subconjunctival and retinal hemorrhages
  - Thrombocytopenia
- Hypopyon (layering of leukemia cells in anterior chamber of eye)
- Papilledema CNS infiltration
- Painless testicular enlargement in boys
  - Testicular infiltration
- Swelling of the face, orthopnea
  - Superior vena cava (SVC) syndrome in presence of mediastinal mass

- Rash, subcutaneous nodules
  - Leukemic infiltration of skin (leukemia cutis)
  - Petechiae
- Extremity weakness; numbness or tingling
  - Spinal cord compression

DIAGNOSTIC TESTS & INTERPRETATION
Lab

- CBC
  - Increased or decreased WBC count: <10,000/μL in 50% of cases, >50,000/μL in 20% of cases
  - Hemoglobin <10 g/dL in 80% of cases
  - Thrombocytopenia (platelets <100,000/μL) in 75% of cases. Think of ITP if platelets <10,000/μL and rest of CBC is normal.
  - Peripheral smear usually shows characteristic leukemic lymphoblasts.
- PT/PTT, DIC panel
- Chemistry panel:
  - Tumor lysis syndrome: elevated uric acid, potassium, and phosphorous with a secondary hypocalcemia.
  - Elevated creatinine secondary to uric acid or calcium phosphate crystal deposition in the renal tubules.
  - Slight abnormality of liver function tests due to leukemic infiltrate
  - Elevated lactic dehydrogenase (LDH)

ALERT
Beware of any machine-generated differential that has a high percentage of atypical lymphocytes. Leukemic blasts can be mistaken for these cell types and the smear should be reviewed by a pathologist or oncologist.

Imaging
- Chest X-ray—5–10% of cases have a mediastinal mass

Diagnostic Procedures/Other
- Bone marrow aspirate and biopsy:
  - Presence of >25% leukemic lymphoblasts is diagnostic.
  - Immunophenotyping, morphology, and cytogenetic studies are diagnostic and prognostic.
- CSF examination for lymphoblasts:
  - >5 blasts/hpf is positive

Pathological Findings
Morphologic confirmation of lymphoblasts in bone marrow with immunophenotyping. May have combinations of:

- Precursor B- CD 10+, 19+, 20+, 22+, TdT +
- Precursor T- CD 2+, 3+, 5+, 7 +, TdT+
- May also have some minimal myeloid marker involvement- CD 13+, 33+, 34+.

DIFFERENTIAL DIAGNOSIS

- Infectious:
  - Pertussis and parapertussis
  - Parvovirus
  - Cytomegalovirus
  - Acute infectious lymphocytosis
  - Infectious mononucleosis (EBV)

- Hematologic:
  - Idiopathic thrombocytopenic purpura
  - Aplastic anemia
  - Evans syndrome
- Rheumatologic:
  - Juvenile idiopathic arthritis
  - Vasculitis
- Malignant conditions:
  - Neuroblastoma with bone marrow involvement
  - Lymphoma with bone marrow involvement
  - Rhabdomyosarcoma
  - Retinoblastoma
  - Acute or chronic myelogenous leukemia
  - Myelodysplastic syndrome
  - Langerhans cell histiocytosis

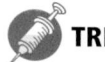 TREATMENT

ISSUES FOR REFERRAL
Patients suspected of having ALL should be referred as soon as possible to a pediatric oncologist for further evaluation.

INITIAL STABILIZATION
Emergency care is required for the following:
- Hyperleukocytosis
- Spinal cord compression
- Mediastinal mass/SVC syndrome
- Tumor lysis syndrome

GENERAL MEASURES
- Therapy stratified according to risk groups (low, standard, high, and very high). Overall, there are several phases of intensive outpatient therapy followed by a prolonged maintenance (2–3 years).
- Remission Induction [to achieve (<5% blasts in bone marrow, minimal residual disease <0.01%)]:
  - Vincristine (VCR)
  - Prednisone or dexamethasone
  - PEG–Asparaginase
  - Anthracycline—if high-risk
  - Intrathecal chemotherapy
- Consolidation/interim maintenance (focusing on CNS prophylaxis): Weekly intrathecal chemotherapy:
  - Low/average-risk patients get mild oral chemotherapy with weekly VCR and lower dose methotrexate (MTX).
  - Higher risk patients get combinations of more intensive chemotherapy with cyclophosphamide, cytarabine, methotrexate, vincristine, and asparginase.
- Delayed intensification (further decrease leukemic burden):
  - Combinations of intensive weekly chemotherapy used in higher risk induction and consolidation.
- Very High risk patients, Ph+ ALL, and infants get extra-intensive cycles, including the above chemotherapy at higher doses and etoposide, before starting Maintenance.

- Maintenance:
  - Length varies by protocol
  - Daily oral 6MP and weekly oral MTX
  - Pulses of VCR and glucocorticoid steroids
  - Periodic intrathecal chemotherapy
- Ph+ ALL also gets treated continuously with molecularly targeted oral tyrosine kinase inhibitors (imatinib or dasatinib).
- Patients with CNS involvement, persistent testicular ALL, and higher risk patients may get treated with prophylactic or therapeutic doses of cranial radiation.
- Very high-risk patients are often treated with bone marrow transplant (BMT) when they are in remission.
- Total duration therapy of varies but the minimum is 2 years, with a maximum of 3.25 years depending upon sex of patient and protocol.

 ONGOING CARE

FOLLOW-UP RECOMMENDATIONS
Patient Monitoring
At completion of therapy:
- CBC every 3 months for 2 years, then every 4–6 months for 2 years, then yearly visits. Liver and renal function tests every 3–6 months
- Cardiac evaluation yearly
- Endocrine evaluation in children close to puberty
- All survivors should be followed in a pediatric oncology survivorship clinic.

PROGNOSIS
- Morphologic remission post-induction in all risk categories, with presently available therapy, is 98%.
- Long-term survival (overall) approaches 80%.
- Long-term survival in low risk patients is 90–95%; standard risk group is about 85%. Long-term survival in high-risk group is about 60–75%.
- Long-term survival in very high-risk group is 20–50% (often with transplant).

COMPLICATIONS
- Due to disease:
  - Hyperleukocytosis (WBC count >100,000): Can lead to stroke, respiratory distress
  - Mediastinal mass (usually T-cell lineage): Can lead to cardiorespiratory arrest
  - Tumor lysis syndrome: Can lead to renal failure, cardiac arrhythmias
  - Coagulopathy: Can lead to stroke and hemorrhage
- Relapse: Approximately 20% of patients who obtain a remission will relapse, usually within 5 years of diagnosis. If the relapse occurs while the patient is actively receiving therapy outcome is poor (<20%), even with BMT. If the relapse is >36 months from diagnosis or isolated to the CNS or testicle, survival is improved (40–70%) with chemotherapy, radiation and/or BMT.
- Potential irreversible toxicity due to therapy:
  - Cranial radiation (XRT): Secondary brain tumors, leukoencephalopathy and deterioration of intellectual functions/learning deficits, growth retardation, decreased bone density
  - L-Asparaginase: thrombosis, stroke
  - Intrathecal chemotherapy: learning disabilities
  - Doxorubicin/daunorubicin: Cardiac toxicity, secondary AML
  - MTX: Stroke, hepatotoxicity
  - Steroids: Avascular necrosis of joints, growth retardation.

ADDITIONAL READING

- Borowitz MJ, Devidas M, Hunger SP, et al. Clinical significance of minimal residual disease in childhood ALL and its relationship to other prognostic factors: a COG study. *Blood*. 2008;111:5477–5485.
- Mullighan CG, Goorha S, Radtke I, et al. Genome-wide analysis of genetic alterations in acute lymphoblastic leukemia. *Nature*. 2007;446: 758–764.
- Nguyen K, Devidas M, Cheng S-C, et al. Factors influencing survival after relapse from acute lymphoblastic leukemia: A COG study. *Leukemia*. 2008;1–9.
- Pui CH, Robison LL, Look AT. Acute lymphoblastic leukemia. *Lancet*. 2008;371:1030–1043.
- Pulte D, Gondos A, Brenner H. Trends in 5- and 10-year survival after diagnosis with childhood hematologic malignancies in the United States, 1990–2004. *J Natl Cancer Inst*. 2008;100(18); 1301–1309.

 CODES

ICD9
- 204.00 Acute lymphoid leukemia, without mention of having achieved remission
- 204.01 Acute lymphoid leukemia, in remission
- 204.02 Acute lymphoid leukemia, in relapse

ICD10
- C91.00 Acute lymphoblastic leukemia not having achieved remission
- C91.01 Acute lymphoblastic leukemia, in remission
- C91.02 Acute lymphoblastic leukemia, in relapse

FAQ

- Q: Can a child on treatment for ALL go to school or leave the house?
- A: Yes. Most centers encourage the child to live a normal life, including school, activities, and travel.
- Q: Will hair fall out and the child be sick for all 3 years on chemotherapy?
- A: The hair usually falls out within a few weeks of initiating therapy and grows back when maintenance therapy begins (6–8 months). Most children feel relatively well during therapy, especially maintenance chemotherapy.
- Q: Does the child need to be isolated from other children?
- A: The most serious infections a child on chemotherapy gets come from bacteria that the child is already colonized with, not community-acquired viruses. That being said, the child should be isolated from any child who has varicella or other known symptomatic infection.

ACUTE MYELOID LEUKEMIA

David T. Teachey

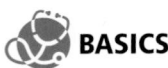 **BASICS**

DESCRIPTION
- Acute myeloid leukemia (AML) is a block in differentiation and an unregulated proliferation of myeloid progenitor cells.
- Classified according to the World Health Organization (WHO) classification (2008)
- Formerly classified by French-American-British (FAB) classification
- WHO classification based on genetic alterations, whereas FAB based on morphology

EPIDEMIOLOGY
- 7th most common pediatric malignancy
- Leukemia in 1st 4 weeks of life is usually AML
- Ratio of AML to acute lymphoblastic leukemia (ALL) throughout childhood is 1:4.
- Boys and girls are equally affected.

Incidence
- Incidence peaks at 2 years and again at 16 years of age.
- 500 children/year in the US

RISK FACTORS
Genetics
- Only 20–30% of pediatric blasts have a normal karyotype, vs. 40–50% in adults.
- 60% of abnormal karyotypes fall into known subgroups.
- Translocations or duplications of the *MLL* gene at 11q23 and monosomy 7 are found in many cases of therapy-induced AML and carry a poor prognosis.
- Translocations t(8;21), t(15;17), and inv(16) carry a better prognosis.

PATHOPHYSIOLOGY
- Principal defect is a block in the differentiation of primitive myeloid precursor cells
- 2 predominant mechanisms have been identified:
  - Defect at the level of transcriptional activation
  - Defects in the signaling pathway of hematopoietic growth factors. The proto-oncogene Ras is mutated in up to 1/3 of patients with AML.

ETIOLOGY
- Exact cause unknown
- Acquired risk factors:
  - Exposure to benzene
  - Exposure to ionizing radiation
  - Therapy induced, from chemotherapy for a prior malignancy
  - Alkylating agents such as cyclophosphamide, nitrogen mustard, chlorambucil, and melphalan (typically presents several years after therapy)
  - Epipodophyllotoxins such as VP16, VM26 (typically occurs within 2 years after therapy and is characterized by rearrangements involving 11q23)

- Certain congenital syndromes that carry an increased risk of AML:
  - Fanconi anemia
  - Bloom syndrome
  - Neurofibromatosis type I
  - Down syndrome
  - Severe congenital anemia (i.e., Kostmann disease treated with granulocyte colony-stimulating factor)
  - Diamond Blackfan anemia
  - Paroxysmal nocturnal hemoglobinemia
  - Li-Fraumeni syndrome

DIAGNOSIS

HISTORY
Children with AML can present with very few symptoms or with life-threatening sepsis or hemorrhage. Common symptoms include the following:
- Fever: 30–40%
- Pallor: 25%
- Weight loss/anorexia: 22%
- Fatigue: 19%
- Bleeding (i.e., cutaneous, mucosal, menorrhagia): 33%
- Bone or joint pain: 18%

PHYSICAL EXAM
- Signs of anemia:
  - Pallor, fatigue, headache, dyspnea, systolic flow murmur
- Signs of thrombocytopenia:
  - Petechiae, bruising, epistaxis, gingival bleeding
- Signs of infection:
  - Fever
  - Lingering bacterial infections of lung, sinuses, gingiva, perirectal area, skin
- Other exam findings:
  - Hepatomegaly
  - Splenomegaly
  - Lymphadenopathy
  - Gingival hyperplasia
  - Papilledema, cranial nerve palsies (rare)
  - Colorless or slightly purple subcutaneous nodules: "Blueberry muffin" lesions of leukemia cutis (more commonly seen in neonates)

DIAGNOSTIC TESTS & INTERPRETATION
Techniques such as fluorescence in situ hybridization, Southern blotting, and reverse transcriptase–polymerase chain reaction are becoming necessary diagnostic tools for AML.

Lab
- CBC:
  - Anemia, thrombocytopenia, elevated or low total WBC peripheral smear
  - Myeloblasts may be seen.
- Prothrombin time (PT)/partial thromboplastin time (PTT) fibrin spit products:
  - Elevated in some cases, especially with acute promyelocytic leukemia (M3)
  - Can have severe, life-threatening disseminated intravascular coagulation (DIC)
- Electrolytes (abnormalities associated with tumor lysis syndrome):
  - Hyperkalemia
  - Hypocalcemia
  - Hyperphosphatemia
  - Hyperuricemia
- CSF analysis for cell count and cytology:
  - >5 WBC/mm^3 is suggestive of CNS disease.
  - 5–15% of cases have CNS involvement at diagnosis.

Diagnostic Procedures/Other
Bone marrow aspirate:
- >20% myeloblasts is diagnostic.
- Confirm with immunophenotyping and cytochemistry.

Pathological Findings
- Immunophenotyping:
  - Blasts positive for myeloid-associated surface antigens (CD11b, CD13, CD14, CD15, CD33, or CD36) in 90% of cases
  - Lymphoid markers: T and B cells may be present in 30–60% of pediatric patients.
  - CD41, CD42, and CD61 (megakaryocytic)
- Morphology:
  - Large blasts with low nuclear/cytoplasmic ratio
  - Multiple nucleoli and cytoplasmic granules
- Cytochemistry:
  - Blasts are positive for myeloperoxidase and Sudan black and usually negative for periodic acid–Schiff (PAS) and terminal deoxynucleotide transferase (TdT).

DIFFERENTIAL DIAGNOSIS
- Myeloid blast crisis of chronic myeloid leukemia (Philadelphia chromosome positive)
- ALL
- Leukemoid reaction
- Exaggerated leukocytosis

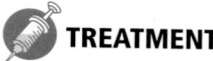

TREATMENT

MEDICATION (DRUGS)
- Patients are treated with 6–9 months of intensive chemotherapy given in cycles.
- The most effective drugs for remission induction in AML are anthracyclines (e.g., doxorubicin, daunomycin, and mitoxantrone) and cytarabine (Ara-C).
- Etoposide (VP-16), gemtuzumab (anti-CD33 monoclonal antibody), dexamethasone, L-asparaginase, and 6-thioguanine are added in some regimens (remission rate is ~70–85%).
- High rate of remission induction with all-*trans*-retinoic acid in acute promyelocytic leukemia
- Intrathecal Ara-C for CNS prophylaxis

ADDITIONAL TREATMENT
General Measures
- Hydration, alkalization, and allopurinol during induction
- Rasburicase should be considered in patients with marked elevations in uric acid and renal compromise (contraindicated in patients with G6PD deficiency).
- Blood product support:
  – Avoid products from family members, owing to the possibility of allogeneic bone marrow transplant.
- Broad-spectrum antibiotics and antifungal therapy for fever and neutropenia
- Prophylactic trimethoprim-sulfamethoxazole for *Pneumocystis* infection

Additional Therapies
Allogeneic bone marrow transplant may be the best treatment for AML in 1st remission.

IN-PATIENT CONSIDERATIONS
Initial Stabilization
Children with suspected AML should have immediate evaluation with physical exam, history, and laboratory data including CBC, PT/PTT, electrolytes, calcium, phosphorus, uric acid, and creatinine.

ONGOING CARE

FOLLOW-UP RECOMMENDATIONS
Patient Monitoring
- Blood counts monthly for 1st year, every 4 months for the 2nd year, and every 6 months thereafter
- Liver and kidney function tests every 3–6 months
- Cardiac function should be checked every 12 months.
- Endocrine function should be tested in pubertal children.

PROGNOSIS
- 85% achieve remission with intensive chemotherapy.
- ~30–60% achieve long-term survival (>5 years after diagnosis).
- Factors associated with poor prognosis:
  – WBC count >100,000/mm^3
  – Monosomy 7
  – Secondary AML or prior myelodysplastic syndrome
  – FLT3 mutation (FLT3-ITD)
  – Poor initial response to therapy (induction failure or MRD positive [>0.01%] at end of induction)
  – MRD (minimal residual disease): Testing that adds sensitivity to identify lesser quantities of residual leukemia not seen on morphologic exam, using flow cytometry or genetic testing

COMPLICATIONS
- Bleeding (usually secondary to thrombocytopenia)
- DIC occurs in some types of AML, including acute promyelocytic leukemia (M3).
- Treat aggressively with fresh frozen plasma and platelet transfusions.
- Infection:
  – 40% of patients are febrile at diagnosis.
  – Empiric antibiotic therapy must be started after blood cultures are obtained.
- Leukostasis:
  – Intravascular clumping of blasts causing hypoxia, infarction, and hemorrhage
  – Usually with WBC >200,000/mm^3
  – Brain and lung are commonly affected organs.
  – Leukapheresis or exchange transfusion may be indicated for patients who are symptomatic with extremely high blast counts.

- Tumor lysis syndrome:
  – Refers to the metabolic consequences from the release of cellular contents of dying leukemic cells
  – Hyperuricemia can lead to renal failure.
  – Hyperkalemia, hyperphosphatemia, and secondary hypocalcemia can be life threatening.
  – Patients should be hydrated with fluid containing bicarbonate and given allopurinol.

ADDITIONAL READING
- Vardiman JW, Thiele J, Arber DA, et al. The 2008 revision of the World Health Organization (WHO) classification of myeloid and acute leukemia: Rationale and important changes. *Blood*. 2009; 114:937–951.
- Pui CH, Carroll WL, Meshinchi S, et al. Biology, risk stratification, and therapy or pediatric acute leukemias: An update. *J Clin Oncol*. 2011;29: 551–565.
- Rubnitz JE, Gibson B, Smith FO. Acute myeloid leukemia. *Hematol Oncol Clin North Am*. 2010;24: 35–63.
- Kersey JH. Fifty years of studies of biology and therapy of childhood leukemia. *Blood*. 1997;90: 4243–4251.

CODES

ICD9
205.0 Myeloid leukemia

ICD10
- C92.00 Acute myeloblastic leukemia, not having achieved remission
- C92.01 Acute myeloblastic leukemia, in remission
- C92.02 Acute myeloblastic leukemia, in relapse

FAQ
- Q: Is an indwelling line required for therapy?
- A: Always
- Q: Are repeated hospitalizations likely?
- A: Repeated hospitalizations are needed for chemotherapy and infectious complications.
- Q: Can the child go to school?
- A: May be able to go intermittently during therapy

ADENOVIRUS INFECTION

Jason Newland
Jessica Newman

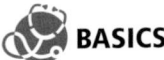

BASICS

DESCRIPTION
Adenoviruses are ubiquitous, nonenveloped, double-stranded DNA viruses. There are at least 51 human serotypes.

GENERAL PREVENTION
See Table 1.

Table 1. Precautions for hospital patients

Symptoms	Type of Precautions
Respiratory disease	Contact and droplet
Gastrointestinal	Contact
Conjunctivitis	Contact

Oral vaccines have been used by the military.

EPIDEMIOLOGY
- Primary infection usually occurs early in life (by age 10 years) and is, most often, characterized by upper respiratory symptoms.
- Military trainees are especially susceptible to infection, probably due to crowded living conditions.
- Respiratory and enteric infections may occur at any time of year. Epidemics of respiratory disease occur in winter and spring.
- Cause 2–5% of all pediatric respiratory tract infections
- Transmission of respiratory disease occurs via contact with infected secretions.
  – Transmission of enteric adenoviruses is via the fecal–oral route.
- Outbreaks of pharyngo-conjunctival fever have been associated with inadequately chlorinated swimming pools and shared towels.
- One of the most common causes of viral myocarditis in children and adults

Incidence
Peaks between 6 months and 5 years of age

RISK FACTORS
Exposure to adenovirus

PATHOPHYSIOLOGY
Adenoviruses may cause a lytic infection or a chronic/latent infection. In addition, they are capable of inducing oncogenic transformation of cells, although the clinical significance of this observation remains unclear.

ETIOLOGY
Infection with adenovirus

COMMONLY ASSOCIATED CONDITIONS
- Respiratory infections:
  – Upper respiratory tract infections: Otitis media, common cold, pharyngitis
  – Lower respiratory tract infection: Pneumonia, pertussis-like syndrome, croup, necrotizing bronchitis, bronchiolitis
- Pharyngoconjunctival fever:
  – Low-grade fever associated with conjunctivitis, pharyngitis, rhinitis, and cervical adenitis
  – 15% of patients may have meningismus.
  – Increased incidence in summer months
  – Common-source outbreaks most often associated with type 3
- Epidemic keratoconjunctivitis:
  – Bilateral conjunctivitis with preauricular adenopathy
  – May persist for up to 4 weeks
  – Corneal opacities may persist for several months.
  – Associated with types 8, 19, and 37
- Myocarditis preceding viral illness:
  – Present with cardiovascular collapse, CHF, respiratory distress, or ventricular tachycardia
  – Prognosis is poor.
  – High mortality; a large number require transplant, and a portion develop dilated cardiomyopathy
- Hemorrhagic cystitis may cause microscopic or gross hematuria:
  – If present, gross hematuria persists on average for 3 days.
  – Often associated with dysuria and urinary frequency
  – More common in males than females
  – Associated with types 11 and 21
  – Can occur in both immunocompetent and immunocompromised hosts
- Infantile diarrhea:
  – Watery diarrhea associated with fever
  – Symptoms may persist for 1–2 weeks
  – Associated with types 40, 41, and less often 31
- CNS-infection epidemics (associated with outbreaks of respiratory disease) and sporadic cases of encephalitis and meningitis have been observed; often associated with pneumonia
- Immunocompromised hosts:
  – Can cause disseminated disease including pneumonia, hepatitis, and gastroenteritis
  – Fatality rates much higher, up to 75% in hematopoietic stem cell transplant patients
  – Observed in transplanted patients; up to 10% of liver/renal transplant patients
- Miscellaneous: Associated with intussusception (isolated in up to 40% of cases) and fatal congenital infection

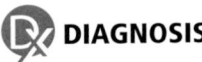

DIAGNOSIS

HISTORY
- Fever:
  – Nonspecific
- Rhinitis:
  – Upper respiratory infection (URI)
- Laryngitis, sore throat:
  – URI
- Nonproductive or croupy cough:
  – Respiratory infection
- Headache, myalgias:
  – CNS infection
- Hematuria (gross or microscopic), dysuria, urinary frequency:
  – Hemorrhagic cystitis
- Watery diarrhea:
  – Enteric adenovirus
- Conjunctivitis, rhinitis, exudative pharyngitis, and meningismus:
  – Typical findings of adenovirus

PHYSICAL EXAM FINDINGS
- Pulmonary tachypnea, wheezing, rales:
  – Pneumonia
- Tachycardia, tachypnea, gallop rhythm, hepatomegaly:
  – Myocarditis
- Abdominal tenderness, distention:
  – Gastroenteritis

DIAGNOSTIC TESTS & INTERPRETATION
Lab
- CBC:
  – Leukocytosis or leukopenia, often with left shift in the differential counts
- ESR:
  – Often elevated
- Viral isolation:
  – From nasopharyngeal secretions, urine, conjunctivae, or stool
- Viral identification:
  – Observe viral antigen in infected cells by immunofluorescence, amplify genome by polymerase chain reaction
  – Stool antigen test for serotypes 40/41
  – Highest yield from nasopharyngeal swab or stool
  – Adenovirus PCR may be helpful in narrowing differential diagnosis; especially with regards to the immunocompromised host
- ECG:
  – Low-voltage QRS
  – Low-amplitude or inverted T waves
  – Small or absent Q wave in V_5 and V_6

Imaging
- Echocardiogram:
  - Poor ejection fraction
- Chest X-ray
  - Bilateral patchy interstitial infiltrates (lower lobes) or enlarged heart
  - Cardiomegaly

DIFFERENTIAL DIAGNOSIS
- Respiratory infection:
  - Influenza
  - Parainfluenza
  - Human metapneumovirus
  - Pertussis
  - Mycoplasma pneumonia
  - Bacterial pneumonia
  - Boca virus
- Pharyngoconjunctival fever:
  - Group A streptococcus
  - Epstein–Barr virus
  - Parainfluenza
  - Enterovirus
  - Measles
  - Kawasaki disease
- Epidemic keratoconjunctivitis:
  - Herpes simplex
  - Chlamydia
  - Enterovirus
- Myocarditis:
  - Enteroviruses
  - Herpes simplex
  - Epstein–Barr virus
  - Influenza
  - Bacterial myocarditis
- Hemorrhagic cystitis:
  - Glomerulonephritis
  - Vasculitis
  - Renal tuberculosis
- Infantile diarrhea:
  - Rotavirus
  - Norwalk agent
  - Astrovirus
  - Salmonella
  - Shigella
  - Campylobacter
- CNS infection:
  - Enterovirus
  - Herpes simplex virus
  - Mycoplasma
  - Bacterial meningitis

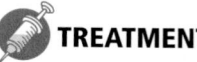
TREATMENT
GENERAL MEASURES
- Supportive care
- Monitor for secondary bacterial infections
- Avoid steroid-containing ophthalmic ointments

MEDICATION (DRUGS)
First Line
Cidofovir has been shown to have benefit in immunocompromised patients with disseminated disease. However, a risk of developing a dose-limiting nephrotoxicity exists. Infusion of AdV-specific cytotoxic T cells or IVIG may have some benefit in immunocompromised patients, particularly hematopoetic stem cell transplant patients.

ONGOING CARE
PROGNOSIS
Most syndromes are self-limited.

COMPLICATIONS
- Bronchiolitis obliterans (rare)
- Corneal opacities with visual disturbance (usually resolves spontaneously)
- Congestive heart failure
- Dilated cardiomyopathy

ADDITIONAL READING
- Bowles NE, Ni J, Kearney KL, et al. Detection of viruses in myocardial tissues by polymerase chain reaction: Evidence of adenovirus as a common cause of myocarditis in children and adults. *J Amer Coll Cardiol*. 2003;42:466–472.
- Hammond S, Chenever E, Durbin JE. Respiratory virus infection in infants and children. *Pediatr Dev Pathol*. 2007;10(3):172–180.
- Krajden M, Brown M, Petrasek A, et al. Clinical features of adenovirus enteritis: A review of 127 cases. *Pediatr Infect Dis J*. 1990;9:636–641.
- Leruez-Ville M, Midard V, Lacaille F, et al. Real-time blood plasma polymerase chain reaction for management of disseminated adenovirus infection. *Clin Infect Dis*. 2004;38:45–52.

- Lindemans CA, Leen AM, Boelens JJ. How I treat adenovirus in hematopoietic stem cell transplant recipients. *Blood*. 2010;116(25):5476–5485. Epub 2010 Sep 13.
- Wirsing von Konig CH, Rott H, Bogaerts H, et al. A serologic study of organisms possibly associated with pertussis-like coughing. *Pediatr Infect Dis J*. 1998;17:645–649.

CODES
ICD9
- 008.62 Enteritis due to adenovirus
- 079.0 Adenovirus infection in conditions classified elsewhere and of unspecified site
- 478.9 Other and unspecified diseases of upper respiratory tract

ICD10
- A08.2 Adenoviral enteritis
- B34.0 Adenovirus infection, unspecified
- J39.8 Other specified diseases of upper respiratory tract

FAQ
- Q: Is there anything one can do to prevent these infections.
- A: Washing hands and avoiding contact with ill persons will help slow the spread of these infections.

ALCOHOL (ETHANOL) INTOXICATION
Ann B. Bruner

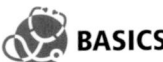 **BASICS**

DESCRIPTION
- Acute ingestion (accidental or intended) of alcohol, resulting in loss of inhibition, often associated with unruly/violent behavior, impaired judgment and/or coordination, diminished alertness/responsiveness, and sedation or coma
- Accidental ingestion is more common in toddlers and younger children.
- Frequency of intentional alcohol use increases with age.
- Alcohol–drug interactions are common because acute intoxication reduces hepatic clearance for other drugs, thereby increasing their serum concentrations.

EPIDEMIOLOGY
Alcohol is 2nd only to caffeine in prevalence and incidence of use among substances of use/abuse.

Prevalence
- >75% of high school students have had more than 1 drink in their lifetime; 37% had their 1st drink before 8th grade.
- Rates of past 30-day alcohol use in 2009 were 3.5% (12–13 yo), 13.0% (14–15 yo), 26.3% (16–17 yo), 49.7% (18–20 yo), and 70.2% (21–25 yo).
- Nearly 50% of high school students report current alcohol use, and 30% report heavy drinking in the past 30 days (>5 drinks).
- Underage (12–20 yo) drinkers are 3 times more likely than adults to use illicit drugs with alcohol.
- Almost 1/3 of high school students have ridden in a car with a driver who has been drinking alcohol.
- Rates of driving under the influence are age-related: in 2009, 6.3% of 16–17 yo, 16.6% of 18–20 yo, and 24.8% of 21–25 yo reported driving under the influence in the past year.
- Rates of binge alcohol use (5 or more drinks in 1 day in past 30 days) in 2009 were 1.6% (12–13 yo), 7.0% (14–15 yo), 17.0% (16–17 yo), 34.7% (18–20 yo), and 46.5% (21–25 yo).
- Among full-time enrolled college students (18–22 yo), 63.9% were current drinkers, 43.5% were binge drinkers, and 16.0% were heavy drinkers (5 or more drinks in 1 day on 5 or more days in past 30 days); full-time college students have higher rates of alcohol use than part-time students or young adults not enrolled in college.

RISK FACTORS
Patients with psychiatric conditions are at an increased risk for abuse of alcohol and other drugs.

GENERAL PREVENTION
- Promote family discussions about alcohol use and abuse.
- Provide safety recommendations to prevent accidental ingestions.

PATHOPHYSIOLOGY
- Effects of alcohol ingestion are related to dose, the time in which alcohol was consumed and then absorbed, and the patient's history of alcohol exposure.
- Alcohol absorption, decreased by the presence of food in the stomach and increased if liquid is carbonated, occurs rapidly and largely in the small intestine.
- Minimal quantities of alcohol are excreted in urine, sweat, and breath.
- >90% of alcohol oxidized in liver follows zero-order kinetics, primarily by alcohol dehydrogenase (ADH) and then acetaldehyde dehydrogenase (ALDH); rate of metabolism is fixed (not related to dose or time) and is proportional to body weight. Ethnic/racial and gender variabilities exist on quantity and efficacy of ADH.
- Ethanol is metabolized by ADH to acetaldehyde, then to acetate, and finally to ketones, fatty acids, or acetone; ketosis and, infrequently, metabolic acidosis can occur.
- Respiratory acidosis can occur secondary to carbon dioxide retention from respiratory depression due to ethanol intoxication.
- Hypoglycemia occurs during acute ethanol intoxication owing to impaired gluconeogenesis resulting from changes in the NADH/NAD+ ratio associated with ethanol metabolism.
- Alcohol affects the CNS primarily through the γ-aminobutyric acid (GABA) and glutamate neurotransmitter systems.

ETIOLOGY
Alcoholic beverages (water and ethanol) are produced from fermentation/distillation of sugar from grapes (wine), grains/corn (beer/whiskey), potatoes (vodka), or sugar cane (rum). After distillation, alcohol is mixed into solution to make specific beverages; products are marketed according to alcohol content or "proof," which is twice the percent. Alcohol content ranges from 3–6% (6–12 proof) in beer to 40–75% (80–150 proof) in vodka/rum/whiskey. Alcohol is often consumed concurrently with other substances (licit and illicit), presenting a mixed clinical picture of intoxication.

COMMONLY ASSOCIATED CONDITIONS
- Alcohol is involved in 30% of all drug overdoses.
- A significant percentage of adolescent trauma patients, especially victims of gunshot wounds, have positive toxicology screens for alcohol and other drugs.

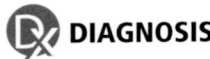 **DIAGNOSIS**

HISTORY
- Medical: Baseline health will affect patient's response to alcohol; diabetics, for example, may have worse hypoglycemia.
- Type and dose of other drugs ingested:
  - Clinical effects of and treatment for other ingestions can vary depending on substance.
  - Polysubstance ingestion is very common.
- Psychiatric history: Evaluate for possible suicidal ideation.
- Gathering details regarding the alcohol consumed (type, amount, and over what time period) may help predict clinical course. For example, blood alcohol concentration (BAC) may continue rising if ingestion occurred recently.
- Intoxication presents clinically with signs ranging from lack of coordination, slurred speech, and confusion (BAC of 20–200 mg/dL) to ataxia and nausea/vomiting (BAC 200–300 mg/dL) to amnesia, seizures, or coma (BAC >300 mg/dL).

PHYSICAL EXAM
- Bruises, lacerations, and fractures may suggest trauma and raise concern about CNS injury.
- Neurologic exam, including mental status, will assess degree of intoxication and consciousness, including patient's ability to protect his or her airway, and risk for aspiration.
- Tachycardia, hypotension may indicate dehydration.
- Fever may suggest infection.
- Average time for normalization of mental status in intoxicated adults is 3–3.5 hours; patients without clinical improvement in 3 hours should be evaluated for other causes of altered mental status.

DIAGNOSTIC TESTS & INTERPRETATION
Lab
- Blood alcohol concentration:
  - Generally correlates with clinical picture.
  - In children, signs of intoxication may be present at levels of 50 mg/dL.
  - Serum levels of 600–800 mg/dL can be fatal.
- Blood and/or urine toxicology screen:
  - Most urine toxicology screens do not test for alcohol.
  - Concurrent ingestions are common.
- Acetaminophen level:
  - Usually not part of the general serum toxicology screen
  - Consider if polysubstance ingestion suspected and/or if patient has suicidal ideation
- Serum electrolytes:
  - Alcohol is a diuretic. The associated nausea and vomiting seen with intoxication may result in severe dehydration.
  - Ketosis and, infrequently, metabolic acidosis can occur.
- Serum glucose level: Ethanol inhibits gluconeogenesis and can be associated with hypoglycemia.
- Blood gas can show both respiratory and metabolic acidosis.

DIFFERENTIAL DIAGNOSIS
- Environmental:
  - Other ingestions (overdose of sedatives or illicit drugs, such as benzodiazepines, marijuana, narcotics, lysergic acid diethylamide [LSD], and phencyclidine [PCP])
  - Toxic exposures (ethylene glycol, methanol, carbon monoxide)
  - Head trauma
- Infection
  - Meningitis
  - Encephalitis
  - Sepsis
- Tumor: Brain tumor
- Metabolic:
  - Hypoglycemia
  - Ketoacidosis
  - Hyperammonemia
  - Electrolyte imbalances (hyponatremia, hypernatremia)
- Miscellaneous:
  - Increased intracranial pressure from hydrocephalus, mass, other
  - Stroke

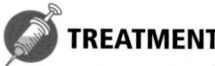

TREATMENT

MEDICATION (DRUGS)
IV dextrose as needed for hypoglycemia

ADDITIONAL TREATMENT
General Measures
- Assess airway, breathing, and circulation (ABC).
- Protect airway: The patient may require intubation and mechanical ventilation.
- Mainstay is supportive therapy, as no specific ethanol antidote exists.
- Appropriate trauma management as needed
- Because alcohol is absorbed rapidly, gastric lavage is indicated only if the patient is seen immediately after ingestion (within minutes).

ISSUES FOR REFERRAL
- Refer to substance abuse specialist (addiction medicine, psychiatrist, or certified addictions counselor) for detailed evaluation and treatment.
- Refer for psychiatric evaluation if depression, anxiety, suicidal ideation, or any other mental health condition is suspected.
- Assess for other risk-taking behaviors, including other substance use, sexual activity, use of motor vehicles while intoxicated, weapon carrying, and delinquency, and their sequelae, including pregnancy, sexually transmitted infections, and violence.

IN-PATIENT CONSIDERATIONS
Initial Stabilization
Keep patient awake; watch for vomiting as patients are at risk for choking owing to depressed gag reflex.

Admission Criteria
- Unstable vital signs (hypotension)
- Persistent CNS depression/impaired mental status
- Potential severity of comorbid psychiatric conditions (depression/suicidality)
- Inability to contact a parent/guardian

IV Fluids
IV fluids for dehydration and hypotension

Nursing
Observe and monitor vital signs and neurologic status.

Discharge Criteria
- Stable vital signs
- Patient awake, alert, responsive, and oriented
- Decreasing BAC
- Parent/guardian fully informed about patient's alcohol use

 ## ONGOING CARE

DIET
NPO secondary to depressed gag reflex

PROGNOSIS
BAC serum levels of 600–800 mg/dL can be fatal.

COMPLICATIONS
- Diuresis and dehydration
- Vasodilation and hypotension
- Vomiting, aspiration, potential respiratory arrest
- Hypoglycemia
- Metabolic acidosis
- Impaired mental status
- Engagement in risk-taking behaviors (e.g., other drug use, unprotected intercourse) while intoxicated
- CNS depression
- Gastritis
- GI bleeding
- Acute pancreatitis
- Motor vehicle collisions associated with driving while intoxicated
- Alcoholism
- Alcohol withdrawal following a period of intoxication in chronic users (symptoms include tachycardia, elevated blood pressure, irritability, nausea, vomiting, and tremor)

ADDITIONAL READING

- Centers for Disease Control and Prevention. National drunk and drugged driving prevention month—December 2003. *MMWR Morb Mortal Wkly Rep.* 2003;52:1185–1186.
- Coupey SM. Specific drugs. In: Schydlower M, ed. *Substance abuse: A guide for health professionals*, 2nd ed. Elk Grove Village, IL: American Academy of Pediatrics; 2002:208–215.

- Foxcroft DR, Ireland D, Lister-Sharp DJ, et al. Longer-term primary prevention for alcohol misuse in young people: A systematic review. *Addiction.* 2003;98:397–411.
- Pitzele HZ, Tolia VM. Twenty per hour: Altered mental state due to ethanol abuse and withdrawal. *Emerg Med Clin N Am.* 2010;28:683–705.
- Porter RS. Alcohol and injury in adolescents. *Pediatr Emerg Care.* 2000;16(5):316–320.
- Substance Abuse and Mental Health Services Administration. *Results from the 2009 National Survey on Drug Use and Health: Volume I. Summary of national findings* (Office of Applied Studies, NSDUH Series H-38A, HHS Publication No. SMA 10-4856 Findings). Rockville, MD: Substance Abuse and Mental Health Services Administration; 2010.

 ## CODES

ICD9
980.0 Toxic effect of ethyl alcohol

ICD10
- F10.920 Alcohol use, unspecified with intoxication, uncomplicated
- F10.929 Alcohol use, unspecified with intoxication, unspecified
- T51.0X1A Toxic effect of ethanol, accidental (unintentional), initial encounter

FAQ

- Q: How quickly does a person metabolize alcohol?
- A: The liver metabolizes ~10 g of ethanol per hour, which corresponds to a decline in BAC of 18–20 mg/dL/hr.
- Q: What is the legal level of BAC that defines driving under the influence of alcohol?
- A: This varies by state, but generally is between 80 and 100 mg/dL.
- Q: Why do some individuals, particularly of Asian descent, turn red or develop signs of pruritus after ingesting alcohol?
- A: Flushing, pruritus, and nausea are due to high levels of acetaldehyde. Variations in the metabolic activity of dehydrogenase enzymes are associated with factors such as gender, history of alcohol use, and genetics. Decreased ALDH activity, which is more common in Native Americans and Asians, can result in increased levels of acetaldehyde (an estimated 50% of Asians).

ALLERGIC CHILD

Matthew Fogg

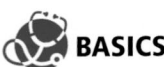 **BASICS**

DEFINITION
- The allergic child tends toward IgE-mediated reactions in response to pollens, molds, environmental allergens, drugs, insect stings, and foods.
- Reactions may manifest as:
  - Eczema
  - Allergic rhinitis
  - Asthma
  - Angioedema
  - Hives
  - Anaphylaxis
- Children may have dark circles under their eyes (allergic shiners) or a nasal crease from the "allergic salute" (upward rubbing of the nose to relieve itch).
- Children inherit the tendency to be allergic, but do not inherit specific allergies.

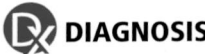 **DIAGNOSIS**

DIFFERENTIAL DIAGNOSIS
- **Eyes**
  - Physical and chemical irritants
  - Viral or bacterial infection
- **Nose**
  - Recurrent upper respiratory tract infections
  - Rhinitis medicamentosa: Reaction to nasal sprays
  - Drugs that cause nasal congestion:
    - Oral contraceptives
    - Reserpine
    - Guanethidine
    - Propranolol
    - Thioridazine
    - Tricyclic antidepressants
    - Aspirin
  - Airway irritants:
    - Smoke
    - Environmental pollution
    - Cold air
  - Kartagener syndrome: Sinusitis, bronchiectasis, immobile cilia
  - Cystic fibrosis
  - Sinusitis
- **Lungs**
  - Airway irritants:
    - Smoke
    - Environmental pollution
    - Cold air
  - Gastroesophageal reflux
  - Foreign body aspiration
  - Anatomic defect in airway
  - Cystic fibrosis
  - Kartagener syndrome
  - Immune deficiency
- **Skin**
  - Viral exanthems
  - Autoimmune disorders
  - Physical and chemical irritants

HISTORY
Careful history of seasonal or year-round symptoms and environmental exposures is essential.

Questions best asked systematically in a review of systems format:
- **Ears**
  - Otitis
  - Myringotomy tubes
  - Hearing loss
- **Nasal**
  - Frequent upper respiratory infections
  - Sinusitis
  - Polyps
  - Epistaxis
  - Snoring
  - Sneezing
  - Rhinitis
  - Deviated septum
  - Obstruction
  - Itch
  - Mouth breathing
  - Nasal discharge
- **Throat**
  - Sore throat
  - Throat clearing
  - Postnasal drip
  - Palate itch
  - Tonsillitis
  - Tonsillectomy
  - Croup
- **Chest**
  - Day cough
  - Night cough
  - Sputum production
  - Pain
  - Wheeze
  - Shortness of breath
  - Cyanosis
- **Eyes**
  - Itching
  - Tearing
  - Discharge
  - Swelling
  - Redness
  - Rubbing
- **Skin**
  - Eczema
  - Hives
  - Angioedema
  - Contact dermatitis
  - Seborrheic dermatitis
  - Skin infections
  - Pruritus

Does the child have food or drug allergies?
- **Question:** What type of reaction does the child have?
- *Significance:* Allergy (IgE-mediated reactions resulting in wheezing, allergic rhinitis, hives, angioedema, eczema, or anaphylaxis) or intolerance (nonspecific rash, diarrhea, gas, headache, or hyperactivity)
- **Question:** Ask about food allergy and anaphylaxis?
- *Significance:* Food allergy or history of anaphylaxis is an indication for an EpiPen and lifelong avoidance.
- **Question:** Has the child ever been stung by a bee, and, if so, what was the reaction?
- *Significance:* Systemic reactions are an indication for referral to an allergist for venom desensitization. Venom desensitization can be potentially lifesaving.
- **Question:** Does anyone in the family have hay fever (allergic rhinitis), asthma, or eczema?
- *Significance:* Familial history of atopy increases the likelihood of atopy in other family members.

Regarding the environment:
- **Question:** Does the child's home have a basement, damp areas, or a humidifier?
- *Significance:* Sources of mold spores; humidity also increases dust mite population.
- **Question:** Is there forced air heat?
- *Significance:* Tends to blow allergen-laden dust around the home
- **Question:** Is home cooled by opening windows?
- *Significance:* Lets pollens into the house
- **Question:** Are there any smokers in the home?
- *Significance:* Airway irritants can exacerbate respiratory difficulties.
- **Question:** Are there any pets in the home, at school, or in daycare?
- *Significance:* Animal dander is a common aeroallergen.
- **Question:** Are there many stuffed animals or books in the bedroom?
- Does the bedroom have carpeting?
- Is bedding washed frequently?
- What type of pillow is used?
- Is the mattress encased in plastic?
- *Significance:* Dust mites
- **Question:** Where does the patient spend most of his or her time? Does the patient attend daycare?
- *Significance:* Upper respiratory tract infections can mimic allergies and exacerbate reactive airway disease.

PHYSICAL EXAM

A complete physical exam is essential to rule out systemic disease that can mimic allergies.

- **Finding:** Ocular allergic signs?
- *Significance:*
  - Allergic shiners due to passive congestion in the nose, which impedes the venous return to the vessels under the eyes
  - Cobblestoning of the conjunctiva
  - Dennie-Morgan line, infraorbital folds associated with suborbital edema secondary to atopy
  - Clear stringy discharge
- **Finding:** Nasal allergic signs?
- *Significance:*
  - Pale edematous nasal mucosa
  - Nasal crease across the bridge of nose secondary to repeated upward rubbing of the nose
  - Clear nasal discharge with or without occlusion
- **Finding:** Ear allergic signs?
- *Significance:* Fluid in the middle ear or retracted tympanic membranes may be associated with eustachian tube dysfunction seen with allergic inflammation.
- **Finding:** Throat allergic signs?
- *Significance:* Cobblestoning of posterior pharynx secondary to submucosal lymphoid hyperplasia
- **Finding:** Lung allergic signs?
- *Significance:* Wheezes, rhonchi, decreased air entry, and chronic obstruction can be secondary to allergic responses.
- **Finding:** Skin allergic signs?
- *Significance:* Eczema, hives, angioedema, and dermatographism

DIAGNOSTIC TESTS & INTERPRETATION

- **Test:** Immediate hypersensitivity
- *Significance:*
  - Skin prick tests to suspected allergens based on history (study of choice)
  - Intradermal skin tests for patients who have a negative prick test and a suspicious history pose a greater risk of systemic reactions (environmental allergens only, not for foods)
  - Radioallergosorbent (RAST) tests measure free serum IgE to a specific antigen to which a particular patient may be sensitized—primarily for patients at risk for a severe systemic reaction from skin testing or in whom skin testing is not feasible.
  - Skin tests are preferable to RAST tests in most cases.
  - Do not screen for food allergy with RAST tests without a significant history of reaction. Many false positives will show up leading to inappropriate dietary restriction and parental anxiety.
  - Eosinophils in the blood or respiratory secretions may be indicative of an allergic diathesis
- **Test:** Baseline pulmonary function studies should be obtained on asthmatic children or in children with an allergic history.
- *Significance:* To evaluate for obstructive disease

 TREATMENT

General Measures

- Specific environmental control (as determined by skin testing)
- Pets should be kept out of the bedroom if a child has allergic stigmata.
- If a child has severe allergies or asthma related to pet exposure, the animal should be removed from the home.
- To keep the dust mite population under control, the bedding should be washed in hot water at least once every 2 weeks, the pillow should be fiber filled, and the mattress should be encased in plastic.

ISSUES FOR REFERRAL

- A patient failing medical management of upper respiratory or ocular allergies with routine antihistamine/decongestant medications may be referred to an allergist who can help identify triggers contributing to the problem.
- Poorly controlled asthma not responding to intermittent inhaled β-agonists or an asthmatic child who is symptomatic between exacerbations, or one who has an atypical pattern of exacerbations.
- Asthma patients with frequent hospitalizations or steroid-dependent asthma patients
- Patients who are absent from school frequently because of allergic or asthmatic symptoms
- Patients with limited activity
- Strong seasonal history of respiratory complaints
- Difficult-to-manage atopic dermatitis
- Recurrent croup
- Food allergy
- History of anaphylaxis
- Egg-allergic patients who require influenza vaccine
- Drug allergy
- Latex allergy

 ONGOING CARE

PROGNOSIS

- In general, environmental allergies that cause rhinitis and asthma persist into adulthood.
- Most children outgrow food allergies to milk, egg, soy, wheat, and other foods.
- Children may rarely outgrow peanut, tree nut, or shellfish allergy.
- Allergic children have the biologic potential to become sensitized to many environmental allergens; limit exposure to prevent sensitization.

ADDITIONAL READING

- Bailey E, Shaker M. An update on childhood urticaria and angioedema. *Curr Opin Pediatr.* 2008;20(4): 425–430.
- Fireman P. Diagnosis of allergic disorders. *Pediatr Rev.* 1995;16:178–183.
- Halken S, Lau S, Valovirta E. New visions in specific immunotherapy in children: An iPAC summary and future trends. *Pediatr Allergy Immunol.* 2008; 19(Suppl 19):60–70.
- Hopkin JM. Asthma and allergy-disorders of civilization? *Q J Med.* 1998;91:169–170.
- Middleton E, Reed CE, Adkinson NF, et al. *Allergic principles and practice,* 4th ed. Philadelphia: Mosby, 1993.
- Sites DP, Terr AI, Parslow TG. *Basic and clinical immunology,* 8th ed. Englewood Cliffs, NJ: Prentice Hall, 1994.

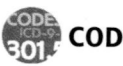 CODES

ICD9

- 477.0 Allergic rhinitis due to pollen
- 692.9 Contact dermatitis and other eczema, unspecified cause
- 995.3 Allergy unspecified

ICD10

- J30.1 Allergic rhinitis due to pollen
- L30.9 Dermatitis, unspecified
- T78.40XA Allergy, unspecified, initial encounter

FAQ

- Q: Do children outgrow allergies?
- A: In general, environmental allergies that cause rhinitis and asthma persist into adulthood. However, most children outgrow food allergies to milk, egg, soy, wheat, and other foods. Children may rarely outgrow peanut, tree nut, or shellfish allergy in ~25% cases.
- Q: Can allergic children have the biologic potential to become sensitized to many environmental allergens?
- A: The goal should be to limit exposure to these antigens to prevent sensitization.
- Q: If a parent is allergic to a specific allergen, can the child inherit this allergy?
- A: Children inherit the tendency to be allergic, but they do not inherit specific allergies.
- Q: What treatments are available?
- A: Specific environmental control, as determined by skin testing, antihistamines, topical steroids, and immunotherapy

ALOPECIA (HAIR LOSS)

Hope Rhodes
Terry Kind

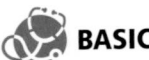 **BASICS**

DEFINITION
- Absence of hair where it normally grows
- Categorized as acquired or congenital
  - Most cases are acquired: Tinea capitis is most common, followed by traumatic alopecia and alopecia areata.
- Also categorized as diffuse or localized
  - Most cases of alopecia are localized and, of these, tinea capitis is the most common.
- Many normal healthy newborns lose their hair in the first few months of life.
  - Hair loss may be exacerbated by friction from bedding/sleep surface, especially in atopic infants.
- Normally, 50–100 hairs are shed and simultaneously replaced every day, on average.
- 90% of alopecia cases are due to the following disorders:
  - Tinea capitis
  - Alopecia areata
  - Traction alopecia
  - Telogen effluvium
    - Alopecia is preceded by a psychologically or physically stressful event 6–16 weeks prior to the onset of hair loss.
    - Growing hairs convert rapidly to resting hairs.

RISK FACTORS
Genetics
- Alopecia areata:
  - Polygenic with variety of triggering factors
  - Family history in 10–42% of cases
  - Males and females equally affected
  - Onset usually before age 30 years
- Monilethrix (also called beaded hair):
  - A rare autosomal dominant disorder

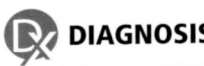 **DIAGNOSIS**

DIFFERENTIAL DIAGNOSIS
Consider the most likely diagnoses first.
- **Infectious**
  - Tinea capitis
  - Varicella
  - Syphilis
- **Congenital**
  - Aplasia cutis congenita
  - Incontinentia pigmenti
  - Oculomandibulofacial syndrome (sparse hair, hypoplastic teeth, cataracts, short stature)
  - Goltz syndrome (alopecia, focal dermal hypoplasia, strabismus, nail dystrophy)
  - Triangular alopecia of the frontal scalp
  - Focal dermal hypoplasia
  - Hair-shaft defects (trichodystrophies)
  - Ectodermal dysplasias
  - Nevi
  - Progeria

- **Nutritional**
  - Zinc deficiency
  - Marasmus
  - Kwashiorkor
  - Anorexia nervosa
  - Hypervitaminosis A
  - Celiac disease
- **Endocrinologic**
  - Androgenetic alopecia
  - Hypothyroidism
  - Hyperthyroidism
  - Hypoparathyroidism
  - Hypopituitarism
  - Diabetes mellitus
- **Rheumatologic**
  - Systemic lupus erythematosus
  - Scleroderma
- **Trauma**
  - Traction alopecia
  - Trichotillomania
  - Scalp electrode scar from in utero monitoring
- **Toxin**
  - Radiation
  - Medications (e.g., anticoagulants, antimetabolites)
  - Heavy metals (e.g., arsenic, lead)
- **Toxic exposures**
  - Antimetabolites
  - Anticoagulants
  - Antithyroid medications
  - Lead
  - Arsenic
- **Stress**
  - Trichotillomania
- **Miscellaneous**
  - Alopecia areata (autoimmune)
  - Telogen effluvium
  - Darier disease (keratotic crusted papules, keratosis follicularis)
  - Lichen planus
  - Burn

Commonly Associated Conditions
- May be associated with a genetic, endocrine, or toxin-mediated condition
  - Look for nail, skin, teeth, or gland involvement
- Trichotillomania is frequently associated with a finger-sucking habit.

APPROACH TO THE PATIENT
- Treatment of alopecia is guided by underlying etiology.
- Other than reassurance and waiting, there is no proven effective long-term therapy for alopecia areata. Topical steroids may show short-term benefit. There are no randomized clinical trials on the use of topical immunotherapy or intralesional steroids.
- Caution regarding side effects of all potential treatments

- Topical antifungals alone are not adequate to treat tinea capitis.
- A topical shampoo, such as selenium sulfide or ketoconazole shampoo, is recommended for tinea capitis to decrease fungal shedding and risk of spread to others.

HISTORY
- **Question:** Attempt to classify the alopecia.
- *Significance:* To aid in diagnosis and subsequent treatment plan
- **Question:** Is the loss acquired or congenital? Is the alopecia treatable or likely to be self-limited?
- *Significance:* Consider most likely diagnoses, including tinea capitis, traumatic alopecia, and alopecia areata
- **Question:** Associated abnormalities?
- *Significance:* May be part of a syndrome
- **Question:** Is there an endocrine abnormality or a toxin/medication effect?
- *Significance:* Some of these would require prompt attention.
- **Question:** Assess hair loss.
- *Significance:*
  - Increased amount of hair in the brush or in the shower/tub drain?
  - Does hair appear or feel thinner?
  - Patches of hair loss or broken hairs noted?
- **Question:** Considering trichotillomania?
- *Significance:* Note that patients often deny hair-pulling. Direct confrontation is rarely helpful.

PHYSICAL EXAM
Assess localized vs. diffuse hair loss
- **Finding:** Associated systemic signs or any nonscalp findings?
- *Significance:* May signify a genetic syndrome or endocrine abnormality
- **Finding:** Scalp?
- *Significance:*
  - Alopecia areata: Except for well-demarcated hair loss, scalp appears normal with smooth surface.
  - Tinea capitis: Scalp is often scaly and may be erythematous; areas of hair loss with broken hair stubs. Referred to as "black-dot" alopecia.
- **Finding:** Bizarre configuration and irregular outline of hair loss. Hairs of varying lengths?
- *Significance:* Distinguishes traction/traumatic alopecia from alopecia areata
- **Finding:** Short broken hairs but not black dots?
- *Significance:* Short hairs are usually associated with trichotillomania, whereas black dot alopecia is seen with tinea capitis.
- **Finding:** Frontal, vertex, or bi-temporal decreased hair density in adolescents?
- *Significance:* May be adolescent-onset, androgenetic alopecia

- **Finding:** Hair shaft varies in thickness, with small node-like deformities (like beads), increased breakage, and partial alopecia?
- *Significance:*
  – Monilethrix
  – Other hair-shaft abnormalities with increased fragility include pseudomonilethrix, trichorrhexis, pili torti, pili bifurcati, Menkes kinky hair syndrome, and trichothiodystrophy.
- **Finding:** Nail defects such as dystrophic changes and fine stippling?
- *Significance:*
  – Nail defects are seen in 10–20% of cases of alopecia areata.
  – Nail defects accompanying localized alopecia along with syndactyly, strabismus, and dermal hypoplasia may be found in Goltz syndrome.
  – In ectodermal dysplasias, nails, hair, teeth, or glands may be affected.
- **Finding:** Pubic hair and eyebrow hair loss?
- *Significance:*
  – Found in a form of alopecia areata called "alopecia universalis," where nearly all body hair is lost (alopecia totalis involves the loss of all scalp hair).
  – Body hair loss such as pubic hair or eyebrow hair may also occur in trichotillomania.

DIAGNOSTIC TESTS & INTERPRETATION
- **Test:** Fungal culture
- *Significance:*
  – Recommended when assessing for tinea capitis as a cause of alopecia
  – Definitive results may take up to several weeks; may treat while awaiting results.
  – Using a cotton-tipped applicator, culturette, toothbrush, or direct plating on Sabouraud dextrose agar, culture will be positive for *Trichophyton tonsurans* in >90% of cases in North America.
  – Less common are *Microsporum canis*, *Microsporum audouinii*, *Trichophyton mentagrophytes*, and *Trichophyton schoenleinii*.
- **Test:** Potassium hydroxide (KOH) exam
- *Significance:*
  – The KOH exam is another way to assess for tinea capitis.
  – Hyphae and spores within hair shaft indicate tinea capitis.
  – With *Microsporum*, spores surround the hair shaft.
  – Endocrine testing
  – With alopecia areata or diffuse alopecia, consider endocrine tests or referral to an endocrinologist or dermatologist for further evaluation.
  – Routine screening for autoimmune disorders is generally not indicated.
- **Test:** Hair-pluck test
- *Significance:*
  – Used to determine the ratio of telogen (resting) to anagen (growing) hairs
  – ~50 hairs are plucked (with 1 firm tug using a hemostat clamped around the hair ~1 cm from the scalp) and examined under the low-power lens of a microscope to determine the percentage of hairs that are telogen and anagen hairs.
  – >25% telogen hairs are indicative of telogen effluvium.

- **Test:** Dermatophyte testing medium (DTM)
- *Significance:*
  – Assessing for tinea capitis
  – Definitive results may take from days to weeks.
  – If dermatophyte colonies grow on the medium, the phenol red indicator in the agar will turn from yellow to red.
- **Test:** Wood's light (lamp) examination
- *Significance:*
  – *M. canis*, *M. audouinii*, or *T. schoenleinii* fluoresces green
  – *T. tonsurans* does not fluoresce
- **Test:** Scalp biopsy
- *Significance:*
  – Can help to distinguish alopecia areata and trichotillomania
  – In alopecia areata, hair follicles become small but continue to produce fine hairs; there is mitotic activity in the matrix, and often inflammation is present.
  – In trichotillomania, follicles are not small. They are usually in a transitional (catagen) phase and no longer produce normal hair shafts. Keratinous debris, fibrosis, and clumps of dark melanin pigment are present. Significant inflammation is absent.
  – In telogen effluvium, follicles remain intact without inflammation.

 TREATMENT

MEDICATION (DRUGS)
First Line
- For tinea capitis: Microsize griseofulvin 10–25 mg/kg/d (maximum 1 g) or ultramicrosize griseofulvin 5–15 mg/kg/d (maximum 750 mg) orally once per day for 4–6 weeks. Approved for children >2 years of age.
- For alopecia areata requiring treatment: Topical corticosteroids may be used for isolated patches for short-term benefit.

Second Line
- For tinea capitis: Terbinafine, itraconazole, or fluconazole may be effective, although only terbinafine is FDA approved for this condition.
- For alopecia areata: There is limited evidence for long-term effectiveness of any treatment. For trial of other therapies (intralesional steroid, topical immunotherapy) seek consultation with a dermatologist.

General Measures
- Treatment of alopecia is guided by the underlying cause.
- If alopecia signifies a toxic exposure or an endocrine abnormality, the underlying condition may require prompt diagnosis and treatment.
- Infectious causes of alopecia (such as with tinea capitis) should be treated promptly.
- Most patients with alopecia areata do not need treatment, as regrowth will occur spontaneously.
- Complementary and alternative medicine (CAM)
  – Hypnotherapy, massage, acupuncture, and onion juice are among the complementary therapies that have been tried for conditions like alopecia areata and trichotillomania. Of note, though many patients try CAM for alopecia, more research is needed.

 ONGOING CARE

PROGNOSIS
- Tinea capitis, alopecia areata, and traction alopecia:
  – Hair will regrow, may take months
  – There is a poorer prognosis with alopecia universalis. <10% have full recovery.
- Telogen effluvium:
  – Spontaneous regrowth is expected unless the stressful event continues/recurs.
- Alopecia areata may spontaneously remit and then recur.

ADDITIONAL READING
- Alkhalifah A, Alsantali A, Wang E, et al. Alopecia areata update. *J Am Acad Dermatol*. 2010;62: 177–188, 191–202.
- FDA. Consumer updates: Lamisil approved to treat scalp ringworm in children. Available at: http://www.fda.gov/forconsumers/consumerupdates/ucm048710.htm
- Haynes JW, Persons R, Jamieson B. Childhood alopecia areata: What treatment works best? *J Fam Pract*. 2011;60(1):45–52.
- Hunt N, McHale S. The psychological impact of alopecia. *BMJ*. 2005;331(7522):951–953.
- National Alopecia Areata Foundation. Website: http://www.naaf.org
- van den Biggelaar FJ, Smolders J, Jansen JF. Complementary and alternative medicine in alopecia areata. *Am J Clin Dermatol*. 2010;11(1):11–20.

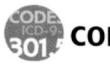 **CODES**

ICD9
- 110.0 Dermatophytosis of scalp and beard
- 704.00 Alopecia, unspecified
- 704.01 Alopecia areata

ICD10
- B35.0 Tinea barbae and tinea capitis
- L63.9 Alopecia areata, unspecified
- L65.9 Nonscarring hair loss, unspecified

FAQ
- Q: When can children with tinea capitis return to school?
- A: Once treatment with a systemic antifungal has begun, the child may return to school. A topical shampoo, such as selenium sulfide or ketoconazole shampoo, is recommended to decrease fungal shedding and the risk of spread to others.
- Q: Will the hair grow back?
- A: For the 3 most common causes of childhood alopecia—accounting for 90% of cases; tinea capitis, alopecia areata, and traction alopecia—hair will regrow, but may take months to do so.

ALPHA-1-ANTITRYPSIN DEFFICIENCY

Melissa Kennedy
Joshua R. Friedman

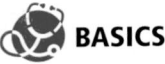 BASICS

DESCRIPTION
- α_1-Antitrypsin deficiency is an autosomal recessive genetic disorder that causes lung and liver disease.
- Classical PiZZ α_1-antitrypsin deficiency is caused by homozygosity for the autosomal recessive Z mutant allele of α_1-antitrypsin.
- α_1-antitrypsin is a 55-kd glycoprotein that is synthesized by the liver and released into the circulation, where it is the main inhibitor of host tissue damage caused by neutrophil proteases.
  – Lung disease begins after the 3rd decade of life and culminates in emphysema.
  – Liver disease may present as neonatal jaundice or in older children with elevated liver enzymes, portal hypertension, or cirrhosis.

EPIDEMIOLOGY
- One of the most common inherited disorders worldwide, although most patients do not have severe disease
- Most common genetic cause of liver disease in children and emphysema in adults

Incidence
- Incidence of the PiZZ genotype is highest in whites in North America, Australia, and Europe, particularly in Scandinavia, the British Isles, Northern France and the Tyrol region of Italy
- In the U.S., the PiZ allele frequency is ~14.5 per 1000, with lower rates among Asians, blacks, and Latinos and higher rates among whites.
- The incidence of classical α1-antitrypsin deficiency (PiZZ) is 1 in 1,500 to 1 in 3,500 live births.
- Only ~10% of PiZZ or PiSZ individuals will develop clinically significant liver disease.

Prevalence
- An estimated 70,000–100,000 individuals are affected in North America.
- As many as 25 million people in the U.S. are carriers of a mutant allele.

RISK FACTORS
Genetics
- α_1-Antitrypsin is a serine protease inhibitor encoded by the SERPINA1 gene. Classic, or PiZZ α_1-antitrypsin deficiency is caused by a homozygous point mutation at position 342 in the α_1-antitrypsin gene encoding a substitution of lysine for glutamate. The 2nd most common mutation, or the S allele, occurs at position 246 and results in the substitution of valine for glutamate. The normal allele is M.
- The Z mutation is associated with the accumulation of α_1-antitrypsin polymers within the endoplasmic reticulum of hepatocytes. These are not secreted into the circulation, resulting in low serum α_1-antitrypsin levels. It is unclear whether polymerization causes retention in the endoplasmic reticulum (ER) or vice versa.

- Patients with PiZZ alleles have the most significant findings, with serum levels of α_1-antitrypsin at levels less than 15% of normal.
- The heterozygous carrier state of the Z allele is found in 1.5–3% of the population and is not by itself a common cause of liver injury, however, it may be a modifier gene for other liver diseases.
- Other intermediate genotypes, PiMS, PiMZ, and PiSS, have not been definitively associated with hepatic disease, although referral center data reports patients with chronic liver disease having a higher frequency of PiMZ than would be predicted by chance.
- Compound heterozygotes with PiSZ phenotype may develop liver disease identical to PiZZ patients.
- Only about 10% of affected individuals experience clinically significant liver disease, indicating that other genetic or environmental factors are important modifiers of the disease.

PATHOPHYSIOLOGY
- Lung disease in PiZZ individuals results from loss of α_1-antitrypsin function. Excessive activity of destructive enzymes, such as elastase, cathepsin G, and proteinase 3, results in progressive emphysema. This is greatly accelerated by cigarette smoking as well as atmospheric pollutants.
- In contrast, liver disease in α_1-antitrypsin deficiency is caused by a gain of function in the Z mutant, which results in intracellular retention of the protein and hepatocellular damage.
  – The mutant Z polypeptide is unable to fold correctly after being translocated into the endoplasmic reticulum. As a result, it is retained in the ER where some molecules aggregate to form large polymers, and others are directed to proteolytic degradation pathways. Very few molecules are secreted.

ETIOLOGY
Mutations in the SERPINA1 gene result in lung disease through unopposed protease activity and in liver disease by intracellular retention of mutant α_1-antitrypsin.

DIAGNOSIS

HISTORY
- Highly variable presentation in neonates and young children
- Most patients with liver disease will have protracted jaundice during the 1st 8 weeks of life, which may be associated with abdominal distention, poor feeding, poor weight gain, hepatomegaly, and splenomegaly.
- Jaundice usually clears by 1 year of age.
- Normal liver function, continued liver disease, or progression to cirrhosis may follow.

- Presentation of liver disease may also occur during childhood or beyond. Symptoms may include hepatomegaly, failure to thrive, jaundice, or complications of portal hypertension and cirrhosis.
- Fulminant hepatic failure is very rare but has been reported.

PHYSICAL EXAM
Evidence of jaundice, hepatosplenomegaly, abdominal distention, and other stigmata of chronic liver disease

DIAGNOSTIC TESTS & INTERPRETATION
Lab
- Elevated total and conjugated bilirubin, elevated serum transaminases, hypoalbuminemia, or coagulopathy.
- Protein electrophoresis to determine the protease inhibitor (Pi) phenotype is the gold standard for diagnosis of α_1-antitrypsin deficiency.
- Serum levels of α_1-antitrypsin can be used as a complementary test to compare phenotype results against or to guide work-up before phenotype results are available.
- Quantitative serum α_1-antitrypsin levels:
  – PiMM: 20–53 mmol/L
  – PiZZ: $\leq$2.5–7 mmol/L
  – Pi null/null phenotype: No measurable levels of α_1-antitrypsin
  – False-negative results may occur because the protein acts as an acute-phase reactant and may rise into the normal range in an ill PiZZ individual.
  – In retrospective studies, low levels of α_1-antitrypsin had a positive predictive value of 94%, whereas normal levels had a negative predictive value of 100%.
- Confirmation is made by serum protein electrophoresis to determine the allele type.

Imaging
Ultrasound with Doppler study for evaluation of portal hypertension and/or for pretransplantation evaluation if liver failure develops.

Diagnostic Procedures/Other
Definitive diagnosis is made by serum protein electrophoresis to determine the α_1-antitrypsin phenotype. The diagnosis should be supported by liver biopsy.

Pathological Findings
- Liver biopsy in infants can show a variety of findings including giant cell transformation, lobular hepatitis, steatosis, inflammation, fibrosis, hepatocellular necrosis, bile duct paucity, or bile duct proliferation
- A diagnostic finding is diastase-resistant, periodic acid-Schiff staining globules in hepatocytes, which represent dilated endoplasmic reticulum membranes engorged with polymerized mutant Z-type α_1-antitrypsin protein.

DIFFERENTIAL DIAGNOSIS

- The differential diagnosis varies with the age at presentation.
- Neonates and infants generally present with jaundice. Other diagnoses to consider in this age group include biliary atresia, anatomic biliary abnormalities, congenital infections, galactosemia, and tyrosinemia. (See "Neonatal Cholestasis and Jaundice" for complete listing.)
- In older children, viral (hepatitis viruses, EBV, and CMV), toxic (ethanol, acetaminophen), metabolic (Wilson disease), and obstructive causes should be considered.

 TREATMENT

- α_1-antitrypsin deficiency does not have a specific treatment.
- Management is based on preventing complications of chronic liver disease.
- Cigarette smoking and hepatotoxins must be avoided.
- Liver transplantation is reserved for severe liver disease. In addition to replacing the diseased liver, the transplant graft will secrete normal α_1-antitrypsin, thereby halting progression of the lung disease.
- Enzyme replacement therapy is used in adults to prevent progression of lung disease. This has no effect on liver disease.
- Screening imaging or α-fetoprotein levels may be monitored due to the concern for an increased risk of hepatocellular carcinoma.
- Annual influenza vaccination and pneumococcal vaccination every 5 years
- Vaccinations against hepatitis A and B

MEDICATION (DRUGS)

- Ursodeoxycholic acid, a choleretic agent, can be used at a dose of 20–30 mg/kg/d to manage the cholestasis and pruritus associated with liver disease.
- Augmentation therapy:
  - Pooled human plasma–derived α_1-antitrypsin has been used to restore circulating levels of the protease inhibitor to levels above the protective threshold.
  - Results in a decrease in the rate of decline in 1-second forced expiratory volume and decreased mortality rate during the period of study
  - Future therapeutics: Various compounds are being investigated for their ability to promote proper folding of the mutant protein, thereby allowing normal secretion and preventing hepatocellular damage. Hepatocyte transplantation and gene therapy strategies are being investigated.

SURGERY/OTHER PROCEDURES

Surgical treatment at this time consists of orthotopic liver transplantation for patients with end-stage liver disease. Disease does not recur following transplantation. For lung disease, volume reduction surgery or lung transplantation may be used.

 ONGOING CARE

FOLLOW-UP RECOMMENDATIONS
Patient Monitoring
Annual liver and pulmonary function testing

PROGNOSIS
Only 10% of PiZZ and PiSZ individuals will have clinically significant liver disease during childhood; ~50% of the remaining individuals will have mildly elevated aminotransferases as the only liver abnormality. More significant liver disease may develop during late adulthood.

COMPLICATIONS
- Cirrhosis and early-onset lower-lobe emphysema.
- The course of liver disease is highly variable in affected individuals:
  - Jaundice, acholic stools, and hepatomegaly may present during the first weeks of life.
  - Jaundice usually clears by the 4th month and complete resolution of symptoms, chronic liver disease, or the development of cirrhosis may follow.
- Older children may present with manifestations of chronic liver disease or cirrhosis, with evidence of portal hypertension.
- Major dermatologic manifestation:
  - Panniculitis, an inflammation of the fat just beneath the skin, causing the skin to harden and form lumps, patches, or lesions
  - Likely that the damage is initiated by the destructive action of unrestrained neutrophils elastase

ADDITIONAL READING

- Coakley RJ. α1-Antitrypsin deficiency: Biological answers to clinical questions. *Am J Med Sci.* 2001;321:33–41.
- de Serres FJ. Worldwide racial and ethnic distribution of α1-antitrypsin deficiency. *Chest.* 2002;122:1818–1829.
- Miranda E, Pérez J, Ekeowa UI, et al. A novel monoclonal antibody to characterize pathogenic polymers in liver disease associated with α1-antitrypsin deficiency. *Hepatology.* 2010;52(3): 1078–1088.
- Perlmutter DH. Alpha-1-antitrypsin deficiency: Diagnosis and treatment. *Clin Liver Dis.* 2004;8: 839–859.
- Perlmutter DH. Pathogenesis of chronic liver injury and hepatocellular carcinoma in alpha-1-antitrypsin deficiency. *Pediatr Res.* 2006;60:233–238.

- Pittulainen E. α1-Antitrypsin deficiency in 26-year-old subjects. *Chest.* 2005;128:2076–2081.
- Steiner SJ. Serum levels of α1-antitrypsin predict phenotype expression of the α1-antitrypsin gene. *Dig Dis Sci.* 2003;48(9):1793–1796.
- Stoller JK. Augmentation therapy with α1-antitrypsin. Patterns of use and adverse effects. *Chest.* 2003;123:1425–1434.
- Sveger T. The liver in adolescents with alpha-1-antitrypsin deficiency. *Hepatology.* 1995;22: 514–517.
- Teckman J. α1-Antitrypsin deficiency in childhood. *Semin Liver Dis.* 2007;27(3):274–281.
- Teckman JH, Lindblad D. Alpha-1-antitrypsin deficiency: diagnosis, pathophysiology, and management. *Curr Gastroenterol Rep.* 2006;8: 14–20.

 CODES

ICD9
273.4 Alpha-1-antitrypsin deficiency

ICD10
E88.01 Alpha-1-antitrypsin deficiency

FAQ

- Do all patients with PiZZ disease get liver involvement?
- A: No. ~10% will have liver disease, and most of these will present with jaundice during the neonatal period. In most of these, the jaundice will resolve during the 1st year of life. The rate of progression of liver disease to cirrhosis in all PiZZ subjects is variable, but overall is low.
- Q: What is the best initial diagnostic test for α_1-antitrypsin deficiency?
- A: The total serum α_1-antitrypsin level is an appropriate screening test. In persons with low levels, the diagnosis must be confirmed via protease inhibitor typing.

ALTITUDE ILLNESS

Patrick B. Solari
Paige L. Wright
George A. Woodward

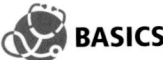 **BASICS**

DESCRIPTION
- Acute mountain sickness (AMS): Failure to adapt to the hypoxic demands of altitude. Includes a group of clinical signs and symptoms seen in travelers to altitudes >2,500 m
- Mild mountain sickness: Headache in morning and on exertion, anorexia, nausea, dizziness, vomiting, shortness of breath on exertion, insomnia, irritability, periodic breathing (Cheyne-Stokes respiration), poor performance
- Moderate mountain sickness: Severe headache, lassitude (weariness, indifference, antisocial), weakness, anorexia, nausea, ataxia, decreased urine output, diminished judgment and coordination. Capable of activities with difficulty.
- Severe mountain sickness: Insidious or acute onset, usually 2–4 days after ascent. Can progress to life-threatening situation within hours. Can include pulmonary and cerebral edema.
- High-altitude cerebral edema (HACE): Develops over 1–3 days after ascent, usually preceded by AMS. Headache, vomiting, lassitude, irritability, drowsiness, ataxia, slurred speech, cranial nerve paralysis, hypo- or hyperreflexia, hemiparesis, hemiplegia, mental status changes (confusion, irrationality, depression, disorientation, amnesia, hallucinations, severe nightmares), decreased urine output, seizures, papilledema, coma, death
- High-altitude pulmonary edema (HAPE): Often develops over several days and may be associated with or exacerbated by concurrent viral illness. Initially with dyspnea on exertion, then at rest, decreased exercise capability, dry cough, fatigue, tachypnea, low-grade fever <38.5°C (99.5°F). Develop pink frothy sputum, cyanosis, wheezing, rales, tachycardia, low-grade fever, and orthopnea
- Other altitude-related issues: High-altitude syncope, amnesia, edema (facial and extremity), retinopathy (hemorrhages), pharyngitis and bronchitis, flatus, immune suppression, thrombosis, coagulation abnormalities (thrombolic events), platelet changes, chronic mountain illness (Monge disease, polycythemia), weight loss

RISK FACTORS
- Travel in high-altitude areas
- Rapid ascent
- Underlying medical conditions, such as sickle cell disease, hypertension, sleep apnea, obstructive lung disease, cerebrovascular disease, or concurrent infections.
- Infants younger than 4–6 weeks have immature circulation and could be more susceptible to altitude illness.

GENERAL PREVENTION
- Avoid rapid ascent:
  – Limit ascents to 300 m (1,000 ft) per day above 3,000 m (>10,000 ft).
- Gradual acclimatization:
  – Do not fly or drive to heights above 3,000 m.
  – Allow at least 24 hours for each 1,000 m (3,300 ft) gained.
  – Exercise is not a substitute for acclimatization (or protection against AMS).
- Early recognition of symptoms (even if minor):
  – Assume symptoms secondary to AMS unless proven otherwise.
  – Go no higher until symptoms resolve.
  – Descend if worsening.
- Climb high, sleep low.
- Avoid alcohol, codeine, sedative-hypnotics, and respiratory depressants.
- Exercise within individual capacity:
  – Avoid heavy exercise after passive ascent for at least 24 hours.

PATHOPHYSIOLOGY
- Complex combination of anatomic factors, as well as physiologic and biochemical responses to hypoxia.
- AMS is thought to be related to rise in intracranial pressure at altitude that is worsened by exertion. Early fluid retention also linked to development of AMS.
- HACE is linked to hypoxia-induced increase in cerebral blood flow and vasogenic edema. Those with a "tight-fitting" brain within the skull may have less ability to buffer edema and may be more susceptible to HACE.
- HAPE is linked to exaggerated pulmonary hypertension, specifically elevated pulmonary artery pressure (PAP) and impaired alveolar fluid clearance. Medications that lower PAP may prevent HAPE.

COMMONLY ASSOCIATED CONDITIONS
Ophthalmologic:
- Retinal vessel engorgement
- Retinal hemorrhages: Usually resolves in 7 to 10 days without symptoms. 100% of people at 6,500 m (21,450 ft)
- Macular hemorrhages: More severe, associated with visual changes
- Ultraviolet keratitis

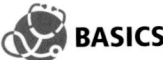 **DIAGNOSIS**

HISTORY
- Previous altitude illness:
  – Suggests symptoms in future with ascent to similar altitude
- Altitude where symptoms occurred, method of arrival at altitude, and rate of ascent.
  – Rapid ascent minimizes time for natural acclimatization and increases risk of developing altitude illness.
- Exertion level:
  – Increased exertion on ascent may increase speed of symptom development.
- Medical history, medications, drug or alcohol use:
  – Pre-existing problems such as asthma, sickle cell disease, hypertension, sleep apnea, obstructive or restrictive lung disease, cerebrovascular disease, or concurrent infections, may predispose one to development of altitude illness.

SIGNS AND SYMPTOMS
- See "Description."
- Symptoms either insidious or acute onset, usually 2–4 days after ascent:
  – Can become life threatening within hours
- Morning headache, progressive with ascent:
  – Suggests HACE
- Insomnia, difficulty falling asleep, frequent waking:
  – Suggests hypoxia, early AMS
- Periodic breathing (hyperpnea to apnea):
  – Suggests moderate to advanced AMS
- GI: Anorexia, nausea, vomiting, abdominal cramps, flatus:
  – Potentially related to ascent
- Pulmonary: Dry cough, shortness of breath, sore throat, dyspnea on exertion and at rest, decreased exercise capability:
  – Potential progression to HAPE
- Neurologic: Lassitude, weariness, indifference, fatigue, irritability, dizziness, ataxia, or weakness:
  – Progression to HACE
- Decreased urine output edema or fluid retention:
  – Indicative of fluid shifts, fluid losses, inadequate replacement, or dehydration

PHYSICAL EXAM
- Normal in early AMS:
  – Abnormalities usually occur after 12–24 hours at altitude (range, 2–96 hours).
- Lake Louise Score (LLS): (0–15)
  – Elevation Gain + Headache + Score >3 is considered diagnostic of AMS.

Score	0	1	2	3
Headache	None	Mild	Mod	Severe
GI	None	Mild upset	Mod upset	Vomiting
Fatigue	None	Mild tired	Mod tired	Incapacitating
Dizziness	None	Mild dizzy	Mod dizzy	Severe dizziness
Sleeping	None	Less sleep	Mod waking	No sleep

- Children's LLS:
  – Used in preverbal children.
  – To calculate Children's LLS, combine the Fussiness score with the Symptom score
  – Children's LLS Score >7 (Fussiness Score >4, Symptom Score >3) is considered diagnostic of AMS.

Fussiness score	0	3	6
Amount	None	Intermittent	Constant
Intensity	Not fussy	Moderately Fussy	Extremely Fussy

Symptom score	0	1	2	3
Eating	Norm	Mild	Mod Eating	Not eating; vomiting
Playing	Norm	Mild less	Play	No play at all
Sleeping	Norm	Mild less	Difficult sleep	Unable to sleep

DIAGNOSTIC TESTS & INTERPRETATION
- ECG: Rule out myocardial etiology of symptoms or consequence of ascent.
- HAPE: May have evidence of RV strain

Lab
- Toxicology screen
- Electrolytes
- Arterial blood gas:
  - Check oxygenation, ventilation, and acid–base status.
- Carbon monoxide level
- CBC:
  - Assess oxygen-carrying capacity of blood.
  - Look for anemia, polycythemia, and platelet abnormalities.

Imaging
- Chest x-ray:
  - Vasocongestion, patchy or diffuse infiltrates, often worse than physical exam suggests.
- Ventilation and perfusion scan:
  - Structural pulmonary assessment
- Brain CT scan:
  - Assess for structural abnormalities and cerebral edema.

DIFFERENTIAL DIAGNOSIS
- Environmental:
  - Alcohol toxicity, hangover, drug effects, hypothermia, carbon monoxide poisoning
- Medical/metabolic:
  - Dehydration, viral illness
- Psychosocial:
  - Exhaustion, sleep deprivation, personality traits (irritability), insomnia

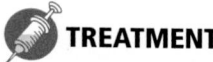 TREATMENT

MEDICATION (DRUGS)
- Acetazolamide (carbonic anhydrase inhibitor):
  - Prevention of AMS:
    - Pediatric dose: 2.5 mg/kg PO q12h
    - Adult dose: PO 125 mg BID
  - Treatment of early AMS
    - Pediatric Dose: 2.5 mg/kg PO q12h
    - Adult dose PO 250 mg BID
  - Caution for those with sulfa allergy.
  - Use in conjunction with (not in place of) gradual ascent, descent if symptomatic
- Dexamethasone (Decadron) PO/IV/IM:
  - Prevention of AMS, HACE:
    - NOT recommend for prophylaxis in pediatrics.
    - Adult dose: 2 mg PO q6h
  - Treatment of AMS, HACE (drug of choice):
    - Pediatric dose: 0.15 mg/kg/dose q6h
    - Adult dose (AMS): 4 mg q6h, (HACE): 8 mg once, then 4 mg q6h
  - Do not use longer than 10 days (glucocorticoid suppression)
- Nifedipine:
  - Prevention and treatment of HAPE:
    - Pediatric dose: 0.5 mg/kg/dose q8h
    - Adult dosage: 20-mg sustained release q8–12h
    - For prevention, start 24 hours prior to ascent and continued for 5 days at altitude.
    - Adjunct to descent, O_2
- Tadalafil:
  - Phosphodiesterase inhibitors, shown to decrease pulmonary artery pressure (PAP) at high altitude and may reduce incidence of HAPE, not studied in children.
  - Prevention of HAPE:
    - Adult dosage: 10 mg PO BID
    - For prevention, start 24 hours prior to ascent and continued for 5 days at altitude.

- Adjunct to descent
- Salmeterol:
  - Long-acting beta-agonist:
    - High dose: 125 mcg q12h (adults)
    - Limited clinical experience
  - Use as adjunct with nifedipine, not as monotherapy.

ADDITIONAL TREATMENT
General Measures
- Mild AMS:
  - Treatment may not be needed.
  - Symptomatic headache relief with ibuprofen, acetaminophen, aspirin, prochlorperazine
  - Temporal artery massage
  - Halt ascent until symptoms improve.
- Moderate to severe AMS:
  - Descent
  - Supplemental oxygen >90% SpO_2 (relieves hypoxia, reduces pulmonary hypertension)
  - Acetazolamide
  - Consider dexamethasone (if allergic to sulfa or cannot take acetazolamide)
  - Vasodilators (nifedipine, morphine)
- HACE:
  - Descend immediately.
  - Supplemental Oxygen to keep SpO_2 >90%
  - Dexamethasone
  - Portable hyperbaric chamber
  - Consider intubation and hyperventilation.
- HAPE:
  - Descend immediately.
  - Supplemental oxygen to keep SpO_2 >90%
  - Acetazolamide
  - Nifedipine
  - B-agonist (Salmeterol, Albuterol)
  - Sildenafil, Tadafil
  - Consider antibiotics
  - Portable hyperbaric chamber
  - CPAP
  - Knee-chest position with abdominal squeeze
  - Pursed-lip breathing, mask, intubation
  - Symptoms may recur when positive pressure is removed.

IN-PATIENT CONSIDERATIONS
Initial Stabilization
- Suspect AMS
- Stop ascent
- Partial or full descent:
  - Gamow portable hyperbaric chamber may be used until descent arranged.
- Oxygen if available
- Fluids
- Consider acetazolamide
- Avoid alcohol, codeine, sedative-hypnotics:
  - Avoid respiratory depressants

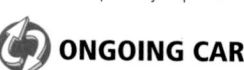 ONGOING CARE

DIET
- Increase fluid and calorie consumption with altitude and exertion.
- Increased carbohydrate diet.
- Avoid alcohol, tobacco, sedatives, and recreational drugs.

PROGNOSIS
- Expect improvement with mild mountain sickness in 1–2 days.
- Moderate mountain sickness clears with descent and acclimation.
- Severe mountain sickness usually clears with descent and therapy.

- Excellent if recognized quickly, ascent stopped, and/or descent and therapy initiated
- Can be poor if symptoms go unrecognized or noted without appropriate descent and therapy

ADDITIONAL READING
- Bärtsch P, Mairbäurl H, Maggiorini M, et al. Physiological aspects of high-altitude pulmonary edema. *J App Physiol*. 2005;98:1101–1110.
- Carpenter TC, Niermeyer S, Durmowicz AG. Altitude-related illness in children. *Curr Probl Pediatr*. 1998;28:177–198.
- Imray C, Wright A, Subudhi A, et al. Acute mountain sickness: Pathophysiology, prevention, and treatment. *Prog Cardiovasc Dis*. 2010;52:467–484.
- Sartori C, Allemann Y, Scherrer U. Pathogenesis of pulmonary edema: Learning from high-altitude pulmonary edema. *Respir Physiol Neurobiol*. 2007;159:338–349.
- Wilson MH, Newman S. The cerebral effects of ascent to high altitude. *Lancet Neurol*. 2009;8(2):175–191.

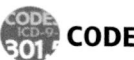 CODES

ICD9
993.2 Other and unspecified effects of high altitude

ICD10
- T70.20XA Unspecified effects of high altitude, initial encounter
- T70.20XD Unspecified effects of high altitude, subsequent encounter
- T70.20XS Unspecified effects of high altitude, sequela

FAQ
- Q: Can one develop AMS at moderate altitudes, such as during a ski vacation?
- A: Yes, although the altitudes encountered rarely lead to the development of severe symptoms in this population.
- Q: Will physical conditioning prior to ascent decrease the risk of developing altitude illness?
- A: No. In fact, better conditioning may inadvertently increase the risk of developing altitude illness, as one may achieve higher altitudes more quickly.
- Q: Are children more likely to develop HAPE than adults?
- A: Children from low altitudes have no greater risk of developing HAPE than adults; however, children who reside at high altitudes are more likely than adults to develop re-entry HAPE.
- Q: Should I give prophylaxis to my child to prevent AMS?
- A: Not usually. Only children with a significant history of AMS or unavoidable significant ascent should be given prophylaxis with acetazolamide. This can often be avoided by good planning with adequate rest and pacing of ascent. Prophylaxis with dexamethasone is not recommended in children.
- Q: Should everyone in whom a headache develops when at a higher than usual altitude be treated with acetazolamide?
- A: Not necessarily. Consider other causes of headaches and other conservative measures like rest and analgesics. The decision to treat should be based on severity of illness and other options available.

AMBLYOPIA
Monte D. Mills

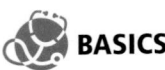 **BASICS**

DESCRIPTION
Amblyopia is generally classified by cause, with 3 primary types:
- Anisometropic amblyopia: Resulting from asymmetric refractive error and resultant unilateral blurring. This is the most common cause of amblyopia.
- Strabismic amblyopia: Resulting from misalignment of the eyes, and subsequent lack of an image that can be "fused", or integrated into a single image in the brain. This is most likely with early-onset, constant strabismus. Up to 60% of patients with strabismus will also have amblyopia.
- Deprivation amblyopia: Resulting from optical imperfection (cataract, ptosis, corneal opacity, prolonged patching or bandage), which prevents the formation of a clear image in one or both eyes. Deprivation, especially if it begins early in life, is associated with the most severe amblyopia.

EPIDEMIOLOGY
Amblyopia is the most common cause of unilateral vision loss in children and young adults.

Prevalence
Large population-based studies indicate that 2–5% of the adult population has amblyopia.

PATHOPHYSIOLOGY
- Asymmetric input between the 2 eyes (unilateral cataract, anisometropia, etc.) is more likely to cause amblyopia than symmetrically poor images, due to competitive influences between the 2 eyes. As a result, amblyopia is usually unilateral.
- Bilateral amblyopia may result from severe, symmetric bilateral image degradation such as bilateral cataract, bilateral high ametropia (high refractive error), etc.
- Visual acuity in amblyopic eyes varies from minimal impairment (20/25) to legal blindness (<20/200). Other significant impairments in amblyopic eyes may include reduced contrast sensitivity, reduced or absent binocularity and depth perception, and impaired or distorted spatial perception. Peripheral visual fields are preserved, and vision is never completely lost (no light perception) from amblyopia alone.

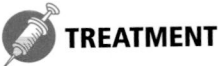 **DIAGNOSIS**

SIGNS AND SYMPTOMS
Poor vision

HISTORY
- Age of onset of vision loss
- Eye trauma, injury, or surgery
- Refractive error or glasses
- Ptosis or ocular occlusion
- Family history of strabismus, anisometropia, or amblyopia

PHYSICAL EXAM
- Visual acuity is the single most significant sign in detection of amblyopia. Vision must be tested in each eye separately, with reliable occlusion (adhesive patch, opaque card, or plastic occluder). Because most amblyopia is monocular, testing vision with both eyes open is inadequate as a screening tool.
- Binocularity tests such as Titmus stereopsis (3D fly) will detect suppression, which is frequently associated with amblyopia.

DIAGNOSTIC TESTS & INTERPRETATION
Vision testing in young children is difficult and, sometimes, unreliable:
- Children must be tested with each eye separately.
- Repeating the tests and adjunctive tests including the Titmus test, cover testing, photoscreening, and Bruchner red reflex test will increase the sensitivity of screening.

Lab
Imaging
Imaging studies of the optic nerves and posterior visual pathways may be useful in selected cases to exclude other causes of vision loss.

DIFFERENTIAL DIAGNOSIS
- Amblyopia is diagnosed by exclusion: Conditions that cause vision loss without easily recognized pathology might be mistaken for amblyopia.
- In children, the differential diagnosis of vision loss in normal-appearing eyes includes the following:
  - Uncorrected refractive error (hyperopia, myopia, astigmatism)
  - Optic nerve hypoplasia
  - Optic atrophy
  - Compressive, toxic or hereditary optic neuropathies
  - Retinopathies, including Leber congenital amaurosis, Stargardt disease, retinitis pigmentosa, and others
  - Central visual impairment (cortical blindness)
  - Glaucoma
  - Factitious or functional causes (hysterical blindness)

TREATMENT

GENERAL MEASURES
- Unilateral amblyopia:
  - Treat underling cause of vision loss (strabismus, anisometropia, optical opacity) and force preferential use of the amblyopic eye.
  - The classic and most common treatment is occlusion with an adhesive patch worn over the opposite eye for several hours per day.
  - The amount of time of occlusion necessary to reverse amblyopia depends on variables including the severity of amblyopia, cause of amblyopia, age, and other associated ocular conditions.
  - Typically worn, from a few weeks to months
  - Infants and very young children require closer observation to prevent reversing the amblyopia to the previously preferred eye (occlusion amblyopia) from excessive patching.
  - Optical penalization of the opposite eye using topical cycloplegic eyedrops, such as atropine 1%. Recent studies suggest that atropine penalization may be as effective as patching to treat mild or moderate amblyopia.
  - Treatment should be attempted in amblyopic children within the "sensitive period" of birth to 8 years of age. Improvement of vision with treatment of older children has been reported, but is much less likely. Treatment is usually continued until visual acuity is equal to the opposite eye, or no further improvement is seen over several examinations with treatment.
  - The primary risk of treatment is overcorrection, with iatrogenic amblyopia in the occluded opposite eye.
- In strabismic amblyopia, initiation of treatment for amblyopia need not wait for correction of the strabismus. In fact, the stability of the surgical strabismus correction is improved if amblyopia therapy is initiated before surgery:
  - Treatment is usually continued until visual acuity in both eyes is equal, or until vision in the amblyopic eye shows no further improvement after several examinations over a period of time.

ISSUES FOR REFERRAL
Prompt referral of failures and children suspected of poor vision for complete ophthalmic examination is essential for successful amblyopia screening programs.

ONGOING CARE

FOLLOW-UP RECOMMENDATIONS
- In general, the younger the patient, the more intensive the patching therapy, and the milder the amblyopia, the more frequent vision testing is necessary to ensure that vision in the opposite, occluded eye is not harmed.
- Children are clever at finding ways to avoid the temporary vision impairment from patching, and will peek or remove patches frequently.
- In younger children, amblyopia may recur after successful treatment.

PATIENT MONITORING
- Children should be retested frequently, and retreated if vision drops after finishing successful initial treatment.
- Testing should continue at least annually until the child is at least 8 years old.

PATIENT EDUCATION
Because the outcome of amblyopia depends entirely on early detection and treatment within the first few years of life, all children should be screened by monocular recognition visual acuity as early as possible (at the 3- or 4-year well-child visit), and testing should be repeated annually until 8 years of age. Children who are not capable of accurate visual acuity testing by 4 years of age should also be referred for complete evaluation

PROGNOSIS
- After treatment, amblyopia may recur and vision should be retested regularly.
- Patients with strabismus, even if previously treated with glasses or surgery, must be followed for amblyopia.
- Vision loss from amblyopia will persist even after the condition that originally caused the amblyopia has resolved. In some cases, when there is no obvious cause, a history of episodes of anisometropia, occlusion, or strabismus must be considered.

COMPLICATIONS
- Left untreated, amblyopia results in irreversible, uncorrectable vision loss after visual maturity (8–10 years of age).
- Usually the vision loss is unilateral, and the functional effects may be minimal if vision in the remaining eye is normal.
- In bilateral cases, or if other diseases or injury affects the remaining eye, the outcome can be significant functional impairment, including legal blindness.

ADDITIONAL READING

- American Academy of Ophthalmology. *Preferred Practice Pattern: Amblyopia*. San Francisco: American Academy of Ophthalmology; 2002.
- American Academy of Ophthalmology. *Preferred Practice Pattern: Pediatric Eye Examination*. San Francisco: American Academy of Ophthalmology; 2002.
- Clarke MP, Wright CM, Hrisos S, et al. Randomised controlled trial of treatment of unilateral visual impairment detected at preschool vision screening. *BMJ*. 2003;327:1251.
- Demirkilinc BE, Uretmen O, Kose S. The effect of optical correction on refractive development in children with accommodative esotropia. *J AAPOS*. 2010;14(4):305–310.
- Holmes JM, Beck RW, Kraker RT, et al. Impact of patching and atropine treatment on the child and the family in the amblyopia treatment study. *Arch Ophthal*. 2003;121:1625–1632.
- Repka MX, Beck RW, Holmes JM, et al. A randomized trial of patching regimens for treatment of moderate amblyopia in children. *Arch Ophthal*. 2003;121:603–611.

 CODES

ICD9
- 368.00 Amblyopia
- 368.01 Strabismic amblyopia
- 368.03 Refractive amblyopia

ICD10
- H53.009 Unspecified amblyopia, unspecified eye
- H53.029 Refractive amblyopia, unspecified eye
- H53.039 Strabismic amblyopia, unspecified eye

FAQ
- Q: How long will patching be necessary?
- A: It is not possible to predict exactly how long treatment will be necessary to restore vision. In general, the younger the patient, the milder the impairment, and the more intensive the patching, the more quickly vision is restored. In general, patching is usually continued for 1–4 months in most cases of anisometropic or strabismic amblyopia. Normalization of vision or lack of further improvement is usually the treatment end point.
- Q: Will vision be normal after treatment?
- A: The degree of recovery with amblyopia therapy depends on the density of the amblyopia, the cause, and the age at which treatment is initiated. In almost all children younger than 6–8 years, some visual improvement can be expected with amblyopia treatment, although not all patients will improve to 20/20 vision.
- Q: Will patching eliminate the need for glasses?
- A: No, patching does not influence the outcome of refractive errors (power of glasses, Refractive Error). Glasses may still be needed after patching is completed.
- Q: Will patching for amblyopia improve the strabismus?
- A: No, in most cases patching for amblyopia will not eliminate strabismus or the need for strabismus surgery. However, in most cases it is best to begin amblyopia treatment before surgery, to improve the surgical outcome.
- Q: Is "vision therapy" without patching an effective treatment for strabismus?
- A: Although eye exercises, pleoptics, and other vision therapies have been used to treat amblyopia, none is as effective as patching or other occlusive therapy. Current vision therapy techniques have not been proven to improve amblyopia.
- Q: My child refuses to wear a patch. Are there alternatives to patching?
- A: Yes, optical penalization with glasses, atropine cycloplegic penalization, and even contact lens occlusion can be effective. However, patching is the most reliable and effective treatment. Parental support, encouragement, and reward are essential for treatment compliance.

AMEBIASIS

Jason Kim

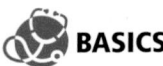 **BASICS**

DESCRIPTION
Clinical syndromes associated with *Entamoeba histolytica* infection

EPIDEMIOLOGY
- Treatment of drinking water
- Hand washing
- Appropriate disposal of human fecal waste
- Use of condoms
- Infection-control measures: Standard precautions are recommended for the hospitalized patient.

Incidence
Amebiasis accounts for 40–50 million cases of colitis worldwide and leads to 40,000–110,000 deaths annually.

Prevalence
- The estimated prevalence in the US is 4% although there have been no recent serosurveys in developed countries.
- Worldwide distribution involving an estimated 10% or more of the world's population. Most common in tropical areas, with infection rates as high as 20–50%. The highest morbidity and mortality are seen in developing countries in Central America, South America, Africa, and Asia.

RISK FACTORS
- The very young, the elderly, and patients with underlying immunosuppression or malnutrition are at highest risk for severe disease.
- Patients in whom the diagnosis should be considered include:
  - Immigrants from or travelers to endemic areas
  - Children with bloody stools or mucus in stools
  - Children with hepatic abscess
  - The febrile child with right upper quadrant pain and tenderness, abdominal pain, or discomfort
  - The child with hepatomegaly, typically without jaundice

PATHOPHYSIOLOGY
- Fecal–oral transmission
- *E. histolytica* is excreted as cysts or trophozoites in the stool of infected patients.
- Ingested cysts are unaffected by gastric acid and become trophozoites that colonize and invade the colon.
- Amebae attach to epithelial cells via a galactose/N-acetylgalactosamine (Gal/GalNac) binding lectin. The parasite has the ability to lyse human epithelial cells, or kill by inducing apoptosis. Then cytokines and chemokines released attract neutrophils, macrophages, and lymphocytes. The host immune response contributes significantly to the reduction of epithelial integrity.

- Amebas then use cysteine protease to cleave extracellular matrix proteins to invade the submucosal layers.
- Amebas can then disseminate directly from the intestine to the liver in up to 10% of patients. Dissemination from the liver to the lung, heart, brain, and spleen has been described.
- The incubation period is typically 1–3 weeks but can range from a few days to months or years.

ETIOLOGY
- *E. histolytica* is nonflagellated protozoan parasite.
- Other species of the *Entamoeba* family are nonpathogenic, including the morphologically identical *Entamoeba dispar*.

DIAGNOSIS

HISTORY
Intestinal disease may be asymptomatic or have mild symptoms such as abdominal discomfort, flatulence, constipation, and occasionally diarrhea.

PHYSICAL EXAM
- The most common clinical manifestation is intestinal amebiasis.
- Nondysenteric colitis is characterized by intermittent diarrhea and abdominal pain.
- Acute amebic colitis (dysenteric) is associated with grossly bloody stools with mucus, abdominal pain, and tenesmus.

DIAGNOSTIC TESTS & INTERPRETATION
The diagnosis of amebiasis depends on the recognition of typical symptoms and routine laboratory tests.

Lab
- CBC typically reveals a leukocytosis.
- Transaminases are often not elevated.
- Occult blood is detected in stool.
- Stool samples:
  - Isolation and visualization:
    - Serial stool samples, usually 3, are recommended.
    - Samples obtained within 1–2 hours of passage should be examined by wet mount and fixed in formalin and polyvinyl alcohol.
    - Serial stool samples are necessary since cysts may be shed intermittently. 3 serial stool samples will detect up to 70% of patients with amebic colitis and 50% of patients with hepatic abscess.
    - Stool samples should not be contaminated by urine, water, barium, enema substances, laxatives, or antibiotics, since these substances may destroy or interfere with identification of the trophozoites.
    - Microscopy has a sensitivity of <60% and specificity of 10–50% on a single sample.
  - Second-generation stool antigen testing kits (commercially available) also have demonstrated excellent sensitivity and specificity comparable to real time PCR.

- Serology:
  - Serum antiamebic antibodies are considered an adjunct to diagnosis.
  - ~85% of patients with amebic dysentery and 99% of patients with liver amebiasis will have positive serology.
  - Molecular testing to differentiate *Entamoeba histolytica* from non-pathogenic *Entamoeba* species is in the research phase.

Imaging
- Ultrasound, CT, or MRI of the liver
- In patients with hepatic amebiasis, chest x-ray may reveal elevation of the right hemidiaphragm.

Diagnostic Procedures/Other
- Note: Amebae are difficult to visualize in abscess aspirates and substantial risk is associated with CT or ultrasound-guided procedures, including bleeding, peritonitis secondary to spillage of amebae, or rupture of echinococcal cysts.
- Colonoscopy

Pathological Findings
- Identification of trophozoites or cysts in the stool
- Colonic or rectal mucosa visualized by colonoscopy reveals ulcerations, and amebae can often be found around these lesions.

DIFFERENTIAL DIAGNOSIS
The diagnosis is often missed in children because the disease is not included in the differential. Because it is not common in the US, amebiasis may initially be misdiagnosed as bacterial dysentery. Differential diagnosis includes the following:

- Infection: *Salmonella* species *Shigella* species, *Campylobacter* species, *Yersinia* species, *Clostridium difficile*, *Escherichia coli* (enteroinvasive and enterohemorrhagic) pyogenic abscess, Echinococcal cyst, inflammatory bowel disease: Crohn disease, ulcerative colitis,
- Miscellaneous: Ischemic colitis, diverticulitis, arteriovenous malformations, hepatoma

TREATMENT

MEDICATION (DRUGS)

First Line

- Asymptomatic intestinal amebiasis: Intraluminal agents:
  - Iodoquinol is the drug of choice. The recommended dosage is 30–40 mg/kg/d (maximum, 1,950 mg) PO in 3 divided doses for 20 days.
- Acute amebic colitis or extraintestinal amebiasis:
  - Metronidazole (a tissue-active agent) 35–50 mg/kg/d PO in 3 divided doses for 10 days (maximum, 2,250 mg/d) plus a course of treatment with an intraluminal active agent (as above). ~1/3 of patients treated with metronidazole alone will relapse.

Second Line

- Asymptomatic intestinal amebiasis:
  - Diloxanide furoate (Furamide) at doses of 20 mg/kg/d (maximum, 1,500 mg/d) PO in 3 divided doses or paromomycin, 25–35 mg/kg/d PO in 3 divided doses for 7 days.
- Acute amebic colitis or extraintestinal amebiasis:
  - One study has reported good efficacy using nitazoxanide in children; however, it was small and combined E. histolytica and E. dispar into one stratum.
  - However, nitazoxanide shows good activity in vitro against E. histolytica.

ADDITIONAL TREATMENT

General Measures

- The goal of treatment is the elimination of tissue-invading trophozoites and intestinal cysts.
- The choice of treatment regimens depends on the clinical presentation.
- Agents that are active against E. histolytica are divided into 2 categories: Drugs with activity against intraluminal amebae and drugs with activity against extraintestinal and invasive amebiasis.

SURGERY/OTHER PROCEDURES

Patients with large liver abscesses or who have failed medical therapy should be considered candidates for surgical or percutaneous drainage.

 ONGOING CARE

FOLLOW-UP RECOMMENDATIONS

Patient Monitoring

- Follow-up stool examination is always necessary to ensure eradication of intestinal amebae.
- For amebic abscesses, drainage should be considered if response to medical therapy has not occurred in 4–5 days.

PROGNOSIS

Clinical improvement is expected within 72 hours of initiation of therapy.

COMPLICATIONS

- Amebic liver abscess:
  - 2nd most common presentation of amebiasis, often not associated with amebic dysentery
- Ameboma:
  - Abdominal mass representing granulation tissue in the colon
- Extraintestinal manifestations of amebiasis are presumed to be a result of direct extension from liver abscesses. These include the following:
  - Pericarditis
  - Pleuropulmonary abscess or empyema
  - Bronchohepatic fistula
  - Genitourinary tract abscess
  - Cerebral abscess
  - Cutaneous amebiasis:
    ○ This is a rare finding in children, with ~6,510 cases reported in the literature.
    ○ Shallow painful cutaneous ulcers in the diaper area, usually found in association with amebic colitis or dysentery
  - Epidemiologic studies from countries with high prevalence of amebiasis show an association between amebic diarrhea and poor growth. The negative effect on growth was significantly more deleterious than diarrhea caused either by Giardia or Cryptosporidium.

ADDITIONAL READING

- Bercu TE, Petri WA, Behm JW. Amebic colitis: New insights into pathogenesis and treatment. Curr Gastroenterol Rep. 2007;9(5):429–423
- Haque R, Huston CD, Hughes M, et al. Amebiasis. N Engl J Med. 2003;348:1565–1573.
- Mangaña ML, Fernández-Díez, Mangaña M. Cutaneous amebiasis in pediatrics. Arch Dermatol. 2008;144:1369–1372
- Mondal D, Petri WA, et al. Entamoeba histolytica associated diarrheal illness is negatively associated with the growth of preschool children: Evidence from a prospective study. Trans Royal Soc Trop Med Hyg. 2006;100:1032–1038.
- Ravdin JI, Stauffer WM. Entamoeba histolytica (amebiasis). In: Mandell GL, Bennett JE, Dolin R, eds. Principles and Practice of Infectious Diseases, vol. 2. 6th ed. Philadelphia: Churchill Livingstone; 2005:3097–3111.
- Stauffer W, Ravdin JI. Entamoeba histolytica: An update. Curr Opin Infect Dis. 2003;16:479–485.
- Tanyukse IM, Petri WA. Laboratory diagnosis of amebiasis. Clin Micr Rev. 2003;16:713–729.

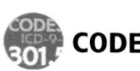 CODES

ICD9
006.9 Amebiasis, unspecified

ICD10
A06.9 Amebiasis, unspecified

AMENORRHEA

Renee K. Kottenhahn
Deborah B. Ehrenthal

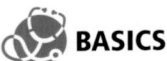 **BASICS**

DESCRIPTION

Amenorrhea is the absence of menstruation. It is divided into 2 categories:

- *Primary amenorrhea* is the failure to begin menstruation by age 16 in girls with otherwise appropriate pubertal development or by age 14 in the absence of secondary sexual characteristics. Evaluation should also be considered if a girl has not menstruated within 2 years of obtaining Tanner IV breast development regardless of her age.
- *Secondary amenorrhea* is the cessation of menstruation for 3 cycles or 6 months in girls and women with previously established regular cycles:
  - Should not be used when referring to girls who are within their 1st 2 years of menarche because regular ovulatory cycles have not yet been established; their periods are unpredictable.
- A regular menstrual cycle is a sign of good health. The absence of menses or disruption of regular cycles once they have been established can result from systemic disease, genetic or anatomic abnormalities, physical or emotional stress, or unrecognized pregnancy. The goal of the evaluation is to identify the underlying cause (see Differential Diagnosis section below)
- Approach to patient:
  - A stepwise approach to the evaluation guided by the history and physical exam is recommend:
    o Phase 1: Exclude pregnancy by urine or serum HCG testing.
    o Phase 2: Obtain a complete history to differentiate between primary and secondary amenorrhea to help identify the underlying cause.
    o Phase 3: Perform a directed physical exam.
    o Phase 4: Initiate stepwise diagnostic testing to assess for causes of amenorrhea.

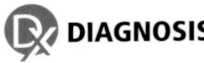 **DIAGNOSIS**

HISTORY

- Age of patient:
  - Genetic abnormalities more common in younger patients
  - Premature ovarian failure found with increasing age
- Past and current medical history
  - Prior/current/chronic illness including autoimmune, renal, thyroid, or liver disease; diabetes, or cancer (radiation or chemotherapy), which may be the underlying cause of amenorrhea
- Stressful life events:
  - A diagnosis of exclusion
- Growth and weight changes
  - Consider endocrinopathy, genetic disease, PCOS, rapid weight gain, eating disorder or other chronic disease
- Behavioral:
  - Eating disorder and/or excessive exercise

- Headaches:
  - Assess for visual field defects, dizziness (suggesting pituitary tumor or other intracranial process)
- Reproductive and menstrual history:
  - Age at menarche
  - Menstrual cycles: regularity, flow, duration; characteristics of last menstrual period (normal or abnormal)
  - Sexual history: Sexual activity, prior pregnancy, current or prior contraceptive use (Depo-Provera can cause amenorrhea for up to 18 months)
  - Presence of symptoms of molimina in the past: menstruation associated with breast tenderness, fluid retention, cramping
  - Risk factors for uterine scarring
- Galactorrhea:
  - Spontaneous milky discharge from the breast suggests elevated prolactin or thyroid abnormality, or may be due to manual stimulation, medications, pituitary tumor, or illicit drug use.
- Abdominal or pelvic pain:
  - Cyclic or intermittent abdominal/pelvic pain suggests a uterine anomaly or obstruction.
- Skin and hair:
  - Excess hair growth (inquire about shaving, plucking, or waxing), acne, balding, and acanthosis nigricans are symptoms of androgen excess and suggest PCOS, congenital adrenal hyperplasia (rare), or a tumor (rare).
  - Easy bruising or pigmented striae suggest Cushing syndrome.
- Medications:
  - Hormonal and cytotoxic medications, illicit drugs, antidepressant drugs, and medications such as opiates.

PHYSICAL EXAM

- General appearance, height, and weight with calculation of BMI (body mass index in kg/m^2):
  - Obesity raises suspicion of PCOS or Cushing syndrome.
  - Athleticism or underweight suggests female athlete triad or eating disorder, respectively.
  - Stigmata of Turner syndrome (short stature, web neck, etc.) or other genetic syndrome
  - Abnormal growth pattern suggests endocrinopathy, dietary restriction, chronic disease, or genetic disorder.

- Skin exam:
  - Acne, hirsutism (increased facial hair, midline hair over sternum and lower abdomen), acanthosis nigricans, and balding are suggestive of virilization or PCOS.
  - Bruises or pigmented striae suggest Cushing syndrome.
- Tanner staging and breast exam:
  - Abnormal Tanner stage for chronologic age suggests an endocrine, metabolic, or genetic abnormality.
  - Galactorrhea suggests abnormalities in prolactin or thyroid.
- Thyroid nodule or enlargement:
  - Evaluate for hyperthyroidism or hypothyroidism.
- Abdominal mass:
  - Evaluate for uterine obstruction, tumor.
- Genitourinary exam:
  - Abnormal external genitalia suggests outflow tract abnormalities.
  - Clitoral enlargement is a sign of virilization and raises suspicion for an androgen-secreting tumor or congenital adrenal hyperplasia.
  - The decision to do a digital or speculum pelvic exam should be based on the patient's age/maturity/gynecologic history/and ability to tolerate the exam. An ultrasound may be a helpful adjunct to evaluate anatomy (see below).

DIAGNOSTIC TESTS & INTERPRETATION

Lab

- Standard initial testing: pregnancy test, FSH/LH, estradiol, TSH, free T4 prolactin (8 a.m.)
- For primary amenorrhea include genetic testing by checking a karyotype to identify sex chromosome abnormalities.
- If PCOS is suspected or virilization is identified also include total and free testosterone, DHEA-S, and 17-hydroxyprogesterone.
- If Cushing syndrome is suspected consider an overnight dexamethasone suppression test or 24-hour urinary free cortisol excretion.

Imaging

- Imaging should be used selectively.
- Transvaginal or Pelvic ultrasound:
  - Confirm presence of normal müllerian structures (uterus and ovaries) for patients with primary amenorrhea.
  - Exclude ovarian mass, renal abnormalities based on abnormal physical exam or laboratory results.
- MRI of the pituitary gland if indicated based on neurologic symptoms, galactorrhea, and/or laboratory results (elevated prolactin)

Diagnostic Procedures/Other

Progesterone challenge: to be used selectively only after primary evaluation completed

DIFFERENTIAL DIAGNOSIS

- Outflow tract abnormalities:
  - Imperforate hymen, transverse vaginal septum, müllerian agenesis, androgen insensitivity syndrome (testicular feminization)
- Ovarian failure:
  - Chromosomal abnormalities, radiation- or chemotherapy-induced ovarian failure, autoimmune premature ovarian failure, idiopathic premature ovarian failure
- Chronic anovulation:
  - Androgen excess: polycystic ovary syndrome (common), congenital adrenal hyperplasia, ovarian or adrenal tumor
  - Elevated prolactin: Prolactinoma, medications, hypothyroidism, others
  - Low or normal LH/FSH: Chronic or systemic illness, psychological stress, eating disorders, extreme obesity, excessive exercise
  - Thyroid disease
  - Other endocrine abnormality: Pituitary insufficiency, Cushing syndrome
- Medications:
  - Cytotoxic, hormonal contraception, opiates, psychiatric medications, and others
- Pregnancy

TREATMENT

- Identification and management of the underlying disorder is key.
- Estrogen/progestin hormonal therapy should not be initiated prior to completing a full evaluation.
- Premature use of hormonal therapy may alter subsequent testing.
- Contraindications to hormone therapy must be ruled out (refer to World Health Organization [WHO] Medical Eligibility Criteria at http://www.who.int/reproductivehealth/publications/family_planning/en/).

ADDITIONAL TREATMENT

Additional Therapies

Behavioral interventions: A family-based approach is recommended for addressing complex behavior problems or emotional symptoms in an adolescent.

ADDITIONAL READING

- Braverman PK, Sondheimer SJ. Menstrual disorders. *Pediatr Rev.* 1997;18(1):17–25.
- Donaldson MD, Gault EJ, Tan KW, et al. Optimizing management in Turner syndrome: From infancy to adult transfer. *Arch Dis Child.* 2006;91(6):513–520.
- LeClair C, Ehrenthal DB, Hillard PJA. Amenorrhea. In: Ehrenthal DB, Hoffman MK, Hillard PJA, eds. *Menstrual disorders.* American College of Physicians Women's Health Series. American College of Physicians: Philadelphia, 2006:51–75.

- Slap GB. Menstrual disorders in adolescence. *Best Pract Res Clin Obstet Gynaecol.* 2003;17(1):75–92.
- Speroff M, Fritz L. *Clinical gynecologic endocrinology and infertility,* 8th ed. Philadelphia: Lippincott Williams & Wilkins; 2011:435–494.

CODES

ICD9
626.0 Primary or secondary amenorrhea

ICD10
- N91.0 Primary amenorrhea
- N91.1 Secondary amenorrhea
- N91.2 Amenorrhea, unspecified

FAQ

- Q: What are the normal benchmarks for evaluating pubertal development in girls?
- A: Normal benchmarks for evaluating pubertal development in girls: Breast development by age 12–13, menarche ~2 years after breast development (by age 14), or menarche within 2 years of achieving Tanner IV breast stage.
- Q: Does a patient who says she has never had sex still need a pregnancy test?
- A: Yes

ANAEROBIC INFECTIONS

Hamid Bassiri
Adam J. Ratner (5th edition)

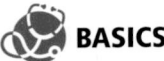 **BASICS**

DESCRIPTION
Anaerobic bacteria are organisms capable of growing in a reduced oxygen environment, either exclusively (obligate anaerobes) or in addition to growing in air (facultative anaerobes). Anaerobic bacteria can cause invasive and sometimes serious disease.

EPIDEMIOLOGY
While anaerobic bacteremia is less frequent in children than in adults, some pediatric anaerobic infections are common at certain sites (e.g., chronic otitis media or sinusitis).

- Anaerobic bacteria most commonly found in polymicrobial infections with other anaerobic and aerobic flora.
- Because of their fastidious nature, the ability of microbiology laboratories to identify anaerobic bacteria is highly dependent on proper collection and transport of culture specimens. As a result, anaerobic bacteria can often be missed.
- The most common anaerobes include various genera of gram-negative rods (*Bacteroides*, *Prevotella*, *Porphyromonas*, *Fusobacteria*, *Bilophila*, and *Sutterella*), gram-positive cocci (*Peptostreptococcus*), spore-forming gram-positive bacilli (*Clostridia*), nonspore-forming gram-positive bacilli (*Eubacterium*, *Bifidobacterium*, *Propionibacterium*, *Actinomyces*, and *Lactobacillus*), and gram-negative cocci (*Veillonella*).

RISK FACTORS
Increased risk is associated with impaired host immunity or presence of devitalized tissue (owing to surgery, trauma, vascular insufficiency, diabetes), or presence of foreign bodies.

PATHOPHYSIOLOGY
- Generally occurs when there is a break in a mucocutaneous barrier.
- Numerous virulence factors have been described, including exotoxins (e.g., *Clostridia* spp.), antiphagocytic capsule (e.g., *Bacteroides* spp.), and endotoxins (e.g., *Fusobacterium* spp.)

ETIOLOGY
Anaerobic infections most commonly derive from the normal flora of the oropharynx, skin, intestines, or the female genital tract. Thus, anaerobic infections are often associated with a loss of integrity of anatomic or epithelial barriers at these sites.

COMMONLY ASSOCIATED CONDITIONS
- CNS infections:
  - Brain abscess
  - Subdural empyema
  - Epidural abscess
- Head and neck infections:
  - Sinusitis (generally polymicrobial)
  - Chronic otitis media
  - Ludwig angina (infection of the submandibular space)
  - Cervical adenitis
  - Peritonsillar abscess
  - Dental abscess
  - Gingivitis
  - Actinomycosis of jaw
  - Lemierre disease (septic thrombophlebitis of the internal jugular vein owing to *Fusobacterium*, often resulting in pulmonary abscess formation)
- Pleuropulmonary infections:
  - Aspiration of oral and/or gastrointestinal fluids
  - Pneumonia, abscess formation
  - Secondary to aspirated foreign bodies
  - Actinomycosis
- Peritonitis/peritoneal abscess:
  - Appendiceal abscess
  - Perforated viscus
  - Postoperative complication
  - Trauma-related
  - Actinomycosis
- Cholangitis:
  - Ascending infection may occur following biliary tract surgery (e.g., Kasai procedure).
  - Infection is often polymicrobial.
- Soft tissue infection:
  - Paronychia
  - Pilonidal cyst
  - Crepitant cellulitis
  - Necrotizing fasciitis
  - Gas gangrene (*Clostridium* spp.)
  - Infected decubitus ulcers (may result in contiguous osteomyelitis)
  - Penetrating wounds (may lead to tetanus)
- Infections of the female genital tract:
  - Endometritis or salpingitis
  - Tubo-ovarian or adnexal abscess
  - Pelvic inflammatory diseases
  - Pelvic abscess
  - Bartholin gland, vulvar, or perineal abscess
  - Bacterial vaginosis
- Infected bite wounds:
  - Anaerobes isolated from 50% of human or animal bites
- Bacteremia:
  - Often associated with focal primary site of involvement (gastrointestinal disease, abscess)
- Neonatal infections:
  - Cellulitis at fetal monitoring sites
  - Aspiration pneumonia
  - Omphalitis
  - Conjunctivitis
  - Infant botulism

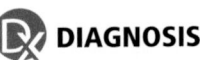 **DIAGNOSIS**

Involvement of anaerobic bacteria should be suspected in infections with suppuration, abscess formation, tissue necrosis, or in hosts with systemic disease.

HISTORY
- Impaired mental status:
  - Increased risk of aspiration
- History of thumb sucking:
  - Anaerobes frequently isolated from paronychia
- History of animal or human bites
- Recent surgery or trauma:
  - Poor drainage or devitalized tissue associated with anaerobic infection
- Underlying immunodeficiency or chronic illness:
  - Impaired phagocytic function
- History of pus that is "sterile" (no growth on routine cultures)

PHYSICAL EXAM
- Location of infection:
  - See "Associated Conditions."
- Poor dentition:
  - Increased colonization of oropharynx with anaerobic organisms
- Necrotic tissue or crepitus
- "Dishwater" pus or discharge with foul odor:
  - Characteristic of anaerobic infections
- Lateral neck pain in association with respiratory distress:
  - Lemierre disease causes septic thrombophlebitis of the internal jugular vein and lung abscess.

DIAGNOSTIC TESTS & INTERPRETATION
Lab
- Gram stains with unique morphology:
  - Small, pleomorphic gram-negative bacilli (*Bacteroides* spp.); large gram-positive organisms with "boxcar" morphology (*Clostridium* spp.)
- Anaerobic cultures:
  - Should be performed on tissue or aspirated fluid obtained in a sterile fashion from the infected site. Anaerobically collected specimens should be transported to the microbiology laboratory promptly.
  - Do not send swabs for anaerobic cultures.

Imaging
- Radiographs:
  - Air–fluid level, cavity formation, gas in tissue
- CT and/or MRI scans:
  - Often important to define anatomic location and extent of disease

DIFFERENTIAL DIAGNOSIS
- Likely pathogens not recovered from aerobic cultures
- Failure of empiric antibiotic coverage that is not active against anaerobes

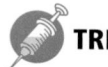 TREATMENT

ADDITIONAL TREATMENT
General Measures
In general, antimicrobials with the best activity against anaerobes include metronidazole, carbapenems, chloramphenicol, and beta-lactam/beta-lactamase inhibitor combinations. Clindamycin, cephamycins, and antipseudomonal synthetic penicillins also have relatively good range of activity. Penicillin, cephalosporins, tetracyclines, macrolides, aminoglycosides, trimethoprim-sulfamethoxazole, and monobactams have either variable or poor activity against anaerobes and should not be used as empiric therapy. Most fluoroquinolones (except moxifloxacin) also have variable activity. Vancomycin has activity against gram-positive but not gram-negative anaerobes.

Empiric drug therapy:
- CNS infections:
  - Vancomycin + cefotaxime + metronidazole
- Head and neck infections:
  - Ampicillin-sulbactam, amoxicillin-clavulanate, or clindamycin
- Pleuropulmonary infections:
  - Ampicillin-sulbactam, amoxicillin-clavulanate, or clindamycin
- Peritonitis/peritoneal abscess:
  - Ampicillin-sulbactam, ticarcillin-clavulanate, piperacillin-tazobactam, or cefoxitin, or meropenem, imipenem
- Cholangitis:
  - Piperacillin-tazobactam, or meropenem, imipenem
- Soft tissue infection:
  - Site dependent
- Infections of the female genital tract:
  - Site dependent
- Infected bite wounds:
  - Ampicillin-sulbactam, piperacillin-tazobactam, amoxicillin-clavulanate
- Bacteremia:
  - Isolate dependent
- Neonatal infections:
  - Site dependent

COMPLEMENTARY & ALTERNATIVE THERAPIES
- Neutralization of toxins, especially in the case of botulism or tetanus
- Hyperbaric oxygen, although still sometimes used (especially in Clostridial infections), has not been shown to be of proven benefit, although it may help define and demarcate the borders of devitalized tissues.

SURGERY/OTHER PROCEDURES
Effective drainage of abscesses and debridement of devitalized tissue is essential.

 ONGOING CARE

PROGNOSIS
- Determined by speed with which infection is appropriately treated with antibiotics and/or drainage.
- High rates of mortality associated with clinically apparent anaerobic bacteremia.
- Specific prognosis depends on the bacterial species involved and the status of the patient's immune system.
- Soft tissue infections caused by *Clostridium* spp. may cause up to 20% mortality despite aggressive therapy.

COMPLICATIONS
Vary with nature of infection, but can include extension of infection to adjacent structures, or development of bacteremia.

ADDITIONAL READING
- Brook I. Anaerobic infections in children. *Adv Exp Med Biol*. 2011;697:117–152.
- Brook I. Clinical review: Bacteremia caused by anaerobic bacteria in children. *Crit Care*. 2002;6:205–211.
- Correa AG. Clostridial intoxication and infection. In: Feigin RD, Cherry JD, Demmler GJ, et al., eds. *Textbook of Pediatric Infectious Diseases*. 5th ed. Philadelphia: WB Saunders; 2004:1751–1758.
- Feingold SM. Anaerobic infections. In: Schlossberg D, ed. *Clinical Infectious Disease*. New York: Cambridge University Press; 2008:887–894.

 CODES

ICD9
- 031.1 Cutaneous diseases due to other mycobacteria
- 040.89 Other specified bacterial diseases
- 041.84 Other specified bacterial infections in conditions classified elsewhere and of unspecified site, other anaerobes

ICD10
- A49.8 Other bacterial infections of unspecified site
- A49.9 Bacterial infection, unspecified
- B96.89 Other specified bacterial agents as the cause of diseases classified elsewhere

ANAPHYLAXIS

Mathew Fogg

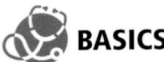 **BASICS**

DESCRIPTION
- Anaphylaxis is an explosive antigen-specific IgE-mediated response resulting in the release of potent biologically active mediators from mast cells and other inflammatory cells. However, non–IgE-mediated direct mast cell degranulation can result in a similar response.
- In fatal anaphylaxis, death may occur from airway obstruction and/or shock. When treating a patient with anaphylaxis, respiratory symptoms and hypotension should be taken very seriously.
- System(s) affected: Heart; lungs; skin; GI tract; upper respiratory tract:
- Any or all of these target organs may be affected.

EPIDEMIOLOGY
Incidence
- 0.4 cases per million individuals annually
- Increased hospital incidence of 0.6 cases per 1,000 patients
- 400–800 deaths annually in the US

RISK FACTORS
Genetics
Atopy can be familial, and atopics are at more risk for anaphylaxis.

PATHOPHYSIOLOGY
- Inducing agents stimulate mast cells to release inflammatory mediators via either an antigen-specific or an antigen-nonspecific manner. These mediators may then act either locally or systemically. Mediator release results are in the table Pathophysiology of Anaphylaxis.

Pathophysiology of anaphylaxis

Pathologic process	Sign or symptom	Putative mediator responsible
Vascular permeability	Urticaria, angioedema, laryngeal edema, abdominal swelling, cramps	Histamine (H1) leukotrienes, prostaglandins
Vasodilation	Flushing, headache	Histamine (H1 and H2), leukotrienes, prostaglandins
Smooth-muscle contraction	Wheezing, gastrointestinal cramps, diarrhea	Histamine (H1), leukotrienes, prostaglandins
Congestion	Rhinorrhea, bronchorrhea	Histamine (H2), prostaglandins, leukotrienes

ETIOLOGY
- IgE mediated:
  - Antibiotics (penicillin and others)
  - Foreign protein agents (insect venom, latex antigens, fire ant venom, blood products, and others)
  - Therapeutic agents (allergen extracts, vaccines, and others)
  - Foods (peanuts, nuts, shellfish, and others)
- Non–IgE-mediated "anaphylactoid" reactions (activates histamine release from mast cells without protein binding to IgE):
  - Radiocontrast media
  - Opiates
  - Dextran
  - Vancomycin
  - Polymyxin B
  - Quaternary ammonium muscle relaxants (i.e., methyl scopolamine bromide, homatropine methylbromide, methantheline bromide, and Pro Banthine bromide)

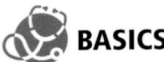 **DIAGNOSIS**

Decide quickly whether the symptoms the patient is experiencing are consistent with anaphylaxis.
- Phase 1: Initiate therapy for anaphylaxis. This generally includes epinephrine 1:1,000 administered SQ, H1 antihistamines, H2 antihistamines, and rapid volume expansion if necessary.
- Phase 2: Attempt to identify the agent that induced the anaphylactic reaction.

HISTORY
- Reaction time to offending allergen:
  - Anaphylactic reactions usually begin within seconds to minutes after contact with offending antigen. This can help the physician identify the antigen responsible.
- History of anaphylaxis:
  - If so, the patient likely knows the allergen responsible.
  - Efforts should be directed toward allergen avoidance.
- Does the patient have autoinjectable epinephrine?
  - Most deaths from anaphylaxis are associated with delayed administration of epinephrine. Most patients with a history of anaphylaxis should have autoinjectable epinephrine.
- Insect sting:
  - Insect or fire ant venom allergy can result in anaphylaxis. It is important to identify the insect if possible (remember that honeybees leave their stinger at the sting site). Immunotherapy is indicated and effective for anaphylaxis in venom-allergic patients.
- Food allergies:
  - Any food can cause anaphylaxis.
  - Dramatic increase in childhood food allergy in past 15 years
  - Cow's milk, egg, soy, peanut, wheat, tree nuts, and shellfish are the most common.

- Medications:
  - Beta-blockers make treatment of anaphylaxis more difficult.
  - Alternative medications (glucagon) should be sought in patients with a history of anaphylaxis.
- Signs And Symptoms
  - Consistent with anaphylaxis:
    - Profuse rhinorrhea
    - Urticaria
    - Wheezing
    - Throat tightness
    - Tachycardia
    - Hypotension
  - Any combination of the following symptoms:
    - Cutaneous: Urticaria/angioedema
    - Respiratory: Bronchospasm/laryngeal edema
    - Cardiovascular: Hypotension, arrhythmias, myocardial ischemia
    - GI: Nausea, vomiting, pain, diarrhea
  - Patients commonly describe a sense of impending doom:
    - May be the 1st sign of an impending anaphylactic reaction

PHYSICAL EXAM
- Angioedema:
  - May be noted anywhere during a systemic allergic reaction
  - Much more significant if it involves the lips, tongue, mouth, or larynx (can result in airway obstruction)
- Urticaria:
  - Cutaneous manifestation of a systemic allergic reaction
- Profuse rhinorrhea:
  - May signal upper respiratory tract involvement in a systemic allergic reaction
- Wheezing:
  - Signals lower respiratory tract involvement in a systemic allergic reaction
- Tachycardia and hypotension:
  - Signals cardiovascular involvement in a systemic allergic reaction
  - Tachycardia usually represents a compensatory mechanism in order to maintain the patient's BP from fluid extravasation.

DIAGNOSTIC TESTS & INTERPRETATION
- Treatment of anaphylaxis should never be withheld while awaiting laboratory confirmation.
- ECG:
  - Anaphylaxis may show rhythm abnormalities, ischemic changes, or infarction on an ECG.

Lab
- Plasma histamine:
  - Plasma histamine is elevated during anaphylaxis, but is difficult to measure because of its extremely short half-life.
  - Useful only in research setting
- Serum tryptase level:
  - Preferred test if available
  - Serum tryptase is elevated during anaphylaxis.
  - Tryptase is elevated for several hours after the onset of anaphylaxis.
  - Tryptase often not elevated in anaphylaxis due to foods

- CBC:
  - Hemoconcentration (as judged by an increased hematocrit or hemoglobin) is common as fluid exits the intravascular space during an anaphylactic reaction.
- Cardiac enzymes:
  - Myocardial ischemia during anaphylaxis may result in a myocardial infarction, and elevated cardiac enzymes.

Note: Skin tests are significantly better than RAST tests for diagnosis of venom and food allergy.

Imaging
Chest radiograph: Bronchospasm associated with anaphylaxis may result in air trapping and hyperinflated lung fields on chest film.

DIFFERENTIAL DIAGNOSIS
- Genetic/metabolic:
  - Hereditary angioedema
  - Systemic mastocytosis
  - Pheochromocytoma
  - Carcinoid
- Allergic/immunologic:
  - Idiopathic
  - Foods
  - Insect stings
  - Drugs
  - Latex
- Nonimmunologic mast cell degranulation
- Exercise-induced (may occur only after ingestion of a specific food)
- Serum sickness
- Miscellaneous:
  - Vasovagal collapse

 TREATMENT

MEDICATION (DRUGS)
First Line
- SQ epinephrine 1:1,000 concentration:
  - Infants to adults: 0.01 mg/kg, maximum of 0.5 mg of 1:1,000 solution, repeated q3–5min
  - Early administration of epinephrine is essential.
- Diphenhydramine IV or PO:
  - Children: 5 mg/kg in 3 or 4 divided doses; maximum 300 mg/d
- Ranitidine IV:
  - 2–4 mg/kg in 2 divided doses
  - H2 blockade may be helpful in refractory anaphylaxis.
- Hydrocortisone or another systemic steroid should be started:
  - 1–5 mg/kg/d in 2–4 divided doses
  - thought to prevent a late-phase reaction
  - Of little help during an immediate anaphylactic reaction
  - Glucagon: Second-line treatment for patients with anaphylaxis on a beta-blocker who are not responding to epinephrine.

ADDITIONAL TREATMENT
General Measures
- Maintain airway.
- A tourniquet may be applied (above the injection or sting site) to decrease venous blood return from the site of antigen entry.

- Supplement with oxygen, place in recumbent position, and elevate legs. Patients have increased oxygen consumption during anaphylaxis.
- Maintain BP with volume expanders or pressors. Hypotension is a serious manifestation of anaphylaxis.

 ONGOING CARE

FOLLOW-UP RECOMMENDATIONS
Patients not admitted to the hospital should be observed for several hours, because late "biphasic" reactions can begin as late as 24 hours after the initial anaphylaxis.

- These patients are at risk for a 2nd episode of anaphylaxis.
- Patients with anaphylaxis should be treated with steroids during the acute treatment, and they should be given a short course of oral corticosteroids to finish at home.
- Must be discharged with autoinjectable epinephrine (this will provide temporary relief so the patient will have time to seek medical assistance).
- Patients must know to seek immediate medical help if symptoms return.

Patient Monitoring
- All patients who have had anaphylaxis should be discharged with epinephrine in an auto-injecting apparatus.

Note: All patients with anaphylaxis would benefit from consultation with an allergist.

- Factors that may help alert you to make a referral include the following:
  - History of idiopathic anaphylaxis:
    - An allergist can help by testing likely triggers.
  - History of anaphylaxis to insect stings or fire ants:
    - Anaphylaxis to insects or fire ants is an indication for venom desensitization.
  - History of food anaphylaxis:
    - The allergist can assist with an appropriate avoidance diet and support resources.
  - History of latex anaphylaxis:
    - The allergist can assist with strict latex-avoidance precautions, and latex testing if the history is unclear.

PATIENT EDUCATION
All patients should follow up with an allergist.

PROGNOSIS
Excellent, provided the trigger can be avoided

COMPLICATIONS
- Pulmonary edema, pulmonary hemorrhage, and pneumothorax
- Laryngeal edema with or without airway obstruction
- Myocardial ischemia and infarction
- Death may result from asphyxiation from upper airway obstruction or profound shock or both.

ADDITIONAL READING

- Bailey E, Shaker M. An update on childhood urticaria and angioedema. *Curr Opin Pediatr.* 2008;20(4):425–430.
- Cahaly RJ, Slater JE. Latex hypersensitivity in children. *Curr Opin Pediatr.* 1995;7:671–675.
- Greenberger PA, Rotskoff BD, Lifschultz B. Fatal anaphylaxis: Postmortem findings and associated comorbid diseases. *Ann Allergy Asthma Immunol.* 2007;98(3):252–257.
- Lane RD, Bolte RG. Pediatric anaphylaxis. *Pediatr Emerg Care.* 2007;23(1):49–56.
- Sicherer SH, Simons FE. Self-injectable epinephrine for first-aid management of anaphylaxis. *Pediatrics.* 2007;119(3):638–646.

 CODES

ICD9
- 977.9 Poisoning by unspecified drug or medicinal substance
- 995.0 Other anaphylactic shock, not elsewhere classified
- 995.60 Anaphylactic shock due to unspecified food

ICD10
- T78.00XA Anaphylactic shock due to unspecified food, initial encounter
- T78.2XXA Anaphylactic shock, unspecified, initial encounter
- T78.09XA Anaphylactic shock due to other food products, initial encounter

FAQ

- Q: Can a patient have an anaphylactic reaction on 1st exposure to an allergen?
- A: A patient must have had a previous exposure to the offending allergen for sensitization to occur. Therefore, anaphylactic reactions should not occur on 1st exposure. Remember: Infants can be sensitized in utero and through breast milk and topically; therefore, a baby may react upon "1st" exposure to a food.
- Q: When should the autoinjectable epinephrine be used?
- A: Immediately at the onset of an anaphylactic reaction. It is recommended to use it for any acute allergic reaction other than isolated hives or skin itching.
- Q: Do patients outgrow this condition?
- A: No. Subsequent reactions tend to have a more rapid onset, and tend to be more severe. Children often outgrow food-induced anaphylaxis.
- Q: Who should be referred to an allergist?
- A: All patients who have experienced anaphylaxis would benefit from consultation with an allergist. Patients with anaphylaxis from insect stings, fire ants, and certain antibiotics can be desensitized. In addition, the allergist can be helpful in identifying obscure triggers of anaphylaxis.

ANEMIA OF CHRONIC DISEASE (ANEMIA OF INFLAMMATION)

Michele P. Lambert

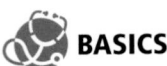 **BASICS**

DESCRIPTION
Anemia that accompanies a variety of systemic diseases, with the common features of chronicity and inflammation. Anemia of chronic disease is more properly called anemia of inflammation (AI) and is the combined result of mildly increased destruction of RBCs, relative erythropoietin resistance, and iron-restricted erythropoiesis.

PATHOPHYSIOLOGY
Typically mild to moderate anemia (Hgb 7–12); develops in the setting of infection, inflammatory disorders, and some malignancies.
- Characterized by inadequate erythrocyte production in the setting of low serum iron and low iron-binding capacity despite normal or increased macrophage iron stores (or increased or normal ferritin as used in clinical practice)
- Typically normochromic, normocytic but, if longstanding, can be hypochromic, microcytic (especially in children)
- Main mechanism appears to be:
  - Iron restriction (limited iron supply to erythropoiesis) Hepcidin is increased by IL-6 and causes depletion of the only known membrane iron transporter (ferroportin) resulting in cellular inability to release stored iron and enterocyte inability to absorb iron.
- Other factors contributing to anemia in various degrees include:
  - Increased red cell destruction
  - Diagnostic phlebotomy or other blood loss
  - Cytokine-mediated interference with erythropoietin signaling
  - Cytokine-mediated suppression of erythropoiesis
  - Cytokines such as interleukin-1 (IL-1) and interleukin-6 (IL-6) can activate ferritin synthesis. The ferritin can lead to sequestration of iron, which eventually is converted into hemosiderin.

ETIOLOGY
Underlying disease process

COMMONLY ASSOCIATED CONDITIONS
- Underlying disease process:
  - Infections, both acute and chronic
  - Inflammatory disease
  - Collagen vascular diseases
  - Malignancies
  - Renal failure
- Anemia of chronic disease often coexists with other causes of anemia, including occult blood loss, hemolysis, dietary iron deficiency, and drug-related marrow suppression

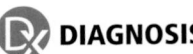 **DIAGNOSIS**

SIGNS AND SYMPTOMS
- Various abnormal physical findings may be present, depending on the underlying chronic disease process.
- May have mild pallor but will not have signs of circulatory collapse.
- Similar disease can be seen more acutely in the setting of anemia of critical illness (also part of AI).

HISTORY
Anemia develops over the first month of the underlying disease process and then remains fairly stable over time.

PHYSICAL EXAM
- Mild pallor
- Mild tachycardia, may be inapparent at rest
- Very rarely more overt signs of anemia such as flow murmur, gallop or hepatomegaly
- Physical findings of the underlying disease

DIAGNOSTIC TESTS & INTERPRETATION
If only the serum iron is obtained, without other iron studies, the child may be inappropriately diagnosed with iron deficiency.

Lab
- CBC with indices
  - Normocytic, normochromic (can be microcytic, hypochromic when very long standing) anemia with hematocrit rarely <20%
  - Reticulocyte count usually in the normal range, but low for the level of anemia
- Iron studies:
  - Low plasma iron, with low total iron-binding capacity
  - Low transferrin saturation by iron
  - Normal or high ferritin level
- Elevated free erythrocyte protoporphyrin
- Hemosiderin in bone marrow macrophages is increased if bone marrow aspiration is done and the aspirate is viewed with iron stains.
- Albumin and transferrin are both low
- Acute-phase reactants such as C-reactive protein may be elevated.

Diagnostic Procedures/Other
Bone marrow aspiration is generally not indicated.

DIFFERENTIAL DIAGNOSIS

Anemia of chronic disease is often confused with iron-deficiency anemia.

- In anemia of chronic disease:
  - Mild to moderate anemia
  - Mild anisocytosis
  - Usually normochromic, normocytic but can be hypochromic with microcytosis
  - Decreased plasma iron
  - Decreased iron-binding capacity
  - Normal or slightly low transferrin saturation
  - Decreased marrow sideroblasts
  - Normal or elevated reticuloendothelial iron
  - Elevated free erythrocyte protoporphyrin
  - Normal or elevated ferritin
- In iron deficiency:
  - Decreased plasma iron
  - Increased iron-binding capacity
  - Decreased transferrin saturation
  - Decreased marrow sideroblasts
  - Decreased reticuloendothelial iron
  - Increased free erythrocyte protoporphyrin
  - Decreased serum ferritin
- In both iron deficiency and anemia of chronic disease:
  - Decreased plasma iron
  - Decreased transferrin saturation
  - Decreased marrow sideroblasts
  - Elevated free erythrocyte protoporphyrin
  - Decreased reticulocyte count
- Tests that help differentiate iron deficiency from anemia of chronic disease:
  - Iron-binding capacity
  - Serum ferritin
  - Reticuloendothelial iron stain in marrow

TREATMENT

GENERAL MEASURES

- Iron:
  - Generally, no role for iron therapy unless there is coexisting iron-deficiency anemia. However, recent studies in patients with renal disease have shown improved response to erythropoietin with coadministration of parenteral iron.
- Recombinant human erythropoietin:
  - Effective, but indications for use are still not universally accepted
  - Often used in chronic renal failure
  - Has been used in inflammatory bowel disease, with good results
  - Should be used for more severe and symptomatic anemia in which the underlying disease is likely to be prolonged and difficult to treat
- Treatment should be directed at the underlying disease process.

SPECIAL THERAPY

Transfusion of packed RBCs is sometimes indicated intermittently in severe anemia with hemodynamic compromise.

ONGOING CARE

FOLLOW-UP RECOMMENDATIONS

Patient Monitoring

Treatment of underlying disease process may promote slow resolution of associated anemia. Hematocrit increases ~6–8 weeks after start of recombinant human erythropoietin therapy; continues to rise over 6 months.

COMPLICATIONS

If severe, patients may be transfusion dependent and, thus, be at risk for complications associated with packed RBC transfusions.

ADDITIONAL READING

- Ganz T, Nemeth E. Iron sequestration and anemia of inflammation. *Sem Hematology.* 2009;46(4): 387–393.
- Ganz T. Molecular pathogenesis of anemia of chronic disease. *Pediatr Blood Cancer.* 2006; 46:554–557.
- Goodnough LT, Skikne B, Brugnara C. Erythropoietin, iron, and erythropoiesis. *Blood.* 2000;96:823–833.

CODES

ICD9

- 281.3 Other specified megaloblastic anemias not elsewhere classified
- 283.0 Autoimmune hemolytic anemias
- 285.29 Anemia of other chronic disease

ICD10

- D53.1 Other megaloblastic anemias, not elsewhere classified
- D59.1 Other autoimmune hemolytic anemias
- D63.8 Anemia in other chronic diseases classified elsewhere

FAQ

- Q: Does anemia that is associated with a chronic disease require further evaluation?
- A: If the anemia fits within the usual expectations for the patient's diagnosis, there is no need to pursue further investigation, except in specific cases. If there is an associated malignancy for which marrow metastasis is possible, a bone marrow aspirate and biopsy should be done. In conditions with malabsorption, nutritional deficiencies, and blood loss should be ruled out.

ANICRYPTOCOCCAL INFECTIONS

Samir S. Shah

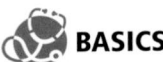
BASICS

DESCRIPTION
Cryptococcosis, an opportunistic fungal infection caused by *Cryptococcus neoformans*, may involve several organ systems, including the CNS, lungs, bones, visceral organs, and skin.

EPIDEMIOLOGY
- Most pediatric infections occur in immunocompromised hosts, including those with malignancy, HIV, and solid organ or bone marrow transplantation; 20% of infections requiring hospitalization occur in normal hosts.
- There is no person-to-person spread of the infection.

Incidence
- Occurs in 5–15% of HIV-infected adults, usually with CD4+ lymphocyte counts <50 cells/mm^3. Occurs in 0.8–2.3% of HIV-infected children. The lower infection rate in children reflects their lower exposure to sources of Cryptococcus neoformans. The overall seroprevalence is 0% in neonates and 4.1% in school-age children, compared to 69% in adults.
- 1–3% of solid-organ transplant recipients develop Cryptococcus neoformans infections; typically >1 year after transplantation.

GENERAL PREVENTION
- Most studies on prevention address HIV-infected patients.
- Use of highly active antiretroviral therapy (HAART) prevents most cases of cryptococcosis in HIV-infected patients.
- Primary prophylaxis with fluconazole prevents new-onset cryptococcal disease in HIV-infected patients. However, primary prophylaxis is not routinely recommended except for those with limited access to HAART and those with high levels of antiretroviral drug resistance.
- Maintenance (suppressive) therapy after completion of therapy for cryptococcal infection is recommended for HIV-infected patients. In those with low CD4+ lymphocyte counts, relapse rates are 100% without maintenance antifungal therapy, 18–25% with amphotericin B or itraconazole, and 2–3% with fluconazole.
  - Prophylaxis may be discontinued in patients receiving HAART with CD4+ lymphocytes >100/mm^3 and undetectable viral loads.
- There is no consensus on the duration of fluconazole suppressive therapy after treatment of cryptococcosis in HIV-negative immunocompromised patients. Most experts provide maintenance (suppressive) antifungal therapy with fluconazole PO (6 mg/kg/d) for at least 1 year after the completion of acute treatment and then reassess its ongoing use based on the level of current immunosuppression.

PATHOPHYSIOLOGY
- Primary infection occurs through the inhalation of aerosolized soil particles containing the yeast forms. The skin and gastrointestinal tract are also portals of entry.
- Protective immune response requires specific T-cell–mediated immunity.
- CNS infection with *Cryptococcus neoformans* results from hematogenous dissemination.

COMMONLY ASSOCIATED CONDITIONS
- *Cryptococcus neoformans* is the most common cause of fungal meningitis in the US.
- Disseminated infection occurs more commonly among immunocompromised hosts.
- Concurrent *Pneumocystis carinii* pneumonia was detected in 13% of adults with cryptococcal meningitis.
- Pulmonary involvement is asymptomatic in up to 50% of cases, and disease may be either focal or widespread.
- Bone involvement occurs in 10% of cases of disseminated cryptococcal infection.
- Cutaneous involvement mimics acne-type eruptions that ulcerate and results from hematogenous spread of the organism or from direct extension of bone infection.

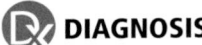
DIAGNOSIS

HISTORY
- Cryptococcal meningitis may present as either an indolent infection or acute illness.
- Symptoms of cryptococcal meningitis include headache, malaise, and low-grade fever. Nausea, vomiting, altered mentation, and photophobia are less common. Stiff neck, focal neurologic symptoms (e.g., decreased hearing, facial nerve palsy, or diplopia), and seizures are rare.
- Primary pulmonary cryptococcal disease is not well described in children because most cases are disseminated at the time of diagnosis. 50% of adults have cough or chest pain, and fewer have sputum production, weight loss, fever, and hemoptysis.
- In immunocompromised hosts, the onset of infection is more rapid and the course more severe. Pulmonary involvement is minimal when dissemination occurs quickly.

PHYSICAL EXAM
- None of the presenting signs of cryptococcal infection are sufficiently characteristic to distinguish it from other infections, particularly in immunocompromised patients.
- CNS involvement: Nuchal rigidity, photophobia, and focal neurologic deficits
- Respiratory tract involvement: Cough, tachypnea, grunting, and subcostal or intercostal retractions. Decreased breath sounds or dullness to percussion may be present, or the lung exam may be normal.
- Cutaneous manifestations: Erythematous or verrucous papules, nodules, pustules, acneiform lesions, ulcers, abscesses, or granulomas. Lesions can occur anywhere on the body, but are found most often on the face and neck.
  - Mucocutaneous findings are present in 10–15% of cases of disseminated disease.

DIAGNOSTIC TESTS & INTERPRETATION
Lab
- Lumbar puncture: Diagnose cryptococcal meningitis:
  - CSF should be sent for cell count and differential; protein; glucose; cultures for bacterial, fungal, and viral pathogens; and cryptococcal antigen (India ink stain is less commonly performed).
  - Examination of the CSF reveals <500 WBC/mm^3 (usually <100 WBC/mm^3), mostly mononuclear leukocytes, with minimal changes in protein. CSF glucose is <50 mg/dL in ~65% of patients.
  - Budding yeast are seen on India ink stain in 50% of cases.
  - CSF cultures are positive in ~90% of patients.
  - The latex agglutination test for cryptococcal polysaccharide antigen is specific, sensitive, and rapid. Titers ≥1:4 suggest the diagnosis of cryptococcal infection if appropriate controls (to exclude the presence of rheumatoid factor or other nonspecific agglutinins) are negative.
  - HIV-infected patients with pneumonia and CD4+ T-lymphocyte counts <200 cells/mm^3 should be evaluated with sputum fungal culture, blood fungal culture, and a serum cryptococcal antigen test. A lumbar puncture to exclude the possibility of occult meningitis should be considered. If any test is positive for *Cryptococcus neoformans*, then a lumbar puncture should be performed to exclude cryptococcal meningitis.
- Blood culture and serum cryptococcal antigen titers: Diagnose disseminated cryptococcal infection. Serum cryptococcal antigen tests are positive in >85% of patients with cryptococcal meningitis.
- Sputum culture: Diagnose cryptococcal pneumonia.
- Skin or bone biopsy: Diagnose cutaneous or osteoarticular cryptococcal infection.
- HIV testing: Evaluation for immunodeficiencies, including HIV, is warranted in any patient with cryptococcosis.
- CBC with differential: May reveal hypereosinophilia (absolute eosinophil count >1,500/mm^3)
- Serum electrolytes: Detect hyponatremia, a complication of cryptococcal meningitis.

Imaging
- Chest x-rays (anteroposterior and lateral): Nodules, diffuse infiltrates, and pleural effusions may be seen in cryptococcal pneumonia.
- Head CT or MRI: May demonstrate granulomatous lesions (cryptococcomas; ~15% of patients with meningitis) or elevated intracranial pressure. MRI reveals dilation of perivascular spaces in almost half the cases.

DIFFERENTIAL DIAGNOSIS

- Although cryptococcosis occurs most commonly in HIV-infected patients with low CD4+ lymphocyte counts, the diagnosis warrants consideration in all febrile immunocompromised children (e.g., solid-organ transplant, leukemia)
- Meningitis: Viruses and *Mycobacterium tuberculosis*
- Pneumonia: Other pulmonary mycoses, including aspergillosis, histoplasmosis, and blastomycosis. Also consider *Mycoplasma pneumoniae* and *Mycobacterium tuberculosis*.
- Bone: Osteogenic sarcoma
- Cutaneous: Molluscum contagiosum, herpes simplex virus infection, pyoderma gangrenosum, and cellulitis

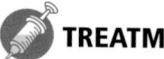 **TREATMENT**

ADDITIONAL TREATMENT
General Measures
- Clinical management depends on extent of disease and immune status of the host.
- Pulmonary and extrapulmonary disease, HIV-negative, nontransplant:
  - Normal hosts with isolated pulmonary nodules may not need treatment if the serum cryptococcal antigen is negative and the patient is asymptomatic.
  - Patients with symptoms, extensive pulmonary disease, or evidence of extrapulmonary disease require treatment.
  - Fluconazole 6–12 mg/kg/d PO (max 400 mg) for 6–12 months for mild/moderate disease. Alternate regimen: Itraconazole 4–10 mg/kg/d PO (max 400 mg) for 6–12 months (monitor drug levels); or amphotericin B 0.7–1 mg/kg/d PO for 3–6 months.
  - Same as CNS for severe disease
  - Maintenance therapy with fluconazole should be considered for immunocompromised patients (see "Prevention").
- CNS, HIV-negative, non-transplant:
  - Induction/consolidation: Amphotericin B (0.7–1 mg/kg/d) plus flucytosine (100–150 mg/kg/d PO, divided q6h) for 4 weeks, then fluconazole PO (10–12 mg/kg/d) for a minimum of 8 weeks followed by maintenance therapy with fluconazole PO (6 mg/kg/d) for 6–12 months. Alternate induction/consolidation regimen: Amphotericin B plus flucytosine for 6–10 weeks.
- Pulmonary and extrapulmonary disease, HIV-infected, or transplant:
  - Fluconazole (PO) 6–12 months for mild/moderate disease; same as CNS infection for severe disease.
  - Consider surgical débridement for patients with persistent or refractory pulmonary or bone lesions.
- CNS disease, HIV-infected or transplant:
  - Induction/consolidation: Amphotericin B (IV) plus flucytosine (PO) for at least 2 weeks, followed by fluconazole PO (10–12 mg/kg/d) for at least 8 weeks; consider subsequent suppressive therapy with fluconazole PO (6 mg/kg/d)
  - Intrathecal amphotericin B is very toxic but may be used in refractory cases.

- HIV-infected patients require continuation of antifungal drugs indefinitely because of the high recurrence rate of cryptococcosis.
- Liposomal amphotericin (5 mg/kg/d) or amphotericin B lipid complex (5 mg/kg/d) IV may be substituted for amphotericin B, especially in patients with pre-existing renal dysfunction and those receiving calcineurin inhibitors.
- Flucytosine is used only in combination with amphotericin B and not as a single agent because of the rapid emergence of drug resistance.
- Voriconazole, a new triazole antifungal agent, demonstrates excellent in vitro activity against *Cryptococcus neoformans* but requires clinical study. Caspofungin, a new echinocandin antifungal agent, is not active against *Cryptococcus neoformans*.

 ONGOING CARE

FOLLOW-UP RECOMMENDATIONS
Patient Monitoring
- Because of the risk of relapse, patients should be seen at 3-month intervals for 12–18 months following treatment. Immunocompromised patients should be evaluated every 2–3 months, even while on suppressive therapy, to monitor clinically for relapse.
- Repeat lumbar punctures documenting a decrease in CSF cryptococcal antigen and sterility of culture are useful in evaluating response to treatment. During therapy for acute meningitis, an unchanged or increased titer of CSF antigen correlates with clinical and microbiologic failure to respond to treatment. Serum antigen titers are not helpful for this purpose.
- Evaluate patients with cryptococcal meningitis for neurologic sequelae.
- HIV-infected patients require suppressive antifungal therapy (see "Prevention").

PROGNOSIS
- Mortality is rare in patients with isolated pulmonary or cutaneous disease.
- In-hospital mortality is ~20% for cryptococcal meningitis and ~8% for non-CNS cryptococcal infections.
  - In normal hosts with meningitis, poor prognostic factors include serum or CSF cryptococcal titers >1:32 or CSF WBC <20/mm^3.
  - In HIV-infected patients with meningitis, poor prognostic factors include hyponatremia, concomitant growth of *Cryptococcus neoformans* from another site, increased intracranial pressure, and any alteration of mental status.
- Up to 40% of patients with cryptococcal meningitis have residual neurologic deficits.
- Relapse rates are high in HIV-infected patients (see "Prevention").

COMPLICATIONS
- Elevated intracranial pressure with meningitis.
- Pulmonary, cutaneous, and bone involvement may occur (see "Associated Conditions").
- In solid-organ transplant patients, those receiving tacrolimus immunosuppression are less likely to have CNS involvement and more likely to have skin, soft tissue, or osteoarticular involvement.

ADDITIONAL READING

- Gonzalez CE, Shetty D, Lewis LL, et al. Cryptococcosis in human immunodeficiency virus-infected children. *Pediatr Infect Dis J*. 1996;15:796–800.
- Joshi NS, Fisher BT, Prasad PA, et al. Epidemiology of cryptococcal infection in hospitalized children. *Pediatr Infect Dis J*. 2010;29:e91–e95.
- Pappas PG, Perfect JR, Cloud GA, et al. Cryptococcosis in human immunodeficiency virus-negative patients in the era of effective azole therapy. *Clin Infect Dis*. 2001;33:690–699.
- Perfect JR, Dismukes WE, Dromer F, et al. Clinical practice guidelines for the management of cryptococcal disease: 2010 update by the Infectious Diseases Society of America. *Clin Infect Dis*. 2010;50:291–322.

 CODES

ICD9
- 117.5 Cryptococcosis
- 321.0 Cryptococcal meningitis

ICD10
- B45.1 Cerebral cryptococcosis
- B45.9 Cryptococcosis, unspecified

FAQ

- Q: What are the sources of *Cryptococcus* in nature?
- A: Pigeon droppings and soil. Naturally acquired infections occur in lower mammals, especially cats. However, neither animal-to-human nor human-to-human infections have been reported.
- Q: Should all children with *Cryptococcus* be evaluated for immunodeficiency?
- A: Yes.

ANKYLOSING SPONDYLITIS

Timothy Beukelman
Randy Q. Cron
Eric Hanson (5th edition)

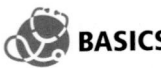 **BASICS**

DESCRIPTION
An inflammatory arthritis that tends to be asymmetric peripherally and involve the insertion of tendons and ligaments and the sacroiliac joints and spine

EPIDEMIOLOGY
• Typically affects adolescent boys
• Much less common in blacks:
  – HLA-B27 occurs in 70–90% of patients, and is present in 8% of whites and 6% of blacks in the general population.

Prevalence
~1/10,000 white boys

RISK FACTORS
Genetics
• HLA-B27 associated
• Usually a family history of a male relative with disease

PATHOPHYSIOLOGY
Inflammatory synovitis of joints and calcification of the anterior and posterior longitudinal ligaments of the spine

ETIOLOGY
Idiopathic

 DIAGNOSIS

• Inflammatory back pain (better with exercise, not relieved by rest) of insidious onset that has been present for at least 6 weeks.
• Inactivity stiffness resulting in gelling of peripheral joints and back

HISTORY
• Pain
• Family history

PHYSICAL EXAM
• Sacroiliac tenderness:
  – Indicates site of inflammation
• Pain on direct palpation at insertion of Achilles tendon and plantar fascia at calcaneal insertion (location of entheses):
  – Indicates site of inflammation

DIAGNOSTIC TESTS & INTERPRETATION
• Schober test of lumbar spine flexibility:
  – Mark 15-cm span at mid-lower back at level of iliac crest while patient is standing.
  – Have patient flex back as far as possible.
  – Re-measure span.
  – Abnormal if <5 cm increase in span

Lab
CBC, erythrocyte sedimentation rate (ESR), HLA-B27, rheumatoid factor (RF), and antinuclear antibody (ANA) tests:
• ESR is occasionally not elevated.
• RF and ANA are typically negative.

Imaging
Sacroiliac views:
• Demonstrate evidence of pseudo-widening, erosions, and/or sclerosis, with fusion being a late finding. Because x-ray findings may take years to develop in the presence of disease, MRI is supplanting x-ray as the initial modality to assess SI involvement in some centers.

DIFFERENTIAL DIAGNOSIS
• Caution:
  – Over-diagnosis in HLA-B27–positive individuals in whom other causes for joint swelling should be considered
• Infection:
  – Reactive arthritis caused by enteric pathogens or *Chlamydia* species
  – Whipple disease
  – Intestinal-bypass–associated arthritis
  – Discitis
  – Pott disease
• Tumors:
  – Osteoid osteoma
• Trauma:
  – Traumatic injury causing lower back pain/spasm
  – Herniated disc
• Metabolic:
  – Ochronosis
• Congenital:
  – Kyphosis
• Immunologic:
  – Inflammatory bowel disease–associated arthropathy
  – Oligoarticular juvenile idiopathic arthritis
• Psychologic:
  – Feigning lower back pain/stiffness
• Miscellaneous:
  – Psoriasis-associated arthritis

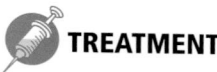 **TREATMENT**

MEDICATION (DRUGS)
- NSAIDs:
  - Naproxen
  - Indomethacin
  - Diclofenac
- Disease-modifying drugs:
  - Sulfasalazine
  - Methotrexate
  - Leflunomide
  - Tumor necrosis factor inhibitors

ADDITIONAL TREATMENT
General Measures
- Therapy may need to be lifelong.
- After initiation of therapy, should see some improvement in stiffness, synovitis, and range of motion over weeks to several months

Additional Therapies
Physical therapy:
- Physical therapy is an essential component of treatment.
- Must encourage range-of-motion exercises and avoid prolonged neck flexion.

SURGERY/OTHER PROCEDURES
In advanced cases, total hip replacement, C-spine fusion, and/or spinal wedge osteotomy (the latter if posture is severely affected).

 ONGOING CARE

DIET
- Food intake should be good with NSAIDs.
- Ensure folate intake with methotrexate.

PATIENT EDUCATION
Activity:
- As tolerated. In cases of severe/advanced disease, modify behaviors accordingly in consideration of reduced spine flexibility and subsequent risk of serious injury.

PROGNOSIS
Poor if disease remains active for 10 years or more

COMPLICATIONS
- Acute anterior uveitis
- Aortic insufficiency
- Worsening stiffness
- Ankylosis with risk of vertebral subluxation, fracture, and nerve damage, including cauda equina syndrome
- Acute or chronic eye pain
- Chest pain or shortness of breath

ADDITIONAL READING
- Colbert RA. Classification of juvenile spondyloarthropathies: Enthesitis-related arthritis and beyond. *Nat Rev Rheumatol*. 2010;6:477–485.
- Colbert RA. Early axial spondyloarthritis. *Curr Opin Rheumatol*. 2010;22:603–607.
- Stoll ML, Lio P, Sundel RP, et al. Comparison of Vancouver and International League of Associations for rheumatology classification criteria for juvenile psoriatic arthritis. *Arthritis Rheum*. 2008;59:51–58.

- Homeff G, Burgos-Vargas R. TNF-alpha antagonists for the treatment of juvenile-onset spondyloarthritides. *Clin Exp Rheumatol*. 2002;20(suppl 28):S137–S142.
- Sherry DD, Sapp LR. Enthesalgia in childhood: Site-specific tenderness in healthy subjects and in patients with seronegative enthesopathic arthropathy. *J Rheumatol*. 2003;30:1335–1340.
- Tse SM, Laxer RM. Juvenile spondyloarthropathy. *Curr Opin Rheumatol*. 2003;15:374–379.
- Tse SM, Laxer RM, Babyn PS, et al. Radiologic improvement of juvenile idiopathic arthritis-enthesitis-related arthritis following anti-tumor necrosis factor-alpha blockade with etanercept. *J Rheumatol*. 2006;33:1186–1188.

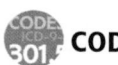 **CODES**

ICD9
720.0 Ankylosing spondylitis

ICD10
- M08.1 Juvenile ankylosing spondylitis
- M45.9 Ankylosing spondylitis of unspecified sites in spine

FAQ
- Q: Should HLA-B27 be checked routinely in boys with back pain?
- A: Detection of HLA-B27 alone should not precipitate an extensive workup because it is so common in the normal healthy population. However, the risk for developing a spondyloarthropathy is 16 times greater than in HLA-B27–negative individuals.
- Q: Can affected individuals play contact sports?
- A: This is probably not a good idea because as the spine fuses, the risk for fracture of the spine (especially the cervical spine) increases. However, children with milder forms of disease, such as enthesitis related arthritis, should not be discouraged.

ANOMALOUS CORONARY ARTERY

Shellie M. Kendall
Geoffrey L. Bird (5th edition)

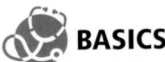 **BASICS**

DESCRIPTION
The anomalous coronary artery arises from the pulmonary artery rather than the aorta. Most commonly, the left coronary is the anomalous artery.

EPIDEMIOLOGY
Incidence
Very rare anomaly. Occurs in 0.25% of congenital heart disease.

Prevalence
The majority of patients present in infancy, at around the age of 2 months. The literature contains case reports of patients presenting as old as during the 4th to 7th decades of life.

PATHOPHYSIOLOGY
- In the neonatal period, pulmonary artery pressure is increased owing to elevated pulmonary vascular resistance. Initially this elevated pulmonary artery pressure provides antegrade flow from the pulmonary artery through the anomalous coronary artery. As pulmonary vascular resistance drops, pulmonary artery pressure drops. When the diastolic blood pressure in the pulmonary artery is lower than the myocardial perfusion pressure (diastolic aortic pressure), pulmonary runoff "steals" blood from the myocardium, resulting in myocardial ischemia.
- The fact that the left ventricle is perfused with desaturated blood plays a less important role than the overall perfusion-related imbalance between myocardial oxygen demand and supply.

ETIOLOGY
- Abnormal septation of the conotruncus into the aorta and pulmonary artery
- Persistence of the pulmonary buds and involution of the aortic buds that will eventually form the coronary arteries
- As-yet-unspecified genetic predisposition

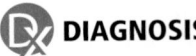 **DIAGNOSIS**

HISTORY
- Typically presents with paroxysms of poor feeding, pallor, tachypnea, and diaphoresis
- Irritability, crying, appearance of being in pain (especially after meals)
- Congestive heart failure
- Can be asymptomatic
- Can be symptomatic in infancy and then gradually improve (with the development of adequate coronary collateralization)
- Older children and adults may have dyspnea, syncope, or angina pectoris
- Sudden death

PHYSICAL EXAM
- Signs of congestive heart failure (e.g., cachexia, tachycardia, tachypnea, lethargy, diaphoresis)
- Loud P_2 component of S
- Gallop rhythm
- Murmur of mitral regurgitation, or a continuous murmur reminiscent of a coronary arteriovenous fistula
- Diagnosis should be entertained in any infant presenting with cardiomegaly or perplexing cardiorespiratory symptoms.

DIAGNOSTIC TESTS & INTERPRETATION
Imaging
- Chest radiograph: Cardiomegaly, pulmonary edema
- Nuclear imaging: Thallium myocardial perfusion imaging shows reduced uptake in ischemic regions.
- Electrocardiography: Anterolateral infarct pattern in an infant (Q in I, aVL, V_4–V_6), abnormal R-wave progression in precordial leads
- Echocardiogram: Attachment of coronary artery to pulmonary artery by 2-dimensional imaging. Doppler interrogation shows flow passing from coronary artery to great artery rather than vice versa.
  - Dilation of the right coronary artery
  - Left ventricular function impairment, wall motion abnormalities, and dilation
  - Mitral regurgitation
  - Echogenic papillary muscles

Diagnostic Procedures/Other
- Cardiac catheterization: Angiographic and hemodynamic parameters may correlate with degree of cardiovascular dysfunction.
  - Low cardiac output
  - High left atrial filling pressures
  - Pulmonary arterial hypertension
- Aortic root angiography shows passage of contrast medium from normally connected right coronary artery to the left coronary arterial system to the pulmonary artery.
- Pulmonary artery angiogram shows reflux of contrast medium into the left coronary artery and/or a "negative wash-in" of unopacified blood flowing from left coronary to pulmonary artery.
- Coronary CT angiography: Excellent diagnostic modality for older patients with slower heart rates allowing better resolution.

DIFFERENTIAL DIAGNOSIS
- Cardiomyopathy
- Mitral valve regurgitation
- Left ventricular failure from other causes
- Colic
- Bronchiolitis

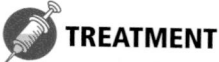 **TREATMENT**

ADDITIONAL TREATMENT
General Measures
The 1st priority is to safely institute supportive care measures while expeditiously planning for surgical intervention. Medical therapy alone has a very limited role in the current era.

SURGERY/OTHER PROCEDURES
- Direct reimplantation of the left coronary artery into the aorta using a button of pulmonary arterial tissue and/or an extension-tube graft of anterior and posterior pulmonary arterial wall tissue sewn into a narrow cylinder to avoid tension, distortion, and stenosis of the coronary
- Creation of an aortopulmonary window and tunnel that directs blood from aorta to the left coronary ostium (Takeuchi procedure).
- Ligation of the origin of the left coronary artery (to prevent flow runoff into the pulmonary artery or "steal") is less frequently used, even in very ill infants.
- Ligation of the origin of the left coronary artery and reconstitution of flow with saphenous or internal mammary graft is less frequently used in the current era.

IN-PATIENT CONSIDERATIONS
Initial Stabilization
Attention to basic life support measures (airway, breathing, and circulation) and prompt referral to a pediatric cardiac center. An excess of procedures, interventions, and manipulation is poorly tolerated by this group of patients. Even with the full support of a tertiary care center's experienced team, these measures are fraught with peril.

 ONGOING CARE

PROGNOSIS
- Untreated, 65–85% of those who present in infancy will die before the age of 1 year, usually after 2 months of age (when pulmonary vascular resistance falls).
- Very few of those who present early improve spontaneously.
- Late results after surgery are excellent in many centers. Hospital mortality in larger selected series of these frequently moribund patients is ≤5%, with very little subsequent attrition.
- Mitral regurgitation usually improves after surgery establishes a patent dual-coronary system, but this may take 6–12 months to be fully realized. Follow-up evaluation is warranted, as mitral regurgitation may progress despite surgery, and valve repair may be required later.

ADDITIONAL READING

- Azakie A, Russell JL, McCrindle BW, et al. Anatomic repair of anomalous left coronary artery from the pulmonary artery by aortic re-implantation: Early survival, patterns of ventricular recovery and late outcome. *Ann Thorac Surg.* 2003;75(5):1535–1541.
- Dodge-Khatami A, Mavroudis C, Backer CL. Anomalous origin of the left coronary artery from the pulmonary artery: Collective review of surgical therapy. *Ann Thorac Surg.* 2002;74(3):946–955.
- Keane JF, Lock JE, Fyler DC, eds. *Nadas' Pediatric Cardiology.* Philadelphia: WB Saunders; 2006.
- Lange R, Vogt M, Horer J, et al. Long-term results of repair of anomalous origin of the left coronary artery from the pulmonary artery. *Ann Thorac Surg.* 2007;83(4):1463–1471.
- Michielon G, Di Carlo D, Brancaccio G, et al. Anomalous coronary artery origin from the pulmonary artery: Correlation between surgical timing and left ventricular function recovery. *Ann Thorac Surg.* 2003;76(2):581–588, discussion 588.
- Pelliccia A. Congenital coronary artery anomalies in young patients: New perspectives for timely identification. *J Am Coll Cardiol.* 2001;37(2):598–600.

 CODES

ICD9
746.85 Coronary artery anomaly

ICD10
- Q24.5 Malformation of coronary vessels
- Q25.8 Other congenital malformations of other great arteries

FAQ
- Q: How do you differentiate crying from the symptoms of myocardial ischemia from crying from colic?
- A: This is not easy, but clinical assessment should manifest the signs of CHF, shock, and low cardiac output, which are decidedly atypical for the usual patient with colic. If the patient is still feeding, the crying in patients with this lesion classically occurs after meals, when blood is shunted to the liver and intestines. This is not a highly sensitive finding, and concern should lead to further objective evaluation.

ANOREXIA NERVOSA

Candice P. Chen

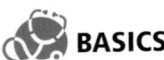 **BASICS**

DESCRIPTION
DSM-IV criteria:
- Refusal to maintain body weight at or above a minimally normal weight (i.e., weight loss or failure to gain weight during a period of growth leading to maintenance of body weight <85% of expected)
- Intense fear of gaining weight or becoming fat, even though underweight
- Disturbance in the way in which one's body weight, shape, or size is perceived; undue influence of body weight or shape on self-esteem; or denial of seriousness of currently low body weight
- In postmenarchal females, amenorrhea
- Types: Restricting (no binge eating or purging) or binge eating/purging

Reprinted with permission from the *Diagnostic and Statistical Manual of Mental Disorders*, 4th ed., text revision (Copyright 2000). American Psychiatric Association.

EPIDEMIOLOGY
Prevalence
- Typically, adolescent girls or young women, although 5–15% of cases are in male patients
- Estimated 0.5–1% of adolescents have an eating disorder.
- Studies indicate that >50% of children and adolescents presenting with a concern of an eating disorder do not meet the full DSM-IV diagnostic criteria but still require treatment.

RISK FACTORS
More prevalent in industrialized societies; occurs in all US household income levels and major ethnic groups.
- Dieting is a possible risk factor for the future development of an eating disorder.
- Adolescents participating in activities that emphasize maintaining a certain weight (e.g., gymnastics, ballet, ice skating, wrestling) are at increased risk.
- Personality traits such as low self-esteem, difficulty expressing negative emotions, difficulty resolving conflict, and perfectionist tendencies are associated with an increased risk.

Genetics
Family and twin studies indicate a genetic component. A relative of a person with an eating disorder has a 10× greater lifetime risk of developing an eating disorder.

GENERAL PREVENTION
When counseling on obesity, take care not to foster overaggressive dieting. Help children and adolescents build self-esteem while addressing their weight concerns.

PATHOPHYSIOLOGY
- Physical manifestations are generally due to weight loss and malnutrition. In an attempt to conserve energy, the body becomes functionally hypothyroid (euthyroid sick syndrome). Body temperature and heart rate decrease. As cardiac function becomes impaired, orthostasis and hypotension occur. Reduced peripheral circulation causes hair thinning, brittle nails, dry skin, and lanugo.
- Hypothalamic hypogonadism results from malnutrition and stress and causes delayed puberty and amenorrhea. Decreased estrogen and testosterone also contribute to osteoporosis.
- Electrolyte abnormalities generally develop as a result of malnutrition. However, sodium abnormalities may develop owing to dehydration or excess water intake, and hypokalemia may develop secondary to vomiting and/or laxative or diuretic use.

ETIOLOGY
Multifactorial including genetic, neurochemical, psychodevelopmental, and sociocultural factors

COMMONLY ASSOCIATED CONDITIONS
- Depression
- Anxiety disorders
- Substance abuse

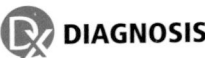 **DIAGNOSIS**

HISTORY
- Question: Have you ever weighed much less than other people thought you should?
  - Patients may try to hide their illness. A negative response does not negate an eating disorder.
- Question: What is the least amount you have weighed in the past year?
  - The reported weight, along with the current height, should be used to calculate a body mass index (BMI).
- Question: Are you afraid of gaining weight?
  - Patients will often report an intense fear of gaining weight.
- Question: How do you think you look?
  - A patient's perceived body image is often distorted. Perceived body image may be significantly misaligned with reality.
- Question in postmenarchal females: Have you ever missed menstrual periods? Have you ever missed 3 in a row?
  - 3 or more missed periods in a row is an indication of amenorrhea.
- Obtain a diet history, including 24-hour diet, history of binge-eating, purging, food restrictions, or calorie counting; use of diuretics, laxatives, diet pills, or emetics; elimination history; exercise history (i.e., how much, intensity); menstrual history; substance use.

PHYSICAL EXAM
- All patients should have a full physical exam with special emphasis on:
  - Vital signs, weight, height, BMI: Patient may have bradycardia, hypotension, orthostasis, or hypothermia; BMI is needed to determine if weight is <85% expected.
  - Physical and sexual growth and development: Patient may be emaciated or have atrophic breasts or delayed puberty.
  - Cardiovascular system: May detect a cardiac arrhythmia, murmur, or evidence of congestive heart failure
  - Dry skin, lanugo, thinning scalp hair, angular stomatitis
  - Salivary gland enlargement or Russell sign (scarring on dorsum of hand): Suggests purging behavior
  - Muscular irritability or weakness: May occur with severe malnutrition or use of an emetic
  - Evidence of self-injurious behavior: May indicate previous suicide attempts
- All patients need dental exam for enamel erosion and tooth loss due to purging behavior or insufficient calcium intake, respectively.

DIAGNOSTIC TESTS & INTERPRETATION
Lab
- All patients with anorexia nervosa:
  - Serum electrolytes, blood urea nitrogen/creatinine: Most are normal, may show dehydration or sodium or potassium abnormalities
  - TSH; if indicated, free T_4, T_3: To rule out thyroid disease
  - CBC with differential: Mild anemia is common due to iron or folate deficiency; WBC count is generally low due to malnutrition.
  - ESR: Generally low due to malnutrition
  - AST, ALT, alkaline phosphatase: Occasionally abnormal due to fatty liver
  - Urinalysis: Evaluate specific gravity to assess for dehydration that may be seen with purging or diuretic use.
- Malnourished and severely symptomatic patients:
  - Complement component 3a: May indicate nutritional deficiencies when other markers are within normal ranges
  - Serum calcium, magnesium, phosphorous: May all be low; in hospitalized patients follow phosphorous daily to assess for refeeding syndrome.
  - Serum ferritin: May be low
  - Electrocardiogram: May have bradycardia, ST-T wave abnormalities with hypokalemia, increased PR interval and 1st-degree heart block, prolonged QTc
  - 24-hour urine for creatinine clearance: Generally low, normal may indicate azotemia
- Patients amenorrheic for >6 months:
  - Dual-energy x-ray absorptiometry (DEXA) scan: Evaluates bone density to determine risk of compression fracture and bone loss
- Nonroutine assessments:
  - Toxicology screen, if suspect substance use
  - Serum amylase, fractionated for salivary gland isoenzyme: If available, with vomiting, will be elevated
  - Serum LH, FSH, prolactin, if persistent amenorrhea with normal weight: LH and FSH will generally be low.
  - β-HCG: Rule out pregnancy.
  - Stool for guaiac, if suspected GI bleed
  - Stool or urine for bisacodyl, emodin, aloe-emodin, and rhein, if suspected laxative abuse

DIFFERENTIAL DIAGNOSIS
- Oncologic: Brain tumor, other cancers
- Gastroenterologic: Inflammatory bowel disease, celiac disease
- Endocrinologic: Diabetes mellitus, thyroid disease, hypopituitarism, Addison disease
- Psychiatric: Depression, obsessive-compulsive disorder, substance abuse
- Other chronic diseases or infections
- Superior mesenteric artery syndrome (can also be a consequence of eating disorder)

TREATMENT

MEDICATION (DRUGS)

Medications should be used in conjunction with nutritional and psychosocial treatment, not as the primary or sole modality of treatment. If possible, defer medications until weight has been restored.

- Antidepressants to treat persistent depression or anxiety:
  - SSRIs have the most evidence for efficacy.
  - Do not use bupropion in patients with eating disorders because of an increased risk of seizures in patients with eating disorders.
  - Avoid tricyclic antidepressants and MAOIs owing to potential lethality and toxicity with overdose.
- Consider 2nd-generation and low-potency antipsychotics for select patients with severe symptoms such as severe resistance to gaining weight, severe obsessive thinking, and/or disease denial that approaches delusional status.

ADDITIONAL TREATMENT

Psychosocial treatment:

- Goals: Understand and change behaviors and attitudes related to eating disorder, improve interpersonal and social functioning, address comorbid psychopathology
- Psychotherapy: Individual, family, group. Evidence suggests outcomes are better for family therapy than individual therapy for adolescents.

ISSUES FOR REFERRAL

The treatment of anorexia generally involves a multidisciplinary team, including a pediatrician, a nutritionist, and a psychiatrist. In some areas, patients may also be referred to pediatricians who specialize in eating disorders.

IN-PATIENT CONSIDERATIONS

Admission Criteria

Criteria for inpatient hospitalization:

- Weight <75% ideal body weight or weight loss despite treatment; food refusal; body fat <10%; daytime heart rate <50 bpm; nighttime heart rate <45 bpm; systolic blood pressure <90 mm Hg; orthostatic hypotension; temperature <96°F; arrhythmia
- Additional factors to consider: Suicidality, other psychiatric disorders requiring hospitalization, severe substance use disorder, uncontrolled vomiting, hematemesis, weight close to previous weight where patient became medically unstable

Discharge Criteria

Patient is medically stable. Evidence indicates that patients who reach 90% of their recommended average body weight before discharge have lower readmission rates.

 ONGOING CARE

DIET

Nutritional treatment:

- Goals: Restore weight, normalize eating patterns, achieve normal perceptions of hunger and satiety, correct malnutrition
- Establish target weight and rate of weight gain: Goal is weight at which menstruation is restored or normal physical and sexual development resume.
- Usually begin intake at 30–40 kcal/kg/d, may increase to 70–100 kcal/kg/d. Weight gain goal 0.25–1 kg/wk is realistic.
- In severely malnourished patients, avoid refeeding syndrome by starting slowly, generally 1,000–1,600 kcal/d, increasing by 200–400 kcal/d.
- Reserve NG feeds for patients with extreme difficulty recognizing their illness, those refusing treatment, or those with eating-associated guilt.
- Evaluate and treat GI symptoms including constipation, bloating, and abdominal pain. Stool softeners and polyethylene glycol are treatments of choice. Avoid stimulant laxatives.
- Add vitamin and mineral supplements (e.g., phosphorous, calcium); may require acute supplementation.
- When desired weight is achieved, calculate ongoing caloric intake based on weight and activity (usually 40–60 kcal/kg/d).

PATIENT EDUCATION

Help limit physical activity and caloric expenditure if exercise is a significant component of the patient's illness.

PROGNOSIS

Adolescent outcomes are better than adult outcomes. One study following adolescents hospitalized for anorexia nervosa showed 86.3% with partial or complete recovery at 10–15-year follow-up. However, the median time to partial recovery was 57.4 months.

COMPLICATIONS

- Fluid and electrolyte imbalances
- Rapid refeeding of severely malnourished patients (refeeding syndrome) can cause hypophosphatemia, leading to cardiac failure, stupor and coma, and hemolytic anemia.
- Cardiovascular: ECG abnormalities (conduction abnormalities are thought to be the most common proximal cause of death), pericardial effusion; and use of ipecac (an emetic no longer available) was associated with irreversible myocardial damage and diffuse myositis
- GI: Delayed gastric emptying, slow GI motility, bloating, constipation, fatty liver, hypercholesterolemia from abnormal lipoprotein metabolism, and esophagitis or Mallory-Weiss tears from chronic vomiting
- Endocrine: Euthyroid sick syndrome, amenorrhea, osteopenia, growth retardation (may have permanent effects in younger patients)

- Renal: Increased risk of renal stones, polyuria due to abnormal vasopressin secretion; in refeeding, 25% develop peripheral edema due to increased renal sensitivity to aldosterone.
- Hematologic: Anemia, leukopenia, thrombocytopenia
- Neuropsychologic: Cortical atrophy, apathy, poor concentration, cognitive impairment, seizures, peripheral neuropathy

ADDITIONAL READING

- American Academy of Pediatrics Committee on Adolescence. Identification and management of eating disorders in children and adolescents. *Pediatrics.* 2010;126(6):1240–1253.
- American Psychiatric Association. *Treatment of patients with eating disorders, 3rd ed. Am J Psychiatry.* 2006;163(7 Suppl):4–54.
- Becker AE, Grinspoon SK, Klibanski A, et al. Eating disorders. *N Engl J Med.* 1999;340:1092–1098.
- Zimmerman M. *Interview guide for evaluating DSM-IV psychiatric disorders and the mental status examination.* East Greenwich, RI: Psych Production Press; 1994.

See Also (Topic, Algorithm, Electronic Media Element)

- National Eating Disorders Association (www.nationaleatingdisorders.org)
- National Association of Anorexia Nervosa and Associated Disorders (www.anad.org)

 CODES

ICD9

307.1 Anorexia nervosa

ICD10

- F50.00 Anorexia nervosa, unspecified
- F50.01 Anorexia nervosa, restricting type
- F50.02 Anorexia nervosa, binge eating/purging type

FAQ

- Q: What is the expected inpatient treatment duration?
- A: Duration of hospitalization varies; average is ~5–6 weeks.
- Q: When may the patient return to school?
- A: Generally, weight should be >85% of expected, the student should be medically stable, and the health professional should work with the school administration to ensure a suitable treatment program.
- Q: When may the athlete return to play?
- A: Generally, when weight is >85% of expected, the patient is medically stable, and a suitable treatment plan is in place.

ANTHRAX
Andrew P. Steenhoff

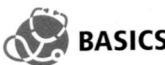 **BASICS**

DESCRIPTION
Bacillus anthracis is a spore-forming, Gram-positive rod that can cause acute infection (anthrax) in humans and animals.

GENERAL PREVENTION
- Antibiotics are effective against germinating *Bacillus anthracis* but not against the spores. Therefore, if prophylactic antibiotics are stopped prematurely, remaining spores can cause disease when they germinate. This phenomenon of delayed-onset disease does not occur with cutaneous or gastrointestinal exposures.
- Where the threat of transmission of *Bacillus anthracis* spores is deemed credible, decontamination of skin and potential fomites (e.g., clothing) may be considered to reduce the risk for cutaneous and gastrointestinal forms of the disease.
- Anthrax vaccine absorbed (AVA) is the only licensed human anthrax vaccine in the USA. Primary vaccination consists of subcutaneous injections at 0, 2, and 4 weeks, and 3 booster vaccinations at 6, 12, and 18 months. Annual booster injections are required to maintain immunity. The most common adverse event is injection-site discomfort (e.g., edema, pain, local hypersensitivity).

ALERT
Pulmonary disease caused by anthrax is a hemorrhagic mediastinitis with pleural effusions and *not* a bronchopneumonia.

EPIDEMIOLOGY
Incidence
- Anthrax is primarily zoonotic. Most naturally acquired anthrax infections are cutaneous (95%). Inhalational (5%) and GI (<1%) forms are particularly rare.
- Prior to October 2001, only 18 cases of inhalational anthrax were reported in the USA during the 20th century.
- No human-to-human spread of inhalational anthrax has been reported.
- Rare cases of human-to-human transmission of cutaneous anthrax have been reported after direct contact with infected skin lesions.
- Anthrax has been used as an agent of bioterrorism.

PATHOPHYSIOLOGY
- After inhalation, wound inoculation, or ingestion, *Bacillus anthracis* spores infect macrophages, germinate, and proliferate.
  - Proliferation occurs at the site of infection and in regional lymph nodes.
  - Replicating bacteria release toxins, leading to edema, hemorrhage, and necrosis.

- Incubation period depends on the route of transmission.
  - Inhalational anthrax: Infection requires inhalation of >8,000 spores; incubation period is 2–60 days.
  - Cutaneous anthrax: Spores enter a cut or abrasion in the skin; incubation period is 1–12 days.
  - Gastrointestinal anthrax: Spores are ingested in undercooked, infected meat; incubation period is 1–7 days; infection occurs in the upper (oropharyngeal lesions) or lower (intestinal lesions) GI tract.
- Hematogenous spread of the bacteria causes infection at other sites, including the CNS, liver, spleen, and kidney.

COMMONLY ASSOCIATED CONDITIONS
If anthrax is intentionally released, physicians must be alert for diseases caused by other potential biologic warfare agents (e.g., plague, tularemia, Q fever, smallpox, and botulism).

 DIAGNOSIS

SIGNS AND SYMPTOMS
HISTORY
- Inhalational anthrax:
  - Clinical presentation is a 2-stage illness.
  - Initial symptoms are nonspecific and last 1–3 days. They include low-grade fever, dry cough, headache, vomiting, chills, weakness, abdominal pain, and substernal discomfort. This stage may be followed by a brief period of apparent recovery.
  - 2nd-stage symptoms develop abruptly 2–5 days later: fever, hemoptysis, dyspnea, chest pain, and profuse diaphoresis. Death may occur within 1–2 days.
- Cutaneous anthrax:
  - Painless lesions develop on affected areas soon after exposure.
  - Systemic symptoms of fever, malaise, and headache may occur.
- GI anthrax:
  - Oropharyngeal form causes sore throat, dysphagia, and fever.
  - Intestinal form also causes nausea, vomiting, anorexia, severe abdominal pain, and bloody diarrhea.

PHYSICAL EXAM
- Clinical presentation of anthrax in children is varied; rapid diagnosis and effective treatment require recognition of the broad spectrum of clinical presentations
- Inhalational anthrax:
  - Tachypnea, hypoxia, cyanosis
  - Stridor, rales, signs of pleural effusion
  - Hemoptysis, hematemesis, melena

- Cutaneous anthrax:
  - Initial painless, pruritic macule or papule enlarges into a 1–3-cm round ulcer by the second day.
  - 1–3-mm vesicles with clear or serosanguineous fluid surround the ulcer.
  - A painless, depressed, black eschar follows, often with extensive local edema.
  - Over 1–2 weeks, the eschar dries, loosens, and falls off, occasionally with scarring.
  - Painful, regional lymphadenopathy may occur.
- GI anthrax:
  - Unilateral oral or esophageal ulcers, cervical lymphadenopathy
  - Cecal or terminal ileal ulcers (Intestinal anthrax progresses to massive ascites and acute abdomen.)
- Disseminated anthrax (potential complication of any of the above forms of anthrax):
  - Sepsis syndrome: Tachycardia, hypotension, septic shock
  - Meningitis: Meningismus, delirium, obtundation

DIAGNOSTIC TESTS & INTERPRETATION
Lab
- Gram-stain smear and culture from vesicular fluid:
  - Diagnose cutaneous anthrax
  - Gram stain reveals large, Gram-positive, boxcar-shaped bacilli.
  - Capsule is visible on polychrome methylene blue stain.
  - *Bacillus anthracis* grows readily on blood agar.
- Anthraxin skin test:
  - Measures anthrax cell-mediated immunity
  - It is positive in 80% of patients within 72 hours of infection and in >95% of cases within 3 weeks.
  - The test was positive in 72% of patients >16 years after recovery.
- Serologic enzyme-linked immunosorbent assay (ELISA):
  - Measures antibodies to the lethal and edema toxins of *Bacillus anthracis*
  - Positive if a single acute-phase titer is >1:32 or if there is a fourfold or greater rise between acute and convalescent titers collected 4 weeks apart
- Polymerase chain reaction, immunohistochemical staining
- Nasopharyngeal swab or induced respiratory secretion culture:
  - Used for epidemiologic investigation
  - The sensitivity, specificity, and predictive value of nasal swab testing are unknown; therefore, this test should not be used to guide the use of postexposure prophylactic antibiotics.
- Blood culture: Patients with cutaneous anthrax may have bacteremia with *Bacillus anthracis* even without significant signs of systemic disease.
- CBC
- Serum electrolytes, glucose, and calcium:
  - Hypokalemia, acidosis, hypoglycemia, and hypocalcemia occurred during experimental anthrax infection in animals.
  - Hemorrhagic meningitis

Imaging

Chest X-ray (or chest CT scan):

- Inhalational anthrax causes a hemorrhagic mediastinitis.
- X-ray shows a widened mediastinum and pleural effusions.
- No infiltrates are present.

DIFFERENTIAL DIAGNOSIS

- The prodromal illness of inhalational anthrax may resemble a lower respiratory tract infection, although upper respiratory infection symptoms are characteristically absent.
- Patients with inhalational anthrax may have a widened mediastinum on chest radiograph which may resemble an aortic aneurysm or bacterial mediastinitis.
- Necrotic skin lesions may resemble plague, tularemia, ecthyma gangrenosum, and brown recluse spider bite.
- GI anthrax may be confused with other infectious causes of enteritis (e.g., *Shigella, Salmonella, Yersinia, Campylobacter,* enterohemorrhagic *Escherichia coli, Clostridium difficile,* colitis), intussusception, Meckel diverticulum, and inflammatory bowel disease.

 TREATMENT

GENERAL MEASURES

Direct physical contact with a substance alleged to be anthrax:

- Wash exposed skin and articles of clothing with soap and water.
- Administer postexposure prophylaxis until the substance is proved not to be anthrax.
- Contact the public health department or the Centers for Disease Control and Prevention (CDC).

MEDICATION (DRUGS)

- Postexposure prophylaxis: Ciprofloxacin 15 mg/kg (up to 500 mg) *or* doxycycline 2 mg/kg (up to 100 mg) or levofloxacin 8 mg/kg (up to 250 mg) PO b.i.d. for 60 days.
  (Pediatric: Use ciprofloxacin for initial prophylaxis. Switch to amoxicillin or penicillin if susceptibility testing permits.)
- Treatment:
  – For all forms of anthrax, begin with IV therapy and switch to oral therapy when clinically appropriate. Treat for 60 days (IV and PO combined).
  – Inhalational or gastrointestinal anthrax: Ciprofloxacin 15 mg/kg (up to 400 mg) *or* doxycycline 2 mg/kg (up to 100 mg) IV q12h *plus* clindamycin or rifampin
  – Cutaneous anthrax: Ciprofloxacin or doxycycline IV. (Pediatric: Begin therapy with ciprofloxacin [plus clindamycin or rifampin for inhalational/gastrointestinal anthrax] and convert to penicillin G IV if susceptibility testing permits and when clinical improvement is documented.)

 ONGOING CARE

FOLLOW-UP RECOMMENDATIONS
PROGNOSIS

- Inhalational anthrax:
  – Case fatality rates were previously estimated to be >85% after symptoms develop. However, early use of appropriate antibiotic therapy appears to improve survival.
  – Survival rate is higher if symptoms develop >30 days after exposure.
- Cutaneous anthrax:
  – Case fatality rate is 20% without antibiotic treatment and <1% with antibiotic treatment.
- GI anthrax: Case fatality rate is 25–60%.

COMPLICATIONS

- Antibiotic therapy of cutaneous anthrax limits the likelihood of developing systemic symptoms but does not change the course of the eschar formation.
- Systemic dissemination of inhalational, cutaneous, or gastrointestinal anthrax may lead to sepsis, meningitis, and death.

ADDITIONAL READING

- Alexander JJ, Colangelo PM, Cooper CK, et al. Amoxicillin for postexposure inhalational anthrax in pediatrics rational for dosing recommendations. *PIDJ.* 2008;27:955–957.
- Bravata DM, Holty JE, Wang E, et al. Inhalational, gastrointestinal, and cutaneous anthrax in children: A systematic review of cases: 1900 to 2005. *Arch Pediatr Adolesc Med.* 2007;161(9):896–905.
- Centers for Disease Control. Update: Investigation of bioterrorism-related anthrax and interim guidelines for exposure management and antimicrobial therapy, October 2001.
- Centers for Disease Control. Use of anthrax vaccine in the United States: Recommendations of the Advisory Committee on Immunization Practices (ACIP). *MMWR Morb Mortal Wkly Rep.* 2000; 49(RR-15):1–20. *MMWR Morb Mortal Wkly Rep.* 2001;50(42):909–919. Erratum in: *MMWR Morb Mortal Wkly Rep.* 2001;50(43):962.
- Kyriacou DN, Adamski A, Khardori N. Anthrax: From antiquity and obscurity to a front-runner in bioterrorism. *Infect Dis N Am.* 2006;20:227–251.
- Li F, Nandy P, Chien S, et al. Pharmacometrics-based dose selction of levofloxacin as a treatment for postexposure inhalational anthrax in children. *Anticrobial Agents Chemotherapy.* 2010;54: 375–379.
- Scorpio A, Blank TE, Day WA, et al. Anthrax vaccines: Pasteur to the present. *Cell Mol Life Sci.* 2006;63:2237–2248.

- Stocker JT. Clinical and pathological differential diagnosis of selected potential bioterrorism agents of interest to pediatric health care providers. *Clin Lab Med.* 2006;26:329–344.

MISCELLANEOUS

Infection control:

- Immediately notify the hospital epidemiologist, infection control department, or local health department of suspected cases.
- No data suggest that patient-to-patient transmission of inhalational anthrax occurs. Standard barrier isolation precautions are recommended for all hospitalized patients with all forms of anthrax infection. High-efficiency particulate air-filter masks or other measures for airborne precautions are not indicated.
- There is no need to immunize or provide prophylaxis to patient contacts unless they, like the patient, were exposed to the aerosol.
- If anthrax is used as a bioweapon, spores may be detected on environmental surfaces. Inhalational anthrax is unlikely to be caused by secondary aerosolization of these spores.

 CODES

ICD9
- 022.0 Cutaneous anthrax
- 022.1 Pulmonary anthrax
- 022.9 Anthrax, unspecified

ICD10
- A22.0 Cutaneous anthrax
- A22.1 Pulmonary anthrax
- A22.9 Anthrax, unspecified

FAQ

- Q: Does the government have a plan in place if there were mass exposure to anthrax?
- A: Yes. Under emergency plans, the federal government would ship appropriate antibiotics from its stockpile to wherever they are needed.
- Q: Should individuals ask their physicians to write a prescription for ciprofloxacin (or other antibiotic) so they have prophylaxis available?
- A: No. Ciprofloxacin and other antibiotics should not be prescribed unless there is a clearly indicated need. In addition, indiscriminate prescribing and widespread use of ciprofloxacin could hasten the development of drug-resistant organisms.
- Q: Can a person get screened or tested for anthrax?
- A: No screening test is available to determine whether anthrax exposure has occurred. The only way exposure can be determined is through a public health investigation.
- Q: What are the clues to differentiate pulmonary or inhalational anthrax from RSV in children?
- A: Children with pulmonary anthrax display a high WCC with left shift compared to the relatively normal WCC of those with RSV. Blood O_2 levels may be severely depressed in inhalational anthrax.

APLASTIC ANEMIA

Alexis Teplick
Janel L. Kwiatkowski (5th edition)

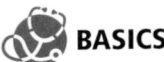

BASICS

DESCRIPTION
- A heterogeneous disorder within the bone marrow failure syndromes
- Characterized by a marked decrease or absence of blood precursors in the bone marrow and peripheral pancytopenia. The disorder exists in both acquired and congenital forms.

EPIDEMIOLOGY
Incidence
- Annual incidence of 2 new cases per 1 million in US and Europe
- Incidence in Asia is ~3-fold higher than in West, likely owing to environmental exposures or infectious agents.
- ~80% of cases are acquired, and 20% of cases are due to inherited bone marrow failure syndromes.

Prevalence
- Two major age peaks: 15–25 years and >60 years
- Male = female in acquired cases; males may be slightly overrepresented in hereditary cases.

RISK FACTORS
Genetics
- Acquired cases have been associated with specific histocompatibility antigens (human leukocyte antigen-DR2 twice as frequent in aplastic anemia patients as in the unaffected population), as well as with polymorphisms in genes encoding cytokines and with upregulation of the transcription factor T-bet.
- May be associated with heritable conditions including Fanconi anemia, dyskeratosis congenita, and others

PATHOPHYSIOLOGY
- An inciting event, such as infection or medication, provokes an aberrant immune response with oligoclonal expansion of cytotoxic T lymphocytes.
- Aberrant cytokine production by T lymphocytes suppresses hematopoietic cell proliferation and triggers apoptosis of CD34– progenitor cells.
- This results in a marked reduction in the number of hematopoietic stem cells (CD34+).
- Stromal (supporting) cells within the bone marrow microenvironment are usually normal.

ETIOLOGY
- Acquired:
  - Idiopathic (70% of cases)
  - Idiosyncratic drug side effects (e.g., chloramphenicol, nonsteroidal anti-inflammatory drugs, antiepileptics, quinacrine, cimetidine)
  - Hepatitis (usually non-A, non-B, and non-C)
  - HIV-1, EBV, human herpes virus-6, CMV
  - Chemicals/toxins such as insecticides (dichlorodiphenyltrichloroethane [DDT], parathion); benzene, carbon tetrachloride
  - Radiation
  - Malnutrition: Kwashiorkor, marasmus, anorexia nervosa
  - Paroxysmal nocturnal hemoglobinuria (PNH)
  - Pregnancy
  - Autoimmune mechanisms
  - Preleukemia, myelodysplastic syndrome (MDS)

- Congenital:
  - Fanconi anemia
  - Dyskeratosis congenita
  - Shwachman-Diamond syndrome
  - Reticular dysgenesis
  - Amegakaryocytic thrombocytopenia
  - Familial

DIAGNOSIS

HISTORY
- Evidence of bone marrow failure:
  - Pallor, lethargy, easy fatigue, weakness, and loss of appetite are signs of anemia. These may not be noticed by patient/parent owing to slow onset of anemia (with compensation).
  - Petechiae, easy and excessive bruising, prolonged epistaxis, gingival bleeding, hematuria, and bloody stools are signs/symptoms of thrombocytopenia.
  - Infections that do not respond to antibiotics, oral ulcers, and gingival hyperplasia may be signs of neutropenia.
- Evidence of cause:
  - Drug or toxin exposure (although usually not identified)
  - History of hepatitis, jaundice, or other viral infections

PHYSICAL EXAM
- Cachexia suggests another etiology, such as malignancy.
- Excessive bruising, petechiae, and pallor as signs of severe thrombocytopenia and anemia. Skin hyper- or hypopigmentation may be seen with Fanconi anemia.
- Oral mucosal ulcerations and bleeding, thrush, palatal petechiae, and gingival hypertrophy as signs of neutropenia and thrombocytopenia
- Tachycardia and systolic ejection murmur from anemia
- Lymphadenopathy and hepatosplenomegaly suggest acute leukemia/malignant process and are not associated with aplastic anemia.
- Perianal ulcerations/infection from neutropenia
- Skeletal anomalies and dysmorphic features may be signs of Fanconi anemia.
- Classic triad of dyskeratosis congenita includes dystrophic nails, lacy reticular pigmentation, and oral leukoplakia (75% of patients with DC will have at least one of these).

DIAGNOSTIC TESTS & INTERPRETATION
Lab
To confirm the diagnosis:
- CBC with differential and reticulocyte count
  - Severe aplastic anemia (at least 2 of the following)
    - Granulocyte count <500/mm³
    - Platelet count <20,000/mm³
    - Reticulocyte count (corrected for hematocrit) <1%
  - Very severe aplastic anemia, as above but granulocyte count <200/mm³
  - Mild or moderate aplastic anemia (hypoplastic anemia), less severe cytopenias

- Supplemental laboratory studies: Liver function tests; hepatitis A, B, and C antibody panel; viral serologies (e.g., Epstein-Barr virus, parvovirus B19 [IgG and IgM], varicella zoster virus, cytomegalovirus, human immunodeficiency virus, human herpes virus-6)

To exclude other causes:
- Bone marrow aspirate for chromosomal analysis to rule out MDS, acute leukemia
- Diepoxybutane chromosome breakage study (on peripheral blood) for Fanconi anemia
- Flow cytometry performed on red cells and granulocytes to exclude PNH
- Telomere length profile to evaluate for dyskeratosis congenita (telomere length extremely short in this disorder)
- Red cell folate and vitamin B₁₂ levels to detect deficiency causing pancytopenia with macrocytosis

Imaging
Usually not needed. Magnetic resonance imaging of thoracic and lumbar spine will show increased fatty infiltration of marrow space; helpful when bone marrow aspirate shows patchy cellularity.

Diagnostic Procedures/Other
Bone marrow aspirate and biopsy

Pathological Findings
Bone marrow aspirate and biopsy in severe aplastic anemia marrow will be hypocellular with fatty infiltration, <25% cellularity on biopsy.

DIFFERENTIAL DIAGNOSIS
- Acute leukemia
- MDS
- PNH
- Folate or B₁₂ deficiency (macrocytic anemia)
- Acute drug reaction with bone marrow suppression
- Acute infection (viral) with bone marrow suppression (e.g., HIV-1, cytomegalovirus, parvovirus B19, EBV)
- Marrow infiltration by malignant tumors (e.g., non-Hodgkin lymphoma, neuroblastoma)
- Hemophagocytic lymphohistiocytosis (i.e., familial erythrophagocytic lymphohistiocytosis)

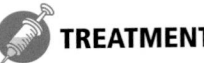

TREATMENT

MEDICATION (DRUGS)
First Line
Antithymocyte globulin (ATG) and cyclosporine are 1st-line medications for treatment of severe aplastic anemia in those without an HLA-identical sibling donor.

Second Line
For refractory aplastic anemia:
- Repeat course of ATG/cyclosporine
- Stem cell transplantation from unrelated donor
- High-dose cyclophosphamide
- Alemtuzumab (a humanized monoclonal antibody specific for CD52, which is present on lymphocytes) is in clinical trials.

ADDITIONAL TREATMENT
General Measures
- Bone marrow transplantation:
  - Treatment of choice for patients <40 years of age with severe aplastic anemia and human leukocyte antigen-identical sibling as marrow donor
  - Transplant early; minimize supportive transfusions.
  - Alternative donor bone marrow transplantation should be used only for patients who have failed immunosuppressive therapy.
  - Peripheral blood stem cell and umbilical cord blood regimens are currently being tested.
- Immunosuppressive therapy:
  - ATG and cyclosporine. Growth factors (G-CSF or granulocyte macrophage colony-stimulating factor) are often given if severely neutropenic, although addition of growth factors has not been shown to improve survival.
  - High-dose cyclophosphamide without bone marrow transplantation. This treatment was associated with a greater number of early deaths from infection than was treatment with antithymocyte globulin/cyclosporine.
- Androgens:
  - Used for the treatment of Fanconi anemia
  - Effective in moderate and mild aplastic anemia, particularly if anemia is the most significant cytopenia
- Supportive therapy:
  - Transfusion support: Family donors should not be used (to avoid alloimmunization); use CMV-safe, irradiated, leukodepleted products; minimize number of transfusions.
  - Infectious disease support: Pan culture and institute broad-spectrum parenteral antibiotics for fever/neutropenia; antifungal therapy for persistent fevers. Adding G-CSF may lead to more rapid rise in neutrophil counts, although there are some reports of increased clonal transformation. Maintain good hand washing and oral hygiene. Avoid rectal temperatures. Long-term prophylactic antibiotics are not recommended.

IN-PATIENT CONSIDERATIONS
Initial Stabilization
- Broad-spectrum antibiotics for febrile neutropenic patients; consider antifungal therapy for patients with prolonged fevers.
- Platelet transfusions for bleeding; maintain platelet count >10,000/mm³ in nonbleeding adolescent/adult patients (single-donor units, irradiated, leukocyte depleted)
- Red cell transfusions in severely anemic patients should be given slowly, to prevent congestive heart failure (unless anemia is acute and due to blood loss rather than lack of production). Use irradiated, leukocyte-depleted, cytomegalovirus-safe red cell product from unrelated donors.

 ONGOING CARE

FOLLOW-UP RECOMMENDATIONS
Patient Monitoring
- Time to recovery: Response to medical therapy is not immediate, but most responses to medical therapy, with some degree of blood count recovery, occur within 3 months of treatment. Hematologic recovery may be incomplete, and some patients may remain cyclosporine dependent.
- Signs of recovery include normalization of mean corpuscular volume (MCV) and increasing reticulocyte, neutrophil, and monocyte counts. Full platelet recovery may take months.
- Other:
  - 8–15% risk of MDS and/or myeloid leukemia at 10 years. May be lower in children
  - 15% risk of PNH at 5 years. May be lower in children
  - Risk of relapse or development of clonal bone marrow disorders is higher in patients treated with immunosuppression than in those treated with stem cell transplantation.

DIET
Avoid raw fish and undercooked meats in neutropenic patients.

PROGNOSIS
- In patients with severe aplastic anemia, 80–90% mortality at 2 years if untreated
- Bone marrow transplant from human leukocyte antigen-identical sibling donor:
  - 79% overall survival in children
  - 80–90% survival at 5 years for the young, uninfected, and minimally transfused patient
- Bone marrow transplant from human leukocyte antigen–identical unrelated donor: 30–55% survival (due to older population, frequent graft rejection, more severe graft-versus-host disease, infection from delayed engraftment with prolonged neutropenia)
- Immunosuppressive therapy:
  - 60–80% response rate (initial treatment)
  - Higher response rate in children
- Factors associated with poor outcome:
  - Bleeding at presentation
  - Severe pancytopenia (absolute neutrophil count <200/mm³, platelet <20,000/mm³)
  - Prolonged pancytopenia (>1 month)
  - Active infection at diagnosis
- Relapse:
  - Risk of relapse is 30–40% at 5 years; many respond to salvage therapy.
  - Salvage therapy: 2nd course of immunosuppressive therapy (50% salvage), matched unrelated-donor bone marrow transplantation (30–55% overall survival)

COMPLICATIONS
- Infection: Overwhelming bacterial sepsis and fungal (Aspergillus) infections are most frequent cause of death.
- Hemorrhage: Intracranial, especially if refractory to platelet transfusions
- Iron overload secondary to long-term RBC transfusions, with subsequent organ dysfunction if untreated

ADDITIONAL READING
- Alter BP. Bone marrow failure syndromes in children. *Pediatr Clin North Am.* 2002;49(5):973–988.
- Brodsky RA, Jones RJ. Aplastic anemia. *Lancet.* 2005;365:1647–1656.
- Frickhofen N, Rosenfeld SJ. Immunosuppressive treatment of aplastic anemia with antithymocyte globulin and cyclosporine. *Semin Hematol.* 2000;37:56–68.
- Guinan EC. Acquired aplastic anemia in childhood. *Hematol Oncol Clin N Am.* 2009;23(2):171–191.
- Shimamura A, Alter BP. Pathophysiology and management of inherited bone marrow failure syndromes. *Blood Rev.* 2010;24(3):101–122.
- Young NS, Calado RT, Scheinberg P. Current concepts in the pathophysiology and treatment of aplastic anemia. *Blood.* 2006;108(8):2509–2519.

 CODES

ICD9
- 284.09 Other constitutional aplastic anemia
- 284.89 Other specified aplastic anemias
- 284.9 Aplastic anemia, unspecified

ICD10
- D61.2 Aplastic anemia due to other external agents
- D61.09 Other constitutional aplastic anemia
- D61.9 Aplastic anemia, unspecified

FAQ
- Q: Can family members donate blood for a child with aplastic anemia?
- A: This is not recommended, as transfusion with blood products from parents or siblings increases the risk of graft rejection of bone marrow in the setting of a related-donor bone marrow transplant.
- Q: What activities should a child with aplastic anemia avoid?
- A: Patients with low RBC counts should avoid excessive exercise or high-altitude exposure. Patients with low WBC counts are more susceptible to bacterial infections. Patients should avoid dental work, as this may introduce bacteria into the bloodstream through the mouth. Patients with low platelet counts should avoid contact sports (e.g., football, hockey, lacrosse, skiing).
- Q: How does one learn more about experimental therapies for the treatment of aplastic anemia?
- A: Inquiries to the National Institutes of Health (NIH) in Bethesda, Maryland, or to the hematology division of the nearest medical school or National Institutes of Health–designated cancer center should result in information about the availability of experimental therapies.

APPENDICITIS

Melissa Kennedy
Joy Collins
Vera de Matos (5th edition)

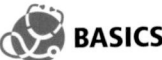 **BASICS**

DESCRIPTION
Acute inflammation of the appendix

EPIDEMIOLOGY
- Most common acute surgical emergency in childhood
- Affects 250,000 people per year in the US
- Peak incidence in 10–19-year-old age group where incidence is 233 per 100,000 children
- Incidence much less in younger children, 1–2/10,000 in children <4 years

PATHOPHYSIOLOGY
- Acute obstruction is caused by obstruction of appendiceal lumen by fecalith, calculi, hyperplastic lymphoid tissue, a worm, or (rarely) a carcinoid tumor.
- Bacteria invade the appendiceal wall at sites of ulceration, producing inflammation.
- Necrosis of appendiceal wall results in perforation with fecal contamination of the peritoneum and localized abscess formation and peritonitis.

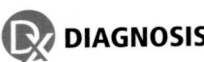 **DIAGNOSIS**

Classic signs and symptoms include right lower quadrant (RLQ) pain, anorexia, nausea, and vomiting.

HISTORY
- Abdominal pain is most common symptom and is virtually always present.
- Classically pain begins in the periumbilical region and then migrates to the right lower quadrant, nausea and vomiting occur next, and fever and leukocytosis occur later.
- Other less specific symptoms include flatulence, diarrhea, change in bowel habits, rectal tenderness, and malaise.
- Patients in the younger age group are more challenging to diagnose as toddlers may not be able to explain onset and location of pain. Delayed diagnosis and perforation is higher in this age group.

PHYSICAL EXAM
- Several findings on the physical exam may indicate appendicitis and peritoneal irritation.
- Pain and tenderness at McBurney point (1.5–2 inches from the anterior superior iliac spine [ASIS] in a line from the umbilicus to the ASIS)
- Rovsing sign is pain in the right lower quadrant with palpation in the left lower quadrant.
- The psoas sign is right lower quadrant pain with passive right hip extension and indicates a retrocecal appendix.
- The obturator sign is right lower quadrant pain with right hip and knee flexion followed by internal rotation of the right hip and indicates a pelvic appendix.
- Other physical exam findings include abdominal rebound tenderness, guarding, and focal tenderness on rectal exam.
- Following perforation, the abdomen becomes rigid and tender with absent bowel sounds.
- Patients are often febrile, tachypneic, and tachycardic.
- Special questions and examining tricks include:
  - Ask patient if the car ride was painful (e.g., going over bumps) as this should elicit peritoneal signs.
  - Palpation of RLQ with stethoscope
  - Jiggling the bed should produce RLQ pain.
  - Pain may be elicited by asking patient to cough or hop on right foot.

DIAGNOSTIC TESTS & INTERPRETATION
Lab
- CBC, expect elevated WBC count with left shift
- Urinalysis to exclude urinary tract pathology
- Pregnancy test in females of child-bearing age

Imaging
The diagnosis of appendicitis can often be made without the use of imaging based on history, physical exam, and laboratory studies with a diagnostic accuracy of 80–90% in some studies.

- Abdominal radiograph:
  - Often normal
  - May show fecalith, indistinct psoas margins, cecal wall thickening
  - Air-fluid levels would suggest a small bowel obstruction.
  - Free air or pneumoperitoneum may indicate a perforation.
- Ultrasound:
  - Findings include edema, inflammation, or abscess formation.
  - Diagnostic accuracy depends on the experience of the sonographer.
  - Most specific finding is maximum outer diameter (MOD) of ≥7 mm and is associated with a sensitivity of 98.7% and a specificity of 95.4%.
  - Currently initial imaging study of choice for the diagnosis of appendicitis
- CT scan:
  - Findings include fat stranding, abscess or phlegmon, appendicolith when present, and focal cecal thickening.
  - High diagnostic accuracy for diagnosis of appendicitis and may have a higher sensitivity than ultrasound; however, exposure to ionizing radiation is a concern

DIFFERENTIAL DIAGNOSIS
- Infection:
  - Gastroenteritis (e.g., *Yersinia*, *Campylobacter*)
  - Constipation
  - Right lower lobe pneumonia
  - Mesenteric adenitis
  - Typhlitis
  - Urinary tract infection
  - Pelvic inflammatory disease, tubo-ovarian abscess, or ectopic pregnancy
  - Parasitic infection (*Trichuris trichiura*, *Ascaris lumbricoides*)

- Inflammatory:
  - Inflammatory bowel disease exacerbation
  - Anaphylactic purpura
  - Cholecystitis
  - Pancreatitis
  - Diverticulitis
- Genetic/metabolic:
  - Diabetes
  - Sickle cell disease
  - Renal stones
  - Hypernatremia
  - Crohn disease
- Miscellaneous:
  - Function abdominal pain
  - Fecalith
  - Torsion of testes or ovaries
  - Ovarian cyst
  - Endometriosis
  - Small bowel obstruction

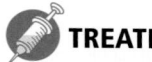 TREATMENT

ADDITIONAL TREATMENT
General Measures
- IV fluids to correct hypovolemia, electrolyte abnormalities
- Broad-spectrum antibiotics should be given, and continued for a longer duration if perforation is suspected.
- Nasogastric tube and pain medications may provide comfort preoperatively.

SURGERY/OTHER PROCEDURES
- After the diagnosis is made by a careful history and repeat clinical exam, diagnostic imaging should not delay the surgery.
- Emergency appendectomy: Laparoscopic technique has comparable results to open technique and is associated with faster recovery to daily activity.
- If abscess is present, alternative treatment option is initial nonoperative management with percutaneous abscess drainage and broad-spectrum antibiotics followed by interval appendectomy.

 ONGOING CARE

PROGNOSIS
- Recovery is rapid.
- Prognosis excellent without perforation
- Pitfalls:
  - Position of appendix may vary (i.e., location of pain may vary).
    - Retroiliac appendix, poorly localized pain
    - Retrocecal appendix, right upper quadrant (RUQ) pain
    - Appendix in gutter, flank pain
    - Pelvic appendix, pain on rectal exam or diarrhea caused by direct irritation of sigmoid colon
  - Appendicitis progresses rapidly in children; perforation often occurs owing to delayed diagnosis.
  - Pain may resolve briefly following perforation.

COMPLICATIONS
- Mostly seen in cases of perforated appendicitis:
  - Abdominal and pelvic abscesses are also more frequent after a perforated appendicitis (1.3%).
- Intestinal obstruction:
  - In patients with perforated appendicitis paralytic ileus may persist after 3–4 days leading to mechanical obstruction. This usually resolves with nasogastric tube decompression.
  - Patients with perforated appendicitis may develop bowel obstruction 4 weeks after the appendectomy due to adhesive bands, requiring emergency surgery.

ADDITIONAL READING

- Andersen BR, Kallehave FL, Andersen HK. Antibiotics versus placebo for prevention of postoperative infection after appendicectomy (Cochrane Review). *Cochrane Database Syst Rev.* 2001;(3):CD001439.
- Emil S. Risk of rupture in appendicitis. *J Am Coll Surg.* 2006;203(2):265–266.
- Goldin AB, Khanna P, Thapa M, et al. Revised ultrasound criteria for appendicitis in children improve diagnostic accuracy. *Pediatr Radiol.* Epub 2011 Mar 16.
- Lintula H, Kokki H, Vanamo K, et al. The costs and effects of laparoscopic appendectomy in children. *Arch Pediatr Adolesc Med.* 2004;158(1):11–12.
- Muehlstedt SG, Pham TQ, Schmeling DJ. The management of pediatric appendicitis: A survey of North American Pediatric Surgeons. *J Pediatr Surg.* 2004;39(6):875–879; discussion 879.16.

 CODES

ICD9
541 Appendicitis, unqualified

ICD10
K37 Unspecified appendicitis

ARTHRITIS, JUVENILE IDIOPATHIC (RHEUMATOID)

Elizabeth Candell Chalom

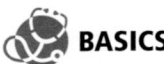 **BASICS**

DESCRIPTION
Chronic synovial inflammation of unknown etiology in at least 1 joint, for at least 6 weeks. Age of onset must be <16 years old. In 1997, a new classification system was introduced to classify juvenile idiopathic arthritis (JIA) into 7 subtypes:
- Oligoarticular arthritis affects <5 joints during the 1st 6 months of the disease. Tends to involve large joints, especially the knee. Peak age of onset is 1–6 years; 80% are antinuclear antibody (ANA) positive:
  - Persistent oligoarticular JIA remains in <5 joints.
  - Extended oligoarticular JIA spreads to involve 5 or more joints. Has worse prognosis than persistent oligoarthritis.
- Polyarticular juvenile idiopathic arthritis affects ≥5 joints. Can occur at any age: Peak ages of onset are 1–4 and 7–10 years.
  - Rheumatoid factor positive (RF+) polyarticular juvenile idiopathic arthritis is like adult-onset idiopathic arthritis that occurs in a child. It is often quite aggressive.
  - Rheumatoid factor negative (RF−) polyarticular juvenile idiopathic arthritis is usually less aggressive and easier to control.
- Systemic-onset idiopathic juvenile arthritis:
  - Characterized by high, spiking quotidian or diquotidian fevers and an evanescent pink/salmon-colored macular rash
  - Affected children may also have lymphadenopathy, hepatosplenomegaly, pericarditis, or pleuritis.
  - Arthritis may not appear until weeks to months after the onset of the systemic symptoms.
  - Can occur at any age
- Enthesitis-related arthritis (ERA) generally affects boys, many of whom are human leukocyte antigen (HLA)-B27 positive, in late childhood or adolescence
- Psoriatic arthritis is associated with psoriasis. It often begins in a few joints and then becomes polyarticular. It often involves small joints of hands and feet, as well as knees. Dactylitis is seen in nearly 50% patients.

EPIDEMIOLOGY
Incidence
- Incidence ranges from 1–22/100,000/year
- Affects ~70,000–100,000 children in the US

Prevalence
- Prevalence ranges from 8–150/100,0000; varies but is thought to be ~1/1,000
- Girls are affected twice as often as boys, but boys are affected more frequently with ERA.
- ~50% of children with JIA have the oligioarticular type.
- 30% have the polyarticular type.
- 10% have systemic-onset JIA.

RISK FACTORS
Genetics
- Rare in siblings, but many studies have demonstrated increased frequencies of various human leukocyte antigen markers in JIA.
- Each marker may be associated with a different subtype of JIA:
  - Human leukocyte antigen-DR4: RF+ polyarticular JIA
  - Human leukocyte antigen-DR1: Oligoarticular disease without uveitis
  - Human leukocyte antigen-DR5: Oligoarticular JIA with uveitis
  - Human leukocyte antigen-B27: ERA
  - Human leukocyte antigen-A2: Early-onset oligoarticular JIA

DIAGNOSIS

HISTORY
- Morning stiffness that improves after a warm shower/bath or with stretching and mild exercise is common in JIA. Many young children do not complain of pain, but walk with a limp or refuse to walk down stairs in the morning.
- Joints often become sore/painful again in the late afternoon or evening.
- Patients with JIA generally do not complain of severe pain, but rather they avoid using joints that are particularly affected. If a child has severe pain in a joint, especially pain that seems out of proportion to the physical findings, diagnoses other than JIA should be entertained.
- In systemic JIA, the fever curve is important to document. Between fever spikes, the child is often completely afebrile. The rash is evanescent and patients often have a history of fatigue, malaise, and weight loss.

PHYSICAL EXAM
- Arthritis must be present not just arthralgias:
  - May be restricted range of motion in the affected joints and soft tissue contractures as well
- Enthesitis and sacroiliac tenderness are often seen in ERA.
- In systemic JIA, the rash, if present, is almost pathognomonic for this disease.
- Lymphadenopathy and hepatosplenomegaly may be seen in systemic JIA.
- A careful cardiac and pulmonary examination must be done to look for pericarditis and pleuritis.

ALERT
Arthritis must be present for at least 6 weeks before a patient can be diagnosed with JIA. Many viral illnesses can produce joint pain and swelling that mimics JIA but resolves within 4–6 weeks.

DIAGNOSTIC TESTS & INTERPRETATION
Lab
- No laboratory finding is diagnostic for JIA.
- Many patients with JIA, especially the polyarticular and systemic types, have elevated sedimentation rates and anemia.
- Antinuclear antibody is a useful test in classifying patients with JIA and determining the risk of uveitis. Positive in:
  - 80% of oligoarticular
  - 40–60% of polyarticular
  - 15–20% of normal population
- Rheumatoid factor will be positive in 15–20% of patients with polyarticular arthritis and usually indicates a more aggressive form of arthritis.

Imaging
- Radiography is often normal early in JIA.
- Later, if arthritis persists, bone demineralization, loss of articular cartilage, erosions, and joint fusion may be seen.

DIFFERENTIAL DIAGNOSIS
- Monoarticular JIA:
  - Septic joint
  - Toxic synovitis
  - Trauma
  - Hemarthrosis
  - Villonodular synovitis
- Monoarticular or oligoarticular JIA:
  - Lyme disease
  - Acute rheumatic fever or poststreptococcal arthritis
  - Viral/postviral arthritis
  - Malignancies
  - Sarcoidosis
  - Inflammatory bowel disease
- Polyarticular JIA:
  - Viral or postviral illness (especially parvovirus)
  - Lyme disease
  - Lupus
- Systemic-onset JIA:
  - Infection
  - Oncologic process (leukemia, lymphoma)
  - Inflammatory bowel disease
  - Lupus

ARTHRITIS, JUVENILE IDIOPATHIC (RHEUMATOID)

A

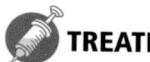 **TREATMENT**

MEDICATION (DRUGS)
First Line
- Steroids: Intra-articular steroids
  - Triamcinolone hexacetonide injections are often used when there is only 1 or 2 active joints
  - Systemic steroids:
    o Systemic steroids are often needed to control flares or with the initial presentation of polyarticular or systemic JIA. Because of the many side effects, patients should be weaned off steroids as soon as possible.
    o Glucocorticoids can be given orally (daily or every other day) or as IV pulses (every 1–8 weeks).
- NSAIDs:
  - First-line therapy for mild JIA
  - If there is no response to the initial NSAID after 4–6 weeks of an adequate dose, a different one should be tried. Patients will often respond differently to the various NSAIDs.
  - If patients experience GI upset or excessive bruising, COX-2 inhibitors may be used. If the arthritis remains active after 2–3 months, a second line treatment should be added.

Second Line
- If NSAIDs are ineffective in controlling the disease, or the patient has moderate to severe arthritis, a second-line agent should be added, such as methotrexate or sulfasalazine.
- Methotrexate: If the arthritis does not respond to NSAIDs, methotrexate is the most common second-line agent for active arthritis in multiple joints. Laboratory values must be monitored closely, in these patients, looking for bone marrow suppression or elevation of transaminase levels.
- Sulfasalazine is most often used in ERA.

Third Line
- Biologic agents are often added when patients do not respond adequately to methotrexate or cannot tolerate its side effects, or the arthritis is severe.
- Antitumor necrosis factor therapy is frequently used: Etanercept is a receptor for tumor necrosis factor that is given SC once or twice a week. Infliximab is a chimeric antibody to tumor necrosis factor that is given IV every 4–8 weeks. Adalimumab is a fully humanized antibody to tumor necrosis factor given SC every other week.
- IL-1 inhibition may work better than TNF inhibition in systemic JIA. Anakinra is a recombinant IL-1 receptor antagonist. It is given as a daily SC injection. Monthly injections with another IL-1 inhibitor are being studied.
- Anti- IL-6 therapy (Tocilizumab) is an IV medication given every other week. It has recently been approved for children with systemic onset JIA.
- Abatacept is a co-stimulation blocker. It blocks the interaction of CD28 on T cells with CD80 and CD86 receptors on antigen presenting cells. It is given IV every 4 weeks. It is currently being tested as a SC injection.
- Rituximab is an antibody to CD20, which is present on all B cells. It is approved for use in adult RA but not in JIA.
- Medications such as cyclophosphamide or thalidomide are sometimes necessary to control severe systemic-onset JIA.

ADDITIONAL TREATMENT
General Measures
- Responses to treatments for juvenile idiopathic arthritis vary tremendously:
  - Some patients may respond to NSAIDs within 1–2 weeks.
  - Others take 4–6 weeks to improve, and some may not respond at all.
  - Steroids usually start to relieve symptoms within a few days.
  - Methotrexate usually takes 4–8 weeks until a benefit is seen.
  - Anti–tumor necrosis factor therapy can start decreasing symptoms in as little as 1–2 weeks, or it may take up to 3 months.
  - Other second-line agents can take up to 16 weeks until the maximum benefit is seen.
- The waxing and waning nature of JIA itself adds to the variability of patient responses to treatments.

Additional Therapies
- Physical and occupational therapy are important in the management of JIA.
- The goal is to maintain range of motion, muscle strength, and function.

 ONGOING CARE

PROGNOSIS
- Varies considerably
- Children with oligoarticular JIA usually do well and often go into remission within a few years of starting treatment. They may have flares, however, even up to 10 years after being symptom free and off all medications.
- Patients with polyarticular JIA who are rheumatoid factor positive often develop a severe arthritis that may persist into adulthood.
- Rheumatoid factor-negative polyarticular patients generally do better, and many outgrow their disease.
- 50% of patients with systemic-onset JIA will develop severe chronic polyarticular arthritis.

COMPLICATIONS
- Joint degeneration with loss of articular cartilage
- Soft tissue contractures
- Leg-length discrepancies
- Micrognathia
- Cervical spine dislocations
- Rheumatoid nodules
- Growth retardation
- Uveitis: oligoarticular JIA, especially with a positive antinuclear antibody, is associated with a chronic uveitis, which can lead to loss of vision if not detected early with routine slit-lamp eye examinations. Uveitis may also be seen in polyarticular JIA but it is less common.

- Pericarditis and pleuritis, as well as severe anemia, may develop in patients with systemic-onset JIA.
- Macrophage activation syndrome, or hemophagocytic syndrome:
  - Rare, but potentially lethal complication of systemic-onset JIA, resulting from an overproduction of inflammatory cytokines
  - May present as an acute febrile illness with pancytopenia and hepatosplenomegaly
  - Diagnosis is made by bone marrow aspiration.
  - Treatment is often with high-dose steroids and cyclosporine.

ADDITIONAL READING
- Andersson GB. Juvenile arthritis—who gets it, where and when? A review of current data on incidence and prevalence. *Clin Exp Rheumatol.* 1999;17(3):367–374.
- Frosch M, Roth J. New insights in systemic juvenile idiopathic arthritis—from pathophysiology to treatment. *Rheumatology (Oxford).* 2008;47(2):121–125.
- Ilowite NT. Update on biologics in juvenile idiopathic arthritis. *Curr Opin Rheumatol.* 2008;20(5):613–618.
- Patel H, Goldstein D. Pediatric uveitis. *Pediatr Clin North Am.* 2003;50(1):125–136.
- Schneider R, Passo MH. Juvenile idiopathic arthritis. *Rheum Dis Clin North Am.* 2002;28(3):503–530.
- Weiss J, Ilowite N. Juvenile idiopathic arthritis. *Pediatr Clin North Am.* 2005;52(2).

 CODES

ICD9
- 714.30 Chronic or unspecified polyarticular juvenile rheumatoid arthritis
- 714.31 Acute polyarticular juvenile rheumatoid arthritis
- 714.32 Pauciarticular juvenile rheumatoid arthritis

ICD10
- M08.3 Juvenile rheumatoid polyarthritis (seronegative)
- M08.89 Other juvenile arthritis, multiple sites
- M08.90 Juvenile arthritis, unspecified, unspecified site

FAQ
- Q: Will the patient outgrow JIA?
- A: Prognosis depends on the type of JIA. In some studies, up to 50% of patients with JIA still had active disease 10 years after diagnosis. Only 15%, however, had any loss of function.
- Q: Will siblings of patients with JIA develop the disease?
- A: Rarely, but it can occur

ASCARIS LUMBRICOIDES

Genevieve L. Buser
Suzanne Dawid (5th edition)

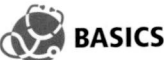
BASICS

DESCRIPTION
Ascaris lumbricoides is a large nematode (roundworm), 15–40 cm in length, which infects humans via eggs found in soil.

EPIDEMIOLOGY
Incidence
- All ages may be affected; however, children are more frequent hosts owing to oral behavior, and tend to have a higher worm burden.
- Ascariasis is more common where sanitation is poor and population dense.
- Eggs are viable in the soil for more than 6 years in temperate climates.

Prevalence
~1/6 of the world's population is infected.

GENERAL PREVENTION
Infection control:
- Sanitary disposal of human excrement, not using human feces as fertilizer and hand washing could eliminate this infection.
- In communities with high *Ascaris* carriage, community-wide recurring administration of anthelmintics is effective.

PATHOPHYSIOLOGY
- Fertilized eggs are ingested from soil contaminated with human feces.
- Larvae are liberated in the small intestine.
- Larvae invade the venous system and travel to the portal circulation, inferior vena cava, and finally, pulmonary capillaries.
- During migration through the pulmonary vessels, an eosinophilic response is evoked.

- Larvae penetrate the alveoli, are expelled by coughing, and swallowed (day 10–14).
- Larvae become adult worms in the small intestine.
- Female worms excrete up to 200,000 eggs per day.
- Fertilized eggs require 2–3 weeks of incubation in soil to become infectious and restart cycle.
- Ingestion to excretion takes 2–3 months.

ETIOLOGY
Children commonly acquire this infection from playing in dirt contaminated with *Ascaris* eggs.

DIAGNOSIS

HISTORY
- Most patients with mild to moderate infections are asymptomatic.
- Moderate to heavy infections may cause malnutrition and non-specific gastrointestinal symptoms.
- History of passage of large worms in the stool or vomitus is suggestive; history of wheezing may precede passage of worms by 2–3 months.
- During the pulmonary migratory stage, larvae cause an inflammatory response (Löeffler's syndrome): Dyspnea, cough, fever, shifting pulmonary infiltrates and eosinophilia.
- During the intestinal phase, symptoms are due to the presence of worms: pain, obstruction (2 per 1000), peritonitis from perforation, and biliary colic, hepatitis or pancreatitis from blockages due to worms.
- Chronic infection can cause nutritive, malabsorptive, and cognitive deficits.

PHYSICAL EXAM
- Chest: May have rales or wheezing if *Ascaris* larvae are in the lungs.
- Abdomen: Auscultate and palpate for signs of obstruction or perforation.

DIAGNOSTIC TESTS & INTERPRETATION
Lab
- Microscopic examination of stool specimens will demonstrate the characteristic ascarid eggs (round with thick shell).
- During the pulmonary phase, may have peripheral eosinophilia and larvae in sputum, but negative stool examinations.
- Serologic tests are unnecessary and are poorly specific to the diagnosis.

Imaging
- Chest radiograph, if cough is present.
- Abdominal imaging, if abdominal signs or symptoms of obstruction or perforation.

DIFFERENTIAL DIAGNOSIS
- Ascariasis should be considered in the differential diagnosis when a patient presents with pneumonia and peripheral eosinophilia.
- The diagnosis of Ascaris infection should be considered whenever intestinal obstruction is seen in an endemic area.
- This infection may be associated with other parasites acquired from contaminated soil: hookworm (*Necator americanus*, *Ancyclostoma duodenale*), *Trichuris trichiura*, *Strongyloides stercoralis*, *Toxocara canis*.

TREATMENT

MEDICATION (DRUGS)

First Line

- Oral:
  – Albendazole 400 mg, single dose
  – Mebendazole 100 mg, BID for 3 days
  – Ivermectin 150–200 mcg/kg, single dose
- For children <2 years old, limited studies suggest medications are safe, although not approved for this age group.
  – For children <1 year old, World Health Organization recommends: Albendazole 200 mg, single dose.
- Alternatives (oral):
  – Pyrantel pamoate 11 mg/kg to max 1 g, single dose; side effects
  – Nitazoxanide 7.5 mg/kg to max 500 mg BID for 3 days; less effective
- Piperazine citrate (75 mg/kg/d for 2 days; maximum, 3.5 g) has been used historically for cases of intestinal obstruction (causes worm paralysis), but it is no longer available in the US.

SURGERY/OTHER PROCEDURES

Surgery or endoscopic retrograde cholangiopancreatography may be required for severe intestinal or biliary tract obstruction.

 ## ONGOING CARE

FOLLOW-UP RECOMMENDATIONS

- Treatment is highly effective.
- Re-examination of stool specimens 2 weeks after therapy can be considered, but is not essential.
- Reinfection is common in endemic areas, and has led to mass drug administration programs.

Patient Monitoring

Warn parents about passage of worms in stool with treatment.

PROGNOSIS

- Once intestinal infection is detected and treated, the prognosis is excellent.
- If obstructive or respiratory complications have occurred, the prognosis is less favorable.
- The case fatality rate in cases with complications is up to 5%, most from obstruction.

COMPLICATIONS

- Bronchopneumonia may be seen during the pulmonary migrational stage, producing fever, cough, dyspnea, wheeze, eosinophilia, and pulmonary infiltrates (Löeffler's syndrome).
- Heavy infestations may cause abdominal pain, malabsorption, and growth failure.
- Children may experience obstruction (ileocecal), malabsorption, or intussusception.
- Perforation of a viscus or migration into the appendix, biliary, or pancreatic ducts may rarely occur.

ADDITIONAL READING

- American Academy of Pediatrics. *Ascaris lumbricoides Infections.* In: Pickering LK, ed. *Red Book: 2009 Report of the Committee on Infectious Diseases,* 28th ed. Elk Grove Village, IL: American Academy of Pediatrics; 2009:221–222.
- CDC. Parasites–Ascaris. Available at http://www.cdc.gov/parasites/ascariasis/index.html. Accessed Aug 22, 2011.
- Dold C, Holland CV. Ascaris and ascariasis. *Microbes Infect.* 2011;13:632–637.
- Hall A, Hewitt G, Tuffrey V, et al. A review and meta-analysis of the impact of intestinal worms on child growth and nutrition. *Matern Child Nutr.* 2008;4(Suppl 1):118–236.
- Katz M, Hotez PJ. Parasitic nematode infections. In: Feigin RD, ed. *Textbook of Pediatric Infectious Diseases,* 5th ed. Philadelphia: Saunders: 2004:2782–2784.
- O'Lorcain P, Holland CV. The public health importance of *Ascaris lumbricoides. Parasitology.* 2000;121(suppl):S51–S71.

 ## CODES

ICD9
127.0 Ascariasis

ICD10
B77.9 Ascariasis, unspecified

ASCITES

Evelyn K. Hsu
Ruben W. Cerri (5th edition)

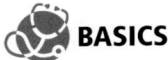 **BASICS**

DESCRIPTION

- Ascites is defined as a pathologic accumulation of intraperitoneal fluid:
  - This can be transudative (thin, low protein count and low specific gravity) or exudative (high protein count and specific gravity)
- Peritoneal fluid formation is a dynamic process of production and absorption.
- See Table 1, Analysis of Ascitic Fluid

- Accumulation of fluid occurs with:
  - Inflammatory conditions (e.g., mesenteric adenitis, tuberculosis, pancreatitis, secondary to inflammation of visceral and/or parietal peritoneum)
  - Portal hypertension or obstruction of portal vein flow and/or lymphatic flow by mass, tumor, or external pressure; tumors of abdominal viscera, retroperitoneum, thorax, or mediastinum (often characterized by chylous ascites)

- Infectious: Abscess, tuberculosis, Chlamydia infection, schistosomiasis
- GI: Infarcted bowel, perforation
- Pancreatic: Pancreatitis, ruptured pancreatic duct
- Neoplastic: Lymphoma, neuroblastoma
- Gynecologic: Ovarian tumors, torsion, or rupture
- Miscellaneous: Systemic lupus erythematous, eosinophilic ascites, chylous ascites, hypothyroidism, ventriculoperitoneal shunt

Table 1. Analysis of ascitic fluid

Condition	Gross appearance	Protein, g/L	Serum-ascites gradient, RBCs, g/dL >10,000	Cell count	Include WBC	Other tests
Cirrhosis	Straw-colored or bile-stained	<25 (95%)	>1.1	1%	<250 (90%); predominantly mesothelial	
Neoplasm	Straw-colored, hemorrhagic, mucinous, or chylous	>25 (75%)	<1.1	20%	>1,000 (50%); variable cell types	Cytology, cell block, peritoneal biopsy
Tuberculous peritonitis	Clear, turbid, hemorrhagic, chylous	>25 (50%)	<1.1	7%	>1,000 (70%); usually >70% lymphocytes	Peritoneal biopsy, stain and culture for acid-fast bacilli
Pyogenic peritonitis	Turbid or purulent	If purulent, >25	<1.1	Unusual	Predominantly polymorphonuclear leukocytes	Positive Gram's stain, culture
CHF	Straw-colored	Variable, 15–53	>1.1	10%	<1,000 (90%); usually mesothelial, mononuclear	
Nephrosis	Straw-colored or chylous	<25 (100%)	<1.1	Unusual	<250; mesothelial, mononuclear	If chylous, ether extraction, Sudan staining
Pancreatic ascites (pancreatitis, pseudocyst)	Turbid, hemorrhagic, or chylous	Variable, often >25	<1.1	Variable, may be blood-stained	Variable	Increased amylase in ascitic fluid and serum

PATHOPHYSIOLOGY

- Development of ascitic fluid may be sudden or insidious, associated with nonhepatic etiologies, or secondary to acute reduction in hepatocellular function in a marginally compensated liver.
- Intra-abdominal factors (resulting in a net flow of fluid and protein out of the mesenteric capillary bed):
  - Decreased plasma colloid osmotic pressure
  - Increased capillary pressure
  - Increased ascitic colloid osmotic fluid pressure
  - Decreased ascitic fluid hydrostatic pressure

  - Primary (congenital) abnormalities of the lymphatics (Milroy disease), congenital neonatal ascites, secondary to abdominal trauma (e.g. ureteral rupture), hematologic diseases (hydrops secondary to hemolysis), congestive heart disease; and lysosomal storage diseases including sialidosis (neuraminidase deficiency), Wolman disease, sialic acid storage disease, GM1 gangliosidosis, Gaucher disease, and Niemann-Pick type C
  - Decreased plasma oncotic pressure secondary to hypoalbuminemia (increased losses from renal and GI tract; decreased production in cases of hepatic failure)
  - Rupture of intra-abdominal viscus or peritoneal/mesenteric cyst, bowel perforation

ETIOLOGY

- Hepatic: Liver cirrhosis with portal hypertension, chronic liver failure, portal vein occlusion, Budd-Chiari syndrome, lysosomal storage disease
- Renal: Nephrotic syndrome, obstructive uropathy, perforated urinary tract, peritoneal dialysis
- Cardiac: CHF, constrictive pericarditis, inferior vena cava web

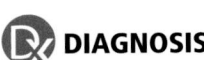 **DIAGNOSIS**

HISTORY

- The etiology for acute decompensation in hepatocellular function (e.g., massive bleeding, sepsis, superimposed infections) should be investigated.
- Use of umbilical catheters in newborn period (increased risk of portal vein thrombosis)
- Evidence of chronic liver disease
- Respiratory distress
- Exposure to hepatotoxins
- Developmental delay or growth failure suggestive of metabolic disease

PHYSICAL EXAM

- Vital signs
- Abdominal circumference
- Weight
- Auscultation of the pericardium
- Neurologic examination to evaluate for encephalopathy

- Skin changes suggestive of chronic liver disease
- Special attention should be directed toward identification of a distended abdomen, fullness in the flanks, inverted umbilicus, and development of hernias, scrotal edema, rectal prolapse, and a prominent anterior wall.
- Techniques to detect free intra-abdominal fluid include presence of a fluid wave or shifting dullness.
- Other physical examination signs include splenomegaly and caput medusae (portal hypertension), cor pulmonale (congestive heart failure), pericardial friction rub (pericarditis), diffuse abdominal pain (peritonitis or visceral perforation), abdominal pain radiating to the back (pancreatitis), lower extremity edema (suggestive of Budd Chiari) and lymphedema (lymphatic obstruction/trauma to the thoracic duct).

DIAGNOSTIC TESTS & INTERPRETATION
Lab
- Complete WBC count
- Electrolytes
- Liver function tests: Transaminases, prothrombin time/partial thromboplastin time, total protein, albumin, total and fractionated bilirubin
- Amylase and lipase (to exclude pancreatitis)
- Creatinine and blood urea nitrogen
- Blood cultures
- Urine for specific gravity
- Viral serologies, including hepatitis A, B and C viruses, CMV, EBV, coxsackievirus, enteroviruses
- Plasma amino acids, urine organic acids, lactate/pyruvate (for evaluation for metabolic disease)
- Specific testing for etiologies of chronic liver disease if suspected

Imaging
- Ultrasound of the abdomen with Doppler study to differentiate between free and loculated fluid collection and the presence of intra-abdominal masses as well as to evaluate patency of hepatic and portal vasculature and directionality of flow
- Abdominal computed axial tomography
- Abdominal radiography

Diagnostic Procedures/Other
- Abdominal paracentesis:
  – Safe procedure in the evaluation of etiologies of ascites. The 2 complications are perforation of the bowel and hemorrhage. With sterile conditions, a narrow-bore angiocatheter, usually 15 or 18 gauge, is inserted through the linea alba 2 cm below the umbilicus, using the Z-technique.
  – Done for: Routine studies, including WBC count, culture, LDH, total protein, albumin, glucose, Gram stain, amylase, cholesterol with triglycerides, and cytology
- Calculate serum–ascites albumin gradient (SAAG): (Serum albumin) – (ascites albumin). SAAG ≥ 1.1 g/dL indicates portal hypertension very likely; SAAG < 1.1 g/dL, suspect other causes. These tests require ~10–20 mL of fluid:
  – When glucose in the ascitic fluid is < 30 mg/dL, tuberculous peritonitis must be excluded.
  – When ascitic amylase is greater than the normal serum amylase, pancreatitis is suggested.

Pathological Findings
Analysis of ascitic fluid:
- The fluid should be examined for its gross appearance; protein content, cell count, and differential cell count should be determined.
- Gram and acid-fast stains and culture should be performed. Cytologic and cell-block examination may disclose an otherwise unsuspected carcinoma or storage disorder.
- See details in Table 1.

DIFFERENTIAL DIAGNOSIS
- Enlarged liver or spleen
- Mesenteric cyst: Does not have shifting dullness when position is changed
- Intestinal obstruction

 TREATMENT

ADDITIONAL TREATMENT
General Measures
- The management of the ascites should be directed toward the underlying etiology. In a patient with cirrhosis, accumulation of ascites should be avoided by preventing complications such as sodium and fluid overload, esophageal hemorrhage, spontaneous bacterial peritonitis, hepatorenal syndrome, inferior vena cava obstruction, and renal and cardiac circulatory disturbances.
- Sodium intake should be restricted to 1–2 mEq/kg/d (low-salt diet). Excess sodium in the form of intravenous normal saline should be avoided. For pressure support, colloid is preferred.
- Water should be restricted to 50–75% of maintenance requirements in patients with significant water excess or profound hyponatremia.
- Diuretic therapy, with the goal of reduction of bodyweight by 0.5–1% daily until ascites is resolved. Spironolactone (2–3 mg/kg/d) most effective in cirrhotic patients, in combination with furosemide. When diuretics are used, urine output and serum electrolytes should be closely monitored to prevent prerenal azotemia and decreased effective blood flow to the kidneys

- Refractory ascites: Diuretic-refractory ascites derives from a lack of response to dietary sodium restriction and maximal diuretic therapy. Treatment options:
  - Therapeutic abdominal paracentesis (large-volume paracentesis) should be used only in resistant cases and for tense ascites, because ascitic fluid tends to reaccumulate. Paracentesis of volumes >1 L should be accompanied by IV infusion of 25% albumin during the procedure.
  - Transjugular intrahepatic portosystemic shunting (TIPS) consists of a metallic stent that bridges the branches of the portal and hepatic veins. May be valuable in cases where portal hypertension is felt to be the underlying etiology of ascitic accumulation.
  - Orthotopic liver transplantation (OLT) is the only curative therapy for refractory ascites from liver disease and the only definitive treatment that has been shown to improve survival.

 ONGOING CARE

FOLLOW-UP RECOMMENDATIONS
Patient Monitoring
- Weight and effects of diuretics should be assessed closely, with attention to preservation of renal function.
- Urine and serum electrolytes should be monitored.
- Abdominal girth should be measured frequently.
- In cases of infection or peritonitis, a repeat paracentesis should be performed ~48 hours after the initiation of antibiotics for culture and WBC count.

ALERT
- With congenital ascites, evaluate for lysosomal storage diseases.
- When performing paracentesis, make certain that the fluid is ascitic and not intraluminal.
- Ultrasonography may be helpful to determine the location of this fluid.
- With new onset of ascites, make certain to evaluate for abdominal neoplasia.
- With marginally compensated liver disease, attempt to identify the source of the patient's acute decompensation.

PROGNOSIS
Dependent upon the etiology:
- Nephrotic syndrome: Will regress as proteinuria clears
- Liver failure: Will depend upon recovery of liver function
- Cirrhosis (complicated by ascites): Associated with significant morbidity and mortality, related in part to the severe underlying liver disease and in part to the ascites per se. Once ascites appears, the expected mortality rate is ~50% in just 2 years. With liver transplantation, survival is improved dramatically.

COMPLICATIONS
- Infection:
  - Ascitic fluid infection can be classified into 3 categories based on ascitic culture results, polymorphonuclear leukocyte count, and presence or absence of a surgical source of infection
  - An abdominal paracentesis must be performed and ascitic fluid must be analyzed before a confident diagnosis of ascitic fluid infection can be made. The blood culture bottle should be injected with peritoneal fluid at the bedside in order to increase the culture's yield.
  - Spontaneous ascitic fluid infection: Infection of the peritoneal fluid of patients with ascites in the absence of secondary causes, such as bowel perforation or intra-abdominal abscess
- Subtypes:
  - Spontaneous bacterial peritonitis (SBP) (65%)
  - Monomicrobial nonneutrocytic bacterascites (MNB)
  - Culture-negative neutrocytic ascites (CNNA)
- Secondary bacterial peritonitis: An identified intra-abdominal surgically treatable primary source of infection (e.g., perforated gut, perinephric abscess) that usually requires emergency surgical intervention

- Polymicrobial bacterascites: This diagnosis should be suspected when the paracentesis is traumatic or unusually difficult because of ileus, or when stool or air is aspirated into the paracentesis syringe (diagnostic of gut perforation by the paracentesis needle). Antibiotic therapy should be started if there is a high index of suspicion and:
  - Polymorphonuclear leukocytes <250/mm³: No treatment
  - Polymorphonuclear leukocytes >250 but <500 mm³: IV antibiotics if clinical suspicion high; or, wait and retap
  - Polymorphonuclear leukocytes >500 mm³: IV antibiotics (e.g., cefotaxime + ampicillin)
  - Polymorphonuclear leukocytes >500 mm³: Rule out secondary peritonitis.
  - An indication of therapeutic response is a decrease in the neutrophil count in the ascitic fluid by 50% from that detected on presentation. It is appropriate to treat according to sensitivities when cultures are available. The length of therapy depends on clinical response but should be a minimum of 10 days.

- Other complications:
  - Respiratory distress from decreased lung volume and diaphragmatic limitation: Hepatic hydrothorax (large symptomatic pleural effusion that occurs in a cirrhotic patient in the absence of primary cardiopulmonary disease); abdominal wall hernias with rupture; tense ascites with leakage (especially after paracentesis)
- Conservative management consists of appropriate initial therapy for most of these except hernia rupture, which requires surgical reduction.
- Consider prophylactic antibacterial therapy to prevent recurrence

ADDITIONAL READING

- Hou W, Sanyal AJ. Ascites: Diagnosis and management. *Med Clin North Am*. 2009;93(4): 801–817.
- Runyon BA. Management of adult patients with ascites due to cirrhosis: An update. *Hepatology*. 200949(6):2087–2107.
- Wongcharatrawee S, Garcia-Tsao G. Clinical management of ascites and its complications. *Clin Liver Dis*. 2001;5:833–850.
- Yu AS, Hu KQ. Management of ascites. *Clin Liver Dis*. 2001;5(2):541–568.
- Zervos EE. Management of medically refractory ascites. *Am J Surg*. 2001;181(3):256–264.

 CODES

ICD9
- 457.8 Other noninfectious disorders of lymphatic channels
- 778.0 Hydrops fetalis not due to isoimmunization
- 789.59 Other ascites

ICD10
- I89.8 Other specified noninfective disorders of lymphatic vessels and lymph nodes
- P56.0 Hydrops fetalis due to isoimmunization
- R18.8 Other ascites

FAQ

- Q: What etiologies are likely in cases of congenital ascites?
- A: Lysosomal storage disorders and/or other metabolic diseases should be excluded. If hepatic function is impaired, causes of neonatal liver failure should also be investigated.
- Q: What is the best test to discriminate the type of ascites?
- A: Analysis of the peritoneal fluid collected by abdominal paracentesis is required for this purpose. The serum: Ascites albumin gradient is helpful to discriminate ascites due to portal hypertension from other etiologies.

ASPERGILLOSIS

Michelle Dunn
Theoklis Zaoutis (5th edition)

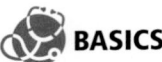

BASICS

DESCRIPTION
- Applied to the wide variety of illnesses caused by fungi in the genus *Aspergillus*
- Most human disease is caused by *Aspergillus fumigatus*, *Aspergillus flavus*, or *Aspergillus niger*; other *Aspergillus* spp. may occasionally cause disease.

EPIDEMIOLOGY
- *Aspergillus* spp. are saprophytic molds that are ubiquitous and worldwide, growing in soil, grain, dung, bird droppings, and decaying plant matter.
- Spores (conidia) are resistant to desiccation, lightweight, and are easily dispersed in air currents.
- Humans breathe in hundreds of conidia daily, which are handled by alveolar macrophages and neutrophils.
- The main route of transmission is via inhalation of airborne spores; person-to-person spread does not occur.
- The incubation period has not been defined.
- Nosocomial outbreaks have occurred when ventilation or heating systems become contaminated, or when large numbers of spores become airborne during building construction or renovation.

Incidence
The incidence of aspergillosis varies by the type of population. The overall incidence in immunocompromised children is ~0.4%. The incidence in bone marrow transplant patients is higher (4.5%).

RISK FACTORS
Other than those with otomycosis or allergic bronchopulmonary disease, most patients infected with *Aspergillus* are immunocompromised in some way. Patients at risk include those with malignancy, solid-organ transplantation, bone marrow transplantation, chronic steroid therapy, HIV, and congenital immunodeficiencies.

GENERAL PREVENTION
Infection control:
- Hospitalized, immunosuppressed patients are at risk for invasive aspergillosis.
- Environmental measures to control airborne spread of spores in hospitals during construction are indicated.
- Laminar-flow rooms with appropriate filters will significantly decrease contact with airborne conidiospores.

PATHOPHYSIOLOGY
- The most common portal of entry for *Aspergillus* is the respiratory tract; however, damaged skin or operative wounds, the cornea, and the ear can also serve as sites of entry.
  - The development of disease depends on the interaction between the organism (virulence) and the host, specifically host defense mechanisms.
  - *Aspergillus* produces toxic metabolites such as elastase, cytotoxins, endotoxins, phospholipases, and various inhibitors of immune function.
  - *Aspergillus* is an unusual pathogen in immunocompetent patients. The first line of defense in the lungs is the macrophages. Neutrophils are also a key part of the host defense against *Aspergillus*.
- Conditions that alter the normal immunologic mechanisms predispose to invasive aspergillosis. Examples include leukemia (neutropenia), corticosteroids (decreased neutrophil mobilization and macrophage killing), and chronic granulomatous disease (decreased oxidative-mediated killing)

ETIOLOGY
Aspergillus sp., most commonly *Aspergillus fumigatus*

COMMONLY ASSOCIATED CONDITIONS
- Allergic bronchopulmonary aspergillosis (ABPA) is characterized by periodic episodes of wheezing, low-grade fever, eosinophilia on peripheral smear, transient infiltrates on chest radiographic film, and a cough productive of brown mucus plugs. ABPA is thought to represent a hypersensitivity response to *Aspergillus* colonization of the lungs. It occurs most commonly in patients with chronic respiratory disease (i.e., in children with cystic fibrosis or asthma).
- Otomycosis is a localized, noninvasive infection of the external ear seen in healthy hosts. It occurs more commonly in warm, wet climates.
- Sinusitis occurs in both healthy and immunocompromised patients. Healthy patients can present with signs and symptoms of chronic sinusitis or a mass (aspergilloma) in the maxillary or ethmoid sinuses. Immunocompromised patients present with invasive disease characterized by bony destruction with extension to contiguous sites such as the orbit or CNS.
  - Noninvasive pulmonary aspergillomas are pulmonary fungus balls that grow in bronchogenic cysts or other lung cavities without invading lung tissue. They are the most frequent form of pulmonary aspergillosis.
- Invasive pulmonary aspergillosis occurs in the immunocompromised host, most commonly in patients with hematologic malignancy, solid-organ transplants, HIV infection, or other patients receiving long-term immunosuppressive therapy. Invasion of blood vessels by *Aspergillus* leads to infarction, necrosis, and hematogenous dissemination.
- Invasive aspergillosis in immunocompromised hosts can also involve the sinuses, brain, or skin. Rarer infections include endocarditis, meningitis, osteomyelitis, esophagitis, or infection of the eye.

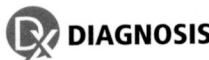

DIAGNOSIS

HISTORY
- Question: Is there a history of chronic otitis externa?
  - Associated with otomycosis
- Question: Is there a history of sinusitis that does not clear?
  - Indolent or noninvasive paranasal sinusitis presents with signs and symptoms of chronic sinusitis that are unresponsive to antibiotic therapy
- Question: Does an asthmatic patient cough up large, dark mucus plugs?
  - ABPA should be considered in the asthmatic patient with a history of expectorating dark mucus plugs, or a history of fleeting pulmonary infiltrates on chest radiography (due to bronchial plugging).
- Question: Is the patient immunocompromised?
  - Immunocompromised patients, especially those with prolonged neutropenia, are at highest risk for invasive aspergillosis. Patients with neutropenia, who are febrile for 1 week despite broad-spectrum antibiotics, are at increased risk of invasive fungal infection.

PHYSICAL EXAM
- Otomycosis is characterized by a mass of black spores (*Aspergillus niger*) that start close to the eardrum and eventually fill the external canal, pain on tragal movement, and occasionally a purulent discharge. It is only rarely an invasive disease.
- Invasive sinus aspergillosis may present with severe pain, proptosis, monocular blindness, and bony destruction on radiographic films, with evidence of direct extension to the anterior fossa or orbit, or with widespread dissemination. The maxillary sinuses are most commonly involved.
- Invasive pulmonary aspergillosis may be indistinguishable from other causes of pneumonia on physical examination. Findings may include fever, tachypnea, rales, hypoxemia, and hemoptysis (secondary to the angioinvasive potential of the organism).

DIAGNOSTIC TESTS & INTERPRETATION
Lab
Initial lab tests
- Isolation of *Aspergillus* sp. by culture is required for definitive diagnosis.
- *Aspergillus* can be recovered from samples of blood, cerebrospinal fluid, sputum, urine, broncho-alveolar lavage sample, or tissue biopsy. Types of specimens collected are guided by history and physical examination.
- *Aspergillus* spp. recovered from cultures of the respiratory tract (e.g., sputum and nasal cultures) are usually a result of colonization in the immunocompetent host but may indicate invasive disease in the immunocompromised host. The positive predictive value may be as high as 80–90% in patients with leukemia or bone marrow transplants.

- Microscopic examination of specially stained tissue samples, or of 10% potassium hydroxide wet-preparation samples, which are positive for branching, septate hyphae are suggestive of *Aspergillus* or other fungal invaders.
- Elevated serum IgE, eosinophilia, *Aspergillus*-specific serum IgE, and an immediate-type skin test response to *Aspergillus* antigen are often present in patients with allergic aspergillosis and are helpful in establishing the diagnosis.
- Radiographic studies may include characteristic findings such as wedge-shaped pleural-based densities or cavities on plain x-rays. Findings on CT scans include the "halo sign" (an area of low attenuation surrounding a nodular lung lesion) initially (caused by edema or bleeding surrounding an ischemic area) and later the "crescent sign" (an air crescent near the periphery of a lung nodule, caused by contraction of infarcted tissue).
- Recent developments in early diagnosis include the use of high-resolution chest CT, new rapid stain techniques and monoclonal antibodies for broncho-alveolar lavage samples, and serum ELISA for *Aspergillus galactomannan*.
- The galactomannan (an aspergillus cell wall component) ELISA may be helpful in diagnosing aspergillosis in immunocompromised children even prior to CT changes

DIFFERENTIAL DIAGNOSIS
- Other bacterial and fungal infections in immunocompromised hosts
- Allergic pneumonitis (other causes):
  – Chronic bacterial sinusitis
- Neoplasm

 TREATMENT

MEDICATION (DRUGS)
First Line
The newer azole antifungal agent voriconazole is considered primary therapy for invasive aspergillosis. Treatment is generally at least 12 weeks.

Second Line
- Amphotericin B and the lipid-based amphotericin preparations remain appropriate second-line therapeutic options for patients who do not tolerate voriconazole or who are not responding to therapy. For patients in whom amphotericin is being considered, the lipid-based formulations may be preferred as initial therapy in those with marginal renal function or in those receiving other nephrotoxic drugs.
- Caspofungin is also effective second line therapy.
- Itraconazole has been shown to be efficacious in the treatment of mild to moderate aspergillosis. The oral form of itraconazole may be considered as an alternative to amphotericin for prolonged treatment once disease progression has been halted with IV amphotericin therapy.

ADDITIONAL TREATMENT
General Measures
- ABPA is frequently managed with oral steroids. In patients with corticosteroid-dependent ABPA, the addition of itraconazole has been shown to be an effective adjunctive agent. Itraconazole is also used when patients have slow or suboptimal response to steroid therapy, relapse, or steroid toxicity.
- If paranasal sinusitis is noninvasive, surgical drainage or débridement usually results in clearance of the infection.
- Otomycosis (most commonly secondary to *Aspergillus niger*) is often found in association with a bacterial external otitis. Débridement of the external canal and treatment of underlying bacterial external otitis usually produces a good therapeutic response.

SURGERY/OTHER PROCEDURES
Surgical excision, in addition to antifungal medication is sometimes required for localized débridement in invasive disease.

 ONGOING CARE

FOLLOW-UP RECOMMENDATIONS
Patient Monitoring
The course of illness is variable, depending on host immune function and the location and invasiveness of disease.

ALERT
- Any immunocompromised patient with persistent fevers or signs of invasive infection who does not improve on treatment with broad-spectrum antibiotics must be evaluated for fungal infection, and the empiric use of antifungal medications should be considered.
- The rare finding of diffuse nodular pneumonia in children may be indicative of an underlying diagnosis of chronic granulomatous disease and aspergillosis.

PROGNOSIS
- Good in noninvasive disease, such as simple otomycosis or paranasal sinusitis
- Immunosuppressed or severely neutropenic patients may have rapid extension or dissemination of disease; prognosis is often very poor. Early recognition and aggressive treatment and débridement are necessary.

COMPLICATIONS
- Disseminated infection, defined as infection of 2 or more organs, can involve any of the previously discussed sites, as well as the CNS, heart, bones, or skin. Invasiveness depends on the immune state of the host, as well as the period of time and number of spores in the exposure.
- Patients with underlying diseases that predispose them to pulmonary cavitations, blebs, or cysts (such as asthma, chronic bronchitis, tuberculosis, sarcoid, histoplasmosis, and bronchiectasis) may develop an aspergilloma (fungus ball) after seeding their pulmonary secretions with *Aspergillus*. When the mass is large enough to be demonstrated on chest x-ray study, serum levels of IgG antibody to *Aspergillus* are characteristically high. Patients may present with hemoptysis, exacerbation of their underlying disease, or, rarely, invasion or dissemination.

ADDITIONAL READING

- American Academy of Pediatrics. *Aspergillosis*. In: Pickering LK, Baker CJ, Kimberlin DW, Long SS, eds. *2009 Red Book: Report of the Committee on Infectious Diseases*, 28th ed. Elk Grove Village, IL: American Academy of Pediatrics; 2009:222–224.
- Arendrup MC, Fisher BT, Zaoutis TE. Invasive fungal infections in the paediatric and neonatal population: Diagnostics and management issues. *Clin Microbiol Infect*. 2009;15(7):613–624.
- Marr KA, Patterson T, Denning D. *Aspergillosis*: Pathogenesis, clinical manifestations, and therapy. *Infect Dis Clin North Am*. 2002;16(4):875–894, vi.
- Moss RB. Allergic bronchopulmonary aspergillosis and *Aspergillus* infection in cystic fibrosis. *Curr Opin Pulm Med*. 2010;16(6):598–603.
- Patterson TF. Combination antifungal therapy. *Pediatr Infect Dis J*. 2003;22(6):555–556.
- Steinbach WJ, Stevens DA. Review of newer antifungal and immunomodulatory strategies for invasive aspergillosis. *Clin Infect Dis*. 2003; 37(suppl 3):S157–S224.
- Steinbach WJ. Pediatric *Aspergillosis*: Disease and treatment differences. *Pediatr Infect Dis J*. 2005; 24(4):358–364.
- Stevens DA, Kan VL, Judson MA, et al. Practice guidelines for diseases caused by *Aspergillus*. *Clin Infect Dis*. 2000;30:696–709.
- Tamma P. The galactomannan antigen assay. *Pediatr Infect Dis J*. 2007;26(7):641–642.
- Zaoutis TE, Heydon K, Chu JH, et al. Epidemiology, outcomes, and costs of invasive aspergillosis in immunocompromised children in the US, 2000. *Pediatrics*. 2006;711(4):711–716.

 CODES

ICD9
- 117.3 Aspergillosis
- 380.15 Chronic mycotic otitis externa
- 518.6 Allergic bronchopulmonary aspergilliosis

ICD10
- B44.81 Allergic bronchopulmonary aspergillosis
- B44.89 Other forms of aspergillosis
- B44.9 Aspergillosis, unspecified

FAQ
- Q: What are rare complications of aspergillosis?
- A: Endocarditis, osteomyelitis, and cutaneous disease
- Q: Does person-to-person spread occur?
- A: No. The principal route of transmission is inhalation of airborne spore

ASPLENIA/HYPOSPLENIA

Matthew J. Ryan

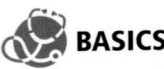 **BASICS**

DESCRIPTION
Asplenia is the absence of the spleen due to either a congenital anomaly or a surgical procedure. Hyposplenia is defined by the impaired functional capacity of the spleen to prevent bacterial infections.

RISK FACTORS
- Risk of bacteremia is highest in younger children and in the years immediately following splenectomy.
- *Streptococcus pneumoniae* is the most common pathogen-causing septicemia in asplenic children followed by *Haemophilus influenzae*, *Neisseria meningitidis*, *Staphylococcus aureus*, and other streptococci.

PATHOPHYSIOLOGY
- Most patients with hyposplenism have no problems handling antigens. However, if the spleen is minimally functional, problems may develop. The major consequence is an inability to handle infections.
- The spleen is a major component of the reticuloendothelial system; it is important both for antibody synthesis (contains nearly 50% of the B lymphocytes) and removal of opsonized organisms (mononuclear phagocytes). The encapsulated microbes such as pneumococcus, meningococcus, and *Haemophilus* are usually eliminated by this mechanism.
- For patients <4 years of age in whom few alternate routes of bacterial clearance exist, significant pathology can result from impaired splenic function.
- Heterotaxy syndrome should be viewed separately because its prognosis is distinctly unfavorable. Heterotaxy syndrome is characterized by complex congenital heart defects, asplenia or polysplenia, and abdominal heterotaxy.
  - Common associated anomalies include atrioventricular canal defects, conotruncal anomalies, anomalous systemic pulmonary venous connections, and abnormalities of visceroatrial situs.
  - The embryologic basis is thought to be a disturbance in embryogenesis in the 5th week of development that results in bilateral right-sidedness with abnormal pulmonary lobation in 80% of patients and abdominal heterotaxy in 72%.
  - Heterotaxy syndrome has an incidence of 1:6000 to 1:20,000 live births.

ETIOLOGY
- Secondary to:
  - Surgical splenectomy
  - Congenital asplenia
- In association with certain diseases or illnesses
- For complete list of causes, see "Differential Diagnosis."

DIAGNOSIS

HISTORY
The history taking should be directed toward the differential diagnosis. However, in the apparently healthy child with no identified risk factors who presents with an overwhelming infection with an encapsulated organism, the blood smear should be examined for signs of hyposplenism (see "Lab" below).

PHYSICAL EXAM
- On physical exam, the spleen may be normal, large, or atretic. Therefore, the size of the spleen cannot be used as an indicator of splenic function.
- The size is most closely linked to the underlying etiology.
  - Complete splenic replacement by cysts, neoplasm, or amyloid is an example of hyposplenic splenomegaly.
  - Sequestration crises such as those associated with sickle cell disease and malaria clog the spleen with cellular debris, which results in increased spleen size and decreased function.
  - Sickle cell disease patients typically have splenomegaly early in life as the spleen tends to sequester the abnormal red cells. With time, the spleen slowly auto-infarcts and eventually becomes nonpalpable. Sickle cell patients have impaired splenic function at all stages and should receive prophylactic antibiotics.

DIAGNOSTIC TESTS & INTERPRETATION
Lab
- The reduction or absence of splenic function can be determined by specific hematologic changes. Examination of a blood smear is essential to evaluate for signs of decreased splenic function.
- The spleen normally removes intracellular debris such as Howell-Jolly bodies (nuclear remnants), Heinz bodies (denatured hemoglobin), and Pappenheimer bodies (iron granules). Findings of target cells (red cells with a bull's eye center due to excessive membrane relative to the amount of iron and hemoglobin), Howell-Jolly bodies, Heinz bodies, Pappenheimer bodies, and pitted erythrocytes are indicative of hyposplenism or asplenia.
- Pits or pox on the red cell surface are the most sensitive indicator of hyposplenism. These are submembranous vacuoles that can be seen only in wet preparations of red cells fixed in 1% glutaraldehyde and viewed using direct interference-contrast microscopy.
- The ^{51}Cr-labeled heat-damaged red cells can be used as a measure of the capacity of the spleen to clear particulate matter from the bloodstream.

Imaging
- Ultrasound with Doppler: Useful to assess spleen size and direction of flow in splenic vein and portal vessels.
- CT scan/abdominal MRI: Aids in the detection of polysplenia
- Radionucleotide liver/spleen scan: Functional reticuloendothelial cells will be seen with this imaging modality.

DIFFERENTIAL DIAGNOSIS
Diminished splenic function found in:

- Congenital:
  - Isolated congenital asplenia
  - Heterotaxy syndrome
- Hematologic:
  - Sequestration crises (e.g., sickle hemoglobinopathies, essential thrombocytosis, malaria)
  - Sickle cell disease
  - Hereditary hemoglobinopathies

- Autoimmune:
  - Glomerulonephritis
  - Systemic lupus erythematosus
  - Rheumatoid arthritis
  - Sarcoidosis
  - Sjögren syndrome
  - Graves disease
  - Graft-versus-host disease
- Gastrointestinal/hepatic:
  - Celiac disease
  - Inflammatory bowel disease
  - Chronic liver disease/portal hypertension
- Space-occupying lesions:
  - Tumors, such as lymphoma
  - Amyloidosis
  - Cysts
- Postsplenectomy:
  - Trauma
  - Beta-thalassemia
  - Hereditary spherocytosis
- Vascular:
  - Splenic artery occlusion
  - Splenic vein thrombosis
- Miscellaneous:
  - Normal infants
  - Elderly
  - Bone marrow transplant
  - HIV infection
- Splenic irradiation

 TREATMENT

ADDITIONAL TREATMENT
General Measures
- Immunization with a pneumococcal conjugate and/or polysaccharide vaccine should be carried out in all patients with hyposplenism. In those patients who will be undergoing a scheduled splenectomy, the *S. pneumoniae*, meningococcus, and *H. influenzae* type b should be given at least 14 days prior to the operation.
- All children between 6 weeks and 59 months of age should receive the 4-dose series of the 13-valent pneumococcal conjugate vaccine (PCV13). A 23-valent pneumococcal polysaccharide vaccine (PPSV23) is available for children >2 years of age. A repeat of the PPSV23 should be administered 5 years after the 1st dose.

- Children should also receive the *Haemophilus influenzae* type b vaccine.
- Tetravalent meningococcal polysaccharide vaccine should be given to all asplenic patients at 2–10 years of age. Meningococcal conjugate vaccine should be administered to adolescents. Revaccination is recommended every 5 years in patients with functional or anatomic asplenia.
- Antimicrobial prophylaxis should be strongly considered in all asplenic children <5 years and for up to 3 years postsplenectomy. Oral penicillin is being replaced by amoxicillin-clavulanic acid, fluoroquinolones, and cefuroxime owing to increasing penicillin resistance.

ALERT
Generally, for patients <4 years, splenectomy is contraindicated because of the risk of developing bacterial infection.

ADDITIONAL READING

- American Academy of Pediatrics. *Red Book: 2009 Report of the Committee on Infectious Diseases.* 28th ed. Elk Grove Village, IL: American Academy of Pediatrics; 2009.
- Brigden ML. Detection, education and management of the asplenic or hyposplenic patient. *Am Fam Physician.* 2001;63:499–506, 508.
- Committee on Infectious Diseases. Recommendations for the Prevention of *Streptococcus pneumoniae* Infections in Infants and Children. Use of 13-valent pneumococcal conjugate vaccine (PCV13) and pneumococcal polysaccharide vaccine (PPSV23). *Pediatrics.* 2010;126(1): 186–190.
- Hirota WK, Petersen K, Baron TH, et al. Guidelines for antibiotic prophylaxis for GI endoscopy. *Gastrointest Endosc.* 2003;58(4):475–482.

- Melles DC, de Marie S. Prevention of infections in hyposplenic and asplenic patients: An update. *Neth J Med.* 2004;62(2):45–52.
- Phoon CK, Neill CA. Asplenia syndrome: Risk factors for early unfavorable outcome. *Am J Cardiol.* 1994;73:1235–1237.
- Sumaraju V, Smith LG, Smith SM. Infectious complications in asplenic hosts. *Infect Dis Clin North Am.* 2001;15:551–565.

 CODES

ICD9
- 289.59 Other diseases of spleen
- 759.0 Anomalies of spleen, congenital

ICD10
- D73.0 Hyposplenism
- Q89.09 Congenital malformations of spleen

FAQ

- Q: What should I do if my child has a fever?
- A: In hyposplenic patients, especially those <4 years of age, all fevers should be taken seriously. Even if the child is being treated with prophylactic penicillin, he or she should be treated for all symptomatic bacterial infections.
- Q: Are there any special times I need to worry about infections?
- A: Asplenic patients receiving dental work or GI endoscopy should be considered on a case-by-case basis. Antibiotic prophylaxis should strongly be considered in asplenic patients undergoing high-risk endoscopic procedures (i.e., sclerotherapy, stricture dilation), as a transient bacteremia can occur in up to 50% of these patients.

ASTHMA
Lee J. Brooks

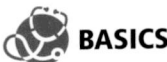 **BASICS**

DESCRIPTION
- Characterized by 3 components:
  - Reversible airway obstruction
  - Airway inflammation
  - Airway hyperresponsiveness to a variety of stimuli
- Diagnosis (the 3 "R"s)
  - Recurrence: Symptoms are recurrent.
  - Reactivity: Symptoms are brought on by a specific occurrence or exposure (trigger).
  - Responsive: Symptoms diminish in response to bronchodilator or anti-inflammatory agent.

ALERT
Pitfalls:
- Not recognizing that asthma can manifest as chronic cough; wheezing may not be evident.
- Reluctance to "label" child with having asthma (using terms such as reactive airway disease or bronchitis)
- Frequent antibiotic or cough medicine use to treat asthma symptoms
- "Recurrent pneumonias" often are actually asthma exacerbations; subsegmental atelectasis on chest radiograph misdiagnosed as an infiltrate
- Underreporting of asthma symptoms; beware the child who "doesn't like to play sports"; he/she may have learned that exercise causes dyspnea.
- Poor adherence with therapy when symptoms are controlled
- Failure to use inhaled medications properly: Inhaled medication use must be taught and reviewed at each visit. A fixed-volume holding chamber should always be used with a pressurized metered-dose inhaler (pMDI), regardless of patient age. pMDIs should be refilled based on the number of doses used, not by estimating contents by shaking or spraying. pMDIs with a built-in dose counter are preferred.

EPIDEMIOLOGY
Incidence
- Most common chronic illness in children
- Death from asthma in children more than tripled from 1979 to 1996, but has been decreasing since then, perhaps owing to better recognition and increased use of anti-inflammatory medications. The incidence of death from asthma does not seem to correlate with severity.

Prevalence
- Wheezing in children is extremely common in the industrialized world (cumulative prevalence, 30–60%).
- In younger children, most episodes occur following viral infections.
- >50% of children who wheeze in early childhood stop wheezing by age 6 years.
- 14% of all young children (40% of those who wheeze during infancy) continue to wheeze.

RISK FACTORS
Genetics
- Children of asthmatics have higher incidence of asthma.
  - 6–7% risk if neither parent has asthma
  - 20% risk if 1 parent has asthma
  - 60% risk if both parents have asthma
- Several genes are known to be associated with the development of atopy and bronchial muscle responsiveness.

GENERAL PREVENTION
- Patient and caregiver education is mandatory to establish provider/caregiver partnership and ensure adherence with treatment plan.
- Every patient/caregiver should be taught that asthma is a chronic, inflammatory condition that can be controlled with proper therapy.
- All medications should be explained and potential risks (side effects) and benefits reviewed.
- A written asthma management plan should be provided, outlining daily therapy and an "action plan" for managing exacerbations of asthma.
- Environmental counseling:
  - Avoid airborne irritants (tobacco smoke, wood stoves, noxious fumes).
  - Minimize dust-mite exposure.
  - Minimize stuffed animals, quilts, books, and clutter.
  - Use dust mite–proof coverings on mattresses, pillows, and box springs.
  - Wash pillows, blankets, and sheets in hot water.
  - Avoid molds by decreasing relative humidity to 50%.
  - Remove pets from child's bedroom and from house if patient is allergic to the animal.

PATHOPHYSIOLOGY
- Immune and inflammatory responses in the airways are triggered by an array of environmental antigens, irritants, or infectious organisms.
- Atopy and asthma are related.
  - Eosinophilia and the ability to make excess IgE in response to antigen are associated with increased airway reactivity.
  - Asthma is more common in children who have allergic rhinitis and eczema.

- Viral infections, particularly respiratory syncytial virus (RSV), during infancy may play a role in the development of asthma or may modify the severity of asthma.
- Exposure to cigarette smoke and other airway irritants influences the development and severity of asthma.
- Airway is stimulated and primary inflammatory mediators released.
- Airway is invaded by inflammatory cells (mast cells, basophils, eosinophils, macrophages, neutrophils, B and T lymphocytes).
- Inflammatory cells respond to and produce various mediators (cytokines, leukotrienes, lymphokines), augmenting the inflammatory response.
- Airway epithelium is inflamed and becomes disrupted, and basal membrane is thickened.
- Airway smooth muscle is hyperresponsive, and bronchoconstriction ensues.
- Airway smooth muscle hypertrophy and airway epithelial hyperplasia are characteristic chronic changes resulting from poorly controlled asthma.

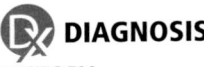 **DIAGNOSIS**

HISTORY
- Inquire about these symptoms: Coughing, wheezing, shortness of breath, chest tightness:
  - Frequency of symptoms defines severity.
  - Precipitating factor (trigger)
  - Response to bronchodilator or anti-inflammatory medication
  - Family history of asthma or atopy
- Pattern of symptoms:
  - Perennial versus seasonal
  - Continuous versus acute
  - Duration and frequency of episodes
  - Diurnal variation/nocturnal symptoms
- Do any of the following set off the breathing difficulty?
  - Infections (upper respiratory, sinusitis)
  - Exposure to dust (mites), animal dander, pollen, mold
  - Cold air or weather changes
  - Exercise or play
  - Environmental stimulants (e.g., cigarette smoke, strong odors, pollutants)
  - Emotional factors (e.g., laughing, crying, fear)
  - Drug intake (aspirin, nonsteroidal anti-inflammatory drugs, β-blockers)
  - Food additives
  - Endocrine factors (e.g., menses, pregnancy, thyroid dysfunction)

- Review of systems:
  - Symptoms of complicating factors (gastroesophageal reflux, sinusitis, allergies)
  - Dyspepsia, sour taste (gastroesophageal reflux); throat clearing, purulent nasal discharge, halitosis, cephalalgia, or facial pain (sinusitis); nasal itching ("allergic salute"), eye rubbing, sneezing, watery nasal discharge (allergies)
- Impact of asthma:
  - Number of hospitalizations/intensive care unit admissions
  - Number of emergency room visits/doctor's office visits
  - Asthma attack frequency
  - Number of missed school days/parent workdays
  - Limitation on activity (may be subtle)
  - Number of courses of systemic steroids needed
- Environmental history:
  - Type of home
  - Location of home (urban, suburban, rural)
  - Heating system/air conditioning
  - Use of humidifier
  - Presence of molds, cockroaches, rodents
  - Fireplace
  - Carpeting
  - Stuffed animals
  - Pets
  - Exposure to cigarette smoke

PHYSICAL EXAM
- Pulmonary exam may be normal when asymptomatic.
- Assess work of breathing:
  - Level of distress
  - Intercostal/supraclavicular muscle retractions
- Chest shape (i.e., normal versus barrel shaped)
- Lung auscultation:
  - Wheezing
  - End-expiratory involuntary cough
  - Prolonged expiratory phase
  - Crackles or coarse breath sounds
  - Stridor (indicates extrathoracic airway obstruction)
- Head, eyes, ears, nose, and throat exam: Signs of allergies or sinusitis:
  - Watery or itchy eyes
  - Allergic shiners
  - Dennie lines
  - Nasal congestion
  - Boggy nasal turbinates
  - Nasal polyps
  - Postnasal drip
- General exam (vital signs):
  - Blood pressure (pulsus paradoxus)
  - Respiratory rate (tachypnea)
- Skin: Evidence of eczema
- Extremities: Digital clubbing (very rare in asthma; suggests alternative diagnosis)
- Physical exam trick: Forced-exhalation maneuver to observe for wheezes or for precipitating coughing

DIAGNOSTIC TESTS & INTERPRETATION
Lab
- Pulmonary function tests:
  - Essential for the assessment and ongoing care of children with asthma
  - Spirometry measures the degree of airway obstruction and the response to bronchodilators.
  - Values obtained can measure absolute degree of airway obstruction.
  - Serial values can follow progress of disease and response to treatment.
  - Children as young as 4–5 years old can usually perform spirometry with practice.
- Provocational testing:
  - Exercise challenge: Determines effect of exercise on triggering airway obstruction
  - Cold-air challenge: Indirect test of airway hyperresponsiveness
  - Methacholine challenge: A positive test supports the diagnosis of asthma (useful in cases for which history is equivocal and pulmonary function test is normal), measures the degree of airway hyperreactivity
- Allergy evaluation:
  - Blood tests (eosinophil count, IgE level)
  - Skin testing (best test for assessing allergen sensitivity)
  - RAST testing (not as accurate as skin testing)
  - Sputum/nasal examination for presence of eosinophilia
- Other studies:
  - Gastroesophageal reflux evaluation
  - pH probe
  - Milk scan
  - Barium swallow (confirms normal anatomy)
- Peak flow meter (home testing):
  - Measures peak flow rate (PEFR)
  - Effort dependent
  - Assesses central, not peripheral, airway obstruction
  - Used with patients who have poor symptom recognition or labile asthma
  - Dips in peak flow rate precede onset of clinical asthmatic symptoms.
  - Peak flow rate should be performed at least once a day.
  - Peak flow rate values are divided into 3 zones:
    - Green: ≥80% of baseline
    - Yellow: 50–80% of baseline
    - Red: 50% of baseline
- Specific peak flow rate guidelines should be individualized for each patient based on the best measurement obtained during a 14-day period when the child is well.

Imaging
- Chest radiograph should be obtained if the diagnosis is uncertain or there is not the expected response to treatment, to rule out congenital lung malformations or obvious vascular malformations:
  - Findings can be normal.
  - Common findings are peribronchial thickening, subsegmental atelectasis, and hyperinflation.
- Sinus CT is useful if symptoms suggest sinusitis.
- Chest CT should be performed if bronchiectasis or anatomic abnormality is suspected.

Diagnostic Procedures/Other
Bronchoscopy can rule out anatomic malformations, foreign bodies, mucous plugging, vocal cord dysfunction, aspiration (lipid-laden macrophages).

DIFFERENTIAL DIAGNOSIS
- Infectious:
  - Pneumonia
  - Bronchiolitis
  - Chlamydia infection
  - Laryngotracheobronchitis
  - Sinusitis
  - Immune deficiency
- Mechanical:
  - Extrinsic airway compression
  - Vascular ring
  - Foreign body
  - Vocal cord dysfunction
  - Tracheobronchomalacia
- Miscellaneous:
  - Cystic fibrosis
  - Bronchopulmonary dysplasia
  - Pulmonary edema
  - Gastroesophageal reflux
  - Recurrent aspiration
  - Bronchiolitis obliterans

TREATMENT

MEDICATION (DRUGS)

- Corticosteroids (anti-inflammatory agents):
  - Most effective anti-inflammatory agents
  - Inhaled: Reduce airway inflammation and hyperresponsiveness more than any other inhaled agents; inhibit production and release of cytokines and arachidonic acid–associated metabolites; enhance β-adrenoreceptor responsiveness; side effects include oral thrush; may minimally affect growth velocity at moderate or high doses
  - Dosage individualized to each patient. Agents vary in topical potency and systemic bioavailability; available as pMDIs, dry-powder inhalers (DPIs), or nebulized. Fluticasone (Flovent) 44, 110, 220 mcg/puff pMDI and 50, 100, 250 mcg DPI; budesonide (Pulmicort) 90, 180 mcg/puff DPI and 250, 500, and 1,000-mcg vials for nebulizer; beclomethasone (Beclovent, Vanceril, Qvar) 40, 42, 80, 84 mcg/puff; triamcinolone (Azmacort) 100 mcg/puff; flunisolide (AeroBid) 250 mcg/puff; mometasone (Asmanex) 220 mcg DPI
  - Oral: Used for asthma exacerbations or for severe asthma that cannot be otherwise controlled. Exacerbations: Prednisone 1–2 mg/kg/d for 3–7 days or longer; usually tapered if >7 days of therapy required or if systemic steroids are used frequently. Ongoing therapy: 0.5–1 mg/kg/d daily or every other day for patients with severe asthma. Undesirable side-effect profile. When used daily, assess bone density and for cataract formation at least yearly.
  - IV: Methylprednisolone (Solu-Medrol) 1–2 mg/kg IV q6–12h until improved and able to take oral medication
- Leukotriene modifiers (anti-inflammatory agents):
  - Block the synthesis and/or action of leukotrienes
  - 5-Lipoxygenase inhibitors, zileuton: May cause hepatic dysfunction
  - Leukotriene receptor antagonists: Zafirlukast (10 mg; Accolate) and montelukast (4, 5, and 10 mg; Singulair)
  - Indicated as monotherapy for mild or exercise-induced asthma and in combination with an inhaled corticosteroid for more effective symptom control or using a lower dose of inhaled corticosteroid
- Mast-cell stabilizers
  - Weak anti-inflammatory agents
  - Preparations: Cromolyn sodium; nedocromil sodium (Tilade, available in Canada)
  - Decrease bronchial hyperresponsiveness
  - Can be used prior to exercise for exercise-induced symptoms
  - No significant side effects
  - Inhaled: Nebulizer; MDI

- β_2-agonists (bronchodilators): Indication is for relief of acute bronchoconstriction (quick-relief medicine); used as needed in people with asthma who have breakthrough symptoms; used prior to exercise in exercise-induced bronchospasm; regular use or overuse associated with worsened control of asthma; routes include inhaled (most effective, metered-dose inhaler or nebulizer) and oral (least effective, most side effects); short-acting (4–6 hours) preparations include albuterol (Ventolin, Proventil, ProAir), terbutaline (Brethaire, Brethine), and metaproterenol (Alupent); a single-isomer preparation of albuterol (Xopenex) may have a slightly longer duration of action and perhaps fewer side effects; longer-acting (up to 12 hours) preparations include salmeterol (Serevent) and formoterol (Foradil) available as pMDI and DPI, can be used daily in conjunction with anti-inflammatory agent for improved symptom control. Fixed combination products of inhaled corticosteroid and a long-acting β-agonist (Advair, Dulera, Symbicort) are available as DPIs and pMDIs.
- There may be an increased risk of asthma-related deaths in patients using long-acting β-agonists (LABA) and it is suggested that LABAs be prescribed only for patients not adequately controlled on other asthma-controller medications or whose disease severity warrants initiation of treatment with 2 maintenance therapies.
  - Theophylline (bronchodilator): 2nd-line agent used when more conventional therapies are unsuccessful; indications are chronic, poorly controlled asthma and nocturnal asthma (if no gastroesophageal reflux); adjunctive therapy with β_2-drugs and steroids in hospitalized patients in selected cases; route (oral or IV); serum levels must be routinely monitored (therapeutic levels are 10–20 mg/mL). Side effects are seen with increased levels. Many factors affect theophylline levels. Increased levels are seen with erythromycin, ciprofloxacin, cimetidine, viral illnesses, fever. Decreased levels are seen with phenobarbital, phenytoin, rifampin. Sustained-release tablets should not be crushed.
- Anticholinergic agents (bronchodilators): Adjunctive bronchodilators, may be useful in patients who only partially respond to β-agonists; preparations include ipratropium bromide MDI or ampule for nebulization (Atrovent).
- Monoclonal antibodies against IgE (Xolair) can be given as a monthly SC injection in severe asthma patients with moderately high IgE levels.

ISSUES FOR REFERRAL

- A patient who requires hospitalization more than once a year, or who has required intensive care
- A patient who requires frequent bursts of systemic corticosteroids
- A patient whose airway obstruction is not easily reversible
- A patient who has clinical features suggesting another pulmonary process

COMPLEMENTARY & ALTERNATIVE THERAPIES

- Miscellaneous drugs used in severe cases
- Steroid-sparing agents:
  - Troleandomycin (TAO): Macrolide antibiotic; decreases clearance of corticosteroids, thus prolonging the effects of corticosteroids on the lung; lower corticosteroid dosing required
  - Methotrexate: Potent immunosuppressive drug; needs further investigation in children
  - Cyclosporine: Shown to have steroid-sparing effect in adult population with asthma; side effects are significant and may limit use
  - Magnesium sulfate (MgSO$_4$): Used intravenously as a smooth muscle relaxer in severe acute asthma exacerbation
- Helium:
  - May improve airflow in severe asthma
  - Can improve ventilation and potentially oxygenation
- Immunotherapy:
  - Efficacy in asthma is controversial
  - Most effective if a single antigen can be identified
  - Used only in select cases if medical management and environmental control measures are ineffective

ONGOING CARE

FOLLOW-UP RECOMMENDATIONS
Long-term follow-up is essential to maintain normal activity and pulmonary function. All patients should use a valved holding chamber with pMDIs, and technique for all inhaled medications should be reviewed regularly.

Patient Monitoring
Signs that may indicate problems: Increased symptoms (cough day or night, wheeze), exercise limitations or symptoms during exercise, decrease in peak flow rate, increasing use of inhaled bronchodilators, subject not improving on enhanced home therapy

DIET
- Avoid foods or food additives (if truly allergic).
- Food-induced asthma is uncommon.

PATIENT EDUCATION
Activity:
- Most patients with asthma can participate fully in sports, even at a high level, with close follow-up. Extra medications such as albuterol and/or cromolyn may be required before vigorous exercise. All athletes should have their quick-relief medications on hand at all times.
- Athletes with asthma may need to report their medications to the governing bodies of their sport.

PROGNOSIS
With proper therapy and good adherence to treatment regimen: Excellent

COMPLICATIONS
Morbidity: Frequent hospitalizations and absence from school. Psychological impact of having a chronic illness. Decline in lung function over time

ADDITIONAL READING

- Allen JL, Bryant-Stephens T, Pawlowski NA. *The Children's Hospital of Philadelphia guide to asthma*. Philadelphia: Wiley-Liss; 2004.
- Bush A, Sagiani S. Management of severe asthma in children. *Lancet*. 2010;376:814–825.
- Ducharme FM, Ni Chroinin M, Greenstone I, et al. Addition of long-acting beta2-agonists to inhaled corticosteroids versus same dose inhaled corticosteroids for chronic asthma in adults and children. *Cochrane Database Syst Rev*. 2010;(5): CD005535.
- Halken S, Lau S, Valovirta E. New visions in specific immunotherapy in children: an iPAC summary and future trends. *Pediatr Allergy Immunol*. 2008; 19(Suppl 19):60–70.
- Kercsmar CM. Current trends in management of pediatric asthma. *Respir Care*. 2003;48:194–205.
- Liu AH, Szefler SJ. Advances in childhood asthma: Hygiene hypothesis, natural history, and management. *J Allergy Clin Immunol*. 2003;111: S785–S792.
- National Asthma Education and Prevention Program. *Expert Panel Report 3: Guidelines for the diagnosis and management of asthma*. NIH-NHLBI publication. Washington, DC: U.S. Government Printing Office; August 2007.
- Reid MJ. Complicating features of asthma. *Pediatr Clin North Am*. 1992;39:1327–1341.
- Salvatoni A, Piantanida E, Nosetti L, et al. Inhaled corticosteroids in childhood asthma: Long-term effects on growth and adrenocortical function. *Paediatr Drugs*. 2003;5:351–361.
- Silverstein MD, Mair JE, Katusic SK, et al. School attendance and school performance: A population-based study of children with asthma. *J Pediatr*. 2001;139(2):278–283.
- Stempel DA. The pharmacologic management of childhood asthma. *Pediatr Clin North Am*. 2003; 50:609–629.

 ## CODES

ICD9
- 493.00 Extrinsic asthma, unspecified
- 493.92 Asthma, unspecified type, with (acute) exacerbation

ICD10
- J45.901 Unspecified asthma with (acute) exacerbation
- J45.909 Unspecified asthma, uncomplicated

FAQ

- Q: Will my child outgrow his or her asthma?
- A: Family history and allergies affect the ultimate outcome. Wheezing during the 1st 3 years of life is extremely common, with 40–50% of all children wheezing at some time. Many of these children do not develop asthma and "outgrow" their illness by school age. Some patients develop asthma again as young adults.
- Q: Can my child become dependent on asthma medications?
- A: Children do not become "dependent" on these medications as they would with narcotic agents. Daily asthma medications are required to maintain airway patency and to control airway inflammation.
- Q: Will my child be on medications for the rest of his or her life?
- A: This depends on the severity of the asthma. The types, doses, and frequency of asthma medications will change over a patient's lifetime.
- Q: Do inhaled steroids affect patient growth?
- A: There is some transient and slight decrease in growth velocity seen in children who receive moderate-dose inhaled corticosteroids (~0.5 mg/d). Ultimate height does not seem to be affected.

ATAXIA

Sunil Thummala
Susan L. Perlman (5th edition)

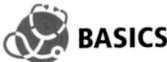 **BASICS**

DESCRIPTION

- Incoordination or clumsiness of movement, disproportionate to weakness
- Most acute ataxias are acquired; chronic ataxias are congenital or hereditary.
- Caused by dysfunction of cerebellum, proprioception, or vestibular system

Clinical presentation:

- Ataxia with fever, rash, GI illness, or recent immunization suggests more benign acute cerebellar ataxia; headache, diplopia, vomiting: More ominous—acute hydrocephalus, tumor, or stroke
- Altered mental status, headache, or seizures raise suspicion for acute disseminated encephalomyelitis (ADEM).
- Brainstem encephalitis: Cranial neuropathies
- Disorders of vestibular pathway: Severe vertigo, nausea, vomiting, and hearing problem
- Toxic/metabolic causes usually alter consciousness.
- Rapidly ascending weakness following infection suggests Guillain Barré (GBS).
- Acute-onset ataxia with diplopia suggests brain stem stroke, tumor.
- Rapidly clearing ataxia with confusion and focal weakness suggests postictal state.
- Headache, visual scintillations, nausea, and dizziness suggest migraine.
- Mitochondrial disorders commonly feature short stature, seizures, retinopathy, heart block, myopathy, and mental retardation.
- Friedreich ataxia is associated with cardiomyopathy, diabetes, scoliosis, pes cavus, and peripheral neuropathy.
- Ataxia telangiectasia: Telangiectasias, frequent bronchopulmonary infection, leukemia/lymphoma, other cancers

EPIDEMIOLOGY

- ~80% of acute ataxias due to postviral, intoxication, GBS.
- ~1 in 1,000 children develops acute ataxia following varicella infection.
- Congenital cerebellar syndromes: Caused by perinatal trauma, vascular events ("ataxic cerebral palsy"). Dandy-Walker syndrome and structural cerebellar abnormalities are rarer.
- Friedreich ataxia: 2–4 in 100,000
- Ataxia with oculomotor apraxia: 5 in 100,000
- Brain gliomas: Common in children

GENERAL PREVENTION

Accidental intoxications, varicella vaccination

PATHOPHYSIOLOGY

- Dysfunction of cerebellum, proprioceptive sensors, and vestibular system causes ataxia.
- Unilateral cerebellar ataxia: Ipsilateral cerebellum or its connections
- The cerebellum can also become the target of autoimmune phenomena.

ETIOLOGY

- Acute-onset ataxias: Postinfectious (ADEM) inflammatory conditions, infection, intoxication, tumors, intracerebral hemorrhage, stroke, trauma, conversion disorder:
  - Intoxication by benzodiazepines, antihistamines, anticonvulsants, lead, CO, alcohol, inhalants
  - Posterior fossa tumors: Medulloblastoma, occult neuroblastoma/opsoclonus-myoclonus-ataxia syndrome
  - Pontine/medullary strokes, strokes involving cerebellum, cerebellar peduncles
  - Acute ataxia with inconsistent findings suggests psychogenic ataxia.
- Episodic: Migraine, seizures, inborn errors of metabolism, familial periodic ataxia (dominant)
- Chronic progressive ataxias: Genetic:
  - Friedreich, ataxia telangiectasia, aminoacidopathies, hexosaminidase A deficiency, abetalipoproteinemia/hypobetalipoproteinemia, Wilson disease, mitochondrial peroxisomal disorders, dominant spinocerebellar ataxias
  - Chiari malformation, Dandy-Walker syndrome, agenesis of cerebellar vermis
- Paraneoplastic: Ataxia may precede opsoclonus/ myoclonus due to neuroblastoma/ganglioneuroma.

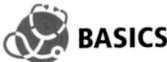 **DIAGNOSIS**

HISTORY

- Acute ataxia:
  - History directed to possible intoxication, head trauma, or migraine
  - Recent infection suggests postviral cerebellar ataxia, labyrinthitis, or Guillain-Barré syndrome, ADEM
  - Access to drugs, altered mental status = possible intoxication
  - Recent trauma: Concussion, vertebral dissection/stroke, intracranial bleed
  - History of congenital heart defect: Cerebellar stroke
  - Severe vertigo, nausea, vomiting, hearing problem: Labyrinthitis
- Episodic ataxias:
  - Headache with nausea, visual changes, focal neurologic findings: Migraine syndrome
- Chronic ataxias:
  - Irritability or progressive macrocephaly or cranial neuropathy suggests posterior fossa pathology (e.g., tumor).
  - Multiple system involvement should raise concern for metabolic/genetic causes (mitochondrial disorders, organic acidurias, Friedreich ataxia, ataxia telangiectasia).

PHYSICAL EXAM

- Abnormalities on cranial nerve exam for posterior fossa pathology
- Ataxia proportional to degree of weakness suggests lesion in motor pathway (e.g., myasthenia gravis, GBS).
- Absent DTR: GBS
- Limb dysmetria (appendicular ataxia), dysdiadochokinesis, hypotonia, tremor
- Vermis: Manifests as truncal ataxia, gait ataxia ("drunken" movements), nystagmus, dysarthria, titubation
- Vestibular: Gait ataxia, nystagmus, abnormal Rinne and Weber tests
- Disorders of proprioception: Positive Romberg test, decreased reflexes

DIAGNOSTIC TESTS & INTERPRETATION
Lab

- Toxicology screen in acute ataxia; drug levels for specific intoxication
- Lumbar puncture for CSF analysis (for ADEM, GBS, infection)
- EEG if postictal ataxia is a possibility
- Full workup for neuroblastoma in ataxia-opsoclonus/myoclonus: Body CT, MIBG scan, serum ferritin, urine (HVA/VMA)
- Metabolic: Lysosomal hydrolases, ammonia, plasma and CSF lactate, pyruvate, long-chain fatty acids, plasma/urine amino and organic acids
- Low cholesterol: Abetalipoproteinemia
- Elevated α-fetoprotein, decreased serum IgA: Ataxia telangiectasia.
- Genetic tests for Friedreich ataxia, ataxia telangiectasia, and the dominantly inherited spinocerebellar ataxias (many subtypes)
- Mitochondrial screening: Plasma or CSF lactate, genetic testing on blood, muscle biopsy

Imaging

- Radiologic studies are necessary when intoxication has been ruled out. Imaging of brain can help rule out tumor, stroke, or demyelination.
- MRI is superior to CT in most cases; however, if intracranial hemorrhage is a concern a noncontrast CT can quickly confirm diagnosis and aid in treatment

Pathological Findings

Pathology is specific to the underlying etiology, although neurodegenerative cerebellar disease may show only nonspecific loss of Purkinje cells.

DIFFERENTIAL DIAGNOSIS

- Movement disorders (exaggerated physiologic tremor, chorea, athetosis) and limb weakness may be mistakenly diagnosed as ataxia.
- Paretic ataxia: Incoordination proportional to the degree of weakness suggests ataxia (GBS, tick paralysis).
- Psychogenic: Variable effort; no pathologic nystagmus; changing character of tremor, excessive swaying while walking but no fall (astasia-abasia); corrective steps before falling

- Acute ataxia:
  - Intoxication: Depressed mental status; toxicology screen; medications at home
  - Posttraumatic: History/physical findings
  - Postinfectious: Acute cerebellar ataxia (with dysarthria, mild hypotonia)
  - Paraneoplastic: Ataxia may precede opsoclonus/myoclonus due to neuroblastoma/ganglioneuroma.
  - Migraine: Resolves in hours; headache may precede ataxia.
  - Labyrinthitis: Fast phase of nystagmus is unidirectional.
  - ADEM: White matter changes on MRI or CT
  - Acute polyneuropathy: Guillain-Barré syndrome (areflexia, signs of sensory ataxia)
  - Stroke: Focal deficits; abnormal imaging studies
  - Postictal: Rapidly resolving ataxia with negative studies, slowing on EEG; history of convulsion
  - Familial periodic ataxia: Family history
  - Metabolic disorders: Pyruvate dysmetabolism (attacks provoked by febrile illness, associated lactic acidosis), biotinidase deficiency (associated seizures, skin rash)
  - Psychogenic: Variable effort; no pathologic nystagmus; gait is grossly unsteady, corrective steps before falling
- Chronic ataxia:
  - Brain tumor (especially in children <10 years of age): Associated cranial neuropathies, papilledema, headache, pyramidal tract signs
  - Friedreich ataxia: Onset 5–15 years of age, other affected siblings, associated cardiomyopathy, diabetes, polyneuropathy, scoliosis, pes cavus
  - Ataxia telangiectasia: Onset <5 years of age, frequent bronchopulmonary infection, and leukemia/lymphoma (elevated -fetoprotein)
  - Ataxia with oculomotor apraxia type 1: Onset 2–18 years of age, associated polyneuropathy, chorea, cognitive difficulty (hypoalbuminemia, hypercholesterolemia)
  - Ataxia with oculomotor apraxia type 2: Onset 2–22 years of age, associated polyneuropathy, chorea (elevated -fetoprotein and CPK)
  - Leukodystrophy: Adreno-, metachromatic, Pelizaeus-Merzbacher (abnormal MRI)
  - Other metabolic diseases: Niemann-Pick type C (bone marrow biopsy); Refsum disease; juvenile-onset Tay-Sachs disease, neuraminidase deficiency (lysosomal disorders); maple syrup urine disease, Hartnup disease (amino acid storage); familial coenzyme Q10 deficiency; familial vitamin E deficiency; cerebral folate transport disorder (low 5-MHTF in CSF)
  - Abetalipoproteinemia: Hypocholesterolemia
  - Mitochondrial disease: Retinopathy, sensorineural hearing loss, diabetes, growth delay, seizures, strokelike episodes, myopathy, elevated pyruvate and lactate levels
  - Congenital disorders of glycosylation
  - Thiamine deficiency
  - Celiac disease
  - Autosomal dominant ataxias
  - Long-term phenytoin use: Primarily adults
  - Rare: Ataxic cerebral palsy, brain dysgenesis, Joubert syndrome, multiple sclerosis, Gerstmann-Sträussler (familial, prion disease)

 TREATMENT

- Treatment of individual disorders associated with ataxia is beyond the scope of this chapter.
- Majority of acute ataxias are self-limited, needing only supportive care.
- Treatment depends on underlying condition (e.g., if due to phenytoin toxicity, adjust phenytoin dose).
- Precautions and limitation of activity to decrease injury
- Early identification and management of aspiration
- Steroids, IVIG, plasma exchange for ADEM (limited evidence)
- Brainstem encephalitis: Antibiotics/antiviral coverage until studies are negative
- Immunomodulatory therapies have been tried (steroids, plasma exchange, IVIG) for paraneoplastic ataxia-opsoclonus/myoclonus, which may persist long after therapy for the tumor.
- Epilepsy, migraine preventive therapy
- Acetazolamide may be helpful in familial periodic ataxia.
- Drugs useful for tremor can be helpful for cerebellar tremor.
- Replacement therapies rarely helpful: Vitamin E, thiamine, B$_{12}$, coenzyme Q10; biotin; folinic acid (cerebral folate disorder).
- Physical and occupational therapy, speech therapy, other rehabilitation interventions

 ONGOING CARE

PROGNOSIS
- Most acute ataxias are postviral and have good prognosis.
- Acute postinfectious cerebellar ataxia resolves over days to weeks; if imaging studies show demyelination, recovery may take longer.
- Behavioral and learning difficulties may persist in 20% of children with postviral acute cerebellar ataxia.
- Most patients with ADEM recover completely.
- Familial periodic ataxia has benign course.

COMPLICATIONS
- Risks of injuries, aspiration, secondary infections, and depression.
- GBS: Monitor for autonomic instability, respiratory failure
- Ataxia telangiectasia: Immunodeficiency, neoplasia

ALERT
- Inadvertent intoxication with anticonvulsants may not be detected on routine toxin screen.
- MRI: Evaluate ataxia and a headache (Arnold-Chiari type 1 malformation, tumor)

ADDITIONAL READING

- Connolly AM, Dodson WE, Prensky AL, et al. Course and outcome of acute cerebellar ataxia. *Ann Neurol.* 1994;35:673–679.
- Dressler D, Benecke R. Diagnosis and management of acute movement disorders. *J Neurol.* 2005; 252(11):1299–1306.
- Mercuri E, He J, Curati WL, et al. Cerebellar infarction and atrophy in infants and children with a history of premature birth. *Pediatr Radiol.* 1997;27: 139–143.
- Palau F, Espinos C. Autosomal recessive cerebellar ataxias. *Orphanet J Rare Dis.* 2006;1:47–65.
- Ryan MM, Engle EC. Acute ataxia in childhood. *J Child Neurol.* 2003;18(5):309–316.
- Salas AA, Nava A. Acute cerebellar ataxia in childhood: Initial approach in the emergency department. *Emerg Med J.* 2010;27(12):956–957.

See Also (Topic, Algorithm, Electronic Media Element)
- National Ataxia Foundation: http://www.ataxia.org
- Friedreich's Ataxia Research Alliance: http://www.curefa.org
- Ataxia-Telangiectasia (A-T) Children's Project: http://www.atcp.org/

 CODES

ICD9
- 334.0 Friedreich's ataxia
- 334.8 Other spinocerebellar diseases
- 438.84 Ataxia

ICD10
- G11.1 Early-onset cerebellar ataxia
- G11.3 Cerebellar ataxia with defective DNA repair
- R27.0 Ataxia, unspecified

FAQ

- Q: What intoxications are most likely to cause ataxia?
- A: Benzodiazepines, the major anticonvulsants (except valproate), psychotropic medications, ethanol, tricyclics, and antihistamines
- Q: How long can postinfectious cerebellar ataxia last?
- A: Rarely, it may last for months, but usually improves during that time.
- Q: What is the role of physical therapy for cerebellar ataxia?
- A: Repetitive exercise balance and coordination may improve ataxia. Vestibular compensation exercise may improve vertigo in patients with vestibular ataxia.

ATELECTASIS

Richard M. Kravitz

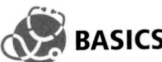 **BASICS**

DESCRIPTION
- State of collapsed and airless alveoli
- May be subsegmental, segmental, or lobar, or may involve the entire lung
- A radiographic sign of an underlying disease and not a diagnosis unto itself

EPIDEMIOLOGY
- Depends on the underlying disease causing atelectasis
- Resorption atelectasis the most common form

RISK FACTORS
Genetics
Depends on the underlying disease causing atelectasis (i.e., cystic fibrosis; primary ciliary dyskinesia)

GENERAL PREVENTION
- Maintaining adequate cough
- Good airway clearance techniques in patients at risk for atelectasis

PATHOPHYSIOLOGY
- Reduced lung compliance
- Loss of alveoli (if extensive) may lead to hypoxia.
- Intrapulmonary shunting develops from hypoxia-induced pulmonary arterial vasoconstriction, which may lead to areas of ventilation/perfusion (V/Q) mismatch and further hypoxia.
- If atelectasis is extensive and long-term, pulmonary hypertension may develop.
- Atelectatic areas are prone to bacterial overgrowth and possible secondary infection.

ETIOLOGY
- Airway obstruction (resorption atelectasis):
  - Most common cause of atelectasis in children
  - Obstructed communication between alveoli and trachea
- Large airway obstruction:
  - Intrinsic: Foreign-body aspiration, mucus plug, tumor, plastic bronchitis
  - Extrinsic: Hilar adenopathy, mediastinal mass, congenital lung malformations

- Small airway obstruction
  - Acute infection: Bronchiolitis, pneumonia (respiratory infections are the most common cause of acute atelectasis)
  - Altered mucociliary clearance: CNS depression, smoke inhalation, pain
- Mechanical compression of the pulmonary parenchyma or pleural space (compressive atelectasis):
  - Intrathoracic compression: Pneumothorax, pleural effusion, lobar emphysema, intrathoracic tumors, cardiomegaly, diaphragmatic hernias
- Abdominal distention: Large intra-abdominal tumors, hepatosplenomegaly, massive ascites, morbid obesity
- Decreased surface tension in the small airways and alveoli (adhesive atelectasis):
  - Stems from surfactant deficiency
  - Diffuse surfactant deficiency (e.g., hyaline membrane disease, acute respiratory distress syndrome, smoke inhalation)
  - Localized surfactant deficiency (e.g., acute radiation pneumonitis, pulmonary embolism)
- Neuromuscular weakness (hypoventilation):
  - Inherent weakness (e.g., Duchenne muscular dystrophy, spinal muscular atrophy, paralysis)
  - Acquired weakness (e.g., postanesthesia hypoventilation)

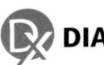 **DIAGNOSIS**

HISTORY
- Dependent on the underlying disease process
- May be asymptomatic
- Cough and/or wheeze can be present
- Dyspnea
- Chest pain
- Special questions:
  - Is the atelectasis acute, recurrent, or chronic in terms of its duration?
  - Is there a history of asthma, chronic lung disease, or exposure to smoke or toxic fumes that would increase the risk for atelectasis?

PHYSICAL EXAM
- May be normal
- Tachypnea
- Rales or rhonchi
- The most specific sign is localized decrease or loss of breath sounds.
- Dullness to percussion if large area involved
- Tracheal deviation and shift of heart sounds toward atelectatic side
- Localized wheezes in cases of partial obstruction
- Cyanosis (seen when extensive atelectasis is present, causing impairment of oxygenation and areas of ventilation/perfusion mismatch)

DIAGNOSTIC TESTS & INTERPRETATION
Lab
Appropriate test is dependent on the underlying etiology:
- Asthma:
  - Spirometry
  - Sweat test (if cystic fibrosis suspected)
- Infection:
  - Cultures (sputum, blood, bronchoalveolar lavage fluid)
  - Nasal washing (especially for viruses)
  - PPD (when tuberculosis is suspected)
- Foreign-body aspiration:
  - Bronchoscopy (to remove the obstructing agent. Rigid bronchoscopy is indicated if the obstructing agent is a foreign body; flexible can be used for mucus plugs, plastic bronchitis, or infectious etiology)
- Immunodeficiency:
  - CBC with differential
  - Immunoglobulins (IgG, IgA, IgM)
  - HIV testing
- Congenital malformations:
  - CT scan of the chest (for lung malformation)
  - Bronchoscopy (for H-type tracheoesophageal fistula [TEF] or bronchial stenosis)

Imaging
- Chest radiograph:
  - Most important diagnostic tool
  - Radiographic signs of atelectasis:
    - ○ Loss of lung volume from the affected lobe
    - ○ Compensatory hyperexpansion of the remaining lobes on the affected side
    - ○ Shift of interlobar fissures
    - ○ Elevation of diaphragm
    - ○ Mediastinal shift toward the affected side
    - ○ Approximation of ribs on the affected side
- CT of chest:
  - Confluence of bronchi and blood vessels converge toward the affected side
  - Provides information with regard to precise location and extent of any obstructing process

DIFFERENTIAL DIAGNOSIS
- Pneumonia:
  - Viral pneumonia versus subsegmental atelectasis
  - Bacterial pneumonia versus segmental or lobar atelectasis
- Thymus (may often be mistaken for atelectasis in an upper lobe)
- Congenital malformations (e.g., sequestration, bronchogenic cyst)
- Pleural effusion

 TREATMENT

ADDITIONAL TREATMENT
General Measures
- Treat underlying disease (i.e., removal of aspirated foreign body; clearance of mucus plugs; treatment of any underlying infection)
- Chest physical therapy with bronchodilators (usually for at least 1 month).
- If no improvement with conservative therapy, a bronchoscopy with lavage to remove possible mucus plug is indicated (lavage may be with saline or, in select cases, with recombinant human DNase or N-acetylcysteine).
- Consider surgery to remove the affected region:
  - Chronic or recurrent atelectasis
  - Unresponsive to therapy
  - Focal bronchiectasis has developed.
  - Significant morbidity is seen.

- Prevention of recurrent or future atelectasis: Directed toward underlying cause, when applicable
- Airway clearance is important in clearing areas of atelectasis.
- Various techniques are available including:
  - Manuel chest physiotherapy
  - Mechanical chest physiotherapy (ThAIRapy vest)
  - Incentive spirometry
  - Acapella or Flutter devices
  - Intermittent positive pressure breathing (IPPB) or intrapulmonary percussive ventilator (IPV)
  - Mechanical insufflator-exsufflator (Cough Assist):
    - ○ For patients with weakened cough (i.e., neuromuscular weakness)

 ONGOING CARE

FOLLOW-UP RECOMMENDATIONS
Patient Monitoring
Expect improvement: 1–3 months in typical, uncomplicated cases

PROGNOSIS
- Dependent on the underlying disease process
- In otherwise healthy individuals: Excellent

COMPLICATIONS
- Recurrent infections
- Bronchiectasis
- Hemoptysis
- Abscess formation
- Fibrosis of the pulmonary parenchyma

ADDITIONAL READING
- Birnkrant DJ, Pope JF, Eiben RM. Management of the respiratory complications of neuromuscular diseases in the pediatric intensive care unit. *J Child Neurol*.1999;14(3):139–143.
- Hough JL, Flenady V, Johnston L, et al. Chest physiotherapy for reducing respiratory morbidity in infants requiring ventilator support. *Cochrane Database Syst Rev*. 2008.

- McCool FD, Rosen MJ. Nonpharmacologic airway clearance therapies: ACCP evidence-based clinical practical guidelines. *Chest*. 2006;129:250S–259S.
- Oermann CM, Moore RH. Foolers: Things that look like pneumonia in children. *Semin Respir Infect*. 1996;11:204–213.
- Redding GJ. Atelectasis in childhood. *Pediatr Clin North Am*. 1984;31:891–905.
- Riethmueller J, Kumpf M, Borth-Bruhns T, et al. Clinical and *in vitro* effect of dornase alfa in mechanically ventilated pediatric non-cystic fibrosis patients with atelectasis. *Cell Physiol Biochem*. 2009;23:205–210.
- Slattery DM, Waltz DA, Denham B, et al. Bronchoscopically administered recombinant human DNase for lobar atelectasis in cystic fibrosis. *Pediatr Pulmonol*. 2001;31:383–388.

 CODES

ICD9
518.0 Pulmonary collapse

ICD10
- J98.11 Atelectasis
- P28.10 Unspecified atelectasis of newborn

FAQ
- Q: When is the optimal time for bronchoscopy?
- A: There are no established criteria for when a bronchoscopy should be performed. A bronchoscopy should be done early in the course of illness when:
  - There is a high suspicion of a foreign body.
  - Significant respiratory distress is present.
  - Cases of acute chest syndrome in patients with sickle cell disease
  - If the atelectasis is extensive and conservative treatment is ineffective
  - Bronchoscopy is infrequently performed in patients with cystic fibrosis secondary to its recurrent nature.

ATOPIC DERMATITIS
Albert C. Yan

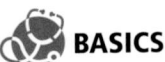 **BASICS**

DESCRIPTION
Atopic dermatitis or eczema is a chronic, recurrent, pruritic skin eruption seen in individuals with associated personal or family history of atopy (e.g., asthma, allergies, hay fever, or rhinitis). The disease is characterized by intermittent acute flares. It most commonly begins in infancy or early childhood.

EPIDEMIOLOGY
Incidence
- Atopic dermatitis is a common disease, occurring in nearly 1 in 5 children.
- ~60% of patients with atopic dermatitis will develop it in the 1st year of life, and 30% between the ages of 1 and 5 years.

Prevalence
- A family history of atopy (e.g., allergies, asthma, eczema, or hay fever) is present in 30–70% of patients.
- Atopic dermatitis is usually worse in the winter, but can flare at any time of year.

RISK FACTORS
Genetics
- There is a genetic trait seen in atopic dermatitis, with 30–70% of family members having atopy (allergies, asthma, eczema, or hay fever).
- The exact mode of inheritance is not well defined and appears to be multifactorial. However, in a subset of patients, studies indicate a strong link to filaggrin mutations among patients suffering from atopic dermatitis, asthma, and ichthyosis vulgaris.

PATHOPHYSIOLOGY
- Histologic findings are dependent on the stage of atopic dermatitis (i.e., acute or chronic).
- Lymphocytes can be seen infiltrating the epidermis.
- The acute form shows spongiosis and intercellular edema that can lead to vesicle formation.
- The chronic form is characterized by epidermal psoriasiform hyperplasia and hyperkeratosis.

ETIOLOGY
- Etiology of atopic dermatitis is multifactorial, with genetic, environmental, physiologic, and immunologic factors.
- Increased viral (warts and molluscum) and dermatophyte infections seen in these patients appears to be related to cytokine-induced suppression of endogenous antimicrobial peptides.
- Patients often have elevated IgE levels and decreased chemotaxis of neutrophils.
- Up to 70% of patients have a family history, but the mode of inheritance is not well defined.

 **DIAGNOSIS**

HISTORY
- Age of onset
- Location
- Prior treatment
- Bathing habits
- Family history of atopy (allergies)
- Asthma
- Eczema
- Hay fever
- Special questions:
  - Excessive dryness exacerbates this disease; therefore, inquiry about bathing habits, frequency, and emollients is helpful.

PHYSICAL EXAM
- Acute flares reveal weeping and crusted erythema.
- Chronic disease is characterized by hyperpigmentation or hypopigmentation, lichenification, and scaling.
- The distribution of the disease is dependent on age.
  - During infancy to ~2 years of age, the disease is widespread and includes cheeks, forehead, scalp, and extensor surfaces.
  - In children from ~3–11 years of age, the disease involves the more characteristic flexural sites with lichenification.
  - The hands and face can also be involved.
  - From adolescence to adulthood, the flexures, neck, hands, and feet are frequently involved, with the face and neck flaring occasionally.
- When the disease is severe, it can present as exfoliative erythroderma with diffuse scaling and erythema.
- Other associated findings include: Dennie-Morgan folds (infraorbital folds), pityriasis alba (dry white patches), hyperlinear palms, facial pallor, infraorbital darkening, follicular accentuation, keratosis pilaris (dry, rough hair follicles on extensor surfaces of upper arms and thighs), and ichthyosis.

DIAGNOSTIC TESTS & INTERPRETATION
Lab
- No tests by themselves are diagnostic of atopic dermatitis.
- Biopsy can be helpful to rule out papulosquamous disease, such as psoriasis.
- IgE levels are often elevated. When extremely high, evaluation for associated comorbidities such as HyperIgE syndrome should be considered
- Bacterial cultures can help identify superinfection during acute flares. Rapid fluorescent antibody studies, polymerase chain reaction studies, or viral cultures, and Tzanck smear can identify complications of eczema herpeticum.
- Patch testing can help differentiate atopic dermatitis from contact dermatitis.

DIFFERENTIAL DIAGNOSIS
- Diagnostic criteria have been established for atopic dermatitis:
  - Severe seborrheic dermatitis
  - Contact dermatitis
  - Allergic or irritant, psoriasis
  - Wiskott-Aldrich syndrome
  - Langerhans cell histiocytosis
  - Acrodermatitis enteropathica
  - Scabies
  - Xerosis
  - Hyper-IgE syndrome (including recently described mutations in STAT3, DOC8, and tyk2)
- Metabolic deficiencies:
  - Carboxylase deficiencies
  - Prolidase deficiencies

TREATMENT
MEDICATION (DRUGS)
- Antihistamines, such as hydroxyzine or diphenhydramine, may help to decrease itching in selected patients.
- Topical steroids control inflammation and mid- to high-potency steroids can be used during acute flares, with tapering of steroids to milder potency when control is achieved. Once cleared, topical steroids can be held and substituted with emollients. Long-term use of steroids can lead to atrophy, telangiectasias, tachyphylaxis, and occasionally, stunting of growth.
- Oral antibiotics are indicated when there is superinfection of lesions. Dilute bleach baths (about 1/4 cup per full tub of water or about 1 tsp per gallon of water) can be used as a once or twice weekly 10-minute soak to help reduce bacterial skin colonization and risk for recurrent skin infection.
- Antivirals are needed for cases of eczema herpeticum. During acute flares with oozing and crusting and when there is superinfection with bacteria or herpes simplex virus, compresses can be helpful.
- Tacrolimus ointment and pimecrolimus cream are topical therapies recently approved for use in children 2 years of age and older. These are calcineurin phosphatase inhibitors that act to suppress T-cell function. Because these agents are not steroids, they are not atrophogenic and do not appear to alter hypothalamic–pituitary axis function. However, less is known regarding its long-term effects in children. Children who receive this medication should receive instructions for diligent sun protection and sunscreen use to minimize potentiation for sun damage.

- Systemic steroids are generally not used because of the chronicity of atopic dermatitis, and are reserved for when control of the eruption is very difficult, and then use should be of short duration.
- Phototherapy with UVB can be used in patients with extensive disease that is resistant to other therapy.
- The use of topical barrier repair agents cleared by the US Food and Drug Administration include N-palmitoylethanolamine cream, MAS063DP cream, and various ceramide formulations and may be useful adjuncts to therapy.

ADDITIONAL TREATMENT
General Measures
- There is no cure for atopic dermatitis.
- Parents must understand that this is a chronic disease with intermittent flares and that control is the aim of treatment.
- Good skin care is critical to maintenance and includes use of mild soaps, frequent use of emollients, and avoidance of excessive bathing.
- Avoidance of irritants from the environment, such as wool sweaters or blankets, is recommended. Protective clothing at night to avoid scratching while sleeping is also helpful, as is trimming the nails.

 ONGOING CARE

FOLLOW-UP RECOMMENDATIONS
Patient Monitoring
It should be emphasized to parents that atopic dermatitis is a chronic disease and that good skin care is necessary to control disease activity. Up to 40–50% of children will outgrow their atopic dermatitis after the age of 5 years.

COMPLICATIONS
- Decreased cell-mediated immunity, decreased chemotaxis, and decreased production of endogenous antimicrobial peptides can result in increased infection (e.g., viral, dermatophyte, bacterial). Patients with atopic dermatitis have a high density of Staphylococcus aureus on their skin, and given the fissures and open excoriations, there is a risk of superinfection of these lesions.
- The decreased integrity of the skin can result in widely spread cutaneous infections such as herpes simplex infection, known as Kaposi varicelliform eruption or eczema herpeticum. Similar problems can also be seen with coxsackievirus or molluscum contagiosum and used to occur with Vaccinia.

- Cataracts can be found in patients with atopic dermatitis.
- Overuse of potent topical steroids can result in hypopigmentation, telangiectasias, atrophy, and striae, as well as excess systemic absorption leading to hypothalamic–pituitary axis suppression and growth retardation.
- Early growth delay is not uncommon among children with atopic dermatitis, although later catch-up growth is generally seen. This may be related to various mechanisms including impaired growth-hormone release. This growth delay can occur independent of topical steroid exposure.
- Pigmentary changes may result from overuse of topical medications; however, the lesions of atopic dermatitis may themselves cause postinflammatory skin color changes independent of topical therapy.

ADDITIONAL READING

- Batchelor JM, Grindlay DJ, Williams HC. What's new in atopic eczema? An analysis of systematic reviews published in 2008 and 2009. Clin Exp Dermatol. 2010;35(8):823–827.
- Burks AW, James JM, Hiegel A, et al. Atopic dermatitis and food hypersensitivity reactions. J Pediatr. 1998;132(1):132–136.
- Eichenfield LF, Hanifin JM, Luger TA, et al. Consensus conference on pediatric atopic dermatitis. J Am Acad Dermatol. 2003;49(6):1088–1095.
- Hill DJ, Hosking CS. Emerging disease profiles in infants and young children with food allergy. Pediatr Allergy Immunol. 1997;8(Suppl 10):21–26.
- Kalavala M, Dohil MA. Calcineurin inhibitors in pediatric atopic dermatitis: A review of current evidence. Am J Clin Dermatol. 2011;12(1):15–24.
- Krakowski AC, Eichenfield LF, Dohil MA. Management of atopic dermatitis in the pediatric population. Pediatrics. 2008;122(4):812–824.
- Lever WF, Schaumberg-Lever G. Histopathology of the Skin, 7th ed. Philadelphia: JB Lippincott; 1990.
- Ong PY, Leung DYM. Immune dysregulation in atopic dermatitis. Curr Allergy Asthma Rep. 2006;6(5):384–389.
- O'Regan GM, Irvine AD. The role of filaggrin in the atopic diathesis. Clin Exp Allergy. 2010;40(7): 965–972.
- Spergel JM. Epidemiology of atopic dermatitis and atopic march in children. Immunol Allergy Clin North Am. 2010;30(3):269–280.

 CODES

ICD9
691.8 Other atopic dermatitis and related conditions

ICD10
- L20.83 Infantile (acute) (chronic) eczema
- L20.89 Other atopic dermatitis
- L20.9 Atopic dermatitis, unspecified

FAQ
- Q: Will the child outgrow this?
- A: Up to 40–50% of children will outgrow their atopic dermatitis after age 5 years. In some patients, however, the disease will persist to variable extents throughout adulthood.
- Q: When atopic dermatitis is controlled, is any treatment necessary?
- A: Excessive dryness can exacerbate or flare disease. Therefore, less frequent use of soaps and frequent use of emollients are recommended.
- Q: Do food hypersensitivities play a role in atopic dermatitis?
- A: This is a debated issue. In general, the majority of patients are probably not adversely affected by foods. However, some individuals, particularly those who are unresponsive to routine therapy, may benefit from screening for food hypersensitivity and a trial of avoidance to any foods that test positive. The most common foods associated with exacerbation when an association can be made are eggs, milk, wheat, soy, peanuts, and fish.

ATRIAL SEPTAL DEFECT
Jonathan Fleenor

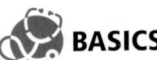 **BASICS**

DESCRIPTION
- An opening in the atrial septum, other than a patent foramen ovale (PFO)
- 4 major types of atrial septal defects (ASDs):
  - Secundum atrial septal defect
  - Primum atrial septal defect
  - Sinus venosus atrial septal defect
  - Coronary sinus atrial septal defect
- A patent foramen ovale usually does not cause a significant intracardiac shunt. A probe patent foramen ovale can be found in up to 15–25% of normal hearts at pathologic exam.
- Secundum defects make up 60–70% of all atrial septal defects. Usually there is a shunt from the left atrium to the right atrium.
- Primum defects occur in ~30% of all atrial septal defects. They are usually associated with a cleft mitral valve. This defect is the result of an abnormality of the endocardial cushions, and therefore is also referred to as an incomplete AV canal defect.
- Sinus venosus defects can be of the superior or inferior vena caval type and occur in ~5–10% of all atrial septal defects. In atrial septal defects of the superior vena caval type, the right pulmonary veins (usually right upper lobe) may drain anomalously to the superior vena cava or right atrium.
- Coronary sinus atrial septal defects are rare and occur in <1% of all atrial septal defects. They are often associated with absence of the coronary sinus and a persistent left superior vena cava that joins the roof of the left atrium (also known as an "unroofed coronary sinus").

EPIDEMIOLOGY
Females > males (2:1)

Incidence
- Difficult to determine
- Occurs in 6–10% of all cardiac anomalies encountered

PATHOPHYSIOLOGY
- A left-to-right shunt occurs through the atrial septal defect. For large defects, this results in right atrial and right ventricular (RV) volume overload.
- There is usually increased pulmonary blood flow.
- The left-to-right shunt generally increases with time as pulmonary resistance drops and right ventricular compliance normalizes.
- Moderate and large defects are associated with a Qp/Qs ratio of >2:1.
- The direction of atrial shunting is determined by the relative compliance of the right and left ventricles.

ETIOLOGY
- Atrial septal defects may be associated with partial or total anomalous pulmonary venous drainage, mitral valve anomalies, transposition of the great arteries, or tricuspid atresia.
- Although usually isolated, atrial septal defects may occur as part of a syndrome (Holt-Oram [autosomal dominant]).

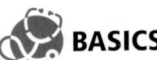 **DIAGNOSIS**

HISTORY
- Most infants are asymptomatic.
- Older children with moderate left-to-right shunts are often asymptomatic, but may have mild fatigue or dyspnea, especially with exercise.
- Children with large left-to-right shunts may complain of fatigue and dyspnea, which may become noticeable as the child gets older.
- Growth failure is uncommon.
- Older patients with large atrial shunts may develop atrial arrhythmias.

PHYSICAL EXAM
- Inspection and palpation of the precordium are usually normal, although older children with a large atrial septal defect may have a hyperdynamic precordium, right ventricular heave, or precordial bulge.
- Auscultation reveals 3 important features:
  - Wide and "fixed" splitting of S_2. Splitting of S_2 (A_2 and P_2 components) is caused by a delay in emptying of a volume-loaded right ventricle.
  - A systolic ejection murmur at the upper left sternal border. This murmur is caused by an increase in blood flow across a normal pulmonary valve. It may be differentiated from the murmur of pulmonary stenosis because there is no click.
  - A diastolic murmur at the lower sternal border, indicating a Qp/Qs ratio of at least 2:1. This murmur is caused by increased flow across the tricuspid valve.

DIAGNOSTIC TESTS & INTERPRETATION
Lab
- ECG:
  - Usually normal sinus rhythm with an rSR' (incomplete right bundle branch block pattern) in lead V_1, V_3R, and V_4R, indicating right ventricular volume overload. For larger shunts, ECG may show evidence of right atrial enlargement as well as 1st-degree AV block. A late finding suggestive of pulmonary hypertension is right ventricular hypertrophy.
- Chest radiograph:
  - Cardiomegaly (right atrium and right ventricle), increased pulmonary vascular markings, and a dilated pulmonary trunk are seen in patients with significant left-to-right shunts.
- Echocardiogram:
  - A 2-D echo study is diagnostic; it reveals the location, size, and associated defects, if any. It may demonstrate dilated right-heart structures. Color Doppler generally permits visualization of the direction of shunt flow. Older children and adolescents may require transesophageal echo to best define the atrial septal defect.
- Cardiac catheterization:
  - Generally unnecessary. It is indicated when pulmonary vascular disease is suspected (determination of pulmonary vascular resistance) or for associated cardiac defects.

DIFFERENTIAL DIAGNOSIS
- Ventricular septal defect
- Patent ductus arteriosus
- AV canal defect
- Valvar pulmonary stenosis

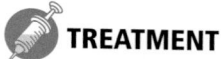 **TREATMENT**

ADDITIONAL TREATMENT
General Measures
- Infants with congestive heart failure should be treated with diuretics.
- Elective closure is indicated for atrial septal defects associated with large left-to-right shunts, cardiomegaly, or symptoms.
  - The timing of closure is usually deferred until 3–5 years of age.
  - For most secundum-type atrial septal defects, device closure of the defect can be performed in the cardiac catheterization laboratory, thus avoiding surgery.
- Prevention of paradoxical emboli and cerebrovascular accidents is an uncommon but possible indication for closure of atrial septal defects or patent foramen ovale.
- Irreversible pulmonary hypertension from a long-term left-to-right shunt usually does not occur until adolescence or young adulthood.
- Sinus venosus, primum, and coronary sinus–type atrial septal defects require surgical closure. The mortality of surgical repair for an uncomplicated ASD approaches 0%.
- There is some anecdotal evidence suggesting that PFOs are a cause of migraine headaches in certain populations. Prospective adult studies are currently ongoing to further investigate this question.

 ONGOING CARE

FOLLOW-UP RECOMMENDATIONS
Patient Monitoring
- Children with typical auscultation, chest radiograph, and ECG findings should undergo an echocardiographic evaluation to determine the location and size of the atrial septal defect.
- Children with atrial septal defects should have regular follow-up to assess for signs of congestive heart failure or right ventricular volume overload. Restriction of activity is unnecessary. SBE prophylaxis is not indicated for an isolated secundum atrial septal defect. Residual atrial septal defect after surgery is rare.
- SBE prophylaxis is indicated for the 1st 6 months (assuming no residual defect) after closure of a secundum defect.
- Complications related to surgery include:
  - Sinus node dysfunction
  - Venous obstruction (facial or pulmonary edema) may occur after a sinus venosus atrial septal defect repair.
  - Postpericardiotomy syndrome, which manifests with nausea, vomiting, abdominal pain, or fever, may occur a few weeks after surgical repair. Although a friction rub may not be present, the chest radiograph may show cardiomegaly and the echocardiogram may reveal a pericardial effusion.

PROGNOSIS
- The prognosis for small atrial septal defects seems excellent without specific therapy.
- Spontaneous closure of small secundum atrial septal defects can occur in up to 80% of infants in the 1st year of life. Isolated secundum atrial septal defects of moderate and large size do not typically cause symptoms in most infants and children.
- Pulmonary hypertension is rare in childhood.
- Atrial flutter and fibrillation occur in up to 13% of unoperated patients older than 40 years.
- Bacterial endocarditis is rare in children with isolated atrial septal defect.
- Paradoxical emboli may occur, and should be considered in patients with cerebral or systemic emboli.

ADDITIONAL READING

- Horton SC, Bunch TJ. Patent foramen ovale and stroke. *Mayo Clin Proc.* 2004;79(1):79–88.
- Kharouf R, Luxenberg DM, Khalid O, et al. Atrial septal defect: Spectrum of care. *Pediatr Cardiol.* 2008;29(2):271–280.
- Meijboom F, Roos-Hesselink J, Sievert H. The role of the atria in congenital heart disease. *Cardiol Clin.* 2002;20(3):351–366.
- Ohye RG, Bove EL. Advances in congenital heart surgery. *Curr Opin Pediatr.* 2001;13(5):473–481.
- Radzik D, Davignon A, van Doesburg N, et al. Predictive factors for spontaneous closure of atrial septal defect diagnosed in the first 3 months of life. *J Am Coll Cardiol.* 1993;22:851–853.
- Rocchini AP. Pediatric cardiac catheterization. *Curr Opin Cardiol.* 2002;17(3):283–288.
- Zanchetta M, Rigatelli G, Pedon L, et al. Role of intracardiac echocardiography in atrial septal abnormalities. *J Interv Cardiol.* 2003;16(1):63–77.

 CODES

ICD9
- 429.71 Acquired atrial septal defect
- 745.4 Ventricular septal defect
- 745.5 Atrial septal (ostium secundum type)

ICD10
- Q21.1 Atrial septal defect
- Q21.2 Atrioventricular septal defect

FAQ

- Q: When should a moderate secundum atrial septal defect be closed?
- A: This can generally be electively performed in children prior to their starting grade school.
- Q: What is the significance of a patient having GI complaints (nausea and vomiting) 2–3 weeks after surgical closure of an atrial septal defect?
- A: This may represent a pericardial effusion (postpericardiotomy syndrome).

ATTENTION-DEFICIT/HYPERACTIVITY DISORDER (ADHD)

William G. McNett

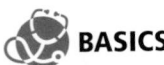

BASICS

DESCRIPTION
- Attention-deficit hyperactivity disorder (ADHD) is a syndrome characterized by persistent and developmentally inappropriate levels of inattention and/or hyperactivity and impulsivity. It can be classified into 3 subtypes:
  - Hyperactive/impulsive
  - Inattentive
  - Combined
- DSM-IV criteria for diagnosis:
  - At least 6 of 9 behaviors in inattention and/or hyperactivity/impulsivity
  - Persisting for at least 6 months that is maladaptive and inconsistent with developmental level
  - Some symptoms present before age 7 years
  - Impairment from symptoms present in 2 or more settings
  - Clear evidence of clinically significant impairment in social, academic, or occupational functioning

Prevalence
- 3–7% of school-age children
- 3–4 times more common in males than females
- Females more likely to have inattentive type

RISK FACTORS
Genetics
- Risk of ADHD in first-degree relatives is ~25%.
- Concordance in monozygotic twins: 59–81%; dizygotic twins: 33%

COMMONLY ASSOCIATED CONDITIONS
- Learning disorders
- School failure
- Tic disorder
- Oppositional defiant disorder and conduct disorder
- Mood disorders: anxiety and depression
- Poor peer relations

DIAGNOSIS

- Typically, patients are brought to medical attention during the early school years because their behavior falls out of normal range in their ability to pay attention in class, to avoid class disruption, and/or to control impulsive behavior.
- Many patients with ADHD can be diagnosed and treated in the pediatrician's office.
- A large percentage of patients with ADHD may have associated conditions and will need multidisciplinary pediatric teams of developmental pediatrics, psychologists, neurologists, and/or psychiatrists for assessment and treatment.

SIGNS AND SYMPTOMS
HISTORY
- A detailed history of the child's behavior at home, school, and with peers is needed.
- Onset and duration of noted behaviors
- Ability to make and keep friends
- Academic progress
- Birth history with details about prematurity, *in utero* drug exposure, and perinatal asphyxia
- Developmental history, specifically language acquisition and fine motor skills
- Sleep history
- Family history of ADHD and/or learning disorders
- Family history of cardiac disease including arrhythmias, hypertrophic cardiomyopathy or sudden cardiac death in children or young adults
- Social history: those who live with patient, recent family discord, separation, recent death in the family, recent change in schools
- Past medical history and medication history

PHYSICAL EXAM
- Hearing and vision testing to rule out vision disturbances or hearing impairment, respectively, as a cause of inattention
- Weight and height measurements for baseline before starting medication and to help rule out thyroid dysfunction as underlying cause
- Vital signs including BP and pulse are important for baseline measurements.
- Examination of neck to ensure no obvious thyroid enlargement or change in thyroid gland
- Skin exam to rule out neurocutaneous syndromes
- Thorough cardiac exam
- Thorough neurological exam to rule out an intracranial process that may cause similar symptoms

DIAGNOSTIC TESTS & INTERPRETATION
- Rating scales:
  - Multiple scales available including Connor Rating Scales-Revised, Vanderbilt ADHD Rating Scales, Child Behavior Checklist
  - Both parent and teacher ratings are routine components of the assessment.
  - Some assess only ADHD (Connor); others include assessment of possible co-morbidities (Vanderbilt and Child Behavior Checklists).
  - Most scales may be used by clinicians for follow-up to assess effectiveness of treatment.
  - All 3 scales have similar reliability and validity; most clinicians choose a single tool and gain familiarity with it.
- IQ and achievement testing:
  - Necessary to rule out mental retardation and learning disorder that may mimic ADHD or be a comorbidity of ADHD
  - An evaluation for an Individual Educational Plan (IEP) should be obtained following parental request of the child's school. Note: Federal law mandates that all school-age children have an IEP based upon written request by the parent. Who administers the IEP depends on whether the school is public or private, and on the school district.

Lab
Based on history and/or physical exam, consider:
- Thyroid function tests: If growth curves show unexpected acceleration or deceleration of growth
- Blood lead level to rule out lead toxicity
- CBC to rule out anemia
- EKG prior to starting stimulant medication if family history is significant

DIFFERENTIAL DIAGNOSIS
- Medical:
  - Seizures
  - Sleep disorder
  - Sensory impairment (vision, hearing)
  - Thyroid disorder
  - Medication side effects
  - Toxins (lead)
  - Iron deficiency anemia
  - Postconcussion syndrome
- Developmental:
  - Mental retardation
  - Autism spectrum disorder
  - Language or speech disorder
- Educational:
  - Learning disabilities
  - Inappropriate school environment
- Psychiatric:
  - Depression
  - Mania
  - Anxiety disorders
  - Obsessive–compulsive disorder
  - Oppositional defiant disorder
  - Conduct disorder
- Social:
  - Disorganized/chaotic family environment
  - Physical abuse/neglect
  - Sexual abuse
  - Psychosocial stressors

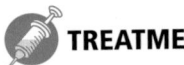

TREATMENT

GENERAL MEASURES
- 3 treatment modalities in combination:
  - Educational support
  - Behavior modification/psychological counseling
  - Medication (usually stimulant)
- Although all 3 modalities may not be necessary, they all should be discussed with the patient and parents.

NON-PHARMACOLOGIC
- Educational:
  - Request a 504 Plan through patient's school to evaluate for possible accommodations (different then an IEP)
  - Proper educational placement
  - Small teacher-to-student ratio in classroom
  - Good communication between school and home
  - Homework log monitored by teacher and parent
- Psychological support may be helpful for:
  - Patient who has poor peer relations
  - Patient with a comorbidity
  - Families that are having difficulty with parenting issues
  - Families that are unstructured and may contribute to patient's symptoms

MEDICATION (DRUGS)

First Line

- **Stimulant:** Methylphenidate (Ritalin, Methylin, Metadate, Focalin, Concerta, Daytrana Patch), dextroamphetamine-amphetamine (Dexedrine, Dextrostat, Adderall)
- **Efficacy:** 80% of children with ADHD show significant improvement with use of stimulant medication soon after proper dosing is achieved.
- **Pharmacokinetics:** Individual response is highly variable. Onset is within 20–30 minutes. Stimulants have different duration of action: Short-acting stimulants last 3–6 hours (Methylphenidate, Ritalin, Methylin, Focalin, Dexedrine, Dextrostat, Adderall) with dosing 2–3 times/d; Long-acting stimulants last 3–8 hours (Methylphenidate SR, Ritalin SR, Methylin ER, Metadate ER, Dexadrine Spanules); and extended-release stimulants last 8–12 hours (Ritalin LA, Metadate CD, Concerta, Focalin XR, Daytrana, Vyvanse, Adderall XR) needing once-a-day dosing.
- **Dose:** Weight-based dosing is not effective because of differences in metabolism. Start with smallest dose and titrate up for effect. Start with short-acting medication. For some younger children, this may provide a sufficient duration of therapy for school. If a second dose is needed, converting to a longer-acting medication is reasonable. Start medication when the parents are available to watch for side effects and duration of action (typically over a weekend). Follow closely with the parents; ask them to get feedback from school on a weekly basis until dose is properly adjusted. This process may take 1–2 months to be completed.
- **Side effects:** Decreased appetite, abdominal pain, weight loss, tics, headache, difficulty falling asleep, and jitteriness. Most stimulant-related side effects are short-lived and are responsive to dose or timing adjustments. Severe movement disorders, obsessive–compulsive ruminations, or psychotic symptoms are very rare and disappear when medication is stopped.
- **Contraindications:** Glaucoma, symptomatic cardiovascular disease, hyperthyroidism, hypertension

Second Line

- Atomoxetine (Strattera): Selective norepinephrine uptake inhibitor. once-a-day dosing, same side-effect profile as stimulants, not as efficacious as a stimulant but may be a viable alternative for patients who do not tolerate stimulant medication or if a patient's family is hesitant to use stimulants. Effects of medication may not be seen for several weeks after starting.
- Others: α-Adrenergic (clonidine, Guanfacine), tricyclic antidepressants (imipramine, nortriptyline, desipramine), atypical antidepressants (Wellbutrin, Effexor). Usually prescribed by specialists, including psychiatrists and behavioral specialists.

ISSUES FOR REFERRAL

- When comorbidities are suspected
- If patient is not responding to increasing dose of medication
- If the patient is having difficulty tolerating different stimulants
- Onset of symptoms beyond grade school

 ONGOING CARE

FOLLOW-UP RECOMMENDATIONS

- Initially, follow-up should be every 1–2 weeks until proper dosing is achieved. Can be done by telephone or e-mail communication.
- After initial stabilization, patients should be seen every 3–6 months.
- Monitor weight, height, BP, and heart rate.
- Assess for change in growth velocity.
- Assess family and peer relationships.
- Assess school performance.
- Check for medication side effects. If onset of sleep is disturbed, consider melatonin for sleep initiation.
- Assess for ongoing need for medication.

ADDITIONAL READING

- American Academy of Pediatrics. Committee on Quality Improvement and Subcommittee on Attention-Deficit/Hyperactivity Disorder. Clinical practice guideline: Diagnosis and evaluation of the child with attention-deficit/hyperactivity disorder. *Pediatrics.* 2000;105:1158–1170.
- American Academy of Pediatrics. Committee on Quality Improvement and Subcommittee on Attention-Deficit/Hyperactivity Disorder. Clinical practice guideline: Treatment of the school-aged child with attention-deficit/hyperactivity disorder. *Pediatrics.* 2001;108:1033–1044.
- Collett BR, Ohan JL, Myers KM. Ten-year review of rating scales. V: Scales assessing attention-deficit/hyperactivity disorder. *J Am Acad Child Adolesc Psychiatry.* 2003;42:1015–1037.
- Perrin JM, Friedman RA, Knilans TK. AAP Policy Statement: Cardiovascular monitoring and stimulant drugs for attention deficit/hyperactivity disorder. *Pediatrics.* 2008;122(2):451–453.
- Pliszka S. Practice parameter for the assessment and treatment of children and adolescents with attention-deficit/hyperactivity disorder. *J Am Acad Child Adolesc Psychiatry.* 2007;46(7):894–921.
- Weber W, Newmark S. Complementary and alternative medical therapies for attention-deficit/hyperactivity disorder and autism. *Pediatr Clin North Am.* 2007;54(6):983–1006.

 CODES

ICD9

- 314.00 Attention deficit disorder without mention of hyperactivity
- 314.01 Attention deficit disorder with hyperactivity

ICD10

- F90.0 Attention-deficit hyperactivity disorder, predominantly inattentive type
- F90.1 Attention-deficit hyperactivity disorder, predominantly hyperactive type
- F90.9 Attention-deficit hyperactivity disorder, unspecified type

FAQ

- Q: Does complementary and alternative medical (CAM) therapies, including diet, play a role in treating ADHD?
- A: Although in the past it has been thought that certain foods and additives caused ADHD, there are no scientific studies that show changes in diet to be of benefit. Frequently, families will want to explore the use of CAM therapies either in conjunction with or instead of treatment with stimulant medication. In addition to not showing benefit, there may be safety issues associated with certain CAM therapies. If safety can be assured, it may be reasonable for patients to try for a finite period of time if it ultimately helps the patient. If CAM therapy fails, the parents may be more willing to try stimulant medication.
- Q: Is medication needed every day?
- A: This depends on the needs of the patient. Some patients need medication in order to function successfully with peers or in structured environments, like team sports or weekend schools. Other patients who need help mainly with focusing attention do well with medication only during learning periods (school days). Many patients will not need medication during the summer holiday or during school breaks.
- Q: How long will my child be on medication?
- A: A large percentage of children with ADHD will continue to have symptoms as adults. Although every patient is different, some patients may need to continue medication through formal learning (high school and college). During this time, they should be able to learn coping strategies to minimize the effects of their symptoms. If treatment goals are being met, it is reasonable to have a trial off medications to see if performance off medications can be sustained (sometimes called a drug holiday).
- Q: Are there support groups available?
- A: An organization that is widely recognized as an advocacy and support group for families is Children and Adults with Attention Deficit/hyperactivity Disorder (www.chadd.org). This organization provides links to local groups that meet regularly, and provides a forum for parents to discuss having a child with ADHD. One should use discretion when using online resources; there are many online websites that are sponsored by pharmaceutical companies and others that encourage alternatives to medication and actively discourage use of currently recommended treatments.

ATYPICAL MYCOBACTERIAL INFECTIONS

Richard M. Rutstein

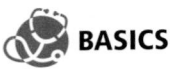 **BASICS**

DESCRIPTION

Atypical mycobacterial (ATM) infection refers to disease caused by *Mycobacterium* other than tuberculosis, bovis, and leprae, and usually involves *Mycobacterium avium intracellulare, M. scrofulaceum, M. kansasii, M. fortuitum,* and *M. chelonae*. These diseases are also referred to as nontuberculous mycobacterial infections, environmental mycobacterial infections, and mycobacteria other than tuberculosis (MOTT) infections.

EPIDEMIOLOGY

- 80–90% of cases of adenitis caused by ATM infection occur in preschool-aged children (ages 1–5 years).
- In children with chronic illness, especially cystic fibrosis, lung disease from ATM may be a factor in progressive lung disease.
- In adults in the US, the prevalence of ATM pulmonary disease is now higher than that caused by *Mycobacterium tuberculosis*.
- Early in the HIV epidemic, the incidence rate of disseminated disease in HIV-infected adults was ~40%; in HIV-infected children, 10–20%. This rate has decreased markedly in recent years through the routine use of prophylaxis and because of the improved immunologic function in HIV-infected individuals on newer antiretroviral agents.
- A rare genetic defect, leading to intraleukin-12 receptor deficiency, has been associated with increased risk of ATM-related disease. Treatment with tumor necrosis factor-alpha–modifying agents (such as infliximab and etanercept) also increases the risk.

PATHOPHYSIOLOGY

- Organisms are ubiquitous in the environment (soil, fresh water, ocean water, home and hospital water, dust, and food [eggs, dairy products, meat]).
- It is spread by aerosol inhalation or ingestion of contaminated food, dust, or water.
- Person-to-person spread has never been documented and is not a concern.

ETIOLOGY

- The most common associated illness is unilateral chronic cervical adenopathy/adenitis in preschool-aged children.
- In adults, ATM infection may cause a chronic single pulmonary nodule or more extensive chronic lung disease.
- In children and adults infected with HIV, disseminated disease is common, yet it is not common in other acquired or congenital immunodeficiencies that affect T-cell function.
- Rarely, it may cause otitis/mastoiditis as well as pulmonary disease in immunocompetent children.
- Chronic skin, bone, or soft tissue infections may develop after trauma/surgery, acupuncture, or application of tattoos, usually with *M. chelonae* or *M. fortuitum* as the etiologic agents.
- Infections of indwelling central venous catheters appear to be on the increase, especially among children on chemotherapy.
- Colonization with this mycobacterium is common among older patients with cystic fibrosis. Whether these organisms play a pathogenic role in ongoing lung damage in this population is an area of intense study.

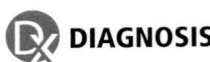 **DIAGNOSIS**

HISTORY

- Region of residence
- Recent travel
- Length of time of adenopathy, associated systemic symptoms
- Contact with cats (for differential of cat-scratch disease or toxoplasmosis)
- Systemic symptoms, such as fever and weight loss, make neoplastic disease more likely.
- Chronic cough would suggest *M. tuberculosis*.
- Recent upper respiratory symptoms/fever suggest viral or bacterial cause.

PHYSICAL EXAM

- Most common: Single or regional cervical adenopathy, 90% of the time, is unilateral, firm, not fixed, and not especially tender or warm; occasionally, there is spontaneous drainage.
- Generalized adenopathy makes ATM disease unlikely.
- Systemic signs of infection are absent.
- Hepatosplenomegaly indicates other diagnosis, especially neoplastic disease or HIV-related illness.
- Normal nutritional status
- In disseminated disease, chronic high fevers, abdominal pain, and wasting are common.
- Occasionally may cause SQ nodules that frequently ulcerate.

DIAGNOSTIC TESTS & INTERPRETATION

Pitfalls: Use of incision and drainage/aspiration for treatment of adenitis, which can lead to chronically draining node. Aspiration may be needed to make the original diagnosis, but total excision results in almost 100% cure rates.

Lab

- Specific PPD tests are not readily available at this time. Many children with ATM adenitis will have 5–10-mm reactions to standard PPD: in one study, 27% of those with culture proven NTM adenitis had a PPD >10 mm.
- Definitive diagnosis is made by isolation and identification of organism. The most frequently identified strains are: *M. avium intracellulare, M. kansasii, M. chelonae, M. fortuitum,* and *M. scrofulaceum*.
- Normal chest radiograph
- In disseminated disease, cultures are positive from blood and bone marrow aspirates.
- Diagnosis using PCR assays under development. May be helpful on staining of biopsied material.

ATYPICAL MYCOBACTERIAL INFECTIONS

DIFFERENTIAL DIAGNOSIS
- For unilateral adenopathy/adenitis:
- Viral/bacterial adenitis—affected nodes are tender, warm, and erythematous; usually associated with upper respiratory symptoms and/or fever.
- Cat-scratch disease (contact with cat, usually kitten). Frequently, child will have scratch/puncture mark on arm. There are rarely any systemic signs/symptoms.
- Neoplastic disease

 TREATMENT

MEDICATION (DRUGS)
For disseminated or pulmonary disease, or when complete surgical excision of an infected node is not possible, 3- or 4-drug treatment regimens based on sensitivity. Combinations generally include several of the following antibiotics: Rifabutin, clarithromycin or azithromycin, ethambutol, ciprofloxacin, and amikacin. Newer antibiotics, such as mefloquine and moxifloxacin, may also have significant activity against atypical mycobacterial strains.

SURGERY/OTHER PROCEDURES
Complete surgical excision for isolated adenopathy secondary to ATM; chemotherapy unnecessary in most cases

 ONGOING CARE

FOLLOW-UP RECOMMENDATIONS
Routine follow-up should be done for 1 year after excision to monitor for possible local/contralateral recurrence.

PATIENT EDUCATION
Prevention: For HIV-infected children with severe immunodeficiency, prophylaxis with once-weekly azithromycin decreases the risk of development of disseminated disease.

PROGNOSIS
- For localized adenopathy: Excellent
- For disseminated disease: Generally treatable in the rare immunocompetent individual
- In patients with AIDS: Generally treatable in terms of symptom relief which required lifelong therapy, but with newer anti-HIV therapies, NTM chemotherapy may be stopped after 1–2 years.

COMPLICATIONS
- Chronic draining of infected cervical nodes
- Rarely, pulmonary disease or dissemination
- Chronic skin/bone infections
- Disseminated disease

ADDITIONAL READING

- Cruz AT, Ong LT, Starke JR. Mycobacterial infections in Texas children. *Pediatr Infect Dis*. 2010;29: 772–774.
- Hazra R, Robsin CD, Perez-Atayde AR, et al. Lymphadenitis due to nontuberculous mycobacteria in children: Presentation and response to therapy. *Clin Infect Dis*. 1999;28:123–129.
- Lee WJ, Kang SM, Sung H, et al. Non-tuberculous mycobacterial infections of the skin: A retrospective study of 29 cases. *J Derm*. 2010;37:965–972.
- Olivier KN, Weber DJ, Wallace RJ Jr, et al. Nontuberculous mycobacteria. I. Multicenter prevalence study in cystic fibrosis. *Am J Respir Crit Care Med*. 2003;167:828–834.
- Reilly AF, McGowan KL. Atypical mycobacterial infections in children with cancer. *Pediatr Blood Cancer*. 2004;43(3):698–702.
- Starke JR. Management of nontuberculous mycobacterial cervical adenitis. *Pediatr Infect Dis J*. 2000;19:674–675.

CODES

ICD9
- 031.0 Pulmonary diseases due to other mycobacteria
- 031.1 Cutaneous diseases due to other mycobacteria
- 031.9 Unspecified diseases due to mycobacteria

ICD10
- A31.0 Pulmonary mycobacterial infection
- A31.8 Other mycobacterial infections
- A31.9 Mycobacterial infection, unspecified

FAQ
- Q: Should all cases of cervical adenitis be tested for ATM?
- A: The typical case of cervical adenitis, presenting with the usual prodrome, responds rapidly to appropriate oral or parenteral antibiotics, which would not be the case if ATM were the culprit. Certainly, a PPD test should be done on all children with cervical adenitis. If the node is aspirated, in addition to routine bacterial cultures, fluid should be sent for mycobacterial culture. Additionally, testing for cat-scratch disease should be part of the evaluation of all cases of cervical adenitis.
- Q: Should patients with disease secondary to ATM undergo a chest radiograph?
- A: Yes. Although uncommon, ATM-related pulmonary disease can be seen in children.
- Q: If the node is excised, should oral therapy be instituted?
- A: Most studies suggest that oral therapy is unnecessary following total excision.

AUTISM/PERVASIVE DEVELOPMENTAL DISORDER (PDD) SPECTRUM

Alisson Richards
David C. Rettew
Jeanne Greenblatt (5th edition)

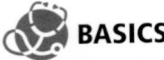 **BASICS**

DESCRIPTION
- Neurodevelopmental syndrome characterized by:
  - Delays/impairments in development of social, communication, play, and behavioral skills
  - Onset usually in 1st years of life
- Spectrum of related disorders:
  - Autistic disorder: Symptoms prior to age 3 years, impairments in social relatedness, communication, and play, and restricted interests/activities
  - Asperger disorder: Social deficits, restricted range of interests, relatively preserved language development, average to above-average cognitive abilities
  - Pervasive developmental disorder not otherwise specified: Subthreshold autism
  - Childhood disintegrative disorder: Developmental deterioration after 24 months of age
  - Note: DSM5 proposal is to combine all diagnoses above into 1 diagnosis, autism spectrum disorder

EPIDEMIOLOGY
Prevalence
- ~1% or 1 child in every 110, with rate possibly increasing
- 4–5 times more common in males than females

RISK FACTORS
Genetics
- Strong genetic influence
- Risk in 1st-degree relatives 2–8%
- Immunizations: Initial association with vaccines not established (multiple studies)

COMMONLY ASSOCIATED CONDITIONS
- Mental retardation
- Gastrointestinal problems
- Seizure disorders
- Sleep disorders
- Attention problems, anxiety, depression, mood disturbances
- Aggression and self-injury

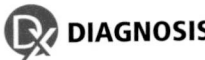 **DIAGNOSIS**

Typically pediatricians are the 1st point of contact and play an important role in early recognition, which is then followed by screening tools and referral for early intervention through a developmental pediatrician, psychologist, child psychiatrist, or neurologist where assessment and treatment plans can be coordinated with the schools.

HISTORY
- A detailed prenatal, neonatal, developmental, medical, family, and social history essential
- Delays/impairments in communication:
  - Rare cases present with "acquired epileptic aphasia" (paroxysmal electroencephalogram in sleep)
  - Marked inability to initiate and sustain conversation (when speech is present)
  - Cognitive delays
- Delays/impairments in reciprocal social interactions:
  - Impairment in eye contact, facial expression, nonverbal social behaviors
  - Impaired social interactions
  - Lack of imaginary play appropriate to developmental level
  - Lack of pointing
  - Doesn't include others in play
- Stereotyped behaviors and restricted interests:
  - Stereotypies (e.g., rocking, hand flapping)
  - Restricted range of interests/activities
  - Attachment to unusual objects, fascination with parts of objects
  - Behavioral rigidity, distress with changes in routine
  - Unusual sensory interests in objects or persons (smelling, touching, sensitivity to clothing)

PHYSICAL EXAM
- Evaluate for growth disturbance
- 20–30% have macrocephaly: Neurocutaneous disorder, storage disease, hydrocephalus, or no identifiable cause
- Signs of self-injurious behavior
- Stereotypical behavior, involuntary movements, motor coordination abnormalities, mirror/overflow movements
- Ophthalmologic/audiologic evaluations to rule out visual or hearing deficits
- Long, thin face, prominent ears: Fragile X (macroorchidism may not be present until after puberty)
- Pigmented lesions: Neurocutaneous syndromes, hypopigmented macules/fibromas suggest tuberous sclerosis
- Microcephaly: Toxoplasmosis, other viruses, rubella, cytomegalovirus, herpes virus (TORCH) infection, Angelman syndrome, Rett disorder
- Look for spasticity, visual loss, ataxia: Leukodystrophy

DIAGNOSTIC TESTS & INTERPRETATION
Lab
- Head MRI/CT: If intellectual or focal neurologic deficit is present, suspect neurocutaneous disease:
  - Electroencephalogram if epilepsy is suspected (~25%)
  - Chromosome studies: If child is intellectually disabled
  - Genetic tests/microarrays: if child is intellectually disabled
  - Toxoplasma, other viruses, rubella, cytomegalovirus, herpesvirus titers: Setting of microcephaly
  - CBC: Evaluation of growth delay and/or pica
  - Blood lead level: R/O lead intoxication
  - Thyroid function tests: R/O hyper-/hypothyroidism
  - Audiogram/brainstem auditory evoked response: For children with speech and language delay and to rule out hearing deficits
  - Ophthalmologic evaluations to rule out visual deficits

Diagnostic Procedures/Other
Screening tools:
- Modified Checklist for Autism in Toddlers (M-CHAT) downloadable at http://www.firstsigns.org/downloads/m-chat.PDF
- Social Responsiveness Scale (SRS)
- Autism Diagnostic Observation Schedule (ADOS) and Autism Diagnostic Interview (ADI-R) are structured interviews and assessments usually performed by a psychologist, developmental pediatrician, psychiatrist, or neurologist: Considered the gold standard

DIFFERENTIAL DIAGNOSIS
- Intellectual impairment: MAY not have pervasive developmental disorder/autism IF communication, behavior, play, and social skills appropriate to developmental age
- Rett syndrome: Females; hand-washing/-wringing movements, head-growth deceleration before 48 months of age
- Deafness: Delayed/absent oral language acquisition; behavioral/social difficulties may relate to language delays
- Mixed receptive-expressive language disorder: No deficits in social interactions or restricted range of interests
- Selective mutism
- Anxiety, obsessive-compulsive disorder, or PTSD

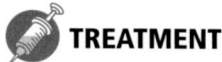

TREATMENT

MEDICATION (DRUGS)

- Pharmacotherapy treats associated symptoms of autism:
- Symptoms/medications to consider:
  - Self-injurious behavior: Atypical/typical antipsychotics, guanfacine, clonidine
  - Sleep disturbances: Melatonin, clonidine, trazodone
  - Seizures: Newer anticonvulsants, carbamazepine, phenytoin, valproate, barbiturates (may worsen hyperactivity/irritability)
  - Hyperactivity/attention difficulties: Psychostimulants, atomoxetine, bupropion, clonidine, guanfacine
  - Obsessive-compulsive disorder symptoms/perseveration: SSRIs, clomipramine
  - Tic disorders: Guanfacine, clonidine, atypical/typical antipsychotics
  - Depression: SSRIs, bupropion, venlafaxine
  - Anxiety: SSRIs, buspirone, venlafaxine, benzodiazepines (rarely as may increase disorganization and agitation)
  - Aggression: atypical antipsychotics, SSRIs, anticonvulsants, guanfacine
- FDA-approved medications include aripiprazole ages 6–17 and risperidone ages 5–16
  - Important to monitor baseline glucose and lipids as atypical antipsychotics are associated with metabolic syndrome
  - Used for associated aggression and irritability

ALERT

- Autism and the pervasive developmental disorder spectrum disorders vary greatly in symptom presentation. Discordancy among clinicians' diagnoses and under- and overdiagnoses of these disorders are common.
- Symptom presentation differs at different stages of development.
- Medication often not helpful for core autistic features and patients often develop side effects
- Subclinical seizure types may be detected only on electroencephalogram

ADDITIONAL TREATMENT
General Measures
Nonpharmacologic

- Psychoeducational assessment: Support cognitive, developmental, adaptive, functional, communication, and social needs:
  - Intensive educational/behavioral interventions should target acquisition of communicative, social, cognitive skills.
- Early sustained structured behavioral intervention using applied behavior analysis (ABA) and behavior modification highly beneficial in many children
- Vocational training important for some adolescents and adults

- Social skills training especially for higher-functioning patients is essential.
- Education and support for parents and siblings integral to treatment
- Conventional psychotherapy not indicated to address core features of autism and pervasive developmental disorder

COMPLEMENTARY & ALTERNATIVE THERAPIES

- Almost 1/3 of children with ASD have received some form of complementary and alternative medicine (CAM).
- Important to ask and understand what is being used

ONGOING CARE

FOLLOW-UP RECOMMENDATIONS
Patient Monitoring

- Prognosis linked to cognitive ability and acquisition of social/communication skills
- Early intervention and provision of services can improve prognosis.
- If no language by 5 years of age, substantial language development unlikely
- Children with autism/pervasive developmental disorder often require lifelong treatment and support.
- Physician should remain active in long-term treatment planning and individual and family support

DIET
Little systematic evidence to support that gluten-free diets are helpful, but there are many claims of their effectiveness

ADDITIONAL READING

- Committee on Children with Disabilities. Technical report: The pediatrician's role in the diagnosis and management of autistic spectrum disorder in children. *Pediatrics*. 2001;107(5):E85.
- Greenspan SI, Brazelton TB, Cordero J, et al. Guidelines for early identification, screening, and clinical management of children with autism spectrum disorders. *Pediatrics*. 2008;121(4): 828–830.
- Gutstein S, Sheely R. *Relationship development intervention activities for young children*. London: Jessica Kingsley Publications; 2002.
- Johnson CP, the Council on Children with Disabilities. Identification and evaluation of children with autism spectrum disorders. *Pediatrics*. 2007; 120:1183–1215.
- Meyers MM, Johnson CP, the Council on Children with Disabilities. Clinical report: Management of children with autism spectrum disorders. *Pediatrics*. 2007;120:1162–1182.

- Moeschler JB, Shevell M, Committee on Genetics. Clinical genetic evaluation of the child with mental retardation or developmental delays. *Pediatrics*. 2006;117:2304–2316.
- Rogers SJ, Vismara LA. Evidence-based comprehensive treatments for early autism. *J Clin Child Adolesc Psychol*. 2008;37(1):8–38.
- Scahill L, Martin A. *Psychopharmacology*. In: Volkmarr FR, Klin A, Paul R, et al., eds. *Handbook of autism and pervasive developmental disorders*. Hoboken, NJ: Wiley; 2005:1102–1122.
- Volkmar F, Cook EH Jr, Pomeroy J, et al. Practice parameters for the assessment and treatment of children, adolescents, and adults with autism and other pervasive developmental disorders. *J Am Acad Child Adolesc Psychiatry*. 1999;38(12 Suppl): 32S–54S.
- Walker DR, Thompson A, Zwaigenbaum L, et al. Specifying PDD-NOS: A comparison of PDD-NOS, Asperger syndrome and autism. *J Am Acad Child Adolesc Psychiatry*. 2004;43(2):172–180.

CODES

ICD9
- 299.00 Autistic disorder, current or active state
- 299.91 Unspecified pervasive developmental disorder, residual state

ICD10
- F84.0 Autistic disorder
- F84.9 Pervasive developmental disorder, unspecified

FAQ

- Q: What are the chances of having a 2nd child with autism?
- A: In families with 1 child with autism, the recurrence risk for subsequent children is 3–7%. This is in contrast to the risk in the general population, which is 0.1–0.2%.
- Q: What is the value of brain imaging in autism?
- A: MRI may help diagnose a heritable syndrome with genetic counseling implications (e.g., leukodystrophy, tuberous sclerosis), but is usually unhelpful in high-functioning cases without severe intellectual impairment and focal neurologic findings.
- Q: Does the MMR vaccine cause autism?
- A: There is no causal association between the MMR vaccine and autism.

AUTOIMMUNE HEMOLYTIC ANEMIA

Michele P. Lambert

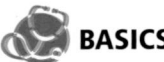 **BASICS**

DESCRIPTION
Autoimmune hemolytic anemia is characterized by shortened red cell survival that is caused by autoantibodies directed against RBCs, with or without the participation of complement on the red cell membrane.

EPIDEMIOLOGY
Incidence
- ~1–3:100,000 persons/year
- Peak incidence in childhood is in first 4 years of life with warm autoimmune hemolytic anemia.

Prevalence
- Less common in children and adolescents than in adults
- No apparent racial or sexual predisposition (in childhood)

PATHOPHYSIOLOGY
- Warm autoantibodies (~80% cases):
  - Maximal activity of *in vitro* antibody RBC binding at 37°C
  - IgG-class antibody usually
  - IgG-coated RBCs cleared, predominantly in the spleen, by macrophages
- Cold autoantibodies (cold agglutinins) (7–25%):
  - Maximal activity of *in vitro* RBC binding at temperatures between 0°C and 30°C
  - Almost always caused by IgM antibody with specificity for antigens of the i/I system on RBCs
  - Anti-I antibodies characteristic of *Mycoplasma pneumoniae*–associated hemolysis
  - Anti-i antibodies are usually found in infectious mononucleosis.
  - Hemolysis is complement dependent.
- Paroxysmal cold hemoglobinuria:
  - IgG autoantibody binds RBC at cooler areas of the body (i.e., extremities), causing irreversible binding of complement components (C3 and C4). When coated RBCs enter warmer areas of the body, IgG falls off and complement causes hemolysis (Donath–Landsteiner biphasic hemolysin).
  - Unusual IgG antibody with anti-P specificity
  - Most frequently found in children with viral infections (30%)

ETIOLOGY
- Idiopathic
- Passive transfer of maternal antibodies
- Secondary to an underlying disorder
  - Infection: Viral (e.g., *Mycoplasma*, Epstein–Barr virus, cytomegalovirus, hepatitis, HIV) or bacterial (e.g., Streptococcus, typhoid fever, *Escherichia coli* septicemia)
  - Drugs: Antimalarials, antipyretics, sulfonamides, penicillin, rifampin
  - Hematologic disorders: Leukemia, lymphoma
  - Immunopathic/autoimmune disorders: Lupus, mixed connective tissue disorders, Wiskott–Aldrich syndrome, ulcerative colitis, rheumatoid arthritis, common variable immunodeficiency, scleroderma, Evans syndrome/ALPS (autoimmune lymphoproliferative syndrome)
  - Tumors: Ovarian, carcinomas, thymomas, dermoid cysts

 DIAGNOSIS

Natural History:
- Acute disease:
  - Onset with rapid fall in hemoglobin level over hours to days
  - Usual course: Complete resolution of disease within 3–6 months
  - Resolution more likely in children who present between 2 and 12 years of age
- Chronic disease:
  - Slower onset of anemia over weeks to months, with some having persistence of hemolysis or intermittent relapses
  - More likely to be associated with underlying chronic Illness
  - More common in adults and children <2 years or >12 years of age

HISTORY
- Pallor
- Jaundice
- Dark urine
- Fever
- Weakness
- Dizziness
- Syncope
- Exercise intolerance

PHYSICAL EXAM
- Pallor
- Jaundice
- Splenomegaly
- Hepatomegaly
- Tachycardia, systolic flow murmur, S3 gallop
- Orthostasis in acute onset

DIAGNOSTIC TESTS & INTERPRETATION
Lab
CBC:
- Hemoglobin level decreased (occasionally, thrombocytopenia seen in Evans syndrome)
- Mean corpuscular volume may be normal.
- Reticulocyte count increased (although may also be decreased if reticulocytes bear the target antigen)
- Peripheral smear: Spherocytes, polychromasia, macrocytes, agglutination
- Direct antiglobulin test (Coombs)—positive (usually):
  - Single most important test
  - Warm autoimmune hemolytic anemia will have IgG ± C3 positive.
  - Cold autoimmune hemolytic anemia and paroxysmal cold hemoglobinuria will have C3 positive.
- Haptoglobin level decreased
- Indirect hyperbilirubinemia
- Elevated lactate dehydrogenase
- Urinalysis: Hemoglobinuria, increased urobilinogen

- Bone marrow aspiration: Erythroid hyperplasia (to rule out leukemia or lymphoma associated with autoimmune hemolytic anemia)
- Cold agglutinin titer: Positive (usually >1:64)
- Donath–Landsteiner test should be performed in cases of suspected paroxysmal cold hemoglobinuria.

ALERT
- A negative Coombs test can occur when small numbers of IgG or C3 molecules are present on the red cell membrane or if most of the coated red cells are cleared from circulation (i.e., in cases of less severe hemolysis, low-affinity antibodies, or in cases of very severe, rapid clearance).
- Radiolabeled Coombs test or enzyme immunoassays are more sensitive diagnostic tests in these circumstances.
- Reticulocytopenia may occur in most severe cases where the antibody coats and removes reticulocytes.

DIFFERENTIAL DIAGNOSIS
- Defects intrinsic to RBC:
  - Membrane defects such as hereditary spherocytosis
  - Enzyme defects including hemolytic episode due to G6PD deficiency
  - Hemoglobin defects
  - Congenital dyserythropoietic anemias
  - Paroxysmal nocturnal hemoglobinuria
- Defects extrinsic to RBC:
  - Immune mediated:
    ○ Isoimmune: Hemolytic disease of the newborn, blood group incompatibility
    ○ Autoimmune (see "Etiology")
    ○ Drug-dependent RBC antibodies
    ○ Hemolytic transfusion reaction
  - Nonimmune-mediated:
    ○ Idiopathic
    ○ Secondary to an underlying disorder (i.e., hemolytic uremic syndrome, thrombotic thrombocytopenic purpura)
    ○ Mechanical: March hemoglobinuria, heart valves

TREATMENT

MEDICATION (DRUGS)
First Line
Corticosteroids:
- Indication:
  - In IgG-mediated disease, steroids have been shown to interfere with macrophage Fc and C3b receptors responsible for RBC destruction. In addition, they have been shown to elute IgG Ab from the RBC surface (improving survival).
  - In chronic, warm, autoimmune hemolytic anemia, pulsed high-dose dexamethasone has been shown to be effective in some cases.
- Complications:
  - Both short- and long-term side effects
  - Generally not effective in cold agglutinin disease

- Dose:
  - Start prednisone PO/methylprednisolone IV at 2 mg/kg/d in divided doses.
  - Tapering of steroids should begin after a therapeutic response is achieved (may take several days to weeks).
- Goal:
  - Initially, to return to normal hemoglobin level with tolerable doses of steroid, or off steroids entirely
  - In some patients, goal may be achieving decreased hemolysis and a clinically asymptomatic state with minimal steroid side effects.
  - Alternative treatments should be considered for patients unresponsive to steroids or who require high doses for maintenance of hemoglobin level.

Second Line
- IV immunoglobulin:
  - Indication:
    - May be useful in selected cases of immune hemolytic anemia unresponsive to steroids
  - Mechanism of action is not entirely clear
  - Effect is usually temporary; retreatment may be required every 3–4 weeks
  - Complications:
    - Red cell antibodies in IVIG preparations may be a confounder
    - Aseptic meningitis.
    - Theoretical risk of transfusion transmitted viral infection
    - Expensive
    - Dose: Up to 1 g/kg/d for 5 days has been required to achieve a beneficial effect.
- Plasmapheresis/exchange transfusion:
  - Indication:
    - Will slow the rate of hemolysis in severe disease, especially if IgM mediated
  - Indicated if thrombotic thrombocytopenic purpura cannot be excluded
  - Complications:
    - Only of short-term benefit
  - Expensive
- Rituximab: monoclonal anti CD20 antibody likely works through depletion of B cells
  - Indicated in refractory AIHA (375 mg/m^2 weekly for 2–4 weeks)
  - Response 40–100%
  - Particularly useful in Warm AIHA
  - Adverse effects: fever, chills, rigors, hypertension, bronchospasm; rare risk of viral infections
- Immunosuppressive agents (antimetabolites and alkylating agents):
  - Indication:
    - When there is a clinically unacceptable degree of hemolysis that is refractory to steroids and splenectomy
  - Some have been effective in cold agglutinin disease.

- Complications:
  - There are varying side effects dependent on the agent used. Therefore, clinical indications must be strong and exposure to drug should be limited.
- Dose:
  - Adjusted to maintain WBC >2,000, absolute neutrophil count (ANC) >1,000, and platelet count at 50,000–100,000 cells/mm^3
- Alemtuzumab (anti CD52): may be effective very refractory AIHA particularly secondary to B-CLL

ADDITIONAL TREATMENT
General Measures
Blood transfusion:
- Indication: Physiologic compromise from the anemia (usually only in severe acute onset)
- Complications:
  - The blood bank may be unable to find compatible blood. In IgG-mediated disease, autoantibody is usually pan reactive; therefore, you must use the least incompatible unit of blood.
  - In cold agglutinin disease, use a blood warmer for all infusions to decrease IgM binding and monitor for acute hemolysis during transfusion.

SURGERY/OTHER PROCEDURES
Splenectomy:
- Indication:
  - Patients unresponsive to medical management, who require moderate- to high-maintenance doses of steroids or who develop steroid intolerance may be candidates.
- Not effective in cold agglutinin disease
- Response rate is 50–70%, with many partial remissions.

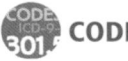 **ONGOING CARE**

FOLLOW-UP RECOMMENDATIONS
Patient Monitoring
- Hemoglobin level q4h to q12h (depending on severity) until stable
- Reticulocyte count: Daily
- Spleen size: Daily
- Hemoglobinuria: Daily

COOMBS TEST: WEEKLY
PROGNOSIS
- Dependent on age, underlying disorder (if any), and response to therapy. See also "Diagnosis" section ("Natural History").
- Mortality in pediatric series ranged from 9% to 19%.

COMPLICATIONS
- May be increased risk of venous thrombosis in patients with AIHA
- May also predispose to lymphoproliferative disorders
- Gallstones related to chronic hemolysis

ADDITIONAL READING
- Barros MMO, Blajchman MA, Borde JO. Warm autoimmune hemolytic anemia: Recent progress in understanding the immunobiology and treatment. *Tran Med Rev.* 2010;24:195–210.
- Hoffman PC. Immune hemolytic anemia – select topics. *Hematology.* 2009;80–86.
- King K, Ness PM. Treatment of autoimmune hemolytic anemia. *Semin Hematol.* 2005;42(3): 131–136.
- Meyer O, Stahl D, Beckhove P, et al. Pulsed high-dose dexamethasone in chronic autoimmune hemolytic anemia. *Br J Haematol.* 1997;98: 860–862.
- Petz LD. Cold antibody autoimmune hemolytic anemia. *Blood Rev.* 2008;22:1–15.

CODES

ICD9
283.0 Autoimmune hemolytic anemias

ICD10
- D59.0 Drug-induced autoimmune hemolytic anemia
- D59.1 Other autoimmune hemolytic anemias

FAQ
- Q: Will the anemia go away?
- A: Children with cold autoantibodies tend to have short-lived illness, whereas children with warm antibodies often have a chronic clinical course characterized by periods of remissions and relapses.
- Q: Is this contagious?
- A: No. Another child may acquire the same viral illness; however, the body's response to produce an autoantibody is dependent on the individual patient.

AVASCULAR (ASEPTIC) NECROSIS OF THE FEMORAL HEAD (HIP)

Ali Al-Omari
Wudbhav N. Sankar
John Dormans

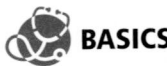 **BASICS**

DESCRIPTION
- Avascular (aseptic) necrosis results from the interruption of the blood supply to bone (either traumatic or nontraumatic occlusion).
- The femoral head is the most common site.
- A particular type of avascular necrosis of the hip that occurs in children is known as Perthes disease (see "Perthes Disease").

RISK FACTORS
Genetics
Variable, depending on cause.

PATHOPHYSIOLOGY
- Death and necrosis of bone with gradual return of blood supply
- Necrotic bone gradually resorbed and replaced by new bone

ETIOLOGY
- Traumatic:
  - Hip fracture
  - Hip dislocation
  - Slipped capital femoral epiphysis
  - Complication of casting, bracing, surgery
- Nontraumatic:
  - Idiopathic (older, after physeal closure); similar to adult avascular necrosis
  - Idiopathic (younger, before physeal closure, Perthes disease)
  - Caisson disease
  - Sickle cell disease
  - Septic arthritis
  - Steroids or chemotherapy
  - Malignancy(Leukemia)
  - Gaucher disease
  - Viral infection (HIV, CMV)
  - Radiation therapy
  - Hypercoagulable states

DIAGNOSIS

HISTORY
- Onset (gradual or after traumatic event)
- Association with:
  - Trauma
  - Medications (steroids or chemotherapy)
  - Casting, splinting, surgery (iatrogenic)
  - Pain, limping
  - Stiffness (decreased range of motion)

PHYSICAL EXAM
- Gait:
  - Limping
  - Antalgic gait (decreased)
  - Trendelenburg gait
- Note range of motion:
  - Flexion and extension
  - Abduction and adduction
  - Internal and external rotation
- Hip joint irritability (short arc rotation)
- Signs of other disease process (e.g., sickle cell disease)
- Physical examination trick: Loss of internal rotation is usually the first and most affected loss of motion seen.

DIAGNOSTIC TESTS & INTERPRETATION
Lab
Initial lab tests
- Laboratory examinations should be normal in most forms of avascular necrosis of the femoral head.
- Exceptions:
  - Sickle cell disease
  - Septic arthritis
  - Chemotherapy

Imaging
- Radiographic findings:
  - Sclerosis
  - Subchondral fracture
  - Collapse
  - Reossification
  - Repair
- Other potential findings:
  - Cysts
  - Physeal growth arrest (young)
  - Early osteoarthritis
  - Subluxation

DIFFERENTIAL DIAGNOSIS
- Trauma:
  - Osteochondral fracture
  - Impaction fracture
  - Epiphyseal/physeal fracture
- Infection:
  - Osteomyelitis
  - Septic arthritis
- Neoplastic process: Epiphyseal tumors (chondroblastoma, Trevor disease, etc.)
- Rheumatologic processes

TREATMENT

MEDICATION (DRUGS)
- NSAIDs may be effective in decreasing associated inflammation.
- If associated with steroid use, discontinuation or elimination if appropriate

ADDITIONAL TREATMENT
General Measures
- Maintain range of motion (physical therapy, traction, continuous passive motion).
- Contain the femoral head in the acetabulum (see "Perthes Disease" treatment principles).
- Duration of therapy variable, depending on cause

SURGERY/OTHER PROCEDURES
Redirectional osteotomy:
- Femoral or acetabular reorientation
- Core decompression to stimulate new blood supply (older patient)

ONGOING CARE

DIET
- Thought not to alter disease process
- Recommend general balanced diet

PROGNOSIS
- Overall, good if mild involvement and patient is young
- See "General Prevention."
- When to expect improvement: Variable, depending on cause
- Moderate to severe cases may end up requiring a total hip replacement

COMPLICATIONS
- Decreased range of motion, pain, limping
- Osteoarthritis
- Physeal arrest with growth disturbance

ALERT
Signs to watch for:
- Subluxation
- Early osteoarthritis
- Growth arrest

ADDITIONAL READING

- Lahdes-Vasama T, Lamminen A, Merikanto J, et al. The value of MRI in early Perthes disease: An MRI study with a 2 year follow up. *Pediatr Radiol.* 1997;27:517–522.
- Mont MA, Jones LC, Hungerford DS. Nontraumatic osteonecrosis of the femoral head: Ten years later. *J Bone Joint Surg Am.* 2006;88(5):1117–1132. Review. Erratum in: *J Bone Joint Surg Am.* 2006; 88(7):1602. (Dosage error in article text.)
- Roposch A, Mayr J, Linhart WE. Age at onset, extent of necrosis, and containment in Perthes disease. Results at maturity. *Arch Orthop Trauma Surg.* 2003;123:68–73.

- Shipman SA, Helfand M, Moyer VA, et al. Screening for developmental dysplasia of the hip: A systematic literature review for the US Preventive Services Task Force. *Pediatrics.* 2006;117(3):e557–e576.
- Tokmakova KP, Stanton RP, Mason DE. Factors influencing the development of osteonecrosis in patients treated for slipped capital femoral epiphysis. *J Bone Joint Surg (Am).* 2003;85-A:798–801.

CODES

ICD9
- 732.1 Juvenile osteochondrosis of hip and pelvis
- 733.42 Aseptic necrosis of head and neck of femur

ICD10
- M87.059 Idiopathic aseptic necrosis of unspecified femur
- M91.80 Other juvenile osteochondrosis of hip and pelvis, unspecified leg

FAQ

- Q: What type of medication is most often associated with avascular necrosis of the hip?
- A: Steroids
- Q: For avascular necrosis in children (Perthes disease of the hip, for example), is younger or older age associated with a better prognosis?
- A: Younger age

BABESIOSIS

Oluwakemi B. Badaki-Makun
Frances M. Nadel

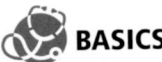 **BASICS**

DESCRIPTION
- Human babesiosis is a tick-borne malarial like illness characterized by fever, malaise, and hemolytic anemia
- Most infected individuals are asymptomatic

EPIDEMIOLOGY
- The 1st human case in the US was reported from California in 1966
- Transmission usually occurs in the summer and early fall
- In the US, most cases have been reported from the Northeast, Midwest, and Pacific Coast
  - Endemic areas include Rhode Island, Massachusetts, and New York
  - Cases have been reported in New Jersey, Maryland, Virginia, Georgia, Wisconsin, and Minnesota

Incidence
There were >450 confirmed cases of human babesiosis diagnosed in the US between 1968 and 1993.

Prevalence
- Difficult to ascertain because asymptomatic infection appears to be common in endemic areas
- It has been reported, for instance, that seroprevalence is as high as 9% in some endemic areas of Rhode Island

RISK FACTORS
- Asplenia (functional or anatomic)
- Malignancy
- HIV/AIDS
- Immunosuppressive medications
- Primary immunodeficiency syndrome
- Extremes of age, especially age >50 years

Genetics
There is no known genetic predisposition.

GENERAL PREVENTION
- Prevention begins with avoidance of tick bites (especially important for high-risk individuals; see "Risk Factors" below)
- Simple measures include wearing long-sleeved shirts and long pants, with pants tucked into the socks in tick-infested areas
- Avoid endemic regions during the peak months of May to September
- Light clothing will make ticks easier to see
- Use DEET-containing insect repellents during outdoor activities
- Spraying one's clothing with a permethrin tick repellent may also be helpful
- Children and dogs should be inspected daily for ticks after being outside
- Currently, there is no universal laboratory screening of blood products
- Prophylaxis is not recommended after a tick bite
- Currently, there is no vaccine available

PATHOPHYSIOLOGY
- A bite from an infected tick transmits the protozoa
- Incubation period:
  - Usually 1–4 weeks
  - Can be as long as 9 weeks
- Infection of the erythrocyte causes membrane damage and lysis, which promotes adherence to the endothelium and microvascular stasis
- The spleen plays an important role in decreasing the protozoal load, through antibody production and filtering abnormally shaped infected red blood cells

ETIOLOGY
- Human babesiosis is caused by the intraerythrocytic parasite of the *Babesia* genus
- In the northeast US, *Babesia microti* is the most commonly isolated agent
- *Babesia divergens* is the responsible agent in Europe
- WA-1 and MO-1 cause babesiosis in western US and Missouri, respectively
- *Ixodes dammini* (*Ixodes scapularis*), the same tick responsible for Lyme disease, is the invertebrate vector for *B. divergens*
- Rarely, the disease has been acquired through transplacental/perinatal transmission or through transfusion of contaminated blood products
  - Babesiosis is the most common tick-borne disease transmitted by contaminated blood transfusions

COMMONLY ASSOCIATED CONDITIONS
It is estimated that 11–23% of patients have concurrent Lyme disease.

DIAGNOSIS

HISTORY
- Few patients recall a tick bite
- Patients live in or have recently traveled to an endemic region
- Initial symptoms begin 1–4 weeks after the tick bite and are vague. They may include progressive fatigue, malaise, headaches, and anorexia, accompanied by intermittent fevers as high as 40°C
- Chills, myalgias, and arthralgias may follow these symptoms
- Less common complaints include cough, sore throat, abdominal pain, and emotional lability

PHYSICAL EXAM
- Fever is often the only finding
- Mild conjunctival injection and pharyngeal erythema
- Some may have mild hepatomegaly and/or splenomegaly
- Jaundice or hematuria may also be seen
- Petechiae and ecchymosis occur in rare cases, most often in the presence of severe illness with associated shock and/or DIC

DIAGNOSTIC TESTS & INTERPRETATION
Lab
- Giemsa- or Wright-stained thick and thin blood smears may demonstrate the intraerythrocytic ring form:
  - This is often confused with the ring form of Plasmodium falciparum, the etiologic agent of malaria
  - Rarely, the pathognomonic "Maltese Cross" forms of the *Babesia* parasite may also be seen on the blood smear
  - Multiple smears should be performed as initial smears may be falsely negative
- Indirect immunofluorescent assay:
  - Antigen-specific for *B. microti*
  - In endemic areas, the test has a sensitivity of 91% and a specificity of 99%
  - Can be used when blood smears are negative
  - In general, a titer = 1:64 indicates exposure
  - Titer = 1:256 suggests acute infection
  - There is little correlation between titer levels and severity of disease
  - Immunoglobulin levels decline rapidly within months of recovery
- Polymerase chain reaction is highly sensitive and specific
- Isolation of the parasite can be done by intraperitoneal injection of a patient's blood into a golden hamster, but results take weeks
- Other tests: Most of the abnormal routine test results are the result of hemolysis
- Urinalysis:
  - Proteinuria
  - Hemoglobinuria
- CBC:
  - Normal leukocyte count/leukopenia
  - Normocytic/normochromic anemia
  - Thrombocytopenia
  - Atypical lymphocytosis
  - Reticulocytosis
- Possible positive Coombs test
- Elevated ESR
- Liver function tests: Elevated bilirubin, lactate dehydrogenase, and liver transaminases
- In asymptomatic patients, these tests are often normal

ALERT
False negatives:
- The blood smears may not demonstrate the protozoan at low levels of parasitemia
- Serologic false positives for *B. microti* include cross-reactivity with other *Babesia* sp. or malarial organisms
- Theoretical serologic false positives for WA1:
  - Rheumatoid factor
  - Antinuclear antibody
  - Antibody to *Toxoplasma gondii*

DIFFERENTIAL DIAGNOSIS
- Nonspecific viral syndrome
- Malaria
- Influenza
- Lyme disease
- Ehrlichiosis

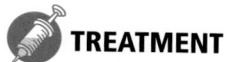 TREATMENT

MEDICATION (DRUGS)
Regardless of regimen, treatment is generally for 7–10 days.

First Line
- Asplenic, immunodeficient, or severely symptomatic patients should be treated with clindamycin and quinine IV
- The pediatric dose of clindamycin is 20–40 mg/kg/day IV/PO divided q6–8h (max 600 mg/dose). The adult dose is 600 mg PO q8h or 300–600 mg IV q6h
- Quinine is dosed 10–25 mg/kg/day PO divided into 3 doses. Adult dose is 650 mg PO q8h

Second Line
- Combination of atovaquone and azithromycin:
  - Has similar treatment effectiveness with fewer side effects (such as vertigo, tinnitus and GI upset) than clindamycin and quinine in adults
  - Use of atovaquone and azithromycin has not been studied in the pediatric population; clindamycin and quinine are the recommended treatment choice for symptomatic children
  - Pediatric dosing: Atovaquone 20 mg/kg (max 750 mg) q12h; azithromycin 10 mg/kg (max 500 mg) PO on day 1 and 5 mg/kg (max 250 mg) daily thereafter
  - Adult dosing: Atovaquone 750 mg q12h; azithromycin 500–1000 mg PO on day 1 and 250–1000 mg PO daily thereafter
- In areas endemic for Lyme disease and Ehrlichiosis, consider adding doxycycline until lab confirmation of absence of either disease in the patient with babesiosis

ADDITIONAL TREATMENT
General Measures
Those with mild clinical disease usually recover without treatment.

Additional Therapies
- For life-threatening infections, exchange transfusion has been successful. Consider in patients with severe parasitemia (≥10%), severe hemolysis or renal/hepatic/pulmonary compromise
- Progressive respiratory distress may require mechanical ventilation

ALERT
- Signs to watch for:
  - Respiratory distress, especially after treatment has begun
  - Pancytopenia and lymphadenopathy: May indicate the development of hemophagocytic syndrome
- Pitfalls:
  - Children who are from endemic areas and have an acute febrile illness may be misdiagnosed with a nonspecific viral illness
  - One should be suspicious for a coinfection with Lyme disease or ehrlichiosis (human anaplasmosis) in those who are not responding to standard therapy
  - Delayed recognition of this uncommon disease may be life threatening in the immunocompromised patient
  - In endemic areas, babesiosis should be considered in a post-transfusion febrile illness in at-risk populations

 ONGOING CARE

FOLLOW-UP RECOMMENDATIONS
When to expect improvement:
- Some improvement of symptoms should be noted within 24–48 hours of onset of therapy
- Those who are only mildly affected usually have resolution of their symptoms over a few weeks
- For severely affected and immunodeficient patients, the convalescent period may be as long as 18 months
- In untreated asymptomatic individuals, parasitemia may persist for months to years
- Long-term complications are rare
- Recrudescence has been reported

COMPLICATIONS
- Rarely fatal in the US
- Pancytopenia and overwhelming secondary bacterial sepsis may occur
- Serious and fulminant complications have been described:
  - Pulmonary edema and adult respiratory distress syndrome, often happening after treatment has begun
  - CHF
  - Renal failure
  - Hemophagocytic syndrome/disseminated intravascular coagulation
  - Seizures/coma
- Those co-infected with Lyme disease are susceptible to more severe disease and complications

ADDITIONAL READING
- Buckingham SC. Tick-borne infections in children: Epidemiology, clinical manifestations, and optimal management strategies. *Paediatr Drugs*. 2005;7(3):163–176.
- Fox LM, Wingerter S, Ahmed A, et al. Neonatal babesiosis: Case report and review of the literature. *Pediatr Infect Dis J*. 2006;25(2):169–173.
- Homer MJ, Aguilar-Delfin I, Telford SR 3rd, et al. Babesiosis.*Clin Microbiol Rev*. 2000;13(3):451–469.
- Krause PJ. Babesiosis. *Med Clin North Am*. 2002;86(2):361–373.
- McGinley-Smith DE, Tsao SS. Dermatoses from ticks. *J Am Acad Dermatol*. 2003;49:363–392.
- Vannier E, Gewurz BE, Krause PJ. Human babesiosis. *Infect Dis Clin North Am*. 2008;22(3):469–488, viii–ix.
- Wormser GP, Dattwyler RJ, Shapiro ED, et al. The clinical assessment, treatment, and prevention of Lyme disease, human granulocytic anaplasmosis, and babesiosis: Clinical practice guidelines by the Infectious Diseases Society of America. *Clin Infect Dis*. 2006;43(9):1089–1134.

 CODES

ICD9
088.82 Babesiosis

ICD10
B60.0 Babesiosis

FAQ
- Q: How long does a tick have to be attached for infection to occur?
- A: In general, successful transmission requires at least 24 hours of attachment.
- Q: How should a tick be removed?
- A: The tick should be grasped with forceps as close to its head as possible and pulled straight up. If possible, it should be saved for identification.
- Q: Does infection confer lifetime immunity?
- A: Reinfection is possible.

BACK PAIN

Heather McKeag
Thomas H. Chun (5th edition)

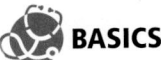 **BASICS**

DEFINITION
Any condition causing pain of the thoracic, lumbar, or sacral spine

EPIDEMIOLOGY
- Recurrent/chronic back pain: 8% of adolescents
- 12–50% lifetime prevalence

RISK FACTORS
- Increased risk with repetitive activity and age
- Role of obesity yet to be determined
- Inheritance patterns for some congenital (scoliosis, Scheuermann kyphosis), inflammatory/rheumatologic causes, and sickle cell disease have been described.

ETIOLOGY
- Back pain can result from a variety of causes involving the bony or muscular structures of the back, intervertebral discs, spinal cord, or peripheral nerves.
- Specific etiology identified ~50% of the time

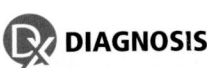 **DIAGNOSIS**

DIFFERENTIAL DIAGNOSIS
- **Mechanical/trauma**
  - Disc herniation
  - Musculotendinous strain
  - Apophyseal ring fracture
- **Developmental**
  - Pars defects: Children usually >10 years
  - Spondylolysis (stress fracture of posterior vertebral elements/pars interarticularis, repetitive-stress injury)
  - Spondylolisthesis (anterior displacement/"slip" of vertebral body, evolution of bilateral spondylolysis)
  - Scheuermann kyphosis: Deformity of thoracic spine associated with vertebral body wedging

- **Inflammatory**
  - Juvenile idiopathic arthritis
  - Ankylosing spondylitis
  - Inflammatory diskitis
- **Neoplastic**
- **Infectious**
  - Diskitis
  - Epidural abscess
- **Other**
  - Sickle cell, abdominal disease (pancreatitis, pyelonephritis), psychogenic
- Age differentiation:
  - <10 years: Diskitis, tumor, epidural
  - >10 years: Pars defects, inflammatory disorders

ALERT
Warning signs of potentially serious causes of back pain in children include:
- Young age: <4 years old
- Duration of pain: >3 weeks
- Chronic interference with normal activity (e.g., school, sports, play)
- Associated fever, weight loss, or other systemic symptoms
- Postural shift of trunk
- Neurologic abnormality
- Limitation of spinal motion (e.g., bending forward, straight leg raise)

HISTORY
- History to include:
  - Onset of symptoms
  - Characteristics of pain
  - History of trauma
  - Pain with activity
  - Inflammatory symptoms
  - Systemic symptoms
  - Neurologic symptoms
- **Question:** Focal pain, neurologic symptoms, interference with activity?
- *Significance:* Increased concern for pathology
- **Question:** Symptoms improved with rest?
- *Significance:* Spondylolysis, Scheuermann kyphosis, muscular strain, overuse
- **Question:** Stable pain or worse at night?
- *Significance:* Tumor, infection, inflammatory

PHYSICAL EXAM
- **Finding:** Inspection—sacral dimples, hair tufts, vascular anomalies, café-au-lait spots, or discrepancies in limb length?
- *Significance:* Occult abnormalities
- **Finding:** Palpation—point or focal tenderness along spine?
- *Significance:* If bony, consider fracture; if paraspinal, consider muscle strain
- **Finding:** Range of motion—forward flexion → increases strain on anterior elements of spine (vertebral bodies and disk spaces)?
- *Significance:* Pain—herniated disk, diskitis, vertebral osteo, vertebral body tumor
- **Finding:** Range of motion—extension→ increases strain on posterior elements of spine (facet joints, pars interarticularis, pedicles)?
- *Significance:* Pain—fracture, spondylolysis, osteoid osteoma, tumor

Also perform:
- FABER test (flexion, abduction, external rotation with foot on opposite knee) → pressure on bent knee and opposite hip strains SI joint.
- Neurologic exam: Reflexes, Babinski, gait, sensation, strength, tone
- Abdominal/pelvic exams

DIAGNOSTIC TESTS & INTERPRETATION
- **Test:** CBC, ESR, CRP, blood culture
- *Significance:* Infection
- **Test:** ANA, RF, HLA B27
- *Significance:* Inflammatory

Imaging
- Plain x-rays (AP and lateral; oblique and flexion/extension if warranted) of the spine:
  – Scottie Dog's Collar: Spondylolysis (stress fracture of the pars interarticularis)
  – If negative, pursue further imaging
- Bone scan: Occult/subtle bony lesions
- CT spine: Spondylosis/spondylolisthesis
- MRI: Tumor, infection, disk injuries

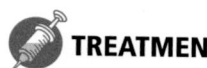 **TREATMENT**

ADDITIONAL TREATMENT
General Measures
- If warning signs are absent, conservative management with NSAIDs, physical therapy, and close follow-up are appropriate.
- Abnormal exam/history warrants imaging.
- Spondylolysis/spondylolisthesis:
  – <50% slip: Conservative medical treatment
  – >50% slip/persistent back pain: Surgical treatment
- Diskitis: Anti-staphylococcal coverage
- Bed rest/activity limitation: Adult data do not support this strategy.
- General Prevention
  – Back muscle strengthening and hamstring stretching exercises may be helpful.
  – Maximum backpack load: 10–15% body weight

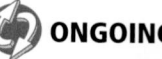 **ONGOING CARE**

FOLLOW-UP RECOMMENDATIONS
- Patients managed conservatively should be re-evaluated within 2 weeks.
- All patients should follow up immediately for any worsening symptoms, especially pain or neurologic symptoms.
- Referral to primary care sports medicine or orthopedic colleagues when necessary

PROGNOSIS
- Dependent on the underlying cause
- The majority, when properly diagnosed and treated, do well, without significant sequelae.
- Not possible to predict future course of spondylolysis, spondylolisthesis, or Scheuermann kyphosis.

COMPLICATIONS
Paralysis, other permanent neuromuscular injury, chronic back pain

ADDITIONAL READING

- Bernstein RM, Cozen H. Evaluation of back pain in children and adolescents. *Am Fam Physician*. 2007;76(11):1669–1676.
- Haidar R, Saad S, Khoury NJ, et al. Practical approach to the child presenting with back pain. *Eur J Pediatr*. 2011;170(2):149–156.

- Houghton KM. Review for the generalist: Evaluation of low back pain in children and adolescent. *Pediatr Rheumatol Online J*. 2010;8:28.
- King HA. Back pain in children. *Orthop Clin North Am*. 1999;30(3):467–474.
- Rodriguez DP, Poussaint TY. Imaging of back pain in children. *Am J Neuroradiol*. 2010;31(5):787–802.

 CODES

ICD9
- 724.1 Pain in thoracic spine
- 724.2 Lumbago
- 724.5 Backache (postural)

ICD10
- M54.5 Low back pain
- M54.89 Other dorsalgia
- M54.9 Dorsalgia, unspecified

FAQ

- Q: Which children should have activity restrictions?
- A: High-risk children (i.e., those with spinal or bony abnormalities of familial histories of spondylolysis) should avoid hyperextension and contact sports.
- Q: When can/should the child resume activities?
- A: Low-risk children with a normal neurologic exam can resume activity or sports when they are pain free.

BAROTITIS
Judith Brylinski Larkin

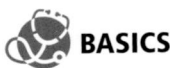 BASICS

DESCRIPTION
- Barotrauma of the middle or inner ear, most commonly caused by flying in an airplane or scuba diving but also caused by elevators and high altitudes
- May also be seen in those who have used a hyperbaric oxygen chamber and in people involved in explosions—blast injuries
- Referred to as "middle ear squeeze" by scuba divers

EPIDEMIOLOGY
- Severe disease uncommon in commercial aircraft because of pressurization
- Significant disease is more common in scuba divers, in those who fly military aircraft, and during use of hyperbaric oxygen chambers.

Incidence
- There is wide variation, with studies reporting an incidence of 8–55% for children after a single flight.
- Most studies agree that the incidence is ~20% in adults after a single flight.
- 40% incidence in scuba diving

RISK FACTORS
- Age: Infants or toddlers are at higher risk because of small eustachian tubes.
- Disease states that impede normal eustachian tube function: Otitis media, upper respiratory tract infection (URI), allergic rhinitis
- Smoking
- Vigorous use of Valsalva maneuver

GENERAL PREVENTION
- Gradual descent during scuba diving—never rapid
- When ascending, divers should avoid rising more quickly than their air bubbles.
- Yawning, swallowing, chewing, or doing Valsalva maneuver during takeoff and landing in planes, and during ascent and descent when scuba diving
- Gentle Valsalva—never vigorous
- Avoid flying or diving when you have a URI or allergic rhinitis.
- Avoid sleeping on plane during takeoff and landing.
- Break seal of wet suit hood to allow water to fill external canal before descent.
- Avoid use of ear plugs.

PATHOPHYSIOLOGY
- Boyle's Law states that as pressure of a gas decreases, volume increases, and as pressure of a gas increases, volume decreases.
- Ambient pressure decreases during airplane/scuba diving ascent and increases during descent.
- During ascent, the tympanic membrane bulges outward and the eustachian tube vents the excess middle ear pressure. Pressure is easily equalized.
- During descent, the TM bulges inward and the eustachian tube resists inward flow of air. Pressure equalization is difficult.
- At a pressure differential of 60 mm Hg (greater ambient to middle ear pressure), subjective discomfort is reported.
- At a pressure differential of 90 mm Hg, the eustachian tube collapses and becomes obstructed. Autoinflation is unsuccessful.
- Tympanic membrane can rupture at pressure differentials >100–400 mm Hg.
- Barotitis is sometimes classified using Teed's classification of disease severity (see "Physical Exam").

ETIOLOGY
Differences in the atmospheric pressure between the inner ear, middle ear, and environment result in injury to the middle and/or inner ear.

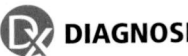 DIAGNOSIS

HISTORY
- Ear pain, pressure sensation, diminished hearing
- Symptoms of inner ear damage may include vestibular and/or auditory complaints including tinnitus, vertigo, nausea, and vomiting.
- History of recent airplane flying, scuba diving, or hyperbaric oxygen chamber use

PHYSICAL EXAM
- Nystagmus
- Hearing loss
- Teed's classification to describe appearance of the tympanic membrane:
  - Grade 0: Symptoms without physical signs
  - Grade 1: Diffuse redness and retraction of TM
  - Grade 2: Grade 1 plus slight hemorrhage into TM
  - Grade 3: Grade 1 plus gross hemorrhage into TM
  - Grade 4: Bulging TM with air-fluid level, blood in TM
  - Grade 5: Free hemorrhage into TM and ear canal with perforation of TM

DIAGNOSTIC TESTS & INTERPRETATION
Imaging
CT of the inner ear may be indicated in patients with vestibular symptoms or hearing loss to rule out inner ear damage.

Diagnostic Procedures/Other
Hearing tests should be performed on all patients who have signs of barotrauma and on patients with normal physical exams but who are symptomatic.

DIFFERENTIAL DIAGNOSIS
- Otitis media with effusion
- Acute otitis media
- Otitis externa
- Blunt trauma to the tympanic membrane
- Exposure to extremely loud noise

 TREATMENT

MEDICATION (DRUGS)
- Nasal decongestant sprays (oxymetazoline [Afrin]):
  - Have been reported by some to be helpful but a randomized clinical trial showed no advantage over placebo
  - Theory: By constricting mucosal arterioles, eustachian tube function is enhanced.
  - Topical decongestants are used 1 hour prior to plane travel/diving and 1/2 hour prior to plane descent.
  - 2 drops/sprays per nostril
  - Use in children over 6 years of age.
- Oral decongestants:
  - 2 randomized controlled trials suggest that oral decongestants may be effective, though a trial in children did not show a beneficial effect.
  - May be helpful through the same physiologic pathway as topical agents
  - Should be initiated 1–2 days prior to the expected pressure change
- Antihistamines:
  - May also be helpful by reducing mucosal edema and enhancing the eustachian tube orifice
  - Can be used on the day of the expected pressure change
- Nasal surfactants may be useful but ongoing studies are needed.
- Pain relievers such as acetaminophen, ibuprofen, and naproxen may be useful for severe pain.

ADDITIONAL TREATMENT
General Measures
- Valsalva maneuver (blowing the nose while pinching the nostrils closed) may be helpful when diving or descending and will force air into the middle ear via the eustachian tube, thereby equalizing the pressure between the middle ear and the environment. This should be done gently.
- Swallowing, yawning, and chewing can help to release pressure through the eustachian tube when descending in an airplane or when returning to the water surface while scuba diving.
- Politzer bag: Instrument used for clearing pressure disequilibrium that has not improved with Valsalva maneuvers and a trial of decongestants.
- Otovent: Another instrument that may be used for treatment or prevention; usage can be taught to children as young as 2–6 years of age.
- Myringotomy with or without tubes may be required to relieve pressure in severe disease. It may also be used as a preventative measure in those with a history of barotitis.
- Myringotomy is effective for the patient with excruciating pain or unrelenting eustachian tube dysfunction; this is best performed by an otolaryngologist.

SURGERY/OTHER PROCEDURES
Rarely, myringotomy with or without tube insertion is required to relieve pressure and pain, as well as prevent complications. Myringotomy is a surgical procedure where a small incision is made in the tympanic membrane. This opens the middle ear space and equalizes the pressure on both sides of the tympanic membrane. Myringotomy without tube insertion will relieve pressure, but the opening may close very quickly and may not allow time for the barotrauma to heal; on occasion, myringotomy with tube insertion is necessary. Tympanostomy tubes are not appropriate for scuba divers.

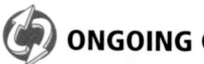 ONGOING CARE

FOLLOW-UP RECOMMENDATIONS
Patient Monitoring
Most patients with barotitis can be managed conservatively. Those with complications noted above require specialist referral.

PROGNOSIS
- Complete spontaneous resolution in mild cases
- Middle ear barotrauma is usually self-limited and correctable with the techniques described in the "General Measures" section. In rare instances, where there is severe pain or eustachian tube dysfunction, myringotomy with or without tube insertion will relieve the pressure differential.

- Pressure differential without damage to the middle or inner ear usually resolves within a few days of returning to normal atmospheric pressure.
- Barotitis that results in injury to the middle or inner ear has a variable rate of improvement; some damage may be permanent (e.g., that to the organ of Corti), while other injury is reversible (e.g., that involving the tympanic membrane).
- Variable outcome for auditory and vestibular symptoms and injuries to the inner ear

COMPLICATIONS
- Vertigo
- Tinnitus
- Hearing loss
- Tympanic membrane rupture
- Oval or round window rupture
- Hemorrhage

ADDITIONAL READING
- Buchanan BJ, Hoagland J, Fischer PR. Pseudoephedrine and air travel associated ear pain in children. *Arch Pediatr Adolesc Med*. 1999;153:466–468.
- Janvrin S. Middle ear pain and trauma during air travel. *Clin Evid*. 2002;7:466–468.
- Jones JS, Sheffeild W, White L, et al. A double blind comparison between oral pseudoephedrine and topical oxymetazoline in the prevention of barotrauma during air travel. *Am J Emerg Med*. 1998;16:262–264.
- Mirza S, Richardson H. Otic barotraumas from air travel. *J Laryngol Otol*. 2005;119(5):366–370.
- Rosenkust L, Klokker M, Katmolm M. Upper respiratory infections and barotraumas in commercial pilots: A retrospective survey. *Aviat Space Environ Med*. 2008;79(10):960–963.
- Stangerup SE, Klokker M, Vesterhauge S, et al. Point prevalence of barotitis and its prevention and treatment with nasal balloon inflation: A prospective controlled study. *Otol Neurotol*. 2004;25(2):89–94.

 CODES

ICD9
- 993.0 Otitic barotrauma

ICD10
T70.0XXA Otitic barotrauma, initial encounter

FAQ
- Q: Is the Valsalva maneuver also effective on plane ascent?
- A: Yes, creating even greater pressure in the middle ear by performing the Valsalva maneuver can overcome a resistant eustachian tube and result in sudden venting of increased middle ear pressure.
- Q: Can children with otitis media travel in airplanes?
- A: Yes, Weiss and Frost (1987) have shown that commercial air travel did not result in worsening of symptoms and, in fact, the presence of otitis media with effusion seemed to be protective against barotitis.
- Q: How can I minimize my child's ear pain when traveling in an airplane?
- A: For infants: Have them nurse, take a bottle, or suck on a pacifier during ascent and descent. Older children may eat or chew gum or suck on hard candies. This will result in pharyngeal movements that will repeatedly open the eustachian tube and equalize middle ear pressure to environmental pressure. Children can also be taught the Valsalva maneuver. If the child is currently experiencing an upper respiratory infection, use of decongestants prior to flight may be helpful.

BELL PALSY

Stephen J. Falchek

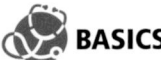 **BASICS**

DESCRIPTION
- This paralysis may involve all of the modalities affected by the 7th cranial nerve:
  - Mimetic facial movement
  - Taste
  - Cutaneous sensation
  - Hearing acuity
  - Lacrimation
  - Salivation

The most important feature in diagnosis and management of Bell palsy is the distinction between a peripheral and a central 7th nerve palsy.

EPIDEMIOLOGY
Incidence
- Annually, incidence ranges from 3/100,000 in patients <10 years to 25/100,000 in adults.
- Only 1% of cases have bilateral involvement.

PATHOPHYSIOLOGY
Nearly all cases of true Bell palsy are believed to arise from a viral infection of the facial nerve and, in particular, the geniculate ganglion.

ETIOLOGY
- Idiopathic: pregnancy related
- Infectious:
  - Herpes simplex virus 1
  - Human herpes virus 6
  - Herpes zoster (without Ramsay–Hunt syndrome)

COMMONLY ASSOCIATED CONDITIONS
Associated illnesses can cause or predispose to an isolated facial nerve palsy, but are important to distinguish from a classic Bell palsy.
- Rubella
- Lyme disease (*Borrelia burgdorferi*): In Lyme neuropathy, early reports indicated a preponderance of tic bite histories involving the ipsilateral face, implying a retrograde migration of the spirochetes into the nerve and resultant nerve root/arachnoid irritation in at least some cases, as opposed to hematogenous dissemination and CNS penetration.
- Epstein–Barr virus (EBV)
- Cytomegalovirus (CMV)
- Mumps
- HIV
- *Mycoplasma pneumoniae*
- Sarcoidosis

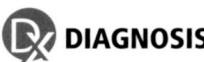 **DIAGNOSIS**

SIGNS AND SYMPTOMS
HISTORY
- Mastoid or retroauricular pain ipsilateral to the side of developing symptoms (40–50% of patients)
- 50% of patients will have no clear sensory prodrome.
- Bell palsy often follows some identifiable infectious illness, such as viral upper respiratory tract infection (URI) symptoms, *Mycoplasma pneumoniae* infection, Lyme disease or infectious mononucleosis. However, an identified antecedent illness is not requisite for the diagnosis.

- The onset is almost always rapid, with progression to a fairly constant state of unilateral paresis or paralysis within hours to 2–3 days.
- As the weakness progresses, the patient (and family members) may note:
  - Difficulty with oral motor tasks (e.g., eating and drinking) due to inability to maintain mouth closure
  - Inability to completely close the eye on the affected side (sometimes leading untrained observers to note an eyelid "droop" on the normal side, due to the contrast with normal eyelid closure and movements)
  - Decreased lacrimation, and eye itching and burning
  - Hyperacusis
  - Ipsilateral facial numbness (less commonly)
  - Distortion of the taste of foods (dysgeusia)
- Bilateral symptoms (<1%) are distinctly rare and suggest an alternative diagnosis, such as Guillain–Barré syndrome or other infectious, inflammatory, or metabolic disease.

PHYSICAL EXAM
- Weakness of all muscles of mimetic facial movement is noted on the affected side.
- A classic feature of peripheral facial nerve palsies is symmetric weakness or paralysis of the upper (frontalis), middle (orbicularis oculi), and lower (orbicularis oris) muscles on voluntary and involuntary mimetic movements. Having the patient wrinkle his or her forehead/raise his or her eyebrows, close his or her eyes tightly, and bare his or her teeth or smile, respectively, tests these.
- Occasionally, slow or absent spontaneous blinking on the affected side.
- The corneal reflex should be decreased or absent on the affected side, but the consensual response on the unaffected side should be preserved.
- The sensory division of the 7th cranial nerve is tested by examining taste perception on the anterior tongue:
  - This is done by applying, ipsilaterally, swabs soaked in a sugar solution and a salt solution to the anterolateral aspect of the tongue, without allowing for mouth closure and dispersion of the substances to the other side. Taste sensation should be ipsilaterally decreased.
  - Despite complaints of retro-auricular pain and unilateral facial "numbness," abnormalities of cutaneous sensation typically are not verifiable by sensory testing in pure 7th-nerve palsies. The presence of true diminution of sensation should raise the question of other cranial nerve involvement (e.g., 5th cranial nerve).
- Examination of the external auditory canal on both sides is crucial.
  - Vesicular lesions of the tympanic membrane indicate a zoster-associated palsy (i.e., Ramsay–Hunt syndrome).
  - Purulent acute otitis media or evidence of trauma mandate aggressive antibiotic treatment and possibly urgent surgical subspecialty evaluation and imaging of the temporal bone.

DIAGNOSTIC TESTS & INTERPRETATION
Imaging
- The decision to defer medical imaging in the evaluation of a typical Bell palsy should be based on a sound clinical history and physical examination. Unusual features should provoke thoughtful review and broader investigation where indicated.
- MRI of the head with gadolinium enhancement: recommended in cases of unusual presentation or progression (e.g., bilateral involvement, slow progression (over >1 week), or other cranial nerve findings). Several small series have proposed that gadolinium enhancement of the involved 7th nerve predicts a slower or less optimal recovery.

DIFFERENTIAL DIAGNOSIS
- Trauma:
  - Birth (especially forceps pressure to lateral face)
  - Congenital facial palsies should not be regarded as Bell palsy, but rather symptomatic of some other cause.
  - Temporal bone/petrous bone fractures
  - Deep lacerations or trauma to parotid region
- Infection:
  - Purulent acute otitis media/mastoiditis
  - Basilar meningitis
  - Petrositis (Gradenigo syndrome)
  - Varicella zoster virus (VZV; Ramsay–Hunt syndrome)
  - Syphilis
  - Trichinosis
  - Tuberculosis
  - Leprosy
- Inflammatory:
  - Sarcoidosis
  - Behçet disease
  - Giant cell arteritis
  - Polyarteritis nodosa
  - Guillain–Barré syndrome
  - Melkersson–Rosenthal syndrome: rare neurologic disorder characterized by recurring facial paralysis, swelling of the face and lips (usually the upper lip), and the development of folds and furrows in the tongue
- Tumors:
  - Cerebellopontine angle tumors, osteosarcomas, cholesteatomas, neurofibromas, lymphoma
  - Hyperostosis cranialis interna, osteopetrosis
- Metabolic:
  - Diabetes (nerve ischemia)
  - Hyperparathyroidism
  - Hypothyroidism
  - Porphyria
- Congenital/Genetic:
  - Congenital absence or hypoplasia of depressor anguli oris muscle
  - Möbius syndrome
  - Chiari malformation
  - Syringobulbia

B

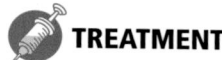 **TREATMENT**

Identifying treatable causes of 7th-nerve palsy (e.g., Lyme borreliosis and Ramsay–Hunt syndrome) is crucial for optimizing outcome and preventing comorbidities of these illnesses.

GENERAL MEASURES
- Eye protection and lubrication: A significant risk for corneal injury is best managed by applying artificial tear solutions at least 3–4 times daily and lubricating gels (e.g., Lacri-Lube) at night. Patching and protective eyewear, during active play and sleep, is usually prescribed on the basis of the degree of remaining eyelid closure.
- Corticosteroids: Prednisone, considered only within the first 72 hours of symptoms. Recommended dose: 1 mg/kg/d (maximum 80 mg) for 5 days, with a taper over the following 5 days.
- Acyclovir: Most clearly indicated for the treatment of Ramsay–Hunt syndrome. It is also used empirically by some practitioners in standard Bell palsy management, although evidence for its supplementary use to corticosteroids is relatively weak; see discussion below. Recommended dose: 20 mg/kg/d, divided into 5 times a day, for 10 days; maximum 400 mg 5 times daily. Generally, any evidence of vesicular eruption in the ear canal or face should be treated promptly with acyclovir, as outcomes from VZV-associated palsies are reported to be worse in general.

Physical Therapy
The benefits of facial muscle physical therapy remain controversial. Despite an increasing number of studies, some with controls, and subsequent meta-analyses, the results are conflicting. At present, there is no incontrovertible evidence for benefit due to facial physical therapy. There is no evidence that facial physiotherapy is harmful. The decision to pursue physical therapy after Bell palsy is a matter of personal preference for the practitioner and family.

MEDICATION (DRUGS)
- Corticosteroids: Recent large series and meta-analyses indicate that treatment with corticosteroids is effective in reducing the risk of incomplete recovery; however, this treatment seems to be only effective if initiated within the first 48 hours of symptoms. Furthermore, statistical significance in treatment versus placebo seems to be most evident only in patients older than 40 years. However, the occurrence of synkinesias does seem to be less in patients treated with steroids within 48 hours across all age groups.
- Antivirals: These same series suggest that there is little or no benefit to therapy with either acyclovir or valacyclovir alone, and that there is at best a non-statistically significant improvement when used in combination with corticosteroids.
- Antibiotics: In areas where Lyme disease is endemic, many practitioners will begin treatment with oral antibiotics presumptively, while awaiting serologies (recall that the IgM titer is the most useful in the acute setting). (See "Lyme Disease" chapter):

First Line
- Prednisone, 60–80 mg/day for 5 days, with a subsequent taper over 5 days; total treatment course 10 days; must be initiated in the first 48 hours for significant results.
- Amoxicillin, 50 mg/kg/d divided in 3 doses for 21–28 days, when Lyme disease suspected

Second Line
For presumed Lyme disease:
- Patients >8 years: doxycycline, 100 mg b.i.d. for 21–28 days
- Patients of all ages: cefuroxime, 30 mg/kg/d in 2 divided doses for 21–28 days

SURGERY/OTHER PROCEDURES
Surgical decompression: Previously, surgical decompression of the 7th nerve had been proposed as a possible treatment in cases where recovery was delayed or the clinical course more severe. No clinical evidence to support the benefit of this strategy has emerged. Surgical decompression is best reserved for "other" cases of facial nerve palsy in which there is a definable syndrome of nerve compression due to extrinsic factors, such as exostoses, tumor, etc.

ISSUES FOR REFERRAL
Subspecialty consultation: In general, patients are referred if their recovery time is prolonged or if there is a relapsing pattern or other deviations from the expected course. However, the presence of other questionable cranial nerve involvement, recent trauma, meningeal symptoms, or neurologic findings (e.g., eye movement abnormalities, acute hemiparesis, etc.) should be viewed with great concern and evaluated in an urgent-care setting.

 ONGOING CARE

DIET
There are no dietary restrictions that affect the outcome of Bell palsy.

PATIENT EDUCATION
Minimizing risk for injury to the cornea ipsilateral to the facial palsy may require either restricting some activities where debris or contusions to the eye are likely, or wearing protective eyewear during such activities. Examples include beach activities and competitive sports. These restrictions only need to be in effect so long as there is inadequate closure of the eyelid on the affected side.

PROGNOSIS
- 60–70% full-recovery rate from isolated 7th-nerve palsy
- Signs of recovering function (generally improving control of mimetic movement) are typically apparent by the 3rd week after onset.
- Prognosis for recovery seems to be worse with either a secondary deterioration in function after 2–4 days, no signs of recovery after three weeks, or demonstrated gadolinium enhancement of the affected facial nerve on MR imaging.
- Of patients with less than total recovery, many will experience at least partial return to normal function; cosmetic results vary in this group.
- Outcome of idiopathic facial palsy as a pregnancy complication seems to be less favorable (~55% full recovery).
- Up to 7% of patients may experience a 2nd occurrence at some point in the future.

COMPLICATIONS
- Corneal injury, due to decreased lacrimation and poor eye closure
- Several sequelae, generally related to aberrant reinnervation of affected end organs, are observed after an episode of Bell palsy.
  - Various synkinesias (abnormal involuntary movements that accompany a normally executed voluntary movement), including the Marin–Amat phenomenon (spontaneous eye closure with mouth opening, or its converse)
  - Blepharospasm, hemifacial spasm, facial contractures
  - The "crocodile tears" phenomenon (eating provokes ipsilateral tearing) results from crossed reinnervation between lacrimal and salivary parasympathetic fibers.

ADDITIONAL READING
- Axelsson S, Berg T, Jonsson L, et al. Prednisolone in Bell's palsy related to treatment start and age. *Otol Neurotol*. 2011;32(1):141–146.
- Numthavaj P, Thakkinstian A, Dejthevaporn C, et al. Corticosteroid and antiviral therapy for Bell's palsy: A network meta-analysis. *BMC Neurol*. 2011;11: 1–10.
- Pereira LM, Obara K, Dias JM, et al. Facial exercise therapy for facial palsy: Systematic review and meta-analysis. *Clin Rehabil*. 2011;25(7):649–658. [Epub 2011 Mar 7].
- Quant EC, Jeste SS, Muni RH, et al. The benefits of steroids versus steroids plus antivirals for treatment of Bell's palsy: A meta-analysis. *BMJ*. 2009; 339:b3354.
- Teixeira LJ, Soares BG, Vieira VP, et al. Physical therapy for Bells' palsy (idiopathic facial paralysis). *Cochrane Database Syst Rev*. 2008;(3):CD006283.

CODES

ICD9
351.0 Bell palsy

ICD10
G51.0 Bell's palsy

FAQ

- Q: How does one differentiate between peripheral facial nerve palsy and a CNS lesion?
- A: A critical step in diagnosis is the differentiation of peripheral from central (upper motor neuron) lesions. With upper motor neuron lesions (above the level of the 7th-nerve nucleus), there is preferential weakness of lower facial musculature and, sometimes, differential paresis of voluntary versus spontaneous emotional mimetic movements. Brainstem lesions, on the other hand, may produce a peripheral-appearing lesion, but almost always have involvement of other pathways and cranial nerve nuclei, e.g., ipsilateral lateral rectus palsy and contralateral somatic hemiplegia (Millard–Gubler syndrome).

BEZOARS

Andrew B. Grossman

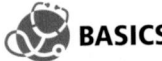 **BASICS**

DESCRIPTION
- Accumulation of foreign material in the GI tract
- Commonly divided into 3 categories based on the substances from which they are derived:
  - Phytobezoar (vegetables/fruits)
  - Trichobezoar (hair)
  - Lactobezoar (milk/formula)
- Documented over 2 millennia and has medical value in some cultures

EPIDEMIOLOGY
- Phytobezoars occur almost exclusively in adults.
- 90% of trichobezoars occur in female patients younger than 20 years.
- Lactobezoars occur mostly in premature, low-birth-weight infants.

PATHOPHYSIOLOGY
- Trichobezoars:
  - Associated with mental retardation, pica, trichotillomania, and trichophagia; may ingest own hair but also rugs and animal or doll hair
  - History of trichophagia is obtained in only 50% of cases.
  - Retention and accumulation of hair strands in the gastric folds
  - Bezoars may become large and form a cast in the stomach leading to abdominal mass.
  - Bezoar may extend through the pylorus into the small bowel. This "tail" may obstruct the ampulla of Vater, leading to jaundice and pancreatitis.
  - Most cases of trichophagia do not result in bezoar formation.

- Phytobezoars:
  - Most common form among adults, rare in children
  - Associated with gastric dysmotility and poor gastric emptying (either primary or following gastric surgery) and hypochlorhydria
  - Composed primarily of cellulose, hemicellulose, lignins, and tannins
- Lactobezoars (milk):
  - Most often reported in premature, low-birth-weight infants being fed high-calorie premature formula (although there are reports in full-term infants and exclusively breast-fed infants)
  - Factors contributing to lactobezoar formation include:
    - Formulas with high casein content
    - Early and rapid feeding advancement in small infants
    - High-caloric-density formulas
    - Formulas with high calcium/phosphate content
    - Continuous tube feedings
    - Altered gastric motility in low-birth-weight infants

ETIOLOGY
Classification of bezoars is dependent on the most prominent substance from which they are formed, including:
- Trichobezoars: Hair, carpet
- Phytobezoars: Indigestible fruit and vegetable matter
- Lactobezoars: Milk

- Less common materials include foreign bodies, gallstones, and medicines, including vitamins, antacids, psyllium, sucralfate, cimetidine, and nifedipine; can occur in CF patients after lung transplantation
- Colonic and rectal bezoars due to indigestible sunflower seeds, popcorn, and gum have been reported in children and adults. These usually present with obstruction, although encopresis and colitis-type symptoms have been described.

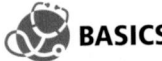 **DIAGNOSIS**

HISTORY
- Signs and symptoms of bezoar formation include:
  - Pain
  - Halitosis
  - Nausea
  - Vomiting
  - Diarrhea
  - Gastric ulceration
  - Upper GI bleeding and perforation
  - Left upper quadrant mass
- Trichobezoars:
  - Unusual patterns of balding
  - Palpable left upper quadrant mass in the abdomen is often detected
  - Hair found in the stool
- Phytobezoars:
  - Abdominal mass is palpable in <50% of patients.
- Lactoezoars:
  - Abdominal distention, diarrhea, emesis, increased gastric residuals

DIAGNOSTIC TESTS & INTERPRETATION
Lab
- Iron-deficiency anemia
- Presence of steatorrhea or protein-losing enteropathy

Imaging
- Plain abdominal x-ray: Heterogenous intragastric mass that could be mistaken for food-filled stomach
- Upper GI barium studies may identify and outline the mass.
- Ultrasound and CT can also be helpful

Diagnostic Procedures/Other
Endoscopy allows for direct visualization, elucidation of composition of bezoar

DIFFERENTIAL DIAGNOSIS
Any gastric foreign body can mimic a gastric mass and may present on palpation.

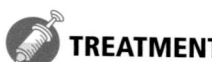 TREATMENT

ADDITIONAL TREATMENT
General Measures
- Trichobezoars:
  – Difficult to remove endoscopically, attempts to fragment may result in migration and small bowel obstruction
  – Solution is surgical removal: They are normally large, and hair is not dissolvable.

- Phytobezoars:
  – Medications such as prokinetic agents to stimulate gastric motility
  – Enzyme therapy to help dissolve the material
  – N-acetylcysteine treatment via nasogastric tube has been documented in one case report
  – Endoscopic fragmentation or extraction
  – Surgical extraction
  – Diet alteration
- Lactobezoars:
  – Withholding feedings for 48 hours while the patient is sustained on IV fluids will resolve most lactobezoars.
  – Gentle gastric lavage may be helpful.

ADDITIONAL READING

- Chen MK, Beierle EA. Gastrointestinal foreign bodies. *Pediatr Ann*. 2001;30:736–742.
- Chogle A, Bonilla S, Browne M, et al. Rapunzel syndrome: A rare cause of biliary obstruction. *J Pediatr Gastroenterol Nutr*. 2010;51:522–523.
- DuBose TM 5th, Southgate WM, Hill JG. Lactobezoars: A patient series and literature review. *Clin Pediatr (Phila)*. 2001;40:603–606.
- Lynch KA, Feola PG, Guenther E. Gastric trichobezoar: An important cause of abdominal pain presenting to the pediatric emergency department. *Pediatr Emerg Care*. 2003;19:343–347.
- Malhotra A, Jones L, Drugas G. Simultaneous gastric and small intestinal trichobezoars. *Pediatr Emerg Care*. 2008;24(11):774–776.
- Taylor JR, Streetman DS, Castle SS. Medication bezoars: A literature review and report of a case. *Ann Pharmacother*. 1998;32:940–946.
- Tsou VM, Bishop PR, Nowicki MJ. Colonic sunflower seed bezoar. *Pediatrics*. 1997;99:896–897.
- Walker-Renard P. Update on the medicinal management of phytobezoars. *Am J Gastroenterol*. 1993;88:1663–1666.

 CODES

ICD9
- 935.2 Foreign body in stomach
- 936 Foreign body in intestine or colon
- 938 Foreign body in digestive system, unspecified

ICD10
- T18.2XXA Foreign body in stomach, initial encounter
- T18.3XXA Foreign body in small intestine, initial encounter
- T18.4XXA Foreign body in colon, initial encounter

FAQ

- Q: What are some commonly used medications that can lead to bezoar formation?
- A: Vitamins, antacids, psyllium, sucralfate, cimetidine, and nifedipine
- Q: What may place an infant at risk for formation of a bezoar?
- A: The literature suggests that formulas with high casein content may be linked with lactobezoar formation. Other possible contributing factors include early and rapid feeding advancement in small infants, high-density formulas, formulas with a high calcium/phosphate content, continuous tube feedings, and altered gastric motility in low-birth-weight infants.

BILIARY ATRESIA

Kathleen M. Loomes

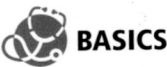 **BASICS**

DESCRIPTION
Biliary atresia is a progressive obliteration of the extrahepatic and intrahepatic biliary ducts of the liver.

EPIDEMIOLOGY
- Extrahepatic biliary atresia accounts for 25–30% of cases of neonatal cholestasis.
- Occurs with a frequency of 1 per 8,000–15,000 live births
- Most common cause of neonatal jaundice for which surgery is indicated

RISK FACTORS
Genetics
- No clear genetic inheritance can be demonstrated.
- Rarely reported to recur in families
- Human genes that determine laterality and genes that affect bile duct development may be important in pathogenesis of some cases.

PATHOPHYSIOLOGY
- Extrahepatic biliary atresia can affect all or part of the extrahepatic biliary tree.
- When only the distal common bile duct, cystic duct, or gallbladder is affected, biliary drainage may be established (<10% of patients).
- Coexisting anomalies are found in ~20% of patients; associations include:
  - Absence of the inferior vena cava with azygous continuation
  - Preduodenal portal vein and symmetric liver
  - Malrotation
  - Situs inversus
  - Bronchial anomalies
  - Multiple spleens (polysplenia)
  - Other anomalies within the spectrum of heterotaxy, including structural congenital heart defects in a minority
- Histology:
  - Extrahepatic biliary obstruction begins near the time of birth and progresses.
  - For approximately the 1st year, liver biopsy shows cholestasis, interlobular bile duct proliferation, and a mononuclear infiltrate invading the periductal tissue:
    - Bile plugs may be present within ducts.
    - Portal tracts are expanded by fibrosis.
    - Some patients may already have well-established cirrhosis.
  - Later biopsies show degeneration and loss of bile ducts.
  - If the biopsy is performed at <4 weeks of age, the pathology may be confused with other causes of neonatal cholestasis, such as giant cell hepatitis.

ETIOLOGY
Etiology is unclear; each of the following has been suggested but has never been substantiated:
- Environmental factors
- Viral infection (Reovirus 3, rotavirus, cytomegalovirus)
- Vascular insufficiency
- Genetic factors: No clear genetic inheritance; likely genetic predisposition
- Immune dysregulation in neonate affecting hepatobiliary system
- Pancreatic reflux
- Defective morphogenesis:
  - Ductal plate malformations have been noted in some biliary atresia liver biopsies.
  - Laterality or developmental genes may play a role in some cases.
- Multifactorial (e.g., in a genetically susceptible host, a viral infection soon after birth could trigger an immune reaction that progressively destroys the biliary tree)

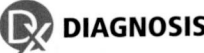 **DIAGNOSIS**

HISTORY
- Typically, the patient is an otherwise healthy infant who develops jaundice within the 1st 90 days of life.
- Stools usually pale, but may have normal color

PHYSICAL EXAM
- Jaundice is best visualized by examination of the hard palate, buccal mucosa, or sclerae.
- Jaundice may not be present until the bilirubin exceeds 5–7 mg/dL in the newborn period and 2 mg/dL in the older child.
- Acholic stools, hepatomegaly, and abnormal liver consistency need not be present to establish the diagnosis.

DIAGNOSTIC TESTS & INTERPRETATION
Diagnostic Procedures/Other
- Conjugated hyperbilirubinemia is defined as a conjugated fraction >2 mg/dL or a conjugated bilirubin >15% of the total.
- Any infant with a conjugated hyperbilirubinemia should be referred for workup:
  - Fractionated bilirubin
  - Aspartate aminotransferase, alanine aminotransferase, alkaline phosphatase, γ-glutamyl transferase, total protein, albumin:
    - CBC, PT/PTT
  - Bacterial cultures (blood, urine, stool)

- Further diagnostic testing should be done as clinically indicated, with early referral to a pediatric gastroenterologist.
  - Viral studies (hepatitis B, hepatitis C, Epstein-Barr virus, TORCH, HIV, adenovirus, enterovirus)
  - α_1-Antitrypsin level with Pi typing
  - Urine and plasma amino acids
  - Urine organic acids and succinylacetone
  - Urine bile acid analysis
  - Urine for reducing substances while the child is ingesting lactose; if positive, assay of galactose-1-phosphate uridylyl transferase activity
  - X-ray studies to exclude evidence of congenital infections and Alagille syndrome (i.e., calcifications of brain and butterfly vertebrae), as indicated
  - Eye exam for congenital infections and eye anomalies associated with Alagille syndrome (posterior embryotoxon)
  - Sweat chloride measurement
  - Thyroid function tests
- Other studies:
  - Abdominal ultrasound to rule out biliary anomalies such as choledochal cyst; also may identify laterality defects, such as polysplenia; although ultrasound findings are not diagnostic, identification of the "triangular cord" sign may be significant.
  - Hepatobiliary scintigraphy
  - Liver biopsy
  - Operative cholangiogram, if liver biopsy is suggestive of biliary obstruction

DIFFERENTIAL DIAGNOSIS
The differential diagnosis includes all causes of neonatal cholestasis:
- Extrahepatic causes of neonatal cholestasis:
  - Biliary atresia
  - Choledochal cyst
  - Neonatal sclerosing cholangitis
  - Bile duct stenosis
  - Anomalies of the choledochopancreaticoductal junction
  - Spontaneous perforation of the common bile duct
    - Obstructing neoplasia or stone
    - Inspissated bile or mucous plug
- Infection
  - Sepsis
  - UTI
  - TORCH infections (*Toxoplasma*, rubella, cytomegalovirus, herpes simplex virus)
  - Coxsackie B virus, echovirus, adenovirus, enterovirus
  - Viral hepatitis
  - HIV

- Epstein-Barr virus
- Metabolic abnormalities:
  - α_1-Antitrypsin deficiency
  - Cystic fibrosis
  - Galactosemia
  - Inborn errors of bile acid metabolism
  - Hereditary fructose intolerance
  - Zellweger syndrome
  - Tyrosinemia
  - Neonatal iron storage disease (likely to present with liver failure)
  - Citrin deficiency
  - Respiratory chain disorders
- Genetic disorders:
  - Alagille syndrome (syndromic bile duct paucity)
  - Trisomy 17, 18, and 21 and Turner syndrome
  - Progressive familial intrahepatic cholestasis:
    - FIC1 deficiency (Byler syndrome)
    - BSEP deficiency (PFIC2)
    - MDR3 deficiency
    - Benign recurrent intrahepatic cholestasis
  - Dubin-Johnson syndrome
  - Rotor syndrome
- Drugs/toxins:
  - Medications
  - Total parenteral nutrition
- Systemic disease:
  - Postshock
  - Postasphyxia
  - CHF
  - Panhypopituitarism
- Other:
  - Idiopathic neonatal giant cell hepatitis
  - Nonsyndromic paucity of interlobular bile ducts

 TREATMENT

ADDITIONAL TREATMENT
General Measures
- After the diagnosis of extrahepatic biliary atresia is established, Kasai portoenterostomy is performed.
- Subsequent management is directed at providing nutrition and monitoring for common problems.
- Recent studies show that average 2-year survival post-Kasai with native liver is ~50%.

SURGERY/OTHER PROCEDURES
- Kasai hepatoportoenterostomy (Kasai procedure) is performed to establish biliary drainage. Corticosteroids are used postoperatively in many centers to improve biliary drainage, but well-controlled studies have not been completed to date.
- Indications for transplantation include persistent cholestasis, life-threatening hemorrhage from portal hypertension, failure to thrive, intractable pruritus, recurrent cholangitis, ascites, and liver failure.

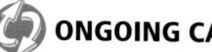 **ONGOING CARE**

FOLLOW-UP RECOMMENDATIONS
- In 1 recent study, the best prognostic factor was a total bilirubin <2 mg/dL at the 3-month follow-up post-Kasai.
- Outcomes are less favorable overall in patients with BA splenic malformation syndrome.
- Development of ascites was associated with a poor outcome (early liver transplantation).
- Common long-term problems:
  - Poor growth
  - Fat-soluble vitamin deficiency
  - Recurrent cholangitis
  - Portal hypertension
  - Pruritus
  - Ascites
  - Progression of liver damage despite a surgical drainage procedure
- The clinician should:
  - Monitor growth parameters and fat-soluble vitamins.
  - Monitor liver span, liver texture, and spleen size to follow progress of disease.
  - Follow liver function tests and CBC.
  - Watch closely for cholangitis: Suggestive findings include fever, elevated transaminases, and γ-glutamyl transferase levels.

ALERT
- Age at the time of surgical intervention is the most important determinant of outcome—delay in diagnosis can be tragic.
- Without surgical intervention, 50–80% of children will die from biliary cirrhosis by age 1 year, and 90–100% by age 3 years.

DIET
- Malabsorption is common and leads to fat-soluble vitamin deficiency and malnutrition; patients receive routine supplementation with vitamins A, D, E, and K.
- Diet should be enriched with medium-chain triglycerides, which do not require bile flow for absorption.
- Nasogastric tube feedings should be implemented if growth is inadequate.

COMPLICATIONS
- Prevention of cholangitis: During the 1st year of life, most children are maintained on daily oral antibiotics to prevent infections from ascending into the liver.
- Pruritus is common and develops when there is increased serum bile acid concentration. Approaches to treatment (with limited success) include ursodeoxycholic acid, antihistamines, cholestyramine, improved nutrition, rifampin, phenobarbital, and naloxone.
- Hyperlipidemia/xanthomas: Hyperlipidemia can be treated with choleretic agents, bile acid–binding resins, and improved nutrition.

- Ascites: Spironolactone, chlorothiazide, and furosemide are commonly used diuretics. Acute changes in fluid balance or a rapid diuresis can be achieved using furosemide with albumin replacement.

ADDITIONAL READING
- Cowles RA, Lobritto SJ, Ventura KA, et al. Timing of liver transplantation in biliary atresia-results in 71 children managed by a multidisciplinary team. *J Pediatr Surg.* 2008 Sep;43(9):1605–1609.
- Davenport M, Tizzard SA, Underhill J, et al. The biliary atresia splenic malformation syndrome: A 28-year single-center retrospective study. *J Pediatr.* 2006;149(3):393–400.
- Hadzic N, Davenport M, Tizzard S, et al. Long-term survival following Kasai portoenterostomy: Is chronic liver disease inevitable? *J Pediatr Gastroenterol Nutr.* 2003;37:430–433.
- Hartley JL, Davenport M, Kelly DA. Biliary atresia. *Lancet.* 2009;374(9702):1704–1713.
- Karrer FM, Bensard DDM. Neonatal cholestasis. *Semin Pediatr Surg.* 2000;9:166–169.
- Mack CL. The pathogenesis of biliary atresia: Evidence for a virus-induced autoimmune disease. *Semin Liver Dis.* 2007;27(3):233–242.
- Shneider BL, Brown MB, Haber B, et al. A multicenter study of the outcome of biliary atresia in the United States, 1997 to 2000. *J Pediatr.* 2006;148:467–474.

 CODES

ICD9
751.61 Biliary atresia

ICD10
- Q44.2 Atresia of bile ducts
- Q44.7 Other congenital malformations of liver

FAQ
- Q: When should a patient with neonatal jaundice have a fractionated bilirubin test?
- A: If hyperbilirubinemia has not resolved by 2 weeks of age. This allows ample time for evaluation of neonatal cholestasis and the possible need for surgical intervention.
- Q: What are the most important factors in success of the Kasai portoenterostomy?
- A: The age at referral of the patient for evaluation and the experience of the center performing the procedure.
- Q: Can the physician prioritize the diagnostic evaluation?
- A: The diagnostic workup for neonatal cholestasis is usually prioritized to investigate the most treatable and dangerous etiologies, taking into account the history, physical exam, and laboratory findings. Since outcomes in biliary atresia depend on age at surgery, the diagnosis must be made early. The full workup should be complete within a few days to 2 weeks, depending on the age of the child.

BLASTOMYCOSIS

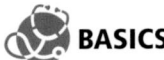

Leonel Toledo
Theoklis Zaoutis (5th edition)

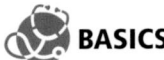 BASICS

DESCRIPTION
- Systemic infection caused by the dimorphic soil fungus *Blastomyces dermatitidis*
- Dimorphism is characterized by a mold phase (mycelial form) that grows at room temperature and a yeast form that grows at body temperature.
- Incubation period estimated at 30–45 days

EPIDEMIOLOGY
- Similar to other dimorphic fungi, *B. dermatitidis* is a soil saprophyte (mycelial form).
- No person-to-person transmission has been documented.
- Congenital infections occur rarely.

Prevalence
- Infection is endemic in the US in the southeast and central states and in the towns bordering the Great Lakes, with the highest incidence in Arkansas, Kentucky, Louisiana, Mississippi, North Carolina, Tennessee, and Wisconsin.
- Other reported areas of infection include parts of Canada (Ontario, Manitoba), Africa, India, and South America.
- Disease may be more severe and chronic in children with T-cell defects (especially HIV infection).
- Children account for 3–11% of cases of blastomycosis.

GENERAL PREVENTION
- No special precautions for hospitalized patients are indicated.
- The natural reservoir is undetermined.

PATHOPHYSIOLOGY
- Inhalation of the fungus into the lung is followed by an inflammatory response with neutrophils and macrophages.
- Blastomycosis most commonly presents as a subacute pulmonary disease, but the clinical spectrum of the disease extends from asymptomatic to disseminated disease that involves the skin, bones, and genitourinary system.
- As many as 50% of infections are asymptomatic.

ETIOLOGY
- Infection is most commonly caused by inhalation of spores from *B. dermatitidis*.
- Less common modes of acquiring the infection include accidental inoculation, dog bites, conjugal transmission, and intrauterine transmission.
- Point-source outbreaks have been associated with occupational and recreational activities that occur in areas with moist soil and decaying vegetation, such as along streams and rivers.
- Natural infection occurs only in 2 mammalian species, humans and dogs.

COMMONLY ASSOCIATED CONDITIONS
- Pulmonary blastomycosis:
  - Most common form of infection by *Blastomyces* in children
  - Can be acute, subacute, or chronic
  - Illness severity can vary greatly, from asymptomatic to presentations of upper respiratory tract infection, bronchitis, pleuritis, pneumonia, or severe respiratory distress.
- Cutaneous blastomycosis:
  - Skin manifestations are variable and include nodules, verrucous lesions, subcutaneous abscesses, or ulcerations.
  - Cutaneous disease occurs following pulmonary inoculation in most cases, but can also occur after direction inoculation into the skin.
- Disseminated blastomycosis:
  - Usually begins as pulmonary infection, with subsequent spread to involve skin (most commonly), bone, genitourinary tract, and CNS.
  - Can disseminate to virtually any organ system.

DIAGNOSIS

HISTORY
- For children with acute pulmonary blastomycosis, the most common presenting symptoms are:
  - Cough (may be productive)
  - Fever
  - Chest pain
  - Malaise
- Children with chronic pulmonary disease present with:
  - Chronic (>2 weeks) nonproductive cough
  - Pleuritic chest pain
  - Poor appetite
  - May also be a history of fever, chills, weight loss, fatigue, night sweats, or, rarely, hemoptysis
- History of residence or travel to an endemic area

PHYSICAL EXAM
- Initial pulmonary infection may present with physical exam findings similar to those of bacterial pneumonia.
- Respiratory signs and symptoms often have resolved by the time cutaneous manifestations are apparent.
- Skin involvement appears as nodules, nodules with ulceration, and, finally, granulomatous lesions with advancing borders.
- Sites in disseminated disease include lung, skin, bone, genitourinary tract, CNS, and, infrequently, liver and spleen, lymph nodes, thyroid, heart, adrenals, omentum, GI tract, muscles, and pancreas.

DIAGNOSTIC TESTS & INTERPRETATION
Diagnostic Procedures/Other
- Definitive diagnosis requires the growth of *B. dermatitidis* from a clinical specimen.
- Direct visualization of the yeast form may be performed on samples of sputum, urine, cerebrospinal fluid, bronchoalveolar lavage sample, or tissue biopsy.

- Culture of the organism from samples can be performed and a DNA probe used to identify *B. dermatitidis*.
- Serologic tests lack sensitivity and specificity and are generally not helpful in establishing blastomycosis.
- A negative serologic test does not rule out infection, and a positive test should not be used as an indication to start treatment with *Blastomyces*.
- The most accurate serologic test is the enzyme immunoassay.
- An assay to detect *Blastomyces* antigen in urine is available, but cross-reactivity occurs in 70–100% of patients with histoplasmosis, paracoccidioidomycosis, and *Penicillium marneffei* infections.
- Chest radiography commonly reveals lobar consolidation. Cavitation, fibronodular patterns, and mass effect may also be seen.

DIFFERENTIAL DIAGNOSIS
- Acute bacterial infection
- Neoplasm
- Tuberculosis
- Sarcoidosis
- Other fungal infections causing pneumonia

 TREATMENT

MEDICATION (DRUGS)
- Though acute pulmonary infections may resolve without treatment, the high rate of progression to extrapulmonary disease leads many experts to recommend treatment for all cases of blastomycosis.
- Mild or moderate pulmonary or extrapulmonary disease:
  - Oral itraconazole
  - Alternative agents include ketoconazole or fluconazole.
- Severe pulmonary disease, other severe infection, or immunosuppression:
  - IV amphotericin B
  - Therapy may be switched to oral itraconazole after clinical stabilization with amphotericin B.

- CNS blastomycosis:
  - Lipid amphotericin B over 4–6 weeks, followed by an oral azole
- During pregnancy:
  - IV amphotericin B
  - Azoles should be avoided owing to potential teratogenicity.
- Length of therapy is site dependent:
  - ≥6 months or longer for pulmonary disease
  - ≥12 months or longer for bone or CNS disease
- Lifelong suppressive therapy with oral itraconazole may be required for immunosuppressed patients and in patients who experience relapse despite appropriate therapy.
- Voriconazole, a new azole agent, has in vitro activity against *B. dermatitidis* and penetrates the CSF better than itraconazole. Anecdotal reports support its use as an option for step-down therapy for CNS infection.

SURGERY/OTHER PROCEDURES
Occasionally drainage of abscesses and debridement of bone are necessary.

 ONGOING CARE

FOLLOW-UP RECOMMENDATIONS
Patient Monitoring
- All azoles can cause hepatitis.
- Hepatic enzymes should be measured before starting therapy, 2–4 weeks after therapy has begun, and every 3 months during therapy.
- All azoles inhibit P-450 enzymes. Consider drug–drug interactions when the patient is taking other medications.

PROGNOSIS
- Before antifungal medications were available, the mortality associated with blastomycosis was up to 90%.
- Appropriate treatment with antifungal medications results in excellent cure rates and mortality rates of <10%.
- The prognosis for chronic cutaneous disease is better than that for systemic disease.

COMPLICATIONS
- Dissemination is the main complication of the infection, occurring in up to 80% of children with blastomycosis.
- Systemic infection may be well advanced before symptoms are noted, making eradication more difficult. Long-term therapy and follow-up may be necessary.

ADDITIONAL READING

- Bradsher RW, Chapman SW, Pappas PG. Blastomycosis. *Infect Dis Clin North Am.* 2003;17: 21–40, vii.
- Chapman SW. Blastomyces dermatitis. In: Mondell GL, et al., eds. *Principles and practice of infectious diseases*, 5th ed. New York: Churchill Livingstone; 2000:2733–2746.
- Chapman SW, Bradsher RW, Campbell GD Jr, et al. Practice guidelines for the management of patients with blastomycosis. *Clin Infect Dis.* 2000;30: 679–683.
- Chapman SW, Dismukes WE, Proia LA, et al. Clinical practice guidelines for the management of blastomycosis: 2008 update by the Infectious Diseases Society of America. *Clin Infect Dis.* 2008;46(12):1801–1812.
- Chu JH, Feudtner C, Heydon KH, et al. Hospitalizations for endemic mycoses: A population based national sample. *Clin Infect Dis.* 2006;42:822–825.
- Montenegro BL, Arnold JC. North American dimorphic fungal infections in children. *Pediatr Rev.* 2010;31(6):e-40–e-48.
- Saccente M, Woods GL. Clinical and laboratory update on blastomycosis. *Clin Microbiol Rev.* 2010; 23(2):367–381.

 CODES

ICD9
116.0 Blastomycosis

ICD10
- B40.2 Pulmonary blastomycosis, unspecified
- B40.3 Cutaneous blastomycosis
- B40.9 Blastomycosis, unspecified

BLEPHARITIS

Lee R. Atkinson-McEvoy

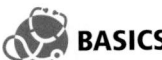 **BASICS**

DESCRIPTION
- Inflammation or infection of the margins of the eyelid
- Hallmark clinical features include redness, itching or burning, and crusting or scaling of the lid margins
- Classified according to location:
  - Anterior blepharitis involves the eyelashes and follicles of the eyelid. It is usually caused by seborrhea and/or infection—bacterial (e.g., *Staphylococcus* infection), viral (e.g., molluscum contagiosum), and parasitic (phthiriasis).
  - Posterior blepharitis involves the meibomian gland openings. This occurs in meibomian gland dysfunction.
- Anterior blepharitis:
  - Seborrheic blepharitis:
    - Notable for easy-to-remove, yellow, greasy scales along the eyelashes
    - Occurs in conjunction with similar seborrheic scales of the eyebrow, scalp, and external ears
  - Staphylococcal blepharitis:
    - Acute, localized infection of the eyelid margin caused by *Staphylococcus aureus* or *S. epidermidis*.
    - Hallmark features of staphylococcal-induced blepharitis are fibrinous, difficult-to-remove scales at the eyelash bases with concomitant inflammation of the lid margin, and occasionally loss of eyelashes
    - Mixed blepharitis: Presence of a staphylococcal infection complicating seborrhea of the eyelids

GENERAL PREVENTION
- Treat seborrheic dermatitis of scalp early.
- Discourage eye rubbing in patients.
- Encourage frequent hand washing for children.
- For children with allergic symptoms, oral antihistamines may decrease eye rubbing.

EPIDEMIOLOGY
Atopic or allergic contact dermatitis as a cause of blepharitis occurs in up to 65% of patients.

Incidence
- No studies that give an exact incidence but is a commonly seen diagnosis
- Up to 30% of patients with trisomy 21 (Down syndrome) have blepharitis

RISK FACTORS
- Presence of atopic, allergic, or seborrheic dermatitis
- Contact lens wearers
- Presence of dry eye

PATHOPHYSIOLOGY
- There are several glands—meibomian glands, pilosebaceous glands of Zeis, and the apocrine glands of Moll—that exit along the eyelid margin. These glands produce the lipid component of tears.
- When these glands become infected or dysfunctional, the clinical features notable for blepharitis may occur.
- Spread of bacteria to the glands of Zeis or the meibomian glands can lead to development of a hordeolum, or stye.
- Staphylococcal exotoxins can lead to conjunctivitis or keratitis.

ETIOLOGY
COMMONLY ASSOCIATED CONDITIONS
- Seborrheic dermatitis
- Allergic or contact dermatitis
- Down syndrome (trisomy 21)
- Ocular rosacea
- Dry eye (keratoconjunctivitis sicca) is associated with staphylococcal blepharitis.

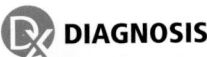 **DIAGNOSIS**

SIGNS AND SYMPTOMS
- Complaints of irritation (burning, pain, or itching sensation) that are worse in the morning
- Eye discharge or crust, particularly along lashes
- Erythema of eyelid margins
- Eyelid sticking
- Eyelash loss

HISTORY
Ask about:
- History of previous inflammation of eyelid margins, or presence of symptoms for a prolonged period of time
- Pruritus
- Use of any medications or products (e.g., contacts lenses, soaps, or makeup) used on or around the eye
- Environmental irritants (e.g., smoke, allergens)
- Frequent rubbing of the eye or contact with eyelids by hands
- Hand-washing practices
- Cleansing of eyelids
- Past medical and family histories of atopy
- Seasonal variation of symptoms (suggests allergic etiology)
- History of lice

PHYSICAL EXAM
- Evaluate eyelid margins and eyelashes for crust, erythema, loss of hair, and ulceration.
- With chronic infection, you may see thickening of the eyelid margin.
- With herpes simplex viral infection, you may see grouped vesicles along the eyelid.
- Evaluate remainder of eye, particularly the conjunctiva and sclera, for evidence of inflammation or infection. A slit-lamp exam is indicated if there seems to be any evidence of involvement of the conjunctiva or sclera.
- Examine the scalp and skin of the head for evidence of seborrhea, atopic dermatitis, contact dermatitis, louse infestation, or rosacea.

DIAGNOSTIC TESTS & INTERPRETATION
Lab
- Laboratory testing is indicated only in cases that do not respond to treatment.
- Bacterial or viral culture of the lid margins can be helpful in cases when the diagnosis is unclear, or in severe cases of blepharitis with ulceration.
- Giemsa staining of conjunctival scrapings may show the presence of neutrophils, which is useful in cases where cultures do not conclusively show signs of infection.

DIFFERENTIAL DIAGNOSIS
- Atopic or contact dermatitis
- Psoriasis
- Rosacea (usually accompanied by dilated telangiectasia of the blood vessels in the lid margins, cheeks, nose, and chin)
- Dacryostenosis
- Acute conjunctivitis (bacteria, viral, or allergic)

 TREATMENT

GENERAL MEASURES
- Eyelid margin cleansing twice daily is considered 1st-line therapy:
  - A warm compress should be placed over closed eyelids for 5–10 minutes to loosen debris.
  - Next, the eyelid margins should be cleansed with a dilute mixture of baby shampoo (brands that do not irritate the eyes) and water.
  - Commercial eyelid cleansers are also available.
  - A cotton swab dipped in the cleansing solution can be used to help release the crust.
- Contact lens use should be avoided until resolution of symptoms.
- Prolonged viewing of television, computer screens, or hand-held games results in decreased blinking and drying of the eye; these should be avoided during symptoms of blepharitis. Excessive use of these should be evaluated in children with recurrent episodes of blepharitis.

MEDICATION (DRUGS)
First Line
- Lid hygiene with dilute baby shampoo or commercial eyelid cleanser
- Topical antibiotic such as bacitracin or erythromycin applied to eyelids 1 or more times per day or at bedtime for at least 1 week

Second Line
- In cases associated with seborrhea, treatment of the accompanying scalp and eyebrow involvement should be initiated with selenium sulfide shampoo once to twice a week, with manual removal of the crusting in those areas with a fine-toothed comb or soft-bristle brush.
- More resistant cases, blepharitis associated with rosacea, or those that fail to improve may be treated with an oral antibiotic such as erythromycin in younger children or doxycycline in older adolescents for 2–4 weeks.
- Any evidence of involvement of the sclera or conjunctiva especially if herpes is suspected should be referred to an ophthalmologist.

 ONGOING CARE

- Once symptoms have resolved, there is no need for routine follow-up of blepharitis.
- If symptoms begin to recur, encourage early initiation of eyelid hygiene with the soap-and-water wash.

ADDITIONAL READING

- Bernardes TF, Bonfioli AA. Blepharitis. *Semin Ophthalmol*. 2010;25(3):79–83.
- Denton P, Barequet IS, O'Brien TP. Ocular infections: Update on therapy. Therapy of infectious blepharitis. *Ophthalmol Clin North Am*. 1999;12:9–14.
- Farpour B, McClellan KA. Diagnosis and management of chronic blepharokeratoconjunctivitis in children. *J Pediatr Ophthalmol Strabismus*. 2001; 38:207–212.
- Hara JH. The red eye: Diagnosis and treatment. *Am Fam Physician*. 1996;54:2423–2430.
- Lemp MA. Contact lenses and associated anterior segment disorders: Dry eye, blepharitis, and allergy. *Ophthalmol Clin North Am*. 2003;16:463–469.
- Nazir SA, Murphy S, Siatkowski RM, et al. Ocular rosacea in childhood. *Am J Ophthalmol*. 2004;137: 138–144.
- Shields SR. Managing eye disease in primary care: Part 2. How to recognize and treat common eye problems. *Postgrad Med*. 2000;108:83–96.

 CODES

ICD9
- 041.10 Staphylococcus infection in conditions classified elsewhere and of unspecified site, staphylococcus, unspecified
- 373.00 Blepharitis, unspecified

ICD10
- B95.8 Unspecified staphylococcus as the cause of diseases classified elsewhere
- H01.009 Unspecified blepharitis unspecified eye, unspecified eyelid
- H01.019 Ulcerative blepharitis unspecified eye, unspecified eyelid

FAQ

- Q: Is blepharitis contagious?
- A: Blepharitis is not spread to other family members. However, the bacteria that can cause the infection may be transmitted by hand contact; thus, frequent hand washing is recommended.
- Q: Does blepharitis recur?
- A: Blepharitis may recur. In cases of children with seborrhea and atopic dermatitis, treatment of these conditions may limit the frequency of flare-ups. Early eyelid hygiene may limit the severity of future recurrences.

BONE MARROW AND STEM CELL TRANSPLANT

Valerie I. Brown

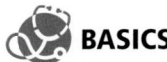 **BASICS**

DESCRIPTION
Reconstitution of damaged, defective, or infiltrated bone marrow with IV infusion of hematopoietic progenitor (stem) cells from:
- The patient (autologous)
- An identical twin (syngeneic)
- A histocompatible donor (allogeneic)

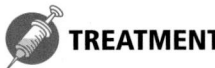 **TREATMENT**

TREATMENT INDICATIONS
- Accepted indications if a human leukocyte antigen (HLA)–identical related donor is available:
  - Acute lymphoblastic leukemia in 2nd complete remission and in certain very high-risk subtypes
  - Acute myelogenous leukemia in 2nd complete remission and in 1st complete remission in certain high-risk subtypes
  - Chédiak-Higashi and other severe neutrophil defects
  - Chronic myelogenous leukemia when in the chronic phase and within a year from time of diagnosis.
  - Congenital bone marrow failure syndromes:
    ○ Diamond-Blackfan anemia
    ○ Shwachman-Diamond syndrome
  - Fanconi anemia
  - Hemophagocytic lymphohistiocytosis (HLH)
  - Inborn errors of metabolism
  - Juvenile myelomonocytic leukemia
  - Lymphoma in 2nd complete remission
  - Myelodysplastic syndromes
  - Myelofibrosis
  - Osteopetrosis
  - Severe aplastic anemia
  - Sickle cell anemia
  - Systemic lupus erythematosus, especially if unresponsive or intolerant to conventional medical therapy
  - Severe combined immunodeficiency and other congenital immunodeficiencies
  - Thalassemia major
  - Wiskott-Aldrich syndrome
- In certain cases, if an HLA-identical related donor is unavailable, then an HLA-identical unrelated donor is used as an alternative.
- Autologous transplantation is an accepted treatment for lymphoma in 2nd complete remission and for high-risk or stage IV solid tumors in complete remission or very good partial response (neuroblastoma) or in 2nd complete remission (germ cell tumor, Wilms tumor, Ewing sarcoma—experimental).

DONOR SELECTION (IN ORDER OF PREFERENCE)
- Identical twin: The increased risk of relapse of leukemia is offset by decreased treatment-related mortality.
- Human leukocyte antigen–identical sibling:
  - <30% of stem cell transplant candidates have an HLA-identical sibling.
- Other family members:
  - Rarely (i.e., in 5% of families), a nonsibling relative who is phenotypically mismatched for 1 antigen will be found.
- Haploidentical transplantations (2 or 3 human leukocyte antigen–antigen mismatches) have been performed but require depletion of T cells from the graft to avoid fatal graft-versus-host disease.
- Unrelated donors: The National Marrow Donor Program (NMDP) has >2 million volunteers registered and maintains a cooperative search agreement with European registries. >60% of preliminary searches yield at least 1 potential donor.
- Autologous (either peripheral stem cells or bone marrow)

PRETRANSPLANT REGIMENS (CONDITIONING)
- The purpose of conditioning (either chemoradiotherapy or chemotherapy alone) is 3-fold:
  - To provide immune suppression to avoid destruction of the allograft by residual immunologically active cells in the host
  - To destroy any residual cancer cells and load antigen-presenting cells with tumor antigens
  - To provide space for the new bone marrow to grow
- Agents used primarily for immunosuppression:
  - Cyclophosphamide
  - Fludarabine
  - Antithymocyte globulin
  - Alemtuzumab (Campath)
- Agents used primarily for antineoplastic effects or bone marrow ablation:
  - Busulfan
  - Cytarabine (ARA-C)
  - Etoposide (VP-16)
  - Carmustine (BCNU)
  - Carboplatin
  - Melphalan
- Agents used for both purposes:
  - Total-body irradiation
  - Thiotepa
- Nonmyeloablative (reduced intensity):
  - Uses less cytotoxic preparative regimens
  - Requires profound immunosuppression of host and a generous infusion of hematopoietic stem cells for donor engraftment to occur
  - Can lead to sustainable mixed chimerism but can also result in complete loss of donor over time
  - Being pursued to reduce risk of organ toxicity and therefore can be offered to patients with nonhematologic malignancies or with malignancies that have been heavily pretreated who would ordinarily not meet the criteria for a myeloablative transplant

STEM CELL COLLECTION METHODS
- Conventional bone marrow
- Peripheral blood stem cells collected via apheresis
- Umbilical cord blood

 ONGOING CARE

TOXICITIES/COMPLICATIONS
- Chemoradiotherapy:
  - Universal: Nausea/vomiting/diarrhea, alopecia, pancytopenia, mucositis
  - Possible and agent specific:
    ○ Total-body irradiation: Skin erythema, parotitis
    ○ Cyclophosphamide: Hemorrhagic cystitis, syndrome of inappropriate secretion of antidiuretic hormone, cardiomyopathy
    ○ ATG: Allergy, serum sickness
    ○ Busulfan: Seizures, pulmonary fibrosis, bronzing of the skin
    ○ ARA-C: Fever, neurologic symptoms, acute respiratory distress syndrome (ARDS)
    ○ Etoposide/Etopophos: Allergic reactions
    ○ BCNU: Pulmonary fibrosis
- Graft failure:
  - Usually due to destruction of the graft by the immunologically active cells in the host or insufficient absolute number of donor stem cells infused
  - Predisposing factors:
    ○ Previous blood transfusions
    ○ Use of reduced-intensity preparative regimens
    ○ Use of methotrexate to prevent graft-versus-host disease
    ○ T-cell depletion of donor cells
  - Can occur early (failure to engraft) or even after successful engraftment
  - Rare in human leukocyte antigen–identical sibling transplantations
  - Risk increases with unrelated donors (6%) or T-cell depletion (14% but depends on the degree of T-cell depletion, and the use of ATG seems to decrease incidence of graft rejection significantly)
  - Usually fatal unless patient receives 2nd transplant emergently
- Graft-versus-host disease: See topic
- Infection:
  - The major cause of nonrelapse mortality
  - Immune dysfunction is caused by a period of severe myelosuppression immediately following stem cell transplant, lack of sustained transfer of clinically significant donor-derived B-cell and T-cell immunity, a recapitulation of normal lymphoid ontogeny, and the effects of graft-versus-host disease and its treatment.
  - In the 1st month posttransplantation, bacterial and fungal infections predominate. Use of prophylactic broad-spectrum antibiotics and antifungal agents during the time of severe myelosuppression has helped considerably.
  - In the 2nd and 3rd months, viral infections predominate, which include cytomegalovirus, adenovirus, herpesvirus (HSV, HHV6), varicella virus, and polyomavirus (BK) as well as *Pneumocystis carinii* pneumonia.
  - After 3 months: Herpes zoster and bacterial infections in patients with chronic graft-versus-host disease

– Acyclovir prophylactically is used in patients who are herpes zoster virus or varicella zoster virus positive. Foscarnet is started prophylactically in cytomegalovirus seropositive recipients receiving a seronegative allograft; use of ganciclovir is avoided for the 1st 100 days posttransplant because of drug-related neutropenia.
  ○ Note: After T-depleted transplantations, the risk of fatal Epstein-Barr virus infection is increased.
• Hemorrhagic cystitis
  – Occurs weeks to months posttransplant
  – Caused by cyclophosphamide, viruses, and GvHD
  – Therapy: IV hydration, antiviral therapy (cidofovir), urology intervention (bladder irrigation, Alum, Formalin)
• Hepatic veno-occlusive disease (sinusoidal obstruction syndrome):
  – Usually occurs within 3 weeks posttransplant
  – Clinical criteria met when 2 of the following are present:
    ○ Hepatomegaly and/or right upper quadrant pain
    ○ Hyperbilirubinemia (>2 mg/dL)
    ○ 5% weight gain and/or ascites
  – Incidence of 25% (range, 5–60%) and mortality of 38% (range, 3–67%) have been reported.
  – Progressive hepatic failure with multiorgan failure (renal insufficiency/failure, respiratory embarrassment, and/or encephalopathy) often develops in severely affected patients.
  – Therapy is largely supportive. Currently, there is no definitive therapy. Use of defibrotide is experimental.
• Interstitial pneumonitis:
  – Typically appears 40–80 days post–bone marrow transplant as rapid-onset tachypnea, fever, and hypoxia associated with bilateral interstitial infiltrates
  – Mortality rate >60%
  – Common causes include:
    ○ Cytomegalovirus
    ○ *Pneumocystis carinii*
    ○ Idiopathic: When no bacterial, viral, fungal, or protozoan cause is identified. Radiation to the lungs probably plays a role in the development of "idiopathic" pneumonitis.

POTENTIAL LONG-TERM SEQUELAE
• Endocrine:
  – Hypothyroidism: Seen in ~20% of patients after total-body irradiation
  – Growth hormone deficiency: Seen in over 1/2 of patients receiving total-body irradiation
  – Primary gonadal failure and absence of development of secondary sexual characteristics are common, especially if the recipient was prepubertal at the time of transplantation or received total-body irradiation.
  – Metabolic syndrome: incidence of insulin resistance is as high as 50%.

• Infertility: Sterility is expected after total-body irradiation; fertility may be preserved after cyclophosphamide alone; if possible, cryopreservation of sperm or oocytes is strongly encouraged prior to transplantation.
• Ophthalmologic: Cataracts are seen in 40% of patients after total-body irradiation and in 20% after chemotherapy alone. A higher incidence is seen in those who also receive steroids.
• Dental: Poor calcification of teeth and root blunting have been seen. The defects are more severe in children younger than age 7 at transplantation.
• Pulmonary: Bronchiolitis obliterans (BO) or bronchiolitis obliterans organizing pneumonia (BOOP)
• Neuropsychological:
  – Intellectual function: Few prospective studies published
  – Long-term depression and anxiety: Have been reported
• Renal:
  – Radiation nephritis
  – Hemolytic uremic syndrome and thrombocytopenic purpura occur, especially during treatment with cyclosporine.
  – Hypertension: Incidence is twice as high than in general population.
• Secondary malignancies: 15-year cumulative incidence rates are 20% and 6% after regimens with and without total-body irradiation, respectively.
• Recurrent leukemia: Current treatment options include donor leukocyte infusions to induce graft versus leukemia effect, nonmyeloablative (reduced intensity) transplants, or full allogeneic bone marrow transplant.

IMMUNIZATIONS POSTTRANSPLANT
• If patients are free of chronic graft-versus-host disease and off all immunosuppression medications for at least 6 months:
  – At 1 year posttransplant, patients should begin primary immunization schedule with DPaT, iPV, HIB, hepatitis A, hepatitis B, Menactra (if >11 years old), Pneumovax, and Prevnar.
  – At 2 years posttransplant, patients should receive measles, mumps, rubella, HPV (females 9–26 years old), and varicella vaccines.
• If patients have chronic graft-versus-host disease:
  – Hold immunizations until patient no longer has graft-versus-host disease and has been off immunosuppression for >6 months except for influenza, Pneumovax, and Prevnar vaccines, which should be given 1 year posttransplantation.
• All patients should receive influenza vaccine after 4 months posttransplant and then annually.

ADDITIONAL READING
• Baker KS, Bresters D, Sande JE. The burden of cure: Long-term side effects following hematopoietic stem cell transplantation. *Pediatr Clin North Am*. 2010; 57:323–342.
• Copelan EA. Hematopoietic stem-cell transplantation. *N Engl J Med*. 2006;354:1813–1826.
• Peters C, Cornish JM, Parikh SH, et al. Stem cell sources and outcome after hematopoietic stem cell transplantation (HSCT) in children and adolescents with acute leukemia. *Pediatr Clin North Am*. 2010;57:27–46.
• Smith AR, Wagner JE. Alternative haematopoietic stem cell sources for transplantation: Place of umbilical cord blood. *Br J Haematol*. 2009;147: 246–261.
• Wayne AS, Baird K, Egler RM. Hematopoietic stem cell transplantation for leukemia. *Pediatr Clin North Am*. 2010;57:1–25.
• Wingard JR, Hsu J, Hiemenz JW. Hematopoietic stem cell transplantation: An overview of infectious risks and epidemiology. *Infect Dis Clin North Am*. 2010;24:257–272.

FAQ
• Q: When can a patient return to school after transplantation?
• A: Typically, patients receiving autologous transplants and those receiving allogeneic transplants can return to school 6 months and 9 months posttransplantation, respectively, depending on the patient's immune reconstitution and function and the season; avoid returning to school during flu season; may need to adjust schedule because of fatigue.
• Q: If my patient relapses after bone marrow transplant, can a 2nd bone marrow transplant be done?
• A: Previously, there were few therapeutic options for patients who relapsed <1 year post–bone marrow transplant. Remissions after an infusion of buffy coat (containing T cells) from the patient's donor, called *donor leukocyte infusion*, have been achieved. Although most successful infusions have been in patients with chronic myelogenous leukemia, success has also been seen in acute leukemia. Chronic graft-versus-host disease will often result.

BOTULISM
Sheila M. Nolan

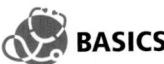

BASICS

DESCRIPTION
- An illness produced by neurotoxins elaborated by *Clostridium botulinum*, which causes an acute, descending, flaccid paralysis
- The neurotoxin may be ingested or absorbed from infected wounds, or ingested spores germinate, producing toxin.
- There are 3 primary types of illness:
  - In infant botulism, ingested spores germinate and colonize the infant's colon and elaborate toxin.
  - In adults, the patient ingests preformed toxin while eating improperly prepared or stored foodstuffs.
  - In wound botulism, spores germinate in an infected wound and toxin is absorbed.

EPIDEMIOLOGY
- Infants are usually white, breast-fed, and from middle-class families.
- There often is a history of a recent change in feeding practice (addition of formula or solids or changing from breast to bottle feeding).
- Honey seems to be a particularly contaminated food and has been implicated in California. Corn syrup has also been reported to contain botulinum spores but much less frequently than honey and has been associated with significantly fewer cases of infant botulism.
- Breastfed infants get ill at an older age than do bottle-fed infants; all cases of sudden infant death syndrome (SIDS) associated with infant botulism have been in bottle-fed infants.
- Food-borne cases are usually associated with the use of home-processed foods—especially vegetables, fruits, and condiments.

Incidence
- Infant botulism occurs in the 1st year of life, with >95% of cases reported in the 1st 6 months.
- Intestinal botulism is the most common form of human botulism in the US, with >100 cases reported annually.
- Wound botulism is very rare.

Prevalence
- Cases are seen more frequently in rural and suburban areas.
- Most cases have been reported in California, Utah, and Pennsylvania.

RISK FACTORS
Infants who have <1 bowel movement per day may be at increased risk.

GENERAL PREVENTION
- Botulinum toxin is heat labile; 5 minutes of boiling will destroy the toxin.
- Home-canned foods should be boiled for ≥10 minutes before serving.
- Spores are more resistant to heat. Home canners must use temperatures well above boiling to destroy spores effectively (120°C for 30 minutes). Pressure cookers are needed to achieve these conditions.

PATHOPHYSIOLOGY
- Neurotoxin is taken up by nerve endings and irreversibly blocks acetylcholine release in peripheral cholinergic synapses.
- Cranial nerves are usually affected first and most severely, leading to difficulty swallowing and loss of airway-protective reflexes. Respiratory failure develops.
- Botulinum toxin does not cross the blood–brain barrier; therefore, the sensorium remains clear.
- Recovery occurs with the regeneration of terminal motor neurons and the formation of new motor end plates.
- Infants are particularly prone to colonic colonization with *C. botulinum*. When foods other than breast milk are introduced in breast-fed infants, changes in flora may be especially important.

ETIOLOGY
C. botulinum, the etiologic agent, is a gram-positive, spore-forming, obligate anaerobic bacteria that is found in soil throughout the world.

DIAGNOSIS

HISTORY
- Usually constipation, with a progressive course of lethargy, weakness, and poor feeding
- Occasionally, progression may be quite rapid, and the abrupt onset of lethargy and weakness may suggest the diagnosis of bacterial sepsis or meningitis.
- Food-borne cases result in complaints of emesis in ~50% of patients.
- There may initially be complaints of diarrhea followed by constipation.
- The incubation period from ingestion to the onset of symptoms is usually 18–36 hours (range, a few hours to several days).
- Patients complain of weakness and dry mouth.
- Visual complaints include blurry vision, loss of accommodation, and diplopia.
- Patients may complain of dysphagia or dysarthria.
- Patients may have urinary retention.
- Fever is absent.
- Within 3 days, there is the onset of the characteristic descending, symmetrical paralysis. The cranial nerves are usually affected 1st.
- Mentation is clear, except for understandable anxiety and agitation.
- Wound botulism:
  - Has an incubation period of 4–14 days
  - Fever may or may not be present.
  - Patients often report constipation, but rarely nausea or vomiting.
  - They may complain of unilateral sensory changes and of purulent discharge from the wound.

PHYSICAL EXAM
- Older children and adults:
  - Often appear alert and are afebrile
  - Ptosis, extraocular palsies, and fixed and dilated pupils are often the 1st signs of descending paralysis.
  - Loss of airway-protective reflexes and respiratory muscle weakness leads to respiratory failure.
  - The triad of bulbar palsies, a lucid sensorium, and the absence of fever should prompt one to consider strongly a diagnosis of botulism.
- Infant botulism:
  - Presents in a similar way
  - Patients are usually afebrile.
  - They are usually weak, with decreased spontaneous activity at presentation.
  - They have an expressionless (masklike) face, ptosis, a weak cry, poor head control, and generalized weakness and hypotonia.
  - Pupils:
    - Often midposition initially and may be at least weakly reactive
    - Pupillary response is fatigable.
    - In many cases, pupils become fixed and dilated for a period.
  - Except for the symmetric, descending paralysis, the remainder of the physical examination is normal.
- Signs of autonomic instability include unexpected fluctuations in skin color, BP, and heart rate.
- Physical examination trick:
  - In infants, early in the course of the disease, pupillary and corneal reflexes may fatigue easily.

DIAGNOSTIC TESTS & INTERPRETATION
Lab
- Tests for the presence of toxin or the organism can be conducted on patient samples (serum, gastric aspirates, feces, or wound exudate) or suspected foodstuffs.
- Anaerobic cultures of a wound or the GI tract may yield the organism.

Imaging
EEG, MRI, and CT are nonspecific and usually normal in the absence of any complications.

Diagnostic Procedures/Other
Requirements for testing:
- Most tests for toxin and cultures are conducted by state health departments.
- The most common test performed is an assay for botulinum toxin in stool.
- Specimens must be shipped in sealed, break-proof, and leak-proof containers. Even small amounts of toxin, if inhaled or ingested, can lead to disease.
- Suspect foods should be shipped refrigerated and in their original containers if possible.
- Electromyography (EMG) shows a characteristic pattern of brief-duration, sharp-amplitude, overly abundant motor unit action potentials (brief short-acting potentials).

DIFFERENTIAL DIAGNOSIS
- Infections:
  - In noninfants, bacterial sepsis, meningitis, poliomyelitis, tick paralysis, and diphtheric polyneuritis
  - In infants, sepsis and meningitis may present in a similar way.
  - Absence of fever and a clear sensorium make sepsis and meningitis less likely.
- Neurologic:
  - Myasthenia gravis usually spares the pupillary response, whereas it is fatigable in botulism, if not absent.
  - In Werdnig-Hoffman disease (type I spinal muscle atrophy), facial muscles are spared.
- Toxins: Drug ingestions may lead to weakness and lethargy.

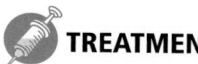 **TREATMENT**

MEDICATION (DRUGS)
- Antibiotics are not helpful in infant botulism:
  - In suspected infant botulism, aminoglycoside antibiotics (e.g., gentamicin) should be avoided, as they may produce an abrupt worsening of the weakness and ensuing respiratory failure.
- Prompt recognition of infant botulism and early treatment with human IV botulism immunoglobulin (BabyBIG®) has been shown to decrease time to recovery and hospital discharge. BabyBIG® is available through the California Department of Public Health's Infant Botulism Treatment and Prevention Program.
- Equine antitoxin is not recommended for infant botulism.
- Antibiotics are indicated only for documented complications such as pneumonia.
- Cathartics are not beneficial, and enemas may cause colonic distention and increased toxin absorption.
- Cases of botulism resulting from ingested toxin or wound infection:
  - Should be treated with heptavalent botulinum antitoxin (HBAT), available from the CDC
  - Antitoxin should not be administered to asymptomatic individuals who have only eaten suspect foods.
- Wound botulism should be treated with IV penicillin G 250,000 U/kg/d.

ADDITIONAL TREATMENT
General Measures
- All patients with suspected botulism should be admitted to the hospital and have continuous monitoring of their heart rate, respiratory rate, and oxygenation, as well as frequent assessment of their respiratory effort and airway-protective reflexes.
- The mainstay of therapy is meticulous supportive care. Particular attention is paid to respiratory and nutritional needs.
- Endotracheal intubation may be necessary both for patients with frank respiratory failure and when airway-protective reflexes are lost.
- Wounds should be explored and débrided, and anaerobic cultures should be obtained.

- Cases of suspected toxin ingestion should be treated early with induced emesis and/or gastric lavage in an attempt to decrease toxin exposure.
- All cases should be reported to the state health department and the Centers for Disease Control (CDC), Atlanta, Georgia.
- Supportive care should be continued until the patient is able to be weaned from respiratory support and begin PO feedings.

IN-PATIENT CONSIDERATIONS
Initial Stabilization
Good supportive care with emphasis on respiratory support, including intubation and mechanical ventilation when needed, is the most important consideration in emergency therapy.

 ONGOING CARE

PROGNOSIS
- Food-borne botulism carries a mortality rate of 20–25%. This rate is lower in patients <20 years old (10%).
- Patients with a shorter incubation period usually have more severe involvement and a worse prognosis, probably related to an increased amount of toxin ingested.
- If recognized early and treated aggressively, botulism carries a good prognosis, and complete recovery can be expected. Fatigability may persist for up to 1 year.
- Infant botulism has an estimated mortality rate of <5% in hospitalized patients. Complete recovery can be expected when disease is recognized early and treated appropriately.

COMPLICATIONS
- The most serious and fatal complication is respiratory failure due to paralysis of the respiratory muscles.
- Bulbar dysfunction in infant botulism may lead to dehydration before presentation.
- The loss of airway-protective reflexes can lead to aspiration and pneumonia.
- Constipation and urinary retention may precede the onset of paralysis and may complicate later management as well. Cases of severe *Clostridium difficile* enterocolitis with hypovolemia, hypotension, and prolonged ICU stays have been reported in infants with botulism.
- The earliest symptoms in adults and older children may be visual changes, including blurred vision, loss of accommodation, and diplopia.
- Syndrome of inappropriate secretion of diuretic hormone and urinary tract infections have been reported in infants with infant botulism.

ADDITIONAL READING

- Arnon SS, Schechter R, Maslanka SE, et al. Human botulism immune globulin for the treatment of infant botulism. *N Engl J Med.* 2006;354(5):462–467.
- Brook I. Infant botulism. *J Perinatol.* 2007;27(3):175–180.
- Centers for Disease Control and Prevention. Infant botulism—New York City, 2001–2002. *JAMA.* 2003;289:834–836.
- Centers for Disease Control and Prevention. Investigational heptavalent botulinum antitoxin (HBAT) to replace licensed botulinum antitoxin AB and investigational botulinum antitoxin E. *MMWR Morb Mortal Wkly Rep.* 2010;59(10):299.
- Muensterer OJ. Infant botulism. *Pediatr Rev.* 2000;21:427.
- Passaro DJ, Werner SB, McgeeJ, et al. Wound botulism associated with black tar heroin among injecting drug users. *JAMA.* 1998;279:859–863.
- Shapiro RL, Hatheway C, Swerdlow DL. Botulism in the United States: A clinical and Epidemiologic review. *Ann Intern Med.* 1998;129:221–228.

 CODES

ICD9
- 005.1 Botulism food poisoning
- 040.41 Infant botulism
- 040.42 Wound botulism

ICD10
- A05.1 Botulism food poisoning
- A48.51 Infant botulism
- A48.52 Wound botulism

FAQ
- Q: Can infant botulism recur?
- A: True recurrence in infant botulism has not been documented.
- Q: Should antitoxin be given to persons who have ingested food that they think might be contaminated with botulinum toxin?
- A: Because the antitoxin carries a significant risk of serum sickness, it should be given only to persons with neurologic symptoms.
- Q: Where is antitoxin obtained?
- A: Antitoxin may be obtained from the Centers for Disease Control and Prevention, Atlanta, Georgia; 770-488-7100.
- Q: Where is human IV botulism immunoglobulin obtained?
- A: Human IV botulism immunoglobulin, which is produced from pooled human plasma from screened individuals, may be obtained from the California Department of Health Services Infant Botulism Treatment and Prevention Program; 510-231-7600.

B

BRAIN ABSCESS

Catherine Zorc
Jeffrey P. Louie (5th edition)

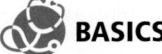 **BASICS**

DESCRIPTION
- Suppurative infection involving the brain parenchyma
- May be a single or multiple lesion

EPIDEMIOLOGY
- Males are affected more than females (2:1 male-to-female predominance).
- Average age of presentation is ~7 years of age.

Incidence
~1,500–2,500 cases (adults and pediatric combined) occur per year.

Prevalence
2–4% of children with cyanotic congenital heart disease will develop a brain abscess (tetralogy of Fallot being the most common).

RISK FACTORS
- Cyanotic congenital heart disease
- Otorhinolaryngologic infections such as sinusitis, mastoiditis, and chronic otitis media
- Meningitis (especially with neonates)
- Penetrating head trauma
- Surgical manipulation of the brain (ventriculoperitoneal shunts, tumor removal)
- Esophageal manipulation (sclerotherapy or dilation)
- Cystic fibrosis
- Dental infections
- Lung infections
- Any site of infection (osteomyelitis, orbital, cellulitis, urinary tract infections)
- Patients who have traveled to endemic areas with neurocysticercosis (Latin America, parts of Africa, Asia, and the Indian subcontinent).
- Congenital or acquired immunocompromised patients
- No definitive etiology occurs in 30% of patients

GENERAL PREVENTION
- During recreational activities, wearing helmets may prevent penetrating head trauma.
- Preventive medicine: Dentistry and otorhinolaryngology

PATHOPHYSIOLOGY
- Microorganisms enter the brain parenchyma through contiguous or hematogenous (metastasis) pathways.
- Location of brain abscesses:
  – Cyanotic congenital heart disease patients tend to have abscesses within the middle meningeal artery distribution: Frontal, parietal, and temporal lobes.
  – Frontal abscesses are commonly seen with sinus and dental infections.
  – Temporal, parietal, or cerebellar abscesses tend to occur with mastoiditis or otitis media.
  – Brain abscesses can occur anywhere in the brain parenchyma, regardless of a predisposing risk factor, secondary to hematogenous metastasis.

ETIOLOGY
- Bacteria are the most common causes.
- *Streptococcus* sp. and *Staphylococcus* sp. are the most commonly cultured microorganisms.
- Neonates may develop abscesses after a Gram-negative meningitis (*Proteus*, *Citrobacter*, and *Enterobacter*).
- A single organism is found in ~70% of patients.
- Anaerobic organisms are being found with increasing incidence with improved laboratory and culture techniques. Common pathogens are *Bacteroides*, *Peptostreptococcus*, *Fusobacterium*, *Propionibacterium*, *Actinomyces*, *Veillonella*, and *Prevotella*.
- No growth of a pathogen occurs in 30% of specimens.
- Parasitic infections are often caused by *Taenia solium* (neurocysticercosis).
- Fungi and protozoa are commonly found in immunocompromised patients.

 DIAGNOSIS

HISTORY
The location of the brain abscess or abscesses will often influence the history of presentation and physical exam.
- Fever, headache, and vomiting each occur in ~60–70% of cases.
- Classic triad of fever, headache, and focal neurologic findings occurs in <30% of cases.
- Headache is the most common complaint.
- Average duration of symptoms prior to diagnosis is ~4 weeks.
- Vomiting and mental-status changes can often be the presenting chief complaints.
- Neonates will often have a history of meningitis before developing a brain abscess.
- Questions should focus on acute or chronic otolaryngologic infections such as sinusitis, chronic otitis media, and mastoiditis, as well as a history of cholesteatomas.
- Cyanotic congenital heart disease should be determined, as well as partially repaired cyanotic congenital heart disease.

PHYSICAL EXAM
- Neonates may present with a full fontanel, increasing head circumference, seizures, or vomiting.
- Older children may have signs of a focal neurologic deficit, hemiparesis, or even papilledema.
- Meningeal symptoms occur in ~30% of patients.
- Ataxia may be found with cerebellar lesions.

DIAGNOSTIC TESTS & INTERPRETATION
Lab
- Routine lab tests are not helpful and cannot rule out the diagnosis.
- <10% of blood cultures are positive.
- CBC may be mildly elevated, and <10% will show a left shift.
- ESR is a poor indicator of brain abscesses.
- Electrolytes may show low sodium, indicating syndrome of inappropriate secretion of diuretic hormone.

- A lumbar puncture is contraindicated if any intracranial mass lesion is suspected, but if CSF is obtained:
  - It may show a mild-to-moderate pleocytosis (20% of patients may have normal values).
  - Opening pressure is always elevated.
  - Glucose may be decreased in 30% of patients.
  - Protein is elevated in 70% of cases.
  - CSF cultures are often sterile, unless the abscess ruptures into the ventricles.

Imaging
- CT with contrast and MRI scans are the studies of choice in diagnosing brain abscesses.
- Cranial ultrasound may be useful in premature neonatal cases.

ALERT
- Not all patients with brain abscesses have fevers.
- Pitfalls:
  - Failing to consider a brain abscess in a child with altered mental status, fevers, and meningismus
  - Performing a lumbar puncture
  - Failing to use contrast with the CT scan

DIFFERENTIAL DIAGNOSIS
- **Infectious**
  - Meningitis
  - Encephalitis
  - Subdural empyema
  - Epidural abscess
- **Vascular**
  - Venous sinus thrombosis
  - Migraine
  - Cerebral infarct
  - Cerebral hemorrhage
- **Miscellaneous**
  - Primary or secondary tumor
  - Pseudotumor cerebri
  - Hydrocephalus

 ## TREATMENT

MEDICATION (DRUGS)
- Broad-spectrum antibiotics should be started at the time of diagnosis, until identification of the microorganism is determined. At that time, the antibiotics can be tailored to the offending microorganism.
- Most brain abscesses are removed surgically. A few may require CT-guided aspiration.
- MRI or CT-guided stereotactic aspiration is encouraged.

- When multiple abscesses are found on CT scan, 1 lesion should be aspirated to identify the microorganism.
- Some patients are managed successfully with antibiotics alone, which may be appropriate in carefully selected patients, especially if there is a single abscess <2 cm. Antiparasitic medications are controversial in the treatment of neurocysticercosis.
- Antifungals should be considered for immunocompromised patients.
- The use of steroids is controversial.
- Antiepileptic therapy may be indicated, but there are no studies that guide use in patients with brain abscess.
- If a patient is manifesting signs and symptoms of increased intracranial pressure (Cushing triad: Bradycardia, hypertension, and abnormal respirations) or if the patient is comatose and is unable to protect his or her airway, the patient should be intubated, hyperventilated, and given mannitol.
- Patients with unknown predisposing factors should be evaluated by cardiology, dental, and otorhinolaryngology. Immunology should be considered in children with significant medical histories of chronic infections.

 ## ONGOING CARE

FOLLOW-UP RECOMMENDATIONS
- A high index of suspicion is required to diagnose a brain abscess. A delay in diagnosis or performing a lumbar puncture for suspected meningitis increases mortality and morbidity.
- With the advent of CT and MRI scans, the mortality rate has dropped from ~30% to <14%.
- Multiple abscesses, coma on presentation, <2 years of age, performance of a lumbar puncture, and rupture of abscess into the ventricle carry a higher mortality rate. 30–40% of patients have some morbidity. This ranges from seizures, hemiparesis, focal neurologic deficits, or hydrocephalus to cognitive/behavioral problems.

PATIENT MONITORING
- Neonates and older patients may be discharged with home physical therapy and home nursing for IV antibiotics.
- Patients will need IV antibiotics for a total of 3–4 weeks. Some may require longer courses of antibiotics.
- Some children will need follow-up CT or MRI scans.
- Follow-up with neurosurgical, rehabilitation, and neurology clinics is usually required.

COMPLICATIONS
- Arise from the location, size, and number of intracranial abscesses
- Can vary from syndrome of inappropriate secretion of diuretic hormone or seizures to focal neurologic deficits

ADDITIONAL READING
- Calfee DP, Wispelwey B. Brain abscess. *Semin Neurol*. 2000;20:353–360.
- Cochrane DD. Brain abscess. *Pediatr Rev*. 1999; 20:209–214.
- Goodkin HP, Harper MB, Pomeroy SL. Intracerebral abscess in children: Historical trends at Children's Hospital Boston. *Pediatrics*. 2004;113:1765–1770.
- Mitchell WG. Neurocysticercosis and acquired cerebral toxoplasmosis in children. *Semin Pediatr Neurol*. 1999;6:267–277.
- Saez-Llorens X. Brain abscess in children. *Semin Pediatr Infect Dis*. 2003;14:108–114.
- Sidaras D, Mallucci C, Pilling D, et al. Neonatal brain abscess-potential pitfalls of CT scanning. *Childs Nerv Syst*. 2003;19:57–59.
- Yogev R, Bar-Meir M. Management of brain abscess in children. *Pediatr Infect Dis J*. 2004;23:157–160.

 ## CODES

ICD9
324.0 Intracranial abscess

ICD10
G06.0 Intracranial abscess and granuloma

FAQ
- Q: Do all brain abscesses require surgery?
- A: No. Select cases will regress with antibiotics and follow-up with MRI.
- Q: What is the best way to diagnose brain abscess?
- A: MRI

BRAIN INJURY, TRAUMATIC

Jerry Larrabee
Karen LeComte (5th edition)

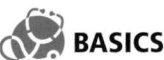 BASICS

DESCRIPTION
Traumatic brain injury (TBI): Damage to the brain from accidental or nonaccidental trauma:
- Children >1 year: GCS <14, amnesia >15 minutes for event, penetrating head injury
- Children <1 year: Any LOC, protracted emesis, suspected abuse
- Severe brain injury: Usually initial GCS <9

EPIDEMIOLOGY
- Trauma, number 1 cause of death of children >1 year. Head injury most common contributor to morbidity and mortality.
- Between 29,000 and 50,000 children in the US <19 suffer permanent disability from TBI each year.
- Age-dependent mechanism of injury and pathophysiology
- <2 years old: Nonaccidental trauma is principle cause of TBI.
- >2 years old: Falls (~37%) are most common cause of trauma.
- For severe TBI, nonaccidental trauma remains principal cause in young children.
- Motor vehicle accidents in older children, although penetrating injuries becoming more common

PATHOPHYSIOLOGY
- Primary:
  - Focally applied forces: Lacerations, penetration injuries, skull fractures
  - Contusions, intracerebral hematomas uncommon. Epidurals, classic subdurals <10% in children
  - Acceleration-deceleration/shearing forces: Cervical spine injuries, diffuse axonal injury (DAI), non-aneurysmal subarachnoid hemorrhage, subdural hematoma (SDH) from shear forces
- Secondary:
  - Extension of injury to viable tissue/entire brain
  - Dysautoregulation of cerebral blood flow, neuroexcitotoxicity and inflammatory mediators. CT or MRI signs of edema may progress over 3–5 days (see "Treatment").
- Age-specific pathophysiology
  - Infants/toddler:
    ○ Shear forces on the brain due to acceleration/deceleration avulse axons from their cell bodies (DAI); often compounded by tearing and bleeding of dural veins.
    ○ Unmyelinated infant brain absorbs rather than transfers impact. Immature, distensible skull renders brain less likely to contuse or herniated, but more likely to sustain diffuse secondary injuries, with swelling.
    ○ Subgaleal hematoma, cephalohematoma (below the periosteum), and caput succedaneum (confined to the superficial scalp) at birth do not predict brain injury.

- More severe birth trauma can result in SDH.
- Bilateral interhemispheric SDH suggests nonaccidental trauma.
- Diffuse injuries secondary to shaken impact syndrome can lead to cerebral swelling with secondary infarction and/or decreased central respiratory control, leading to apnea, hypoxia, and cerebral edema.
- Children <3 at risk of growing skull fracture when leptomeningeal cyst protrudes through a dural tear (late effect).
- Suspect nonaccidental trauma with growing skull fracture, if >1 cranial bone involved, or if other injuries are present.
  - Older children/adolescents:
    ○ Still more subject to DAI than adults due to incomplete myelination
    ○ Projectile injuries in adolescent population
    ○ Can result from nonaccidental trauma (usually with other stigmata of assault)

 DIAGNOSIS

HISTORY
- Eyewitness accounts are invaluable.
- Details of who was caring for the child
- Falls: Did loss of consciousness precede fall? Height of fall, surface of impact
- History of epilepsy, cardiac problems
- History of previous concussions (consider "second impact syndrome") or trauma
- Intoxication (of child, caregiver, others in the environment)
- Prior physical abuse/neglect?
- Restrained motor vehicle passenger? Angle of impact
- How did patient act or change over time? Unresponsive? Confused? Headache? Visual changes? Vomiting? Seizure?

PHYSICAL EXAM
Rapid neurologic exam in trauma:
- Can derive some of these by observation. Note presence of neuromuscular blockers/sedation
  - Level of arousal: Awake, lethargic, stuporous, unresponsive
  - Resting posture: Spontaneous, restless, still normal, flexor, extensor
  - Respiration: In context of arousal and posture, hyperpnea or Cheyne-Stokes respiration
  - Response to stimulation: Voice, pain (of earlobe to avoid spinal withdrawal response); note localization, withdrawal, posturing
  - Pupils: Equal, anisocoria >1 mm, unequal/sluggish pupil, unequal/wide/fixed pupil
  - Extraocular movements: Disconjugate gaze nonlocalizing with drugs/trauma, 3rd nerve palsy uncal herniation sign, 4th nerve palsy common in head injuries, 6th nerve palsy from trauma or increased ICP

  - Brainstem reflexes: Corneals (V & VII), oculocephalic if patient unable to cooperate with eye exam and cervical spine cleared. Avoid gag—raises ICP
  - Muscle reflexes/motor exam: Lateralizing signs may indicate contralateral hemispheric lesion, with ipsilateral dilated pupil may indicate uncal herniation
  - Sensory: Brief for 4 limbs/spinal level if indicated
- This exam should be repeated often according to the patient's level of acuity. A more detailed exam tailored to degree of arousal can be done as the patient is stabilized.

DIAGNOSTIC TESTS & INTERPRETATION
Lab
In all patients with suspected TBI, consider:
- CBC (infants can have a large amount of intracranial blood loss)
- PT/PTT (to evaluate a possible bleeding disorder as a possible preoperative laboratory test)
- Electrolytes
- Toxin screen

Imaging
- Unenhanced CT scan of the brain is the imaging study of choice for initial evaluation of a patient with suspected TBI.
- Abnormal CT: Lesion density, midline shift, compression of cisterns, bone fragments
- MRI: Useful for DAI (with a negative head CT) as well as showing small lesions (e.g., punctate contusions)
- In suspected cervical spine injury where patient is unresponsive, MRI of the spine to rule out noncontiguous unstable ligamentous injury
- Long-bone films if degree of injury is not consistent with history or history of fall from unclear height
- With CT scan showing normal brain/ventricular spaces: Consider EEG and lumbar puncture if a nontraumatic etiology for altered mental status is suspected.

DIFFERENTIAL DIAGNOSIS
Neurologic presentation varies in severity from a normal examination through coma similar to hypoxic-ischemic brain injuries (e.g., near-drowning), other causes of stupor/coma, seizure activity (postictal encephalopathy).
- Distinction between simple concussion, DAI, and hypoxic-ischemic injury may be difficult at initial presentation, becoming clear as clinical picture/neuroimaging evolves.

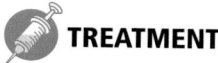 TREATMENT

- Airway, breathing, circulation
- Prehospital stabilization: Avoid hypoxemia and hypotension (strong, possibly modifiable, independent predictors of outcome in TBI)

ADDITIONAL TREATMENT
General Measures

- Maintenance of CPP >50 positively influences outcome in TBI (MAP – ICP = CPP), especially in first 48 hours.
- A rapid neurologic exam repeated over time is instrumental in directing the patient's care.
- Secondary survey: External evidence of head injury/deformities, ecchymoses (periorbital-orbital roof fracture; mastoid-petrous temporal fracture), lacerations, penetrations. CSF leak nasal/otic.
- Seizures: Ativan 0.1–0.2 mg/kg IV at 2 mg/min or rectal Diastat 0.3–0.5 mg/kg if no IV access. Then load fosphenytoin 15–20 mg/kg IV. Important to treat to avoid increased ICP, neurotoxicity, hypoxia.
- No evidence that seizure prophylaxis >1 week post-trauma prevents late seizures
- No evidence that steroids improve outcome
- Hypothermia may be protective, no difference in long-term outcome.
- No evidence for prophylactic use of mannitol, though it is effective for control of increased ICP. Bolus doses 0.25 g/kg of body weight to 1 g/kg of body weight to goal ICP <20 mm Hg
- Hypertonic saline for increased ICP as above under fluid resuscitation
- The postresuscitation GCS score should be recorded in all trauma patients.
- Involvement of neurosurgery with moderate GCS <13 injury, even if patient initially stable
- Survival for children with severe TBI is greater when treated in pediatric ICU.
- Decompressive craniectomy may be considered given the following conditions:
  – Diffuse cerebral swelling on cranial CT imaging
  – Within 48 hours of injury
  – No episodes of sustained ICP >40 mm Hg before surgery
  – GCS >3 at some point subsequent to injury
  – Secondary clinical deterioration
  – Evolving cerebral herniation syndrome
- AAP guidelines set conditions for return to play depending on severity of concussion:
  – Grade I—mild; no LOC, amnesia, or confusion; return to play after 20 minutes
  – Grade II—moderate; no LOC, some confusion and amnesia >15 minutes; return to play after 1 week
  – Grade III—severe; LOC; return to play after 1 month; assume cervical spine injury/stabilize no return to play unless symptoms resolved, including exertional symptoms
  – An AAP concussion statement outlines graded return activities barring symptoms and suggests (a) no same-day return; (b) and consider removal from season play for 3 concussions in one season or postconcussive symptoms >3 months

IN-PATIENT CONSIDERATIONS
Initial Stabilization

- Cervical spine stabilization and clearance; in severe TBI, entire spine is stabilized:
  – If necessary, orotracheal intubation with rapid sequence induction; avoid hypotension
  – Hyperventilation may induce regional cerebral ischemia in children, especially in first 24 hours.
  – Increased ICP managed by bed elevation of 30 degrees, hypertonic fluids, sedation
- Hemodynamic stabilization (normal high systolic BP ~135) predictor of better outcome in TBI (Median systolic BP = 90 mm Hg + [2 × age in years])
  – Hemodynamic instability indicative of systemic hemorrhage (abdomen, long-bone fractures). Pericardial tamponade (narrow pulse pressure). Neurogenic shock.
  – Hypotension late sign. Early: ↑HR, ↓capillary refill, ↓urine output
  – Fluid resuscitation: Consider hypertonic saline. Mounting evidence of improved outcomes especially with hemorrhagic shock and TBI (titrate continuous 3% saline infusion 0.1–1 mL/kg/h).
  – Fluid bolus may worsen intracranial hypertension (ICP).
  – Consider monitoring ICP to maintain <20 mm Hg for abnormal admission CT scan, and GCS 3–8 after CPR, or normal CT and GCS 3–8, and posturing, or hypotension, or if serial neurologic exams precluded by sedation.

 ONGOING CARE

PROGNOSIS

- Presence of both hypoxemia and hypotension on arrival to ER bode poorly.
- 24-hour GCS better predictor of outcome than postresuscitation; PRISM score also helpful
- GCS <3 poor prognosis unless secondary to epidural hematoma; rapid evacuation can minimize permanent deficits
- Diffuse white matter, subcortical gray or brainstem lesions on MRI portend long periods of coma and poorer outcome
- Somatosensory evoked potentials (VEPS or BAEPs) are less sensitive but have high specificity in predicting neurologic outcome.
- Degree of injury on head CT can be predictive.
- Patients who have sustained moderate-to-severe head injury (GCS = 13) often have academic difficulties, memory abnormalities, and disinhibition.
- Monitoring for cognitive difficulties, hyperactivity, seizures, hydrocephalus, movement disorders, paralysis, visual/hearing disturbance, headache; psychologists, neurologists, neurosurgeons, ophthalmologists, audiologists, and physical therapists may be helpful.
- Leptomeningeal cyst (especially in children <3 years old) almost always develops within 6 months of injury.
- Refer any patient with known skull fracture who manifests a new swelling in area of old fracture to neurosurgery for 3D CT imaging of the head.
- ~10% of patients with severe head injury will develop epilepsy.

ADDITIONAL READING

- Adelson PD, Bratton SL, Carney NA, et al. Critical pathway for the treatment of established intracranial hypertension in pediatric traumatic brain injury. *Pediatr Crit Care Med*. 2003;4(Suppl 3):S65–S67.
- American College of Radiology. *Suspected cervical spine trauma*. Reston, VA: American College of Radiology, 2002.
- Halstead ME, Walter KD, Council on Sports Medicine and Fitness. Clinical report—sport-related concussion in children and adolescents. *Pediatrics*. 2010;126:597–615.
- Hymel KP, Makoroff KL, Laskey AL, et al. Mechanisms, clinical presentations, injuries, and outcomes from inflicted versus noninflicted head trauma during infancy: Results of a prospective, multicentered, comparative study. *Pediatrics*. 2007;119(5):922–929.
- Jagannathan J, Okonkwo DO, Dumont AS, et al. Outcome following decompressive craniectomy in children with severe traumatic brain injury: A 10-year single-center experience with long-term follow-up. *J Neurosurg*. 2007;106(Suppl 4):268–275.
- Jayawant S, Parr J. Outcome following subdural haemorrhages in infancy. *Arch Dis Child*. 2007; 92(4):343–347.
- White JR, Farukhi Z, Bull C, et al. Predictors of outcome in severely head-injured children. *Crit Care Med*. 2001;29:534–540.
- Information on head injury:
  – Centers for Disease Control and Prevention: www.cdc.gov/concussion/HeadsUp/high_school.html
- Sources of online cognitive testing:
  – Computerized neuropsychological tests—US Army Medical Department: www.armymedicine.army.mil/prr/anam.html
  – CogState: www.cogstate.com/go/sport
  – ImPACT: www.impacttest.com

 CODES

ICD9

- 854.00 Intracranial injury of other and unspecified nature without mention of open intracranial wound, unspecified state of consciousness
- 854.01 Intracranial injury of other and unspecified nature without mention of open intracranial wound, with no loss of consciousness
- 854.02 Intracranial injury of other and unspecified nature without mention of open intracranial wound, with brief [less than one hour] loss of consciousness

ICD10

- S06.9X0A Unsp intracranial injury w/o loss of consciousness, init
- S06.9X1A Unsp intracranial injury w LOC of 30 minutes or less, init
- S06.9X2A Unsp intracranial injury w LOC of 31–59 min, init

BRAIN TUMOR
Michael J. Fisher

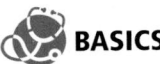

BASICS

DESCRIPTION
A primary neoplasm arising in the CNS

EPIDEMIOLOGY
Incidence
- Most common solid neoplasm of childhood (2nd to leukemia in overall incidence)
- Incidence rising (>3,000 new cases/year)
- 4.5 cases/100,000 children/year
- Peak incidence in children ≤7 years of age

Prevalence
- Slight male predominance
- Majority arise infratentorially (within cerebellum or brainstem) in children 1–11 years of age
- Majority arise supratentorially in children <1 year of age

RISK FACTORS
Genetics
- Not a heritable condition
- Primary CNS tumors are associated with several familial syndromes:
  - Neurofibromatosis with optic pathway gliomas (NF1) and meningiomas (NF2)
  - Tuberous sclerosis with gliomas and rarely ependymomas
  - Li–Fraumeni syndrome with astrocytomas
  - Von Hippel–Lindau with cerebellar hemangioblastoma
  - Turcot syndrome with primitive neuroectodermal tumor

PATHOPHYSIOLOGY
The majority of tumors are classified based on their histology. The most common are:
- Glioma:
  - Arises from astrocytes (supportive tissue)
  - >50% of childhood CNS tumors
  - Ranges from low grade (often in the cerebellum or optic pathway) to high grade (grade III to IV; in the cerebrum or brainstem)
  - Locally recurrent and invasive when high grade
- Primitive neuroectodermal tumor/medulloblastoma:
  - Malignant embryonal tumor arising from unknown cell type
  - Comprises ~20% of childhood CNS tumors
  - Most common malignant brain tumor in children
  - Majority arise in the midline of the cerebellum (referred to as medulloblastoma)
  - Predisposition for leptomeningeal dissemination
- Ependymoma:
  - Arises from ependymal cells that line the ventricular system
  - 8–10% of childhood CNS tumors
  - Most commonly occurs in the 4th ventricle; may arise in the spinal cord
  - Locally recurrent and invasive; spinal metastases rare at initial diagnosis

- Germ cell tumor:
  - Derived from totipotent germ cells
  - 3–5% of childhood CNS tumors
  - Majority are located in the pineal or suprasellar region
- Atypical teratoid/rhabdoid tumor:
  - Rare embryonal tumor arising from unknown cell type; often misdiagnosed as primitive neuroectodermal tumor
  - <3% of childhood CNS tumors
  - Majority arise in children <5 years of age
  - Propensity to arise in the posterior fossa with frequent leptomeningeal dissemination; reported in association with malignant rhabdoid tumors of the kidney
- Craniopharyngioma: 6–9% of childhood CNS tumors
- Tumors of the choroid plexus
- Ganglioglioma
- Meningioma and hemangioblastoma, rare in children

ETIOLOGY
- No specific causative agents are known, but there is an association with radiation, chemical exposure, other malignancies, familial/heritable diseases, immunosuppression (lymphoma)
- Molecular markers and variants of individual tumor types are being identified.

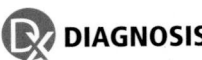

DIAGNOSIS

Tumor location dictates symptoms and signs.

HISTORY
- Headache and vomiting (particularly in the morning), irritability, and lethargy are associated with increased intracranial pressure.
- Difficulty swallowing, slurred speech, and diplopia may indicate brainstem tumor.
- Visual-field deficits (bumps into things) could indicate optic tract lesion.
- Focal weakness hints at pyramidal tract lesion.
- Ataxia may be a sign of cerebellar lesion.
- Changes in behavior or school performance, new-onset seizures, and weakness could be signs of supratentorial lesion.
- Polyuria/polydipsia may indicate hypothalamic/pituitary lesion.
- Failure to thrive, emaciation, euphoria, and increased appetite in an infant may indicate hypothalamic lesion (diencephalic syndrome).
- Back pain, extremity weakness, and bowel/bladder dysfunction could signify spinal cord metastases (often seen with primitive neuroectodermal tumor/medulloblastoma and germ cell tumors).

PHYSICAL EXAM
- Papilledema, impaired upgaze and/or lateral gaze, macrocephaly (infants), and bulging fontanelle are signs of increased intracranial pressure.
- Focal deficit on neurologic exam helps localize the mass lesion:
  - Isolated cranial nerve VI and VII palsies may indicate brainstem tumor.
  - Ataxia and dysmetria could indicate cerebellar mass.
  - Decreased visual acuity, visual-field deficit, absent pupillary light response, and strabismus may all be signs of optic tract tumor.
  - Changes in cognitive function, mood, and affect could indicate supratentorial lesion.
  - Impaired upgaze, convergence nystagmus, and pupils respond to accommodation but poorly to light are signs of pineal lesion (Parinaud syndrome).
- Signs of neurocutaneous disease (e.g., café-au-lait spots, Lisch nodules) may indicate a syndrome such as neurofibromatosis type 1.

DIAGNOSTIC TESTS & INTERPRETATION
Imaging
- MRI with and without gadolinium enhancement is the "gold standard" for identification, localization, and characterization of tumors.
- CT can be used as an initial study, but if negative and a high index of suspicion, follow with MRI. Useful to evaluate for hydrocephalus and hemorrhage.

Diagnostic Procedures/Other
Staging of tumor:
- Postoperative head MRI within 24–48 hours to determine residual disease before postoperative inflammatory changes are prominent
- Spine MRI and CSF cytology required for neuraxis staging of tumors with high risk of leptomeningeal dissemination
- Elevated α-fetoprotein and quantitative β-human chorionic gonadotropin in CSF and serum are markers for germ cell tumors.

DIFFERENTIAL DIAGNOSIS
- Infection: Cerebral abscess
- Tumors: Metastatic tumor to brain, uncommon with childhood solid tumors
- Trauma: Hemorrhage unlikely to be confused with tumor
- Congenital:
  - Arteriovenous malformation
  - Hamartoma
  - Dysplastic brain

- Psychosocial: Some patients with nausea, vomiting, or behavior changes are first diagnosed with psychiatric disorders, GI disorders, failure to thrive, or anorexia nervosa prior to discovery of a brain tumor.

ALERT
New onset of psychoses should prompt imaging to rule out tumor.

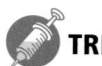 TREATMENT

SURGERY/OTHER PROCEDURES
- Both for histology and to attempt maximal tumor debulking; should be performed by experienced pediatric neurosurgeon
- Rarely indicated in intrinsic pontine (brainstem) glioma
- Ventriculoperitoneal shunt when needed for obstructive hydrocephalus (risk of peritoneal seeding minimal)

ALERT
Patient should be referred to a pediatric brain tumor/oncology center at diagnosis (preoperatively).

Radiotherapy
- Volume and dose vary depending on histology.
- Radiation therapy to the tumor bed is used for most patients with brain tumors.
- Medulloblastoma/primitive neuroectodermal tumor patients need craniospinal radiation therapy. The one exception is infants and young children (<3 years of age), in whom cognitive deficits from radiation therapy can be devastating.
- Duration of radiation therapy: Usually 6 weeks
- Newer approaches to limit exposure of normal brain include intensity modulated and proton radiotherapy.

MEDICATION (DRUGS)
- Dexamethasone to control increased intracranial pressure (0.5 mg/kg divided q6h)
- Chemotherapy:
  - Drugs are most often used in combination:
    ◦ Carboplatin, vincristine, or 6-thioguanine, procarbazine, CCNU, vincristine for low-grade glioma
    ◦ Cisplatin, CCNU, vincristine, etoposide, and cyclophosphamide are active agents for primitive neuroectodermal tumor/medulloblastoma
    ◦ Temozolomide for high-grade glioma
  - New protocols currently being evaluated:
    ◦ High-dose chemotherapy with stem cell rescue for high-risk primitive neuroectodermal tumor/medulloblastoma
    ◦ Targeted therapies, angiogenesis inhibitors
  - Duration of chemotherapy: 6 months to 2 years

ALERT
Possible conflict with other treatments: Chemotherapy can alter anticonvulsant levels.

ONGOING CARE

- Neurologic deficits can take months to improve or stabilize with permanent deficit.
- Any worsening or relapse of symptoms must be evaluated for tumor recurrence.
- MRI every 3 months the 1st year, every 6 months for the next 2 years, and annually thereafter. Benefit of routine surveillance imaging is controversial.

PROGNOSIS
- Dependent on histology of tumor, location, and extent of initial resection
- Glioma:
  - Low grade: ≥90% 5-year progression-free survival (PFS) following gross total resection; 45–65% for subtotal resection
  - High grade: Median survival 8–31 months; depends on grade and extent of resection
  - Intrinsic pontine: Median overall survival of 9–13 months from diagnosis
- Medulloblastoma:
  - 79–83% PFS at 5 years if localized, gross total resection achieved, and >3 years old at diagnosis
  - <50% PFS if disseminated
- Ependymoma:
  - 50–70% survival at 5 years with total resection
  - <30% survival with subtotal resection
- Infants overall have a worse prognosis, possibly due to the limitations of therapy and/or the aggressiveness of the tumor.

ALERT
Even benign tumors may be life-threatening if their location precludes resection.

COMPLICATIONS
- Secondary to disease:
  - Increased intracranial pressure:
    ◦ Obstruction of CSF flow
    ◦ Requires immediate neurosurgical evaluation
- Secondary to radiotherapy:
  - Neurocognitive sequelae (age and dose related)
  - Endocrinopathy (growth hormone deficiency, hypothyroidism, gonadal dysfunction)
  - Risk of second malignancies (meningioma, glioma, sarcoma)
- Secondary to chemotherapy:
  - Risks associated with bone marrow suppression (infection, bleeding, anemia)
  - Hearing loss
  - Risk of secondary leukemia

ADDITIONAL READING

- Abdullah S, Qaddoumi I, Bouffet E. Advances in the management of pediatric central nervous system tumors. *Ann N Y Acad Sci.* 2008;1138:22–31.
- Blaney SM, Haas-Kogan D, Poussaint TY, et al. Gliomas, ependymomas, and other nonembryonal tumors. In: Pizzo PA, Poplack DG, eds. *Principles and Practice of Pediatric Oncology*, 6th ed. Philadelphia, PA: Lippincott Williams & Wilkins, 2011:717–824.
- Central Brain Tumor Registry of the United States. CBTRUS 2007–2008 Primary brain tumors in the United States statistical report, 2000–2004 (years of data collected). Available at: http://www.cbtrus.org [Accessed November 2008].
- Packer RJ. Brain tumors in children. *Arch Neurol.* 1999;56:421–425.
- Phillips PC, Grotzer MA. Brain tumors in children. In: Asbury AK, McKhann GM, McDonald WI, et al., eds. *Diseases of the nervous system: Clinical neuroscience and therapeutic principles*, 3rd ed. Cambridge, UK: Cambridge University Press, 2002:1448–1461.
- Sievert AJ, Fisher MJ. Pediatric low-grade gliomas. *J Child Neurol.* 2009;24(11):1397–1408.
- Valentino TL, Conway EE, Jr, Shiminski Maher T, et al. Pediatric brain tumors. *Pediatr Ann.* 1997;26: 579–587.

CODES

ICD9
- 191.9 Malignant neoplasm of brain, unspecified
- 225.9 Benign neoplasm of nervous system, part unspecified
- 239.6 Neoplasm of unspecified nature of brain

ICD10
- C71.9 Malignant neoplasm of brain, unspecified
- D33.9 Benign neoplasm of central nervous system, unspecified
- D43.9 Neoplasm of uncertain behavior of cnsl, unsp

FAQ

- Q: Are my other children at risk for getting a brain tumor?
- A: No (except in rare cases of certain familial syndromes).
- Q: Did something I do cause this?
- A: No. In addition, the claims made about high-power lines and cellular phones causing brain tumors or cancer are unproven.

BRANCHIAL CLEFT MALFORMATIONS

Anita Bhandari
Raezelle Zinman

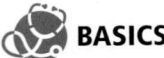 **BASICS**

DESCRIPTION
- The fetal branchial apparatus is a foregut derivative and develops in the 2nd fetal week.
- 5 paired pharyngeal arches are separated by 4 endodermal pouches internally and 4 ectodermal clefts externally.
- Overgrowth of the 2nd through 4th cleft creates the cervical sinus and occurs during weeks 4 and 5.
- Persistence of the cervical sinus produces a spectrum of cysts, sinus tracts, and fistulas.
- **Classification:**
  - 1st branchial cleft anomalies:
    - Site: anywhere from external auditory canal to angle of mandible, usually superior to or within parotid
    - Fistula tract: External auditory canal
  - 2nd branchial cleft anomalies
    - Site: Ventral to anterior border of sternocleidomastoid muscle, lateral to carotid sheath, and dorsal to submandibular gland
    - Fistula tract: Palatine tonsil
  - 3rd branchial cleft anomalies:
    - Site: Posterior triangle in middle to lower left side of the neck near level of upper thyroid lobe
    - Fistula: Upper lateral piriform sinus wall to lower lateral neck posterior to sternocleidomastoid muscle
  - 4th branchial cleft anomalies:
    - Site: Close association to thyroid gland associated with clinical thyroiditis if cyst infected
    - Fistula: Apex of piriform sinus to base of neck anterior to sternocleidomastoid muscle

EPIDEMIOLOGY
- Overwhelming majority of cysts in newborns and infants are developmental, whereas in children and adults they are inflammatory or neoplastic.
- Midline malformations are most often thyroglossal duct cysts or dermoids.
- Cysts occurring in the laterocervical region are usually branchial cleft malformations, the most common of these are derivatives of the 2nd cleft, followed by those of the 1st cleft, of the 4th pouch and thymic cysts.
- 3rd and 4th branchial cleft anomalies are rare, with most presenting as sinus tracts rather than cysts.
- Suspect congenital anomaly in the clinical setting of recurrent infection.

RISK FACTORS
Genetics
Familial history of branchial defects occasionally noted

 DIAGNOSIS

HISTORY
- Present since birth
- Recurrent neck infections
- Intermittent discharge from neck
- Fever
- Tenderness

PHYSICAL EXAM
- Mass usually mobile
- Usually a single lesion
- Nonpulsatile
- Lesion usually nontender (unless actively infected)
- Assess for sites of drainage:
  - At the anterior or posterior border of the sternocleidomastoid muscle
  - In the posterior pharynx at the tonsillar fossa or piriform sinus

DIAGNOSTIC TESTS & INTERPRETATION
Lab
- CBC with differential: Increased WBC with left shift seen with infection
- Tuberculin test to rule out tuberculosis
- Microbiology: oral cavity flora in neck abscess suspicious for branchial pouch anomaly

Imaging
- Chest radiography to assess for hilar adenopathy, suggesting a systemic process (such as tuberculosis or malignancy)
- Lateral neck radiography to assess for airway compromise (not usually seen)
- Ultrasound to help differentiate solid masses from cystic masses
- Fistulogram to inject contrast into the fistula to delineate its course
- CT scan of neck for superior spatial delineation and definition of anatomic compartment of the lesion
- MRI for more detailed soft tissue characterization and recognition of solid components within cystic masses

DIFFERENTIAL DIAGNOSIS
- Congenital:
  - Anterior triangle of neck:
    - Thymic cyst
  - Midline and anterior triangle of neck:
    - Ranula
    - Laryngocele
    - Sialocele
    - Thyroglossal cyst
  - Dermoid/teratomatous cyst:
    - Bronchogenic cyst
  - Posterior triangle of neck:
    - Lymphangioma
    - Hemangioma

- Inflammatory:
  – Adenitis
  – Granulomatous disease (sarcoidosis, tuberculosis)
  – Lymphoepithelial cysts (HIV)
  – Otorrhea
  – Parotiditis
  – Retropharyngeal abscess
  – Thyroiditis
- Tumors:
  – Lymphoma
  – Rhabdomyosarcoma
  – Cystic schwannoma (anterior triangle of neck)
  – Pilomatrixoma

TREATMENT

MEDICATION (DRUGS)
Antibiotics are indicated if the lesion is infected.

SURGERY/OTHER PROCEDURES
- Excision of the entire lesion is the standard approach.
- Novel endoscopic and marsupialization approaches have recently been reported.
- Surgery should be delayed if infection present.

ONGOING CARE

FOLLOW-UP RECOMMENDATIONS
- Postoperative follow-up as outpatient for wound inspection
- Observation for recurrence or reinfection

ALERT
- Lesion may recur if not completely excised.
- High incidence of reinfection if not properly treated.

PROGNOSIS
If lesion completely excised: Excellent. Many patients require multiple procedures.

COMPLICATIONS
- Cysts, sinus tracts, and fistulaes can become recurrently infected (especially with abscess formation).
- Surgery is more difficult if there have been previous infections or previous surgery.
- Damage to facial, hypoglossal, and glossopharyngeal nerves or carotid artery can occur during surgical repair.
- Recurrence of the lesion seen if not fully removed.
- Thyroiditis
- Parotiditis (more common in first branchial arch malformation)

ADDITIONAL READING

- Acierno SP, Waldhausen JH. Congenital cervical cysts, sinuses and fistulae. *Otolaryngol Clin North Am*. 2007;40:161–176.
- Graham A. Development of the pharyngeal arches. *Am J Med Genet*. 2003;119A:251–256.
- Mandell DL. Head and neck anomalies related to the branchial apparatus. *Otolaryngol Clin North Am*. 2000;33:1309.
- Nicoucar K, Giger R, Jaecklin T, et al. Management of congenital third branchial arch anomalies: A systematic review. *Otolarngolo Head Neck Surg*. 2010;142:21–28.
- Nicoucar K, Giger R, Jaecklin T, et al. Management of congenital fourth branchial arch anomalies: A review and analysis of published cases. *J Pediatr Surg*. 2009;44:1432–1439.
- Nicollas R, Guelfucci B, Roman S, et al. Congenital cysts and fistulas of the neck. *Int J Pediatr Otorhinolaryngol*. 2000;55:117–124.
- Prabhu V, Ingrams D. First branchial arch fistula: Diagnostic dilemma and improvised surgical management. *Am J Otolaryngol*. 2010 Oct 28. (Epub)

 CODES

ICD9
744.41 Branchial cleft sinus or fistula

ICD10
- Q18.0 Sinus, fistula and cyst of branchial cleft
- Q18.2 Other branchial cleft malformations

FAQ

- Q: Can the cyst, fistula, or sinus recur?
- A: Only a 3% recurrence rate is seen if the lesion is completely excised. A higher rate of recurrence is seen in cases of incomplete excision or with previous surgeries.
- Q: Should the lesion be removed as soon as it is discovered?
- A: The lesion should not be removed if there is an active infection present; treat the infection first and then schedule elective surgery.

BREAST ABSCESS
Charles A. Pohl

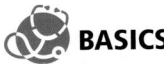 **BASICS**

DESCRIPTION
- Breast abscess: Infection of the breast bud or tissue associated with localized pus and inflammation
- Mastitis: Infection of the breast tissue observed primarily during lactation

EPIDEMIOLOGY
Incidence
5–11% of women with breastfeeding mastitis develop a breast abscess.

Prevalence
- Affects primarily infants (peak age 1–6 weeks) and adolescents
- Bilateral abscesses, seen among neonates, are rare.
- Male-to-female ratio is 1:2 in neonates.

RISK FACTORS
- In lactating teens, primiparity
- Gestational age >40 weeks
- Mastitis

GENERAL PREVENTION
- Avoid breast manipulation (including piercing).
- In lactating teens, establish good breastfeeding techniques.
- Recognize and treat mastitis early.

PATHOPHYSIOLOGY
- Newborns:
  - Trauma, breast hypertrophy from maternal estrogen, or compromised host defenses enable spread of bacteria that are often colonized in the nasopharynx and umbilicus.
  - The bacteria and/or its toxin, in turn, cause(s) subcutaneous destruction and loculated pus formation.
- Adolescents/adults: Trauma (e.g., sexual manipulation, nipple rings, tight-fitting bras, incorrect latching during breastfeeding), contiguous spread of a local infection (e.g., mastitis, acne), or underlying structural abnormalities (e.g., mammary duct ectasia, epidermal cysts) cause breast tissue edema and destruction by bacteria and/or its toxin.
- When mastitis is associated with breastfeeding, the inflammation inhibits milk release. The stasis of milk, in turn, may allow for bacterial proliferation.

ETIOLOGY
- Newborn infection: *Staphylococcus aureus* (most common), group A or B streptococcus, and Gram-negative enteric bacteria, including *Escherichia coli*, *Pseudomonas aeruginosa*, *Proteus mirabilis*, salmonella species
- Adolescent/adult infection: *S. aureus* (most common) with up to 19% being methicillin-resistant; *E. coli*, *P. aeruginosa*, *Mycobacterium tuberculosis*, *Neisseria gonorrhoeae*, and *Treponema pallidum* are infrequent pathogens.

DIAGNOSIS

HISTORY
- Ask about history of breast trauma or manipulation, concomitant illness or infections, and patient's immunologic status.
- Constitutional symptoms including irritability and lethargy usually are absent unless the infection involves deeper tissue or the bloodstream (1/3 of cases).
- Low-grade fever
- Salmonella infections generally present with GI symptoms.

PHYSICAL EXAM
- Firm, tender breast mass with overlying erythema and warmth. Fluctuant mass may be present.
- Regional adenopathy
- Purulent nipple discharge (rare)
- Necrotizing fasciitis is distinguished from breast abscess by pain out of proportion to the cutaneous signs, crepitus, or presence of straw-colored bullae.

DIAGNOSTIC TESTS & INTERPRETATION
Lab
- Gram stain and culture of nipple discharge, needle aspirate, and/or surgical incision and drainage help(s) guide therapeutic decisions if a fluctuant mass or discharge is present.
- Blood culture:
  - Useful in neonates
  - Consider full sepsis work-up if patient is febrile and toxic-appearing.
- CBC: Leukocytosis (>15,000 cells/mm³) is present in 1/2–2/3 of patients.
- Surveillance cultures of nasopharynx and umbilicus should be considered in neonates to rule out colonization with *S. aureus*.

Imaging
Ultrasound may be useful if fluctuant mass is suspected or if poor response to antimicrobial therapy.

Diagnostic Procedures/Other
If fluctuant, needle biopsy may be diagnostic and therapeutic.

DIFFERENTIAL DIAGNOSIS
- Physiologic conditions:
  - Breast engorgement (usually bilateral; absence of fever and erythema)
  - Mastodynia (painful breast engorgement; associated with ovulatory cycles; cyclic pattern)
- Infectious: Cellulitis including mastitis (absence of a loculated breast mass)
- Tumors (rare):
  - Fibroadenomas
  - Rhabdomyosarcoma
  - Non-Hodgkin lymphoma
  - Fibrocystic disease
  - Intraductal papilloma
  - Cystosarcoma phyllodes
  - Hemangioma
- Trauma:
  - Contusion (firm, tender, poorly defined mass)
  - Hematoma (sharply defined mass with ecchymosis)
  - Fat necrosis (firm, nontender, circumscribed, mobile mass)
- Miscellaneous: Mondor disease (thrombophlebitis of the subcutaneous veins in the breast)
  - Typically seen in adults
  - Presents with tenderness and pain
  - Associated with trauma
  - Spontaneously resolves
- Vascular malformation

ALERT
- Neonatal infections require prompt recognition, intervention, and identification of other involved sites to avoid widespread infection and poor outcome.
- Unrecognized fluctuant mass and its subsequent drainage will delay therapeutic response.
- Incidence of community-acquired methicillin-resistant *Staphylococcus aureus* (CA-MRSA) is increasing in many regions of the country.

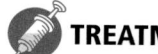 **TREATMENT**

MEDICATION (DRUGS)
- Neonatal infection:
  - Parenteral β-lactamase-resistant antistaphylococcal antibiotics (e.g., Nafcillin 100 mg/kg/24 h) or ceftriaxone 50–75 mg/kg/24 h)
  - Aminoglycosides (e.g., gentamicin 2.5 mg/kg/dose q8–12h) should be included if the infant appears ill or if the Gram stain reveals Gram-negative bacilli.
  - Consider vancomycin (40 mg/kg/24 h) if MRSA suspected in neonate over 1 month of age.
- Adolescent infection:
  - Parenteral antistaphylococcal antibiotics (e.g., nafcillin 50–100 mg/kg/24 h; maximum 12 g/24 h)
  - Consider amoxicillin–clavulanic acid (45 mg/kg/24 h) or clindamycin (450–1,800 mg/24 h orally with max dose 1.8 g/24 h; 1,200–1,800 mg/24 h parenterally with max dose 4.8 g/24 h) in patients with penicillin allergies and those who are well appearing and without systemic symptoms.
  - Consider adding aminoglycosides in situations as described above.
- Duration:
  - Usually for 10–14 days
  - Length of parenteral treatment is based on isolate and the clinical response. Oral agents may be used after a few days if a good clinical response occurs.

ADDITIONAL TREATMENT
General Measures
- Warm compresses
- Nonsteroidal anti-inflammatory agents (NSAIDs) help control the inflammation and pain in older children.
- Continuation of breastmilk expression helps prevent engorgement and further milk stasis.

ISSUES FOR REFERRAL
Consider referral to an infectious disease specialist if recurrent.

SURGERY/OTHER PROCEDURES
- Incision and drainage if a fluctuant mass is present
- Surgical exploration is necessary if necrotizing fasciitis is suspected.

IN-PATIENT CONSIDERATIONS
Admission Criteria
- Ill appearance
- Neonates
- Inability to tolerate oral medications
- Concern for medication nonadherence

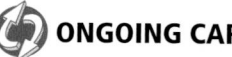 **ONGOING CARE**

FOLLOW-UP RECOMMENDATIONS
Clinical improvement should be evident after 48 hours of parenteral antibiotics.

ALERT
Signs to watch for:
- A poor or delayed clinical response to antibiotic therapy suggests a resistant organism, an unusual pathogen, or a different diagnosis.
- An evolving fluctuant mass warrants surgical intervention.
- Reaccumulation of fluctuant mass
- Toxic appearance, prolonged fever, purulent discharge, or progressive erythema postoperatively
- Crepitus associated with excessive pain and/or straw-colored bullae suggests necrotizing fasciitis.

PATIENT EDUCATION
- Continue breastfeeding.
- Establish good breastfeeding techniques.

PROGNOSIS
- Most children recover without any sequelae.
- Neonates are more likely to have bilateral abscesses (<5% cases).
- Neonates have higher morbidity and complications.

COMPLICATIONS
- Cellulitis (most common; 5–10%)
- Abscess rupture with disseminated infection (e.g., bacteremia, pneumonia)
- Septicemia
- Toxin syndromes (e.g., toxic shock syndrome)
- Necrotizing fasciitis
- Scar formation from mammary gland destruction (associated with a reduced breast size after puberty)

ADDITIONAL READING

- Barbosa-Cesnik C, Schwartz K, Foxman B. Lactation mastitis. *JAMA*. 2003;289:1609–1612.
- Fortunov RM, Hulten KG, Hammerman WA, et al. Community-acquired Staphylococcus aureus infections in term and near-term previously healthy neonates. *Pediatr*. 2006;1188:874–881.
- Michie C, Lockie F, Lynn W. The challenge of mastitis. *Arch Dis Child*. 2003;88:818–821.
- Moazzez A, Kelso RL, Towfigh S, et al. Breast abscess bacteriologic features in the era of community-acquired methicillin-resistant Staphylococcus aureus epidemics. *Arch Surg*. 2007;142(9):881–884.
- Strickler T, Navratil F, Foster I, et al. Nonpuerperal mastitis in adolescents. *J Ped*. 2006;148:278–281.
- Stricker T, Navratil F, Sennhauser FH. Mastitis in early infancy. *Acta Paediatr*. 2005;94(2):166–169.

 CODES

ICD9
- 611.0 Inflammatory disease of breast
- 675.11 Abscess of breast associated with childbirth, delivered, with or without mention of antepartum condition
- 675.12 Abscess of breast associated with childbirth, delivered, with mention of postpartum complication

ICD10
- N61 Inflammatory disorders of breast
- O91.119 Abscess of breast associated with pregnancy, unsp trimester
- O91.12 Abscess of breast associated with the puerperium

FAQ
- Q: How can you differentiate a breast abscess from mastitis?
- A: Although both illnesses involve signs of inflammation (i.e., warmth, erythema, swelling, tenderness), a breast abscess is distinguished from mastitis in that the former presents as a firm, well-defined mass (with or without fluctuant material).
- Q: Should a mother discontinue breastfeeding if she has a breast abscess?
- A: To avoid milk stasis, breastfeeding should be continued unless impeded by a surgical incision site or the overall clinical condition of the mother.
- Q: What is the role of homeopathic remedies (e.g., belladonna, Phytolacca) in the treatment of mastitis and breast abscess?
- A: Currently, there is insufficient scientific evidence to support their routine use.
- Q: Are anaerobic organisms common pathogens for breast abscesses?
- A: No. Although anaerobic pathogens are isolated in up to 40% of infections, their role is controversial, and therapy directed at them is unnecessary.

BREASTFEEDING

Amy E. Renwick

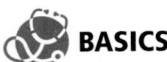 **BASICS**

DESCRIPTION
Breast milk is recognized by the American Academy of Pediatrics (AAP), the World Health Organization (WHO), and many other groups as the optimal nutrition for human infants.

- Physiology:
  - Milk secretion becomes possible near the middle of pregnancy. After delivery, production increases, starting with colostrum. Transitional milk "comes in" with a rapid increase in volume within ~2–5 days of delivery.
  - Prolactin produced in response to nipple stimulation (i.e., suckling, pumping, etc.) causes the continuous secretion of milk into the lumen of breast alveoli.
  - The volume of milk produced appears to be a function of frequency of removal rather than serum levels of prolactin. Inhibitory factors in the milk provide negative feedback to decrease milk production when the breast is not drained. Mechanical pressure from engorgement may also decrease production.
  - Oxytocin released from the posterior pituitary gland causes ejection of milk into the ducts and sinuses of the breast (let-down), making the milk available for removal.
  - Let-down can be triggered by physical stimulation of the breast or by mental stimulation such as hearing a baby's cry or looking at a picture of an infant.
- Composition:
  - Largely independent of maternal diet, with the exception of fatty acids and water-soluble vitamins.
  - Colostrum is particularly high in proteins, including secretory immunoglobulin A.
  - Hindmilk, expressed as the breast is nearing emptying, has a significantly higher fat content than foremilk from the beginning of the feeding.
- Benefits of breastfeeding:
  - For child:
    ○ Decreases risk of postneonatal death; reduces incidence and severity of gastroenteritis, respiratory infections, acute otitis media, bacterial meningitis, obesity, sudden infant death syndrome (SIDS), asthma, leukemia and UTIs
    ○ May decrease risk of high cholesterol, diabetes, hypertension, lymphoma, and celiac disease
  - For mother: Decreases risk of ovarian and breast cancer, hastens return to prepregnancy weight, decreases postpartum bleeding
  - For family: Cost savings over buying formula, fewer workdays lost to care for ill child, assists with optimal child spacing (via lactational amenorrhea)
  - For society: Improved public health, lower health expenditures, decreased environmental impact

EPIDEMIOLOGY
Prevalence
- 75% of infants in the US begin breastfeeding (according to Centers for Disease Control and Prevention [CDC] data from 2007)
- At 3 months, 33% breastfeed exclusively
- At 6 months, 43% breastfeed, 13% exclusively
- Only 22% of infants breastfed at 12 months of age
- Racial disparities in breastfeeding exist, with lower rates of initiation found among blacks when compared with whites.

RISK FACTORS
- Contraindications to breastfeeding:
  - Infant with classic galactosemia
  - Maternal conditions:
    ○ HIV (in developed countries)
    ○ Illicit drug use
    ○ Active, untreated tuberculosis
    ○ Herpes simplex virus lesions on breast (may use other breast if unaffected)
    ○ HTLV-I or -II positive
    ○ Exposure to radioactive material, while there is radioactivity in the milk
    ○ Use of some medications, such as cytotoxic drugs
- Maternal risk factors for not initiating or not continuing breastfeeding:
  - Not planning to breastfeed prior to delivery
  - Young age (<25 years)
  - Low education (less than high school education)
  - Being single
  - Cigarette smoking
  - Participation in WIC (Special Supplemental Nutrition Program for Women, Infants and Children)
- Infant conditions that may interfere with breastfeeding:
  - Prematurity
  - Low birth weight
  - Hyperbilirubinemia, if infant is treated with phototherapy, or if mother is asked to stop breastfeeding by health care professional
  - Hypotonia
  - Cleft lip or palate
  - Ankyloglossia (tongue-tie)
- Maternal conditions that may interfere with breastfeeding:
  - History of breast surgery
  - Abnormal breast shape
  - Inverted nipples
  - Use of medications that inhibit lactation (e.g., antihistamines, oral contraceptives)
  - Severe or chronic illness
- Common reasons cited for breastfeeding cessation:

  - Inadequate milk production, or infant not seeming satisfied with breast milk
  - Infant having difficulty feeding
  - Sore nipples
  - Returning to work or school

 DIAGNOSIS

HISTORY
- Maternal breastfeeding experience with previous children?
- Frequency and duration of feedings:
  - Should feed at least 8–12 times a day in the 1st weeks of life, with no more than 4 hours between feedings
  - Time needed to empty the breast varies from ~5–20 minutes.
- Signs that infant is satisfied afterward: Is the infant calm, not rooting or sucking, sleepy?
- Does mother feel sensation of let-down (by ~2 weeks postpartum)?
- Do breasts feel full prior to a feeding, and less full afterward?
- Any sustained pain during feeding? Initial discomfort should resolve within about a minute. Continued pain may indicate an improper latch, injured nipple, candidal infection of the nipple, or mastitis.
- Number of wet diapers and bowel movements each day? By 3–5 days, infants should have 3–5 wet diapers and bowel movements each day. By 5–7 days, expect about 6 wet diapers and 3–6 bowel movements. It is important to note that this stooling pattern may change for breastfed babies, who may only stool once every 4–5 days by ~4 weeks of life.
- Family support? Support from partners, other family members, and friends may increase the likelihood of breastfeeding success.

PHYSICAL EXAM
- Direct observation of a feeding:
  - Is mother alert to infant's cues? Alertness, restlessness, rooting, lip smacking, and sucking are early signs of hunger; crying is a late sign.
  - Are mother and infant positioned comfortably? Mother should not have to bend down. Infant should be well supported, with head, shoulders, and hips aligned.
  - For an effective latch, lips should be everted and mouth wide open, with lips approaching a 180° angle. As much as possible of the areola, especially the lower portion, should be in the infant's mouth.
  - Signs of a good suck and milk transfer include deep, rhythmic movement of the jaw; frequent sounds of swallowing; and milk visible in the infant's mouth.
- Weight:
  - Newborns should lose no more than 7–10% of their birth weight in the few days following delivery, and should return to birth weight within 2 weeks.
  - Expect initial weight gain of ~20–30 g/d in the 1st 2 months of life.
  - Be aware that standard CDC growth charts are not based predominantly on breastfed infants, who may weigh less than formula-fed infants from 3–12 months of age. The CDC and the AAP now recommend using WHO growth charts rather than the CDC growth charts for all children 0–2 years.

- Oropharynx, for thrush or anatomic abnormalities
- Jaundice
- Hydration status
- Mother's nipples:
  – Inversion
  – Cracking or bleeding may result from improper latch, removal of infant from nipple without breaking suction, or prolonged exposure to moisture.
  – Erythema: Seen with candidal infection; often accompanied by a burning sensation

DIAGNOSTIC TESTS & INTERPRETATION
Lab
- Bilirubin level, if clinically indicated
- Sodium level in infant, if there is concern for dehydration
- Sodium level in breast milk, if infant is hypernatremic

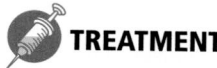 TREATMENT

MEDICATION (DRUGS)
- Vitamin D, 400 IU/d, beginning as early as the 1st few days of life and by 2 months. Continue even if supplementing with formula, unless getting at least 1 L of formula daily. May be given in the form of a daily multi- or tri-vitamin, or as vitamin D drops.
- Fluoride, beginning at 6 months, when indicated.
- Iron, 1 mg/kg/d, from age 4 months until taking iron-rich complementary foods, has been recommended for term infants who are exclusively or primarily breastfed; 2 mg/kg/day starting by age 1 month is recommended for preterm infants.
- Thrush or candidal infection of the nipples requires simultaneous treatment of both mother and infant with a topical antifungal agent, such as Lotrimin cream in the mother and oral nystatin solution in the baby, in addition to washing of any objects that have contact with the infant's mouth.

ADDITIONAL TREATMENT
General Measures
- Cracked nipples may be treated by applying breast milk and allowing nipples to air dry, or by applying purified lanolin. Nipples should be kept dry. If the infant must be removed from the breast while sucking, the mother should slide a clean finger into the mouth to break the suction 1st.
- Engorgement can be relieved by frequent feeding or pumping, or by the application of cool compresses. If engorgement causes difficulty with latching, some milk can be pumped or expressed manually prior to putting the child to the breast.
- Clogged milk ducts may be addressed with warm compresses, frequent emptying of the breast, massaging the area, and varying feeding positions.
- Pumping or breast shells may help with inverted nipples.

COMPLEMENTARY & ALTERNATIVE THERAPIES
- Herbs traditionally used to try to increase milk supply (galactagogues) include:
  – Fenugreek (*Trigonella foenum-graecum*): Usually taken as tea or capsules. May be effective (limited evidence); thought to be safe. Maternal side effects may include asthma symptoms, diarrhea, allergic reaction, decreased blood sugar, and maple syrup odor.
  – Milk thistle (*Silybum marianum*): Usually taken as a tea. Not studied
  – Goat's rue (*Galega officinalis*): Usually taken as a tea. Not studied

 ONGOING CARE

FOLLOW-UP RECOMMENDATIONS
Patient Monitoring
- 2–3 days after newborn hospitalization: Weight check, physical exam, and observation of feeding
- At age 2–3 weeks: Weight check and breastfeeding support

DIET
- For the infant:
  – No food or fluid other than breast milk is needed for the 1st 6 months of life.
  – After 6 months, iron-rich foods should be part of the diet, and other complementary foods may be introduced.
- For the mother:
  – ~500 kcal/d are used for breastfeeding.
  – Women should avoid breastfeeding for at least 2 hours after alcohol consumption; the level in milk correlates with the level in blood. Ethanol also inhibits let-down.
  – If infant has G6PD deficiency, mother should avoid fava beans and certain medications.

COMPLICATIONS
- Infant:
  – Hyperbilirubinemia
  – Dehydration
  – Hypernatremia
  – Failure to thrive
- Mother:
  – Engorgement
  – Clogged milk duct
  – Mastitis
  – Candidal nipple infection
  – Cracked nipples

ADDITIONAL READING
- The Academy of Breastfeeding Medicine. Available at: http://www.bfmed.org. Accessed March 20, 2011.
- Hale T. *Medications and mothers' milk*, 14th ed. Amarillo, TX: Hale Publishing; 2010.
- Kleinman RE. *Pediatric nutrition handbook*, 6th ed. Elk Grove Village, IL: American Academy of Pediatrics; 2009.
- Kramer MS, Kakuma R. Optimal duration of exclusive breastfeeding. *Cochrane Database Syst Rev.* 2009;(1).
- Lawrence RA, Lawrence RM. *Breastfeeding: A guide for the medical profession*, 7th ed. Philadelphia: Saunders; 2011.
- Meek JY, ed. *American Academy of Pediatrics new mother's guide to breastfeeding.* New York: Bantam Books; 2002.
- Neville MC. Anatomy and physiology of lactation. *Pediatr Clin North Am.* 2001;48:13–34.
- Resources for patients:
  – www.lalecheleague.org
  – www.womenshealth.gov/breastfeeding

FAQ
- Q: How do I know if my baby is getting enough milk?
- A: Look for signs of effective feeding as described above. Your baby should suck deeply and rhythmically during a feeding, seem satisfied after a feeding, make at least 6 wet diapers a day after the 1st week, and gain weight.
- Q: How can I increase my milk supply?
- A: Increase the frequency of feeding or pumping. Offer the 2nd breast after your baby finishes with the 1st. Alternate the side that is offered 1st. Pump after nursing sessions. If pumping often, use a hospital-grade double pump. Get plenty of sleep and fluids, and try to reduce stress.
- Q: How long can expressed breast milk be stored safely?
- A: At room temperature (up to 77°F) for 3–8 hours. In a refrigerator, for 3–8 days. In a freezer, for 6–12 months. Thawed breast milk should be refrigerated and used within 24 hours of thawing.
- Q: How long should breastfeeding be continued?
- A: The AAP recommends breastfeeding at least until 12 months of age, and as long afterward as is mutually desired. The WHO recommends breastfeeding for at least 2 years. Exclusive breastfeeding is nutritionally adequate for the 1st 6 months.
- Q: Can adoptive mothers breastfeed?
- A: Induced lactation is possible. Lactation experts should be consulted.

BREASTFEEDING JAUNDICE AND BREAST MILK JAUNDICE

John I. Takayama

 BASICS

DESCRIPTION
Early-onset breastfeeding jaundice (BFJ) and late-onset breast milk jaundice (BMJ) are the 2 major overlapping causes of jaundice in otherwise healthy breastfed infants:

- BFJ: Associated with inadequate breastfeeding; exaggerated early onset (3–5 days), unconjugated hyperbilirubinemia (>12 mg/dL)
- BMJ: Associated with being fed breast milk; late onset (1–6 weeks), unconjugated hyperbilirubinemia (>10 mg/dL)

EPIDEMIOLOGY
Incidence
BMJ affects 10–30% of breastfed newborns during the 2nd to 6th weeks of life.

RISK FACTORS
For Jaundice
- Blood group incompatibility with positive direct antiglobulin test
- Other known hemolytic disease (e.g., glucose-6-phosphate dehydrogenase [G6PD] deficiency)
- Gestational age
- Previous sibling received phototherapy
- Exclusive breastfeeding
- Race (e.g., East Asian)

Genetics
- BFJ: Subsequent siblings of infants with jaundice are more likely to develop jaundice.
- BMJ: Mutations in the bilirubin uridine diphosphate-glucuronosyltransferase gene (UGT1A1) have been identified in a Japanese population and were felt to be associated with BMJ.

PATHOPHYSIOLOGY
- Bilirubin is a breakdown product of hemoglobin and other heme-containing proteins. In newborns, shorter lifespan of a larger number of erythrocytes, immaturity of the bilirubin uptake and conjugation system in the liver, and increased enterohepatic circulation (initiated by a more rapid hydrolysis of conjugated bilirubin to the unconjugated form) contribute to hyperbilirubinemia and jaundice.
- BFJ: Inadequate intake of milk and calories with or without relative dehydration, leading to increased intestinal bilirubin absorption and enterohepatic circulation
- BMJ: Several hypotheses proposed, but remain unproven. Factors found in the milk of some mothers of infants with BMJ include:
  - Pregnanediol isomer: Steroid metabolite of progesterone, competitive inhibitor of hepatic glucuronyl transferase
  - Increased concentrations of nonesterified (free) fatty acids that inhibit hepatic glucuronyl transferase
  - Factors that increase enterohepatic circulation of bilirubin (e.g., β-glucuronidase)
- Defects in bilirubin UGT1A1 may be associated with BMJ.

ETIOLOGY
BFJ is likely to be the predominant cause of early-onset jaundice; however, it is often difficult to distinguish from jaundice related to other causes because of considerable overlap.

 DIAGNOSIS

HISTORY
Ask the following questions:
- How is the infant feeding?
  - Infrequent and difficult breastfeeding are predictors of BFJ.
  - Many BFJ infants have increased enterohepatic circulation and dehydration, reflected by delayed passage of meconium and significant weight loss.
  - Poor intake also delays stooling, which contributes to increased enterohepatic circulation of bilirubin.
- Is there a family history of jaundice in a sibling?
  - Prior history may indicate similar risk factors and genetic propensities for developing jaundice.
  - Severe neonatal jaundice suggests familial or inherited hemolytic disease.
- Are there relatives with a history of anemia, gallbladder disease, or splenectomy? Hemolytic anemias constitute an inheritable cause of severe and prolonged jaundice.
- Are there maternal risk factors?
  - Maternal illness (e.g., diabetes) and medication use (e.g., oxytocin) are associated with jaundice.
  - Infants born to mothers positive for group B streptococcus are at increased risk for neonatal sepsis.
  - Recent epidemiologic studies indicate a positive relationship between maternal age and hyperbilirubinemia.
- Are there birth-related risk factors?
  - Sepsis should be included in the differential diagnosis. Assess for presence of fever, prolonged rupture of amniotic membranes, or cloudy or malodorous amniotic fluid.
  - Traumatic delivery, including the use of instruments, such as forceps or vacuum, may result in jaundice because of associated bruising and cephalohematomas.
- When did jaundice become noticeable?
  - Jaundice before 24 hours of age suggests a hemolytic process or infection.
  - Early jaundice beyond 24 hours is associated with BFJ.
  - Prolonged jaundice beyond 1–2 weeks suggests BMJ.
- How is the infant doing? Infants with BMJ are in good health, vigorous, eating well, and gaining weight.

PHYSICAL EXAM
Jaundice generally progresses from the face to the lower extremities in proportion to rising serum bilirubin concentrations. Look for the following:
- Cephalohematoma, facial bruising: May contribute to hyperbilirubinemia
- Increased respirations, cyanosis, grunting, nasal flaring, intercostal retractions: May suggest infection

- Hepatosplenomegaly: Suggests infectious, metabolic, or severe hemolytic causes of hyperbilirubinemia
- Abdominal distention: Suggests intestinal obstruction
- Dry mucous membranes and skin tenting: Consistent with dehydration which may contribute to BFJ
- Well-appearing older infant who is gaining weight: Consistent with BMJ

DIAGNOSTIC TESTS & INTERPRETATION
Lab
Generally, minimal laboratory evaluation is necessary in a healthy breastfed infant with mild to moderate jaundice in the absence of risk factors for other causes of jaundice. However, BFJ and BMJ are diagnoses of exclusion. The following tests should be considered, depending on the clinical presentation:
- Total serum bilirubin (or transcutaneous bilirubin), with level interpreted by age:
  - May assist in diagnosis and choice of therapy
  - Must be measured in all infants with very early jaundice <24 hours of age
  - Recommended in all infants with persistent jaundice
- Conjugated or direct serum bilirubin: Elevated level (>1 mg/dL or 10% of total serum bilirubin) may indicate infection, biliary obstructive disease, cholestasis, metabolic disease, or severe hemolysis.
- Maternal blood type and Rh status in all cases; infant blood type, Coombs test, and/or Rh test on cord blood if indicated (mother's blood type is O and/or Rh is negative): Identifies risk for hemolytic anemia from blood type and/or Rh incompatibility, with considerations for treatment at lower levels of total serum bilirubin
- CBC and smear:
  - Abnormal hematocrit assists in diagnosis of polycythemia or anemia; the smear is helpful to look for signs of hemolysis.
  - Decreases in hematocrit over time may reflect ongoing hemorrhage or hemolysis.
  - Abnormal white cell count may indicate infection.
- G6PD quantitative test:
  - G6PD deficiency is common worldwide, and a rapid increase in bilirubin may occur later than in other types of hemolytic disease.
  - Risk of kernicterus seems to be higher in infants with G6PD deficiency, indicating consideration of treatment at lower levels of total serum bilirubin.

DIFFERENTIAL DIAGNOSIS
- Infection: Sepsis (jaundice is usually not the sole presenting sign)
- Hematologic:
  - ABO or Rh isoimmunization
  - Erythrocyte enzyme defects (e.g., G6PD deficiency)
  - Erythrocyte membrane defects (e.g., hereditary spherocytosis)
  - Polycythemia

- GI: Intestinal obstruction (e.g., meconium ileus, Hirschsprung disease, pyloric stenosis)
- Congenital: Transient familial neonatal hyperbilirubinemia
- Metabolic:
  – Hypothyroidism
  – Galactosemia
  – Gilbert syndrome
  – Crigler-Najjar syndrome
- Miscellaneous:
  – Dehydration
  – Cephalohematoma
  – Maternal oxytocin use

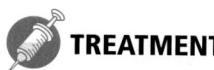 TREATMENT

ADDITIONAL TREATMENT
General Measures
- BFJ:
  – Increase frequency of breastfeeding to 10–12 times during the 1st 3 days of life.
  – Supplement with formula if significant feeding problems or poor milk production
  – Phototherapy if serum bilirubin levels exceed the American Academy of Pediatrics (AAP) recommended threshold levels for phototherapy for full-term healthy infants based on infant's age in hours, gestational age, and neurotoxicity risk factors (i.e., implement phototherapy for infants 25–48 hours old if total serum bilirubin $\geq$12–15 mg/dL; 49–72 hours old if bilirubin $\geq$15–18 mg/dL; >72 hours old if bilirubin $\geq$18–20 mg/dL)
  – Phototherapy may contribute to dehydration; therefore, it is essential to monitor hydration status.
  – Consider partial exchange blood transfusion for full-term healthy infants 25–48 hours old with total serum bilirubin >19–22 mg/dL and for infants $\geq$48 hours old with total serum bilirubin >22–25 mg/dL. Exchange transfusion should be considered in conjunction with phototherapy.
  – Home phototherapy poses less of an obstruction to effective breastfeeding than does hospitalization, and may be an option in certain circumstances (e.g., bilirubin levels close to the threshold for hospital phototherapy according to AAP practice guidelines).
- BMJ:
  – Continue observation.
  – Refrain from complete or partial interruption of nursing and the feeding of formula.
  – If bilirubin >20 mg/dL consider supplementation with formula or interruption of breastfeeding temporarily and substitute with formula and/or administration of phototherapy.
- Supportive therapy:
  – BFJ and BMJ: Monitor serum bilirubin levels closely.
  – BFJ: Lactation consultation
  – BMJ: Close observation
- BFJ and BMJ: Continue treatment until serum bilirubin levels are consistently within acceptable levels.

 ONGOING CARE

FOLLOW-UP RECOMMENDATIONS
- Pitfalls:
- Visual assessment of jaundice may be inaccurate.
- Thresholds for starting phototherapy are lower for infants with hemolytic diseases, including G6PD deficiency and Rh incompatibility, and for premature infants and infants who are ill because kernicterus occurs at lower levels of bilirubin than in newborns without these risk factors.
- Discharge follow-up at 72–120 hours of age, especially for breastfed infants, is important to identify significant hyperbilirubinemia, given decreasing duration of postpartum hospital stay.
- Follow-up assessment should include infant weight, oral intake, pattern of voiding and stooling, and jaundice.

Patient Monitoring
When to expect improvement:
- BFJ: If phototherapy is instituted, expect significant improvement in jaundice within 24 hours.
- BMJ: After temporary interruption of breastfeeding for 24–48 hours, though interruption of breastfeeding is rarely necessary

PROGNOSIS
- BFJ and BMJ: Generally excellent if hyperbilirubinemia is identified and treated appropriately; however, both evaluation and treatment may contribute to disruption of breastfeeding and increased parental anxiety, resulting in breastfeeding cessation.
- Bilirubin encephalopathy (kernicterus) is extremely rare if serum bilirubin $\leq$30 mg/dL in infants who are otherwise well.
- Increased risk for hyperbilirubinemia in subsequent siblings

COMPLICATIONS
- BFJ and BMJ: Kernicterus (bilirubin encephalopathy; extremely rare), characterized acutely by lethargy, hypotonia, opisthotonus, and seizures, and on a more chronic basis by hearing loss, upward gaze palsy, and cerebral palsy
- Cessation of breastfeeding
- Parental and health care provider anxiety

ADDITIONAL READING

- American Academy of Pediatrics Subcommittee on Hyperbilirubinemia. Management of hyperbilirubinemia in the newborn infant 35 or more weeks of gestation [see comment] [erratum, *Pediatrics*. 2004;114(4):1138]. *Pediatrics*. 2004;114:297–316.
- Gartner LM. Breastfeeding and jaundice. *J Perinatol*. 2001;21:S25–S29.
- Hannon PR, Willis SK, Scrimshaw SC. Persistence of maternal concerns surrounding neonatal jaundice. *Arch Pediatr Adolesc Med*. 2001;155:1357–1363.
- Maisels MJ, Bhutani VK, Bogen D, et al. Hyperbilirubinemia in the newborn infant > or = 35 weeks' gestation: An update with clarifications. *Pediatrics*. 2009;124(4):1193–1198.
- Newman TB, Liljestrand PJ, Escobar GJ. Hyperbilirubinemia benchmarking. *Pediatrics*. 2004;114:323.
- Ross G. Hyperbilirubinemia in the 2000s: What should we do next? *Am J Perinatol*. 2003;20:415–424.
- Watchko JF. Hyperbilirubinemia and bilirubin toxicity in the late preterm infant. *Clin Perinatol*. 2006;33:839–852.

 CODES

ICD9
774.39 Breast milk jaundice

ICD10
P59.3 Neonatal jaundice from breast milk inhibitor

FAQ

- Q: Will my baby have developmental or neurologic problems afterward?
- A: Not from jaundice, if hyperbilirubinemia is appropriately monitored and treated
- Q: Will exposure to sunlight decrease the level of jaundice?
- A: Yes; however, avoid prolonged exposure and direct sunlight to prevent sunburn. Periodic indirect sunlight (e.g., exposure in a warm sunlit room) is sufficient.
- Q: Should I stop breastfeeding?
- A: The frequency of breastfeeding should be increased and appropriate lactation consultation obtained for BFJ. Early, frequent breastfeeding may decrease the risk. For BMJ, temporary cessation of breastfeeding will lower the total serum bilirubin; however, this recommendation should only be considered along with supplementation with formula and phototherapy if total serum bilirubin is $\geq$20 mg/dL.

BREATH-HOLDING SPELLS

Neera Goyal
Paul S. Matz

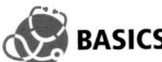 **BASICS**

DESCRIPTION
- Breath-holding spells (BHS) are benign, non-epileptic events in young children. May be associated with color change, loss of consciousness, and tonic and/or clonic movements.
- Can be frightening for parents and caregivers
- Classified into two main types: cyanotic and pallid.
  - Cyanotic BHS: Involuntary and reflexive expiratory apnea resulting in cerebral anoxia.
  - Pallid BHS: Vagal-mediated bradycardia or asystole resulting in cerebral anoxia (breath holding only a minor component).
- True epileptic events, called anoxic-epileptic seizures, may be triggered by either type.

GENERAL PREVENTION
- Toddlers may learn that intense crying can lead to a cyanotic BHS, followed by secondary gain of an action or object. Caregivers should minimize giving in to what the child wants so as not to reinforce the BHS.
- Main injury risk associated with BHS is head trauma. Children should be lowered to the floor and away from sharp or hard surfaces.

EPIDEMIOLOGY
- 50–60% of children with BHS have the cyanotic type; 20–30% have the pallid type; and 20% are mixed or unclassifiable
- Occur primarily between ages 1 and 5 years and resolve by school age. Rare before 6 months of age.
- Boys and girls affected equally, although boys may peak earlier (13–18 months) than girls (19–24 months).
- Most children with BHS have multiple episodes per week. Frequency of spells may range from multiple episodes daily to once yearly.

Incidence
BHS are relatively common among young children, with an estimated prevalence of 5%.

RISK FACTORS
Genetics
- There is a familial tendency for BHS.
- Approximately one third of children have a family member with a history of BHS in childhood.
- Within families, multiple children may have different types of BHS.
- Some data indicate autosomal dominant inheritance with reduced penetrance; however, no gene has been identified.

ETIOLOGY
- Cyanotic:
  - Usually triggered by violent crying
  - Breath holding is reflexive and occurs on expiration.
  - Trigger leads to hypocapnic cerebral ischemia and reflexive Valsalva, causing increased intrathoracic pressure, expiratory apnea, and hypoxemia.
- Pallid:
  - The trigger is usually a sudden, unexpected stimulus, frequently a mild head injury.
  - Excessive vagal response, resulting in severe bradycardia or asystole and cerebral anoxia.
- Anoxic–epileptic seizures:
  - Occasionally both types may lead to anoxic-epileptic seizures with/without status epilepticus
  - In contrast to idiopathic epilepsy, these occur secondary to cerebral anoxia.

COMMONLY ASSOCIATED CONDITIONS
- Iron deficiency anemia has been associated with BHS. However, the precise mechanism for this association is unclear.
- Sleep-disordered breathing may have an association with cyanotic BHS.

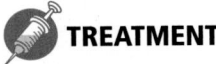 **DIAGNOSIS**

SIGNS AND SYMPTOMS
HISTORY
- Clinical history is the key to diagnosis and will distinguish BHS from epileptic seizures:
  - BHS are provoked by a situation or event.
  - BHS seizures are brief and recovery is rapid.
  - Changes in skin color and loss of consciousness occur before seizure activity
- Cyanotic type:
  - Intense crying followed by forced expiration and apnea.
  - Rapid onset of cyanosis followed by loss of consciousness, generalized clonic jerks, opisthotonus, and/or bradycardia.
- Pallid type:
  - Triggered by a startle or minor trauma
  - Crying is not prominent, but pallor is common.
  - Followed by loss of consciousness, loss of muscle tone, and a fall to the ground.
  - Bradycardia with periods of asystole longer than 2 seconds may be observed.
- A family history of sudden death should prompt further cardiac investigation.

PHYSICAL EXAM
Physical examination, including neurologic and cardiovascular exam, should be normal.

DIAGNOSTIC TESTS & INTERPRETATION
Lab
- Evaluation for iron deficiency anemia, including CBC, MCV, and TIBC may be helpful.
- Low serum ferritin may be an early indicator of iron deficiency.
- No other laboratory studies, including serum electrolytes, are routinely indicated.

Imaging
- Neuroimaging is not routinely indicated.

Diagnostic Procedures/Other
- 12-lead ECG to evaluate for long QT syndrome and other abnormalities should be strongly considered, particularly for pallid BHS.
- EEG should be considered for children with prolonged loss of consciousness, suspected epileptic activity, or significant post-ictal symptoms
- If EEG is requested, ocular compression with ECG may provide additional useful information in confirming the diagnosis of BHS.

DIFFERENTIAL DIAGNOSIS
- Behavioral:
  - Voluntary breath holding (characterized by prolonged inspiratory phase)
  - Psychogenic seizures
- Neurologic:
  - Epilepsy
- Cardiac:
  - Long QT syndrome
  - Wolff–Parkinson–White syndrome
  - Complete heart block
  - Supraventricular tachycardia
  - Hypertrophic cardiomyopathy
  - Vasovagal syncope

TREATMENT

INITIAL STABILIZATION
- Children should be lowered to the floor and away from sharp or hard surfaces.
- Airway clearance and cardiopulmonary resuscitation may be necessary for prolonged events.
- Most events are self-limited.

MEDICATION (DRUGS)
First Line
- Iron therapy may be beneficial, particularly for those with concomitant iron deficiency anemia
  - Ferrous sulfate, 5–6 mg/kg/day. Recommended course of treatment is ~8 weeks.

Second Line
- Anticholinergic therapy has been used for severe, frequent pallid BHS to reduce vagal activity:
  - Oral atropine sulfate or atropine methonitrate
  - Transdermal scopolamine patches
- Piracetam, a derivative of the inhibitory neurotransmitter GABA, has been demonstrated to be effective in preventing BHS. The mechanism of action for this drug remains unclear.
- Antiepileptic medication may be used to prevent anoxic-epileptic seizures associated with BHS.

SURGERY/OTHER PROCEDURES
In rare cases of severe BHS with significant bradycardia or asystole, pacemaker implantation may successfully prevent recurrent events. However, the vast majority of patients can be managed without surgery.

ISSUES FOR REFERRAL
- Protracted seizure activity or significant post-ictal symptoms may require further neurologic investigation and intervention.
- Prolonged loss of consciousness with hypotension or family history of sudden death may suggest life-threatening cardiac dysrhythmias and require further cardiac investigation.
- Children with severe cyanotic BHS and anatomic or functional airway abnormalities may be at risk for life-threatening events; referral for tracheostomy or ventilator assistance may be necessary.

IN-PATIENT CONSIDERATIONS
Admission Criteria
Children with bradycardia, asystole, or epileptic activity requiring cardiopulmonary resuscitation should be admitted for stabilization and further evaluation.

Discharge Criteria
Discharge from the hospital is appropriate once other causes, including neurologic and cardiovascular abnormalities, have been ruled out.

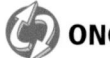 ONGOING CARE

FOLLOW-UP RECOMMENDATIONS
Only routine follow-up is indicated for uncomplicated BHS.

PATIENT EDUCATION
- An important part of managing children with BHS is counseling parents with regard to the expected benign course for these events.

DIET
An iron-rich diet may prevent iron deficiency anemia, which has been associated with BHS.

Activity
- No specific precautions for activity
- Parents should not avoid regular discipline in an attempt to prevent BHS.

Prevention
- Most events triggered by a minor injury or crying cannot be prevented.
- Special treatment or attention should be avoided to minimize secondary gain.
- Children having a BHS should be lowered to the floor and away from sharp or hard surfaces.
- Cardiopulmonary resuscitation should generally be avoided.
- Prolonged unconsciousness (>1 minute) warrants more complete medical evaluation.

PROGNOSIS
Prognosis is excellent. BHS generally occur in otherwise healthy children and spontaneously resolve by 4–7 years of age.

COMPLICATIONS
- Not associated with significant long-term complications
- Approximately 20% of children with a history of BHS may experience syncope in later childhood
- Reports of death consequent to BHS are exceedingly rare.

ADDITIONAL READING

- Boon R. Does iron have a place in the management of breath holding spells? *Arch Dis Child*. 2002;87(1):77–78.
- Breningstall GN. Breath-holding spells. *Pediatr Neurol*. 1996;14:91–97.
- Daoud AS, Batieha A, Al-Sheyyab M, et al. Effectiveness of iron therapy on breath-holding spells. *J Pediatr*. 1997;130:547–550.
- DiMario FJ. Prospective study of children with cyanotic and pallid breath-holding spells. *Pediatrics*. 2001;107(2):265–269.
- Donma MM. Clinical efficacy of piracetam in treatment of breath-holding spells. *Pediatr Neurol* 1998;18(1):41–45.
- Guilleminault C, Huang YS, Chan A, et al. Cyanotic breath-holding spells in children respond to adenotonsillectomy for sleep-disordered breathing. *J Sleep Res*. 2007;16(4):406–413.
- Horrocks IA, Nechay A, Stephenson JB, et al. Anoxic–epileptic seizures: observational study of epileptic seizures induced by syncopes. *Arch Dis Child*. 2005;90(12):1283–1287.
- Kelly AM, Porter CJ, McGoon MD, et al. Breath-holding spells associated with significant bradycardia: successful treatment with permanent pacemaker implantation. *Pediatrics*. 2001;108(3):698–702.

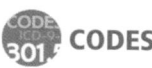 CODES

ICD9
786.9 Breath holding

ICD10
R06.89 Other abnormalities of breathing

FAQ

- Q: Are children with BHS at risk for any permanent neurologic or developmental problems?
- A: Children with BHS are not at increased risk for developing epilepsy. Normal cognitive development is expected.
- Q: Should all patients with BHS have an ECG and EEG?
- A: ECG should be strongly considered for children with BHS, particularly those with pallid type, to evaluate for long QT syndrome and other cardiac abnormalities that could be potentially fatal. Routine EEG is not warranted for these patients unless the history or exam is not consistent with a diagnosis of BHS.
- Q: How often should a child with BHS be evaluated by a physician?
- A: Once an initial evaluation has been completed and the diagnosis of BHS has been confirmed, only routine follow-up is necessary.

BRONCHIOLITIS (SEE ALSO: RESPIRATORY SYNCYTIAL VIRUS)

Howard B. Panitch

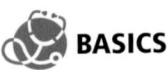 **BASICS**

DESCRIPTION
Acute lower respiratory tract infection causing obstruction of the small to medium conducting airways of the lung

EPIDEMIOLOGY
- In the US, occurs from late fall through the winter and early spring. The respiratory syncytial virus (RSV) epidemic season begins earlier in the southeastern US, and in some areas (e.g. Florida, Hawaii) can occur throughout the year. Parainfluenza 3 occurs throughout the year, as does adenovirus. Influenza virus epidemics usually begin in late fall, peak in January/February, and wane by April. Human metapneumovirus peaks slightly later in the year (March) than does RSV (January).
- RSV infects most children within the 1st 2 years of life; 57% of those hospitalized are <6 months.
- RSV reinfection occurs in 50–75% of children followed, and reinfection within the same RSV season is possible.
- ~1/2 of all children experience an infection with parainfluenza 3 before 1 year of age.
- Mortality associated with primary RSV infection in otherwise healthy children has been estimated to be 3.1 deaths per 100,000 person-years in infants <1 year of age, and is ~1–3% among children with underlying conditions. It is the most common viral cause of death in infants <1 year old.
- Up to 50% of infants with bronchiolitis develop subsequent wheezing.
- Patient groups at high risk of severe RSV disease:
  – Premature infants (<36 weeks' gestation)
  – Infants ≤10 weeks of age at time of RSV infection
  – Congenital heart disease
  – Chronic lung disease (including bronchopulmonary dysplasia [BPD])
  – Low birth weight
  – Cystic fibrosis
  – Compromised immune function (from chemotherapy, transplant, congenital or acquired immunodeficiencies)
  – Neuromuscular diseases
  – Trisomy 21

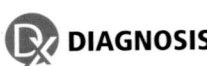 **DIAGNOSIS**

HISTORY
- Rhinorrhea with clear to white copious nasal secretions
- Initial hoarse cough for 3–5 days; progresses to deep, wet cough of increased frequency
- Poor feeding is an early sign of respiratory fatigue; may lead to dehydration
- Low-grade fever is characteristic but not a reliable marker of severity of disease; contributes to increased insensible fluid loss
- Restlessness or lethargy may indicate impending respiratory failure (hypoxemia and/or CO_2 retention).
- Apnea can be sole presenting sign in younger infants.
- Cyanosis/color change or increased work of breathing may suggest impending respiratory failure.

PHYSICAL EXAM
- General appearance:
  – Interactive versus ill appearing
  – Paroxysmal cough (most common sign), not associated with a "whoop"
- HEENT exam
  – Nasal flaring
  – Nasal congestion with copious secretions
- Pulmonary exam
  – Pattern of breathing: Apnea or periodic breathing
  – Tachypnea: >70/min is associated with severe illness
  – Intercostal retractions (increased resistance, decreased compliance); subcostal retractions (hyperinflation)
  – Thoracoabdominal asynchrony
  – Hyperresonance to percussion
  – Diffuse, high-pitched heterophonic wheezing
  – Prolonged expiratory phase
  – Fine inspiratory crackles (may be heard in both bronchiolitis and pneumonia)
  – Diffuse rhonchi
- Other findings:
  – Signs of dehydration
  – Low-grade fever
  – Tachycardia
  – Bradycardia associated with apnea
  – Possible cyanosis of nail beds and oral mucosa
  – Liver and spleen typically caudally displaced by hyperinflated lungs

DIAGNOSTIC TESTS & INTERPRETATION
Lab
- Pulse oximetry: To assess oxygenation
- Arterial blood gas:
  – Degree of hypoxemia (determine A-a gradient)
  – Evidence of respiratory failure and respiratory acidosis with CO_2 retention (late finding)
- Serum electrolytes: Sickest patients may have syndrome of inappropriate antidiuretic hormone release and hyponatremia.
- RSV serology (acute and convalescent serum samples): No practical application for clinical use
- Rapid viral identification:
  – Best samples for testing:
    ○ Nasopharyngeal aspirate
    ○ Nasopharyngeal wash
  – Adequate samples for testing:
    ○ Nasal swab
    ○ Tracheal aspirate
    ○ BAL fluid
- Rapid tests:
  – Immunofluorescence assay (direct or indirect):
    ○ >85% sensitivity and specificity
    ○ Results in 45 minutes
    ○ Negative predictive value >87%
  – Enzyme immunoassay (EIA):
    ○ 60–90% sensitivity
    ○ 70–95% specificity
    ○ Negative predictive value 75–98%
    ○ Results in 15–30 minutes
    ○ Does not require the presence of viable virus
  – Reverse transcriptase polymerase chain reaction (RT-PCR):
    ○ 93.5–100% sensitivity
    ○ 63.9–100% specificity
    ○ Results in <1 hour

- Viral culture:
  – Culture of nasopharynx
  – Considered "gold standard." May take up to 14 days for results
  – Sensitivity and specificity highly dependent on quality of sample, handling of specimen, and time to delivery to virology laboratory

Imaging
Chest radiography findings include:
- Hyperinflation, flattened diaphragms
- Peribronchial thickening
- Patchy or more extensive atelectasis
- Possible collapse of a segment or a lobe
- Diffusely increased interstitial markings commonly seen

DIFFERENTIAL DIAGNOSIS
- Pneumonia (viral or bacterial)
- Asthma
- Gastroesophageal reflux (GER)
- Foreign body aspiration
- Exposure to noxious agents (chemicals, fumes, toxins)
- CHF
- Cystic fibrosis

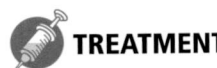 **TREATMENT**

ADDITIONAL TREATMENT
General Measures
- Most cases are mild and may be treated at home.
- Adequate fluid intake
- Maintenance of nasal airway patency:
  – Short-term nasal decongestant
  – Suction secretions with suction bulb.

Additional Therapies
- Careful fluid hydration; deficit plus ~2/3 maintenance fluids
- Supplemental oxygen:
  – Given to any patient with hypoxemia
  – Preferably warmed and humidified by nasal cannula, head box, or tent
- Management to overcome airway obstruction:
  – Bronchodilators:
    ○ Some (but not all) infants with bronchiolitis will improve clinically with bronchodilator administration. A trial of an aerosolized β-adrenergic agent with critical assessment to see if there is any relief of symptoms is reasonable.
    ○ Infants with a prior history of wheezing or familial history of asthma or atopy are more likely to respond to bronchodilators.
    ○ Theophylline is not usually useful as a bronchodilator in bronchiolitis, and may potentially worsen GER, if present.
  – Nebulized epinephrine:
    ○ Potentially beneficial in infants with moderate to severe bronchiolitis. It is both an α- and β-receptor agonist.
    ○ Both racemic epinephrine (0.1 mL/kg of 2.25% solution) and L-epinephrine have been studied separately and showed beneficial results compared with β-agonists.

– Anticholinergic agents: Ipratropium bromide has not been shown to be effective in the treatment of bronchiolitis.
– Corticosteroids:
  ○ In previously healthy infants, corticosteroids are not routinely recommended. Use of systemic (oral or parenteral) steroids may confer a small benefit in shortening duration of hospital stay or symptoms (<1/2 day).
  ○ The combination of inhaled epinephrine with oral dexamethasone in children cared for in an emergency room may decrease the need for hospitalization.
  ○ Use of inhaled corticosteroids does not decrease duration of symptoms or recurrence of cough and wheezing after acute bronchiolitis resolves.
– Leukotriene modifiers:
  ○ Infants who develop wheezing with RSV infection have high concentrations of cysteinyl leukotrienes and histamine in respiratory secretions.
  ○ The role of montelukast in acute bronchiolitis remains unclear.
  ○ Use of montelukast to prevent postbronchiolitis wheezing does not appear to be effective.
– Mucolytics:
  ○ Recombinant human DNase and N-acetylcysteine are not effective in shortening the duration of symptoms in infants with bronchiolitis.
  ○ Hypertonic saline (3%) aerosolized in combination with epinephrine shortens length of hospitalization compared to use of epinephrine alone.
  ○ Hypertonic saline can be used safely without pretreatment with a bronchodilator.
– Surfactant:
  ○ Shown to prevent progression of deterioration in lung mechanics in a small number of infants with respiratory failure requiring mechanical ventilation secondary to RSV bronchiolitis
– Heliox:
  ○ Helium–oxygen mixtures used in place of nitrogen–oxygen (air) have been shown to improve clinical score and shorten ICU stays in small series of infants with severe bronchiolitis.
  ○ The gas does not alter the course of the underlying illness, but because helium is less dense than nitrogen, resistance in areas of turbulent flow is decreased.
  ○ This in turn can decrease breathing effort, respiratory rate, and heart rate.
– Antibiotics:
  ○ Not usually indicated
  ○ Other than otitis media or urinary tract infection, the incidence of concurrent serious bacterial infection (pneumonia, meningitis, sepsis) is <7% in healthy infants with no underlying disease who have RSV bronchiolitis.
– Antiviral agents (ribavirin): See Respiratory Syncytial Virus
– Immunoprophylaxis: See Respiratory Syncytial Virus

IN-PATIENT CONSIDERATIONS
Admission Criteria
- Historical risk factors for severe disease:
- <2 months of age
  – Gestational age <36 weeks
  – Underlying cardiopulmonary disease (e.g., hemodynamically significant heart disease, BPD)
- Immunodeficiency or other high-risk group for developing severe disease
- Presence of apnea, tachypnea (respiratory rate >70/min), retractions, poor feeding, pallor, lethargy, or agitation (signs of impending respiratory failure)
- Pulse oximetry <95% in room air
- Atelectasis on chest radiograph

 ## ONGOING CARE

FOLLOW-UP RECOMMENDATIONS
Patient Monitoring
- Most infants with no underlying disease improve within 3–5 days. In some, nasal congestion and cough may continue for 1–3 weeks. Premature infants and those with underlying cardiopulmonary disease typically experience a protracted illness.
- Those who need mechanical ventilation may have difficulties with extubation owing to excessive secretions and atelectasis.
- As many as 50% of infants will have recurrent wheezing through the 1st decade of life.

PROGNOSIS
- For most previously healthy infants, the prognosis is good.
- Premature infants of 32–35 weeks' gestation hospitalized for bronchiolitis have been shown to have an increased number of subsequent hospitalizations for respiratory problems, a greater number of outpatient visits, and an increased risk of sudden death compared with those who were not hospitalized for bronchiolitis.
- Mortality associated with primary RSV infection in otherwise healthy infants is 0.005–0.02%.
- Up to 50% of infants with bronchiolitis develop subsequent episodes of recurrent wheezing until 11 years of age.
- Bronchiolitis obliterans may be a sequela in patients infected with adenovirus or Mycoplasma pneumoniae.

COMPLICATIONS
- Impending respiratory failure (increased breathing effort, retractions, hypoxemia, CO_2 retention, lethargy)
- Sudden deterioration suggesting atelectasis due to mucous plugging
- Fatigue may occur in infants who have prolonged and extensive disease.
- Fatigue will manifest with increased pCO_2 and worsening hypoxemia.

ALERT
- Hypoxemia is common, so always monitor oxygen saturation.
- Be aware of apnea.
- In cases of clinical bronchiolitis, causes of false-negative ELISA tests:
  – Poor quality of sample
  – Sample contamination
  – Insufficient sample
  – Non-RSV bronchiolitis

ADDITIONAL READING

- Garcia CG, Bhore R, Soriano-Fallas A, et al. Risk factors in children hospitalized with RSV bronchiolitis versus non-RSV bronchiolitis. Pediatrics. 2010;126:e1453–e1460.
- Hall CB. Respiratory syncytial virus and parainfluenza virus. N Engl J Med. 2001;44:1917–1928.
- Plint AC, Johnson DW, Patel H, et al. Epinephrine and dexamethasone in children with bronchiolitis. N Engl J Med. 2009;360:2079–2089.
- Subcommittee on Diagnosis and Management of Bronchiolitis. Diagnosis and management of bronchiolitis. Pediatrics. 2006;118:1774–1793.
- Yanney M, Vyas H. The treatment of bronchiolitis. Arch Dis Child. 2008;93:793–798.

 ## CODES

ICD9
- 079.6 Respiratory syncytial virus (RSV)
- 786.07 Wheezing

ICD10
- J20.5 Acute bronchitis due to respiratory syncytial virus
- J21.9 Acute bronchiolitis, unspecified

FAQ

- Q: How did my child get bronchiolitis?
- A: RSV bronchiolitis is a common, seasonal, lower respiratory tract infection that is easily transmissible.
- Q: Can my child become reinfected?
- A: Children can become reinfected with RSV bronchiolitis, and infection can occur more than once during the same respiratory season.
- Q: Do patients with bronchiolitis need to be isolated?
- A: RSV-positive patients need to be isolated with other RSV-positive patients and from uninfected patients.
- Q: Will my child develop asthma?
- A: Recurrent wheezing has been described in up to 50% of infants with RSV bronchiolitis. However, most data are retrospective and observational. Whether RSV per se can contribute to the development of asthma and allergic sensitization remains unclear.

BRONCHOPULMONARY DYSPLASIA (CHRONIC LUNG DISEASE OF PREMATURITY)

John M. Good

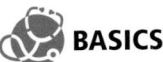 **BASICS**

DESCRIPTION
A chronic lung disease, seen mainly in premature infants, characterized by inflammation and scarring in the lungs.

GENERAL PREVENTION
- Prevention of prematurity
- Antenatal steroids
- Early use of surfactantLimited use of high pressure ventilation

EPIDEMIOLOGY
Prevalence
BPD is one of the most common chronic lung diseases in children.

RISK FACTORS
- Birth weight of <1250 g
- Infants who were born at >30 weeks' gestation.

PATHOPHYSIOLOGY
- Remains complex and poorly understood
- Lung damage caused by a variety of toxic factors which interferes with alveolarization (septation), leading to alveolar simplification with a reduction in the overall surface area for gas exchange as well as damage to the developing pulmonary vasculature.

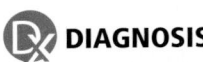 **DIAGNOSIS**

SIGNS AND SYMPTOMS
HISTORY
- Maternal use of antenatal steroids
- Gestational age, birth weight, APGAR score
- Initial resuscitative efforts, need for intubation, use of surfactant, duration in intubation, type of ventilation, duration of supplemental oxygen therapy, and other factors: These may have influenced the type and degree of lung injury.
- Familial history of asthma, atopy, or other children with bronchopulmonary dysplasia
- Social support structure
- Any potentially exacerbating factors, such as exposure to smoking
- Feeding and sleeping history

PHYSICAL EXAM
- Review of systems, including careful assessment of work of breathing both at rest and during activity
- A review of growth charts
- Vitals including respiratory rate and pulse oximetry both at rest and with activity
- Signs of pulmonary hypertension, including peripheral edema, hepatomegaly, and venous distention

DIAGNOSTIC TESTS & INTERPRETATION
Lab
- Electrocardiogram: Often followed serially to assess for right ventricular hypertrophy
- Echocardiogram: Often, a useful adjunct to follow patients with right ventricular hypertrophy
- Cardiac catheterization: Reserved for patients with evidence of pulmonary hypertension and cardiac dysfunction
- Pulmonary function testing: Often used to follow patients and evaluate responsiveness to interventions
- Blood gases: Useful in acute and chronic management of bronchopulmonary dysplasia to follow the degree of hypoxia and hypercapnia

Imaging
Changes on chest radiography include hyperinflation, emphysema, cyst formation, pulmonary edema, fibrosis, and cardiovascular changes. Severity of these changes may help predict the severity of the disease.

Diagnostic Procedures/Other
Bronchoscopy, barium swallow, pH probe, and sleep studies may reveal underlying conditions contributing to pulmonary dysfunction.

DIFFERENTIAL DIAGNOSIS
- Asthma
- Atelectasis
- Bronchiolitis obliterans
- Congenital heart disease
- Cystic adenomatoid malformation
- Cystic fibrosis
- Idiopathic pulmonary fibrosis
- Infections
- Meconium aspiration syndrome
- Patent ductus arteriosus
- Pneumonia
- Recurrent aspiration
- Subglottic stenosis
- Tracheomalacia http://www.emedicine.com/ped/topic158.htm

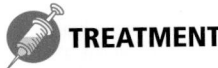 **TREATMENT**

GENERAL MEASURES
Diet
- Infants with bronchopulmonary dysplasia may have increased caloric needs as much as 150 kcal/kg/d.
- Premature and critically ill infants may be deficient in antioxidants. Supplementation has not yet been shown to affect outcomes.

MEDICATION (DRUGS)
- Diuretics:
  - Used for treating pulmonary edema, often improving lung mechanics and gas exchange
  - Furosemide may have other benefits, including effects on prostaglandin synthesis, direct vasodilatation, and improved surfactant production.
  - Side effects from long-term furosemide therapy include azotemia, ototoxicity, electrolyte abnormalities, excessive urinary calcium loss, osteopenia, and nephrocalcinosis.
  - Thiazide diuretics, usually used with a potassium-sparing diuretic such as spironolactone, are not as effective as furosemide.
  - Routine monitoring of electrolytes is recommended for patients on long-term diuretic therapy.
  - Electrolyte supplementation is often required with long-term diuretic usage.
- Bronchodilators:
  - Inhaled β-agonists are effective treatment for reversible bronchospasm, although safety and efficacy of long-term use has yet to be established.
  - Albuterol is often the drug of choice, although longer-acting agents are often used as well.
  - Muscarinic antagonists may be useful adjuncts, especially in patients who are not significantly responsive to albuterol. Believed to work on large- and medium-sized airways
  - Cromolyn, though not a bronchodilator, is often used for its anti-inflammatory effects and has a low side-effect profile.
  - Methylxanthines are often used in the treatment of apnea, have a mild diuretic effect, and help improve diaphragmatic contractility, making them potentially useful in bronchopulmonary dysplasia.
- Pulmonary vasodilators:
  - Supplemental oxygen is an effective vasodilator and remains a mainstay of treatment for infants with hypoxia.

- Steroids:
  - Steroid usage is controversial.
  - Increased risk for sepsis has probably been overstated.
  - Often used successfully in short regimens to wean ventilatory support and hasten extubation
  - No long-term benefits of steroid therapy have been demonstrated.
  - Inhaled steroids may provide anti-inflammatory effects without systemic side effects, making them attractive as both prevention and treatment.
  - Routine use in premature infants is an active area of investigation.
  - Linear growth retardation has been a concern.
  - Newer agents that can be nebulized are now available, improving drug delivery in small infants.

 ONGOING CARE

FOLLOW-UP RECOMMENDATIONS
- A multidisciplinary approach is recommended for all patients with moderate and severe disease.
- Team may include primary care physician, pediatric pulmonologist, pediatric cardiologist, nutritionist, and speech, respiratory, occupational, and physical therapists.
- Monitor growth and nutritional status.
- Monitor neurodevelopmental status, including NICU "high-risk" follow-up.

ALERT
- Ensure adequate calcium and phosphorus intake in patients at risk for hyperparathyroidism and rickets.
- Patients <2 years of age are candidates for respiratory syncytial virus immune globulin injections (palivizumab; Synagis), if not contraindicated.
- Patients >6 months are candidates for influenza vaccine, if not contraindicated.
- Chest physiotherapy may cause pathologic fractures in patients with osteopenia.

PROGNOSIS
- Most survivors demonstrate slow, steady improvement.
- High death rate (17–47%) for patients with severe disease requiring prolonged mechanical ventilation
- No treatment modality has shown significant impact on the long-term outcome of chronic bronchopulmonary dysplasia.
- Survivors often have long-term pulmonary sequelae including hyperinflation, reactive airways, and exercise intolerance.
- Even older children and young adults who were thought to be asymptomatic can have abnormal responsiveness to exercise.
- Newer technologies, in particular high-frequency ventilation and exogenous surfactant, have improved survival rates for premature infants; however, reduction in the incidence and severity of bronchopulmonary dysplasia has been difficult to demonstrate.

COMPLICATIONS
- Prolonged intubation may cause subglottic stenosis and tracheomalacia.
- Pulmonary hypertension may occur as a result of vasculature damage and subsequent intimal proliferation, which may, in turn, produce right ventricular hypertrophy and, if severe enough, cor pulmonale.
- Pulmonary edema often occurs secondary to increased pulmonary capillary permeability and increased pulmonary pressures.
- Reactive airways, bronchospasm, and altered pulmonary mechanics owing to a poorly compliant lung may result in abnormal pulmonary function testing and increased work of breathing.
- Malnutrition and growth failure may occur as a result of increased work of breathing and a subsequently high caloric expenditure.
- Impaired lung defenses result in an increased susceptibility to infection, especially respiratory syncytial virus.

ADDITIONAL READING

- Bancalari E, Claure N, Sosenkol R. Bronchopulmonary dysplasia: Changes in pathogenesis, epidemiology and definition. *Semin Neonatol.* 2003;8:63–71.
- Jobe AH, Ikegami M. Prevention of bronchopulmonary dysplasia. *Curr Opin Pediatr.* 2001;13:124–129.
- Hayes D Jr., Feola DJ, Murphy BS, et al. Pathogenesis of bronchopulmonary dysplasia. *Respiration.* 2010;79(5):425–436.
- Van Marter LJ. Epidemiology of bronchopulmonary dysplasia. *Semin Fetal & Neonatal Med.* 2009;14(6):358–366.
- Doyle LW, Anderson PJ. Long-term outcomes of bronchopulmonary dysplasia. *Semin Fetal & Neonatal Med.* 2009;14(6):391–395.

 CODES

ICD9
770.7 Bronchopulmonary dysplasia

ICD10
P27.1 Bronchopulmonary dysplasia origin in the perinatal period

FAQ

- Q: Will antibiotics help my child?
- A: Some evidence indicates that infection with ureaplasma may be important in the pathogenesis of bronchopulmonary dysplasia. It remains to be seen whether treatment affects outcome. Overuse of antibiotics increases occurrence of antibiotic resistance.

- Q: Which babies should get respiratory syncytial virus immunoglobulin injections (palivizumab; Synagis)?
- A: The AAP Committee on Infectious Diseases recommends immunoprophylaxis for infants with bronchopulmonary dysplasia who are <2 years of age at the onset of respiratory syncytial virus season. Other premature infants may be candidates as well, with or without bronchopulmonary dysplasia:
- Infants born at ≤28 weeks at the onset of respiratory syncytial virus season and who are ≤12 months should receive immunoprophylaxis monthly for the entire season.
- Infants born at 29–32 weeks' gestation and who are ≤6 months at the beginning of respiratory syncytial virus season should also receive immunoprophylaxis.
- Infants born between 32 and 35 weeks may or may not be candidates for palivizumab (Synagis) depending on the presence or absence of other risk factors, such as day-care attendance, school-aged siblings, exposure to environmental air pollutants, congenital abnormalities of the airways, or severe neuromuscular disease.
- Q: Will anti-respiratory syncytial virus immunoprophylaxis (palivizumab; Synagis) prevent my baby from getting respiratory syncytial virus?
- A: It will not prevent respiratory syncytial virus infection, but it will help your child's own immune system attack the virus.
- Q: Will my child have asthma when he grows up?
- A: Asthma occurs in >50% of older children who survived bronchopulmonary dysplasia.
- Q: What types of additional therapies can help my child?
- A: Such therapies include the following:
- Chest physiotherapy may help to mobilize secretions and to prevent atelectasis.
- Speech and occupational therapy may help infants who have had prolonged intubation or other interventions that interfere with oral functioning (and, therefore, may have some degree of oral-motor dysfunction and oral aversion).
- Other infants simply with increased work of breathing may have discoordinated suck and swallow, making oral feedings difficult.
- Physical therapy may help infants with gross and fine motor delays, poor tone, and abnormal posture.
- Parents can learn many of the therapies to incorporate therapeutic exercises and positioning into their daily routines.

BRUISING
Julie W. Stern

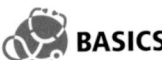

BASICS

DEFINITION
Bruises are the result of extravasation of blood into the skin. Conventional usage often groups petechiae and bruises (or ecchymoses) together as purpura and defines them as follows:
- Petechiae: Flat, red, or reddish purple, 1–3 mm, nonblanching
- Ecchymoses: Larger than petechiae, local extravasation, nonpulsatile, sometimes palpable, color depends on age of lesion

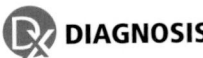

DIAGNOSIS

DIFFERENTIAL DIAGNOSIS
- **Congenital/anatomic**
  - Coagulation factor abnormality: Hemophilia, von Willebrand disease
  - Platelet defect: Bernard–Soulier syndrome, Glanzmann thrombasthenia, and storage pool defects
  - Congenital alloimmune or isoimmune thrombocytopenia
  - Neonatal extramedullary hematopoiesis
  - Hereditary hemorrhagic telangiectasia
- **Infectious**
  - Meningococcemia
  - Viral infections (coxsackievirus, echovirus)
  - Rocky Mountain spotted fever
  - Syphilis
  - Pertussis—secondary to severe cough
  - Septic or fat emboli
  - Disseminated intravascular coagulation—acquired factor deficiency
- **Toxic, environmental, drugs**
  - Warfarin—acquired factor deficiency
  - Corticosteroids—striae caused by increased capillary fragility
  - Aspirin and ibuprofen—cause a qualitative platelet abnormality
  - Sulfonamides
  - Bismuth
  - Chloramphenicol
- **Trauma**
  - Normal activity
  - Child abuse
  - Valsalva, crying, forceful coughing
  - Cupping or coin rubbing
  - Tight garments
- **Tumor (quantitative platelet abnormality): Bone marrow replacement**—leukemia, myelofibrosis, or (rarely) metastatic solid tumors
- **Genetic/metabolic**
  - Uremia
  - Vitamin C deficiency
  - Vitamin K deficiency—owing to antibiotics, biliary atresia, malabsorption (acquired factor deficiency)
- **Allergic/inflammatory/vasculitic**
  - Henoch–Schönlein purpura
  - Bone marrow failure: Aplastic anemia (including Fanconi, paroxysmal nocturnal hemoglobinuria)
  - Increased destruction: Idiopathic thrombocytopenic purpura, Evans syndrome, lupus
  - Nephrotic syndrome
  - Collagen vascular disease
  - Ehlers–Danlos syndrome
  - Snake bite (copperhead)
- **Miscellaneous (disorders that simulate bruises)**
  - Ataxia telangiectasia
  - Cherry angiomas
  - Kaposi sarcoma

DIAGNOSIS TO THE PATIENT
General goal is to determine if the cause of the bruising is thrombocytopenia, a coagulation disorder, or an extrinsic factor (such as trauma, infection).
- **Phase 1:** Determine if the history of bruising and/or petechiae is acute or chronic in onset and if there is known trauma vs. spontaneous lesions (see Table 1)

Table 1. How to estimate the age of bruises

1. New	Purple, dark red
2. 1–4 days	Dark blue to brown
3. 5–7 days	Greenish to yellow
4. >7 days	Yellow

- Acute onset of diffuse subcutaneous bleeding with bruises of different ages may indicate severe thrombocytopenia.
- Generally, children will not bruise or develop petechiae spontaneously until the platelet count is <20,000/mm^3.
- Idiopathic thrombocytopenic purpura, leukemia, aplastic anemia, and so forth, can cause this bleeding.
- A hematologist should be consulted because of the risk of potentially life-threatening bleeding.
- Chronic history of recurrent bleeding may indicate an inherited coagulation defect such as von Willebrand disease or hemophilia. Familial history may be positive, although von Willebrand disease often goes undiagnosed into adulthood if there has been no challenge such as surgery.
- **Phase 2:** Perform screening tests for bleeding disorders to categorize the abnormality
  - Platelet count to assess level of thrombocytopenia
  - PT/PTT: Prolongation of either one or both of these may aid in diagnosis of von Willebrand disease, coagulation factor deficiencies, liver disease, and vitamin K deficiency.
  - Bleeding time: Prolongation may indicate a platelet aggregation disorder or von Willebrand disease. Use as a screening test is controversial and rarely used routinely in pediatrics.
  - PFA-100: Value as screening test for bleeding disorders controversial

HISTORY
- **Question:** Significant bruising in the neonatal period?
- *Significance:* May indicate neonatal thrombocytopenia, congenital infections, and sepsis with disseminated intravascular coagulation
- **Question:** Bleeding in the neonatal period?
- *Significance:* Hemophilia. Other inherited disorders of coagulation may not be diagnosed until a child is older; tend to be mild, may be uncovered with preoperative testing or postoperative bleeding complications. Idiopathic thrombocytopenic purpura may occur at any age.
- **Question:** Pattern of bruising?
- *Significance:* In a younger child, may indicate normal toddler activity, child abuse, or religious practices such as coining (common among Southeast Asians).
- **Question:** Use of aspirin, ibuprofen, cough syrups with guaifenesin, and/or antihistamines?
- *Significance:* Platelet dysfunction; use of these drugs may also unmask an otherwise mild inherited bleeding disorder.
- **Question:** Ecchymosis or petechiae?
- *Significance:* Infections such as meningococcemia or viruses and collagen vascular diseases may present with these.
- **Question:** Familial history?
- *Significance:* Positive familial history of inherited disorders of coagulation factors or platelet aggregation may aid in directing the workup. Negative familial history does not rule out any of these disorders.

PHYSICAL EXAM
- **Finding:** Good appearance, with a history of an antecedent viral illness?
- *Significance:* Those with idiopathic thrombocytopenic purpura often appear well, though often with a history of an antecedent viral illness.
- **Finding:** Ill appearance?
- *Significance:* It should raise concerns about malignancy, infection (especially meningococcemia), or other acquired coagulation factor deficiencies such as those seen with liver failure.
- **Finding:** Bruising in unusual locations (back, genitalia, thorax)?
- *Significance:* Should raise suspicions of child abuse, especially if lesions are in different stages of healing or suggest the pattern of a hand or belt.
- **Finding:** Purpura confined mostly to the legs?
- *Significance:* Typical of Henoch–Schönlein purpura
- **Finding:** Multiple ecchymoses in the pretibial regions?
- *Significance:* Most toddlers will have that occur with normal activity.

- **Finding:** Petechiae entirely above the nipple line?
- *Significance:* Consistent with Valsalva maneuver, severe cough, and viral infections
- **Finding:** Deeper bleeding in muscles and joints?
- *Significance:* Hemophilia
- **Finding:** Bleeding in mucous membranes?
- *Significance:* Severe thrombocytopenia, streptococcal pharyngitis, varicella, measles, and other viral infections can cause this.
- **Finding:** Gingival and/or mucous membrane bleeding?
- *Significance:* Von Willebrand disease can present with this.
- **Finding:** Involvement of the reticuloendothelial system?
- *Significance:* Can be found with malignancies such as leukemia or with viral or bacterial infections, indicated by hepatosplenomegaly or lymphadenopathy.
- **Finding:** Upper extremity limb malformations and bruising?
- *Significance:* May present with syndromes such as Fanconi anemia and thrombocytopenia absent radii (TAR)

ALERT
Factors that make this an emergency include:
- Severe thrombocytopenia below 10,000–20,000/mm³ carries a higher risk of spontaneous internal bleeding including intracranial bleeding.
- Bleeding or bruising accompanied by evidence of leukemia or other malignancy
- Evidence of sepsis (disseminated intravascular coagulation) or meningococcemia

DIAGNOSTIC TESTS & INTERPRETATION
- **Test:** CBC
- *Significance:* Platelet count is the most important; abnormalities of WBC or Hgb may aid in diagnosis of bone marrow infiltration or failure.
- **Test:** PT
- *Significance:* Elevation may indicate warfarin ingestion or factor VII deficiency or vitamin K deficiency.
- **Test:** aPTT
- *Significance:* Prolongation is seen with hemophilia and may be seen in von Willebrand disease.
- **Test:** Both PT and PTT
- *Significance:* Both are prolonged in disseminated intravascular coagulation, liver failure, and severe vitamin K deficiency.
- **Test:** Bleeding time
- *Significance:* Lengthened in platelet aggregation disorders and with drug effects
- **Test:** Fibrinogen
- *Significance:* Decreased in liver failure, disseminated intravascular coagulation
- **Test:** Urinalysis
- *Significance:* Hematuria and/or proteinuria may indicate Henoch–Schönlein purpura, nephrotic syndrome, or other vasculitis.

 TREATMENT

General Measures
Thrombocytopenia precautions for platelets <20,000–50,000—toddlers may need a helmet until platelet count recovers; patients with hemophilia may need restricted activity, generally not needed for patients with von Willebrand disease. Depends on underlying cause:
- Factor replacement for hemophilia
- Platelet transfusion for thrombocytopenia due to decreased production
- IVIG/steroids/Rh immune globulin for ITP

ISSUES FOR REFERRAL
- Outpatient evaluation for bruising without significant thrombocytopenia, family history of bleeding disorder
- Suspected child abuse

Admission Criteria
Severe thrombocytopenia, suspected child abuse, significant bleeding, significant head trauma

 ONGOING CARE

FOLLOW-UP RECOMMENDATIONS
Patient-Monitoring
Recurrent and chronic ITP possible

COMPLICATIONS
Significant bleeding with a bleeding disorder, thrombocytopenia

ADDITIONAL READING

- Berntorp E. Progress in haemophilic care: Ethical issues. *Haemophilia.* 2002;8:435–438.
- Buchanan GR. Bleeding signs in children with idiopathic thrombocytopenic purpura. *J Pediatr Hematol Oncol.* 2003;25(Suppl 1):S42–S46.
- Geddis AE, Balduini CL. Diagnosis of immune thrombocytopenic purpura in children. *Curr Opin Hematol.* 2007;14(5):520–525.
- Horton TM, Stone JD, Yee D, et al. Case series of thrombotic thrombocytopenic purpura in children and adolescents. *J Pediatr Hematol Oncol.* 2003;25:336–339.
- Khair K, Liesner R. Bruising and bleeding in infants and children—a practical approach. *Br J Haematol.* 2006;133(3):221–231.
- Kos L, Shwayder T. Related articles, cutaneous manifestations of child abuse. *Pediatr Dermatol.* 2006;23(4):311–320.
- Wight J, Paisley S. The epidemiology of inhibitors in haemophilia A: A systematic review. *Haemophilia.* 2003;9:418–435.

 CODES

ICD9
- 287.2 Other nonthrombocytopenic purpuras
- 459.89 Other specified disorders of circulatory system
- 782.7 Spontaneous ecchymoses

ICD10
- D69.2 Other nonthrombocytopenic purpura
- R23.3 Spontaneous ecchymoses
- R58 Hemorrhage, not elsewhere classified

CLINICAL PEARLS
- The amount of bruising may not correlate with the amount of internal bleeding that has occurred. Hemophiliacs can significantly drop their hemoglobin during a thigh or psoas bleed without having much in the way of ecchymosis.
- A child presenting with idiopathic thrombocytopenic purpura may have bruises and petechiae from head to toe without changing the hemoglobin much at all.

FAQ
- Q: Is hemophilia always diagnosed in the newborn period?
- A: No. A familial history may provide clues, but a significant number of patients represent a spontaneous mutation. Additionally, not all boys with hemophilia will bleed with circumcision, and the diagnosis may not be made until the infants become more active.
- Q: What is a common cause of bruising among girls?
- A: Girls may first come to attention at menarche and be diagnosed at that time with von Willebrand disease. Rarely, girls whose fathers have hemophilia may be unfavorably lyonized and, therefore, have decreased factor levels consistent with mild hemophilia.
- Q: Can boys with a family history of von Willebrand disease be circumcised?
- A: Yes, but only within the first few days of life and testing does not need to be completed prior to procedure. If procedure is not completed in the neonatal period, testing may need to be delayed until 6 months of life or later.

BRUXISM

Howard M. Rosenberg
Rochelle G. Lindemeyer
Zuhair Sayany (5th edition)

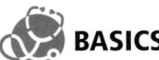 **BASICS**

DESCRIPTION
- Nonfunctional grinding of the teeth
- Poorly understood phenomenon with many suggested etiologies
- Usually a subconscious activity that may occur during the day or night
- Clenching is a related condition which is also considered to be a nonfunctional habit.
- Nonfunctional (or "parafunctional") habits include mandibular movements not involved with normal chewing, swallowing, or speaking, e.g., chewing pencils, nails, or cheek, or biting lip.
- If made aware of their tooth grinding while awake, children can often stop. However, bruxism while asleep is more difficult to modify and has become classified with restless leg syndrome and sleep walking.

EPIDEMIOLOGY
- May occur throughout life, but frequency tends to peak up to the ages of 7–10 years, then decreases with age
- Infants have been known to grind their teeth with the eruption of the first primary tooth.
- May sometimes be temporarily or intermittently present, making diagnosis difficult
- Girls may be affected more frequently, but there are not adequate studies on the role of gender.
- More common in children with developmental disabilities, principally severe mental retardation, Down syndrome, and some autism spectrum disorders
- Recent literature implicates genetics in bruxism, but no genetic mechanism has been explained.

Prevalence
In children, prevalence has been reported to be from 7% to 88% (with most reports indicating an average of 15–30%).

ETIOLOGY
The exact cause is not known, but several factors have been implicated and most feel that it is multifactorial:
- Dental (local) factors (current evidence is that they play only a small role, about 10%):
  - Occlusal interferences, including malocclusions, in which teeth do not interdigitate smoothly
  - High dental restorations (e.g., fillings or crowns)
  - Intraoral irritation (e.g., sharp tooth cusp)
  - Teething

- Psychological factors:
  - Nervous tension (related to stress, anger, and aggression)
  - Personality disorders
  - Mental retardation
  - Post-traumatic stress disorder
- Common systemic factors:
  - Moving between levels of sleep
  - Neuromuscular disorders (e.g., cerebral palsy)
  - Brain injury
  - Burn injuries
  - Hyperactivity
- Uncommon or rare systemic factors:
  - Asthma
  - Obstructed breathing (as with large tonsils and adenoids)
  - Genetics
  - Allergies
  - Nutritional and vitamin deficiencies
  - Intestinal parasites
  - Endocrine disorders
  - Restricted mobility of the cervical spine
  - Posture of the head
  - Mouth breathing
  - Medications (amphetamines, antidepressants—particularly serotonin reuptake inhibitors)

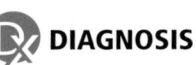 **DIAGNOSIS**

- Teeth:
  - Wear facets, abraded areas
  - Extreme wear of primary teeth is occasionally observed, but it is extremely rare that pulp becomes exposed or nerve damage occurs.
  - Broken dental restorations
  - Loosening
  - Exacerbation of pre-existing periodontal disturbances (gingival inflammation and recession, alveolar bone loss)
  - Pain or sensitivity
- Muscular symptoms in any of the head and neck muscles most often seen in the lateral pterygoids followed by the medial pterygoids and masseters:
  - Pain
  - Trismus
  - Spasm

- Headache especially in the morning
- Temporomandibular joint (TMJ) disorders:
  - Pain in the TMJ area
  - Symptoms (pain, trismus, spasm) in the masticatory muscles
  - Limited mandibular range of motion
- Grinding sounds, nocturnal (at night) and/or diurnal (during the day), which may be extremely distressing to parents and caregivers

DIFFERENTIAL DIAGNOSIS
- Dental problems
- Seizures
- Drug reaction
- Stress

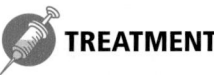 **TREATMENT**

MEDICATION (DRUGS)
Rarely used:
- Analgesic for symptoms
- Anti-inflammatory (e.g., ibuprofen) for symptoms
- Muscle relaxants for symptoms
- Mild tranquilizers if anxiety plays an etiologic role

ADDITIONAL TREATMENT
General Measures
- Patient and family education: Ensure that the bruxism itself does not become an issue generating stress for the child.
- Behavior (habit) therapy
- Stress counseling:
  - Identify and address sources of stress
  - Biofeedback exercises
- Counseling/psychotherapy
  - Hypnosis

Additional Therapies
- Uncommonly used:
  - Plastic or vinyl bite guard (must not interfere with normal dental growth and development)
  - Occlusal adjustment (selective tooth grinding to balance the bite): There is no evidence-based support.
  - Dental restorations: Treat and restore carious lesions. Stainless steel crowns may be used for extreme wear in primary teeth to stop tooth sensitivity and/or prevent pulpal exposure.
- Rarely used:
  - Orthodontics
    - Tonsillectomy and adenoidectomy

COMPLEMENTARY & ALTERNATIVE THERAPIES

Rarely used:

- Warm compresses for muscle or TMJ symptoms
- Limit affected muscle activity (e.g., "do not open wide," "take very small bites," "do not chew gum")
- Ultrasound
- Transcutaneous electrical nerve stimulation (TENS)
- Acupressure and/or acupuncture
- Correct cervical spine dysfunction (particularly head position) or posture

IN-PATIENT CONSIDERATIONS
Initial Stabilization

- Treatment for bruxism is rarely indicated in children.
- Therapy is justified if damage to the permanent dentition or periodontal structures is observed (occasionally in adolescents).
- Limit treatment to the most simple and reversible measures. There are inadequate data to support the efficacy of irreversible treatment (e.g., selective tooth grinding, orthodontics) in children.
- For comatose patients with self-injurious issues, various mouth guards or mouth props have been protective; intraoral botulinum-A injections have relieved the spasticity.

 ONGOING CARE

FOLLOW-UP RECOMMENDATIONS
Patient Monitoring

Continue to monitor for significant associated problems; intercede if damage to permanent dentition and/or periodontal structures is observed.

PROGNOSIS

- Although associated problems are well documented, there are no data that establish cause-and-effect relationships for bruxism in childhood continuing into adulthood.
- Preschool children:
  – Typically ceases without therapeutic intervention
  – Associated problems are rare.
- School-aged children:
  – Typically ceases without therapeutic intervention
  – Monitor for associated conditions without treatment
- Adolescents:
  – More commonly benefit from therapeutic intervention
  – Associated problems may also require therapy (e.g., abrasion of teeth; muscular, TMJ symptoms).

- Special-needs children:
  – Long-term prognosis is poor.
  – Acute situations in children who are comatose or those who have suffered traumatic brain injuries or severe burns may be managed by the use of prefabricated bite blocks, or in rare cases, by the fabrication of custom-fitted mouth guards. These appliances are used primarily to prevent self-injurious soft-tissue damage from parafunctional reactions such as lip, cheek, and tongue biting.

ADDITIONAL READING

- American Academy of Pediatric Dentistry. Guidelines on acquired temporomandibular disorders in infants, children and adolescents. Reference manual 2010–2011. *Pediatr Dent*. 2010;32:232–237.
- Barbosa TDS, Miyakoda LS, Pocztaruk RDL, et al. Temporomandibular disorders and bruxism in childhood and adolescence: Review of the literature. *Int J Pediatr Otorhinolaryngol*. 2008;72:299–314.
- Cheifetz AT, Osganian SK, Allred EN, et al. Prevalence of bruxism and associated correlates in children as reported by parents. *J Dent Child (Chic)*. 2005;72:67–73.
- DiFrancesco RC, Junqueira PA, Trezza PM, et al. Improvement of bruxism after T & A surgery. *Int J Pediatr Otorhinolaryngol*. 2004;68:441–445.
- Lang R, White PJ, Machalicek W, et al. Treatment of bruxism in individuals with developmental disabilities: A systematic review. *Res Dev Disabil*. 2009;30:809–818.
- Lavigne GJ, Khoury S, Abe S, et al. Bruxism physiology and pathology: An overview for clinicians. *J Oral Rehabil*. 2008;35:476–494.
- Lindemeyer RG. Bruxism in children. *Dim Dntl Hyg*. 2011;9:60–63.
- Manfredini D, Lobbezoo F. Role of psychosocial factors in the etiology of bruxism. *J Orofac Pain*. 2009;23:153–166.
- Motta LJ, Martins MD, Fernandes KP, et al. Craniocervical posture and bruxism in children. *Phyiother Res Int*. 2011;16:57–61.
- Restrepo C, Gomez S, Manrique R. Treatment of bruxism in children: A systematic review. *Quintessence Int*. 2009;40:849–855.

 CODES

ICD9
- 306.8 Other specified psychophysiological malfunction
- 327.53 Sleep related bruxism

ICD10
- F45.8 Other somatoform disorders
- G47.63 Sleep related bruxism

FAQ

- Q: How should bruxism in a preschool child be treated?
- A: The great majority of bruxism in children stops without any therapy. Considering the controversial nature of treatment modalities, it is prudent to advise no treatment for childhood bruxism and to advise the parents that the condition is common and is usually outgrown.
- Q: What about treating bruxism in adolescence?
- A: Because damage to the permanent teeth or periodontal structures may have long-term consequences, bruxism in adolescence may be a concern. Still, treatment should be limited to the most simple and reversible approaches. Careful dental evaluation would be an important first step.
- Q: Does damage to the primary teeth result in problems with the permanent teeth or with the TMJ?
- A: There is no evidence that bruxism in children leads to problems during adolescence or later.
- Q: Should custom-fitted mouth guards be fabricated for children with traumatic brain or burn injuries who engage in lip or tongue biting?
- A: The long-term prognosis is often poor in these patients. For patients with transitory soft-tissue injuries, conservative measures such as prefabricated bite blocks to get through the acute stage should be tried first. Patients who exhibit chronic chewing may require the fabrication of custom-fitted mouth guards, which may require the use of deep sedation or general anesthetic procedures to construct the appliance. The risk of these procedures would need to be weighed against the benefit of the bite guard.

BULIMIA
Nadja Peter

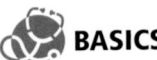 **BASICS**

DESCRIPTION
Bulimia nervosa is an eating disorder characterized by:
- Recurrent episodes of binge eating characterized by rapid consumption of large amounts of food in discrete periods of time, usually <2 hours
- Compensatory behavior such as self-induced vomiting, laxative or diuretic use, strict dieting, or vigorous exercise to induce weight loss
- Minimum average of 2 binge-eating episodes per week for at least 3 months
- Feeling of lack of control over eating behavior during eating binges
- Frenzied quality, often occurring alone and secretively
- Associated feelings of guilt, anxiety, low self-esteem, and depression
- Persistent overconcern with body shape and weight
- Symptoms and psychopathology may overlap with anorexia nervosa and eating disorder not otherwise specified, but does not occur exclusively during episodes of anorexia nervosa.

EPIDEMIOLOGY
- Onset in late adolescence to early adulthood (range: 13–28 years of age)
- Age of onset has been decreasing in recent generations.
- Females account for 85–90% of cases.
- 83% of patients have lifetime history of an anxiety disorder, 63% have a lifetime history of depression.

Prevalence
- Affects 1–3% of young females in Western countries
- Affects 4–10% of adolescent and college-aged females
- 10× more common than anorexia nervosa

RISK FACTORS
Genetics
Recent studies, including twin studies, suggest that bulimia nervosa and binge eating may be familial.

GENERAL PREVENTION
- Emphasize healthy self-esteem and body image during visits with preadolescents and adolescents
- There is some evidence that regular family dinners may have some protective effect.

ETIOLOGY
- Personality traits of low self-esteem, self-regulatory difficulties, frustration, intolerance, and impaired ability to recognize and express feelings directly have been described in patients with bulimia nervosa.
- There appears to be a small positive association between childhood sexual abuse, traumatic events, PTSD, and the development of an eating disorder, but the size and nature of this association is as yet unknown.
- May be 2 subtypes:
  - Multi-impulsive: Patient relies on bingeing and purging as a way of regulating intolerable states of tension, anger, and fragmentation.
  - Postdieting: Binge eating is precipitated by dietary restraint with compensatory behaviors maintained by reduction of guilty feelings associated with fears of weight gain.

- Neuroendocrine abnormalities may also play a role: Abnormalities in serotonergic and vagal function have been demonstrated in patients with bulimia nervosa.
- Cholecystokinin response to a meal is decreased in patients with bulimia nervosa, which may also indicate abnormal satiety signaling.
- May be abnormalities in other hormones or neurotransmitters, such as leptin, dopamine, and endorphins, but unclear if these are cause or effect

DIAGNOSIS

HISTORY
- Eating-disorder specific:
  - Eating habits
  - Rituals, behaviors
  - Body image
  - Actual and desired weights, minimum and maximum weights
  - Use of laxatives, diuretics, diet pills, emetics
  - Presence of binge or purge behavior
  - Menstrual history
  - History of exercise
  - Unease with other people watching them eat
  - Preoccupation with food/eating
  - Preoccupation with body weight/shape
  - Fear of loss of control over one's body
- General:
  - Weakness or fatigue, or hyperactivity
  - Thirst, frequent urination
  - Headaches
  - Abdominal pain, fullness, or bloating; nausea
  - Constipation or diarrhea
- Psychiatric:
  - Mood disorder
  - Substance abuse
  - Anxiety
  - Personality disorders
  - Suicidal tendencies
  - Low self-esteem
  - Feelings of ineffectiveness
- Family:
  - Medical and psychiatric histories

PHYSICAL EXAM
- Vital signs: Check for hypotension
- Weight: May be normal, overweight, or underweight
- Edema of hands and feet: Evidence of low albumin or compensatory renal sodium and water retention
- Calluses on knuckles or hands: Russell sign secondary to inducing vomiting
- Erosion of dental enamel: Exposure to gastric juices secondary to frequent vomiting
- Muscle cramps or weakness: Hypokalemia
- Special questions:
  - How much do you want to weigh?
  - How do you control your weight?
  - How do you feel about yourself?
  - How often do you vomit, use diuretics or laxatives?

DIAGNOSTIC TESTS & INTERPRETATION
Lab
- Perform a laboratory evaluation as part of the diagnostic workup. Laboratory evaluation is most useful for assessing complications; there is no diagnostic or confirmatory laboratory test for bulimia nervosa. Many patients have normal laboratory studies.
- CBC: Iron-deficiency anemia
- Electrolytes, including calcium, magnesium, and phosphate: Abnormalities may occur as a result of prolonged vomiting or use of laxatives.
- BUN and creatinine: Renal function usually normal, but BUN may be elevated secondary to dehydration or low secondary to protein loss
- Glucose: Patient may be hypoglycemic.
- Cholesterol, lipids: May be elevated in starvation states
- Amylase: Pancreatitis
- Total protein, albumin, prealbumin: Usually normal, but may be low as evidence of malnutrition
- Liver function tests: Transaminases may be mildly elevated (up to twice normal).
- ESR: Almost invariably normal; if elevated, consider occult organic process
- Total carbon dioxide: Metabolic alkalosis from vomiting or metabolic acidosis if using laxatives
- Urine toxicology screen (optional): May be positive, as this disorder often is associated with substance abuse

Imaging
- Electrocardiogram with rhythm strip: May reveal U waves associated with hypokalemia
- Consider upper GI series with small-bowel follow-through
- Consider dual-energy x-ray absorptiometry (DEXA) scan if prolonged amenorrhea, to evaluate bone density

Diagnostic Procedures/Other
Eating disorder questionnaires: Questionnaire assessments appear to be equivalent to diagnostic interview in diagnosing bulimia nervosa.

DIFFERENTIAL DIAGNOSIS
- Psychogenic vomiting
- Drug abuse
- GI obstruction
- Hiatal hernia

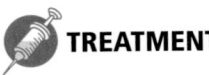 **TREATMENT**

MEDICATION (DRUGS)
- Antidepressants:
  - Decrease the binge–purge behavior
  - Improve attitudes about eating
  - Lessen preoccupation with food and weight
  - Fluoxetine (Prozac), sertraline (Zoloft), desipramine, citalopram, and fluvoxamine (Luvox) have been used with good results in patients with bulimia nervosa.
  - Effect of antidepressant may diminish over time, and patient may relapse when drug is stopped.
  - Psychotherapy combined with antidepressant therapy appears to have the best outcome.

– Response rate to alternative treatments after cognitive behavioral therapy and antidepressant first-line therapy is generally low.
– Few studies either of medication or psychotherapy have included patients under 18 years of age, so preferred therapy in these patients is still uncertain.
• Stool softeners: Often of little use for constipation; consider nonstimulating osmotic laxatives if severe
• Ondansetron: Shown in 1 study to decrease vomiting frequency; may help normalize the physiologic mechanism controlling satiation

ADDITIONAL TREATMENT
General Measures
• Outpatient psychotherapy
• Cognitive behavioral therapy (CBT):
– More effective than interpersonal psychotherapy or behavioral therapy alone. The psychotherapy with the best evidence of efficacy
– Helps patients determine other ways to cope with the feelings that precipitate purging and to try to correct maladaptive beliefs about body image
– May also be done in a self-help format, which may be effective as well. Self-help manual format also showing promise
– 1 study of CBT in adolescents showed considerable promise.
• Individual interpersonal psychotherapy also helpful in longer term
• Family treatment (to help with dysfunctional family dynamics)
• Group therapy
• During treatment, patients and their families may cause "splitting" of the hospital staff. To avoid this, always be supportive and maintain consistency in stating goals.

Additional Therapies
Physical activity was shown in 1 study to reduce the pursuit of thinness and to decrease bingeing/purging behavior. Both physical activity and yoga have shown promise as adjunct treatments.

IN-PATIENT CONSIDERATIONS
Initial Stabilization
Hospitalize in cases of:
• Hypovolemia
• Severe electrolyte disturbances
• Intractable vomiting
• Acute psychiatric emergencies (e.g., suicidal ideation, acute psychosis)
• Medical complication of malnutrition (e.g., aspiration pneumonia, cardiac failure, pancreatitis, Mallory–Weiss syndrome)
• Comorbid diagnosis that interferes with the treatment of the eating disorder (e.g., severe depression, obsessive-compulsive disorder, severe family dysfunction)
• Failure of outpatient therapy

 ONGOING CARE

FOLLOW-UP RECOMMENDATIONS
• Reduction in binge and purge episodes may take months or years.
• Behavioral and thought disorders associated with bulimia nervosa may be of long duration.

Patient Monitoring
Signs to watch for:
• Weight loss or major weight fluctuations
• Electrolyte abnormalities
• Muscle cramps
• Fatigue
• Depression or mood disturbance
• Willful behavior or acting out

PROGNOSIS
• Very low mortality: 0.3% (but may be underestimated secondary to poor follow-up in studies)
• Most patients have episodic course with trend toward improvement.
• No studies of long-term prognosis in adolescents
• Adult studies: 5–10-year follow-up:
– 50% made full recovery
– 30% relapsed
– 20% still met full criteria for bulimia nervosa
• Poor prognostic indicators:
– Concomitant depression, personality disorder, or substance abuse
– Frequent vomiting
– History of substance abuse
• Good prognostic indicators:
– High motivation for treatment
– No concurrent disruptive psychopathology
– Good self-esteem

COMPLICATIONS
• Pulmonary:
– Aspiration pneumonia
– Pneumomediastinum
• GI:
– Pancreatitis
– Parotid or salivary gland enlargement
– Gastric and esophageal irritation and gastroesophageal reflux
– Mallory–Weiss tears
– Paralytic ileus (due to laxative abuse and hypokalemia)
– Severe constipation (due to laxative abuse and subsequent dependence)
• Metabolic:
– Hypokalemia (due to laxative abuse or vomiting)
– Secondary cardiac dysrhythmias, myopathy, ileus
– Electrolyte imbalances, including hypomagnesemia; acid–base disturbances
– Fluid imbalances
– Hyperamylasemia
– Edema (secondary to hypoproteinemia or renal sodium and water retention secondary to hypovolemia and secondary hyperaldosteronism)
– Bone loss (if amenorrhea; significantly more common in anorexia nervosa)
• Dental:
– Enamel erosion
– Caries and periodontal disease

ADDITIONAL READING
• Abraham SF, von Lojewski A, Anderson G, et al. Feelings: What questions best discriminate women with and without eating disorders? *Eat Weight Disord*. 2009;14:e6–e10.
• Agras WS, Walsh BT, Fairburn CG, et al. A multicenter comparison of cognitive-behavioral therapy and interpersonal psychotherapy for bulimia nervosa. *Arch Gen Psychiatry*. 2000;57:459–466.
• Carei TR, Fyfe-Johnson AL, Breuner CC, et al. Randomized controlled clinical trial of yoga in the treatment of eating disorders. *J Adolesc Health*. 2010;46:346–351.
• Faris PL, Eckert ED, Kim SW, et al. Evidence for a vagal pathophysiology for bulimia nervosa and the accompanying depressive symptoms. *J Affective Dis*. 2006;92:79–90.
• Favano A, Caregaro L, Tenani E, et al. Time trends in age of onset of anorexia nervosa and bulimia nervosa. *J Clin Psychiatry*. 2009;70:1715–1721.
• Haines J, Gillman MW, Rifas-Shiman S, et al. Family dinner and disordered eating behaviors in a large cohort of adolescents. *Brunner-Mazel Eating Disorders Monograph Series*. 2010;18(1):10–24.
• Hay PP, Bacatchuk J, Stefano S, et al. Psychological treatment for bulimia nervosa and binging. *Cochrane Database Syst Rev*. 2009;4:CD000562.
• Kreipe RE, Birndorf SA. Eating disorders in adolescent and young adults. *Med Clin North Am*. 2000;84:1027–1049.
• Mehler PS. Clinical practice: Bulimia nervosa. *N Engl J Med*. 2003;349:875–881.
• Schapman-Williams AM, Lock J, Courturier J. Cognitive-behavioral therapy for adolescents with binge eating syndromes: A case series. *Int J Eat Disord*. 2006;39:252–255.
• Smolak L, Murnen SK. A meta-analytic examination of the relationship between childhood sexual abuse and eating disorders. *Int J Eat Disord*. 2002;31:136–150.

 CODES

ICD9
307.51 Bulimia nervosa

ICD10
• F50.2 Bulimia nervosa
• F50.9 Eating disorder, unspecified

FAQ
• Q: How do I determine if a patient has anorexia with vomiting or bulimia?
• A: The key feature of bulimia nervosa is the binge episode, which distinguishes it from anorexia nervosa. If there are not at least 2 binge eating episodes per week for at least 3 months, the diagnosis is not bulimia.
• Q: What laboratory abnormalities should I look for in my patients with bulimia?
• A: Electrolyte abnormalities, particularly hypokalemia. Patients may develop a hypochloremic metabolic alkalosis. If electrolytes are significantly abnormal, the patient should be hospitalized until they have normalized.

C1 ESTERASE INHIBITOR DEFICIENCY

Judith Kelsen

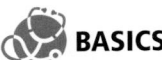 **BASICS**

DESCRIPTION

- A hereditary and acquired form of recurrent angioedema. The attacks are usually without urticaria.
- Has been classified into a number of types, including:
  - Hereditary angioedema (HAE) type I (transmitted as autosomal dominant)
  - HAE type II (transmitted as autosomal dominant)
  - Acquired angioedema (AAE) type I, II, III, IV
  - AAE type II
- HAE type I accounts for ~85% of the C1 esterase deficiencies and is a genetic alteration that leads to impairment of mRNA transcription or translation and, therefore, decreased enzyme synthesis. Often thought of as quantitative deficiency.
- HAE type II is a genetic alteration that leads to production of an inactive protein. May be thought of as a qualitative deficiency.
- HAE type III is an estrogen-dependent form; typical clinical features of type I with normal C1 INH level and function and normal C4. These cases are all female and have dominant mode of inheritance.
- In acquired deficiency of C1 esterase inhibitor, (C1-INH) there appears to be a normal ability to synthesize the enzyme; however, the enzyme is metabolized at an increased rate. This syndrome may be seen in patients with autoimmune diseases or malignancy and usually occurs after the 4th decade of life.
- AAE type I is a very rare syndrome usually associated with lymphoproliferative (usually B-cell) carcinomas, autoimmune diseases, and paraproteinemias. Because of the other disease processes, complement-activating factors and idiotype–anti-idiotype complexes act to increase consumption of C1-INH.

- AAE type II develops when an autoantibody is produced against the C1-INH protein. When these antibodies adhere to the C1 esterase molecule, conformational change occurs, leading to decreased function or enhanced metabolism. This type is often associated with autoimmune disorders.
- AAE type III: Associated with sex hormones (specifically in pregnancy).
- AAE type IV: Drug-induced AAE, particular associated with ACE inhibitors or angiotensin receptor blockers.
- AAE forms may be differentiated from HAE by genetic studies and serologically by significantly decreased C1q, C1r, and C1s levels, and decreased functional activity of the enzyme in AAE

EPIDEMIOLOGY

Incidence
1:50,000

Genetics
HAE type I and II are transmitted as autosomal dominant.

PATHOPHYSIOLOGY

- C1-INH is a single-chain polypeptide with a molecular weight of 108 kd. The gene has been identified on chromosome 11 (11q12–q13.1). It is involved in the control of vascular permeability.
- C-INH is a member of the serpin family of serine protease inhibitors, produced in the liver.
- This protein inhibits the classic complement pathway by inhibiting activation of C2 and C4. In the fibrinolytic system, C1-INH inhibits formation of plasmin, the activation of C1r and C1s, and the formation of bradykinin from kininogen.
- Deficiency of this enzyme results in activation of the classic complement system along with fibrinolysis and kinin formation, which is felt to participate in the production of angioedema.
- Kinin is known to cause similar histologic lesions to histamine, but without pruritus.
- The complement activation leads to production of C2b, a product that also has kininlike activity, and bradykinin, a vasoactive peptide that may also participate in the formation of angioedema.

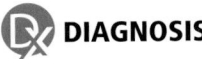 **DIAGNOSIS**

HISTORY

- Presentation: Patients with HAE usually present in the 2nd decade of life with angioedema involving the subcutaneous tissues (mostly involving the extremities).
- Attacks can be precipitated by trauma, infection, or pregnancy.
- Classically the edema develops gradually over several hours and increases slowly over 12–36 hours.
- However, patients may experience abdominal attacks with sudden and very severe onset without visible edema.
- GI effects: Predominant symptom in 25% of patients: Angioedema involving the GI tract may lead to severe pain, vomiting, and diarrhea as well as ascites. Secondary to transient edema of small bowel resulting in intestinal obstruction, ascites and hemoconcentration.
- Respiratory complications: 2 of 3 patients will have orofacial or laryngeal swelling.
- Hives: The edema usually occurs without evidence of inflammation; rash resembles urticaria (however, episodes of urticaria have also been documented).
- The variability of clinical manifestations, even among individuals with the same genetic mutation, is striking, implicating nongenetic factors or other genes as possible mediators of clinical presentation.
- Emesis
- Diarrhea
- Hypotension from extravasation of plasma into the skin
- Hemoconcentration
- Azotemia
- CNS complaints, including headache, hemiparesis, and seizures, may be triggered by trauma or stress.
- AAE presents similarly, in the same way but usually in the 4th decade of life; not associated with a familial history.

PHYSICAL EXAM

Depending on the clinical features, angioedema causes pale, well-demarcated, tense, brawny, nonpruritic, and nonpitting single or multiple localized swellings. These may involve the periorbital tissues, genitalia, face, tongue, lips, larynx, extremities, and GI tract.

DIAGNOSTIC TESTS & INTERPRETATION

Lab

- C1-INH concentration
- C1-INH activity
- C4 concentration: Low serum level
- C4D: Cleavage product of C4, low even when C4 is normal
- C1q concentration (usually lower in patients with AAE)

DIFFERENTIAL DIAGNOSIS

- IgE mediated:
  - Episodic angioedema
  - Allergic reactions to food and drugs
  - Physically induced angioedema
- Hypocomplementemic HAE
- Idiosyncratic:
  - NSAIDs
  - Other drugs
- Lupus erythematosus
- Idiopathic

 TREATMENT

ADDITIONAL TREATMENT

General Measures

- During an acute episode, management focuses on adequate respiratory and fluid resuscitation and the treatment of pain.
- In HAE, acute attacks are treated with replacement of the C1-INH with IV concentrates. Fresh frozen plasma may also be used.
- A recent study has demonstrated that the time to onset of symptom relief is an appropriate end point for assessing the efficacy of C1-INH therapy.
- For prophylaxis, androgens (such as danazol and stanozolol) are used in postpubertal patients with HAE of both types. These androgens stimulate the synthesis of C1 inhibitor, and although the level of activity is not normalized, it is increased sufficiently to be clinically efficacious.

- In prepubertal children, androgens are used only in those with severe attacks; purified C1-INH can be used if available. Antifibrinolytics should be used in prepubertal children over androgens.
- Patients should avoid estrogen OCP or use with caution.
- For patients who do not tolerate androgens, tranexamic acid and ε-aminocaproic acid (antifibrinolytic inhibitors or plasmin activity) may be used, although they carry the risk of significant side effects.
- AAE type I patients may respond to epinephrine for reversal of airway compromise.
- AAE type I requires an intensive search for malignancy, although this form of AAE occasionally appears before the development of clinical signs of the malignancy.
- Androgens are also effective in preventing attacks in individuals with this syndrome.
- AAE type II requires immunosuppression to decrease formation of the autoantibody.
- These patients may respond to C1-INH concentrate.
- Androgen treatment has not led to good clinical response.
- Prophylaxis prior to dental procedures or surgery: High-dose danazol
- Potential treatment: Plasma kallikrein antagonists Bradykinin antagonists Serine protease inhibitors
- Genetic counseling: Given autosomal dominant inheritance, family counseling is important.

IN-PATIENT CONSIDERATIONS

Initial Stabilization

Therapy is divided into management of the acute attack, maintenance therapy for HAE, and more specific interventions for those with AAE.

ADDITIONAL READING

- Agostoni A, Aygoren-Pursun E, Binkley KE, et al. Hereditary and acquired angioedema: Problems and progress: Proceedings of the third C1 esterase inhibitor deficiency workshop and beyond. *J Allergy Clin Immunol*. 2004;114(3 Suppl):S51–S131.
- Bernstein J. Hereditary Angioedema: Validation of the endpoint time to onset of relief by correlation with symptom intensity. *Asthma Allergy Proc*. 2011;32(1):36–42.
- Csepregi A, Nemesanszky E. Acquired C1 esterase inhibitor deficiency. *Ann Intern Med*. 2000;133: 838–839.
- Frank MM. Update on preventive therapy (prophylaxis) of hereditary angioedema. *Asthma Allergy Proc*. 2011;32(1):17–21.
- Gompels M, Lock R, Abinun M. C1 inhibitor deficiency: Consensus document. *Clin Exp Immunol*. 2005;139:379–394.
- Riedll MA. Update on the acute treatment of hereditary angioedema. *Asthma Allergy Proc*. 2011;32(1):11–16.
- Weiler C, Van Dellen R. Genetic tests indications and interpretations in patients with hereditary angioedema. *Mayo Clin Proc*. 2006;81(7):958–972.

 CODES

ICD9

- 277.6 Other deficiencies of circulating enzymes
- 279.8 Other specified disorders involving the immune mechanism

ICD10

D84.1 Defects in the complement system

FAQ

- Q: What are other causes of angioedema?
- A:
  - Classic allergic reactions to food and drugs
  - Physically induced angioedema
  - IgE-mediated episodic angioedema
  - Idiosyncratic reactions to nonsteroidal anti-inflammatory and other drugs
  - Lupus erythematosus
  - Idiopathic causes
- Q: What are the usual precipitating factors in causing reactions?
- A: Recurrent episodes of angioedema, abdominal pain, nausea, and vomiting that occur spontaneously or after local trauma, especially to the upper respiratory tract:
  - Vigorous exercise
  - Emotional stress
  - Menstruation

CAMPYLOBACTER INFECTIONS

Matthew P. Kronman
Eric J. Haas (5th edition)
Louis M. Bell, Jr. (5th edition)

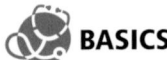 **BASICS**

DESCRIPTION
- *Campylobacter* is a motile, curved, microaerophilic, non–lactose-fermenting, oxidase-positive Gram-negative rod that requires oxygen and carbon dioxide for optimal growth.
- Three main *Campylobacter* species involved in human infections include *C. jejuni* and *C. coli* (which cause enteritis) and *C. fetus* (implicated in systemic illness). Rarer human pathogens include *C. concisus*, *C. curvus*, *C. hyointestinalis*, *C. lari*, *C. rectus*, *C. sputorum*, and *C. upsaliensis*.

EPIDEMIOLOGY
- *Campylobacter* infections are among the most common causes of enteritis worldwide, with the highest attack rates observed in children <4 years.
- More than 2 million cases of *Campylobacter* infection are estimated to occur in the U.S. annually.
- Estimated rates of *Campylobacter* infection vary widely worldwide. In the U.S., the estimated annual rate is 12.7/100,000, and the highest rate is in New Zealand at 396/100,000.
- 30–100% of chickens, turkeys, and water fowl are infected asymptomatically. Other reservoirs of infection include swine, cattle, sheep, horses, rodents, household pets (especially young pets), and contaminated water and milk.
- Transmission of disease is by the fecal-oral route from contaminated food and water or by direct contact with fecal material from animals or persons infected with the organism.
- 40% of *Campylobacter* enteritis is estimated to be attributable to chicken consumption; other risk factors for *Campylobacter* enteritis include use of acid-suppressive medications and consumption of chicken prepared outside the home.
- Frequent exposure to *Campylobacter* (e.g., among food handlers and abattoir workers), may protect against disease.
- Person-to-person transmission of *C. jejuni* has been reported when the index cases were young children who were incontinent of feces; vertical transmission from mother to neonate has also been reported.
- Asymptomatic hospital personnel or food handlers have not been implicated as sources.
- The peak rate of isolation occurs in the warmer months of the year (late summer, early fall).
- *Campylobacter* is the most common cause of travelers' diarrhea in Southeast Asia, accounting for a third of all infections.

- Compared with 1996–1998, foodborne illnesses caused by *Campylobacter* in the U.S. decreased 30% in 2009.
- Resistance to fluoroquinolones and macrolides is becoming increasingly common—both ranging from ~20–40% in the U.S. and as high as >80% in some parts of the world—and thought to be related to both human and agricultural use of antibiotics.

GENERAL PREVENTION
- Hand washing after contact with animals or animal products, cleaning cooking utensils and cutting boards after contact with raw poultry, proper cooling and storage of foods, pasteurization of milk, and chlorination of water supplies will decrease the overall risk for infection.
- Diapered infants with symptomatic infection should be excluded from child care until resolution of diarrhea.
- In the hospital setting, contact precautions are recommended for infected infants and children who are incontinent of stool and should be maintained until the patient receives at least 48 hours of antibiotic treatment.
- Certain *C. jejuni* strains with decreased risk of secondary Guillain-Barré syndrome (GBS) are being considered as candidates for vaccine development.

PATHOPHYSIOLOGY
- *Campylobacter* spp. possess 1 or 2 flagella that provide the organism's motility and facilitate intestinal colonization.
- *C. jejuni* adheres to epithelial cells and mucus, secretes cytotoxins (which play a role in the development of watery diarrhea), can invade intestinal epithelial cells, and induces an inflammatory ileocolitis.
- As few as 500 organisms may be required to produce infection.
- Bacteremia, although uncommon, can occur, especially in the neonate and immunocompromised host; *C. fetus* is the species most likely to be isolated. *C. fetus* can also cause neonatal meningitis.
- *C. upsaliensis*, *C. lari*, and *C. hyointestinalis* have been identified in immunocompromised individuals and are usually associated with a self-limiting enteritis but can occasionally cause systemic illness.

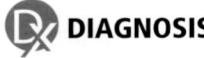 **DIAGNOSIS**

HISTORY
- Fever, abdominal pain, bloody diarrhea? Illness is characterized by fever, abdominal pain, and bloody diarrhea. Symptoms can last for 24 hours and be indistinguishable from a viral gastroenteritis, or can be relapsing, thus mimicking inflammatory bowel disease.
- Abdominal pain, diarrhea, malaise, and fever: Signs and symptoms of *C. jejuni* infection.
- Duration of symptoms? Incubation period is 1–7 days and is usually self-limited by 5–7 days.
- Inflammatory ileocolitis? The most common manifestation in children.
- If the infection establishes a chronic phase (20% of infected patients), symptoms may mimic inflammatory bowel disease and other immunoreactive complications may occur.

Exposures:
- Inadequately cooked poultry or poultry prepared outside the home? Chickens are asymptomatic carriers.
- Exposure to unpasteurized milk products? Unpasteurized milk is a source of *Campylobacter* infection.
- Well water used? Contaminated water serves as a reservoir.
- New pets or young pets? Young animals (dogs and cats) may be reservoirs of infection.

DIAGNOSTIC TESTS & INTERPRETATION
Diagnostic Procedures/Other
- Examination of fecal specimen for darting motility of *C. jejuni* by darkfield or phase-contrast microscopy, if examined within 2 hours of passage, can permit presumptive diagnosis.
- Stool culture: Can be used, but selective media (Skirrow, Butzler, or campy-BAP), microaerophilic conditions, and an incubation temperature of 42°C must be used to isolate *Campylobacter* species.
- DNA-based testing: Development of this diagnostic tool will improve the ability to detect and differentiate *Campylobacter* spp. much faster than the current gold standard of stool culture.

ALERT
Not all bacterial colitis presents with blood or mucus in the stool. Therefore, increased suspicion for bacterial colitis should exist if the diarrhea is prolonged or the patient has significant environmental exposures.

DIFFERENTIAL DIAGNOSIS

- *Campylobacter* infection should be considered in all patients with a diarrheal illness, especially those with a history of bloody or mucous stools, recurrent gastritis, or in immunocompromised hosts.
- Other important intestinal and foodborne bacterial pathogens include *Aeromonas, C. difficile, E. coli, Listeria, Plesiomonas, Salmonella, Shigella, Vibrio* species, and *Yersinia*.
- Viral and parasitic pathogens to consider include Rotavirus, Norovirus, Adenovirus types 40 and 41, *Giardia, Cyclospora,* and *Cryptosporidium*.

TREATMENT

MEDICATION (DRUGS)

- Immunocompetent children with diarrhea usually improve with rehydration alone.
- Select patient populations (HIV and other immunocompromised individuals, pregnant women) may benefit from early therapy.
- If treated early in the course of enteritis (<4 days), erythromycin or azithromycin appear to be effective in eradicating the organism from the stool within 2–3 days.
- Ciprofloxacin, tetracycline, aminoglycosides, and imipenem are alternative antimicrobials if resistant or bacteremic strains are present, although fluoroquinolone resistance in particular is rising.
- Treatment duration for enteritis is 5–7 days.
- Appropriate treatment of bacteremia should be based on antimicrobial susceptibility testing.

ONGOING CARE

FOLLOW-UP RECOMMENDATIONS

- When treated, symptoms should improve in 2–3 days.
- In the untreated patient, the median excretion of organism is to 2–3 weeks, but can be as long as 3 months. Asymptomatic carriage is uncommon in humans.

PROGNOSIS

For patients with enteritis, the prognosis is very good, regardless of whether antibiotic treatment is given.

COMPLICATIONS

- Postinfectious immunologic complications include reactive arthritis, GBS, Miller-Fisher syndrome (a GBS variant predominantly affecting eye movement), Reiter syndrome, and erythema nodosum.
- GBS is estimated to affect 1 in 1000 patients with *Campylobacter* infection.

- *C. jejuni* is the most frequently identified cause of GBS with serotypes O:19 and O:41, and is responsible for up to 40% of GBS cases.
- HLA-B27 antigen is associated with reactive arthropathy. The estimated incidence of reactive arthritis after *Campylobacter* infection ranges from 0% to 7%.
- Seizures may develop in young children with enteritis and high fevers.
- A typhoidlike syndrome and meningitis have also been reported in patients with *Campylobacter* infection.
- Spontaneous abortion and hemolytic-uremic syndrome have been described with *C. upsaliensis*.

ADDITIONAL READING

- Centers for Disease Control and Prevention. Preliminary FoodNet data on the incidence of infection with pathogens transmitted commonly through food—10 states, 2009. *MMWR Morb Mortal Wkly Rep.* 2009;59:418–422.
- Janssen R, Krogfelt KA, Cawthraw SA, et al. Host-pathogen interactions in Campylobacter infections: The host perspective. *Clin Microbiol Rev.* 2008;21(3):505–518.
- Luangtongkum T, Jeon B, Han J, et al. Antibiotic resistance in *Campylobacter*: Emergence, transmission and persistence. *Future Microbiol.* 2009;4(2):189–200.
- Shah N, DuPont HL, Ramsey DJ. Global etiology of travelers' diarrhea: Systematic review from 1973 to the present. *Am J Trop Med Hyg.* 2009;80(4):609–614.
- Tam CC, Higgins CD, Neal KR, et al. Chicken consumption and use of acid-suppressing medications as risk factors for *Campylobacter enteritis*, England. *Emerg Infect Dis.* 2009;15(9):1402–1408.
- van Putten JP, van Alphen LB, Wosten MM, et al. Molecular mechanisms of campylobacter infection. *Curr Top Microbiol Immunol.* 2009;337:197–229.

 CODES

ICD9
008.43 Intestinal infection due to campylobacter

ICD10
A04.5 Campylobacter enteritis

FAQ

- Q: Is treatment necessary if the child is asymptomatic by the time the *Campylobacter* is isolated as the pathogen causing the enteritis?
- A: No treatment is needed in this situation. Therapy for symptomatic patients, although it may be of benefit, has not been proven efficacious.
- Q: Are there any risks of *Campylobacter* infection to pregnant patients?
- A: Women infected symptomatically or asymptomatically may experience recurrent abortions or preterm deliveries. Life-threatening infections to the fetus or newborn are also possible.
- Q: Can one develop immunity to *Campylobacter* infections?
- A: Immunity to *C. jejuni* is acquired after 1 or more infections. For children living in endemic areas, effective natural immunity is a result of significant repeated early exposure with a progressive decrease in the illness/infection ratio as age increases.
- Q: What is the relationship between GBS and *C. jejuni* infection?
- A: Many strains of *C. jejuni* have surface glycolipids that are similar to gangliosides, which are abundant in the central and peripheral nervous systems. Antibody formation from this infection binds to the gangliosides, causing the demyelinating process characteristic of GBS.

C

CANDIDIASIS

Michelle Dunn
Theoklis Zaoutis (5th edition)

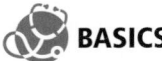 **BASICS**

DESCRIPTION

A spectrum of diseases caused by *Candida* species (yeasts):

- In immunocompetent children, most candidiasis is manifested as superficial mucosal (oropharyngeal candidiasis or thrush) and cutaneous (diaper dermatitis) infection.
- In immunocompromised children, *Candida* may cause invasive and disseminated disease.

EPIDEMIOLOGY

Incidence

Incidence of nosocomial *Candida* infections has risen over the past 20 years, and *Candida* spp. are currently the 3rd most commonly recovered isolates in cases of nosocomial bloodstream infection in premature infants and older children.

RISK FACTORS

Surgery, central venous catheters, prematurity, neonates, total parenteral nutrition, transplant recipients, malignancy, neutropenia, corticosteroid use, antibiotic therapy, and burn patients

GENERAL PREVENTION

- Sterilize bottle nipples and toys to prevent reinoculation of oral candidiasis.
- Avoid unnecessarily long courses of broad-spectrum antibiotics.
- Maintain IV catheters and catheter–skin insertion sites appropriately.
- Some evidence exists for using prophylactic fluconazole in high-risk preterm infants

ETIOLOGY

- Neonatal colonization is acquired from infected vaginal mucosa during birth. Incidence of colonization increases with age of the infant. Transmission also occurs during nursing from the mother's breast or from imperfect sterilization of bottle nipples. Colonization is an important risk factor for invasive infection.
- *C. albicans* is the most common species isolated in children; the remaining infections are caused by other *Candida* spp., including *C. glabrata*, *C. parapsilosis*, and *C. tropicalis*.

COMMONLY ASSOCIATED CONDITIONS

Candida spp. may cause disease at any site.

- Mucosal candidiasis:
  - Oropharyngeal candidiasis (thrush) occurs in up to 40% of healthy newborns. Patches of white, curdish material are visible on the buccal and gingival mucosa. It may cause mouth pain and poor nursing. In older children, it is associated with the use of antibiotics or immunosuppressive drugs, conditions of endocrine or immune dysfunction, and malignancy.

  - Candidal glossitis occurs secondarily to antibiotic therapy. The tongue is smooth and erythematous, and patients complain of glossodynia (painful tongue). Perlèche (angular cheilosis) results from chronic licking of the corners of the mouth and is characterized by fissuring, erythema, and pain.
  - Esophageal candidiasis occurs in HIV-infected patients and those on immunosuppressive therapy; 30% have associated thrush.
- Cutaneous candidiasis:
  - Diaper dermatitis is most common during infancy because of predisposing factors found with diaper use.
  - Intertriginous candidiasis is characterized by a confluent, erythematous, weeping rash with a scaling edge found at skin folds: Axillae, groin, gluteal folds, intramammary region, interdigital spaces, and umbilicus. Predisposing factors in healthy patients include chronic moisture, recent antibiotic use, and obesity.
- Vaginal candidiasis: Characterized by vaginal discharge (curdlike or mucoid), pruritus, vulvar burning, and dysuria. Oral contraceptives, antibiotics, pregnancy, corticosteroids, and immunodeficiency are predisposing conditions. Classified as uncomplicated or complicated:
  - Uncomplicated: 90% of patients; condition is mild to moderate; frequency is sporadic; organism is *C. albicans*; the host is immunocompetent.
  - Complicated: 10% of patients; presence of any one of the following factors defines a complicated infection: Severe, recurrent infection by non-*albicans Candida* spp.; or predisposing host factor
  - The reliability of self-diagnosis is poor (<50% correct); therefore, potassium hydroxide (KOH)/pH testing is suggested for diagnosis.
- Congenital candidiasis: Cutaneous infection acquired from contaminated amniotic fluid that is usually treated with topical antifungal agents and has an excellent prognosis
- Invasive candidiasis:
  - Defined as candidemia and disseminated candidiasis
  - Occurs in the immunocompromised host. Risk factors include prematurity, malignancy, immunodeficiency syndromes, diabetes mellitus, broad-spectrum antibiotic therapy, corticosteroids, chemotherapy, hyperalimentation, indwelling catheters, recent complex surgery, and stem cell or organ transplantation.
  - The most frequent sites of involvement are the GI tract, lungs, kidneys (pyelonephritis, mycetoma), liver, spleen, eyes, and brain (meningoencephalitis). Fungal sepsis may occur. Peritoneal, urinary tract, and cardiac valve candidal infections are most often related to instrumentation or catheterization in the immunocompromised host.

- Chronic mucocutaneous candidiasis:
  - Noninvasive infection of the skin, hair, mucous membranes, and nails
  - Typically seen in the 1st year of life, and almost all cases occur within the 1st decade
  - Caused by a T-cell immunodeficiency resulting in a poor response to candidal antigens. Patients lack a delayed-type hypersensitivity reaction to intradermal injection of candidal antigens.

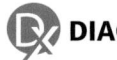 **DIAGNOSIS**

HISTORY

- Recurrent infection:
  - In oral thrush, reinfection may occur from nipples, pacifiers, or toys (see "General Prevention" and "Alert").
  - In recurrent vaginitis, bacterial or non-*albicans Candida* spp. infections are possible.
- Recent antibiotic use: Oral thrush often occurs in infants, but may occur in normal older children after treatment with systemic antibiotics.
- Predisposing conditions: Systemic dissemination of infection is more likely with impaired immunity.
- Visual changes or discomfort: Features of endophthalmitis include eye pain, blurred vision, scotomata, and photophobia.

PHYSICAL EXAM

- Oral lesions: Buccal or lingual mucosa, gingiva, and tongue lesions have a characteristic white, friable pseudomembrane that when scraped away, reveals reddened, denuded, and sometimes ulcerated mucosa.
- Rash:
  - The rash of monilial diaper dermatitis is initially scattered.
  - Erythematous papules progress and coalesce into a deeply erythematous, weeping, confluent rash with a scaling border and satellite lesions.
  - In neonates with congenital candidiasis, skin findings include vesicles, pustules, or a diffuse macular rash.
  - Patients with invasive candidiasis may also present with a diffuse, erythematous rash.

DIAGNOSTIC TESTS & INTERPRETATION

Dilated retinal examination (by an ophthalmologist): Endophthalmitis, a sight-threatening complication, should be excluded in all patients with candidemia.

Lab

- Direct light microscopic examination of specimen:
  - Clinical diagnosis of mucosal, cutaneous, and vaginal candidiasis can be confirmed by microscopic examination of material scraped gently from lesions.
  - KOH preparation (10% or 20% potassium hydroxide) allows visualization of the long, branching, hyphae of *C. albicans*.
  - Vaginal pH remains normal (<4.5) with vaginal candidiasis.

- Fungal culture:
  - *Candida* spp. can be isolated from culture of mucosal or cutaneous scrapings, blood, urine, CSF, bone marrow, tissue biopsy, abscess aspirate, and bronchoalveolar lavage fluid.
  - However, the sensitivity of blood culture is only 50–60% in patients with invasive candidiasis.

Imaging
CT scan, ultrasound, and echocardiogram: Important to identify deep organ lesions (liver, spleen, brain, kidney, or heart) associated with disseminated infection

DIFFERENTIAL DIAGNOSIS
- Oral lesions:
  - Aphthous stomatitis
  - Acute necrotizing gingivitis
  - Herpes gingivostomatitis
  - Other viral causes of stomatitis (e.g., coxsackievirus)
- Diaper dermatitis: Atopic, seborrheic, bacterial, or occlusional
- Intertriginous infections: Seborrheic and atopic dermatitidis
- Vaginitis
- Congenital candidiasis:
  - Viral infections (especially herpes viruses)
  - Bacterial infections
  - Benign neonatal skin conditions
- Invasive candidiasis: Bacterial infection or other fungal infection
- Chronic mucocutaneous candidiasis: HIV

 TREATMENT

MEDICATION (DRUGS)
- Oral candidiasis: Nystatin suspension until 2 days after lesions have cleared. In older patients, nystatin as a swish-swallow suspension or in oral tablet form for >7 days is effective. Clotrimazole lozenges are also effective; 10 mg dissolved in mouth 5 times daily for 7 days.
  - Fluconazole and ketoconazole are effective for infections that are persistent or occur in immunocompromised hosts. Azole-resistant *C. albicans* has been described in HIV-infected individuals with recurrent infection.
- Esophageal candidiasis:
  - A therapeutic trial with fluconazole for patients with presumed esophageal candidiasis is a cost-effective alternative to endoscopy;
    ○ Symptoms should resolve within 7 days after the start of therapy.
    ○ A 14–21-day course is recommended. Itraconazole solution and IV amphotericin B are acceptable alternatives.

- Cutaneous or intertriginous candidiasis and candidal diaper dermatitis:
  - Both are treated by keeping the area dry and using nystatin (100,000 U/g q.i.d.) until the rash has cleared.
  - Topical regimens of clotrimazole 1%, miconazole 2%, ketoconazole 2%, and econazole 1% are also effective.
- Uncomplicated vaginal candidiasis:
  - Topical agents are highly effective in uncomplicated infections (cure rates >80%): clotrimazole, miconazole, butoconazole, and terconazole (dose varies with 1-, 3-, or 7-day treatment).
  - Oral agents are also effective: Fluconazole (10 mg/kg up to 150 mg as a single dose), ketoconazole (400 mg daily for 5 days), and itraconazole (200 mg b.i.d. for 1 day or 200 mg daily for 3 days)
- Complicated vaginal candidiasis:
  - Extend antimycotic therapy to 7–14 days
  - Non-*albicans* species of *Candida* usually respond to topical boric acid (600 mg/d for 14 days). Azole-resistant *C. albicans* infections are extremely rare in the immunocompetent host.
- Recurrent vaginitis (more than 4 episodes of proven infection during a 12-month period):
  - Usually caused by azole-susceptible *C. albicans*
  - Induction therapy with 2 weeks of a topical or oral azole is followed by a maintenance regimen for 6 months.
  - Suitable maintenance regimens include fluconazole (150 mg weekly), ketoconazole (100 mg daily), itraconazole (100 mg every other day), or daily therapy with a topical azole.
- Systemic or disseminated candidiasis:
  - Begin treatment in hospital because of severity of illness, underlying disease process, and need for the IV route of drug administration.
  - Address predisposing factors (e.g., removal of indwelling catheters).
  - Antifungal agents commonly used in children include amphotericin B, fluconazole, or the combination of fluconazole plus amphotericin B (with the amphotericin B administered for the 1st 5 or 6 days only).
- Fluconazole may be used in those infected with a *Candida* sp. known to be fluconazole susceptible. Many *C. glabrata* and *C. krusei* are resistant.
- Flucytosine could be considered in combination with amphotericin B for more severe infections. It should not be used alone because resistance quickly develops.
- Lipid-based amphotericin B: 3–6 mg/kg/d IV. Appropriate for patients who are refractory to, intolerant of, or at high risk of being intolerant of conventional amphotericin B preparations
- Intolerance to conventional amphotericin B is usually defined as initial renal insufficiency (creatinine clearance <25 mL/min), significant rise in creatinine during therapy (to 2.5 mg/dL in adults or 1.5 mg/dL in children), or severe acute administration-related toxicity. The toxicity of amphotericin (rigors, anemia, thrombocytopenia, and renal failure) requires close monitoring and may limit its use.

- Caspofungin, only available IV, is approved for candidal esophagitis, candidemia, and other invasive candidal infections.
- Duration of therapy is longer for candidal meningitis (4 weeks), endophthalmitis (6–12 weeks), endocarditis (>6 weeks following surgical therapy), and osteomyelitis (6–12 months).

ALERT
Pitfalls:
- Failure to eliminate source of reinfection. Recurrent thrush in a breast-fed infant may indicate *C. albicans* colonization of the mother's nipples; this can be eliminated by treatment of the nipples with nystatin cream.
- Failure to consider that symptoms of persistent vaginitis may be caused by non-*albicans Candida* spp. or by bacteria (see "Vaginitis")
- Failure to maintain a high index of suspicion for invasive candidiasis in an immunocompromised patient. Persistent fevers despite antibiotic therapy, diffuse rash, and visual complaints are important clues.

ADDITIONAL READING

- Fisher BT, Zaoutis TE. Caspofungin for the treatment of pediatric fungal infection. *Pediatr Infect Dis J.* 2008;27:1099–1102.
- Maródi L, Johnston RB Jr. Invasive *Candida* species disease in infants and children: Occurrence, risk factors, management, and innate host defense mechanisms. *Curr Opin Pediatr.* 2007;19(6): 693–697.
- Pappas PG, Rex JH, Sobel JD, et al. Guidelines for the treatment of candidiasis. *Clin Infect Dis.* 2004;38:161–189.
- Zaoutis TE, Argon J, Berlin JA, et al. The epidemiology and attributable outcomes of candidemia in adults and children hospitalized in the United States: A propensity analysis. *Clin Infect Dis.* 2005;41:1232–1239.
- Zaoutis T, Walsh TJ. Antifungal therapy for neonatal candidiasis. *Curr Opin Infect Dis.* 2007;20:592–597.

 CODES

ICD9
- 112.0 Candidiasis of mouth
- 112.89 Other candidiasis of other specified sites
- 771.7 Neonatal Candida infection

ICD10
- B37.0 Candidal stomatitis
- P37.5 Neonatal candidiasis
- B37.9 Candidiasis, unspecified

FAQ

- Q: When should an older child with thrush be worked up for possible immunodeficiency?
- A: Thrush in the older child is usually caused by recent antibiotic or steroid treatment. If no apparent cause is found, an immunologic evaluation that includes HIV testing should be considered.

CARBON MONOXIDE POISONING

Kevin Osterhoudt

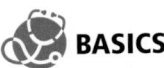 **BASICS**

DESCRIPTION
- Carbon monoxide (CO) is an odorless gas produced via incomplete combustion of carbonaceous fuels.
- CO poisoning occurs when carboxyhemoglobin and CO accumulation leads to impaired physiologic function.

EPIDEMIOLOGY
CO poisoning is the leading cause of death by poisoning within the US.

Incidence
- More than 136,000 CO exposures were reported to the American Association of Poison Control Centers in 2009, with ~1/3 of such exposures occurring in children.
- Seasonal cold weather leads to increases in incidence of exposure.

GENERAL PREVENTION
- Furnaces should receive regular maintenance by skilled technicians.
- Automobiles, gas-powered machinery, and nonelectrical space heaters should only be used with proper ventilation.
- CO detectors should be installed within living spaces.

PATHOPHYSIOLOGY
- On inhalation, some CO binds to hemoglobin to form carboxyhemoglobin.
- Carboxyhemoglobin does not carry oxygen.
- Carboxyhemoglobin produces an allosteric leftward shift of the oxyhemoglobin dissociation curve.
- Carboxyhemoglobin elimination half-life:
  - ~4 hours in room air
  - 1–2 hours in 100% oxygen
  - 20 minutes in 100% oxygen at 3 atmospheres
- CO interacts with cellular proteins, leading to impaired mitochondrial function.
- CO is a source of oxidative stress and poisoning may begin a cascade of inflammatory vasculitis within the CNS.

ETIOLOGY
- Common sources of CO exposure include:
  - Automobile or boat exhaust
  - Smoke inhalation from house fires
  - Oil, gas, or kerosene space heaters or cooking stoves
  - Portable electricity generators and construction equipment
  - Faulty home furnaces
- The solvent methylene chloride is metabolized to CO by the liver after ingestion, inhalation, or dermal absorption.

COMMONLY ASSOCIATED CONDITIONS
Victims of house fires may suffer from thermal injury and/or cyanide poisoning.

 DIAGNOSIS

Many emergency medical services crews carry CO detectors.

HISTORY
- Health of family members?
  - CO is an environmental gas that often sickens multiple household members.
- Use of furnace or space heaters?
  - May suggest source of exposure
- Time of exposure?
  - Carboxyhemoglobin levels must be interpreted with consideration to their timing.
- Duration of exposure?
  - Toxicity is related to both magnitude and duration of exposure.
- Loss of consciousness?
  - Syncope appears to be the best clinical predictor of delayed neurologic sequelae.
- Signs and symptoms:
  - Mild CO intoxication:
    - Malaise
    - Nausea
    - Light-headedness
    - Headache
    - Vomiting
  - Moderate to severe CO intoxication:
    - Confusion
    - Syncope
    - Weakness
    - Angina

PHYSICAL EXAM
- Soot on nasal mucosa: Suggests possibility of thermal pulmonary injury
- Hypotension: Suggests severe CO poisoning
- Cherry red skin: This classic sign is mostly a postmortem finding.

DIAGNOSTIC TESTS & INTERPRETATION
Lab
- Co-oximetry: Allows quantitation of carboxyhemoglobin
- Arterial blood gas: Allows accurate assessment of oxygenation
- Hemoglobin quantitation: The percent carboxyhemoglobin concentration must be considered in relation to the total hemoglobin.
- Serum bicarbonate: A wide anion gap metabolic acidosis suggests the accumulation of lactate, which may result from severe CO poisoning or concomitant cyanide poisoning.
- Creatine kinase: CO poisoning victims are susceptible to rhabdomyolysis.
- Troponin: CO poisoning may lead to myocardial injury.
- ECG: Hypoxemia and metabolic poisoning may lead to cardiac ischemia.

Imaging
- Neuroimaging:
  - Not routinely helpful in acute management
- Globus pallidus and subcortical white matter changes may be seen after severe or chronic CO poisoning.

ALERT
Pitfalls:
- Pulse oximetry frequently overestimates the percentage of oxyhemoglobin.
- Smokers may have carboxyhemoglobin levels up to 10%.
- Hemolysis, or the presence of fetal hemoglobin, may lead to mild elevation of carboxyhemoglobin.
- In-hospital carboxyhemoglobin levels are not good at predicting risk of delayed neurologic sequelae.

DIFFERENTIAL DIAGNOSIS
- Influenza
- Gastroenteritis
- Vasomotor syncope
- Asphyxia
- Stroke

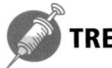

TREATMENT

General Measures
- Recognize CO exposure.
- Remove patient from source of CO.

ADDITIONAL TREATMENT
- Consider hyperbaric oxygen treatment referral to prevent delayed neurologic sequelae.
- Relative indications:
  - Loss of consciousness
  - Seizures
  - Pregnancy
  - Persistent neurologic symptoms
  - CO concentration >25%
- Contraindications:
  - Concurrent illness or injury requiring ongoing acute care
  - Unvented pneumothorax
  - Lack of accessible hyperbaric oxygen chamber
- Complications:
  - Barotitis media
  - Tympanic membrane rupture
  - Claustrophobic anxiety
  - Seizure
  - Pneumothorax

ALERT
Pitfalls:
- Failure to differentiate CO poisoning from winter viral illness
- Syncope may be hard to discern in young infants
- Undue delay in hyperbaric oxygen therapy, which is most effective in 1st 6 hours after exposure

ISSUES FOR REFERRAL
- Neuropsychological testing may benefit individuals with perceived neurocognitive deficits.
- Cardiac evaluation for those with myocardial ischemia

IN-PATIENT CONSIDERATIONS
Initial Stabilization
Administer 100% oxygen at least until patient is asymptomatic and carboxyhemoglobin level is <5–10%.

Admission Criteria
- Perceived merit of hyperbaric oxygen therapy
- Persistent neurologic symptoms
- Evidence of myocardial ischemia
- Associated injuries that merit hospitalization

Discharge Criteria
- Conclusion of hyperbaric therapy
- Stable cardiovascular and neurologic systems after elimination of excess carboxyhemoglobin

ONGOING CARE

FOLLOW-UP RECOMMENDATIONS
Delayed neurologic sequelae may develop 2–40 days after exposure.

PROGNOSIS
- Acute mortality appears to be caused by carboxymyoglobin formation and ischemic ventricular dysrhythmia.
- Patients stable on presentation to medical care have a good prognosis for recovery.
- Delayed neurologic sequelae may manifest in as many as 10–40% of patients after a CO-mediated syncopal episode.

COMPLICATIONS
- Death
- Delayed neurologic sequelae, e.g.:
  - Neurocognitive deficits
  - Personality changes
  - Parkinsonism

ADDITIONAL READING

- Buckley NA, Isbister GK, Stokes B, et al. Hyperbaric oxygen for carbon monoxide poisoning: A systematic review and critical analysis of the evidence. *Toxicol Rev*. 2005;24:75–92.
- Martin JD, Osterhoudt KC, Thom SR. Recognition and management of carbon monoxide poisoning in children. *Clin Ped Emerg Med*. 2000;1:244–250.
- Teksam O, Gumus P, Bayrakci B, et al. Acute cardiac effects of carbon monoxide poisoning in children. *Eur J Emerg Med*. 2010;17:192–196.
- Weaver LK. Clinical practice. Carbon monoxide poisoning. *N Engl J Med*. 2009;360:1217–1225.
- Weaver LK, Hopkins RO, Chan KJ, et al. Hyperbaric oxygen for acute carbon monoxide poisoning. *N Eng J Med*. 2002;347:1057–1067.

CODES

ICD9
986 Inhalation of carbon monoxide

ICD10
- T58.94XA Toxic effect of carbon monoxide from unspecified source, undetermined, initial encounter
- T58.94XD Toxic effect of carbon monoxide from unspecified source, undetermined, subsequent encounter
- T58.94XS Toxic effect of carbon monoxide from unspecified source, undetermined, sequela

FAQ

- Q: At what carboxyhemoglobin level should hyperbaric oxygen therapy be recommended?
- A: In practice, most dissociation of carboxyhemoglobin occurs with administration of normal-pressure oxygen before hyperbaric therapy can be administered.
- The advocated value of hyperbaric oxygen is to limit cerebral ischemic reperfusion injury in an effort to ameliorate delayed neurologic sequelae.
- Carboxyhemoglobin levels may not directly correlate in this risk stratification, and the occurrence of syncope or seizure may be used as a surrogate marker.
- Currently, patients with CO concentrations >25% may be considered as potential candidates for hyperbaric oxygen.
- Q: In a household, which family member is at greatest risk of CO poisoning?
- A: Smaller and younger children have greater minute ventilation rates and may attain higher carboxyhemoglobin concentrations at a given exposure level.
- It is unclear whether it is possible that developing brain tissue is more susceptible to the deleterious effects of CO poisoning.

C

CARDIOMYOPATHY

Kimberly Molina
Nelangi Pinto

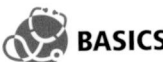 **BASICS**

DESCRIPTION

Cardiomyopathy (CM) is defined as a disease of the heart muscle which results in impaired function (systolic, diastolic, or both). It is classified based on structural and functional abnormalities:

- Dilated cardiomyopathy (DCM): The key finding in DCM is impairment of ventricular systolic function with cardiac dilation. Predominantly involves the left ventricle (LV), and manifests as CHF.
- Hypertrophic cardiomyopathy (HCM): Excessive thickening of the LV that is not secondary to load conditions such as aortic stenosis or hypertension. Up to 20–25% of the patients exhibit LV outflow tract obstruction.
- Restrictive cardiomyopathy (RCM): A myocardial disease in which there is impairment of ventricular diastolic function (or relaxation) from an increased stiffness of the ventricle. This results in decreased ventricular filling while systolic function is generally preserved.
- Left ventricular noncompaction (LVNC): A disease where the myocardium of the LV has not completely compacted resulting in persistence of trabeculations and myocardial dysfunction.

EPIDEMIOLOGY

Incidence

- Overall incidence of cardiomyopathy is 1–2 cases per 100,000 people. There is a peak incidence during the 1st year of life and a 2nd peak in adolescence.
- DCM: Studies have reported the incidence to range from 0.3–2.6 cases per 100,000 people.
- HCM: Reported incidence is 0.3–0.5 cases per 100,000 people.

Prevalence

- DCM: 36 cases per 100,000 people
- HCM: Estimated to be 10–20 cases per 100,000 people
- RCM: Least common form of CM (<5%)
- LVNC: ~9% of CM cases

RISK FACTORS

Genetics

- DCM: Familial DCM accounts for ~20% of cases.
  - Autosomal dominant inheritance remains the most common pattern. Although no specific gene has been identified as the cause of familial DCM, 6 genes have been localized in different family cohorts.
  - DCM has also been seen in association with diseases of X-linked inheritance, such as Duchenne and Becker muscular dystrophy, and Barth syndrome.
  - May also be inherited via mitochondrial DNA, with differing penetrance.
- HCM: ~60% of reported cases are thought to be inherited. Traditionally, HCM is inherited in an autosomal dominant pattern with incomplete penetrance.
- RCM: Idiopathic cases may have a familial occurrence and may be associated with a skeletal myopathy. An autosomal dominant form of the disease with variable penetrance has been associated with Noonan syndrome.
- LVNC: Familial in 20–30%. May be X-linked, mitochondrial, autosomal recessive or dominant

ETIOLOGY

- DCM: There are many etiologies for DCM. Etiology is identified only ~30% of the time:
  - Of known causes, the most common is myocarditis (coxsackievirus B, echovirus, adenovirus). DCM can also occur from toxin exposure (anthracyclines), ischemic coronary artery disease (anomalous left coronary artery from the pulmonary artery, coronary aneurysms), and chronic tachyarrhythmias
  - Can occur as a finding associated with another disease or syndrome. These include X-linked muscular dystrophies, inborn errors of fatty-acid oxidation, disorders of mitochondrial oxidative phosphorylation, nutritional deficiencies, primary and secondary carnitine deficiency.
  - It may be familial and genetically inherited.
  - DCM is most commonly idiopathic.
- HCM: Etiology is known about 25% of the time. Often genetically inherited. Caused by myocyte hypertrophy with fibrillin disarray.
- RCM: Most commonly idiopathic, although known causes include:
  - Systemic disease such as lupus erythematosus, sarcoidosis, amyloidosis, infiltrative diseases (Gaucher disease, Hurler syndrome), storage diseases (Fabry disease), carcinoid syndrome, and radiation-induced fibrosis
  - Familial forms of RCM

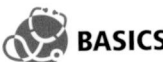 **DIAGNOSIS**

In the early stages of all 3 forms of cardiomyopathy, the symptoms are nonspecific and can mimic other disease processes. The cardiac examination can be completely normal. Therefore, those patients who raise suspicion for this disease either by family history or clinical presentation should be carefully evaluated.

HISTORY

- DCM: Symptoms usually develop slowly although they may also be of sudden onset:
  - Irritability
  - Respiratory distress
  - Dyspnea with exertion
  - Anorexia, abdominal pain, nausea
  - Failure to thrive
  - Exercise intolerance
  - Syncope
  - Palpitations
- HCM: Children are often asymptomatic and are first referred for evaluation based on family history or for murmur evaluation. Of those with symptoms, the following may be present:
  - Chest pain with exertion
  - Dizziness
  - Syncope
  - Palpitations
- RCM: Symptoms are usually due to systemic and pulmonary congestion from high atrial pressures. They are usually more evident late in the disease:
  - Dyspnea with exertion
  - Abdominal pain
  - Chest pain
  - Palpitations

PHYSICAL EXAM

- Cardiac:

- DCM: Tachycardia, cardiomegaly, hepatomegaly, S3 or S4 gallop; evidence of congestive heart failure, and decreased cardiac output
- HCM: Can be normal or have systolic murmur owing to mitral regurgitation and/or LV outflow tract obstruction. The presence of outflow tract obstruction produces a systolic ejection murmur of variable intensity related to the degree of obstruction; the murmur increases in intensity with Valsalva and decreases in magnitude with squatting. A parasternal or carotid thrill may be present, as may an S4 gallop.
- RCM: Jugular venous pulse either fails to fall or rises during inspiration (Kussmaul sign): The presence of S3 or S4. Advanced cases may exhibit weak peripheral pulses as evidence of low cardiac output.
- Respiratory (DCM and RCM): Tachypnea, rales, wheezing
- Abdominal (DMC and RCM): Hepatomegaly, ascites, tenderness to palpation

DIAGNOSTIC TESTS & INTERPRETATION

Lab

Initial lab tests

DCM: In addition to routine inflammatory markers, specific tests should be obtained to establish the cause:

- Metabolic: Carnitine level, serum organic acids, and urine organic and amino acids, pyruvate, lactate, thyroid function tests
- Genetic: Chromosomal analysis, mutations of the dystrophin gene
- Infectious: Enterovirus, coxsackievirus A/B, hepatitis, cytomegalovirus, Epstein-Barr virus, adenovirus, parvovirus, herpes simplex virus, and human immunodeficiency virus
- Brain natriuretic peptide (BNP) is often used to follow heart failure in patients with CM.

Imaging

Echocardiogram:

- Allows for assessment of systolic function, ventricular dimensions, outflow tract obstruction, and diastolic filling properties
- DCM: Significant dilation of left (and right) ventricle with decreased systolic function
- HCM: Gold standard for diagnosis: LV hypertrophy, intraventricular pressure gradient, and systolic anterior motion of the mitral valve
- RCM: Disproportionately dilated atria with impaired diastolic filling by Doppler. LV function is normal until late stages.
- LVNC: Deep trabeculations and intertrabecular recesses in the LV, ventricular hypertrophy and systolic dysfunction

Diagnostic Procedures/Other

- Nonspecific tests:
  - Chest radiograph: Cardiomegaly, pulmonary venous congestion, pulmonary edema, and pleural effusions; segmental atelectasis from compression of the bronchioles

– EKG: Supraventricular or ventricular arrhythmia may be seen.
  ○ DCM: Sinus tachycardia, nonspecific ST segment and T-wave changes;
  ○ HCM: Hypertrophy, deep Q waves;
  ○ RCM: Atrial enlargement, nonspecific ST and T-wave changes;
  ○ LVNC: Marked ventricular hypertrophy, T-wave inversion.
• Cardiac catheterization:
  – DCM: Rarely used as the primary diagnostic tool in this disease; the procedure is used to delineate coronary anatomy and to perform endomyocardial biopsies.
  – HCM: Determination of the presence or absence of LV outflow tract obstruction, evaluation of diastolic dysfunction, classic spike and dome arterial pulse tracing, Brockenbrough phenomenon (a beat following a premature ventricular contraction exhibits an arterial pulse pressure less than that of a control beat).
  – RCM: Atrial pressures are elevated from increased LV and RV end-diastolic pressures. Ventricular pressures exhibit a rapid and deep early decline at the onset of diastole followed by a rapid rise to a plateau in early diastole (dip and plateau or square-root sign).

DIFFERENTIAL DIAGNOSIS
• DCM: Children and young adults often present with symptoms that mimic other disease states:
  – For example, abdominal distention, right upper quadrant pain, nausea, and anorexia indicate right heart failure, but could be mistaken for hepatic or gallbladder disease.
  – Wheezing, tachypnea, and dyspnea on exertion may be diagnosed as bronchitis or asthma.
  – Cardiomegaly on chest radiograph may be mistaken for a large pericardial effusion.
• HCM: This disease must be differentiated from the LV hypertrophy that is seen in a well-trained athlete.
• RCM: Should be distinguished from constrictive pericarditis because the latter is usually a remediable process. A history of tuberculosis, trauma, or cardiac surgery may suggest constrictive pericarditis.

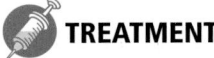 **TREATMENT**

ADDITIONAL TREATMENT
General Measures
• DCM:
  – At the time of diagnosis, a trial of IV γ-globulin and/or other immunomodulators (prednisone, azathioprine) to treat possible myocarditis though impact on outcomes is unclear.
  – Diuretics
  – Afterload reduction (enalapril, captopril)
  – Inotropic agents (milrinone, dobutamine, digoxin)
  – Aldactone (improves New York Heart Association [NYHA] functional class)
  – Anticoagulation to avoid embolic complications
  – Antiarrhythmics as needed, β-adrenergic blockers (metoprolol, carvedilol)
  – Ventricular assist devices have been used in those with end-stage heart failure either as a bridge to recovery or to transplantation.
• HCM: β-adrenergic blockers remain 1st-line medical therapy. Calcium channel blockers or disopyramide may also be used. Antiarrhythmics may also be part of the medical regimen. There is no evidence that prophylactic medical treatment will reduce the risk of sudden death.

– If medical therapy is not effective, other options may include septal myectomy (for severe outflow obstruction) and atrioventricular sequential pacing.
  – The placement of an implantable cardioverter defibrillator (ICD) may be indicated.
• RCM: The mainstay of medical therapy is symptomatic treatment:
  – Diuretics can be used with caution to treat venous congestion without reducing the ventricular filling pressure.
  – Antiarrhythmics are used to treat the high incidence of atrial arrhythmias.
  – ICDs have also been used to treat life-threatening ventricular arrhythmias.
  – Anticoagulation is used owing to the high risk of thrombus formation and embolic complications from hemostasis in the dilated atrium.
  – Because of the natural history of this disease, most patients eventually require a cardiac transplant.
• Patients with cardiomyopathies are generally restricted from strenuous exercise due to increased risk of sudden cardiac death.

SURGERY/OTHER PROCEDURES
• DCM or RCM: Heart or heart–lung transplantation (if the pulmonary vascular resistance is elevated); transplantation may be necessary if all therapeutic endeavors prove to be futile.
• HCM: Septal myectomy if indicated

IN-PATIENT CONSIDERATIONS
Initial Stabilization
Patients with DCM may present critically ill requiring intubation and inotropic support.

 ONGOING CARE

PROGNOSIS
• DCM: The rate of death or transplant is ~30% at 1-year and 46% at 5-year follow-up. Age (>6 years), ventricular function, and symptoms of congestive heart failure at diagnosis are risk factors for a worse outcome.
• HCM: Overall incidence of sudden death is 4–6% in children and adolescents, and as low as 1% in adults. Between the ages of 12 and 35 years and in young athletes, HCM is the most common cause of sudden death. Obstruction may slowly develop or progress. Heart failure symptoms usually do not occur until adulthood. Survival is poorer (82%) for those diagnosed at <1 year of age.
• RCM: The reported median survival in RCM is 1.4 years in children with <20% freedom from death or transplant at 5 years.
• LVNC: 5-year survival free of death or transplantation is 75%.

COMPLICATIONS
• CHF can occur in all forms of cardiomyopathy.
• Arrhythmias may be seen and are frequently ventricular in origin.
• Thrombus formation can be seen owing to the stasis of blood in dilated cardiac chambers and the hypocontractile ventricle. Therefore, systemic or pulmonary emboli are possible.

ADDITIONAL READING
• Ammash NM, Seward JB, Bailey KR, et al. Clinical profile and outcome of idiopathic restrictive cardiomyopathy. *Circulation*. 2000;101:2490–2496.
• Silva JN, Canter CE. Current management of pediatric dilated cardiomyopathy. *Curr Opin Cardiol*. 2010;25:80–87.
• Towbin JA. Hypertrophic cardiomyopathy. *PACE*. 2009;32:S23–S31.
• Towbin JA, Lowe AM, Colan SD, et al. Incidence, causes, and outcomes of dilated cardiomyopathy in children. *JAMA*. 2006;296:1867–1876.
• Wilkinson JD, Landy DC, Colan SD, et al. The pediatric cardiomyopathy registry and heart failure: Key results from the first 15 years. *Heart Failure Clin*. 2010;6:401–413.

 CODES

ICD9
425.4 Other primary cardiomyopathies

ICD10
• I42.0 Dilated cardiomyopathy
• I42.8 Other cardiomyopathies
• I42.9 Cardiomyopathy, unspecified

FAQ
• Q: Should family members be evaluated once a cardiomyopathy is diagnosed in a 1st-degree relative?
• A: Yes. In some forms of cardiomyopathy, there is a strong genetic component and family members should be evaluated. If the cardiomyopathy is known to be acquired, evaluation of relatives is not required.
• Q: Does the cardiomyopathy of infants of diabetic mothers carry the same clinical course and outcome as that of patients with HCM?
• A: No. The pathophysiology is initially similar in that asymmetric hypertrophy of the ventricular septum is often seen with or without LV outflow obstruction. However, the clinical course of the cardiomyopathy in these infants is usually benign and resolves within the 1st 6 months of life.
• Q: What are the differentiating features of HCM and the benign physiologic hypertrophy of an athlete's heart?
• A: Several criteria are used to make this distinction. For example, a familial history of HCM raises the suspicion of this entity. Studies have suggested specific echocardiographic LV dimensions to differentiate benign hypertrophy and HCM (i.e., a wall thickness of ≥15 mm or LV cavity dimension <45 mm are more consistent with HCM). Also, evidence of abnormal mitral valve inflow is suggestive of HCM.

CATARACT

Gil Binenbaum
Anne K. Jensen
William Anninger
Brian J. Forbes (5th edition)

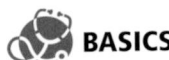 **BASICS**

DESCRIPTION
Any opacification of the normally clear crystalline lens of the eye. While many cataracts are small and nonprogressive and do not cause visual symptoms, visually significant cataracts represent a major challenge and require prompt diagnosis and management for optimal visual outcome.

EPIDEMIOLOGY
- Accounts for between 10% and 40% of childhood blindness worldwide.
- Ranges from 1 to 15 per 10,000 children worldwide, and 1 to 3 per 10,000 children in developed countries.

GENERAL PREVENTION
There is currently no known way to prevent congenital cataracts other than correcting any underlying metabolic abnormality if present. It is essential, however, that all newborns (and all children) receive screening eye examinations by healthcare providers. In much of the world, early diagnosis and referral is still the limiting factor for a child's ultimate visual prognosis.

PATHOPHYSIOLOGY
- Derangement of the normal developmental growth of the crystalline fibers of the central lens nucleus or peripheral lens cortex. The location of the opacity often suggests the gestational age at which it occurred.
- Frequently classified according to morphology or etiology.
- Dense central opacities of ≥3 mm are visually significant and may produce visual disability

ETIOLOGY
- Congenital: About 1/3 are inherited, 1/3 are associated with systemic disorders, and 1/3 are idiopathic.
- Familial: May be inherited as autosomal dominant, autosomal recessive, or X-linked recessive traits. Autosomal dominant cataracts are most commonly bilateral nuclear opacities but marked variability can be present even within the same pedigree. Multiple contributing genetic loci have been identified.
- Acquired:
  – Toxic: May result from chronic steroid use or radiation exposure
  – Traumatic: May result from either blunt or penetrating ocular trauma. Often stellate or rosette shaped
  – Inflammatory: From chronic uveitis
- Ocular Abnormalities: May be associated with other primary ocular abnormalities, including aniridia and various anterior chamber dysgenesis syndromes
- Systemic Conditions: See below.

COMMONLY ASSOCIATED CONDITIONS
- Prenatal factors: Intrauterine infection (toxoplasmosis, syphilis, rubella, cytomegalovirus, or herpes simplex, collectively known as TORCH infection), fetal alcohol syndrome
- Metabolic and endocrine: Galactosemia, neonatal hypoglycemia, hypoparathyroidism, diabetes mellitus
- Chromosomal: Trisomy 21 (Down syndrome), 13 or 15; Turner syndrome
- Dermatologic: Congenital ichthyosis, hereditary ectodermal dysplasia, infantile poikiloderma
- Renal: Lowe and Alport syndromes
- Skeletal: Marfan and Conradi syndromes
- Rheumatologic: Juvenile idiopathic arthritis, other uveitis (psoriatic, HLA-B27, etc.)
- Other: Craniofacial and mandibulofacial syndromes, neurofibromatosis, myotonic dystrophy, Fabry disease

 DIAGNOSIS

HISTORY
- Decreased visual responses? Cataracts may decrease vision.
- Sun sensitivity or squinting in bright light? Cataracts may cause glare and light sensitivity.
- Strabismus (ocular misalignment)? May indicate loss of vision in one eye
- White pupil? Cataracts may appear as a white object in or under the pupil.
- Asymmetric or abnormal pupillary reflections (red eyes) with flash photography? Cataract may block the normal red reflex.
- Nystagmus? May be an ominous sign for the degree of vision loss
- Ocular trauma? Can cause traumatic cataract
- Delayed development? Especially with significant bilateral congenital cataracts, patients may fail to attain developmental milestones.
- Careful family and prenatal history? Up to 1/3 of congenital cataracts are inherited. Also assess for history of intrauterine infection or alcohol exposure
- Positive family history or known history of an associated systemic condition? See "Associated Conditions."

PHYSICAL EXAM
- Decreased visual acuity: In preverbal child, assess via fix and follow. In verbal child, assess with Snellen chart.
- Strabismus: May indicate loss of vision
- Leukocoria: White pupil
- Absent, asymmetric or irregular red reflex: Use direct ophthalmoscope. Most sensitive method to detect cataract
- Nystagmus: Very poor prognostic sign
- Laterality of disease: Bilateral cataracts are more likely due to systemic disease.
- Globe (eyeball) size: Microphthalmia (small eye) suggests congenital cataracts..
- Complete physical exam: To assess for associated conditions

DIAGNOSTIC TESTS & INTERPRETATION
Lab
For cases with a definitive etiology, laboratory evaluation is typically not necessary. For bilateral cataracts without a clear cause, a selective workup to rule out associated conditions may be indicated.
- Serologies: Titers to rule out TORCH infections and syphilis; blood glucose, calcium, and phosphate to exclude metabolic disorders such as diabetes and hypoparathyroidism
- Urine tests: Reducing substances to rule out galactosemia; protein, amino acids, and pH to rule out Lowe syndrome
- Red blood cell enzyme levels: Galactokinase and gal-1-uridyltransferase as part of galactosemia workup
- Karyotype: In conjunction with genetic consultation and ocular examination of parents and siblings

Imaging
Ocular ultrasonography if unable to visualize structures posterior to the opacity.

Diagnostic Procedures/Other
- Complete, timely ophthalmic evaluation by a pediatric ophthalmologist, including slit-lamp biomicroscopy and dilated fundus examination.
- Electrophysiologic testing of the visual system may be helpful to evaluate visual potential.

DIFFERENTIAL DIAGNOSIS
- The differential diagnosis of childhood cataracts is more concerned with the underlying cause of leukocoria (white pupil) rather than the presence of some other entity, as the cataract itself is readily identified on examination.
- Leukorrhea or poor red reflex DDX: Retinoblastoma, retinopathy of prematurity, persistent fetal vasculature, uveitis, retinal detachment, Coats disease, others
- Cataracts may also be an expression of an underlying systemic disease, which must be diagnosed for the child's overall benefit.

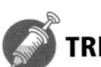 **TREATMENT**

ADDITIONAL TREATMENT
General Measures
- Importance of timely referral:
  – Congenital cataracts may require surgical removal by 4–6 weeks of age to prevent irreversible deprivation amblyopia, so quick referral is critical.
  – Acquired pediatrics cataracts may also cause amblyopia, typically prior to 7 years of age.
- Conservative management:
  – Partial cataracts with good visual acuity that do not block the visual axis may be managed conservatively with observation, pharmacologic pupillary dilatation, and/or amblyopia treatment as needed (occlusion of the contralateral eye). Glasses may or may not be of additional help.
  – Small cataracts may progress, so nonsurgical cases require close follow-up.

SURGERY/OTHER PROCEDURES

- Visually significant cataracts must be removed surgically, followed by optical correction for aphakia (lacking a lens), pseudophakia (artificial lens), and/or inability to accommodate (focus in), and amblyopia treatment.
- Successful treatment may be extremely difficult, and intervention must occur very early in life in the case of congenital cataracts or as soon as possible in later-onset cataracts.
- To prevent deprivation amblyopia in bilateral cases, both cataracts are typically removed within 1 or 2 weeks of each other, if not simultaneously.
- Postoperative care:
  – Overview: Removing the lens leaves the child aphakic (without a lens). Postoperative optical correction with contact lens, glasses, and/or intraocular lens (pseudophakic) and amblyopia treatment are essential for optimal visual prognosis.
  – Contact lens: In children <1 year, optical correction of bilateral aphakia is most frequently accomplished with contact lenses or spectacles. In unilateral cases, a contact lens is best if tolerated.
  – Intraocular lens (IOL): In children >1 year, IOLs are frequently placed. Timing and willingness to place IOLs varies depending on surgeon and family preference.
  – Amblyopia therapy: In unilateral cataract cases, successful visual rehabilitation usually requires aggressive occlusion therapy to the normal eye, possibly for years. Even when treatment is successful, normal binocular vision with preserved depth perception is unlikely.
  – Contact VS IOL: The Infant Aphakia Treatment Study Group recently reported no difference in visual grating acuity at 1 year for 114 infants aged 1–6 months with unilateral cataract randomized to IOL placement or aphakia with contact lens. However, an increased rate of additional procedures was reported for the IOL group (63% vs. 12%).

ONGOING CARE

FOLLOW-UP RECOMMENDATIONS

- Without treatment, visually significant cataracts result in progressive visual loss. When an opacity that is present at birth or very early in life is not promptly addressed, the visual loss quickly becomes irreversible.
- Once surgical removal is performed and optical correction is started, the child, parents, and ophthalmologist enter into an intensive and long rehabilitation period, lasting until visual maturity and stability are reached (usually 7–10 years of age). Afterward, yearly eye examinations are a minimum requirement.
- Parental and educational support services, as well as special local, state, and federal services for the visually handicapped and blind may be required, as not all children with successful surgical results will have good vision.

ALERT
PITFALLS include (i) lack of early diagnosis, referral, and treatment, (ii) lack of understanding of irreversible deprivation amblyopia, and (iii) lack of compliance with postoperative optical correction and occlusion therapy.

PROGNOSIS

- Before 1980, most children treated for monocular cataracts had a best corrected vision <20/200, and children with bilateral cataracts had 20/80–20/200 acuities.
- Earlier surgery, better surgical techniques, and rapid postsurgical optical correction now frequently result in best-corrected visual acuities of 20/40–20/200 for monocular cataracts and 20/40 or better for bilateral cataracts.
- Useful vision can be restored or obtained in newborns with unilateral cataracts if the surgery is completed within the 1st 6 weeks of life. After this time, visual restoration becomes progressively more difficult, because of irreversible deprivation amblyopia.
- The prognosis for visual rehabilitation in children with bilateral congenital cataracts is slightly better, providing surgical removal and optical correction are accomplished early, preferably prior to 8 weeks of age.
- Although later-onset cataracts have a better prognosis because the visual system has developed to some degree, these children still require immediate evaluation and treatment.
- In all cases, the onset or presence of nystagmus before the cataract is removed is an ominous sign of poor outcome and adds further urgency to the need for surgical removal.
- Family compliance with both postsurgical optical correction and amblyopia treatment is critical and directly affects the child's ultimate visual outcome later in life.

COMPLICATIONS

- Lack of removal of a visually significant cataract at the appropriate time leads to irreversible deprivation amblyopia, in which case no amount of surgery, optical correction, or amblyopia therapy is of benefit.
- Cataract removal in children leaves the eye without a lens (aphakic), with an IOL (pseudophakic), and/or unable to focus without some type of optical correction (spectacles or contact lenses). Unless rapid restoration of optical correction occurs, irreversible refractive amblyopia may still occur after the cataract is removed, particularly if the cataract is unilateral.
- Short- and long-term postoperative complications also include visual axis reopacification, glaucoma (elevated intraocular pressure with optic nerve damage), retinal detachment, and very rarely endophthalmitis (intraocular infection). These complications may lead to vision loss or loss of the eye, and long-term ophthalmology follow-up is required.

ADDITIONAL READING

- Amaya L, Taylor D, Russell-Eggitt I, et al. The morphology and natural history of childhood cataracts. *Surv Ophthalmol*. 2003;48:125–144.
- Childhood cataracts and other lens disorders. In: Simon JW, et al., eds. *Pediatric Ophthalmology and Strabismus: Basic and Clinical Science Course*, Section 6. San Francisco: American Academy of Ophthalmology; 2010–2011.
- Gimbel HV, Basti S, Ferensowicz M, et al. Results of bilateral cataract extraction with posterior chamber intraocular lens implantation in children. *Ophthalmology*. 1997;104:1737–1743.
- Infant Aphakia Treatment Study Group. A randomized clinical trial comparing contact lens with intraocular lens correction of monocular aphakia during infancy. *Arch Ophthal*. 2010;(128)7: 810–818.
- Lambert SR, Drack AV. Infantile cataracts. *Surv Ophthalmol*. 1996;40:427–458.
- Levin AV. Congenital eye anomalies. *Pediatr Clin North Am*. 2003;50:55–76.
- Wilson ME Jr, Trivedi RH, Hoxie JP, et al. Treatment outcomes of congenital monocular cataracts: The effects of surgical timing and patching compliance. *J Pediatr Ophthalmol Strabismus*. 2003;40:323–329; quiz 353–354.
- Wilson ME, Pandey SK, Thakur J. Pediatric cataract blindness in the developing world: Surgical techniques and intraocular lenses in the new millennium. *BJO* 2003;87:14–19.
- Zetterstrom C, Lundvall A, Kugelberg M. Cataracts in children. *J Cataract Refract Surg*. 2005;31:824–840.
- Zwann J, Mullaney PB, Awad AA, et al. Pediatric intraocular lens implantation: Surgical results and complications in more than 300 cases. *Ophthalmology*. 1998;105:112–119.

CODES

ICD9
- 366.04 Nuclear cataract
- 366.9 Unspecified cataract
- 743.30 Congenital cataract, unspecified

ICD10
- H25.10 Age-related nuclear cataract, unspecified eye
- H26.9 Unspecified cataract
- Q12.0 Congenital cataract

FAQ

- Q: Is surgical removal of the cataract a visual cure?
- A: No. Surgery is only the beginning of treatment, which also includes optical correction and amblyopia therapy.
- Q: Once the cataract is removed, will intensive, extensive follow-up be needed?
- A: Yes. The visual prognosis is directly related to postsurgical treatment compliance.
- Q: Is the cataract easier to treat when the child is older?
- A: No. Irreversible deprivation amblyopia develops as the child grows, precluding any chance for normal vision. In newborns, cataracts must typically be removed at 4–6 weeks of age.

C

CAT-SCRATCH DISEASE

Laura K. Brennan
Louis M. Bell (5th edition)

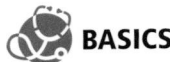 **BASICS**

DESCRIPTION
Cat-scratch disease (CSD) is a subacute, regional lymphadenitis syndrome that occurs following cutaneous *Bartonella henselae* inoculation, usually from a cat scratch or bite.

EPIDEMIOLOGY
Incidence
- There are ~24,000 cases and 2,000 hospital admissions each year; CSD likely represents the most common cause of chronic benign regional adenopathy.
- CSD occurs in patients of all ages, with the majority of cases being in those <21 years old.
- CSD is more common when one is scratched by a cat <12 months of age and/or a cat with fleas.

GENERAL PREVENTION
- Preventive measures should be directed toward minimizing contact between infected cats and people.
- Keeping kittens and older cats indoors and avoiding rough play may decrease the likelihood of infection.
- Avoidance of stray animals and good local care of any sustained bite or scratch are essential.
- Care of cats should involve effective flea control.

PATHOPHYSIOLOGY
- Following infection, the primary inoculation site shows acellular areas of necrosis in the dermis, surrounded by multiple layers of histiocytes and epithelioid cells; a zone of lymphocytes surrounds the histiocytes and some giant cells may be present.
- Involved nodes initially develop generalized lymphoid hyperplasia, followed by the development of stellate granulomas; the centers are acellular and necrotic, and may be surrounded by histiocytes and peripheral lymphocytes.
- Progression leads to microabscesses, which may become confluent and lead to pus-filled sinuses within the infected nodes.

ETIOLOGY
The etiologic agent is now referred to as *Bartonella henselae* (previously, *Rochalimaea henselae*), a fastidious, slow-growing, pleomorphic gram-negative bacillus.

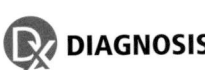 **DIAGNOSIS**

HISTORY
- Cat contact:
  - >90% of patients have an antecedent cat contact.
- A skin rash:
  - A papule generally appears on the skin at the site of inoculation 3–12 days after the initial cat scratch.
  - This papule then often progresses through a vesicular and crusty stage.

- Appearance of large lymph nodes:
  - Within 1–2 weeks after appearance of a skin lesion, lymphadenopathy in the region of drainage (generally immediately proximal to the skin lesion) may be noted.
- Other symptoms:
  - Fever and mild systemic symptoms (such as generalized achiness, malaise, and anorexia) may also be present in up to 30% of patients.

PHYSICAL EXAM
- ≥1 red papule at the inoculation site may be detectable.
- The true sign of CSD (present in ~90% of cases) is chronic or subacute lymphadenitis involving the 1st or 2nd set of nodes draining the inoculation site:
  - The groups affected, in decreasing order of frequency, are the axillary, cervical, submandibular, periauricular, epitrochlear, femoral, and inguinal lymph nodes.
  - Affected nodes are usually tender, with overlying erythema, warmth, and induration.
  - ~10–30% spontaneously suppurate or form a sinus tract to the skin.

DIAGNOSTIC TESTS & INTERPRETATION
Lab
- Indirect fluorescence antibody (IFA) testing:
  - For detection of serum antibodies to *B. henselae*
  - Available at many commercial laboratories, state public health laboratories, and the Centers for Disease Control and Prevention
  - Should be used to confirm a CSD diagnosis
  - In general, IFA IgG titers <1:64 suggest no current infection; titers between 1:64 and 1:256 represent possible early or old infection (and should be rechecked in 1–2 weeks); titers >1:256 strongly suggest active or recent infection.
  - There is less sensitivity with IgM titers, which may not always be positive at diagnosis, even in acute disease.
  - A single IgG titer of ≥1:512, a 4-fold rise in titer, or seroconversion is necessary for serologic diagnosis of CSD.
- Enzyme immunoassay (EIA) testing:
  - Also for detection of serum antibodies to *B. henselae*
  - Similar sensitivity and specificity to IFA
- Blood cultures:
  - Using lysed or centrifuged blood may at times yield *B. henselae* growth from infected individuals in whom bacteremia is suspected.
  - Growth typically is obtained on blood agar after 12–15 days, but may require incubation period of up to 45 days.
- Polymerase chain reaction (PCR):
  - Available in some commercial and research laboratories
  - Sensitive and specific method for diagnosis of *Bartonella* infection in tissue specimens (e.g., needle aspiration of lymph node)
  - PCR+ serum samples have been reported in several patients, but serum PCR is likely less sensitive than IFA serology.

- Warthin-Starry silver stain:
  - May demonstrate *B. henselae* bacilli in chains, clumps, or filaments within necrosed areas of lymph node or within primary inoculation site of the skin.
  - Not specific for *B. henselae* and not definitively diagnostic of CSD, but is strongly suggestive in conjunction with compatible clinical findings

DIFFERENTIAL DIAGNOSIS
Most known causes of lymphadenopathy (see "Neck Masses"). Location of the abnormal lymph nodes may supply a strong clue.

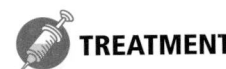 **TREATMENT**

MEDICATION (DRUGS)
- Antibiotics shown to be effective against *B. henselae* include:
  - Trimethoprim-sulfamethoxazole (TMP-SMX), the macrolides, rifampin, doxycycline, ciprofloxacin, and gentamicin.
  - A recommended regimen for uncomplicated CSD would include azithromycin 500 mg initially then 250 mg daily for a total of 5 days in patients >45.5 kg and 10 mg/kg on the 1st day and 5 mg/kg for the subsequent 4 days.
  - Alternatively, trimethoprim-sulfamethoxazole (TMP-SMX) 6–8 mg/kg of TMP 2 or 3 times daily for 7 days in children may be used.
- For immunocompromised patients and those with severe or systemic disease (including encephalitis), azithromycin, erythromycin, or doxycycline should be administered; gentamicin sulfate 5 mg/kg/d divided q8h IM or IV for at least 2 weeks should also be administered in cases of endocarditis. Optimal duration of treatment is unclear, but may need to be up to several months in immunocompromised patients to prevent relapse.

ADDITIONAL TREATMENT
General Measures
Antibiotic therapy for CSD in immunocompetent hosts is somewhat controversial as the disease is self-limited and most reports suggest little or no overall improvement with antibiotics. Many experts suggest conservative, symptomatic treatment only, except in severe or systemic disease or in immunocompromised patients.

ISSUES FOR REFERRAL
- Consider infectious disease consult to aid in evaluation and diagnosis.
- Consider general surgery consult for needle aspiration if needed.

SURGERY/OTHER PROCEDURES

- Percutaneous needle aspiration of painful, fluctuant nodes can be performed for relief of pain.
- Incision and drainage should be avoided to reduce the risk of sinus tract formation, and surgical excision is generally not necessary.

IN-PATIENT CONSIDERATIONS

Admission Criteria

- Severe pain refractory to oral analgesics
- Workup to rule out serious other causes of lymphadenopathy or symptomatology
- Severe or unusual complications of CSD

Discharge Criteria

- Pain under adequate control
- No concern for serious or life-threatening complications or other disorders requiring further evaluation or treatment

 ONGOING CARE

FOLLOW-UP RECOMMENDATIONS

- Most patients will have a benign course and may expect resolution of systemic symptoms in <2 weeks.
- Slow resolution of enlarged or painful lymph nodes will occur over weeks to months (usually ≤4 months).
- ~10–30% of affected lymph nodes will spontaneously suppurate.
- 5–15% of patients will have disseminated disease; the course for patients with severe complications, including encephalitis, will be more prolonged, but without lasting sequelae.

PROGNOSIS

- Most patients have a benign course with complete recovery.
- Patients with significant complications, such as encephalopathy, thrombocytopenic purpura, or bone lesions, usually have a more prolonged course but still have a good long-term prognosis.

COMPLICATIONS

- Regional lymphadenitis
- Fever of unknown origin
- Osteolytic bone lesions
- Parinaud oculoglandular syndrome:
  - Occurs when the site of primary inoculation is the conjunctiva or eyelid
  - A mild to moderate conjunctivitis develops along with ipsilateral preauricular lymphadenopathy.

- Encephalopathy/encephalitis:
  - May occur suddenly 2–6 weeks after the initial symptoms of CSD, and seizures may be the heralding symptom
  - Patients may become delirious and then comatose for several days before recovering.
  - Spinal fluid is typically normal or shows minimal WBC and protein elevation.
  - Recovery is generally complete.
- Neuroretinitis:
  - Acute (usually unilateral) vision loss from optic nerve edema
  - Associated with stellate macular exudates
- Visceral organ involvement:
  - Occasionally hepatosplenic involvement with multiple hypoechoic lesions will be found on abdominal ultrasound exam.
- Erythema nodosum:
  - Likely represents a delayed hypersensitivity reaction to the infection
  - Most often involves the subcutaneous fat of the legs and, at times, dorsum of arms, hands, and feet
- Osteolytic bone lesions occur as a rare complication.
- Other, rare complications:
  - Thrombotic thrombocytopenic purpura
  - Henoch-Schönlein purpura
  - Erythema marginatum
  - Mesenteric lymphadenitis
  - Pneumonia
  - Arthralgias
  - Osteomyelitis
  - Hypercalcemia
  - Guillain-Barré Syndrome
  - Transverse myelitis
- Endocarditis

ADDITIONAL READING

- Agan BK, Dolan MJ. Laboratory diagnosis of Bartonella infections. *Clin Lab Med*. 2002;22: 937–962.
- Bass JW, Freitas BC, Freitas AD, et al. Prospective randomized double blind placebo-controlled evaluation of azithromycin for treatment of cat-scratch disease. *Pediatr Infect Dis J*. 1998;17: 447–452.
- Baylor P, Garoufi A, Karpathios T, et al. Transverse myelitis in 2 patients with Bartonella henselae infection (cat scratch disease). *Clin Infect Dis*. 2007; 45(4):e42–e45. Epub 2007 Jul 5.
- Biswas S, Rolain JM. Bartonella infection: Treatment and drug resistance. *Future Microbiol*. 2010; 5(11):1719–1731.

- Ciervo A, Mastroianni CM, Ajassa C, et al. Rapid identification of Bartonella henselae by real-time polymerase chain reaction in a patient with cat scratch disease. *Diagn Microbiol Infect Dis*. 2005;53:75–77.
- Durá-Travé T, Yoldi-Petri ME, Gallinas-Victoriano F, et al. Neuroretinitis caused by Bartonella henselae (cat-scratch disease) in a 13-year-old girl. *Int J Pediatr*. 2010;2010:763105. Epub 2010 Jun 15.
- English R. Cat-scratch disease. *Pediatr Rev*. 2006; 27:123–127.
- Heye S, Matthijs P, Wallon J, et al. Cat scratch disease osteomyelitis. *Skeletal Radiol*. 2003;32: 49–51.
- Massei F, Gori L, Taddeucci G, et al. Bartonella henselae infection associated with Guillain-Barré syndrome. *Pediatr Infect Dis J*. 2006;25:90–91.
- Schutze GE. Diagnosis and treatment of Bartonella henselae infections. *Pediatr Infect Dis J*. 2000;19: 185–187.

 CODES

ICD9

078.3 Cat-scratch disease

ICD10

A28.1 Cat-scratch disease

FAQ

- Q: Can a sibling develop CSD from an infected patient?
- A: No; person-to-person transmission is not reported.
- Q: Should the parents of a child with CSD get rid of the cat?
- A: In general, this is not recommended. These animals are not ill; the capacity to transmit disease appears to be transient, and recurrent disease is rare.

CAVERNOUS SINUS SYNDROME

Sabrina E. Smith
Dennis J. Dlugos

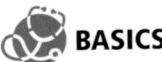 **BASICS**

DESCRIPTION
- Cavernous sinus syndrome comprises disease processes that localize to the cavernous sinus—a venous plexus that drains the face, mouth, tonsils, pharynx, nasal cavity, paranasal sinuses, orbit, middle ear, and parts of the cerebral cortex.
- Small lesions in this region may produce dramatic neurologic signs.

EPIDEMIOLOGY
Incidence
Cavernous sinus syndrome is a rare but serious condition.

PATHOPHYSIOLOGY
- The cavernous sinus is located lateral to the pituitary gland and sella turcica, superior to the sphenoid sinus, and inferior to the optic chiasm.
- Within the cavernous sinus are the carotid artery, the pericarotid sympathetic fibers, and the abducens nerve (VI); within its lateral wall are the oculomotor nerve (III), the trochlear nerve (IV), and the ophthalmic and maxillary divisions of the trigeminal nerve (V1, V2).
- Cavernous sinus syndrome is typically caused by septic or aseptic sinus thrombosis, neoplasm, or trauma. Acute obstruction by mass or thrombosis may progress rapidly if not diagnosed and treated quickly.

ETIOLOGY
- Infectious agents include *Staphylococcus aureus*, *Streptococcus pneumoniae*, Gram-negative rods, and anaerobes; *Mucormycosis* and *Aspergillus* in immunocompromised patients.
- Aseptic venous thrombosis has been associated with sickle cell anemia, trauma, dehydration, vasculitis, pregnancy, oral contraceptive use, congenital heart disease, inflammatory bowel disease, and hypercoagulable states.
- Neoplasms involving the cavernous sinus include pituitary adenomas, meningiomas, trigeminal schwannomas, craniopharyngiomas, lymphomas, neuromas, chordomas, chondrosarcomas, nasopharyngeal carcinomas, and very rarely teratomas. Neoplasms may present with diplopia, visual-field deficits, headache, or isolated cranial nerve deficits.
- The lateral extension of pituitary neoplasms into the cavernous sinus usually affects the 3rd cranial nerve, with the 4th and 6th nerves less commonly involved. Rupture of a cystic craniopharyngioma may present as acute cavernous sinus syndrome.
- Carotid-cavernous fistulas, often with a more chronic course, are direct high-flow shunts between the internal carotid artery and the cavernous sinus. Most often sequelae of trauma, they may present with a history of ocular motility deficits, arterialization of conjunctival vessels, and a bruit usually heard best over the orbit. Less commonly, rupture of a carotid cavernous aneurysm may lead to fistula formation.

- Nonspecific and idiopathic inflammation of the cavernous sinus, also called idiopathic cavernous sinusitis or Tolosa–Hunt syndrome, has been reported in patients as young as 3 1/2 years. This is a diagnosis of exclusion. However, MRI may show enlargement of the affected cavernous sinus with an adjacent soft-tissue mass that resolves after treatment with steroids.

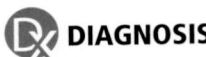 **DIAGNOSIS**

HISTORY
- Recent facial furuncle or cellulitis, sinusitis, dental infection, otitis, or orbital cellulitis may predispose to cavernous sinus syndrome.
- Fever, headache, eye pain, diplopia, and facial paresthesias may be present.

PHYSICAL EXAM
- Conjunctival injection with lid swelling and proptosis indicates cavernous sinus venous congestion.
- Ptosis, anisocoria, ophthalmoparesis, and facial sensory changes are signs of cranial nerve involvement.
- Horner syndrome: Sympathetic nerve fibers traveling with V1 may be affected. Usually occurs in conjunction with an abducens nerve (CN VI) palsy with an inability to abduct the eye.
- Signs and symptoms begin unilaterally, but may rapidly spread bilaterally.
- The optic nerve and visual acuity are spared early in cavernous sinus syndrome, but can be affected as it progresses.
- Funduscopic findings include venous dilatation and hemorrhages.
- Ocular bruit may be heard in any acute cavernous sinus syndrome, but especially in carotid-cavernous fistula.
- Signs of meningitis and systemic toxicity rapidly evolve if infections are untreated.

DIAGNOSTIC TESTS & INTERPRETATION
Lab
- CBC, ESR, PT/PTT, blood culture: Basic studies in any child with suspected acute cavernous sinus syndrome. Blood cultures are positive in 70% of cases of septic venous sinus thrombosis.
  - Lumbar puncture should be performed if there is no contraindication and infection is suspected.
  - ~35% of patients with septic cavernous sinus thrombosis have CSF findings consistent with bacterial meningitis—excess neutrophils, increased protein, and/or decreased glucose.
- Evaluation for a prothrombotic state should be considered in patients with cavernous sinus thrombosis, especially in the absence of infection or trauma. Specific labs include protein C activity, protein S functional, antithrombin III activity, Factor V Leiden gene mutation, prothrombin gene mutation, anticardiolipin antibodies, β-2-glycoprotein antibodies, dilute Russell viper venom time, homocysteine, lipoprotein(a), and Factor VIII activity.

- Antinuclear antibody panel, angiotensin-converting enzyme level, and HIV test should be obtained before diagnosis of Tolosa–Hunt syndrome (diagnosis of exclusion).

Imaging
Any child with proptosis, cranial nerve findings, or an ocular bruit should have an urgent MRI or CT.
- MRI, with and without gadolinium, with special attention to the cavernous sinus and parasellar region, is the imaging study of choice.
- Magnetic resonance venography may be helpful.
- CT angiography may be the preferred study to evaluate for carotid-cavernous fistula.

Diagnostic Procedures/Other
- Diagnosis of carotid-cavernous fistulas requires angiography.
- Nasopharyngeal biopsy and culture if *Mucormycosis* or *Aspergillus* is suspected

DIFFERENTIAL DIAGNOSIS
Other disorders that may resemble cavernous sinus syndrome include:
- Orbital cellulitis
- Sphenoid sinusitis
- Thyroid eye disease
- Cavernous carotid aneurysm
- Orbital apex tumor
- Orbital pseudotumor
- Ocular migraine
- Ocular trauma
- Burkitt lymphoma

ALERT
- Ophthalmoplegic migraine or cluster headache must be distinguished from cavernous sinus syndrome by neuroimaging studies and history.
  - Proptosis does not occur in migraine or cluster headache.
  - Ophthalmoplegic migraine is a diagnosis of exclusion, especially on first presentation.
- Acute infection and hemorrhage of the pituitary gland—pituitary apoplexy—may present with acute bilateral ophthalmoplegia and signs of acute pituitary insufficiency; most commonly occurs with pituitary neoplasms, but may also occur in pregnant women at the time of delivery.
- Chronic granulomatous disorders such as sarcoid and tuberculosis may underlie cavernous sinus syndrome.

TREATMENT

First priority is to rule out septic cavernous sinus thrombosis, life-threatening infections of the face, sinuses, middle ear, teeth, and orbit.

MEDICATION (DRUGS)
First Line
- For septic cavernous sinus thrombosis, broad-spectrum antibiotics (including coverage of penicillinase-resistant staphylococci and anaerobes) are begun immediately. Duration of therapy is usually 2–4 weeks beyond the resolution of symptoms.
- Amphotericin B if *Mucormycosis* or *Aspergillus* is suspected.
- Idiopathic cavernous sinusitis, a diagnosis of exclusion, responds to corticosteroids. Treatment should not be started until neoplasm and infection have been ruled out.

Second Line
Anticoagulation is controversial, but 1 study in adults found that heparin reduced morbidity from septic cavernous sinus thrombosis.

SURGERY/OTHER PROCEDURES
- Surgical drainage of the primary infection (i.e., sinusitis) may be indicated (avoiding surgical manipulation of the cavernous sinus itself).
- Post-traumatic carotid-cavernous fistulas rarely close spontaneously and have been treated with endoarterial balloon embolization.

ONGOING CARE

- Septic cavernous sinus thrombosis may relapse or embolic abscesses may develop 2–6 weeks after therapy has been stopped.
- Repeat MRI with gadolinium should be considered, especially if symptoms recur or new symptoms develop.
- Mortality remains 13–30%, and <40% of patients recover fully from cranial nerve deficits.
- Patients with carotid-cavernous fistulas frequently have persistent cranial nerve deficits even after embolization.

- Idiopathic cavernous sinusitis responds to steroids, but relapses can be problematic. Clinical follow-up and serial MRI scans are indicated to rule out a low-grade neoplasm or fungal infection.
- Consultation with a neuro-oncologist and a neurosurgeon is important for suspected neoplasms or surgical lesions.

PROGNOSIS
- Prognosis depends on the underlying cause.
- Bacterial infections usually respond if diagnosed and treated promptly.

COMPLICATIONS
- Vary with the cause of cavernous sinus syndrome. Septic cavernous sinus syndrome thrombosis and fungal infections may rapidly evolve to bilateral thrombosis, life-threatening sepsis, and meningitis.
- Visual impairment and cranial nerve palsies may persist.
- Mucormycosis, usually seen in patients with diabetic ketoacidosis, is especially dangerous.
- Carotid arteritis with resulting stenosis, occlusion, or embolism may occur, resulting in focal neurologic deficits.
- Aseptic cavernous sinus syndrome thrombosis may evolve to more extensive intracranial venous sinus thrombosis.
- Local spread of neoplasms will continue if not treated appropriately.

ADDITIONAL READING

- Chen CC, Chang PC, Shy CG, et al. CT angiography and MRI angiography in the evaluation of carotid-cavernous sinus fistula prior to embolization: A comparison of techniques. *Am J Neuroradiol*. 2005;26:2349–2356.
- Ebright JR, Pace MT, Niazi AF. Septic thrombosis of the cavernous sinuses. *Arch Int Med*. 2001;161: 2671–2676.
- Eisenberg MB, Al-Mefty O, DeMonte F, et al. Benign nonmeningeal tumors of the cavernous sinus. *Neurosurgery*. 1999;44:949–955.
- Keane JR. Cavernous sinus syndrome: Analysis of 151 cases. *Arch Neurol*. 1996;53:967–971.
- Lee AG, Quick SJ, Liu GT, et al. A childhood cavernous conundrum. *Surv Ophthalmol*. 2004; 49(2):231–236.

 CODES

ICD9
- 325 Phlebitis and thrombophlebitis of intracranial venous sinuses
- 437.6 Nonpyogenic thrombosis of intracranial venous sinus
- 671.50 Other phlebitis and thrombosis complicating pregnancy and the puerperium, unspecified as to episode of care or not applicable

ICD10
- O22.50 Cerebral venous thrombosis in pregnancy, unsp trimester
- I67.6 Nonpyogenic thrombosis of intracranial venous system
- G08 Intracranial and intraspinal phlebitis and thrombophlebitis

FAQ

- Q: Will my child's eye movements return to normal?
- A: In most cases, oculomotor nerves regain function as other signs improve, although they may take the longest to recover.
- Q: Can more pain medicine be given?
- A: There is often an attempt to balance side effects of sedation and hypoventilation against the need for pain control, especially when intracranial pressure is a concern.

CAVERNOUS TRANSFORMATION AND PORTAL VEIN OBSTRUCTION

Vani V. Gopalareddy
John Y. Tung

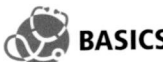 **BASICS**

DESCRIPTION
- Major cause of prehepatic portal hypertension
- Cavernous transformation: The collection of collaterals that develop around an obstructed vessel
- Portal vein obstruction:
  - In pediatrics, obstruction is most typically of the portal vein.
  - Main portal vein or splenic vein is obstructed anywhere along its course, between the hilum of the spleen and the porta hepatis.
  - In cirrhosis and hepatic malignancies, the thromboses usually begin intrahepatically and spread to the extrahepatic portal vein. In most other etiologies, the thromboses usually start at the site of origin of the portal vein. Occasionally, thrombosis of the splenic vein propagates to the portal vein, most often resulting from an adjacent inflammatory process such as chronic pancreatitis.

EPIDEMIOLOGY
- Most children with portal vein thrombosis present between birth and 15 years of age.
- Acute presentation is rare.
- Chronic cases present with complications of portal hypertension.
- Bleeding is more typical in patients presenting <7 years of age.
- Splenomegaly in the absence of symptoms is more typical for patients ages 5–15.

RISK FACTORS
Genetics
A genetic basis of this problem has not been identified, although congenital abnormalities of the heart, major blood vessels, biliary tree, and renal system are often found.

PATHOPHYSIOLOGY
Asymptomatic splenomegaly or upper gastrointestinal hemorrhage, resulting from extrahepatic portal hypertension. Less commonly, the patient presents with ascites or failure to thrive.

ETIOLOGY
50% of portal vein obstructions are idiopathic. Identified causes include:
- Congenital vascular anomaly:
  - Portal vein malformation
  - Webs or diaphragms within the portal vein
- Clot resulting from a hypercoagulable state
- Clot from other causes:
  - Omphalitis
  - Umbilical-vein catheterization
  - Portal pyelophlebitis
  - Intra-abdominal sepsis
  - Surgery near the porta hepatis
  - Sepsis
  - Cholangitis
  - Dehydration
  - Trauma
- Other causes for portal vein obstruction in older children:
  - Ascending pyelophlebitis from perforated appendicitis
  - Primary peritonitis, cholangitis, and pancreatitis causing a splenic vein thrombosis
  - Inflammatory bowel disease

 DIAGNOSIS

HISTORY
- Other causes of splenomegaly (see "Splenomegaly" topic for complete differential):
  - Exposure to infectious mononucleosis
  - Metabolic storage disease (e.g., Gaucher disease)
  - Malignancy (e.g., chronic myelogenous leukemia)
- History of prematurity and admission to NICU should alert the clinician to previous umbilical catheterization and increased risk of portal vein thrombosis.

SIGNS AND SYMPTOMS
- Clinical history and examination should concentrate on identifying possible causes predisposing to portal vein obstruction.
- Portal vein obstruction does not affect liver function unless the patient has an underlying liver disease such as cirrhosis. This is partially due to a compensatory increased flow of the hepatic artery maintaining the total hepatic blood flow.

PHYSICAL EXAM
Splenomegaly and possible hemorrhoids: Spleen is measured from the left anterior axillary line at the costal margin diagonally toward the umbilicus and inferiorly toward the iliac crest.

DIAGNOSTIC TESTS & INTERPRETATION
Lab
- CBC: Leukopenia and thrombocytopenia will be present if there is hypersplenism.
- Aspartate aminotransferase/alanine aminotransferase/γ-glutamyl transferase: Should be normal
- PT/PTT: May be abnormal if malabsorption is present
- Additional testing associated with hypercoagulable states (as clinically indicated):
  - Protein C
  - Protein S
  - Anti–thrombin III levels
  - Factor V Leiden mutation
  - Activated protein C resistance
  - Lupus anticoagulation evaluation
  - Anticardiolipin antibodies (IgA, IgG, IgM)
  - Antinuclear antibody
  - Blood homocysteine
  - Prothrombin 20-21-0 mutation
  - Methylene tetrahydrofolate reductase mutation evaluation
  - Factor VIII coagulant
  - Reptilase time
  - Heparin cofactor II
  - Tissue plasminogen activator
  - Plasminogen activator inhibitor-1
  - Sticky platelet evaluation
  - Paroxysmal nocturnal hemoglobinuria (genetics or flow cytometry evaluation)

Imaging
- Ultrasound with Doppler:
  - To examine portal vein flow and to identify collateral veins if there is cavernous transformation of the portal vein
  - Liver may be slightly small, but may be normal in texture.
  - Remains the most useful imaging study
- CT or MRA can give additional information if needed.

Diagnostic Procedures/Other
- Liver biopsy:
  - Exclude other etiologies
  - Not done as a routine
- Upper endoscopy and sigmoidoscopy: To define extent of varices

Pathological Findings
- Portal hypertension: Spider nevi, prominence of abdominal veins, splenomegaly
- Bruising: Prominent especially when there is a coexistent consumption of clotting factors
- Normal liver palpation and percussion
- Ascites rarely present

DIFFERENTIAL DIAGNOSIS
The differential diagnosis must exclude other causes of splenomegaly and portal hypertension.

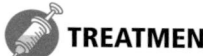 TREATMENT

ADDITIONAL TREATMENT
General Measures
Therapy is designed to manage variceal hemorrhage and to identify an underlying cause to determine if the patient is at risk for additional venous thrombosis or malignancy.
Therapy for GI hemorrhage:
- Prophylactic variceal banding for large varices
- β-Blocker therapy in older children
- Rex shunt (mesenterico–left intrahepatic portal vein shunt):
  - Created using the internal jugular vein, internal iliac vein, or dilated coronary vein, which is used to connect the superior mesenteric vein and the umbilical portion of the left portal vein (in the liver)
  - Restores the physiologic intrahepatic portal vein perfusion
  - Avoids the consequences of long-term portosystemic shunting, especially hepatic encephalopathy
- Portosystemic shunts: Divert portal blood into the low-pressure systemic venous circulation. Classified into:
  - Nonselective shunts: These communicate the entire portal venous system to a systemic venous circulation such as the mesocaval shunt, proximal splenorenal shunt, and portacaval shunts. Nonselective shunts divert more blood into the systemic venous system, and patients are more likely to have encephalopathy.
  - Selective shunts: These divert the gastrosplenic portion of the portal venous flow into the left renal vein or the inferior vena cava. The most common selective shunt is the distal splenorenal shunt (also known as the Warren shunt).

 ONGOING CARE

FOLLOW-UP RECOMMENDATIONS
Focus on growth parameters, early detection of malabsorption, presence of GI hemorrhage, and nutritional intervention.

Patient Monitoring
Pitfalls:
- Patient should be advised about activity restrictions owing to splenomegaly. Spleen guards are recommended.
- Patient should be told to avoid medicines that interfere with platelet function.
- Medications that increase BP that are sometimes found in over-the-counter cold medications (e.g., phenylephrine) can increase splanchnic pressures and may provoke variceal bleeds.
- Aggressive contact sports are actively discouraged in children with hepatosplenomegaly.

PROGNOSIS
Long-term prognosis is good:
- Upper GI hemorrhage becomes less problematic as the child becomes older.
- Rex shunt restores normal physiology and decreases portal pressure. It is the 1st-line therapy in experienced centers.
- Most patients receive β-blockers or undergo prophylactic banding. If the liver function remains normal as in most cases, it is rare for encephalopathy to develop unless a large portosystemic shunt is created.

COMPLICATIONS
- Variceal hemorrhage from the upper tract or from the perianal varices
- Splenomegaly with hypersplenism: Thrombocytopenia, consumption coagulopathy, leukopenia
- Steatorrhea and protein-losing enteropathy occur secondary to venous congestion of the intestinal mucosa.

- Degree of portal hypertension is variable and depends on the formation of spontaneous shunts that may decompress the portal hypertension. These autoshunts may predispose to the development of complications such as hepatic encephalopathy or hepatopulmonary syndrome.
- Spleen can undergo autoinfarction, resulting in intermittent episodes of pain.
- A large spleen is susceptible to traumatic rupture, and spontaneous rupture may occur with infectious mononucleosis.

ADDITIONAL READING
- Fuchs J, Warmann S, Kardorff R, et al. Mesenterico—left portal vein bypass in children with congenital extrahepatic portal vein thrombosis: A unique curative approach. *J Pediatr Gastroenterol Nutr*. 2003;36:213–216.
- Mowat AP. *Liver Disorders in Childhood*. Boston: Butterworths; 1987.
- Ryckman FC, Alonso MH. Causes and management of portal hypertension in the pediatric population. *Clin Liver Dis*. 2001;5:789–818.
- Superina RA, Alonso EM. Medical and surgical management of portal hypertension in children. *Curr Treat Options Gastroenterol*. 2006;9(5):432–443.
- Superina R, Shneider B, Emre S, et al. Surgical guidelines for the management of extra-hepatic portal vein obstruction. *Pediatr Transplant*. 2006;10(8):908–913.

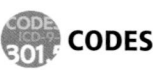 CODES

ICD9
- 452 Portal vein thrombosis
- 453.79 Chronic venous embolism and thrombosis of other specified veins
- 572.3 Portal hypertension

ICD10
- I81 Portal vein thrombosis
- I82.890 Acute embolism and thrombosis of other specified veins
- I82.891 Chronic embolism and thrombosis of other specified veins

FAQ
- Q: Should I restrict my child's activities?
- A: Contact sports should be limited or a spleen guard used. NSAIDs, including aspirin, should be avoided because of the risk of hemorrhage.

CELIAC DISEASE

Alycia A. Leiby
Vani V. Gopalareddy

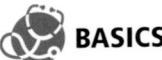

BASICS

DESCRIPTION
Celiac disease (CD) can be defined as a lifetime sensitivity to the gliadin fraction of the wheat protein gluten, (gluten consists of 4 gliadin fractions), and related alcohol-soluble proteins (called *prolamines*) found in rye and barley. CD occurs in genetically susceptible individuals who ingest these proteins, leading to chronic intestinal inflammation, epithelial damage, villous atrophy, and decreased absorptive surface. The mucosal lesions and symptoms resolve upon withdrawal of gluten-containing foods.

- Other names: Celiac sprue, nontropical sprue, and gluten-sensitive enteropathy
- The presentations of CD can be divided into the following categories:
  - Classic GI form: Typical presentation is younger than the age of 2 years, within a few months after the introduction of gluten-containing foods in the diet. The child presents with diarrhea, failure to thrive, anemia, fat malabsorption, wasting of muscles, bloated abdomen, fractious and unhappy behavior. The stools are explosive and foul, and half of the young children may have vomiting.
  - Celiac crisis: A rare presentation with explosive watery diarrhea, marked abdominal distention, dehydration, hypotension, lethargy, and electrolyte abnormalities
  - Late-onset GI form: Presentations in children older than 2 years include recurrent abdominal pain, bloating, constipation, mild or intermittent diarrhea, weight loss, and (rarely) nausea and vomiting.
  - Extraintestinal form
- Strong to moderate evidence:
  - Dental enamel defects: Caries of permanent dentition in all 4 quadrants (30%), hypoplasia of permanent teeth
  - Skin: Dermatitis herpetiformis in 5% of patients >15 years of age. The lesions are severely pruritic with erythematous blisters distributed symmetrically over the external surface of the extremities and on the trunk. Urticaria (hives) and psoriasis are also described.
  - Osteopenia/Osteoporosis
  - Short stature: 8–10% of children with short stature have CD.
  - Reproductive system: Delayed puberty, infertility, and spontaneous abortion, low-birth-weight infants
  - Hematological system: Anemia (iron-deficiency anemia unresponsive to treatment with oral iron)
  - Arthritis

- Evidence less strong:
  - Hepatic system: Cryptogenic hepatitis, autoimmune hepatitis, and chronic hypertransaminasemia, hepatic failure
  - CNS: Epilepsy, depression, dementia, schizophrenia, ataxia ("gluten-associated ataxia" due to cerebellar degeneration), migraine headaches. Behavioral changes such as irritability
  - Silent/Asymptomatic: Patients lack any GI or extraintestinal signs and symptoms. They are usually identified by population serologic screening or have the family history of CD. The small intestinal biopsy reveals mucosal damage in this group of individuals.
  - Potential/Latent CD: These patients have positive serology for the disease; however, the small intestine reveals normal histology. Over time, with further ingestion of gluten, it is believed that some of these individuals will develop CD.

EPIDEMIOLOGY
Incidence
- CD can present at any age after the introduction of gluten containing cereals.
- Women are more affected than men

Prevalence
- The prevalence of CD in children is between 3 and 13 per 1000 patients.
- Prevalence varies with the population studied; in the U.S. it is ~1 in 130.

RISK FACTORS
Risk increased by:
- Syndromes: Down (17-fold) Turner, and Williams
- Selective IgA deficiency (31-fold)
- 1st-degree relatives of patients with CD (18-fold)
- Diabetes Type 1: (4-fold)
- Repeat testing may be needed for at-risk patients who have negative initial serology and are HLA DQ2 and/or DQ8 positive.
- Breastfeeding, especially through the introduction of gluten may decrease the risk of celiac disease.

Genetics
- There is a 5–15% prevalence in 1st-degree relatives with CD. The concordance in monozygotic twins is supportive of a genetic role.
- 86–90% of patients have the HLA-DQ2, and ~5% carry the HLA-DQ8 allele.
  - 30% of general population in North America is HLA-DQ2 positive
  - Absence of DQ2 and DQ8 tests have a high negative predictive value.

COMMONLY ASSOCIATED CONDITIONS
- Autoimmune thyroiditis
- Type 1 diabetes mellitus
- Sjögren syndrome
- Selective IgA deficiency
- Williams syndrome
- Down syndrome
- Turner syndrome

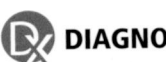

DIAGNOSIS

Failure to thrive, weight loss, abdominal pain, vomiting, diarrhea, constipation, abdominal distention

HISTORY
- Diet? Determine the relationship between initiation of gluten and the manifestation of symptoms.
- Description of stools? Stools tend to be explosive and foul smelling.
- Description of behavior? Young children tend to be irritable, older children may complain of fatigue, joint pains.

PHYSICAL EXAM
- Growth pattern: Some may have short stature and failure to thrive.
- Classic presentation is a large abdomen with wasted buttocks. Most patients do not have that appearance.
- Signs of anemia, dental enamel defects, dermatitis herpetiformis.

DIAGNOSTIC TESTS & INTERPRETATION
Diagnostic Procedures/Other
- Specific tests:
  - Serology, including tissue transglutaminase antibody IgA (tTG IgA), antiendomysial antibody (AEA), antigliadin antibody IgA/IgG (AGA IgA/IgG)
  - IgA quantification: 0.2–0.4% of the general population and 2–7% of patients with CD are IgA deficient; therefore, it is recommended to check serum IgA concurrently with the serology tests. If patients are IgA-deficient, then the IgA-type CD tests are unreliable.
  - Antigliadin antibody (AGA) IgA and IgG: 50–90% with active CD are positive. Unfortunately, many normal individuals without CD will have an elevated AGA IgG causing much confusion. This test is not recommended in population screening because of low specificity.
  - Deamidated antigliadin antibody IgA and IgG (D-AGA): Newer serologic test with 85% sensitivity and 95% specificity
  - tTG IgA: The autoantigen responsible for the endomysial pattern is tTG (90–100% sensitive and specific). The tTG assay correlates well with antiendomysial antibody (AEA) and biopsy. It is less expensive, rapid, and not a subjective test as opposed to the AEA assay.

- Nonspecific tests:
  - Laboratory tests for vitamin and mineral deficiency states, tests of absorption (fecal fat, D-xylose uptake), bone densitometry, class II HLA genotyping (DQ2 and DQ8), CBC, iron panel
- It is recommended to obtain multiple small bowel biopsies during endoscopy due to the patchy distribution of lesions.
  - Before the biopsy is done, check all the celiac antibodies as a screening test.
  - Separate biopsy from the duodenal bulb should also be taken
  - Biopsy should be done on an unrestricted diet.
  - The current recommendation is to obtain a small bowel biopsy on a gluten-containing diet. Symptoms should resolve on a glutenfree diet (GFD) with normalization of serology tests and the restoration of small bowel histology. Routine repeat biopsy is not necessary in children.

Pathological Findings
Features that characterize CD are:
- Partial, subtotal, or total villous atrophy
- Increased intraepithelial lymphocytes (>30%)
- Crypt hyperplasia
- Increased crypt cell mitosis
- Infiltration of lamina propria with excess lymphocytes (CD4 T cells mainly) and plasma cells

DIFFERENTIAL DIAGNOSIS
- Presumed infectious causes:
  - Giardiasis
  - Rotavirus, parasites
  - Chronic gastroenteritis
  - Postenteritis enteropathy
  - Intractable diarrhea of infancy
  - Tropical sprue
  - Intestinal bacterial overgrowth
  - Immunodeficiency syndromes (HIV)
- Presumed noninfectious:
  - Milk or soy protein intolerance
  - Protein-calorie malnutrition
  - Eosinophilic gastroenteritis
  - Autoimmune enteropathy
  - Graft-versus-host disease
  - Collagenous sprue
  - Peptic duodenitis
  - Immunodeficiency syndromes
  - Crohn disease
  - Congenital enteropathies (microvillus inclusion disease, tufting enteropathy)
  - Bowel ischemia
  - Radiation
  - Chemotherapy

 TREATMENT

MEDICATION (DRUGS)
- Lactase enzyme replacement at the beginning of GFD
- Calcium and vitamin D for osteopenia
- Iron for iron deficiency anemia

 ONGOING CARE

FOLLOW-UP RECOMMENDATIONS
Patient Monitoring
tTG and AGA titers are useful monitoring for recovery. A decrease in these antibodies is expected with a GFD, accompanied by improvement of presenting symptoms.
- It is suggested to recheck tTG after 6 months of GFD, then yearly in asymptomatic patients.

DIET
- GFD with resolution of GI symptoms within weeks:
  - Within 2 weeks of commencing a GFD, 70% of patients will note symptomatic improvement.
  - May need to restrict lactose initially due to secondary lactase deficiency
- GFD:
  - Avoidance of all wheat, rye, barley
  - Consider avoiding oats, secondary to cross-contamination with wheat proteins

PROGNOSIS
In patients on a strict GFD, there is very little risk of malignant lymphoma and other malignancies. In patients with CD, it is strongly recommended to remain on a GFD for life.

COMPLICATIONS
- Intestinal lymphoma has been reported in 10–15% of adult patients (>40 years of age) with CD who were noncompliant with GFD.
- Other complications (described mostly in adults) include other GI malignancies including carcinoma as well as strictures, ulcerative jejunoileitis, splenic atrophy, and skeletal disorders.
- Refractory CD
- Note: This has not been reported in childhood.
  - A diagnosis of exclusion defined by persistent symptoms of malabsorption despite a strict GFD for at least 6 months with continued villous atrophy on duodenal biopsy
  - This should provoke a workup for other causes of villous atrophy.
  - Affects up to 5% of adult patients with CD

- 75% of these patients harbor an abnormal clonal intraepithelial T-lymphocyte population, which is associated with a condition currently classified as "cryptogenic enteropathy-associated T-cell lymphoma."
- Complications of refractory sprue: Enteropathy-associated T-cell lymphoma, ulcerative jejunoileitis, and collagenous sprue.
- Treatment: Immunosuppressives including corticosteroids, azathioprine, cyclosporin, total parenteral nutrition, in addition to GFD

ADDITIONAL READING
- Fasano A, Catassi C. Coeliac disease in children. *Best Pract Res Clin Gastroenterol*. 2005;19:467–478.
- Hill ID, Dirks M, Liptak G, et al. Guideline for the diagnosis and treatment of celiac disease in children: Recommendations of the North American Society for Pediatric Gastroenterology, Hepatology and Nutrition. *J Pediatr Gastroenterol Nutr*. 2005;40:1–19.
- Leffler DA, Schuppan D. Update on serologic testing in celiac disease. *Am J Gastroenterol*. 2010;105(12):2520–2524.
- Olsson C, Hernell O, Hörnell A, et al. Difference in celiac disease risk between Swedish birth cohorts suggests an opportunity for primary prevention. *Pediatrics*. 2008;122(3):528–534.
- Rodrigues AF, Jenkins HR. Investigation and management of coeliac disease. *Arch Dis Child*. 2008;93(3):251–254.

 CODES

ICD9
579.0 Celiac disease

ICD10
K90.0 Celiac disease

FAQ
- Q: Are oats included in the gluten-containing cereal group?
- A: Strictly speaking, wheat, rye, and barley are more closely related in their development from the primitive grains than are oat, rice, corn, sorghum, and millets, which do not activate CD. Gluten free means a diet devoid of all wheat, rye, and barley. Several studies have shown that ingestion of oats did not cause histologic or clinical deterioration. However, it is important to use a brand of oats that has been tested and shown not have any gluten contaminants.

CELLULITIS
Nicholas Tsarouhas

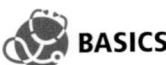 **BASICS**

DESCRIPTION
- Cellulitis is an acute, spreading pyogenic inflammation of the dermis and subcutaneous tissue, often complicating a wound or other skin condition.
- Cellulitis may be further classified by the unique area of the body it affects (e.g., periorbital or orbital cellulitis, peritonsillar cellulitis, etc.).

EPIDEMIOLOGY
- The most common cause of cellulitis in children is *Staphylococcus aureus* or *Streptococcus pyogenes* infection, which develops secondary to local trauma of the integument.
- Community-acquired methicillin-resistant *S. aureus* (CA-MRSA) infections continue to rise but are not seen as commonly with cellulitis as they are with purulent abscesses.
- The prevalence of CA-MRSA among purulent skin and soft tissue infections is >60% in some communities.
- Clinical failures with penicillin-resistant *S. pneumoniae* have not yet become a significant problem in cases of uncomplicated cellulitis.
- Bacteremic disease is uncommon owing to the tremendous efficacy of vaccines against both *Haemophilus influenzae* type b (HIB) and *Streptococcus pneumoniae*.

GENERAL PREVENTION
- Good wound care can prevent most cases.
- All wounds should be cleaned with soap and water, then covered with a clean, dry cloth.
- Topical antibiotic ointment is optional.

PATHOPHYSIOLOGY
- Cellulitis usually occurs after local trauma that breaches in the integument (abrasions, lacerations, bite wounds, excoriated dermatitis, varicella, etc.).
- May develop secondary to local invasion or infection (e.g., sinusitis leading to orbital cellulitis)
- Hematogenous dissemination (rarely)

ETIOLOGY
- *S. aureus*: MSSA (methicillin-susceptible *S. aureus*) and MRSA
- Group A β-hemolytic streptococci (GABHS, or *S. pyogenes*)
- *S. pneumoniae* (uncommon)
- Group B streptococci (GBS), gram-negative rods (GNRs): In neonates
- HiB (rare)
- *Pseudomonas aeruginosa*, anaerobic bacteria: In immunocompromised children
- *Pasteurella* species: From cat and dog bites
- *Eikenella corrodens*: From human bites

COMMONLY ASSOCIATED CONDITIONS
- Periorbital:
  - Usually from local trauma (scratch, impetigo, eczema, excoriated varicella, etc.)
  - Hematogenous spread is very uncommon.
  - Rarely associated with infectious conjunctivitis
- Orbital:
  - Commonly associated with severe sinusitis
  - Less commonly: Dental abscess, trauma, hematogenous spread
- Buccal: Usually from local trauma; hematogenous seeding also very rare.
- Peritonsillar:
  - Commonly secondary to GABHS pharyngitis
  - Cellulitis may progress to a peritonsillar abscess.
- Extremity: Usually secondary to local trauma
- Breast: Usually with mastitis (neonates)
- Perianal:
  - Seen in infants and young children
  - Etiology: GABHS
  - Perianal pain, pruritus, and erythema; sometimes associated with bloody stools
- Cellulitis–adenitis syndrome:
  - Uncommon infection of neonates and infants
  - Etiology: GBS, *S. aureus*, GNRs
  - Bacteremia/Meningitis commonly associated

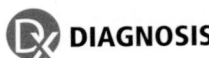 **DIAGNOSIS**

HISTORY
- An expanding, red, painful area of swelling is the most common presentation.
- Mild constitutional symptoms (with or without fever) are commonly associated with cellulitis.
- A history of local trauma to the integument is the clue to the portal of bacterial entry.
- Visual changes, proptosis, or painful or limited eye movements are classic findings in orbital cellulitis.
- Painful swallowing, pain with opening the mouth (trismus), and muffled ("hot potato") voice are classic presenting symptoms of peritonsillar cellulitis/abscess.

PHYSICAL EXAM
- Erythema, edema, tenderness, and warmth: Usual clinical findings of cellulitis
- Distinct demarcation of raised erythema: Classic description of erysipelas, a superficial cellulitis usually associated with *S. pyogenes*
- A red streak extending proximally from the extremity: Lymphangitis, which usually implies more serious involvement
- Regional adenopathy: Commonly associated with minor cellulitis; occasionally complicated by lymphadenitis

DIAGNOSTIC TESTS & INTERPRETATION
Lab
- WBC: Normal or elevated
- Blood culture: Rarely positive. Ill-appearing children and children with extensive areas of cellulitis may warrant a blood culture.
- Wound culture: As resistance continues to rise (especially MRSA), wound cultures are useful.

Imaging
- Radiographs: Sometimes helpful to rule out complications such as osteomyelitis. Also useful in cases of suspected foreign bodies
- Ultrasound: Often useful to distinguish cellulitis from abscess, which might need incision and drainage (I & D).
- Head CT scan: Important in cases when clinical distinction between periorbital and orbital cellulitis is difficult. Useful in orbital cellulitis to delineate extent of disease

Diagnostic Procedures/Other
In some cases, a cutaneous biopsy, examined by an experienced pathologist, may be needed to identify the correct diagnosis.

DIFFERENTIAL DIAGNOSIS
- *Allergic angioedema* can be excluded by its lack of tenderness and the absence of fever.
- Allergic reactions to *insect stings* are usually pruritic and may present with mild-to-severe local erythema; a bite history should be sought.
- Red giant *urticarial* lesions, similarly, may masquerade as cellulitis.
- *Contact dermatitis* is distinguished by its painlessness, pruritus, and the Koebner phenomenon (appearance of isomorphic lesions in the lines of scratching).
- A *traumatic contusion* may be mistaken for cellulitis, but the history should be confirmatory.
- Severe *conjunctivitis* presents with conjunctival injection, chemosis, and discharge.
- "*Popsicle panniculitis,*" a cold-induced fat injury to the cheeks of infants, mimics buccal cellulitis; a history of cold weather exposure, eating ice, or popsicle sucking should be sought.
- *Erythema nodosum*, a panniculitis, consists of raised, tender lesions that are frequently over the shins; it may present as a single erythematous lesion. It is associated with systemic disorders, including inflammatory bowel disease.
- *Superficial thrombophlebitis* is distinguished by a tender cord palpable along the course of the affected superficial vein.
- An *eye malignancy* (retinoblastoma), invasive *tumor* (rhabdomyosarcoma), or *metastatic disease* (neuroblastoma, leukemia, lymphoma) may simulate periorbital or orbital cellulitis.

TREATMENT

MEDICATION (DRUGS)

- Most cases of uncomplicated, superficial cellulitis may still be treated with β-lactam oral antibiotics active against *Staphylococcus* and *Streptococcus* (e.g., amoxicillin—clavulanate or cephalexin).
- Cephalexin may be the most cost-effective option in the routine outpatient management of uncomplicated cellulitis, especially in areas where MRSA prevalence is low (<10%).
- Alternatively, in areas where the local prevalence of community-associated MRSA is very high, empiric therapy for skin and soft tissue infections might include an antibiotic with MRSA coverage, such as clindamycin or trimethoprim-sulfamethoxazole.
- Abscesses, in which *S. aureus* is a likely pathogen, should be treated with clindamycin or trimethoprim-sulfamethoxazole; importantly, however, the mainstay of therapy is I & D.
- Trimethoprim-sulfamethoxazole, importantly, does not cover GABHS, a known important pathogen in some skin and soft tissue infections.
- Erythromycin may be used in patients allergic to penicillin.
- Isolates resistant to erythromycin may be cross-resistant to clindamycin as well.
- Tetracycline, doxycycline, and minocycline are additional alternatives, especially in the penicillin-allergic patients.
- Ill-appearing children or those with extensive cellulitic lesions require IV antibiotics.
- As MRSA infections continue to rise, many experts now recommend clindamycin as initial parenteral therapy.
- Oxacillin, nafcillin, cefazolin, and ampicillin—sulbactam are reasonable alternatives when MRSA is not strongly suspected.
- Vancomycin is used as empiric therapy in ill-appearing children or with severe or rapidly progressive infections.
- Linezolid, a newer antibiotic that can be given IV or PO, is very effective against MRSA, but it is expensive and should mostly be reserved for multiresistant organisms.
- If hematogenous dissemination is a strong possibility, an agent active against HiB also should be added (e.g., ceftriaxone, cefotaxime).
- The duration of antibiotics (IV and PO) should generally be 7–10 days.
- Bite wounds should have tetanus and rabies prophylaxis issues addressed.

ALERT

- Remember to consider the possibility of MRSA in all deep, invasive, or persistent infections (i.e., consider clindamycin).
- Penicillin and amoxicillin are never good empiric choices for cellulitis owing to their poor *S. aureus* coverage.

ADDITIONAL TREATMENT
General Measures
Local care of cellulitis involves elevation and immobilization of the limb to reduce swelling and cool sterile saline dressings to remove purulence from open lesions.

SURGERY/OTHER PROCEDURES
Abscesses should always be drained.

ONGOING CARE

FOLLOW-UP RECOMMENDATIONS
- Steady improvement should be expected.
- If daily improvement is not noted, consider:
  - Inappropriate antimicrobial coverage
  - A deeper infection or abscess that needs drainage
  - Foreign body

PROGNOSIS
The prognosis for complete recovery is good as long as appropriate antimicrobials are administered in a timely fashion.

COMPLICATIONS
- Local or distant spread of infection is possible.
- Suppuration and abscess formation may occur (e.g., peritonsillar abscess).
- Extremity cellulitis may extend into the deep tissues to produce an arthritis or osteomyelitis, or it may extend proximally as a lymphangitis.
- Orbital cellulitis may be complicated by visual loss and/or cavernous sinus thrombosis.
- Prior to widespread immunization against HiB, the bacteremia associated with facial cellulitis was associated with pneumonia, meningitis, pericarditis, epiglottitis, arthritis, and osteomyelitis.

ADDITIONAL READING

- Elliott DJ, Zaoutis TE, Troxel AB, et al. Empiric antimicrobial therapy for pediatric skin and soft-tissue infections in the era of methicillin-resistant Staphylococcus aureus. *Pediatrics.* 2009;123(6):e959–e966. Epub 2009 May 26.
- Falagas ME, Vergidis PI. Diseases that masquerade as infectious cellulitis. *Ann Intern Med.* 2005;142(1): 47–55.
- Hazin R, Abuzetun JY, Khatri KA. Derm diagnoses you can't afford to miss. *J Fam Pract.* 2009;58(6): 298–306.
- Hersh AL, Weintrub PS, Cabana MD. Antibiotic selection for purulent skin and soft-tissue infections in ambulatory care: A decision-analytic approach. *Acad Pediatr.* 2009;9(3):179–184.
- Hyun DY, Mason EO, Forbes A, et al. Trimethoprim-sulfamethoxazole or clindamycin for treatment of community-acquired methicillin-resistant Staphylococcus aureus skin and soft tissue infections. *Pediatr Infect Dis J.* 2009; 28(1):57–59.
- Khawcharoenporn T, Tice A. Empiric outpatient therapy with trimethoprim-sulfamethoxazole, cephalexin, or clindamycin for cellulitis. *Am J Med.* 2010;123(10):942–950.
- Odell CA. Community-associated methicillin-resistant Staphylococcus aureus (CA-MRSA) skin infections. *Curr Opin Pediatr.* 2010;22(3):273–277.
- Phillips S, MacDougall C, Holdford DA. Analysis of empiric antimicrobial strategies for cellulitis in the era of methicillin-resistant Staphylococcus aureus. *Ann Pharmacother.* 2007;41(1):13–20. Epub 2007 Jan 2.
- Rudloe TF, Harper MB, Prabhu SP, et al. Acute periorbital infections: Who needs emergent imaging? *Pediatrics.* 2010;125(4):e719–e726. Epub 2010 Mar 1.
- Stevens DL, Eron LL. Cellulitis and soft-tissue infections. *Ann Intern Med.* 2009;6:150(1):ITC11.

CODES

ICD9
- 041.00 Streptococcus infection in conditions classified elsewhere and of unspecified site, streptococcus, unspecified
- 682.9 Cellulitis and abscess, unspecified site

ICD10
- B95.5 Unspecified streptococcus as the cause of diseases classified elsewhere
- L03.90 Cellulitis, unspecified

FAQ

- Q: Should MRSA be considered only in patients with risk factors such as recent hospitalization, chronic illness, health care worker contact, and recent antibiotic use?
- A: No. MRSA is commonly isolated now from patients with no identified risk factors.
- Q: Is ophthalmology consultation necessary in all cases of periorbital cellulitis?
- A: Ophthalmology consultation is not necessary in simple, uncomplicated cases of periorbital cellulitis that clearly have no associated proptosis, limitation in extraocular eye movement, or visual impairment that would suggest a more serious orbital cellulitis.

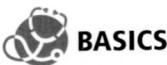

CEREBRAL PALSY

Stephen Contompasis

BASICS

DESCRIPTION
Cerebral palsy (CP) describes a group of disorders of movement and posture, limiting activity, attributed to nonprogressive underlying brain pathology. The motor disorders of CP are often accompanied by disturbances of sensation, cognition, communication, perception, and/or behavior, or by a seizure disorder:

- Spastic (pyramidal; 75%): Increased deep tendon reflexes, sustained clonus, hypertonia, and the clasp-knife response:
  - Spastic diplegia: Lower extremity involvement
  - Spastic hemiplegia: 1 side of the body involved
  - Spastic quadriplegia: Total body involvement; usually associated with dystonia
- Dyskinetic (10%): Fluctuating tone, rigid total body involvement by definition. Persistent primitive reflex patterns (asymmetric tonic neck reflex, labyrinthine)
  - Athetoid: Slow writhing movements (or chorea; rapid, random, jerky movements)
  - Dystonic: Posturing of the head, trunk, and extremities
- Ataxic (<10%): Characterized by cerebellar signs (ataxia, dysmetria, past pointing, tremor, nystagmus) and abnormalities of voluntary movement
- Mixed (10%): 2 or more types codominant, most often spastic and dyskinetic
- Other (10%): Criteria for CP met, but specific subtype cannot be defined
- Extrapyramidal: Sometimes applied to nonspastic types of CP as a group

EPIDEMIOLOGY
- ~50% of cases are associated with prematurity.
- Increased concordance among monozygotic versus dizygotic twins in some studies (not in others)
- Intrauterine growth retardation (IUGR) more common in CP than controls, especially for full-term infants in whom CP develops
- Male > female (1.3:1)
- Inconsistent relationship to maternal age, socioeconomic status, and parity
- Prenatal factors are more strongly associated with subsequent CP than are perinatal or postnatal factors; however, individual risk factors are poorly predictive of subsequent CP in the individual child.
- Perinatal asphyxia accounts for only ~9% of CP; diagnosis requires evidence of hypoxic-ischemic insult, severe encephalopathy (e.g., neonatal seizures, severe hypotonia), and consistent laboratory/radiologic findings.
- Increased with multiple gestation (10% were twins in 1 study)
- Prevalence ~2/1,000

ETIOLOGY
- Not apparent in most cases. A more recently recognized perinatal factor is the presence of chorioamnionitis; mild or even subclinical infection may have increased association with CP.
- Epidemiologic studies indicate 2 types of vulnerability to CP:
  - Prematurity: Vulnerability of the periventricular white matter between 28 and 32 weeks of gestation results in periventricular leukomalacia.
  - IUGR: Fetal growth retardation associated with CNS dysgenesis, non-CNS malformation, teratogens, growth retardation, evidence of hypoxic-ischemic encephalopathy

COMMONLY ASSOCIATED CONDITIONS
- Sensory:
  - Sensorineural and conductive hearing loss
  - Impaired visual acuity
  - Oculomotor dysfunction
  - Strabismus
  - Cortical visual impairment
  - Somatosensory impairments
- Cognitive/developmental:
  - Intellectual disability in ~50%, especially in spastic quadriparesis
  - Autism, ADHD
  - Language and learning disabilities
  - Dysarthria
  - Sleep and behavioral disturbances
- Neurologic:
  - Seizures
  - Hydrocephalus
- Musculoskeletal:
  - Contractures
  - Hip subluxation/dislocation
  - Scoliosis
- Cardiorespiratory:
  - Upper airway obstruction
  - Aspiration pneumonitis
  - Restrictive lung disease/thoracic deformity
  - Reactive airway disease
- GI/nutritional:
  - Poor growth
  - Gastroesophageal reflux
  - Constipation
  - Oral motor dysfunction/dysphagia
- Urinary: Neurogenic bladder
- Skin: Decubitus ulcers
- Dental:
  - Malocclusions
  - Caries
  - Gingival hyperplasia
  - Abnormalities of enamel (congenital)

DIAGNOSIS

HISTORY
- Prenatal:
  - Exposure to toxins/drugs
  - Infections or fever
  - HIV/STD risk
  - Vaginal bleeding
  - Abnormal fetal movement
  - Preeclampsia (especially proteinuria)
  - Breech position
  - Poor maternal weight gain
  - Premature labor
  - Fetal distress
  - IUGR
  - Prenatal testing
  - Placental disorders
- Perinatal:
  - Premature delivery
  - Neonatal resuscitation
  - Low Apgar scores (<5 at 5 minutes)
  - Birth trauma
  - Evidence of neonatal encephalopathy (seizures, lethargy, hypotonia)
  - Complicated neonatal course (intraventricular hemorrhage, prolonged respiratory support, meningitis, sepsis, hyperbilirubinemia)
- Postnatal:
  - Hospitalization for severe infection or trauma
  - Periodic or persistent deterioration in function (suggests neurodegenerative/metabolic disease)
- Development:
  - Significant delay in motor milestones/motor quotient (age of typical skill attainment/age of attainment <0.5) (e.g., not rolling at 10 months, not sitting at 12 months, not walking at 24 months)
  - Associated with persistent primitive reflexes (e.g., prominent tonic neck and labyrinthine responses at 1 year of age) and delayed or absent development of protective reactions (e.g., lateral prop at 7 months, parachute at 13 months)
  - Associated delays in language, play, social, and adaptive behavior

PHYSICAL EXAM
- General observation: Evidence of dysmorphism/pigmentary skin changes and growth abnormalities (clues to etiology)
- Head circumference: To evaluate for microcephaly/macrocephaly/hydrocephaly; growth velocity points to timing of brain pathology.
- Strabismus/cataracts/iris or retinal abnormalities: Eye exam: Cranial nerve damage, muscle imbalance, metabolic disease, or congenital infection
- Musculoskeletal:
  - Decreased range with contractures
  - Leg-length discrepancy: Hip dislocation
  - Spinal curvature/scoliosis

- Neurologic:
  - Documentation of best level of visual motor/manipulative skills (transfer, hold a cup): To follow course of motor impairment
  - Cranial nerves: Strabismus, speech and swallowing, vision and hearing
  - Tone: Spasticity versus rigidity versus hypotonia
  - Strength: Often decreased
  - Hyperactive deep tendon reflexes and clonus in spasticity; Babinski reflex (extensor response to plantar stimulation)
  - Persistent primitive reflexes
  - Protective reactions: Head and trunk righting, prop reactions, parachute; cerebellar signs
  - Balance, stability

ALERT
Pitfalls:
- Overdiagnosis of CP in premature infants with spastic hypertonia; normalization of tone/function may take up to 2 years.
- False or premature assumption of cognitive deficit in children with severe dysarthria. May take years of augmentative communication supports to determine true potential
- Slowly progressive neurodegenerative disease and pediatric neurotransmitter disorders may masquerade as CP.
- Cervical cord lesions may masquerade as quadriparetic spastic CP.
- Determination of ideal body weight/caloric requirements may be complex in CP; skinfold measuring <10th percentile best indicator of poor nutrition
- Pain is a common problem, with more than half of adults and children with CP reporting pain as an ongoing health concern.

DIAGNOSTIC TESTS & INTERPRETATION
Lab
- Genetic and metabolic studies: If history or physical suggests a progressive or hereditary disorder
- Blood chemistries, liver function studies, cell counts: Evaluate nutritional/metabolic status, anticonvulsant levels

Imaging
- Brain imaging: Perform when hydrocephalus is suspected; can help determine etiology
- Radiography: Should be done routinely in spastic diparesis for hip dislocation; consider scoliosis films.
- Radionuclide studies to evaluate gastroesophageal reflux, gastric emptying, aspiration

Diagnostic Procedures/Other
- Hearing and vision: All in 1st year, with regular follow-up exams
- Audiologic evaluation required per guidelines
- Urodynamic studies: Spastic bladder in those with recurrent UTIs or voiding dysfunction
- Sleep study: May disclose treatable obstructive sleep apnea in those with somnolence or abnormal sleep–wake cycles

- Pulmonary function studies: Document progressive restrictive pulmonary dysfunction (e.g., in severe scoliosis)
- Consider bone density: Liability to fractures
- Brain wave (EEG): If seizure suspected

DIFFERENTIAL DIAGNOSIS
- Motor syndromes related to spinal cord, lower motor neuron, peripheral nerve, primary muscular disease, or progressive disorders of the basal ganglia (dopa-responsive dystonia)
- Connective tissue disorders (primary and secondary) resulting in musculoskeletal abnormalities (e.g., arthrogryposis multiplex, skeletal dysplasias)
- Inborn errors of metabolism and CP: Protean manifestations, dyskinesia, ataxia, postnatal growth failure, neurologic deterioration, recurrent vomiting

 TREATMENT

ADDITIONAL TREATMENT
General Measures
- Family-centered care is directed toward optimizing activity and participation.
- Interdisciplinary clinics: Services (medical, surgical, therapy) coordinated with primary physician
- More frequent health maintenance visits and coordination meetings from a medical home practice may assist in managing multiple chronic associated heath conditions.
- Spasticity reduction with IM injections of botulinum toxin and oral or intrathecal Baclofen used increasingly, though consensus on functional improvement long term is variable
- Orthopedic management with directed procedures to reduce contractures and improve posture has more evidence on improving functional outcomes long term.
- Education services: Recent emphasis on inclusion/mainstreaming; for many, special education services are still required.
- Augmentative communication supports especially for nonverbal/dysarthric children
- Physical, occupational, speech/language therapy, other allied health professionals: Therapy provided in home, school, and hospital settings; directed primarily at improved mobility, self-care, and communication; orthodontists for braces
- Counseling support for children coping with chronic disability
- Social services: Provided in a variety of contexts to aid in the coordination of care
- Vocational counseling and employment options, assistance with transition to adulthood, self-advocacy, self-determination
- Transition to adult health care system

 ONGOING CARE

FOLLOW-UP RECOMMENDATIONS
- Requirements for follow-up vary greatly with the degree of disability and impairment. An interdisciplinary clinic setting may be more appropriate for a child with severe CP.
- Early referral to a pediatric orthopedist is indicated, especially for monitoring of the hip.
- Early referral for developmental assessment: Need for early intervention, to optimize development and promote family coping

DIET
Nutritional assessment and support for those with dysphagia or poor growth (especially calcium, vitamin D intake)

ADDITIONAL READING
- Ashwal S, Russman BS, Blasco PA, et al. Practice parameter: Diagnostic assessment of the child with cerebral palsy. Report of the Quality Standards Subcommittee of the American Academy of Neurology and the Practice Committee of the Child Neurology Society. *Neurology.* 2004;62:851–863.
- Cooley WC. Providing a primary care medical home for children and youth with cerebral palsy. *Pediatrics.* 2004;114(4):1106–1113.
- Pakula AT, Van Naarden Braun K, Yeargin-Allsopp M. Cerebral palsy: Classification and epidemiology. *Phys Med Rehabil Clin N Am.* 2009;20(3):425–452.
- Rosenbaum P, Paneth N, Leviton A, et al. A report: The definition and classification of cerebral palsy April 2006. *Dev Med Child Neurol.* 2007;49:8–14. doi:10.1111/j.1469-8749.2007.tb12610.x
- Strauss D, Brooks J, Rosenbloom L, et al. Life expectancy in cerebral palsy: an update. *Dev Med Child Neurol.* 2008;50(7):487–493.

 CODES

ICD9
- 333.71 Athetoid cerebral palsy
- 343.9 Infantile cerebral palsy, unspecified
- 344.89 Other specified paralytic syndrome

ICD10
- G80.0 Spastic quadriplegic cerebral palsy
- G80.3 Athetoid cerebral palsy
- G80.9 Cerebral palsy, unspecified

FAQ
- Q: Is severe clumsiness a form of CP?
- A: Mild spastic diplegia or hemiplegia may present this way, but tone abnormalities and significant functional impairments distinguish CP from milder developmental coordination disorders.
- Q: Do all children with CP also have intellectual disability?
- A: Only ~50% have intellectual disability.

CERVICITIS

Sarah E. Winters
Elizabeth M. Wallis
Jane Lavelle (5th edition)

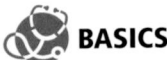

BASICS

DESCRIPTION
Infection of the endocervix resulting in inflammation, leading to mucopurulent cervical discharge, edema, erythema, bleeding, and friability of the cervix and endocervical canal

EPIDEMIOLOGY
- The true incidence of cervicitis is unknown, but the primary causes (gonorrhea/chlamydia) are more common in adolescents and young adults than any other age group.
- Because many patients are asymptomatic and the interpretation and presence of the clinical signs is quite variable, many cases go undiagnosed.

RISK FACTORS
- Early age of coitarche
- Multiple sexual partners
- Absent/Inconsistent condom use

ETIOLOGY
In most cases of cervicitis, no pathogen is isolated. Common causes include:
- Chlamydia trachomatis
- Neisseria gonorrheae
- Herpesvirus hominis
- Trichomonas vaginalis
- Mycoplasma genitalium

COMMONLY ASSOCIATED CONDITIONS
The presence of other sexually transmitted infections (STIs) must be considered, including:
- Syphilis
- Hepatitis B
- HIV
- Bacterial vaginosis

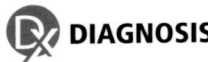

DIAGNOSIS

HISTORY
- Often asymptomatic
- If symptomatic: Symptoms consistent with but not diagnostic of cervicitis:
  - Abnormal vaginal bleeding and/or discharge? Inflamed cervix may bleed spontaneously or following sexual intercourse
  - Dysuria? May indicate urethritis or bladder infection
  - Vulvar itching? May be associated discharge from cervical inflammation or a coexisting vaginal infection
  - Dyspareunia? Common complaint owing to the sensitive cervix

- Past medical history—important to evaluate risk factors related to sexual health, but not diagnostic of cervicitis:
  - Previous STI? Identifies patients at increased risk for reinfection
  - Last menstrual period? Symptomatic infection often occurs within 7 days of the last menstrual period because of loss of the protective endocervical mucous plug.
  - Birth control method? Condoms are protective.
  - Exposure to infected partner? Identifies patient at increased risk
  - Gravity?
  - Parity?

PHYSICAL EXAM
- Abdominal: No tenderness on palpation of the abdomen—infection is limited to the cervix.
- Vaginal: Signs of vaginal/external lesions consistent with herpes simplex virus (HSV)
- Pelvic:
  - Mucopurulent discharge from the cervical os or yellow exudative discharge present on a cotton-tipped swab from the endocervical canal: Clinical evidence of cervical infection
  - No cervical motion or adnexal tenderness or masses: Pathology has not extended beyond the cervix to the upper genital tract.
  - Friability of the exocervix: Easily induced bleeding from the cervical canal, not to be confused with normal cervical ectopy (area of columnar epithelium around the cervical os presenting as a discrete, nonfriable, reddish circle)

ALERT
Pitfalls:
- Failure to recognize the importance of evaluating the internal pelvic organs by physical examination with the presenting symptoms of dysuria, vaginal discharge, or abnormal menstrual bleeding in the postpubertal female.
- Imperative not to confuse normal cervical ectropion in an adolescent with cervicitis.

DIAGNOSTIC TESTS & INTERPRETATION
Lab
- Nucleic acid amplification tests done on the patient's urine offers the least invasive method to detect chlamydia and/or gonococcal infection. Cervical or vaginal swabs may also be used for nucleic acid amplification tests provided that there is no bleeding:
  - Cervical swabs, vaginal swabs obtained by the health care provider, and urine have similar sensitivity and specificity.
  - Cervical cultures for chlamydia and gonorrhea will also identify the pathogen, but require a speculum examination.
  - Identifies the pathogen, which is important for patient and partner treatment and disease surveillance

- HSV culture if vesicular rash or ulcers are present: Important to identify the cause of the ulcers for treatment and patient counseling
- Wet preparation, culture or antigen testing for T. vaginalis: Often coexisting infection when other STIs are identified.

DIFFERENTIAL DIAGNOSIS
- It is helpful to consider cervicitis/vaginitis as a single disease in the evaluation process because the symptoms of these two entities are the same.
- Inflammation of the vulva, urethra, and/or bladder, and vagina
- In patients presenting with abnormal menstrual bleeding, these infectious causes are common.
- Pregnancy is a frequent cause of abnormal vaginal bleeding.
- Foreign body can be associated with both discharge and bleeding.
- PCOS, thyroid dysfunction, and hyperprolactinemia can all present with abnormal vaginal bleeding.

TREATMENT

MEDICATION (DRUGS)
- Gonorrhea:
  - Ceftriaxone 250 mg IM or, if not available, cefixime 400 mg PO in a single dose PLUS azithromycin 1 g PO, single dose or doxycycline 100 mg PO b.i.d. for 7 days
  - Recently noticed patterns of resistance to fluoroquinolones have caused the CDC to no longer recommend this class as 1st line of treatment of gonococcal cervicitis in the U.S. If fluoroquinolones are used, a test of cure is necessary.
- C. trachomatis:
  - Azithromycin 1 g PO, single dose
  - Doxycycline 100 mg PO b.i.d. for 7 days
  - Erythromycin base 500 mg PO q.i.d. for 7 days
- T. vaginalis:
  - Metronidazole 2 g PO, single dose
  - Metronidazole 500 mg PO b.i.d. for 7 days
  - Tinidazole 2 g PO in a single dose
- H. hominis:
  - Acyclovir 400 mg PO t.i.d. for 7–10 days or until resolution
  - Acyclovir 200 mg PO 5 times daily for 7–10 days or until resolution
  - Famciclovir 250 mg PO t.i.d. for 7–10 days or until resolution
  - Valacyclovir 1 g PO b.i.d. for 7–10 days or until resolution

IN-PATIENT CONSIDERATIONS
Initial Stabilization
Patients meeting the criteria for the clinical diagnosis of cervicitis or those who have a high likelihood of infection should receive presumptive therapy for *N. gonorrheae* and *C. trachomatis*. Treat other pathogens if clinically indicated or if documented by laboratory studies.

 ## ONGOING CARE

FOLLOW-UP RECOMMENDATIONS
- The recommended treatment regimens have an excellent cure rate.
- The patient should have resolution of symptoms 3–5 days after starting therapy.
- Routine follow-up cultures are not necessary unless the patient remains symptomatic or in the case of pregnancy.
- Nucleic acid amplification tests done <6 weeks following treatment may yield false-positive results because of persistence of dead organisms.
- Detection of an STI at follow-up is most likely the result of re-exposure and reinfection.

Patient Monitoring
- Partners should be referred for evaluation and treatment if laboratory diagnosis of GC/Chlamydia or *Trichomonas* is made
- GC/Chlamydia are reportable STIs

PROGNOSIS
If treated appropriately, patients are cured and have no sequelae from the infection.

COMPLICATIONS
The patient with endocervical infection is at risk for:
- Reinfection
- Other STIs
- Pregnancy

- Symptomatic or asymptomatic upper genital tract disease, (pelvic inflammatory disease), with all its sequelae:
  – Tubo-ovarian abscess
  – Infertility
  – Ectopic pregnancy
  – Chronic pelvic pain

ADDITIONAL READING
- American Academy of Pediatrics. Sexually transmitted diseases. In: Pickering LK, eds. *2007 Red Book: Report of the Committee on Infectious Diseases*, 27th ed. Elk Grove Village, IL: American Academy of Pediatrics; 2007.
- Centers for Disease Control and Prevention. Sexually transmitted diseases treatment guidelines, 2010. *MMWR*. 2010;59(RR-12).
- Centers for Disease Control and Prevention. Update to CDC's sexually transmitted diseases treatment guidelines, 2006: Fluoroquinolones no longer recommended for treatment of gonococcal infections. *MMWR Morb Mortal Wkly Rep.* 2007; 56(14):332–336.
- Emans JS, Laufer MR, Goldstein DP. *Pediatric and Adolescent Gynecology*, 5th ed. Philadelphia: Lippincott Williams & Wilkins; 2005.
- Holmes KK. Lower genital tract infection syndromes in women. In: Holmes KK, Sparling PF, Stamm WE, et al., eds. *Sexually Transmitted Diseases*, 4th ed. New York: McGraw-Hill; 2007:987–1016.
- Neinstein LS. *Adolescent Health Care: A Practical Guide*, 5th ed. Philadelphia: Lippincott Williams & Wilkins; 2007.

 ## CODES

ICD9
- 098.15 Gonococcal cervicitis (acute)
- 099.53 Other venereal diseases due to chlamydia trachomatis, lower genitourinary sites
- 616.0 Cervicitis and endocervicitis

ICD10
- A54.03 Gonococcal cervicitis, unspecified
- A56.01 Chlamydial cystitis and urethritis
- N72 Inflammatory disease of cervix uteri

FAQ
- Q: How much cervical motion tenderness is present in patients with cervicitis?
- A: None. Patients with cervicitis have inflammation and infection of the cervix only. They do not have any evidence of peritoneal inflammation on physical examination; therefore, patients with tenderness should be treated with the protocols recommended by the Centers for Disease Control and Prevention for pelvic inflammatory disease. This does not include the use of a single dose of azithromycin.
- Q: Which partners should be referred for treatment?
- A: Sex partners from the preceding 60 days should be referred for evaluation and treatment. Treatment is based on documented or presumptive etiologies.
- Q: What is the appropriate treatment for *M. genitalium*?
- A: *M. genitalium* has clearly been implicated in the development of urethritis in males and is thought to play some role in the development of cervicitis in females (although that role is not entirely clear). Data suggests that azithromycin may be the best treatment for this infection.
- Q: How often should asymptomatic sexually active adolescents be screened for STIs?
- A: Sexually active men and women under 25 should be screened annually for STIs.

CHANCROID

Heather McKeag
Christine S. Cho (5th edition)

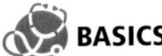 **BASICS**

DESCRIPTION
Infection with the gram-negative coccobacillus *Haemophilus ducreyi*, resulting in necrotizing, purulent, painful genital ulcers that may be associated with regional lymphadenitis.

EPIDEMIOLOGY
- Probably underrecognized and underreported
- In underdeveloped countries, it is a major cause of genital ulcer syndrome.
- Major cofactor in the transmission of HIV
- Seen more commonly in males; females are more likely to be asymptomatic.
- Occurs in discrete outbreaks; endemic in some areas of the U.S.
- Sexual contact is the only known route of transmission.
- If diagnosed in children, sexual abuse should be considered.

Incidence
Cases in the U.S. steadily declined until 2000, since then the incidence has fluctuated. In 2009, there were 28 reported cases.

RISK FACTORS
Increased association with individuals involved in drug use and prostitution

GENERAL PREVENTION
- Condom use
- Treatment of partners whether or not they have symptoms
- Evaluation for the presence of other sexually transmitted diseases

PATHOPHYSIOLOGY
- Trauma and abrasion allow the organism to penetrate the epidermis.
- 3–10 days later, an erythematous, tender papule develops and progresses to a pustule.
- The pustule ruptures after 2–3 days, leaving a shallow ulcer with a painful, necrotic base with undermined edges.
- Single or multiple ulcers may be present.

ETIOLOGY
The most common causes of genital ulcer syndrome include syphilis, HSV, and chancroid.

COMMONLY ASSOCIATED CONDITIONS
- Associated with HIV transmission and infection
- Coinfection with syphilis and human herpesvirus may occur (10%).

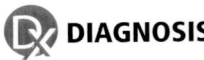 **DIAGNOSIS**

Diagnosis of chancroid routinely based on clinical findings after the exclusion of other causes of genital ulcer disease.

HISTORY
- Males usually present with symptoms referable to an acute painful genital ulcer.
- Females may be asymptomatic or present with nonspecific symptoms (dysuria, vaginal discharge, pain with stooling or sexual intercourse, rectal pain, or bleeding).

PHYSICAL EXAM
Classic findings:
- Extremely painful ulcer with an irregular, undermined border and a gray, necrotic center:
  - In males: Found on prepuce or coronal sulcus
  - In females: Found on the vulva, cervix, or perianal area
- Painful, unilateral, inguinal lymphadenopathy in 50%: May spontaneously drain (bubo)
- Extragenital sites are rare and include the inner thigh area, breasts, fingers, mouth.

DIAGNOSTIC TESTS & INTERPRETATION
Diagnosis is made by clinical findings and exclusion of other causes of genital ulcers.

Lab
- Gram stain from the base of the ulcer: May show short gram-negative coccobacilli in parallel "school of fish" arrangement. This finding does not compare favorably with culture-proven or clinically diagnosed cases, so routine use is not helpful.
- Cultures from the ulcer:
  - *H. ducreyi* is a fastidious organism and requires specialized media and technique for successful isolation.
  - Compared with newer amplification techniques, it has been proven to be 75% sensitive
  - Currently the only method routinely available for the definite diagnosis of chancroid
- DNA amplification:
  - A genital ulcer multiplex polymerase chain reaction (GUM) test has been developed for simultaneous amplification of DNA targets from *H. ducreyi*, *T. pallidum*, and HSV types 1 and 2; offers improved sensitivity when compared with culture
  - This technology is not routinely available

- Monoclonal antibody:
  - Monoclonal antibody against the outer membrane protein of *H. ducreyi* using immunofluorescent antibody has also proven to be more sensitive than culture.
  - Could provide easy, rapid, inexpensive, sensitive testing, but not available currently
- Additional testing:
  - Culture and PCR for HSV 1 & 2, RPR: Evaluation for the common causes of genital ulcer syndrome should be done routinely.
  - HIV test: Genital ulcers are a significant cofactor for HIV infection.

DIFFERENTIAL DIAGNOSIS
- Chancroid must be distinguished from the other causes of genital ulcers, including syphilis, herpes simplex virus (HSV), lymphogranuloma venereum, and granuloma inguinale. More than one of these pathogens may be present in individual cases.
- Uncommon etiologies include:
  - Trauma
  - Fixed drug eruptions
  - Lymphogranuloma venereum
  - Inflammatory bowel disease
  - Behçet syndrome

 TREATMENT

MEDICATION (DRUGS)
- Azithromycin 1 g PO, once
- Ceftriaxone 250 mg IM, once
- Ciprofloxacin 500 mg b.i.d. for 3 days (patients >18 years)
- Erythromycin 500 mg q.i.d. for 7 days
- One-time directly observed dosing with azithromycin or ceftriaxone recommended.

SURGERY/OTHER PROCEDURES
Persistent inguinal fluctuant adenitis may be treated with either needle aspiration or incision and drainage.

 ONGOING CARE

FOLLOW-UP RECOMMENDATIONS
- Symptoms improve within 3–7 days.
- Ulcers heal between 1 and 4 weeks.
- Lymphadenopathy may take longer to regress; may progress to fluctuance in spite of adequate therapy.
- Patients should be followed weekly until symptoms resolve.
- For patients who do not follow the typical course, consider other causes of genital ulcers; noncompliance; presence of a coexisting sexually transmitted disease, especially HIV infection; and, rarely, presence of a resistant organism.
- Recent sexual partners (within the preceding 10 days) should be treated.
- If initial HIV and syphilis test results are negative, they should be repeated in 3 months following diagnosis of chancroid.

PATIENT EDUCATION
Prevention: Condom use with all sexual activity

COMPLICATIONS
- Draining bubo
- Coinfection with syphilis and HSV
- HIV infection

ADDITIONAL READING
- American Academy of Pediatrics. Chancroid. In: Pickering LK, Baker CJ, Kimberlin DW, Long SS, eds. *Red Book: 2009 Report of the Committee on Infectious Diseases*, 28th ed. Elk Grove Village, IL: American Academy of Pediatrics; 2009:250–252.
- Centers for Disease Control and Prevention. STD Surveillance 2009. Available at: http://www.cdc.gov/std/stats09/tables/1.htm Accessed February 26, 2011.
- Karthikeyan K. Recent advances in management of genital ulcer disease and anogenital warts. *Dermatol Ther*. 2008;21(3):196–204.
- Lewis DA. Chancroid: Clinical manifestations, diagnosis and management. *J Sex Health HIV*. 2003;79:68–71.
- Mackay IM, Harnett G, Jeoffreys N, et al. Detection and discrimination of herpes simplex viruses, *Haemophilus ducreyi*, *Treponema pallidum*, and Calymmatobacterium (*Klebsiella*) granulomatis from genital ulcers. *Clin Infect Dis*. 2006;42(10):1431–1438.
- Trager JD. Sexually transmitted diseases causing genital lesions in adolescents. *Adolesc Med Clin*. 2004;15(2):323–352.

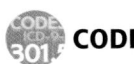 **CODES**

ICD9
099.0 Chancroid

ICD10
A57 Chancroid

C

CHEST PAIN

Steven M. Selbst

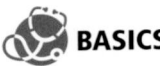 **BASICS**

DEFINITION
Chest pain is a common pain syndrome in childhood. It is less common than abdominal pain and headache. Commonly Associated Conditions

COMMONLY ASSOCIATED CONDITIONS
- Asthma
- Cystic fibrosis
- Diabetes mellitus (long-standing)
- Hypertrophic cardiomyopathy
- Kawasaki disease
- Marfan syndrome
- Sickle cell disease
- Systemic lupus erythematosus

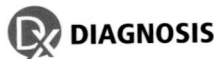 **DIAGNOSIS**

DIFFERENTIAL DIAGNOSIS
- **Musculoskeletal disorders**
  - Chest wall strain
  - Costochondritis
  - Direct chest trauma
  - Slipping rib syndrome
- **Cardiac pathology**
  - Arrhythmia (supraventricular tachycardia, premature ventricular contractions)
  - Coronary artery anomalies
  - Coronary artery aneurysms (Kawasaki disease)
  - Infections (myocarditis, pericarditis)
  - Myocardial infarction/ischemia
  - Structural abnormalities: Aortic stenosis, hypertrophic cardiomyopathy, pulmonic stenosis, mitral valve prolapse, severe coarctation of the aorta
- **GI disorders**
  - Caustic ingestions
  - Esophageal foreign bodies
  - Esophagitis (sometimes tetracycline, "pill," induced)
- **Psychogenic causes**
  - Anxiety
  - Hyperventilation
- **Respiratory disorders**
  - Asthma
  - Cough (prolonged)
  - Pleural effusion
  - Pneumonia
  - Pneumothorax: Spontaneous, trauma related, drug related (cocaine)
  - Pneumomediastinum
  - Pulmonary embolism
- **Miscellaneous**
  - Breast mass
  - Cigarette smoke
  - Pleurodynia
  - Precordial catch syndrome
  - Shingles
  - Sickle cell crises
  - Thoracic tumor

APPROACH TO THE PATIENT
Identify the rare child with a serious cause for chest pain (see table in "Physical Exam"—[Important Physical Findings on General Examination of Child with Chest Pain])
- **Phase 1:** Is the patient in acute distress? If so, begin emergency management and proceed rapidly to find the cause of pain.
- **Phase 2:** For most stable children with chest pain, determine whether laboratory tests are needed to help identify the cause.
- **Phase 3:** Treat specific conditions as appropriate. Begin analgesics, reassure the family, and arrange for follow-up care.

Hints for Screening Problems
Take a thorough history and perform a careful physical exam. Examine the chest last—do not focus only on this area. Use laboratory tests sparingly, only to confirm clinical suspicions.

HISTORY
- **Question:** How severe, how often is the pain?
- *Significance:* Constant, frequent severe pain is more likely to be distressing, interruptive of daily activity. Serious etiology is not well correlated with frequency, severity of pain.
- **Question:** What is the type of pain? Its location?
- *Significance:* Burning pain is associated with esophagitis. Sharp, stabbing pain relieved by sitting up or leaning forward is typical of pericarditis. Young children do not describe or localize chest pain well.
- **Question:** When was the onset of pain?
- *Significance:* Acute pain (<48 hours) is more likely to have an organic cause. Chronic pain (>6 months) is more likely to be psychogenic, idiopathic. In an older child with sudden onset of pain, consider an arrhythmia, pneumothorax, or musculoskeletal injury. In a young child with sudden onset of pain, consider a foreign body (coin) in the esophagus, or injury.
- **Question:** Is the pain induced by exercise?
- *Significance:* Exercise-induced chest pain may be related to serious cardiac disease or asthma.
- **Question:** Recent trauma, rough play, or muscle overuse?
- *Significance:* Musculoskeletal (chest wall) pain
- **Question:** Eaten spicy foods? Taken tetracycline or other pills?
- *Significance:* Esophagitis. Teens often take pills with little water and then lie down. The undissolved pill may lodge in the esophagus and cause pain.
- **Question:** Recent use of cocaine?
- *Significance:* Hypertension, tachycardia, myocardial ischemia, or pneumothorax
- **Question:** Use of oral contraceptives or recent leg trauma?
- *Significance:* Pulmonary embolism. This is rare in the pediatric age group.

- **Question:** Recent significant stress (e.g., move, death of loved one, serious illness)?
- *Significance:* Psychogenic pain. We know children have headaches and abdominal pain related to stress. Chest pain may also relate to unusual stress.
- **Question:** Associated complaints?
- *Significance:* Fever may imply pneumonia, myocarditis, and pericarditis. Syncope, palpitations may imply cardiac arrhythmias or severe anemia. Joint pain, rash may relate chest pain to collagen vascular disease. Pain that resolves with parental attention may indicate an emotional cause.
- **Question:** Positive familial history?
- *Significance:* Hypertrophic cardiomyopathy is often familial. Those with this disorder may have familial history positive for sudden death. When there is a positive familial history of heart disease or chest pain, the parents may be unusually concerned about the symptom in a child. The child often has a nonorganic cause.
- **Question:** Past medical history?
- *Significance:* Previous Kawasaki disease, long-standing insulin-dependent diabetes mellitus, and sickle cell disease may have serious cardiac or pulmonary complications leading to chest pain. Marfan syndrome has increased risk for aortic dissection, pneumothorax. Asthma has increased risk for pneumonia, pneumothorax. Collagen vascular disease has increased risk for pleural effusion, pericarditis. Most underlying structural cardiac lesions rarely produce chest pain.

PHYSICAL EXAM
- **Important physical findings on general examination of child with chest pain**
  - Severe distress
  - Chronically ill appearance
  - Fever
  - Skin rash or bruising
  - Abdominal pathology
  - Arthritis present
  - Anxiety apparent
- **Finding:** Child is in significant distress?
- *Significance:* Requires emergency care; stabilization. Consider pneumothorax, arrhythmia.
- **Finding:** Child appears chronically ill?
- *Significance:* Chest pain may be found in serious illnesses such as malignancy (Hodgkin lymphoma) or systemic lupus erythematosus.
- **Finding:** Fever?
- *Significance:* Consider pneumonia, myocarditis, pericarditis
- **Finding:** Skin bruising present?
- *Significance:* Chest pain may be related to unrecognized trauma. Osteomyelitis of the rib is a rare cause.
- **Finding:** Abdominal pathology?
- *Significance:* Pain may be referred to the chest.
- **Finding:** Arthritis present?
- *Significance:* Collagen vascular disease may manifest as pleural effusion, chest pain.
- **Finding:** Unusually anxious child?
- *Significance:* Underlying stress may lead to pain.

- **Important physical findings on chest examination of child with chest pain**
  - Breast abnormality
  - Subcutaneous emphysema
  - Heart murmur, rub, arrhythmia
  - Chest wall tenderness
- **Finding:** Breast enlargement, asymmetry, tenderness?
- *Significance*: Physiologic breast changes in young teens may be painful. Consider pregnancy in teenage girls. *
- **Finding:** Decreased breath sounds, wheezing?
- *Significance*: May suggest pneumonia, asthma with overuse of chest wall muscles.
- **Finding:** Subcutaneous emphysema palpable on chest or neck?
- *Significance*: Pneumothorax, pneumomediastinum
- **Finding:** Heart murmur, rub, arrhythmia?
- *Significance*: Congenital heart disease, cardiac infections such as myocarditis, pericarditis, supraventricular tachycardia, ventricular tachycardia
- **Finding:** Tenderness of chest wall, costochondral junctions?
- *Significance*: Musculoskeletal pain

ALERT
Factors that make this an emergency include:
- Pneumothorax: May present with severe sudden chest pain, respiratory distress, cyanosis, hypotension
- Cardiac arrhythmia: Ventricular tachycardia or supraventricular tachycardia in an older child may progress to heart failure or a lethal rhythm.
- Cocaine intoxication: May present with pneumothorax, cardiac arrhythmia, hypertension
- Direct chest trauma: May lead to cardiac contusion and arrhythmia
- Caustic ingestions or esophageal foreign bodies require prompt attention.

DIAGNOSTIC TESTS & INTERPRETATION
- **Test:** EKG
- *Significance*:
  - Obtain if history suggests cardiac pathology (e.g., acute onset of pain, pain on exertion, pain associated with syncope, dizziness, palpitations, history of congenital heart disease, serious associated medical problems [Kawasaki disease, diabetes mellitus], use of cocaine)
  - Obtain also if physical exam is abnormal. For instance, respiratory distress, cardiac abnormality, fever, significant trauma
- **Test:** Holter monitor
- *Significance*: Arrange for this study if cardiac arrhythmia suspected. Electrocardiogram may fail to detect intermittent arrhythmia.
- **Test:** Exercise stress test, pulmonary function tests
- *Significance*: Obtain if pain induced by exertion
- **Test:** Drug screen
- *Significance*: Obtain if cocaine use suspected

Imaging
Chest radiograph:
- Same as for EKG
- Obtain also if history suggests cardiac or pulmonary pathology, tumor, Marfan syndrome, or foreign body (coin ingestion)
- Obtain also if physical exam suggests decreased breath sounds or palpation of subcutaneous air

 TREATMENT

ADDITIONAL TREATMENT
General Measures
Chest pain in children is rarely related to cardiac pathology: Not all children with chest pain have a benign etiology; pain associated with exertion, syncope, dizziness is concerning for heart disease; if the child is febrile, consider pneumonia or viral myocarditis. Treat specific cause when found. OTC analgesics (acetaminophen, ibuprofen) suffice for most pain. Antacids may be diagnostic and therapeutic for esophagitis pain. Rest, heat, relaxation techniques may be useful. Avoid expensive, invasive laboratory studies with chronic pain and normal physical exam, benign history.

ISSUES FOR REFERRAL
- Acute distress
- Significant trauma
- History of heart disease or related serious medical problem
- Pain with exercise, syncope, palpitations, dizziness
- Serious emotional disturbance
- Esophageal foreign body, caustic ingestion
- Pneumothorax, pleural effusion

 ONGOING CARE

PROGNOSIS
40% will have continued chest pain for 6–24 months. Most have an excellent prognosis.

ADDITIONAL READING

- Bullaro FM, Bartoletti SC. Spontaneous pneumomediastinum in children—a literature review. *Pediatr Emerg Care*. 2007;23:28–30.
- Danduran MJ. Chest pain: Characteristics of children and adolescents. *Pediatr Cardiol*. 2008;29: 775–781.
- Durani Y, Egan M, Baffa J, et al. Pediatric myocarditis: Presenting clinical characteristics. *Am J Emerg Med*. 2009;27:942–947.
- Galioto FM. Child chest pain: A course of action. *Contemp Pediatr*. 2007;24(5):47–57.
- Gokale J, Selbst SM. Chest pain and chest wall deformity. *Pediatr Clin North Am*. 2009;56:49–65.
- Gumbiner CH. Precordial catch syndrome. *South Med J*. 2003;96:38–41.
- Lipsitz JD, Masia-Warner C, Apfel H, et al. Anxiety and depressive symptoms and anxiety sensitivity in youngsters with noncardiac chest pain and benign heart murmurs. *J Pediatr Psychol*. 2004;29: 607–612.

- Madhok AB, Boxer R, Green S. An adolescent with chest pain-sequela of Kawasaki disease. *Pediatr Emerg Care*. 2004;20:765–768.
- Massin MM, Bourguignont A, Coremans C, et al. Chest pain in pediatric patients presenting to an emergency department or to a cardiac clinic. *Clin Pediatr*. 2004;43:231–238.
- Rajpurkar M, Warrier I, Chitlur M, et al. Pulmonary embolism—experience at a single children's hospital. *Thromb Res*. 2007;119:699–703.
- Selbst SM. Approach to the child with chest pain. In: Eslick G, Selbst SM, eds. *Pediatric chest pain*. Philadelphia, PA: Elsevier, 2010:1221–1234.

 CODES

ICD9
- 277.00 Cystic fibrosis without mention of meconium ileus
- 493.90 Asthma, unspecified type, unspecified
- 786.50 Chest pain, unspecified

ICD10
- E84.9 Cystic fibrosis, unspecified
- J45.909 Unspecified asthma, uncomplicated
- R07.9 Chest pain, unspecified

FAQ
- Q: How common is chest pain in children?
- A: Chest pain is a common pain syndrome reported in 6/1,000 children who present to an urban emergency department. The complaint is less common than abdominal pain or headache. Although children of all ages may complain of chest pain, the mean age is about 12 years.
- Q: Is follow-up important?
- A: Yes. Serious pathology is unlikely to be found if not diagnosed initially. However, watch for signs of exercise-induced asthma or for emotional problems that were not obvious initially. Ensure that the child returns to normal activity when appropriate.
- Q: What is the prognosis for most children with chest pain?
- A: Most children with chest pain have an excellent prognosis. ~40% of children with chest pain will have continued symptoms for 6–24 months.

CHICKENPOX (VARICELLA, HERPES ZOSTER)

Genevieve L. Buser
Barbara M. Watson (5th edition)

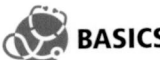 **BASICS**

DESCRIPTION
Varicella-zoster virus (VZV) is a highly contagious neurotropic herpesvirus.

EPIDEMIOLOGY
- Person-to-person transmission occurs by droplet and airborne transmission of infectious respiratory secretions or direct contact with vesicles and respiratory secretions.
- Incubation 10–21 days (usually 14–16 days) after exposure; cases most contagious 2 days before the rash appears until 5 days after new lesions stop appearing.
  - Immunocompromised patients may have longer or shorter incubation.
  - Post-IVIG, incubation may be up to 28 days.
- Neonates born to mothers with active VZV develop rash 9–15 days (range 1–16) later.
- Immunity from natural disease is usually lifelong; but symptomatic and asymptomatic re-infections do occur, boosting antibody levels.
- Cell-mediated immunity (especially NK cells) is more important than humoral immunity in limiting primary and zoster forms of VZV.
- Disease is more severe in immune-compromised persons, infants >3 months, adolescents, adults, persons with pulmonary disorders (asthma), persons with chronic skin disorders (eczema), and persons on oral and/or IV steroids or long-term aspirin therapy.
- Congenital varicella embryopathy: Risk is 1–2% when maternal primary VZV infection occurs before the 20th week of gestation.
- Since wild-type VZV decreased by 85% from 1995 to 2004, breakthrough VZV or reinfection now represents 62% of all reported VZV cases.

GENERAL PREVENTION
- Since 1995, varicella has been a vaccine-preventable disease and it has been incorporated in the harmonized immunization schedule recommended by the American Academy of Pediatrics (AAP) and American Committee on Immunization Practices (ACIP). Please refer to www.cdc.gov for most up-to-date information.
- Active immunization:
  - Live-attenuated Oka strain vaccine.
  - The vaccine is recommended for routine immunization of all healthy susceptible children, adolescents, and adults.
- Immunogenicity: ~85% of immunized children developed protective levels of humoral and cellular immunity after 1 dose; ~100% with 2 doses. 3 × less likely to have breakthrough disease when 2 doses of vaccine were administered.
- Effectiveness: 70–90% effective against all VZV disease; 100% effective against severe disease (e.g., median number of vesicles was 50 in vaccinated children and 250 in unvaccinated children).
- Duration of immunity >10 years.

- Contraindications:
  - Anaphylaxis to vaccine components (e.g., neomycin, gelatin)
  - Pregnant, immunocompromised, or <12 months of age.
  - HIV is an exception: It is recommended to vaccinate HIV-positive children if CD4+ T-cell counts are ≥15%. Give doses 3 months apart.
  - High-dose corticosteroid doses of >2 mg/kg/d or >20 mg/d of prednisone, or its equivalent, for ≥14 days are considered immunosuppressive doses: VZV vaccine should not be given until corticosteroid therapy has been discontinued for at least 1 month.
  - This does not apply to topical, inhaled, nasal or physiologic replacement corticosteroids.
- Postexposure prophylaxis:
  - If no contraindication to VZV vaccine: Administer VZV vaccine to susceptible hosts (1st or 2nd dose) within 72 hours (up to 120 hours) of exposure.
  - See "General Measures" for isolation.
  - If contraindications to VZV vaccine: Consider passive immunization.
- Passive immunization if:
  - (i) No evidence of immunity in exposed person, and (ii) probability that exposure will result in infection, and (iii) likelihood of complications of VZV in the exposed person due to risk factors.
  - Administer varicella immunoglobulin (VariZIG) or intravenous immunoglobulin (IVIG) as per protocol within 96 hours of exposure.
  - If VariZIG or IVIG is unavailable, or >96 h have passed, some experts recommend post-exposure prophylaxis with oral acyclovir (20 mg/kg q6h, for 7 days), beginning 7–10 days after exposure.
  - See "General Measures" for isolation.

 DIAGNOSIS

HISTORY
- Chickenpox:
  - Fever *concurrent* with rash.
  - Rash: Pruritic maculopapular to vesicles "dew drop on a rose petal"; appear in crops, begin on trunk/back, then to extremities, face. Vesicles break and crust over 3–5 days. Lesions in all stages on same child.
  - Headache, malaise, decreased appetite.
- Zoster:
  - Prodrome of pain, pruritus, paresthesias, allodynia in 1–3 dermatomes 1–3 days prior to appearance of vesicles. Scab in 5–10 days.
  - No systemic symptoms unless dissemination outside of dermatome (e.g., viremia)

PHYSICAL EXAM
- Chickenpox:
  - Pathognomonic rash: May be scant or atypical in immunocompromised hosts
  - Vesicles may appear in the mouth, conjunctiva, vagina, and urethra.
  - Assess for complications: Interstitial pneumonia, encephalitis, secondary bacterial infection (especially group A streptococcus).

- Zoster:
  - Chest > ophthalmic branch of trigeminal (V1)
  - Ramsey-Hunt: Zoster oticus and ipsilateral lower motor neuron palsy (7th, geniculate).
  - Hutchinson sign: Zoster on medial side of nose and herpes zoster ophthalmicus
  - Assess for extra-dermatomal lesions to suggest dissemination, and infection.

DIAGNOSTIC TESTS & INTERPRETATION
Lab
- Immunofluorescence: Vesicular fluid, bronchoalveolar lavage (BAL)
- PCR: Vesicular fluid, blood, CSF, BAL
- Culture: Vesicular fluid, blood, CSF, BAL
- Serology:
  - Acute and convalescent sera: Enzyme immunoassay (EIA), immunofluorescence assay (IFA), latex agglutination (LA), fluorescent antibody to membrane antigen (FAMA), and enzyme-linked immunosorbent assay (ELISA).
  - The complement-fixation test is not reliable in determining immunity and has been abandoned.

DIFFERENTIAL DIAGNOSIS
The differential diagnosis includes other causes of vesicular rash:
- Coxsackie virus infection (hand, foot, mouth)
- Eczema herpeticum
- Herpes zoster with dissemination
- Impetigo
- Insect bites
- Monkeypox
- Mycoplasma (erythema multiforme)
- Pseudomonas (ecthyma gangrenosum)
- Rickettsial pox
- Scabies
- Toxic epidermal necrosis, Stevens-Johnson, and various noninfectious vesicular conditions of the skin.

TREATMENT

MEDICATION (DRUGS)
- Acyclovir, valacyclovir, famciclovir, foscarnet, and vidarabine have been shown in clinical trials to be effective against VZV.
- Acyclovir is the drug of choice in children.
- Any child who is ill enough to warrant hospitalization and whose rash demonstrates new vesicle formation should be treated with IV acyclovir, including immunocompromised hosts:
  - <1 year: 10–20 mg/kg q8h
  - ≥1 year: 500 mg/m^2 q8h, or 10–20 mg/kg q8h
  - ≥12 years: 10 mg/kg q8h
- Because of poor oral bioavailability, use IV route in immunocompromised hosts.
- Treat for 7–10 days, or until no new lesions for 48 hours.
- Chickenpox or zoster in outpatient immunocompetent patient requiring treatment because of risk factors:
  - Acyclovir (PO): (>2 years old): 20 mg/kg q6h, to max of 800 mg q6h, for 5 days.
  - Valacyclovir (PO): (≥12 years old) 1000 mg q8h, for 5 days. Better bioavailability.

- Children with VZV should not receive salicylates because of the association with Reye syndrome. Use acetaminophen to control fever.
  - Consider treatment in immunocompetent patients if there is an increased risk of complications: ≥12 years old, secondary household case, chronic cutaneous or pulmonary disease, newborn infants, or persons on short or intermittent or inhaled corticosteroids, or long-term salicylate therapy.
- In the era of a preventable disease, acyclovir should be considered before complications of varicella warrant hospitalization.

ADDITIONAL TREATMENT
General Measures
- Isolation of hospitalized patients with chickenpox:
  - Contact and Airborne Precautions of the index case for the duration of vesicular eruption and all vesicles crusted (usually 5 days, longer in immunocompromised patients)
  - Use negative-pressure rooms, if possible.
  - Exposed susceptible persons should be in Contact and Airborne precautions from day 8 to 21 after the onset of rash in the index patient.
  - Neonates born to mother with VZV: Contact and Airborne precautions until day 28.
  - Embryopathy does not require precautions if there are no active lesions.
  - Persons who received VariZIG or IVIG should be kept in Contact and Airborne precautions for 28 days after exposure.
- Isolation of hospitalized patients with zoster:
  - Immunocompromised patients who have zoster (localized or generalized) and immunocompetent patients with disseminated zoster should remain in Contact and Airborne Precautions for the duration of the illness, as above.
  - Immunocompetent patients with localized zoster: Contact Precautions until all lesions crusted.
- Isolation of outpatients with chickenpox:
  - Child should remain at home, away from susceptible and high-risk persons, until no new eruptions and all vesicles have crusted.
- Isolation of outpatients with zoster:
  - For immunocompetent patients with localized zoster, Contact Precautions are recommended until all lesions are crusted. If lesions can remain completely covered, child may return to school; however, active lesions are infectious.
  - Antivirals such as acyclovir, valacyclovir, or famciclovir may shorten the duration of outpatient VZV disease and shedding to others.

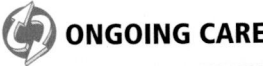

ONGOING CARE

FOLLOW-UP RECOMMENDATIONS
Patient Monitoring
For normal healthy individuals, follow-up is not necessary.

PROGNOSIS
- For most children, this childhood exanthema is a benign disease that lasts 6–8 days.
- Postherpetic neuralgia can cause significant morbidity following zoster.

COMPLICATIONS
Complications are associated with significant morbidity and may occur regardless of the use of acyclovir:

- Secondary bacterial infection—especially group A streptococcal infections and *Staphylococcus aureus*
- CNS (1 in 4000): Transverse myelitis, myelopathy, encephalitis (60 cases/yr prevaccine), meningo-encephalitis, acute cerebellar ataxia, necrotizing retinitis
- Varicella interstitial pneumonitis (more common in adults and infants)
- GI: Pancreatitis, appendicitis, and hepatitis
- Heme: Idiopathic thrombocytopenia, disseminated intravascular coagulation (hemorrhagic VZV)
- Nephritis
- Vasculopathy of small and large cerebral vessels causing strokes
- Zoster sine herpete: Radicular pain without rash, but virologic confirmation of reactivation. Can be dermatomal or CNS.
- Individuals with AIDS may have chronic VZV, including progressive myelopathy.
- Congenital varicella syndrome: Characterized by limb atrophy and scarring of the extremity (cicatrices), CNS, and eye manifestations.
- Postherpetic neuralgia: neuropathic pain more common in zoster patients >60 years.
- Death: 1–2 deaths per week in the US; between 1990 and 1994, varicella was the most common vaccine-preventable cause of death in individuals <20 years. However, the universal immunization program has reduced this to 4 deaths in the year 2001.

ADDITIONAL READING

- American Academy of Pediatrics. *Varicella-Zoster Infections.* In: Pickering LK, ed. *Red Book: 2009 Report of the Committee on Infectious Diseases,* 28th ed. Elk Grove Village, IL: American Academy of Pediatrics; 2009:714–727.
- CDC. Varicella-zoster virus infection. http://www.cdc.gov/ncidod/diseases/list_varicl.htm
- Macartney K, McIntyre P. Vaccines for post-exposure prophylaxis against varicella (chickenpox) in children and adults. *Cochrane Database Syst Rev.* 2008;16:CD001833.
- Seward JF, Marin M, Vázquez M. Varicella vaccine effectiveness in the US vaccination program: A review. *J Infect Dis.* 2008;197(Suppl 2):S82–89.

 # CODES

ICD9
- 052.7 Chickenpox with other specified complications
- 052.8 Chickenpox with unspecified complication
- 052.9 Varicella without mention of complication

ICD10
- B01.89 Other varicella complications
- B01.9 Varicella without complication
- B02.9 Zoster without complications

FAQ

- Q: What do you do for a patient on corticosteroids who has not had VZV and is exposed to VZV?
- A: The patient is considered immunosuppressed if he is receiving >2 mg/kg/d or >20 mg/d of prednisone or its equivalent. If the child is susceptible, had sufficient exposure, and is at risk for serious disease, he is a candidate for passive immunization with VariZIG or IVIG, or acyclovir post-exposure prophylaxis, because a vaccine is contraindicated now. Also, he should be on Contact and Airborne precautions (if inpatient) from day 8 to 28 from the exposure.
- Q: What about asthmatic patients on inhaled steroids? Can they be immunized safely, and are they at risk of more severe varicella if not immunized?
- A: Yes, asthmatics on inhaled steroids can be safely immunized because the dose of inhaled steroid is not immunosuppressive. Recent data show that asthmatic children who are unimmunized get more severe wild-type varicella disease.
- Q: Is there any patient who should not receive VZV vaccine?
- A: Yes. Immunosuppressed individuals, pregnant patients, and infants <1 year old should not receive the VZV vaccine. HIV patients can get VZV vaccine if CD4+ T-cell counts are ≥15%.
- Q: How contagious is breakthrough (reinfection) varicella disease?
- A: Surveillance studies have demonstrated that the secondary attack rate from breakthrough (re-infection) varicella is 30% in individuals with >50 lesions. Hence, when such individuals can expose high-risk susceptible patients in health care settings, infection control precautions should be observed. Public health investigation of outbreaks has demonstrated transmission of varicella from vaccinated individuals to high-risk, susceptible individuals (e.g., acute lymphocytic leukemia, transplant recipients, or HIV).
- Q: If a child gets zoster, with wild-type or vaccine strain, should she or he be treated with antiviral drugs?
- A: Maybe, surveillance studies have demonstrated that adolescents and children who develop herpes zoster after wild-type varicella infection have more pain and hospitalizations due to secondary infection than those with vaccine-strain varicella. Treatment of herpes zoster in children (as has been demonstrated in adults) shortens the course of illness and, more importantly, in school-aged children, decreases shedding. Since active surveillance has demonstrated that herpes zoster cases can be index cases in outbreaks, it is a public health option to treat herpes zoster in children who are going back to school.
- Q: I carry both the varicella-zoster and the zoster vaccine in my office, as I see both children and adults. Can I use the zoster vaccine in a child, instead of the varicella-zoster vaccine?
- A: No. The zoster vaccine is formulated very differently than the varicella-zoster vaccine, and should only be given to in adults >60 years old, as indicated.

C

CHILD ABUSE, PHYSICAL

Sarah M. Frioux
Cindy W. Christian

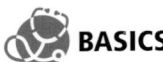 BASICS

DESCRIPTION
Injuries or illnesses that occur to children as a result of family dysfunction. In practice, child abuse is considered nonaccidental injury of children at the hands of their caregivers. Physical abuse is legally defined by state laws.

EPIDEMIOLOGY
- Abuse may occur in families from any socioeconomic class, ethnicity, or community.
- The recognition of child physical abuse begins with the clinician's acknowledgement that child abuse occurs commonly.
- Parents who were abused as children are at much greater risk for abusing their own children. It is estimated that 30% of abused children go on to be abusive parents.

Incidence
- In 2008, there were 3.3 million referrals to child welfare agencies in the US for child abuse and neglect. ~702,000 children were determined to be victims of child maltreatment.
- The child abuse victimization rate was 9.3 per 1,000 children in the national population.
- Almost 1,800 abusive deaths per year, by conservative estimates

Prevalence
Domestic violence and child abuse have a 50% concurrence.

GENERAL PREVENTION
- Much of what is considered prevention is actually early intervention in high-risk families.
- Primary prevention would include universal parenting education and home visitation for all families. Currently, families thought to be at risk for abuse are identified and offered services.
- Home visitation by nurses for low-income, 1st-time mothers has been shown to decrease the risk for child abuse.
- Screening families for domestic violence can be the 1st clue to child victimization.

ALERT
Pitfalls:
- Failing to consider abuse in the differential diagnosis of all pediatric trauma
- Failing to consider abuse in the differential diagnosis of all infants and toddlers with mental status changes (especially apparent life-threatening events [ALTEs]), even in the absence of bruising
- Failing to consider alternative medical diagnoses in children for whom you suspect abuse
- Acute (<10 days) rib fractures are easily missed on radiographs.

ETIOLOGY
Multifactorial:
- Includes societal, familial, and individual factors
- Associated with poverty, family stress, family isolation

COMMONLY ASSOCIATED CONDITIONS
- Domestic violence
- Sexual abuse
- Neglect
- Emotional abuse
- Juvenile delinquency
- Poverty
- Parental substance abuse, including alcohol

 DIAGNOSIS

HISTORY
- A detailed history of injury is essential for comparing the mechanism provided by the historian with the injuries identified.
- The following historical features should raise the question of child physical abuse:
  - History provided does not correlate with findings.
  - Child's development is not compatible with mechanism described.
  - History of events changes with time.
  - Unexpected delay in seeking care
  - No history of trauma is provided. In such cases, ask when the child was last well, and who was caring for the child at that time. This may be helpful in identifying when the child was injured and by whom.
  - Search for indications of family stress, isolation, substance abuse, and violence, including domestic violence.

PHYSICAL EXAM
- Always perform a complete exam in a well-lit room.
- Assess for:
  - Growth failure
  - Bruises: Any inflicted injury that lasts >24 hours constitutes significant injury.
  - Burns
  - Oral injuries
  - Palpable rib fractures
  - Abdominal injuries
  - Genital injuries
  - Retinal hemorrhages: Children with suspected abusive head trauma should have a dilated eye exam by an ophthalmologist.
- Are the findings explained by any medical condition? Examples would include multiple bruises in a patient with a bleeding disorder or long bone fractures in a patient with a metabolic bone disease (such as rickets).

DIAGNOSTIC TESTS & INTERPRETATION
Lab
For children with bruising and/or bleeding:
- CBC, including a platelet count: Evaluate for anemia and thrombocytopenia.
- Prothrombin time/partial thromboplastin time, INR: Evaluate for hemophilia and other bleeding disorders.
- Platelet function evaluation (PFA-100): Evaluate for von Willebrand disease.
- Liver function tests: Evaluate for liver injury.
- Amylase, lipase: Evaluate for pancreatic injury.
- Urinalysis: Screen for genitourinary injury, abdominal trauma, or myoglobinuria.
- Creatine kinase (if muscle injury or extensive soft tissue injury): Evaluate for muscle injury, possible myoglobinuria.
- Lumbar puncture: Evaluate for meningitis; identify bloody CSF.
- Toxicology screen: For unexplained altered mental status or if it is suspected that the child may have been poisoned

Imaging
- Skeletal survey: Recommended for all children <2 years old and for occasional children 2–5 years old with suspected abusive injuries. Repeat skeletal surveys 2–3 weeks after initial presentation often reveal additional fractures that were not visible at the time of acute injury.
  - Not generally used for children >5 years
  - Bony injuries highly suggestive of physical abuse include posterior rib, metaphyseal (also known as bucket-handle or corner fractures), scapular, sternal, and spinous process fractures.
- Other radiography: Clavicle, long bone shaft, and linear skull fractures are common accidental fractures that have low specificity for physical abuse.
- Radionuclide bone scan: Serves as an adjunct to skeletal survey
- CT and MRI:
  - For suspected head, thoracic, or abdominal trauma
  - MRI or head CT should be considered in all children <1 year with other concerning/suspicious injuries, such as unexplained bruises or fractures.
  - Subdural hemorrhage is a hallmark of abusive head trauma. Subdural hemorrhages associated with abuse can be located anywhere around the brain, but are often found in the posterior interhemispheric fissure.

Pathological Findings
In cases of child death due to suspected physical abuse, a full autopsy must be completed by a qualified examiner.

DIFFERENTIAL DIAGNOSIS
- Varies depending on injury sustained
- Bruises:
  – Accidental injury
  – Dermatologic disorders: Mongolian spots, erythema multiforme, phytophotodermatitis
  – Hematologic disorders: Idiopathic thrombocytopenic purpura (ITP), leukemia, hemophilia, vitamin K deficiency, disseminated intravascular coagulopathy (DIC), platelet disorders, hemophilia
  – Cultural practices: Cao gio (coining; practice of rubbing the skin with a coin to alleviate various symptoms of illness); quat sha (spoon rubbing)
  – Infection: Sepsis, purpura fulminans (e.g., with meningococcemia)
  – Genetic diseases: Ehlers-Danlos, familial dysautonomia (with congenital indifference to pain)
  – Vasculitis: Henoch-Schönlein purpura
- Burns:
  – Accidental burns
  – Infection: Staphylococcal scalded skin syndrome, impetigo
  – Dermatologic: Phytophotodermatitis, Stevens-Johnson syndrome, fixed drug eruption, epidermolysis bullosa, severe diaper dermatitis
  – Cultural practices: Cupping (process by which a small amount of alcohol is heated in a cup and inverted over the skin. As the heated air cools, a vacuum is produced causing ecchymotic lesions. It is believed that this suction from the cup will draw out illness. Moxibustion (Chinese folk remedy in which cones or balls of the moxa herb are burned on the skin at therapeutic points)
- Fractures:
  – Accidental injury
  – Birth trauma
  – Metabolic bone disease: Osteogenesis imperfecta, copper deficiency, rickets
  – Infection: Congenital syphilis, osteomyelitis
- Head trauma:
  – Accidental head injury
  – Hematologic disorders: Vitamin K deficiency (hemorrhagic disease of the newborn), hemophilia, DIC
  – Intracranial vascular abnormalities
  – Infection
  – Metabolic diseases: Glutaric aciduria type I

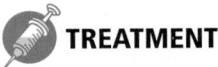 **TREATMENT**

ADDITIONAL TREATMENT
General Measures
- Report all suspected abuse to local child welfare agency.
- Report abuse to law enforcement when injuries warrant police investigation.
- Consult social worker.

IN-PATIENT CONSIDERATIONS
Admission Criteria
- Hospitalization is primarily for the treatment of the identified injuries.
- Admission to the hospital to ensure the protection of the child during initial investigation by child welfare is sometimes necessary.

Discharge Criteria
Discharge disposition is generally dependent on determinations from child welfare agencies regarding the safety and welfare of the child victim.

 ONGOING CARE

FOLLOW-UP RECOMMENDATIONS
Patient Monitoring
- Cases will be investigated by child welfare agents and/or the police.
- Need for foster care placement and/or ongoing supervision decided by child welfare investigators
- Improvement of individual injuries varies according to the injury.
- Family functioning may improve with intervention for some families, but may never improve for others. Changes in family functioning often require intensive, long-term intervention.
- Noncompliance with medical follow-up or additional injuries to child may indicate ongoing abuse or parental substance abuse.

PROGNOSIS
Varies greatly depending on injuries sustained, family problems, available support systems

COMPLICATIONS
- Death
- Mental retardation
- Cerebral palsy
- Seizures
- Learning disabilities, school failure
- Emotional problems

ADDITIONAL READING
- American Academy of Pediatrics Committee on Child Abuse and Neglect. Evaluating infants and young children with multiple fractures. *Pediatrics.* 2006;118:1299–1303.
- American Academy of Pediatrics, Section on Radiology. Diagnostic imaging of child abuse. *Pediatrics.* 2009;123:1430–1435.
- Kellogg ND, the Committee on Child Abuse and Neglect. Evaluation of suspected child physical abuse. *Pediatrics.* 2007;119:1232–1241.
- U.S. Department of Health and Human Services. *Administration on Children, Youth and Families. Child maltreatment 2008.* Washington, DC: U.S. Government Printing Office; 2010.

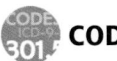 **CODES**

ICD9
995.50 Child abuse, unspecified

ICD10
T74.12XA Child physical abuse, confirmed, initial encounter

FAQ
- Q: What are the signs of abusive head trauma?
- A: Abusive head trauma is a clinical diagnosis based on history, physical exam findings, and radiologic data. The hallmark of abusive head trauma is subdural hemorrhage, which is often a marker for diffuse, deceleration brain injury. Most victims (80%) have retinal hemorrhages, which tend to be bilateral, multilayered, and sometimes severe. Some, but not all, children have old and/or new skeletal or skin injuries, although these are not always identified. The symptoms of head trauma in young children are nonspecific and include mental status changes, apparent life-threatening events, vomiting, lethargy, irritability, and seizures. Abusive head injury in infants is often missed by physicians who fail to consider the diagnosis in babies with the above-mentioned symptoms, leading to further injury or death of abused infants.
- Q: Are retinal hemorrhages pathognomonic for physical abuse?
- A: No. Retinal hemorrhages may be seen in a variety of diseases and in many newborn infants. They occur in ~30% of newborns delivered vaginally. In these children they usually resolve in a few days, but may rarely last for 5–6 weeks. Outside of the newborn period, severe inflicted injury is the leading cause of retinal hemorrhages in children. Retinal hemorrhages may also result from increased intracranial pressure, severe hypertension, carbon monoxide poisoning, meningitis, vasculitis, endocarditis, and coagulopathy. Severe, bilateral hemorrhages are often related to abuse.
- Q: When is a child abuse report filed?
- A: Whenever there is a suspicion, based on the history, physical exam, laboratory data, and/or psychosocial assessment, that a child's injuries or illnesses were a result of abuse or neglect. Certainty regarding the diagnosis is not needed.
- Q: Can I be held liable for reports that are made that are not substantiated?
- A: No. Health care workers who report suspected abuse in good faith are protected by state laws that mandate physicians to report suspected abuse.

CHLAMYDIAL INFECTIONS

Marleine Ishak
Sumit Bhargava

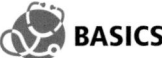 **BASICS**

DESCRIPTION

Chlamydiae are obligate intracellular bacteria responsible for pulmonary infections, ocular trachoma, STDs, and infections of the genital tract in the pediatric and adult population.

- The genus *Chlamydophila* has 3 species known to affect humans:
  - *C. trachomatis*
  - *C. psittaci*
  - *C. pneumoniae*
- All 3 species can produce the clinical picture of the so-called atypical or interstitial pneumonia.
- *C. trachomatis* can cause afebrile pneumonia in 10–20% of infants born to infected mothers. Infected infants usually present prior to 2 months of age. Up to 50% of patients have a history of inclusion conjunctivitis.
- *C. psittaci* is mainly pathogenic for birds and occasionally affects humans, typically causing interstitial pneumonitis with associated fever, headache, malaise, and nausea.
- *C. pneumoniae* causes pneumonia, pharyngitis, sinusitis, and bronchitis in humans. Along with *Mycoplasma pneumoniae*, *C. pneumoniae* probably accounts for most of the community-acquired pneumonias (CAP) in school-age children and adolescents.

ALERT
- *C. trachomatis*:
  - Infection can occur in infants delivered by cesarean section, even without rupture of amniotic membranes.
  - Ocular prophylaxis at birth does not reliably prevent conjunctivitis or extraocular infection, even if erythromycin ointment is used. Topical treatment alone is not recommended because it does not eradicate the nasopharyngeal colonization.
- *C. pneumoniae*:
  - Lack of a commercially reliable test for diagnosis. Microimmunofluorescence (MIF) is proven diagnostic in >50% of infected children. An increase in antibody titer may be delayed for several weeks after onset of symptoms. Early antimicrobial therapy may interfere with the development of detectable antibodies.
  - Sometimes, it is difficult to differentiate between infection and carrier state, and between recent and past infection.
  - Recurrent infections are common. Prolonged nasopharyngeal shedding can occur for months after acute disease.
- Isolation: Standard precautions for both *C. pneumoniae* and *C. trachomatis*
- Control measures: In infants infected with *C. trachomatis*, the mother and her sexual partner should be treated. None for *C. pneumoniae*

GENERAL PREVENTION

Adequate surveillance and treatment of *C. trachomatis* colonizing the genital tract of pregnant women is the best way of preventing disease in the infant.

EPIDEMIOLOGY
- *C. trachomatis*:
  - There are at least 18 serologically distinct variants (serovars A through K).
  - *C. trachomatis* is the most frequent cause of epididymitis in sexually active young men.
  - Incubation period: 5–14 days after delivery for conjunctivitis
  - The possibility of sexual abuse should be considered in older infants and children with vaginal, urethral, or rectal *C. trachomatis*.
- *C. psittaci* (psittacosis/ornithosis):
  - Both healthy and sick birds can transmit the bacteria via the airborne route by their excrement or secretions.
  - Important sources of human disease are parakeets, parrots, macaws, pigeons, and turkeys.
  - Workers in poultry slaughter plants, poultry farms, pet shops, laboratory workers, and pet owners are at high risk.
  - Although usually rare in children, it should be considered in any child with environmental exposure who develops an atypical pneumonia. The incubation period is 7–14 days.
- *C. pneumoniae*: Antigenically, morphologically, and genetically distinct from other chlamydiae
  - It is assumed to be transmitted from person to person through aerosolized respiratory secretions.
  - *C. pneumoniae* has recently been associated with atherosclerotic cardiovascular disease. Limited evidence associates *C. pneumoniae* with asthma and bronchospasm, Alzheimer disease, multiple sclerosis, Kawasaki disease, HIV and other immune disorders, malignancy, otitis media, and episodes of acute chest syndrome in patients with sickle cell disease.
  - Coinfection with other respiratory pathogens, especially *M. pneumoniae* and *Streptococcus pneumoniae*, is frequent.
  - Incubation period: ~21 days

Incidence
C. trachomatis:
- This is the most common reportable sexually transmitted infection in the USA. The number of new infections exceeds 4 million annually.
- *C. trachomatis* is responsible for neonatal conjunctivitis, trachoma, pneumonia in young infants, genital tract infection, and lymphogranuloma venereum (LGV).
- Rates of infection in adolescent girls are 15–20%.
- 23–55% of all cases of nongonococcal urethritis in men are caused by *C. trachomatis*. Up to 50% of men with gonorrhea may be coinfected with *C. trachomatis*.
- *C. trachomatis* pneumonia usually develops in infected infants <2 months of age (2 weeks to 5 months). The contagiousness of pulmonary disease is unknown, but is considered low.
- Half of the neonates born to infected mothers via vaginal delivery will acquire *C. trachomatis*. Conjunctivitis may develop in 30–50%.
- Pneumonia may develop in up to 30% of infants with nasopharyngeal infection.

- Ocular trachoma caused by serovars A, B, Ba, and C is the most common cause of preventable blindness in the world, but is rare in the USA.

Prevalence
C. pneumoniae:
- Increased prevalence rates of *C. pneumoniae* specific antibody have been documented in school-age children, reaching 30–45% in adolescents.
- Studies of CAPs in children have found *C. pneumoniae* in 6–19% of cases. Evidence of lower respiratory tract infection has been found in 0–18% of the pediatric population.
- Most infections are mild or asymptomatic. Acute infection does not appear to vary by season. A carriage state has been detected in 2–5% of patients. Recurrent infection is common, especially in adults.

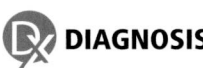 **DIAGNOSIS**

HISTORY
- *C. trachomatis*:
  - Presents between 4 and 12 weeks of age
  - Insidious onset
  - Afebrile illness
  - Rhinorrhea
  - Repetitive cough: Staccato type in >50% of infants; sometimes, pertussis-like coughing spells
  - Conjunctivitis in up to 50% of infants
  - Mild-to-moderate respiratory distress
- *C. pneumoniae*:
  - Often insidious onset
  - May manifest as pharyngitis, sinusitis, bronchitis, or pneumonia
  - Fever
  - Hoarseness
  - Prolonged cough; can be productive
  - Biphasic course

PHYSICAL EXAM
- *C. trachomatis*:
  - Afebrile
  - 50% of patients will have conjunctivitis with discharge (can be seen up to several weeks after birth).
  - Rhinitis with mucoid discharge or nasal stuffiness, sometimes causing significant airway obstruction
  - Hypoxia is frequently present
  - Apneic episodes may be seen in preterm infants
  - Moderate tachypnea (50–60 breaths/min)
  - Staccato cough
  - Scattered rales on chest auscultation
  - Wheezing is an uncommon finding.
- *C. pneumoniae*:
  - Patients may be asymptomatic or mildly to moderately ill.
  - Prolonged cough (2–6 weeks)
  - Cervical lymphadenopathy
  - Postnasal discharge
  - Nonexudative pharyngitis: Wheezing, frequently without rales, on chest auscultation
- *C. psittaci*:
  - Abrupt onset of fever.
  - Nonproductive cough
  - Malaise

DIAGNOSTIC TESTS & INTERPRETATION
Lab
- C. trachomatis:
  - Definitive diagnosis is by isolation of the organism in tissue culture. Confirmation is by microscopy of the characteristic inclusions by fluorescent antibody staining. Specimens are obtained from the nasopharynx, conjunctiva, vagina, or rectum. Dacron polyester–tipped swabs should be used for collection.
  - FDA-approved nucleic acid amplification methods such as polymerase chain reaction (PCR), strand displacement amplification (SDA), and transcription-mediated amplification (TMA) are more sensitive (98%) than cell culture and more specific and sensitive than DNA probe, direct fluorescent antibody (DFA), or enzyme immunoassay (EIA). In addition, these have been approved for urine studies in both men and women, making them useful noninvasive tests for adolescents.
  - DNA probe, DFA, and EIA are the most common nonculture direct antigen-detection tests approved by the FDA. These are most sensitive (90%) and specific (95%) in conjunctival specimens. These methods can have false-positive results when used for vaginal or rectal specimens.
  - Serum antibody detection is difficult to perform, and tests are not widely available.
  - Eosinophilia of 300–400/mm³, hyperinflation, bilateral diffuse infiltrates on chest radiograph, and elevation of IgM (>110 mg/dL) and IgG (>500 mg/dL) are indirect evidence that indicate C. trachomatis pneumonia.
  - Only culture should be used for sexual abuse or other forensic purposes.
  - Annual Chlamydia screening for all sexually active women younger than age 25 and for all pregnant women in the first trimester of pregnancy is recommended.
- C. pneumoniae:
  - No reliable test is available commercially. Serologic testing is the primary laboratory means of diagnosis.
  - The nasopharynx is the optimal site for recovery of C. pneumoniae. It is also isolated from sputum and pleural fluid.
  - Serologic diagnosis by MIF is the most sensitive and specific test. Evidence of acute infection: 4-fold elevation of IgG titers, specific IgM titer of ≥1:16, specific IgG titer of ≥1:512, WBC count is usually normal.
- C. psittaci:
  - 4-fold increase in acute and convalescent serum antibodies concentrations.

Imaging
Chest radiography:
- C. trachomatis: Hyperinflation with bilateral diffuse infiltrates
- C. pneumoniae: Focal to bilateral infiltrates; pleural effusions

DIFFERENTIAL DIAGNOSIS
- C. trachomatis:
  - Viral respiratory pathogens: Respiratory syncytial virus (RSV), adenovirus, influenza A and B, parainfluenza
  - Other agents that can cause pneumonitis: cytomegalovirus, Pneumocystis carinii, Ureaplasma urealyticum, Bordetella pertussis

- C. pneumoniae:
  - M. pneumoniae
  - Influenza A and B
  - Parainfluenza
  - Adenovirus
  - Respiratory syncytial virus
  - Can resemble typical bacterial pneumonia
  - Less frequently: C. psittaci, Coxiella burnetii, or Legionella pneumophila

 TREATMENT
MEDICATION (DRUGS)
- C. trachomatis:
  - Erythromycin, 50 mg/kg/d divided q.i.d. for 14 days (therapy is effective in 80–90% of cases). Additional topical therapy is unnecessary. An association between oral erythromycin and infantile hypertrophic pyloric stenosis (IHPS) has been reported in infants <6 weeks of age. Parents should be informed of the possible risk of IHPS and its signs.
  - If the patient does not tolerate erythromycin, oral sulfonamides may be used after the immediate neonatal period. Children >8 years can be treated with tetracycline, 25–50 mg/kg/d divided q.i.d. for 7 days
  - A single 1-g oral dose of azithromycin may be used in children ≥45 kg or ≥8 years of age.
  - In adults and adolescents, a single 1-g dose of azithromycin or doxycycline 100 mg b.i.d. orally for 7 days is first-line treatment.
- C. pneumoniae:
  - Erythromycin suspension: 50 mg/kg/d divided q.i.d. for 14 days. For adolescent patients, erythromycin 500 mg q.i.d. for 14 days or 250 mg q.i.d. for 21 days. An alternative for children >9 years is doxycycline 100 mg b.i.d. for 14 days.
  - Clarithromycin: 15 mg/kg/d divided b.i.d. for 10 days is as effective as erythromycin.
  - Azithromycin: 10 mg/kg on day 1 (maximum, 500 mg) followed by 5 mg/kg days 2–5 (maximum, 250 mg) is as effective as erythromycin in pediatric studies.
  - Adolescents can be treated with doxycycline 100 mg b.i.d. for 14–21 days, tetracycline 250 mg q.i.d. for 14–21 days, azithromycin 1.5 g for 5 days, levofloxacin 500 mg/d PO or IV for 7–14 days, or moxifloxacin 400 mg/d PO for 10 days.
  - Antibiotic treatment failure rate is ~20%. A second course of therapy is sometimes needed. Follow-up should be recommended.

 ONGOING CARE
PROGNOSIS
- In general, good
- Infection with C. trachomatis has been associated with long-term respiratory sequelae, such as an increased incidence of reactive airway disease and abnormal pulmonary function tests.
- Slow recovery
- Cough and malaise may persist for several weeks.

COMPLICATIONS
- In very young infants, chlamydial pneumonia can lead to apnea or respiratory failure. If untreated, infection can persist for weeks to months and can lead to persistent hypoxemia

- Complications of psittacosis include myocarditis, hepatitis, pancreatitis, and secondary bacterial pneumonia.
- 40% of women whose chlamydial infection is untreated develop pelvic inflammatory disease. 20% of these women may become infertile.
- Role of Chlamydia in pathogenesis of asthma and atherosclerosis is under investigation.

ADDITIONAL READING
- Centers for Disease Control and Prevention. Sexually transmitted disease guidelines 2002. MMWR. 2002;519(No:RR-6):1–75.
- Chlamydial infections in Children and Adolescents. Pediatr Rev. 2009;30(7).
- Geisler WM. Management of uncomplicated Chlamydia trachomatis infections in adolescents and adults: Evidence reviewed for the 2006 Centers for Disease Control and Prevention sexually transmitted diseases treatment guidelines. Clin Infect Dis. 2007;44(Suppl 3):S77–S83.
- Harris JA, Kolokathis A, Campbell M, et al. Safety and efficacy of azithromycin in the treatment of community acquired pneumonia in children. Pediatr Infect Dis J. 1997;16:293–297.
- US Preventative Services Task Force. Screening for Chlamydial infection: US Preventative Services Task Force recommendation statement. Ann Intern Med. 2007;147:128–133.

CODES

ICD9
- 077.98 Unspecified diseases of conjunctiva due to chlamydiae
- 079.98 Unspecified chlamydial infection
- 483.1 Pneumonia due to chlamydia

ICD10
- A74.0 Chlamydial conjunctivitis
- A74.9 Chlamydial infection, unspecified
- J16.0 Chlamydial pneumonia

FAQ

- Q: If the mother has an untreated genital infection, should we treat the asymptomatic newborn?
- A: Yes. The child should receive oral erythromycin for 14 days.
- Q: Do we need to pursue the diagnosis of other STDs?
- A: Yes. Gonorrhea, syphilis, hepatitis B, and human immunodeficiency virus infection need to be ruled out. If conjunctivitis is present, an ocular swab to exclude Neisseria gonorrhoeae infection must be included.
- Q: When do we need to suspect C. trachomatis pneumonia?
- A: In any infant <4 months of age who presents with cough, tachypnea, and rales on examination, when the chest radiograph shows bilateral infiltrates with hyperinflation.

CHOLELITHIASIS

Michelle T. Rook
Vera de Matos (5th edition)

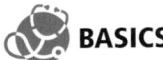 **BASICS**

DESCRIPTION
Cholelithiasis is defined by the presence of cholesterol and/or pigment stones in the gallbladder. Rare in infancy and childhood, it is usually found incidentally on an ultrasound. Risk factors in children include obesity, hemolytic disease, cystic fibrosis (CF), Crohn disease, and long-term total parenteral nutrition (TPN).

EPIDEMIOLOGY
- Cholelithiasis is relatively uncommon in childhood and adolescence; however, the incidence is increasing.
- Gallstones occurring in utero and in infancy have been described.
- Obesity accounts for up to 1/3 of the gallstones observed in all children and the majority of children with no underlying medical conditions. Obesity is estimated to increase the risk of gallstones in children by over 4-fold.
- Canadian Eskimos and Native Africans have the lowest risk of cholelithiasis.
- Native Americans, Swedes, Scandinavians, and Czechs have the highest risk.
- Pigment stones are more prevalent in prepubertal children, whereas cholesterol stones are predominant in adolescence and adulthood.

Incidence
- Prior to puberty the incidence of gallstones is equal in males and females. After puberty the incidence increases in females.
- In females, the incidence of cholelithiasis is 0.27% between the ages of 6 and 19 years, increasing to 2.7% between the ages of 18 and 29 years.
- There is an increased incidence in sickle cell disease, with up to 50% having gallstones by 22 years of age.

Prevalence
- The prevalence of cholelithiasis in children and adolescents reported in the literature is ~0.1–0.6%.
- In obese children, the prevalence is 2%.
- In children with sickle cell disease, the prevalence is 17–29%.
- The prevalence of gallstones in North American and European adults is 10–20%.

RISK FACTORS
- Acute renal failure
- Anatomic abnormalities (biliary stricture, duodenal diverticulum)
- CF
- Chronic hemolysis (sickle cell disease, thalassemia, spherocytosis, malaria)
- Chronic overnutrition with carbohydrate and triglyceride-rich, low-fiber diet
- Down syndrome
- Family history
- Female gender
- Hepatobiliary disease/cirrhosis

- Ineffective erythropoiesis (vitamin B_{12} and folate deficiencies)
- Medications (estrogens, octreotide, clofibrate, furosemide, cyclosporine, ceftriaxone, oral contraceptives)
- Necrotizing enterocolitis
- Obesity
- Pregnancy/Parity
- Prematurity
- Prolonged fasting/low-calorie diets/rapid weight loss
- Severe Crohn disease of the ileum and/or ileal resection
- TPN
- Trauma/Abdominal surgery

Genetics
- Mutations have been identified in genes encoding the ABC transporters for phosphatidylcholine (adenosine triphosphate–binding cassette, subfamily B), for bile salts (*ABCB11*), or for cholesterol 7a-hydroxylase (*CYP7A1*), the CCK-A receptor (*CCKAR*) and the CF gene (*CFTR*).
- *ABCB4* is also known as *MDR3* (multidrug-resistant 3 glycoprotein). *MDR3* is a phospholipid translocator in the hepatocyte membrane, involved in biliary phosphatidylcholine excretion. MDR3 deficiency can cause severe neonatal liver disease, but mutations in MDR3 have also been associated with cholelithiasis, cholestasis of pregnancy, and biliary cirrhosis.
- Variants of ABCG8 and UGT1A1, associated with bile acid metabolism and Gilbert syndrome, are risk factors for cholelithiasis
- Other gene polymorphisms are currently under investigation in humans.

GENERAL PREVENTION
Exercise and dietary modifications can decrease gallstone formation.

PATHOPHYSIOLOGY
- Bile is an aqueous solution of lipids, with bile salts, phospholipids, and cholesterol. Changes in the proportion of bile constituents, nucleation (aggregation of cholesterol crystals), changes in gallbladder motility, or infection can lead to stone formation.
- Stones are of 3 types: pigment (5–50% in pediatric patients), cholesterol stones, and mixed.
- Black pigment stones are associated with increased unconjugated bilirubin:
  – Hemolytic diseases
  – Abnormal erythropoiesis
  – Enterohepatic circulation of unconjugated bilirubin:
    ○ Ileal resection, Crohn disease
    ○ CF
- Brown pigment stones are associated with infection.
- The solubility of cholesterol in bile depends on bile salts and phospholipid concentrations. Cholesterol stones are associated with:
  – A decrease in bile salt pool
  – Decreased bile acid synthesis
  – Hypersecretion of cholesterol into the bile
  – Gallbladder stasis (weight loss, pregnancy, long-term TPN)
  – Increased biliary mucus secretion
  – Medications: Furosemide, ceftriaxone, cyclosporine

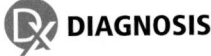 **DIAGNOSIS**

HISTORY
- Gallstones in children are most commonly incidental findings on abdominal ultrasound.
- Biliary colic, pancreatitis, obstructive jaundice, cholangitis, or other complications should be excluded.
- Intolerance to fatty food rarely exists in children.
- The history should always include questions concerning:
  – Previous episodes of right upper quadrant (RUQ) abdominal pain
  – Any risk factors for hemolysis
  – History of prematurity and necrotizing enterocolitis
  – Nutritional history
  – Medication use
  – Surgical history
  – Associated medical conditions (e.g., short gut syndrome, ileal disease)

PHYSICAL EXAM
- The physical exam may be completely normal or may uncover the acute abdomen of pancreatitis.
- Murphy sign (tenderness on palpation of the RUQ of the abdomen associated with inspiration) may be elicited in adolescents.
- Silent gallstones present coincidentally in infants and young children.
- Classic symptoms of RUQ pain (Murphy sign) and vomiting are more common in older children and adolescents.
- Younger children present with nonspecific symptoms, including obstructive jaundice, and mild elevation in transaminases.
- Fever is unusual in all age groups and often indicates the development of rare complications in children:
  – Cholecystitis
  – Choledocholithiasis
  – Cholangitis
  – Gallbladder perforation:
    ○ Pancreatitis develops in 8% of patients with gallstones and is the most common complication.
    ○ Pancreatitis is more common in obese adolescents who have undergone rapid weight reduction, as reported in the adult population.

DIAGNOSTIC TESTS & INTERPRETATION
Lab
- Laboratory tests should include a complete blood count, urinalysis, amylase, lipase, fractionated bilirubin, alkaline phosphatase, γ-glutamyltransferase (GGT), and transaminase levels.
- Results should typically be within normal ranges.
- Abnormal results may suggest infection, obstruction, or another disease process.

Imaging
- Ultrasound is the diagnostic procedure of choice: Noninvasive with high sensitivity and specificity
- Plain radiography may not be useful, as the majority of gallstones in children are not radio-opaque.
- Magnetic resonance cholangiopancreatography (MRCP) is useful to define anatomy in hepatobiliary disease and identify choledocholithiasis.

Diagnostic Procedures/Other
- Endoscopic retrograde cholangiopancreatography (ERCP) is diagnostic for evaluation of choledocholithiasis and therapeutic for removal of stones, stenting, or decompression of the biliary tree.
- Surgery should be considered for symptomatic patients.

Pathological Findings
Pigment stones may be black or brown. Black stones are associated with hemolysis or cirrhosis. Brown stones are associated with biliary tract infection.

DIFFERENTIAL DIAGNOSIS
- Acalculous gallbladder disease
- Biliary dyskinesia
- Cholecystitis
- Common bile duct stones
- Congenital biliary anomalies
- Hydrops of the gallbladder (may be associated with Kawasaki disease)

 TREATMENT

MEDICATION (DRUGS)
- Spontaneous resolution in asymptomatic children is common, without the need for frequent medication use.
- Ursodeoxycholic acid (UDCA) suppresses hepatic cholesterol synthesis and secretion and can improve gallbladder muscle contractility by decreasing muscle cell cholesterol content in the plasma membranes.

ADDITIONAL TREATMENT
General Measures
- Primary prevention: High fiber intake, diet low in saturated fatty acid and nuts, and moderate physical activity. Children with asymptomatic gallstones should only be observed. During infancy, there is a chance for spontaneous stone dissolution, especially if cholelithiasis is linked to TPN.
- In children who are dependent on TPN and in patients with short bowel syndrome, pseudo-obstruction, inflammatory bowel disease, and with a hemoglobinopathy, gallstones should be removed.
- Laparoscopic cholecystectomy is the procedure of choice in symptomatic children.

- Prevention of gallstone formation is done by treating underlying risk factors (small enteral feeds in addition to TPN, early pancreatic enzyme supplements in patients with CF, using alternative forms of contraception in high-risk populations, and weight control in obese infants and children with known hemolytic disease).
- Pigment stone formation increases with age. Sickle cell patients should have the gallbladder removed when stones are identified. This will decrease the risk of cholecystitis and other complications and will also help to differentiate between biliary colic and sickle cell crisis.
- Patients with a history of cholecystitis are at increased risk for further episodes (69% will have biliary colic within 2 years, and 6% will require cholecystectomy).

SURGERY/OTHER PROCEDURES
- Indicated in symptomatic gallstones
- Laparoscopic cholecystectomy is the procedure of choice.

ALERT
Lithotripsy using shock waves has not been approved for use in children.

 ONGOING CARE

FOLLOW-UP RECOMMENDATIONS
Patient Monitoring
- Asymptomatic patients: Monitor for onset of symptoms; no utility for repeat imaging or labs unless symptomatic
- Symptomatic patients: Consider cholecystectomy.

ADDITIONAL READING

- Buch S, Schafmayer C, Volzke H, et al. Loci from a genome-wide analysis of bilirubin levels are associated with gallstone risk and composition. *Gastroenterology.* 2010;139(6):1942–1951.
- Guarino MP, Cong P, Cicala M, et al. Ursodeoxycholic acid improves muscle contractility and inflammation in symptomatic gallbladders with cholesterol gallstones. *Gut.* 2007;56(6):815–820.
- Irish MS, Pearl RH, Caty MG, et al. The approach to common abdominal diagnosis in infants and children. *Pediatr Clin North Am.* 1998;45:729–772.
- Kaechelev V, Wabitsch M, Thiere D, et al. Prevalence of gallbladder stone disease in obese children and adolescents: Influence of the degree of obesity, sex and pubertal development. *J Pediatr Gastroenterol Nutr.* 2006;42(1):66–70.

- Kasirajan K, Obermeyer RJ, Kehris J, et al. Microinvasive laparoscopic cholecystectomy in pediatric patients. *J Laparoendosc Adv Surg Tech A.* 1998;8(3):131–135.
- Lobe TE. Cholelithiasis and cholecystitis in children. *Semin Pediatr Surg.* 2000;9:170–176.
- Lucena JF, Herrero JI, Quiroga J, et al. A multidrug resistance 3 gene mutation causing cholelithiasis, cholestasis of pregnancy, and adulthood biliary cirrhosis. *Gastroenterology.* 2003;124(4):1037–1042.
- Rosmorduc O, Hermelin B, Boelle PY, et al. ABCB4 gene mutation-associated cholelithiasis in adults. *Gastroenterology.* 2003;125(2):452–459.
- Stringer MD, Taylor DR, Soloway RD. Gallstone composition: Are children different? *J Pediatr.* 2003;142:435–440.

 CODES

ICD9
- 574.20 Calculus of gallbladder without mention of cholecystitis, without mention of obstruction
- 574.21 Calculus of gallbladder without mention of cholecystitis, with obstruction

ICD10
- K80.20 Calculus of gallbladder without cholecystitis without obstruction
- K80.21 Calculus of gallbladder without cholecystitis with obstruction

FAQ

- Q: Does my child with CF have a greater problem with gallstones?
- A: Yes. Children with CF may have more frequent development of gallstones than will normal children. Reports of gallstones while on UDCA therapy have also been noted.
- Q: Why does my child with sickle cell disease have gallstones?
- A: Because the hemolytic process involves breakdown of hemoglobin, which produces bilirubin. This process may accelerate the formation of pigmented gallstones.
- Q: If my child has repeated attacks of abdominal pain and there are gallstones in the gallbladder, should he have surgery? What kind?
- A: Yes. Laparoscopic cholecystectomy is typically recommended.

CHOLERA

Matthew P. Kronman

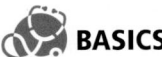 **BASICS**

DESCRIPTION

- *Vibrio cholerae* is a curved, motile gram-negative rod. Many serogroups exist, but only serogroups O1 and O139 cause epidemic clinical cholera.
- *V. cholerae* serogroup O1 is divided into 2 biotypes: Classical and El Tor. The classical biotype was formerly predominant, but currently the El Tor biotype is more commonly observed, having achieved worldwide spread since the 1960s.
- *V. cholerae* serogroup O139 was 1st identified in 1992 and resembles the O1 El Tor biotype, but possesses a distinct lipopolysaccharide and capsule.
- Humans are the only known host for *V. cholerae*, but organisms can also exist freely in water, thereby potentially contaminating fish and shellfish.

EPIDEMIOLOGY

- Diarrheal disease, including cholera, is the 2nd leading cause of mortality in children <5 years worldwide.
- Reporting systems for cholera are not robust, in part owing to national fears concerning travel and trade restrictions. Accurate incidence rates are therefore not available, but the World Health Organization (WHO) estimates 3–5 million cases of cholera occur annually, resulting in as many as 100,000 deaths.
- The 1st 6 recorded cholera pandemics occurred prior to 1923, but the current 7th pandemic began in 1961.
- Most cholera occurs in Asia and Africa, but *V. cholerae* is now endemic in many countries secondary to the 7th pandemic and increasing globalization. Regions previously free of cholera have become susceptible to severe outbreaks, as occurred in Haiti in 2010.
- In the US, most cases result from travel, but the Gulf Coast of Louisiana and Texas have an endemic focus of cholera, resulting in disease related to undercooked shellfish consumption.

- Inadequate drinking water and sanitation create an environment for increased transmission; peri-urban slums, refugee camps, areas of recent disaster, etc., are high-risk areas for cholera epidemics.
- The typical incubation period is usually 2–3 days but ranges from ~12 hours to 5 days.
- People with low gastric acidity (which decreases killing of ingested organisms) and those with blood group O are at increased risk of cholera.
- Young children are at increased risk of severe cholera.
- 75% are infected asymptomatically; of those with symptoms, the range of illness can be moderate to severe.
- Case fatality rates are ~1% when timely treatment is available, but can rise as high as 50% in severe cases in extremely resource-limited settings.
- Secondary transmission can occur in households with affected members if strict handwashing and hygiene is not followed.
- *V. cholerae* isolates resistant to tetracyclines, fluoroquinolones, sulfonamides, and β-lactams are increasingly reported worldwide.

GENERAL PREVENTION

- Transmission:
  - Handwashing after defecation and before food preparation is essential. Boiling or disinfection of water also prevents infection.
  - Thorough cooking of shellfish (which can be naturally contaminated) prevents infection.
  - During travel to endemic areas, avoidance of swimming or bathing in fresh water is recommended.
  - In the hospital setting, contact precautions are recommended for infected infants and children who are incontinent of stool for the duration of illness.
  - Confirmed cases of cholera must be reported to the local department of health.
  - Prophylaxis of contacts of confirmed cases is not currently recommended by the WHO, but hygiene teaching and anticipatory guidance are crucial.
- Vaccines:
  - No cholera vaccines are available in the US.
  - Two whole cell killed oral cholera vaccines have ~50% efficacy in preventing cholera over the subsequent 2-year period.
  - Whole cell killed injectable cholera vaccines provide a similar efficacy to oral vaccines but are generally not recommended owing to increased side effects.

PATHOPHYSIOLOGY

- Infection follows ingestion of large numbers of organisms from contaminated water or food (particularly raw or undercooked shellfish and fish, but also room temperature damp vegetables).
- The infectious dose for severe cholera is ~10^8 organisms, but can be as little as 10^4 organisms in young children or those with decreased gastric acidity, such as those on acid suppression or after certain meals.
- The key virulence factor responsible for the profuse watery diarrhea seen in cholera is cholera toxin.
- Cholera toxin is made up of 1 A and 5 B subunits. The B subunits facilitate attachment of toxin to intestinal cells, and the A subunit activates adenylate cyclase, increasing intracellular levels of cyclic adenosine monophosphate (cAMP), which causes chloride and sodium to be secreted into the gut lumen. Water follows via osmosis.
- Those with severe illness can progress rapidly to severe dehydration, circulatory collapse, and death.
- Symptomatic patients may shed as many as 10^{10} to 10^{12} organisms per liter of stool and will shed organisms for 1–2 weeks.

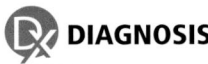 **DIAGNOSIS**

HISTORY

- Fever, vomiting, profuse watery diarrhea? Severe illness is characterized by voluminous watery diarrhea (at times up to 1 liter per hour) flecked with mucus ("rice-water stools").
- Sick contacts with similar symptoms? Cholera epidemics can spread rapidly.
- Exposures:
  - Return from travel within the last 5 days? Cholera is endemic in many parts of the world, and the incubation period is typically 2–3 days.
  - What is the patient's water source? Contaminated water serves as a reservoir.
  - Inadequately cooked shellfish? Shellfish such as oysters and crabs can harbor the organism.

C

DIAGNOSTIC TESTS & INTERPRETATION
Diagnostic Procedures/Other
- Selective media (thiosulfate citrate bile salts sucrose agar) must be used to isolate *V. cholerae*. This selective media is not typically used for routine stool culture, so clinicians must alert the microbiology laboratory if culture testing for *V. cholerae* is desired.
- Serologic testing on acute and convalescent sera is also available through the Centers for Disease Control and Prevention (CDC).
- Stool culture may not always be positive in suspected cases of cholera, and rapid dipstick methods to identify cholera toxin and lipopolysaccharide, direct fluorescent antibody assays, and polymerase chain reaction (PCR)–based diagnostic methods also exist.

DIFFERENTIAL DIAGNOSIS
- Other *Vibrio* species can cause gastroenteritis (commonly caused by *V. parahaemolyticus* but also by *V. fluvialis*, *V. hollisae*, and *V. mimicus*) or wound infections and sepsis (*V. vulnificus*). Of these, only *V. parahaemolyticus* and *V. vulnificus* cause outbreaks.
- Additional important intestinal bacterial pathogens include *Aeromonas*, *Campylobacter*, *Clostridium difficile*, *Escherichia coli*, *Listeria*, *Plesiomonas*, *Salmonella*, *Shigella*, *Vibrio* species, and *Yersinia*.
- Viral and parasitic pathogens to consider include rotavirus, norovirus, adenovirus types 40 and 41, *Giardia*, *Cyclospora*, and *Cryptosporidium*.

 TREATMENT

ADDITIONAL TREATMENT
General Measures
- The mainstay of treatment for cholera is rapid institution of rehydration.
- Patients with moderate disease may require only oral rehydration solutions, but those with more severe disease (volume loss >10%) require intravenous fluids.
- Oral rehydration solutions should be administered in frequent small sips to those with vomiting, and should contain at minimum 75 mEq/L of sodium to replete the significant sodium losses associated with cholera.

- Antibiotics are recommended for those with severe cholera; debate exists as to whether those with moderate cholera ought to receive antibiotics.
- Sensitive strains of *V. cholerae* are susceptible to doxycycline, ciprofloxacin, azithromycin, and trimethoprim-sulfamethoxazole, though there are increasing reports of resistance worldwide.
- Single-dose azithromycin can reduce the duration of symptoms by 50% and may reduce excretion of the organism to 1–2 days.
- During outbreaks, rapid institution of improved sanitation and safe water availability are critical to decrease the extent of the outbreak.

 ONGOING CARE

FOLLOW-UP RECOMMENDATIONS
In the untreated patient, the typical period of *V. cholerae* shedding is 1–2 weeks. Asymptomatic carriage is uncommon.

PROGNOSIS
For patients with prompt rehydration, the prognosis is very good, regardless of whether antibiotic treatment is given.

COMPLICATIONS
- The main complications of cholera are those of severe dehydration, such as renal failure, thrombosis, and cardiovascular collapse.
- There are no significant long-term complications of cholera.

ADDITIONAL READING
- Alam M, Hasan NA, Sultana M, et al. Diagnostic limitations to accurate diagnosis of cholera. *J Clin Microbiol*. 2010;48(11):3918–3922.
- Graves PM, Deeks JJ, Demicheli V, et al. Vaccines for preventing cholera: Killed whole cell or other subunit vaccines (injected). *Cochrane Database Syst Rev*. 2010;(8):CD000974.
- Kitaoka M, Miyata ST, Unterweger D, et al. Antibiotic resistance mechanisms of Vibrio cholerae. *J Med Microbiol*. 2011;60:397–407.

- Nelson EJ, Harris JB, Morris JG Jr, et al. Cholera transmission: The host, pathogen and bacteriophage dynamic. *Nat Rev Microbiol*. 2009;7(10):693–702.
- Saha D, Karim MM, Khan WA, et al. Single-dose azithromycin for the treatment of cholera in adults. *N Engl J Med*. 2006;354(23):2452–2462.
- Sur D, Lopez AL, Kanungo S, et al. Efficacy and safety of a modified killed-whole-cell oral cholera vaccine in India: An interim analysis of a cluster-randomised, double-blind, placebo-controlled trial. *Lancet*. 2009;374(9702):1694–1702.
- Weil AA, Khan AI, Chowdhury F, et al. Clinical outcomes in household contacts of patients with cholera in Bangladesh. *Clin Infect Dis*. 2009;49(10):1473–1479.
- *The World Health Organization cholera fact sheet*. June 2010. Available at http://www.who.int/mediacentre/factsheets/fs107/en/index.html. Accessed March 4, 2011.

 CODES

ICD9
001.9 Cholera, unspecified
ICD10
A00.9 Cholera, unspecified

FAQ
- Q: What foods should I avoid while traveling to cholera-endemic regions?
- A: Foods that incur a risk of cholera transmission include untreated or unboiled water and ice, undercooked fish and shellfish, raw vegetables, food and beverages from street vendors, and cooked food stored at ambient temperature.
- Q: Does cholera pose a risk to pregnant patients?
- A: Given the severe fluid losses, cholera can be a life-threatening infection to the fetus, with fetal loss occurring in as many as 50% of women in their 3rd trimester despite aggressive fluid resuscitation.
- Q: What is the risk of developing cholera among household contacts of those with disease?
- A: Up to 50% of household contacts may develop diarrheal symptoms, typically within 2 days of exposure to the index case.

CHRONIC DIARRHEA
Edisio Semeao

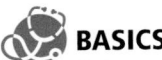 **BASICS**

DESCRIPTION
- Diarrhea lasting >2–4 weeks, whereas acute diarrhea, generally caused by enteric pathogens, is self-limiting and duration of symptoms <1 week
- Stool output >200 g/d in children and adults or 10 g/kg/d in infants is considered diarrhea.
- The initial focus is to establish the pattern of stool output with regard to:
  - Volume
  - Frequency
  - Consistency
  - Gross appearance

EPIDEMIOLOGY
- Chronic diarrhea seen in the tropics and developing countries is more likely infectious in nature than in the US.
- Gender and genetic factors do not play a significant role in most cases of chronic diarrhea.

PATHOPHYSIOLOGY
The major categories are osmotic and secretory. Inflammatory and motility disorders are smaller but important subcategories to consider.
- Osmotic diarrhea occurs when unabsorbable solute accumulates in the lumen of the small intestine and colon:
  - This increases the intraluminal osmotic pressure and results in excessive fluid and electrolyte losses in stool.
  - Osmotic diarrhea will improve with fasting.
  - Osmotic diarrhea is usually related to malabsorption of dietary products or to the presence of congenital or acquired disaccharidase deficiency or glucose-galactose defects.
- Secretory diarrhea occurs when the net secretion of fluid and electrolyte is in excess of absorption in the intestine:
  - The intestinal mucosa is normally very active in both of these processes.
  - The diarrhea occurs independently of the osmotic load in the intestinal lumen and does not improve with fasting.
  - The mechanisms for secretory diarrhea include the activation of intracellular mediators such as cAMP, cGMP, and calcium-dependent channels.
  - These mediators stimulate active chloride secretion from the crypt cells and inhibit the neutral coupled sodium chloride absorption.
- Inflammation in the intestine can cause an alteration in mucosal integrity resulting in exudative loss of mucus, blood, and/or protein. Increased permeability and altered mucosal surface area may affect absorption and result in diarrhea owing to a malabsorptive process.
- Motility disorders will affect the intestinal transit time. Hypomotility states such as stasis from bacterial overgrowth can lead to diarrhea.

DIAGNOSIS

HISTORY
- Evaluation of the stool pattern, including consistency, frequency, and appearance:
  - The history of blood and mucus in stool is strongly suggestive of inflammation.
  - Large-volume stools (>750 mL/d) imply small bowel disease and/or a secretory process.
  - Watery stools tend to be more associated with carbohydrate malabsorption, small bowel processes, medications, and functional processes.
  - Steatorrhea (fatty stools) can be greasy, oily, foul smelling, and bulky and are usually associated with pancreatic disease, bacterial overgrowth, and short bowel syndrome.
- Dietary intake including the types of food and the occurrence of diarrhea in close relationship to specific foods (e.g., dairy products) may be diagnostic. The amount and type of liquid ingested may also be helpful in diagnosis.
- Nutritional status and growth parameters need to be assessed. The presence of growth failure or malnutrition has considerable implications compared with a child with normal growth and no history of weight loss.
- Onset of diarrhea such as abrupt or gradual is important to determine. Overall duration of the diarrhea and pattern of intermittent versus continuous may also help in determining the underlying process.
- Other symptoms associated with the diarrhea are important to assess and include abdominal pain, fever, bloating, tenesmus, soiling, rashes, and joint complaints.
- Exposure to medications (antibiotics, laxatives, chemotherapeutic agents) or herbal therapies
- History of abdominal surgery
- Inquire about travel history.
- Family history of certain disorders may raise the level of suspicion in the patient. These include celiac disease, inflammatory bowel disease, cystic fibrosis, and other pancreatic processes.

PHYSICAL EXAM
- Nutritional status: Compare height, weight, and head circumference with normal standards and previous exam measurements.
- Anthropometric measurements are important in assessing loss of body fat and muscle mass.
- Peripheral edema, ascites, rash, dystrophic nails, alopecia, chronic chest findings, and pallor may all be indicative of nutritional deficiencies secondary to chronic diarrhea.
- A rectal exam may reveal stool impaction with overflow diarrhea:
  - Is there blood in the stool?
  - Perianal disease (fistula, skin tags, abscess)
- Evidence of infection should be considered with symptoms such as fever, bloody diarrhea, and vital sign instability.
- Aphthous lesions, arthritis, and clubbing
- The abdominal exam in most patients is generally nonspecific.

DIAGNOSTIC TESTS & INTERPRETATION
Lab
- Stool samples:
  - Stool should be tested for occult blood and for the presence of fecal leukocytes.
  - Stool pH and reducing substances: If stool is positive for reducing substances and/or the pH is <5.5, carbohydrate malabsorption with or without proximal small bowel injury is likely. (Note: Sucrose is not a reducing substance. If sucrose malabsorption is suspected, stool sample has to be hydrolyzed with hydrochloric acid and heat before analysis.)
  - A positive Sudan stain of the stool is indicative of fat malabsorption. However, a 72-hour fecal fat collection remains the gold standard to diagnose fat malabsorption.
  - Stool for fecal elastase to assess fat malabsorption
  - Stool should be cultured for bacteria, ova and parasites, and viral organisms. *Clostridium difficile* toxins A and B are heat labile, and stool must be kept cool during transport. Collect stool in the correct containers to ensure accurate and reliable analysis.
  - Stool may be collected for electrolyte and osmolality measurements. Osmotic gap >100 mOsm/kg is indicative of an osmotic diarrhea.
  - Spot or 24-hour collection for fecal α_1-antitrypsin to assess protein loss
  - Stool collection for fecal calprotectin to assess for IBD—protein found in neutrophils that enter the bowel during an inflammatory process
- Blood samples:
  - Hemoglobin and RBC
  - Prealbumin and albumin are good parameters of protein and overall nutritional status.
  - Electrolytes
  - Erythrocyte sedimentation rate and C-reactive protein (CRP) can serve as markers for inflammatory conditions.
  - Hormonal studies to assess for secretory tumors (vasoactive intestinal peptide [VIP], gastrin, secretin, urine assay for 5-HT)
  - In the evaluation for celiac disease, serum antitissue transglutaminase antibody and antiendomysial antibodies as long as the total serum IgA is normal
  - Hepatic panel, coagulation profile, and fat-soluble vitamin levels (25 OH vitamin D; vitamins E, A, K) may be helpful to assess fat malabsorption.
  - Viral serologies such as HIV and cytomegalovirus need to be considered in the immunocompromised host with diarrhea.
  - Thyroid studies in patients with large-volume watery diarrhea
- Specialized studies:
  - A D-xylose absorption test is helpful in screening for small bowel injury. Timed serum D-xylose following oral ingestion is significantly lower in diseases causing diffuse mucosal damage to the small bowel (i.e., postviral enteropathy, celiac disease).
  - A hydrogen breath test may be helpful in evaluating the possibility of small bowel bacterial overgrowth.
- Sweat chloride if cystic fibrosis is suspected

Imaging

- Plain radiograph studies usually not helpful
- Upper GI series with small bowel follow-through may show partial small bowel obstruction, strictures, or evidence of inflammatory bowel disease.
- Abdominal CT scan may help in assessing the pancreas for calcifications and inflammation.

Diagnostic Procedures/Other

- Endoscopy with small bowel biopsy and small bowel aspirate for culture to help diagnose certain congenital, immunologic, or infectious causes of diarrhea:
  - Small bowel disaccharidase studies will help detect carbohydrate malabsorption.
- Colonoscopy will diagnose colitis related to inflammatory bowel disease or infection.
- Video capsule endoscopy may also be used to further evaluate the small bowel for evidence of inflammation.

DIFFERENTIAL DIAGNOSIS

- Infants (<1 year of age):
  - Cow's milk and/or soy protein intolerance
  - Intractable diarrhea of infancy is associated with diffuse mucosal injury beginning at <6 months of age resulting in malabsorption and malnutrition.
  - Infectious/protracted postinfectious diarrhea
  - Microvillus inclusions disease
  - Autoimmune enteropathy
  - Hirschsprung disease with enterocolitis
  - Transport defects (e.g., congenital chloridorrhea)
  - Nutrient malabsorption (e.g., congenital glucose-galactose malabsorption and congenital lactase deficiency, sucrase-isomaltase deficiency)
  - Cystic fibrosis
  - AIDS enteropathy
  - Primary immune defects
  - Munchausen syndrome by proxy (factitious)
  - Drug, toxin induced
- Children (1–5 years of age):
  - Chronic nonspecific diarrhea of infancy (toddler's diarrhea)
  - Infectious/postinfectious enteritis
  - Giardiasis
  - Eosinophilic gastroenteritis
  - Sucrase-isomaltase deficiency
  - Tumors (neuroblastoma, VIPoma with secretory diarrhea)
  - Inflammatory bowel disease
  - Celiac disease
  - Cystic fibrosis
  - Small bowel bacterial overgrowth
  - AIDS enteropathy
  - Constipation with (overflow) encopresis
  - Acquired short bowel syndrome
  - Shwachman syndrome
  - Factitious
- Children (>5 years of age):
  - Similar to above
  - Acquired lactose deficiency (early adolescent)
  - Inflammatory bowel disease
  - Celiac disease
  - Constipation with (overflow) encopresis
  - Irritable bowel syndrome (adolescent)
  - Laxative abuse (adolescents)
  - Infection

- Bacterial (*Aeromonas, Plesiomonas, Campylobacter, Salmonella, Mycobacterium tuberculosis, Yersinia,* recurrent *C. difficile*)
- Viral (rotavirus, adenovirus, Norwalk virus, Noro virus)
- Parasites (amoeba, trichuris, cryptosporidium, *Giardia, Schistosoma, Cyclospora*)
- Small bowel bacterial overgrowth
- Tumors (neuroblastoma, VIPoma with secretory diarrhea)
- Primary bowel tumors (rare, adolescent)
- Complex congenital heart disease with protein-losing enteropathy
- Pancreatic insufficiency/chronic pancreatitis
- Hyperthyroidism
- Diabetes

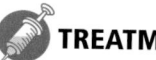 TREATMENT

MEDICATION (DRUGS)

- The use of antimotility agents such as loperamide and Lomotil, and antisecretory agents, such as octreotide, may have a role in noninfectious causes of diarrhea. However, identification and treatment of the underlying cause of diarrhea is always preferable.
- Pancreatic enzymes may be used in specific patients.
- Luminal (nonabsorbed) antibiotics for small bowel bacterial overgrowth

ALERT

- In certain cases in which the diet is altered as a therapeutic intervention, the physician must ensure that the patient is still absorbing adequate calories and micronutrients so that the nutritional status of the patient is not further compromised.
- Avoid the reinstitution of a regular diet too quickly following a severe and/or protracted insult to the gut since this may further exacerbate the diarrhea.
- The use of antimotility and antisecretory agents should be judicious and as an adjunct to other therapy, but not as the mainstay in the treatment regimen.
- In patients with cow's milk and/or soy allergy, rechallenge after 12 months of age in a controlled environment in case anaphylaxis occurs.
- Children with the following symptoms should see a health care provider:
  - Signs of dehydration
  - Diarrhea for more than 24–48 hours
  - A fever of 102°F or higher
  - Stools containing blood or pus
  - Stools that are black and tarry

ADDITIONAL TREATMENT

- The 1st goal is to ensure adequate hydration status, nutritional intake and to permit normal growth and development.
- Antibiotics when infection is suspected
- Many causes of congenital diarrhea do not have specific therapy available, and treatment is supportive.

- Diet: If infection is severe or protracted, a predigested formula may be necessary early in the recovery phase. If oral nutrition appears inadequate, the formula can be given in a slow, continuous fashion via a nasogastric/jejunal tube. Remove offending agent (e.g., cow's milk protein, soy protein, lactose, or gluten). In cases in which there is increased motility and thus rapid transit time, such as in chronic nonspecific diarrhea, alterations in the diet can be very helpful. Elimination of sorbitol-containing juices, which increases the osmotic load, and low-carbohydrate diet will help to lower the osmotic load delivered to the intestine. Furthermore, a high-fat diet will slow the intestinal transit time and increase the time available to absorb fluid, electrolytes, and nutrients from the intestinal tract.

ADDITIONAL READING

- Bhutta ZA, Nelson EA, Lee WS, et al. Recent advances and evidence gaps in persistent diarrhea. *J Pediatr Gastroenterol Nutr.* 2008;47(2):260–265.
- Lee SD, Surawicz CM. Infectious causes of chronic diarrhea. *Gastroenterol Clin North Am.* 2001;30: 679–692, viii.
- Pawlowski SW, Warren CA, Guerrant R. Diagnosis and treatment of acute or persistent diarrhea. *Gastroenterology.* 2009;136(6):1874–1886.
- Salvilahti E. Food-induced malabsorption syndromes. *J Pediatr Gastroenterol Nutr.* 2000; 30(Suppl):S61–S66.

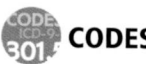 CODES

ICD9

- 009.2 Infectious diarrhea
- 787.91 Diarrhea

ICD10

- A07.9 Protozoal intestinal disease, unspecified
- K52.89 Other specified noninfective gastroenteritis and colitis
- R19.7 Diarrhea, unspecified

FAQ

- Q: If my infant has cow's milk allergy, when can he have cow's milk?
- A: In patients with cow's milk and/or soy allergy, rechallenge should be after 12 months of age and should be in a controlled environment in case anaphylaxis occurs. If the testing is negative, ingestion of cow's milk can be recommended.
- Q: What are the best markers for success in management of chronic diarrhea?
- A: If weight and height normalize, the chances of continued malabsorption are unlikely.

CHRONIC GRANULOMATOUS DISEASE

Mathew Fogg

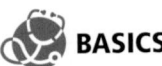 **BASICS**

DESCRIPTION
Rare inherited defect involving phagocytes. The defective phagocytes (neutrophils and monocytes) have a decreased or absent ability to generate reactive oxygen intermediates, leaving the host susceptible to recurrent bacterial and fungal infections.

EPIDEMIOLOGY
Prevalence
~1 in 500,000 individuals

RISK FACTORS
Genetics
- Gene mutations may occur spontaneously and are inherited as an X-linked variant or autosomal recessive variant.
- Mutations may occur in any 1 of the 4 subunits of the neutrophil NADPH oxidase complex.

PATHOPHYSIOLOGY
- Associated defects involve the NADPH oxidase complex of the neutrophil.
- Neutrophils in chronic granulomatous disease (CGD) have an impaired ability to combat infection via an impaired respiratory burst.
- The NADPH oxidase complex is composed of 4 subunits, any of which may be defective in CGD:
  - 60% of patients with CGD have a defect in the gp91-phox subunit, which is inherited in an X-linked manner.
  - 33% of patients have a defect in the p47-phox subunit, which is inherited in an autosomal recessive manner.
  - Defects occur less frequently in the p22-phox and p67-phox subunits.

ETIOLOGY
CGD is not acquired; it is inherited as an X-linked variant or as an autosomal variant.

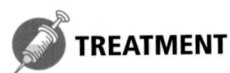 **DIAGNOSIS**

HISTORY
- Usually present <2 years of age with marked lymphadenopathy, hepatosplenomegaly, draining lymph nodes, and pneumonias
- Tend to develop infections with unusual organisms, such as *Staphylococcus aureus*, *S. epidermidis*, *Serratia marcescens*, *Pseudomonas*, *Escherichia coli*, *Candida*, *Aspergillus*, *Nocardia*, and *Salmonella*
- Disease is inherited in an X-linked and autosomal recessive pattern. Therefore, there may be other affected family members.
- Mother with lupus: There is a higher incidence of lupus in females who are carriers for CGD.

SIGNS AND SYMPTOMS
- General goal: Decide whether the patient's type of infections (osteomyelitis, perirectal abscess) and infecting organisms are consistent with the diagnosis of CGD.
- Order a DCF or DHR assay.
- If abnormal, initiate sulfamethoxazole/trimethoprim prophylaxis.

PHYSICAL EXAM
- Skin abscess or boils: Patients develop frequent skin infections.
- Mucous membrane and perirectal infections: Patients commonly develop infections at mucous membrane and epidermal junctions, especially in the perirectal area.
- Lymphadenopathy: Patients commonly develop lymphadenopathy and draining lymph nodes.
- Hepatosplenomegaly: Common finding in patients with CGD
- Abnormal lung examination: Pulmonary disease common in patients with CGD

DIAGNOSTIC TESTS & INTERPRETATION
Lab
- Nitroblue tetrazolium test:
  - Older test for CGD, no longer widely used by immunologists
  - Neutrophils from normal individuals can reduce the dye, resulting in a color change. Neutrophils from patients with CGD cannot reduce the dye, and it remains colorless.
  - Neutrophils and monocytes from patients with CGD have an impaired hexose monophosphate shunt. Therefore, they have a decreased conversion of NADP to NADPH and a decreased oxidative burst, which results in an inability to reduce the nitroblue tetrazolium in this study.
  - Results may be inaccurate if not performed by experienced technician.
- DCF or DHR assay:
  - Can directly measure the production of hydrogen peroxide using a fluorescent label and flow cytometry
  - Patients with CGD have decreased hydrogen peroxide production.
  - DHR and DCF are very similar tests.
- Immunoblotting: Can be used to quantify the amount of each NADPH subunit present

DIFFERENTIAL DIAGNOSIS
- Infectious: Infections are related to the immunodeficiency.
- Genetic/Metabolic:
  - Leukocyte glucose-6-phosphate dehydrogenase deficiency
  - Myeloperoxidase deficiency
  - Humoral immunodeficiencies
  - Complement deficiencies

TREATMENT
MEDICATION (DRUGS)
- Antibiotic prophylaxis: Trimethoprim-sulfamethoxazole is the antibiotic of choice, because both components are concentrated in the neutrophil and for its bacterial spectrum.
- Recombinant interferon-γ:
  - Reserved for patients with severe disease
  - May decrease the incidence of infection

- Acute infections:
  - Broad-spectrum IV antibiotics: Should be a low threshold to start this therapy. Severe infections should be treated with broad-spectrum IV antibiotics until an organism is identified. Good initial antibiotics include IV penicillins, aminoglycosides, and antipseudomonal antibiotics.
  - Amphotericin B: Should not be withheld if a fungal infection is suspected or if the patient's clinical status is deteriorating despite broad-spectrum antibiotics.
  - Leukocyte transfusions: Reserved for severe infections; efficacy is controversial.

ISSUES FOR REFERRAL

Factors that may help alert you to make a referral:
- New diagnosis of CGD:
  - Immunologists can assist with antibiotic prophylaxis and with parameters for when to seek medical attention.
  - Can help identify which genetic variant is responsible for the patient's disease
- Pregnant carrier for CGD:
  - Immunologists can help with prenatal diagnosis.
  - Some centers may consider in utero bone marrow transplantation for an affected fetus.
- Fever or suspected infection: Patients with CGD tend to develop infections in unusual sites with unusual organisms. An immunologist can help with the evaluation and appropriate antibiotic coverage.

COMPLEMENTARY & ALTERNATIVE THERAPIES

Bone marrow transplant: CGD has been cured in patients with matched transplants.

 ONGOING CARE

FOLLOW-UP RECOMMENDATIONS
Patient Monitoring
- CGD is a lifelong disease.
- Patients tend to develop chronic lung disease; therefore, pulmonary function studies should be followed at least annually.
- Liver disease is also common; therefore, liver function studies should also be followed at least annually.
- Female carriers should be observed for signs of lupus erythematosus.

PROGNOSIS
- Survival beyond the 4th decade is common.
- Bone marrow transplantation is curative.

COMPLICATIONS

These patients have an increased susceptibility to bacterial and fungal infections that usually are not pathogenic in normal hosts:
- Recurrent skin infections
- Sepsis
- Chronic lung disease (secondary to recurrent infections)
- Chronic liver disease (secondary to recurrent infections)
- Chronic osteomyelitis of large and small bones
- Malabsorption
- Systemic and discoid lupus erythematosus: Increased incidence in female carriers
- The diagnosis of CGD should be considered in patients with:
  - Recurrent lymphadenitis
  - Staphylococcal hepatic abscess
  - *Aspergillus* or *Nocardia* pneumonia
  - *Serratia marcescens* osteomyelitis
  - Infections with *Pseudomonas cepacia*
  - *Salmonella* sepsis
  - Perirectal abscesses
  - Brain abscesses

ADDITIONAL READING

- Fleisher TA. Back to basics: Primary immune deficiencies: Windows into the immune system. *Pediatr Rev.* 2006;27(10):363–372.
- Hernandez M, Bastian JF. Immunodeficiency in childhood. *Curr Allergy Asthma Rep.* 2006;6(6): 468–474.
- Horwitz ME, Barrett AJ, Brown MR, et al. Treatment of chronic granulomatous disease with nonmyeloablative conditioning and a T-cell-depleted hematopoietic allograft. *N Engl J Med.* 2001;344: 881–888.

- Jirapongsananuruk O, Malech HL, Kuhns DB, et al. Diagnostic paradigm for evaluation of male patients with chronic granulomatous disease, based on the dihydrorhodamine 123 assay. *J Allergy Clin Immunol.* 2003;111:374–379.
- Kamani N, Douglas SD. Natural history of chronic granulomatous disease. *Diagn Clin Immunol.* 1988;5:314–317.
- Schappi MG, Klein NJ, Lindley KJ, et al. The nature of colitis in chronic granulomatous disease. *J Pediatr Gastroenterol Nutr.* 2003;36:623–631.

 CODES

ICD9
288.1 Functional disorders of polymorphonuclear neutrophils

ICD10
D71 Functional disorders of polymorphonuclear neutrophils

FAQ

- Q: What do the infecting organisms have in common?
- A: Patients with CGD are most susceptible to catalase-positive organisms.
- Q: Are all CGD patients with fever admitted automatically?
- A: No. It is true that these patients are more prone to invasive and systemic infections, but these patients are not admitted with every febrile episode (especially if there is evidence of a minor bacterial or viral infection). However, subtle signs of an invasive infection must be taken very seriously, and these patients are certainly admitted.
- Q: Can a prenatal diagnosis be made?
- A: Yes. However, currently this can be done only in a limited number of research laboratories, and the testing is not commercially available. Testing involves chorionic villus sampling, and it can be done only on families in which the specific mutation has been mapped.

C

CHRONIC HEPATITIS

John Y. Tung MB
Vani V. Gopalareddy

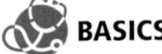 **BASICS**

DESCRIPTION
- Chronic hepatitis is a continuing inflammation of the liver that may lead to cirrhosis.
- Features include inflammation not caused by acute self-limiting infection or past drug exposure with raised transaminases and histologic evidence of hepatitis.

EPIDEMIOLOGY
Depends on the cause of the underlying disease:
- Nonalcoholic steatohepatitis (NASH) is a leading cause of elevated AST/ALT.
- Hepatitis B: Common in immigrant children from Asia and Eastern Europe
- Hepatitis C: Common in those who had blood transfusions and blood products before screening became available, users of IV drugs, nasal cocaine users
- Wilson disease presents mainly in older children (>2 years) and adults.
- Autoimmune liver disease is more common in females and older children.(suspect in >6 months age)
- Autoimmune hepatitis (AIH) may be associated with other autoimmune conditions such as diabetes, ulcerative colitis, autoimmune thyroiditis, and celiac disease.
- Cystic fibrosis and α_1-antitrypsin deficiency: Predominantly white patients but may occur in other ethnic groups.

PATHOPHYSIOLOGY
Pathology has been traditionally classified as chronic persistent hepatitis, chronic aggressive hepatitis, and chronic lobular hepatitis. The hepatocytes are damaged, with inflammatory cellular infiltration accompanied by liver regeneration.
- Chronic persistent hepatitis:
  - Minimal portal tract fibrosis
  - Slightly widened portal tracts
  - Limiting plate is intact and inflammation does not extend beyond this.
  - No bridging fibrosis between portal tracts
- Chronic aggressive hepatitis:
  - Perilobular hepatitis, with inflammatory cells extending from portal tracts into parenchyma with fibrosis
  - Piecemeal necrosis: Necrotic hepatocytes surrounded by lymphocytes and fibroblasts
  - In advanced disease, fibrosis bridges the portal tracts (bridging fibrosis).
  - Cirrhosis occurs when there is loss of architecture owing to fibrosis.
- Chronic lobular hepatitis:
  - Liver architecture is preserved with scattered changes of acute hepatitis with hepatocyte necrosis in the lobules (perivenular regions).
- These changes are most often associated with hepatitis B and non-A, non-B hepatitis.

ETIOLOGY
- Autoimmune liver disease
- Viral hepatitis
- Obesity (NASH)
- Progressive familial intrahepatic cholestasis syndromes (PFIC)
- Congenital hepatic fibrosis
- Cystic fibrosis
- Metabolic disease:
  - Mitochondrial disease
  - Lysosomal storage disorders
  - Peroxisomal disease
  - Lipid storage disease
  - Glycogen storage disease
  - Wilson disease and others
- Drug hepatotoxicity:
  - Methotrexate
  - Isoniazid
  - Thioguanine
  - 6-Mercaptopurine
  - Valproate
- Liver disease associated with other chronic diseases:
  - Cardiac disease
  - Autosomal recessive polycystic kidney disease
  - Diabetes mellitus
  - Langerhans cell histiocytosis
  - Immunodeficiency
  - Total parenteral nutrition cholestasis

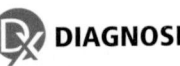 **DIAGNOSIS**

HISTORY
- Preceding clinical signs and symptoms for at least 6 months and complete medical history:
  - History of blood transfusions
  - Surgery
  - Medications
  - Foreign travel
  - Social circumstances that predispose to liver diseases
- Symptoms of chronic illness can be nonspecific:
  - Poor growth
  - Intermittent jaundice
  - Abdominal pain
  - Bleeding
  - Malabsorption
  - Fever
  - Amenorrhea
  - Poor school achievement
  - Itching
- Variceal bleeding may be a presenting syndrome in patients with portal hypertension.
- A history of jaundice in infancy, family history of liver disease or autoimmune liver disease, blood transfusions, IV drug use, or multiple sexual partners can suggest an etiology of hepatitis.

PHYSICAL EXAM
Stigmata of chronic liver disease are:
- Spider nevi
- Cutaneous shunts
- Palmar erythema
- Cyanosis (hepatopulmonary syndrome)
- Jaundice
- Itching
- Enlarged liver or small, shrunken liver
- Splenomegaly
- Ascites
- Rickets
- Mental changes
- Fetor associated with high ammonia
- Obesity

DIAGNOSTIC TESTS & INTERPRETATION
Lab
- Albumin, creatinine, γ-glutamyl transferase, aspartate aminotransferase, alanine aminotransferase, bilirubin, PT, CBC, blood group, Coombs test
- Other testing as indicated by the specific clinical presentation:
  - Viral serologies: Hepatitis B, hepatitis C, hepatitis D
  - Autoantibodies: Type 1: Smooth muscle (also called antiactin), antinuclear, antisoluble liver antigen, Type 2: Liver kidney microsomal, primary sclerosing cholangitis: pericytoplasmic antineutrophil (p-ANCA)
  - Immunoglobulins: IgG elevated in autoimmune liver disease
  - Fasting glucose, insulin levels, CRP, lipid profile (suspected NASH)
  - alpha1-Antitrypsin level and phenotype
  - Serum ceruloplasmin, serum copper, 24-hour urine copper (+/?penicillamine challenge), quantitative liver copper (Wilson disease)
  - Cholesterol, triglycerides elevated in cholestatic syndromes, glycogen storage, Alagille syndrome, certain lysosomal disease, steatohepatitis
  - Metabolic workup as indicate
  - CPK level to rule out muscle source of elevated ALT/AS
  - Urinary succinylacetone: Tyrosinemia
  - Urinary bile acids: Bile acid synthetic defects and some progressive intrahepatic cholestatic syndrome
  - Sweat test and cystic fibrosis genotyping
  - Alpha-1-fetoprotein
  - Fibrosis markers (FibroSURE; FibroTest; ActiTest) are not validated for children but may be useful in older patients.

Diagnostic Procedures/Other
- Ultrasound: Focus on liver, spleen with Doppler flow studies. This may also demonstrate steatosis.
- Other testing as indicated by specific clinical presentation:
  - MRI can demonstrate percentage steatosis
  - Fibroscan can measure liver stiffness/fibrosis.
  - Liver biopsy

- Percutaneous transhepatic cholangiography, endoscopic retrograde cholangiopancreatography or magnetic retrograde cholangiopancreatography may be useful if primary sclerosing cholangitis is suspected
- Colonoscopy: Sclerosing cholangitis, inflammatory bowel disease
- Bone marrow aspirate to exclude Niemann-Pick type C or other storage disorders
- Enzyme from white cells or cultured fibroblasts (skin biopsy) to exclude lysosomal storage disease, glycogen storage disease
- Angiography: Congenital or acquired venous or arterial malformations, assessment of portosystemic shunt
- Cardiac catheterization to assess pulmonary hypertension and cardiac status
- Macroaggregated albumin scan to assess hepatopulmonary syndrome and hepatic encephalopathy
- Muscle biopsy to assay respiratory chain enzymes in mitochondrial disorders
- Genotyping: Wilson disease, cystic fibrosis, and others

DIFFERENTIAL DIAGNOSIS
Nonhepatic etiologies of lab or physical exam abnormalities:

- Hepatomegaly: Elevated right-sided cardiac pressures, such as patients with Fontan operations, right-sided heart failure; respiratory diseases with lung hyperexpansion
- Splenomegaly:
  - Blood malignancies
  - Storage diseases
  - Hematologic disease with hemolysis
  - Infection
  - Vascular
- Jaundice: Often confused with hypercarotenemia
- Elevated transaminases: Consider nonhepatic sources such as skeletal muscles in myopathies. With jaundice, consider hypopituitarism in infancy.
- Alkaline phosphatase: May be elevated in growing children and in rickets; may not indicate biliary obstruction.
- γ-Glutamyl transferase:
  - Produced in choroid plexus, renal tubules, pancreatic and biliary ducts
  - Often elevated in patients on antiepileptic drugs and in alcoholics
- Abnormal coagulation: Anticoagulant medications, bacterial overgrowth with malabsorption, inherited disorders of coagulation, sepsis

 TREATMENT

ADDITIONAL TREATMENT
General Measures
The management of patients is dictated by the underlying diagnosis.

- General management:
  - Maintaining growth and development is paramount.
  - Fat-soluble vitamins (A, D, E, K) given orally are poorly absorbed in cholestasis, and levels must be monitored.
  - Anthropometric parameters must be recorded, including skinfold thickness.
  - Body mass index
  - Medium-chain triglyceride–rich formulas can reduce fat malabsorption.
  - Branched-chain amino acids may be useful in patients with hepatic encephalopathy.
  - Ursodeoxycholic acid: Choleretic
  - Encourage bolus feedings; minimizing continuous feeding and total parenteral nutrition may reduce gallbladder sludge.
  - Proactive involvement of clinical psychologist, play therapist can help alleviate problems such as depression and fear.
  - Aggressive weight management in patients with obesity/hypermetabolic syndrome with steatohepatitis. Curbing passive activities such as television, computer games.
  - Chronic debilitating pruritus: Indication for liver transplantation after failure of medical therapy. Treatment for pruritus includes:
    ○ Antihistamines
    ○ Cholestyramine
    ○ Naltrexone
    ○ Rifampicin
    ○ Ursodeoxycholic acid
  - Monitoring portal hypertension: Assessment of portal flow on ultrasound and splenic size may provide some indication of disease progression.
  - Treatment of recurrent cholangitis may decelerate the progression of liver disease.
  - Aggressive treatment for spontaneous bacterial peritonitis in patients with ascites
  - Early referral to a liver transplant center
  - Complete immunization schedule including hepatitis A
- Specific management depends on the underlying liver disease.

 ONGOING CARE

FOLLOW-UP RECOMMENDATIONS
Patient Monitoring
- Look for hepatocellular carcinoma developing in patients with chronic liver disease, an ultrasound scan of liver and AFP every 6 months is a reasonable schedule.
- Advise patients with enlarged spleens to wear a spleen guard and avoid activities that can cause splenic rupture.

PROGNOSIS
Some diseases are treatable while others are progressive and not amenable to treatment. A subset of patients will progress to end-stage liver disease and regular liver transplantation.

ADDITIONAL READING
- Geller SA. Hepatitis B and hepatitis C. *Clin Liver Dis.* 2002;6:317–334.
- Murray KF, Shah U, Mohan N, et al. Chronic hepatitis. *J Pediatr Gastroenterol Nutr.* 2008; 47(2):225–233.
- Zein NN. Hepatitis C in children: Recent advances. *Curr Opin Pediatr.* 2007;19(5):570–574.

 CODES

ICD9
- 571.40 Chronic hepatitis, unspecified
- 571.41 Chronic persistent hepatitis
- 571.42 Autoimmune hepatitis

ICD10
- K73.0 Chronic persistent hepatitis, not elsewhere classified
- K73.9 Chronic hepatitis, unspecified
- K75.4 Autoimmune hepatitis

FAQ
- Q: What are the risks of providing very young patients with a liver transplant?
- A: Although transplant in the very young is more difficult, with the increased use of split liver techniques, outcomes of orthotopic liver transplantation in infants have improved.
- Q: Why should we be aggressive with vitamin supplementation?
- A: There is significant malabsorption of vitamins A, D, E, and K. Vitamins D and E deficiencies are the most significant, causing rickets and neuropathy.
- Q: Oral supplements of vitamins are sometimes very difficult to administer in the very young. How can I overcome this problem?
- A: It is common practice in some centers to give vitamins D and E as an intramuscular injection on a monthly basis, with levels done in between.
- Q: Why do jaundiced children scratch?
- A: The accumulation of bile salts causes pruritus.
- Q: Are the stigmata of chronic liver disease also seen in children?
- A: Spider nevi, liver palms, splenomegaly, cutaneous shunts, and clubbing are very common.

CHRONIC KIDNEY DISEASE

Rebecca Ruebner
Lawrence Copelovitch

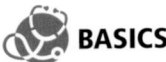 **BASICS**

DESCRIPTION
- Chronic kidney disease (CKD), previously referred to as chronic renal failure: The Kidney Disease Outcomes Quality Initiative (K/DOQI) of the National Kidney Foundation (NKF) defines CKD as either kidney damage or a decreased glomerular filtration rate (GFR) for 3 or more months
- Kidney damage is defined as pathological abnormalities or markers of kidney injury, including abnormalities in the composition of the blood or urine, or abnormalities in imaging tests.
- CKD is stratified from stages 1–5:
  - Stage 1: normal GFR (>90) but some evidence of kidney damage
  - Stage 2: GFR 60–89
  - Stage 3: GFR 30–59
  - Stage 4: GFR 15–29
  - Stage 5: GFR <15 or dialysis/transplant (end-stage)

EPIDEMIOLOGY
Incidence
~3–8 new cases of end-stage renal failure are reported per 1 million children per year.

Prevalence
- Among children in the US with CKD entered into the North American Pediatric Renal Transplant Cooperative Study, 65.9% are boys and 63.9% are white.
- Prevalence of CKD has been reported to be 32.4 per 1 million children in western Europe, with 6% <3 years of age, 30% between 3 and 9 years of age, and 64% between 9 and 15 years of age.

RISK FACTORS
Genetics
Several hereditary diseases can cause CKD, including:
- Alport disease (partially X-linked dominant)
- Polycystic kidney disease (autosomal recessive or dominant)
- Familial juvenile nephronophthisis (autosomal recessive)
- Cystinosis (autosomal recessive)
- Hyperoxaluria (autosomal recessive)
- Congenital nephrotic syndrome (autosomal recessive)
- Nail patella syndrome (autosomal dominant)
- Sickle cell disease (autosomal recessive)

PATHOPHYSIOLOGY
- Infants <2 years of age develop CKD due to either obstructive uropathy or renal hypodysplasia.
- Children 2–5 years of age develop CKD secondary to neonatal vascular accidents and hemolytic-uremic syndrome, obstructive uropathy, or renal hypodysplasia.
- More common causes of CKD in older children and adolescents include various types of glomerulonephritis (e.g., focal segmental glomerulosclerosis, crescentic glomerulonephritis, lupus nephritis), reflux nephropathy, or hereditary causes (e.g., Alport syndrome).

ETIOLOGY
- Congenital:
  - Renal dysplasia/hypoplasia
  - Obstructive uropathy (posterior urethral valves, prune belly syndrome)
  - Polycystic kidney disease
- Acquired:
  - Nephrotic syndrome (FSGS)
  - Glomerulonephritis (lupus, vasculitis)
  - Chronic interstitial nephritis

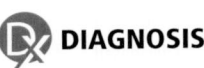 **DIAGNOSIS**

HISTORY
- Past history:
  - Perinatal complications
  - Oligohydramnios
  - Single umbilical artery
  - Recurrent UTIs
  - Enuresis
- Familial history:
  - Renal disease
  - Hearing impairment

SIGNS AND SYMPTOMS
- Malaise
- Poor appetite
- Vomiting
- Bone pain
- Headache (if hypertensive)
- Polyuria
- Polydipsia

PHYSICAL EXAM
- General:
  - Short stature
  - Retarded weight gain
  - Dermatologic pallor
  - Fetid breath
- Head, ears, eyes, nose, and throat:
  - Retinal changes
  - Presence of preauricular sinus
  - Hearing deficit
- Chest:
  - Rales
- Heart:
  - Flow murmur
  - Gallop
  - Rub
- Abdomen:
  - Palpable kidneys
  - Suprapubic mass
- Extremities:
  - Rachitic changes
  - Edema
  - Absent patella
- Neurologic system:
  - Developmental delay
  - Altered mental status
  - Hypotonia
  - Irritability

DIAGNOSTIC TESTS & INTERPRETATION
Lab
- Serum chemistries: Azotemia, hyperkalemia (if advanced), acidemia, hypocalcemia, hyperphosphatemia, elevated alkaline phosphatase (Onset of these electrolyte abnormalities is CKD stage 4, GFR <30.)
- CBCs: Normocytic anemia with low reticulocyte count (CKD stage 3, GFR <60)
- Urinalysis: Isosthenuria, proteinuria
- Intact parathyroid hormone: Elevated
- 25-Vitamin D: often low
- 24-hour urine collection: GFR can be estimated with concomitant blood sampling by calculating the creatinine clearance: Ucreat × (volume voided/1,440)/Pcreat × 1.73/body surface area. The resultant value is expressed as mL/min/1.73 m^2. Normal range is 90–140 mL/min/1.73 m^2 above age 2
- A simpler and more commonly used method to estimate GFR in children >1 year of age with CKD is the CKiD bedside equation, an update to the traditional Schwartz formula. The calculation is already corrected for surface area and does not require a urine collection: Height (cm) × 0.413 correction factor/Pcreat. Plotting the reciprocal of the serum creatinine versus time can approximate the rate of decline of renal function. This may be useful in determining when renal replacement therapy will be necessary.

Imaging
- Chest x-ray: Pulmonary edema, cardiomegaly
- Bone films: Delayed bone age, rickets, osteomalacia, osteitis fibrosa
- Renal ultrasound: Small echogenic kidneys, cystic kidneys, hydronephrosis
- EKG, in hyperkalemic patients: Peaked T waves

DIFFERENTIAL DIAGNOSIS
- Differentiate acute kidney injury from CKD
- Usually, CKD is insidious and associated with poor growth, delayed puberty, rickets, polyuria, and anemia. The kidneys may be smaller on renal ultrasound. A renal biopsy may be indicated to determine the cause of renal failure if genetic causes are suspected (for family counseling) or if treatment is being considered.

 ## TREATMENT

MEDICATION (DRUGS)
- Phosphate binders (e.g., calcium carbonate, calcium acetate, sevelamer; avoid aluminum if possible)
- 1,25-dihydroxy vitamin D and/or 25-hydroxy vitamin D
- Alkali therapy (e.g., sodium bicarbonate/citrate)
- Antihypertensive therapy
- ACE inhibitors (renoprotection)
- Recombinant erythropoietin
- Ferrous sulfate (if iron deficient)
- Recombinant human growth hormone

ADDITIONAL TREATMENT
ISSUES FOR REFERRAL
Pediatric primary care physicians should observe patients with CKD in consultation and with assistance from a pediatric nephrologist.

COMPLEMENTARY & ALTERNATIVE THERAPIES
Dialysis: Indications similar to those for acute renal failure or when GFR <10 mL/min/1.73 m^2 and patient is experiencing fatigue, poor school performance, or weight loss due to severe dietary restrictions.

ALERT
During episodes of gastroenteritis, infants with CKD may be prone to dehydration because they have obligatory polyuria due to a concentrating defect. Do not use urine output level or specific gravity of urine as indices for hydration. If hospitalized, fluid levels considered "maintenance" may be insufficient due to polyuria.

SURGERY/OTHER PROCEDURES
- Transplantation: In some cases, a preemptive transplant may be offered instead of dialysis.
- Consider arteriovenous fistula or graft placement for patients who will require long-term hemodialysis.

 ## ONGOING CARE

DIET
Restrictions mandated by condition:
- Protein (not less than RDA in children)
- Phosphate
- Potassium
- Sodium (indicated if patient swollen)
- Fluid (indicated in conditions related to oliguria)

PROGNOSIS
Depends on underlying cause, child's age, degree of renal insufficiency, and need for dialysis or transplantation. There is a significantly increased risk of cardiovascular morbidity and mortality in young adults with CKD.

COMPLICATIONS
- Growth retardation is particularly severe when CKD develops in the 1st year of life. Growth failure may be secondary to poor nutrition, bone disease, acidosis, or a direct effect on the growth hormone-IGF-1 axis.
- Renal osteodystrophy may be seen early in association with CKD, taking the form of growth failure, bowing of the lower extremities, and slipped epiphysis. Vitamin D deficiency and secondary hyperparathyroidism are the major factors leading to bone disease.
- Anemia develops secondary to decreased erythropoietin secretion and decreased erythrocyte survival. The anemia is a normocytic variant associated with a low reticulocyte count.
- Cardiovascular disease including LVH, and coronary artery disease often develops in early adulthood. Uncontrolled hypertension, anemia, hyperlipidemia, and hyperparathyroidism all contribute to this leading cause of death in adults with CKD.
- Neurodevelopmental delay increases in children with CKD. This is probably due to uremic effects on the development of the brain.
- Hypertension may be seen in some patients with CKD, due either to hyperreninemia or hypervolemia.
- Platelet abnormalities, protein-calorie malnutrition, and immunologic disturbances are also seen in patients with uremia.

ADDITIONAL READING

- Friedman AL. Etiology, pathophysiology, diagnosis, and management of chronic renal failure in children. *Curr Opin Pediatr*. 1996;8:148–151.
- KDOQI Clinical Practice Guideline for Nutrition in Children with CKD: 2008 update. Executive summary. KDOQI Work Group. *Am J Kidney Dis*. 2009;53(3 Suppl 2):S11–S104
- Mahan JD, Patel HP. Recent advances in pediatric dialysis: A review of selected articles. *Pediatr Nephrol*. 2008;23(10):1737–1747.
- Schwartz GJ, Munoz A, Schneider MF, et al. New equations to estimate GFR in children with CKD. *J Am Soc Nephrol*. 2009;20:629–637.

 ## CODES

ICD9
- 585.1 Chronic kidney disease, Stage I
- 585.2 Chronic kidney disease, Stage II (mild)
- 585.9 Chronic kidney disease, unspecified

ICD10
- N18.1 Chronic kidney disease, stage 1
- N18.2 Chronic kidney disease, stage 2 (mild)
- N18.9 Chronic kidney disease, unspecified

FAQ

- Q: Which OTC medications should be avoided in children with CKD?
- A: NSAIDs, pseudoephedrine (if patient hypertensive), enemas containing phosphate, and antacids containing magnesium or aluminum should not be taken.
- Q: Can children with CKD receive immunizations?
- A: Children with CKD should especially receive all necessary immunizations, because some vaccines are contraindicated after transplantation. In some cases, booster immunizations are necessary because of an inadequate response to the initial series (e.g., hepatitis B virus, measles, mumps, rubella; varicella).
- Q: When is recombinant human erythropoietin indicated?
- A: Generally, this medication should be considered when the hematocrit level is <33% (hgb <11.0 g/gL).

CIRRHOSIS
Rose C. Graham

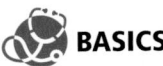

BASICS

DESCRIPTION
Cirrhosis is the end stage of progressive hepatic necrosis, fibrosis, and regenerative nodule formation that may occur as a result of many different liver diseases. It results in distortion of liver architecture and compression of hepatic vascular and biliary structures. In its advanced form, it is irreversible and often requires liver transplantation for survival of the patient.

EPIDEMIOLOGY
- On the basis of varying causes, no specific epidemiologic pattern can be identified.
- Cirrhosis due to chronic HCV infection is the most common indication for liver transplantation in adults.
- Biliary cirrhosis due to biliary atresia is the most common indication for liver transplantation in children.

Genetics
- Many distinct genetic disorders can cause cirrhosis, such as Wilson disease and hereditary hemochromatosis.
- Human leukocyte antigen (HLA) associations have been identified in several autoimmune disorders, including sclerosing cholangitis.

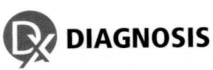

DIAGNOSIS

SIGNS AND SYMPTOMS
- Compensated (latent) cirrhosis: Asymptomatic, with no signs or symptoms of liver disease. Discovered incidentally either during routine physical examinations with an enlarged liver and/or palpable spleen, or as a result of an investigation for an unrelated condition.
- Decompensated (active) cirrhosis: As cirrhosis progresses, overt signs and symptoms may occur including failure to thrive, muscle weakness, fatigue, fever, jaundice, pruritus, edema, abdominal pain, ascites, steatorrhea, spontaneous bleeding (i.e., epistaxis) or bruising, and deterioration in school performance or depression. In addition, this stage may present with acute, precipitous liver failure or a life-threatening complication such as an esophageal variceal hemorrhage.

HISTORY
Based on the varying etiologic agents, one should elicit pertinent historical features characteristic of each specific problem, as detailed:
- Exposure to infectious hepatitis, antecedent viral illnesses
- Exposure to hepatotoxins
- Family or personal history of genetic, metabolic, or autoimmune diseases
- Neurologic problems, deteriorating school performance, depression (Wilson disease)

PHYSICAL EXAM
- General: Poor growth, malnutrition, fever, cachexia, obesity [Nonalcoholic steatohepatitis (NASH)]
- Skin: Jaundice, flushing, pallor, cyanosis, palmar erythema, spider angiomata, fine telangiectasia (face and upper back), easy bruising
- Abdomen: Ascites (distention, fluid wave, shifting dullness), caput medusa (prominent periumbilical veins), splenomegaly, rectal varices, hepatomegaly, or a shrunken liver
- Extremities: Digital clubbing, hypertrophic osteoarthropathy, muscle wasting, peripheral edema
- Endocrine: Gynecomastia, testicular atrophy, delayed puberty
- Central nervous system: Asterixis, positive Babinski sign, mental status changes, hyperreflexia, muscle wasting
- Eyes: Kayser–Fleischer rings (Wilson disease)

DIAGNOSTIC TESTS & INTERPRETATION
Lab
These tests focus on determining the etiology and the severity of liver disease prior to a liver biopsy.
- Tests of liver cell injury: Alanine aminotransferase (ALT), aspartate aminotransferase (AST), lactic dehydrogenase (LDH)
- Tests of synthetic function: Albumin and other serum proteins, prothrombin time (PT), partial thromboplastin time (PTT), international normalized ratio (INR), ammonia, plasma and urine amino acids, serum lipids and lipoproteins, cholesterol and triglycerides
- Tests of cholestasis: Fractionated bilirubin, alkaline phosphatase, γ-glutamyltransferase, cholesterol, serum and urine bile acids
- Tests of fibrosis: Serum markers may be useful to evaluate hepatic fibrosis noninvasively; however, these are still being investigated for clinical utility. Possible markers include procollagen III peptide, tissue inhibitor of metalloproteinase, type IV collagen, laminin, hyaluronic acid, and prolyl-hydroxylase.
- Miscellaneous disease-specific serum tests:
  - Viral serologies: Toxoplasma, rubella, cytomegalovirus, herpesvirus, hepatitis B, hepatitis C, Epstein–Barr virus, other viruses
  - Wilson disease: Serum ceruloplasmin, 24-hour urine copper, and slit-lamp exam for Kaiser–Fleischer rings
  - α_1-Antitrypsin deficiency: α_1-Antitrypsin serum level and protease inhibitor (Pi) phenotype
  - Autoimmune hepatitis: Sedimentation rate, autoantibodies (antinuclear, anti-smooth muscle, anti-liver kidney microsomal, anti-F-actin), serum immunoglobulins
  - Hemochromatosis: Serum iron, total iron binding capacity, ferritin
  - Metabolic/genetic: Fasting blood sugar, lactate, pyruvate, uric acid, sweat test, carnitine, creatine phosphokinase (CPK), porphyrins, serum amino acids, urine organic acids, urine reducing substances, urine succinylacetone, fatty acid degeneration products, α-fetoprotein

Imaging
- Ultrasound with Doppler images: Evaluates for anatomic variation or obstruction of the biliary tree, presence of ascites, portal hypertension, and vascular obstruction
- Hepatobiliary radioisotope scanning: Assess for biliary excretion in neonatal cholestasis.
- Cholangiography [magnetic resonance cholangiopancreatography (MRCP)]: Assess for intra- and extrahepatic biliary disease (stones, choledochal cyst, sclerosing cholangitis).
- Elastography by ultrasound or magnetic resonance imaging is a newer technique still being studied that may be useful in quantifying liver fibrosis noninvasively.

Diagnosis Procedures/Surgery
- Liver biopsy:
  - Percutaneous needle biopsy, intraoperative wedge biopsy, transjugular liver biopsy
  - Confirm the presence, type, and degree of activity of cirrhosis.
  - Various hepatic diseases that progress to cirrhosis have characteristic histologic findings. However, the process of cirrhosis may obscure the nature of the original insult, rendering morphologic and histologic classifications unhelpful.
- Cholangiography:
  - Intraoperative cholangiography: Assess for extrahepatic biliary atresia in neonates.
  - Endoscopic retrograde cholangiopancreatography (ERCP): Assess for extrahepatic biliary disease in older patients where MRCP is not helpful or therapeutic interventions possible (i.e., stent placement).

DIFFERENTIAL DIAGNOSIS
- Biliary:
  - Extrahepatic biliary atresia
  - Choledochal cyst
  - Tumors
  - Common bile duct and biliary lithiasis
  - Alagille syndrome
  - Biliary hypoplasia
  - Sclerosing cholangitis
  - Graft-versus-host disease
  - Vanishing bile duct syndrome due to drugs (e.g., trimethoprim–sulfamethoxazole)
  - Langerhans cell histiocytosis
- Hepatic:
  - Infectious hepatitis, including toxoplasma, rubella, cytomegalovirus, herpes virus (TORCH) infections, viral hepatitis B, C, D; Epstein–Barr virus, other viruses
  - Autoimmune hepatitis
  - NASH, associated with obesity
  - Drugs/toxins and alcohol

C

- Genetic/metabolic (examples for each category, not a complete list):
  – Cystic fibrosis
  – α_1-Antitrypsin deficiency
  – Congenital hepatic fibrosis
  – Progressive familial intrahepatic cholestasis (PFIC)
  – Wilson disease
  – Hereditary hemochromatosis
  – Carbohydrate defects: Galactosemia, hereditary fructose intolerance, glycogen storage III and IV
  – Amino acid defects: Tyrosinemia
  – Lipid storage diseases: Gaucher disease, Niemann–Pick type C
  – Mitochondrial disorders: Fatty acid oxidation defects, respiratory chain defects
  – Peroxisomal disorders: Zellweger syndrome
  – Porphyrias: Erythropoietic protoporphyria
- Vascular:
  – Budd–Chiari syndrome
  – Veno-occlusive disease
  – Congestive heart failure

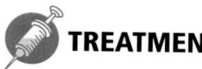 **TREATMENT**

MEDICATION (DRUGS)
First Line
- Fat-soluble vitamin supplementation: Vitamins A, D, E, and K
- Diuretic therapy (furosemide, spironolactone, chlorothiazide) for patients with ascites
- Albumin infusions for patients with refractory ascites
- Beta-blockers have been shown to decrease portal pressure and reduce the risk of variceal bleeding in adults with portal hypertension.
- Antibiotics, if suspicious for spontaneous bacterial peritonitis (avoid nephrotoxic agents)
- Lactulose, lactitol, and neomycin are used for patients with hepatic encephalopathy.

SURGERY/OTHER PROCEDURES
- Endoscopic variceal band ligation or sclerotherapy for variceal GI bleeding
- Paracentesis for refractory ascites or diagnosis of spontaneous bacterial peritonitis
- Portosystemic shunt placement [surgical or radiologic transjugular intrahepatic portosystemic shunting (TIPS) procedure] for complications of uncontrolled portal hypertension
- Liver transplantation

 ONGOING CARE

DIET
- Malnutrition is common in chronic liver diseases because of several metabolic derangements, fat malabsorption, anorexia, and increased energy requirements.
- Adequate caloric intake is critical and, often, will require supplemental nasogastric tube feedings.
- Some of the dietary fat should be provided as medium-chain triglycerides, which do not require bile for absorption.
- Fat-soluble vitamin levels should be monitored and supplemented, if necessary.
- Careful attention must also be paid to fluid and electrolyte balance; sodium restriction (<2 mEq/kg/d) may be necessary in the presence of ascites.

Activity
Spleen guard and avoidance of abdominal trauma if significant splenomegaly

PROGNOSIS
- The prognosis for cirrhosis leading to decompensation depends on the underlying cause.
- The underlying condition should be treated where possible (e.g., Wilson disease, autoimmune hepatitis)
- Poor prognostic features in children include prolonged INR unresponsive to vitamin K, ascites, malnutrition, low plasma cholesterol, elevated bilirubin level, and presence of hepatorenal syndrome.

COMPLICATIONS
- Malnutrition and growth failure
- Malabsorption (diarrhea, steatorrhea, fat-soluble vitamin deficiencies)
- Portal hypertension and variceal bleeding
- Chronic gastritis, peptic ulcer disease, gastroesophageal reflux
- Ascites
- Encephalopathy
- Hypersplenism (associated with anemia, thrombocytopenia, and neutropenia)
- Anemia
- Coagulopathy
- Hepatopulmonary syndrome (hypoxemia, cyanosis, dyspnea, digital clubbing)
- Hepatorenal syndrome (rapidly progressive renal failure in patients with cirrhosis)
- Bacterial infections, spontaneous bacterial peritonitis
- Hepatocellular carcinoma

ADDITIONAL READING
- Feldstein AE, Charatcharoenwitthaya P, Treeprasertsuk S, et al. The natural history of non-alcoholic fatty liver disease in children: A follow-up study for up to 20 years. *Gut.* 2009; 58:1538–1544.
- Kamath BM, Olthoff KM. Liver transplantation in children: Update 2010. *Pediatr Clin N Am.* 2010;57:401–414.
- Leonis MA, Balistreri WF. Evaluation and management of end-stage liver disease in children. *Gastroenterology.* 2008;134(6):1741–1751.
- Lewindon PJ, Shepherd RW, et al. Importance of hepatic fibrosis in cystic fibrosis and the predictive value of liver biopsy. *Hepatology.* 2011;53: 193–201.
- Mencin AA, Lavine JE. Nonalcoholic fatty liver disease in children. *Curr Opin Clin Nutr Metab Care.* 2011;14:151–157.
- Poupon R, Chazouilleres O, Poupon RE. Chronic cholestatic diseases. *J Hepatol.* 2000;32(1 suppl): 129.

 CODES

ICD9
- 571.5 Cirrhosis of liver without mention of alcohol
- 571.6 Biliary cirrhosis

ICD10
- K74.5 Biliary cirrhosis, unspecified
- K74.60 Unspecified cirrhosis of liver

FAQ
- Q: Will my child with cystic fibrosis develop cirrhosis?
- A: The medical literature cites a 5–10% incidence of cirrhosis in children with cystic fibrosis. Children with cystic fibrosis liver disease who develop cirrhosis are at risk for complications of portal hypertension.
- Q: Will every child with cirrhosis need a liver transplant?
- A: Most children who develop cirrhosis from causes such as biliary atresia or metabolic disease will ultimately require a liver transplant.

CLEFT LIP AND PALATE

Oksana A. Jackson
Jesse A. Taylor
Christine A. Carman (5th edition)
David W. Low (5th edition)

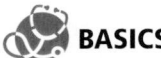 **BASICS**

DESCRIPTION
- Cleft lip:
  - Deformity of the upper lip that may include a discontinuity of vermilion, skin, muscle, and mucosa, as well as the underlying gingiva and bone
  - May be unilateral or bilateral
  - A complete cleft extends into the nose. An incomplete cleft has a bridge of intact tissue between the oral and nasal cavities.
- Cleft palate:
  - May involve the gingiva, hard palate, and/or soft palate
  - Represents a visible separation between the 2 halves of the roof of the mouth, involving mucosa, muscle, and often the bones of the hard palate
  - A submucous cleft palate has intact mucosa, but the underlying muscle and bone are at least partially divided.

EPIDEMIOLOGY
Incidence
- Incidence of cleft lip with or without cleft palate is 1 in 700 births
- Incidence of cleft lip with or without cleft palate increases with parental (especially paternal) age >30 years. Some association with low socioeconomic class may be nutrition related.

Prevalence
- Racial heterogeneity noted in cleft lip and cleft palate (Asians, 2.1 in 1,000 births; whites, 1 in 1,000; blacks, 0.41 in 1,000)
- Isolated cleft palate is present in 1 in 2,000 births across races.

Genetics
- 1/3 of patients with cleft lip and/or cleft palate have a positive family history; positive family history is noted twice as often in cleft lip with or without cleft palate as in cleft palate alone.
- Some recognized patterns of malformation that include cleft lip and/or cleft palate may be caused by exposure to teratogens, but there is little evidence linking isolated clefts to exposure to any single teratogenic agent.
  - A notable exception is phenytoin; use during pregnancy has been associated with a 10-fold increase in the incidence of cleft lip.
- Incidence of cleft lip in infants born to mothers who smoke during pregnancy is twice that in those born to nonsmoking mothers.

PATHOPHYSIOLOGY
- Muscle fibers are atrophic and disorganized in the region of the cleft.
- Mitochondrial abnormalities are noted at the cleft margins by histochemical and electromyographic studies.

ETIOLOGY
- Cleft lip may result from failure of the medial nasal and maxillary processes to join *in utero*, or possibly from lack of adequate mesenchymal reinforcement, leading to subsequent breakdown and separation.
- Cleft palate results from failure of the palatal shelves to fuse.
- Prenatal dietary supplementation with folic acid and vitamin B_6 has led to lower-than-expected incidence of cleft lip and cleft palate and to a decreased incidence of neural tube defects.
- Bilateral cleft lip is associated with cleft palate in 86% of cases. Unilateral cleft lip is associated with cleft palate in 68% of cases.
- Cleft lip/cleft palate is more common on the left, particularly in boys.

COMMONLY ASSOCIATED CONDITIONS
- Among patients with clefts of the secondary palate alone, syndromes associated with microdeletions of chromosome 22q11.2 are currently the most common syndromic diagnoses.
  - Collectively known as 22q11.2 deletion syndrome, includes velocardiofacial syndrome, DiGeorge syndrome, and conotruncal anomaly face syndrome
  - Inheritance is autosomal dominant with considerable variability in phenotypic expression, which may include facial dysmorphism, developmental delay, cardiovascular anomalies, immunologic abnormalities, cleft palate, and velopharyngeal dysfunction.
- Next most common syndrome associated with palatal clefts is Stickler syndrome:
  - Characterized by autosomal dominance, cleft palate, epicanthal folds, flat facies, joint hyperflexibility, severe myopia, retinal detachment, and glaucoma
  - Caused by a mutation of the gene for type 2 collagen (chromosome 12q)
- Most common syndrome associated with clefts of the lip and/or palate is Van der Woude (autosomal dominant, lower lip pits, 1q32)
- Other genetic syndromes associated with cleft lip and/or palate:
  - CHARGE syndrome (pattern of malformation with majority of patients having CHD7 mutation)
  - Smith–Lemli–Opitz (defect in cholesterol synthesis, 7q34) Pierre Robin Sequence is a condition usually associated with a wide U-shaped cleft palate.
  - Characterized by a small mandible, retropositioned tongue, and subsequent upper airway obstruction
  - May occur in infants with or without genetic syndromes (Stickler most common)
  - Most clefts are nonsyndromic and may be either multifactorial in origin or the result of changes at a major single-gene locus

DIAGNOSIS

HISTORY
- Prenatal exposure to alcohol, cigarettes, phenytoin, and isotretinoin
- Family history of cleft lip or cleft palate
- Speech problems in first-degree relative

PHYSICAL EXAM
- Incomplete or complete cleft of lip, alveolus, hard and soft palate, or uvula. Soft palate and uvula clefts are always midline, whereas lip, alveolar, and hard palatal clefts can be unilateral or bilateral.
- A bifid uvula or a notch in the bone at the posterior hard palate may indicate a submucous cleft.
- A small mandible and retropositioned tongue may indicate a risk for airway obstruction (Pierre Robin sequence).
- Look for associated anomalies of the face, heart, and extremities that may indicate a clefting syndrome.
- Tricks:
  - Examine the palate from the top of the patient, with the head in your lap, using a tongue depressor and flashlight.
  - Palpate the posterior hard palate for a possible notch in the bone.
  - Palpate the gums and maxilla for a possible notch in the floor of the nose.

DIAGNOSTIC TESTS & INTERPRETATION
- Complete ophthalmologic examination to check for myopia, glaucoma, and retinal detachment
- Pulse oximetry to check for desaturation while feeding or while supine
- Polysomnography to distinguish central from obstructive apnea
- Hearing evaluation
- Increased serum 7-dehydrocholesterol and decreased serum cholesterol to rule out Smith–Lemli–Opitz syndrome
- Karyotype to rule out specific genetic abnormalities
- Fluorescence *in situ* hybridization to rule out a chromosome 22q11.2 deletion
- Echocardiography, renal ultrasound, and endocrine laboratory studies if indicated

Imaging
Prenatal diagnosis of cleft lip is reliable by ultrasound; prenatal diagnosis of cleft palate remains unreliable by ultrasound. 3D ultrasound has improved the reliability of prenatal diagnosis. Fetal MRI provides excellent soft tissue definition and can be used when the diagnosis is uncertain on ultrasound or to better delineate the severity of the cleft. After birth, no additional radiologic imaging is indicated in patients with isolated cleft lip and/or palate.

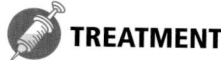

TREATMENT

ADDITIONAL TREATMENT
General Measures
Airway management
- Prone positioning if the tongue is causing airway obstruction
- Plastic surgery and ENT consultation if airway obstruction persists

ORTHODONTICS
Preoperative orthodontics may include: Obturators to facilitate feeding and speech, nasoalveolar molding and palatal reposition before lip and palate repair, palatal expansion prior to bone grafting, conventional orthodontics, including braces, maxillary appliances, prosthetic teeth, bridgework, maxillary and/or mandibular distraction to advance the mid- or lower face

SURGERY/OTHER PROCEDURES
- Significant airway obstruction and desaturation in the neonatal period refractory to prone positioning may indicate the need for a tongue-lip adhesion, release of the floor of the mouth musculature, mandibular distraction, or tracheostomy.
- Wide clefts of the lip may benefit from preliminary lip adhesion at 2–3 months of age. Timing of definitive lip repair varies from 2 to 6 months of age.
- Palate repair is generally done at <1 year of age to decrease speech and language difficulties.
- Otitis media is more common with cleft palate, and bilateral myringotomy tubes can be inserted at the time of cleft repair.
- Correction of secondary deformities may include:
  – Lip scar revision
  – Cleft nasal deformity correction (infancy to adulthood)
  – Alveolar bone grafts (usually when permanent canines are erupting)
  – Pharyngoplasty for soft palate–velopharyngeal incompetence
  – Closure of palatal fistulas
  – Orthognathic surgery for severe jaw deformities

Admission Criteria
Airway obstruction or severe feeding difficulties in the neonate

Discharge Criteria
- Stable airway
- Tolerating feedings

ONGOING CARE

FOLLOW-UP RECOMMENDATIONS
Multidisciplinary team:
- Pediatrician
- Plastic surgeon
- Speech pathologist
- Orthodontist
- Pediatric dentist
- Psychologist
- Social worker
- Nurse practitioner
- Anthropologist (facial growth specialist)
- Geneticist
- Support groups

DIET
Cleft patients may have significant feeding problems because of an inability to generate negative intraoral pressure necessary to feed efficiently.
- Premie nipples with enlarged or cross-cut openings, or soft plastic squeezable bottles, can facilitate milk flow.
- Poor weight gain may necessitate nasogastric tube feedings.

PROGNOSIS
Good. Most patients undergo normal growth and development. Long-term follow-up by a multidisciplinary team and parental support are critical to optimization of outcomes.

COMPLICATIONS
- Airway obstruction and feeding disorders, particularly with Pierre Robin sequence
- Chronic otitis media
- Speech problems, including hypernasality and articulation errors
- Associated malformations:
  – ~1/3 of patients with cleft palate has associated anomalies, with isolated cleft palates having the highest. CNS, cardiac, urinary tract malformations, and clubfoot are commonly associated with clefting.
- Potential problems:
  – Hypernasal resonance and nasal air emission during speech may indicate velopharyngeal incompetence or palatal fistula. Up to 30% of patients may require additional palatal or pharyngeal surgery following initial palate repair.
  – Multiple ear infections may require prolonged use of myringotomy tubes to prevent hearing impairment. Audiograms should be obtained regularly.
  – Delays in speech and language development may require detailed evaluation, early intervention programs, and speech therapy.
  – Poor dentition, occlusal problems (crossbite), gingivitis, and crowding
  – Behavior disorders and psychosocial adjustment disorders
  – ~25% of affected individuals will manifest maxillary hypoplasia that requires jaw surgery to correct occlusal abnormalities.

ALERT
- Failure to diagnose airway obstruction in infants with Pierre Robin sequence may lead to failure to thrive or, in severe cases, death.
- Failure to diagnose associated anomalies may lead to missed syndromes and inaccurate genetic counseling.
- A submucous cleft palate can be easily missed until hypernasal speech is noted later in life.

ADDITIONAL READING
- Heinrich A. Prenatal diagnosis of cleft deformities and its significance for parent and infant care. *J Craniofac Surg*. 2006;34(supp 2):14–16.
- Mulliken JB, Wu JK, Padwa BL. Repair of bilateral cleft lip: Review, revisions, and reflections. *J Craniofac Surg*. 2003;14:609–620.

- Murray JC. Gene/environment causes of cleft lip and/or palate. *Clin Genet*. 2002;61:248–256.
- Nasser M, Fedorowicz Z, Newton JT, et al. Interventions for the management of submucous cleft palate. *Cochrane Database Syst Rev*. 2008;23;(1):CD006703.
- Redford-Badwal DA, Mabry K, Frassinelli JD. Impact of cleft lip and/or palate on nutritional health and oral-motor development. *Dent Clin North Am*. 2003;47:305–317.
- Strong EB, Buckmiller LM. Management of the cleft palate. *Facial Plast Surg Clin North Am*. 2001;9:15–25, vii.

CODES

ICD9
- 749.11 Cleft lip, unilateral, complete
- 749.12 Cleft lip, unilateral, incomplete
- 749.13 Cleft lip, bilateral, complete

ICD10
- Q36.0 Cleft lip, bilateral
- Q36.1 Cleft lip, median
- Q36.9 Cleft lip, unilateral

FAQ

- Q: will there be a scar
- A: All cleft lip repairs will leave some type of permanent scar, with potential asymmetry that may benefit from later additional lip scar revision.
- Q: What is the goal of surgery
- A: Goal is to create a lip that does not attract undue attention.
- Q: What is the most difficult part of surgery
- A: The nose is often the most difficult to correct, because of asymmetry in cartilage and skin contour.
- Q: Will my child be able to speak clearly?
- A: Most children will achieve velopharyngeal competence and normal speech, but may require additional speech therapy to achieve this goal.
- Q: Is cleft palate inherited?
- A: For nonsyndromic cleft lip with or without cleft palate:
- Risk of having a second child with a cleft, if neither parent has a cleft: 4%
  – Child's risk of later having a child with a cleft: 4%
  – Risk of having a third child with a cleft, if parents have 2 affected children but neither parent is affected: 9%
  – Risk of having a second child with a cleft, if 1 parent also has a cleft: 17%
- For nonsyndromic isolated cleft palate:
  – Risk of having a second child with a cleft, if neither parent has a cleft: 2%
  – Child's risk of later having a child with a cleft: 3%
  – Risk of having a third child with a cleft, if parents have 2 affected children but neither parent is affected: 1%
  – Risk of having a second child with a cleft, if 1 parent also has a cleft: 15%

C

CLUBFOOT

Richard S. Davidson

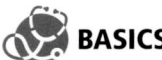 **BASICS**

DESCRIPTION
Clubfoot is a congenital or neuromuscular deformity in which the hindfoot is fixed in equinus and varus and the forefoot is fixed in varus, equinus, and often cavus.

EPIDEMIOLOGY
- The risk of deformity increases by 20–30 times when there is an affected 1st-degree relative.
- Male > female (2:1)

Incidence
Incidence is 1–1.4/1,000 live births, but can vary among different ethnic groups.

PATHOPHYSIOLOGY
- Many anatomic abnormalities have been postulated as causing clubfoot:
  - Anomalous or deficient muscles, myoblasts, mast cells, abnormal primary bone formation, joint and muscle contractures, vascular anomalies (absent dorsalis pedis artery), nerve anomalies
  - Abnormalities of the fibrous connective tissue
- Interruption of the development of the embryonic foot has also been suggested.

ETIOLOGY
- Most cases are idiopathic (multifactorial inheritance pattern with significant environmental influence).
- Infrequently, neuromuscular imbalance may underlie the deformity (cerebral palsy, myelomeningocele, lipomas of the cord, caudal or sacral agenesis, polio, arthrogryposis, fetal alcohol syndrome).
- Rapid recurrence should prompt a thorough examination for possible underlying etiologies.

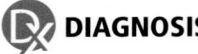 **DIAGNOSIS**

HISTORY
- Family history of clubfoot (3%)
- Onset of deformity (congenital or developmental)

PHYSICAL EXAM
- Careful examination of:
  - The neuromuscular system for neuromuscular etiologies such as lumbosacral sinuses, dimples, and lipomas as well as spasticity, asymmetry, and muscle imbalance
  - The hips for hip dysplasia
  - The neck for torticollis
- Physical exam trick:
  - Push the foot into a corrected position. Is the deformity fully correctable? Overcorrectable?

DIAGNOSTIC TESTS & INTERPRETATION
Lab
- The diagnosis is clinical.
- Radiographs (after 3 months of age) may confirm bone position but cannot make the diagnosis.
- At 3–6 months of age, anteroposterior (AP) and lateral radiograph films in dorsiflexion (maximal correction) may help in defining residual deformity. The beam should be focused on the hindfoot for both the anteroposterior and lateral radiographs, as the measured angles will be hindfoot angles.
- Decreased talocalcaneal angle on the anteroposterior and lateral views ($\leq25°$) confirm persistent deformity.
- Medial displacement of the cuboid on the calcaneus and persistent plantar flexion of the forefoot on the hindfoot (talar to 1st metatarsal angle) indicate more complex deformities.

DIFFERENTIAL DIAGNOSIS
Distinguish other deformities of the foot:
- Metatarsus adductus or varus (heel is in neutral position, no fixed equinus)
- Calcaneovalgus (foot is in valgus, no fixed heel equinus)
- Vertical talus (foot is in valgus, heel in equinovalgus)
- Many children with clubfoot also have tibial torsion, which is a normal variant in our society that rarely requires treatment.

 TREATMENT

ADDITIONAL TREATMENT
General Measures
- Ponseti method and its variations have become the standard of initial treatment.
- Initial treatment:
  - Care can begin in the 1st week after birth though later treatment is generally successful as well.
- Initial treatment is serial (weekly) manipulation and casting with long leg casts 1st correcting abduction, then rotation, then dorsiflexion. The talar head is stabilized with the casting physician's thumb while the contralateral hand manipulates the foot.
- Taping may be useful for treatment of the infant requiring ICU care; access to the feet should be maintained for blood tests.
- Failure to correct the deformity completely by manipulation within 8–12 weeks of casting should lead to surgical intervention.
- Long leg serial casting by the Ponseti technique improves results so that in most clubfeet little more than heel cord lengthening and possibly posterior ankle release is required. The operated foot is stabilized for healing for 1 month in a Ponseti-type cast.
- Following surgery, bracing with bars and shoes for 3 months full time and then 3 years nights and naps is an integral part of the Ponseti method.
- With the Ponseti method, 30–45% of patients my have various forms of recurrence requiring repeated casting and/or surgical release through maturity.

ONGOING CARE

FOLLOW-UP RECOMMENDATIONS

Patient Monitoring

- Realignment of the deformity is the goal and should be achieved with casting and surgery.
- Most surgeons cast the feet for 1 month postoperatively.
- With the Ponseti method, bars and shoes are recommended full time for 3 months and nights for 3 years to maintain the correction.
- Remember, the cause of the deformity is not corrected. Only the alignment of the bones and lengthening of the soft tissues are corrected.
- Depending on the severity of the deformity, all corrected clubfeet can be expected to demonstrate varying amounts of calf narrowing and weakness, ankle and subtalar stiffness, a difference between the feet of 1–2 shoe sizes, and even a leg-length discrepancy, usually <2 cm.
- There also will be decreased ankle and subtalar motion as compared to normal.
- Adolescent children with clubfeet often will get leg cramps and will tire easily while doing sports.
  - Recurrence of heel cord tightness is common, especially during periods of rapid growth. Additional heel cord stretching and casting and, infrequently, additional surgery may be needed.
- All true recurrences should lead to further evaluation for neuromuscular or syndromic causes that might have been missed in the infant.

ADDITIONAL READING

- Hamel J, Becker W. Sonographic assessment of clubfoot deformity in young children. *J Pediatr Orthop B*. 1996;5:279–286.
- Roye BD, Hyman J, Roye DP Jr. Congenital idiopathic talipes equinovarus. *Pediatr Rev*. 2004;25:124–130.
- Scher DM. The Ponseti method for treatment of congenital club foot. *Curr Opin Pediatr*. 2006;18(1):22–25.
- Scherl SA. Common lower extremity problems in children. *Pediatr Rev*. 2004;25:52–62.
- Yamamoto H, Muneta T, Morita S. Nonsurgical treatment of congenital clubfoot with manipulation, cast, and modified Denis Browne splint. *J Pediatr Orthop*. 1998;18:538–542.

CODES

ICD9

- 754.51 Talipes equinovarus
- 754.62 Talipes calcaneovalgus
- 754.70 Talipes, unspecified (Congenital deformity of foot not otherwise specified)

ICD10

- Q66.0 Congenital talipes equinovarus
- Q66.1 Congenital talipes calcaneovarus
- Q66.8 Other congenital deformities of feet

FAQ

- Q: How can a rigid clubfoot be distinguished from a positional clubfoot?
- A: During initial evaluation of the child, it is important to assess the amount of flexibility in a clubfoot. This can be most easily done by flexing the hip to 90°, flexing the knee to 90°, and then gently trying to turn the forefoot into a straight position lined up with the thigh. If the foot easily spins around into a normal position, it can be assumed that this is a flexible or positional clubfoot. If deformity persists, this is a rigid deformity. If possible, the examining physician should palpate the heel to see if the os calcis comes out of its equinus position filling the heel pad. In some children, particularly with a rocker bottom sole, the heel pad looks as if it is in the correct position, but the os calcis remains in equinus with the posterior aspect of the os calcis proximal to the heel pad.
- Q: What percentage of clubfeet is successfully treated by casting?
- A: To some extent, the amount of success depends on how much correction is desired. Occasionally, cast correction will provide a partial correction. Some feet, after casting, can be held in the corrected position, only to spin back to the clubfoot deformity when released. Positional clubfeet are likely to improve with casting in perhaps 98% of cases. Rigid clubfeet are much less likely to be corrected by casting. The success rate with casting alone in the rigid feet is likely to be ~10%. It is important to remember that casting and surgery cannot make the clubfoot normal.

- Q: What will be the permanent disability of a congenital clubfoot deformity?
- A: Although casting and surgical correction of a congenital clubfoot can realign the bones, the surgery does little to correct the underlying neuromuscular problems. As a result, all children with rigid clubfeet are likely to have a leg-length inequality (usually <1.5 inches), a smaller foot (usually 1–2 sizes), calf narrowing that cannot be significantly improved with exercise, and joint stiffness (ankle, subtalar, and midfoot). Even children with optimal realignment of the deformity will notice their inability to perform gymnastic activities or running activities requiring normal range of motion of the ankle and foot. Many will complain of the inability to keep up with their peer group during adolescent and young adult sports activities.
- Q: How soon should an infant with congenital clubfoot be referred to an orthopedic surgeon?
- A: Casting begins within the 1st to 2nd week of life. Clearly, medical and life-threatening conditions will take precedence over the treatment of the clubfoot. Access to the feet for IV or blood studies will interfere with a casting regimen. Casting should begin as soon as is practical. It may even be possible to begin taping of the foot as an alternative to casting, which will still allow IV access to the feet. Referral to an orthopedic surgeon should, therefore, follow as soon as is practical. Studies have shown that excellent results can be obtained from the Ponseti method even when initiated after the 1st year of life.

C

COARCTATION OF AORTA

Luz Natal-Hernandez
Geoffrey L. Bird (5th edition)

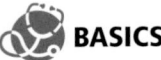

BASICS

DESCRIPTION
- Discrete stenosis of the upper thoracic aorta, usually just opposite the site of insertion of the ductus arteriosus (juxtaductal). A segment of tubular hypoplasia and/or a remnant of ductal tissue gives rise to a prominent posterior infolding ("the posterior shelf").
- The hemodynamic lesion is most often discrete, but may be long segment or tortuous in nature. It is usually juxtaductal but may occur in other sites (i.e., the abdominal aorta). The prevalence of other associations (bicuspid aortic valve) and long-term complications (hypertension) indicate the possibility that this lesion is part of a broader spectrum arteriopathy and/or endothelial disorder.

EPIDEMIOLOGY
Prevalence
- ~6–8% of patients with congenital heart disease have coarctation.
- Male > Female (1.5–4.0:1)

RISK FACTORS
Genetics
- Multifactorial: Occurs in 35% of patients with Turner syndrome (XO)
- Has been described in cases of monozygotic twins
- Many studies document the prevalence of a microdeletion at 22q11 in patients with arch anomalies and ventricular septal defects.

PATHOPHYSIOLOGY
- Decreased systemic blood flow to lower extremities after ductal closure
- Increased resistance to left ventricular (LV) outflow causes LV hypertrophy. Relative underperfusion of the renal vessels, baroreceptors, and multiple other mechanisms combine to induce a compensatory systolic hypertension.
- If the coarctation is severe, LV dysfunction and CHF result, with low cardiac output and increased LV end diastolic pressure.
- Decreased myocardial perfusion may be present in cases of very low output.

DIAGNOSIS

HISTORY
There are 2 typical patterns for the clinical presentation of coarctation:
- An infant with CHF or shock—a small, pale, irritable child in respiratory distress. Typically precipitated by ductal closure, this presentation is more common in infants with coarctation and other intracardiac malformations (20–30%):
  - Poor feeding
  - Dyspnea
  - Diaphoresis
  - Poor weight gain
  - Oliguria
- An otherwise asymptomatic child or adolescent with systolic hypertension and/or a heart murmur (70–80%):
  - Lower-extremity claudication
  - Headaches

PHYSICAL EXAM
- Tachypnea and tachycardia
- Discrepant arterial pulses and systolic blood pressure in the upper and lower extremities
- Weak, "thready" pulses
- Grades 2–3/6 systolic ejection murmur
- Gallop rhythm in an infant with CHF
- Ejection click of a bicuspid aortic valve
- The most important finding is decreased or absent lower extremity pulses. Are pulses present? Is there a delay between the brachial and femoral pulses?
- Heart murmur: Best heard at the upper left sternal border, at the base and radiating to the left interscapular area posteriorly
- An infant with severe coarctation and a patent ductus arteriosus (PDA) may have "differential cyanosis." The lower part of the body appears cyanotic because the descending aortic flow is provided by the right ventricle (RV) through the PDA (check postductal saturation).

ALERT
- The most reliable clinical findings to diagnose native, residual, or recurrent coarctation are the presence of pressure differences in the upper and lower extremities and decreased or absent femoral pulses. Palpable pulses do not exclude coarctation. What one palpates is pulse pressure, not absolute systolic pressure.
- 4-extremity BP measurement is very important in assessing infants and children with possible congenital heart disease. Proper cuff size must be used.
- Bowel ischemia can be present in the ill patient, and emesis or poor feeding are hallmark signs.

DIAGNOSTIC TESTS & INTERPRETATION
Lab
- EKG: RV hypertrophy is usually present in symptomatic infants. EKG is often normal in children. LV hypertrophy is apparent with more severe coarctation or coarctation of longer standing, particularly in older children.
- Blood tests: In the patient presenting in extremis, management, initial therapy, and timing of surgery can be aided or guided by arterial blood gas analyses and markers of end organ dysfunction.

Imaging
- Chest x-ray: In the infant, moderate to severe cardiomegaly with increased pulmonary vascular markings (PVMs). In an asymptomatic child, the heart size is often normal, with normal PVMs. Rib notching may be seen in older children secondary to dilated intercostal collateral vessels.
- Echocardiography: Localization, degree of coarctation, and associated findings (PDA, arch hypoplasia, ventricular septal defect). Assessment of associated left-sided obstruction: Mitral valve abnormality, LV outflow obstruction, and aortic stenosis (bicuspid aortic valve)
- MRI: Clearly defines the location and severity of coarctation. Useful for serial follow-up postoperatively (especially aortic aneurysms)

Diagnostic Procedures/Other
Cardiac catheterization and angiography: Usually not indicated unless there are further questions to be answered and/or a planned intervention

DIFFERENTIAL DIAGNOSIS
- Other left-sided heart obstructive lesions
- Hypoplastic left heart syndrome
- Cardiomyopathy and/or myocarditis
- Critical aortic stenosis (aortic obstruction to a degree that adequate systemic perfusion depends upon patency of the ductus arteriosus)
- Shock from sepsis, metabolic disease, or other entities

TREATMENT

ADDITIONAL TREATMENT
General Measures
- For the sick neonate who presents with severe congestive heart failure or shock (possible ductal-dependent obstruction to systemic blood flow):
  - Prostaglandin infusion: 0.1 mcg/kg/min (anticipating adverse effects including apnea)
  - Inotropic support: 3–5 mcg/kg/min dopamine
  - Diuretics for pulmonary venous hypertension or pulmonary edema
  - Surgical intervention should follow as soon as possible.

- For the asymptomatic child, elective repair and assessment of hypertension are appropriate; however, aggressive antihypertensive pharmacotherapy is not indicated prior to surgical intervention.
- Other:
  - Interventional cardiology:
    - Percutaneous balloon angioplasty of native coarctation in infants and children is pursued in some centers. Others have concern about rates of recurrent stenosis, hypertension, aneurysm formation, and iliofemoral arterial injury.
    - Use of vascular stents to relieve the area of stenosis, particularly in older children and adolescents, have provided an alternative to surgical intervention. May increase the need for reintervention in the future when compared to the surgical approach.

SURGERY/OTHER PROCEDURES

- Infancy:
  - Surgical repair of severe coarctation and coarctation associated with intracardiac anomalies
  - The surgical mortality rate for infants with coarctation and a large ventricular septal defect ranges from 5–15% and is higher for children with more complex intracardiac anomalies.
- Childhood:
  - Elective coarctation repair between ages 18 months and 3 years in asymptomatic children without severe upper extremity hypertension. Later repair is associated with an increased risk of sustained hypertension and other late complications.
- Types of surgical repair: End-to-end anastomosis, subclavian flap aortoplasty, prosthetic patch aortoplasty, bypass graft

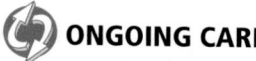 **ONGOING CARE**

FOLLOW-UP RECOMMENDATIONS
Patient Monitoring

- Re-examine every 12 months with 4-extremity pulse and BP assessment.
- Residual or recurrent coarctation occurs most commonly in those patients requiring repair in early infancy and can depend on the method of intervention (e.g., higher incidence with patch aortoplasty and coarctation ridge resection); some centers delay percutaneous balloon angioplasty of residual or recurrent lesions until 2 months postoperatively.
- Persistent systemic hypertension: Most common in patients whose coarctation repair is delayed beyond late childhood
- Aortic aneurysm formation
- Intracranial aneurysms and/or cerebrovascular accidents
- Antibiotic prophylaxis to prevent endocarditis or endarteritis
- May have hypertension with exercise, even if normotensive at rest
- Exercise-induced hypertension without anatomic stenosis may respond to beta-blocker therapy.

PROGNOSIS

- Untreated coarctation has a poor natural history with the onset of CHF, especially in those patients with other intracardiac malformations. Claudication is common in older children with previously undiscovered coarctation. Generally, the short-term prognosis following successful intervention for isolated coarctation in infancy or childhood is excellent. Procedure-related mortality in every modern series is very near zero.
- Clinical conditions that may affect long-term prognosis after repair of coarctation include:
  - Residual or recurrent coarctation
  - Hypertension (rest and exercise)
  - Aortic aneurysm (associated with repair technique)
  - Associated intracardiac lesions
  - Intracranial aneurysms
  - Occurrence or progression of aortic valve disease
  - Premature coronary arterial and cerebrovascular disease
- Associated lesions:
  - Bicuspid aortic valve occurs in 85% of patients with coarctation.
  - PDA
  - Ventricular septal defect
  - Valvar or subvalvar aortic stenosis
  - Mitral stenosis: Often associated with structural mitral valve abnormalities (i.e., supravalvar mitral ring, thickening of mitral leaflet, single papillary muscle with parachute deformity, or short dysplastic chordae tendinea)
  - Shone syndrome: Multiple left-sided obstructive lesions, including supravalvular mitral ring, parachute mitral valve, subaortic obstruction, and coarctation
  - Berry aneurysm of the circle of Willis
  - Renal artery stenosis associated with abdominal coarctation
  - Congenital diaphragmatic hernia

COMPLICATIONS

- Shock, if severe untreated obstruction
- CHF, if severe untreated obstruction
- Systemic hypertension, before and after intervention
- Intracranial aneurysms
- Mesenteric ischemia
- Paraplegia
- Postoperative complications:
  - Bleeding
  - Postcoarctectomy syndrome/mesenteric ischemia
  - Paradoxical hypertension
  - Spinal cord ischemia (0.4%)
  - Residual coarctation
  - Chylothorax
  - Stridor
  - Diaphragm paralysis
  - Aortic aneurysm or dissection
  - Paralysis

ADDITIONAL READING

- Carr JA. The results of catheter based therapy compared with surgical repair of adult aortic coarctation. *J Am Coll Cardiol.* 2006;47(6): 1101–1107.
- Celermajer DS, Greaves K. Survivors of coarctation repair: Fixed but not cured. *Heart.* 2002;88(2): 113–114.
- Cowley CG, Orsmond GS, Feola P, et al. Long-term randomized comparison of balloon angioplasty and surgery for native coarctation of the aorta in childhood. *Circulation.* 2005;111(25):3453–3456.
- Kanter KR. Management of infants with coarctation and ventricular septal defect. *Semin Thorac Cardiovasc Surg.* 2007;19(3):263–268.
- Shah L, Hijazi Z, Sandhu S, et al. Use of Endovascular Stents for the Treatment of Coarctation of the Aorta in Children and Adults: Immediate and Midterm Results. *J Invasive Cardiol.* 2005;17(11):614–618.
- Toro-Salazar OH, Steinberger J, Thomas W, et al. Long-term follow-up of patients after coarctation of the aorta repair. *Am J Cardiol.* 2002;89(5):541–547.

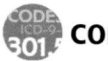 **CODES**

ICD9
747.10 Coarctation of aorta (preductal) (postductal)

ICD10
Q25.1 Coarctation of aorta

FAQ

- Q: When is the most appropriate time to perform surgical repair of simple coarctation?
- A: Recommendations vary regarding the age at which asymptomatic children (without severe upper-extremity hypertension) should undergo intervention. Advances in technique no longer require patients to be "grown" to a threshold size or weight, and there is increasing evidence that severity and incidence of late complications correlate directly with older age at repair. While some authors mention 3–5 years of age, others recommend repair as early as 18 months to 2 years of age.
- Q: What is the incidence of systemic hypertension after surgical repair of coarctation?
- A: Greatly depends on age at repair, surgical method or technique, length of follow-up interval, and how one defines or measures hypertension. In no situation is the answer zero, and this important complication is one of several reasons patients require life-long detailed follow-up. 1 year after a technically perfect repair via resection with end-to-end anastomosis, the patient operated on in early childhood is unlikely to have hypertension at rest. However, 20 years further along, a patient of older age at repair is quite likely to have significant hypertension on exercise stress testing.

COCCIDIOIDOMYCOSIS

Leonel Toledo
Theoklis Zaoutis (5th edition)
Samir S. Shah (5th edition)

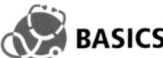 **BASICS**

DESCRIPTION
Coccidioidomycosis is an infection caused by the dimorphic fungi *Coccidioides immitis* and *Coccidioides posadasii*.

EPIDEMIOLOGY
- Primary infection is most commonly seen in the summer and fall months.
- The average incubation period is 10–16 days (range 1–4 weeks).
- There is no person-to-person spread.
- 60% of acute infections are subclinical (asymptomatic).
- Clusters of cases can involve dust storms, earthquakes, and occupational or recreational exposure.
- Congenital infection is rare.

Prevalence
C. immitis is found in the soil and is endemic in the southwestern US (western Texas, New Mexico, Arizona, California), northern Mexico, and parts of South and Central America. Up to 1/3 of the population in endemic areas has been infected.

RISK FACTORS
- Risk factors for disseminated coccidioidomycosis include immunosuppression, male gender, extremes of age (neonates and elderly), African or Filipino descent, and pregnancy.
- The course of illness is highly variable and dependent on host immune response and amount of exposure. HIV-infected patients and other patients with immunosuppression owing to T-lymphocyte dysfunction (lymphoma, organ transplantation, high-dose corticosteroids, receipt of immunomodulators) are particularly susceptible to severe forms of pulmonary and extrapulmonary coccidioidomycosis.

GENERAL PREVENTION
Infection control:
- No special isolation or precautions for the hospitalized patient
- Contaminated dressings from skin lesions should be handled and discarded with care.
- Inhalation of aerosolized spores from culture can be hazardous to laboratory personnel.
- Preventive efforts are aimed at dust control and trials to eliminate organisms from soil.
- Immunocompromised people should be counseled to avoid activities that may expose them to aerosolized spores in endemic areas.

PATHOPHYSIOLOGY
- In soil *Coccidioides* organisms exist in the hyphal phase. The hyphae produce spores called arthroconidia. Inhalation of arthroconidia from disturbed, arid soil is the major route of infection. In tissues arthroconidia enlarge to form spherules. Mature spherules release endospores that develop into new spherules and continue the tissue cycle.
- Most patients have infection limited to a localized area of lung and hilar nodes after mounting an intense inflammatory response with granuloma formation.
- Primary cutaneous coccidioidomycosis rarely occurs by direct inoculation of the skin (trauma). A relatively painless, indurated nodule with occasional central ulceration develops at the site of injury. Regional lymphadenopathy is often present.
- Extrapulmonary dissemination occurs via lymphatic or hematologic spread and usually involves the skin, bones and joints, and central nervous system, but can spread to virtually any organ system.

ETIOLOGY
- Osteomyelitis is subacute or chronic and frequently involves more than 1 bone (40%). Common sites are the hands, feet, ribs, and vertebrae.
- Meningitis develops within 6 months of initial infection. Hydrocephalus is a common complication. CNS vasculitis and intracerebral abscesses are rare.

DIAGNOSIS

HISTORY
- Travel or residence in an endemic area is typical. Risk factors for disseminated infection should be sought.
- Acute pneumonia:
  - Fever, dry or productive cough, and pleuritic chest pain
  - Systemic symptoms include headache, malaise, arthralgias, sore throat, and fatigue.
  - Also known as "valley fever"
- Hemoptysis, although rare in children, is reported in 15% of adults with symptomatic pulmonary infection.
- Trauma precedes primary cutaneous disease.
- Myalgias, arthralgias, chills, night sweats, and anorexia suggest systemic dissemination.
- Headache, vomiting, and altered mental status suggest meningitis.
- Most infections (60%) are asymptomatic.

PHYSICAL EXAM
- Signs of pneumonia and pleural effusions are often present with symptomatic pulmonary infection. Indurated nodules and regional lymphadenopathy are seen with primary cutaneous infection.
- Reactive rashes:
  - Contain no live organisms
  - Erythematous maculopapular rash is seen in 50% of symptomatic children.
  - Erythema nodosum and erythema multiforme occur later in the course of infection.
  - Erythema nodosum correlates with the development of cell-mediated immunity and is associated with a low incidence of dissemination.

- Hematogenous dissemination to the skin:
  - Lesions may consist of papules, nodules, abscesses, pustules, sinus tracts, and verrucous ulcers.
  - May be single or multiple
  - Can occur anywhere, but are most common on the nasolabial fold
- Chorioretinal lesions are present in ≤40% of patients with disseminated disease.
- Stridor is present with infection of the subglottic tissues.
- Signs of increased intracranial pressure are seen with central nervous system infection. Classic signs of meningeal irritation are usually absent.

ALERT
- Clinicians in endemic areas should maintain a high level of clinical suspicion.
- Diagnosis in nonendemic areas may be missed owing to low clinical suspicion or missed travel history.
- False-negative serologic results may occur during the initial weeks of infection or in an immunocompromised host.

DIAGNOSTIC TESTS & INTERPRETATION
Lab
- Direct examination and culture:
  - Cytologic examination of bronchoalveolar fluid is diagnostic in only about 1/3 of persons and is less sensitive than culture. Visualization of large spherules is possible in stained specimens of sputum, tracheal aspirates, urine, or tissue biopsy. They are rarely seen in CSF.
  - The organisms can be detected by culture in experienced laboratories. The yield is highest from purulent material. The yield from other sources, such as pleural fluid, blood, and gastric aspirates, is lower.
  - A DNA probe can identify *Coccidioides* species in cultures.
- Coccidioidin or spherulin skin intradermal testing has been used as an epidemiologic tool in the past but is no longer commercially available.
- Serologic studies:
  - *C. immitis*–specific IgM antibody is detectable in 75% of patients 1–3 weeks after symptom onset and usually is absent after 6 months. False-positive results are seen in 15% of patients with cystic fibrosis.
  - IgG is detected by the complement fixation (CF) assay from serum or CSF. It is positive in 50% of patients at 4 weeks and 83% at 3 months following symptomatic primary infection. In general, higher titers reflect more extensive infection and rising complement fixation antibody concentrations are associated with worsening disease.

– Enzyme immunoassay (EIA) for qualitative detection of IgM and IgG is sensitive but can yield false-positive results. It can be useful for screening, but a positive EIA should be confirmed with another test.

– Hematologic findings include elevated erythrocyte sedimentation rate, leukocytosis, and eosinophilia (in 10%).

- Other studies:
  – CSF findings in meningitis include hypoglycorrhachia and pleocytosis with mononuclear cell predominance.

Imaging
Radiologic studies:

- Chest radiograph may reveal well-circumscribed nodules, lobar or patchy pulmonary infiltrates, pleural effusions, cavitary lesions, and hilar adenopathy.
- Radiographs of involved bones may reveal lytic lesions. Scintigraphy or MRI of bone is more sensitive for the diagnosis of osteomyelitis.

DIFFERENTIAL DIAGNOSIS

- Other pulmonary mycoses (e.g., *Histoplasma capsulatum*, *Aspergillus fumigatus*, and *Blastomyces dermatitidis*)
- *Mycobacterium tuberculosis* (lung or CSF)
- *Mycoplasma pneumoniae*
- Influenza and other viral infections that present as bronchopneumonia
- Skin lesions may mimic other endemic mycoses, tuberculosis, actinomycetes, or syphilis.

 TREATMENT

ADDITIONAL TREATMENT
General Measures

- Uncomplicated or minor disease is self-limited and should not be treated with antifungal therapy (>95% of cases).
- Treatment of uncomplicated respiratory infection is recommended for infants, pregnant women, and patients with continuous fever for >1 month, >10% weight loss, extensive or progressive pulmonary disease, or immunodeficiency (either from HIV or as a result of immunosuppressive medications). Use either oral fluconazole or itraconazole for 3–6 months.
- Diffuse pneumonia or immunocompromised host: Start therapy with amphotericin B and replace with oral fluconazole or itraconazole when clinical improvement is demonstrated. The total length of therapy should be at least 1 year, and for patients with severe immunodeficiency, oral azole therapy should be continued as secondary prophylaxis.
- Disseminated infection, nonmeningeal: Treat with oral fluconazole or itraconazole. Amphotericin B is alternative therapy, especially if lesions worsen or are at critical locations, such as the vertebral column. The duration of therapy may be longer than for those with pneumonia only.
- Meningitis: Oral fluconazole is preferred (800–1,000 mg/d). Itraconazole (400–600 mg/d) is also effective. Therapy should be continued indefinitely.
- Intrathecal amphotericin B may be useful in central nervous system infections.

- Voriconazole and posaconazole, new azole agents, have been shown to be effective in a few case reports.
- Surgical débridement is used for localized and persistent lesions in bone and lung.

 ONGOING CARE

FOLLOW-UP RECOMMENDATIONS
Patient Monitoring

- Rising or unchanging CF titers while the patient is receiving treatment may indicate treatment failure, most often due to noncompliance or an occult focus that may require surgical drainage.
- All azoles inhibit P-450 enzymes. Consider drug–drug interactions when the patient is taking other medications.

PROGNOSIS

- Most infections are asymptomatic (60%) or mild (35%) and self-limited.
- Primary infection of the lungs is usually self-limited, with a course of illness lasting 1–3 weeks; complications (see above) may prolong the course.
- Fatigue can last for several months.
- Dissemination is infrequent (see above for risk factors). Morbidity and mortality have improved with use of antifungal therapy, but immunocompromised patients still have a poor prognosis after the development of disseminated infection. The mortality rate is 70% in HIV-infected patients with diffuse pulmonary coccidioidomycosis.
- Meningitis, untreated, is nearly always fatal within 2 years of diagnosis.

COMPLICATIONS

- Localized complications of primary pulmonary infection are infrequent and include pleural effusions and pericarditis.
- ~5% of lung infections result in residual pulmonary sequelae, usually nodules or abscess cavities. 1/3 of these cavities spontaneously resolve within 2 years. Hemoptysis and rupture of the abscess, with formation of an empyema, are potential complications in patients with unresolved cavities.
- Extrapulmonary dissemination usually develops within a year after the initial infection, but may appear much later if immunity is impaired (e.g., HIV infection, malignancy, immunosuppressive therapy).
- Hospital admission seems to be more common in patients with comorbid conditions and frequently necessitates surgical intervention.
- Hydrocephalus may occur with central nervous system involvement.

ADDITIONAL READING

- Ampel NM. New perspectives on coccidioidomycosis. *Proc Am Thorac Soc.* 2010;7:181–185.
- Chu JH, Feudtner C, Heydon KH, et al. Hospitalizations for endemic mycoses: A population based national sample. *Clin Infect Dis.* 2006;42:822–825.
- Deresinski SC. Coccidioidomycosis: Efficacy of new agents and future prospects. *Curr Opin Infect Dis.* 2001;14:693–696.

- Fisher BT, Chiller TM, Prasad PA, et al. Hospitalizations for coccidioidomycosis at forty-one children's hospitals in the United States. *Pediatr Infect Dis J.* 2010;29(3):243–247.
- Galgiani JN, Ampel NM, Catanzaro A, et al. Practice guidelines for the treatment of coccidioidomycosis. *Clin Infect Dis.* 2000;30:658–661.
- Galgiani JN, Catanzaro A, Cloud GA, et al. Comparison of oral fluconazole and itraconazole for progressive, nonmeningeal coccidioidomycosis: A randomized, double-blind trial. *Ann Intern Med.* 2000;133:676–686.
- Montenegro BL, Arnold JC. North American dimorphic fungal infections in children. *Pediatr Rev.* 2010;31(6):e-40–e-48.
- Shehab ZM. Coccidioidomycosis. *Adv Pediatr.* 2010;57(1):269–286.
- Stevens DA. Coccidioidomycosis. *N Engl J Med.* 1995;332:1077–1082.

 CODES

ICD9
- 114.3 Other forms of progressive coccidioidomycosis
- 114.5 Pulmonary coccidioidomycosis, unspecified
- 114.9 Coccidioidomycosis, unspecified

ICD10
- B38.2 Pulmonary coccidioidomycosis, unspecified
- B38.7 Disseminated coccidioidomycosis
- B38.9 Coccidioidomycosis, unspecified

FAQ

- Q: Do all patients with symptomatic primary respiratory infection due to *C. immitis* require treatment?
- A: No. Since >95% of initial pulmonary infections are self-limited, treatment is not always required. Patients with concurrent risk factors (e.g., HIV, organ transplant, or high doses of corticosteroids) or evidence of unusually severe infections should always be treated. Factors suggesting increased severity of infection include weight loss of >10%, night sweats, infiltrates involving more than half of 1 lung or portions of both lungs, and complement fixation antibody to *C. immitis* >1:16.
- Q: How should pregnant women with coccidioidomycosis be managed?
- A: Diagnosis of primary infection during the 3rd trimester of pregnancy or immediately in the postpartum period should raise consideration for treatment. During pregnancy, amphotericin B is the treatment of choice because fluconazole and other azole antifungals are likely teratogenic.

COLIC

William B. Carey

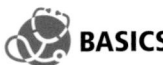 **BASICS**

DESCRIPTION

- A poorly defined and incompletely understood state of prolonged or excessive crying in young infants who are otherwise well
- No standard definition of this phenomenon
- Best definition available: >3 hours a day of irritability, fussing, or crying on >3 days in any 1 week during the 1st 3–4 months of life in an infant who is otherwise healthy and well fed. Some add the criterion of a duration ≥3 weeks.
- Crying is not qualitatively different, but quantitatively. It is considerably more than the average.
- Lack of a firm, standard definition means that varying groups of subjects have been studied and limits our certainty as to incidence and causes of prolonged crying and as to effectiveness of management plans.

ALERT
Numerous pitfalls await the unprepared physician:
- Overdiagnosing the condition of the infant or caregiving inadequacies of parents
- Overtreatment of the infant with changes of feedings, medications, and various inappropriate procedures such as enemas and rectal manipulations. Despite the widely held, popular view that cow's milk allergy is a principal reason for excessive crying, no study of acceptable double-blind design has demonstrated its occurrence in infants who are free of respiratory, gastrointestinal (GI), or cutaneous manifestations of allergy.
- Unnecessary laboratory tests
- Colic is defined as a pattern of recurring episodes of crying. Other explanations should be carefully considered 1st for an acute bout of crying.
- The physician should be wary of enthusiastic reports in the popular press or the medical literature that "at last there is a cure for colic." Certainty is not easily achieved in an area where there is such a problem with definitions and with methodologic problems like achieving truly double-blind trials.

EPIDEMIOLOGY
Incidence and prevalence estimates difficult due to lack of standard definition. Incidence figures of 10–15% typically cited in texts.

RISK FACTORS
Genetics
No genetic influence has been discovered, but it has not been investigated. Temperamental traits are known to be largely inborn, however.

GENERAL PREVENTION
No study has yet demonstrated any certain way of preventing this prolonged or excessive crying. Methods that are likely to be helpful are:
- Education of all parents about infant crying and soothing.
- Informing them of the expected average number of hours per day.
- Most parents do not know that one of the common reasons for an infant to cry is fatigue, and that stimulation at these times is not helpful.
- Dealing with various pertinent parental anxieties when they occur should be undertaken.

PATHOPHYSIOLOGY
- No single cause is always found.
- Typically, the problem lies in the interaction between factors in the infant and the environment at a unique time of biological vulnerability:
  - In the infant there is a normal physiologic or temperamental predisposition to be more sensitive, irritable, intense, less rhythmical, or harder to soothe than average for the age.
  - Parents generally have not yet learned how to read the infant's individual needs correctly and respond appropriately. They may be manipulating the infant in ways that increase rather than decrease the amount of crying.
  - This interaction takes place at a time in the 1st 3–4 months when the immature central nervous system (CNS) makes the infant temporarily more vulnerable to the disorganizing effects of this poor fit.
- Colic generally occurs in the absence of any abnormality in the infant or the parents, but rather when the parents have not yet learned to interact harmoniously with the infant.
- There is no evidence that the bowel is at fault; flatus is more likely to be the result of the crying than the cause.
- Psychosocial risk factors, such as poor support for the mother and various stressors, are probably more common than in noncolicky infants, but they are not necessary.
- When such external factors are present, they seem to exert their effects primarily by reducing the parent's ability to respond appropriately to the infant.
- Physical problems in the infant, such as milk allergy or gastric reflux, probably account for no >10% of all prolonged crying at this time, and would exclude an infant from this diagnosis of colic, which requires that the infant be physically well.

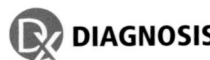 **DIAGNOSIS**

HISTORY
- Define symptoms: Intensity, duration, and frequency of crying. Some parents complain more than others about the crying.
- Colic typically begins shortly after a baby comes home from a newborn nursery.
- It can last until 3–4 months of age if not successfully managed.

ALERT
- If excessive crying lasts after 4 months, other diagnoses should be considered.
- Ask parents to describe a typical day:
  - Description of a typical day or keeping a crying diary is helpful.
  - This will give insights into the daily routine, feeding, rest, interpretive skills and responses of the parents.
- Ask parents to describe and demonstrate their soothing techniques.
- Information on the baby's temperament can be obtained by asking the parents to describe the baby's typical reaction patterns to stimuli.
- Medical history should include concerns about the pregnancy and the newborn period, anxieties related to parents' own experiences as children or with previous children, and the quality of family supports and other stressors.

PHYSICAL EXAM
- No findings are expected if the child has colic. However, examination should always be performed to reassure both parents and physician.
- Attempts at management over the telephone without a physical examination are likely to be unsuccessful.

DIAGNOSTIC TESTS & INTERPRETATION
Lab
No tests are indicated unless specifically suggested by history or physical examination.

DIFFERENTIAL DIAGNOSIS
- Normal crying:
  - Average, normal infants cry about 2 hours a day at 2 weeks of age, just under 3 hours at 6 weeks, and then decrease to ~1 hour by 12 weeks.
  - Normal crying, like colic, tends to occur predominantly in the evening and can vary from day to day.

- Prolonged or excessive crying from physical causes:
  - Faulty feeding techniques: Overfeeding or underfeeding and inadequate burping or sucking
  - Physical problems in the infant: Acute disorders such as otitis media, intestinal cramping with diarrhea, corneal abrasion, and incarcerated hernia; or chronic ones such as gastroesophageal reflux
  - Cow's milk allergy, lactose intolerance, or transmission of irritating substances such as caffeine via breast milk

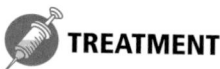

TREATMENT

MEDICATION (DRUGS)
- Drugs, such as phenobarbital or diphenhydramine, are seldom necessary.
- Some observers have reported beneficial effects when used for 1 or 2 weeks in conjunction with counseling, but these results have not as yet been subjected to double-blind studies.
- Simethicone has not been shown to be helpful. Herbal teas should not be recommended because of their varied and often unknown contents.

ADDITIONAL TREATMENT
General Measures
- The most effective form of treatment at present is counseling the parents about the interaction.
- Main points:
  - The infant is not sick.
  - Crying may be persistent, but there is no evidence of a physical problem.
  - There is no proof the infant is having pain, just distress. Avoid iatrogenic problems caused by suggesting that something is wrong with the infant.
  - The infant is probably overaroused and tired.
  - Education about infant crying.
  - Parents need to know how much normal infants cry and how they vary in sensitivity, irritability, and soothability.
  - The way parents react to their infants can affect the amount of crying.
  - Parents often do not understand that a common reason for infant crying is fatigue and a need to be left alone.
  - The excessive crying can be reduced.
  - Parents have to learn to tune in more sensitively to infants' needs and to be more appropriately and effectively responsive to them.
- Basic strategy:
  - Soothe more, as by a pacifier, repetitive sound, swaddling, swinging, or a hot water bottle, and stimulate less by decreasing the picking up, holding, and feeding the infant when it is not appropriate.
  - Contrary to popular opinion, there is no evidence that there is a better behavioral outcome at the present or later from the parents' always responding immediately to every cry.
  - A quiet environment, correction of any faulty feeding techniques, and a minimum of unnecessary handling without changing the composition of the feedings. Pertinent psychosocial issues should be dealt with.

- Expression of optimism by the pediatrician about the immediate outcome is justified and in itself improves chances of success. Simply saying that the colic will be gone by 3–4 months of age is not comforting and may be quite the opposite.
- Extra carrying does not help.
- Almost any procedure done with conviction is likely to be followed by a temporary reduction in crying because of the placebo effect.
- The normal trend toward diminished crying over time has given some forms of treatment an undeserved reputation of effectiveness.

ONGOING CARE

FOLLOW-UP RECOMMENDATIONS
Patient Monitoring
- It is important to keep in close touch with parents of an excessively fussy baby. Telephone contact every 2–3 days is essential until improvement. Re-examination is rarely needed.
- Standard pediatric textbooks state that little can be done to change the pattern. However, several studies report that colic can be sharply reduced within 2–3 days if management such as that described above is used. Some infants take longer, but virtually all respond to suitable management.

DIET
Formula changes are frequently attempted by physicians hoping for a simple solution, but they rarely are effective. Sometimes they seem to be helpful for a few days, only to cease being so soon after that.

PROGNOSIS
Without intervention, this prolonged crying usually diminishes somewhere around 3–4 months. Some recent studies have reported a variety of possible long-term outcomes such as continued aversive temperaments, more behavior problems, and diminished parental self-confidence. More investigations with attention to methodologic details are needed to clarify these matters. Particularly deserving attention is the possible pathogenic role of the physician in incorrectly informing the parents that there is something physically wrong with the infant.

COMPLICATIONS
- Excessive crying does not turn into any other condition, but the factors that caused it may contribute to sleep problems and other behavioral concerns in the infant after the colic has gone.
- Parents are usually exasperated by it.
- The most serious outcome is that, owing to parental exasperation, the infant may be physically abused.
- The infant is likely to be overfed.

ADDITIONAL READING

- Blum NJ, Taubman B, Ttretina LL, et al. Maternal ratings of infant intensity and distractibility. *Arch Pediatr Adolesc Med.* 2002;156:286–290.
- Carey WB. "Colic": Prolonged or excessive crying in young infants. In: Carey WB, Crocker AC, Coleman WL, et al. (eds). *Developmental-Behavioral Pediatrics*, 4th ed. Philadelphia: Saunders Elsevier; 2009.
- Carey WB. The effectiveness of parent counseling in managing colic. *Pediatrics.* 1994;94:333–334.
- Lester BM, Barr RG. *Colic and Excessive Crying.* 105th Ross Conference on Pediatric Research. Columbus, OH: Ross Products Division, Abbott Laboratories; 1997.
- St. James-Rboerts I. Summary: What do we know? What are the implications of the findings for practitioners? What do we need to know? In: Barr RG, St. James-Roberts I, Keefe MR, eds. *New Evidence on Unexplained Early Infant Crying: Its Origins, Nature and Management.* Skillman, NJ: Johnson & Johnson Pediatric Institute; 2001: 327–333.
- Van Ijzendoorn MH, Hubbard FOA. Are infant crying and maternal responsiveness during the first year related to infant-mother attachment at 15 months? 2000;2(3):371–391.
- Wessel MA, Cobb JC, Jackson EB, et al. Paroxysmal fussing in infants, sometimes called "colic." *Pediatrics.* 1954;14:421–434.

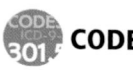 # CODES

ICD9
- 780.92 Excessive crying of infant (baby)
- 789.7 Colic

ICD10
- R10.83 Colic
- R68.11 Excessive crying of infant (baby)

FAQ

- Q: What is wrong with my baby? What can we do to relieve the pain? Why is he/she so gassy? How do you know that it is not due to an allergy? Shouldn't we strengthen the formula? You mean it's all my fault? Will this ever stop? What will he/she be like later?
- A: All the answers are to be found above.

COMA

Daniel Shumer
Amy R. Brooks-Kayal (5th edition)
Eric Marsh (5th edition)

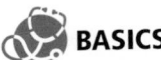 **BASICS**

DEFINITION
Coma is defined as a state in which the patient appears to be asleep, shows no awareness of their surroundings, and cannot be aroused. Coma is a transient state, whereby patients recover, die, or progress to a permanent state of impairment. Often a medical emergency, immediate intervention may be required to preserve life and brain function (e.g., abnormalities in breathing, circulation, glucose, or electrolytes).

- Coma is at the far end of a spectrum of acute impaired consciousness, which also includes:
  - Lethargy or stupor: Patient arousable, but does not stay awake; impaired responses to commands
  - Delirium: A confused, agitated patient with fragmented attention, concentration, and memory
- Coma may progress to:
  - Persistent vegetative state: Chronic state of unconsciousness with no awareness or cognition, no voluntary responses, and no language abilities. Preserved autonomic functions and sleep/wake cycles.
  - Brain death: Coma, apnea, and no brainstem reflexes

ALERT
- Be aware of psychogenic coma and locked-in states (see "Differential Diagnosis").
- Loss of protective airway reflexes signals impending respiratory failure.

EPIDEMIOLOGY
Traumatic and non-traumatic comas have similar annual incidences of about 30/100,000 children. Boys are more often victims of trauma and near drowning than are girls. Infants and young children are more likely to have a non-traumatic etiology; traumatic causes are more common in older childhood and adolescence.

PATHOPHYSIOLOGY
Dysfunction of the reticular activating system in the brainstem or bilateral cerebral dysfunction causes impaired arousal and consciousness.

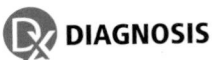 **DIAGNOSIS**

DIFFERENTIAL DIAGNOSIS
- **Trauma**
  - Perform imaging for epidural/subdural or intracerebral bleeding, cerebral swelling, and/or diffuse axonal injury
- **Intoxication**
  - Household drug ingestion including barbiturates, opiates, psychotropics, and salicylates, street drugs, alcohol, smoke or carbon monoxide inhalation, ethylene glycol, lead and others

- **Hypoxia/diffuse ischemia**
  - Drowning, suffocation, myocardial infarction, heart failure, arrhythmia, hypotension
- **Infection**
  - Bacterial or viral meningitis, encephalitis, postinfectious encephalomyelitis, toxic shock, subdural empyema, systemic shock/sepsis. The most common pathogen leading to coma is *Neisseria meningitidis.*
- **Metabolic disorders**
  - Hypoglycemia (salicylate or ethanol intoxication, insulin overdose/hyperinsulinemia), diabetic ketoacidosis (DKA) (neurologic deterioration on initiation of insulin therapy), hyperglycemic nonketotic coma, Reye syndrome, electrolyte abnormalities (Na, K, Ca, Mg); hepatic/uremic encephalopathy; inborn errors of metabolism; endocrine abnormalities (hypothyroidism, Addisonian crisis); hypothermia/hyperthermia
- **Tumor**
  - Can cause increased intracranial pressure and herniation
- **Seizure**
  - Nonconvulsive status, spike and wave stupor
- **Vascular**
  - Hemorrhage from arteriovenous malformation (AVM), aneurysm, coagulopathy, infarction, cerebral venous thrombosis, hypertensive encephalopathy
- **Hydrocephalus**
  - Ventriculoperitoneal (VP) shunt obstruction, mass/bleed obstructing ventricular outflow

Disorders mimicking coma:

- **Psychogenic coma**
  - Patient may resist passive eye opening, regard self in a mirror, and avoid passive arm fall over face and other noxious stimuli.
- **Catatonia**
  - A form of psychogenic coma, patients may hold a posture, sit or stand.
- **Locked-in state/complete paralysis**
  - Patient is paralyzed with intact cerebral function. May occur in severe neuromuscular disorders (acute polyneuropathy) or in ventral pontine lesions (hemorrhage, demyelination).

HISTORY
- **Question:** Evidence or history of head trauma, drowning, or other trauma?
- *Significance:* Are there concerns for nonaccidental trauma?
- **Question:** What medications are in the home? Has the patient been depressed or displayed suicidal behaviors?
- *Significance:* Ingestion/drugs/toxins
- **Question:** Recent fevers, viral or bacterial illnesses, mental status changes, sick contacts, immunosuppression, infectious risk factors?
- *Significance:* Infection

- **Question:** Medical history?
- *Significance:* Seizure disorder, diabetes, heart disease, neurologic disease including previous episodes of coma
- **Question:** Recent nausea, vomiting, mental status change?
- *Significance:* Increased intracranial pressure

PHYSICAL EXAM
- **Finding:** Vital sign changes?
- *Significance:* Hyperthermia suggests infection. Tachycardia suggests fever, pain, hypovolemia, arrhythmia, heart failure. Bradycardia suggests . . . etc.
- **Finding:** Signs of head trauma?
- *Significance:* Raccoon eyes (suggests fracture of frontal skull base), Battle's sign (ecchymosis at mastoid suggests basilar skull fracture), retinal hemorrhages, bulging fontanelle, CSF leak from the nose or ear(s)
- **Finding:** Nuchal rigidity, Kernig and Brudzinski signs (often absent in infants with open fontanelles)?
- *Significance:* Signs of meningitis
- **Finding:** Papilledema?
- *Significance:* Suggests increased ICP
- **Finding:** Skin?
- *Significance:* Pallor (anemia), jaundice (liver failure), cyanosis (hypoxia), flushing (warm shock), bruising (trauma), rashes (infection)
- **Finding:** Neurologic—assess level of consciousness, verbal or motor response to voice, touch, and painful stimuli. Assess pupil size, symmetry and reflexes.
- *Significance:* Anisocoria suggests compression of oculomotor nerve or brainstem nucleus. Small reactive or large reactive pupils suggest intoxication. Fixed and dilated pupils suggest a brainstem injury or brain death. Assessment of eye movements can provide information about the function of cranial nerves. A persistent conjugate eye deviation suggests an injury to ipsilateral cerebrum or a contralateral seizure. Oculocephalic (doll's eye), oculovestibular (caloric), pupillary, and gag reflex can assess cranial nerves and their brainstem nuclei. Asses muscle tone, motor responses to stimuli, and deep tendon reflexes. Abnormal motor responses: Decerebrate posturing (extension and internal rotation of the extremities), decorticate posturing (adduction and flection at the elbows).
- Glasgow Coma Scale/Pediatric Glasgow Coma Scale—associated with prognosis in certain situations
  - Eye opening (score range 1–4)
  - Verbal response (score range 1–5)
  - Motor response (score range 1–6)

DIAGNOSTIC TESTS & INTERPRETATION

Initial blood studies obtained with placement of an IV line include:

- Glucose, electrolytes, blood urea nitrogen/creatinine, calcium, magnesium
- CBC and blood culture
- Arterial blood gas
- Toxicology screen
- Ammonia, liver transaminases

Other helpful studies based on the clinical picture may include:

- Metabolic labs (urine organic acids, serum amino acids), urinalysis, urine culture, thyroid function tests, cortisol, coagulation studies, carboxyhemoglobin (CO poisoning), LP with CSF protein, glucose, cell count and culture
- **Test:** LP
- *Significance*: To rule out infection, bleed; defer until after CT if focal exam or signs of increased ICP. If question of traumatic tap, spin out red cells promptly and examine fluid for xanthochromia.
- **Test:** EEG
- *Significance*: Helpful to rule out nonconvulsive status epilepticus
- **Test:** Electrophysiologic studies
- *Significance*: Somatosensory evoked, brainstem auditory evoked, and visual evoked potentials may be helpful for diagnosis and prognosis.

Imaging

- CT head: Quick noncontrast scan can detect hemorrhage, hydrocephalus, herniation, and masses. May be followed by contrasted images or MRI. Should be done prior to LP to rule out a mass (risk for herniation from LP).
- Cervical spine series (CT or lateral and anterior–posterior radiograph studies): Indicated if evidence of trauma by history or on physical exam. Spine must be stabilized until injury is ruled out.
- MRI brain: To look for causes if other workup is unrevealing.

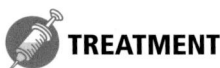 TREATMENT

SURGERY/OTHER PROCEDURES

Neurosurgical intervention may be required in cases of head trauma, hemorrhage, mass lesion, or hydrocephalus. Neurology consultation is usually indicated.

IN-PATIENT CONSIDERATIONS
Initial Stabilization

- First priority is stabilization of respiratory and hemodynamic status (airway, breathing and circulation management).
- If head trauma is suspected, stabilize the cervical spine with a collar while securing the airway.
- Endotracheal intubation: Often required for airway protection and adequate oxygenation
- Large-bore IV lines should be placed and isotonic fluids administered as needed to replace intravascular volume and maintain adequate blood pressure.

- Evidence of increased ICP:
  - Hyperventilate to decrease blood carbon dioxide to 30–35 torr
  - Give mannitol (0.5–1 g/kg IV). Can also give dexamethasone, 1–2 mg/kg IV
  - Fluids given should be isotonic and the volume limited to maintain adequate perfusion
  - Treat fever with antipyretics and environmental cooling methods
  - Elevate head to 30 degrees above horizontal, avoid head-turned posture to maximize cerebral venous drainage
  - Hospitalization in the intensive care unit for close monitoring of changes in respiratory status or signs of increased ICP
  - Neurosurgical consultation
- If finger-stick glucose determination is low, give 2–4 mL/kg of 25% dextrose (D25) IV (D10 if young infant).
- If opiate ingestion is suspected, administer naloxone (0.1 mg/kg IV for infants <5 years or <20 kg, 2 mg for older, larger children).
- Correct electrolyte and acid–base abnormalities
- Empiric treatment with IV antibiotics (ceftriaxone, vancomycin, and acyclovir, for example) should be given if bacterial or viral meningitis is suspected.

 ONGOING CARE

PROGNOSIS

Prognosis depends on underlying etiology. Complete recovery is frequently seen after ingestions or metabolic comas. In contrast, patients with coma resulting from severe head trauma or hypoxic injury have lower survival rates and survivors often have significant neurologic sequelae and require long-term physical, occupational, and cognitive therapies. The Glasgow Coma Score has been shown to correlate with outcomes in some situations such as *traumatic brain injury* and viral encephalitis.

COMPLICATIONS

Acute coma:

- Brain injury
- Respiratory failure/aspiration
- Deep venous thrombosis
- Pneumonia (aspiration and infectious)

ADDITIONAL READING

- Jacinto SJ, Gieron-Korthals M, Ferreira JA. Predicting outcome in hypoxic-ischemic brain injury. *Pediatr Clin North Am*. 2001;48:647–660.
- Kirkham FJ, Newton CR, Whitehouse W. Paediatric coma scales. *Dev Med Child Neurol*. 2008;50(4): 267–274.
- Martin C, Falcone RA Jr. Pediatric traumatic brain injury: An update of research to understand and improve outcomes. *Curr Opin Pediatr*. 2008; 20(3):294–299.
- Tasker RC. Neurolocal critical care. *Curr Opin Pediatr*. 2000;12:222–226.
- Trubel HK, Novotny E, Lister G. Outcome of coma in children. *Curr Opin Pediatr*. 2003;15:283–287.

 CODES

ICD9

- 779.2 Cerebral depression, coma, and other abnormal cerebral signs in fetus or newborn
- 780.01 Coma

ICD10

- P91.5 Neonatal coma
- R40.20 Unspecified coma

FAQ

- Q: What is the value of the Pediatric Glasgow Coma Scale?
- A: The PGCS is helpful in predicting prognosis but not for diagnosing the cause of coma. However, the etiology of the coma can impact the usefulness of the scale. For example, PGCS has a better correlation with outcomes following traumatic brain injury than it does for cold-water drowning episodes.
- Q: When a bacterial infection is suspected as a potential etiology of coma, should antibiotic therapy be delayed until CSF has been obtained for testing?
- A: Starting antibiotic therapy prior to obtaining CSF may lead to a false-negative CSF culture. However, if there is any concern for increased ICP or mass effect from tumor or abscess causing coma, a CT should be obtained prior to an LP, and antibiotics should be started meanwhile. LP in the setting of mass effect can cause herniation. Therefore, if bacterial CSF infection is suspected, antibiotic therapy should not be delayed while stabilizing the patient and obtaining a head CT. Peripheral blood culture can be obtained at the time of IV placement.

COMMON VARIABLE IMMUNODEFICIENCY

Elena Elizabeth Perez

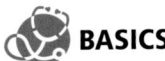 **BASICS**

DESCRIPTION
- A rare heterogeneous immunodeficiency syndrome characterized by:
  - Low IgG, A, and/or IgM
  - Recurrent infections
  - A wide spectrum of immunologic abnormalities including autoimmune disease, inflammatory conditions, and the development of lymphomas
- The most common clinically important primary immunodeficiency
- Other terminology for this disease include:
  - Acquired hypogammaglobulinemia
  - Adult-onset hypogammaglobulinemia
  - Dysgammaglobulinemia
  - Common variable hypogammaglobulinemia
- Diagnosis of exclusion, requiring variable reduction in 1 or more immunoglobulin classes (IgG, IgA, and/or IgM), impaired specific antibody responses, and in some cases reduction of B-cell number

EPIDEMIOLOGY
- Incidence is estimated to be 1 in 25,000 to 1 in 66,000 in the general population.
- Can present at any age
  - Most diagnosed between 20 and 40 years of age
  - Described in patients as young as 6 months
- Diagnosis is usually made several years after the onset of recurrent infections (pneumonia, sinusitis, otitis).
- A subgroup of children has been described in which the onset of disease was most often <5 years of age. This group was characterized by a relapsing and remitting course in which autoimmune disease predominated.
- About 20–25% of patients with common variable immunodeficiency have 1 or more autoimmune conditions at the time of diagnosis.
- Affects males and females equally.

RISK FACTORS
Genetics
- Complex genetics, likely multifactorial
- Rare recessive mutations described in:
  - T cell, inducible costimulatory (ICOS) I none kindred
  - CD19 in few unrelated families
  - B-cell activating factor (BAFF) in 2 siblings
  - CD20 and CD81 in 1 patient each
  - TACI (transmembrane activator and calcium-modulating cyclophilin ligand interactor (TNFRSF13B) in 8% of patients, associated with autoimmunity and lymphoid hyperplasia; heterozygous mutation more common than homozygous, significance not clear due to similar mutation found in healthy family members
- IgA deficiency more likely in offspring of parents with common variable immunodeficiency
- Incidence of IgA deficiency, autoimmune disease, malignancies increased in family members of patients with common variable immunodeficiency

PATHOPHYSIOLOGY
- Hypogammaglobulinemia is the main characteristic.
- Impaired immunoglobulin and specific antibody production despite normal B-lymphocyte numbers.
- An increased proportion of immature B cells is often present.
- Deficiency of class switched memory B cells associated with more complex disease (autoimmunity, granulomatous disease, hypersplenism, and lymphoid hyperplasia
- Functional defects of both B and T lymphocytes are described.

ETIOLOGY
- The primary immunologic defect(s) leading to this syndrome is unknown: Multiple defects have been associated with common variable immunodeficiency including:
  - Lack of somatic mutation within variable region genes
  - Lack of memory B cells
- Some genetic defects have been described but do not account for the majority of cases. These include:
  - Inducible costimulatory receptor (ICOS) deficiency, <1% of patients
  - Mutations in TNF receptor family member transmembrane activator and calcium-modulator and cyclophilin ligand interactor (TACI). TACI is involved in isotype switching of B cells. Only 1 TACI allele is mutated in majority of patients studied.
  - Mutation in TACI has also been observed in relatives of CVID patients who have IgA deficiency B-cell defects include inability to secrete antibodies, and impaired upregulation of CD70 and CD86 (co-stimulatory molecules), and reduction of switched CD27+ B cells.
    ○ Impaired maturation, IL-12 secretion, and upregulation of costimulatory molecules by antigen presenting cells may impair T cells, which are important for providing help to B cells for antibody production.
    ○ Toll-like receptor 9 (TLR9) response and expression by B cells may also be impaired. TLR signaling pathways are being investigated for their potential role in pathogenesis of CVID.
    ○ Mutations in CD19, CD20, CD81 and BAFF are described in few cases

 DIAGNOSIS

HISTORY
- Recurrent sinopulmonary infections, especially sinusitis and pneumonia, with encapsulated bacteria
- Autoimmune diseases such as autoimmune hemolytic anemia, idiopathic thrombocytopenic purpura, thyroid disease, and chronic active hepatitis
- Localized or systemic granulomatous disease that can be diagnosed years before low IgG is considered. Lungs, spleen, lymph nodes are most commonly affected. Can be misdiagnosed as sarcoidosis.
- Persistent diarrhea of infectious (e.g., *Giardia lamblia*) or noninfectious causes
- Inflammatory bowel diseaselike disorder in 6–10% of patients
- Noninfectious, diffuse pulmonary complications described as granulomatous-lymphocytic interstitial lung disease (GLILD) exhibit granulomatous and lymphoproliferative histologic patterns (lymphocytic interstitial pneumonia [LIP], follicular bronchiolitis, and lymphoid hyperplasia).
- Severe or unusual viral infections with herpes simplex, cytomegalovirus, and varicella, such as pneumonitis, hepatitis, or encephalitis. Chronic meningoencephalitis can be seen with enteroviral infection.

PHYSICAL EXAM
- Evaluation should focus on the presence of infection.
- 30% of patients will have lymphadenopathy and/or splenomegaly.

DIAGNOSTIC TESTS & INTERPRETATION
Lab
- IgG, IgA, IgM below age-appropriate norms
- CBC with differential: Examine smear for evidence of hemolysis in autoimmune hemolytic anemia.
- Autoimmune antibody screen: Antinuclear antibody, autoantibody panel
- Stool culture for bacteria and ova/parasites to evaluate chronic diarrhea
- Isohemagglutinins as well as functional antibody titers to bacterial antigens such as tetanus, diphtheria, and pneumococcus are usually low to absent.
- Spirometry may be helpful in following chronic lung disease.
- Mitogen/Antigen stimulation studies will help assess lymphocyte function.
- T- and B-lymphocyte enumeration by flow cytometry
- B-cell phenotyping becoming more available
- Absent B lymphocytes suggests X-linked agammaglobulinemia rather than common variable immunodeficiency.
- Appropriate cultures based on site of infection

Imaging
Chest and sinus x-ray studies/CT scans may be warranted for evaluation of chronic disease.

Diagnostic Procedures/Other
- GI endoscopy with biopsies for cases of idiopathic persistent diarrhea
- Lymph node biopsy in suspected malignancy

DIFFERENTIAL DIAGNOSIS
- Other primary antibody-deficiency disorders: X-linked agammaglobulinemia and transient hypogammaglobulinemia of infancy
- Severe malabsorption with protein-losing enteropathy
- HIV infection
- Chronic lung disease: Cystic fibrosis, immotile cilia syndrome, and α_1-antitrypsin deficiency
- Primary autoimmune diseases: Immune idiopathic thrombocytopenic purpura, autoimmune hemolytic anemia, systemic lupus erythematosus, thyroiditis

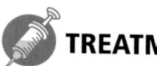
TREATMENT

MEDICATION (DRUGS)
First Line
Immunoglobulin replacement therapy

Second Line
Antibiotics as needed for infection, may also be used as adjunct to immunoglobulin replacement as prophylaxis.

ADDITIONAL TREATMENT
General Measures
- Monthly IV immunoglobulin replacement:
  – Starting dose is usually 400–600 mg/kg/month IV or FDA-approved formulation(s) for SC administration, given weekly.
- Appropriate antibiotics for acute infections. Prophylactic antibiotics may be helpful in chronic/recurrent infections.
- Cautious use of corticosteroids may be necessary in the treatment of gastrointestinal (GI) and autoimmune manifestations.

ISSUES FOR REFERRAL
- Autoimmune manifestations
- GI: Chronic abdominal pain or signs of possible lymphoid hyperplasia

IN-PATIENT CONSIDERATIONS
Nursing
- Supervision during IVIG administration
- Monitor for side effects of therapy
- Have anaphylaxis medications available

ONGOING CARE

FOLLOW-UP RECOMMENDATIONS
- Close and frequent follow-up is warranted for patients with severe, recurrent symptoms. It may be as frequent as monthly, depending on symptoms.
- Signs and symptoms suggesting malignancy (e.g., persistent adenopathy in absence of infection, significant weight loss, or abdominal mass) should be evaluated expeditiously. Abdominal pain may indicate infection or lymphoid hyperplasia.

Patient Monitoring
CBC with differential, ALT, Creatinine, IgG level

DIET
Normally no restriction

PATIENT EDUCATION
Several Web sites available to patients and families:
- Immune deficiency Foundation: http://primaryimmune.org
- International Patient Organization for Primary Immunodeficiencies: www.ipopi.org
- The Jeffrey Modell Foundation: www.jmfworld.org
- National Institute of Allergy and Immunology: www.niaid.nih.gov

PROGNOSIS
Immunoglobulin replacement therapy, prophylactic antibiotics when necessary, and close follow up by immunology have greatly improved the overall prognosis. The newer challenge with this disease is detection and management of autoimmune and other disease associated complications.

COMPLICATIONS
- Autoimmune disease in 20% of common variable immunodeficiency patients. Most common are autoimmune hemolytic anemia and idiopathic thrombocytopenia purpura.
- GI complications include chronic diarrhea, malabsorption, and weight loss. Inflammatory bowel disease and *Helicobacter pylori* infection have also been observed.
- Granulomatous infiltrations may mimic sarcoidosis.
- Lymphoproliferative disease: Overall risk is 8–10%. The most common are lymphomas, usually non-Hodgkin lymphoma, well differentiated, mostly Epstein-Barr virus negative.
- Chronic sinusitis and lung disease with abnormal pulmonary function tests
- Progressive decline in T-lymphocyte function

ADDITIONAL READING
- Agarwal S, Cunningham-Rundles C. Autoimmunity in common variable immunodeficiency. *Curr Allergy Asthma Rep.* 2009;9(5):347–352.
- Ballow M. Primary immunodeficiency disorders: Antibody deficiencies. *J Allergy Clin Immunol.* 2002;109:581–591.
- Brant D, Gershwin M. Common variable immune deficiency and autoimmunity. *Autoimmun Rev.* 2006;5:465–470.
- Castigli E, Geha R. Molecular basis of common variable immunodeficiency. *J Allergy Clin Immunol.* 2006;117(4)740–746.
- Cunningham-Rundles C. Immune deficiency: Office evaluation and treatment. *Allergy Asthma Proc.* 2003;24:409–415.
- Moratto D, Gulino AV, Fontana S, et al. Combined decreased of defined B and T cell subsets in a group of common variable immunodeficiency patients. *Clin Immunol.* 2006;121:203–214.
- Park JH, Levinson AI. Granulomatous-lymphocytic interstitial lung disease (GLILD) in CVID. *Clin Immunol.* 2010;134(2):97–103.
- Puck JM. Neonatal screening for severe combined immune deficiency. *Curr Opin Allergy Clin Immunol.* 2007;7(6):522–527.
- Salzer U, Grimbacher B. Common Variable immunodeficiency: The power of costimulation co-stimulation. *Semin Immunol* 2006;18:337–346.
- Simonte S, Cunningham-Rundles C. Update on primary immunodeficiency: Defects of lymphocytes. *Clin Immunol.* 2003;109:109–118.

CODES

ICD9
- 279.00 Hypogammaglobulinemia, unspecified
- 279.06 Common variable immunodeficiency
- 279.10 Immunodeficiency with predominant T-cell defect, unspecified

ICD10
- D83.0 Common variable immunodeficiency with predominant abnormalities of B-cell numbers and function
- D83.2 Common variable immunodeficiency with autoantibodies to B- or T-cells
- D83.9 Common variable immunodeficiency, unspecified

FAQ
- Q: What is the life expectancy of patients with the diagnosis of common variable immunodeficiency?
- A: Because the clinical presentations and symptoms are variable, it is difficult to predict the life expectancy in individual patients. Intravenous immunoglobulin replacement, in addition to antibiotic therapy, has greatly improved the outlook for these patients. However, despite adequate therapy, a large percentage of patients with common variable immunodeficiency have a progressive decline in immune function. Major morbidity and mortality usually result from the associated complications of malignancy, chronic lung disease, and severe autoimmune disease. In one study, the mortality is estimated at 23–27% over a median follow-up of 7 years (0–25 years). The 20-year survival after diagnosis for males is 64% and for females 67% versus 92% and 94%, respectively, for the general population. Main causes of death include respiratory complications, granulomatous disease of organs, liver disease, malnutrition due to GI pathology, uncontrolled autoimmune manifestations and lymphoma.
- Q: Should patients with common variable immunodeficiency receive live viral vaccines?
- A: In general, patients receiving IVIG replacement therapy do not require any vaccinations. Live viral vaccines should be avoided in these patients, especially if they have deteriorating immune function.
- Q: Can common variable immunodeficiency be diagnosed prenatally?
- A: Because there are no clear genetic inheritance patterns, prenatal diagnosis is unavailable.

COMPLEMENT DEFICIENCY

Erin E. McGintee

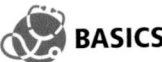 **BASICS**

DESCRIPTION

- Complement consists of >30 plasma and cell membrane proteins that function as cofactors in defense against pathogenic microbes and in the generation of many immunopathogenic disorders.
- Biologic actions include:
  - Cytolysis: Destruction of cells by disrupting cell membrane
  - Opsonization of organisms, which facilitates phagocytosis
  - Inflammation by generation of peptides, which can upregulate chemotaxis and can cause vasodilatation
  - Clearance of immune complexes and apoptotic cells
  - Interaction and augmentation of adaptive immune response

EPIDEMIOLOGY

- Prevalence of known primary immunodeficiency is 1 per 100,000.
- Complement accounts for ~2% of all primary immunodeficiencies.

RISK FACTORS

Genetics

- Most complement deficiencies are autosomal recessive traits.
- Properdin deficiency is X-linked.
- C1 inhibitor deficiency is autosomal dominant.
- Heterozygotes are usually phenotypically normal.

PATHOPHYSIOLOGY

Table 1. Complement deficiency and related clinical problems

Deficiency	Clinical Manifestations
C1(qrs), C2, C4	Systemic lupus erythematosus, vasculitis, glomerulonephritis, pyogenic infections
C3	Glomerulonephritis, pyogenic infections, neisserial infections, immune complex disease
C1 inhibitor	Hereditary angioedema
Factor H, I	Hemolytic uremic syndrome, glomerulonephritis
Properdin	Neisserial infections
Factor B, D	Neisserial infections
MBL, MASP	Repeated infections, accelerated course of systemic lupus erythematosus, rheumatoid arthritis
C5, C6, C7, C8, C9	Disseminated neisserial infections
CD55, CD59	Paroxysmal nocturnal hemoglobinuria

ETIOLOGY

- 3 pathways (the classic, the alternative, and the mannose-binding lectin) converge on same terminal pathway—the membrane attack complex
- Classic pathway requires antibody for initiation, whereas alternative and mannose-binding lectin pathways can be activated without antibody.
- Complement deficiencies may be primary or secondary.
- Secondary deficiencies of complement are usually owing to a consumptive or decreased productive state:
  - Newborn state
  - Malnutrition, anorexia nervosa
  - Liver cirrhosis
  - Reye syndrome
  - Nephrotic syndrome

See the table "Complement Deficiency and Related Clinical Problems."

 **DIAGNOSIS**

HISTORY
Indications for evaluating complement system:
- Systemic lupus erythematosus, juvenile rheumatoid arthritis, or other immune complex disease
- Recurrent pyogenic infections
- 2nd episode of bacteremia at any age
- 2nd episode of meningococcal meningitis or gonococcal arthritis
- Recurrent angioedema without urticaria
- Pneumococcal bacteremia after infancy

PHYSICAL EXAM
Depends on suspected complement defect, but may see any of the following:
- Failure to thrive
- Scars from various infections
- Joint destruction
- Angioedema

DIAGNOSTIC TESTS & INTERPRETATION
Diagnostic Procedures/Other
- CH50: To assess integrity of classical pathway:
  - The quantity of serum required to lyse 50% of an aliquot of antibody-sensitized sheep RBC
  - Specimen handling: Complement components are thermolabile; common cause of abnormal values is improper handling. Procedure may require use of dry ice.
- APH50: To assess integrity of alternate pathway
- C3, C4, and other individual components based on clinical history
- C1 esterase inhibitor level and function to evaluate for HAE.

DIFFERENTIAL DIAGNOSIS
- Humoral deficits such as immunoglobulin deficiency or dysfunction
- Consumptive process such as sepsis

ALERT
- Special care is required for the proper handling of blood test to prevent falsely low values.
- Sometimes the complement cascade can be activated and consume the complement factor, leading to the improper diagnosis of a complement deficiency.

 TREATMENT

ADDITIONAL TREATMENT
General Measures
- Fresh-frozen plasma for acute severe infections
- Aggressive workup and management of infections
- Prophylactic antibiotics may be useful for recurrent infections.
- Immunization for pneumococci, *Haemophilus influenzae*, and *Neisseria meningitidis* for patient and household members
- Close monitoring for onset of autoimmune disease
- Study other family members for genetic counseling.
- Attenuated androgens and fibrinolysis inhibitor aminocaproic acid can be used as prophylaxis for HAE
- HAE can also be treated prophylactically or acutely with purified C1-INH concentrate, and acute attacks can also be treated with kallikrein antagonist given SC.

 ONGOING CARE

COMPLICATIONS
Deficiencies can lead to:
- Recurrent infection
- Immune complex disease
- Autoimmunity

ADDITIONAL READING
- Frank M. Complement disorders and hereditary angioedema. *J Allergy Clin Immunol*. 2010;125:S262–71.
- Bonilla FA, Geha RS. Primary immunodeficiency diseases. *J Allergy Clin Immunol*. 2003;111(2 Suppl):S571–S581. Erratum in *J Allergy Clin Immunol*. 2003;112:267.
- Frank MM. Complement deficiencies. *Pediatr Clin North Am*. 2000;47:1339–1354.
- Frieri M. Complement-related diseases. *Allergy Asthma Proc*. 2002;23:319–324.
- Hackett SJ, Flood TJ. Selective screening for complement deficiencies in patients with meningococcal disease. *Pediatr Infect Dis J*. 2004;23(1):87–88.
- O'Bier A, Muniz AE, Foster RL. Hereditary angioedema presenting as epiglottitis. *Pediatr Emerg Care*. 2005;21(1):27–30.
- Walport MJ. Complement: First of two parts. *N Engl J Med*. 2001;344:1058–1066.
- Walport MJ. Complement: Second of two parts. *N Engl J Med*. 2001;344:1140–1144.

CODES

ICD9
279.8 Other specified disorders involving the immune mechanism

ICD10
D84.1 Defects in the complement system

FAQ
- Q: How common are complement deficiencies?
- A: Very uncommon. They account for 2% of all immunodeficiencies.
- Q: When should I evaluate for a complement deficiency?
- A: Any child with recurrent sinopulmonary infections or >1 episode of a neisserial infection.

CONCUSSION

Nicole Ryan
Daniel Licht
Nicholas S. Abend

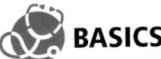 BASICS

DESCRIPTION

- Concussion is a complex pathophysiological process affecting the brain, induced by traumatic biomechanical forces.
- There are a graded set of clinical symptoms that may or may not involve a loss of consciousness.
- Concussion may be caused by either a direct blow to the head, face, neck, or elsewhere on the body with an "impulsive" force transmitted to the head.
- Concussion typically results in the rapid onset of short-lived impairment of neurologic function that resolves spontaneously. In a small percentage of children, postconcussive symptoms may be prolonged.
- Concussion may result in pathological changes, but the acute clinical symptoms largely reflect a functional rather than structural injury and no abnormality is seen on standard neuroimaging studies.

EPIDEMIOLOGY

- A recent review estimated that up to 3.8 million recreation- and sport-related concussions occur annually in the U.S.
- Concussion is underreported.
- Most common sports include football, ice hockey, soccer, wrestling, lacrosse, basketball, baseball, softball, field hockey, and volleyball.
- Girls have higher rates of concussion than boys in similar sports.
- Risk of injury depends on game, position, and use of helmet.

GENERAL PREVENTION

Given that children may have a sense of invulnerability and desire to return to usual activities quickly, preparticipation medical visits should emphasize that reporting concussion immediately is essential and loss of consciousness is not the only manifestation of concussion. Helmet use is essential at reducing the severity of a blow to the head. Seatbelt use has dramatically reduced head trauma in motor vehicle accidents.

PATHOPHYSIOLOGY

- The brain is buoyed in the cranium by cerebrospinal fluid that acts as protective insulation. With acceleration–deceleration, the brain continues to experience momentum and strikes against bone. The temporal and frontal lobes are particularly prone to injury because of their location adjacent to irregular parts of the skull.
- Depressed level of consciousness is thought to be the result of rotational stretch injury to the reticular activating system in the dorsal aspect of the brain stem.

- Changes after concussion include changes in neuronal depolarization and neurotransmitter release, impaired axonal function, and altered brain autoregulation and glucose metabolism.
- Children may respond to brain trauma differently than adults due to developmental factors such as brain size, brain water content, myelination level, skull and suture geometry and elasticity, and differential skull to body proportions.

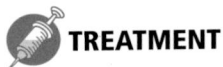 DIAGNOSIS

HISTORY

- Detailed symptom evaluation.
- Information regarding prior concussions.
- History of pre-existing cognitive or attention problems should be elicited to help guide interpretation of postinjury testing.

SIGNS AND SYMPTOMS

- Postconcussive symptoms may be divided into 4 domains:
- Somatic: Headaches, fatigue, decreased energy, nausea, vision change, tinnitus dizziness, incoordination and balance difficulty.
- Emotional/Behavioral: Irritability, increased emotionality, personality change, depression, or anxiety.
- Cognitive: Slowed thinking and response time, impaired concentration, learning, memory, and problem solving ability.
- Sleep disturbances are common.

PHYSICAL EXAM

- A detailed neurological examination should be performed to detect worrisome signs and to allow accurate observation over time.
- Mental status: Orientation (person, place, time), concentration (digit span), and memory (anterograde and retrograde).
- Cranial nerves: Pupil reactivity, eye movements (particularly smooth pursuit and saccadic movements), visual fields, face movement and sensation, tongue protrusion.
- Motor
- Sensory
- Cerebellar: Agility: Finger-to-nose-to-finger, rapid alternating movements (finger tapping, toe tapping), tandem gait (forwards and backwards, eyes open and closed).
- Exertion provocative tests: 5 push-ups, 5 sit-ups, 5 knee bends, 40-yard sprint; look for change in exam.

DIAGNOSTIC TESTS & INTERPRETATION
Imaging

- Computed tomography of the head (HCT) is the test of choice to evaluate for intracranial hemorrhage or skull fracture 24–48 hours after injury. There is increased suspicion of intracranial injury in patients with severe headache, seizures, focal neurologic findings, repeated emesis, changes in alertness, slurred speech, poor orientation, neck pain, loss of consciousness >30 seconds, or significant irritability.
- Clear indications for HCT have not been elucidated and children may have intracranial lesions with asymptomatic head injury, so a relatively low threshold for neuroimaging is appropriate.
- Children <1 year of age should be imaged because symptoms may be difficult to detect and nontraumatic etiologies must be considered.
- Children <2 years of age should be imaged unless there was a low-energy mechanism and no symptoms/signs for at least 2 hours.
- MRI is more appropriate if imaging is needed >48 hours after injury. Newer MRI modalities such as functional MRI, gradient echo, perfusion, and diffusion tensor imaging may be more informative but research to date is lacking. Susceptibility-weighted imaging (SWI) or echo gradient sequences can highlight small hemorrhages that are evidence of diffuse axonal injury (DAI). DAI is associated with more severe injury.

Diagnostic Procedures/Other
Neuropsychological testing:

- Computerized testing is now widely available and baseline testing is being performed by many school athletic departments. Research is still needed as to the optimum timing of this testing and whether it improves outcome.

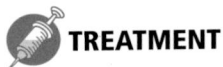 TREATMENT

- Onsite acute evaluation should include the usual ABCs and evaluation for potential associated injuries such as cervical spinal injury.
- Standardized, validated instruments for mental status testing are available and can be administered quickly on the sideline (i.e., SCAT-2).

ADDITIONAL TREATMENT
General Measures

- Remove the child from the contest with no return to play if concussion is suspected.
- Monitor the athlete for several hours after the injury to evaluate for any deterioration.

- Consider referral to the emergency department if there is repeated vomiting, severe or worsening headache, seizure, unsteady gait, slurred speech, weakness or numbness in the extremities, unusual behavior, signs of a basilar skull fracture, or a GCS <15.
- Children <2 years of age may need more prolonged observation in an ED or inpatient setting.
- There is currently no evidence-based research on the use of any medication in the treatment of the concussed pediatric athlete.

ISSUES FOR REFERRAL
- Neuropsychological evaluation should be considered in children with multiple concussions or when recovery is not progressing as expected to document impairment, identify factors contributing to persisting difficulties, and guide school accommodations or formal intervention.
- If admitted for observation, consults by speech therapy, physical therapy, and physiatry should be considered to evaluate subtle sequelae.

SURGERY/OTHER PROCEDURES
Neurosurgical evaluation or transfer to a trauma center should be considered for symptoms of prolonged unconsciousness, persistent mental status alterations, worsening postconcussive symptoms, abnormalities on neurologic examination, or abnormalities on neuroimaging.

IN-PATIENT CONSIDERATIONS
Admission Criteria
Consider admission if the child continues to have altered level of consciousness, if focal neurologic signs are present, or if patient remains severely symptomatic.

Nursing
If observation is required, nursing staff must be able to perform neurological assessments at regular intervals.

Discharge Criteria
- Planning must be individualized if intracranial lesions are present.
- The child and guardian should receive return to play guidelines focused on avoiding second impact syndrome, in which a second concussion occurs soon after a first concussion. Concussions have a cumulative effect and result in increased vulnerability to future injuries.

- No athlete should return to play while still symptomatic from a concussion. This includes physical, cognitive, or behavioral symptoms. There must be no symptoms or signs at rest or during exertion.
- Activities with a high cognitive demand should be limited while symptomatic, including television, computer, videogames, and texting. School accommodations may be needed.
- Before considering return to play, any medication to reduce symptoms must be stopped and the athlete must be symptom-free off medications.
- Return to play should occur in a gradual fashion because symptoms may be aggravated with exertion. Consider in sequence light aerobic activity, noncontact sport related activity, full practice, and then game play.
- Retirement should be considered for any athlete who has sustained 3 concussions in an individual season, has had postconcussive symptoms for more than 3 months, when recovery requires an increasing amount of time, or when concussions occur with less forceful injury.

 ONGOING CARE

FOLLOW-UP RECOMMENDATIONS
Patient Monitoring
If the patient is discharged home for observation, the guardian should have detailed instruction regarding reasons to return to the ED. These include difficult to awaken or quickly falls back asleep, worsening headache or dizziness, emesis, seizures, blood or clear fluid from the ears or nose, major changes in behavior, any focal weakness/sensory/vision changes.

PROGNOSIS
- In general, the prognosis is excellent, but depends on the severity of the injury.
- The typical adult patient with a concussion will recover to baseline function in 6–12 weeks.
- Athletes and children usually recover in 48 hours. However, children with previous head injury, learning difficulties, or neurologic, psychiatric, or family problems may continue to show significant ongoing problems at 3 months.
- Chronic headaches, persistent difficulty with short- and long-term memory and episodic confusion are common sequelae of the cumulative damage that occurs with repeated concussive injuries.

COMPLICATIONS
- Postconcussion symptoms such as confusion, altered concentration, memory and problem solving, irritability, emotional changes, and headaches may take several months to resolve.
- Serious head injury may occur and requires immediate neurosurgical evaluation, neurocritical care, and often serial HCT imaging because intracranial lesions, such as contusion or hemorrhages (epidural, subdural, intraparenchymal), can expand. These may occur with or without skull fracture, and may occur without an initial loss of consciousness.

ADDITIONAL READING
- Halstead ME, Walter KD, The Council on Sports Medicine and Fitness. Clinical report–sport-related concussion in children and adolescents. *Pediatrics.* 2010;126(3):597–615.
- Kelly JP, Rosenberg JH. Diagnosis and management of concussion in sports. *Neurology.* 1997;48: 575–580.
- McCrory P, Meeuwisse W, Johnston K, et al. Consensus statement on Concussion in Sport 3rd International Conference on Concussion in Sport held in Zurich, November 2008. *Clin J Sports Med.* 2009;19(3):185–200.
- US Department of Health and Human Services, *Centers for Disease Control and Prevention. Heads Up Toolkits.* Atlanta, GA: Centers for Disease Control and Prevention; 2005.
- Report of the Quality Standards Subcommittee. Practice parameter: The management of concussion in sports. *Neurology.* 1997;48:581–585.

CODES

ICD9
- 850.5 Concussion with loss of consciousness of unspecified duration
- 850.9 Concussion, unspecified

ICD10
- S06.0X0A Concussion without loss of consciousness, initial encounter
- S06.0X9A Concussion with loss of consciousness of unspecified duration, initial encounter

CONGENITAL HEPATIC FIBROSIS

Jessica Wen
J. Fernando del Rosairo (5th edition)

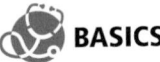

BASICS

DESCRIPTION
- Congenital hepatic fibrosis (CHF) is an inherited, noncirrhotic liver disease associated with cystic disease of the kidneys.
- Prominent clinical features include:
  – Portal hypertension
  – Increased risk of ascending cholangitis
- Liver biopsy shows the classic lesion of ductal plate malformation.
- Majority of patients with CHF have associated autosomal recessive polycystic kidney disease (ARPKD). However, several other genetic diseases also result in CHF.

EPIDEMIOLOGY
Incidence
The incidence of ARPKD is 1/20,000–1/40,000 live births.

RISK FACTORS
Genetics
- Inheritance is autosomal recessive in most families.
- PKHD1, the ARPKD/CHF disease gene, is located on chromosome 6p12. The gene is large, consisting of at least 86 exons extending over 469 kb of genomic DNA. It is expressed at high levels in fetal and adult kidneys and at lower levels in the liver and pancreas.
- Mutations of the PKHD1 gene include frameshift, nonsense, and out-of-frame splicing alterations that are consistent with a loss of function mechanism.
- The presence of 2 truncating mutations leads to the most severe phenotype, associated with death in the neonatal period.
- The PKHD1 gene product is a protein called polyductin or fibrocystin. It is a transmembrane protein located mostly on the primary cilia and apical surface of renal tubular cells and cholangiocytes. It complexes with polycystin 1 and polycystin 2, the mutated proteins in ADPKD. Together, the complex is thought to function as mechanotransducer, detecting the shear force from urine and bile flow. Further studies will be needed to identify the biologic function of polyductin and to determine how mutations of the protein cause disease.

PATHOPHYSIOLOGY
- Ductal plate malformation is a characteristic histologic lesion of the liver, implying a disturbance of the normal development of the bile ducts.
- Hallmarks on pathology include:
  – Dilated intrahepatic bile ducts, often described as staghorn shaped
  – Increased amounts of noninflammatory fibrosis in the portal tracts
  – Normal appearance of hepatocytes and lobular architecture
- The primary defect in ARPKD may be linked to ciliary dysfunction. The ciliary structure is abnormal in ARPKD renal tubule cells and cholangiocytes.
- Developmental abnormalities involve the liver and kidneys, and less commonly, the vasculature and the heart.
- Portal hypertension is thought to result from the fibrosis in the portal tracts, as well as, in some patients, from portal vein abnormalities.

COMMONLY ASSOCIATED CONDITIONS
- Hepatomegaly
- Hypersplenism
- Portal hypertension
- Conditions associated with the finding of ductal plate malformation:
  – CHF
  – ARPKD
  – Autosomal dominant polycystic kidney disease (ADPKD)
  – Caroli syndrome
  – CHF-nephronophthisis
  – Congenital disorder of glycosylation type 1b (phosphomannose isomerase deficiency)
  – Congenital malformation syndromes:
    ○ Meckel Gruber syndrome
    ○ Joubert syndrome
    ○ Jeune syndrome
    ○ Bardet-Biedl syndrome

DIAGNOSIS

HISTORY
- Severely affected patients are usually diagnosed in utero or shortly after birth, due to massively enlarged cystic kidneys. Prenatal renal dysfunction may result in pulmonary hypoplasia.
- Older patients may present with systemic hypertension or signs of portal hypertension and esophageal variceal bleeding
- Patients may present with fever and jaundice (cholangitis) or, rarely, with signs of liver failure.

PHYSICAL EXAM
- Firm, enlarged liver with a prominent left lobe
- Splenomegaly
- Kidneys may be palpable on abdominal exam.

DIAGNOSTIC TESTS & INTERPRETATION
Lab
Initial lab tests
- Thrombocytopenia and leukopenia are associated with hypersplenism.
- Liver enzymes and bilirubin are typically normal; transaminases may be mildly elevated in some patients.
- Usually hepatic synthetic function (albumin, prothrombin time) is normal.
- May see elevated blood urea nitrogen and creatinine with renal involvement
- Genetic testing is available.

Imaging
Ultrasound with Doppler:
- Increased hepatic echogenicity
- Splenomegaly
- Evidence of portal hypertension
- Cystic kidneys

Diagnostic Procedures/Other
Liver biopsy:
- Characteristic histology of ductal plate malformation
- If cholangitis is suspected clinically, send specimen for bacterial culture

DIFFERENTIAL DIAGNOSIS
Varies with presentation. Usually differential diagnosis is that of cirrhosis.

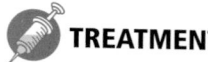

TREATMENT

MEDICATION (DRUGS)
Choleretic agents, including ursodeoxycholic acid, are used in bile stasis and refractory cholangitis.

ADDITIONAL TREATMENT
General Measures
- Suspected cholangitis should be managed with liver biopsy, culture, and appropriate antibiotics. Some patients with chronic cholangitis may require antibiotic prophylaxis.
- Endoscopic sclerotherapy and/or variceal banding provide relief from variceal hemorrhage in many cases.
- Activity:
  – No contact sports if splenomegaly is present.
  – Spleen guard may be used to protect against injury from abdominal trauma.

SURGERY/OTHER PROCEDURES
- Portosystemic shunting may be required.
- Liver transplant may be indicated for chronic cholangitis, recurrent bleeding, or progressive hepatic disease.
- Some children may require combined liver and renal transplantation.

ONGOING CARE

FOLLOW-UP RECOMMENDATIONS
Patient Monitoring
- Watch for recurrent upper GI tract bleeding.
- Morbidity occurs mainly from portal hypertension and cholangitis.
- There is an increased incidence of portal hypertension with age.
- Mortality may result from ascending cholangitis associated with sepsis and hepatic failure.
- Those presenting during childhood have better prognosis compared to those presenting within neonatal period

DIET
No restrictions are needed.

PROGNOSIS
- Good for older children who present with CHF.
- Ascending cholangitis with resultant sepsis and hepatic failure is a major cause of morbidity and mortality.

COMPLICATIONS
- Portal hypertension with hypersplenism and variceal bleeding
- Cholangitis
- Renal and/or hepatic failure
- Associated vascular anomalies in the liver and brain
- Increased risk of hepatocellular or cholangiocarcinoma
- Systemic hypertension owing to renal involvement

ADDITIONAL READING

- Badano JL, Mitsuma N, Beales PL, et al. The ciliopathies: An emerging class of human genetic disorders. *Annu Rev Genomics Hum Genet.* 2006;7:125–148.
- Guay-Woodford LM, Desmond RA. Autosomal recessive polycystic kidney disease: The clinical experience in North America. *Pediatrics.* 2003;111(5 Pt 1):1072–1080.
- Gunay-Aygun M, Avner ED, Bacallao RL, et al. Autosomal recessive polycystic kidney disease and congenital hepatic fibrosis: Summary statement of a first National Institutes of Health/Office of Rare Diseases conference. *J Pediatr.* 2006;149(2):159–164.
- Harris PC, Rossetti S. Molecular genetics of autosomal recessive polycystic kidney disease. *Mol Genet Metab.* 2004;81:75–85.
- Harris PC, Torres VE. Polycystic kidney disease. *Annu Rev Med.* 2009;60:321–337.

CODES

ICD9
777.8 Other specified perinatal disorders of digestive system

ICD10
P78.89 Other specified perinatal digestive system disorders

FAQ
- Q: Will other children of mine be affected?
- A: Maybe. The inheritance pattern is autosomal recessive, with the possibility of an affected sibling being 1:4.
- Q: Is my child at increased risk if he contracts viral hepatitis?
- A: Yes, the underlying liver disease places these patients at increased risk. They should be immunized against hepatitis A and B.
- Q: If my child has a fever, does she need to be seen by her doctor?
- A: Yes. Patients with CHF who have fever without an obvious source should be evaluated for possible cholangitis, at least by obtaining a blood culture and liver enzymes.

CONGENITAL HYPOTHYROIDISM

Adda Grimberg

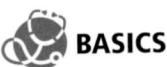 **BASICS**

DESCRIPTION
Primary thyroid failure that is present at birth

EPIDEMIOLOGY
Incidence
- Increasing trend in the US of unclear etiology (definitional issues related to newborn screening vs. true increase from unidentified risk factors)
  - Had been 1 in 3,000–4,000 births, US and worldwide
  - In 2007, US incidence 1 in 2,370 births
- Male/female ratio is 1:2–1:3.
- 80% dysgenesis or agenesis; 20% dyshormonogenesis

Prevalence
- Racial differences: Prevalence in black infants ~1/3 that in whites
- Higher prevalence of congenital hypothyroidism in low-birth-weight (>2,000 g) and macrosomic (≥4,500 g) babies

RISK FACTORS
Genetics
- Dysgenesis is usually sporadic.
  - Familial occurrence in 2%
  - Mutations have been found in the TSH-receptor gene and in the transcription factors PAX-8, TTF-1, and TTF-2 (FOXE1).
- Dyshormonogenesis is inherited in an autosomal recessive pattern. Most commonly:
  - Chromosome 2p: Mutations in the thyroid peroxidase gene result in partial or complete loss of iodide organification.
  - Chromosome 19p: Mutations in the sodium-iodide symporter gene result in an inability to maintain the normal thyroid-to-plasma iodine concentration difference.
- Pendred syndrome (chromosome 7q): Mutations in PDS gene cause the most common syndromal form of deafness; a mild organification defect leads to goiter, usually in childhood.
- Down syndrome neonates have lower T_4 (left-shifted normal distribution) and mildly elevated TSH, suggesting a mild hypothyroid state.

ETIOLOGY
- Thyroid gland malformation:
  - Agenesis: Absent thyroid gland
  - Dysgenesis: Ectopic (e.g., sublingual) or incorrectly formed (e.g., hemigland) thyroid
- Dyshormonogenesis:
  - 15 known defects of thyroxine (T_4) synthesis, including those in iodide transport and iodide organification
- Transient hypothyroidism:
  - Maternal ingestion of antithyroid drugs
  - Transplacental transfer of maternal antithyroid antibodies (transient or permanent damage)
  - Exposure to high levels of iodine-povidone, Betadine in neonatal period

DIAGNOSIS

HISTORY
- Symptoms that may relate to hypothyroidism:
  - Prolonged jaundice
  - Poor feeding
  - Constipation
  - Sedate or placid child
  - Poor linear growth
- Family history of thyroid disorders:
  - Autoimmune thyroid disease
  - Vague histories of "mild hypothyroidism" not requiring treatment are often found in families with thyroid-binding globulin deficiency.
- Maternal medications
- Birth history
- Results of the newborn screen
- Signs and symptoms:
  - Most children are diagnosed by the neonatal screening program:
    - 5–10% false-negative rate
    - Neonatal screening protocols differ state to state (i.e., may screen T_4, TSH, or both).
    - In severely ill neonates who are transferred from 1 unit or hospital to another, be sure the state screen is not overlooked! If missed by the state screening procedure, the symptoms above are seen within the 1st 2 months of life.

PHYSICAL EXAM
- Signs that may relate to hypothyroidism:
  - Hypothermia
  - Large fontanelles (especially posterior) with wide cranial sutures
  - Coarse facial features, including macroglossia
  - Hoarse cry
  - Hypotonia
  - Delayed deep tendon reflex release
  - Distended abdomen
  - Umbilical hernia
- Examine for possible goiter; helpful tricks:
  - Inspect the base of tongue for ectopic gland.
  - While supporting the posterior neck and occiput, allow the infant's head to hang back over a parent's arm or exam table. This will extend the neck and allow better visualization of the anterior region.

DIAGNOSTIC TESTS & INTERPRETATION
Lab
- Neonatal screening program (filter card):
  - Methods vary from state to state; screen for T_4 and then run TSH levels on the lowest 10th percentile of that day's T_4 values or screen for TSH elevations.
  - Abnormal results on state screen should prompt *immediate* examination and confirmatory tests.
  - Because of delayed TSH elevations, very low-birth-weight babies and those with congenital cardiac anomalies may need rescreening for diagnosis.

- Confirmatory tests:
  - Serum T_4 and TSH are preferable to a repeated filter screen, which may result in delayed diagnosis and treatment.
  - If abnormalities in binding are suspected, also check thyroid-binding globulin level and free T_4 level or tri-iodothyronine (T_3) resin uptake.
  - Free T_4 level is the most sensitive indicator of secondary or tertiary hypothyroidism (hypopituitarism).
- Antenatal tests:
  - Fetal goiter can be detected by prenatal ultrasound.
- Reference ranges for 3rd trimester amniotic fluid concentrations of TSH and total and free T_4 are established for diagnosis of fetal hypothyroidism among those with goiters. Otherwise, cordocentesis is needed.

Imaging
- ^{123}I or technetium thyroid scan to define gland anatomy (agenesis, dysgenesis, ectopic gland)
- ^{123}I scan with perchlorate washout to help identify dyshormonogenesis
- ^{123}I scan must be obtained before beginning thyroxine replacement therapy. If this delays treatment, defer scanning until brain growth is complete (2 years of age), when a period off medication is safer.
- Ultrasonography can also evaluate thyroid anatomy (but not dyshormonogenesis) and does not require deferral of treatment.

DIFFERENTIAL DIAGNOSIS
- Developmental:
  - Transient hypothyroxinemia in the 1st weeks of life in premature babies
- Metabolic:
  - Sick euthyroid syndrome in severely ill neonates
- Secondary or tertiary:
  - Panhypopituitarism
  - Congenital isolated central hypothyroidism (a "hot spot" mutation in the TSH-β gene)
  - Central congenital hypothyroidism due to maternal Graves disease during pregnancy (estimated incidence 1:35,000; thought to indicate impaired maturation of the fetal hypothalamic–pituitary–thyroid system from a hyperthyroid fetal environment)
- Genetic:
  - Thyroid-binding globulin deficiency (X-linked recessive)
- Environmental:
  - Iodine exposure (e.g., delivery by cesarean section, surgery in the neonatal period)
  - Maternal iodine deficiency (American Thyroid Association has recommended that pregnant and lactating women take prenatal vitamins containing 150 mcg of iodine daily)
  - Maternal use of antithyroid drugs or lithium

- Immunologic:
  - Transfer of maternal antithyroid and TSH-receptor blocking antibodies

ALERT

False positives:
- X-linked thyroid-binding globulin deficiency: Low total T_4, normal TSH, and normal free T_4. Diagnose with low thyroid-binding globulin level or high T_3 resin uptake. No treatment is necessary!
- Panhypopituitarism: Low T_4 and low or low-normal TSH (i.e., loss of the negative feedback loop). Screen with free T_4. Treat with L-thyroxine as for primary hypothyroidism, and investigate for other pituitary hormone deficiencies.
- Blood specimens obtained before 48 hours of life may have "elevated" TSH as a result of the normal postnatal surge.

False negatives:
- Normal newborn screening can be falsely reassuring in babies with congenital central hypothyroidism.

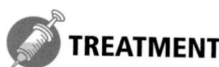 **TREATMENT**

MEDICATION (DRUGS)

L-Thyroxine:
- 10–15 mcg/kg/d once a day. Titer dose to keep T_4 in the upper range of normal.
- TSH levels may not normalize for several weeks, even with good T_4 values.
- A minority of infants have variable pituitary–thyroid hormone resistance, with relatively elevated serum levels of TSH for their free T_4 that improves with age.
- Starting dose of 50 mcg daily (12–17 mcg/kg/d) may provide more rapid normalization (free T_4 by 3 days and TSH by 2 weeks).
- Duration: Lifelong:
  - If medication is started without imaging studies and diagnosis is not clear, can stop L-thyroxine after completion of brain growth (2–3 years of age). Re-evaluate need for supplementation after a 6-week trial off.

 ONGOING CARE

FOLLOW-UP RECOMMENDATIONS

- When to expect improvement:
  - Most children are asymptomatic at diagnosis.
  - Parents may note an increase in activity, improvement in feeding, and increase in urination and bowel movements soon after starting treatment.
- Signs to watch for: Poor growth and low T_4 and elevated TSH values suggest poor compliance or undertreatment. Neuropsychologic sequelae:
  - IQ scores are predominantly in the normal range, but subtle impairments in language and motor skills and specific learning disabilities may occur despite early treatment. Neurocognitive evaluation and rehabilitation should be provided.
  - Maternal hypothyroxinemia during early gestation can lead to neurodevelopmental delays if not corrected during pregnancy.

DIET

- No restrictions
- Soybean flour (as in some formulas) can decrease gastrointestinal absorption of L-thyroxine.
- Pharmacies in recent years have been recommending that L-thyroxine be administered on an empty stomach. The Drugs and Therapeutics Committee of the Pediatric Endocrine Society recommended that consistency in administration, coupled with regular dose titration to thyroid function tests, is more important than improving absorption by restricting intake to only times of empty stomach.

PATIENT EDUCATION

- Whether the child will be retarded depends on when the diagnosis was made and how quickly treatment was started. There may be an increase in learning disabilities when compared with siblings, even in patients treated within the 1st 4 weeks of life.
- If a dose is forgotten, it should be given as soon as it is remembered. If it is the next day, 2 doses should be given.
- L-Thyroxine is available only in tablet form. The tablet should be crushed between 2 spoons and the powder dissolved in a small amount of formula or breast milk and offered to the baby at the *start* of a feeding to ensure complete ingestion.
- There are no side effects from the medication. The tablet contains only the hormone that the child's thyroid is not making. It is synthetically produced, so there are no infectious risks.

PROGNOSIS

- Excellent, if treatment is started within the 1st 2 weeks of life
- Level of T_4 at birth is an important indicator of long-term sequelae.

COMPLICATIONS

- If untreated:
  - Severe mental retardation (cretinism)
  - Poor motor development
  - Poor growth
- Children with hypothyroidism as part of hypopituitarism do not seem to be as significantly affected by their low thyroid hormone levels as do those with primary hypothyroidism.

ADDITIONAL READING

- American Academy of Pediatrics, Rose SR, Section on Endocrinology and Committee on Genetics, et al. Update of newborn screening and therapy for congenital hypothyroidism. *Pediatrics*. 2006;117: 2290–2303.
- Bubuteishvili L, Garel C, Czernichow P, et al. Thyroid abnormalities by ultrasonography in neonates with congenital hypothyroidism. *J Pediatr*. 2003;143: 759–764.
- Delahunty C, Falconer S, Hume R, et al. Levels of neonatal thyroid hormone in preterm infants and neurodevelopmental outcome at 5 1/2 years: Millennium Cohort Study. *J Clin Endocrinol Metab*. 2010;95:4898–4908.
- Fisher DA, Schoen EJ, La Franchi S, et al. The hypothalamic-pituitary-thyroid negative feedback control axis in children with treated congenital hypothyroidism. *J Clin Endocrinol Metab*. 2000; 85:2722–2727.

- Fu J, Jiang Y, Liang L, et al. Risk factors of primary thyroid dysfunction in early infants born to mothers with autoimmune thyroid disease. *Acta Paediatr*. 2005;94:1043–1048.
- Kempers MJ, Ozgen HM, Vulsma T, et al. Morphological abnormalities in children with thyroidal congenital hypothyroidism. *Am J Med Genet A*. 2009;149A:943–951.
- Kempers MJ, van Tijn DA, van Trotsenburg AS, et al. Central congenital hypothyroidism due to gestational hyperthyroidism: Detection where prevention failed. *J Clin Endocrinol Metab*. 2003;88:5851–5857.
- Larson C, Hermos R, Delaney A, et al. Risk factors associated with delayed thyrotropin elevations in congenital hypothyroidism. *J Pediatr*. 2003;143: 587–591.
- Leung AM, Pearce EN, Braverman LE. Iodine content of prenatal multivitamins in the United States. *N Engl J Med*. 2009;360:939–940.
- Nebesio TD, McKenna MP, Nabhan ZM, et al. Newborn screening results in children with central hypothyroidism. *J Pediatr*. 2010;156:990–993.
- Ng SM, Anand D, Weindling AM. High versus low dose of initial thyroid hormone replacement for congenital hypothyroidism. *Cochrane Database Syst Rev*. 2009;(1):CD006972.
- Oerbeck B, Sundet K, Kase BF, et al. Congenital hypothyroidism: Influence of disease severity and L-thyroxine treatment on intellectual, motor, and school-associated outcomes in young adults. *Pediatrics*. 2003;112:923–930.
- Olney RS, Grosse SD, Vogt RF Jr. Prevalence of congenital hypothyroidism—current trends and future directions: Workshop summary. *Pediatrics*. 2010;125(Suppl 2):S31–S36.
- Park SM, Chatterjee VK. Genetics of congenital hypothyroidism. *J Med Genet*. 2005;42:379–389.
- Raymond J, LaFranchi SH. Fetal and neonatal thyroid function: Review and summary of significant new findings. *Curr Opin Endocrinol Diabetes Obes*. 2010;17:1–7.
- van Trotsenburg AS, Vulsma T, van Santen HM, et al. Lower neonatal screening thyroxine concentrations in Down syndrome newborns. *J Clin Endocrinol Metab*. 2003;88:1512–1515.

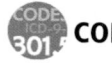 **CODES**

ICD9

- 243 Congenital hypothyroidism (disorder)
- 269.3 Mineral deficiency, not elsewhere classified
- 759.89 Other specified congenital anomalies

ICD10

- E03.0 Congenital hypothyroidism with diffuse goiter
- E03.1 Congenital hypothyroidism without goiter
- E00.9 Congenital iodine-deficiency syndrome, unspecified

FAQ

- Q: What are some of the reasons that a normal newborn will have an abnormal thyroid screen?
- A: Blood tests obtained prior to 48 hours of age may have an elevated TSH from newborn surge; some states (for quality control) will ask to have a certain percentage of tests repeated, even though they are normal.

CONGESTIVE HEART FAILURE

Jondavid Menteer

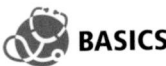 **BASICS**

DESCRIPTION

Heart failure (HF) is the pathophysiologic state in which the heart is unable to pump sufficient blood to meet the metabolic demands of the body.

- Right heart failure:
  - Hepatomegaly
  - Jugular venous distension
  - Edema
  - Right ventricular/parasternal heave
  - Ascites, pleural effusions
- Left Heart Failure:
  - Tachypnea, retractions, grunting
  - Pulmonary edema, rales
  - Orthopnea
  - Shock/depressed perfusion
  - Diffuse/displaced point of maximum impulse (PMI)
- Either left or right heart failure:
  - Exercise intolerance
  - Tachycardia
  - Sweating, especially. when supine/sleeping
  - Poor perfusion/pulses
  - Poor feeding/GI symptoms
  - Growth failure (primarily weight)

RISK FACTORS

- In Utero
  - Arrhythmias: Supraventricular or ventricular tachycardia, complete heart block (CHB)
  - Volume overload: Atrioventricular (AV) valve regurgitation or arteriovenous malformation (AVM)
  - Primary myocardial disease: Cardiomyopathy (dilated, hypertrophic), myocarditis
  - Anemia: Rh isoimmune disease, thalassemia, and twin-twin transfusion
  - Premature closure of ductus arteriosus with isolated right ventricular failure
- In Neonates
  - Myocardial dysfunction: Asphyxia, acidosis, myocarditis, hypoglycemia, cardiomyopathy (dilated, hypertrophic, ventricular noncompaction), ischemia (anomalous left coronary artery from the pulmonary artery), metabolic defects, or pressure overload imposed by aortic stenosis, pulmonary hypertension, or coarctation of the aorta.
  - Volume overload: atrial septal defect (ASD) (large), ventricular septal defect (VSD) (large), patent ductus arteriosus (PDA) (moderate to large), truncus arteriosus, aortopulmonary window, anomalous pulmonary venous return, AVM in any location.
  - Arrhythmias: supraventricular or ventricular tachycardia, CHB.
  - Left heart inlet obstruction: Mitral stenosis, cor triatriatum, pulmonary venous obstruction.
  - Note: Certain cyanotic heart diseases such as hypoplastic left heart syndrome may present with elevated pulmonary blood flow or depressed systemic blood flow, and minimal desaturation. These patients may have HF in the first days of life due to increased pulmonary circulation or due to shock from ductal closure.
- In Infants
  - Myocardial dysfunction: Cardiomyopathy (dilated, hypertrophic, restrictive, ventricular noncompaction), endocardial fibroelastosis, metabolic/mitochondrial diseases, myocarditis, Kawasaki disease, anomalous left coronary artery

from pulmonary artery, or chronic pressure overload due to coarctation of the aorta or aortic stenosis.
  - Volume overload: ASD (large), VSD, PDA, common AV canal defect, partial anomalous pulmonary venous connections.
  - Secondary causes: renal disease (volume overload, electrolyte disturbance), hypertension, hypothyroidism, sepsis.
  - Arrhythmias: supraventricular or ventricular tachycardia, CHB.
  - Pericardial effusion due to juvenile rheumatoid arthritis (JRA), systemic lupus erythematosus (SLE), other inflammatory diseases, or following repair of congenital heart disease (CHD).
- In Childhood and Adolescence
  - Unrepaired CHD with volume and/or pressure overload.
  - Repaired CHD with residual defects that result in volume and/or pressure overload.
  - Acquired heart disease: Pericarditis, myocarditis, endocarditis, acute rheumatic fever.
  - Cor pulmonale (pulmonary hypertension, Eisenmenger syndrome, chronic lung disease).
  - Cardiomyopathy due to primary myocardial disease (dilated, hypertrophic, restrictive, ventricular noncompaction), chemotherapy (anthracyclines), radiation therapy, sickle cell anemia, thalassemia, neuromuscular disease (e.g., Duchenne or Becker muscular dystrophy).

GENERAL PREVENTION

- Limited use of cardiac anthracycline drugs in cancer therapy
- Prompt treatment (within 1 week) of streptococcal pharyngitis to prevent rheumatic fever
- SBE prophylaxis to prevent infective endocarditis

ALERT

- In patients with HF due to large left-to-right shunts, long-term spontaneous clinical improvement of HF with decreased murmur may indicate the development of pulmonary vascular disease (Eisenmenger syndrome), leading to cyanosis eventually.
- Care must be used in the administration of oxygen to the undiagnosed infant with heart disease. A patient with single-ventricle physiology (e.g., hypoplastic left heart syndrome) can have manifestations of heart failure and mild desaturation (92–98%). Providing oxygen in this situation can result in shock due to excessive pulmonary blood flow and inadequate systemic blood flow.

ETIOLOGY

- Low cardiac output HF (e.g., all cardiomyopathy, severe atrioventricular valve regurgitation)
- High cardiac output HF
  - Left-to-right shunts (e.g.,t ASD, VSD, PDA)
  - AVM
  - Anemia and other non-cardiovascular causes

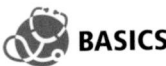 **DIAGNOSIS**

HISTORY

- Infants and Neonates
  - Prolonged feedings associated with tachypnea, retractions, or diaphoresis.

  - Emesis, inadequate caloric intake, irritability with feeding, and failure to thrive.
  - Frequent respiratory infections.
  - Orthopnea – "spoiled baby" becomes distressed when supine.
  - Family history of HF or sudden unexpected deaths.
- Childhood and Adolescence
  - Exercise intolerance with exertional dyspnea.
  - Palpitations or chest pain, especially during exercise.
  - Chronic cough, wheezing, orthopnea, fatigue, weakness, anorexia, nausea, and edema.
  - Gradual weight loss (anorexia, nausea, and increased metabolic demands).
  - Sudden weight gain (fluid retention).
  - Family history of HF or unexpected deaths at a young age.

PHYSICAL EXAM

- Infants And Neonates
  - Tachycardia
  - Gallop rhythm
  - Murmur of outflow obstruction, elevated flow, AV valve regurgitation, VSD, or semilunar valve incompetence.
  - Systolic click (semilunar valve abnormalities)
  - Abnormal second heart sound (fixed split, loud P2 component)
  - Tachypnea, wheezing, crackles, rales
  - Nasal flaring/grunting/retractions
  - Abdominal or cranial bruit
  - Hepatomegaly +/− splenomegaly
  - Edema (periorbital)
  - Cool and/or mottled extremities
  - Poor capillary refill or pulses
- Children And Adolescents
  - Tachycardia
  - Gallop rhythm
  - Murmur of outflow obstruction, elevated flow, AV valve regurgitation, VSD, or semilunar valve incompetence.
  - Loud second heart sound (P2 component)
  - Hyperactive precordium, displaced PMI
  - Tachypnea, retractions
  - Wheezing ("cardiac asthma") or rales
  - Jugular venous distension
  - Hepatomegaly +/− splenomegaly
  - Edema (periorbital, peripheral)
  - Pulsus alternans, pulsus paradoxus
  - Cool extremities, poor pulses, poor capillary refill
  - Evaluation of mucus membranes, skin, and extremities for manifestations of Kawasaki disease, rheumatic fever, or endocarditis

DIAGNOSTIC TESTS & INTERPRETATION
Diagnostic Procedures/Other

- Chest X-ray
- Cardiomegaly, increased pulmonary vascular markings, hyperinflation, pleural effusion, Kerley-B lines.
- Electrocardiography
  - Abnormal P-waves
  - ST-T wave changes (ischemia, strain, inflammation/myocarditis)
  - Heart block (1st, 2nd, 3rd degree) or tachyarrhythmia.
  - Characteristic ECG findings such as anomalous left coronary artery from the pulmonary artery (Q waves and/or inverted T waves in leads I and aVL, left ventricular hypertrophy, right ventricular hypertrophy, and/or lateral Q waves with or without active ischemic changes)

- Pericarditis pattern (diffuse ST elevation and/or low QRS voltage)
- Hypertrophy (cardiomyopathy, CHD, storage disease)
• Echocardiography
  - Rule out CHD, evaluate coronary origins
  - Assessment of cardiac systolic and diastolic function
• Cardiac Catheterization (for selected cases)
  - Assessment of cardiac hemodynamics and anatomy.
  - Endomyocardial biopsy may be helpful in the diagnosis of myocarditis, storage disease, or cardiomyopathy.
  - Electrophysiologic study to evaluate for the induction of arrhythmia.
  - Therapy (see later)
• Cardiac MRI or CT (for selected cases)
  - Delineation of complex anatomic abnormality
  - Right ventricular performance
• Other Laboratory Abnormalities
  - Blood gas: Metabolic acidosis with elevated lactate.
  - Chemistry: Hyponatremia (dilutional), pre-renal state
  - Blood counts: Anemia, leukocytosis, or leukopenia (e.g., viral myocarditis)
  - ESR elevation (e.g., acute rheumatic fever or Kawasaki disease)
  - B-type natriuretic peptide (BNP or NT-BNP) elevation
  - Urine: Proteinuria, high urine specific gravity, microscopic hematuria
  - Evaluation for metabolic causes of cardiomyopathy may include pyruvate, amino acid quantification, urine organic acids, carnitine, selenium, acylcarnitine profile, liver function tests
  - Viral evaluation (adenovirus, coxsackievirus, Epstein–Barr virus, cytomegalovirus, parvovirus, echovirus, etc.)

DIFFERENTIAL DIAGNOSIS
• Tachycardia:
  - Fever
  - Dehydration
  - Anemia
  - Supraventricular tachycardia or ventricular tachycardia without heart failure
  - Hyperthyroidism
  - Pericardial effusion
• Tachypnea:
  - Respiratory disease or infection
  - Pulmonary venous obstruction
  - Acidosis (metabolic disease, poisoning, etc)
  - Pneumothorax/pleural effusion
  - Carbon monoxide poisoning
• Edema:
  - Hypoalbuminemia
  - Systemic inflammatory conditions / allergies
  - Hypothyroidism
• Sepsis
  - Hepatomegaly:
  - Liver disease
  - Storage disease
  - Extramedullary hematopoiesis

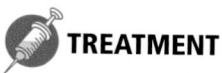

TREATMENT

ADDITIONAL TREATMENT
General Measures
Treatment of Underlying Cause
• Surgical palliation or correction of structural abnormality.

• Interventional cardiac catheterization (e.g., balloon dilation of aortic or pulmonary stenosis, coil embolization of patent ductus arteriosus, device closure of ASD, dilation, or stenting of coarctation of the aorta).
• Carnitine, Coenzyme Q10, riboflavin, antioxidant replacement for select cardiomyopathies.
• Targeted medical treatment of endocarditis, myocarditis, anemia, rheumatic fever, Kawasaki disease, or hypertension.
• Radiofrequency ablation of tachyarrhythmia.
• Medical therapy for patients, or mothers of fetuses with tachyarrhythmia.
• Pacing for bradyarrhythmias (e.g., heart block).
• Control of chronic inflammatory conditions, such as SLE or JRA.

COMPLEMENTARY & ALTERNATIVE THERAPIES
Management
• Assessment of degree of illness:
  - If perfusion is compromised or acidosis is present, ICU care is indicated.
  - Hospitalization may be necessary to initiate treatment or prepare for surgery in some cases (coronary abnormalities, aortic coarctation, myocarditis).
  - Many patients diagnosed as outpatients with CHD or cardiomyopathy may not require inpatient treatment. Immediate consultation with a pediatric cardiologist should be arranged.
• Immediate Management:
  - General measures: Activity restriction as indicated, oxygen as needed (not for patients with pulmonary overcirculation),
  - Sometimes: Tube feedings or parenteral nutrition if there is concern for splanchnic circulation or severe failure to thrive.
  - Drainage of pericardial effusion, if needed.
  - Inotropic agents (digoxin, milrinone, dobutamine in refractory cases, etc)
  - Intravenous immunoglobulin (IVIG) for myocarditis or Kawasaki disease
  - Loop diuretics (e.g., furosemide)
  - Nesiritide (synthetic BNP) for refractory fluid overload
  - Mechanical respiratory or circulatory support, if necessary (ventilator, extracorporeal membrane oxygenation, ventricular assist device)
• Chronic therapy:
  - Digoxin
  - Loop diuretics (e.g., furosemide) for fluid overload/edema
  - Afterload reduction [e.g. angiotensin-converting enzyme (ACE) inhibitors]
  - Antagonism of activated neurohormonal systems: ACE inhibitor or angiotensin receptor blocker, spironolactone, beta-blocker
  - Anticoagulation or anti-platelet therapy (especially in restrictive and severe dilated cardiomyopathy)
  - Biventricular pacing/resynchronization in some cases
  - Heart and heart/lung transplantation in select cases

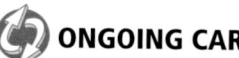 ONGOING CARE

FOLLOW-UP RECOMMENDATIONS
• Dependent on the etiology and degree of HF. Generally, initial follow-up of a patient with heart failure should be intensive, focussed on assessing response to therapy. Initial follow-up generally weekly, spreading to monthly or quarterly over time, under the supervision of a pediatric cardiologist.

• Depending on the etiology and degree of HF, echocardiography, ECG, blood chemistry, BNP levels, INR, Holter monitoring, and chest radiographs will be evaluated.

ADDITIONAL READING
• Aurbach SR, Richmond ME, Lamour JM, et al. BNP Levels Predict Outcome in Pediatric Heart Failure Patients: Post-hoc Analysis of the Pediatric Carvedilol Trial. *Circulation Heart Fail.* 2010;3:616–611.
• Hetzer R, Potapov EV, Stiller B, et al. Improvement in survival after mechanical circulatory support with pneumatic pulsatile ventricular assist devices in pediatric patients. *Ann Thorac Surg.* 2006;82: 917–925.
• Kay JD, Colan SD, Graham Jr TP. Congestive heart failure in pediatric patients. *Am Heart J.* 2001; 142(5):923–928.
• Shaddy RE. Optimizing treatment for chronic congestive heart failure in children. *Crit Care Med.* 2001;29(10 Suppl):S237–S240.

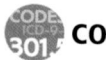 CODES

ICD9
• 428.0 Congestive heart failure, unspecified
• 428.1 Left heart failure
• 428.9 Heart failure, unspecified

ICD10
• I50.1 Left ventricular failure
• I50.9 Heart failure, unspecified
• Q24.9 Congenital malformation of heart, unspecified

FAQ
• Q: My child has a large VSD and is prescribed digoxin and furosemide. Should I take salt out of his diet?
• A: No. Excessive salt restriction is seldom enforceable and is not necessary. A no-added-salt diet is generally sufficient.
• Q: What is the importance of tachycardia and bradycardia in heart failure?
• A: Tachycardia limits diastolic filling time and may result in a decreased output. However, bradycardia may be poorly tolerated in patients with heart failure and a relatively fixed stroke volume who are dependent on heart rate to maintain an appropriate output. Either may be problematic for a patient in chronic heart failure. Most HF patients do not have as much heart rate variation as healthy people.
• Q: What are the major causes of death to heart failure patients?
• A: Younger children tend to die of progressive heart failure. Ventricular arrhythmias are the most common cause of sudden death in older children and adults with HF. Other causes of mortality include infection and stroke.
• Q: My patient has a normal blood pressure, but the cardiologist says more ACE inhibition is necessary. Why?
• A: Blood pressure is the weight that the myocardial muscle must "lift" with every beat. By decreasing the blood pressure as much as possible (short of causing dizziness or syncope), the work done by the heart and myocardial oxygen consumption are reduced. Reduction of the systemic blood pressure also potentially reduces the amount of left-to-right shunting through a VSD, PDA, and AP window.

CONJUNCTIVITIS

Anne K. Jensen
Brian J. Forbes
William R. Katowitz (5th edition)

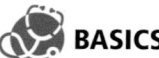 **BASICS**

DESCRIPTION
An inflammatory process of the conjunctiva, the membrane covering the eye and inside of the eyelids, manifested by redness and edema, frequently with associated discharge. It is critical to rule out *Gonococcus* infection because of the destructive nature of the eye disease and associated systemic infection.

EPIDEMIOLOGY
Incidence
- Children: Viral infection is the most common cause and is highly contagious.
- Neonates: Ophthalmia neonatorum, conjunctivitis in the 1st month of life, is the most common infection in neonates. Remains a significant cause of blindness in children worldwide. *Chlamydia trachomatis* is the most common infectious cause.

PATHOPHYSIOLOGY
- Results from bacterial, viral, allergic, or toxic activation of the inflammatory response that causes dilation and exudation from conjunctival blood vessels
- Pathology involves dilated conjunctival capillaries with leukocytic infiltration and edema of conjunctiva and substantia propria.

ETIOLOGY
- Ophthalmia neonatorum
  - In the 1st 24 hours of life, most likely due to irritation from silver nitrate or Betadine eyedrops.
  - *Gonococcus* conjunctivitis is treatable if recognized early but devastating if diagnosis is delayed or missed.
  - Chronic *Chlamydia* infection can lead to scarring and corneal opacity. *Chlamydial pneumonia* develops in 20% of patients with chlamydial conjunctivitis.
- Bacterial
  - Agents include staphylococci, streptococci, *Pseudomonas*, and *Haemophilus*, and serious complications of these are rare.
- Viral
  - Adenovirus is the most common agent.
  - Recurrent herpes simplex virus infection can lead to significant visual loss from corneal scarring, even with proper therapy.
  - Other viral etiologies usually follow a benign course, but may rarely lead to conjunctival scarring.
- Allergic
  - Histamine-mediated response

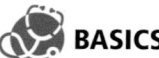 **DIAGNOSIS**

HISTORY
- Ophthalmia neonatorum
  - *Gonococcus:* Typically presents 2–4 days after birth with mucopurulent discharge.
  - *Chlamydia:* Typically presents 4–10 days after birth with mucopurulent discharge.
- Bacterial
  - Eye redness and mucopurulent discharge. Patient may complain of sticky eyelids upon waking. Mild photophobia and discomfort may be present but are typically not painful.
- Viral
  - HSV ocular infection may present as conjunctivitis. Often associated with corneal anesthesia, so painless. In neonates, occurs 1–2 weeks after birth as unilateral serous discharge and conjunctival injection.
  - Other viral causes often present with upper respiratory symptoms, fever, sore throat, eye redness, tearing, serous discharge, eyelid edema, and photophobia. Typically begins in one eye but spreads to the other within a few days. History of similar infection in siblings or contacts is common.
- Allergic
  - Bilateral itching and tearing. Classically, a complaint of itching or foreign body sensation in an older child with red eyes

PHYSICAL EXAM
- General
  - Cornea is clear.
  - Vision, pupils, and motility are normal.
  - Refer to an ophthalmologist for vesicular rash on eyelids or corneal changes, as the condition may be caused by herpes simplex virus and can be vision threatening.
- Bacterial
  - Mucopurulent discharge (opaque and thick)
  - Injected conjunctiva, episcleral vessels, palpebral conjunctival papillae
  - Preauricular lymphadenopathy less common
- Viral
  - HSV ocular infection may involve corneal ulceration or dendritic or disciform keratitis.
  - Serous discharge (clear and watery)
  - May involve pseudomembrane formation, pinpoint subconjunctival hemorrhages, and palpable preauricular lymph nodes
- Allergic
  - Bilateral conjunctival edema and chemosis

ALERT
- Failure to diagnose *Gonococcus* conjunctivitis may lead to corneal perforation.
- HSV ocular infection is associated with a significant risk of blindness. Have high suspicion for HSV with any recurrent unilateral eye redness, corneal changes, or vesicular rash on eyelids.
- Steroids can activate or accelerate unrecognized herpes simplex virus infection, and chronic use can lead to raised intraocular pressure or cataract formation.
- Chronic use of empiric broad-spectrum antibiotics for self-limited conjunctivitis can promote bacterial resistance though less so than for systemic antibiotic administration.

DIAGNOSTIC TESTS & INTERPRETATION
Lab
- Gram stain
  - Note: Always for ophthalmia neonatorum
  - *Gonococcus:* Gram-negative intracellular diplococcus
  - *Chlamydia:* Intracytoplasmic, paranuclear inclusion bodies on Gram stain and conjunctival scraping with Giemsa stain for basophilic intracytoplasmic inclusion bodies
  - Viral or chemical: Polymorphonuclear leukocytes without bacteria.
- Culture
  - Viral: Cultures for HSV and adenovirus are not clinically useful.
  - Bacterial: Blood agar and chocolate agar
  - *Gonococcus:* Thayer-Martin media
  - *Chlamydia:* Culture techniques are not widely available. However, they remain the gold standard for diagnosis. Specimens should be obtained using an aluminum shafted Dacron-tipped swab and processed within 24 hours. A positive test is confirmed when the organism is identified using fluorescein-conjugated monoclonal antibody. Other equally effective methods involve polymerase chain reaction or direct fluorescent antibody.
- Conjunctival scrapings
  - Allergic: Mast cells and eosinophils
- Serum tests
  - Allergic: Immunoglobulin E may be elevated.
  - *Chlamydia:* The diagnosis of *Chlamydial* pneumonia can be made with a serum test, but is not reliable for *Chlamydial* conjunctivitis.

DIFFERENTIAL DIAGNOSIS
- Ophthalmia neonatorum
  - Chemical conjunctivitis: Noninfectious, mild, self-limited. Result of silver nitrate or povidone-iodine administration
  - Birth trauma: Unilateral, often with associated eyelid contusion, history of forceps use or difficult delivery
  - Congenital glaucoma: Mild redness, minimal discharge. Look for enlarged eye, cloudy cornea, tearing, and photophobia.
  - Nasolacrimal duct obstruction: Unilateral or bilateral discharge, may be clear to mucopurulent with reflux from nasolacrimal sac. Conjunctiva is usually white and nonerythematous.
- All conjunctivitis

- Preseptal cellulitis: Early eyelid edema/erythema. Looks like conjunctivitis, especially in young children with a difficult exam. Motility deficit, proptosis, decreased vision, and afferent pupillary defect are consistent with orbital cellulitis.
- Keratitis: Signifies corneal infection. May have associated conjunctivitis. Primary herpes keratitis is associated with vesicular eyelid rash and pain. Consult an ophthalmologist. Bacterial keratitis may be caused by staphylococci, streptococci, and *Pseudomonas*; Lyme spirochete; or vitamin A deficiency.
- Episcleritis: Inflammation of the thick loose connective tissue between the clear conjunctiva and the white-appearing stroma of the sclera. Rare disease in childhood. Can be associated with rheumatologic disease
- Scleritis: Presents as red eye. Severe disease involving inflammation of the sclera. Rare in childhood. Associated with systemic disease. Requires oral or IV steroids
- Iritis: Frequently unilateral, with or without a history of trauma. Photophobia, decreased vision, and constant pain (except if associated with juvenile rheumatoid arthritis). Contagious history is rare. Consult an ophthalmologist for full evaluation, including pupillary dilation.
- Systemic diseases with red eye
  - Varicella: Ocular involvement in rare cases. Treat with antiviral medications.
  - Stevens-Johnson syndrome: Secondary to viruses, mycoplasma, or adverse drug reaction. Mucous membrane involvement may lead to conjunctival bullae with risk of rupture and subsequent scarring.
  - Kawasaki disease: Acute vasculitis. Classic symptoms include (1) fever, (2) bilateral nonexudative conjunctivitis, (3) strawberry tongue, (4) oropharyngeal changes, (5) cervical adenopathy, (6) trunk rash, and (7) erythematous palms and soles with peeling around nail beds.

 TREATMENT

MEDICATION (DRUGS)
- Ophthalmia neonatorum
  - *Gonococcus*: Ceftriaxone, 30–50 mg/kg/d IV q8–12h and ocular irrigation followed by topical 0.5% erythromycin or 1.0% tetracycline ophthalmic ointments q.i.d. for 14 days. Also treat for *Chlamydia*.
  - *Chlamydia*: Oral erythromycin syrup, 12.5 mg/kg/d in 4 doses for 14 days. Topical 0.5% erythromycin or 1.0% tetracycline ophthalmic ointment q.i.d. both eyes for 14 days as above. (Povidone-iodine 1.25% ophthalmic drops q.i.d. can be used if other antibiotics are not readily available.)
- Bacterial
  - Empiric antibiotic treatment if bacterial infection is suspected, including erythromycin ointment, sulfacetamide 10%, polymyxin-trimethoprim, fluoroquinolone, or azithromycin drops
- Viral
  - Herpes simplex: Topical trifluorothymidine (Viroptic solution), 9 times a day for at least 14 days with or without systemic acyclovir
  - Other viral: Over-the-counter antihistamine or decongestant drops for comfort. Cidofovir has recently been considered as a potential antiadenoviral therapy, but its clinical use is limited by local toxicity to the skin, eyelids, and conjunctiva.
- Allergic

- A new class of topical mast cell stabilizers such as olopatadine b.i.d. is effective for more involved cases.

ADDITIONAL TREATMENT
General Measures
- Ophthalmia neonatorum
  - Cases of suspected gonococcal conjunctivitis should be hospitalized for IV antibiotics and workup for sepsis.
  - For suspected chlamydial infection topical and oral therapy is usually appropriate.
- Bacterial
  - Usually self-limited, but treatment may help shorten course and prevent spread of infection. Contact lens users should remove lenses until infection clears and consider use of fluoroquinolone.
- Viral
  - Suspected HSV warrants hospitalization for intravenous antiviral therapy.
  - For suspected adenovirus, children should stay home from school until no additional discharge. Cool compresses for comfort
- Allergic
  - Remove offending allergen if possible.
  - Mild symptoms can be treated with preservative-free artificial tears. Consider topical antiallergy medicine if symptoms persist
- Chemical
  - Close observation only. Self-limited

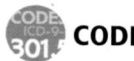 ONGOING CARE

FOLLOW-UP RECOMMENDATIONS
Patient Monitoring
- Daily follow-up is necessary for *Gonococcus*, *Chlamydia*, and herpes simplex virus.
- For epidemic viral conjunctivitis, frequency is dictated by severity (daily to weekly).
- For allergic conjunctivitis, follow-up can be made after a few weeks of treatment.
- No office follow-up is recommended for routine conjunctivitis.
- Follow atypical conjunctivitis closely until a more serious disease can be excluded.
- A nonresponsive or worsening condition needs ophthalmic consultation.

COMPLICATIONS
- Significant complications are extremely rare for common bacterial, viral, or allergic conjunctivitis.
- Blindness may result from untreated neonatal conjunctivitis, or from recurrent HSV ocular infection.

ADDITIONAL READING
- Bielory L, Mongia A. Current opinion of immunotherapy for ocular allergy. *Curr Opin Allergy Clin Immunol.* 2002;2:447–452.
- Brook I. Ocular infections due to anaerobic bacteria in children. *J Pediatr Ophthalmol Strabismus.* 2008;45(2):78–84.
- Crede CSF. Reports from the obstetrical clinic in Leipzig: Prevention of eye inflammation in the newborn. *Am J Dis Child.* 1971;121:3–4.
- Doreen TL, Reynolds S. Diagnosis and management of pediatric conjunctivitis. *Pediatr Emerg Care.* 2003;19:48–55.

- Greenberg MF, Pollard ZF. The red eye in childhood. *Pediatr Clin North Am.* 2003;50:105–124.
- Hillenkamp J, Reinhard T, Ross RS, et al. The effects of cidofovir 1% with and without cyclosporin a 1% as a topical treatment of acute adenoviral keratoconjunctivitis. *Ophthalmology.* 2002;109(5):845–850.
- Isenberg SJ, Apt L, Valenton M, et al. A controlled trial of povidone-iodine to treat infectious conjunctivitis in children. *Am J Ophthalmol.* 2002;134:861–868.
- Rietveld RP, van Weert HC, ter Riet G, et al. Diagnostic impact of signs and symptoms in acute infectious conjunctivitis: Systematic literature search. *BMJ.* 2003;327:789.
- Sethuraman US, Kamat D. The red eye: Evaluation and management. *Clin Pediatr.* 2009;48:588–600.
- Strauss EC, Foster CS. Atopic ocular disease. *Ophthalmol Clin North Am.* 2002;15:1–5.
- Trocme SD, Sra KK. Spectrum of ocular allergy. *Curr Opin Allergy Clin Immunol.* 2002;2:423–427.

CODES

ICD9
- 077.99 Unspecified diseases of conjunctiva due to viruses
- 372.30 Conjunctivitis, unspecified
- 771.6 Neonatal conjunctivitis and dacryocystitis

ICD10
- B30.9 Viral conjunctivitis, unspecified
- H10.9 Unspecified conjunctivitis
- P39.1 Neonatal conjunctivitis and dacryocystitis

FAQ
- Q: Is conjunctivitis contagious?
- A: All infectious conjunctivitis is contagious, but to varying degrees. Viral or epidemic keratoconjunctivitis (EKC) is the most contagious. Careful handling of secretions, tissues, towels, and bed linens and strict handwashing usually prevent spread. Wipe surfaces with isopropyl alcohol or dilute bleach to prevent recontamination. *Gonococcus*, *Chlamydia*, and herpes simplex virus can be transmitted through infected discharge or secretions, but this is less common. The most common source is the infected birth canal.
- Q: Should the patient with "pink eye" (non-*Gonococcus*, non-*Chlamydia*, non–herpes simplex virus conjunctivitis) be treated with empiric antibiotics?
- A: Empiric treatment with topical antibiotics can cause harm in the case of sulfa-containing compounds. Antibiotic toxicity, including Stevens-Johnson reactions, can occur from sulfa antibiotics, and use of antibiotics long term promotes selection of resistant strains of bacteria. Empiric treatment also increases manipulation of the infected eye and thus increases the risk of spread.
- Q: How long is the patient with "pink eye" (non-*Gonococcus*, non-*Chlamydia*, non–herpes simplex virus conjunctivitis) contagious and when can the patient return to school?
- A: The organism can be recovered from the eye for up 2 weeks after onset of symptoms, demonstrating that patients are infectious during this time. Practically, children should probably be kept out of school for at least 1 week.

CONSTIPATION

Kristin N. Fiorino
Maria R. Mascarenhas

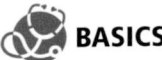 **BASICS**

DESCRIPTION
Delay or difficulty in defecation to <2–3 stools per week, which may result in pain, rectal bleeding, and encopresis or soiling. May also refer to a decrease in frequency of bowel movements compared with the patient's usual bowel pattern.

GENERAL PREVENTION
Dietary measures: High-fiber diet, plenty of fluids, fruits and vegetables, avoidance of excessive caffeine and milk (calcium) intake, plus regular physical activity.

PATHOPHYSIOLOGY
- Retention of stool allows water to move out of stool, increasing size and firmness.
- Decreased motility leads to a buildup of desiccated stool causing painful defecation that leads to ongoing stool retention. As the rectosigmoid enlarges, a child's ability to sense rectal fullness diminishes, and he or she may not appreciate the need to defecate. Often there is a family history of motility disturbances or constipation.

ETIOLOGY
- Most patients will have idiopathic or functional constipation with no identifiable cause: Usually an acute event followed by chronicity.
- Intentional or unintentional withholding of stool may result in hard stools, anal pain, and fissures that perpetuate and lead to constipation: Rectal dilatation, decreased sensation of the urge to defecate, shortening of the anal canal, decreased tone of the external anal sphincter, and encopresis can result.
- Precipitating events include:
  – Transition from breast milk to cow's milk
  – Excessive cow's milk intake
  – Insufficient water intake
  – Power struggle in toddlers
  – Refusal to use toilets outside the home
  – Zealous toilet training
  – Perianal streptococcal infection
  – Transient viral illness (diarrhea followed by constipation)
- Constipation also can be caused by anatomic anomalies in the lower GI tract, decreased propulsion, increased rectal sensitivity threshold, a functional outlet obstruction (muscular spastic levator ani or impaired relaxation of the puborectalis).
- Neurologic causes:
  – Abnormalities of the myenteric plexus
  – Intestinal pseudoobstruction
  – Congenital aganglionosis
  – Visceral neuropathies
  – Visceral myopathies
  – Familial dysautonomia

- Lesions of the spinal cord result in loss of rectal tone and sensation and reduced anal closure, affecting the sacral reflex center (e.g., meningocele, myelomeningocele, tethered cord).
- Anatomic disorders of anus and rectum (stricture, stenosis, mass, ectopic anus, imperforate anus, fistula).
- Endocrine abnormalities (hypothyroidism), drugs, electrolyte abnormalities

DIAGNOSIS

HISTORY
- Question: What is the timing of the passage of meconium?
  – If it is delayed for >48 hours, consider Hirschsprung disease.
- Is the child able to pass a bowel movement unaided by a suppository or enema?
  – If rectal stimulation is required for passage of a bowel movement, consider Hirschsprung disease or habituation to rectal stimulation.
- What are the size, frequency, and consistency of bowel movements?
  – 1–3 normal (in size and consistency) painless bowel movements may be passed every 1–3 days. The size of bowel movements reflects the caliber of the colon.
- Does the child experience frequent urination, bed-wetting, or urinary tract infections?
  – Frequently linked to chronic constipation.
- Is there soiling?
  – Soiling occurs with stool impaction or with nerve damage involving the anus.
- Is there the presence of rectal sensation?
  – Patients with long-standing constipation or withholding who develop a dilated rectum may lose the sensation of rectal distention.
- Is there a history of painful bowel movements or rectal fissure?
  – This could be the cause of withholding secondary to fear of painful bowel movements.
- Is the child experiencing any stressful events (i.e., new sibling, family death)?
  – Stress can precipitate stool withholding.
- Is there an unsteady gait?
  – This may suggest neuromuscular problems.
- Did the child experience difficult toilet training?
  – May be associated with encopresis.

PHYSICAL EXAM
- General: Look for evidence of systemic illness and alarm signals: Weight loss, anorexia, delayed growth, delayed passage of meconium, urinary incontinence, passage of bloody stools (in the absence of anal fissure), fever, vomiting, and diarrhea.
- Abdomen: Abdominal distention (indicative of the presence of stool or gas), presence of stool masses (size, location), distended bladder, and bowel sounds (may be decreased in intestinal pseudoobstruction)

- Rectal examination:
  – Perianal soiling
  – Size and position of anus (may suggest imperforate or ectopic anus)
  – Presence of skin tags and fissures
  – Perianal or anal erythema (streptococcal proctitis)
- Evidence of child abuse
- On digital examination, assess anal tone (decreased in functional constipation; long and tight anal canal in Hirschsprung); amount and consistency of stool; size of rectum (dilated rectum with chronic constipation; tight and empty anus with Hirschsprung disease); presence of blood
- Absence of anal wink or cremasteric reflex suggests neurologic abnormalities.
- Neurologic examination: Decreased reflexes in the lower extremities
- Back: Check for sacral dimple, tuft of hair (underlying sacral abnormality), flat buttocks, and patulous anus.

ALERT
- Grunting baby syndrome: Infants cry, scream, and draw up their legs during a bowel movement. They respond to rectal distention by contracting their pelvic floor. This is not constipation.
- Always rule out an organic cause.
- Always consider medications as a cause.

DIAGNOSTIC TESTS & INTERPRETATION
Lab
Water soluble contrast enema: An unprepped study is useful to diagnose Hirschsprung disease. A prepped study is useful to diagnose a stricture. Most patients with constipation will not require this test.

Imaging
Abdominal radiograph study: Look for evidence of bowel obstruction. Measurement of abdominal transit time with radio-opaque markers is useful for efficacy of cleanout and presence of a megarectum.

Diagnostic Procedures/Other
Anorectal manometry: Analyzes rectal sensation, resting and squeezing pressures, and pelvic floor dyssynergia (anismus)

DIFFERENTIAL DIAGNOSIS
- Hirschsprung disease: Congenital aganglionic megacolon
- Neuromuscular causes: Tethered spinal cord, spinal muscular atrophy
- Anal abnormalities: Anteriorly displaced anus (ectopic anus), imperforate anus, anal stenosis
- Endocrine abnormalities: Hypothyroidism, hyperparathyroidism, adrenal insufficiency
- Electrolyte imbalance: Hypokalemia, hyponatremia, hypomagnesemia, hypercalcemia
- Lead ingestion: Anemia, constipation, and abdominal pain
- Infant botulism: Constipation, aphonia, and weakness
- Infection: Chagas, tetanus
- Meconium ileus: Inspissated stool at birth in cystic fibrosis
- Inflammatory bowel disease (IBD)
- Celiac disease (gluten enteropathy)

- Abdominopelvic mass: Can cause constipation by pressure (i.e., distended bladder or pelvic tumor); pregnancy can also cause constipation.
- Chronic intestinal pseudoobstruction: Abdominal distention, diarrhea, and constipation
- Surgical conditions: Malrotation, congenital intestinal bands, intestinal stenoses, acquired colonic strictures resulting from IBD, necrotizing enterocolitis (NEC), pyloric stenosis
- Drugs: Calcium supplements, iron, barium, opiates, anticholinergic agents, antispasmodics

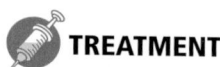 TREATMENT

ADDITIONAL TREATMENT
General Measures
- Treatment of functional constipation:
  - Disimpaction: If patient is impacted, 3–5 hypertonic phosphate enemas may be required for initial disimpaction. Children >2–3 years of age require adult-size enemas, whereas younger children require pediatric-size enemas.
  - Evacuation: Following rectal disimpaction, evacuation can be achieved by using polyethylene glycol solution (Go-Lytely), orally or via nasogastric tube over 6–8 hours until the effluent is clear. Alternatively, MiraLAX can be used on a daily basis to achieve evacuation over 1–2 weeks. Doses are given in 4–8 oz of liquid once or twice daily. Maximum dose of MiraLAX or Go-Lytely 1.5 g/kg.
- Maintenance stool softeners:
  - Infants ≤6 months of age may be given sorbitol containing juices, lactulose, or Karo syrup. Children >6 months of age may be given lactulose (0.7–2 g/kg/d (1–3 mL/kg/d), max 40 g/d (60 mL/d)) or MiraLAX (0.5–1 g/kg, max 17 g/d).
  - Mineral oil or Kondremul (>1 year of age 1–3 mL/d, >6 years 10–25 mL/d) is added as an adjunctive lubricant to aid in the passage of stool but contraindicated in children <12–15 months as well as in children at risk for aspiration.
- Rescue stimulant laxatives: Bisacodyl or senna may be used as a stimulant laxative for short periods of time. Long-term use has been associated with colonic nerve damage in adults.
- Diet: A balanced diet of whole grains, fruits, and vegetables is recommended. A high-fiber diet is recommended (toddler 14 g/d; school-aged 17–25 g/d; adolescent 25–31 g/d). Fiber should be increased gradually to minimize side effects of flatulence. Caffeine and excessive milk-product intake (>16 oz/d of milk) may be constipating.
- Fluid intake: High fluid intake is important.
- Toilet sitting: Regular toilet sitting twice a day for 10 minutes, preferably 15–20 minutes after meals, is necessary to help retrain the bowel.
- Calendar: It is important to keep a record of stools, accidents, toilet sitting, and medications in order to identify causes of failure.
- Biofeedback can be helpful in patients who fail conventional therapy and who have the following abnormalities on anorectal manometry: Decreased sensory threshold to rectal distention, paradoxical contraction of the external anal sphincter and puborectalis muscle during simulated defecation (pelvic floor dyssynergia)

- Treatment of complications:
  - Encopresis (soiling or diarrhea): Abdominal radiographs with radio-opaque markers show large amounts of stool in the colon, including a dilated rectum and markers mainly in the rectosigmoid. Disimpaction or clean-out, followed by treatment of constipation, is recommended (see above).
  - Intestinal obstruction: Vomiting, abdominal pain, and constipation. Abdominal radiograph film shows intestinal obstruction. Make nil per os, (NPO) provide IV fluids, and rule out an acute abdomen. Then give enemas and clear out stool from below. Never give oral laxatives or a polyethylene glycol solution in a case of obstruction.
  - Sigmoid volvulus: Chronically constipated child with symptoms of acute abdomen, fever, tender abdomen, and palpable mass. Abdominal radiograph shows obstruction in the colon. Contrast enema may reveal and possibly reduce a volvulus.

 ONGOING CARE

FOLLOW-UP RECOMMENDATIONS
Patient Monitoring
- Schedule regular visits to make certain therapy is maintained, decreasing the frequency of visits when patient is doing well.
- Parents should call when problems develop.
- Compliance and good follow-up are key to successful management of constipation.

PROGNOSIS
For functional constipation, the success rate is variable (45–90%). Presence of abdominal pain at the time of presentation, close follow-up, and use of mineral oil are good prognostic factors. Presence of soiling, use of stimulant laxatives, and lack of follow-up were associated with failure.

COMPLICATIONS
- Anal fissures: Infrequent hard stools can cause a tear of the anal mucosa, causing pain and withholding.
- Encopresis: Chronic constipation leads to progressive rectal dilatation and decreased rectal sensation. Fecal impaction results in secondary soiling or encopresis.
- Intestinal obstruction: Manifests as vomiting, abdominal pain, and constipation. Abdominal radiograph films show intestinal obstruction and presence of large amounts of stool.
- Sigmoid volvulus: A chronically constipated child may present with symptoms of acute abdomen, fever, tender abdomen, and palpable mass. Abdominal radiograph shows obstruction in the colon. Barium enema may be both diagnostic and therapeutic by achieving reduction.

ADDITIONAL READING
- Baker SS, Liptak GS, Colletti RB, et al. Evaluation and treatment of constipation in infants and children: Recommendations of the North American Society for Pediatric Gastroenterology, Hepatology and Nutrition. J Pediatr Gastroenterol Nutr. 2006; 43:e1–e13.
- Bekkali NLH, van den Berg MM, Dijkgraaf MGW, et al. Rectal fecal impaction treatment in childhood constipation: Enemas versus high doses oral PEG. Pediatrics. 2009;124(6):e1108–e1115.
- Croffie JM, Fitzgerald J. Idiopathic constipation. In: Walker WA, Kleinman RE, Sherman PM, et al. Pediatric Gastrointestinal Disease, 4th ed. Philadelphia: BC Decker; 2004:1000–1055.
- Hyman PE, Milla PJ, Benninga MA, et al. Childhood functional gastrointestinal disorder: Neonate/ toddler. Gastroenterology. 2006;130:1519–1526.
- Lewis LG, Rudolph CD. Practical approach to defecation disorders in children. Pediatr Ann. 1997;26:4260–4268.
- LexiComp Online. www.lexi.com
- Rasquin A, DiLorenzo C, Forbes D, et al. Childhood functional gastrointestinal disorders: Child/ adolescent. Gastroenterology. 2006;130: 1527–1537.
- US Department of Health and Human Services. Dietary Guidelines for Americans, 2010. Available at: http://www.health.gov/dietaryguidelines/ 2010.asp.

 CODES

ICD9
- 564.00 Constipation, unspecified
- 564.01 Slow transit constipation
- 564.09 Other constipation

ICD10
- K59.00 Constipation, unspecified
- K59.01 Slow transit constipation
- K59.09 Other constipation

FAQ
- Q: When is constipation an emergency?
- A: When intestinal obstruction, sigmoid volvulus, or Hirschsprung enterocolitis occurs.
- Q: Does MiraLAX have a taste?
- A: MiraLAX advantages include its lack of taste, smell, or odor and that it can be mixed in any liquid.

CONTACT DERMATITIS

Kara N. Shah

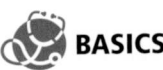 **BASICS**

DESCRIPTION
- An acute or chronic eczematous eruption that may result from either direct irritation to the skin (irritant contact dermatitis) or from a delayed-type (type IV) hypersensitivity reaction to a contact allergen (allergic contact dermatitis).
- Most cases of contact dermatitis are irritant contact dermatitis (>80%).

EPIDEMIOLOGY
Incidence
The incidence of contact dermatitis in children is not known.

Prevalence
- The prevalence of allergic contact dermatitis increases with age.
- Contact dermatitis can occur at any age but is relatively uncommon in infants.
- Infants are more likely to develop an irritant contact dermatitis.
- In children, the overall prevalence of allergic contact dermatitis is ~20%.

RISK FACTORS
- Susceptibility to certain contact allergens for delayed-type hypersensitivity is in part genetically determined.
- It is unclear whether atopic dermatitis is associated with an increased risk of developing contact dermatitis.
- Increased exposure to potential irritants and allergens and the chronic or intermittent development of an impaired skin barrier are predisposing factors.

GENERAL PREVENTION
Minimize contact exposure to known or potential irritants and allergens.

PATHOPHYSIOLOGY
- Allergic contact dermatitis requires initial exposure and sensitization to an allergen and only occurs in susceptible individuals. Repeated exposure to the allergen leads to the development of a T-cell-mediated delayed-type (type IV) hypersensitivity reaction.
- Irritant contact dermatitis does not involve an immunologic response and can occur in anyone, even after the 1st exposure to the irritant. It commonly results from frequent or chronic exposure to moisture and/or friction such as from water, saliva, or urine or to acidic or alkaline chemicals such as soaps and detergents.
- Both processes result in nonspecific findings of dermal and epidermal edema and inflammation and may be indistinguishable from other forms of eczematous dermatitis.

ETIOLOGY
- Irritant contact dermatitis:
  – Frequent handwashing or water immersion
  – Soaps and detergents
  – Saliva (lip licking)
  – Urine and feces (diaper dermatitis)
- Allergic contact dermatitis:
  – Nickel and other metals (cobalt, chromate)
  – Rubber/elastic (Thiuram)
  – Fragrances (e.g., Balsam of Peru)
  – Clothing dyes
  – Formaldehydes and formaldehyde-releasing products
  – Lanolin (wool alcohol)
  – Topical antibiotics (neomycin, bacitracin)
  – Rubber and rubber accelerators
  – Plants (*Toxicodendron* species, e.g., poison ivy, poison oak, and poison sumac, which contain the allergen urushiol)

 DIAGNOSIS

HISTORY
- Patients may present with either the acute development of a pruritic inflammatory dermatitis or with the chronic persistence of a localized, mildly pruritic dermatitis.
- Many patients are unable to associate a specific allergen with the development of symptoms. With regard to acute allergic contact dermatitis, this is often due to the latency between the exposure and the development of symptoms (usually 48–72 hours but occasionally as long as several days).
- Patients with either an irritant contact dermatitis or a chronic contact dermatitis should be asked about all chemicals and other potential contact irritants or allergens to which they are intermittently or frequently exposed.

PHYSICAL EXAM
- Acute allergic contact dermatitis manifests as erythematous edematous papules and plaques, often with vesicles and crusting.
- Chronic allergic contact dermatitis manifests as erythematous and often hyperpigmented patches and plaques, usually with lichenification (accentuation of skin markings) as a result of chronic rubbing.
- Irritant contact dermatitis more commonly manifests as erythematous papules and patches with less prominent edema, vesiculation, and crusting.
- The morphology of contact dermatitis commonly consists of geometric, angulated, or asymmetric lesions that correlate with the pattern of allergen exposure.
- The distribution of the dermatitis may suggest particular allergens, such as the dorsum of the feet (shoe rubber) or earlobes and/or periumbilical area (nickel).
- In older children a perioral rash often signifies an irritant contact dermatitis from lip licking.

DIAGNOSTIC TESTS & INTERPRETATION
Lab
In general, routine laboratory testing is not helpful in confirming the diagnosis of contact dermatitis.

Diagnostic Procedures/Other
Formal epicutaneous patch testing to evaluate suspected contact allergens may be performed by a dermatologist or allergist. The patch test involves the controlled exposure of multiple allergens to the skin. Positive reactions manifest with the development of erythema, edema, and vesicles at the site of exposure, usually within 48–96 hours. It may be performed using a standard panel of allergens (the T.R.U.E. Test) or by the application of selected allergens at the discretion of the specialist.

Pathological Findings
- Skin biopsy findings may not be specific and often overlap with other eczematous dermatoses.
- Acute contact dermatitis shows edema of the epidermis and dermis with a mixed inflammatory infiltrate. There may be intraepidermal vesicles and a prominence of eosinophils in the dermal inflammatory infiltrate.
- Chronic contact dermatitis usually shows prominent hyperkeratosis (thickening) of the stratum corneum and epidermal rete ridges with minimal edema. A sparse inflammatory infiltrate may be present.

DIFFERENTIAL DIAGNOSIS
- Infection:
  – Impetigo and cellulitis: Bacterial infections of the skin, usually caused by *Staphylococcus aureus* or group A *Streptococcus*, may manifest as erythematous, edematous crusted patches and plaques. Pustules and/or deep-seated inflammatory nodules may also be present. Infection is usually associated more with pain and tenderness than with pruritus.
  – Scabies: Intensely pruritic papules and nodules with a predilection for the hands and feet (especially the web spaces), the axillae, and the groin. There are often multiple affected family members.
- Neoplastic:
  – Langerhans cell histiocytosis: The skin manifestations may present as scaling red-brown papules and petechial macules that favor the scalp and the intertriginous areas, including the diaper area. Affected infants and children may also manifest gingival inflammation, hepatosplenomegaly, and adenopathy.
- Metabolic:
  – Acrodermatitis enteropathica: A genetic or acquired deficiency of zinc that usually presents with characteristic bullae and erosions involving the hands and feet and periorificial areas (perioral, periocular, and perineal). These patients also develop failure to thrive, diarrhea, and alopecia.

- Immunologic:
  - Atopic dermatitis: Infantile atopic dermatitis usually begins within the 1st 6 months of life. It may favor the face and extremities or occur more diffusely with truncal involvement but usually spares the diaper area and the perinasal and periocular areas. It is associated with erythematous, excoriated, and crusted papules, patches, and plaques and with chronic pruritus, which is often worse at night. Atopic dermatitis is often accompanied by a personal or family history of atopy (reactive airways disease and/or allergic rhinitis).
  - Seborrheic dermatitis: Usually affects infants <1 year of age or adolescents. It manifests as erythema and greasy scaling patches that favor the scalp, face, ears, and intertriginous areas. It is usually asymptomatic.
  - Nummular eczema: A chronic, often intensely inflammatory and pruritic dermatitis that presents with multiple round, crusted, edematous, erythematous patches and plaques. Lesions often favor the extremities.
  - Psoriasis vulgaris: A chronic dermatitis that presents with recurrent well-defined erythematous plaques with silvery scale. Commonly affected areas include the scalp, elbows, knees, and genital regions.

 TREATMENT

MEDICATION (DRUGS)
First Line
- Topical corticosteroids help with the pruritus and inflammation associated with both acute and chronic contact dermatitis. Use of a medium- to high-potency topical corticosteroid (class 2–4) for a short duration (1–2 weeks) is usually more effective than prolonged treatment with low-potency topical corticosteroids. The use of medium- to high-potency fluorinated topical corticosteroids should be avoided on the face, axillae, and groin. The skin of these areas is thinner and more susceptible to side effects. A low-potency topical corticosteroid such as hydrocortisone (class 6–7) should be used instead.
- Systemic antihistamines are generally not necessary for treating contact dermatitis, but can be considered if pruritus is extreme. The use of topical antihistamines is not recommended.
- In severe cases involving a large body surface area or associated with significant facial edema, a short course (14–21 days) of systemic corticosteroids may be appropriate, with tapering over 1–2 weeks to avoid a rebound of the dermatitis.

Second Line
The intermittent use of a topical calcineurin inhibitor such as tacrolimus ointment or pimecrolimus cream, which have anti-inflammatory and steroid-sparing properties, may be considered as adjunctive therapy in patients with chronic contact dermatitis.

ADDITIONAL TREATMENT
General Measures
- The most effective treatment involves identification and elimination of the offending allergens or exposures. This often requires extensive education of the patient and family regarding potential sources of exposure.
- Mild cases of acute contact dermatitis may not require treatment and will resolve within 1–2 weeks.
- Moderate to severe cases of acute contact dermatitis and most cases of chronic contact dermatitis often require treatment to reduce symptoms and hasten resolution.
- Prompt bathing with soap and water immediately after exposure to poison ivy, poison oak, or poison sumac may help to reduce exposure to the allergen in susceptible individuals. Zanfel is an OTC cleanser that reportedly binds to and eliminates the urushiol allergen from the skin if used immediately after contact with poison ivy, poison oak, and poison sumac.
- Acute allergic contact dermatitis: Application of cool compresses and shake lotions with drying properties (i.e., Caladryl) can be helpful. Products containing colloidal oatmeal, such as Aveeno oatmeal bath and Aveeno lotion, may also be helpful in soothing inflamed skin.

 ONGOING CARE

FOLLOW-UP RECOMMENDATIONS
Patient Monitoring
- Follow-up depends on the severity of the dermatitis and elimination of continued exposure to the allergen.
- Patients who do not improve after 1–2 weeks of therapy should be re-evaluated.

PATIENT EDUCATION
- Prevention:
  - Patients should be instructed on allergen avoidance, including the use of protective gloves and clothing where appropriate.
  - Ivy Block contains quaternium-18 bentonite (bentoquatam 5%), a barrier lotion that prevents exposure to the allergen in poison ivy if applied prior to anticipated exposure.

PROGNOSIS
Complete resolution can be expected after appropriate treatment and elimination of further exposure to the allergen.

COMPLICATIONS
Generally, there are no long-term complications, although secondary bacterial infections may occur.

ADDITIONAL READING

- Bruckner AL, Weston WL. Beyond poison ivy: Understanding allergic contact dermatitis in children. *Pediatr Ann.* 2001;30(4):203–206.
- Jacob SE, Brod B, Crawford GH. Clinically relevant patch test reactions in children – a United States based study. *Pediatr Dermatol.* 2008;25:520–527.
- Lee PW, Elsaie ML, Jacob SE. Allergic contact dermatitis in children: Common allergens and treatment: A review. *Curr Opin Pediatr.* 2008; 21:491–498.
- Militello G, Jacob SE, Crawford GH. Allergic contact dermatitis in children. *Curr Opin Pediatr.* 2006; 18(4):385–390.
- Weston WL, Bruckner A. Allergic contact dermatitis. *Pediatr Clin North Am.* 2000;47:4.

 CODES

ICD9
692.9 Contact dermatitis and other eczema (unspecified cause)

ICD10
- L23.9 Allergic contact dermatitis, unspecified cause
- L24.9 Irritant contact dermatitis, unspecified cause
- L25.9 Unspecified contact dermatitis, unspecified cause

FAQ
- Q: Can the fluid from blisters caused by poison ivy spread the rash to other parts of the body?
- A: The contents of the vesicles and bullae from rhus dermatitis are not contagious. After exposure to poison ivy is eliminated, new lesions appear because of the variable sensitivity of various areas of the body to the allergen.
- Q: After making lemonade at a picnic on the beach, my child developed a red, blistering rash on his face. What was the cause?
- A: A phototoxic form of contact dermatitis can result from exposure to plant compounds (psoralens) and ultraviolet light (sunlight). The condition is called phytophotodermatitis, and the plants that can cause this include lime and lemons, celery, dill, parsnip, and carrot juices.
- Q: Is it possible to avoid contact dermatitis using protective clothing or skin barrier creams?
- A: Yes. Proper-fitting protective gloves and clothing are a highly effective means of decreasing irritant exposure. However, gloves permeable to irritants such as organic solvents may increase the exposure to the irritant. Some contact allergens can also permeate rubber gloves, which therefore are of no benefit. Rubber gloves are contraindicated in individuals with immediate and delayed-type allergy to latex and rubber additives. With the exception of Ivy Block lotion, the use of barrier creams in the prevention of contact dermatitis is not effective.
- Q: How does saliva cause a perioral rash in some kids? Is there something unusual in the saliva that is causing this?
- A: "Lip-licker dermatitis" is an irritant dermatitis that results from chronic and/or excessive exposure to moisture. It is not caused by any specific substances in the saliva.

C

CONTRACEPTION

Molly J. Richards
Daniel H. Reirden

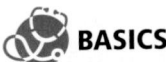 **BASICS**

DESCRIPTION
The prevention of conception or pregnancy. The "ideal" contraceptive is 100% effective, has no side effects, can easily be reversed, and can easily be used by adolescents.
Contraceptive types
- Abstinence: Refraining from intercourse
  - Most effective way to prevent transmission of HIV, viral hepatitis, human papilloma virus (HPV), herpes simplex virus (HSV), syphilis, *Neisseria gonorrhoeae*, and *Chlamydia trachomatis*
- Barrier methods to sperm entry (male and female condoms, diaphragm):
  - Male condoms: 85% effective with typical use. The female condom and diaphragm with spermicide are 79% and 84% effective, respectively.
  - Proper use of the male and female condoms can prevent transmission of HIV, HPV, HSV, syphilis, *N. gonorrhoeae*, and *C. trachomatis.*
- Spermicidal agents (foam, film, vaginal inserts):
  - Nonoxynal-9 is the active agent most widely used.
  - 73% effective in preventing pregnancy with typical use
  - Reduced transmission of *C. trachomatis* and *N. gonorrhoeae*
  - Spermicides used with condoms will increase overall efficacy to 93% with typical use.
- Hormonal agents (oral contraceptive pills, transdermal patch, vaginal ring, and emergency contraception [EC]):
  - Oral contraceptive pills: Include combination estrogen and progestin pills (COC) and the progestin-only pill (POP)
  - Monophasic COCs contain a fixed dose of estrogen and progestin, whereas phasic COCs may vary the doses of estrogen, progestin, or both.

- COC pills are 94.5–97% effective in preventing pregnancy with typical use (99.9% effective with perfect use) and have been shown to reduce the incidence of endometrial and ovarian cancers after as little as 3 months of use, protect against salpingitis (PID) and subsequent ectopic pregnancies, and decrease incidence of benign breast disease and dysmenorrhea. They are used effectively to treat problems including dysfunctional uterine bleeding and polycystic ovary syndrome.
- The POP contains progesterone only. It is sometimes referred to as the "mini-pill." Effectiveness is highly dependent on perfect use.
- Transdermal patch: Contains ethinyl estradiol and norelgestromin. Each patch is left in place for 7 days and changed weekly, allowing 1 patch-free week per month to allow menses to occur; efficacy is comparable to that of oral contraceptive pills; convenient due to once-weekly change; may be less effective in women weighing >90 kg
- Vaginal ring: A soft, flexible, polymer ring containing ethinyl estradiol and etonogestrel that is inserted into the vagina for 3 weeks and then removed for 1 week to allow menses to occur; benefits include once-a-month insertion, avoidance of 1st-pass liver effects, and lower hormone doses.
- EC: Also called postcoital contraception; safe method of contraception that employs either COCs or POPs:
  - COC pills can reduce the risk of pregnancy by 75% after unprotected intercourse, if taken in correct doses within 72 hours.
  - The progesterone-only method may reduce the risk of pregnancy by 88%; although most effective when used within 72 hours of intercourse, some data suggest that treatment is effective up to 5 days after unprotected intercourse.

- Long-acting reversible contraceptive methods:
  - Depo-medroxyprogesterone acetate (Depo-Provera): Effective contraceptive administered IM once every 3 months
  - Etonogestrel implant: Single rod subdermal implant containing 68 mg of progestin etonogestrel providing contraception for up to 3 years. Benefits include long-term pregnancy prevention with little effort needed for compliance and high efficiency rates. May also decrease dysmenorrhea
  - Levonorgestrel-releasing intrauterine device (IUD): T-shaped polyethylene intrauterine device containing 52 mg of levonorgestrel. FDA approved for use for up to 5 years but may be effective up to 7 years. The annual failure rate is 0.1%. Has been shown to significantly reduce menstrual bleeding and dysmenorrhea
  - Copper T380 IUD: Contraceptive effect related to in utero oxidation with release of copper ions. The annual failure rate is reported to be as low as 0.8%. FDA approved for use up to 10 years but may be effective for up to 12 years

ALERT
- Advising teenagers to abstain from all forms of physical intimacy may be counterproductive in the context of their psychosocial development.
- Contraceptive use may lead to patients' discontinuing use of condoms. Providers should emphasize at every visit that only condoms protect against sexually transmitted diseases.

GENERAL PREVENTION
- Encourage the consistent use of latex condoms.
- Patients using oral contraceptive pills must be strongly encouraged to cease tobacco use. Methods of treating nicotine dependence should be employed if indicated.

PATHOPHYSIOLOGY

- The spermicides nonoxynol-9 and octoxynol-9 act by destroying sperm cell membranes.
- Most spermicidal preparations contain an inert base (foam, cream, or jelly) to support the spermicidal agent and provide a barrier to sperm entry.
- Hormonal therapy suppresses ovulation by directly decreasing release of gonadotropin-releasing hormone (GnRH) from the hypothalamus and follicle-stimulating hormone (FSH) and luteinizing hormone (LH) from the pituitary gland.
- Progesterone causes thickening of the cervical mucus, thinning of the endometrium, and decreased tubal motility.
- Copper: Copper ions may inhibit transtubal sperm migration, thus preventing zygote formation.
- EC: Mechanisms of action include disruption of ovulation, impairment of the endometrium to prevent implantation, and possibly alteration of sperm or ova transport.

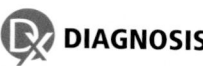 **DIAGNOSIS**

HISTORY

General considerations in method selection include:

- What is the teen's sexual history?
- Is sexual activity spontaneous or planned?
- Does the patient feel that she or he can be compliant with a daily pill or barrier methods?
- Does the patient require absolute confidentiality?
- Is the patient comfortable inserting a diaphragm or applying a condom?
- Does the patient have open communication with his or her partner?
- Does the patient desire pregnancy? Does his or her partner?
- Are there any other barriers to compliance with the chosen contraceptive method?

PHYSICAL EXAM

- Obtain baseline weight and BP.
- It is not necessary to perform a pelvic exam on young women initiating hormonal contraception. Biannual screening for STIs and regular Papanicolaou smears beginning at 21 years of age should be recommended.

DIAGNOSTIC TESTS & INTERPRETATION
Lab
Pregnancy test prior to initiating hormonal contraceptives

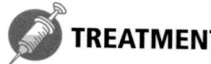 **TREATMENT**

ADDITIONAL TREATMENT
General Measures

- Barrier methods: Trained personnel can teach the proper technique for application of the diaphragm and male and female condoms.
- Spermicides:
  - These must be inserted near the time of intercourse; some formulations require 10–15 minutes for activation, and most have an unpleasant taste.
  - Trained office personnel can teach the proper technique for insertion.
- Oral contraceptive pills:
  - Monthly packages of oral contraceptive pills contain 3 weeks of hormone, followed by 1 week of placebo or a pill-free interval.
  - Menstruation begins after 2–3 days of placebo.
  - Oral contraceptive pills are taken as a daily pill, preferably at the same time every day (to minimize nausea, some users find bedtime helpful).
  - The optimal time to start oral contraceptive pills is within 5 days after the start of the menstrual period. A "same-day" start method may be used to promote immediate use of pills provided the young woman is not pregnant at the visit.

- Oral contraceptive pills may not offer protection during the 1st cycle; therefore, a back-up barrier method should be used. Instructions for missed pills should be explained and given to all adolescents initiating oral contraceptive pills.
  - Fertility returns, on average, 2–3 months after discontinuation. 1–2% of patients will experience a delay in fertility for up to 1 year.
- EC: 3 types of EC are available in the US: COCs (also known as the Yuzpe regimen), POPs, and the copper-releasing IUD:
  - The Yuzpe regimen is safe and well studied. It consists of two doses of COCs containing at least 100 mcg of estrogen with 0.5 mg of levonorgestrel each. The 2 doses should be taken 12 hours apart and within 72 hours of unprotected intercourse.
    ○ This dose of estrogen will often cause nausea and vomiting; therefore, pretreatment with an antiemetic, such as meclizine, is recommended.
  - POP methods: Only levonorgestrel has been studied as a nonestrogen-containing EC.
  - Plan B: Contains 0.75 mg of levonorgestrel per tablet and, although initially approved as 2 doses separated by 12 hours, subsequent studies have confirmed efficacy with both pills being taken at the same time (1.5 mg total dose). Additional studies have indicated efficacy up to 5 days after the unprotected coitus.
    ○ The FDA recently approved Plan B for over-the-counter status for women aged ≥17 years. Adolescents <17 years will still require a prescription.
- Long-acting reversible contraceptive methods:
  - Depo-Provera is given IM in the deltoid or gluteus maximus muscle:
    ○ Each injection has a 12-week duration and must be repeated every 12 weeks to ensure protection against pregnancy.
    ○ The initial injection is optimally given within 5 days after the start of the last menstrual period or when the provider can be reasonably assured that the patient is not pregnant.
    ○ Fertility (and ovulatory cycles) should return within 6 months of the last injection.

- Etonogestrel implant is inserted subdermally in the medial aspect of the nondominant arm 6–8 cm above the elbow. Training is required for insertion:
  ○ Implant provides contraception for up to 3 years.
  ○ Insertion should be scheduled when one can be as certain as possible that the adolescent is not pregnant.
  ○ Implant will offer contraceptive protection immediately if inserted at right time of cycle.
- Most adolescents (more than 90%) ovulate within 3–4 weeks of removal of implant.
- Levonorgestrel and Copper T380 IUDs are inserted into the uterus during an office pelvic exam by a trained provider:
  ○ Insertion should be scheduled when one can be as certain as possible that the adolescent is not pregnant; this is best achieved during the 5 days after the start of the last menstrual period or when switching from another effective hormonal contraceptive method.
  ○ Discomfort during IUD insertion is common, with 86% of adolescents reporting mild to severe pain with insertion.
  ○ Return to fertility is rapid following removal of either intrauterine device.

ALERT

Drug interactions:
- Drugs that activate the cytochrome P-450 enzyme will diminish the efficacy of hormonal contraceptives. This is of greatest concern with low-dose preparations and can be remedied by using higher doses.
- Drugs that diminish hormonal contraceptive effects include phenobarbital, carbamazepine, primidone, rifampin, griseofulvin, HIV protease inhibitors, and tetracyclines (including doxycycline). Hormonal contraceptives can increase levels of phenytoins, benzodiazepines, antidepressants, corticosteroids, β-blockers, theophylline, and alcohol. Hormonal contraceptives can decrease the efficacy of acetaminophen, oral anticoagulants, hypoglycemics, and methyldopa.

ONGOING CARE

FOLLOW-UP RECOMMENDATIONS
Patient Monitoring
- Patients using hormonal contraceptives should be seen within 6 weeks to 2 months of initiation, to evaluate compliance and side effects.
- BP should be monitored at every visit.

PROGNOSIS
- Within 3 months of oral contraceptive pill use, only 44–45% of patients remain compliant.
- After 1 year, only 33% are compliant.

COMPLICATIONS
- Barrier methods:
  - Latex allergy: Patients may use polyurethane rather than latex condoms.
  - Breakage or permeability: Oil-based lubricants and most intravaginal medications used with latex condoms will increase the risks of these complications. Animal skin condoms are permeable to viral pathogens.
  - Irritation, UTIs, and toxic shock syndrome (if the diaphragm is left in place longer than 24 hours) may be seen with diaphragm use.
- Spermicides:
  - Local irritation or allergic reaction
  - May increase the risk of HIV infection in adolescents with high-risk sexual partners
- Hormonal contraceptives:
  - Mortality from gynecologic and related causes was 7/100,000 in 15–19-year-old adolescents per year. If no fertility control measures were used, the mortality is 0.3/100,000 in nonsmoking oral contraceptive pill users and 2.2/100,000 in smoking oral contraceptive pill users.
  - Minor side effects of COC pills include menstrual spotting, nausea, breast changes, fluid retention, leukorrhea, minor headache, and depression.
  - Thromboembolic events and liver disease are extremely rare in nonsmoking adolescents using estrogen-containing oral contraceptive pills.
  - Contraindications to COC pills include history of thromboembolic event, structural heart disease, breast cancer, pregnancy, active liver disease, migraine headaches with an aura, prolonged immobilization, or severe hypertension. Caution should be taken when prescribing COC pills to adolescents with undiagnosed abnormal uterine bleeding, those <6 weeks postpartum, those who use medications that affect liver enzymes, and those with gallbladder disease.

– Minor side effects of POPs include weight gain, rapid hair turnover, and menstrual irregularities.
– Depo-medroxyprogesterone acetate has been shown to reduce bone mineral density in several studies. Because adolescence is the period of peak bone mass accretion, there is concern that its use during adolescence may increase the risk for osteopenia or osteoporosis later in life. Until more studies are available, it is probably advisable to avoid its use in those adolescents at high risk for osteoporosis, such as adolescents with anorexia nervosa or chronic renal failure.
– Nausea and/or vomiting occur in most patients using estrogen-based EC or "doubling up" on oral contraceptive pills.
– Most common side effect reported with etonogestrel implant is abnormal bleeding. A wide range of bleeding patterns may be experienced and it is not possible to predict the bleeding pattern for any individual.
– Overall, in the 90-day reference periods of clinical trial experience, 33.3% had infrequent bleeding, 21.4% had amenorrhea, 6.1% had frequent bleeding, and 16.9% had prolonged bleeding.
– The lower androgenic effect of etonogestrel may make side effects of acne and weight gain less frequent than with other progestins.
– Contraindications to IUD placement are those who are pregnant or suspected to be pregnant; have PID, either currently or in the past 3 months; have puerperal or postabortion sepsis (currently or in past 3 months); or have undiagnosed abnormal vaginal bleeding, malignancy of the genital tract, uterine abnormalities that distort the uterine cavity, an allergy to any component of IUDs, or Wilson disease (for the Copper T IUD only).

– Intrauterine devices have been associated with a slightly higher risk of PID within the 1st 20 days after insertion, especially if cervical infection is present. IUDs do not increase risk of PID above baseline after this time.
– Younger age may confer an increased risk of IUD failure from expulsion because of smaller uterus and higher incidence of nulliparity.
– The Copper T IUD has been associated with increased menstrual bleeding and spotting, especially in 1st 3–6 months after insertion. In addition, some women may experience menstrual pain and heavy bleeding throughout use.

ADDITIONAL READING

- Calderoni ME, Coupey SM. Combined oral contraception. *Adolesc Med.* 2005;16:517–537.
- Conard LE, Gold MA. Emergency contraception. *Adolesc Med.* 2005;16:585–602.
- Deans EI, Grimes DA. Intrauterine devices for adolescents: A systematic review. *Contraception.* 2009;79:418–423.
- Gold MA, Johnson LM. Intrauterine devices and adolescents. *Curr Opin Obstet Gynecol.* 2008;20:464–469.
- Isley M. Implanon: The subdermal contraceptive implant. *J Pediatr Adolesc Gynecol.* 2010;23:364–367.
- Rimsza M. Counseling the adolescent about contraception. *Pediatr Rev.* 2003;24:162–169.

 CODES

ICD9
- V25.8 Other specified contraceptive management
- V25.09 Other general counseling and advice on contraceptive management
- V25.9 Unspecified contraceptive management

ICD10
- Z30.8 Encounter for other contraceptive management
- Z30.09 Encounter for other general counseling and advice on contraception
- Z30.9 Encounter for contraceptive management, unspecified

FAQ

- Q: My patient asks for confidentiality regarding contraception. Should I comply?
- A: Yes. Teenagers have the right to confidentiality regarding contraception and treatment of STDs. Every state has a law or provision for confidential access to contraceptive services. Importantly, it may be in the patient's best interest to have a caring adult involved. Which adult and how he or she is involved should be negotiated with the adolescent.
- Q: One of my patients has asked me to prescribe EC in advance for her. Is this something that I should do?
- A: Studies done thus far have shown that use of EC is safe. In fact, there are no absolute contraindications to using progestin-only EC. Because unprotected sexual encounters often take place at a time when adolescents do not have access to their health care providers (e.g., evenings or weekends), advanced prescription is of benefit for many adolescents.
- Q: What should I tell my patient if she misses a dose of her oral contraceptive?
- A: If she has missed 1 pill, she should take it as soon as she remembers, then take the next pill at the regular time. If she has missed 2 doses, she should take 2 when she remembers, and then 2 the next day. She should use a back-up method during the cycle in which she had to "double up." If she has missed 3 or more pills, she will probably menstruate. After discarding the last pack, she should start a new pack on the 1st Sunday after the start of her next period. She is not protected during the remainder of this cycle.

COR PULMONALE

Brian D. Hanna
Heather L. Meluskey

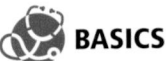 **BASICS**

DESCRIPTION
- Cor pulmonale is right ventricular (RV) failure secondary to an altered pulmonary process that results in a loss of functional capillary vascular bed and in excessive pulmonary artery pressure and pulmonary vascular resistance (PVR).
- Cor pulmonale is not the result of a primary congenital heart defect.

ALERT
- In newborns, the RV muscle mass is comparable to that of the left ventricle.
- RV failure from pulmonary hypertension (PH) occurs but is rare in newborns.
- RV failure in newborns is usually a consequence of hypoxemia, ischemia, metabolic acidosis (e.g., persistent fetal circulation), and/or premature restriction/closure of the intrauterine ductus arteriosus.

EPIDEMIOLOGY
- Cor pulmonale may be found at any age but is typically a result of a long-standing pulmonary process. However, severe bronchopulmonary dysplasia (BPD) is an increasingly common cause of neonatal PH.
- Primary pulmonary hypertension (PPHN) is most often diagnosed in the 2nd or 3rd decade of life with a female predominance, and it is often diagnosed during pregnancy.

Incidence
- PPHN has a yearly incidence of 2 per million.
- The incidence of cor pulmonale is dependent on the severity of the underlying lung pathology.

Prevalence
- Upwards of 2/1,000 neonatal intensive care unit patients will develop significant cor pulmonale.
- 2% of infants undergoing cardiac surgery will have PH, with an associated mortality of 10–20%.

RISK FACTORS
Genetics
- Pediatric patients with trisomy syndromes are at high risk for PH.
- Familial PH has been mapped to chromosome 2q32, but this is less frequently found in patients with secondary etiologies of PH.
- Region 2q32 point mutations encode for a defective bone morphogenic receptor 2, a pulmonary vascular smooth muscle receptor that mediates proliferation.

PATHOPHYSIOLOGY
- Chronic hypoxia is the principal factor, resulting in a cascade of endothelial dysfunction with pulmonary vasoconstriction, followed by the development of PH.
- A variety of vasoactive mediators may be responsible for the effect on vasomotor tone.
- Alveolar hypoventilation, hypoxemia, hypercarbia, and/or acidemia all result in increased RV afterload and decreased RV systolic function.

ETIOLOGY
- Parenchymal lung disease (most common)
- Chronic obstructive pulmonary disease:
  – Cystic fibrosis
  – Asthma
- Restrictive lung disease:
  – Infectious
  – Pulmonary toxins
  – Pulmonary fibrosis
  – Bronchopulmonary dysplasia (combined)
- Upper airway diseases: Tonsillar/adenoidal hypertrophy
- Syndromes (Down, Treacher Collins)
- Neuromuscular disorders: Duchenne muscular dystrophy
- Chest wall deformities

COMMONLY ASSOCIATED CONDITIONS
- Pulmonary vascular abnormalities
- Collagen vascular diseases
- Pulmonary veno-occlusive disease
- Pulmonary thromboembolism
- PPHN

 DIAGNOSIS

HISTORY
- Fatigue
- Failure to thrive/weight loss
- Dizziness
- Syncope
- Exercise intolerance
- Chest pain (secondary to RV ischemia)
- Palpitations
- Hemoptysis

ALERT
Hemoptysis is a life-threatening emergency and heralds a poor prognosis for any patient with PH.

PHYSICAL EXAM
- Tachycardia
- Parasternal RV impulse
- Cyanosis may be evident.
- Hepatomegaly, jugular venous distention, peripheral edema
- A loud, narrowly split or single 2nd heart sound (P_2), RV gallop, holosystolic murmur right of the sternum (tricuspid regurgitation), and/or diastolic murmur at the left upper sternal border (pulmonary insufficiency)

ALERT
In the newborn period to puberty, an abnormally increased RV impulse is best felt under the xiphoid sternum.

DIAGNOSTIC TESTS & INTERPRETATION
Lab
- Brain-type natriuretic peptide is an excellent biomarker of RV diastolic dysfunction and is elevated with worsening cor pulmonale.
- Decreased PaO_2, increased $PaCO_2$, and a compensatory metabolic alkalosis
- Polycythemia may be consistent with chronic hypoxemia.

Imaging
- Chest radiograph: Cardiomegaly from RV dilation and main pulmonary artery enlargement
- Echo: RV dilation, RV hypertrophy, pulmonic insufficiency, and RV pressure estimate from tricuspid regurgitation and/or intraventricular septal position
- V/Q scan is beneficial to rule out thromboembolic disease.

Diagnostic Procedures/Other
- ECG: May show right atrial enlargement, RV hypertrophy, and T-wave inversion
- 6-minute walk: Measures functional capacity and limitations
- Cardiac catheterization, although invasive, remains the gold standard.
- Lung biopsy is usually contraindicated in the face of PH and significant lung disease.

Pathological Findings

- Vascular lesions (plexiform lesions)
- Parenchymal fibrotic lesions
- Concentric and eccentric remodeling

DIFFERENTIAL DIAGNOSIS

- Congenital heart disease with PH and right-to-left shunt (Eisenmenger syndrome)
- Obstruction of pulmonary venous return, both anatomic obstruction and left ventricular failure
- Pulmonary veno-occlusive disease
- Alveolar capillary dysplasia

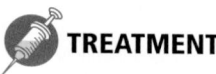 TREATMENT

MEDICATION (DRUGS)

First Line

- Oxygen to keep saturations >90%
- Anticongestive medications (digoxin, diuretics)

Second Line

Vasodilator therapy with care not to worsen the intrapulmonary shunt

ADDITIONAL TREATMENT

General Measures

- The primary goal is reduction of the abnormally elevated pulmonary artery pressure and the RV workload.
- If at all possible, address the primary etiology (i.e., tonsillectomy/adenoidectomy in a patient with obstructive upper airway disease).
- Fluid boluses are poorly tolerated and rarely augment systemic BP.
- Oxygen (nocturnal oxygen)
- Diuretics (if pulmonary congestion)
- Bronchodilators (theophylline)
- Digoxin (may improve RV contractility)
- Anticoagulants

- Pulmonary vasodilators:
  - Nitric oxide
  - Calcium channel blockers (only if >1-year-old and cardiac output is not compromised)
  - Phosphodiesterase-5 inhibitors
  - Endothelin receptor antagonists
  - Prostanoid
- Atrial septostomy (in select cases, may improve cardiac output but at the expense of hypoxemia)
- Lung or heart–lung transplantation
- Usually self-limited activity
- No competitive sports
- Arginine, a nitric oxide donor, has been used; however, the increased amino acid concentrations are proliferative and may worsen the long-term prognosis.

SURGERY/OTHER PROCEDURES

Consider tracheostomy, Nissen fundoplication, and G-tube early

 ONGOING CARE

FOLLOW-UP RECOMMENDATIONS

Patient Monitoring

Home oxygen saturation monitoring is indicated when night O_2 is necessary to keep saturations >90%.

PROGNOSIS

- Patients with reversible lung disease usually have a better prognosis.
- Patients with cor pulmonale are at risk for sudden death because of the inability to augment cardiac output with exercise, growth, or febrile illnesses.
- Numerous medical therapies and lung transplantation may improve long-term survival.
- Long-term survival is variable and depends on the age at onset of pulmonary changes and the underlying conditions (e.g., Down syndrome) that may adversely affect survival.
- Death often occurs in the 2nd or 3rd decade of life.

COMPLICATIONS

Aside from the underlying lung process, the chronic hypoxia results in polycythemia, decreased systemic oxygen delivery, and RV failure secondary to the inability of the RV to handle the excessive afterload.

ADDITIONAL READING

- Bandla HP, Davis SH, Hopkins NE. Lipoid pneumonia: A silent complication of mineral oil aspiration. *Pediatrics*. 1999;103(2):E19.
- Brouillette RT, Fernback SK, Hunt CE. Obstructive sleep apnea in infants and children. *J Pediatr*. 1982;100(1):31–40.
- Perkin RM, Anas NG. Pulmonary hypertension in pediatric patients. *J Pediatr*. 1984;105(4):511–522.
- Proceedings of the 4th World Symposium on Pulmonary Hypertension, February 2008, Dana Point, California, USA. *J Am Coll Cardiol*. 2009; 54(Suppl 1):S1–S117.
- Rashid A, Ivy D. Severe paediatric pulmonary hypertension: New management strategies. *Arch Dis Child*. 2005;90:92–98.
- Simonneau G, Robbins M, Beghetti M, et al. Updated clinical classification of pulmonary hypertension. *J Am Coll Cardiol*. 2009;54(Suppl 1): S43–S54.

 CODES

ICD9

- 415.0 Acute cor pulmonale
- 416.9 Chronic pulmonary heart disease, unspecified

ICD10

- I26.09 Other pulmonary embolism with acute cor pulmonale
- I27.81 Cor pulmonale (chronic)

FAQ

- Q: Is cardiac catheterization indicated in all patients with cor pulmonale?
- A: Yes. Although a great deal of information can be learned from echocardiogram, direct pulmonary artery pressure/resistance measurements require an invasive procedure. In addition, assessment of the reactivity of the pulmonary vascular bed to various agents (oxygen, prostacyclin, and calcium channel blockers) is best performed in the catheterization laboratory.
- Q: Is nocturnal oxygen therapy beneficial?
- A: Nocturnal oxygen has been speculated to delay the progression of cor pulmonale in some select patients with obstructive sleep hypoxemia.

COSTOCHONDRITIS

Richard M. Kravitz

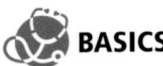 **BASICS**

DESCRIPTION
Costochondritis is chest pain that emanates from a costal cartilage and is reproducible on compression of that cartilage.

ALERT
- Inflammatory costochondritis:
  - Important cause of school absence
  - Adolescents tend to limit physical activity unnecessarily for long periods.
  - Restriction of activities is usually not required.
  - Most adolescents still worry about cardiac problems, even after the diagnosis has been made.
- Infectious costochondritis:
  - Long-term IV antibiotics alone do not resolve the problem; surgical resection and repair also are required.
  - There is a tendency for the infection to spread to adjacent costal cartilages and across the sternum to the contralateral chest wall.
  - In general, avoid costochondral junctions when performing surgical procedures in the chest (i.e., chest-tube placement).

EPIDEMIOLOGY
Incidence
Incidence of sternal wound infections following median sternotomy is 0.1–1.6%.

Prevalence
- Costochondritis accounts for 10–31% of all pediatric chest pain.
- Peak age for chest pain in children is 12–14 years.

PATHOPHYSIOLOGY
- Inflammation of unknown etiology (histologic examination is usually normal)
- Infection:
  - Can present months to years after surgery (the costal cartilage is avascular, making it vulnerable to infection if it has been exposed, injured, or denuded of perichondrium)
  - Complication of median sternotomy
  - Occurs by spread from adjacent osteomyelitis or may arise de novo during surgery

ETIOLOGY
- Infectious:
  - Bacterial:
    - *Staphylococcus aureus* (especially after thoracic surgery)
    - *Salmonella* (in sickle cell disease)
    - *Escherichia coli*
    - *Pseudomonas* sp.
    - *Klebsiella* sp.
  - Fungal:
    - *Aspergillus flavus*
    - *Candida albicans*
- Posttraumatic injury

DIAGNOSIS

HISTORY
- Inflammatory costochondritis:
  - Pain usually preceded by exercise or an upper respiratory tract infection
  - Description of pain:
    - Usually sharp
    - Affects the anterior chest wall
    - Localized or radiates to the back or abdomen
    - Usually unilateral (left side greater than right side)
  - The 4th to 6th costochondral junction is the usual site of pain.
  - Motion of the arm and shoulder on the affected side elicits the pain.
  - Girls are affected more often than are boys.
- Tietze syndrome:
  - Onset is usually abrupt, but can be gradual.
  - Believed to be caused by a minor trauma, though etiology is unknown
  - Description of pain:
    - Radiates to arms or shoulder
    - May last up to several weeks
    - Swelling at the sternochondral junction may persist for several months to years
  - Usually affects the 2nd or 3rd costochondral joint
  - Pain is aggravated by sneezing, coughing, deep inspiration, or twisting motions of the chest
  - No differences in frequency between sexes
- Infectious costochondritis:
  - Slow, insidious course
  - Usually unimpressive clinical symptomatology

PHYSICAL EXAM
- Usually normal
- Inspect for evidence of trauma, scars, bruising, and swelling
- Palpation and percussion of the costochondral and costosternal junctions should reproduce and localize the pain.
- In Tietze syndrome, spindle-shaped swelling is visible at the sternochondral junction.

DIAGNOSTIC TESTS & INTERPRETATION
Lab
- WBC count not helpful (even when infection present)
- EKG (may be helpful if cardiac etiology is being considered)

Imaging
- Radiologic studies (chest x-ray, CT) usually not helpful
- Gallium scan:
  - May be useful in some cases of infectious origin
  - Not highly specific
  - May show increased radionuclide uptake
  - No evidence of osteomyelitis of the sternum in most cases
- Technetium bone scan:
  - Not highly specific

DIFFERENTIAL DIAGNOSIS
- Cardiovascular:
  - Myocardial infarction
  - Pericarditis
  - Pericardial effusion
  - Myocarditis
  - Endocarditis
  - Cardiomyopathy
  - Premature ventricular contractions
  - Supraventricular tachycardia
  - Dissecting aneurysm
- Pulmonary:
  - Asthma
  - Exercise-induced bronchospasm
  - Pneumonia
  - Pleural effusion
  - Pneumothorax
  - Pulmonary embolism

- GI:
  - Gastroesophageal reflux
  - Esophagitis
  - Gastritis
  - Achalasia
- Mechanical:
  - Muscle strain
  - Stress fractures
  - Precordial catch syndrome
  - Trauma
- Rheumatologic:
  - Rheumatoid arthritis
  - Ankylosing spondylitis
- Oncologic:
  - Rhabdomyosarcoma
  - Leukemia
  - Ewing sarcoma
- Miscellaneous:
  - Tietze syndrome
  - Psychogenic chest pain
  - Breast tissue pain (both sexes)

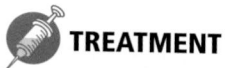 TREATMENT

ADDITIONAL TREATMENT
General Measures
- Inflammatory costochondritis:
  - Anti-inflammatory and analgesic agents
  - Reassurance
  - If pain disturbs normal activities and sports, infiltration with local anesthetic may prove useful.
- Infectious costochondritis:
  - Prolonged course of IV antibiotics
  - Prompt surgical resection of all involved cartilage
  - Reconstructive surgery with muscular flaps should be done.

 ONGOING CARE

FOLLOW-UP RECOMMENDATIONS
Patient Monitoring
- Inflammatory costochondritis:
  - Long-lasting condition
  - Follow-up once a year is recommended.
- Infectious costochondritis:
  - Long-term follow-up after surgery is mandatory.

PROGNOSIS
- Inflammatory costochondritis: Excellent
- Infectious costochondritis: Prognosis relates to:
  - Underlying clinical condition of the patient (i.e., immunocompromised, postradiation therapy for cancer, postcardiac surgery)
  - Extent of surgery required to reconstruct the area damaged by the infection

ADDITIONAL READING

- Brown RT, Jamil K. Costochondritis in adolescents: A follow-up study. *Clin Pediatr*. 1993;32:499–500.
- Fraz M. *Pediatric Respiratory Disease: Diagnosis and Treatment*. Philadelphia: WB Saunders; 1993: 62–172.
- Kocis KC. Chest pain in pediatrics. *Pediatr Clin North Am*. 1999;46:189–203.
- Mendelson G, Mendelson H, Horowitz SF, et al. Can 99mtechnetium methylene diphosphate bone scans objectively document costochondritis? *Chest*. 1997;111:1600–1602.
- Selbst DM. Chest pain in children: Consultation with the specialist. *Pediatr Rev*. 1997;18:169–173.
- Son MB, Sundel RP. Musculoskeletal causes of pediatric chest pain. *Pediatr Clin North Am* 2010; 57:1385–1395.

 CODES

ICD9
- 733.6 Tietze's disease
- 786.50 Chest pain, unspecified
- 786.59 Other chest pain

ICD10
- M94.0 Chondrocostal junction syndrome [Tietze]
- R07.89 Other chest pain
- R07.9 Chest pain, unspecified

FAQ
- Q: Am I having or will I have a heart attack?
- A: Chest pain does not imply a heart problem. This pain arises from the chest wall; there is no risk of a myocardial infarction. A cardiac etiology to chest pain in an adolescent is usually uncommon.
- Q: Is costochondritis related to arthritis?
- A: There is no relation to any form of arthritis.

COUGH

Margaret McNamara

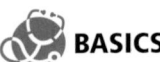 **BASICS**

DEFINITION
The result of a high-velocity expiration, which removes airway secretions, is generally reflexive, but may sometimes be voluntarily initiated or suppressed.

EPIDEMIOLOGY
Cough is the most common symptom presenting to primary care physicians in the US and worldwide, and chronic cough accounts for up to 9% of chief complaints to US pediatricians. In the US, billions of dollars are spent yearly on over-the-counter (OTC) cough and cold medications.

PATHOPHYSIOLOGY
Cough is a symptom of a variety of underlying conditions, which results from a complex reflex phenomenon initiated by cough receptors and mediated in the brainstem's cough center. These receptors are located throughout the large- to medium-sized airways (but not the lower airways), pharynx, paranasal sinuses, external auditory canal, and stomach, and are triggered by thermal, chemical, mechanical, or inflammatory stimuli. The resultant high-velocity expiration, which removes airway secretions, is generally reflexive, but may sometimes be voluntarily initiated or suppressed.

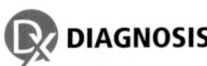 **DIAGNOSIS**

DIFFERENTIAL DIAGNOSIS
Infection and asthma are the most common causes of cough in all pediatric age groups and should always be considered.

- **Causes of acute (<2 weeks) or subacute/ protracted (2–4 weeks) cough**
  - Infection
  - Reactive airway disease (RAD)
  - Sinusitis
  - Irritants
  - Allergy
  - Foreign body
- **Causes of chronic (>4 weeks) cough**
  - Infection
  - Asthma or asthmatic bronchitis
  - Sinusitis
  - Irritants (postinfectious, air pollution)
  - Allergy
  - Foreign body
  - Gastroesophageal reflux (GER)
  - Habitual or psychogenic
  - Anatomic abnormalities: Tracheoesophageal fistula, tracheobronchomalacia, laryngeal cleft, polyps, adductor vocal cord paralysis, pulmonary sequestration, bronchogenic cyst, cystic hygroma, vascular ring, tumor
  - Cystic fibrosis (CF)
  - Ciliary dyskinesia syndromes
  - Immunodeficiency states: HIV, immunoglobulin deficiencies (IgA, IgG), phagocytic defects, complement deficiency
  - Pulmonary hemosiderosis
  - Angiotensin-converting enzyme inhibitors
  - External auditory canal irritation

APPROACH TO THE PATIENT
Given the common nature of cough and the large differential diagnosis it generates, an extremely thorough history and physical exam (H&P) should direct a rational, stepwise approach. ACCP evidence-based clinical practice guidelines for evaluating chronic cough in pediatrics were published in 2006. In general, children with chronic cough should have a chest radiograph, and spirometry should be considered for children >3 years.

- Wright peak flow (WPF) rate; complete pulmonary function tests:
  - Easy to perform WPF in the primary care office with the proper flow meter
  - Helpful to get prebronchodilator and postbronchodilator rates if RAD suspected
  - Standardized tables available with values based on height and race
- Pulmonary function tests may be indicated for diagnosis as well as for assessment of severity or treatment of asthmatics.
- Mantoux test: Purified protein derivative (PPD) to rule out tuberculosis (TB).

HISTORY
- **Question:** Is the cough acute or chronic?
- *Significance:* Pediatric chronic cough is defined as daily cough that lasts for >4 weeks. Although there is significant overlap, differential diagnosis varies depending on the time course.
- **Question:** How is this problem different in children as compared with adults?
- *Significance:* Differential diagnosis varies considerably based on the patient's age.
- **Question:** Is there a recent history of upper respiratory infection (URI)?
- *Significance:* Serial URIs, the most common cause of chronic cough in children, can be diagnosed by a careful history that elucidates waxing and waning symptoms, and will avoid unnecessary tests. Children have an average of 6–8 URIs per year, with each lasting up to 2–3 weeks. Also consider postinfectious/irritative cough, or sinusitis (which complicates up to 5% of URIs). Overall, 8–12% of children with URIs develop complications.
- **Question:** What are the associated symptoms?
- *Significance:*
  - Fever, nasal discharge suggest infection.
  - Fever with chills or night sweats suggests TB; may also have weight loss with TB.
  - Sputum production indicates bronchiectasis or other lower airway pathology.
  - With rhinorrhea, halitosis, headache or facial edema, consider sinusitis.
  - With respiratory distress, suspect RAD, infection, or foreign body.
- **Question:** What is the quality of the cough?
- *Significance:*
  - Chronic wet cough suggests lower airway infection, CF, or bronchiectasis.
  - Dry cough suggests RAD, fungal infection.
  - Barking cough is usually associated with croup.
  - Honking cough is typical in psychogenic cough.
  - Brassy cough may be associated with tracheomalacia or habit cough.
  - Staccato cough suggests Chlamydia in infants.
  - Paroxysmal cough, with or without whoop, suggests pertussis, parapertussis.

- **Question:** What is the pattern of the cough?
- *Significance:*
  - Chronic nighttime cough suggests RAD.
  - With nighttime/early morning cough, consider sinusitis.
  - Seasonal cough suggests allergy.
- **Question:** Are there any known triggers of cough (e.g., smoke, cold air, dust, URI)?
- *Significance:* Consider irritant, allergy, or RAD
- **Question:** Is there any personal or familial history of atopy?
- *Significance:* Consider RAD
- **Question:** Is there a history of recurrent infections?
- *Significance:* Consider immunodeficiency, CF. Also consider pulmonary sequestration if patient has recurrent pneumonias in same location.
- **Question:** Is there any relation of cough to feedings?
- *Significance:* Consider aspiration, GER, and tracheoesophageal fistula in infants.
- **Question:** Is there a history of a choking episode?
- *Significance:* Consider retained foreign body, although there may not be a history of a choking episode in this case, and cough may be episodic as foreign body moves along respiratory tract.
- **Question:** Is there failure to thrive?
- *Significance:* Rule out TB, CF, immunodeficiency
- **Question:** What is the parental level of concern?
- *Significance:* Children's cough generates significant parental stress and concerns, and appreciation of parental worries is valuable when addressing this problem.

PHYSICAL EXAM
- Assess patient's general appearance
- **Finding:** Evidence of failure to thrive?
- *Significance:* Consider TB, CF, immunodeficiency
- **Finding:** Cyanosis or pallor?
- *Significance:* Rule out hypoxemia
- **Finding:** Signs of respiratory distress such as tachypnea, accessory muscle use?
- *Significance:* Most likely RAD or infection
- **Finding:** Barrel chest?
- *Significance:* Suggests air trapping due to chronic disease
- **Finding:** Clubbing?
- *Significance:* May be seen with bronchiectasis
- **Finding:** Nasal polyp?
- *Significance:* May be associated with allergic conditions or CF
- **Finding:** Tracheal deviation?
- *Significance:* Suggests mediastinal mass or foreign body aspiration
- **Finding:** Signs of atopic disease such as eczema, allergic shiners, transverse nasal crease, rhinitis, mucosal cobblestoning, injected conjunctivae?
- *Significance:* Suggest allergy, RAD.
- **Finding:** Rhinorrhea/purulent posterior pharyngeal drainage, sniffling, halitosis, periorbital edema, sinus tenderness?
- *Significance:* Suggest sinusitis
- **Finding:** Wheezing?
- *Significance:*
  - Polyphonic inspiratory or expiratory wheezes suggest RAD.
  - Monophonic or fixed wheezes should make one consider foreign body or mass/congenital lesion.

DIAGNOSTIC TESTS & INTERPRETATION

- Laboratory investigation should reflect a rational, stepwise approach based on likely etiologies after a thorough H&P.
- **Test:** Microbiology workup as indicated (e.g., polymerase chain reaction [PCR] for pertussis, direct fluorescent antibody [DFA] for viral panel, culture for *Chlamydia*).
- *Significance:* Aids in precise diagnosis and treatment as needed
- **Test:** Paranasal sinus CT scan
- *Significance:* Should be used judiciously to evaluate sinus disease.
- **Test:** CBC
- *Significance:* Eosinophilia suggests atopic disease or, rarely, parasitic infection; anemia should prompt one to consider chronic disease or, rarely, pulmonary hemosiderosis.
- **Test:** Sputum sample must contain alveolar macrophages to be adequate.
- *Significance:*
  – Eosinophils suggest asthmatic process or hypersensitivity reaction of lung.
  – Elevated polymorphonuclear cells suggest infection.
  – Predominance of macrophages suggests postinfectious hyper-responsive cough receptors.
  – Hemosiderin staining suggests pulmonary hemosiderosis.
  – Lipid-laden macrophages suggest recurrent aspiration.
  – Routine or special cultures based on likely pathogens
- **Test:** Serum IgE
- *Significance:* Significant elevation indicates allergy or, rarely, parasites.
- **Test:** CFTR mutation panel
- *Significance:* To diagnose CF. Alternatively, sweat chloride test, but need to be sure that laboratory has experience with this test.
- **Test:** Immune workup
- *Significance:* HIV; immunoglobulins
- **Test:** pH probe (or barium swallow)
- *Significance:* GER
- **Test:** Bronchoscopy
- *Significance:* To remove foreign body or obtain tissue samples
- **Test:** High-resolution CT scan of the thorax, video fluoroscopy, echocardiogram, sleep polysomnography, or nuclear medicine scans
- *Significance:* May be judiciously used and are generally reserved until after referral to a specialist

Imaging

Chest x-ray:

- Infiltrates may suggest pneumonia, bronchiolitis, pneumonitis, TB, CF, bronchiectasis, foreign body.
- Volume loss may be seen with foreign body aspiration; sometimes need to obtain lateral decubitus views in young children who cannot cooperate with inspiratory/expiratory views.
- Hyperinflation suggests RAD or CF.
- Mediastinal nodes may indicate infection (especially tuberculosis or fungal) or malignancy.

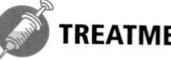 **TREATMENT**

ADDITIONAL TREATMENT
General Measures

- The goal is to treat the underlying cause of the cough, not the symptom.
- To avoid overuse of antibiotics, parents should be informed that viral URI can cause cough that commonly lasts up to 2–3 weeks.
- Educate parents about the beneficial function of cough to remove irritants and about the potential harm of suppressing a productive cough or cough secondary to RAD.
- Honey may be used in children over 1 year old. Acute cough from URI or chronic nonspecific cough (i.e., dry cough in the absence of asthma or other identifiable disease) may be safely, effectively, and inexpensively treated with honey.
- Specific pharmacologic interventions:
  – RAD: Bronchodilators $\pm$ inhaled anti-inflammatory agents, oral or inhaled steroids, removal of irritants
  – Infection: Appropriate antibiotics as indicated. May be considered in cases of chronic moist cough
  – Antihistamines (nonsedating) should be used only when cough coexists with rhinitis.
  – OTC cough medicines are widely prescribed and overused. Systematic reviews conclude that OTC preparations have not been shown to be efficacious in children <5 years of age, have been associated with significant toxicity in this age group, and should be avoided.
- Self-hypnosis is a safe, effective treatment for children with habitual cough.
- Children with "nonspecific cough" (i.e., without specific indicators by H&P as noted above) generally do not derive much benefit from medications and may undergo a period of "watchful waiting." If medications are used, patients need to be reassessed in 2–3 weeks.

ISSUES FOR REFERRAL

- The vast majority of cases of cough, even when chronic, can be diagnosed and managed by the primary care physician.
- Factors in making a referral:
  – The cough is unresponsive to treatment.
  – The cause is likely to be an anatomic malformation or foreign body aspiration.
  – There appears to be involvement of other organ systems (e.g., failure to thrive, GER, congestive heart failure, immunodeficiency, unusual infection).
- Hemoptysis

Initial Stabilization

- Cough should be considered an emergency if there are associated signs or symptoms of respiratory distress.
- Routine emergency airway assessment should be undertaken on presentation and appropriate supportive measures started in cases in which there is concern.

ADDITIONAL READING

- Anbar RD, Hall HR. Childhood habit cough treated with self-hypnosis. *J Pediatr.* 2004;144(2):213–227.
- Carr BC. Efficacy, abuse, and toxicity of over-the-counter cough and cold medicines in the pediatric population. *Curr Opin Pediatr.* 2006; 18(2):184–188.
- Chang AB. American College of Chest Physicians cough guidelines for children: Can its use improve outcomes? *Chest.* 2008;134(6):1111–1112.
- Chang AB. Cough. *Pediatr Clin North Am.* 2009;56:19–31.
- Chang AB, Glomb WB. Guidelines for evaluating chronic cough in pediatrics: ACCP evidence-based clinical practice guidelines. *Chest.* 2006; 129(Suppl 1):260S–283S.
- Marchant JM, Morris PS, Gaffney J, et al. Antibiotics for prolonged moist cough in children (Review). *The Cochrane Library.* 2011;2:1–25.
- Marchant JM, Newcombe PA, Juniper EF, et al. *Chest.* 2008;134(2):303–309.
- Mulholland S, Chang AB. Honey and lozenges for children with non-specific cough (Review). *The Cochrane Library.* 2011;2:1–14.

 CODES

ICD9
- 490 Bronchitis, not specified as acute or chronic
- 493.90 Asthma,unspecified type, unspecified
- 786.2 Cough

ICD10
- J40 Bronchitis, not specified as acute or chronic
- J45.909 Unspecified asthma, uncomplicated
- R05 Cough

FAQ

- Q: Is whooping cough still a problem despite routine childhood immunization?
- A: Yes. Pertussis often goes unrecognized as a cause of acute and chronic cough, particularly in infants who have not completed their immunization series and in older children, adolescents, and adults. Immunity from vaccination or natural infection may wane within 5 years, thus providing a constant reservoir of pertussis in the community.

CROHN DISEASE

Douglas Jacobstein
Robert Baldassano
Petar Mamula

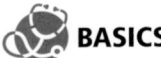 BASICS

DESCRIPTION
Crohn disease (CD) is a chronic inflammatory bowel disease (IBD) that can affect any part of the GI tract.

EPIDEMIOLOGY
- ~20–25% of patients 1st present in childhood or adolescence.
- Family history is present in 30% of patients <30 years old.
- In adulthood, Male = Female; in childhood, Male > Female (1.6:1)

Incidence
- The incidence rate in children is 4.56/100,000 in North America.
- Highest incidence in the white population

RISK FACTORS
Genetics
- 1st-degree relatives have a 5–25% higher risk than the normal population.
- Family members of patients with CD have increased risk for both CD and ulcerative colitis.
- Offspring and siblings have an 8% risk of developing IBD.
- Concordance in monozygotic twins is 50%; in dizygotic twins, 38%.
- CD is complex genetic disease
- 71 CD susceptibility loci have been found on multiple chromosomes.
- CARD15 mutation is present in ~14–18% of patients. Homozygotes carry 2–4% lifetime risk of developing CD.
- Additional genetic links found to possibly predict responses to corticosteroids, anti-TNF agents

PATHOPHYSIOLOGY
- Interaction and combination of environmental factors, genetic susceptibility, host's intestinal flora, and a yet-unspecified triggering factor (likely bacterial products) lead to a dysregulated immune response, causing chronic intestinal inflammation.
- Patients with the CARD15/NOD2 mutation have dysregulated response to bacterial products, which changes innate low-grade to a high-grade inflammatory response.
- There is highly significant association between CD and the IL23R gene on chromosome 1p31, which encodes a subunit of the receptor for the pro-inflammatory cytokine interleukin-23.
- Initially, the T-helper-1 lymphocyte pathway is activated, causing inflammatory cytokines to generate microscopic inflammation, which infiltrates all layers of intestine with cryptitis or crypt abscesses, and distortion of crypt architecture.
- Macroscopically, the intestinal wall is edematous, mesentery may be thickened, local lymph nodes enlarged, and fat extends from the mesentery and "creeps" over the serosal surface.
- Granulomas are found in 20–40% of biopsies and, if found, are pathognomonic.
- Normal bowel can exist in continuity with affected bowel (skip areas).

Rx DIAGNOSIS

HISTORY
- Frequency of signs and symptoms:
  - Weight loss: 85%
  - Diarrhea: 80%
  - Abdominal pain: 85%
  - Fever: 40%
  - Rectal bleeding: 50%
  - Growth failure: 35%
  - Nausea and vomiting: 25%
  - Rectal disease: 25%
  - Extraintestinal signs: 25%
  - Perianal disease: 25%
- Symptoms depend on the intestinal site and the disease activity.
- Sites most often affected, in decreasing frequency, are terminal ileum, right colon, isolated colon, proximal small bowel, and upper GI tract (i.e., stomach, duodenum, esophagus).
- Chronic diarrhea
- Weight loss
- Growth failure (Careful charting of recent growth parameters, especially growth velocities from school or medical records, is essential.)
- Delayed puberty
- Recent travel (enteric infections)
- Antibiotic use (Clostridium difficile)
- Family history of IBD
- Extraintestinal disease:
  - Arthritis
  - Erythema nodosum
  - Pyoderma gangrenosum
  - Mouth ulcers
  - Episcleritis
  - Uveitis
  - Thromboembolic disease
  - Vasculitis
  - Renal stones
  - Amyloidosis
  - Sclerosing cholangitis
  - Pancreatitis

PHYSICAL EXAM
- Growth delay and weight loss, delayed puberty
- Abdominal examination:
  - Hyperactive bowel sounds
  - Right lower quadrant (RLQ) mass and tenderness
  - Palpable thickened loop of intestine
- Rectal and perianal examination: Skin tag, fissure, fistula, and abscess

DIAGNOSTIC TESTS & INTERPRETATION
Lab
- CBC; microcytic anemia due to iron deficiency, normocytic anemia due to chronic disease, macrocytosis suggesting nutrient deficiency: Iron, B_{12}, folate, zinc
- ESR, C-reactive protein, stool calprotectin (disease activity)
- Electrolytes (hydration, renal function)
- Transaminases, alkaline phosphatase, γ-glutamyl transpeptidase (hepatobiliary disease)

- Stool for occult blood and presence of white cells
- Stool cultures, Clostridium difficile toxin A and B
- Perinuclear antineutrophil cytoplasmic antibody (pANCA) and anti-Saccharomyces cerevisiae antibody (ASCA) may be helpful in differentiating among types of IBD.
- Genetic screening among healthy, asymptomatic patients is not recommended.

Imaging
- Consider plain abdominal x-ray in acute presentation to rule out obstruction or perforation.
- Barium upper GI and small bowel follow-through to evaluate extent of disease in small bowel not accessible to endoscopy
- Barium enema has been replaced by colonoscopy in acute colitis and is useful in evaluation of complications such as strictures and fistulas.
- CT scan and ultrasound are useful for evaluation of complications (abscess, phlegmon).
- MRI and abdominal ultrasound are increasingly being used for assessment of disease extent and activity.
- Colonoscopy and upper endoscopy with multiple biopsies are the gold standard tests for initial evaluation and diagnosis of CD.
- Video capsule endoscopy can be used to access small bowel not visualized at the time of endoscopy.

DIFFERENTIAL DIAGNOSIS
- Ulcerative colitis
- Appendicitis
- Infection:
  - Mycobacterium tuberculosis
  - Salmonella
  - Shigella dysenteriae
  - Campylobacter jejuni
  - Aeromonas spp.
  - Yersinia enterocolitica
  - Clostridium difficile
  - Escherichia coli
  - Giardia lamblia
  - Cryptosporidium
  - Strongyloides
- Hemolytic-uremic syndrome
- Henoch-Schönlein purpura
- Irritable bowel syndrome
- Peptic ulcer disease
- Autoimmune enteropathy, immunodeficiency
- Cow's milk protein allergy
- Small intestinal lymphoma

TREATMENT

MEDICATION (DRUGS)

- The goal of therapy is resolution of all symptoms, appropriate growth, and good quality of life. The therapy is used in a stepwise fashion.
- Several 5-aminosalicylic acid (5-ASA) preparations are being used according to their intestinal site of activation because of their anti-inflammatory properties:
  - Mesalamine (Asacol; terminal ileum, colon): 50–100 mg/kg/d (max 4.8 g/d for active disease and 3.2 g/d to maintain remission)
  - Mesalamine (Pentasa; duodenum, jejunum, ileum, colon): 50–100 mg/kg/d (max 4 g/d for active disease and 3 g/d to maintain remission)
  - Balsalazide (Colazal; 6.75 g/d; 110–170 mg/kg/d): Can be given to small children as liquid preparation
  - Mesalamine (Rowasa): 4-g enemas and 500-mg suppositories daily to b.i.d. PR
- Corticosteroids can control intestinal inflammation: 1–2 mg/kg/d oral prednisone (max 60 mg). Initially, patient is treated for several weeks and tapered off within several weeks. Topical hydrocortisone is useful in localized left-sided colonic disease and is available in liquid and foam enemas. Corticosteroid with controlled ileal release, budesonide (9 mg/d) is available.
- Nutritional therapy is frequently used in Europe and Canada as a 1st-line therapy:
  - Elemental and polymeric diet is reported to be effective in inducing remission in active disease.
  - To correct growth failure, an increase in caloric intake is recommended and can be given as overnight nasogastric feeding if oral supplements are not tolerated.
- Azathioprine, 2–3 mg/kg/d, and its metabolite 6-mercaptopurine, 1–1.5 mg/kg/d, are used for the immunomodulatory properties in patients who are unresponsive to corticosteroids or who are dependent on them, and for perianal disease. Adverse events include liver toxicity and leukopenia.
- Frequent laboratory follow-up is necessary, and WBC should be maintained >3–4 × 109/L and platelets >100 × 109/L.
- Methotrexate, 15–25 mg IM or PO once a week
- Other immunomodulatory therapy used infrequently: Cyclosporine, tacrolimus (FK-506), thalidomide, etc.
- Antibiotics:
  - Metronidazole: 15 mg/kg/d
  - Ciprofloxacin: 20 mg/kg/d
- Infliximab, a biologic, chimeric anti–tumor necrosis factor-α antibody (5 mg/kg IV infusion, given every 2–3 months, after initial 3-dose induction therapy at 0, 2, and 6 weeks) for severe and fistulizing disease unresponsive to other therapy
- Other biologic therapies including anti-TNF-α antibodies adalimumab and certolizumab and the antiadhesion molecule natalizumab are available, but not yet approved for use in pediatric CD.
- Complementary therapy (probiotics, prebiotics)

SURGERY/OTHER PROCEDURES

- Surgery is used in patients with localized disease that is unresponsive to other therapy, intractable bleeding, stricturizing disease, especially in case of proximal intestinal dilatation, and perforation. Several types of procedures are available: Strictureplasty, abscess drainage, and intestinal resection (side-to-side anastomosis is widely accepted).
- Most of these procedures are performed laparoscopically, which reduces recovery time.
- Surgery is not curative, and postoperative recurrence at the site of anastomosis is common.

 ## ONGOING CARE

FOLLOW-UP RECOMMENDATIONS
Patient Monitoring
- The morbidity of this disease is high. The majority of patients experience recurring disease.
- Most patients have good general health in between disease and go on to lead productive lives.
- Carcinoma surveillance is necessary on a regular basis.
- After 5 and 20 years of disease, the probability of survival is 98% and 89% of expected survival, respectively.
- Death is a rare complication (2.4% in a large series).

COMPLICATIONS
- Intestinal obstruction due to strictures, or adhesions
- Abscess or phlegmon formation
- Enteroenteric, enterovesical, enterovaginal, and enterocutaneous fistulas
- Perforation
- Gallstones, kidney stones
- Intestinal lymphoma, colon cancer
- Malabsorption resulting in deficiency (e.g., vitamin B_{12} and bile salt deficiency, iron deficiency)
- Massive hemorrhage is rare (1%).
- Growth failure is frequent; final height is reduced and puberty is delayed in CD affecting prepubertal children.
- Osteopenia and osteoporosis secondary to inflammation, nutritional deficiency, and therapeutic side effects (corticosteroids)
- Toxic megacolon is a rare but serious complication.

ADDITIONAL READING

- Benchimol EI, Fortinsky KJ, Gozdyra P, et al. Epidemiology of pediatric inflammatory bowel disease: A systematic review of international trends. *Inflamm Bowel Dis.* 2011;17:423–439.
- Cabre E, Gassull MA. Nutritional and metabolic issues in inflammatory bowel disease. *Curr Opin Clin Nutr Metab Care.* 2003;6(5):569–576.
- Henderson P, van Limbergen JE, Wilson DC, et al. Genetics of childhood-onset inflammatory bowel disease. *Inflamm Bowel Dis.* 2011;17:346–361.
- Hildebrand H, Karlberg J, Kristiansson B. Longitudinal growth in children with IBD. *J Pediatr Gastroenterol Nutr.* 1994;18(2):165–173.
- Kugathasan S, Baldassano RN, Bradfield JP, et al. Loci on 20q13 and 21q22 are associated with pediatric-onset inflammatory bowel disease. *Nat Genet.* 2008;40:1211–1215.
- Mamula P, Markowitz JE, Baldassano RN. Inflammatory bowel disease in early childhood and adolescence: Special considerations. *Gastroenterol Clin North Am.* 2003;32(3):967–995, viii.
- Navarro F, Hanauer SB. Treatment of inflammatory bowel disease: Safety and tolerability issues. *Am J Gastroenterol.* 2003;98(12 suppl):S18–S23.
- Seidman E, Leleiko N, Ament M, et al. Nutritional issues in pediatric inflammatory bowel disease. *J Pediatr Gastroenterol Nutr.* 1991;12:424.
- Spray C, Debelle GD, Murphy MS. Current diagnosis, management and morbidity in paediatric inflammatory bowel disease. *Acta Paediatr.* 2001;90(4):400–405.

CODES

ICD9
- 555.0 Regional enteritis of small intestine
- 555.1 Regional enteritis of large intestine
- 555.9 Regional enteritis of unspecified site

ICD10
- K50.019 Crohn's disease of small intestine with unspecified complications
- K50.119 Crohn's disease of large intestine with unspecified complications
- K50.919 Crohn's disease, unspecified, with unspecified complications

FAQ

- Q: Should the diet of patients with CD be restricted?
- A: Balanced nutrition is required to assure appropriate growth and development. The only foods not recommended are poorly digestible vegetables (if eaten raw), nuts, and popcorn, which can cause obstruction in the narrowed, inflamed intestine. Patients with secondary lactose intolerance should use lactase supplements or avoid milk products while ensuring adequate calories and calcium intake.
- Q: What is the cause of CD?
- A: Both genetic and environmental factors are important in the development of CD. Possible environmental factors include aseptic environment in the 1st few years of life, lack of breast-feeding, frequent use of antibiotics or aspirin, and diet.
- Q: Where can I learn more about CD?
- A: The Crohn and Colitis Foundation of America (CCFA, www.CCFA.org) is a nonprofit organization dedicated to the care of people with CD and ulcerative colitis.
- Q: What new therapies will be used in the near future?
- A: Biologic agents, which use our recently improved knowledge of the immune system either to downregulate inflammatory mediators or upregulate immunomodulatory mediators. It is hoped that this new class of therapies will greatly improve our care of people with CD.

CROUP

Daniel Walmsley

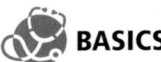 **BASICS**

DESCRIPTION

- Croup (laryngotracheobronchitis) is a common respiratory illness in children that presents with hoarseness, a characteristic barking cough, rhinorrhea, and fever.
- Spasmodic croup (subglottic allergic edema) refers to an illness characterized by sudden inspiratory stridor at night followed by sudden resolution. Mild cold symptoms may be present but are often absent. The child can have frequent attacks on the same night or for multiple, successive nights.

EPIDEMIOLOGY

- Accounts for 15% of the respiratory illnesses seen in children.
- Most commonly occurs in children between 6 and 36 months of age. Although cases can be seen up to 6 years of age, it is uncommon in children older than 6 years.
- Most prevalent in the fall to early winter
- More common in males
- ER visits for croup are most frequent between the hours of 10 pm and 4 am.

RISK FACTORS

- Age: mean age at presentation is 18 months.
- Season: fall or winter
- Anatomic narrowing of the airway (subglottic stenosis, Down syndrome)
- Prior history of croup
- Hyperactive airway (atopic children)
- Pre-existing airway swelling

ETIOLOGY

In children, the cricoid ring of the trachea, located in the immediate subglottic area, is the narrowest part of their upper airway. A small amount of edema in this region can lead to significant airway obstruction; which is what makes them especially susceptible to this illness.

Caused mainly by respiratory viruses including:

- Parainfluenza virus types 1–3, most commonly; accounting for 65% of cases
- Adenovirus
- RSV
- Influenza virus A,B
- Rhinoviruses
- Enteroviruses
- Metapneumovirus
- Enteric cytopathogenic human orphan virus (echovirus)
- Measles—in areas where measles is prevalent
- *Mycoplasma pneumoniae*
- Bacterial infection may occur secondarily by *Staph. aureus*, *S. pyogenes*, and *S. pneumoniae*

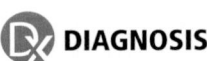 **DIAGNOSIS**

HISTORY

- Croup typically starts with rhinorrhea, cough, coryza, and congestion.
- After a short period (12–48 hours), upper airway obstruction occurs resulting in hoarseness, "barky cough", and inspiratory stridor.
- Fever is often present.
- Symptoms persist for 3–7 days.

- The sudden development of inspiratory stridor without other upper respiratory tract infection (URI) symptoms or fever should prompt the consideration of a foreign body aspiration.
- Recurrent episodes of stridor should lead to the consideration of spasmodic croup, an anatomical abnormality, or an underlying condition such as atopy.
- In a child with truncal or multiple strawberry hemangiomas, a sudden episode of stridor without fever or URI symptoms should raise the concern for a hemangioma in the child's airway.
- Bacterial tracheitis should be suspected in a child who develops marked worsening of symptoms with a high fever after having 5–7 days of mild croup symptoms.

PHYSICAL EXAM

- Examine in a comfortable position and every effort should be taken to minimize anxiety as this can often worsen the symptoms.
- Observe for stridor at rest, irritability, and fatigue. Assess respiratory status and level of consciousness.
- Vital signs: Fever and tachypnea may be present. A child with croup is usually not hypoxic because croup affects the upper airway. Hypoxia is seen only when complete airway obstruction is imminent.
- A child with croup will likely have a hoarse voice, coryza, inflamed pharynx, and varying degrees of respiratory distress.
- The degree of respiratory distress should be observed by assessing for tachypnea, nasal flaring, retractions, grunting, and use of accessory muscles.
- Children with significant upper airway obstruction may sit in a "sniffing" position with their neck mildly flexed and head mildly extended. This is in contrast to the "tripod" position noted in epiglottitis where the child is in a sitting position with the chin pushed forward and refusing to lie down.
- The presence of inspiratory stridor should be determined. Stridor may be present at rest or only with agitation and this difference will affect the patient's management. Stridor at rest is a sign of significant upper airway obstruction and needs urgent treatment.
- The hydration status of the child should be assessed. Drooling should not be present with croup and, if present, may indicate a different diagnosis such as epiglottitis or peritonsillar abscess.
- The severity of croup can be determined by a clinical scoring system know as the modified Westley Croup Score (see Table 1). A score <3: mild disease; a score of 3–6: moderate disease; and a score >6: severe disease.

DIAGNOSTIC TESTS & INTERPRETATION
Lab

- Croup is a clinical diagnosis and laboratory tests are not needed.
- The anxiety associated with blood draws may actually worsen the child's condition.
- Rapid antigen tests to determine the viral agent responsible for the illness may be helpful if the child has an atypical presentation or for infection control if the child requires admission.

Imaging

- Radiographs may be helpful to rule out other causes of stridor; they should be considered in children with atypical courses, recurrent episodes, failure to

Table 1. Croup (laryngotracheobron-chitis)—severity score for croup patients

Indicator of severity of illness	Score
Inspiratory stridor	
None	0
At rest, with stethoscope	1
At rest, w/o stethoscope	2
Retractions	
None	0
Mild	1
Moderate	2
Severe	3
Air entry	
Normal	0
Decreased	1
Severely decreased	2
Cyanosis	
None	0
With agitation	4
At rest	5
Level of consciousness	
Normal	0
Altered mental status	5

respond to treatment, or if a foreign body is suspected (although most are not radio-opaque).
- Classically, an anteroposterior view demonstrates the "steeple" sign; which is a narrowed air column in the subglottic area.

Diagnosis Procedures/Surgery

- Pulse oximetry
- Visual inspection of the airway via bronchoscopy and direct or fiberoptic laryngoscopy may be helpful in cases of recurrent croup to rule out an anatomical abnormality.

Pathological Findings

- Gross pathology: edema and erythema of the subglottic trachea; occasionally, pseudomembranes or exudate are noted.
- Microscopic: edema of airway lining with infiltration of neutrophils, histiocytes, plasma cells, and lymphocytes

DIFFERENTIAL DIAGNOSIS

- Mainly includes other causes of acute stridor with or without respiratory distress.
- Historically, distinguishing croup from epiglottitis was very significant in that the latter could lead to life-threatening airway obstruction. However, the introduction of the HiB vaccine in 1990 led to a marked decline in epiglottitis. Cases of epiglottitis still occur in unimmunized and underimmunized children; therefore, it is important to check the child's immunization status.

Other important diseases to consider in the differential include:

- **Infectious:**
  - Acute epiglottitis
  - Bacterial tracheitis
  - Retropharyngeal abscess
  - Adenotonsillitis
  - Diphtheria

- Pneumonia
- Ulcerative laryngitis
- **Allergic/inflammatory:**
  - Asthma
  - Anaphylaxis (angioneurotic edema)
  - Microaspiration secondary to gastroesophageal reflux or hypotonia
- **Environmental:**
  - Foreign body aspiration
  - Caustic ingestion or burn
  - Smoke inhalation
  - Paraquat poisoning
- **Traumatic:**
  - Subglottic edema/stenosis postintubation
  - Laryngeal or subglottic hematoma
  - Laryngeal fracture
  - Papillomatosis
  - Hemangioma
  - Cystic hygroma
  - Lymphoma
  - Rhabdomyosarcoma
  - Thymoma
  - Teratoma
  - Thyroglossal duct cyst
  - Branchial cleft cyst
- **Congenital anomalies of the upper airway**
  - Tracheomalacia
  - Vascular ring
  - Laryngeal web
- **Genetic/metabolic:** Hypocalcemia

TREATMENT

INITIAL STABILIZATION
- Racemic epinephrine (see below)
- Corticosteroids
- Oxygen (if needed)
- Endotracheal intubation is very rarely required.

General Measures
- Children with mild symptoms can be treated with humidity, antipyretics, and oral hydration at home. However, RCTs have not shown benefit for the use of humidity.
- Short, acute episodes of stridor can be treated with cool mist, a bathroom filled with steam from a shower or cold night air. If the stridor persists, worsens or occurs at rest, the child should be seen in the emergency room.
- It is important to try to keep the child calm as agitation or anxiety can worsen symptoms and increase work of breathing.
- In the child with impending respiratory failure, prompt intubation and direct visualization of the airway in the operating room is imperative. Do not wait for X-rays to confirm a diagnosis.

MEDICATION (DRUGS)
- Corticosteroids and nebulized racemic epinephrine, the main treatments for croup, have resulted in a dramatic reduction in the number of admissions and length of hospital stays in patients with croup.
- Dexamethasone (PO or IM; half-life 36–54 hours) 0.15–0.6 mg/kg single dose has been shown to reduce symptoms in patients with moderate to severe croup. Oral dexamethasone is the most cost-effective steroid treatment available.
- Alternatively prednisolone 1–2 mg/kg for 1–3 daily doses can be given to a patient with croup, although there is no RCT evidence for this method. A recent double-blinded randomized trial demonstrated that a single dose of 1 mg/kg of prednisolone was NOT

as effective at keeping children from emergency medical care as 0.15 mg/kg of dexamethasone.
- Budesonide given via nebulizer at a dose of 2 mg administered q12h—shown in recent studies to be as effective as dexamethasone in reducing symptoms; less systemic absorption compared with dexamethasone, with maximum deposition of drug in the upper airway. Although widely accepted, budesonide is not as readily used as dexamethasone because it is not as cost-effective.
- Racemic epinephrine: A nebulized racemic epinephrine treatment offers immediate reduction in swelling of the laryngeal airway in children who present in extreme respiratory distress. Dose: 0.5 mL of 2.25% solution (D- and L-isomers) in 2.5 mL normal saline delivered via nebulizer as needed.
- L-epinephrine: If racemic epinephrine is not available, 5 mL of L-epinephrine 1:10,000 delivered via nebulizer is effective.

IN-PATIENT CONSIDERATIONS
Admission Criteria
- Severe respiratory distress on presentation (Croup score of >3)
- Persistent hypoxia despite treatment with steroids and racemic epinephrine
- Requirement of treatment of racemic epinephrine more than once over a 3- to 4-hour period
- Dehydration or risk for dehydration
- Admission should be strongly considered for children who present symptomatically to an ER more than once and have significant stridor on day 1 of illness as croup is usually worse on days 2–3.

Discharge Criteria
- Croup score of ≤3 over a 1- to 3-hour period of observation
- Does not require racemic epinephrine in the 3–4 hours prior to discharge
- Able to take adequate PO fluids

Issues for Referral
- The vast majority of children with croup do well. However, transfer to a facility where trained individuals can address pediatric airway problems should be considered if the patient is inadequately responding to treatment or has increasing respiratory distress.

PROGNOSIS
- The vast majority of patients do not require hospitalization.
- Almost all patients go on to complete recovery.

COMPLICATIONS
- Poor oral intake/dehydration
- Hypoxia
- Upper airway obstruction
- Respiratory failure (rare)

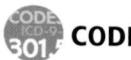

ONGOING CARE

FOLLOW-UP RECOMMENDATIONS
Patient Monitoring
- In most cases, the illness is self-limited, lasting 3–5 days
- A "rebound phenomenon" with worsening of stridor and respiratory distress after initial relief with the racemic epinephrine treatment may be seen up to 2 hours post treatment in some patients.
- Several studies have shown that children can be safely discharged 3–4 hours after racemic epinephrine treatment.

ALERT
Recurrent croup may signal an underlying anatomic problem and needs evaluation for other causes.

ADDITIONAL READING
- Cetinkaya F, Tufekci BS, Kutluk G. A comparison of nebulized budesonide, and intramuscular, and oral dexamethasone for treatment of croup. *Int J Pediatr Otorhinolaryngol.* 2004;68:453–456.
- Cherry JD. Clinical practice croup. *N Engl J Med.* 2008;358(4):384–391.
- Donaldson D, Poleski D, Knipple E, et al. Intramuscular versus oral dexamethasone for the treatment of moderate-to-severe croup: A randomized, double-blind trial. *Acad Emerg Med.* 2003;10:16–21.
- Geelhoed GC, Turner J, Macdonald WB. Efficacy of a small single dose of oral dexamethasone for outpatient croup: A double blind placebo controlled clinical trial. *BMJ.* 1996;313:140–142.
- Malhotra A, Krilov L. Viral croup. *Pediatr Rev.* 2001;(22):5–12.
- Scolnik D, Coates AL, Stephens D, et al. Controlled delivery of high vs low humidity vs mist therapy for croup in emergency departments: A randomized controlled trial. *JAMA.* 2006;295:1274–1280.
- Sparrow A, Geelhoed G. Prednisolone versus dexamethasone in croup: A randomized equivalence trial. *Arch Dis Child.* 2006;91:580–583.
- Westley C, Ross C, Brooks J. Neublized racemic epinephrine by IPPB for the treatment of croup: a double-blind study. *Am J Dis Child.* 1978;132:484–487.

CODES

ICD9
464.4 Croup

ICD10
J05.0 Acute obstructive laryngitis [croup]

FAQ
- Q: Is humidity currently recommended for a patient presenting with croup?
- A: In the previous year, the first randomized controlled trial of mist in the emergency department setting showed no improvement in symptoms in patients with moderate croup.
- Q: Should all children with croup receive steroids?
- A: Steroids are now the first-line treatment for croup. Meta-analysis review strongly supports the use of dexamethasone (PO or IM) or nebulized budesonide for children with moderate to severe croup scores. This analysis showed that steroids result in significant clinical improvement in the first 24 hours after treatment. Increasingly, studies of patients with mild croup are indicating these children may benefit from a single dose of dexamethasone.

CRYING

Mark F. Ditmar

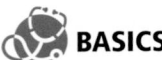 **BASICS**

DEFINITION
- Crying is usually a normal physiologic response to stress, discomfort, unfulfilled needs such as hunger, pain, over- or under-stimulation, or temperature change.
- Crying is felt to be potentially pathologic if it is interpreted by caregivers as differing in quality and duration without apparent explanation and/or persists without consolability beyond a reasonable time (generally 1–2 hours).

ETIOLOGY
- The most likely cause of inconsolable crying in the first few months of life is, without question, infantile colic. Practitioners must be familiar with the clinical pattern of infantile colic, so that deviations are readily recognized.
- Patients' families often suggest teething as a cause of excessive crying (as well as fever, diarrhea, rashes, etc.). Objective data do not support a strong association.
- Be careful in ascribing symptoms and signs to teething.

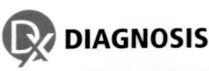 **DIAGNOSIS**

DIFFERENTIAL DIAGNOSIS
- **Congenital/anatomic**
  - Intussusception
  - Gastroesophageal reflux/esophagitis
  - Volvulus
  - Gaseous distention (secondary to improper feeding or burping)
  - Incarcerated inguinal hernia
  - Peritonitis (acute abdomen)
  - Testicular/ovarian torsion
  - Constipation
  - Anal fissure
  - Meatal ulceration
  - Glaucoma
  - Urinary retention (secondary to posterior urethral valves)
  - Cardiac—anomalous coronary artery, hypoxia, congestive heart failure (CHF)
  - Increased intracranial pressure (hydrocephalus, tumor)
- **Infectious**
  - Otitis media/externa
  - Urinary tract infection (UTI)/pyelonephritis
  - Stomatitis/gingivitis
  - Meningitis/encephalitis
  - Discitis
  - Gastroenteritis
  - Mastitis
  - Arthritis, septic
  - Osteomyelitis
  - Perianal cellulitis
  - Balanitis
  - Dermatitis (especially pruritic as in scabies or painful as in staphylococcal scalded skin syndrome)

- **Toxic, environmental, drugs**
  - Neonatal drug withdrawal
  - Prenatal/perinatal cocaine exposure
  - Immunization reactions (especially DPT)
  - Isolated fructose intolerance
  - Drug reactions (especially antihistamines, pseudoephedrine, phenylpropanolamine), including maternal medications in breast milk
  - Vitamin A toxicity
  - Carbon monoxide exposure
  - Emotional/physical neglect
  - Foreign body ingestion (coin, pin)
  - Ear foreign body (e.g., cockroach)
- **Trauma**
  - Corneal abrasion
  - Foreign body (hypopharynx, eye, ear, nose)
  - Skull fracture/subdural hematoma
  - Intracranial hemorrhage
  - Retinal hemorrhage (e.g., shaken baby syndrome)
  - Other fractures (especially extremities)
  - Hair tourniquet syndrome (encircling finger, toe, penis, clitoris)
  - Open diaper pin
  - Bite (human, animal, insect)
- **Genetic/metabolic**
  - Sickle cell crisis
  - Phenylketonuria
  - Hypothyroidism
  - Electrolyte abnormalities (especially sodium)
  - Hypoglycemia
  - Hypocalcemia
  - Hypercalcemia
  - Inborn error of metabolism
- **Allergic/inflammatory**
  - Cow milk allergy
  - Celiac disease (gluten enteropathy)
  - Hemolytic-uremic syndrome
  - Henoch–Schönlein purpura
  - Kawasaki disease
- **Functional**
  - Parental expectations/responses
- **Miscellaneous**
  - Overstimulation
  - Persistent night awakening
  - Night terrors
  - Caffey disease (infantile cortical hyperostosis)
  - Dysrhythmia (especially supraventricular tachycardia)
  - IV infiltration
  - Autism
  - Teething
  - Headache/migraine
  - Temperament
  - Colic
  - Discomfort (cold, heat, itching, hunger)

ALERT
Factors that make this an emergency include:
- Suspicion of meningitis: Stiff neck, bulging fontanel, fever (especially infants <2–3 months)
- Suspicion of intestinal obstruction: Vomiting (especially bilious or projectile), mass on abdominal palpation, and/or bloody stools
- Suspicion of incarcerated hernia or testicular/ovarian torsion
- Evidence of cardiac compromise (CHF, supraventricular tachycardia): Tachycardia, poor perfusion (capillary refill >3 seconds, poor distal pulses), rales
- Evidence of acute dehydration: Weight loss, decreased urine output, orthostatic changes, poor perfusion
- Evidence of child abuse or neglect

APPROACH TO THE PATIENT
General goal is to decide if the crying represents a normal physiologic response, a protracted multifactorial physiologic/developmental response (colic), or a potentially pathologic problem.
- **Phase 1:** How urgent is the need for evaluation? A classic and difficult triage issue. One must identify the periodicity of the problem, associated symptoms, impression of wellness, and parental anxiety/reliability.
- **Phase 2:** When in doubt, particularly if colic seems unlikely, see the patient as soon as possible.

HISTORY
- **Question:** Colic?
- *Significance*:
  - Colic less likely as a cause if onset after 1 month of age or persistent in infants >4 months
  - Recurrent episodes, particularly with a diurnal or evening pattern, are more likely due to colic.
  - Crying shortly after feeding suggests aerophagia or gastroesophageal reflux; 1 hour after feeding suggests formula intolerance. A rare cause of postprandial crying is anomalous coronary arteries.
  - Overfeeding or underfeeding, excessive air swallowing, inadequate burping, and improper formula preparation may contribute to excessive crying.
- **Question:** Fever?
- *Significance*: Indicates potential need for evaluation of meningitis, other infections
- **Question:** Paradoxically increased crying (attempts at consolation make the crying worse, especially with lifting, rocking)?
- *Significance*: Can be seen in meningitis, peritonitis, long-bone fractures, arthritis

- **Question:** Stridor?
- *Significance:* Implies possible upper airway obstruction (mechanical, functional)
- **Question:** Expiratory grunting?
- *Significance:* Indicates higher likelihood of significant pathologic cause of crying (especially cardiac, respiratory, and/or infectious disease)
- **Question:** Cold symptoms and/or daycare attendance?
- *Significance:* Increase likelihood of otitis media
- **Question:** Vomiting?
- *Significance:* Increases likelihood of pathologic GI cause (e.g., obstruction, gastroesophageal reflux with possible esophagitis), particularly in infant <3 months, or CNS disease
- **Question:** Recent fall or trauma?
- *Significance:* May indicate possible fracture, increased intracranial pressure, abuse
- **Question:** Documented weight loss outside of the 2 week neonatal period?
- *Significance:* Suggests an organic cause

PHYSICAL EXAM

- **Finding:** Tympanic membrane with loss of landmarks, poor mobility, and swollen canal?
- *Significance:* Indicate otitis media, otitis externa, foreign body
- **Finding:** Tenderness on palpation of extremities, clavicle, or scalp, or painful or decreased range of motion of joints?
- *Significance:* Suggests fracture, subluxation, osteomyelitis, septic arthritis
- **Finding:** Conjunctival redness, eye tearing, scratches near the eye?
- *Significance:* Suggest corneal abrasion (fluorescein testing of eye warranted) or foreign body in eye (eversion of lid recommended)
- **Finding:** Impacted or bloody stool on rectal exam, abdominal mass?
- *Significance:* Suggest constipation or intussusception
- **Finding:** Geographic scars, frenulum tears, retinal hemorrhages, suspicious bruises, burns, decreased weight/height ratio?
- *Significance:* Suggest neglect/abuse (physical, emotional)
- **Finding:** Bulging or full fontanel (especially in upright, quiet infant)?
- *Significance:* Indicates possible increased intracranial pressure (meningitis, subdural hematoma, vitamin A toxicity)
- **Finding:** Edema of individual toes, fingers, or penis?
- *Significance:* Suggest hair tourniquet syndrome

- **Finding:** Tender swelling in inguinal or scrotal area?
- *Significance:* May indicate incarcerated hernia, testicular torsion
- **Finding:** Heart rate >200 with minimal variability?
- *Significance:* Indicates possible supraventricular tachycardia
- **Finding:** Hypothermia?
- *Significance:* Suggests infections or hypothyroidism

DIAGNOSTIC TESTS & INTERPRETATION

- **Test:** Stool for occult blood
- *Significance:* Possible intussusception, anal fissure
- **Test:** Fluorescein testing of eye
- *Significance:* Corneal abrasion (may occur without significant conjunctival redness)
- **Test:** Urinalysis/urine culture
- *Significance:* UTI
- **Test:** Urine toxicology screen
- *Significance:* Drug withdrawal (neonatal), ingestions, passive exposures (e.g., cocaine)
- **Test:** Pulse oximetry
- *Significance:* Hypoxia (from cardiac causes) may cause increased irritability.
- **Test:** Electrolyte panel/blood glucose
- *Significance:* Endocrine or metabolic disturbance, especially if abnormal sodium, hypoglycemia, significant acidosis, or elevated anion gap

ADDITIONAL READING

- Bolte R. The crying child: What are they trying to tell you? Parts I and II. *Contemp Pediatr.* 2007;24: 74–81, 90–95.
- Douglas P, Hill P. Managing infants who cry excessively in the first few months of life. *BMJ.* 2011;343:1265–1269.
- Freedman SB, Al-Harthy N, Thull-Freedman J. The crying infant: Diagnostic testing and frequency of serious underlying disease. *Pediatrics.* 2009;123: 841–848.
- Herman M, Le A. The crying infant. *Emerg Med Clin North Am.* 2007;25:1137–1159.
- Poole SR. The infant with acute, unexplained, excessive crying. *Pediatrics.* 1991;88:450–455.
- Reijnveld SA, vanderWal MF, Brugman E, et al. Infant crying and abuse. *Lancet.* 2004;364: 1340–1342.

 CODES

ICD9
- 780.92 Excessive crying of infant (baby)
- 789.7 Colic

ICD10
- R10.83 Colic
- R68.11 Excessive crying of infant (baby)

C

CLINICAL PEARLS

- History and physical exam, rather than extensive lab testing, is the key to the diagnosis. In Freedman's ED study of 237 excessively crying infants, fewer than 1% had testing contribute to the diagnosis in the absence of a suggestive clinical picture.
- Be certain that the infant or child is completely undressed so that dermatologic clues will not be missed.
- Quality of cry: Subjective interpretation can be helpful.
  – High-pitched (shrill, piercing) crying in short bursts: Associated with CNS pathology, especially with increased intracranial pressure
  – High-pitched crying in longer bursts: Seen in small-for-gestational age infants, neonatal drug withdrawal
  – Hoarse crying: Seen in hypothyroidism, laryngeal diseases, hypocalcemic tetany
  – Weak crying: May be seen in neuromuscular disorders, infant botulism, and/or the very ill infant
  – Catlike cry: Can be associated with cri du chat syndrome (5p syndrome or absence of short arm of chromosome 5)
- Cessation of crying with ophthalmic anesthetic drops while doing fluorescein staining suggests corneal injury as a cause.
- Bruises are rare in preambulatory children (particularly <6 months); if present, consider inflicted injuries.
- Colic is a diagnosis of exclusion. Be wary of the infant who, despite a period of observation, is not noted at any point to be awake and calm.
- Factors that may help alert you to make a referral include:
  – Infant appears ill (e.g., pallor, grunting, poor arousability, poor response to social overtures)
  – Weight loss or abnormal development (implies much higher likelihood of an organic cause)

CRYPTOCOCCAL INFECTIONS

Samir S. Shah

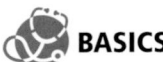

BASICS

DESCRIPTION
Cryptococcosis, an opportunistic fungal infection caused by *Cryptococcus neoformans*, may involve several organ systems, including the CNS, lungs, bones, visceral organs, and skin.

EPIDEMIOLOGY
- Most pediatric infections occur in immunocompromised hosts, including those with malignancy, HIV, and solid-organ or bone marrow transplantation; 20% of infections requiring hospitalization occur in normal hosts.
- There is no person-to-person spread of the infection.

Incidence
- Occurs in 5–15% of HIV-infected adults, usually with CD4+ lymphocyte counts <50 cells/mm^3. Occurs in 0.8–2.3% of HIV-infected children. The lower infection rate in children reflects their lower exposure to sources of *C. neoformans*. The overall seroprevalence is 0% in neonates and 4.1% in school-aged children, compared to 69% in adults.
- 1–3% of solid-organ transplant recipients develop *C. neoformans* infections; typically >1 year after transplantation.

GENERAL PREVENTION
- Most studies on prevention address HIV-infected patients.
- Use of highly-active antiretroviral therapy (HAART) prevents most cases of cryptococcosis in HIV-infected patients.
- Primary prophylaxis with fluconazole prevents new-onset cryptococcal disease in HIV-infected patients. However, primary prophylaxis is not routinely recommended except for those with limited access to HAART and those with high levels of antiretroviral drug resistance.
- Maintenance (suppressive) therapy after completion of therapy for cryptococcal infection is recommended for HIV-infected patients. In those with low CD4+ lymphocyte counts, relapse rates are 100% without maintenance antifungal therapy, 18–25% with amphotericin B or itraconazole, and 2–3% with fluconazole.
  - Prophylaxis may be discontinued in patients receiving HAART with CD4+ lymphocytes >100/mm^3 and undetectable viral loads.
- There is no consensus on the duration of fluconazole suppressive therapy after treatment of cryptococcosis in HIV-negative immunocompromised patients. Most experts provide maintenance (suppressive) antifungal therapy with fluconazole PO (6 mg/kg/d) for at least 1 year after the completion of acute treatment and then reassess its ongoing use based on the level of current immunosuppression.

PATHOPHYSIOLOGY
- Primary infection occurs through the inhalation of aerosolized soil particles containing the yeast forms. The skin and GI tract are also portals of entry.
- Protective immune response requires specific T-cell-mediated immunity.
- CNS infection with *C. neoformans* results from hematogenous dissemination.

COMMONLY ASSOCIATED CONDITIONS
- *C. neoformans* is the most common cause of fungal meningitis in the US.
- Disseminated infection occurs more commonly among immunocompromised hosts.
- Concurrent *Pneumocystis carinii* pneumonia was detected in 13% of adults with cryptococcal meningitis.
- Pulmonary involvement is asymptomatic in up to 50% of cases, and disease may be either focal or widespread.
- Bone involvement occurs in 10% of cases of disseminated cryptococcal infection.
- Cutaneous involvement mimics acne-type eruptions that ulcerate, and results from hematogenous spread of the organism or from direct extension of bone infection.

DIAGNOSIS

HISTORY
- Cryptococcal meningitis may present as either an indolent infection or acute illness.
- Symptoms of cryptococcal meningitis include headache, malaise, and low-grade fever. Nausea, vomiting, altered mentation, and photophobia are less common. Stiff neck, focal neurologic symptoms (e.g., decreased hearing, facial nerve palsy, or diplopia), and seizures are rare.
- Primary pulmonary cryptococcal disease is not well described in children because most cases are disseminated at the time of diagnosis. 50% of adults have cough or chest pain, and fewer have sputum production, weight loss, fever, and hemoptysis.
- In immunocompromised hosts, the onset of infection is more rapid and the course more severe. Pulmonary involvement is minimal when dissemination occurs quickly.

PHYSICAL EXAM
- None of the presenting signs of cryptococcal infection are sufficiently characteristic to distinguish it from other infections, particularly in immunocompromised patients.
- CNS involvement: Nuchal rigidity, photophobia, and focal neurologic deficits
- Respiratory tract involvement: Cough, tachypnea, grunting, and subcostal or intercostal retractions. Decreased breath sounds or dullness to percussion may be present, or the lung exam may be normal.
- Cutaneous manifestations: Erythematous or verrucous papules, nodules, pustules, acneiform lesions, ulcers, abscesses, or granulomas. Lesions can occur anywhere on the body, but are found most often on the face and neck.
  - Mucocutaneous findings are present in 10–15% of cases of disseminated disease.

DIAGNOSTIC TESTS & INTERPRETATION
Lab
- Lumbar puncture: Diagnose cryptococcal meningitis
  - CSF should be sent for cell count and differential; protein; glucose; cultures for bacterial, fungal, and viral pathogens; and cryptococcal antigen (India ink stain is less commonly performed).
  - Examination of the CSF reveals <500 WBC/mm^3 (usually <100 WBC/mm^3), mostly mononuclear leukocytes, with minimal changes in protein. CSF glucose is <50 mg/dL in ~65% of patients.
  - Budding yeast are seen on India ink stain in 50% of cases.
  - CSF cultures are positive in ~90% of patients.
  - The latex agglutination test for cryptococcal polysaccharide antigen is specific, sensitive, and rapid. Titers ≥1:4 suggest the diagnosis of cryptococcal infection if appropriate controls (to exclude the presence of rheumatoid factor or other nonspecific agglutinins) are negative.
  - HIV-infected patients with pneumonia and CD4+ T-lymphocyte counts <200 cells/mm^3 should be evaluated with sputum fungal culture, blood fungal culture, and a serum cryptococcal antigen test. A lumbar puncture to exclude the possibility of occult meningitis should be considered. If any test is positive for *C. neoformans*, then a lumbar puncture should be performed to exclude cryptococcal meningitis.
- Blood culture and serum cryptococcal antigen titers: Diagnose disseminated cryptococcal infection. Serum cryptococcal antigen tests are positive in >85% of patients with cryptococcal meningitis.
- Sputum culture: Diagnose cryptococcal pneumonia
- Skin or bone biopsy: Diagnose cutaneous or osteoarticular cryptococcal infection
- HIV testing: Evaluation for immunodeficiencies, including HIV, is warranted in any patient with cryptococcosis.
- CBC with differential: May reveal hypereosinophilia (absolute eosinophil count >1,500/mm^3)
- Serum electrolytes: Detect hyponatremia, a complication of cryptococcal meningitis

Imaging
- Chest x-rays (anteroposterior and lateral): Nodules, diffuse infiltrates, and pleural effusions may be seen in cryptococcal pneumonia.
- Head CT or MRI: May demonstrate granulomatous lesions (cryptococcomas; ~15% of patients with meningitis) or elevated intracranial pressure. MRI reveals dilation of perivascular spaces in almost half the cases.

DIFFERENTIAL DIAGNOSIS
- Although cryptococcosis occurs most commonly in HIV-infected patients with low CD4+ lymphocyte counts, the diagnosis warrants consideration in all febrile immunocompromised children (e.g., solid-organ transplant, leukemia)
- Meningitis: Viruses and *Mycobacterium tuberculosis*
- Pneumonia: Other pulmonary mycoses, including aspergillosis, histoplasmosis, and blastomycosis. Also consider *Mycoplasma pneumoniae* and *M. tuberculosis*.
- Bone: Osteogenic sarcoma
- Cutaneous: Molluscum contagiosum, herpes simplex virus infection, pyoderma gangrenosum, and cellulitis

 ## TREATMENT
- Clinical management depends on extent of disease and immune status of the host.
- Pulmonary and extrapulmonary disease, HIV-negative, nontransplant:
  - Normal hosts with isolated pulmonary nodules may not need treatment if the serum cryptococcal antigen is negative and the patient is asymptomatic.
  - Patients with symptoms, extensive pulmonary disease, or evidence of extrapulmonary disease require treatment.
  - Fluconazole 6–12 mg/kg/d PO (max. 400 mg) for 6–12 months for mild/moderate disease. Alternate regimen: Itraconazole 4–10 mg/kg/d PO (max. 400 mg) for 6–12 months (monitor drug levels); or amphotericin B 0.7–1 mg/kg/d PO for 3–6 months.
  - Same as CNS for severe disease
  - Maintenance therapy with fluconazole should be considered for immunocompromised patients (see "Prevention").
- CNS, HIV-negative, nontransplant:
  - Induction/consolidation: Amphotericin B (0.7–1 mg/kg/d) plus flucytosine (100–150 mg/kg/d PO, divided q6h) for 4 weeks, then fluconazole PO (10–12 mg/kg/d) for a minimum of 8 weeks followed by maintenance therapy with fluconazole PO (6 mg/kg/d) for 6–12 months. Alternate induction/consolidation regimen: Amphotericin B plus flucytosine for 6–10 weeks.
- Pulmonary and extrapulmonary disease, HIV-infected or transplant:
  - Fluconazole (PO) 6–12 months for mild/moderate disease; same as CNS infection for severe disease.
  - Consider surgical debridement for patients with persistent or refractory pulmonary or bone lesions.

- CNS disease, HIV-infected or transplant:
  - Induction/consolidation: Amphotericin B (IV) plus flucytosine (PO) for at least 2 weeks, followed by fluconazole PO (10–12 mg/kg/d) for at least 8 weeks; consider subsequent suppressive therapy with fluconazole PO (6 mg/kg/d).
  - Intrathecal amphotericin B is very toxic but may be used in refractory cases.
  - HIV-infected patients require continuation of antifungal drugs indefinitely because of the high recurrence rate of cryptococcosis.
  - Liposomal amphotericin (5 mg/kg/d) or amphotericin B lipid complex (5 mg/kg/d) IV may be substituted for amphotericin B, especially in patients with pre-existing renal dysfunction and those receiving calcineurin inhibitors.
  - Flucytosine is used only in combination with amphotericin B and not as a single agent because of the rapid emergence of drug resistance.
- Voriconazole, a new triazole antifungal agent, demonstrates excellent in vitro activity against *C. neoformans* but requires clinical study. Caspofungin, a new echinocandin antifungal agent, is not active against *C. neoformans*.

 ## ONGOING CARE

FOLLOW-UP RECOMMENDATIONS
Patient Monitoring
- Because of the risk of relapse, patients should be seen at 3-month intervals for 12–18 months following treatment. Immunocompromised patients should be evaluated every 2–3 months, even while on suppressive therapy, to monitor clinically for relapse.
- Repeat lumbar punctures documenting a decrease in CSF cryptococcal antigen and sterility of culture are useful in evaluating response to treatment. During therapy for acute meningitis, an unchanged or increased titer of CSF antigen correlates with clinical and microbiologic failure to respond to treatment. Serum antigen titers are not helpful for this purpose.
- Evaluate patients with cryptococcal meningitis for neurologic sequelae.
- HIV-infected patients require suppressive antifungal therapy (see "Prevention").

PROGNOSIS
- Mortality is rare in patients with isolated pulmonary or cutaneous disease.
- In-hospital mortality is ~20% for cryptococcal meningitis and ~8% for non-CNS cryptococcal infections.
  - In normal hosts with meningitis, poor prognostic factors include serum or CSF cryptococcal titers >1:32 or CSF WBC <20/mm^3.
  - In HIV-infected patients with meningitis, poor prognostic factors include hyponatremia, concomitant growth of *C. neoformans* from another site, increased intracranial pressure, and any alteration of mental status.
- Up to 40% of patients with cryptococcal meningitis have residual neurologic deficits.
- Relapse rates are high in HIV-infected patients (see "Prevention").

COMPLICATIONS
- Elevated intracranial pressure with meningitis
- Pulmonary, cutaneous, and bone involvement may occur (see "Associated Conditions").
- In solid-organ transplant patients, those receiving tacrolimus immunosuppression are less likely to have CNS involvement and more likely to have skin, soft-tissue, or osteoarticular involvement.

ADDITIONAL READING
- Gonzalez CE, Shetty D, Lewis LL, et al. Cryptococcosis in human immunodeficiency virus-infected children. *Pediatr Infect Dis J*. 1996;15:796–800.
- Joshi NS, Fisher BT, Prasad PA, et al. Epidemiology of cryptococcal infection in hospitalized children. *Pediatr Infect Dis J*. 2010;29:e91–e95.
- Pappas PG, Perfect JR, Cloud GA, et al. Cryptococcosis in human immunodeficiency virus-negative patients in the era of effective azole therapy. *Clin Infect Dis*. 2001;33:690–699.
- Perfect JR, Dismukes WE, Dromer F, et al. Clinical practice guidelines for the management of cryptococcal disease: 2010 update by the Infectious Diseases Society of America. *Clin Infect Dis*. 2010;50:291–322.

 ## CODES

ICD9
117.5 Cryptococcosis

ICD10
- B45.0 Pulmonary cryptococcosis
- B45.8 Other forms of cryptococcosis
- B45.9 Cryptococcosis, unspecified

FAQ
- Q: What are the sources of *Cryptococcus* in nature?
- A: Pigeon droppings and soil. Naturally acquired infections occur in lower mammals, especially cats. However, neither animal-to-human nor human-to-human infections have been reported.
- Q: Should all children with *Cryptococcus* be evaluated for immunodeficiency?
- A: Yes

CRYPTORCHIDISM

Hsi-Yang Wu
Thomas F. Kolon

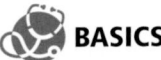 **BASICS**

DESCRIPTION

An undescended testis is one that does not remain at the bottom of the scrotum after the cremaster muscle has been fatigued by overstretching. This is commonly confused with a retractile testis, one that may not always lie in the scrotum, but that will stay in the bottom of the scrotum after overstretching the cremaster.

EPIDEMIOLOGY

Incidence
- 3% of full-term boys have cryptorchidism.
- This percentage falls to 1% by 3 months of age.

Prevalence
- There are 2 peaks for detection of undescended testes: At birth, and at 5–7 years of age. The latter group probably represents those patients with low undescended testes that become apparent with linear growth.
- Bilateral undescended testes occur in 10% of patients with undescended testicles.
- Unilateral anorchia is found in 5% of patients.

Genetics
Of boys with undescended testes, 4% of their fathers and 6–10% of their brothers also had undescended testes. There is a 23% prevalence of cryptorchidism in family members of cases compared to 7.5% of relatives of controls. Androgen receptor gene mutations are not linked to isolated cryptorchidism. Abnormalities in *HOXA10, HOXA11, HOXD13, ESR1, INSL3*, and the *LGR8/GREAT* receptor genes are being investigated in patients with cryptorchidism.

PATHOPHYSIOLOGY
- Normal descent occurs during the 7th month of gestation.
- The majority of testes that will descend spontaneously do so by 3 months of age, possibly due to the gonadotropin surge that is responsible for maturation of the germ cells.
- The undescended testis fails to show normal maturation at both 3 months and 5 years of age.
  – At 3 months of age, the fetal gonocytes are transformed into adult dark spermatogonia.
  – At 5 years of age, the adult dark spermatogonia become primary spermatocytes.
  – Both of these steps are abnormal in the undescended testis, and to a lesser extent, the contralateral descended testis.
  – Previous beliefs that the undescended testis was normal between birth and 1 year of age are incorrect, since they were derived from counts of all germ cells without taking into account whether maturation was occurring.
  – After 2 years of age, thermal effects on the testis being left out of position are seen independent of the endocrinologic effects.

ETIOLOGY
- A multifactorial mechanism of occurrence involving 2 types of theories have been postulated:
  – Hypogonadotropic hypogonadism
  – Abnormal mechanical factors (gubernaculum, epididymis, genitofemoral nerve innervation, intra-abdominal pressure)
- Although boys with undescended testes do have abnormal attachment of the gubernaculum, the mechanical theories do not consistently explain the testis histology found in cryptorchidism.
- Many boys with cryptorchidism have lower morning urinary luteinizing hormone and a decreased luteinizing hormone/follicle-stimulating hormone response to gonadotropin-releasing hormone, corresponding to the abnormal germ cell development in both the undescended and contralateral descended testis.
- The normal initial postnatal gonadotropin surge at 60–90 days of age is absent or blunted in some boys with cryptorchidism. Without this surge, Leydig cells do not proliferate, testosterone does not increase, germ cells do not mature, and infertility may develop. This indicates that a mild endocrinopathy is responsible, and cryptorchidism may be a variant of hypogonadotropic hypogonadism.
- Secondary undescended testes can occur after inguinal surgery, either due to scar tissue or difficulty in diagnosing an undescended testis in a young boy with a hernia.
- Patients with prune belly, Klinefelter, Noonan, and Prader–Willi syndromes have undescended testes.

DIAGNOSIS

HISTORY
- Prematurity
- Exogenous maternal hormones (used in infertility treatments)
- Use of oral contraceptives
- CNS lesions
- Previous inguinal surgery
- Family history for urologic abnormalities
- Neonatal deaths
- Precocious puberty
- Infertility
- Consanguinity

PHYSICAL EXAM
- The undescended testis may be found at the upper scrotum, in the superficial inguinal pouch, or in the inguinal canal. For treatment purposes, the main distinction that needs to be made is whether or not the testis is palpable.
- The patient should be examined sitting in the frogleg position.
  – With warmed hands, check the size, location, and texture of the contralateral descended testis.
  – Begin the examination of the undescended testis at the anterior superior iliac spine.
  – Sweep the groin from lateral to medial with the nondominant hand.
  – Once the testis is palpated, grasp it with the dominant hand, and continue to sweep the testis toward the scrotum with the other hand.
  – With a combination of sweeping and pulling, it is sometimes possible to bring the testis to the scrotum.
  – Maintain the position of the testis in the scrotum for a minute so that the cremaster muscle is fatigued.
  – Release the testis, and if it remains in place, it is a retractile testis.
  – If it immediately pops back, it is an undescended testis.
- For the difficult-to-examine patient (chubby 6-month-olds or obese youths), having them sit with heels together and knees abducted can help relax the cremaster. Wetting the fingers of the nondominant hand with lubricating jelly or soap can increase the sensitivity of the fingers in palpating the small, mobile testis.

DIAGNOSTIC TESTS & INTERPRETATION
Lab
- For the typical patient with a unilateral palpable or nonpalpable undescended testis, no further laboratory evaluation is necessary.
- For the patient with bilateral undescended testis, with 1 testis palpable, no further workup is necessary.
- The patient with bilateral nonpalpable testes should have a chromosomal and endocrinologic evaluation, as should the patient with 1 or 2 undescended testes and hypospadias.
- If the patient has bilateral nonpalpable testes and is <3 months of age, serum luteinizing hormone, follicle-stimulating hormone, and testosterone levels will determine whether testes are present.
- After that age, human chorionic gonadotropin stimulation will result in a measurable serum testosterone if testes are present. A failure to respond to human chorionic gonadotropin stimulation in combination with elevated luteinizing hormone/follicle-stimulating hormone levels is consistent with anorchia.

Imaging

Ultrasound, CT, and MRI can detect testes in the inguinal region, but this is also the region where they are most easily palpable. They are only 50% accurate in showing intra-abdominal testes. Imaging is rarely necessary preoperatively, because, for nonpalpable testes, exam under anesthesia, open inguinal exploration, or laparoscopy is necessary to confirm the presence of testes.

DIFFERENTIAL DIAGNOSIS

- Retractile testes are commonly confused with undescended testes. The key to distinguishing them from undescended testes is the physical exam. All retractile and many undescended testes can be delivered into the scrotum. The retractile testis will stay in the scrotum after the cremaster muscle has been overstretched. The low undescended testis will immediately pop back to its undescended position after being released.
- Atrophic or "vanishing" testes are found anywhere along the normal path to the scrotum. They are believed to be due to neonatal vascular ischemia. The contralateral testis can be hypertrophied in these boys, but this is not a reliable diagnostic sign.
- On evaluation, 80% of nonpalpable testes are present in either the abdomen or in the inguinal canal. A child with bilateral nonpalpable testes should have an endocrine evaluation to rule out anorchia or disorder of sex development (DSD).
- Cryptorchidism associated with hypospadias should also raise the possibility of DSD states, which occurs in 30–40% of patients, mainly consisting of defects in gonadotropin or testosterone synthesis.

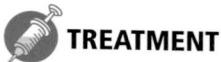 TREATMENT

ADDITIONAL TREATMENT

General Measures

- Patients with undescended testes should be referred for surgical evaluation no later than 3 months of age.
- Hormonal therapy:
  - This was widely used in Europe for inducing descent of undescended testes. Both gonadotropin-releasing hormone and human chorionic gonadotropin were used, with long-term success rates of 20%. Treatment is most successful for low undescended testes, but there is a 25% relapse rate. More recent recommendations from European pediatric endocrinologists indicate that surgery is the preferred therapy.
  - For these reasons, as well as the fact that gonadotropin-releasing hormone and human chorionic gonadotropin are not approved for this indication in the USA, most therapy in the USA aimed at bringing the testis down to the scrotum is surgical (orchiopexy).
  - The use of hormonal therapy after orchiopexy to improve semen analyses in high-risk patients is in its preliminary stages of investigation in Europe and the USA.

SURGERY/OTHER PROCEDURES

Goals in bringing the testis into the scrotum:
- Prevent ongoing thermal damage to the testis.
- Treat the associated hernia sac.
- Prevent testis torsion/injury against the pubic bone.
- Achieve a good cosmetic result/avoid psychological effects of empty scrotum.
- Allow the older child to perform testicular self-exam for cancer.

 ONGOING CARE

FOLLOW-UP RECOMMENDATIONS

Patient Monitoring

After successful orchiopexy, patients are examined at 6–12 months to check on testicular size and position. They are rechecked at puberty to explain the technique and need for monthly testis self-exam concerning early recognition of testis cancer. Patients with retractile testes should be examined annually until age 7, because ~5% will be found to have a testis out of the scrotum.

PROGNOSIS

- Surgery cannot reverse the maturational failure of the undescended testis, but it can prevent ongoing thermal injury.
- Parents are often concerned about future fertility:
  - In patients who have undergone orchiopexy at an early age, it appears that 90% of boys with unilateral cryptorchidism and 65% with bilateral cryptorchidism will achieve paternity.
  - Patients who are interested in their risk for infertility may have a semen analysis performed at age 18.
- Surgery decreases the relative risk of testicular cancer from 5.4 to 2.2 if the surgery is performed before 13 years of age.
  - All patients should be taught proper monthly testicular self-exam at the time of puberty. Some patients with cryptorchidism are at a higher risk of cancer (prune belly syndrome, ambiguous genitalia, karyotypic abnormalities, or the postpubertal boy).

ADDITIONAL READING

- Callaghan P. Undescended testis. *Pediatr Rev.* 2000;21:395.
- Lee PA, Coughlin MT. Fertility after cryptorchidism: Epidemiology and other outcome studies. *Urology.* 2005;427–431.
- Petterson A, Richiardi L, Nordenskjold A, et al. Age at surgery for undescended testis and risk for testicular cancer. *N Engl J Med* 2007;356(18): 1835–1841.

- Pyorala S, Huttunen N-P, Uhari M, et al. A review and meta-analysis of hormonal treatment of cryptorchidism. *J Clin Endocrinol Metab.* 1995;80: 2795–2799.
- Ritzen EM. Undescended testes: A consensus on management. *Eur J Endocrinol.* 2008;159:S87–90.
- Virtanen HE, Cortes D, Rajpert-De Meyts E, et al. Development and descent of the testis in relation to cryptorchidism. *Acta Paediatr.* 2007;96(5): 622–627.
- Virtanen HE, Bjerknes R, Cortes D, et al. Cryptorchidism: Classification, prevalence and long-term consequences. *Acta Paediatr.* 2007; 96(5):611–616.

 CODES

ICD9
752.51 Undescended testis

ICD10
- Q53.9 Undescended testicle, unspecified
- Q53.10 Unspecified undescended testicle, unilateral
- Q53.20 Undescended testicle, unspecified, bilateral

FAQ

- Q: If there is only 1 testicle in the scrotum, will fertility be affected?
- A: In general, the outlook for paternity is good in a patient with only 1 descended testicle. Paternity is more significantly affected with a history of 2 undescended testicles.
- Q: Why do patients with retractile testes require follow-up?
- A: The ability to distinguish between retractile and undescended testes can be difficult in some patients. Some of the patients will be found to have true undescended testes as they grow. Boys should be taught how to perform a monthly testicular self-exam at puberty.

C

CRYPTOSPORIDIOSIS

Abby M. Green
Jane Gould (5th edition)

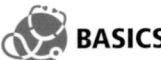 **BASICS**

DESCRIPTION
Cryptosporidiosis is a diarrheal illness caused by a gastrointestinal parasite. In an immunocompetent patient, disease is manifested as a self-limiting gastroenteritis. However, immunocompromised patients can develop protracted severe gastroenteritis, which can lead to severe malnutrition and is potentially life-threatening.

ETIOLOGY
Gastrointestinal illness is caused by ingestion of oocysts of the coccidian protozoa, *Cryptosporidium hominis* (formerly *Cryptosporidium parvum* human genotype or genotype I) which can only infect humans or *C. parvum* (genotype II) which can infect humans, cattle, and other mammals.

EPIDEMIOLOGY
- Oocysts of *Cryptosporidium* shed in stool. They are infectious, thus person-to-person transmission occurs.
- Water sources—drinking or recreational—contaminated with oocysts provide reservoirs for transmission.
- Infection may be transmitted from animals, especially young mammals, to humans via fecal–oral route.
- *Cryptosporidium* has been found in all parts of the world and is a cause of traveler's diarrhea.
- Cryptosporidiosis is self-limited based on host immune response, but without a competent immune system, infection may become severe as in the case of patients with HIV, innate immune defects, or immune-suppressing medications.
- Young children are more often affected, possibly due to a relatively immature immune system.
- Between 2005 and 2007, 8,000 cases per year were reported in the US.

RISK FACTORS
- Outbreaks have been associated with swimming pools, lakes, water recreation parks, drinking water supplies, day camps, contaminated food products, and daycare centers.
- Other risk factors include exposure to livestock, dogs, cats, reptiles, and traveling abroad.

GENERAL PREVENTION
- Isolation of hospitalized patient:
  - Contact precautions (i.e., gown and gloves for all patient contact) are recommended for the length of the hospital stay. Bathrooms should not be shared.
- Community prevention:
  - Public water supplies should be adequately filtered in order to ensure oocyst removal.
    ○ Communities without filtration devices equipped to filter a particle size of 1 μm or smaller are at increased risk for outbreaks.
  - Homeowners with well water should consider installing drinking water filtration systems.
  - Symptomatic patients should not swim in public pools until 2 weeks after symptoms have resolved since chlorine is not effective in disinfecting the water. If a recreational water supply becomes contaminated, it should be closed for proper decontamination measures.
  - Good handwashing after contact with animals
- Control measures:
  - Handwashing, especially after changing diapers
  - Disinfection of diapering areas after each use and frequent disinfection of toys, tabletops, and highchairs during outbreaks is recommended.
  - Oocysts can survive for long periods and are resistant to many disinfectants including chlorine, iodine, and dilute bleach. Boiling water or full-strength bleach disinfectant is most effective.
  - Daycare outbreaks are common; children should not return until diarrhea has resolved.
- Immunocompromised persons:
  - Avoid contact with any person or animal with cryptosporidiosis.

PATHOPHYSIOLOGY
- Transmission occurs when oocysts contaminating food or water are ingested, or through fecal–oral transmission from person to person.
- The infectious dose for humans is low, possibly as little as 10 or fewer oocysts. The incubation period is 1–30 days with a median of 7 days, and oocyst shedding may occur for weeks to months after symptoms resolve. In the majority of people, shedding stops after 2 weeks. Immunocompromised patients can shed for several months.
- Invasion of intestinal epithelial cells—of primarily the small intestines and proximal colon—leads to a secretory diarrhea. Intestinal destruction occurs with villous atrophy and subsequent malabsorption and increased intestinal permeability.
- Parasites may be found in the epithelium of the biliary and respiratory tracts of immunocompromised individuals.
  - Respiratory tract disease is often asymptomatic.
  - Biliary tract involvement may be manifested as sclerosing cholangitis, acalculous cholecystitis, or pancreatitis.

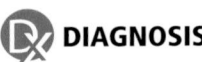 **DIAGNOSIS**

HISTORY
- Acute onset of watery, nonbloody diarrhea, crampy abdominal pain, low-grade fever, and occasionally nausea and vomiting. Other symptoms can include fatigue, anorexia, and weight loss. Fever and vomiting are symptoms more commonly found in children and can lead to the misdiagnosis of viral gastroenteritis.
- Exposure to any of the transmission sources discussed above
- Primary immunodeficiency, HIV, or immune suppression secondary to medications

PHYSICAL EXAM
- Acute weight loss
- Fever
- Tenderness to palpation of abdomen
- Dehydration as manifested by tachycardia, dry mucous membranes, sunken eyes, poor capillary refill
- Immunocompromised patients may exhibit respiratory symptoms such as dyspnea or biliary tract involvement such as colicky right upper quadrant pain.

DIAGNOSTIC TESTS & INTERPRETATION

- Detection of organism in stool specimen is diagnostic. Oocysts are small and may be missed on routine microscopic examination of stool.
  - Modified acid-fast stains detect oocysts as red or pink.
  - Fluorescent stains such as auramine O are fast but have a high rate of false-positives.
  - Immunofluorescent assays and enzyme-linked immunosorbent assays for antigen detection are being used more frequently for detection of oocysts.
- For routine stool culture, laboratory staff should be notified that *Cryptosporidium* is a possible diagnosis so special staining and examination is done.
- Organisms may be identified in intestinal biopsy specimens.
- In immunocompromised hosts, consider:
  - Examination of respiratory secretions for oocysts
  - Abdominal ultrasound, bilirubin measurement, diagnostic endoscopic-retrograde cholangiopancreatography (ERCP)

DIFFERENTIAL DIAGNOSIS

- Other infectious etiology of diarrheal illness:
  - Viral gastroenteritis including rotavirus, adenovirus, astrovirus, Norwalk virus, cytomegalovirus
  - Bacterial gastroenteritis including *Salmonella*, *Shigella*, *Yersinia*, *Campylobacter*, enterotoxigenic *Escherichia coli*, *Vibrio cholerae*
  - *Clostridium difficile* enterocolitis
  - Parasitic gastroenteritis including *Giardia*, *Entamoeba*, *Cyclospora*, *Isospora*, *Microsporidia*
- Noninfectious etiology of diarrheal illness:
  - Allergic colitis, inflammatory bowel disease, irritable bowel syndrome, appendicitis, intussusception, malrotation/volvulus

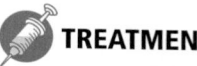 TREATMENT

MEDICATION (DRUGS)

- Disease is often self-limited, and no treatment is necessary for immunocompetent patients.
- Nitazoxanide, a broad-spectrum oral antiparasitic medication, has been licensed by the Food and Drug Administration (FDA) for treatment of children ≥12 months of age with the disease.
- A 3-day course is recommended.
- Dosage for children 1–3 years old is 100 mg b.i.d.; for children 4–11 years old, 200 mg b.i.d.; and for adults, 500 mg b.i.d.
- Paromomycin, a nonabsorbed oral aminoglycoside antibiotic, has not been definitively shown to be efficacious in reducing symptoms or fecal shedding in any patients, regardless of immune status.
- For immunosuppressed patients, oral administration of human immune globulin or bovine immune globulin may reduce symptoms, though no studies definitively prove benefit with this treatment. Improving the CD4 T lymphocyte count in HIV-positive patients with antiretroviral therapy can improve the course of cryptosporidial disease in these patients.

ADDITIONAL TREATMENT
General Measures

- Fluid and electrolyte replacement. For protracted cases, patients may eventually require parenteral nutrition.

 ONGOING CARE

FOLLOW-UP RECOMMENDATIONS
Patient Monitoring

- Because the oocysts can be shed in the stool for a long time after clinical resolution, it is not necessary to check follow-up convalescent stools. However, it is important to realize that asymptomatic patients can still transmit the infection to household and daycare contacts.
- Requiring patients whose diarrhea has resolved to have a negative stool test for *Cryptosporidium* before re-entry to daycare has not been evaluated as an outbreak control measure. Repeated testing is expensive.

PROGNOSIS

- For immunocompetent hosts, gastrointestinal disease is self-limited, usually lasting approximately 10 days. Supportive therapy is usually all that is necessary.
- For immunocompromised patients, diarrhea can be severe, debilitating, and often life-threatening. Aggressive supportive therapy is usually required, along with antimicrobial therapy and immune reconstitution.

ADDITIONAL READING

- American Academy of Pediatrics. Cryptosporidium. In: 2009 *Red book: Report of the Committee on Infectious Diseases*, 28th ed. Elk Grove Village, IL: American Academy of Pediatrics, 2009:272–273.
- Centers for Disease Control and Prevention. Outbreak of cryptosporidiosis at a day camp. *MMWR*. 1996;45(21):442–444.
- Centers for Disease Control and Prevention. Parasites—cryptosporidiosis. Available at: http://www.cdc.gov/parasites/crypto.html [Accessed March 14, 2011].
- Yoder JS, Beach MJ. Cryptosporidiosis surveillance—United States, 2003–2005. *MMWR Surveill Summ*. 2007;56:1–10.

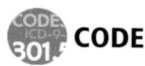 CODES

ICD9
007.4 Cryptosporidiosis

ICD10
A07.2 Cryptosporidiosis

FAQ

- Q: For whom should cryptosporidiosis be considered as a differential diagnosis?
- A: For anyone with acute onset of watery diarrhea with any of the mentioned risk factors
- Q: When is it safe for a child with cryptosporidiosis to return to daycare?
- A: When the diarrhea has resolved

C

CUSHING SYNDROME (ADRENAL EXCESS)

J. Nina Ham
Lorraine E. Levitt Katz

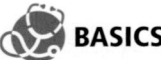 **BASICS**

DESCRIPTION
Cushing syndrome is a state of cortisol or glucocorticoid excess. This may be caused by exogenous steroid use or endogenous production. Endogenous hypercortisolism may be associated with excess production of other adrenal hormones, such as androgens and mineralocorticoids.

EPIDEMIOLOGY
- Cushing disease: Female > male in adults, but prepubertally, male > female
- Adrenocortical carcinoma: Female > male
- Cushing disease: Most common cause of endogenous Cushing syndrome, accounting for 80% of Cushing syndrome in adults and children >7 years of age
- Adrenal tumor: Adrenocortical carcinomas account for >50% of Cushing syndrome in children <7 years of age. These tumors are less common in adults and children >7 years of age.

Incidence
- 0.1–0.5/1,000,000 new pediatric cases per year
- 10 times more common in adults

PATHOPHYSIOLOGY
- Cushing disease: Pituitary ACTH oversecretion, usually due to pituitary adenoma, with resultant bilateral adrenal hyperplasia
- Primary nodular adrenal hyperplasia: Rare cause of Cushing syndrome, can be seen in association with multiple endocrine neoplasia syndrome type 1, McCune-Albright syndrome, Carney complex
- Adrenal tumors
- Adrenal adenomas: Benign tumors that secrete mainly cortisol
- Adrenal cortical carcinomas: Usually large, rapidly growing tumors, which produce a variety of hormones including cortisol and androgens. Children with adrenocortical tumors should be evaluated for Li-Fraumeni syndrome (p53 mutation).
- Ectopic ACTH production: A rare cause of Cushing syndrome in pediatrics. Small cell carcinoma, pheochromocytomas, medullary thyroid carcinoma, and carcinoid tumors can all secrete ectopic ACTH.
- Exogenous steroids: Iatrogenic Cushing syndrome is the most common cause in pediatrics. Cushing syndrome can be caused by chronic systemic, topical, or intranasal steroid use, or ACTH use.

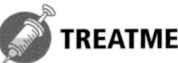 **DIAGNOSIS**

HISTORY
- Growth arrest
- Weight gain, gradual onset
- Weakness and fatigue
- Emotional or mental changes
- Use of oral, topical, inhaled, or intranasal steroids

PHYSICAL EXAM
- Growth arrest: Most consistent finding
- Obesity: Cervicodorsal fat; localized (e.g., moon facies, truncal obesity)
- Thin skin with striae, facial plethora: Sign of cortisol excess
- Hirsutism, acne: Sex hormone effect
- Pubertal arrest/menstrual disorders: Common finding
- Hypertension: Mineralocorticoid effect
- Bruising: Capillary friability
- Hyperpigmentation: Seen in association with high ACTH levels
- Virilization/feminization: Sex hormone effect

DIAGNOSTIC TESTS & INTERPRETATION
Lab
- Diagnostic tests:
  - Midnight salivary cortisol level: Patients are instructed to collect saliva by chewing a commercially available cotton swab at midnight. This provides a convenient, 1st-line screening test. Establishes hypercortisolism, but positive results should be confirmed with urine free cortisol level.
  - Urinary 24-hour free cortisol: Correct for creatinine and body surface area. 2 or 3 separate collections are preferable. Establishes the diagnosis of hypercortisolism with high sensitivity, but lower specificity. False positives may be seen with pseudo-Cushing states, obesity, and depression.
  - Urinary 24-hour 17-hydroxysteroids >6 mg/g creatinine: Establishes the diagnosis of hypercortisolism
  - Overnight dexamethasone suppression test: Dexamethasone 15 mcg/kg (max 1 mg) given at 11 p.m.; check cortisol level at 8:00 a.m. the following morning. Plasma cortisol >5 mcg/L suggests hypercortisolism, but can be falsely negative.
  - Low-dose dexamethasone suppression test: Dexamethasone 0.5 mg q6h × 48 hours (<40 kg, give 30 mcg/kg/d), with serum cortisol measured at 0 and 48 hours.
  - Loss of diurnal variation of plasma cortisol in older children: Normally, the 11:00 p.m. cortisol is <50% of the 8:00 a.m. value. The majority of patients with Cushing syndrome have mean elevated plasma cortisol, without diurnal variation.

- Differentiate causes:
  - ACTH level: Cushing disease (increased ACTH with increased cortisol level), adrenal tumor (low ACTH and increased cortisol)
  - Androgen levels: Often high in adrenocortical carcinoma. Androgen levels are low in benign, cortisol-secreting adenomas.
  - Dexamethasone suppression tests. Low-dose dexamethasone (30 mcg/kg/d) divided q6h PO for 2 days, followed by high-dose (120 mcg/kg/d) divided q6h PO for 2 days. Collect 24-hour urine for cortisol and 17-hydroxysteroids throughout. Non-Cushing states usually suppress urine free cortisol and 17-hydroxysteroids to 50–90% of baseline values after low dose. Majority of pituitary tumors are suppressible after high dose. Adrenal source: Hypercortisolism will not suppress.

Imaging
Tumor location:
- Abdominal CT/MRI will demonstrate adrenal carcinoma, adrenal adenomas, or bilateral hyperplasia/nodules resulting from Cushing disease.
- Abdominal ultrasound may be useful as initial imaging for adrenal tumor.
- Pituitary MRI with gadolinium may demonstrate a pituitary adenoma.
- Cavernous sinus sampling for ACTH: Utility in lateralizing pituitary microadenoma in pediatric patients may be limited.

DIFFERENTIAL DIAGNOSIS
- Cushing disease: Pituitary ACTH oversecretion
- Adrenal tumors:
  - Adrenal adenomas
  - Adrenal cortical carcinomas
- Exogenous glucocorticoid treatment
- Exogenous obesity can cause false elevation of urine free cortisol.

TREATMENT

ADDITIONAL TREATMENT
General Measures
- Cushing disease:
  - Transsphenoidal pituitary surgery: 70–80% success, may be less in some series, perioperative glucocorticoid replacement required, postoperative complications can include transient diabetes insipidus and, rarely, hypopituitarism or permanent diabetes insipidus
  - Pituitary radiation: 6–18 months for effect: Remission in 45–85% of individuals. Remission rate improved if combined with o,p'DDD. Hypopituitarism is the most common side effect.
  - Bilateral adrenalectomy: Indicated in patients with Cushing disease who fail surgery or radiotherapy. May result in Nelson syndrome (i.e., pituitary adenoma growth and hyperpigmentation); long-term glucocorticoid and mineralocorticoid replacement required

- Drug therapy: Ketoconazole (inhibits multiple adrenal enzymes), o,p'DDD (mitotane, an adrenolytic agent), metyrapone (11-hydroxylase inhibitor), aminoglutethimide (20,22-desmolase inhibitor), trilostane (3 -hydroxysteroid dehydrogenase inhibitor), RU-486 (glucocorticoid receptor antagonist). Drug combinations may reduce individual doses and lessen side effects.
- Bilateral nodular hyperplasia:
  - Bilateral adrenalectomy: High rate of surgical complications. Long-term glucocorticoid and mineralocorticoid replacement will be needed.
- Adrenal tumor:
  - Aggressive surgical resection, chemotherapy for carcinoma: Cyclophosphamide (Cytoxan), doxorubicin (Adriamycin), 5-fluorouracil (5-FU), methotrexate (MTX)
  - Drug therapy to control hypercortisolism: o,p'DDD at high doses may lower recurrence risk in patients with complete tumor resection. In those with residual or recurrent disease, it may improve hypercortisolism, but not survival.
  - Glucocorticoid and possibly mineralocorticoid replacement

 ## ONGOING CARE

FOLLOW-UP RECOMMENDATIONS
Patient Monitoring
- Acute glucocorticoid replacement: 10–12 mg/m^2/d divided as b.i.d. to t.i.d. until recovery of hypothalamic/pituitary function (6–12 months). Parents should be taught to triple the dose for stress, fever, illness, or vomiting. Injectable hydrocortisone should be given for emergency use. Taper corticosteroid treatment gradually.
- Chronic glucocorticoid replacement: Patients treated with bilateral adrenalectomy or with o,p'DDD require lifelong steroid replacement and stress-dose steroids.
- Reassess 24-hour urinary cortisol/ketosteroid secretion during the 1st week after treatment and at 6 weeks.
- In the week after effective pituitary surgery, cortisol should be undetectable and ACTH <5 pg/mL, 24 hours after last hydrocortisone dose. Stimulation and suppression tests are performed 6 weeks after surgery (holding hydrocortisone dose).

- Frequent follow-up to monitor for recurrence. Monitor for cortisol withdrawal symptoms, hypopituitarism. Consider medical treatment for persistent hypercortisolism.
- Monitor growth carefully. Linear growth is often compromised in Cushing syndrome. Growth hormone deficiency can result from transsphenoidal surgery or pituitary irradiation.

ALERT
- False-positive tests for hypercortisolism: Stress, lack of suppression, depression, anorexia, primary glucocorticoid resistance
- False-negative tests: Incomplete urine collection, periodic or intermittent cortisol hypersecretion, slow metabolism of dexamethasone
- Aberrant renal metabolism
- Repeat if suspicion is strong.

PROGNOSIS
- The prognosis for cure is good with Cushing disease and adrenal adenoma.
- The prognosis for adrenal carcinoma is poor because of the frequency of micrometastases and high recurrence rate.

COMPLICATIONS
- Growth arrest
- Obesity
- Pubertal arrest
- Glucose intolerance
- Osteoporosis
- Adrenal carcinomas: Metastatic spread

ADDITIONAL READING

- Arnaldi G, Angeli A, Atkinson AB, et al. Diagnosis and complications of Cushing's syndrome: A consensus statement. *J Clin Endocrinol Metab*. 2003;88:5593–5602.
- Atkinson AB, Kennedy A, Wiggam M, et al. Long-term remission rates after pituitary surgery for Cushing's disease. *Clin Endocrinol*. 2005;63(5): 549–559.
- Batista D, Gennari M, Riar J, et al. An assessment of petrosal sinus sampling for localization of pituitary microadenomas in children with Cushing disease. *J Clin Endocrinol Metab*. 2006;91(1):221–224.
- Gomez MT, Malozowski S, Winterer J, et al. Urinary free cortisol values in normal children and adolescents. *J Pediatr*. 1991;118(2):256–258.
- Magiakou MA, Chrousos GP. Cushing's syndrome in children and adolescents: Current diagnostic and therapeutic strategies. *J Endocrinol Invest*. 2002; 25:181–194.
- Putignano P, Toja P, Dubini A, et al. Midnight salivary cortisol versus urinary free and midnight serum cortisol as screening tests for Cushing's syndrome. *J Clin Endocrinol Metab*. 2003;88(9): 4153–4157.
- Savage MO, Chan LF, Grossman AB, et al. Work-up and management of paediatric Cushing's syndrome. *Curr Opin Endocrinol Diabetes Obes*. 2008;15(4): 346–351.
- Savage MO, Scommegna S, Carroll PV, et al. Growth in disorders of adrenal hyperfunction. *Horm Res*. 2002;58(Suppl 1):39–43.

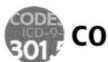 ## CODES

ICD9
255.0 Cushing syndrome

ICD10
E24.9 Cushing's syndrome, unspecified

FAQ

- Q: What clinical features help distinguish patients with pituitary Cushing disease from patients with adrenal tumors?
- A: Cushing syndrome and hyperpigmentation suggest an ACTH effect. Cushing syndrome and virilization suggest adrenal carcinoma.
- Q: What physical characteristics most clearly differentiate children with exogenous obesity from those with Cushing syndrome?
- A: Exogenous obesity is associated with robust linear growth, while Cushing syndrome is associated with growth failure.

CUTANEOUS LARVA MIGRANS

Ross Newman
Jason Newland

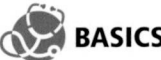 **BASICS**

DESCRIPTION
Infestation of the epidermis by the infectious larvae of certain nematodes. Humans are accidental hosts, with the primary hosts being dogs and cats.

EPIDEMIOLOGY
Worldwide distribution, but most frequent in warmer climates, including the Caribbean, Africa, South America, Southeast Asia, and southeastern USA

RISK FACTORS
• Contracted from soil contaminated with dog and cat feces
• Occupational exposures occur from crawling under buildings, such as among plumbers and pipefitters.
• Route of spread:
  – Primary host (dog or cat) passes eggs to ground through feces
  – Warm, sandy soil acts as an incubator
  – Eggs mature into *rhabditiform larvae* (noninfectious), which molt in 5 days to *filariform larvae* (infectious)
  – Incubation period from infection to symptoms usually 7–10 days, although can range up to several months

PATHOPHYSIOLOGY
• Humans are accidental hosts.
• *Filariform larvae* penetrate the epidermis either through hair follicles or fissures or through intact skin with the use of proteases.
• Larvae are unable to penetrate the basement membrane of the dermis; therefore, the infection remains limited to the epidermis.

• Larvae cannot complete their life cycle in the human host and die within weeks to months.
• Diagnosis is usually clinical. Organisms are rarely recovered from biopsy and antibody titers are unreliable because symptoms are due to hypersensitivity to the organism or its excreta, and immunity usually does not develop.

ETIOLOGY
• Most common organism is the dog or cat hookworm, *Ancylostoma braziliense*.
• Other species include *Ancylostoma canium*, *Uncinaria stenocephala*, and *Bunostomum phlebotomum*.

COMMONLY ASSOCIATED CONDITIONS
• Most common manifestation is an intensely pruritic, linear, reddened, elevated, serpiginous skin lesion known as a "creeping eruption"
• Most common complication is secondary bacterial infection of the involved skin
• Rare cases of a peripheral eosinophilia with pulmonary infiltrates (Loffler syndrome) occur when the larvae invade the bloodstream..

 DIAGNOSIS

HISTORY
• Incubation period
  – Usual time from infection to symptoms is 7–10 days, but may last for up to several months.
• Rash:
  – It is intensely pruritic, raised, serpiginous, and linear. Most commonly located on feet, buttocks, and abdomen. Also found on face, extremities, and genitalia.
• Pruritus:
  – Symptoms typically begin with some tingling in the affected area with the development of the typical rash with intense pruritus.

• Speed at which rash spreads:
  – Rash typically lengthens by a few millimeters to 2–3 cm daily.
• Source of infection:
  – Most frequently contracted from beaches in tropical countries where dogs are frequently found. In the USA, most frequently contracted from moist soil in the southeastern USA contaminated with animal feces.

PHYSICAL EXAM
The classic rash is described as an erythematous, raised, serpiginous rash. In addition, it may begin as vesicular and/or form bullae along the track. Tracks under the skin reflect the course of the larvae. The active end is not part of the track.

DIAGNOSTIC TESTS & INTERPRETATION
Lab
• Biopsy: Not indicated, because it rarely yields organisms
• Serologic testing: Not helpful
• Diagnosis based on clinical presentation

DIFFERENTIAL DIAGNOSIS
• Cutaneous larva migrans should be considered in anyone with an intensely pruritic, raised, serpiginous, linear cutaneous eruption.
• Hookworm infections (*Strongyloides stercoralis*, *Uncinaria stenocephala*, *Bunostomum phlebotomum*, *Gnathostoma spinigerum*)
• Free-living nematodes (*Pelodera strongyloides*), and insect larvae
• Other cutaneous eruptions that may mimic cutaneous larva migrans include scabies, tinea pedis, erythema chronicum migrans of Lyme disease, jelly fish stings, contact dermatitis, and photosensitivity.

TREATMENT

General Measures

- First-line treatment is topical thiabendazole: 10% suspension of 500 mg/5 mL applied four times a day for 10 days
- Alternatively, oral thiabendazole: 25–50 mg/kg/d q12h for 2 days. Not well tolerated
- Ivermectin: 12 mg in a single dose. May repeat if symptoms persist
- Albendazole: Not approved for use in the USA, is available in other countries and is administered as 400 mg/day for 3 days in adults

 ONGOING CARE

FOLLOW-UP RECOMMENDATIONS
Patient Monitoring

- Symptoms persist for 8 weeks, but up to 1 year in untreated patients.
- Those with extensive involvement should be seen after treatment to be certain of improvement in symptoms.

PROGNOSIS

- This is a self-limited disease and will resolve without treatment when the larvae die.
- There is a 98% response rate to topical thiabendazole, a 97% cure rate with ivermectin, and an 89% response rate reported with oral thiabendazole.

COMPLICATIONS

- Most common complication is secondary bacterial infection of the skin.
- Self-limited disease: If untreated, larvae die within 2–8 weeks, but may persist for up to 1 year.
- Rarely, the larvae can invade the dermis and, subsequently, the bloodstream, leading to a peripheral eosinophilia and pulmonary infiltrates (Loffler syndrome).

ADDITIONAL READING

- Blackwell V, Vega-Lopez F. Cutaneous larva migrans: Clinical features and management of 44 cases presenting in the returning traveller. *Brit J Dermatol*. 2001;145:434–437.
- Bouchaud O, ne Houze S, Schiemann R, et al. Cutaneous larva migrans in travelers: A prospective study, with assessment of therapy with ivermectin. *Clin Infect Dis*. 2000;31:493–498.
- Brenner MA, Patel MB. Cutaneous larva migrans: The creeping eruption. *Cutis*. 2003;72(2):111–115.
- Caumes E. Treatment of cutaneous larva migrans. *Clin Infect Dis*. 2000;30(5):811–814.
- Van den Enden E, Stevens A, Van Gompel A. Treatment of cutaneous larva migrans. *N Engl J Med*. 1998;339(17):1246–1247.

 CODES

ICD9
- 126.2 Ancylostomiasis due to ancylostoma braziliense
- 126.9 Ancylostomiasis and necatoriasis, unspecified (cutaneous larva migrans not otherwise specified)

ICD10
- B76.0 Ancylostomiasis
- B76.9 Hookworm disease, unspecified

FAQ

- Q: Can children spread the infection to each other?
- A: The usual spread of infection is from direct contact with the larvae. Spread from 1 individual to another does not occur.

C

CYCLOSPORA

Jessica Newman
Jason Newland

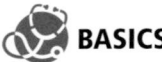 **BASICS**

DESCRIPTION
Cyclospora catayensis, a coccidian protozoan, causes a diarrheal illness first described in humans in 1979.

GENERAL PREVENTION
Fresh produce, especially raspberries, should be washed thoroughly before being eaten, although this still may not entirely eliminate the risk of transmission.

EPIDEMIOLOGY
- Worldwide distribution, with areas of endemic infection (Nepal, Peru, Haiti, Guatemala, Indonesia)
- People living in endemic areas have a shorter illness or may be asymptomatic carriers.
- Cyclospora is an opportunistic infection in human immunodeficiency virus patients.
- In the USA, infection occurs primarily in spring and summer.
- In the USA and Canada, cases are associated with consumption of imported fresh produce.

PATHOPHYSIOLOGY
- Infected patients excrete noninfectious unsporulated oocysts in their stool.
- Sporulation then occurs days to weeks after release into the environment.
- Ingestion of sporulated oocysts occurs and sporozoites are released that invade the intestinal epithelial cells.
- Sporozoites develop into trophozoites which undergo schizogony and form merozoites.
- Merozoites may develop into macro- or microgametes which become fertilized, resulting in oocysts.
- Entire life cycle is completed in the host.
- Incubation period is between 1 and 11 days, with an average of 7 days.

ETIOLOGY
- Outbreaks have been associated with the consumption of raspberries, mesclun (young salad greens), and basil.
- Infection occurs through the consumption of contaminated food and water.
- Transmission does not occur through person-to-person spread.

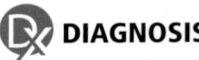 **DIAGNOSIS**

HISTORY
- Fever:
  - Fever is present in ~50% of cases.
- Clinical prodrome:
  - Acute onset of diarrhea is typical, but a flulike prodrome may occur.
- Nature of the diarrhea:
  - Profuse, nonbloody, watery diarrhea that may be foul smelling. Can alternate with constipation.
- Other symptoms experienced:
  - Abdominal cramping, fatigue, anorexia, flatulence and vomiting
- Foods that have been consumed in the past 2 weeks:
  - Illness has been attributed to contaminated raspberries, water, mesclun, snow peas and basil.

PHYSICAL EXAM
Dehydration:
- Due to profuse diarrhea, signs of dehydration (tachycardia, dry mucous membranes, sunken eyes, poor skin turgor, and weight loss) may be present.

DIAGNOSTIC TESTS & INTERPRETATION
Lab
- Ova and parasites with modified acid fast staining: Identification of *Cyclospora, Isospora,* and *Cryptosporidium*
- PCR testing available from the CDC.
- Ova and parasites: Identify common protozoans including *Giardia*
- *Cryptosporidium* and *Giardia* antigen test: Immunoassay with high sensitivity and specificity
- Electron microscopy of stool: Gold standard for diagnosing microsporidia
- Bacterial stool cultures: Identify common bacterial pathogens
- Stool for *Clostridium difficile* PCR: Identify a common cause of diarrhea
- Electrolytes, blood urea nitrogen, creatinine: Determine extent of dehydration

DIFFERENTIAL DIAGNOSIS
- *Cryptosporidium*:
  - Outbreaks associated with contaminated water sources (municipal pools)
  - Person-to-person transmission may occur.
  - Clinically indistinguishable from *Cyclospora*
- *Isospora belli*:
  - Outbreaks associated with food and water
  - Clinically indistinguishable from *Cyclospora,* though fever may be more common
- *Microsporidium*:
  - Outbreaks associated with contaminated water sources
  - Chronic diarrhea occurs in immunocompromised patients, especially HIV patients.
  - Fever is uncommon.

- *Giardia lamblia*:
  - Community epidemics associated primarily with contaminated water sources
  - Person-to-person transmission may occur and has led to outbreaks in day care centers.
  - Clinical presentation may vary from occasional acute watery diarrhea to a severe, protracted diarrheal illness.
- Viral gastroenteritis:
  - Rotavirus
  - Adenovirus 40/41
- Bacterial gastroenteritis:
  - *Clostridium difficile*
  - *Vibrio cholera* and noncholera *Vibrio* species
  - *Escheria coli* (especially toxin-producing strains)
  - *Shigella* species
  - *Salmonella* species
  - *Yersinia enterocolitica*
  - *Campylobacter* species

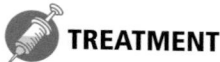 TREATMENT

ADDITIONAL TREATMENT
General Measures
- Immunocompetent patient: Trimethoprim (5 mg/kg)–sulfamethoxazole twice a day for 7–10 days
- HIV patient: Trimethoprim–sulfamethoxazole four times a day for 10 days and then prophylactic dosing 3 times per week to prevent relapse
- Ciprofloxacin or nitazoxanide for 7 days may be alternatives in patients with sulfa allergy.
- Based on severity of dehydration, treatment with IV fluids may be indicated.

IN-PATIENT CONSIDERATIONS
Admission Criteria
Moderate to severe dehydration

 ONGOING CARE

PROGNOSIS
- Most cases are self-limited.
- Diarrhea may last up to 3 months in untreated patients who acquired the parasite in a foreign country where *Cyclospora* is endemic.
- In US outbreaks, the average duration of diarrhea ranged from 10 to 24 days.
- Relapses may occur in untreated patients.
- Patients with HIV have more severe and prolonged diarrhea, which may recur.

COMPLICATIONS
- Dehydration and weight loss are the most common complications.
  - Severe, prolonged diarrhea may lead to dehydration.
  - Malabsorption of D-xylose and excretion of fecal fat occurs, leading to weight loss.
- May cause ascending biliary tract disease in AIDS patients
- Rare associated complications:
  - Guillain–Barré syndrome
  - Reactive arthritis

PATIENT MONITORING
- Infected patients need to be observed closely for dehydration.
- Relapse may occur in HIV patients, so close follow-up is essential.

ADDITIONAL READING
- American Academy of Pediatrics. Cyclospora. In: Pickering LK, ed. *2006 Red Book: Report of the Committee on Infectious Diseases*. 27th ed. Elk Grove Village, IL: American Academy of Pediatrics; 2006:273.
- Herwaldt BL. *Cyclospora cayetanensis*: A review, focusing on the outbreaks of cyclosporiasis in the 1990s. *Clin Infect Dis*. 2000;31:1040–1057.
- Ortega YE, Sanchez R. Update on *Cyclospora cayetanensis*, a food-borne and waterborne parasite. *Clin Microbiol Rev*. 2010:218–234.

 CODES

ICD9
007.5 Cyclosporiasis
ICD10
A07.4 Cyclosporiasis

FAQ
- Q: Does routine ova and parasites testing detect *Cyclospora*?
- A: Rarely; therefore, modified acid–fast staining must be done to improve the laboratory's ability to detect the oocysts
- Q: Can person-to-person transmission occur in cyclospora illness?
- A: No. It takes days to weeks for oocysts to sporulate and become infectious.

CYSTIC FIBROSIS

Samuel B. Goldfarb
Bruce A. Ong

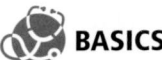 **BASICS**

DESCRIPTION
Cystic fibrosis (CF) is an inherited, autosomal recessive disorder, characterized by chronic obstructive lung disease, pancreatic exocrine insufficiency, and elevated sweat chloride concentration.

ALERT
- Most common pitfall is failure to diagnose. Neonatal screening is not performed in all states.
- Not uncommon to delay making the diagnosis in patients with mild symptoms

EPIDEMIOLOGY
- Most common lethal inherited disease in the Caucasian population
- Carrier frequency of mutations in the CF transmembrane conductance regulator (CFTR) gene:
  - 1:29 in Caucasians
  - 1:49 in Hispanics
  - 1:53 in Native Americans
  - 1:62 in African Americans
  - 1:90 in Asians

Incidence
- 1:3,300 in Caucasians
- 1:9,500 in Hispanics
- 1:11,200 in Native Americans
- 1:15,300 in African Americans
- 1:32,100 in Asians

RISK FACTORS
Genetics
CFTR gene:
- Located on the long arm of chromosome 7
- Most common mutation results in deletion of phenylalanine at position 508 in the CFTR glycoprotein.
- The Δ508 mutation occurs in ~70% of CF patients.
- >1,500 mutations have been reported in the CFTR gene.
- Presence of gene modifiers may cause incomplete phenotypic presentations.

GENERAL PREVENTION
Prepregnancy carrier detection

PATHOPHYSIOLOGY
- CFTR:
  - Membrane glycoprotein, which functions as a cyclic AMP-activated chloride channel at the apical surface of epithelial cells
  - An abnormality in CFTR results in defective chloride conductance.
  - May have other roles in the regulation of membrane channels and the pH of intracellular organelles. May affect cell apical sodium channel regulation
  - CFTR abnormalities may act as binding sites for *Pseudomonas aeruginosa*, promoting proinflammatory responses in the lung.

- In the respiratory system:
  - Lungs are morphologically normal at birth.
  - Increased mucus viscosity
  - Early bacterial colonization despite a robust neutrophilic inflammatory response
  - Mucous plugging and atelectasis
  - Bronchiectasis and emphysema develop.
  - Abnormal nasal sinus development
- In the GI tract:
  - Progressive pancreatic damage from ductal and acinar secretions lead to exocrine pancreatic insufficiency
  - Endocrine pancreatic dysfunction
  - Focal biliary cirrhosis of the liver
  - Hypoplasia of the gallbladder and impaired bile flow

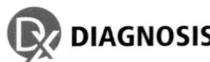 **DIAGNOSIS**

HISTORY
- Most common presenting respiratory symptoms: Chronic cough, recurrent pneumonia, nasal polyps, chronic pansinusitis
- Most common presenting GI symptoms:
  - Meconium ileus (15–20% of patients present with this symptom); pancreatic insufficiency occurs in 85% of patients. In infants, fat malabsorption may lead to chronic diarrhea and failure to thrive.
  - In older patients, pancreatitis, rectal prolapse (occurs in 2% of the patients, must consider CF until proven otherwise, commonly seen between 1 and 5 years of age)
  - Distal obstruction of the small intestine (meconium ileus equivalent, seen in older children and adults)
- Evidence of heat intolerance: In summer, increased sweating may lead to dehydration with hyponatremia or hypochloremic metabolic alkalosis.

PHYSICAL EXAM
- Respiratory findings:
  - Frequent cough, often productive of mucopurulent sputum
  - Rhonchi, crackles, wheezing, hyperresonance to percussion
  - Nasal polyposis
- Other common findings:
  - Digital clubbing
  - Hepatosplenomegaly in patients with cirrhosis
  - Growth retardation
  - Hypertrophic osteoarthropathy
  - Delayed puberty
  - Osteoporosis

DIAGNOSTIC TESTS & INTERPRETATION
Lab
- Sweat test: Keystone for the diagnosis of CF; sweat chloride >60 mEq/L is abnormal.
- Sweat test: keystone for diagnosis of CF:
  - <40 mmol/L – Negative
  - 40 mmol/L to 60 mmol/L – borderline
  - >60 mmol/L – Consistent with CF
  - In infants up to 6 months of age:
    - 30 mmol/L to 60 mmol/L – borderline
    - 60 mmol/L – Consistent with CF

- Diagnostic criteria include:
  - One or more phenotypic features of CF
  OR
  - Sibling with CF
  OR
  - Positive newborn screening test
  AND
  - 2 positive sweat tests
  OR
  - 2 CF mutations on genetic screening
  OR
  - Nasal potential difference (NPD) consistent with CF
- Other causes of elevated sweat chloride:
  - Malnutrition
  - Adrenal insufficiency
  - Nephrogenic diabetes insipidus
  - Ectodermal dysplasia
  - Fucosidosis
  - Hypogammaglobulinemia
  - False negatives seen in CF patients with edema
- Mutation analysis: Can detect >90% of CF patients. Failure to identify 2 mutations reduces, but does not eliminate, the possibility of CF. Immunoreactive trypsinogen test (IRT) is used for newborn screening. In the IRT test, blood drawn 2–3 days after birth is analyzed for trypsinogen. Positive IRT tests must be confirmed by sweat test and/or genetic testing.
- Frequently recovered organisms in sputum cultures:
  - *Haemophilus influenzae*
  - *Staphylococcus aureus*
  - MRSA (methicillin-resistant *S. aureus*)
  - *P. aeruginosa* (nonmucoid and mucoid)
  - *Burkholderia cepacia*
  - *Stenotrophomonas maltophilia*
  - *Aspergillus* species
- Pulmonary function test: Usually reveals obstructive lung disease, although some patients may have a restrictive pattern
- Analysis of stimulated pancreatic secretions: Degree of pancreatic exocrine deficiency
- Fecal elastase measurements can detect pancreatic insufficiency.
- 72-hour fecal fat measurement: Fat malabsorption

Imaging
- Chest radiography:
  - Typical features include hyperinflation, peribronchial thickening, atelectasis, and bronchiectasis.
- CT scan:
  - Early bronchiectasis

DIFFERENTIAL DIAGNOSIS
- Pulmonary:
  - Recurrent pneumonia or bronchitis
  - Asthma
  - Aspiration pneumonia
  - Ciliary dyskinesia
  - Airway anomalies
  - Chronic sinusitis
  - Chronic Aspiration
  - Non-CF bronchiectasis
  - Allergic Bronchopulmonary Aspergillosis
  - Alpha-1 antitrypsin disease

- GI:
  - Failure to thrive
  - Celiac disease
  - Protein-losing enteropathy
  - GERD
  - Chronic pancreatitis
- Other:
  - Metabolic alkalosis
  - Immune deficiency
  - Shwachman-Diamond Syndrome

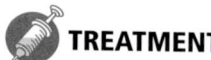 **TREATMENT**

MEDICATION (DRUGS)
First Line
- Antibiotic therapy based on sputum culture results and clinical improvement:
  - Oral antibiotics:
    - Cephalexin
    - Linezolid
    - Trimethoprim-sulfamethoxazole
    - Ciprofloxacin, inhaled tobramycin, colistin, or aztreonam in selected patients
  - IV antibiotics:
    - To treat *S. aureus*, consider oxacillin, ticarcillin with clavulanic acid, linezolid, or vancomycin.
    - To treat *P. aeruginosa* and *B. cepacia*, consider aminoglycoside plus ticarcillin, ceftazidime, or piperacillin.
  - Severe cases with resistant strains may benefit from aztreonam, imipenem, or meropenem.
  - Synergistic antibiotic studies can be performed in patients with multiresistant organisms.
  - Regular azithromycin treatment may be used for both anti-inflammatory purposes to improve lung function.
- Clearance of pulmonary secretions:
  - Chest physical therapy, or with high-frequency oscillatory vest device. Adjunct therapy such as Flutter valve, Acapella, or PEP mask may also be used.
  - Bronchodilator: Aerosol or metered-dose inhaler (β_2-agonist)
  - Mucolytics: RhDNase
  - Anti-inflammatory: Short-term oral steroid course. Inhaled corticosteroids may benefit patients with asthma and/or demonstrating an oral steroid response.
  - Hypertonic saline
- GI disease:
  - Pancreatic enzyme replacement therapy: Used in CF patients who are pancreatic insufficient; dosage adjusted for frequency and character of the stools and for growth pattern; generic substitutes are not bioequivalent to name brands. The maximum recommended dose is 2,500 U of lipase/kg per meal.
  - Vitamin supplements: Multivitamin supplement, fat-soluble vitamins A, D, E, and K
  - Patients with cholestasis may benefit from therapy with ursodeoxycholic acid.

 ONGOING CARE

FOLLOW-UP RECOMMENDATIONS
Patient Monitoring
- Specialized care should be at a CF center.
- Frequency of visits depends on age and severity of illness:
  - Infants should be seen at least once monthly for 1st 12 months, then every 2–3 months thereafter.

DIET
- High-calorie diet with added salt
- Lifelong nutritional support usually required
- Duration of antibiotic therapy is controversial; more frequent use is required as pulmonary function deteriorates.

PROGNOSIS
- Current median survival is ~38 years.
- Variable course of the disease
- The median survival has been increasing for the past 4 decades, although the rate of increase in age has slowed in the past decade.

COMPLICATIONS
- Respiratory complications:
  - Recurrent bronchitis and pneumonia
  - Atelectasis
  - Bronchiectasis
  - Pneumothorax
  - Hemoptysis
  - Chronic sinusitis and nasal polyps
- GI complications:
  - Pancreatic insufficiency in 85–90% of CF patients
  - Patients usually have steatorrhea, poor growth, and poor nutritional status.
  - Decreased levels of vitamins A, E, D, and K
  - Rectal prolapse
  - 10–15% of patients have meconium ileus.
  - Distal intestinal obstruction syndrome
  - Clinically significant focal biliary cirrhosis; hepatobiliary disease in 5% of CF patients
  - Esophageal varices
  - Splenomegaly
  - Hypersplenism
  - Cholestasis
- Reproductive complications:
  - Sterility in 98% of males, due to absence or atresia of the vas deferens
  - Slight decrease in fertility for females secondary to abnormalities of cervical mucus
- Endocrine complications:
  - Glucose intolerance
  - CF-related diabetes occurs with increasing frequency in adolescent and adult patients.
- Skeletal complications:
  - Osteoporosis

ADDITIONAL READING

- Baumer JH. Evidence based guidelines for the performance of the sweat test for the investigation of cystic fibrosis in the UK. *Arch Dis Child.* 2003;88(12):1126–1127.
- Farrell MH, Farrell PM. Newborn screening for cystic fibrosis: Ensuring more good than harm. *J Pediatr.* 2003;143(6):707–712.
- Flume PA, O'Sullivan BP, Robinson KA, et al. Cystic fibrosis pulmonary guidelines: Chronic medications for maintenance of lung health. *AJCCM.* 2007; 176(10):957–969.
- LeGrys VA, Yankaskas JR, Quittell LM, et al. Diagnositc sweat testing: The Cystic Fibrosis Foundation Guidelines. *J Pediatr.* 2007;151(1): 85–89.
- Pier GB. CFTR mutations and host susceptibility to Pseudomonas aeruginosa lung infection. *Curr Opin Microbiol.* 2002;5(1):81–86.
- Ryan G, Mukhopadhyay S, Singh M. Nebulised anti-pseudomonal antibiotics for cystic fibrosis. [update, *Cochrane Database Syst Rev.* 2000;(2):CD001021; PMID: 10796732]. *Cochrane Database Syst Rev.* 2003;(3):CD001021.
- Smyth A, Walters S. Prophylactic antibiotics for cystic fibrosis. *Cochrane Database Syst Rev.* 2000;(2):CD001912.
- Southern KW, Barker PM. Azithromycin for cystic fibrosis. *Eur Respir J.* 2004;24(5):834–838.
- Stallings VA, Stark LJ, Robinson KA, et al. Evidence-based practice recommendations for nutrition-related management of children and adults with cystic fibrosis and pancreatic insufficiency: Results of a systematic review. *J Am Diet Assoc.* 2008;108(5):832–839.
- Yankaskas JR, Marshall BC, Sufian B, et al. Cystic fibrosis adult care: Consensus conference report. *Chest.* 2004;125:1S–39S.

 CODES

ICD9
- 277.01 Cystic fibrosis with meconium ileus
- 277.02 Cystic fibrosis with pulmonary manifestations
- 277.09 Cystic fibrosis with other manifestations

ICD10
- E84.0 Cystic fibrosis with pulmonary manifestations
- E84.9 Cystic fibrosis, unspecified
- E84.11 Meconium ileus in cystic fibrosis

FAQ
- Q: Should relatives be tested?
- A: All siblings should have a sweat test.
- Q: How well will a child with CF do?
- A: The course of the illness is variable. It is difficult to predict the course of disease in an individual.
- Q: How should a borderline sweat test be interpreted?
- A: Borderline sweat tests should always be correlated with other findings such as physical exam, sputum cultures, pulmonary function, radiographic findings, nutritional evaluation, and/or mutation analysis.

CYTOMEGALOVIRUS INFECTION

Sujit S. Iyer
Rakesh D. Mistry

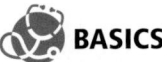 **BASICS**

DESCRIPTION
Cytomegalovirus (CMV) is a ubiquitous double-stranded DNA virus that is a member of the herpesvirus family. Establishes latency in peripheral mononuclear cells.

EPIDEMIOLOGY
- Increased rates of primary infection are seen in early childhood, adolescence, and childbearing years.
- Transmission may occur by contact with infected respiratory secretions, urine, or breast milk, sexual contact, solid-organ transplantation, or transfusion of infective blood products.

Prevalence
Seroprevalence varies with socioeconomic status; 50% of middle- and 80% of lower-socioeconomic-status adults are seropositive.

GENERAL PREVENTION
- Drainage and secretion, and pregnant women precautions, should be instituted for hospitalized patients known to be shedding CMV.
- Seriously ill neonates should receive blood products from cytomegalovirus-negative donors.
- CMV-seronegative solid-organ or bone marrow transplantation recipients should receive organs (and all blood products) from CMV-negative donors whenever possible.
- Controversy exists over the role of hyperimmune globulin to prevent disseminated CMV disease in CMV-negative recipients of CMV-positive transplantation.

PATHOPHYSIOLOGY
Infection leads to intranuclear inclusions with massive enlargement of cells. Almost any organ may become infected with CMV in severe disseminated infection.

COMMONLY ASSOCIATED CONDITIONS
- Congenital infection:
  - Occurs in 1% of newborns
  - Intrauterine transmission more common in mothers with primary infection during pregnancy (40–50%) compared to recurrent infection (<1%). Controversy over postnatal acquisition of CMV via breast milk and whether it precludes breastfeeding in premature infants (has a lower risk for neurologic sequelae)
  - 10% of infected infants are symptomatic at birth, with severe disease characterized by growth retardation, hepatosplenomegaly, thrombocytopenia, and CNS involvement.
  - 10–20% of infants who are asymptomatically infected at birth will develop long-term sequelae.
  - Of symptomatically infected infants, 90% will have neurologic sequelae. Degree of impairments may be predicted by CT findings and FOC at birth.

- Mononucleosis syndrome:
  - CMV can cause a mononucleosis-like syndrome similar to that caused by Epstein–Barr virus (EBV) infection.
  - The most common symptoms are malaise (67%) and fever (50%). ~70% of patients have abnormal liver enzymes.
  - Pharyngitis and splenomegaly less common and severe than observed with EBV-induced mononucleosis.
- Interstitial pneumonitis:
  - Seen primarily in immunosuppressed children and adults
  - Begins with fever and nonproductive cough, but may progress to dyspnea and severe hypoxia over 1–2 weeks
  - Mild, self-limited pneumonitis may occur in immunocompetent patients.
- Retinitis:
  - Seen in ~30% of infants with symptomatic congenital infection
  - Immunosuppressed children should have regular eye exams.
- Hepatitis:
  - Occurs in healthy individuals with primary infections and in immunosuppressed patients with either primary or reactivated disease
  - Fever, mild elevation of liver enzymes and hepatomegaly, are typical. Jaundice and severe hepatitis are uncommon.
- GI disease:
  - Severely immunosuppressed patients may experience esophagitis, gastritis, colitis, or pancreatitis.
  - Diagnosis requires endoscopy with biopsy.
- CNS disease:
  - Commonly seen in infants with symptomatic congenital infection
  - Characterized by microcephaly, periventricular calcifications, seizures, developmental delay, and sensorineural hearing loss
  - Encephalitis or meningoencephalitis may occur postnatally in either healthy or immunocompromised patients.
- Deafness:
  - CMV is the most common cause of congenital deafness.
  - Onset of deafness often seen after first month of life and is progressive. May be missed by newborn hearing screen (if only done in 1st 2 weeks of life)

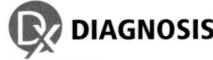 **DIAGNOSIS**

HISTORY
- Day care attendance:
  - Increased risk of infection
- Recent blood transfusion:
  - Transfusion-associated CMV
- Use of immunosuppressive medications:
  - Increased use of serious infection
- Prolonged fever:
  - Mononucleosis-like syndrome
- Blurred vision:
  - CMV retinitis
- Cough, dyspnea, wheezing:
  - CMV pneumonitis
- Vomiting, abdominal pain, diarrhea (watery or bloody):
  - CMV colitis

PHYSICAL EXAM
- Microcephaly:
  - Congenital infection
- White, perivascular retinal infiltrates and hemorrhage:
  - Retinitis
- Deafness (may require audiogram, brainstem evoked auditory responses):
  - Congenital infection
- Photophobia, headache, nuchal rigidity:
  - Meningitis
- Tachypnea, rales:
  - Pneumonitis
- Hepatomegaly and/or splenomegaly:
  - Mononucleosis-like syndrome
- Rash:
  - Petechiae, purpura, "blueberry muffin" lesions, rubelliform rash
- Adenopathy:
  - Mononucleosis-like syndrome

DIAGNOSTIC TESTS & INTERPRETATION
Lab
- Viral culture: Virus may be isolated from nasopharyngeal/oropharyngeal secretions, urine, stool, WBC. Isolation may take up to 4 weeks. Urine or saliva samples are most common way to diagnose congenital disease.
- Shell-vial assay system (staining for early antigen production) allows detection of virus 24–72 hours after inoculation

- Quantitative antigenemia assay: Detection of circulating CMV-infected mononuclear cells by indirect immunofluorescence. In an immunocompromised patient, may monitor response to therapy or identify viral reactivation
- Serology: Enzyme-linked immunosorbent assay or indirect fluorescent antibody assay to detect the presence of CMV IgM or IgG. CMV IgM usually persists for 6 weeks following primary infection, although it may persist up to 6 months.

ALERT
- Due to frequency of asymptomatic shedding, mere isolation of virus does not necessarily establish an etiologic association.
- Severely immunocompromised patients who are actively infected with CMV may be seronegative. 4-fold rise in CMV IgG is not diagnostic of primary infection. Increased antibody titers may occur with reactivation.

Imaging
Noncontrast head CT:
- Periventricular calcifications, cystic abnormalities, ventriculomegaly, periventricular leukomalacia
- Fetal Brain MRI has higher sensitivity than ultrasound for brain abnormalities, and greater predictor of symptomatic infection.

DIFFERENTIAL DIAGNOSIS
- Congenital infection:
  – Congenital rubella syndrome
  – Toxoplasmosis
  – Syphilis
  – Neonatal herpes simplex virus
  – Human immunodeficiency virus
  – Enteroviral infection
- Mononucleosis syndrome:
  – EBV infection
  – Toxoplasmosis
  – Hepatitis A or B infection
- Interstitial pneumonitis:
  – Respiratory syncytial virus
  – Adenovirus
  – Measles
  – Varicella
  – Pneumocystis carinii
  – Chlamydia
  – Mycoplasma
  – Fungal
  – Drug/toxin-induced pneumonitis
- Retinitis:
  – Ocular toxoplasmosis
  – Candidal retinitis
  – Syphilis
  – Herpes simplex virus
- Hepatitis:
  – EBV infection
  – Hepatitis A, B, or C infection
  – Enterovirus
  – Adenovirus
  – Herpes simplex virus
  – Drug/toxin-induced

- GI disease:
  – Herpes simplex virus
  – Adenovirus
  – Salmonella
  – Shigella
  – Campylobacter
  – Yersinia
  – Clostridium difficile
  – Giardia
  – Cryptosporidium
- CNS disease:
  – Congenital disease (see "Congenital Infection," above)
  – Meningoencephalitis in immunocompetent host: Herpes simplex virus, EBV, varicella-Zoster virus, enterovirus, arbovirus
- Meningoencephalitis in immunocompromised host: In addition to organisms listed previously, should include HIV encephalitis, fungal meningitis, toxoplasmosis

 ## TREATMENT

Majority of transplant experts prefer prophylaxis over preemptive therapy in high risk patients (Donor CMV positive, recipient negative).

MEDICATION (DRUGS)
First Line
- Ganciclovir will suppress viral replication but not eradicate virus (virostatic agent)
  – Indications: CMV chorioretinitis in immunocompromised patients; tissue diagnosis (hepatitis, enteritis, pneumonitis) of CMV infection or isolation of CMV from buffy coat of immunocompromised patient; consider for neonate with documented CNS disease to prevent progressive postnatal hearing loss
  – Side effects: Neutropenia (50%), thrombocytopenia (~5%)
- Foscarnet—virostatic agent
  – Indications: CMV chorioretinitis, pneumonitis, hepatitis, enteritis (biopsy proven) in immunocompromised patient who has failed to improve on ganciclovir therapy or who has experienced significant bone marrow toxicity related to ganciclovir use
  – Side effects: Renal impairment (25%), headache (25%), seizures (10%)

 ## ONGOING CARE

PROGNOSIS
Varies with nature of infection (see "Associated Conditions")

COMPLICATIONS
Varies with nature of infection (see "Associated Conditions")

ADDITIONAL READING

- Dollard SC, Schleiss MR, Grosse SD. Public health and laboratory considerations regarding newborn screening for congenital cytomegalovirus. *J Inherit Metab Dis.* 2010;33(Suppl 2):S249–S254. Epub 2010 Jun 8. Review.
- Doneda C, Parazzini C, Righini A, et al. Early cerebral lesions in cytomegalovirus infection: Prenatal MR imaging. *Radiology.* 2010;255(2): 613–621.
- Foulon I, Naessens A, Foulon W, et al. Hearing loss in children with congenital cytomegalovirus infection in relation to the maternal trimester in which the maternal primary infection occurred. *Pediatr.* 2008;122(6):e1123–e1127.
- Kimberlin DW, Lin CY, Sanchez PJ, et al. Effect of ganciclovir therapy on hearing in symptomatic congenital cytomegalovirus diseases involving the central nervous system: A randomized controlled trial. *J Pediatr.* 2003;143:16–25.
- Kurath S, Halwachs-Baumann G, Müller W, et al. Transmission of cytomegalovirus via breast milk to the prematurely born infant: A systematic review. *Clin Microbiol Infect.* 2010;16(8):1172–1178. Review.
- Lawrence RM. Cytomegalovirus in human breast milk: Rrisk to the premature infant. *Breastfeed Med.* 2006;1(2):99–107. Review.
- Noyola DE, Demmler GJ, Nelson CT, et al. Early predictors of neurodevelopmental outcome in symptomatic congenital cytomegalovirus infection. *J Pediatr.* 2001;138(3):325–331.

 ## CODES

ICD9
- 078.5 Cytomegaloviral disease
- 771.1 Congenital cytomegalovirus infection

ICD10
- B25.8 Other cytomegaloviral diseases
- B25.9 Cytomegaloviral disease, unspecified
- P35.1 Congenital cytomegalovirus infection

FAQ

- Q: Should children with congenital cytomegalovirus infection be excluded from day care settings?
- A: No. Due to the high frequency of shedding of cytomegalovirus in the urine and saliva of asymptomatic children, especially those under 2 years of age, exclusion from out-of-home care is not justified for any child known to be infected with cytomegalovirus. Careful attention to hygienic practices, especially hand washing, is important.

DAYTIME INCONTINENCE

Amanda K. Berry
Michael Carr
Seth L. Schulman (5th edition)

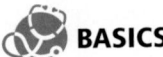 **BASICS**

DESCRIPTION
- Daytime wetting in a child ≥ 5 years of age warrants evaluation.
- Causes of functional incontinence include an array of bladder storage and voiding disorders.
- Voiding dysfunction is abnormal behavior of the lower urinary tract without a recognized organic cause, generally in the form of pelvic floor hyperactivity or bladder–sphincter uncoordination.
- Dysfunctional elimination syndrome describes the association between abnormal bladder and bowel behavior.

ALERT
- Failure to recognize and manage constipation before attempting to manage wetting
- Failure of anticholinergic medication in children with significant postvoid residuals or with constipation
- Use of anticholinergic medications in children with benign frequency of childhood is generally ineffective.
- Increased risk of urinary tract infections (UTIs) when child is placed on anticholinergic medication, due to infrequent voiding/incomplete emptying

EPIDEMIOLOGY
Prevalence
- Studies in children 6–7 years of age have shown that 3.1% of girls and 2.1% of boys had an episode of wetting at least once per week.
- Spontaneous cure rate of 14% per year without treatment
- Of all children who wet, 10% have only daytime wetting, 75% wet only at night, and 15% wet during the day and at night.

RISK FACTORS
- Constipation
- Recurrent UTIs
- Diabetes mellitus/diabetes insipidus
- Attention deficit disorder/attention deficit hyperactivity disorder (ADD/ADHD)
- Developmental delay

Genetics
- Only anecdotal relationships have been seen in functional daytime incontinence, unlike studies showing genetic tendencies in nocturnal enuresis.
- Increased rates of daytime wetting have been reported in urofacial (Ochoa) syndrome, an autosomal-recessive condition, and Williams syndrome which is the result of a deletion involving the elastin gene in chromosome #7.

ETIOLOGY
- Neurogenic bladder (e.g., myelomeningocele)
- Anatomic anomalies (e.g., ectopic ureter)
- Obstructive uropathy (e.g., posterior urethral valves)
- Bladder irritability caused by UTI
- Constipation
- Increased urinary output—polyuria
- Infrequent or deferred voiding
- Overactive bladder
- Low functional bladder capacity, with detrusor instability during filling
- Temperamental factors (e.g., short attention span, inattentiveness to body signals) in children who ignore the urge to void
- Developmental differences in age at which toilet training is achieved
- Vaginal reflux with subsequent leakage of urine
- Giggle incontinence

COMMONLY ASSOCIATED CONDITIONS
- Constipation
- Nocturnal enuresis
- UTIs
- Vesicoureteral reflux is more common in children with voiding dysfunction, due to elevated detrusor pressures that overcome a marginal vesicoureteral junction.

DIAGNOSIS

HISTORY
- Onset (primary vs. secondary)
- Frequency of voiding
- Frequency and degree of wetting
- Presence or absence of any dry interval
- Signs of urgency; use of hold maneuvers; waiting until the last minute to void

- Description of stream (i.e., strong/weak, continuous/interrupted)
- Straining or pushing during voiding
- Frequency and description of bowel movements
- Quality and quantity of fluid intake
- History of soiling
- History of UTIs, vesicoureteral reflux
- ADD/ADHD, learning disabilities, or developmental delays
- Level of concern on part of child/family
- Medications
- Signs and symptoms:
  - Urgency:
    - Posturing; Vincent's curtsy
  - Frequent urination
  - Deferred voiding
  - Weak or intermittent stream
  - Large, hard, or infrequently passed bowel movements
  - Recurrent UTIs

PHYSICAL EXAM
- Abdomen: Signs of constipation; distended bladder
- Rectal: If constipation is suspected
- Spine: Sacral abnormalities
- Genitalia: Labial adhesions, labial erythema, phimosis, urethral stenosis
- Neurologic: Sensation, reflexes, and gait

DIAGNOSTIC TESTS & INTERPRETATION
Lab
- First morning urinalysis to check concentrating ability, rule out occult renal disease
- Urine culture to rule out infection

Imaging
- Renal and bladder ultrasound in children who wet with a history of UTIs and in children with persistent wetting despite regular voiding
- Kidneys, ureter, and bladder (KUB) x-ray to assess for constipation
- MRI of lumbosacral spine if sacral abnormality or refractory to treatment

Diagnostic Procedures/Other
- Uroflowmetry and assessment of postvoid residual urine
- Invasive urodynamic testing is not indicated in neurologically normal children unless refractory to treatment.

DIFFERENTIAL DIAGNOSIS
- UTI
- Constipation
- Developmental variations in toilet training
- Neurogenic bladder
- Spinal cord abnormality
- Giggle incontinence
- Genitourinary tract abnormality (posterior urethral valve, ectopic ureter)
- Vaginal reflux
- Benign increased urinary frequency (pollakiuria)
- Sexual abuse

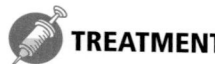 TREATMENT

ADDITIONAL TREATMENT
General Measures
- Aggressive management of bowels so that child is passing at least 1 soft bowel movement daily (see "Constipation")
- Elimination schedule, with voids every 2–3 hours and time to defecate at least once a day. A reminder watch may be helpful.
- Voiding diary provides concrete data and focus for child.
- Positive reinforcement for regular voiding
- Avoid acidic/diuretic beverages (caffeine, carbonation, chocolate, citrus)
- Adequate hydration
- Local management of perineal irritation/vulvovaginitis to ensure comfort during voiding
- Girls with postvoid dribbling due to vaginal reflux should void with their legs wide apart, sitting backward on the toilet when possible, to minimize backflow of urine into the vagina. Wipe after standing up.

MEDICATION (DRUGS)
- A trial of an anticholinergic may be indicated if the child wets despite conservative medical/behavioral management.
- Extended-release formulations are available.
- Common side effects include dry mouth, decreased diaphoresis with flushing, and constipation. Blurred vision and dizziness are less common.

First Line
- Oxybutynin (Ditropan/Ditropan XL): 5–15 mg/d
- Tolterodine (Detrol/Detrol LA): 2–4 mg/d
- Solifenacin (Vesicare): 5–10 mg/d
- Darifenacin (Enablex): 7.5–15 mg/d

ISSUES FOR REFERRAL
Referral to pediatric urologist:
- When wetting is refractory to behavioral management, child may benefit from a noninvasive urodynamic evaluation to assess flow pattern, voiding mechanics, and ability to empty the bladder.

ONGOING CARE

PROGNOSIS
- Spontaneous cure rate of 14% per year without treatment
- 72% of patients sustained improvement 1 year after simple behavioral therapy.

COMPLICATIONS
- Local irritation and inflammation of the perineum
- Functional daytime incontinence is primarily a social problem that affects children's self-esteem and interactions with peers.

ADDITIONAL READING

- Bael A, Lax H, de Jong TP, et al. The relevance of urodynamic studies for urge syndrome and dysfunctional voiding: A multicenter controlled trial in children. *J Urol.* 2008;180(4):1486–1493; discussion 1494–1495.
- Bael A, Winkler P, Lax H, et al. Behavior profiles in children with functional urinary incontinence before and after incontinence treatment. *Pediatrics.* 2008;121(5):e1196–1200.
- Herndon CDA, Joseph DB. Urinary incontinence. *Pediatr Clin North Am.* 2006;53:363–377.
- Loening-Baucke V. Urinary incontinence and urinary tract infection and their resolution with treatment of chronic constipation of childhood. *Pediatrics.* 1997; 100:228–231.

- Saedi N, Schulman SL. Natural history of voiding dysfunction. *Pediatr Nephrol.* 2003;18:894–897.
- Schulman SL. Voiding dysfunction in children. *Urol Clin North Am.* 2004;31:381–390.
- Wiener JS, Scales MT, Hampton J, et al. Long-term efficacy of simple behavioral therapy for daytime wetting in children. *J Urol.* 2000;164:786–790.

CODES

ICD9
- 307.6 Enuresis
- 788.30 Urinary incontinence, unspecified
- 788.91 Functional urinary incontinence

ICD10
- F98.0 Enuresis not due to a substance or known physiol condition
- R32 Unspecified urinary incontinence
- R39.81 Functional urinary incontinence

FAQ

- Q: What findings can distinguish functional incontinence from an ectopic ureter?
- A: An ectopic ureter usually empties below the sphincter or elsewhere, such as in the vagina. Therefore, these girls wet all the time, with no dry period. They do not have symptoms such as urgency. Because in most cases the ureter draining the kidney is duplicated, an ultrasound or IV pyelogram (IVP) may provide more information.
- Q: What is a normal bladder capacity for a child?
- A: Normal bladder capacity (in mL) can be estimated as the child's weight (in kg) × 7. A child's bladder capacity can be determined by measuring voided volumes for 2 consecutive days when the child is well hydrated. The largest voided volume is considered the child's maximum functional capacity.
- Q: When is an MRI of the spine indicated?
- A: Spinal cord imaging should be considered in children with refractory daytime wetting and signs and symptoms suggestive of neuropathic voiding dysfunction, including difficulty voiding, significant postvoid residual urine, or impaired bladder sensation. It should also be considered when ultrasound reveals a thickened bladder wall and hydroureteronephrosis is present in the absence of an obstruction such as posterior urethral valves.

DEHYDRATION
Marc H. Gorelick

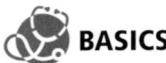 **BASICS**

DESCRIPTION
- Dehydration is a negative balance of body fluid, usually expressed as a percentage of body weight. Mild, moderate, and severe dehydration correspond to deficits of <5%, 5–10%, and >10%, respectively.
- Dehydration is classified into 3 types on the basis of serum sodium concentration: Isotonic (Na 130–150 mmol/L), hypotonic (Na <130 mmol/L), and hypertonic (Na >150 mmol/L)

GENERAL PREVENTION
Many cases of frank dehydration may be prevented by early institution of adequate oral maintenance fluid therapy in children with gastroenteritis, with particular attention to replacement of ongoing stool losses and slow administration of fluids to children with vomiting. Use of appropriate solutions is essential to prevent electrolyte disturbance and worsening of diarrhea.

EPIDEMIOLOGY
Incidence
- ~10% of children in the USA with acute gastroenteritis develop at least mild dehydration.
- Although it accounts for 10% of all nonsurgical hospital admissions for children younger than 5 years, up to 90% of cases can be managed on an outpatient basis.

PATHOPHYSIOLOGY
- Dehydration is caused by either excessive fluid losses or inadequate intake of fluids.
- Some conditions leading to dehydration include:
  - GI losses: Vomiting, diarrhea (most common cause of dehydration in pediatric patients)
  - Renal losses: Diabetes mellitus, diabetes insipidus, diuretic agents
  - Insensible losses: Sweating, fever, tachypnea, increased ambient temperature, large burns
  - Poor oral intake: Stomatitis, pharyngitis, anorexia, oral trauma, altered mental status
  - Note that infants and debilitated patients are at particular risk due to lack of ability to satisfy their thirst freely.

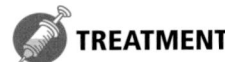 **DIAGNOSIS**

HISTORY
- Frequency and duration of emesis and/or diarrhea will give a rough estimate of risk of dehydration.
- If there were large quantities of water taken, be alert for hypotonic dehydration. If inadequate free water is used for hydration, patient may have hypertonic dehydration
- Frequency and quantity of urination may be difficult to estimate in infants with diarrhea.
- Decreased urination indicates possibility of dehydration.
- Fever increases insensible water loss.
- Exertion or heat exposure increases insensible water loss.

PHYSICAL EXAM
- Acute change in weight is the best indicator of fluid deficit. If the child's recent preillness weight is not available for comparison, a reasonable estimate of the degree of dehydration may be made from physical findings.
- General appearance: Lethargy, irritability, thirst
- Vital signs: Tachycardia; orthostatic increase in heart rate or hypotension; hyperpnea
- Skin: Prolonged capillary refill at fingertip (<2 sec is normal in warm environment); mottling; poor turgor
- Eyes: Decreased or absent tears; sunken eyes
- Mucous membranes: Dry or parched
- Anterior fontanelle: Sunken

ALERT
Diagnostic pitfalls:
- Physical signs generally appear when the deficit is as small as 2%.
- No single finding is pathognomonic of dehydration. A reasonable guideline is that the presence of 3 or more findings indicates at least mild dehydration. The number and severity of physical signs increase with the degree of dehydration.
- Urine output decreases early in the course of dehydration, and a history of decreased urination is a sensitive but nonspecific finding.
- Capillary refill time is a specific but insensitive indicator. It may be falsely prolonged by cool ambient temperature [<20°C (<68°F)]. It is not affected by fever.
- Children with a deficit >15% will show signs of cardiovascular instability such as severe tachycardia and hypotension.
- Physical findings may be more significant for a given degree of dehydration in children with hyponatremia, leading to overestimation of the deficit. Conversely, the clinical picture is reported to be somewhat moderated in hypernatremia.

DIAGNOSTIC TESTS & INTERPRETATION
Lab
- Diagnosis of dehydration is best made on clinical grounds. The following laboratory tests are sometimes helpful adjuncts.
- Serum sodium:
  - Classifies type of dehydration
  - Hyponatremia and hypernatremia are uncommon in dehydration due to gastroenteritis (<5% of cases).
  - Measure sodium levels in cases of clinically severe disease, or if risk factors are present (e.g., infant <2 months, history of excessive free water intake, children with significant neurologic impairment limiting their ability to regulate their own intake).
- Rapid glucose test or serum glucose: To detect hypoglycemia due to prolonged fasting
- Urine specific gravity: This is elevated early in dehydration, but may not become elevated at all in young infants or in children with sickle cell disease.
- Serum bicarbonate: This is frequently low with diarrheal illness, even in the absence of dehydration. Useful to detect significant acidosis when dehydration is clinically severe
- Blood urea nitrogen (BUN): May rise late in dehydration in children

TREATMENT

ADDITIONAL TREATMENT
General Measures
Oral rehydration therapy (ORT):
- Most children can be managed successfully with oral rehydration therapy, either at home or in a health care setting.
- Use rehydration solution containing 2.0–2.5% glucose and 75 mmol/L Na (e.g., WHO solution), or 45–50 mmol/L Na [e.g., Pedialyte (Ross Laboratories, Columbus, OH), Infalyte (Mead Johnson, Evansville, IN)].
- Replace entire deficit in 4–6 hours: For mild dehydration, 50 mL/kg; for moderate to severe dehydration, 80–100 mL/kg. Include ongoing losses, ~5 mL/kg for each diarrheal stool.
- Begin with slow administration, with strict limits when vomiting is present: 5 mL q1–2min. For infants, use a syringe or spoon rather than a bottle. After 1 hour, if the oral liquids have been tolerated, increase the volume and rate.
- Have the child's caregiver participate in giving the fluids, and provide education with regard to fluid replacement and signs of dehydration.
- Monitor weight, intake and output, and clinical signs. Failure of oral rehydration therapy includes intractable vomiting, clinical deterioration, or lack of improvement after 4 hours.

IV Fluids
- IV fluids are required when ORT fails or is contraindicated, such as in severe dehydration or shock, poor gag or suck, depressed mental status, severe hypernatremia (Na > 160 mmol/L), suspected surgical abdomen.
- Administer IV bolus of normal saline or Ringer lactate, 20 mL/kg, over 10–30 minutes. Repeat as needed to restore cardiovascular stability. Avoid dextrose-containing solutions for boluses except to correct documented hypoglycemia.
- Calculate maintenance fluid requirements: 100 mL/kg for the 1st 10 kg, plus 50 mL/kg for the next 10 kg, plus 20 mL/kg over 20 kg.
- Calculate fluid deficit based on clinical estimate or known weight loss. For isotonic or hypotonic dehydration, give 1/3–1/2 normal saline with 5% dextrose, at a rate adequate to provide maintenance and replace deficit over 24 hours. For hypertonic dehydration, replace deficit over 48 hours, using 1/5–1/4 normal saline with 5% dextrose.
- Monitor weight, intake and output, and clinical signs. With hypernatremia, measure serum sodium q4–6h; do not exceed rate of fall of 1 mmol/L/h.
- For mild to moderate isonatremic dehydration, rapid replacement of deficit over 2–6 hours may be possible. Give normal saline at a rate to replace the estimated deficit at a rate of 25–50 cc/kg/h.

MEDICATION (DRUGS)
First Line
Most children with dehydration do not require specific medication therapy. For children with significant vomiting, several studies indicate that ondansetron 0.15 mg/kg PO decreases vomiting and facilitates oral rehydration.

IN-PATIENT CONSIDERATIONS
Admission Criteria
- Failure of oral or IV rehydration within 4 hours
- Severe hypernatremia
- Substantial ongoing losses indicating a high likelihood of recurrence of dehydration

Discharge Criteria
After initiating ORT, children who are tolerating oral fluids at an acceptable rate to replace their deficit over 4–6 hours may be discharged with a willing and reliable caregiver and complete the ORT at home.

 ONGOING CARE

PROGNOSIS
Excellent with appropriate rehydration therapy

COMPLICATIONS
- Severe dehydration may lead to hypovolemic shock and acute renal failure.
- Hyponatremia is associated with hypotonia, hypothermia, and seizures.
- Overly rapid correction of hypernatremia can produce cerebral edema.

PATIENT MONITORING
- After rehydration, children with ongoing losses, as in gastroenteritis, should receive a maintenance solution in addition to regular feedings to maintain a positive fluid balance.
- Recommend 5–10 mL/kg for each diarrheal stool. Avoid clear liquids with excessive glucose, such as fruit juices, punches, and soft drinks, as these can promote osmotic fluid losses in the stool.
- In infants <6 months old, do not give large amounts of plain water, which can lead to hyponatremia.

ADDITIONAL READING
- Armon K, Stephenson T, MacFaul R, et al. An evidence and consensus based guideline for acute diarrhea management. *Arch Dis Child.* 2001;85(2):132–142.
- Centers for Disease Control and Prevention. Managing acute gastroenteritis among children: Oral rehydration, maintenance, and nutritional therapy. *MMWR.* 2003;52 (No. RR-16).
- DeCamp LR, Byerley JS, Doshi N, Steiner MJ. Use of antiemetic agents in acute gastroenteritis: A systematic review and meta-analysis. *Arch Pediatr Adolesc Med.* 2008;162(9):858–865.
- Hartling L, Bellemare S, Wiebe N, et al. Oral versus intravenous rehydration for treating dehydration due to gastroenteritis in children. *Cochrane Library* 2009;(3):CD004390.
- Holliday MA, Ray PE, Friedman AL. Fluid therapy for children: Facts, fashions and questions. *Arch Dis Child.* 2007;92(6):546–550.
- Steiner MJ, DeWalt DA, Byerley JS. Is this child dehydrated? *JAMA.* 2004;291(22):2746–2754.

 CODES

ICD9
- 276.51 Dehydration
- 775.5 Other transitory neonatal electrolyte disturbances

ICD10
- E86.0 Dehydration
- P74.1 Dehydration of newborn

22Q11.2 DELETION SYNDROME (DIGEORGE SYNDROME)

Erin E. McGintee

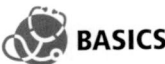 **BASICS**

DESCRIPTION

22q11.2 deletion syndrome, formerly known as DiGeorge syndrome, is characterized by thymic and parathyroid aplasia or hypoplasia, cardiac outflow tract abnormalities, cleft palate, velopharyngeal insufficiency, speech delay, and facial dysmorphism. T-cell immunodeficiency is observed in 80% of children with DiGeorge syndrome:

- Patients with complete DiGeorge syndrome have a severe T-cell defect.
- Partial DiGeorge syndrome occurs when the T-cell defect is partial or transient.

RISK FACTORS

Genetics

- Heterogeneous
- 6–10% of cases are familial.
- Most common associated chromosomal abnormalities are heterozygous microdeletions of 22q11.2.

PATHOPHYSIOLOGY

DiGeorge is believed to be a developmental defect of the 3rd and 4th pharyngeal arches.

 DIAGNOSIS

HISTORY

- Neonatal hypocalcemia secondary to hypoparathyroidism
- Recurrent viral and opportunistic infections: Diarrhea, candidiasis, respiratory infections, *Pneumocystis carinii* pneumonia (PCP)
- Cardiac defects, particularly interrupted aortic arch, septal defects, tetralogy of Fallot, and truncus arteriosus
- Failure to thrive

PHYSICAL EXAM

Facial dysmorphism (micrognathia; low, rotated ears; fish-shaped mouth; short philtrum, anteverted nares, broad nasal bridge, and hypertelorism):

- Cleft lip and palate
- Heart murmur
- Renal abnormalities
- Skeletal abnormalities
- Central nervous system malformations
- Cognitive/behavioral disorders
- Major immunologic features present at birth: Lymphopenia, T-cell dysfunction; antibody levels and function are variable.

DIAGNOSTIC TESTS & INTERPRETATION

Lab

- CBC with differential:
  - Immediately after birth, a lymphocyte count of <1,200/mm^3 is suspicious.
  - Serum calcium
  - Evaluation of parathyroid function, if necessary
- Lymphocyte markers:
  - To determine absolute numbers of T and B cells and their subsets
- Mitogen studies:
  - To study the functional abilities of T and B cells. In DiGeorge syndrome, you may see a variably depressed response to phytohemagglutinin, concanavalin A, and pokeweed mitogen.
- Quantitative immunoglobulins (IgG, IgA, IgM, and IgE):
  - Often the humoral system will be abnormal if there is helper T-cell dysfunction.
- Fluorescence in situ hybridization (FISH) for 22q11 deletion:
  - Most common chromosomal defect

Imaging

Chest radiograph study to evaluate for cardiac malformation and also for the presence of a thymic shadow

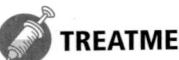 **TREATMENT**

ADDITIONAL TREATMENT

General Measures

- Depending on the defects or deficiencies the child manifests, some issues may need to be addressed:
  - Cardiology for the cardiac malformations
  - Otolaryngology and feeding specialist for cleft palate
  - Endocrinology for follow-up of hypoparathyroidism
  - Speech and cognitive intervention for speech delay
  - Immunology to monitor T-cell disorder and recurrent infections
  - Severe immunodeficiency may require matched sibling bone marrow transplant or thymic transplant.

- Special consideration with infections: Children with the complete DiGeorge syndrome are at increased risk of morbidity and mortality from viral infections either from vaccines or natural infections:
  – Avoid live viral vaccines in cases of severe T-cell dysfunction. These patients may need immunoglobulin replacement therapy to protect from infections.
  – Most patients with CD4+ cell counts >500 cells/mm^3 can be safely and effectively vaccinated with live viral vaccines.
  – Consider varicella immune globulin in a patient with either unknown humoral immunity status or definitive humoral abnormalities and a history of exposure. IV acyclovir may be necessary if varicella develops and patient has severe T-cell defect.
- Special consideration with blood transfusions:
  – Because these patients are at risk for graft-versus-host disease, it is best to use cytomegalovirus-negative, irradiated blood.

 ## ONGOING CARE

FOLLOW-UP RECOMMENDATIONS
Patient Monitoring
- Monitor growth.
- Monitor hearing.
- Monitor development.

PROGNOSIS
Prolonged survival is seen in most patients after the spontaneous improvement of T-cell numbers and function. Patients with complete DiGeorge syndrome may have more severe and persistent T-cell dysfunction. Complications may include an increase in autoimmune phenomena and neurologic sequelae.

COMPLICATIONS
In the newborn period, patients present with hypocalcemic tetany, manifestation of cardiac abnormality, and recurrent infections. Later on, patients present more commonly with neurologic and developmental or behavioral issues. Patients are at increased risk for development of autoimmune disease.

ADDITIONAL READING

- Al-Sukaiti N, Reid B, Lavi S, et al. Safety and efficacy of measles, mumps, and rubella vaccine in patients with DiGeorge syndrome. *J Allergy Clin Immunol*. 2010;126(4):868–869.
- Carotti A, Digilio MC, Piacentini G, et al. Cardiac defects and results of cardiac surgery in 22q11.2 deletion syndrome. *Dev Disabil Res Rev*. 2008; 14(1):35–42.
- Emanuel BS. Molecular mechanisms and diagnosis of chromosome 22q11.2 rearrangements. *Dev Disabil Res Rev*. 2008;14(1):11–18.
- Goldmuntz E. DiGeorge syndrome: New insights. *Clin Perinatol*. 2005;32(4):963–978.
- McLean-Tooke A, Barge D, Spickett GP, et al. Immunologic defects in 22q11.2 deletion syndrome. *J Allergy Clin Immunol*. 2008;122:362–367.
- Perez EE, Bokszczanin A, McDonald-McGinn D, et al. Safety of live viral vaccines in patients with chromosome 22q11.2 deletion syndrome (DiGeorge syndrome/velocardiofacial syndrome). *Pediatrics*. 2003;112(4):e325.
- Perez E, Sullivan KE. Chromosome 22q11.2 deletion syndrome (DiGeorge and velocardiofacial syndromes). *Curr Opin Pediatr*. 2002;14:678–683.
- Radford DJ. The DiGeorge syndrome and the heart. *Curr Opin Pediatr*. 1991;3:828–831.
- Sullivan KE. DiGeorge syndrome/chromosome 22q11.2 deletion syndrome. *Curr Allergy Asthma Rep*. 2001;1(Sep):438–444.

 ## CODES

ICD9
279.11 DiGeorge syndrome

ICD10
D82.1 Di George's syndrome

FAQ

- Q: Is there a definitive test to distinguish between partial and complete DiGeorge syndrome?
- A: Over time, patients with partial DiGeorge syndrome will reconstitute their T cells and acquire improved function based on mitogen and antigen studies.

D

DENTAL/ORAL PAIN AND URGENCIES

Hugh Silk
Sheila Stille
Ciarán DellaFera

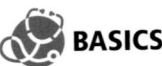

BASICS

DESCRIPTION
Dental urgencies consist of a number of acute issues that occur in the mouth. These include dental caries, cavities, worsening infections, such as abscesses and cellulitis, trauma, and other sources of referred pain.

EPIDEMIOLOGY
- Dental caries are the most common chronic disease of childhood: 19% of 2–5 year olds and 52% of 5–9 year olds
- 30% of preschoolers have suffered a dental trauma to primary teeth
- 25% of 12 year olds have injured their permanent teeth

Incidence
- Peak incidence of dental injury occurs between ages 2 and 4 years
- 80% of caries in children between ages 5–17 occur in 25% of all children, those with the most risk factors

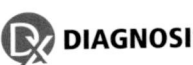

DIAGNOSIS

HISTORY
- Details of when, where and mechanism of injury or infection; determine tetanus status
- Assess symptoms: Pain, swelling, change in occlusion, difficulty opening mouth
- Children may not be able to localize pain and may exhibit vague symptoms (e.g., not eating second to pain or dysphagia or trismus)

PHYSICAL EXAM
- Urgency/emergency Triage
  - Airway first (ABCs)
  - Assess for other life-threatening injuries
  - Assess the Cervical Spine
  - Neurologic exam
  - Check for skull, orbit, or zygomatic fractures
  - Ask/assess primary versus permanent teeth
  - Note availability of dental care
- Examine mouth – systematic approach
  - Irrigate to remove blood, clots, and debris
  - Soft tissues
  - Teeth: Primary or Permanent
  - Bony structures
- Specifically assess for:
  - Tenderness, swelling, erythema
  - Lacerations or ulcers
  - Damaged or mobile teeth
  - Occlusion
  - Mobile jaw segments/step-off abnormalities
  - Pain or limitation on opening
  - Referred pain sources (ear, sinus)

DIAGNOSTIC TESTS & INTERPRETATION
Lab
Rare; culture and sensitivity for complicated infection

Imaging
- See 'Treatment' below for specifics
- May require individual periapical films, panoramic views or CT

Diagnostic Procedures/Other
- General Goals
  - PHASE ONE: Stabilize patient (if necessary)
  - PHASE TWO: Make specific diagnosis; rule out differential diagnoses
  - PHASE THREE: Create patient-centered management plan focusing on alleviating pain/disease
- Hints for Screening Problems
  - Screening/education is key for prevention:
  - Ask and advise about oral hygiene promotion and dental surveillance
  - Education about medical/dental connections
  - Educate about mouth guard use; consult against oral piercings/secondary prevention (remove piercing for sports, don't click on teeth, treat infected piercing early)

DIFFERENTIAL DIAGNOSIS
- INFECTIONS
  - Reversible pulpitis: A carious lesion (cavity) which approaches the dental pulp
  - Irreversible pulpitis: A carious lesion which continues into the dental pulp
  - Periapical abscess: A localized purulent erosive area of bone at apex of tooth root secondary to necrotic pulp of tooth
  - Periodontal abscess: A localized purulent form of periodontitis secondary to loss of supporting structure (ligament, gum)
  - Cellulitis/facial abscess: Second to progression of periapical abscess
  - Pericoronitis: Gum flap traps food and plaque over partially erupted molar or impacted wisdom teeth leading to local inflammation and infection

ALERT
Secondary infections: Submental, sublingual, and submandibular space (Ludwig's angina); fistulas; facial cellulitis; meningitis
- TRAUMA
  - To the teeth
    - Concussion: Tooth is tender but not displaced or mobile
    - Intrusion: Tooth pushed deep into gum/socket
    - Extrusion: Tooth is partially displaced (outward) from the gum/socket
    - Subluxation: Tooth is mobile but majority of ligament attachment is in place
    - Luxation: Tooth is mobile; no or some displacement; ligament support is severely damaged
    - Avulsion: Tooth is completely detached and extruded from mouth
    - Tooth fracture: Four basic types based on depth of break: Enamel only; enamel and dentin; enamel, dentin and pulp; root
  - To the jaw:

- Mandible fracture: Suspect in chin trauma; can break in 2 places along arch
- Maxillary fracture: Alveolar versus LeFort
- ALLERGY/INFLAMATION/VASCULITIS
  - Gingivitis: Superficial inflammation of gums second to poor oral hygiene and plaque irritation, foreign body (food) between teeth and gum, or hormonal changes (OCPs, pregnancy)
  - Periodontitis: Inflammation of bone and supporting ligaments and gum resulting in bone loss
  - Acute necrotizing ulcerative gingivitis (Vincent's angina): Edematous, ulcerated gingival; bacterial etiology
  - Ulcers: Aphthous; infectious (viral: Herpetic, coxsackie; bacterial); traumatic (e.g., biting gum); drug reaction
  - Temporomandibular joint inflammation (TMJ)
- MISCELLANEOUS
  - Bruxism leading to teeth erosion or TMJ
  - Referred pain: Otitis media/externa, sinusitis

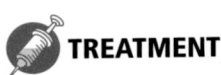

TREATMENT
Emergency Care
- Triage as above in "Physical Exam"
- Address pain early and often

ADDITIONAL TREATMENT
General Measures
- PAIN MANAGEMENT:
  - Acetaminophen, NSAIDs, with or without opioids (note mouth pain can be significant) based on body weight
  - Avoid irritating cold/hot drinks, food
- INFECTIONS:
  - Reversible pulpitis: Restoration (filing)
  - Irreversible pulpitis: Root canal and restoration or extraction
  - Periapical abscess: Local or regional anesthesia, incision and drainage, antibiotics if cellulitis; definitive treatment is root canal and restoration or extraction; antibiotics—penicillin 50 mg/kg/day divided tid, max 1.5 g/day for 10 days; clindamycin 10–25 mg/kg/day divided tid for penicillin allergy
  - Facial cellulitis second to dental infection: outpatient therapy with antibiotics (as above) for mild cases with adherent patients; close follow-up and dental referral for root canal, restoration or extraction
  - Pericoronitis: Irrigate under gum flap; removal of gum flap; extraction if impacted wisdom tooth

ALERT

Inpatient care for extensive cellulitis as spread to deep tissues can result in trismus, sepsis, or airway occlusion; consult Surgery/Oral Surgery, Infectious Diseases; IV broad spectrum antibiotics and analgesics; CT imaging; root canal, restoration or extraction

- TRAUMA
  - Don't assume missing teeth were lost at scene: Consider swallowed, aspirated, in sinus
- Primary Teeth:
  - Luxated teeth: Minimal mobility – monitor; very loose or interfere with occlusion – referral for extraction
  - Intrusion: Don't reposition, will re-erupt; requires imaging to assess damage to underlying permanent tooth; monitor
  - Avulsion: Do NOT re-implant
- Permanent Teeth:
  - Concussion of tooth: Monitor with dentist
  - Subluxation: Usually reposition, splint
  - Extrusion or lateral luxation: Reposition, splint, +/– root canal
  - Intrusion: Do not reposition, often associated with alveolar bone fracture; usually needs extraction after bone heals (4 months later)

ALERT

- Avulsion: A true dental emergency!
  - Hold tooth by crown, DO NOT touch root; Rinse off debris with saline or milk; Re-implant immediately; Bite on gauze or hold tooth in place; See dentist immediately for x-ray, splinting, and root canal treatment.
  - If can't re-implant on scene, transport in saline, milk, or buccal sulcus (not water!)
  - Fractures: Save all fragments for dentist; although, restoration of fragments may not be possible
    - Enamel only: Non-urgent dental referral to smooth rough edges
    - Enamel and dentin: Referral within 12 hours for restoration to protect pulp
    - Enamel, dentin, and pulp: Immediate referral for root canal, restoration or extraction
    - Root fracture: Immediate referral for imaging, root canal, restoration, or extraction
    - Mandibular condyle or alveolar bone fracture: Refer to oral surgeon within 1 hour for reduction; swelling makes more difficult
- ALLERGY/INFLAMMATION/VASCULITIS
  - Gingivitis: Remove any foreign bodies between teeth or in gingival crevice; advise to improve dental hygiene including brushing bid with fluoridated toothpaste and daily flossing; warm saline rinses; regular dental visits for cleaning, prevention. For necrotizing gingivitis refer for debridement; 0.012% chlorhexidine mouth rinses
- PREVENTION
  - Tetanus prophylaxis for intrusion, avulsion, deep laceration or contaminated wound if not updated in past 5 years
  - Remind patient – wear a mouth guard; avoid mouth piercings/jewelry; if already pierced, remove if possible for sports and avoid clicking on teeth; daily dental hygiene; regular dental visits

- High risk sports for dental trauma include: Hockey, football, soccer, boxing, wrestling, basketball, baseball, skateboarding, skiing, bicycling, in-line skating trampoline use
- Mouth guards come in many colors, styles; custom/fitted are better than boil and bite, which are better than stock, however custom are expensive

ISSUES FOR REFERRAL

- See "Treatment" for specifics
- Definitive treatment for ANY tooth-based infection is root canal or extraction of tooth
- Note: Pregnant teenagers can have dental x-rays, restoration, extractions, appropriate antibiotics and analgesics throughout pregnancy; all non-urgent treatment is best done during second trimester due to lowest risk for miscarriage and most comfortable in dental chair; first trimester, schedule appointments in afternoon due to nausea; third trimester, position patient on left side and keep visits short, avoid full recline of chair

SURGERY/OTHER PROCEDURES

Permanent teeth avulsion, tooth fractures involving the pulp or root, jaw fractures, extensive cellulitis require emergent referrals; all other emergencies can be referred next day or later

ADDITIONAL READING

- American Association of Endodontists. Recommended Guidelines of the American Association of Endodontists for the Treatment of Traumatic Dental Injuries. Chicago; 2004.
- Bastone EB, Freer TJ, McNamara JR. Epidemiology of dental trauma: A review of the literature. *Aust Dent J.* 2000;45(1):2–9.
- Bratton TA, Jackson DC, Nkungula-Howlett T, et al. Management of complex multi-space odontogenic infections. *J Tenn Dent Assoc.* 2002;82(3):39–47.
- Cameron A. *Handbook of Pediatric.* 2nd ed. United States: Mosby, 2003.
- Dental care of the medically complex patient. Lockhart PB, editor. Edinburgh (UK): Elsevier Science Limited; 2004.
- Flynn TR, Shanti RM, Levi MH, et al. Severe odontogenic infections, part 1: Prospective report. *J Oral Maxillofac Surg.* 2006;64(7):1093–1103.
- Holmgren EP, Dierks EJ, Homer LD, et al. Facial computed tomography use in trauma patients who require a head computed tomogram. *J Oral Maxillofac Surg.* 2004;62(8):913–918.
- Levin L, Zadik Y, Becker T. Oral and dental complications of intra-oral piercing. *Dent Traumatol* 2005;21(6):341–343.
- McTigue DJ. Diagnosis and management of dental injuries in children. *Pediatr Clin North Am.* 2000;47(5):1067–1084.
- Newsome PR, Tran DC, Cooke MS. The role of the mouth guard in the prevention of sports-related dental injuries: A review. *International J Paediatr Dent.* 2001;11(6):396–404.
- Oral Health Care During Pregnancy and Early Childhood Practice Guidelines. New York Public Health Department 2006. http://www.health.state.ny.us/publications/0824.pdf.
- Walker J, Jakobsen J, Brown S. Attitudes concerning mouthguard use in 7- to 8-year-old children. *J Dent Child.* 2002;69(2):207–211, 126.

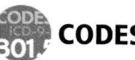 **CODES**

ICD9
- 521.00 Dental caries, unspecified
- 522.4 Acute apical periodontitis of pulpal origin
- 959.09 Injury of face and neck

ICD10
- K02.9 Dental caries, unspecified
- K04.7 Periapical abscess without sinus
- S09.93XA Unspecified injury of face, initial encounter

CLINICAL PEARLS

- Very few true dental emergencies: Spreading cellulitic dental infection; avulsed or fractured permanent tooth or jaw bone
- Definitive treatment for tooth infections is restorative root canal or extraction; must follow up all infections with dental referral
- Dental urgencies can be prevented with proper oral hygiene, preventive dental visits, avoidance of mouth piercings and use of mouth guards

DERMATOMYOSITIS/POLYMYOSITIS

Timothy Beukelman
Randy Q. Cron

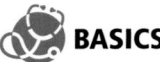
BASICS

DESCRIPTION
The dermatomyositis/polymyositis complex includes a number of conditions in which muscle becomes damaged by a non-suppurative lymphocytic inflammatory process. Juvenile dermatomyositis (JDM) is the most common seen in the pediatric population.

EPIDEMIOLOGY
- The average age of onset is 7 years.
- Overall male-to-female ratio is 1:1.7; however, equal in children <10 years of age.

Incidence
- 1:200,000

RISK FACTORS
Genetics
HLA-DQ0301

ETIOLOGY
- Unknown
- Several potential mechanisms include:
  - Abnormal cell-mediated immunity
  - Immune-complex formation
  - Immunodeficiency
  - Infection
  - Microchimerism
  - Interferon-alpha

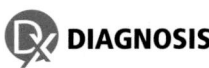
DIAGNOSIS

HISTORY
- Fever: Evidence of systemic illness
- Anorexia and weight loss: GI involvement
- Fatigue: Sign of muscle weakness
- Weakness: Difficulty rising from floor, climbing stairs, swallowing, regurgitation through nose
- Dysphonia: Sign of muscle weakness
- Rash could contain clue to diagnosis.

- Signs and symptoms:
  - Diagnosis requires the presence of the pathognomonic rash plus 3 additional criteria:
    ○ Progressive symmetric weakness of proximal muscles
    ○ Dermatitis-heliotrope rash over eyelids, Gottron papules over extensor surfaces of joints
    ○ Elevated serum level of muscle enzymes
    ○ Electromyograph (EMG) findings of myopathy and denervation
    ○ Biopsy demonstration of inflammatory myositis
    ○ Although not a criterion, T2-weighted MRI is useful in establishing active myositis.

PHYSICAL EXAM
- Muscle weakness/tenderness: Proximal and symmetric
- Rash:
  - 75% have pathognomonic rash, which usually appears several weeks after muscle weakness.
- Facial rash:
  - Violaceous, heliotropic changes over eyelids
- Extremities:
  - Gottron papules over extensor surfaces
- Nailfold telangiectasia:
  - Simultaneous dilated loops, dropout, and arborized capillary loops
- Physical exam tricks:
  - Gower sign: Inability to rise from floor without using hands
  - Use ophthalmoscope to examine nailfold for telangiectasia
  - Objective measure of strength: Duration of straight leg raise (normal = 20 seconds)

DIAGNOSTIC TESTS & INTERPRETATION
Lab
- Autoantibodies:
  - Normal rheumatoid factor, complement, and double-stranded DNA (dsDNA)
  - Antinuclear antibody: 10–50%
  - PM-1: 60% adult polymyositis; however, rare in children
  - Jo-1: Associated with interstitial lung disease

- Muscle enzymes:
  - Elevated in 95% cases
  - Creatine kinase
  - Aspartate aminotransferase
  - Aldolase
  - Lactate dehydrogenase

Imaging
- MRI:
  - Inflamed muscles are identified by signal enhancement.
  - Useful to direct biopsy
- Video swallow study:
  - To identify palatal or proximal esophageal weakness
- Pulmonary function tests/peak flow:
  - To evaluate pulmonary musculature and interstitial lung disease

Pathological Findings
- Skeletal muscle:
  - Group atrophy or perifascicular myopathy
  - Variation in fiber size due to concomitant degeneration and regeneration
  - Inflammatory exudate in perivascular distribution
  - Necrotizing vasculitis of arterioles, capillaries, and venules; probably due to immune-complex deposition
- Skin:
  - Epidermal atrophy
  - Vascular dilatation
  - Lymphocyte infiltration of the dermis

DIFFERENTIAL DIAGNOSIS
- Postinfectious:
  - Influenza A and B, coxsackievirus B, schistosomiasis, trypanosomiasis, toxoplasmosis
  - Bacterial/pyomyositis-focal
- Myositis with other connective tissue diseases:
  - Malignancy (rare in childhood)
  - Mixed connective tissue disease
  - Systemic lupus erythematosus

- Childhood neuromuscular diseases:
  - If no rash, consider muscular dystrophy, congenital myopathies, metabolic disorders (glycogen storage disease, carnitine deficiency, myoadenylate deaminase)
  - Neurogenic atrophies (spinal muscular atrophy and anterior horn, peripheral nerve dysfunction)
  - Neuromuscular transmission disorders
  - Inclusion body myositis

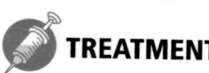 TREATMENT

MEDICATION (DRUGS)
- Aggressive early therapy
- 2 mg/kg/d of prednisone for 1 month, taper over months to years
- IV gamma globulin, efficacious for rash
- Plaquenil, particularly useful for the rash
- Methotrexate (PO, SC, or IV); avoid IM, which may alter serum levels of muscle enzymes
- Cyclosporine
- Mycophenolate mofetil
- Rituximab (experimental for refractory disease)

ALERT
- Steroid-induced myopathy
- Insidious onset
- Proximal and distal muscles, often large muscle groups such as hip flexors
- Normal serum muscle enzymes
- Minimal myopathic changes on electromyograph
- Type II fiber atrophy on muscle biopsy

ADDITIONAL TREATMENT
General Measures
Supportive care:
- Monitor for swallowing difficulty
- Respiratory compromise occasionally requires mechanical ventilation.
- Treatment of calcinosis may include colchicine, diltiazem, and bisphosphonates, but most are generally ineffective.

Additional Therapies
- Physical therapy
  - Initially to maintain range of movement
  - Strengthening only after acute inflammation resolves

 ONGOING CARE

FOLLOW-UP RECOMMENDATIONS
Patient Monitoring
- Function
- Muscle strength
- Joint range of movement
- Development of calcinosis
- Muscle enzyme levels

PROGNOSIS
- Normal to good: 65–80%
- Minimal atrophy and joint contractures: 24%
- Calcinosis: 20–40%
- Wheelchair dependent: 5%
- Death: 3%

COMPLICATIONS
- Myositis
- Rash
- Arthritis
- Calcinosis
- Raynaud syndrome
- Dysphagia and dysphonia
- Restrictive lung disease and aspiration pneumonia
- Myocarditis (rare)
- GI tract vasculitis
- Osteoporosis
- Joint contractures
- Skin infections
- Lipoatrophy

ADDITIONAL READING

- Feldman BM, Rider LG, Reed AM, et al. Juvenile dermatomyositis and other idiopathic inflammatory myopathies of childhood. *Lancet*. 2008;371: 2201–2212.
- Huber AM. Juvenile dermatomyositis: Advances in pathogenesis, evaluation, and treatment. *Paediatr Drugs*. 2009;11:361–374.
- Khanna S, Reed AM. Immunopathogenesis of juvenile dermatomyositis. *Muscle Nerve*. 2010; 41:581–592.
- Kim S, El-Hallak M, Dedeoglu F, et al. Complete and sustained remission of juvenile dermatomyositis resulting from aggressive treatment. *Arthritis Rheum*. 2009;60:1825–1830.
- Niewold TB, Kariuki SN, Morgan GA, et al. Elevated serum interferon-alpha activity in juvenile dermatomyositis: Associations with disease activity at diagnosis and after thirty-six months of therapy. *Arthritis Rheum*. 2009;60:1815–1824.
- Ravelli A, Trail L, Ferrari C, et al. Long-term outcome and prognostic factors of juvenile dermatomyositis: A multinational, multicenter study of 490 patients. *Arthritis Care Res*. 2010;62:63–72.
- Wedderburn LR, Rider LG. Juvenile dermatomyositis: New developments in pathogenesis, assessment and treatment. *Best Pract Res Clin Rheumatol*. 2009; 23:665–678.

 CODES

ICD9
- 710.3 Dermatomyositis
- 710.4 Polymyositis

ICD10
- M33.90 Dermatopolymyositis, unsp, organ involvement unspecified
- M33.00 Juvenile dermatopolymyositis, organ involvement unspecified

FAQ
- Q: Is it mandatory to perform a muscle biopsy to confirm the diagnosis?
- A: No. MRI (T2 or STIR imaging) can suffice.
- Q: Is there an associated risk of malignancy as for adults with this disorder?
- A: Extremely rare.

DEVELOPMENTAL DISABILITIES

Rita Panoscha

 BASICS

DESCRIPTION

- Developmental delay is a descriptive term, not a specific diagnosis, comprising many disorders and encompassing a broad category of etiologies.
- The term describes any situation where a child is not meeting age-appropriate milestones as expected in 1 or more streams of development. These streams of development include gross motor, fine motor, receptive and expressive language, adaptive, and social.
- The key feature is that the rate of progress has been slow over time in the area(s) of delay.

ALERT

- Children with behavioral problems may also be masking developmental delays.
- Children with delays in 1 stream of development may also have delays in other areas of development. For example, language delay may be an indication of general cognitive delays.
- Hearing impairment may present as a delay in development.

EPIDEMIOLOGY

Found in both sexes and all racial and socioeconomic groups

Prevalence

This is a heterogeneous group of disorders with different prevalence rates.

GENERAL PREVENTION

There is no known prevention of developmental delays, although prevention of some of the underlying causes is possible.

PATHOPHYSIOLOGY

- This is highly variable depending on etiology, which can include genetic, familial, metabolic, infectious, endocrinologic, traumatic, anatomic brain malformations, environmental toxins, and degenerative disorders as causes. These disorders often result in some neurologic or neuromuscular injury causing the delay. In many cases, the etiology is never determined.
- Prevalence of this group of disorders may vary depending on how inclusive the definition is. The milder delays are quite common and can be found in any pediatric practice. Some disorders in this grouping are more prevalent in boys. The long-term outcome depends on the severity and type of delay, with the more involved children usually having lifelong disability.

ETIOLOGY

Specific etiologies are too numerous to list completely but a partial list of the more common causes includes:

- Genetic/familial:
  - Fragile X syndrome
  - Trisomy 21 (Down syndrome)
  - Other chromosomal abnormalities
  - Tuberous sclerosis
  - Neurofibromatosis
  - Phenylketonuria
  - Muscular dystrophy
- Nervous system anomalies:
  - Hydrocephalus
  - Lissencephaly
  - Spina bifida
  - Seizures
- Infections:
  - Prenatal cytomegalovirus
  - Rubella
  - Toxoplasmosis
  - HIV
  - Postnatal bacterial meningitis
  - Neonatal herpes simplex
- Endocrinologic:
  - Congenital hypothyroidism
- Environment:
  - Heavy metal poisoning such as lead
  - In utero drug or alcohol exposure
- Trauma/injury:
  - Closed head trauma
  - Asphyxia
  - Stroke
  - Perinatal cerebral hemorrhages

COMMONLY ASSOCIATED CONDITIONS

- There are numerous associated findings including seizures, sensory impairments, feeding disorders, psychiatric disorders (especially depression), and behavioral disorders.
- Having a child with significant developmental delays can also add stress to the family in terms of time, finances, and emotions.

 DIAGNOSIS

HISTORY

A complete and detailed history is needed, including:

- Pregnancy history:
  - Maternal age and parity
  - Maternal complications (including infections and exposures)
  - Medications/drugs used
  - Tobacco or alcohol used, along with quantities
  - Fetal activity

- Birth history:
  - Gestational age
  - Birth weight
  - Route of delivery
  - Maternal or fetal complications/distress
  - Apgar scores
- General health:
  - Significant illnesses, hospitalizations, or surgeries
  - Accidents or injuries
  - Hearing and vision status
  - Medications used
  - Known exposures to toxins
  - Any new or unusual symptoms
- Developmental history:
  - Current developmental achievement in each stream of development
  - Age when developmental milestones were achieved
  - Any loss of skills
  - Where parents think their child is functioning developmentally
- Educational history:
  - Type of schooling and services received, if any
  - Any previous educational/developmental testing
- Behavioral history:
  - Any perseverative or stereotypical behaviors
  - Interaction skills
  - Attention and activity level
- Family history:
  - Anyone with developmental delays, neurologic disorders, syndromes, consanguinity

PHYSICAL EXAM

- A complete physical exam including growth perimeters is needed looking for etiology.
- Key features to include:
  - Observation of interactions and behavior: Any atypical behaviors and general impression
  - Head circumference: Looking for macrocephaly or microcephaly
  - Skin exam: Looking for neurocutaneous lesions
  - Major or minor dysmorphic features: Any indication of a syndrome or anatomic malformation
  - Neurologic examination: Looking for cranial nerve deficits, neuromuscular status, reflexes, balance and coordination, and any soft signs
  - Developmental testing: Although considerable information will already be available on history and observation, a more formal developmental screening or testing should be done. Possible office tests would be the Ages & Stages Questionnaires, Denver-II Developmental Screening Test, the CAT/CLAMS, or the ELM. The latter test is basically for language screening. Referral to a specialist or a multidisciplinary team for more detailed testing is indicated when delay is suspected.

DIAGNOSTIC TESTS & INTERPRETATION
Lab
Initial lab tests
- There is no specific laboratory test battery for general developmental delays. The testing needs to be tailored to the individual situation based on the history and physical exam. A high index of suspicion should be maintained for any associated findings and delays in the other streams of development.
- Some of the more common studies ordered for developmental delay workup:
  - Genetic testing: Warranted for any dysmorphic features, a family history of delays or genetic disorder. A karyotype and fragile X DNA should be considered, particularly for significant cognitive delays. The comparative genomic hybridization (CGH) microarray is now increasingly recommended as a first-line test for developmental delays.
  - Metabolic tests: Tests such as quantitative plasma amino acids, quantitative urine organic acids, lactate, pyruvate, or ammonia should be considered if there is any loss of skills or indication of a metabolic disorder.
  - Thyroid function tests: Most infants will have had screening for hypothyroidism shortly after birth. This should be rechecked if symptoms indicate.

Imaging
Head MRI: Consider a head MRI for head abnormalities, significant neurologic findings, loss of skills, or for workup of a specific disorder such as trauma or leukodystrophy.

Diagnostic Procedures/Other
- Audiologic: Hearing should be checked in any child with speech and language and/or cognitive delays.
- EEG: An EEG should be considered if there is any concern about seizures.
- Subspecialists: Referral to other medical specialists may also be indicated. These specialists may include developmental pediatrics, neurology, genetics, orthopedics, or ophthalmology.

DIFFERENTIAL DIAGNOSIS
- The differential can be extensive and may become more evident with further workup.
- Broad diagnoses include:
  - Mental retardation
  - Developmental language disorder
  - Autism
  - Learning disability
  - Cerebral palsy
  - Attention deficit hyperactivity disorder
  - Significant visual or hearing impairment
  - Degenerative disorders

TREATMENT

ADDITIONAL TREATMENT
General Measures
- Therapy should include appropriately treating any medical conditions and associated findings, for example, anticonvulsants for seizures or hearing aids when appropriate for hearing impairment. In addition, traditional therapy has included early intervention or special education services specifically addressing the areas of delay.
- Therapy could include physical therapists, occupational therapists, speech/language therapists, special educators, psychologists, and audiologists, depending on the needs of the child.

ONGOING CARE

FOLLOW-UP RECOMMENDATIONS
Patient Monitoring
- General pediatric care for well-child visits and to monitor any underlying medical conditions is indicated.
- These children need ongoing monitoring of their therapy and educational programs to ensure that it is still meeting their individual needs, as these needs change over time.
- The families will also need ongoing counseling and support in dealing with a child having special needs.

PROGNOSIS
Variable depending on the type and severity of delay and the etiology

ADDITIONAL READING

- Battaglia A, Carey JC. Diagnostic evaluation of developmental delay/mental retardation: An overview. *Am J Med Genet C Semin Med Genet*. 2003;117C(Feb 15):3–14.
- Council on Children with Disabilities. Identifying infants and young children with developmental disorders in the medical home: An algorithm for developmental surveillance and screening. *Pediatrics*. 2006;118:405–420.
- Feldman HM. Evaluation and management of language and speech disorders in preschool children. *Pediatr Rev*. 2005;26:131–140.
- Gilbride KE. Developmental testing. *Pediatr Rev*. 1995;16:338–345.
- Gropman AL, Batshaw ML. Epigenetics, copy number variation, and other molecular mechanisms underlying neurodevelopmental disabilities: New insights and diagnostic approaches. *J Dev Behav Pediatr*. 2010;31:582–591.
- Johnson CP, Blasco PA. Infant growth and development. *Pediatr Rev*. 1997;18:224–242.
- Liptak GS. The pediatrician's role in caring for the developmentally disabled child. *Pediatr Rev*. 1996;17:203–210.
- Mendola P, Selevan SG, Gutter S, et al. Environmental factors associated with a spectrum of neurodevelopmental deficits. *Ment Retard Dev Disabil Res Rev*. 2002;8(3):188–197.
- Moeschler JB, Shevell M, Committee on Genetics. Clinical genetic evaluation of the child with mental retardation or developmental delays. *Pediatrics*. 2006;117:2304–2316.
- Shevell M. Global developmental delay and mental retardation or intellectual disability: conceptualization, evaluation and etiology. *Pediatr Clin North Am*. 2008;55:1071–1084.
- Simms MD, Shum RL. Preschool children who have atypical patterns of development. *Pediatr Rev*. 2000;21:147–158.

CODES

ICD9
- 315.8 Other specified delays in development
- 315.9 Unspecified delay in development (developmental disorder not otherwise specified)

ICD10
- F89 Unspecified disorder of psychological development
- F88 Other disorders of psychological development

FAQ

- Q: When do you test a child for delays?
- A: A child can have developmental assessments at any age, including infancy. Making a specific diagnosis, for example, for level of mental retardation, may need to wait until the child is older.
- Q: When can a child start receiving services?
- A: Children who qualify can receive therapy services starting at birth and in some cases extending up to age 21 years.
- Q: The parents are raising a concern about delays, but the general impression in the office is that the child is doing okay. What should be done next?
- A: Parents or grandparents may be the first to express concerns, especially in a child with milder delays. A more detailed developmental history and more formal developmental screening or testing would be indicated as an initial step.

DEVELOPMENTAL DYSPLASIA OF THE HIP

John M. Flynn

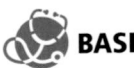 **BASICS**

DESCRIPTION
A range of congenital hip disorders: From mild acetabular dysplasia to dislocation of the femoral head from the acetabulum

ALERT
Pitfalls:
- Missed early diagnosis can result in more complicated management and less favorable outcome.
- Missing an associated syndrome or condition (e.g., tethered cord, arthrogryposis)
- Mistaking a "click" for instability

Incidence
Incidence of hip dysplasia is 0.5–2% of live births; however, true dislocation occurs in 0.1–0.2% of live births.

Genetics
Many patients are first-born females, with familial history of affected first-degree relative.

PATHOPHYSIOLOGY
Owing to mechanical forces, abnormal growth, or underlying laxity, the spatial and biomechanical relationship between the femoral head and the acetabulum is altered.

ETIOLOGY
- Mechanical factors:
  - Breech position
  - Oligohydramnios
  - Packing phenomenon (e.g., first-born child)
  - Postnatal positioning (e.g., swaddling in extension and adduction)
- Laxity or genetic factors:
  - Female
  - Family history (~20%)
  - Certain ethnic groups
  - Generalized ligamentous laxity

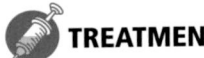 **DIAGNOSIS**

HISTORY
- Much higher incidence of developmental dysplasia of the hip in breech delivery
- 10–20% of patients have familial history.

PHYSICAL EXAM
- Infants are tested with the Ortolani and Barlow tests. These maneuvers involve feeling a "clunk" with either gentle reduction of the dislocated femoral head with abduction and anterior force (Ortolani) or gentle dislocation or an unstable femoral head with adduction with posterior force (Barlow).
- Check for torticollis, metatarsus adductus, and other "packaging" abnormalities.
- Check for an abnormal sacral dimple.
- Although a baby with a dislocated hip may have asymmetric thigh or gluteal folds, many babies with normal hips have such asymmetry.
- Children >4–6 months may have a negative Ortolani, but have limited abduction on the affected hip. The Galeazzi sign may be positive (comparing the femoral lengths by flexing the hip and knee in the supine position).
- Walking-age children may have a Trendelenburg gait (lurching to the side) and a leg length inequality.
- Physical examination tricks:
  - The infant should be as relaxed as possible, preferably sleeping. Check the hips first. When the baby is active or crying, it is difficult to get a good exam.
  - The infant should be examined on a firm surface. The pelvis is stabilized with the opposite hand.

ALERT
- Examination may be normal initially. Consequently, hip evaluation should be performed as part of infant physical examination through 12 months of age.
- Many babies have "clicks" when their hips or knees are manipulated. These high-pitched snapping sensations should not be mistaken for the instability felt on a properly performed Ortolani or Barlow test.

DIAGNOSTIC TESTS & INTERPRETATION
Imaging
- AP pelvis radiograph
  - Recommended after 6 months of age; prior to 6 months of age, radiographs may appear normal because of difficulty determining hip/acetabulum relation in cartilaginous femoral head
- Hip ultrasound:
  - Best test for infants 0–6 months old
  - Can determine hip laxity, subluxation, dislocation, reducibility, presence of interposed tissue, and status of the acetabulum. Can request ultrasound of the lumbosacral spine if there is a deep, abnormal sacral dimple raising concern about tethered cord
  - False positives: Hip "clicks" will be present in 10% of infants; only a small percentage will have hip dysplasia.

DIFFERENTIAL DIAGNOSIS
- Infection
- Spastic hip dislocation due to cerebral palsy, closed head injury, or anoxic brain injury

TREATMENT

ADDITIONAL TREATMENT
General Measures
- Triple diaper:
  - No longer considered to be effective treatment
  - Expensive for parents
- Pavlik harness:
  - Up to 95% effective if used <6 months of age
  - Harness is worn 24 h/d.
  - Exam or ultrasound should be performed 2–3 weeks after initiating the harness for a dislocated hip to prove that the hip is reduced in the harness.
  - Adjust straps every 3 weeks to accommodate growth.
  - After 6 consecutive weeks of treatment, reassess with physical examination and ultrasound. Wean if hip is then stable.
  - Complications include avascular necrosis of proximal femur, femoral nerve palsy (resolves spontaneously), skin irritation
- Closed or open reduction:
  - For patients who present >6 months of age

ONGOING CARE

FOLLOW-UP RECOMMENDATIONS
Patient Monitoring
- When to expect improvement:
  - Usually after ~6 weeks of treatment in the Pavlik harness
- Signs to watch for:
  - A plain radiograph (anteroposterior pelvis X-ray view) is performed at 6 and 12 months. Measure the acetabular index and check for subluxation or dislocation. Depending on the presence of residual dysplasia, later annual visits may be appropriate.

PROGNOSIS
If diagnosed in infancy, prognosis is generally excellent.

COMPLICATIONS
- When congenital hip dysplasia results in hip subluxation or dislocation, complaints include limp, pain, and accelerated degenerative disease of the hip.
- Avascular necrosis of the femoral head is a complication of treatment.

ADDITIONAL READING

- American Academy of Pediatrics. Clinical practice guideline: Early detection of developmental dysplasia of the hip (AC0001). *Pediatrics*. 2000; 105:896–905.
- Bauchner H. Developmental dysplasia of the hip (DDH): An evolving science. *Arch Dis Child*. 2000;83:202.

- Bialik V, Bialik GM, Blazer S, et al. Developmental dysplasia of the hip: A new approach to incidence. *Pediatrics*. 1999;103:93–99.
- Forlin E, Munhoz da Cunha LA, Figueiredo DC. Treatment of developmental dysplasia of the hip after walking age with open reduction, femoral shortening, and acetabular osteotomy. *Orthop Clin North Am*. 2006;37(2):149–160, vi.
- Goldberg MJ. Early detection of developmental hip dysplasia: Synopsis of the AAP Clinical Practice Guideline. *Pediatr Rev*. 2001;22:131–134.
- Guille JT, Pizzutillo PD, MacEwen GD. Development dysplasia of the hip from birth to six months. *J Am Acad Orthop Surg*. 2000;8:232–242.
- Hubbard AM. Imaging of pediatric hip disorders. *Radiol Clin North Am*. 2001;39:721–732.
- Murray KA, Crim JR. Radiographic imaging for treatment and follow-up of developmental dysplasia of the hip. *Semin Ultrasound CT MR*. 2001;22:306–340.
- Portinaro NM, Pelillo F, Cerutti P. The role of ultrasonography in the diagnosis of developmental dysplasia of the hip. *J Pediatr Orthop*. 2007;27(2):247–250.
- Vitale MG, Skaggs DL. Developmental dysplasia of the hip from six months to four years of age. *J Am Acad Orthop Surg*. 2001;9:401–411.

CODES

ICD9
- 754.30 Congenital dislocation of hip, unilateral
- 755.63 Other congenital deformity of hip (joint)

ICD10
- Q65.2 Congenital dislocation of hip, unspecified
- Q65.89 Other specified congenital deformities of hip

FAQ

- Q: Why is follow-up needed if the looseness disappears on examination?
- A: Follow-up examinations and radiographs periodically detect late instability or acetabular dysplasia.
- Q: How effective is the Pavlik harness if used within the first 4 months of life?
- A: In patients with reducible hip dysplasia, the current success rate of the Pavlik harness is ~95%.

DIABETES INSIPIDUS

Sogol Mostoufi-Moab
Sheela N. Magge

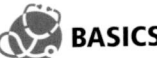 **BASICS**

DESCRIPTION
Polyuria and polydipsia caused by inability to produce or respond to antidiuretic hormone (ADH); also called arginine vasopressin

EPIDEMIOLOGY
Incidence
Because most cases are secondary to another disease, the incidence depends on the primary cause.

RISK FACTORS
Genetics
- Rare genetic causes of central diabetes insipidus (DI) are usually autosomal dominant mutations, and rarely recessive.
- Nephrogenic DI is usually familial (autosomal recessive or dominant and X-linked).

PATHOPHYSIOLOGY
- Antidiuretic hormone stimulates the formation of cyclic adenosine monophosphate (cAMP) in the renal collecting ducts, thereby increasing water permeability and increasing reabsorption of free water.
- Lack of antidiuretic hormone effect results in urinary loss of free water.
- Patients with an intact thirst mechanism drink copiously (polydipsia) to compensate for free water loss.
- If the thirst mechanism is not present or if access to free water is limited (e.g., infants or vomiting), severe dehydration can occur.

ETIOLOGY
- Insufficient antidiuretic hormone secretion:
  - Traumatic or postsurgical
  - Nonaccidental injury in children
  - Related to tumor invasion of posterior pituitary
  - Extension from anterior pituitary/suprasellar: Optic glioma, rarely adenomas
  - Hypothalamic: Germinoma, craniopharyngioma, meningioma
  - Lymphoma
  - Granulomas: Histiocytosis X, sarcoidosis
  - Metastatic carcinoma
  - Post–severe ischemic or hypoxic injury to the brain
  - Familial (autosomal dominant)
  - Congenital malformation of CNS
  - Infection
  - Viral encephalitis
  - Meningitis
  - Tuberculosis
  - Increased metabolic clearance of antidiuretic hormone (gestational diabetes insipidus)
  - Drug or toxin related: Snake venom, tetrodotoxin
  - Autoimmune disorders: Hypophysitis
  - Psychogenic: Excessive water drinking
  - Idiopathic: Must observe for many years to exclude slow-growing tumors

- Unresponsive to antidiuretic hormone:
  - Familial or nephrogenic (X-linked dominant and autosomal recessive forms)
  - Tumor related
  - Urinary tract obstruction, especially in utero
  - Renal medullary cystic disease
  - Electrolyte disturbances: Hypokalemia, hypercalcemia (hypercalciuria)
  - Drugs: Usually reversible (diuretics, diphenylhydantoin, reserpine, cisplatin, rifampin, lithium [may become permanent], demeclocycline, ethanol, chlorpromazine, volatile anesthetics, foscarnet, amphotericin B)
  - Loss of the medullary concentrating gradient due to excessive free water intake relative to solute intake

ALERT
Pitfalls:
- Management of patients without an intact thirst mechanism and of newborns is difficult.
- Patients with psychogenic polydipsia may fail a water deprivation test because prolonged excessive water intake can wash out the renal medullary gradient required for concentrating the urine.
- Surreptitious water intake during water deprivation test
- Idiopathic, acquired diabetes insipidus can be caused by slowly growing brain tumors not visible on the initial magnetic resonance image.

DIAGNOSIS

HISTORY
- Abnormal growth can be a sign of diabetes insipidus.
- Waking up during the night to drink or void:
  - True diabetes insipidus is associated with polyuria throughout the day and night. Enuresis may be the 1st sign in a child who previously acquired bladder control. Patients, including infants, prefer cold water to other liquids such as juice, soda, or milk.
- Number of hours the patient goes without drinking:
  - Patients with complete diabetes insipidus do not voluntarily stop drinking for >1–2 hours unless the thirst mechanism is also abnormal.
  - Patients with diabetes insipidus have such overwhelming thirst, they will drink anything, including bath and toilet water.
- Volume of urine output in a day (not just frequency of urination):
  - The daily volume of urine can be as high as 4–10 L. Younger or dehydrated children with diabetes insipidus tend to make less urine daily than older or hydrated children with diabetes insipidus.

- Familial history of diabetes insipidus:
  - Nephrogenic diabetes insipidus will typically affect maternal uncles during infancy, and mothers may have a mild form
- Frequent episodes of dehydration requiring medical attention:
  - Families may disregard the polydipsia as normal behavior. Repeated episodes of severe dehydration can damage the brain.
- Treatment of adrenal insufficiency in a patient with panhypopituitarism can unmask diabetes insipidus.

PHYSICAL EXAM
- Signs of dehydration:
  - Diabetes insipidus is typically associated with dry, pale skin and mucous membranes. Because this is hyperosmolar dehydration, the patient may not look as severely dehydrated as she or he is.
- Complete neurologic exam:
  - Check for impaired visual fields, which can be the 1st sign of brain tumor.

DIAGNOSTIC TESTS & INTERPRETATION
Lab
- Morning urinary osmolality with simultaneous serum sodium and serum osmolality:
  - If urine osmolality is at least 2 times higher than serum osmolality, patient does not have complete diabetes insipidus, but may still have partial diabetes insipidus.
- Water deprivation test:
  - Though definitive, it requires admission to the hospital for controlled testing under the close supervision of a pediatric endocrinologist. Patient fails test if urinary osmolality cannot concentrate more than twice serum osmolality at the same time that serum osmolality exceeds 305 mOsm/kg; serum osmolality exceeds 305 mOsm/kg at any time; patient loses >5% of body weight and becomes symptomatic from hypovolemia.
  - Once patient fails the water deprivation test, a dose of aqueous vasopressin should be given followed by close monitoring of urinary osmolality to document responsiveness to antidiuretic hormone.
  - Never attempt a water deprivation trial at home. Tell parents to allow free access to water at home in any suspected cases.
- Urinary specific gravity (nonspecific):
  - Insufficient by itself and nondiagnostic during a water deprivation test
- 24-hour urine collection (home testing):
  - To obtain accurate urinary volume while patient has free access to water

Imaging

MRI of the brain with and without contrast, with special cuts of the pituitary and hypothalamus - to confirm the bright spot normally seen in the posterior pituitary and to search for tumors. Its absence is not pathognomonic of diabetes insipidus.

ALERT

Do not restrict water intake unless the patient is in the hospital under close surveillance!

DIFFERENTIAL DIAGNOSIS

- Psychogenic polydipsia
- Abnormal thirst mechanism (dipsogenic diabetes insipidus)
- Hypernatremic dehydration
- Diabetes mellitus
- Polyuric renal failure (e.g., renal tubulopathy)
- Hypercalcemia
- Adrenal insufficiency
- Cerebral salt wasting

TREATMENT

MEDICATION (DRUGS)

- DDAVP: Intranasal spray or oral tablets
- Aqueous vasopressin: SC:
  - Comes as 4 mcg/mL solution and doses range from 0.05 mcg up to 1 mcg SC b.i.d. daily. Titrate dose as you would with DDAVP.
- Duration of action of DDAVP is variable from patient to patient. Titration and frequency of dosing should be made by the family under the supervision of an endocrinologist.
- Control of diabetes insipidus in infants is more difficult because these patients may increase fluid intake because of hunger or increase caloric intake because of thirst, thereby causing an imbalance between free water intake and output. Infants can be treated with diluted formula—the volume and frequency of feedings will be increased, but intake of free water will better match urine output. DDAVP should not be used in infants. In some cases, low renal solute load formula (e.g., Similac PM 60/40) and/or thiazide diuretics have been used in infancy. Strict record keeping of intake/output and accurate daily weighing are usually necessary for infants or patients without an intact thirst mechanism. All infants with diabetes insipidus must be treated by providers experienced with diabetes insipidus of infancy.
- Nephrogenic diabetes insipidus may be treated with diuretics and solute restriction as these patients are resistant to DDAVP.

- Side effects:
  - Facial flushing
  - Increased BP
  - Headache
  - Nasal congestion
  - Hyponatremia: Caused by water overdose (intoxication), not by overdose of drug. Taking a higher dose of DDAVP will generally extend the period of antidiuresis, but will not cause hyponatremia. Drinking too much water in the setting of antidiuresis causes hyponatremia. Water intoxication most often occurs in antidiuresed patients who also are on intravenous fluids, lack an intact thirst mechanism, or have psychogenic polydipsia.
- Duration:
  - Lifelong generally. Some tumors regress with radiation, allowing recovery of antidiuretic hormone secretion.
- Possible conflicts with other treatments:
  - Nasal congestion or GI illness can affect the absorption of DDAVP administered.

ONGOING CARE

FOLLOW-UP RECOMMENDATIONS
Patient Monitoring

- Depends on the patient and underlying disease causing diabetes insipidus
- When to expect improvement:
  - Effects of DDAVP are immediate.
  - Most cases of diabetes insipidus are lifelong. 1 exception is diabetes insipidus that occurs during the 7–10 days immediately after neurosurgery, since this postsurgical diabetes insipidus may resolve spontaneously within 1–2 weeks after surgery (part of triple-phase response).
- Signs to watch for:
  - Lethargy
  - Somnolence
  - Irritability
  - Hyperpyrexia
  - Any sign of dehydration
  - Seizures

DIET
- Patients with an intact thirst mechanism should drink only when thirsty.
- Patients without an intact thirst mechanism should drink only a carefully calculated fluid volume.

PROGNOSIS
- Generally good, but depends on the primary cause
- May cause developmental delay if the hypernatremia is prolonged

COMPLICATIONS
- Without treatment and without access to water:
  - Hypernatremia
  - Dehydration
  - Coma
- When overdosed with water:
  - Hyponatremia
  - Seizures
  - Cerebral edema

ADDITIONAL READING

- Ghirardello S, Garre ML, Rossi A, et al. The diagnosis of children with central diabetes insipidus. *J Pediatr Endocrinol Metab*. 2007 Mar;20(3):359–375.
- Linshaw MA. Back to basics: Congenital nephrogenic diabetes insipidus. *Pediatr Rev*. 2007; 28(10):372–380.
- Majzoub JA, Srivatsa A. Diabetes insipidus: Clinical and basic aspects. *Pediatrc Endocrinol Rev*. 2006; 4(Suppl 1):60–65.
- Ranadive SA, Rosenthal SM. Pediatric disorders of water balance. *Endocrinol Metab Clin North Am*. 2009;38(4):663–672.
- Rivkees SA, Dunbar N, Wilson TA. The management of central diabetes insipidus in infancy: Desmopressin, low renal solute load formula, thiazide diuretics. *J Pediatr Endocrinol Metab*. 2007; 20(4):459–469.

CODES

ICD9
- 253.5 Diabetes insipidus
- 588.1 Nephrogenic diabetes insipidus

ICD10
- E23.2 Diabetes insipidus
- N25.1 Nephrogenic diabetes insipidus

FAQ

- Q: In a patient with an intact thirst mechanism and partial diabetes insipidus, is the use of DDAVP necessary?
- A: No, as long as the patient has constant access to free water.
- Q: How does therapy of diabetes insipidus affect daily life? Is it easily integrated into normal activity and eating patterns?
- A: DDAVP is used in a patient with an intact thirst mechanism to facilitate the daily routine as well as to allow patients to sleep without the need to void frequently during the night.
- Q: Is there a longer-acting preparation or an implantable pump for dosing?
- A: The longest-acting form of antidiuretic hormone is an injected medication and can have effects for 3 days, increasing the risks of hyponatremia. Home use of the nasal spray or tablets, therefore, is easier and safer than the use of injections.

DIABETES MELLITUS

David R. Langdon

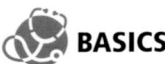 **BASICS**

DESCRIPTION

Diabetes mellitus (DM) is a disorder of absolute or relative insulin deficiency that results in hyperglycemia and disrupts energy storage and metabolism. Severe insulin deficiency can lead to ketosis, acidosis, dehydration, shock, and death.

EPIDEMIOLOGY

- Most common endocrine disorder of childhood
- Type 1 DM: More common in whites of Northern European descent
- Type 2 DM: More common in obese African Americans, Latinos, and Native Americans with strong family history

Incidence

- Type 1 DM:
  - Annual US incidence is ~19/100,000 in children 10–19 years old.
  - Incidence of type 1 DM is rising by 3% per year, but faster in young children.
- Type 2 DM:
  - Incidence is increasing rapidly in adolescents.
  - May be 8–45% of new cases of diabetes in youth, depending on location

Prevalence

- Type 1 DM: Prevalence of type 1 diabetes in youth 0–19 years in US is ~2/1,000.
- Type 2 DM:
  - Estimated prevalence of type 2 DM in youth of 4.1/1,000
  - Estimated prevalence of impaired glucose tolerance (IGT) in youth at least 2/1,000
  - At least 2% of diabetes in children may be due to monogenic diabetes of youth (MODY) or other genetic forms

RISK FACTORS

Genetics

- Susceptibility to type 1 diabetes associated with HLA region of chromosome 6, 5-fold greater risk with MHC antigen types DR3 and DR4
- Multiple genetic defects associated with type 2 diabetes have been identified.
- MODY is a group of autosomal dominant syndromes of partial insulin deficiency due to monogenic defects of pancreatic development or insulin secretion; they make up a small fraction of childhood diabetes.

PATHOPHYSIOLOGY

- Type 1 DM:
  - Loss of pancreatic β cells results in insulin deficiency, leading to hyperglycemia, and predominance of catabolic processes.
  - Hyperglycemia causes hyperosmolality, polyuria, and damage to small blood vessels.
  - Catabolic processes produce ketosis, weight loss, and metabolic acidosis.
- Type 2 DM: Insulin resistance and relative deficiency lead to hyperglycemia, β-cell exhaustion, and changes similar to those in type 1, but initially with greater potential for temporary reversibility.

ETIOLOGY

- Type 1 DM:
  - In genetically susceptible child, an environmental trigger (likely viral) induces expression of DR antigens on β-cell surface.
  - Recruitment of cytotoxic lymphocytes
  - Production of anti-insulin and anti-islet cell antibodies (GAD65, ICA512)
  - Progressive inflammatory, autoimmune loss of β-cell mass results in insulin deficiency.
- Type 2 DM:
  - Insulin sensitivity diminishes owing to obesity and other factors.
  - Insulin resistance leads to compensatory hyperinsulinemia to maintain euglycemia.
- In genetically susceptible persons, insulin secretion fails to match demand, resulting in relative deficiency and hyperglycemia.

COMMONLY ASSOCIATED CONDITIONS

- Type 1 DM: Autoimmune thyroid disease
- Type 2 DM:
  - Obesity
  - Depression
  - Hypertension
  - Fatty liver
  - Hyperlipidemia
  - Sleep apnea
  - Polycystic ovary syndrome

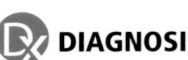 **DIAGNOSIS**

HISTORY

- Polyuria, nocturia, and enuresis are related to hyperglycemia >180 mg/dL.
- Polydipsia: Due to polyuria, hyperosmolality
- Duration of symptoms varies by age: May be days in toddlers, months in adolescents
- Polyphagia: Appetite amplified by loss of calories from glycosuria; this is often absent.
- Weight loss: Dehydration, loss of calories
- Malaise, nausea, vomiting, abdominal pain, hyperventilation, lethargy due to ketosis, acidosis, electrolyte depletion, hyperosmolality
- Type 2 diabetes may present like type 1 or may be entirely asymptomatic.
- MODY is usually asymptomatic.

PHYSICAL EXAM

- Weight loss may occur in type 1 diabetes.
- Candidal vaginitis and balanitis common in young children with type 1 diabetes
- In ketoacidosis: Dehydration, hyperventilation
- Obesity and acanthosis nigricans (hypertrophic skin pigmentation of neck) in type 2

DIAGNOSTIC TESTS & INTERPRETATION
Lab

- Diagnosis based on blood glucose (BG) level: Fasting BG $\geq$126, random BG $\geq$200 mg/dL, or 2-hour BG $\geq$200 on oral glucose tolerance test (OGTT), and exclusion of stress hyperglycemia
- Glycosuria may be intermittent.
- Ketonuria may occur with both types 1 and 2.
- Hemoglobin A1c reflects BG levels of previous 2–3 months and is nearly always elevated at diagnosis of both types.
- GAD, islet cell, and/or insulin autoantibodies nearly always positive in type 1 diabetes, but sometimes in type 2 as well
- In some patients presenting with hyperglycemia and ketosis, it is not possible to distinguish type 1 or type 2 until the course over several months has been followed.
- Some, but not all, adolescents with IGT or impaired fasting glucose (IFG) will progress to type 2 diabetes.
  - IGT is 2-hour glucose between 140 and 200 during OGTT.
  - IFG is fasting glucose between 100 and 125.

DIFFERENTIAL DIAGNOSIS

- UTI (polyuria)
- Renal glycosuria
- Stress-related hyperglycemia
- Drug-induced hyperglycemia (steroids)
- Psychogenic polydipsia
- Pneumonia (in diabetic ketoacidosis [DKA])
- Sepsis (in DKA)
- Acute surgical abdomen (in ketoacidosis)

 TREATMENT

MEDICATION (DRUGS)

(See insulin regimens under "General Measures.")
  In type 2 diabetes, insulin is usually used for symptomatic hyperglycemia. Oral antidiabetic agents may be effective for milder hyperglycemia:

- Metformin is the only oral agent approved for children; it reduces hepatic glucose output.
- Other agents may be useful in certain circumstances: Sulfonylureas, glinides, thiazolidinediones, α-glucosidase inhibitors, exendin, dipeptidyl protease inhibitors.

ADDITIONAL TREATMENT
General Measures

Insulin is given as a fixed or flexible regimen:

- Total daily dose (TDD) usually ~0.7–1.2 U/kg/d; choose higher range for ketoacidosis presentation, obesity, and puberty.
- Dose may decline during "honeymoon period."
- Fixed insulin regimens require fewer shots, but consistent schedule and eating.

- Common fixed regimen is split-mixed: 2/3 of TDD in morning (1/3 as short acting and 2/3 long acting), and 1/3 of TDD in evening (with 1/2 as short acting and 1/2 as long acting), either at dinner or split between dinner and bedtime.
- Flexible insulin regimens consist of basal insulin plus a short-acting bolus for every carbohydrate meal and for high blood sugar.
- Basal dosing: 40–50% of TDD is given as 1 injection of a long-acting insulin such as glargine (Lantus) or detemir (Levemir).
- Boluses of short-acting insulin (lispro or aspart) are given for meals and snacks based on carbohydrate content and BG. Carbohydrate coverage (grams of carbohydrate covered by 1 unit) can be estimated by dividing the TDD into 500. Hyperglycemia coverage can be estimated by dividing the TDD into 1,800 to find how much 1 unit may lower blood sugar.
- SC insulin infusion by pump is another flexible method: Dosing is similar.

SURGERY/OTHER PROCEDURES
Weight loss from bariatric surgery may reverse type 2 diabetes.

 ONGOING CARE

FOLLOW-UP RECOMMENDATIONS
Patient Monitoring
- Regular appointments with diabetes specialist every 3 months to assess management:
  – Is diabetes interfering with emotional health, family relationships, school attendance, athletic activities, or social development?
  – Is family minimizing hospitalization risks from hypoglycemia or DKA with appropriate adjustment of insulin, recognition of lows, glucagon availability, ketone testing, and telephone contact?
  – Is family reducing long-term complication risk by keeping HbA1c lower and by avoiding or treating other risk factors?
  – Exam: Growth, weight, pubertal status, blood pressure, thyromegaly, liver size, injection sites, feet, skin lesions
- Meet with nutritionist periodically or as needed to reassess meal plan.
- Meet with psychologist or social worker as needed to address psychosocial issues.
- Annual screening for long-term complications:
  – Urine for microalbumin
  – Lipid profile, T_4, TSH, celiac screen
  – Eye exam to detect early retinopathy

DIET
- Dietary education for type 1 diabetes is directed toward healthy distribution and matching of carbohydrate intake with insulin action:
  – Recommended distribution of calories: 55% from carbohydrates (mostly complex); 30% from fats; 15% from protein
  – Fixed insulin regimens require snacks spaced between meals and before bedtime.
  – Carbohydrate counting is essential for flexible insulin regimens and helpful for maintaining consistency for fixed regimens.

- In type 2 diabetes, dietary education is directed toward promoting weight loss.
- Reduction of saturated and trans fats, rapidly digested carbohydrates, and salt may be beneficial in both types of diabetes.

PATIENT EDUCATION
- Home BG monitoring before meals, when feeling hypoglycemic or ill
- Insulin injection and site rotation
- Oral carbohydrate for mild hypoglycemia; glucagon 1 mg IM for severe hypoglycemia
- Activity:
  – Frequent exercise reduces BG and insulin requirements in both types of diabetes.
  – Exercise may require extra eating or reduced insulin to prevent hypoglycemia in type 1 diabetes.
  – Detecting or preventing hypoglycemia during or after physical exercise
- Diet: Carbohydrate counting
- Prevention: Checking urine for ketones when blood sugar is high or child feels ill; extra insulin for ketones

COMPLICATIONS
- DKA: Most common cause of hospitalization and death in type 1 diabetes in childhood. See "Diabetic Ketoacidosis."
- Hypoglycemia: This most common acute complication limits achievable glycemic control. If severe, may cause seizure, unconsciousness
- Long-term harm may be reduced by better glycemic control:
  – Nephropathy: Microalbuminuria and hypertension are 1st manifestations before adulthood.
  – Retinopathy: Blood vessel changes may occur in childhood, but not vision loss.
  – Neuropathy: Diminished nerve conduction velocity common; paresthesias are earliest symptoms.
  – Vasculopathy: Large-vessel disease begins in childhood, but clinical effects occur in adults.
  – Prenatal harm to infants of diabetic mothers: Birth defects occur early, large size late.
  – Growth failure (Mauriac syndrome) and delayed sexual maturation
- Depression, family stress, higher divorce rate

ADDITIONAL READING
- American Diabetes Association. Clinical practice recommendations: 2011. *Diabetes Care*. 2011;34:S1.
- American Diabetes Association. Type 2 diabetes in children and adolescents. *Pediatrics*. 2000;105: 671–680.
- Juvenile Diabetes Research Foundation Continuous Glucose Monitoring Study Group, Tamborlane WV, Beck RW, Bode BW, et al. Continuous glucose monitoring and intensive treatment of type 1 diabetes. *N Engl J Med*. 2008;359(14):1464–1476.

- Karam JG, McFarlane SI. Prevention of type 2 DM: Implications for adolescents and young adults. *Pediatr Endocrinol Rev*. 2008;5(Suppl 4): 980–988.
- Nguyen TM, Mason KJ, Sanders CG, et al. Targeting blood glucose management in school improves glycemic control in children with poorly controlled type 1 diabetes mellitus. *J Pediatr*. 2008;153(4):575.
- Pinhas-Hamiel O, Zeitler P. Acute and chronic complications of type 2 diabetes mellitus in children and adolescents. *Lancet*. 2007;369:1823–1831.
- Sperling M, ed. *Diabetes mellitus in children: Pediatric clinics of North America*. Philadelphia: WB Saunders; 2005:1533–1872.
- Steinke JM, Mauer M. Lessons learned from studies of the natural history of diabetic nephropathy in young type 1 diabetic patients. International Diabetic Nephropathy Study Group. *Pediatr Endocrinol Rev*. 2008;5(Suppl 4):958–963.
- Weiss R, Dufour S, Taksali SE, et al. Prediabetes in obese youth: A syndrome of impaired glucose tolerance, severe insulin resistance, and altered myocellular and abdominal fat partitioning. *Lancet*. 2003;362:951–957.

 CODES

ICD9
- 250.00 Diabetes mellitus without mention of complication, type II or unspecified type, not stated as uncontrolled
- 250.01 Diabetes mellitus without mention of complication, type I [juvenile type], not stated as uncontrolled
- 250.02 Diabetes mellitus without mention of complication, type II or unspecified type, uncontrolled

ICD10
- E10.8 Type 1 diabetes mellitus with unspecified complications
- E10.9 Type 1 diabetes mellitus without complications
- E11.8 Type 2 diabetes mellitus with unspecified complications

FAQ
- Q: What is the newest management tool?
- A: Continuous glucose sensors allow patients to avoid symptomatic high and low glucoses by detecting trends, to see the outcome of management decisions, and to reduce the risk of severe nocturnal hypoglycemia.
- Q: What is the risk of diabetes in a sibling or child of a person with type 1 DM?
- A: It is 5–10% in 1st-degree relatives (siblings, offspring) and 40–50% in identical twins.

D

DIABETIC KETOACIDOSIS

David R. Langdon

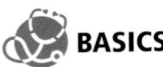 **BASICS**

DESCRIPTION
- Severe metabolic derangement that occurs in patients with diabetes mellitus, either type 1 or untreated type 2, secondary to insulin deficiency and stress hormone excess
- Principal features are hyperglycemia, ketosis, metabolic acidosis, dehydration, and electrolyte deficits.

EPIDEMIOLOGY
Incidence
- Up to 67% of diabetic ketoacidosis (DKA) occurs at diabetes onset; higher percentage in children <4 years and in families with lower socioeconomic status (SES)
- Annual hospitalization rates for DKA are around 10/100,000 children per year.
- Risk of DKA in established type 1 diabetes is 1–10% per patient per year.
- DKA accounts for 65% of all hospital admissions in diabetic children <19 years old.
- DKA accounts for >50% of childhood deaths from diabetes.

RISK FACTORS
- Poor metabolic control
- Previous episodes of DKA
- Adolescent girls
- Lower SES

GENERAL PREVENTION
- Timely recognition of new diabetes in children, especially toddlers, with polyuria and polydipsia
- Anticipatory illness management education to check ketones when feeling ill or glucose is high, to take extra insulin, and to call if ketones persist
- Parental supervision of insulin injections and early ketone testing can prevent most recurrent DKA. Psychosocial assessment and family counseling may be useful but are no substitute for parental participation in the diabetes care.
- Recognition of insulin omission to control weight, and appropriate education or counseling
- Understanding by patient and family that interruption of insulin pump for more than 8 hours may result in DKA.

PATHOPHYSIOLOGY
- DKA results from a combination of insulin deficiency and metabolic stress effects.
- Insulin deficiency may be absolute (new diabetes or omitted insulin) or relative (insufficient dose to offset illness stress).
- Metabolic stress involves counterregulatory hormones glucagon, cortisol, and epinephrine, triggered by acute illness or insulin deficiency.

- Counterregulatory hormones amplify glucose production, impair peripheral uptake, and increase proteolysis and lipolysis.
- Lipolysis and ketosis produce metabolic acidosis. Hyperglycemia produces hyperosmolality, leading to osmotic diuresis, dehydration, and urinary electrolyte loss.
- Approximate deficits per kilogram of body weight:
  – Water: 100 mL/kg
  – Na: 6–10 mEq/kg, K: 3–5 mEq/kg
  – Cl: 3–5 mEq/kg, PO$_4$: 5–7 mmol/kg

ETIOLOGY
- Insulin deficiency due to unrecognized development of either type 1 or type 2 diabetes
- Inappropriate withholding or reduction of insulin during acute illness
- Overwhelming acute illness
- Insulin omission due to parental disengagement, eating disorder, psychosocial stress, substance abuse, or interruption of insulin pump

COMMONLY ASSOCIATED CONDITIONS
Candidal vaginitis or balanitis

 DIAGNOSIS

HISTORY
- Polyuria, polydipsia from hyperosmolality
- Nausea, vomiting, and abdominal pain are related to acidosis and electrolyte disturbance.
- Precipitating event (e.g., intercurrent illness) should be identified if possible.

PHYSICAL EXAM
- Dehydration effects: Tachycardia, dry mucous membranes, sunken eyes, poor skin turgor, poor distal perfusion, hypotension
- Acetone odor to breath from ketosis
- Deep Kussmaul hyperventilation is respiratory compensation for metabolic acidosis.
- Abdominal tenderness due to ketosis, acidosis
- Altered mental status, obtundation due to hyperosmolality, dehydration
- Body temperature is typically low.

DIAGNOSTIC TESTS & INTERPRETATION
Lab
- Glucose: >200 mg/dL (typically 400–1,200)
- Urinalysis: Marked glycosuria and ketonuria
- Sodium: Initial Na may be low, normal, or high:
  – Serum Na reflects duration and severity of hyperglycemia, duration and degree of dehydration, and degree of hyperlipidemia.
  – Prolonged hyperglycemia depresses Na by about 1.6 mEq/L for every 100 mg/dL of elevation, but Na may rise as dehydration becomes extreme (BUN >30 mg/dL).
  – Disproportionately low initial Na may indicate severe hyperlipidemia or adrenal crisis.
  – Whole-body Na is depleted.

- Potassium: Initial serum levels are usually elevated but may be normal or low. Regardless of initial K, body K is depleted.
- Total CO$_2$ or bicarbonate reflects degree of metabolic acidosis and is a useful index of severity:
  – HCO$_3$ <4 mmol/L is severe, reflects pH <7
  – HCO$_3$ 4–14 mmol/L is moderate, will require >8 hours of treatment to reverse
  – HCO$_3$ 15–20 mmol/L is mild, may respond to a few hours of fluids and insulin
- Phosphate: Initially normal, high, or low:
  – Despite initial level, whole-body P is depleted.
- Arterial blood gas reflects metabolic acidosis, with low pH (<7.3) and low pCO$_2$ (10–20 mmol/L).
- CBC: Stress may increase white cell count to 35,000/mm^3 even without infection.
- β-Hydroxybutyrate and serum ketones are elevated (BOHB typically >5 mmol/L).
- Hypertriglyceridemia may be high enough to depress electrolyte levels in unseparated plasma.
- Liver enzymes (ALT, AST) may be mildly elevated.
- Amylase and lipase are often mildly elevated.
- Plasma osmolality is high, and can be estimated by 2(Na + K) + (BUN/2.6) + (glucose/18).

DIFFERENTIAL DIAGNOSIS
- Gastroenteritis
- Acute abdomen (pancreatitis, appendicitis)
- UTI
- Pneumonia
- Stress hyperglycemia
- Salicylate ingestion
- Inborn error of metabolism
- Nonketotic hyperosmolar coma
- Adrenal crisis

 TREATMENT

ADDITIONAL TREATMENT
General Measures
Use of a DKA protocol improves outcomes.

ISSUES FOR REFERRAL
Refer to a pediatric endocrine service for initial diabetes education or for recurrent DKA.

IN-PATIENT CONSIDERATIONS
Initial Stabilization
- Assess and ensure airway and breathing.
- Restore circulation: Normal saline bolus of 10–20 mL/kg; repeat as needed to maintain perfusion:
  – Urine output and specific gravity do not reflect hydration because of osmotic diuresis.
  – Avoid giving more fluids than necessary to reverse or prevent shock. Rapid osmolar correction may incur cerebral edema risk.
  – Determine adequacy of hospital support or arrange transfer. Management of moderate or severe DKA requires frequent nursing attention and rapid availability of physician.

IV Fluids
- Amount and rate of IV fluids:
  - Assume 10% dehydration, 15% in infants.
  - Replace evenly over 24–48 hours.
  - Add maintenance rate to rehydration rate for total IV rate but do not add additional fluid to replace ongoing urine output.
  - Increase rate for inadequate renal or body perfusion. Decrease rate for suspected cerebral edema or pulmonary edema.
- Composition of IV fluids: Tonicity and Na:
  - Start with normal saline. Change to 1/2 normal when circulation is secure and Na is >130.
  - IV fluids should contain K after the 1st hour, or when anuric renal failure or extreme hyperkalemia is ruled out.
- Composition of IV fluids: Potassium:
  - Should contain K at 40 mEq/L, often 1/2 KCl and 1/2 K phosphate (never all phosphate)
  - Problems from inadequate or excessive K are rare if K replacement is begun early by gradual infusion without boluses, riders, or high central line concentrations.
- Composition of IV fluids: Glucose:
  - Add 5% dextrose to IV stock when blood glucose <300 mg/dL.
  - Change to 10% dextrose when glucose <200 mg/dL so that full insulin rate can continue.

ONGOING CARE

FOLLOW-UP RECOMMENDATIONS
Patient Monitoring
For severe DKA, the following monitoring measures are usually warranted:
- Nearly continuous observation to detect changes of mental status or respiration or perfusion
- Cardiorespiratory monitor with hourly blood pressure
- Hourly intake and output
- Hourly glucose checks
- Electrolytes every few hours

PROGNOSIS
Mortality of DKA in children is ~0.2–0.3%.

COMPLICATIONS
- Death in childhood DKA results from cerebral edema (57–87%) or cardiovascular collapse.
- Cerebral edema refers to several forms of acute neurologic catastrophe, especially brainstem herniation and stroke:
  - Highest-risk patients are youngest, and those with most severe dehydration and acidosis.
  - Cause of brain swelling still unsettled: Hypotheses include water influx as osmolality falls or excessive blood flow.
  - Commonly occurs 6–18 hours into treatment, often as patient is improving
  - Heralded as headache, change in mental status, focal neurologic signs, rising blood pressure, or unexpected drop of serum Na
  - From neurologic changes, brain herniation and respiratory arrest may occur rapidly.
  - Treatment of suspected cerebral edema includes slowing of IV fluids, mannitol 0.5–1.0 g/kg by IV infusion over 15 minutes.
  - Obtain CT scan to confirm brain swelling only if patient can be treated during procedure.
  - Prepare to intubate and ventilate if arrest occurs.

- Cardiovascular collapse and death from shock usually due to delay or interruption of IV fluids, or to inadequate fluid rates:
  - Leads to hypovolemic shock and shock damage to kidneys, other organs
  - Give isotonic IV fluid to restore perfusion.
- Some complications are largely avoidable:
  - Hypo- and hyperkalemia can cause arrhythmias. Hypokalemia often from delayed K replacement. Hyperkalemia can occur if K boluses given as "catch-up," or renal failure or rhabdomyolysis.
  - Hypoglycemia can be avoided with frequent glucose checks.
  - Hypocalcemic tetany usually results from excessive phosphate replacement.
  - Hypernatremia reflects prolonged normal saline or bicarbonate, or inadequate water.
- Other complications, not directly attributable to treatment, can occur in severe cases:
  - Pulmonary edema or acute respiratory distress syndrome (ARDS)
  - Pneumomediastinum from hyperventilation
  - Rhabdomyolysis
  - Thrombosis, especially at central line site
  - Disseminated intravascular coagulation (DIC)
  - Rhinocerebral mucormycosis
  - Gastric atony and dilatation
  - Pancreatitis

ADDITIONAL READING

- Dunger DB, Sperling MA, Acerini CL, et al. European Society for Paediatric Endocrinology/Lawson Wilkins Pediatric Endocrine Society consensus statement on diabetic ketoacidosis in children and adolescents. *Pediatrics.* 2004;113:e133–e140.
- Glaser N. Pediatric diabetic ketoacidosis and hyperosmolar state. *Pediatr Clin North Am.* 2005;52:1611–1635.
- Glaser N, Barnett P, McCaslin I, et al. Risk factors for cerebral edema in children with diabetic ketoacidosis. *N Engl J Med.* 2001;344:264–269.
- Green SM, Rothrock SG, Ho JD, et al. Failure of adjuvant bicarbonate to improve outcome in severe pediatric diabetic ketoacidosis. *Ann Emerg Med.* 1998;31:41–48.
- Orlowski JP, Cramer CL, Fiallos MR. Diabetic ketoacidosis in the pediatric ICU. *Pediatr Clin North Am.* 2008;55(3):577–587, x.

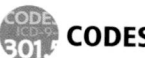

CODES

ICD9
- 250.10 Diabetes with ketoacidosis, type II or unspecified type, not stated as uncontrolled
- 250.11 Diabetes with ketoacidosis, type I [juvenile type], not stated as uncontrolled

ICD10
- E10.10 Type 1 diabetes mellitus with ketoacidosis without coma
- E13.10 Other specified diabetes mellitus with ketoacidosis without coma
- E13.11 Other specified diabetes mellitus with ketoacidosis with coma

FAQ
- Q: What are the usual triggers for DKA?
- A: Mismanagement of minor illness, or omissions of insulin due to lack of parental education or participation.
- Q: What are the most common management errors that contribute to a poor outcome?
- A: Failure to recognize early DKA, prolonged telephone management, delayed fluid start, excessive fluid in emergency department, delayed K replacement, bolus bicarbonate use, inadequate fluids for fear of cerebral edema, failure to monitor closely, failure to respond quickly to mental status changes.
- Q: Does an episode of DKA mean that the usual daily insulin regimen is inadequate?
- A: No. The usual regimen is best assessed by hemoglobin A1c and hypoglycemia frequency. DKA indicates missed insulin or a failure to respond to an unusual situation.

DIAPER RASH

Kara N. Shah

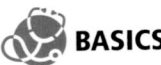 **BASICS**

DESCRIPTION

Also known as diaper or napkin rash, diaper dermatitis is a general term that encompasses a spectrum of skin disorders of varying etiologies that share a common distribution. Diaper dermatitis is not necessarily associated with wearing diapers.

ALERT
- Often the caretaker believes the rash is a result of inadequate cleansing of the skin and subsequently attempts to wash the skin more. This causes additional irritation and exacerbates the underlying dermatitis.
- Severe cases of diaper dermatitis may be complicated by bacterial or fungal infection and may require treatment with topical or systemic antibiotics.

EPIDEMIOLOGY
Prevalence
- Diaper dermatitis is significantly more common in infants and children who are still in diapers and generally resolves when diapers are no longer worn.
- It affects 7–35% of the infant population at any given time and is most commonly found in the 9–12-month age group.

RISK FACTORS
- Concomitant skin disease, such as seborrheic dermatitis and atopic dermatitis
- Acute or chronic conditions associated with increased stooling, diarrhea, or urinary incontinence, such as infectious gastroenteritis and enuresis

GENERAL PREVENTION
- Proper skin care with gentle cleansing with a mild, nonsoap cleanser such as Cetaphil should be encouraged.
- The use of superabsorbent diapers may be suggested along with frequent diaper changes. It is unclear whether there is any difference in the prevalence of diaper dermatitis when disposable versus cloth diapers are used.
- Use of infant wipes may aid in the removal of urine and feces from the skin and they are generally less irritating than use of water and washcloths, although irritant and allergic contact dermatitis has been reported with several of the chemicals used in these products.
- The regular use of barrier creams containing zinc oxide helps to protect the skin from external irritants, including urine and feces.

PATHOPHYSIOLOGY
Diaper rashes are the result of several different processes, alone and in combination:
- Friction and maceration: Rubbing of wet diapers against exposed skin in areas such as the inner surface of the thighs, genitals, buttocks, and abdomen may result in chafing and irritation.
- Irritation: Prolonged exposure to irritants such as feces, urine, and skin cleansers can cause skin breakdown that predominantly affects exposed areas under the diaper, sparing intertriginous areas. Occlusion potentiates the effects of irritants.
- Inflammation: Both infectious and noninfectious processes can trigger an acute or chronic inflammatory response in the diaper area.

ETIOLOGY
- Infection:
  - *Candida albicans*: Infection is common during or immediately after use of systemic antibiotics and with any moderate to severe diaper dermatitis. It is often seen in combination with oral candidal infections (thrush).
  - Group A β-hemolytic *Streptococcus*: The most common bacteria associated with diaper dermatitis
  - *Staphylococcus aureus*: Increasingly recognized as a potential cause of infection in the diaper area
- Inflammation:
  - Seborrheic dermatitis: In infants, usually involves the scalp (cradle cap) and face as well as the diaper area and other intertriginous areas. It is presumably related to an inflammatory response to skin colonization with the common skin yeast *Malassezia*.
  - Allergic contact dermatitis: May be caused by exposure to detergents, fragrances, or dyes in diapers, wipes, or topical medications used in the diaper area
  - Granuloma gluteale infantum: Believed to be caused by chronic application of topical steroids to the diaper area, this self-limiting inflammatory dermatitis is rarely seen today.
- Irritant:
  - Jacquet erosive dermatitis: A severe erosive form of diaper dermatitis that results from chronic and severe inflammation and can be confused with herpes simplex infection

DIAGNOSIS

HISTORY
- A history of acute or chronic diarrhea should suggest a primary irritant dermatitis.
- Antecedent use of oral antibiotics can change the normal bowel and skin flora and may cause diarrhea, which can irritate the skin and predispose to infection with *C. albicans*.
- Prolonged use of topical corticosteroids may modify the appearance of the rash, mask superficial infections, or cause skin atrophy. It can also contribute to the development of granuloma gluteale infantum.

- Chemicals, dyes, and fragrances in lotions, wipes, diapers, and detergents can cause irritant or allergic contact dermatitis.
- Frequent bathing can lead to worsening of a pre-existent dermatitis. Parents often think a diaper rash represents poor hygiene and as a result increase the cleansing of the affected area, further contributing to irritation.
- Signs and symptoms:
  - Irritant diaper dermatitis and that caused by group A β-hemolytic *Streptococcus* or *S. aureus* can be painful.
  - Rarely, seborrheic dermatitis and psoriatic dermatitis can be mildly pruritic but are generally asymptomatic.

PHYSICAL EXAM
- The location of the rash should be carefully noted:
  - Exposed surfaces: Allergic or irritant contact dermatitis, *S. aureus* infection
  - Intertriginous areas: Seborrheic dermatitis, candidal infection, group A β-hemolytic *Streptococcus* infection
  - Perianal: Group A β-hemolytic *Streptococcus* (more common); *S. aureus* (less common)
- The morphology of the dermatitis is of primary importance:
  - Greasy erythema and scaling suggests seborrheic dermatitis.
  - Well-demarcated, shiny, erosive erythematous perianal patches suggest group A β-hemolytic *Streptococcus*.
  - Scattered inflammatory papules or pustules suggest *S. aureus*.
  - Erythematous patches with peripheral erythematous papules with scaling suggest a candidal infection.
  - Indurated red-brown subcutaneous nodules suggest granuloma gluteale infantum.
- A complete physical exam may reveal other features of the underlying diagnosis:
  - The presence of scalp seborrhea (cradle cap) suggests seborrheic dermatitis.
  - The presence of thrush (oral candidiasis) should raise the possibility of a candidal infection.

DIAGNOSTIC TESTS & INTERPRETATION
Lab
- Rarely helpful
- Candidal infections may be verified by a potassium hydroxide preparation of a skin scraping or by a fungal culture.
- Group A β-hemolytic *Streptococcus* and *S. aureus* infection can be confirmed by a bacterial culture obtained by swabbing the affected area.

Pathological Findings
- Skin biopsy is rarely required.
- Can be helpful in diagnosing psoriasis, Langerhans cell histiocytosis, or a nutritional deficiency. Skin biopsy may be nondiagnostic in the case of allergic or irritant contact dermatitis and seborrheic dermatitis.

DIFFERENTIAL DIAGNOSIS
- Scabies: Pruritic, erythematous papules and nodules may involve the diaper area; often there is a family history of multiple affected family members and more widespread involvement.
- Psoriasis: May involve the diaper area either exclusively in infants or may occur in the setting of more diffuse presentation, including other intertriginous areas and the face and scalp. A family history of psoriasis or the presence of psoriasiform plaques elsewhere may suggest the diagnosis.
- Herpes simplex virus: Can present with multiple punched-out erosions in the diaper area, which can be confirmed by specific viral studies such as PCR or DFA. If confirmed, an evaluation for child abuse is mandatory.
- Langerhans cell histiocytosis: Usually presents with multiple reddish-brown crusted papules and/or vesicles and petechiae in conjunction with hepatosplenomegaly. Oral lesions may also be present.
- Nutritional and metabolic disorders: Acrodermatitis enteropathica, which is caused by impaired zinc metabolism (either inherited or acquired), leads to an erosive acrodermatitis involving the face in a perioral and periocular distribution, the diaper area, and the hands and feet. Multiple carboxylase deficiency, essential fatty acid deficiency, and biotinidase deficiency can also present in a similar manner.
- Kawasaki disease: The characteristic diaper rash appears as a scaling, desquamative erythema.
- Child abuse: An unusual history or morphology should suggest the possibility of abuse, especially if the lesions appear geometric or resemble scalds or burns.

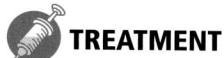

TREATMENT

ADDITIONAL TREATMENT
General Measures
- Proper skin care is the primary treatment modality.
- When soiled, the skin should be gently washed with a mild cleanser and/or infant wipe and patted dry or air dried. Vigorous rubbing of the skin or use of washcloths may cause further irritation and skin breakdown.
- Frequent diaper changes are helpful in minimizing exposure to irritants. The diaper should be kept off and the skin exposed to air as much as possible.
- Routine use of a bland barrier ointment containing zinc oxide with each diaper change is recommended.
- Candidal infections should be treated with topical nystatin cream or a topical antifungal cream such as econazole, ketoconazole, or clotrimazole cream. There is some evidence to suggest that topical clotrimazole may be less efficacious than the use of other topical antifungal agents.

- If the skin is very inflamed or if there is evidence of an allergic contact dermatitis or seborrheic dermatitis, use of a small amount of a low-potency topical corticosteroid such as 1% hydrocortisone cream for a few days can be helpful.
- Topical application of sucralfate suspension or 10% cholestyramine in petrolatum has been used in severe cases. These agents function as a physical barrier and may neutralize bile acids and pepsin.

ALERT
- The prolonged use of topical corticosteroids in the diaper area in contraindicated. The side effects of topical steroids, including skin atrophy, are potentiated when used under occlusion as occurs in the diaper area.
- When topical steroids are required, they are best given as a separate prescription that can be stopped at an earlier time (usually when the rash starts to improve) as opposed to a prescription for a combination product should use of a topical antibacterial or antifungal agent also be required.
- Talcum powder can worsen skin irritation and may be aspirated by both baby and caretaker. Its use should be discouraged.
- If a candidal diaper infection is resistant to topical treatment and thrush (monilia infection of the mouth) is present, oral nystatin or fluconazole may be considered. An evaluation of the mother for a candidal infection of the nipples should also be considered since the mother may transmit the infection to her infant.

ONGOING CARE

FOLLOW-UP RECOMMENDATIONS
Patient Monitoring
With proper treatment, the rash should improve within 4–7 days. Failure of resolution of rash indicates that another process may be complicating the diaper rash, and further evaluation is warranted.

PROGNOSIS
- Diaper dermatitis usually resolves with the institution of appropriate skin care and the treatment of any underlying cause.
- Irritant diaper dermatitis completely resolves once the child is potty trained and out of diapers.

COMPLICATIONS
- Generally none, although secondary bacterial or fungal infections may lead to ulceration.
- The chronic use of topical corticosteroids in the diaper area may lead to skin atrophy and striae.

ADDITIONAL READING
- Adam R. Skin care of the diaper area. *Pediatr Dermatol*. 2008;25:427–433.
- Akin F, Spraker M, Aly R, et al. Effects of breathable disposable diapers: Reduced prevalence of Candida and common diaper dermatitis. *Pediatr Dermatol*. 2001;18:282–290.
- Alberta L, Sweeney SM, Wiss K. Diaper dye dermatitis. *Pediatrics*. 2005;116:e450–e452.
- Heath CH, Desai N, Silverberg NB. Recent microbiological shifts in perianal bacterial dermatitis: Staphylococcus aureus predominance. *Pediatr Dermatol*. 2009;26:696–700.
- Kazaks EL, Lane AT. Diaper dermatitis. *Pediatr Clin North Am*. 2000;47:909–919.
- Odio M, Friedlander SF. Diaper dermatitis and advances in diaper technology. *Curr Opin Pediatr*. 2000;12:342–346.
- Scheinfeld N. Diaper dermatitis: A review and brief survey of eruptions of the diaper area. *Am J Clin Dermatol*. 2005;6:273–281.
- Ward DB, Fleischer AB Jr, Feldman SR, et al. Characterization of diaper dermatitis in the United States. *Arch Pediatr Adolesc Med*. 2000; 154:943–946.

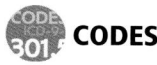 **CODES**

ICD9
691.0 Diaper rash

ICD10
L22 Diaper dermatitis

FAQ
- Q: Should I switch from cloth to disposable diapers (or vice versa)?
- A: This is controversial, although there are some studies that indicate that the superabsorbent disposable diapers may be better for preventing diaper rashes. Cloth diapers used with plastic overpants probably irritate the skin more because they trap moisture against the skin. Frequent changing of diapers is very helpful, along with not wearing diapers at all when practical.
- Q: Is the diaper rash due to not keeping the skin clean enough?
- A: Although the combination of stool and urine may release enzymes that help break down skin integrity, probably more harmful to skin is vigorous and frequent scrubbing with relatively abrasive materials on the macerated, easily damaged skin typically found in the diaper area. This rough cleaning allows introduction of bacteria and yeast into the skin and results in a diaper rash. Parents should be advised to use soft cleaning materials (such as cotton balls) to gently clean stool from the diaper area. It is not usually necessary to clean the skin of urine every time; rather, patting the infant dry with a soft cloth and then replacing the diaper is all that is generally required.

DIAPHRAGMATIC HERNIA (CONGENITAL)

Howard B. Panitch
Gordana Lovrekovic

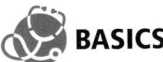 **BASICS**

DESCRIPTION

- Defect in the diaphragm allowing herniation of abdominal contents into the thoracic cavity, causing varying degrees of pulmonary hypoplasia
- 4 types of congenital diaphragmatic hernia (CDH):
  - Bochdalek hernia (posterolateral location)
  - Morgagni hernia (lateral retrosternal location)
  - Pars sternalis (medial retrosternal)
  - Anterolateral

EPIDEMIOLOGY

- Bochdalek hernia:
  - ~90% of all CDHs
  - 70–90% are left-sided
  - May be more common in males
  - 40% of cases associated with some type of other congenital malformation:
    - Heart defect in 10–35%
    - Genitourinary system abnormalities in 23%
    - GI malformations (e.g., malrotation) in 14%
    - CNS abnormalities (e.g., hydrocephalus, spina bifida, anencephaly) in 10%
    - Recognizable syndromes (Beckwith-Wiedemann, Fryns, PAGOD, etc.) in 10%
    - Chromosomal abnormalities (trisomy 13, 18, or 21; Turner syndrome; tetrasomy 12p) in 33%
- Morgagni hernia:
  - Accounts for 2–5% of all diaphragmatic hernias
  - More common in females in series where it is not discovered until adulthood

Incidence
1:2,500–4,000 live births, or 3.3–3.8/10,000 total births

RISK FACTORS
Genetics
- As isolated condition, usually sporadic
- Estimated recurrence rate <2% in 1st-degree relatives: Isolated series in consanguineous families suggest an autosomal recessive inheritance pattern, whereas others have described autosomal dominant or X-linked patterns.
- When associated with syndromes, inheritance pattern is that of the syndrome.
- When CDH detected prenatally, amniocentesis for fetal karyotype contributes important prognostic information for nondirectional prenatal counseling

PATHOPHYSIOLOGY
- Bochdalek hernia more commonly (70–90%) left-sided: Left pleuroperitoneal folds close later than right sided
- Morgagni hernia more commonly right sided: Left-sided defects covered by the heart
- Mortality and morbidity of CDH, in absence of nonpulmonary defects, relate to the degree of pulmonary hypoplasia and pulmonary hypertension.
- Pulmonary hypoplasia:
  - Degree of hypoplasia variable, from mild to incompatible with life
  - Worse on ipsilateral side, but also present on contralateral side
  - Associated with smaller lungs, fewer airway branches, fewer alveoli per terminal lung unit, and decreased surfactant production
  - Less severe in Morgagni hernias than in Bochdalek hernias

- Unclear if hypoplasia is the result of lung compression by herniated abdominal viscera or a primary event that occurs before gastrointestinal contents enter the thorax
- Pulmonary hypertension:
  - Smaller arterioles with excessive muscularization
  - Abnormal response to oxygen (failure to dilate)
  - Can lead to persistence of the fetal circulation postnatally

ETIOLOGY
- True cause: Unknown
- Diaphragm forms between 4 and 12 weeks gestation
- Diaphragm arises from 4 elements:
  - Septum transversum, which becomes the central tendon of the diaphragm
  - Pleuroperitoneal membranes, which extend from the lateral body wall and grow medially and ventrally to fuse with the septum transversum and esophageal mesentery
  - Mesentery of the esophagus, which becomes the crura of the diaphragm
  - Lateral body wall, from which myocytes migrate to muscularize the diaphragm
- Anything that interferes with formation of the diaphragm can result in herniation of abdominal contents into the thorax.
- Bochdalek hernia develops when the pleuroperitoneal membranes fail to fuse before return of the midgut to the abdominal cavity. Failure of fusion of the pleuroperitoneal membranes with other components of the diaphragm results in a communication between thoracic and abdominal cavities.
- Morgagni hernia develops when a defect develops in the septum transversum.
- Pars sternalis hernia usually also includes pericardioperitoneal and sternal defects, as well as omphalocele; may also have cardiac defect

Dx DIAGNOSIS

HISTORY
- Prenatal imaging:
  - CDH is frequently detected by fetal ultrasonography during a routinely scheduled exam or by ultrafast fetal MRI.
  - Herniation of the liver into the chest is the single most reliable predictor of severity, including need for ECMO, and mortality.
  - Some data suggest a sonographically determined lung area–to–head circumference ratio (LHR) <1.4 mm in infants with a left-sided CDH is associated with higher postnatal mortality and overall poorer outcome.
- Bochdalek hernia: Usually presents at birth; patient typically presents with severe cardiorespiratory distress. Rarely can present late (>1 month of age)
- Morgagni hernia:
  - Usually asymptomatic in the newborn period
  - If symptomatic, most commonly presents with recurrent chest infections, but rarely can present with neonatal respiratory distress
  - Older child or adult presentation usually includes vague abdominal discomfort, vomiting, growth failure, chest pain, dyspnea, cough, and recurrent respiratory infections

PHYSICAL EXAM
- Bochdalek hernia:
  - Severity of illness manifests within hours of birth.
  - Neonatal presentation:
    - Polyhydramnios
    - Scaphoid abdomen (abdominal contents in thoracic cavity)
    - Respiratory distress
    - Decreased breath sounds on the affected side
    - Dullness to percussion on the affected side
    - Bowel sounds heard in the chest
    - Heart sounds shifted to the contralateral chest
    - Cardiac point of maximal impulse shifted away from affected side
    - Asymmetry of chest wall
    - Tachypnea, tachycardia, cyanosis
  - Late presentation (>1 month of age):
    - Cough
    - Recurrent chest infections
    - Feeding intolerance
    - Vomiting, abdominal pain, diarrhea
    - Growth failure
    - Intestinal malrotation
    - Gastric volvulus
- Morgagni hernia: Exam may be normal.

DIAGNOSTIC TESTS & INTERPRETATION
Lab
- Arterial blood gas:
  - Significance:
    - pO_2 low: Reflects significant hypoxemia
    - pCO_2 high: Reflects inadequate ventilation
    - pH, bicarbonate, lactate: Reflect significant respiratory and metabolic acidosis
- Karyotype:
  - Significance: 1/3 of neonates with CDH are reported to have chromosomal abnormalities.

Imaging
- Chest radiograph:
  - Bochdalek hernia:
    - Loops of bowel in the thoracic cavity
    - Heart and mediastinal structures shifted away from the affected side
    - Decreased lung volumes (ipsilateral lung more than contralateral lung)
    - Atelectasis of the contralateral lung
    - Unable to visualize diaphragm on the ipsilateral side
    - In left-sided hernias, a nasogastric tube inserted into the stomach will be seen in the thoracic cavity.
    - Bowel remaining in the abdomen usually gasless
  - Morgagni hernia:
    - A mass can be seen in the anterior mediastinum: May be solid or gas-filled
    - Lesion better seen on lateral view
- Echocardiogram: Reduced left ventricular mass in left-sided hernias; can estimate the degree of pulmonary hypertension and exclude congenital heart defects
- Ventilation/perfusion scan: Reduced ventilation and perfusion, especially to the ipsilateral lung. Ventilation increases to a greater degree than does perfusion to the ipsilateral lung over time.
- Fetal ultrasound: Abdominal viscera in the thoracic cavity; polyhydramnios. Can be used to estimate severity of lesion (liver in chest, low LHR portend more severe disease). Also important to rule out other lesions (congenital heart defect, CNS abnormality)

- Ultrafast fetal MRI: Useful when the diagnosis is suspected but cannot be confirmed by fetal ultrasound

DIFFERENTIAL DIAGNOSIS
- Pulmonary:
  - Congenital cystic adenomatoid malformation
  - Pulmonary cyst
  - Pneumatocele
  - Congenital lobar emphysema
  - Pulmonary sequestration
  - Diaphragmatic eventration
  - Hiatal hernia
  - Atelectasis
  - Pulmonary agenesis
  - Pneumothorax
  - Anterior mediastinal mass
  - Pneumonia
  - Pleural effusion
- Cardiac:
  - Dextrocardia
  - Congenital heart disease

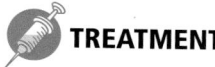 TREATMENT

ADDITIONAL TREATMENT
General Measures
Bochdalek hernia:

- Endotracheal intubation; minimal bag mask ventilation to avoid distension of bowel and further pulmonary compromise
- Decompression of the intrathoracic bowel (placement of a nasogastric tube to low suction allows the bowel to decompress, thus letting the ipsilateral hypoplastic lung expand)
- Oxygenation: Preductal saturation >85%
- Ventilation: Permissive hypercapnia with spontaneous assisted breaths, pressure control ventilation with peak pressures ≤25 cm H_2O and low mandatory rates; avoidance of paralysis
- Correction of acidosis; pH >7.30
- Normalization of BP

ISSUES FOR REFERRAL
- Pulmonary:
  - Chronic lung disease:
    ○ ~25% have obstructive lung disease at age 5 years.
    ○ ~50% have airway hyperreactivity.
  - Diminished perfusion in the ipsilateral lung with progressive increase in ventilation, as detected by ventilation/perfusion scans
  - Lung function can be normal or show a mild restrictive or obstructive pattern.
  - Recurrent respiratory infections
- GI/nutrition:
  - Gastroesophageal reflux (45–90%): May need surgical repair
  - Oral aversion
  - Failure to thrive (>40% at 2 years of age)
- Neurodevelopmental:
  - Greater risk in those with large defects or those requiring ECMO
  - Hypotonia
  - Motor delays (tend to improve with time)
  - Sensorineural hearing loss
- Chest wall: Pectus deformity and scoliosis
- Recurrence of hernia (in up to 50%): Risk greater in those who required patch closure

SURGERY/OTHER PROCEDURES
- Surgical repair of the defect:
  - Decreased morbidity and mortality if the patient is stabilized prior to surgical repair

- Large defects require placement of a prosthetic patch
- Therapies of possible but not proven benefit:
  - ECMO (extracorporeal membrane oxygenation)
  - Inhaled nitric oxide
  - Sildenafil and other pulmonary vasodilators
  - High-frequency oscillatory ventilation
  - Liquid ventilation
- Fetal surgery (either tracheal occlusion or primary repair of the diaphragmatic hernia) has not been shown to improve outcomes
- Morgagni hernia: Surgical repair indicated, even if the patient is asymptomatic, because of the high rate of strangulation of the intrathoracic bowel (10%)

 ONGOING CARE

FOLLOW-UP RECOMMENDATIONS
Patient Monitoring
- Development of pulmonary hypertension in the postoperative period
- Sudden development of hypoxemia in association with pneumothorax
- Bronchospasm
- Worsening course resulting from gastroesophageal reflux and recurrent aspiration

ALERT
- Bochdalek hernias:
  - Inability to stabilize the patient (suggestive of severe pulmonary hypoplasia and/or pulmonary hypertension)
  - Iatrogenic injury to hypoplastic lungs; aggressive ventilation causing barotrauma
  - Delay in transferring patient to an appropriate medical center
  - Lack of recognition of other congenital malformations or chromosomal abnormalities that may affect the patient's ultimate outcome or represent a contraindication to surgical repair
- Morgagni hernias: Not considering the diagnosis when abnormalities are seen on chest radiograph

PROGNOSIS
- Bochdalek hernia:
  - Dependent on the degree of pulmonary hypoplasia and pulmonary hypertension
  - If the patient survives the perioperative period, 55–65% survival (as high as 90% in the most advanced centers)
  - Poor prognostic factors:
    ○ Polyhydramnios
    ○ Liver herniation into the chest
    ○ LHR <1.4 mm (<1.0 mm in some studies)
    ○ Early postnatal presentation (i.e., presenting in the 1st 6 hours vs. after 24 hours)
    ○ Coexistence of cardiac, CNS, or chromosomal abnormalities
    ○ Persistently elevated pCO_2 or decreased pO_2
- Morgagni hernia: Excellent

COMPLICATIONS
- Perinatal:
  - Pulmonary hypoplasia
  - Pulmonary hypertension
  - Persistence of the fetal circulation
  - Chylothorax
  - Chronic respiratory failure
  - Gastroesophageal reflux
  - Death
- Long term:
  - Chronic lung disease
  - Bronchospasm
  - Pneumonia

- Pulmonary hypertension
- Growth failure
- Gastroesophageal reflux, oral aversion, feeding difficulties
- Developmental delay and behavioral disorders
- Sensorineural hearing loss
- Recurrence of the diaphragmatic hernia
- Chest wall deformities (e.g., pectus excavatum, pectus carinatum, asymmetry) and scoliosis

ADDITIONAL READING

- Colvin J, Bower C, Dickinson JE, et al. Outcomes of congenital diaphragmatic hernia: A population-based study in Western Australia. *Pediatrics*. 2005;116:e356–e363.
- Doyle NM, Lally KP. The CDH Study Group and advances in the clinical care of the patient with congenital diaphragmatic hernia. *Semin Perinatol*. 2004;28:174–184.
- Hedrick HL. Management of prenatally diagnosed congenital diaphragmatic hernia. *Semin Fetal Neonat Med*. 2010;15:21–27.
- Kamata S, Usui N, Kamiyama M, et al. Long-term follow-up of patients with high-risk congenital diaphragmatic hernia. *J Pediatr Surg*. 2005;40: 1833–1838.
- Keijzer R, Puri P. Congenital diaphragmatic hernia. *Semin Pediatr Surg*. 2010;19:180–185.
- Muratore CS, Kharasch V, Lund DP, et al. Pulmonary morbidity in 100 survivors of congenital diaphragmatic hernia monitored in a multidisciplinary clinic. *J Pediatr Surg*. 2001;36:133–140.
- Muratore CS, Utter S, Jaksic T, et al. Nutritional morbidity in survivors of congenital diaphragmatic hernia. *J Pediatr Surg*. 2001;36:1171–1176.
- Trachsel D, Selvadurai H, Bohn D, et al. Long-term pulmonary morbidity in survivors of congenital diaphragmatic hernia. *Pediatr Pulmonol*. 2005;39: 433–439.
- van den Hout L, Sluiter I, Gischler S, et al. Can we improve outcome of congenital diaphragmatic hernia? *Pediatr Surg Int*. 2009;25:733–743.

 CODES

ICD9
756.6 Congenital diaphragmatic hernia

ICD10
- Q79.0 Congenital diaphragmatic hernia
- Q79.1 Other congenital malformations of diaphragm

FAQ

- Q: What is the long-term pulmonary function in survivors of Bochdalek hernias?
- A: Most studies report evidence of a mild obstructive process in adolescents or young adults with a history of CDH, with up to 50% also demonstrating significant bronchodilator responsiveness. Less commonly, reports of a mild restrictive defect or normal lung function have been reported. Follow-up ventilation-perfusion studies demonstrate reduced perfusion to the ipsilateral lung.
- Q: What is the optimal time for surgical repair in neonates with Bochdalek hernias?
- A: Delayed surgical repair until the patient is stabilized, avoidance of hyperventilation to achieve alkalinization, and use of pressure-controlled ventilation have been shown to decrease mortality significantly in neonates who meet ECMO criteria (up to 90%).

DIARRHEA
Daniel H. Leung
Sabina Mir

 BASICS

DEFINITION
- Diarrhea is an increase in frequency, volume, or fluidity of a patient's stool as compared to the normal bowel movement pattern.
- Diarrhea can be classically categorized as acute or persistent.
- Acute diarrhea typically presents abruptly with increased fluid content of the stool >10 mL/kg/d and lasts <14 days.
- Persistent diarrhea can also begin acutely and last for ≥14 days. Tenesmus, perianal discomfort, and incontinence may occur.
- Diarrhea is caused whenever there is disruption of the normal absorptive and secretory functions of intestinal mucosa resulting in water and electrolyte imbalance. Malabsorption, maldigestion, cellular electrolyte pump dysfunction, and intestinal colonization or invasion by microorganisms can cause diarrhea.

 DIAGNOSIS

DIFFERENTIAL DIAGNOSIS
Acute diarrhea:
- **Dietary causes**
  - Sorbitol, fructose, lactose, and intolerance to specific foods (beans, fruit, peppers, etc.)
- **Infectious causes**
  - Bacterial (e.g., *Escherichia coli, Clostridium difficile*) and viral (e.g., rotavirus, Norwalk agent, adenovirus)
  - Parasites (*Giardia, Cryptosporidium, Entamoeba*)
- **Medications**
  - Antibiotics, laxatives
- **Vitamin deficiency**
  - Zinc, niacin

Chronic diarrhea:
- **Allergic/autoimmune**
  - Milk/soy protein allergy, eosinophilic enteritis, Henoch–Schönlein purpura (HSP), celiac disease, or autoimmune enteropathy
- **Immunodeficiency**
  - HIV/AIDS, chronic granulomatous disease, hyper IgM, severe combined immunodeficiency
- **Anatomic abnormalities**
  - Short intestinal tract (e.g., h/o necrotizing enterocolitis or Hirschsprung s/p repair), malrotation
- **Bile salt malabsorption**
- **Congenital**
  - Cystic fibrosis, microvillus inclusion disease, tufting enteropathy, or IPEX syndrome
- **Encopresis**
- **Endocrine disorders**
  - Hyperthyroidism, diabetes, congenital adrenal hyperplasia
- **Bacterial overgrowth (e.g., blind loop, ostomy)**
- **Inflammatory bowel disease**
  - Ulcerative colitis, Crohn's disease
- **Intestinal lymphangiectasia**
  - Primary and secondary
- **Irritable bowel syndrome**
- **Lactose intolerance**
  - Primary, secondary, and congenital
- **Pancreatic exocrine dysfunction**
  - Shwachman–Diamond syndrome, cationic trypsinogen deficiency, Jeune syndrome, Pearson syndrome, and Johanson–Blizzard syndrome
- **Postinfectious enteropathy**
- **Secretory tumors**
  - VIPoma, somatostatinoma, gastrinoma

APPROACH TO THE PATIENT
It is important to determine the type of diarrhea (osmotic vs. secretory) as this will alter your diagnostic and therapeutic plan.
- **Phase 1:** Secretory diarrhea: Absorption of intestinal fluid and electrolytes is accomplished through multiple cellular pumps transporting sodium, glucose, and amino acids. Factors that interrupt these pumps (e.g., cholera toxin, prostaglandin E, vasoactive intestinal peptide, secretin, acetylcholine) can cause a severe active isotonic secretory state manifested by profuse diarrhea, dehydration, and acidosis.
- **Phase 2:** Osmotic diarrhea: In general, the solute composition of intestinal fluid is similar to that of plasma. Osmotic diarrhea occurs when poorly absorbed or nonabsorbable solute is present in the intestinal lumen. This can occur with the ingestion of nonabsorbable sugars (e.g., sorbitol), cathartics (e.g., magnesium citrate), carbohydrate malabsorption secondary to mucosal damage (e.g., lactose), maldigestion (e.g., pancreatic dysfunction), rapid transit of intestinal fluid, or with a rare congenital transport defect.

HISTORY
- **Question:** Duration?
- *Significance*: A distinction should be made between acute and chronic diarrhea. The cause of acute diarrhea is almost always related to an infection, a medication, or the addition of a new food.
- **Question:** Travel history?
- *Significance*: Questions should be asked regarding travel to areas where drinking water is contaminated (e.g., *Entamoeba* in Mexico) or food handling/preparation is prolonged or unsanitary (e.g., *Campylobacter, Bacillus cereus,* or *E. coli*). Exposure to freshwater streams or ponds (e.g., *Cryptosporidium, Giardia*) may also be important to address.
- **Question:** Recent use of antibiotics?
- *Significance*: A variety of antibiotics cause *C. difficile* colitis or antibiotic-related diarrhea.
- **Question:** Adolescents?
- *Significance*: Questions should be asked regarding body image and weight. Laxative abuse causing an osmotic diarrhea is common among adolescents who have an eating disorder or athletes attempting to lose weight rapidly.
- **Question:** Family history?
- *Significance*: Conditions with genetic susceptibility (e.g., inflammatory bowel disease, celiac disease)
- **Question:** Systemic symptoms?

- *Significance*: Questions regarding fever, GI bleeding, rashes, or vomiting are vital. Certain GI infections and inflammatory bowel disease have specific associated systemic symptoms.
- **Question:** Hematochezia?
- *Significance*: The occurrence of acute, bloody stools and fever generally indicates a bacterial infection. However, these same symptoms coupled with fatigue, poor urine output, and history of easy bruising may suggest hemolytic uremic syndrome. Bloody stools in combination with a history of crampy abdominal pain, arthritis, and purpuric rash can indicate HSP, a completely different entity. The quantification and description of the bloody stool may also be helpful (e.g., currant jelly-like stools of intussusception vs. bright red blood from milk protein allergy). Chronic bloody diarrhea, abdominal pain, and weight loss are characteristic of inflammatory bowel disease.
- **Question:** Steatorrhea?
- *Significance*: Indicates fat malabsorption (e.g., cystic fibrosis)
- **Question:** Age?
- *Significance*: The age of the child is important because a number of diseases present between birth and 3 months of life including cystic fibrosis, milk or soy protein allergy, and congenital enteropathies.
- **Question:** Previously well infant with recent viral illness and subsequent protracted diarrhea?
- *Significance*: Postviral enteritis should be suspected. This disorder is characterized by severe mucosal injury resulting in transient disaccharidase deficiency and potentially prolonged malabsorption.
- **Question:** Normal preschool-aged children who have 2–10 watery stools per day without other symptoms and/or cause who have increased juice intake?
- *Significance*: Chronic nonspecific diarrhea of childhood or "toddler's diarrhea" should be considered.
- **Question:** Lactose intolerance?
- *Significance*: Commonly occurs in many older children and adults, with >95% occurrence rate in some ethnic groups.
- **Question:** Chronic diarrhea with weight loss?
- *Significance*: Inflammatory or immunologic disorders such as ulcerative colitis, Crohn's disease, and celiac disease must be ruled out. Celiac disease is an immune-mediated enteropathy caused by a permanent sensitivity to gluten and related prolamine in genetically susceptible individuals. It occurs in roughly 1:130 of the US population with a genetic predisposition and should be considered in any child with chronic diarrhea and poor weight gain.

PHYSICAL EXAM
- **Finding:** Child's growth parameters?
- *Significance*: Previous measurements and growth curves are necessary to make an accurate evaluation. Findings of a chronically malnourished child with years of weight loss or poor growth velocity would indicate a divergent differential diagnosis from that of a healthy-appearing child with a history of normal growth.

- **Finding:** Arthritis and rash?
- *Significance:* Diarrhea accompanied by these signs can occur in diseases such as inflammatory bowel disease, celiac disease, HSP, and specific bacterial infections.
- **Finding:** Oral ulcers?
- *Significance:* Occur in inflammatory bowel disease and celiac disease
- **Finding:** Hydration?
- *Significance:* Capillary refill >3 seconds, tachycardia without pain or fever, and dry mucous membranes provide clues to dehydration.
- **Finding:** Nail bed clubbing?
- *Significance:* This finding may direct questioning to rule out cystic fibrosis or chronic inflammatory bowel disease.
- **Finding:** Masses?
- *Significance:* A right lower quadrant mass could suggest an abscess (e.g., terminal ileitis in Crohn's disease or appendiceal abscess) or intussusception (e.g., irritable child with currant jelly-like stools).

DIAGNOSTIC TESTS & INTERPRETATION

- **Test:** Stool culture
- *Significance:* Stool examination for blood, mucus, inflammatory cells, and microorganisms is an important first step in determining the cause of the diarrhea. Stool cultures for parasites (e.g., *Giardia, Cryptosporidium, Entamoeba*), bacterial pathogens (e.g., *Salmonella, Campylobacter, Shigella, Yersinia, Aeromonas, Plesiomonas*), viral particles, and *C. difficile* toxin should be appropriately obtained in all children with unexplained diarrhea.
- **Test:** Stool pH and reducing substances
- *Significance:* These tests are useful in identifying carbohydrate malabsorption. A stool pH <5–6 and stool reducing substances >0.5–1% is suggestive.
- **Test:** Stool osmolality and electrolytes
- *Significance:*
  – Stool osmolality, stool Na, and stool K can be used to calculate an ion gap and differentiate between secretory and osmotic diarrhea.
  – Stool osmotic gap = measured stool osmolality – estimated stool osmolality
    ∘ Estimated stool osmolality = 2 (Na stool + K stool)
    ∘ An increased stool osmotic gap is >50 mOsm/kg.
- **Test:** Hemoccult
- *Significance:* Sensitive and specific test is helpful in distinguishing truly heme + stools from ingested foods/drinks with artificial or natural red coloring. Stool positive for blood is suggestive of infectious (C diff) and organic etiologies (Inflammatory bowel disease)
- **Test:** 72-hour quantitative fecal fat evaluation
- *Significance:* This is a sensitive test for steatorrhea. Patients need to be placed on a high-fat diet (2–4 g/kg) for a minimum of 1 day prior to testing. Over 3 days, all stool is collected, refrigerated, and tested. A diet record needs to be performed for the 3 days that correspond to the stool collection period. The coefficient of fat absorption is calculated: Grams of fat ingested – grams of fat excreted/grams of fat ingested × 100. Normal values are as follows: Premature infants: 60–75%; newborns: 80–85%; children 10 months to 3 years: 85–95%; children >3 years: 93%. When fat malabsorption is present, disorders of pancreatic function (e.g., cystic fibrosis, Shwachman syndrome) or severe intestinal disease should be suspected.

- **Test:** Lactose breath test
- *Significance:* This noninvasive test measures hydrogen levels. It is based on the principle that hydrogen gas is produced by colonic bacterial fermentation of malabsorbed carbohydrates. When abnormal in older healthy-appearing children, primary lactase deficiency is likely. However, in young children, a secondary lactase deficiency should be considered and small-bowel disease should be ruled out.
- **Test:** D-xylose test
- *Significance:* This serum test is an indirect measure of functional small bowel surface area. D-xylose absorption in the blood occurs independent of bile salts, pancreatic enzymes, and intestinal disaccharidases. A specific dose of D-xylose (1 g/kg, maximum 25 g) is given orally after an 8-hour fast, and the serum level of D-xylose is determined after 1 hour. Levels <15–20 mg/dL in children is abnormal and suggestive of disorders that alter or disrupt intestinal mucosa absorption.
- **Test:** Fecal calprotectin
- *Significance:* Calprotectin is a neutrophilic protein detected in stools in inflammatory conditions.
- **Test:** Endoscopy and colonoscopy (optional)
- *Significance:* Direct visualization of the intestinal mucosa as well as intestinal culture, disaccharidase collection, and biopsies can provide clues to diagnosis.
- **Test:** Celiac panel
- *Significance:* This includes a tissue transglutaminase, IgA level, and endomysial antibody.

 TREATMENT

ADDITIONAL TREATMENT
General Measures
- The key elements in treatment of diarrhea are: (a) correction of hydration, (b) correction of electrolytes, and (c) specific treatment of underlying cause when indicated.
- Rehydration is the cornerstone of treatment.
- Oral rehydration therapy with glucose concentrations of 111 mmol/L and 90 mmol/L sodium is recommended.
- IV rehydration is indicated for patients who are severely dehydrated and unable to tolerate oral feedings.

ISSUES FOR REFERRAL
Children who present with growth failure, noninfectious heme-positive diarrhea, or unexplained chronic diarrhea should be considered for referral to a pediatric gastroenterologist.

IN-PATIENT CONSIDERATIONS
Initial Stabilization
Diarrhea can lead to significant dehydration and electrolyte imbalance. Any child suspected of clinical dehydration should be closely observed. Only if oral rehydration is ineffective is IV therapy indicated. Culture-negative GI bleeding associated with severe abdominal pain and diarrhea should always be treated urgently.
- **Antibiotics**
  – *Vibrio cholerae, Shigella,* and *Giardia lamblia* require antimicrobial therapy (i.e., trimethoprim/sulfasoxazole, azithromycin, tetracycline, ciprofloxacin, metronidazole).
  – Prolonged courses of enteropathogenic *E. coli, Yersinia* in sickle cell patients, and *Salmonella*

species infections in the very young febrile or bacteremic infant require antimicrobial therapy.

 ONGOING CARE

DIET
- Breastfeeding should continue during episodes of gastroenteritis, as it promotes mucosal healing and recovery.
  – It was traditionally believed that bowel rest was beneficial for formula-fed infants. Many studies have now shown that return feeding after 4–6 hours promotes a faster recovery.
- **Micronutrient supplementation**
  – Zinc supplementation during episodes of acute diarrhea has been shown to decrease severity and duration as well as preventing future episodes in malnourished children.
- **Probiotics**
  – *Lactobacillus rhamnosus GG* has been shown to shorten the duration of diarrheal illness and viral shedding (e.g., rotavirus).

ADDITIONAL READING

- Ali SA, Hill DR. Giardia intestinalis. *Curr Opin Infect Dis.* 2003;16:453–460.
- Aomatsu T, et al. Fecal Calprotectin Is a Useful Marker for Disease Activity in Pediatric Patients with Inflammatory Bowel Disease. *Dig Dis Sci.* 2011;56(8):2372–2377.
- Castelli F, Saleri N, Tomasoni LR, et al. Prevention and treatment of traveler's diarrhea: Focus on antimicrobial agents. *Digestion.* 2006; 73(Suppl 1):109–118.
- Gore JI, Surawicz C. Severe acute diarrhea. *Gastroenterol Clin North Am.* 2003;32:1249–1267.
- Hartling L, Bellemare S, Wiebe N, et al. Oral versus intravenous rehydration for treating dehydration due to gastroenteritis in children. *Cochrane Database Syst Rev.* 2006;3:CD004390.
- Patel K, Thillainayagam AV. Diarrhea. *Medicine.* 2009;37(1):23–27.
- Surawicz CM. Mechanisms of diarrhea. *Curr Gastroenterol Rep.* 2010;12(4):236–241.
- Thielman NM, Guerrant RL. Clinical practice: Acute infectious diarrhea. *N Engl J Med.* 2004;350:38–47.

 CODES

ICD9
- 008.8 Intestinal infection due to other organism, not elsewhere classified
- 008.61 Enteritis due to rotavirus
- 787.91 Diarrhea

ICD10
- A08.0 Rotaviral enteritis
- K52.9 Noninfective gastroenteritis and colitis, unspecified
- R19.7 Diarrhea, unspecified

DIPHTHERIA

Michael J. Smith

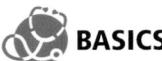 **BASICS**

DESCRIPTION
Acute infectious disease caused by *Corynebacterium diphtheriae*; affects primarily the membranes of the upper respiratory tract with the formation of a gray-white pseudomembrane

EPIDEMIOLOGY
- The single known reservoir for *C. diphtheriae* is humans; disease is acquired by contact with either a carrier or a diseased person.
- Most cases occur during the cooler autumn and winter months in individuals <15 years who are unimmunized.
- Recent outbreaks have occurred, most notably in the new independent states of the former Soviet Union, and supply additional evidence that disease occurs among the socioeconomically disadvantaged living in crowded conditions.

Incidence
Though the disease is distributed throughout the world, it is endemic primarily in developing regions of Africa, Asia, and South America. In the Western world, the incidence of diphtheria has changed dramatically in the past 50–75 years as a result of the widespread use of diphtheria toxoid after World War II. The incidence has declined steadily and is now a rare occurrence.

GENERAL PREVENTION
Active immunization with diphtheria toxoid is the cornerstone of population-based diphtheria prevention. Current recommendations from the Advisory Committee on Immunization Practices (ACIP) of the Centers for Disease Control and Prevention:
- Ages 2 months to 7 years: 5 doses of diphtheria vaccine (with tetanus toxoid and acellular pertussis):
  - First 3 given as DTaP vaccine 0.5 mL IM at 2-month intervals beginning at 2 months of age
  - 4th dose of DTaP should be given at 15–18 months of age.
  - 5th dose of DTaP or DTP at 4–6 years of age
- In 2005, 2 tetanus toxoids, reduced diphtheria toxoid, and acellular pertussis (TdaP) vaccines were licensed for use in adolescents 11–18 years of age.
- 1 booster dose of TdaP should be given to all adolescents at the 11–12-year-old visit, provided they have completed the childhood series. Subsequent tetanus and diphtheria (Td) boosters should be administered every 10 years.
- TdaP should replace the 1st dose of Td in children 7–10 years of age who are undergoing primary immunization
- Isolation of patients with diphtheria is required until culture from the site of infection is negative on 3 consecutive specimens.

PATHOPHYSIOLOGY
- The initial entry site for *C. diphtheriae* is via airborne respiratory droplets, typically the nose or mouth but occasionally the ocular surface, genital mucous membranes, or pre-existing skin lesions.
- Following 2–4 days of incubation at one of these sites, the bacterium elaborates toxin.
- Locally, the toxin induces formation of a necrotic coagulation of the mucous membranes (pseudomembrane) with underlying tissue edema; respiratory compromise may ensue.
- Elaborated exotoxin may also have profound effects on the heart, nerves, and kidneys in the form of myocarditis, demyelination, and tubular necrosis, respectively.

ETIOLOGY
C. diphtheriae, a Gram-positive pleomorphic bacillus

 DIAGNOSIS

- Respiratory tract diphtheria:
  - Nasal diphtheria starts with mild rhinorrhea that gradually becomes serosanguineous, then mucopurulent and often malodorous; occurs most often in infants.
  - Tonsillar and pharyngeal diphtheria begin with anorexia, malaise, low-grade fever, and pharyngitis. A membrane appears within 1–2 days. Cervical lymphadenitis and edema of the cervical soft tissues may be severe. Disease course varies with extent of toxin elaboration and membrane production. Respiratory and cardiovascular collapse may occur.
  - Laryngeal diphtheria most often represents extension of a pharyngeal infection and clinically presents as typical croup. Acute airway obstruction may occur, and in severe cases, the membrane may invade the entire tracheobronchial tree.
  - Cutaneous diphtheria occurs in warmer tropical regions. It is characterized by chronic nonhealing ulcers with gray membrane and may serve as a reservoir in endemic and epidemic areas of respiratory diphtheria.
- Other sites: Rarely vulvovaginal, conjunctival, or aural forms occur.

HISTORY
- Exposure to an individual with diphtheria is not necessarily elicited because contact with an asymptomatic carrier may be the only source of infection.
- Incubation period:
  - Incubation period is 1–6 days.
  - Respiratory diphtheria, depending on the site of infection, may begin with nasal discharge alone or with pharyngitis accompanied by mild systemic symptoms.
  - Progression of symptoms thereafter occurs as outlined above (see "Diagnosis").
- Previous diphtheria immunization history, diphtheria exposure

PHYSICAL EXAM
- Classic findings:
  - Nasal discharge
  - Nasal or pharyngeal membrane
  - Heart rate out of proportion to body temperature
  - Respiratory distress
  - Stridor
  - Cough
  - Hoarseness
  - Palatal paralysis
  - Neck swelling
  - Cervical lymphadenitis
  - Attempt to remove any membrane present results in bleeding.
- Conjunctival diphtheria: Palpebral conjunctival involvement with a red, edematous, membranous appearance
- Aural diphtheria: Otitis externa with a purulent, malodorous discharge
- Cutaneous diphtheria: See "Diagnosis."

DIAGNOSTIC TESTS & INTERPRETATION
Diagnosis should be on clinical grounds: Delay in treatment increases morbidity and mortality.

Lab
- Culture of material from the membrane or beneath the membrane: If a strain of *C. diphtheriae* is isolated, additional testing for presence or absence of toxin production should be done by a laboratory prepared to conduct an animal neutralization test or, alternatively, neutralization (with antitoxin) in tissue culture.
- Examination of a methylene blue-stained lesion: Metachromatic granules may be helpful if performed by an experienced technician.
- Fluorescent antibody testing and counterimmunoelectrophoresis: Previously performed in state laboratories; no longer widely available

DIFFERENTIAL DIAGNOSIS
- Nasal diphtheria:
  - Common cold
  - Nasal foreign body
  - Sinusitis
  - Adenoiditis
  - Snuffles (congenital syphilis)

- Tonsillar or pharyngeal diphtheria:
  - Streptococcal pharyngitis
  - Infectious mononucleosis
  - Primary herpetic tonsillitis
  - Thrush
  - Vincent angina
  - Post-tonsillectomy faucial membranes
  - Oropharyngeal involvement caused by toxoplasmosis, cytomegalovirus, tularemia, and salmonellosis
- Laryngeal diphtheria:
  - Croup
  - Acute epiglottitis
  - Aspirated foreign body
  - Peripharyngeal and retropharyngeal abscess
  - Laryngeal papillomas
  - Other masses

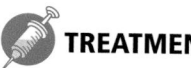 TREATMENT

MEDICATION (DRUGS)
Antibiotic therapy: Use in addition to, not in place of, diphtheria antitoxin (DAT)

- Respiratory diphtheria:
  - Penicillin G
  - Aqueous crystalline 100,000–150,000 U/kg/d in 4 divided doses for 14 days
  - Procaine 25,000–50,000 U/kg/d in 2 divided doses for 14 days or
  - Erythromycin 40–50 mg/kg (maximum 2 g/d) PO or parenterally for 14 days
- Cutaneous diphtheria: Requires local care of the lesion with soap and water and administration of antimicrobials for 10 days

IN-PATIENT CONSIDERATIONS
Initial Stabilization
- DAT antiserum, produced in horses, must be administered as soon as possible. DAT is available from the CDC. (Note: For patients with known horse serum sensitivity, a test dose should be administered first, and if positive, the patient should be desensitized.)
- Pharyngeal or laryngeal disease of <48 hours duration: 20,000–40,000 units IV
- Nasopharyngeal lesions: 40,000–60,000 units IV
- Extensive disease of ≥3 days duration or diffuse neck swelling: 80,000–120,000 units IV

 ONGOING CARE

FOLLOW-UP RECOMMENDATIONS
- Mild cases: After membrane sloughs off in 7–10 days, recovery is usually uneventful.
- More severe cases: Recovery may be slower; serious complications may occur.

PROGNOSIS
- Most strongly dependent on the immunization status of the host. Those without prior adequate immunization have significantly higher morbidity and mortality.
- Delay in onset of treatment also increases mortality. When appropriate treatment has been administered on day 1 of illness, mortality may be as low as 1%. When treatment has been delayed until day 4, the mortality rate is ≤20-fold higher.
- Organism virulence: Toxigenic strains are associated with more severe disease and a poorer prognosis.
- Location of membrane: Laryngeal diphtheria has a higher mortality due to airway obstruction.
- A megakaryocytic thrombocytopenia and WBC count <25,000 are associated with poor outcome.

COMPLICATIONS
- Cardiac toxicity: Myocarditis may develop secondary to elaborated toxin anytime between the 1st and 6th week of illness. Though cardiac failure may occur, most cases are transient.
- Neurologic toxicity occurs secondary to toxin elaboration and mainly reflects bilateral motor involvement.
- Paralysis of the soft palate is most common, but ocular paralysis, diaphragm paralysis, peripheral neuropathy of the extremities, and loss of deep tendon reflexes also occur.
- The frequency of all complications, including those listed above, increases with increasing time between symptom onset and antitoxin administration and also with extent of membrane formation.

ADDITIONAL READING
- American Academy of Pediatrics. Diphtheria. In: Pickering LK, Baker CJ, Long SS, et al., eds. *2009 Red book: Report of the Committee on Infectious Diseases*, 28th ed. Elk Grove Village, IL: American Academy of Pediatrics, 2009:280–283.
- Broder KR, Cortese MM, Iskander JK, et al. Preventing tetanus, diphtheria, and pertussis among adolescents: Use of tetanus toxoid, reduced diphtheria toxoid and acellular pertussis vaccines recommendations of the Advisory Committee on Immunization Practices (ACIP). *MMWR Recomm Rep.* 2006;55(RR-3):1–34.

- Centers for Disease Control and Prevention. Updated recommendations for use of tetanus toxoid, reduced diphtheria toxoid and acellular pertussis (Tdap) vaccine from the Advisory Committee on Immunization Practices, 2010. *MMWR.* 2011;60(1):13–15.
- Enhanced surveillance of non-toxigenic *Corynebacterium diphtheriae* infections. *Commun Dis Rep CDR Wkly.* 1996;6:29–32.
- Galazka A. The changing epidemiology of diphtheria in the vaccine era. *J Infect Dis.* 2000;181(Suppl 1):52–59.

 CODES

ICD9
- 032.1 Nasopharyngeal diphtheria
- 032.85 Cutaneous diphtheria
- 032.9 Diphtheria, unspecified

ICD10
- A36.1 Nasopharyngeal diphtheria
- A36.3 Cutaneous diphtheria
- A36.9 Diphtheria, unspecified

FAQ
- Q: What is the incidence of diphtheria in the US?
- A: No locally acquired case of respiratory diphtheria has been reported in the US since 2003.
- Q: Are there currently places in the world where diphtheria is a problem?
- A: Yes, an epidemic began in 1990 in Russia, spread in 1991 to Ukraine, and during 1993 and 1994, spread to the remaining new independent states of the former Soviet Union. Other endemic regions include the Middle East and Asia, and some countries in Africa and Central and South America. Travelers to these regions should check the CDC website for the latest information.
- Q: What precautions should be taken by travelers to areas of the world with diphtheria outbreaks?
- A: The ACIP recommends that travelers to such areas be up-to-date with diphtheria immunization. Infants traveling to areas where diphtheria is endemic or epidemic should ideally receive 3 doses of DTaP before travel.

DISKITIS

Timothy Beukelman
Randy Q. Cron

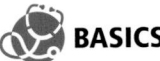 **BASICS**

DESCRIPTION
Often benign, self-limited inflammatory process of an intervertebral disk

EPIDEMIOLOGY
>50% of the cases occur in children <4 years.

Incidence
Peak incidence is between 1 and 3 years of age.

Prevalence
Rare

PATHOPHYSIOLOGY
- Probably of infectious etiology by an indolent organism
- Usually none identified; occasionally *Staphylococcus aureus*, *Moraxella*, or the Enterobacteriaceae are cultured.

ETIOLOGY
Idiopathic or initiated by low-grade infection

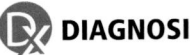 **DIAGNOSIS**

HISTORY
- Uncomfortable child
- Refusal to walk
- Fever
- Back or abdominal pain
- Symptoms of short duration prior to presentation

PHYSICAL EXAM
- Usually, rigid posture and pain elicited on movement (sits in tripod position)
- Focal tenderness to palpation
- Most common locations: L4–5 and L3–4

DIAGNOSTIC TESTS & INTERPRETATION
Lab
Initial lab tests
- Purified protein derivative (PPD)
- WBC count
- Erythrocyte sedimentation rate (ESR)
- Blood cultures

Imaging
- Plain radiographic studies: Usually normal, though may demonstrate disk narrowing as illness progresses
- Bone scan: Demonstrates increased uptake at affected area
- MRI: Useful in atypical situations to confirm location of pathology (demonstrates disk edema)

DIFFERENTIAL DIAGNOSIS
- Infection:
  - Vertebral osteomyelitis (e.g., *Staphylococcus*, *Salmonella*)
  - Potts disease (tuberculous spondylitis)
- Environmental trauma:
  - Fracture
  - Disk herniation
- Tumors: Osteoid osteoma
- Vascular: Avascular necrosis of vertebral body
- Congenital: Spondylolisthesis
- Immunologic: Ankylosing spondylitis
- Miscellaneous: Scheuermann disease (osteochondritis of the vertebral bodies)

ALERT
Difficulty separating early vertebral body osteomyelitis from diskitis

TREATMENT

MEDICATION (DRUGS)
- Usually quite responsive to NSAIDs
- Rarely, antibiotics are indicated.

COMPLEMENTARY & ALTERNATIVE THERAPIES
- Physical therapy
  - Patient should be immobilized during acute period.
  - Casting may be required.

IN-PATIENT CONSIDERATIONS
Initial Stabilization
Duration:
- Follow CBC and ESR
- Continue treatment until child is asymptomatic

 ONGOING CARE

FOLLOW-UP RECOMMENDATIONS
Patient Monitoring
- When to expect improvement: Most patients are asymptomatic in 6–8 weeks.
- Signs to watch for:
  - Recurrence of symptoms due to reactivation of the disease
  - Progressive loss of disk height
  - Destruction of adjacent vertebral bodies

PROGNOSIS
- Usually excellent
- Scoliosis may occur.
- Rarely, facet joint symptoms occur years later.

COMPLICATIONS
- Occasionally, scoliosis or kyphosis
- Rarely, facet joint degenerative disease

ADDITIONAL READING

- Arthurs OJ, Gomez AC, Heinz P, et al. The toddler refusing to weight-bear: A revised imaging guide from a case series. *Emerg Med J*. 2009;26:797–801.
- Early SD, Kay RM, Tolo VT. Childhood diskitis. *J Am Acad Orthop Surg*. 2003;11:413–420.
- Fernandez M, Carrol CL, Baker CJ. Discitis and vertebral osteomyelitis in children: An 18-year review. *Pediatrics*. 2000;105:1299–1304.
- Garron E, Viehweger E, Launay F, et al. Nontuberculous spondylodiscitis in children. *J Pediatr Orthop*. 2002;22:321–328.
- Karabouta Z, Bisbinas I, Davidson A, et al. Discitis in toddlers: A case series and review. *Acta Paeditr*. 2005;94:1516–1518.
- Karadimas EJ, Bunger C, Lindblad BE, et al. Spondylodiscitis: A retrospective study of 163 patients. *Acta Orthop*. 2008;79:650–659.

- Kayser R, Mahlfeld K, Greulich M, et al. Spondylodiscitis in childhood: Results of a long-term study. *Spine*. 2005;30:318–323.
- Marin C, Sanchez-Alegre ML, Gallego C, et al. Magnetic resonance imaging of osteoarticular infections in children. *Curr Probl Diagn Radiol*. 2004;33:43–59.
- McCarthy JJ, Dormans JP, Kozin SH, et al. Musculoskeletal infections in children: Basic treatment principles and recent advancements. *Instr Course Lect*. 2005;54:515–528.

CODES

ICD9
- 722.90 Discitis
- 722.91 Cervical, cervicothoracic
- 722.92 Thoracic, thoracolumbar

ICD10
- M46.40 Discitis, unspecified, site unspecified
- M46.42 Discitis, unspecified, cervical region
- M46.43 Discitis, unspecified, cervicothoracic region

FAQ

- Q: When are a biopsy and tissue culture indicated?
- A: If there is bony destruction of adjacent vertebral bodies or if clinical course is prolonged.
- Q: When are antibiotics indicated?
- A: Obviously, in situations with positive cultures, or if course is atypical or prolonged.

DISORDERS OF SEX DEVELOPMENT

Thomas F. Kolon

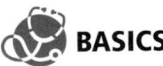 **BASICS**

DESCRIPTION

Chromosomal sex is established at fertilization, which then directs the undifferentiated gonads to develop into testes or ovaries. Phenotypic sex results from the differentiation of internal ducts and external genitalia under the influence of hormones and transcription factors. If there is any discordance among these three processes (i.e., chromosomal, gonadal, or phenotypic sex determination), then ambiguous genitalia develop.

RISK FACTORS

Genetics

- Inactivating or loss-of-function mutations in 5 genes involved in steroid biosynthesis can cause congenital adrenal hyperplasia (CAH): CYP21, CYP11B1, CYP17, HSD3B2, and StAR. Each of these genetic defects is inherited in an autosomal recessive pattern.
- 46XY disorders of sex development (DSD) can result from Leydig cell unresponsiveness to human chorionic gonadotropin luteinizing hormone (hCG-LH) because the production of testosterone by the Leydig cells is critical to male differentiation of the wolffian ducts and the external genitalia. Familial studies are consistent with autosomal recessive transmission. Multiple cases have been described, and conversion and nonsense mutations have been identified in homozygous and compound heterozygous individuals.
- The androgen receptor (AR) gene is located on the long arm of chromosome X. The majority of AR gene mutations affect the steroid-binding domain and result in receptors unable to bind androgens or that bind androgens but exhibit qualitative abnormalities.
- The SRD5A2 gene, which accounts for most fetal 5α-reductase activity, is on chromosome 2. 5α-Reductase 2 deficiency is heterogeneous, and >40 mutations have been reported. Consanguinity has also been described in up to 40% of patients' families. Three genetic isolates of this disorder have been described in the Dominican Republic, the New Guinea Samba Tribe, and Turkey.
- Persistent Müllerian duct syndrome (PMDS) is inherited in a sex-limited autosomal recessive manner caused by a mutation in the antimüllerian hormone (AMH) or AMH-receptor genes. These mutations are most common in Mediterranean or Middle Eastern countries with high rates of consanguinity.
- Mutations or deletions of any of the genes involved in the testis determination cascade (SRY, DSS, DAX1, XH2, SOX9, SF1, WT1) have been identified in dysgenetic 46XY DSD.
- 47XXY males may develop through nondisjunction of the sex chromosomes during the 1st or 2nd meiotic divisions in either parent or, less commonly, through mitotic nondisjunction in the zygote at or after fertilization. These abnormalities almost always occur in parents with normal sex chromosomes.

- Categories of 46XX sex reversal include classic XX male individuals with apparently normal phenotypes, nonclassic XX males with some degree of sexual ambiguity, and XX true hermaphrodites. 80–90% of 46XX males result from an anomalous Y to X translocation involving the SRY gene during meiosis. However, 8–20% of XX males have no detectable Y sequences, including SRY.
- XY gonadal dysgenesis (GD; XY sex reversal or Swyer syndrome) is a heterogeneous condition that can result from deletions of the short arm of the Y chromosome, SRY gene mutations, alterations in autosomal genes, or duplications of the DSS locus on the X chromosome.
- A 45X karyotype may be due to nondisjunction or chromosome loss during gametogenesis in either parent resulting in a sperm or ovum without a sex chromosome. 45X/46XX mosaicism may be present in up to 75% of Turner syndrome patients.
- In true hermaphroditism (TH), the most common karyotype is 46XX followed by 46XX/46XY chimerism, mosaicism, and 46XY. Most 46XX ovotesticular DSDs are SRY negative, and the genes responsible have not yet been identified. A mutated downstream gene in the sex determination cascade likely allows for testicular determination.

PATHOPHYSIOLOGY

- A testis that is poorly formed is called a dysgenetic testis, and an ovary that is poorly formed is called a streak gonad.
- A dysgenetic testis usually has discontinuity of the tunica albuginea with hilar disorganization, hypoplastic or disordered tubules, and fibrotic stroma.
- Streak gonads contain ovarianlike stroma with occasional primordial follicles.
  - A patient with a Y chromosome is at high risk to develop a tumor in a streak or dysgenetic gonad.
  - Gonadoblastoma is the most common tumor. Although it is a benign growth, it can give rise to a malignant tumor called a dysgerminoma. The risk of tumor formation can be up to 35% and is age related (older more at risk).
- An ovotestis has evidence of both seminiferous tubules and ovarian stroma and follicles.

ETIOLOGY

- Currently, 4 main categories of DSDs are described: 46XX DSD; 46XY DSD; gonadal dysgenesis—pure GD (PGD) or mixed GD (MGD); and ovotesticular DSD.
- 46XX DSD is the most common DSD disorder. The ovaries and Müllerian derivatives are normal, and the sexual ambiguity is limited to masculinization of the external genitalia. A female fetus is masculinized only if exposed to androgens, and the degree of masculinization is determined by the stage of differentiation at the time of exposure. These changes may also be secondary to exogenous maternal steroids. Congenital adrenal hyperplasia (CAH) accounts for the majority of 46XX DSD patients (most commonly 21α-hydroxylase or 11β-hydroxylase deficiencies).

- 46XY DSD is a heterogeneous disorder in which testes are present but the internal ducts and/or the external genitalia are incompletely masculinized. The phenotype ranges from completely female external genitalia to mild male ambiguity (such as hypospadias or cryptorchidism). 46XY DSD can result from 8 basic etiologic categories:
  - Testicular unresponsiveness to hCG and LH (Leydig cell agenesis/hypoplasia due to hCG/LH receptor defect)
  - Enzyme defects in testosterone biosynthesis, some of which are common to CAH (StAR, HSD3B2, CYP17, 17β-HSD3)
  - Defects in androgen-dependent target tissues (androgen insensitivity syndrome)
  - Defect in the enzymatic conversion of testosterone (T) to dihydrotestosterone (DHT) (5α-reductase deficiency)
  - Defects in the synthesis, secretion, or response to Müllerian-inhibiting substance (MIS or antimüllerian hormone), resulting in persistent müllerian duct syndrome
  - Aberrations in testicular gonadogenesis (testicular dysgenesis)
  - Primary testicular failure (vanishing testes)
  - Exogenous insults (maternal ingestion of progesterone/estrogen or environmental hazards)
- GD disorders comprise a spectrum of anomalies ranging from complete absence of gonadal development to delayed gonadal failure. Complete or pure GD includes failed gonadal development in genetic males and females due to abnormalities of sex or autosomal chromosomes. Partial GD refers to disorders with partial testicular formation at some point in development including MGD, dysgenetic testes, and some forms of testicular or ovarian regression.
- Ovotesticular DSD requires the presence of both ovarian and testicular tissue in the individual and can result from sex chromosome mosaicism, chimerism, or Y-chromosomal translocation. This uncommon condition may be classified into three groups: Lateral (testis and ovary, usually left), bilateral (ovotestis and ovotestis), and unilateral (most common; ovotestis and testis or ovary). The genital development is ambiguous with hypospadias, cryptorchidism, and incomplete fusion of labioscrotal folds. Genital duct differentiation generally follows that of the ipsilateral gonad.

DIAGNOSIS

HISTORY

Prematurity, exogenous maternal hormones (used in infertility treatments), use of oral contraceptives, CNS lesions, and family history for urologic abnormalities, neonatal deaths, precocious puberty, infertility, or consanguinity.

PHYSICAL EXAM

- Any abnormal virilization or cushingoid appearance of the child's mother should be noted.
- The patient should be examined supine in the frog-leg position with both legs free.
  - Note any dysmorphic features including a short, broad neck or widely spaced nipples. Abnormal phallic size should be documented by width and stretched length measurements.

- Describe the position of the urethral meatus and amount of chordee (ventral curvature):
  - Note the number of orifices: 3 in normal girls (urethra, vagina, and anus) or 2 in boys (urethra, anus). A rectal exam should always be performed for palpation of a uterus.
- With warmed hands, begin the inguinal exam at the anterior superior iliac spine. Sweep the groin from lateral to medial with the nondominant hand:
  - When a gonad is palpated, grasp it with the dominant hand, and continue to sweep toward the scrotum with the other hand to attempt to bring the gonad to the scrotum.
    - Check the size, location, and texture of both gonads if palpable. Wetting the fingers of the nondominant hand with lubricating jelly or soap can increase the sensitivity of the fingers.
  - The undescended testis may be found in the inguinal canal, in the superficial inguinal pouch, at the upper scrotum, or (rarely) in the femoral, perineal, or contralateral scrotal regions. For differential diagnosis and treatment purposes, the distinction needs to be made whether or not the testis is palpable. Unless associated with a patent processus vaginalis, ovaries and streak gonads do not descend, although testes, and rarely ovotestes, may be palpable.
  - Document development and pigmentation of the labioscrotal folds.

DIAGNOSTIC TESTS & INTERPRETATION
Lab
All patients require serum electrolytes, 17OH progesterone (17OHP), T, LH, follicle-stimulating hormone (FSH), karyotype. If 17OHP is elevated, 11 deoxycortisol and deoxycortisol (DOC) will help differentiate 21α- from 11β-hydroxylase deficiency. If 17OHP is normal, T/DHT ratio along with androgen precursors pre-/post-hCG stimulation (if >3 months) will help elucidate the 46XY DSD etiology. A failure to respond to hCG in combination with elevated LH/FSH levels is consistent with anorchia.

Imaging
- Ultrasound can detect gonads in the inguinal region (where they are also most easily palpable) but are only 50% accurate in showing intra-abdominal testes:
  - These tests are also helpful in identifying a uterus.
- A genitogram may be performed to evaluate a urogenital sinus including the entry of the urethra and vagina:
  - A cervical impression can be identified on the vaginogram.
- Although more expensive, a gadolinium-enhanced MRI may also help to delineate the anatomy.

DIFFERENTIAL DIAGNOSIS
The differential diagnosis initially depends on the palpability of gonads on presentation:
- If no gonads are palpable, all 4 categories are possible:
  - Of these, 46XX DSD is most commonly seen, followed by MGD.
- If 1 gonad is palpable, 46XX DSD and PGD are ruled out because ovaries and streak gonads do not descend. MGD, ovotesticular, and 46XY DSD remain possibilities.

- If 2 gonads are palpable, 46 XY DSD and (rarely) ovotesticular DSD are the most likely diagnoses:
  - In 46XY boys, hypospadias and cryptorchidism without an underlying intersex etiology would be a diagnosis of exclusion after a full evaluation.

TREATMENT

Much current research is aimed at understanding the influence of androgens on the fetal/newborn brain and its relationship to gender identity. Diagnosis and management of these children is individualized and should always involve a "team effort" including the pediatric urologist, endocrinologist, geneticist, and psychologist and the child's parents immediately after birth.

ADDITIONAL TREATMENT
General Measures
- Treatment of the newborn with CAH involves correction of dehydration and salt loss by electrolyte and fluid therapy with mineralocorticoid replacement. Glucocorticoid replacement is generally added upon confirmation of the diagnosis.
- Estrogen replacement is begun after puberty in girls with complete AIS.
- Testosterone replacement may be needed in some cases of XY DSD (partial AIS, testicular dysgenesis, primary testicular, or Leydig cell failure) to aid in pubertal changes and for maintenance through adulthood.

SURGERY/OTHER PROCEDURES
- Until further data are available, the current recommendation for a girl with CAH is to continue a female sex of rearing and perform a feminizing genitoplasty depending on the degree of masculinization:
  - This surgery has 3 main aims: Increasing the opening of the vagina with separation from the urethra, reconstructing the female labia, and reducing the size of the enlarged, masculinized clitoris if significant.
  - Most cases need early surgery to separate the urinary system from the genital system for technical and psychological reasons.
- Some gonads need to be removed owing to the risk of tumor formation. Controversy exists concerning the best time to perform orchiectomies in a child with complete AIS reared as female (at diagnosis vs. after puberty). Streak gonads in the presence of a Y chromosome and dysgenetic abdominal testes should be removed. All other undescended testes need to be anchored in the scrotum by abdominal or inguinal orchidopexy. Dysgenetic testes in the scrotum need to be followed closely.
- Urethral reconstruction of hypospadias is performed in all children raised as boys at about 6 months of age.

ONGOING CARE

PROGNOSIS
- The overall prognosis for somatic, sexual, and psychosocial growth and development is good with careful management of most of these children. Any thoughts of gender reassignment should only be entertained after thoughtful discussion with the child's parents and all medical staff involved.
- Except for girls with CAH, many of these patients are infertile.
- Long-term management of mineral and glucocorticoids is by the pediatric endocrinologist. The vaginal introitus in CAH should be re-examined after puberty to assess adequacy of width and depth.
- Undescended testes, especially dysgenetic testes, have an increased risk of tumor formation even after orchidopexy (seminoma-UDT, gonadoblastoma/dysgerminoma-dysgenetic testis). These boys need to learn testis monthly self-exam after puberty.
- Hypospadias repairs are followed at least through potty training to ensure good voiding habits and absence of meatal stenosis or urethrocutaneous fistulae.

ADDITIONAL READING

- Brown J, Warne GJ. Practical management of the intersex infant. *Pediatr Endocrinol Metab*. 2005;18:3–23.
- Diamon DA, Burns JP, Mitchell C, et al. Sex assignment for newborns with ambiguous genitalia and exposure to fetal testosterone: Attitudes and practices of pediatric urologists. *J Pediatr*. 2006; 148:445.
- Hughes IA, Houk CP, Ahmed SF, et al. Consensus statement on management of intersex disorders. International Consensus Conference on Intersex. *Arch Dis Child*. 2006;91(7):554–563.
- Lambert SM, Villain EJ, Kolon TF. A practical approach to ambiguous genitalia in the newborn period. *Urol Clin North Am*. 2010;37(2):195–205.

CODES

ICD9
752.7 Indeterminate sex and pseudohermaphroditism

ICD10
- Q56.3 Pseudohermaphroditism, unspecified
- Q56.4 Indeterminate sex, unspecified

DISSEMINATED INTRAVASCULAR COAGULATION

Char Witmer

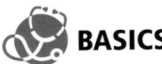 **BASICS**

DESCRIPTION
- Disseminated intravascular coagulation (DIC) is an acquired syndrome that is always secondary to an underlying etiology.
- It is a systemic life-threatening process characterized by an uncontrolled activation of the coagulation and fibrinolytic systems with excessive thrombin generation and the consumption of coagulation factors and platelets.
- Widespread deposition of microthrombi can compromise perfusion and lead to organ failure.
- Ongoing activation and consumption of coagulant factors and platelets can result in diffuse and profuse bleeding.

EPIDEMIOLOGY
- Most commonly secondary to infections
- Overall incidence is difficult to determine secondary to the many conditions that cause DIC.

PATHOPHYSIOLOGY
- Not a disorder in itself; occurs as a result of various initiating events
- Characterized by microvascular thrombosis and hemorrhage
- May be acute (e.g., meningococcemia) or chronic (e.g., malignancy/leukemia)
- There is a systemic intravascular deposition of fibrin as a result of increased thrombin generation, suppression of anticoagulant pathways, impaired fibrinolysis, and activation of inflammatory pathways.
- The initiation of coagulation activation leading to thrombin formation in DIC is mediated via the tissue factor/factor VIIa pathway.
- The tissue factor/factor VIIa pathway is activated via tissue factor expression from damaged endothelial cells.
- Anticoagulant pathways are diminished because of a decrease in the plasma levels of antithrombin and the protein C system through impaired production and increased destruction.
- The increase in fibrinolytic activity is likely secondary to the release of plasminogen activators from damaged endothelial cells.

ETIOLOGY
Most common causes are sepsis (particularly Gram-negative), hypotensive shock, and trauma (particularly head trauma).

- Sepsis/severe infection:
  - Bacterial Gram-negative and -positive sepsis
  - Meningococcemia
  - Malaria: Plasmodium falciparum
  - Fungal: Aspergillus
  - Rickettsial: Rocky Mountain spotted fever
  - Viral
- Trauma:
  - Multiple fractures with fat emboli
  - Massive soft tissue injury
  - Severe head trauma
  - Multiple gunshot wounds
- Malignancies:
  - Acute promyelocytic leukemia
  - Acute monoblastic or myelocytic leukemia
  - Widespread solid tumors (e.g., neuroblastoma)
- Obstetric:
  - Retained intrauterine fetal death
  - Preeclampsia/eclampsia
  - Amniotic fluid embolism
  - Abruptio placentae
  - Post hemorrhagic shock
- Neonatal:
  - Necrotizing enterocolitis
  - Perinatal asphyxia
  - Amniotic fluid aspiration
  - Obstetric complications (placenta abruption, preeclampsia, intrauterine twin demise)
  - Sepsis (bacterial and viral) Erythroblastosis fetalis
  - Respiratory distress syndrome
- Vascular Malformations:
  - Kasabach–Merritt syndrome
  - Large vascular aneurysms
- Miscellaneous:
  - Acute hemolytic transfusion reaction
  - Snake bite
  - Homozygous protein C deficiency (purpura fulminans)
  - Transplant rejection
  - Severe collagen vascular disease
  - Recreational drugs
  - Profound shock or asphyxia
  - Hypothermia or hyperthermia
  - Extensive burn injuries
  - Fulminant hepatitis/hepatic failure
  - Severe pancreatitis

DIAGNOSIS

HISTORY
- Presence of one of the underlying conditions (see "Etiology")
- Abrupt onset of bleeding
- Prolonged bleeding from venipuncture sites
- Bleeding from multiple sites, especially venipunctures, cutdown sites, mucous membranes, skin, GI tract, and genitourinary tract
- Pulmonary or intracranial hemorrhage
- Major organ dysfunction: Pulmonary, renal, hepatic

PHYSICAL EXAM
- Signs of underlying disease
- Generally, a very toxic-appearing patient
- Ecchymosis and petechiae
- Bleeding from previously intact venipuncture sites
- Skin infarctions (purpura fulminans) secondary to thrombosis of dermal vessels
- Pulmonary hemorrhage, gastrointestinal bleeding, bleeding from surgical wounds, hematuria
- Intraperitoneal and pleural hemorrhages

DIAGNOSTIC TESTS & INTERPRETATION
Lab
The following should be followed closely because results change rapidly:
- CBC: Decreased platelet count is often the earliest abnormality.
- Peripheral smear: Schistocytes, microspherocytes (50% of cases)
- PT, aPTT, and thrombin times: Prolonged
- Fibrinogen: in the initial phase could be increased as an acute-phase reactant and then decrease with consumption
- Fibrin degradation products or fibrin split products: Increased
- Soluble fibrin monomer complexes (D-dimers): Increased
- Antithrombin or protein C levels: Decreased
- Factor VIII: In the initial phase could be increased as an acute-phase reactant and then decrease with consumption. Factor VIII should be normal in coagulopathy associated with liver disease.

- There is no single test that can reliably diagnose DIC.
- The following lab abnormalities can be seen:
  - Prolonged PT in 50–75% of patients with DIC
  - Prolonged aPTT in 50–60% of patients with DIC
  - Elevated fibrin degradation products sensitivity 90–100%, but low specificity
  - Elevated d-dimer in 93–100% of patients with DICThrombocytopenia: Range 20–100 × 109/L
- Additional findings include decreased coagulation factors, fibrinogen, antithrombin, and protein C/S
- Multiple scoring systems utilizing common laboratory results have been developed to help determine if a patient is in DIC. These scoring systems have not been validated in pediatric patients.

DIFFERENTIAL DIAGNOSIS
- Coagulopathy of liver disease
- Vitamin K deficiency
- Pathologic fibrinolysis
- Microangiopathic disease, e.g., thrombotic thrombocytopenic purpura or hemolytic uremic syndrome

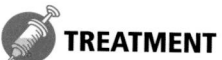

TREATMENT

ADDITIONAL TREATMENT
General Measures
- The most important therapy for DIC is to treat the underlying disorder.
- Supportive therapy may be required to treat symptomatic coagulation abnormalities.
- Replacement therapy:
  - Cryoprecipitate, platelets, and fresh frozen plasma to control bleeding.
  - Fresh frozen plasma also replaces anticoagulants–antithrombin, protein C and S.
- The role of heparin for DIC is controversial. It has been used in chronic DIC, arterial thromboses, or large-vessel venous thromboses.
- Antithrombin at supraphysiologic dosing has been studied with mixed results. Antithrombin is currently not recommended for the treatment of DIC in pediatric patients.

- In pediatric DIC recombinant activated protein C has not been shown to be beneficial.
- Off label use of recombinant activated factor VII has been reported for patients with severe bleeding that is refractory to replacement therapy. There are significant concerns about the prothrombotic potential of this medication.
- Antifibrinolytic agents (aminocaproic or tranexamic acid) have been used for patients with intense fibrinolysis (e.g., Kasabach Merritt or acute promyelocytic leukemia). There are concerns about the prothrombotic potential of this medication.
- Supportive care: Manage other organ system failure.

 ONGOING CARE

PROGNOSIS
- Poor unless underlying disease is treated
- The intensity and duration of DIC depend on the degree of activation of the coagulation system, liver function, blood flow, and ability to reverse underlying etiology that has led to DIC.

COMPLICATIONS
- Hemorrhage:
  - Pulmonary
  - Intracranial
- Thrombosis
- Multiorgan system failure

ADDITIONAL READING
- Favaloro EJ. Laboratory Testing in Disseminated Coagulation. *Seminars in Thrombosis & Hemostasis.* 2010;36(4):458–467.
- Levi M. Disseminated intravascular coagulation. *Crit Care Med.* 2007;35(9):2191–2195.
- Levi M. Disseminated intravascular coagulation: What's new? *Crit Care Clin.* 2005;21:449–467.
- Montagnana M, Franchi M, Danese E, et al. Disseminated Intravascular Coagulation in Obstetric and Gynecologic Disorders. Seminars in Thrombosis & Hemostasis. 2010;36(4):404–418.
- Pipe SW, Goldenberg N. Acquired disorders of hemostasis. In: Orkin SH, Nathan DG, Ginsburg D, A. Thomas Look, David E. Fisher, Samuel E. Lux, eds. *Nathan and Oski's Hematology of Infancy and Childhood.* 7th ed. Philadelphia: Saunders Elsevier; 2009:1591–1620.
- Veldman A, Fischer D, Nold MF, et al. Disseminated intravascular Coagulation in Neonates and Preterm Neonates. *Seminars in Thrombosis & Hemostasis.* 2010;36(4):419–428.

 CODES

ICD9
- 286.6 Defibrination syndrome
- 776.2 Disseminated intravascular coagulation in newborn

ICD10
- D65 Disseminated intravascular coagulation
- P60 Disseminated intravascular coagulation of newborn

D

DOWN (TRISOMY 21) SYNDROME
Esther K. Chung

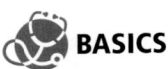 **BASICS**

DESCRIPTION
Syndrome 1st described by John Langdon Down in 1866 consisting of multiple abnormalities, including hypotonia, flat facies, upslanting palpebral fissures, and small ears; also called "Trisomy 21." Other abnormalities include:
- Congenital heart disease (40–50%; most not symptomatic as newborn):
  - Atrioventricular (AV) canal (60% of those with congenital heart disease)
  - Ventriculoseptal defect (VSD)
  - Patent ductus arteriosus (PDA)
  - Atrioseptal defect (ASD)
  - Aberrant subclavian artery
  - Tetralogy of Fallot
- Hearing loss (66–75%): Sensorineural and conductive
- Strabismus (33–45%)
- Nystagmus (15–35%)
- Fine lens opacities (by slit-lamp exam, 59%), cataracts (1–15%)
- Refractive errors (50%)
- Nasolacrimal duct stenosis
- Delayed tooth eruption
- Tracheoesophageal fistula
- GI atresia (12%)
- Celiac disease
- Meckel diverticulum
- Hirschsprung disease (<1%)
- Imperforate anus
- Renal malformations
- Hypospadias (5%)
- Cryptorchidism (5–50%)
- Testicular microlithiasis
- Thyroid disease (15%): Congenital hypothyroidism, hyperthyroidism
- Transient myeloproliferative disorder, neonatal (leukemoid reaction)
- Neonatal polycythemia
- Leukemia (<1%; 10–30 times greater risk than in general population)
- Retinoblastoma and testicular germ cell tumors (slightly greater risk than in general population)
- Infertility, especially in males
- Obesity
- Alopecia areata (10–15%)
- Seizures (5–10%), usually myoclonic
- Alzheimer disease (nearly all age >40 years)
- Mild to moderate mental retardation (IQ range 25–70)
- Dry, hyperkeratotic skin (75%)

EPIDEMIOLOGY
- Male > female (1.3:1)
- Best recognized and most frequent chromosomal syndrome of humans
- 1 of the 3 most common autosomal trisomies in humans (others are Trisomy 18 and 13)
- Most common autosomal chromosomal abnormality causing mental retardation
- >50% of Trisomy 21 fetuses are spontaneously aborted in early pregnancy.

Incidence
1/600–1/800 live births, although incidence varies with maternal age:
- 1/1,500 for maternal ages 15–29 years
- 1/800 for maternal ages 30–34 years
- 1/270 for maternal ages 35–39 years
- 1/100 for maternal ages 40–49 years

RISK FACTORS
Genetics
- 94–97% of cases are the result of chromosomal nondisjunction (failure to segregate during meiosis) in the maternal DNA.
- <5% of cases are the result of paternal nondisjunction.
- Of live births, 2.4% are mosaic (nondisjunction occurs after conception; 2 cell lines are present); generally less severely affected.
- Remainder of cases are the result of translocations between chromosome 21 and 14 [t(14q21q)]; rarely between 21 and 13 or 15; 50% of translocations are sporadic de novo events; 50% result from balanced translocations in 1 parent.

DIAGNOSIS

HISTORY
- Check for previous history of infant with Down syndrome in the family.
- Growth and developmental status
- Feeding problems
- Snoring, signs of sleep apnea (e.g., restless sleep)
- Stool habits
- Hearing concerns

PHYSICAL EXAM
The phenotype is variable from person to person.
- General:
  - Short stature
  - Hypotonia (80–100%), with an open mouth and a protruding tongue
  - Midface hypoplasia
- Head:
  - Brachycephaly with a flattened occiput
  - Microcephaly
  - False fontanel (95%)
- Eyes:
  - Upslanting palpebral fissures (98%)
  - Inner epicanthal folds
  - Brushfield spots (speckling of the iris)
  - Fine lens opacities on slit-lamp exam
  - Cataracts, refractive error, strabismus, and nystagmus
- Ears: Small, prominent, low set; overfolding of upper helix and small canals
- Nose: Small (85%); flat nasal bridge
- Tongue:
  - Relative but not true macroglossia (tongue mass is normal)
  - Fissuring
- Mouth: High-arched or abnormal palate
- Teeth:
  - Missing (50%), small, hypoplastic
  - Irregular placement

- Neck:
  - In infancy, excess skin at the nape
  - Short appearance
  - Occasionally webbed
- Heart: Assess for murmur, arrhythmia, cyanosis.
- Abdomen:
  - In neonate, distention may be present due to obstruction or atresia.
  - Diastasis recti
- Genitals:
  - In adolescents, straight pubic hair
  - In males, small penis, cryptorchidism
- Extremities:
  - Broad hands, with short metacarpals and phalanges
  - 5th finger with hypoplasia of the midphalanx (60%) and clinodactyly (50%)
  - Simian crease (single transverse palmar crease) in ~50%. A newborn with a simian crease has a 1 in 60 chance of having Down syndrome.
  - Wide gap between the 1st and 2nd toes (96%)
  - Syndactyly of 2nd and 3rd toes
  - Hyperflexibility of joints
- Skin:
  - Cutis marmorata (43%)
  - In older children, hyperkeratotic dry skin (75%)
  - Fine, soft, sparse hair

DIAGNOSTIC TESTS & INTERPRETATION
- ECG: Done within the 1st month of life to rule out cardiac disease
- Auditory brainstem response: Done within the 1st 3 months of life to rule out hearing loss

Lab
- 2nd-trimester prenatal triple screen test (α-fetoprotein [AFP], unconjugated estriol, and human chorionic gonadotropin [hCG]):
  - Performed at 15–18 weeks
  - These 3 serum markers together can detect ~60% of the pregnancies affected by Trisomy 21, with a false positive of ~5%.
  - A positive test is an indication for karyotyping with amniocentesis.
- 1st-trimester maternal serum screening (pregnancy-associated plasma protein A and free β-hCG): When these 2 tests are conducted together, it has been shown in multiple studies to have higher sensitivity than 2nd-trimester prenatal screens (91% vs. 70%).
- Chromosomal karyotype on cultured lymphocytes from peripheral blood: May be performed postnatally for confirmation if there is a clinical suspicion of Down syndrome.
- CBC:
  - In the newborn period to check for polycythemia and transient myeloproliferative disorder; repeat test in adolescence.
  - Down syndrome patients may have an increased mean corpuscular volume (MCV), making the diagnosis of iron deficiency anemia difficult.
- Thyroid function tests: To rule out hypothyroidism or hyperthyroidism

Imaging

- 1st-trimester ultrasound measurement of nuchal translucency: Performed in the 1st trimester along with maternal serum screening (see "Lab")
- Fetal ultrasound:
  - May show polyhydramnios if bowel obstruction is present
  - A thickened nuchal fold, an absent nasal bone in the 1st trimester, and echogenic intracardiac foci have been associated with an increased risk for Down syndrome.
- Echocardiography and chest radiography: Done in the 1st month of life to rule out cardiac disease
- Lateral cervical spine radiographs in flexion, neutral, and extension: To rule out atlantoaxial instability, defined as >5-mm space between atlas and odontoid process of the axis. Important measures include:
  - Atlantodens interval (ADI; normal <4.5 mm): The distance between the posterior surface of the anterior arch of C1 and the anterior surface of the dens
  - Neural canal width (NCW; normal ≥14 mm): The distance between the posterior surface of the dens and the anterior surface of the posterior arch of C1
  - Distance of subluxation at the occipitoatlantal joint: Normally ≥7 mm

Diagnostic Procedures/Other

- Prenatal karyotyping via amniocentesis (16–18 weeks' gestation) or chorionic villus sampling (9–11 weeks' gestation):
  - Performed for any woman who presents with a positive triple or quad screen
  - May be offered if prenatal ultrasound reveals a finding associated with Down syndrome
  - Because this test fails to detect 10–15% of Down syndrome cases in older women, amniocentesis is typically offered to all women >35 years.
- Tissue sample other than blood (usually skin): To check for mosaicism

 ONGOING CARE

FOLLOW-UP RECOMMENDATIONS

- Genetic counseling is recommended.
- Many organizations (e.g., Down Syndrome International) are available to families of children with Down syndrome.

Patient Monitoring

- Growth and development:
  - Specific growth charts for Down syndrome should be used.
  - Average age for acquiring developmental milestones differs from normal population.
  - Late closure of fontanelles
  - Consider Early Intervention program for hypotonia and developmental delay.
- Cardiac:
  - Early evaluation in newborn period, with follow-up until the presence or absence of disease is evident.
  - Subacute bacterial endocarditis prophylaxis for patients with certain types of cardiac disease.

- Ophthalmologic:
  - Early evaluation for cataracts and glaucoma
  - Visit to ophthalmologist by 6 months, then every 2 years
- Ear, nose, and throat (ENT)/audiologic:
  - Annual audiologic evaluation in the 1st 3 years of life, then every other year
- Orthopedic: Screen for atlantoaxial instability with radiography in preschool years, then every decade; evaluate for atlantoaxial instability prior to participation in contact sports (e.g., Special Olympics).
- Endocrine: Thyroid function tests in newborn period, ages 6 months and 12 months, then yearly

ALERT

- Use caution with endotracheal intubation if absence or presence of atlantoaxial instability is unknown to avoid spinal cord injury, which may be seen in rare cases.
- Hearing loss may be misinterpreted as a behavioral problem.
- Use care with atropine and pilocarpine for ophthalmologic evaluation because of possible cholinergic hypersensitivity.

PROGNOSIS

- Life expectancy is mildly decreased, with many living into the 6th decade; median age of death is 49 years.
- Alzheimer disease affects ~15% after the 4th decade.
- As adults, most patients with Down syndrome can work in supported positions.

COMPLICATIONS

- Otitis media with effusion (50–70%)
- Sinusitis
- Tonsillar and adenoidal hypertrophy
- Obstructive airway disease with associated sleep apnea (33–75%), cor pulmonale
- Obstructive bowel disease (12%, newborn period)
- Constipation (due to low tone and decreased gross motor mobility)
- Subluxation of the hips (secondary to ligamentous laxity)
- Atlantoaxial instability (10–20%; secondary to ligamentous laxity, which is most severe prior to age 10 years)

ADDITIONAL READING

- American Academy of Pediatrics. Health supervision for children with Down syndrome. *Pediatrics.* 2001;107:442–449.
- Crissman BG, Worley G, Roizen N, et al. Current perspectives on Down syndrome: Selected medical and social issues. *Am J Med Genet Part C Semin Med Genet.* 2006;142C:127–130.
- Dykens EM. Psychiatric and behavioral disorders in person with Down syndrome. *Ment Retard Dev Disabil Res Rev.* 2007;13(3):272–278.

- Mik G, Gholve PA, Scher DM, et al. Down syndrome: Orthopedic issues. *Curr Opin Pediatr.* 2008;20(1): 30–36.
- Roizen NJ, Patterson D. Down's syndrome. *Lancet.* 2003;361:1281–1289.
- Rosen T, D'Alton ME. Down syndrome screening in the first and second trimesters: What do the data show? *Semin Perinatol.* 2005;29:367–375.
- Vachon L, Fareau GE, Wilson MG, et al. Testicular microlithiasis in patients with Down syndrome. *J Pediatr.* 2006;149:233–236.

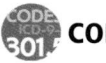 **CODES**

ICD9
758.0 Down's syndrome

ICD10
Q90.9 Down syndrome, unspecified

FAQ

- Q: Why was Down syndrome referred to as mongolism in the past?
- A: There was a mistaken notion about a racial cause for this syndrome because of the facial appearance, which was thought to be similar to that of those of Mongoloid origin.
- Q: Do all children with Down syndrome have mental retardation?
- A: No. Though all persons with nonmosaic Down syndrome have some degree of cognitive disability, some have IQs >70 and are not considered to have mental retardation.
- Q: Can a normal cardiac exam rule out the presence of a cardiac anomaly?
- A: No. The American Academy of Pediatrics recommends that all patients with Down syndrome have a cardiology consultation within the 1st month of life. Timely surgery may be necessary to prevent serious complications.
- Q: Are patients with atlantoaxial instability symptomatic?
- A: No. Most are asymptomatic, but symptoms of cord compression may be seen in 1–2% of patients.
- Q: I have seen growth charts for Down syndrome patients that allow for plotting of lengths, heights, and weights. Are there special growth charts available for plotting head circumference?
- A: Yes. If appropriate growth charts are not used for plotting head circumference, head growth may appear abnormal. Head circumference growth charts are available through the Internet: http://www.growthcharts.com/

DROWNING

Mercedes M. Blackstone

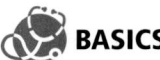 **BASICS**

DESCRIPTION
- Drowning is defined as respiratory impairment from submersion in a liquid medium.
- The term "drowning" does not imply outcome; a victim may live or die after a drowning incident.
- Historically "near drowning," or submersion injury, was defined as survival, at least temporarily, after suffocation by submersion in water.
  - The World Congress on Drowning and the World Health Organization advocate abandoning confusing terms such as "near drowning," "wet drowning," and "dry drowning"; they suggest that the literature should only use the term "drowning."

EPIDEMIOLOGY
- Drowning is second only to motor vehicle collisions as the most common cause of death from unintentional injury in childhood.
- For every drowning death, several children are hospitalized and many more have submersion events with no significant morbidity.
- Bimodal age distribution with peak in children <5 years and again among adolescents 15–19 years
- Bathtub drowning is common in babies, and child neglect or abuse should be considered.
- Adolescent submersion injuries usually involve substance abuse or risk-taking behavior.
- Highest incidence in males, African Americans, children of low socioeconomic status, and residents of southern states.

RISK FACTORS
- Children <5 years of age, especially toddlers and boys, who cannot swim and have direct access to swimming pools, are at highest risk.
- Use of alcohol and illicit drugs
- Inadequate adult supervision
- Children with seizure disorders
- Children with primary cardiac arrhythmias such as long QT syndrome

GENERAL PREVENTION
- Most drownings are preventable.
- Legislation to require adequate 4-sided isolation fencing and rescue equipment for public and residential pools
- Restriction of sale and consumption of alcohol in boating areas, pools, and beaches
- Life vests for children of all ages near bodies of water
- Parental education regarding adequate supervision during bathing and around swimming pools
- Cardiopulmonary resuscitation (CPR) courses for pool owners, parents and older children
- Swimming lessons for young children may also be helpful

PATHOPHYSIOLOGY
- Drowning begins with a loss of the normal breathing pattern as panic ensues and subsequent apnea, laryngospasm, or aspiration occurs.
- Water aspirated into the trachea and lungs washes out surfactant, and leads to atelectasis, intrapulmonary shunting, poor lung compliance, increased capillary permeability, and hypoxemia ultimately resulting in acute respiratory distress syndrome (ARDS).
- Severe hypoxemia is the final common pathway and results in multisystem organ failure
- Cerebral hypoxia results in cerebral edema and increased intracranial pressure and causes the majority of morbidity and mortality associated with drowning.

COMMONLY ASSOCIATED CONDITIONS
- Cervical spine injuries should be considered in older children who have experienced diving accidents.
- Signs of child abuse or neglect should be sought in young children.
- Adolescents may have associated toxic ingestions.
- Comorbid conditions such as epilepsy, long QT syndrome, and autism with mental retardation may be associated with an increased risk of drowning.

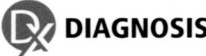 **DIAGNOSIS**

HISTORY
- Mechanism:
  - History of diving or other high-impact injury
  - Intoxication
  - Seizure disorder
  - Cardiac arrhythmia
  - Child abuse
- Prognostic indicators; the following have been correlated with a poor prognosis:
  - Age <3 years
  - Length of submersion >5 minutes
  - Time to effective CPR >10 minutes
  - Lack of vital signs at the scene
  - Length of resuscitation >25 minutes
  - Warmer water: Submersion in very cold water (<5°C [41°F]) may have a good prognosis despite submersion time >5 minutes

PHYSICAL EXAM
- Vital signs with core temperature
- Drowning victims with unclear histories must be treated as trauma victims
- Neurologic:
  - Pupillary response, cranial nerve findings, Glasgow coma scale (GCS) score, gag reflex
  - Serial neurologic exams should be performed to assess neurologic outcome. Children with a GCS score <5 after resuscitation usually have a poor neurologic outcome.
- Respiratory:
  - Lower airway findings (rales, tachypnea, wheezing, retractions, nasal flaring)
  - Drowning victims may have deteriorating pulmonary involvement despite an initially normal exam. Watch closely for signs of lower airway involvement.

- Circulation:
  - Perfusion, strength of distal pulses, capillary refill, urine output
- GI tract:
  - Abdominal distention from swallowed water or ventilation
- Musculoskeletal:
  - Neck injuries in high impact drownings

DIAGNOSTIC TESTS & INTERPRETATION
Lab
- Arterial blood gases:
  - To detect and facilitate treatment of metabolic acidosis in the child with respiratory distress or apnea
- Electrolytes:
  - Not indicated in the seemingly well child; aspiration of huge amounts of water are required to generate electrolyte shifts
- Blood glucose:
  - An elevated level correlates with poor outcome for comatose submersion victims
- Anticonvulsant levels for victims with seizure disorders
- Toxicology screening when ingestion suspected

Imaging
- A chest radiograph is indicated for children with any signs of pulmonary involvement and following intubation
  - Caution: Initial chest radiographs may be normal in the drowning victim.
- Cervical spine films are indicated for victims of high-impact events.
- Neuroimaging for cerebral anoxic injury

Diagnostic Procedures/Other
- ECG to document normal function and evaluate for prolonged QT_C if indicated by history
- Serial pulse oximetry to detect early signs of pulmonary involvement

DIFFERENTIAL DIAGNOSIS
Children with smoke inhalation or hydrocarbon ingestion may have similar presentations. However, the history and the physical exam should easily determine the diagnosis.

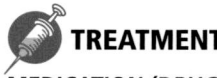 **TREATMENT**

MEDICATION (DRUGS)
- Prophylactic antibiotics or steroids are not indicated.
  - In patients that do develop pneumonia, antimicrobial therapy should cover water-borne pathogens such as *Pseudomonas* and *Aeromonas*.
- Seizures should be aggressively controlled with antiepileptics since they increase oxygen consumption.

ADDITIONAL TREATMENT
General Measures
- Attempts to remove water from the lungs such as abdominal thrusts are not helpful and should not delay administration of rescue breaths.
- Patients who are breathing spontaneously should be placed in the right lateral decubitus position to prevent aspiration.

- Even patients who respond well to bystander resuscitation need to be transported to an emergency department for further monitoring.
- Search for pulses carefully since they may be very weak and slow due to hypothermia; some common arrhythmias such as sinus bradycardia and atrial fibrillation need no immediate treatment.
- The hypothermic patient who is a warm-water (>20°C [86°F]) drowning victim does not have a good prognosis or need vigorous rewarming.

IN-PATIENT CONSIDERATIONS
Initial Stabilization
- Airway:
  - Protect the cervical spine if indicated by history.
  - Ensure a patent airway in the comatose victim or patient in cardiac arrest.
- Breathing:
  - Supplemental oxygen for oxygen saturations by pulse oximetry <95%
  - The drowning victim should be intubated if apneic, unable to maintain a PaO_2 >60 mm Hg on high fractions of supplemental oxygen, or for airway protection
  - Treatment of bronchospasm
- Circulation:
  - For the victim with cardiopulmonary arrest, the asystole protocol should be followed
  - Since capillary leak may occur after an ischemic/anoxic episode, isotonic fluids (e.g., normal saline solution or Ringer lactate, 10-mL/kg aliquots) should be given for signs of intravascular volume depletion (tachycardia, poor perfusion) until normalized.
  - ECG monitoring should be provided with appropriate response to dysrhythmias, especially for the hypothermic, cold-water drowning victim.
  - For severely hypothermic patients with a core temperature <28°C (82.4°F), aggressive rewarming is indicated. Electrical defibrillation and pharmacotherapy may not be successful.
- Disability:
  - Maintenance of eucapnia and adequate oxygenation to prevent further hypoxemia
  - Elevate the head of the bed once c-spine is cleared
- Other measures for reducing intracranial pressure (ICP) have not proven effective, likely because the brain injury and swelling is secondary to hypoxic cell injury as opposed to a traumatic lesion.
- Exposure:
  - The drowning victim should be dried and warmed.
  - Most thermometers do not register temperatures below 34°C (93.2°F) so a hypothermia thermometer may be necessary:
    ○ For core temperatures 32°C (89.6°F) to 35°C (90.5°F), active external rewarming with heating blankets or radiant warmers
    ○ For <32°C (89.6°F), active internal rewarming added (heated aerosolized oxygen and IV fluids, gastric and bladder lavage with warm saline)
    ○ For severe hypothermia (<28°C [82.4°F]) and where available, peritoneal dialysis or hemodialysis, mediastinal irrigation, and cardiac bypass
    ○ The cold-water drowning victim with hypothermia must be rewarmed to a temperature >34°C (89.6°F) before CPR is terminated.
- Remember: The saying, "The patient is not dead until he or she is warm and dead" only applies to drownings in very cold water.

Admission Criteria
- Severely ill children require admission to the intensive care unit
- Children who were apneic, cyanotic, or pulseless at the scene should be admitted to the hospital for close observation even if they appear well.
- A subset of well appearing children may be discharged from the emergency department after being monitored for 6–8 hours

ONGOING CARE

FOLLOW-UP RECOMMENDATIONS
- Long-term follow-up of apparently neurologically intact survivors has shown mild coordination or gross-motor deficiencies.
- Drowning victims may be at increased risk for chronic lung disease, depending on the degree of pulmonary involvement.

Patient Monitoring
- Victims who appear well:
  - Monitor with pulse oximetry for progressive respiratory distress
  - If asymptomatic at 6–8 hours postimmersion, can be discharged
- Victims with significant neurologic injury: Key is to prevent secondary injury:
  - Maintain euvolemia and euglycemia

PROGNOSIS
- Most children (about 75%) recover with intact neurologic survival.
- Duration and severity of initial hypoxic insult are most important determinants of brain injury and death.
- See prognostic factors above under History section. Additional indicators of poor prognosis include:
  - Coma on arrival
  - Needing CPR in the emergency department
  - Initial arterial blood pH <7.1
- Children with warm-water submersion time >4 minutes, who do not receive CPR at the scene, and who have absent vital signs or a GCS score <5 in the emergency department, usually have a poor prognosis.
- Victims who have prolonged submersions in very cold water (<5°C [41°F]) may have a good prognosis because of core cooling with a concomitant decrease in metabolic rate while the brain is still being perfused.
- A good prognostic indicator is continuing improvement in the neurologic examination over the first several hours.

COMPLICATIONS
- Pneumonia
- Pneumomediastinum or pneumothorax in the patient undergoing ventilation therapy
- Brain injury secondary to hypoxia
- Pulmonary injury with intrapulmonary shunting secondary to damage of the alveoli
- ARDS
- Metabolic acidosis secondary to hypoxemia
- Ischemic injury to organs such as liver, kidneys, and intestines

- Disseminated intravascular coagulation secondary to ischemia
- Electrolyte abnormalities uncommon; may occur if a large volume of freshwater is in the stomach and not removed
- Hypothermia in cold water drowning

ADDITIONAL READING
- American Academy of Pediatrics Committee on Injury, Violence, and Poison Prevention. Prevention of drowning. *Pediatr.* 2010;126(1):178–185.
- Hwang V, Shofer FS, Durbin DR, et al. Prevalence of traumatic injuries in drowning and near drowning in children and adolescents. *Arch Pediatr Adolesc Med.* 2003;157:50–53.
- Meyer RJ, Theodorou AA, Berg RA: Childhood drowning. *Pediatr Rev.* 2006;27(5):163–168.
- Noonan L, Howrey R, Ginsburg CM: Freshwater submersion injuries in children: A retrospective review of seventy-five hospitalized patients. *Pediatrics.* 1996;98(3):368–371.
- Papa L, Hoelle R, Idris A. Systematic review of definitions for drowning incidents. *Resuscitation.* 2005;65(3):255–264.
- Thompson DC, Rivara F. Pool fencing for preventing drowning of children. *Cochrane Database Syst Rev.* 2010:CD001047.

CODES

ICD9
994.1 Drowning and nonfatal submersion

ICD10
- T75.1XXA Unsp effects of drowning and nonfatal submersion, init
- T75.1XXD Unsp effects of drowning and nonfatal submersion, subs
- T75.1XXS Unsp effects of drowning and nonfatal submersion, sequela

FAQ
- Q: Should the drowning victim who arrives at the hospital with cardiopulmonary arrest be resuscitated?
- A: Yes, a brief (10–15 minutes) attempt at resuscitation is indicated until circumstances of the drowning and core temperature are known. Warm-water drowning victims who require CPR in the emergency department may rarely (0–25%) have good neurologic recovery, but these patients usually respond quickly (<15 minutes) to therapy.
- Q: Is artificial surfactant useful in drowning victims?
- A: Although useful in neonates, surfactant has not been found to be beneficial for acute lung injury. Further investigation is needed before it can be recommended for clinical use.

DYSFUNCTIONAL UTERINE BLEEDING

Leonard J. Levine
Jonathan R. Pletcher

 BASICS

DESCRIPTION
- Bleeding beyond the range of normal menses, with "normal" defined as duration of 2–8 days, occurring every 21–40 days, with blood loss of 20–80 mL/cycle
- May vary in presentation from heavy, long menses followed by long periods of amenorrhea to short, heavy menses occurring every 1–2 weeks
- Most commonly results from anovulatory cycles, which are secondary to an immature hypothalamic–pituitary–ovarian axis

EPIDEMIOLOGY
- Most commonly occurs within the first 2 years of menarche when >50% of cycles are anovulatory
- Later age at menarche results in longer duration of anovulation
- Most females who experience anovulatory cycles do not develop dysfunctional uterine bleeding (DUB).

RISK FACTORS
Genetics
- Familial history of anovulatory cycles is common.
- Patients with disorders, such as blood dyscrasias and polycystic ovary syndrome (PCOS), usually have familial histories including these disorders.

PATHOPHYSIOLOGY
- In most cases presenting within 2 years of menarche, anovulation (failure to ovulate) results in absence of the corpus luteum. Without the secretory effect of progesterone from the corpus luteum, endometrial proliferation continues because of unopposed estrogen.
- The thickened endometrium eventually outgrows support from the basal endometrium, resulting in sloughing of the highest endometrial levels. Alternatively, cyclic estrogen withdrawal may occur, which will lead to sloughing of the endometrium in the absence of progesterone.
- As subsequent levels of endometrium are shed, bleeding increases. Profuse bleeding may result when the basal endometrium is exposed.

DIAGNOSIS

HISTORY
- Abnormal bleeding:
  - Assessing the amount and site of bleeding will help determine the nature and extent of the problem.
  - Important to know when bleeding began and how much bleeding has occurred to know if the patient is at risk for hemodynamic instability
- The pattern of DUB in relation to the menstrual cycle can help guide the diagnostic workup:
  - Normal cyclic intervals with increased bleeding during each cycle may suggest a bleeding disorder.
  - Normal intervals with bleeding between cycles may suggest infection or foreign body.
  - Abnormal intervals with no cycle regularity may suggest anovulatory cycles, endocrinopathy, or hormonal contraception.
- Cramping suggests ovulation and the presence of progesterone; anovulatory cycles are thus less likely.
- Increased time lapse between menarche and onset of DUB lessens the likelihood of anovulatory cycles.
- Easy bruisability, epistaxis, and/or bleeding gums may be suggestive of a bleeding disorder.
- A family history of thyroid disease, bleeding disorder, PCOS, or DUB will help guide the laboratory workup.
- Ask about sexual abuse when conducting the sexual history. Sexual abuse not only may result in bleeding from trauma but also may be a source of sexually transmitted diseases and pregnancy.

PHYSICAL EXAM
- Often normal in patients with DUB
- Assess vital signs, including orthostatic BPs, for signs of cardiac instability resulting from severe blood loss.
- Skin or mucosal pallor, elevated heart rate, or flow murmur may be indicative of anemic state.
- Assess sexual maturity rating (SMR, or Tanner stage). Menarche usually does not occur before SMR 3, so bleeding before this stage suggests a nonmenstrual source of bleeding.
- Look for signs of androgen excess (e.g., hirsutism, acne), which may be reflective of disrupted ovulatory function.
- Bitemporal hemianopsia is suggestive of a pituitary adenoma leading to hyperprolactinemia. Only 1/3 of adolescents with hyperprolactinemia will experience galactorrhea.
- Assess for evidence of thyroid disease, hematologic disorder (e.g., bruising, petechiae), or systemic disease (e.g., poor nutritional status).
- Speculum-assisted pelvic examination may help determine source of bleeding. Bimanual examination is helpful in assessing ovarian or uterine masses, cervical motion or adnexal tenderness, and uterine sizing.

DIAGNOSTIC TESTS & INTERPRETATION
Lab
- Obtain urine or serum-human chorionic gonadotropin (β-HCG), regardless of sexual history. Urine-HCG testing can reliably detect pregnancy as early as 2 weeks postconception; however, it may be positive for up to 2 weeks following an abortion.
- CBC: Degree of anemia guides treatment plan. Assess for thrombocytopenia. In the setting of acute blood loss, a normal hemoglobin may be falsely reassuring. It is wise to recheck hemoglobin after IV hydration as decreases may be dramatic.
- For *Chlamydia trachomatis* and *Neisseria gonorrhoeae*, obtain cervical cultures or use nucleic acid amplification tests (e.g., PCR or LCR) on urine, vaginal, or cervical swabs. Be careful to check with laboratory or NAAT manufacturers' information as to reliability with blood in sample and based on collection site.
- Wet mount or vaginal swab may be unreliable but should be attempted for presence of WBCs and trichomonas. In some labs *Trichomonas vaginalis* antigen tests may be available.
- Consider prolactin level and thyroid function tests: Hyperprolactinemia may have several causes, including pituitary microadenoma, and result in amenorrhea or DUB.
- Prothrombin and partial thromboplastin time, von Willebrand factor: To assess for hematologic causes of bleeding
- Androgen levels, including testosterone (total and free); dehydroepiandrosterone sulfate (DHEAS); androstenedione: Abnormal levels are supportive of PCOS or other hyperandrogenic state.

Imaging
- Pelvic ultrasound:
  - Indicated when pregnancy is suspected (ectopic or intrauterine)
  - Consider when a pelvic mass is felt, uterine anomaly is being considered, or bimanual examination cannot be completed.
- MRI of the pelvis: Indicated for patients with a suspected pelvic mass when ultrasonography does not clearly define the anatomy

DIFFERENTIAL DIAGNOSIS
~80% of abnormal uterine bleeding in adolescents can be attributed to anovulatory cycles. However, it is important to rule out other causes of irregular or heavy vaginal bleeding.

- Pregnancy: Should be considered and ruled out in every patient, regardless of patient's reported sexual history
  - Ectopic pregnancy
  - Threatened abortion, incomplete abortion
  - Placenta previa
  - Hydatidiform mole
- Infection:
  - Vaginitis (e.g., trichomoniasis)
  - Cervicitis or endometritis (e.g., gonorrhea or chlamydia)
  - Pelvic inflammatory disease
- Hematologic conditions:
  - Bleeding disorders often present as heavy periods from time of menarche.
  - Thrombocytopenia (e.g., immune thrombocytopenic purpura [ITP], leukemia)
  - Platelet dysfunction
  - Coagulation defect (e.g., von Willebrand disease)
- Endocrinologic disorders:
  - Thyroid disease, especially hypothyroidism
  - Hyperprolactinemia
  - PCOS
  - Adrenal disorders
- Trauma: Laceration to vagina or cervix
- Foreign body: Usually associated with strong, foul odor

- Medications:
  - Direct effect on hemostasis (e.g., Coumadin, chemotherapeutic agents)
  - Hormonal effects (e.g., oral contraceptives, Depo-Provera)
- Systemic disease:
  - Disruption of hypothalamic–pituitary–ovarian axis
  - Other examples include systemic lupus erythematosus and chronic renal failure.
- Primary gynecologic disorders:
  - Endometriosis
  - Uterine polyps, submucosal myomas
  - Hemangioma, arteriovenous malformation

ALERT

Pitfalls:

- Neglecting to perform pregnancy testing in an adolescent who denies sexual activity
- Neglecting to reassess hemoglobin concentration after volume expansion
- Neglecting to consider a retained foreign body (e.g., tampon)
- Neglecting to provide both estrogen and progesterone in a timely fashion
- If there is a recurrent course of DUB, consider PCOS, thyroid disease, or other endocrinopathy.

 TREATMENT

ADDITIONAL TREATMENT
General Measures

- For mild DUB (inconvenient, unpredictable bleeding, and the patient has a normal hemoglobin in setting of hemodynamic stability):
  - Reassurance until ovulatory cycles resume. Encourage maintenance of a menstrual calendar, with follow-up in 3–6 months.
  - Iron supplementation
  - If inconvenience and anxiety are unresponsive to reassurance, hormonal therapy with a daily combined oral contraceptive pill (OCP), 1 tablet daily, should be considered to regulate menstrual cycle. If estrogen is contraindicated, may use progesterone-only pill, medroxyprogesterone acetate 10 mg/d PO for 10–14 days every month.
- For moderate DUB (irregular, prolonged, heavy bleeding with a hemoglobin >10 g/dL):
  - Hormonal therapy, as described previously. May start OCP containing 35 μg of ethinyl estradiol twice a day until bleeding stops, then taper to once a day.
  - Menstrual calendar with follow-up every 1–3 months
- For severe DUB (i.e., heavy, prolonged bleeding with a hemoglobin <10 g/dL), treatment depends on the presence of active bleeding:
  - If no active bleeding, hemodynamically stable patients can be started on daily OCPs and iron supplementation, with follow-up in 1–2 months.
  - In the presence of active bleeding: Hormonal therapy, using combined OCP containing higher dose of estrogen (50 mg ethinyl estradiol)—1 pill q.i.d. until bleeding stops, followed by pill taper (q.i.d. for 4 days, t.i.d. for 3 days, b.i.d. for 2 weeks, then 1 pill daily); switch to lower-dose pill

(30–35 mg) after taper complete—antiemetic therapy necessary for high doses of estrogen. Hospitalization of patient during treatment if severe anemia (hemoglobin <7 g/dL), if hemodynamically unstable, or compliance concerns. Blood transfusion as necessary. If patient is unstable and unable to tolerate oral pill regimen, can give IV conjugated estrogen q4h for 24 hours to stop bleeding. Add OCP with progesterone as soon as patient is able to tolerate oral regimen to prevent excessive withdrawal bleeding.
  - Iron supplementation
  - Dilation and curettage rarely necessary, although may be needed if hormonal therapy fails
- Possible side effects:
  - Estrogen, given in high doses, will cause nausea and/or vomiting. An appropriate antiemetic should be used for prophylaxis against these symptoms.
  - High-dose estrogen may have vascular side effects and should be used with caution in patients particularly at risk for vascular events (e.g., patients with a history of lupus, stroke, or thrombotic phenomena; and those who smoke cigarettes). In these cases, consult a gynecologist or adolescent medicine specialist for an alternative progesterone-only therapy.

IN-PATIENT CONSIDERATIONS
Initial Stabilization

If DUB is attributed to anovulatory cycles, or if a complete workup fails to yield a diagnosis, treatment is guided by the severity of DUB and the presence of active bleeding.

 ONGOING CARE

FOLLOW-UP RECOMMENDATIONS
Patient Monitoring

When to expect improvement:

- Bleeding usually tapers after the first few doses of hormone therapy.
- After 6–12 months, if patient does not wish to remain on OCPs, a trial off medication might reveal normal ovulatory cycles.

PROGNOSIS

DUB persists for 2 years in 60% of patients, 4 years in 50%, and up to 10 years in 30%.

COMPLICATIONS

Mild-to-severe anemia resulting from blood loss

ADDITIONAL READING

- Casablanca Y. Management of dysfunctional uterine bleeding. *Obstet Gynecol Clin N Am.* 2008;35: 219–234.
- LaCour DE, Long DN, Perlman SE. Dysfunctional uterine bleeding in adolescent females associated with endocrine causes and medical conditions. *J Pediatr Adolesc Gynecol.* 2010;23:62–70.
- Levine LJ, Catallozzi M, Schwarz DF. An adolescent with vaginal bleeding. *Pediatr Case Rev.* 2003; 3:83–90.
- Rimsza ME. Dysfunctional uterine bleeding. *Pediatr Rev.* 2002;23:227–233 [erratum appears in *Pediatr Rev.* 2002;23].

 CODES

ICD9

- 626.2 Excessive or frequent menstruation
- 626.4 Irregular menstrual cycle
- 626.6 Metrorrhagia

ICD10

- N92.0 Excessive and frequent menstruation with regular cycle
- N93.8 Other specified abnormal uterine and vaginal bleeding
- N93.9 Abnormal uterine and vaginal bleeding, unspecified

FAQ

- Q: If most girls have anovulatory cycles, why do only some present with DUB?
- A: Most girls do have an irregular menstrual cycle during the first 2 years after menarche. However, in most of those girls, the negative-feedback system of estrogen will lead to cyclic endometrial shedding in an anovulatory pattern.
- Q: If DUB from anovulatory cycles is caused by lack of progesterone, why does the initial treatment of severe DUB with active bleeding involve large doses of estrogen?
- A: Estrogen has procoagulation effects that promote hemostasis (e.g., effects on platelet aggregation and levels of fibrinogen and clotting factors). In addition, severe DUB may lead to an exposed endometrial base that bleeds profusely; for progesterone to exhibit its secretory effects, the endometrium in that area must be restored by estrogen.
- Q: When hormonal therapy fails, and the basal endometrium continues to bleed, how does a dilation and curettage act as the final treatment?
- A: The curettage removes any remaining bleeding vessels and stimulates local prostaglandins to create a uterine contracture that inhibits bleeding. This is rarely needed in adolescent patients, as they usually respond to hormonal therapy.

D

DYSMENORRHEA

Esther K. Chung
Marney Gundlach (5th edition)

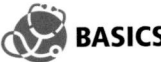

BASICS

DESCRIPTION
Painful menses, usually presenting as cramping pain in the lower abdomen or back:
- Primary dysmenorrhea—in absence of any hormonal or pelvic disease
- Secondary dysmenorrhea—due to hormonal or pelvic disease, most commonly endometriosis

EPIDEMIOLOGY
- Primary dysmenorrhea
  - Typically begins in adolescence; prevalence rates decrease progressively after age 24 years.
  - Less common in the first 2–3 years following menarche; more prevalent in mid- to late-adolescence when cycles are ovulatory.
- Secondary dysmenorrhea is less common in adolescence, and more common in adults.

Prevalence
- Affects up to 90% of adolescents
- 15% of adolescents report that the pain is "severe"

RISK FACTORS
- Young age (<20 years)
- Family history of dysmenorrhea
- Early menarche
- Menorrhagia (heavy menstrual flow)
- Nulliparity
- Smoking
- Long menstrual periods
- Alcohol use
- Depression
- Anxiety

Genetics
- Dysmenorrhea is more common in patients with a positive family history.
- Certain polymorphisms are associated with higher rates of dysmenorrhea.

PATHOPHYSIOLOGY
- Ovulation leads to increased progesterone release in the second half of the menstrual cycle. Progesterone levels fall prior to menstruation, increasing prostaglandin (PG) synthesis.
  - After menarche, anovulatory cycles are common; dysmenorrhea is typically absent in the first few cycles.
- Endometrial PGs cause uterine contractions, increased uterine muscle tone, and blood vessel constriction, resulting in hypoxia, ischemia, and pain.
  - PGF_{2alpha} is thought to stimulate the myometrium and cause vasoconstriction. Severity of dysmenorrhea is directly proportional to endometrial PGF_{2alpha} concentrations.
  - PGs can stimulate the GI tract, causing nausea, diarrhea, and vomiting.
- Leukotrienes are thought to increase uterine pain fiber sensitivity, vasoconstriction, and cause uterine hypercontractility. Leukotrienes are elevated among women with dysmenorrhea.
- Vasopressin, also elevated among women with dysmenorrhea, may play a secondary role by potentiating uterine contractions and ischemic pain.

- Women may have increased uterine basal tone, elevated pressures during contractions, increased frequency of contractions, and uncoordinated contractions. Any combination of these may lead to poor reperfusion and oxygenation, leading to pain.

DIAGNOSIS

- Primary dysmenorrhea: Painful, often spasmodic cramps in the lower abdomen or back, of varying severity, starting hours to a few days prior to menses lasting up to 2–3 days after the start of menses. Pain is strongest in intensity initially, waning by the end of menses. Referred pain to lower back or thighs may occur.
- Secondary dysmenorrhea: May present with similar pain and symptoms but starts 1–2 weeks earlier in the cycle, and often lasts through the entire menses.

HISTORY
- Given the high prevalence, screen all adolescent females for dysmenorrhea; <15% will seek medical attention.
- Pain: Ask about quality and intensity of pain (use pain scales); constant or intermittent occurrence; location; onset, timing, and duration; aggravating or alleviating factors; extent to which the pain limits activities (social, school, sports, work).
- Menstrual:
  - Age at menarche: More common in girls with earlier menarche (more time to progress to ovulatory cycles)
  - Menstrual flow: More common in women with heavy menstrual flow (menorrhagia)
  - Last menstrual period (and previous one, if known)
  - Length of menstrual flow and total cycles
  - Cycle regularity
  - Amount of menstrual flow
- Sexual history: Parity, current sexual activity, contraception, and history of STDs or pelvic inflammatory disease (PID). Adhesions may cause painful menses.
- Associated symptoms: Missing school; nausea, vomiting, diarrhea, headache, irritability, fatigue, breast tenderness, dizziness, weakness, or bloating
- History of sexual, physical, or emotional abuse
- Family history of GYN diseases, including dysmenorrhea, GYN or breast cancer, and complications with oral contraceptive pills (OCPs) including deep vein thrombosis (DVT), stroke, or myocardial infarction
- Medications (including OCPs) including name, dose, when taken in relation to pain, if scheduled or taken as needed, perceived effectiveness
- Diet: Higher intake of polyunsaturated fatty acids correlates with increased menstrual pain.

ALERT
- Pain that started at menarche is not likely primary dysmenorrhea, as most girls are still having anovulatory cycles.
- Progressively worsening pain with each subsequent cycle may indicate endometriosis.
- Cigarette smoking may increase the duration of dysmenorrhea.

PHYSICAL EXAM
- Abdominal exam:
  - Lower abdomen/suprapubic pain
  - Periumbilical pain suggests a GI, not a GYN, source.
  - Enlarged uterus can be palpated in vaginal outlet obstruction.
- Inspection of external genitalia
- Imperforate hymen/hematocolpos
- Pelvic exam:
  - Typically normal in primary dysmenorrhea; may have mild diffuse uterine tenderness
  - Consider deferring in younger girls with mild, classic symptoms and normal external genitalia who have never been sexually active
  - Perform in women with history suggesting secondary dysmenorrhea, a history of sexual intercourse, and those who need a Pap smear, or who have failed NSAIDs

DIAGNOSTIC TESTS & INTERPRETATION
- Lab studies are generally not warranted.
- Consider testing for STIs, pregnancy, PID, or inflammatory bowel disease (IBD) as indicated by history and physical exam.

Imaging
- Consider ultrasound (US) for patients who fail a trial of NSAIDs. US can rule out genital tract abnormalities, ovarian pathologies, or obstructive lesions.
- Transvaginal US provides better images of pelvic anatomy:
  - Discuss the expectations, especially with teens who have never been sexually active or ever used tampons.

Diagnostic Procedures/Other
Consider laparoscopy to establish the diagnosis for patients with adnexal or cul-de-sac pelvic tenderness, first-degree relative with endometriosis, persistent pain despite treatment with NSAIDs and OCPs, significant disability due to pain, or plans for another surgical procedure

DIFFERENTIAL DIAGNOSIS
Primary dysmenorrhea is a diagnosis of exclusion; secondary dysmenorrhea should be ruled out based on history and physical exam, and imaging if warranted.

- Genital: Adenomyosis, congenital vaginal or uterine anomalies, ectopic pregnancy, endometriosis, Mittelschmerz, ovarian cysts or tumors, pelvic adhesions, PID, uterine adhesions, fibroids, or polyps
- GI: Constipation, diverticulitis, IBD, irritable bowel syndrome (IBS)
- Urologic: Interstitial cystitis, kidney stones, urinary tract infection
- Neurologic: Fibromyalgia, herniated disk, lower back pain

TREATMENT

MEDICATION (DRUGS)

First Line

- NSAIDs: PG synthetase (cyclo-oxygenase) inhibitors. In randomized controlled trials (RCTs), NSAIDs are superior to placebo at relieving pain and reducing activity restrictions and school/work absenteeism. Ibuprofen, naproxen sodium, and mefenamic acid are considered to be effective.
- If a patient fails to respond to the first choice at a therapeutic level, try a different NSAID.
- 90% of patients have relief with proper dosing.
- Most effective when used on a regular and not PRN basis for the first 2–3 days of menses
- Start 1 day prior or at the onset of menses
- Choices:
  - Ibuprofen: 400–600 mg PO q6–8h
  - Naproxen: 500 mg PO then 250 mg PO q6–8h
  - Mefenamic acid: 500 mg PO then 250 mg PO t.i.d.; approved for children ≥14 years
- Side effects:
  - Black-box warnings: Increased risk of adverse cardiovascular events, including myocardial infarction, stroke, and new onset or worsening of pre-existing hypertension; increased risk of GI irritation, ulceration, bleeding, and perforation
  - Other side effects include drowsiness, dizziness, headache, mouth dryness, nausea, and indigestion.

Second Line

- OCPs:
  - OCPs suppress ovulation and decrease uterine PG secretion following reduction in progesterone levels.
  - OCPs with medium-dose estrogen (~35 mcg) and first- or second-generation progestogens (levonorgestrel, norethisterone, norgestrel) are more effective than placebo at pain relief and reducing school/work absenteeism. There are few studies on lower dose estrogen and newer progestin formulations.
  - Patients may need 3 months to see improvement. Patients with improvement are more likely to be compliant with OCPs.
  - Good choice for patients who fail NSAIDs as monotherapy, desire pregnancy prevention, or who have acne
  - Extended cycling OCPs: Can prescribe Seasonale (91-day cycle) or use multiple OCP packs to achieve same effect
  - Side effects:
    - Nausea, vomiting, breast tenderness, weight gain, break-through menstrual bleeding, headaches from the estrogen
    - Acne, hirsutism, and depression from the progestogen
    - Rare: DVT, stroke, myocardial infarction
- Secondary dysmenorrhea is treated by addressing the underlying cause.

ISSUES FOR REFERRAL

Consider referral to adolescent gynecologist for consideration of laparoscopy or management of endometriosis, including gonadotropin-releasing hormone (GnRH) agonist treatment

COMPLEMENTARY & ALTERNATIVE THERAPIES

- Stronger evidence exists for:
  - Vitamin B1:
    - Vitamin B1 deficiency can cause muscle cramps, fatigue, and decreased pain tolerance.
    - 100 mg/d PO shown in a single large RCT to be effective at reducing pain
  - Magnesium:
    - Thought to inhibit synthesis of PGF_{2alpha}, promote vasodilation and muscle relaxation
    - May reduce pain and need for additional medication
    - No consistent dose used in studies; consider 500 mg/d PO
  - Transcutaneous electrical nerve stimulation (TENS): Electrodes on the skin stimulate nerves at different current frequencies and intensities. Thought to alter pain perception, rather than to directly affect uterine contractions.
    - High-frequency TENS (low-intensity pulses at a frequency of 50–120 Hz): Effective at pain relief compared to placebo (but not at reducing need for analgesics); not superior to ibuprofen.
    - Low-frequency TENS is no more effective than placebo.
    - Side effects: Headaches, muscle twitches, and localized redness, burning, or pain
- According to a recent Cochrane review, acupuncture may reduce pain in primary dysmenorrhea.
- Exercise may help to reduce symptoms of dysmenorrhea but more research is needed.
- Weaker evidence exists for Vitamin B6, fish oil, and vitamin E. No evidence exists for spinal manipulation, biofeedback, black cohosh, fennel oil, or evening primrose oil.

SURGERY/OTHER PROCEDURES

Laparoscopy may be used as treatment for primary dysmenorrhea:

- Laparoscopic uterine nerve ablation (LUNA) is effective for long-term (≥12 month) pain relief in primary dysmenorrhea.
- Laparoscopic presacral neurectomy is more effective than LUNA for pain relief at ≥6 months follow-up but has significant side effects (especially constipation); should only be performed with pelvic laparoscopic surgeons with special training.

ALERT

There are a number of OTC medicines that are marketed for treating cramps in women. Only those formulations that contain NSAIDs are effective in treating dysmenorrhea. Encourage patients to read labels looking for medications containing ibuprofen or naproxen.

ONGOING CARE

PATIENT EDUCATION

- Stress to patients the importance of keeping a pain diary indicating days of menses, days of pain, pain ratings (0–10 scale), days of limited activities (school or work) due to pain, and associated symptoms.
- Websites for Patient Education Materials:
  - ACOG. Dysmenorrhea. http://www.acog.org/~/media/For%20Patients/faq046.pdf?dmc=1&ts=20120215T1659240616
  - ACOG. Chronic pelvic pain. http://www.acog.org/~/media/For%20Patients/faq099.pdf?dmc=1&ts=20120215T1700537765

PROGNOSIS

Improvement in symptoms may occur after child birth.

COMPLICATIONS

Missed school or work; decreased academic performance, sports participation, and peer socialization

ADDITIONAL READING

- Adams Hillard PJ. Consultation with the specialist: Dysmenorrhea. *Pediatr Rev.* 2006;27:64–71.
- Dawood MY. Primary dysmenorrhea: Advances in pathogenesis and management. *Obstet Gynecol.* 2006;108:428–441.
- Harel Z. Dysmenorrhea in adolescents. *Ann N Y Acad Sci.* 2008;1135:185–195.
- Mannix LK. Menstrual-related pain conditions: Dysmenorrhea and migraine. *J Women Health.* 2008;17:879–891.
- Marjoribanks J, Proctor ML, Farquhar C. Nonsteroidal anti-inflammatory drugs for primary dysmenorrhoea. *Cochrane Database Syst Rev.* 2003;4:CD001751.
- Proctor ML, Murphy PA. Herbal and dietary therapies for primary and secondary dysmenorrhoea. *Cochrane Database Syst Rev.* 2001;2:CD002124.
- Proctor ML, Roberts H, Farquhar CM. Combined oral contraceptive pill (OCP) as treatment for primary dysmenorrhoea. *Cochrane Database Syst Rev.* 2001;2:CD002120.
- Smith CA, Zhu X, He L, et al. Acupuncture for primary dysmenorrheal. *Cochrane Database Syst Rev.* 2011;1:CD007854.

CODES

ICD9

625.3 Dysmenorrhea

ICD10

- N94.4 Primary dysmenorrhea
- N94.5 Secondary dysmenorrhea
- N94.6 Dysmenorrhea, unspecified

FAQ

- Q: What percentage of patients report dysmenorrhea?
- A: Although dysmenorrhea affects up to 90% of adolescents, <15% will seek medical care. It is important to screen all adolescent women for dysmenorrhea. Barriers for seeking physician advice include fears of pelvic exam, lack of knowledge of effective treatments, and confidence in home remedies.

DYSPNEA
Charles Schwartz

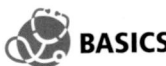 **BASICS**

DEFINITION
Shortness of breath. A subjective feeling of having difficulty breathing.

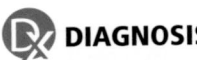 **DIAGNOSIS**

DIFFERENTIAL DIAGNOSIS
- **Congenital**
  - Subglottic stenosis
  - Vocal cord paralysis
  - Macroglossia
  - Pierre Robin sequence
  - Laryngeal atresia
  - Pulmonary sequestration
  - Pulmonary hypoplasia
- **Infectious**
  - Lower airway: Bronchiolitis, pertussis, pneumonia, tuberculosis
  - Upper airway: Croup, epiglottitis, tracheitis, peritonsillar abscess
- **Toxic, environmental, drugs: Aspiration**
  - Fluid
  - Foreign body
  - Carbon monoxide poisoning
  - Methemoglobinemia
  - Smoke inhalation
- **Tumors/cysts**
  - Head/neck: Dermoid cysts, branchial cleft cysts, lingual thyroid, hemangioma, teratoma, papilloma, brainstem tumor
  - Thoracic: Teratoma, cystic hygroma, bronchogenic cyst, pericardial cyst, neurogenic tumor, lymphoma, leukemia
  - Abdominal mass: Hepatic mass, hepatoblastoma, neuroblastoma
- **Allergy: Anaphylaxis**
- **Pulmonary**
  - Asthma
  - Atelectasis
  - Pneumothorax
  - Pleural effusion
  - Hemorrhage
  - Embolism
- **Cardiac**
  - Pulmonary edema

- **Renal**
  - Renal failure causing fluid overload
  - Metabolic acidosis
- **Hematologic**
  - Anemia
  - Sickle cell crisis/acute chest syndrome
- **Muscle weakness**
  - Duchenne muscular dystrophy
  - Spinal muscle atrophy
- **Miscellaneous**
  - High altitude
  - Exercise
  - Psychogenic hyperventilation
  - Anxiety/panic disorders

ALERT
In a child who presents with dyspnea, anxiety or panic disorder should be considered only after the more serious causes have been ruled out.

APPROACH TO THE PATIENT
General goal is to identify the organ system responsible for the dyspnea and to determine whether the process is acute or chronic:
- **Phase 1:** Determine if the cause is respiratory or cardiac in nature. If it is 1 of these 2, is the patient clinically stable and can he or she protect his or her airway? It is important to identify those who will need intensive/emergency care and those who can be worked up in the office.
- **Phase 2:** Inquire about the duration of symptoms and the circumstances around the onset of the dyspnea. History and physical exam should focus on respiratory and cardiology. If these 2 have been ruled out, other causes must be evaluated.
- **Phase 3:** Inquire about other medical problems of the patient.

HISTORY
- **Question:** Onset of dyspnea and what the patient was doing at the time of onset (if acute)?
- *Significance:*
  - In a small child, acute onset may be related to aspiration of a foreign body or liquid.
  - If the patient was unsupervised, foreign body is a high probability.
  - If the dyspnea occurred over days, other respiratory, cardiac, or renal causes should be suspected.

- **Question:** Any fever, cough, chest pain, or runny nose?
- *Significance:* Suggests an infectious cause. Chest pain could be related to a pneumothorax, which may occur spontaneously in some individuals.
- **Question:** Anyone at home who is sick or has respiratory problems/illness?
- *Significance:* Leads toward infection; however, in some cases of congenital heart disease, a respiratory virus such as respiratory syncytial virus can make an otherwise stable patient into a critically ill child.
- **Question:** Children who have a history of wheezing or asthma?
- *Significance:* Likely to re-exacerbate their lung disease
- **Question:** Children who have been hospitalized for respiratory problems in the past?
- *Significance:* Likely to have subsequent difficulty with other respiratory problems
- **Question:** Has the patient ever been diagnosed with a murmur or has a history of cardiac problems?
- *Significance:* In the absence of an infectious type or wheezing type of history, it may help the examiner focus on the cardiac exam.

PHYSICAL EXAM
Lungs
- **Finding:** Crackles or rhonchi on auscultation?
- *Significance:* Lower lung disease such as pneumonia or bronchiolitis. Fluid overload may cause bilateral crackles.
- **Finding:** Wheezing on auscultation?
- *Significance:* Usually heard on expiration; suggests an obstructive lung disease such as asthma or reactive airways disease, or anaphylaxis.
- **Finding:** Distant or absent breath sounds?
- *Significance:* Foreign body aspiration blocking air movement. Pneumothorax should also be suspected.
- **Finding:** Barking cough?
- *Significance:* Croup is usually cased by parainfluenza virus.
- **Finding:** Symptoms worse in supine position?
- *Significance:* May be secondary to pulmonary edema or compression by a mediastinal mass.
- **Finding:** Egophony on auscultation?
- *Significance:* Suspect pleural effusion

Heart

- **Finding:** Loud murmur or gallop on auscultation?
- *Significance*: Cardiac disease in which pulmonary edema may be cause of the dyspnea
- **Finding:** Cyanosis?
- *Significance*: Poor oxygen perfusion
- **Finding:** Low BP and poor skin perfusion?
- *Significance*: The patient may be in shock. Quick identification of the type of shock is needed to correct the underlying problem.
- **Finding:** Clubbing of the digits?
- *Significance*: Suggests chronic disease such as cystic fibrosis or cardiac disease
- **Finding:** Drooling with mouth open in an ill-appearing child?
- *Significance*: Suggests epiglottitis and need for careful evaluation (see "Epiglottitis")
- **Finding:** Abdominal mass palpated?
- *Significance*: May cause compression of lungs
- **Finding:** Ascites or edema?
- *Significance*: Fluid overload from either renal or cardiac cause.

DIAGNOSTIC TESTS & INTERPRETATION

- **Test:** Arterial blood gases
- *Significance*:
  - More detailed assessment of oxygenation and acidosis
  - Delineates metabolic vs. respiratory acidosis
  - May show if compensation has occurred
- **Test:** CBC with differential
- *Significance*:
  - Elevated WBC count with a left shift differential may be a sign of infection.
  - If the patient has pallor, evaluate the hemoglobin to see if the patient is anemic.
  - May be helpful in patients in whom leukemia or other oncologic diseases are suspected
- **Test:** Mantoux test with purified protein derivative
- *Significance*: Include with anergy panel for patients with family history of tuberculosis or who are immigrants from countries where tuberculosis is prevalent
- **Test:** Pulse oximetry
- *Significance*: Rapid assessment of oxygen perfusion

Imaging
Chest radiograph

- Look for appearance of the lung fields for the different types of pneumonia
- Evaluate heart size and pulmonary vascularity for fluid overload
- Hyperinflation suggests an obstructive pulmonary disease such as asthma. A hyperinflated (usually right lobe), darkened lobe is suspicious for foreign body.
- A shift in the heart and presence of a lung edge are common in pneumothorax or effusion.
- Fluid in the costophrenic angle suggests an effusion.

 TREATMENT

ADDITIONAL TREATMENT
General Measures
If hyperventilation is suspected, having the patient breathe into a brown paper bag can be useful in breaking the cycle of hypocarbia.

ISSUES FOR REFERRAL
- Unstable vital signs, inability to oxygenate, and need for critical care services
- Suspected foreign body aspiration; needs a surgical consultation for bronchoscopy
- If asthma is suspected, use criteria in the chapter on asthma.
- Patients with epiglottitis need an otolaryngologist to evaluate the patient under general anesthesia (see "Epiglottitis").
- Suspected oncologic process: Referral to a tertiary care center with a critical care unit staffed by a pediatric oncologist (see "Leukemia")

SURGERY/OTHER PROCEDURES
Patients with pneumothorax may need surgical aspiration or chest tube placement.

Initial Stabilization
Anaphylaxis is a medical emergency and mandates immediate action. Epinephrine, Benadryl, and possibly steroids are the drugs of choice for treatment.

ADDITIONAL READING

- Adinoff A. Obesity is a risk factor for dyspnea but not for airflow obstruction. *Pediatrics*. 2003;112:473–474.
- Denny FW. Acute respiratory infections in children: Etiology and epidemiology. *Pediatr Rev*. 1987;9:135–146.
- Gaston B. Pneumonia. *Pediatr Rev*. 2002;23:132–140.
- Holroyd HJ. Foreign body aspiration: Potential cause of coughing and wheezing. *Pediatr Rev*. 1988;10:59–63.
- Lasley M. New treatments for asthma. *Pediatr Rev*. 2003;24:222–232.
- McIntosh K. Respiratory syncytial virus infections in infants and children: Diagnosis and treatment. *Pediatr Rev*. 1987;9:191–196.

- McIntosh K. Community-acquired pneumonia in children. *N Engl J Med*. 2002;346(6):429–437.
- Rocha G. Pleural effusions in the neonate. *Curr Opin Pulm Med*. 2007;13(4):305–311.
- Segal GB. Anemia. *Pediatr Rev*. 1988;10:77–88.
- Skolnick H. Exercise-induced dyspnea in children and adolescents: If not asthma then what? *Pediatrics*. 2006;118:S35–S36.
- Tan Q, Mason EO, Wald ER, et al. Clinical characteristics of children with complicated pneumonia caused by streptococcus pneumoniae. *Pediatrics*. 2002;110:1–6.

 CODES

ICD9
- 478.5 Other diseases of vocal cords
- 748.3 Other anomalies of larynx, trachea, and bronchus
- 786.09 Other respiratory abnormalities

ICD10
- J38.00 Paralysis of vocal cords and larynx, unspecified
- Q31.1 Congenital subglottic stenosis
- R06.00 Dyspnea, unspecified

FAQ

- Q: In most cases, is dyspnea pulmonary in nature?
- A: Yes, it is in most cases. However, if infectious, foreign body, and asthma causes are ruled out, nonrespiratory causes must be investigated.

D

DYSURIA

Rebecca Ruebner
Lawrence Copelovitch

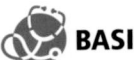

BASICS

DEFINITION
Painful urination

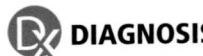

DIAGNOSIS

DIFFERENTIAL DIAGNOSIS
- **Congenital/anatomic**
  - Meatal stenosis
  - Urethral stricture
  - Posterior urethral diverticula
  - Urethral stones
  - Vesicovaginal fistula
- **Infectious**
  - Viral infection
  - Gonorrhea
  - Chlamydia
  - Herpes simplex
  - Tuberculosis
  - Cystitis
  - Candidiasis
  - Urethritis
  - Pinworms
  - Prostatitis
- **Toxic, environmental, drugs**
  - Bubble bath urethritis
  - Spermicides, douches
  - Cytoxan
- **Trauma**
  - Diaper dermatitis
  - Foreign body
  - Bicycle injury
  - Masturbation
  - Sexual abuse
  - Irritation, e.g., from sand, tight pants
- **Tumor**
  - Sarcoma botryoides
- **Genetic/metabolic**
  - Cystinuria
- **Allergic/inflammatory**
  - Food allergy
  - Stevens–Johnson syndrome
  - Contact dermatitis, e.g., poison ivy
- **Functional**
  - Attention mechanism
- **Miscellaneous**
  - Appendicitis

APPROACH TO THE PATIENT
General goal: Determine the cause and begin treatment.
- **Phase 1:** Rule out common causes such as trauma, infection, chemical irritant, constipation, and masturbation.
- **Phase 2:** Continue investigation—look for congenital or acquired problems that cause infection, strictures, or calculi.
- **Phase 3:** Begin treatment.

Hints for Screening Problems
- Ask about medications and food allergies.
- Ask about special situations, e.g., sand in bathing suit causing irritation.

HISTORY
- **Question:** Do the symptoms occur any special time of day?
- *Significance:* May indicate an attention mechanism if occurs before school
- **Question:** What kinds of medication do you take?
- *Significance:* Some medications, e.g., Cytoxan, may cause irritation of the urethra.
- **Question:** Have there been any new foods or known food allergens?
- *Significance:* Milk and citrus fruits may cause dysuria in certain patients. Best to determine whether symptoms regress on elimination of possible offending food.
- **Question:** Do you use bubble bath?
- *Significance:* Bubble bath may deplete the protective lipids in the urethra.
- **Question:** Any signs of bleeding?
- *Significance:* May indicate trauma, infection, or congenital anomalies. Calcium excretion may cause dysuria as well as hematuria.
- Use of spermicides or douches
- Family history of kidney stones
- **Question:** Fever?
- *Significance:* Fever is a common sign of urinary tract infection (UTI).
- **Question:** Frequency?
- *Significance:* Both frequency and dysuria are common findings in UTIs.
- **Question:** Past history of urologic operations?
- *Significance:* Antireflux surgery may have a side effect of dysuria.
- **Question:** What have you taken for discomfort?
- *Significance:* Although cranberry juice is used for many urinary problems, the volume needed is usually more than what can be easily ingested.
- **Question:** Quality and strength of the urinary stream?
- *Significance:* Patients with posterior urethral valves have small, frequent voidings, with low pressure because of the obstruction in the posterior urethra.
- **Question:** Sexual activity?
- *Significance:* Urethritis from gonorrhea or chlamydia

PHYSICAL EXAM
- **Finding:** Any signs of redness or ecchymoses?
- *Significance:* May indicate trauma from masturbation or abuse
- **Finding:** Any bleeding?
- *Significance:* Seen in trauma, tumors, and infection

- **Finding:** Any change in behavior?
- *Significance:* May be an attention-seeking device
- **Finding:** Abnormal swelling?
- Significance: May occur in trauma or rare tumors
- **Finding:** Abnormal urethra?
- *Significance:* Prolapsed urethra or diverticula
- **Finding:** Grapelike structures in vagina?
- *Significance:* Sarcoma botryoides
- **Finding:** Abdominal pain?
- *Significance:* Intra-abdominal abscess or low-lying inflamed appendix may cause dysuria.

DIAGNOSTIC TESTS & INTERPRETATION
Lab
- **Test:** Urinalysis
- *Significance:* In most UTIs, there are WBCs in the urine.
- **Test:** Urine culture
- *Significance:* Check for infection
- **Test:** Metabolic screens
- *Significance:* If sediment shows crystals or if familial history of metabolic disease
- **Test:** Urinary screen for gonorrhea and chlamydia
- *Significance:* DNA amplification by polymerase or ligase chain reaction on freshly voided urine has 95% sensitivity and 100% specificity.

Imaging
Ultrasound: Not routinely requested unless a congenital anomaly is suspected

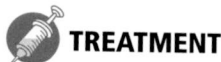 **TREATMENT**

ADDITIONAL TREATMENT
General Measures
- See treatment of UTI, vaginitis, urethritis
- Phenazopyridine (Pyridium) may be used for symptomatic relief while documenting cause of dysuria.
- Warm water sitz baths may be helpful for symptomatic treatment.

ISSUES FOR REFERRAL
- Evidence of congenital anomaly
- Increasing severity of symptoms
- Failure to respond to symptomatic or specific treatment

ADDITIONAL READING
- Claudius H. Dysuria in adolescents. *West J Med*. 2000;172:201–205.
- Hellerstein S, Linebarger JS. Voiding dysfunction in pediatric patients. *Clin Pediatr (Phila)*. 2003;42:43–49.
- Lee HJ, Pyo JW, Choi EH, et al. Isolation of adenovirus type from the urine of children with acute hemorrhagic cystitis. *Pediatr Infect Dis J*. 1996;15:633–634.
- Rushton HG. Urinary tract infections in children: Epidemiology, evaluation, and management. *Pediatr Clin North Am*. 1997;44:1133–1169.

 CODES

ICD9
- 598.9 Urethral stricture, unspecified
- 753.6 Atresia and stenosis of urethra and bladder neck
- 788.1 Dysuria

ICD10
- N35.9 Urethral stricture, unspecified
- Q64.39 Other atresia and stenosis of urethra and bladder neck
- R30.0 Dysuria

FAQ
- Q: How does bubble bath cause dysuria?
- A: The bubble bath depletes lipids that protect the urethra, causing the tissue to swell and become inflamed.
- Q: Can allergies cause dysuria?
- A: It is difficult to directly prove allergies as a cause of dysuria. However, in some cases, elimination of certain foods such as spices, citrus fruits, or known skin allergens has improved symptoms.
- Q: How do children get infected with gonorrhoea?
- A: This is a red flag for sexual abuse, which must be investigated.
- Q: Which viruses cause dysuria?
- A: Adenovirus has been identified.

CLINICAL PEARLS
- Sometimes difficult to differentiate dysuria from frequency, which may cause an uncomfortable feeling or pressure that is described by the child as pain.
- Discharge with dysuria suggests gonococcal or chlamydial infection.
- Low-lying inflamed appendix may cause bladder irritation and dysuria.
- Urethral prolapse may present as hematuria or frequency.

D

EARACHE
Vanessa S. Carlo

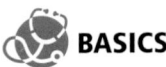

BASICS

DEFINITION
- Otalgia, classified as primary or secondary, means ear pain or an earache.
- Primary otalgia is ear pain that originates inside the ear, either from the external auditory canal or from the middle ear structures.
- Secondary (or referred) otalgia is ear pain that originates from outside of the ear. Any anatomic area that shares innervation with the ear can be the primary source of perceived ear pain.

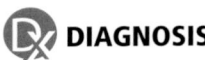

DIAGNOSIS

DIFFERENTIAL DIAGNOSIS
Primary otalgia:
- **Infectious**
  - Acute otitis media (AOM)—most common cause of otalgia in children
  - Otitis externa—inflammation of external auditory canal, usually associated with swimming and/or localized trauma; second most common cause of otalgia in children
  - Cellulitis of the auricle—usually caused by *Streptococcus pyogenes*; typically involves the earlobe
  - Perichondritis—inflammation of the auricle without earlobe involvement
  - Furunculosis—infection of the cartilaginous portion of the external auditory canal. Most commonly caused by *Staphylococcus aureus*. Pain is usually made worse by chewing.
  - Mastoiditis—now a rare complication of AOM, characterized by the auricle being pushed out and forward, away from the head
  - Myringitis (bullous myringitis)—inflammation of the tympanic membrane, usually with painful blisters on the eardrum
  - Varicella and herpes zoster infection within the ear
  - Herpes simplex virus infection within the ear
- **Trauma**
  - Blunt trauma
  - Laceration or abrasion—if inside the ear canal, usually due to cleaning with cotton swabs
  - Thermal injury—frostbite of the ear or burn from a heat source
  - Barotrauma—associated with airplanes and scuba diving
  - Traumatic perforation of the tympanic membrane—frequently presents with tinnitus
- **Tumors**—rare; usually associated with weight loss, voice changes, dysphagia, and persistent cervical lymphadenopathy
- **Allergic/inflammatory**
  - Otitis media with effusion
  - Eczema
  - Psoriasis
  - Allergic reaction to topical antibiotics and cerumenolytic agents
- **Functional**
  - Eustachian tube dysfunction—symptoms are due to pressure differences between the middle ear and the Eustachian tube
- **Miscellaneous**
  - Foreign body—can lead to pain, fullness, and minor hearing loss
  - Impacted cerumen—may cause pain if the cerumen presses against the tympanic membrane

Note: Serous otitis media or otitis media with effusion (OME) is common in pediatrics but is usually painless. Children usually complain of fullness or hearing loss.

Secondary otalgia:
- **Infectious**
  - Dental infections—cavities, abscesses, gingivitis
  - Pharyngitis
  - Parotitis
  - Tonsillitis
  - Peritonsillar abscess
  - Retropharyngeal abscess
  - Sinusitis
  - Cervical lymphadenitis
  - Neck abscess
  - Stomatitis
  - Sialadenitis
  - Ramsay Hunt syndrome—viral neuritis of the facial nerve secondary to herpes zoster infection
- **Trauma**
  - Dental trauma
  - Postsurgical—tonsillectomy, adenoidectomy
  - Oropharyngeal trauma—penetrating injuries, burns
  - Neck and cervical spine injuries
- **Allergic/inflammatory**
  - Allergic rhinitis
  - Cervical spine arthritis
  - Subacute thyroiditis
  - Esophagitis—secondary to gastroesophageal reflux
  - Bell palsy
- **Functional**
  - Temporomandibular joint (TMJ) dysfunction—less common in children. Pain is usually unilateral and aggravated by chewing and biting.
- **Miscellaneous**
  - Foreign body—in oropharynx or esophagus
  - Aphthous ulcers
  - Esophagitis
  - TMJ disease
  - Migraine
  - Aural neuralgia
  - Pillow otalgia (otalgia from sleep position)
  - Psychogenic pain

APPROACH TO THE PATIENT
The first decision that must be made is whether the patient's symptoms require emergent, urgent, or non-urgent intervention. Emergency treatment is rarely required for pediatric patients with otalgia.
- **Phase 1:** Thorough history—must include a full assessment of ear symptoms, followed by questions to determine possible involvement of other head and neck structures
- **Phase 2:** Physical exam—thorough examination of external and internal ear, followed by inspection of the head, neck, and inside of the mouth
- **Phase 3:** Treatment of identifiable conditions
- **Phase 4:** Referral to otolaryngologist (ENT physician), dentist, or other specialist as needed

HISTORY
- **Question:** Duration of symptoms?
- *Significance:* Acute (more likely infection or trauma) vs. chronic
- **Question:** Quality of the pain?
- *Significance:*
  - Constant (more likely otogenic) vs. intermittent (more likely referred)
  - Dull (more likely due to inflammation) vs. sharp (more likely due to trauma or neuralgia)
- **Question:** Severity of pain?
- *Significance:*
  - Severe—usually otogenic
  - Mild to moderate—more likely to be referred

Worsening factors
- **Question:** Movement of auricle or pressure on tragus?
- *Significance:* Characteristic of otitis externa; can also be associated with furunculosis.
- **Question:** Movement of the jaw (biting, chewing)?
- *Significance:* TMJ dysfunction; furunculosis

Associated symptoms
- **Question:** Fever?
- *Significance:* Infection
- **Question:** URI symptoms?
- *Significance:* AOM or OME
- **Question:** Sore throat?
- *Significance:* Referred otalgia
- **Question:** Ear discharge, tinnitus, or vertigo?
- *Significance:* Otogenic causes
- **Question:** Mouth pain?
- *Significance:* Dental issues or stomatitis
- **Question:** Hoarseness?
- *Significance:* Gastroesophageal reflux
- **Question:** Multiple somatic complaints?
- *Significance:* Psychogenic
- **Question:** Recent swimming?
- *Significance:* Otitis externa

- **Question:** Recent travel? Hobbies?
- *Significance:*
  - Barotrauma from scuba diving or air travel
  - Wrestling—auricular trauma
- **Question:** History of recurrent AOM or OME?
- *Significance:* Cholesteatoma

PHYSICAL EXAM
- **Finding:** Erythematous, dull, bulging tympanic membrane, with decreased mobility?
- *Significance:* Suggestive of AOM
- **Finding:** Retracted, immobile tympanic membrane?
- *Significance:* Suggestive of OME or Eustachian tube dysfunction
- **Finding:** Pain with pressure on the tragus or traction on the pinna?
- *Significance:* Suggestive of otitis externa or furunculosis
- **Finding:** Erythema and edema of the external auditory canal?
- *Significance:* Suggestive of otitis externa
- **Finding:** Purulent discharge in external auditory canal?
- *Significance:* Suggestive of otitis externa or AOM with a ruptured tympanic membrane
- **Finding:** Redness, swelling, and/or tenderness of the auricle?
- *Significance:*
  - With earlobe involvement—cellulitis
  - Without earlobe involvement—perichondritis
- **Finding:** Swelling behind the pinna with its lateral displacement?
- *Significance:* Suggestive of mastoiditis
- **Finding:** Normal ear exam?
- *Significance:* Suggestive of secondary otalgia, thus other possible sources must be carefully examined
- **Finding:** Multiple dental caries?
- *Significance:* May be the source of pain; can indicate the presence of a dental abscess
- **Finding:** Foreign body within the ear or in the oropharynx?
- *Significance:* May be the source of pain from direct pressure or secondary to inflammation
- **Finding:** Enlarged, asymmetrical tonsils or uvular deviation from midline?
- *Significance:* Suggestive of tonsillitis or peritonsillar abscess

Look for signs of trauma, inside or outside of the ear.

DIAGNOSTIC TESTS & INTERPRETATION
Labs, imaging studies, and other diagnostic tests are usually unnecessary as a thorough history and physical exam can lead to a diagnosis in the majority of cases.
- **Test:** Culture of ear discharge
- *Significance:* Indicated when otitis externa or AOM with perforation of the tympanic membrane does not resolve as expected with routine antibiotic treatment

- **Test:** Audiometry
- *Significance:* Evaluate for hearing loss, which would suggest primary otalgia
- **Test:** Tympanometry
- *Significance:* Evaluate for OME, Eustachian tube dysfunction, or tympanostomy tube obstruction

Imaging
- CT scan
  - CT of neck—evaluate for retropharyngeal abscess, mass, or hematoma
  - CT of sinuses—evaluate for sinusitis
  - CT of temporal bone—evaluate for AOM, mastoiditis, and other bony pathology
- MRI: Rarely needed unless intracranial lesion is suspected

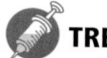 **TREATMENT**

ADDITIONAL TREATMENT
General Measures
- Therapy is directed at the identified underlying cause.
- Pain medications, such as topical benzocaine, acetaminophen, and ibuprofen, are always important since many of the infectious causes are exquisitely painful.
- Observation without antibiotic therapy ("watchful waiting") is indicated in certain groups of children with AOM.

EMERGENCY CARE
- Rarely needed with most causes of otalgia but may be required if:
  - Potential airway compromise from foreign body, mass, or abscess
  - Significant trauma—possible basilar skull fracture
  - Infection with a toxic-appearing child
- For all of the above situations, first establish "ABC's" as needed, hospitalize and consult ENT promptly.

ISSUES FOR REFERRAL
Alerts to make a referral to ENT when otalgia is primary in origin:
- Pain with unexplained hearing loss, vertigo, or tinnitus
- Unexplained or persistent otorrhea
- Suspected neoplasm
- History suggestive of severe barotrauma
- AOM with complications
- Foreign bodies that cannot be removed easily from the ear
- Potential for auricle destruction (e.g., perichondritis may lead to permanent deformation, cauliflower ear)
- Persistent ear pain without an identifiable source should prompt a referral.

ADDITIONAL READING
- American Academy of Pediatrics Subcommittee on Management of Acute Otitis Media. Diagnosis and management of acute otitis media. *Pediatrics.* 2004;113(5):1451–1465.
- Leung AK, Fong JH, Leong AG. Otalgia in children. *J Natl Med Assoc.* 2000;92:254–260.
- Licameli GR. Diagnosis and management of otalgia in the pediatric patient. *Pediatr Ann.* 1999;28: 364–368.
- Majumdar S, Wu K, Bateman N, et al. Diagnosis and management of otalgia in children. *Arch Dis Child Educ Pract Ed.* 2009;94:33–36.
- Shah RK, Blevins NH. Otalgia. *Otoralygol Clin North Am.* 2003;36(6):1137–1151.

 CODES

ICD9
- 388.70 Otalgia, unspecified
- 388.71 Otogenic pain
- 388.72 Referred otogenic pain

ICD10
- H92.01 Otalgia, right ear
- H92.02 Otalgia, left ear
- H92.09 Otalgia, unspecified ear

FAQ
- Q: What are the most common organisms that cause AOM?
- A:
  - *Streptococcus pneumoniae*
  - *Haemophilus influenzae*
  - *Moraxella catarrhalis*
  - Viruses
- Q: What are the most common organisms that cause otitis externa?
- A:
  - *Pseudomonas aeruginosa*
  - *S. aureus*
  - *Staphylococcus epidermidis*
  - Gram-negative rods
  - Fungal (*Aspergillus*) or yeast (*Candida*)—rare
- Q: What is the most common cause of referred ear pain?
- A: Dental disease

EDEMA

Rebecca Ruebner
Lawrence Copelovitch

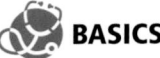 **BASICS**

DEFINITION
Presence of abnormal amount of fluid in the extracellular spaces of the body; usually secondary to low albumin, obstruction of venous or lymphatic channels, or trauma

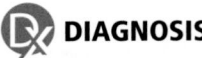 **DIAGNOSIS**

DIFFERENTIAL DIAGNOSIS
- **Localized**
  - Trauma: Pressure or sun damage
  - Infection
  - Allergy
  - Lymphatic obstruction (less common):
    ○ Filariasis
  - Bee stings or insect bites
  - Sickle cell dactylitis
- **Generalized**
  - Congenital: Lymphatic obstruction of legs or thoracic duct
  - Infection: Hepatitis and liver failure; pericarditis
  - Toxic, environmental, drugs:
    ○ Sodium poisoning
    ○ Toxic effect on liver and/or heart (chemotherapy)
    ○ Cirrhosis
    ○ Drug reaction
  - Tumor:
    ○ Obstruction of venous return from enlarged abdominal lymph nodes or tumor
  - Allergic/inflammatory: Protein-losing enteropathy
  - Renal:
    ○ Nephrotic syndrome
    ○ Renal failure
  - Cardiac:
    ○ Congestive heart failure (CHF)
    ○ Pericarditis
  - GI:
    ○ Intestinal protein loss
    ○ Postpericardiotomy or congenital heart surgery
    ○ Hepatobiliary diseases
  - Endocrine: Sodium retention, hypothyroidism

ETIOLOGY
- **Excessive losses of protein**
  - Renal losses
  - GI losses
- **Inadequate production of protein**
  - Liver disease
  - Malnutrition
- **Local trauma**
- **Increased hydrostatic pressure**
  - CHF
  - Cirrhosis
  - Pericardial effusion
  - Postcardiac surgery
  - Venous obstruction
    ○ Superior vena caval syndrome
    ○ Deep vein thrombosis
- **Lymphatic obstruction**

APPROACH TO THE PATIENT
Determine the cause of swelling: Is it localized? Are there any losses of protein? Is there underproduction of protein?
- **Phase 1:** Is the swelling localized as seen in trauma, lymphatic, or venous obstruction?
- **Phase 2:** Are there urinary or GI losses?
  - Associated with decreased serum albumin
  - Most likely source of loss is renal disease, less frequently GI losses
- **Phase 3:** Search for other causes of edema, such as CHF, cirrhosis, lymphatic obstruction

HISTORY
- **Question:** Is the edema localized or generalized?
- *Significance:* See "Differential Diagnosis"
- **Question:** Is the patient asymptomatic or in some distress specifically because of the edema?
- *Significance:* Determine treatment urgency
- **Question:** Evidence of cardiac, renal, or GI disease?
- *Significance:* Major causes of edema
- **Question:** Waist size has become larger, difficulty putting shoes on?
- *Significance:* Evidence of edema in body
- **Question:** Excess salt intake in diet?
- *Significance:* In some patients, contributes to edema
- **Question:** Shortness of breath?
- *Significance:* There may be ascites, which compresses the diaphragm or causes pleural effusions.
- **Question:** Chronic diarrhea?
- *Significance:* Seen in protein-losing enteropathy or lymphatic obstruction
- **Question:** Has any urinalysis been performed in the past?
- *Significance:* May help date the onset of the problem
- **Question:** Swelling around the eyes or face?
- *Significance:* Allergies

PHYSICAL EXAM
- **Finding:** Lumbosacral area, pretibial, scrotum/labia?
- *Significance:* Dependent edema
- **Finding:** Percussion of chest?
- *Significance:* Pleural effusion
- **Finding:** Shifting dullness?
- *Significance:* Early sign of ascites

- **Finding:** Soft ear cartilage?
- *Significance:* Common finding in nephrotic syndrome
- **Finding:** Pitting edema?
- *Significance:* Seen in cases of protein loss
- **Finding:** Venous/lymphatic obstruction or salt poisoning?
- *Significance:* May cause non-pitting edema

DIAGNOSTIC TESTS & INTERPRETATION
- **Test:** Dipstick urinalysis
- *Significance:* If there is generalized edema with heavy proteinuria and hypoalbuminemia, the presumptive diagnosis is always nephrotic syndrome until proven otherwise.
- **Test:** Serum albumin
- *Significance:*
  - If there is generalized edema with no proteinuria but hypoalbuminemia, consider cardiac, GI, or hepatobiliary disease and direct additional studies to evaluate these 3 organ systems specifically.
  - If there is either localized edema or generalized edema but a normal urinalysis and a normal serum albumin, consider other unusual causes for edema, such as mechanical or lymphatic obstruction, certain endocrine disorders, or the effects of drugs or toxins.
- **Test:** Stool albumin
- *Significance:* Seen in protein-losing enteropathy
- **Test:** Cholesterol
- *Significance:* Only high in hypoalbuminemia associated with nephrotic syndrome

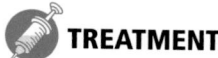 TREATMENT

ADDITIONAL TREATMENT
General Measures
- Moisturize skin
- Avoid pressure sores
- Decrease sodium intake
- Active or passive leg exercise to avoid venous thromboses

- If edema is massive, the patient may awaken with swollen eyelids. Place blocks under the head of the bed to keep the patient's head elevated.
- If there is scrotal edema, jockey shorts will help support the scrotum and protect the skin from breaking down.
- For severe edema with respiratory distress, severe abdominal discomfort, or severe scrotal edema, consider treatment with albumin and/or lasix infusion.

ISSUES FOR REFERRAL
- Nephrotic syndrome—pediatric nephrologist
- Protein-losing enteropathy or hepatobiliary disease—pediatric gastroenterologist
- CHF—pediatric cardiologist
- Endocrine-mediated edema—pediatric endocrinologist
- Lymphatic or other mechanical obstructions—vascular surgeon or pediatric surgeon

INITIAL STABILIZATION
Any child or adolescent with an edema-forming state that compromises either cardiorespiratory function or the vascular integrity of a peripheral organ or limb should be referred immediately to an appropriate specialist for emergency care.

ADDITIONAL READING
- Holliday MA, Segar WE. Reducing errors in fluid therapy management. *Pediatrics.* 2003;111: 424–425.
- Jacobs ML, Rychik J, Byrum CJ, et al. Protein-losing enteropathy after Fontan operation: Resolution after baffle fenestration. *Ann Thorac Surg.* 1996;61:206–208.
- Molina JF, Brown RF, Gedalia A, et al. Protein losing enteropathy as the initial manifestation of childhood systemic lupus erythematosus. *J Rheumatol.* 1996;23:1269–1271.

- Moritz ML, Ayus JC. Prevention of hospital acquired hyponatremia: A case for using isotonic saline. *Pediatrics.* 2003;111:227–230.
- Rosen FS. Urticaria, angioedema, anaphylaxis. *Pediatr Rev.* 1992;13:387–390.
- Vande Walle JG, Donckerwolcke RA. Pathogenesis of edema formation in the nephrotic syndrome. *Pediatr Nephrol.* 2001;16:283–293.

 CODES

ICD9
782.3 Edema

ICD10
- R60.0 Localized edema
- R60.1 Generalized edema
- R60.9 Edema, unspecified

FAQ
- Q: At what level of serum albumin does edema occur?
- A: Edema is generally associated with serum albumin <2.5 g/dL.
- Q: Why does pericardial effusion cause edema?
- A: Pericardial effusion is associated with decreased lymphatic flow and increased venous pressure.
- Q: Is there a certain group of allergens that cause edema?
- A: No, special allergens are associated with edema. The usual causes include foods such as peanuts and drugs such as penicillin.

E

EHRLICHIOSIS AND ANAPLASMOSIS

Senbagam Virudachalam
Jeffrey P. Louie (5th edition)

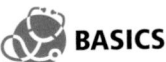 **BASICS**

DESCRIPTION
Zoonotic infection caused by 4 microorganisms of the family Anaplasmataceae. The 2 most common clinically described infections are human monocytic ehrlichiosis (HME), caused by *Ehrlichia chaffeensis*, and human granulocytic anaplasmosis, caused by *Anaplasma phagocytophilum*. *Ehrlichia ewingii*, causes a milder form of ehrlichiosis in immunocompromised patients. A 4th organism, *Neorickettsia sennetsu*, causes a mononucleosis-like syndrome, but rarely causes disease in humans.

GENERAL PREVENTION
- Avoid tick-infested areas.
- Clothes should cover arms and legs.
- Use tick repellents, but with caution in young children.
- A thorough body search should always be done after returning from a tick-infested area:
  - If a tick is found, the area should be cleaned with a disinfectant, and the tick should be removed immediately.
  - To remove the tick, grasp the tick at the point of origin with forceps, staying as close to the skin as possible.
  - Applying steady, even pressure, slowly pull the tick off the skin. After the tick has been removed, clean the skin with a disinfectant.
- Instruct parents to seek medical attention only if symptoms develop.
- No vaccine is available.

EPIDEMIOLOGY
- HME typically occurs in the mid-Atlantic, south central, and southeastern USA, mirroring the pattern of Rocky Mountain spotted fever (RMSF). In addition, it has been found in Europe, South America, Asia, and Africa.
- HGA typically occurs in the northern north central and northeastern USA. In addition, it has been found in northern CA, the mid-Atlantic, and Europe.
- *E. ewengii* only occurs in regions where *E. chaffeensis* occurs.
- *N. sennetsu* has been described in south and Southeast Asia.
- Most patients are infected during April through September, the months of greatest tick and human outdoor activity.
- A second peak of HGA occurs from late October to December.

Incidence
- Varies by state.
- HME: 3.4 cases per million persons (US average, 2008)
- HGA: 4.2 cases per million persons (US average, 2008)
- Incidence is underestimated because 2/3 of both HME and HGA cases are asymptomatic, or only mildly symptomatic.

Prevalence
- Again, difficult to estimate because majority of illnesses are asymptomatic or mild.
- A sero-prevalence study showed that, in endemic areas, 20% children without a history of clinical illness had antibodies to *E. chaffeensis*.

PATHOPHYSIOLOGY
- Obligate intracellular bacteria, pleomorphic, Gram-negative
- Transmission to humans by a tick vector
- Incubation period from 2 to 21 days
- HME infects monocytes and macrophages, whereas HGA infects neutrophils.
- The bacteria reside and divide within cytoplasmic vacuoles of circulating leukocytes, called morulae.
- There is over-induction of the inflammatory and immune response, resulting in clinical manifestations of disease, including multi-organ-system involvement.

ETIOLOGY
- HME is transmitted by *Amblyomma americanum*, the Lone Star tick. The White-tailed deer is the major reservoir.
- HGA is transmitted by *Ixodes scapularis*, a deer tick, or *Dermacentor variabilis*, a brown dog tick. Small mammals such as the white-footed mouse are the major reservoirs.
- Congenital infection is very rare, but has been described in case reports.

🔍 DIAGNOSIS

SIGNS AND SYMPTOMS
- Classic presentation: Fever, headache, and myalgias, followed by the development of a progressive leukopenia, thrombocytopenia, and anemia.
- Fevers are found in all children.
- A pleomorphic rash occurs in ~66% of pediatric patients:
  - Rash is described as macular, maculopapular, petechial, erythematous, vesicular, or a combination of these.
  - Usually distributed on the trunk and extremities; spares palms, soles, and face.
- Chills and myalgia are found in most children.
- Severe headache is often described.
- Abdominal pain, vomiting, anorexia, and diarrhea can be noted.
- Arthralgia (without arthritis) is often described.
- Cough and sore throat are often described.
- Mental status change due to meningoencephalitis is a less common, but potentially fatal, presentation.

HISTORY
History of tick bite or exposure to wooded areas that are endemic for tick-borne diseases is helpful, but is not always present.

PHYSICAL EXAM
- Mental status changes/irritability
- Nuchal rigidity
- Cardiac murmur (II/VI systolic ejection murmur at the left lower sternal border)
- Hepatosplenomegaly
- Poor perfusion with hypotension (shock) has been described in a few children as a presenting symptom.
- Conjunctival or throat injection
- Rash as described

DIAGNOSTIC TESTS & INTERPRETATION
Lab
- CBC with differential (with smear):
  - Thrombocytopenia, $<150,000/mm^3$ (77–92% incidence)
  - Lymphopenia, $<1,500/mm^3$ (75%)
  - Neutropenia, $<4,000/mm^3$ (58–68%, and is more indicative of HGA)
  - Anemia, hematocrit $<30\%$ (38–42%)
  - Intracytoplasmic morulae within leukocytes (20–60%)
- Electrolytes with BUN and creatinine: Hyponatremia (33–65%)
- Liver function tests: Elevated alanine aminotransferase, >55 U/L (90%)
- Coagulation labs, type and cross, as indicated
- CSF:
  - Leukocytosis, with an average cell count of $100/mm^3$
  - Lymphocytic predominance
  - Elevated protein and borderline low glucose (less common in children, more common in adults)
  - Microbiology cultures are negative.
  - Intraleukocytoplasmic *Ehrlichia* micro-organisms (morulae) have been described on CSF smears.
- Serum studies:
  - HME and HGA titers are available through state health departments, the Centers for Disease Control and Prevention, or a reference laboratory.
  - Acute and convalescent antibody titers of *Ehrlichia* (a 4-fold rise or fall is considered positive), obtained 2–4 weeks apart
  - An acute antibody titer of $\geq 1:128$ is considered diagnostic.
  - Polymerase chain reaction is also available for both HME and HGA.
  - The detection of intraleukocytoplasmic *Ehrlichia* microcolonies (morulae) on peripheral blood monocytes or granulocytes is diagnostic, but is not present in all patients.

Diagnosis Procedures/Surgery

- Bone marrow biopsy is not necessary to diagnose the Ehrlichioses, but may be carried out amid concern for other hematologic diseases.
- Bone marrow is usually hypercellular, but normocellularity and hypocellularity have also been found.

ALERT

- Failing to consider the diagnosis of ehrlichiosis or a delay in treatment pending confirmatory serum titers increases morbidity and mortality.
- Thus, treatment should be started if infection is suspected on the basis of history, physical, and initial laboratory data.
- Alternative diagnoses should be considered in children who do not rapidly improve with doxycycline.
- Simultaneous infections have been documented with ehrlichiosis and Lyme disease. Therefore, in patients diagnosed with ehrlichiosis, Lyme titers should also be measured to determine whether there is a dual infection. A study from Wisconsin documented a 12% coinfection rate.
- Other coinfections with ehrlichiosis have also been documented with either RMSF or babesiosis.

DIFFERENTIAL DIAGNOSIS

- Tick-borne infection:
  – RMSF
  – Tularemia
  – Relapsing fever
  – Lyme disease
  – Colorado tick fever
  – Babesiosis
- Other infection:
  – Toxic shock syndrome
  – Kawasaki disease
  – Meningococcemia
  – Pyelonephritis
  – Gastroenteritis
  – Hepatitis
  – Leptospirosis
  – Epstein–Barr virus
  – Influenza
  – Cytomegalovirus
  – Enterovirus
  – Streptococcus pharyngitis
- Miscellaneous:
  – Leukemia
  – Idiopathic thrombocytopenia purpura
  – Hemolytic uremic syndrome

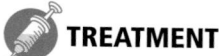 TREATMENT

ADDITIONAL TREATMENT
General Measures

- Volume and BP medications as needed
- Intubation for respiratory failure
- Dialysis for renal failure
- Platelets for thrombocytopenia
- Packed red blood cells for anemia
- Fresh frozen plasma, cryoprecipitate, and vitamin K for DIC
- Antifungal or antibiotics for secondary infections

MEDICATION (DRUGS)
First Line

- Doxycycline, either PO or IV
- Drug of choice regardless of age of child who is severely ill
- Dose: 4.4 mg/kg/day divided q12h (max dose 200 mg q12h)
- Treatment duration: minimum 5–10 days. Continue for 3–5 days after defervescence, longer if there is CNS involvement.

Second Line

- Rifampin has been reported to be an effective antibiotic for children <8 years of age who are less toxic and are experiencing an HGA infection.
- Dose: 20 mg/kg/day divided q12h for 5–10 days.
- This is also the drug of choice for pregnant mothers.
- Unlike Lyme disease, neither amoxicillin nor ceftriaxone has been shown to be effective for the treatment of ehrlichiosis.

 ONGOING CARE

PROGNOSIS

- >60% of patients are hospitalized.
- Case fatality rate for HME is 2–5%; for HGA, 7–10%.
- Elevated BUN and creatinine have been associated with a more severe course.
- Children appear to have an excellent outcome: Blood, renal, and liver abnormalities resolve in 1–2 weeks after initiating antibiotics.
- Cognitive and behavioral problems have been reported.
- Neuropathy has been described.

COMPLICATIONS

- Neurologic:
  – Headache, described as severe
  – Mental status changes
  – Seizures
  – Coma
  – Focal neurologic findings
  – Cognitive learning deficits
- Hematologic:
  – Disseminated intravascular coagulopathy (DIC)
  – Thrombocytopenia
  – Leukopenia
  – Lymphopenia
  – Anemia
- GI:
  – Hemorrhage
  – Elevated liver enzymes
  – Hepatosplenomegaly
- Respiratory:
  – Pulmonary hemorrhage
  – Interstitial pneumonia
  – Pleural effusions
  – Noncardiogenic pulmonary edema

- Infectious:
  – Fungal superinfection
  – Nosocomial infections
  – Opportunistic infections
- Renal:
  – Renal failure
  – Proteinuria
  – Hematuria
- Cardiac:
  – Cardiomegaly
  – Murmurs

ADDITIONAL READING

- Dumler JS, Madigan JE, Pusterla N, et al. Ehrlichioses in humans: Epidemiology, clinical presentation, diagnosis, and treatment. *Clin Infect Dis.* 2007;45(Suppl 1):S45–S51.
- Ismail N, Bloch KC, McBride JW. Human ehrlichiosis and anaplasmosis. *Clin Lab Med.* 2010;30(1): 261–292.
- Jacobs RF, Schultze GE. Ehrlichiosis in children. *J Pediatr.* 1997;131:184–192.
- Krause PJ, Corrow CL, Bakken JS. Successful treatment of human granulocytic ehrlichiosis in children using rifampin. *Pediatrics.* 2003: e252–e253.
- Lantos P, Krause PJ. Ehrlichiosis in children. *Sem Infect Dis.* 2002;13:249–256.

CODES

ICD9

- 082.40 Ehrlichiosis, unspecified
- 082.41 Ehrlichiosis chafeensis [E. chafeensis]
- 082.49 Other ehrlichiosis

ICD10

- A77.40 Ehrlichiosis, unspecified
- A77.41 Ehrlichiosis chafeensis [E. chafeensis]
- A77.49 Other ehrlichiosis

FAQ

- Q: If a tick is removed from my child, should antibiotics be started?
- A: Unlike with Lyme disease, this has yet to be defined. Antibiotics should be started if a child becomes symptomatic.
- Q: What is the most common chief complaint in children with ehrlichiosis?
- A: Intense, unremitting headache:
  – In patients with fever, headache, and flulike illness in the spring to early fall, consider the diagnosis.
  – Laboratory abnormalities of leukopenia, thrombocytopenia, and hepatitis should lead to presumptive therapy until the diagnosis is clear.

ENCEPHALITIS

William V. Raszka, Jr.
A. G. Christina Bergqvist (5th edition)

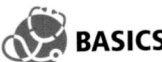 **BASICS**

DESCRIPTION
Encephalitis inflammation of the brain parenchyma with neurologic dysfunction. Rarely confirmed histologically, encephalitis is suggested by clinical evidence of brain dysfunction coupled with laboratory or neuroimaging findings suggestive of inflammation. Causes are myriad and include infection, neoplasia, and autoimmune disease. This chapter will focus on infectious and postinfectious causes.

EPIDEMIOLOGY
Incidence
As encephalitis is not reportable and a specific diagnosis infrequently made, the exact incidence is unknown. Reported incidence rates vary with age, geographic location, season, type of exposure, and immunologic status. In the US ~1,400 deaths/year are attributed to encephalitis. Children, the elderly, immunocompromised hosts, and individuals with significant arbovirus exposure have the highest reported incidence rates.

GENERAL PREVENTION
- Immunization against measles, mumps, rubella, and varicella zoster virus (VZV)
- Avoidance of exposure to arthropod vectors during transmission seasons (summer months in US temperate zones)
- Use of insect repellants and topically applied insecticides if exposed to arthropod vectors in hyperendemic areas (e.g., DEET or permethrin)
- Immunocompromised hosts should avoid consuming high-risk foods (e.g., undercooked beef or pork products).
- Cesarean section for women with 1st-time herpes genitalis at the time of parturition
- Travelers or individuals with unique exposures may benefit from specific vaccines (e.g., Japanese encephalitis or rabies).

PATHOPHYSIOLOGY
- Infecting organisms may (1) always cause encephalitis in the absence of systemic findings (e.g., rabies), (2) infrequently but reliably cause encephalitis (e.g., Eastern equine encephalitis), or (3) frequently cause localized or systemic disease and infrequently, as part of the infection, cause encephalitis (enterovirus and herpes simplex virus [HSV]).
- Organisms may invade the brain parenchyma via the systemic circulation, following meningitis, or through retrograde spread along neural pathways (e.g., rabies, HSV).
- Invasion/infiltration leads to activation of the host immune response and cytokine release.
- Light microscopy may show neuronal involvement and inclusion bodies.
- In postinfectious encephalitis, usually diagnosed as acute disseminated encephalomyelitis, no organism can be identified in the brain parenchyma. Histopathologic exam usually demonstrates perivascular inflammation and evidence of demyelination, suggesting that a host immune response is responsible for the clinical findings.

ETIOLOGY
- In the majority of patients, no etiologic agent is identified. In patients with confirmed encephalitis, a specific infectious agent has been either confirmed or deemed probable in 16% and thought possible in another 13%. In the US, viruses are the most common infectious agents (70%) followed by bacteria (20%).
- The most commonly isolated viruses are enterovirus and HSV. Other common viral agents not listed below include Epstein-Barr virus (EBV) and influenza. Worldwide, measles, mumps, and rubella remain important pathogens.
- Viral pathogens associated with specific seasons (summer and fall) are enterovirus, Eastern equine, Western equine, St. Louis, La Crosse, and West Nile viruses.
- Viral pathogens causing sporadic disease include HSV, HIV, VZV, and rabies.
- Pathogens associated with disease in immunocompromised hosts include cytomegalovirus (CMV), JC virus, and VZV.
- Nonviral causes include *Mycoplasma pneumoniae*, *Bartonella henselae*, *Listeria monocytogenes*, *Mycobacterium tuberculosis*, *Borrelia burgdorferi*, *Rickettsia*, *Toxoplasma gondii* (in immunocompromised), and *Taenia solium* (more commonly in immigrants). *Mycoplasma* is the most common possible bacterial cause (usually diagnosed on a single elevated IgM).
- A specific causal organism is infrequently identified in postinfectious encephalitis.

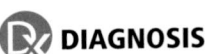 **DIAGNOSIS**

HISTORY
- Inquire about fever, headache, photophobia, increased somnolence, depressed or altered mental status, irritability, confusion, gait disturbance, seizures, and personality changes.
- Ask for symptoms suggestive of a recent or ongoing viral illness such as cough, coryza, malaise, anorexia, diarrhea, nausea, vomiting, and rashes.
- Inquire about recent travel, animal exposures, tick or mosquito bites, immunizations, and immune status, and in neonates, symptoms of HSV in the mother.

PHYSICAL EXAM
- A complete neurologic exam is critical. Abnormal brain function is a hallmark of encephalitis (and helps distinguish it from meningitis). Patients may present with anything from mild confusion to stupor and coma. Distinguishing infectious from postinfectious encephalitis usually cannot be done on clinical grounds particularly as some viral agents can cause both (e.g., measles, VZV, influenza).
- Specific neurologic findings that may suggest an etiologic agent include the following: focal seizures and focal neurologic findings (HSV); hydrophobia, pharyngeal spasms, and mood disturbance (rabies); facial nerve palsy (Lyme disease); flaccid paralysis or poliolike syndrome (West Nile virus); and ataxia (VZV).

- Nonneurologic findings that may suggest an etiologic agent or syndrome include meningismus or positive Kernig or Brudzinski signs (meningoencephalitis); pulmonary rales or rhonchi (*Mycoplasma*); adenopathy and splenomegaly (EBV); petechial skin rash (*Rickettsia*); morbilliform rash (measles); erythematous maculopapular rash (enterovirus); and parotitis (mumps).
- Hypertension, bradycardia, or apnea may suggest impending herniation due to brain swelling.

DIAGNOSTIC TESTS & INTERPRETATION
Lab
- Routine labs such as serum electrolytes, glucose, BUN, creatinine, liver function tests, calcium, magnesium, and complete blood count with differential are recommended, although they infrequently help confirm or exclude a diagnosis.
- Ammonia and blood pH
- Serologic testing (depending on the suspected agent (e.g., West Nile virus and *Mycoplasma*)
- Toxicology screen

Imaging
MRI (or if not available, CT) of the brain with and without contrast medium. Imaging is performed urgently to rule out surgically remediable conditions (e.g., abscess or hematoma). While neuroimaging can be normal in patients with encephalitis, studies often help exclude particular conditions or demonstrate findings suggestive of encephalitis. Typical changes in encephalitis include focal or diffuse parenchymal enhancement (HSV has a preference for the medial temporal lobe).

Diagnostic Procedures/Other
Lumbar puncture:
- Often performed emergently. Defer until the airway, gas exchange, and circulation have been stabilized or if clinical signs and symptoms suggest increased intracranial pressure.
- Measure opening pressure (frequently elevated).
- Send for cell count and differential (lymphocytic predominance suggests a viral process while neutrophilic predominance suggests bacterial or early viral processes). The presence of red blood cells is suggestive of necrotizing encephalitis (often associated with HSV).
- Measure protein (usually elevated) and glucose.
- Send CSF for Gram stain and bacterial culture (20% of patients with suspected encephalitis are diagnosed with bacterial meningitis).
- In immunocompromised hosts, fluid should be sent for fungal stains and culture (and serum for cryptococcal serum antigen).
- In most patients with suspected encephalitis and particularly if there is a lymphocytic CSF pleocytosis, CSF should be sent for HSV polymerase chain reaction (PCR) assay. Other PCR-based tests on CSF, including assays for enterovirus, *Borrelia burgdorferi*, and West Nile virus, may be considered depending on the situation.

- EEG: Performed nonurgently. Findings of periodic lateralizing epileptiform discharges (PLEDs) are suggestive but not diagnostic of herpes.
- Brain biopsy: Now rarely performed

ALERT
- Never assume that a CSF pleocytosis is secondary to seizures.
- Institute antiviral and/or antibacterial therapy promptly; it can always be discontinued after an organism is identified or cultures/PCR are negative.
- The absence of CSF pleocytosis does not exclude encephalitis.
- Save extra CSF and serum obtained at the time of presentation for future testing (very useful if the initial tests are nondiagnostic).
- Children with immunodeficiency or unique exposures (e.g., travel) have an expanded differential diagnosis and may require serologic, culture, or PCR testing not commonly performed to reach a diagnosis.

DIFFERENTIAL DIAGNOSIS
Several toxic, metabolic, vascular, and epileptic syndromes may resemble encephalitis:
- Acute electrolyte disturbance, especially hyponatremia
- Acute obstructive hydrocephalus or ventriculoperitoneal shunt obstruction
- Bacterial meningitis
- Brain abscess
- Cerebral vasculitis, stroke, or septic embolization (endocarditis)
- Hypothyroid crisis
- Ingestions
- Intracranial hemorrhage
- Malignant hyperthermia
- Pituitary infarction
- Reye syndrome
- Sinus thrombosis
- Status epilepticus
- Subdural empyema
- Viral meningitis

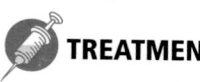 **TREATMENT**

MEDICATION (DRUGS)
- Almost all patients with suspected encephalitis should be started on empiric intravenous acyclovir unless the history, clinical findings, and initial laboratory tests either exclude the diagnosis of HSV or strongly point to an alternative diagnosis.
- Patients with confirmed HSV encephalitis are continued on IV acyclovir for 21 days.
- Patients with suspected encephalitis of unknown etiology and CSF pleocytosis (particularly if the CSF shows a predominance of neutrophils) are usually started on empiric antibiotic therapy for possible bacterial meningitis (the combination of ceftriaxone and vancomycin for all children outside the neonatal age group) until bacterial culture results are negative or a viral cause confirmed.

- Specific anti-infective therapy is available for neuroborreliosis (ceftriaxone), rickettsial disease (doxycycline regardless of age), and toxoplasmosis (pyrimethamine plus sulfadiazine). Whether acyclovir is beneficial in VZV is controversial as in most situations, VZV leads to a postinfectious syndrome. Ganciclovir is used in CMV encephalitis but the outcome remains dismal.
- Anticonvulsants are reserved for clinical or electrographic evidence of seizure/epileptic activity:
  – Choices include lorazepam, phenytoin, phenobarbital, and carbamazepine.

IN-PATIENT CONSIDERATIONS
Initial Stabilization
Most patients are admitted to the hospital and often the intensive care unit for initial stabilization and management.

IV Fluids
- Correct any fluid deficits; thereafter, maintain a euvolemic state. Avoid hypotonic fluids.
- Closely monitor electrolytes, anticipating possible syndrome of inappropriate antidiuretic hormone or diabetes insipidus.

 ONGOING CARE

FOLLOW-UP RECOMMENDATIONS
- Physical and occupational therapists should be consulted early in the course and will be helpful during the convalescence.
- Neuropsychologic testing is helpful to identify cognitive deficits and direct appropriate services.
- Follow-up with speech pathologists and developmental pediatricians may be indicated.

PROGNOSIS
Outcome varies greatly and depends on age, etiologic agent, and disease severity at the time of presentation (e.g., patients presenting in coma do worse). Outcomes range from complete recovery to focal neurologic deficits, persistent vegetative state, and death.

COMPLICATIONS
- Aphasias
- Ataxia
- Developmental delay
- Learning disabilities
- Quadriparesis/hemiparesis
- Seizure disorders, focal or generalized

ADDITIONAL READING
- Chang LY, Huang LM, Gau SS, et al. Neurodevelopment and cognition in children after enterovirus 71 infection. N Engl J Med. 2007; 356(12):1226–1234.
- Elbers JM, Bitnun A, Richardson SE, et al. A 12-year prospective study of childhood herpes simplex encephalitis: Is there a broader spectrum of disease? Pediatrics. 2007;119(2):e399–e407.
- Glaser CA, Honarmand S, Anderson LJ, et al. Beyond viruses: Clinical profiles and etiologies associated with encephalitis. Clin Infect Dis. 2006;43(12):1565–1577.
- Long S. Encephalitis diagnosis and management in the real world. Adv Exp Med Biol. 2011;697: 153–173.
- Redington J, Tyler K. Viral infections of the nervous system, 2002: Update on diagnosis and treatment. Arch Neurol. 2002;59:712–718.
- Sampathkumar P. West Nile virus: Epidemiology, clinical presentation, diagnosis, and prevention. Mayo Clin Proc. 2003;78:1137–1144.
- Silvia MT. Licht DJ. Pediatric central nervous system infections and inflammatory white matter disease. Pediatr Clin North Am. 2005;52:1107–1126.
- Tenembaum S, Chitnis T, Ness J, et al. International Pediatric MS Study Group. Acute disseminated encephalomyelitis. Neurology. 2007;68:S23–S36.

 CODES

ICD9
- 049.9 Unspecified non-arthropod-borne viral diseases of central nervous system
- 062.0 Japanese encephalitis
- 323.9 Unspecified causes of encephalitis, myelitis, and encephalomyelitis

ICD10
- A83.0 Japanese encephalitis
- A86 Unspecified viral encephalitis
- G04.90 Encephalitis and encephalomyelitis, unspecified

FAQ
- Q: My child has been diagnosed with encephalitis; will he be mentally retarded?
- A: The complications following encephalitis vary greatly from severe mental retardation and cerebral palsy to full recovery. There is a correlation between degree of brain destruction and outcome; however, children frequently recover better than adults with a similar degree of illness.

E

ENCOPRESIS

Victor M. Pineiro-Carrero (5th edition)
Amanda Muir

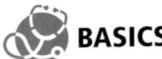 **BASICS**

DESCRIPTION
- Repeated unintentional soiling of underwear
- Most commonly associated with functional constipation with severe stool retention and subsequent overflow incontinence:
  - 90% of cases of encopresis fall into this category
- Another less common type of encopresis refers to the entity of repeated passage of feces into inappropriate places (usually clothing or floor) after the age of 4 years in the absence of constipation and structural or inflammatory diseases, also known as functional nonretentive fecal incontinence (FNRFI).

EPIDEMIOLOGY
- The reported ratio of boys to girls ranges from 2:1 to 6:1. Boys are more likely to experience nonretentive fecal incontinence than girls at a ratio of 9:1.
- There is no association with family size, ordinal position in the family, age of parents, or socioeconomic status.

Prevalence
Encopresis is reported in 1.5–2.8% of children >4 years. Between 10% and 30% of children with encopresis have nonretentive fecal incontinence.

RISK FACTORS
Genetics
Monozygotic twins have a 4-fold higher incidence than do dizygotic twins.

ALERT
- Constipation with a rectal fecal mass is most common risk for encopresis.
- Children with FNRFI have more behavioral problems, poor self-esteem, and higher prevalence of attention deficit disorder.

PATHOPHYSIOLOGY
Chronic constipation with fecal impaction results in overflow incontinence and reduced sensation secondary to rectal distention. The pattern of holding fecal matter, leading to chronic constipation and overflow incontinence, may result from a variety of causes, such as a painful experience from a fissure, difficult toilet training, or refusal to use school bathrooms. However, the history often does not reveal a triggering event.

ETIOLOGY
- Chronic constipation leads to a dilated rectum, decreased rectal sensation, shortening of the anal canal, and decreased anal sphincter tone in some patients.
- Findings on anorectal manometry include increased rectal sensory threshold and paradoxic contraction of the external anal sphincter during attempts at defecation (known as *anismus*).

- FNRFI occurs in children without constipation. The soiling may be a manifestation of an emotional disturbance, and it may be associated with specific triggers (person or place) or may represent an impulsive action triggered by unconscious anger. All studies in these patients are normal, including normal anorectal manometry and normal colonic transit times.

COMMONLY ASSOCIATED CONDITIONS
Enuresis is more frequently seen in patients with FNRFI (45% have daytime and 40% have nighttime enuresis) compared to constipated children.

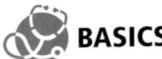 **DIAGNOSIS**

HISTORY
- Toileting habits:
  - Constipation: Frequency and size of bowel movements (large-diameter bowel movements are common in children with encopresis associated with functional constipation)
  - Bowel movements that obstruct the toilet and/or chronic abdominal pain relieved by enemas or laxatives
  - Retentive posturing: Avoiding defecation by contraction of pelvic floor, squeezing the buttocks together (leg scissoring, crossing the legs, standing on tiptoes)
- Irritability, abdominal cramps, decreased appetite (symptoms improve after passage of large stool)
- Onset: Elicit history of triggering events (perianal infection, diet changes, toilet training, avoidance of school bathrooms, sexual abuse, or other stressful events).
- Enuresis (secondary daytime enuresis may occur in patients with megarectum compressing the bladder)
- Timing in the neonatal period of meconium passage, as well as past surgeries, medical history, and medications, are relevant.
- Unsteady or clumsy gait may suggest a neuromuscular disorder.
- Children with FNRFI do not have any history of constipation and have daily bowel movements. The incontinence is diurnal, usually in the afternoon.

PHYSICAL EXAM
- Encopresis with functional constipation:
  - Fecal mass palpable in 40% of patients; fecal soiling in the perianal region
  - Dilated rectum but a normally positioned anus
  - Anal sphincter tone may be normal or slightly decreased; the anal canal is usually shorter than normal.
  - Hard stool or a large amount of "mushy" stool present in rectal vault

- FNRFI:
  - No palpable fecal mass
  - Normal-size rectum
  - Normal sphincter length
- Examine deep tendon reflexes, anal wink, rectal exam, lumbosacral spine exam to look for sacral dimpling, and documentation of normal growth.
- In patients with extreme fear of anal exam, attempt a perianal inspection and obtain a plain radiograph of the abdomen to establish a fecal impaction. In children who fear painful defecation, the necessity of a rectal exam remains debatable.

DIAGNOSTIC TESTS & INTERPRETATION
Referral to a pediatric gastroenterologist for further evaluation, including anorectal manometry, is often a useful adjunctive modality for patients recalcitrant to standard management.

Lab
No tests are needed if both the history and physical exam are consistent with functional constipation and associated encopresis. If the patient's history or physical exam is atypical and a systemic disorder is suspected, appropriate diagnostic tests should be done.

Imaging
- Abdominal radiography is often necessary for patients who refuse a rectal exam, or when a rectal impaction is not palpable on abdominal exam (e.g., in obese patients).
- Enema with water soluble contrast material can be both helpful diagnostically to look for areas of narrowing and therapeutically as a clean-out procedure.
- MRI of the spine can be done for children with suspected spinal abnormalities. This is rarely necessary if the neurological exam is normal.
- Colonic transit study with radio-opaque markers to confirm the patients complaints or assess for slow transit constipation

Diagnostic Procedures/Other
- Rectal suction biopsy can be performed to evaluate for ganglion cells within the colonic mucosa and evaluate for Hirschsprung disease.
- Anorectal manometry can be done in selected cases to evaluate anorectal function. The main indication is to demonstrate the rectoanal inhibitory reflex to exclude Hirschsprung disease and ultra-short-segment Hirschsprung disease. It may also show an increased threshold to rectal sensation, providing important information to the patient and the parents.

DIFFERENTIAL DIAGNOSIS

Determine whether stool leakage is caused by functional constipation or an underlying anatomic, metabolic, or neurologic abnormality. Fecal incontinence may be secondary to diarrheal diseases or defective neuromuscular control, such as in children with spinal defects.

- Neuromuscular:
  - Spinal cord tumor
  - Tethered spinal cord
  - Meningomyelocele
- Anal abnormalities:
  - Anteriorly displaced anus
  - Ectopic anus
- Inflammatory:
  - Proctitis (infectious or ulcerative)
  - Fistula secondary to Crohn disease
  - Celiac disease
- Stricture (after necrotizing enterocolitis or inflammatory bowel disease)
- Abdominal pelvic mass (sacral teratoma, meningomyelocele)
- Hypotonia (cerebral palsy, amyotonia congenita, familial visceral myopathy)
- Hirschsprung disease (constipation common, fecal incontinence rarely seen) or ultra-short-segment Hirschsprung disease
- Postsurgical repair of imperforate anus or Hirschsprung disease
- Endocrine:
  - Hypothyroidism
  - Panhypopituitarism
  - Diabetes mellitus
- Constipating drugs:
  - Opiates
  - Calcium supplements
  - Psychotropics

 **TREATMENT**

MEDICATION (DRUGS)

- Disimpaction must be achieved with either enemas or sedated manual disimpaction to avoid increased encopresis and abdominal pain:
  - Severe cases may require polyethylene glycol ingestion by NG tube after disimpaction in a hospital setting.
- Stimulant laxatives:
  - Magnesium citrate
  - Bisacodyl
  - Senna
- Stool softeners:
  - MiraLAX (0.75 mg/kg/d) is the preferred agent because of its palatability and lack of taste.
  - Milk of magnesia (0.5–1 mL/kg/d) is a good option.
  - Mineral oil (5–20 mL in divided doses) may also be used in older children who have no risk of aspiration.
  - Lactulose(2.5–10 mL/d for infants and 40–90 mL/d in older children)

ISSUES FOR REFERRAL

Patients with nonretentive fecal incontinence usually require referral to a mental health professional for more intensive behavioral intervention.

COMPLEMENTARY & ALTERNATIVE THERAPIES

Behavior modification: Decrease family stress. Have the child sit on toilet for defined amount of time (1 minute/year of age to a maximum of 10 minutes) 1–2 times per day (ideally after a meal, tailored to the age of the child) and try to perform a Valsalva maneuver. Have young children blow into a pinwheel or a balloon to try to make them bear down. Delay toilet training if the child is in diapers (to reduce stress). Motivate using positive reinforcement strategies. Biofeedback can be successful in some cases.

IN-PATIENT CONSIDERATIONS
Initial Stabilization

Management combines pharmacology, behavioral modification, and dietary alterations.

 ONGOING CARE

FOLLOW-UP RECOMMENDATIONS
Patient Monitoring

- 1st follow-up visit is at 2 weeks to ensure compliance and success with the initial management.
- If the fecal impaction has been successfully removed, a reward system is started.
- The patient is followed at monthly intervals to ensure motivation and to be supportive.
- Treatment with stool softeners is needed until behavior and diet have improved and until rectal dilation has resolved.
- Medication is often needed for 6 months or longer.

ALERT

- Parents may misconstrue stool-withholding behavior as an attempt to defecate.
- Parents may think that the soiling represents diarrheal illness, causing a delay in diagnosis and treatment.
- Parents may think their child's soiling is deliberate. They may not understand that the child can neither feel the passage of stool nor prevent it. The usual urge to defecate, which comes from stretching of the ampulla and internal anal sphincter, is not felt because the rectal ampulla is massively distended.
- Patients or their parents often stop stool softeners as soon as a normal stool pattern starts. If therapy has been ended prematurely, the patient's constipation and encopresis returns immediately because rectal tone is still poor and no other behavior or dietary modifications have been made.

DIET
- High fiber
- Adequate fluid

COMPLICATIONS
- Social problems
- UTIs, especially in girls
- Abdominal discomfort
- Decreased appetite and weight loss

ADDITIONAL READING

- Burgers RB, Benninga MA. Functional nonretentive fecal incontinence in children: A frustrating and long-lasting clinical entity. *J Pediatr Gastroenterol Nutr*. 2009;48(Suppl 2):S98–S100.
- Desantis DJ, Leonard MP, Preston MA, et al. Effectiveness of biofeedback for dysfunctional elimination syndrome in pediatrics: A systematic review. *J Pediatr Urol*. 2011;7(3):342–348.
- Di Lorenzo C, Benninga MA. Pathophysiology of pediatric fecal incontinence. *Gastroenterology*. 2004;126(Suppl 1):S33–S40.
- Griffiths DM. The physiology of continence: Idiopathic fecal constipation and soiling. *Semin Pediatr Surg*. 2002;11:67–74.
- Har AF, Croffie JM. Encopresis. *Pediatr Rev*. 2010;31:368–374.
- Loening-Baucke V. Encopresis. *Curr Opin Pediatr*. 2002;14:570–575.
- Loening-Baucke V. Functional fecal retention with encopresis in childhood. *J Pediatr Gastroenterol Nutr*. 2004;38:79–84.
- Rasquin A, Di Lorenzo C, Forbes D, et al. Childhood functional gastrointestinal disorders: Child/adolescent. *Gastroenterology*. 2006:130; 1527–1537.

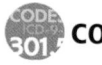 **CODES**

ICD9
- 307.7 Encopresis
- 787.60 Full incontinence of feces
- 787.62 Fecal smearing

ICD10
- F98.1 Encopresis not due to a substance or known physiological condition
- R15.1 Fecal smearing
- R15.9 Full incontinence of feces

FAQ

- Q: Is the medicine addictive?
- A: Stool softeners, rather than cathartics, are chosen for long-term therapy because the colon does not become dependent.
- Q: Will my child become sick if this problem is not resolved?
- A: Most children with chronic constipation and encopresis grow well and do not develop other health problems. The major problems are social and should be taken seriously. Social development is crucial for the school-aged child.

E

ENDOCARDITIS

Jenifer A. Glatz

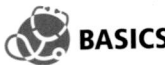 **BASICS**

DESCRIPTION
Infective endocarditis (IE) is a microbial infection of the endocardium of the heart.

EPIDEMIOLOGY
Incidence
- IE is relatively uncommon. The estimated incidence is 0.3 per 100,000 children per year.
- The overall incidence of endocarditis decreased with the advent of antibiotics. However, a recent increase in frequency has been associated with improved survival of patients with congenital heart disease and the more widespread and often prolonged use of central vascular catheters, especially in premature infants.

RISK FACTORS
- Preexisting heart disease (congenital or acquired)
- Prior history of endocarditis
- Cardiac surgery
- Intracardiac pacemakers and implantable cardioverter-defibrillators
- Prosthetic valves or conduits
- Indwelling catheters/IV drug use

GENERAL PREVENTION
- Dental hygiene
- Minimal use of central lines
- Correction of the cardiovascular anomaly by surgery or interventional catheterization techniques
- Subacute bacterial endocarditis (SBE) prophylaxis regimes as per the 2007 American Heart Association recommendations. Give as a single dose 30–60 minutes prior to procedure:
  - Oral: Amoxicillin (50 mg/kg, max 2.0 g)
  - IV or IM: Ampicillin (50 mg/kg, max 2.0 g) or ceftriaxone/cefazolin (50 mg/kg, max 1.0 g)
  - Oral for penicillin-allergic patients: Cephalexin, if no history of urticaria, angioedema, or anaphylaxis (50 mg/kg, max 2.0 g), clindamycin (20 mg/kg PO/IV, max 600 mg) or azithromycin/clarithromycin (15 mg/kg PO, max 500 mg)
  - IV or IM for penicillin-allergic patients: Cefazolin, ceftriaxone, or clindamycin (doses as above)
- SBE prophylaxis is recommended by the AHA only for the following cardiac conditions:
  - Prosthetic cardiac valve or prosthetic material used for cardiac valve repair
  - Prior history of infective endocarditis
  - Unrepaired cyanotic congenital heart disease, including palliative shunts and conduits
  - Congenital heart defect repaired with prosthetic material or device for the 1st 6 months after the procedure
  - Repaired congenital heart disease with residual defect near the site of prosthetic patch or device
  - Cardiac transplantation recipients with cardiac valvulopathy
- SBE prophylaxis is recommended only for the following procedures:
  - Dental procedures involving manipulation of the gingival or periapical region of teeth or perforation of the oral mucosa
  - Invasive respiratory tract procedures involving incision or biopsy, such as tonsillectomy/adenoidectomy or abscess drainage
  - Surgery involving prosthetic intravascular or intracardiac material, including heart valves
- Procedures that do not require SBE prophylaxis:
  - Placement of removable prosthodontic or orthodontic appliances
  - Bleeding from trauma to the lips or oral mucosa or shedding of deciduous teeth
  - Routine anesthetic injections through noninfected oral mucosa tissues
  - Bronchoscopy without a biopsy
  - GI or GU procedures: Prophylaxis solely to prevent IE is not recommended

PATHOPHYSIOLOGY
- Infective endocarditis is primarily seen in patients with preexisting heart disease (congenital or acquired) who develop bacteremia with organisms that are likely to cause infection.
- IV drug abusers and patients with indwelling central venous catheters may develop endocarditis even in the absence of prior heart disease.
- Local turbulence secondary to the cardiovascular abnormality is thought to result in damage of the endocardial surface. The development of a fibrin and platelet network occurs in which bacteria may then become entrapped, causing infection.
- Bacteremia may be a complication of focal infection (e.g., pneumonia, cellulitis, or UTI) or may be associated with various dental and surgical procedures. Bacteremia, however, also occurs spontaneously with usual activities, such as chewing, flossing, and brushing teeth.
- Peripheral manifestations in chronic endocarditis are mediated by immune complex reactions.

ETIOLOGY
- Gram-positive cocci account for 90% of culture-positive endocarditis. There has been a recent shift in the microbial etiology, corresponding with a more acute presentation:
  - *Staphylococcus aureus* is now responsible for most cases of infective endocarditis in all age groups.
  - α-Hemolytic streptococci (*Streptococcus viridans*) are the 2nd most common pathogen in children >1 year.
  - Other organisms that can cause endocarditis are coagulase-negative staphylococci, β-hemolytic streptococci, enterococci, the HACEK group (*Haemophilus aphrophilus, Haemophilus paraphrophilus, Haemophilus parainfluenzae, Actinobacillus actinomycetemcomitans, Cardiobacterium hominis, Eikenella corrodens, Kingella species*), *Candida* species, *Aspergillus* species, *Pseudomonas* species, pneumococci, and *Neisseria* species.
- <20% of endocarditis cases are reported as culture negative.

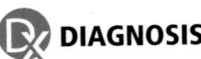 **DIAGNOSIS**

- The Modified Duke Criteria define diagnostic categories (definite endocarditis, possible endocarditis, and rejected cases) based on combinations of major and minor criteria.
- Criteria:
  - Major: Organism specific for IE demonstrated by positive blood culture or histologic specimen and definitive echocardiographic data.
  - Minor: Predisposing heart disease, fever, vascular/immunologic phenomena, or microbiologic evidence not within major criteria.
- Definitive endocarditis requires 2 major, or 1 major plus 3 minor, or 5 minor criteria.
- Several studies have confirmed the high sensitivity and specificity of these criteria.

HISTORY
- Fever
- Malaise
- Anorexia
- Weight loss
- Heart failure symptoms
- Arthralgia/Myalgia
- Neurologic symptoms
- GI symptoms
- Chest pain
- Occasionally, a recent infection, dental visit, or surgical procedure can be identified.
- Acute endocarditis is associated with a more rapidly progressive, fulminant course.

PHYSICAL EXAM
- General:
  - Fever (usually low grade with α-hemolytic streptococci and high grade with *S. aureus*)
  - Petechiae (occurring in 1/3 of cases)
- Embolic or immunologic phenomena:
  - Renal: Glomerulonephritis, infarct
  - Splinter hemorrhages
  - Retinal hemorrhages (Roth spots)
  - Osler nodes (painful)
  - Janeway lesions (painless)
  - Splenomegaly (occurring in about 50% of cases)
  - Arthralgia/Arthritis
  - Neurologic: Cerebral infarction, embolism or hemorrhage. Mycotic aneurysms may also occur.
- Cardiac/Valvulitis:
  - New or change in heart murmur
  - Signs of CHF
- Newborns with IE may present with feeding difficulty, respiratory distress, tachycardia, hypotension, seizures, apnea, and septic emboli.

DIAGNOSTIC TESTS & INTERPRETATION
Lab
- Blood cultures:
  - Most important diagnostic test for endocarditis
  - Positive in 85–90% of reported cases
  - Obtain 3–5 sets from different sites during the 1st 24 hours of suspected endocarditis.
  - Collect the largest volume that is clinically reasonable.
  - The bacteremia of endocarditis is continuous; therefore, it is not necessary to wait to obtain the blood cultures during a fever spike.
- Nonspecific data:
  - Elevated ESR (80%) and C-reactive protein
  - Anemia (44%)
  - Positive rheumatoid factor (38%)
  - Hematuria (35%) and red cell casts
  - Leukocytosis
  - Decreased complement

Imaging
- Echocardiography, transthoracic:
  - Valuable noninvasive technique in the identification of vegetations
  - Specificity is 98% but sensitivity is <60%, so a negative echocardiogram does not rule out endocarditis.
  - Also invaluable for follow-up, including evaluation for potential cardiac complications
- Echocardiography, transesophageal:
  - Especially in older or obese patients, provides better visualization of smaller vegetations, with sensitivity of 76–100%.
  - Recommended in patients with an inconclusive transthoracic study but a high index of suspicion for endocarditis.

ALERT
- The absence of vegetation(s) by echocardiography does not rule out endocarditis.
- In patients with a prosthetic valve, echocardiography is not always helpful, as there is frequently artifact from the prosthetic valve. Abnormal movements of the valve leaflets may suggest a vegetation.
- The ESR may remain elevated for some time, even after cessation of bacteremia.

Diagnostic Procedures/Other
ECG: New-onset abnormalities such as atrioventricular block (even 1st-degree) may represent conduction system and myocardial involvement from invasive disease.

DIFFERENTIAL DIAGNOSIS
- Other infections
- Acute rheumatic fever
- Malignancy
- Connective tissue disorders

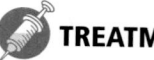

TREATMENT

MEDICATION (DRUGS)
Antibiotics:
- Prolonged IV therapy (at least 4 weeks) is needed.
- Choice of antibiotic(s) and duration of treatment depend on the infecting organism, sensitivity pattern, and patient risk factors.
- For staphylococcal or fungal endocarditis, IV therapy is given for at least 6–8 weeks.

SURGERY/OTHER PROCEDURES
Potential indications (mostly adult data):
- Severe/worsening CHF
- Valvar disease with unstable hemodynamics
- Failing medical therapy
- Large (>10 mm), mobile vegetations
- ≥2 major embolic events
- Fungal endocarditis
- Abscess formation/periannular extension
- Prosthetic valve endocarditis

IN-PATIENT CONSIDERATIONS
Initial Stabilization
- Rest
- Antipyretics
- Optimal nutrition and hydration
- Careful dental hygiene

ONGOING CARE

FOLLOW-UP RECOMMENDATIONS
Patient Monitoring
- Obtain repeat blood cultures after a few days of antibiotic or antifungal therapy to ensure the eradication of bacteria.
- Obtain blood cultures again 2 months after completion of a full course of antibiotic therapy.

PROGNOSIS
If diagnosed in a timely fashion and appropriate therapy is instituted, prognosis is relatively good for bacterial endocarditis. *S. aureus* and fungal endocarditis are associated with higher morbidity and mortality.

COMPLICATIONS
Despite improvements in diagnosis and treatment, IE continues to be a disease with significant morbidity and mortality (~10–20%):
- Cardiac: Valve destruction and perforation leading to incompetence, abscess and fistula formation, heart failure, or conduction abnormalities.
- Embolic events (22–50%) may occur to multiple organ systems (CNS, bowel, coronary arteries, kidneys, spleen, skin, lungs).

ADDITIONAL READING
- Ferrieri P, Gewitz MH, Gerber MA, et al. Unique features of infective endocarditis in childhood. *Circulation*. 2002;105:2115–2127.
- McDonald JR. Acute infective endocarditis. *Infect Dis Clin N Am*. 2009;23(3):643–664.
- Milazzo AS Jr, Li JS. Bacterial endocarditis in infants and children. *Pediatr Infect Dis J*. 2001;20:799–801.
- Wilson W, Taubert KA, Gewitz M, et al. Prevention of infective endocarditis: Guidelines from the American Heart Association. *Circulation*. 2007; 116:1736–1754.

 CODES

ICD9
- 421.0 Acute and subacute bacterial endocarditis
- 421.9 Acute endocarditis, unspecified
- 424.90 Endocarditis, valve unspecified, unspecified cause

ICD10
- I33.0 Acute and subacute infective endocarditis
- I33.9 Acute and subacute endocarditis, unspecified
- I38 Endocarditis, valve unspecified

FAQ
- Q: I forgot to give my child antibiotics prior to the procedure. Should I give him a dose afterward?
- A: The dosage may be administered up to 2 hours after the procedure.
- Q: My child has an innocent heart murmur. Does he need SBE prophylaxis?
- A: SBE prophylaxis is not indicated.
- Q: SBE prophylaxis is recommended for my child, but she already is on long-term antibiotic therapy with that recommended antibiotic. Should she use an additional antibiotic or increase her current dose for the procedure?
- A: An antibiotic from a different class should be selected.

E

ENURESIS
Eugene R. Hershorin
Alicia Edwards-Richards

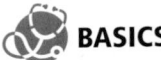 **BASICS**

DESCRIPTION
Involuntary micturition after age of expected bladder control; generally reserved for children ≥6 years:

- Generally refers to monosymptomatic nocturnal enuresis or bedwetting–urinary incontinence only at night.
- ~20% of children may also exhibit both daytime symptoms (urgency, frequency, incontinence) and nighttime wetting, and this is termed dysfunctional voiding
- Monosymptomatic nocturnal enuresis may be primary or secondary:
  – Primary enuresis: Never continent of urine on consecutive nights for at least 6 months (daytime, nocturnal, or both)
  – Secondary enuresis: Had continent period of at least 6 months, then relapse of enuresis
- Most (80%) of nocturnal enuresis is primary.

EPIDEMIOLOGY
- Male > Female (3:1)
- Frequency, severity, longevity of primary nocturnal enuresis (PNE) increases with positive family history.

Incidence
- 43–47% if 1 parent was enuretic
- 15% if neither parent was enuretic
- Twice as high in monozygotic twins as dizygotic twins
- Incidence increased among children also diagnosed with ADHD

Prevalence
- At age 5, 15% of children have PNE.
- ~15% of children with enuresis spontaneously remit each year:
  – By age 10, only 5% still have nocturnal enuresis.
- ~1% of adolescents have nocturnal enuresis.

RISK FACTORS
Genetics
- An autosomal dominant variant of nocturnal enuresis is described in a Danish population.
- Generally, however, no specific genetic abnormality is identified.

ETIOLOGY
- PNE:
  – Underlying treatable cause uncommon
  – Any condition causing polyuria (e.g. diabetes insipidus, diabetes mellitus)
  – Theories: Deep sleep with failure of signal of increased bladder pressure to reach consciousness; maturational delay with bladder emptying at lower volume secondary to small bladder capacity; failure to concentrate urine or to decrease urinary volume at night compared with dry peers

- Daytime incontinence and enuresis, day and night:
  – As above. More concerning for underlying urologic and neurologic disorder
  – Urinary reflux into vagina with seepage after conclusion of voiding
  – Insertion of ureter into urethra or vagina
  – Incontinence with increased abdominal pressure (laughing, coughing, increased intravesicular pressure)
- Secondary enuresis:
  – Any condition causing polyuria
  – UTI
  – Encopresis
  – Emotional stress or trauma including physical and sexual abuse, divorce, depression, new sibling, household moving, new school

DIAGNOSIS

HISTORY
- Onset:
  – Nocturnal versus diurnal
  – Dry period (even if only weeks)
  – Frequency
  – Pattern of urination:
    ○ Constantly wet pants (dribbling)
    ○ Frequent small amounts of urine
    ○ Dysuria
    ○ Frequency
    ○ Hesitancy
    ○ Dry when sleeping away from home
- Past medical history:
  – Obstipation/constipation/stool incontinence (encopresis)
  – Behavioral/developmental history
  – Toilet training history
  – Medications
  – Neurologic symptoms
  – Other medical problems
- Family history:
  – 1 parent or 2
  – Child awareness
- Social history:
  – For whom does this pose problem—parent or child?
  – Effect on child:
    ○ Ability to sleep away from home without embarrassment
    ○ Teasing at school
    ○ Emotional effects
- Social changes:
  – Divorce
  – New significant other for parent
  – New sibling
  – Household move
  – Change in school
  – Death or illness in family
  – Other change in home environment
- Past interventions and effectiveness:
  – Attempt at treatment or punishment and its effectiveness

PHYSICAL EXAM
- Vital signs
- Growth parameters and pattern
- Neurologic exam:
  – Gait, tone, sensory, motor, deep tendon reflexes, cremasteric reflex
  – With funduscopy: To rule out intracranial pressure
- Abdominal exam: To rule out masses, especially renal mass
- Genitalia: Rule out adhesions, vulvovaginitis, balanitis, stenosis, foreign bodies.
- Urinary stream
- Rectal exam: Tone, perianal sensation, anal wink
- Spine: Bony defects, cutaneous signs of underlying spinal defects

DIAGNOSTIC TESTS & INTERPRETATION
Lab
- Urinalysis:
  – Specific gravity
  – Glucose
  – Protein
  – Blood
  – Urine:
    ○ 1st morning void for specific gravity and protein
- Urine culture: Usually not necessary if no symptoms

Imaging
- Rarely necessary in monosymptomatic primary enuresis
- Only if suggestion of anatomic or functional abnormality of genitourinary system

> **ALERT**
> Laboratory evaluation rarely yields specific diagnosis. Balance risks and costs with unlikelihood of yield. Evaluation should generally involve no more than urinalysis.

DIFFERENTIAL DIAGNOSIS
- UTI/Urethritis
- Obstipation/constipation
- Water intoxication
- Diabetes mellitus
- Diabetes insipidus
- Sickle cell disease or trait
- Nephritis/Nephrosis
- Anatomic abnormalities of the urinary tract
- Sleep disorders
- Depression
- Anxiety
- Behavioral disorders
- Medications (sedatives, soporifics, antihistamines, diuretics, caffeine, methylxanthines)
- Spinal cord disease
- Cognitive disorders
- Seizure disorders
- Legitimate safety issues in going to bathroom alone
- Substandard living conditions (cold bathrooms, poor facilities)

TREATMENT

MEDICATION (DRUGS)
- Avoid medication intervention before age 6–8 years
- Desmopressin (DDAVP):
  - Can be used intermittently only on sleep-out nights
  - Effective in 70% of PNE
  - If used chronically, monitor electrolytes and fluid status appropriately.
  - Oral formulation only (nasal formulation associated with increased risk of hypontremia and seizures)
- Imipramine:
  - Tricyclic antidepressant
  - 80% effective
  - No longer 1st- or 2nd-line choice for benign condition because of risk of QTc prolongation and controversial risk of sudden cardiac death and risk of ingestion in siblings
- Oxybutynin: Used in patients with documented detrusor instability

ADDITIONAL TREATMENT
General Measures
- If the problem is affecting only the parents and child is not affected, the treatment should be education and support for the parents:
  - Prognosis for self-resolution
  - Benign nature
  - Available interventions if child becomes concerned
- Avoid all negative interventions.
- Fluid restriction before bed—controversial:
  - May create arguments with parents
  - Success rate low
- Retention training/bladder stretching exercises—controversial
- Cognitive behavioral interventions:
  - Formal programs developed and used by pediatric psychologists: High rate of success; involve "Over Correction Techniques"—frequent practice and rewards for voiding procedures along with enuresis alarm
  - Positive reinforcement for dry nights
  - Use of praise, stickers, token economies
  - Bell-and-pad alarm systems: Most effective of behavioral interventions more effective in conjunction with formal behavioral program; high relapse rate after remission and cessation of alarm usage; 2nd remission very frequent with reintroduction of alarm system; 2nd relapse rare

- Hypnotism:
  - Appears to work by increasing subconscious awareness of bladder pressure during sleep, allowing increased awareness during sleep of intravesicular pressure
  - Use of bell-and-pad alarm may increase success rate

IN-PATIENT CONSIDERATIONS
Initial Stabilization
Specific therapy to address specific anatomic, infectious, or functional renal problems

> **ALERT**
> Decision to treat is a balance of the effect on the child of nontreatment (social, emotional) with the potential side effects of medication.

ONGOING CARE

PROGNOSIS
- 99% percent of cases resolve without treatment.
- Spontaneous resolution is ~15% per year after age 5.

COMPLICATIONS
- Physical:
  - Vulvovaginitis
  - Diaper dermatitis
- Emotional:
  - Embarrassment
  - Poor self-esteem
  - Reluctance to sleep out with peers or nonimmediate family
  - Depression

ADDITIONAL READING
- Bosson S, Lyth N. Nocturnal enuresis. *Clin Evid.* 2002;7:341–348.
- Glazener CM, Evans JH, Peto RE. Tricyclic and related drugs for nocturnal enuresis in children. *Cochrane Database Syst Rev.* 2003:CD002117.
- Graham KM, et al. *Pediatr Review.* 2009;30:165–173.
- Jalkut MW. Enuresis. *Pediatr Clin North Am.* 2001;48:1461–1488.
- Meadow R. Childhood enuresis. *BMJ.* 1970;4:787–789.

CODES

ICD9
- 307.6 Enuresis
- 788.30 Urinary incontinence, unspecified
- 788.36 Nocturnal enuresis

ICD10
- N39.44 Nocturnal enuresis
- R32 Unspecified urinary incontinence

FAQ
- Q: Do the medications cure the enuresis?
- A: None of the medications cures the problem. DDAVP increases reabsorption of water in the kidney, resulting in decreased bladder volumes. Tricyclic antidepressants cause urinary retention by the noradrenergic effects on bladder contraction and detrusor relaxation. Oxybutynin decreases detrusor irritability, resulting in larger bladder capacity before emptying. The medications result in nonemptying of the bladder during sleep, but do not affect the underlying cause. Any resolution that occurs after cessation of medication treatment is probably from the natural resolution of the problem with age.
- Q: Isn't it important to cure the enuresis when the parents bring it up as a problem?
- A: Developmental resolution of nocturnal enuresis occurs at a range of ages, and in almost all cases, the enuresis resolves spontaneously. The most important historical point is for whom is the enuresis is a problem. If the child is not affected by the enuresis, and it is only the parents who desire a cure, the important intervention is to educate them on the natural history of the problem and to let them know about the available interventions and their success rates, for when the child desires a cure.
- Q: Are there any other interventions available for use only on sleep-out nights?
- A: One helpful tip is to allow the child to take a sleeping bag with him or her on sleep-outs. Inside the sleeping bag is a pull-up. When the child gets into the sleeping bag, he or she can change into the pull-up without anyone knowing. In the morning, the child puts his or her underwear back on, leaving the damp pull-up in the sleeping bag; the parent can take it out when the child gets home.

E

EOSINOPHILIC ESOPHAGITIS

James P. Franciosi
Chris A. Liacouras

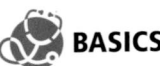 **BASICS**

DESCRIPTION
- Eosinophilic esophagitis (EoE) is clinical, pathologic diagnosis characterized by a localized eosinophilic inflammation of the esophagus.
- Esophageal endoscopic biopsies are required to establish the diagnosis.
- On endoscopic mucosal biopsies, EoE is defined as the presence of at least 15 eosinophils per high-powered field isolated to the esophagus that does not respond to acid blockade medication or with a normal pH/impedance probe test.
- EoE has been associated with variants at chromosome 5q22.

EPIDEMIOLOGY
The incidence and prevalence of EoE in children 0–19 years of age is thought to be respectively 1 and 10 per 10,000 children

PATHOPHYSIOLOGY
The pathophysiology EoE is unknown; however, it has been linked to an allergic response to food antigens that does not follow a typical IgE mediated pattern.

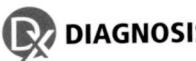 **DIAGNOSIS**

- Symptoms can be similar to gastroesophageal reflux (GERD).
- Typically occurs in toddlers and older children, and is considered distinct from infant milk protein allergy:
  - Vomiting
  - Regurgitation
  - Dysphagia
  - Nausea
  - Epigastric pain
  - Heartburn
  - Chest pain
  - Esophageal food impaction
  - Irritability/feeding difficulties
  - Nighttime cough
  - Abdominal pain
- Complications that can occur with EoE include:
  - Failure to thrive
  - Malnutrition
  - Feeding intolerance
  - Esophageal strictures
  - Hiatal hernia
  - Small-caliber esophagus
  - Esophageal perforation
  - Esophageal fungal or viral superinfection

ALERT
Any patient who is being considered for surgical correction of gastroesophageal reflux (fundoplication) should first be evaluated endoscopically for EoE to prevent unnecessary surgery.

HISTORY
- Eosinophilic Esophagitis EoE in the infant and younger child:
  - Irritability
  - Weight
  - Vomiting
  - Feeding difficulties
  - Personal or family history of atopic disease (asthma, allergic rhinitis, eczema)
- Special questions:
  - Personal or family history of atopic disease?
  - Family history of EoE, dysphagia, severe GERD, esophageal food impactions or dilations?
  - No relief/response to acid blockade medication (minimum of 6–8 weeks)?
- EoE in the older child and adolescent:
  - Heartburn
  - Nausea
  - Vomiting
  - Epigastric pain
- EoE should be considered in any child presenting with dysphagia or food impaction, particular foods avoided or difficulty with eating, personal and family history of atopic disease, and food allergy and esophageal food impaction or dilation.
- Special questions:
  - Personal or family history of atopic disease?
  - Family history of EoE?
  - No relief/response to acid blockade medication?
  - Slow eater? Does the child avoid specific foods?
  - Any sensation of food sticking or difficulty swallowing?
  - Personal or family history of esophageal food impaction?

PHYSICAL EXAM
- Typically normal
- Growth failure (rare, occurs if appetite decreased significantly)
- Allergic shiners, reactive airway disease
- Eczema

DIAGNOSTIC TESTS & INTERPRETATION
Diagnostic Procedures/Other
- Upper endoscopy (esophagastroduodenoscopy, EGD):
  - The gold standard for diagnosis of eosinophilic esophagitis. Typically performed after a trial of acid blockade medication for 6–8 weeks.
  - Endoscopic mucosal biopsies should be obtained from the proximal and distal esophagus (minimum of 2 from each location), the stomach and duodenum. A pathologist who has experience with EoE should examine the mucosal biopsies for the presence of $\geq$15 eosinophils per high-powered field isolated to the esophagus.
- Upper GI series radiography:
  - Typically performed before endoscopy to exclude other etiologies of vomiting. May demonstrate esophageal stricture, corrugated esophagus, foreshortened esophagus, hiatal hernia, a small caliber esophagus, or esophageal perforation. However, none of these findings is specific to EoE.
- pH/Impedance probe:
  - Should be normal in patients with EoE. Considered a gold standard for evaluation of acid reflux disease, but of limited role in the evaluation of EoE
- Blood tests:
  - Peripheral eosinophilia is present in <50% of patients. Currently, there are no widely available serum markers for EoE.
- Food allergy testing:
  - Radio-allergosorbent test (RAST): Serum testing for food specific IgE antibodies; low sensitivity, limited role
  - Skin testing: Percutaneous prick puncture testing for food-specific IgE-mediated reactions
  - Patch testing (atopy patch testing): Allergen in prolonged contact with the skin in patches with the same concentration of food that is ingested
  - Tests for food-specific non–IgE-mediated reactions
  - Food allergy testing is typically only performed after endoscopic confirmation of EoE. Causative food antigens can be identified in 70% of patients through skin prick and patch testing. Although EoE is considered a mixed IgE- and non–IgE-mediated disease, most reactions occur through non–IgE-mediated pathways.

DIFFERENTIAL DIAGNOSIS
- GERD
- Inflammatory bowel disease
- Eosinophilic gastroenteritis
- Celiac disease
- Parasitic infection
- Connective tissue disease
- Drug allergy
- Hypereosinophilic syndrome
- Autoimmune enteropathy
- Candida esophagitis
- Viral esophagitis (herpes or CMV)
- Should exclude other causes of vomiting, failure to thrive

TREATMENT

MEDICATION (DRUGS)

- Fluticasone propionate:
  - A topical or ingested steroid that is an alternative to dietary therapy. Aerosolized fluticasone spray is swallowed instead of being inhaled. Patients do not eat, drink, or rinse their mouth for 30 minutes after using this medication. Achieves histologic remission in >50% of patients. However, with discontinuation of the medication, almost all patients relapse. Reported side effects include esophageal candidiasis, epistaxis, and dry mouth. Long-term effects on growth, bone health, and esophageal fibrosis currently not known. Recommended doses are 110–220 μg (swallowed) b.i.d. for children <6 years of age, and 440–880 μg b.i.d. for children >6 years of age.
- Oral viscous budesonide (OVB):
  - An equally effective alternative swallowed steroid administered in a slurry formulation that is made using Splenda (5 packets/500 mcg) to improve taste and consistency for topical esophageal administration. Pediatric randomized, double-blind, placebo-controlled trial using OVB showed 86.7% histologic response rate in the OVB group compared to none of the controls. Symptom scores were also significantly improved. Dosing of the budesonide was 1 and 2 mg divided b.i.d. based on the respective height classification of <or >5 feet.
- Corticosteroids:
  - An effective treatment for EoE, but symptoms and histologic eosinophilia return when these medications are discontinued. Given the extensive side-effect profile, long-term corticosteroids are not considered an ideal treatment option for EoE. Short courses of oral steroids may have a role in treating emergent EoE patients who present with significant esophageal strictures, severe weight loss, or the inability to eat most foods/liquids. The recommended dose of prednisone is 1–2 mg/kg/d (maximum 60 mg/d).

ADDITIONAL TREATMENT
General Measures

- Several modes of dietary and medication therapy are available depending on disease presentation and therapy.
- Proton pump inhibitors (PPI):
  - 2007 Consensus Guidelines for EoE define this condition as persistent clinicopathologic findings consistent with EoE despite 6–8 weeks of PPI therapy. Retrospective data and adult studies suggest a PPI response rate of 25–40%. No pediatric clinical trials have been conducted to date.

COMPLEMENTARY & ALTERNATIVE THERAPIES

- Endoscopic therapy: Esophageal dilatation is a useful therapy for EoE patients with fixed esophageal strictures. Care must be taken when performing dilatation as significant esophageal mucosal lacerations, tearing, and perforation have been reported. Whenever possible, diagnostic endoscopy followed by a trial of dietary or steroid therapy is recommended prior to esophageal stricture dilation.
- Patients presenting with esophageal food impaction should have the food bolus removed endoscopically, and esophageal biopsies should be obtained to investigate for EoE.

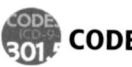 **ONGOING CARE**

DIET

- Elimination diet has been shown to be effective for treatment of eosinophilic esophagitis. Whenever possible, specific allergen testing (skin and patch testing) should be performed to identify and remove specific causative food antigens. However, food allergen testing may be falsely negative, and empiric removal of highly antigenic foods is reported to be successful in >75% of children. The 6 foods that are considered the most antigenic for EoE include milk, soy, nuts, egg, wheat, and fish/shellfish.
- Some patients require an elemental diet. Patients are allowed to drink only water and an amino acid-based formula until the esophageal eosinophilia resolves; subsequently, food is gradually reintroduced. This method frequently requires nasogastric tube feeding as these formulas are often unpalatable. Success with the elemental diet occurs in >95% of patients.

ADDITIONAL READING

- Aceves SS, et al. Topical viscous budesonide suspension for treatment of eosinophilic esophagitis. *J Allergy Clin Immunol*. 2005; 116(3):705–706.
- DeBrosse CW, Collins MH, Buckmeier Butz BK, et al. Identification, epidemiology, and chronicity of pediatric esophageal eosinophilia, 1982–1999. *J Allergy Clin Immunol*. 2010;125(1):112–119.
- Franciosi JP, Fiorino K, Ruchelli E, et al. Changing indications for upper endoscopy in children during a 20-year period. *J Pediatr Gastroenterol Nutr*. 2010;51(4):443–447.
- Furuta GT, Liacouras CA, Collins MH, et al. Eosinophilic esophagitis in children and adults: A systematic review and consensus recommendations for diagnosis and treatment. *Gastroenterology*. 2007;133:1342–1363.
- Kagalwalla AF, et al. Effect of six-food elimination diet on clinical and histologic outcomes in eosinophilic esophagitis. *Clin Gastroenterol Hepatol*. 2006;4(9):1097–1102.
- Liacouras CA. Eosinophilic esophagitis: Treatment in 2005. *Curr Opin Gastroenterol*. 2006;22(2): 147–152.
- Spergel JM, et al. Treatment of eosinophilic esophagitis with specific food elimination diet directed by a combination of skin prick and patch tests. *Ann Allergy Asthma Immunol*. 2005;95(4): 336–343.

CODES

ICD9
530.13 Eosinophilic esophagitis

ICD10
K20.0 Eosinophilic esophagitis

E

FAQ

- Q: Is EoE considered a life-long disease or will it resolve over time?
- A: The long-term outcome for children with EoE is currently unknown. Currently, the natural history of the disease suggests that EoE is a chronic disease that can be controlled with diet or medical therapy.
- Q: Is there any harm in not treating asymptomatic patients with ongoing histologic EoE?
- A: There is much debate about the progression of untreated EoE. The concerns are that, if left untreated, ongoing esophageal eosinophilic may lead to dysphagia, strictures, and esophageal fibrosis.
- Q: Is EoE a genetic or environmental disease?
- A: EoE is more common white males, >50% of patients have atopic disease (such as asthma, eczema, or allergic rhinitis), and 30–50% of patients with EoE have a family history of EoE or atopic disease.
- Q: Is the incidence of EoE increasing?
- A: There has been a significant rise in the number of pediatric and adult EoE diagnoses over the last 5 years. The most likely reason is an improved recognition of this disease among gastroenterologists, allergists, and pathologists. A rising incidence of new cases may also be occurring that is similar to the increase seen in other allergic disorders.

EPIGLOTTITIS

Mark L. Bagarazzi

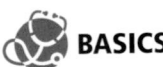 **BASICS**

DESCRIPTION
Acute life-threatening bacterial infection consisting of cellulitis and edema of the epiglottis, aryepiglottic folds, arytenoids, and hypopharynx, resulting in narrowing of the glottic opening.

EPIDEMIOLOGY
Disease due to *Haemophilus influenzae* type B occurs most often between the ages of 2 and 7 years (overall range: infancy to adulthood).

- Epiglottitis and other invasive disease secondary to *H. influenzae* have been reduced by 99% since the introduction of the conjugate vaccines in 1989 (approved at 15 months) and 1990 (approved at 2, 4, and 6 months).
- Nontypeable *H. influenzae* now appears to be a more common cause of invasive disease than type B.
- Year-round occurrence
- Affects males and females equally
- All geographic areas
- Rare in populations in which the peak incidence of meningitis is shifted toward infancy (e.g., Alaskan Eskimos, Native Americans)
- Occasionally secondary cases in households or child care centers
- May be more frequent in children with sickle cell anemia, asplenia, immunoglobulin defects, or hematologic malignancies (e.g., leukemia)
- Disease due to *Streptococcus pyogenes* occurs most often in early school-age children during the winter and early spring and has now been seen as a complication of varicella infection.

Incidence
- Incidence of epiglottitis due to any organism has declined substantially (e.g., 20.9/100,000 per year to 0.9/100,000 per year from 1987 to 1996 in Sweden)
- Incidence rate in children 18 and younger is also on the decline in the US based on data through 2006, although overall rates are steady. Rates in infants may be on the rise.

GENERAL PREVENTION
- Rifampin: 20 mg/kg/d in single dose for 4 days to eradicate *H. influenzae* type B colonization (see "Control measures").
- Universal immunization with *H. influenzae* type B capsular polysaccharide conjugate vaccines at 2, 4, and 6 months, with booster at 12 to 18 months
- Isolation of hospitalized patient: Droplet precautions should be continued for at least 24 hours from the initiation of effective therapy.
- Control measures: Prophylaxis for *H. influenzae* type B index case and susceptible children in household and child care setting, and intimate contacts

PATHOPHYSIOLOGY
Erythema and edema of the uvula, aryepiglottic folds, arytenoids, epiglottis, and vocal cords include an exudate rich in neutrophils and fibrin, which usually proceeds to organization and fibrous scarring.

ETIOLOGY
- *H. influenzae*, nontypeable and type B (accounted for >90% of cases prior to the introduction of HiB vaccine)
- *Staphylococcus aureus*
- *Streptococcus pneumoniae*
- *S. pyogenes* (group A β-hemolytic streptococcus)
- Group C and G β-hemolytic streptococcus (rare)
- *Candida albicans* may be an etiologic agent in immunocompromised patients.
- *Pasteurella multocida* has been implicated in a few cases after exposure to nasopharyngeal secretions from a cat.
- There have been recent reports of epiglottitis due to *Neisseria meningitidis*.
- Other rare isolates: *Moraxella catarrhalis, Klebsiella pneumoniae, Pseudomonas* species
- The inhaled anesthetic sevoflurane has been implicated in a few cases of epiglottitis.

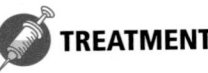 **DIAGNOSIS**

HISTORY
- Abrupt onset of high fever (39–40°C), sore throat, and dysphagia
- Very limited or no prodrome of mild upper respiratory tract infection (URI)
- "Hot potato" voice
- Rapid onset of toxicity and respiratory distress
- Cough and hoarseness are late symptoms, if they occur at all.
- Time from onset of symptoms to presentation with progressive respiratory distress is generally <12 hours.
- Immunization against *H. influenzae* type B
- Child's preferred way of sitting or positioning himself or herself (i.e., sitting upright, leaning forward with chin hyperextended)
- Exposure to cats

PHYSICAL EXAM
- Extremely anxious appearance
- Child prefers to remain sitting up.
- Child often leaning forward with chin hyperextended to maintain airway in a "tripod" position
- Slow and labored respiratory effort
- Drooling is seen as a manifestation of dysphagia.
- Inspiratory stridor, retractions, and late cyanosis
- Diagnosis can be suspected on history and observation of child's appearance alone.
- Do *not* attempt to examine the throat if epiglottitis is a serious consideration.

DIAGNOSTIC TESTS & INTERPRETATION
Lab
- Complete blood count: Increased white blood cell count with left shift
- Cultures of blood (positive in up to 90%) and epiglottis (performed only in the operating room): May be positive for the causative organism

Imaging
Lateral neck radiography: Characteristic "thumb sign" of edematous epiglottis, with narrowing of the posterior airway and ballooning of the hypopharynx (should not be performed until airway team is in place)

ALERT
- A radiograph is indicated only when the diagnosis is in doubt and should not delay airway management.
- Avoid blood collection until the airway has been secured so as not to upset the child unnecessarily.
- Ensure appropriate airway management prior to any other interventions, including laryngeal exam, radiographs, and laboratory studies.
- Finding of stridor in a child with varicella infection may indicate epiglottitis due to *S. pyogenes* (group A β-hemolytic streptococcus).

DIFFERENTIAL DIAGNOSIS
- Viral laryngotracheobronchitis (croup) with or without secondary bacterial tracheitis
- Severe parainfluenza or influenza infection
- Uvulitis
- Peritonsillar, retropharyngeal, or lingual abscess
- Foreign body aspiration in a child with URI
- URI, including croup, in a child with a congenital or acquired airway problem (e.g., premature infant with subglottic stenosis, laryngeal web, vascular ring, tracheal stenosis)
- Hereditary angioedema (deficiency of complement C1 esterase inhibitor) can present with edema of the airway including the epiglottis.
- Diphtheria: Rare in US
- Laryngeal infections, including laryngeal tuberculosis

TREATMENT

MEDICATION (DRUGS)
First Line
- Empiric antibiotic coverage to include gram-positive cocci and β-lactamase–producing *H. influenzae* type B:
  - Cefuroxime: 150 mg/kg/d divided q8h
  - Ampicillin/Sulbactam: 200 mg/kg/d divided q6h
  - Duration of therapy: 7–10 days for all but staphylococcal disease (14–21 days)
- Switch may be made to oral medication after extubation and resumption of feeding.

Second Line
- Chloramphenicol: 75–100 mg/kg/d divided q6h
- Ampicillin: 100–200 mg/kg/d divided q6h for non-β-lactamase–producing *H. influenzae* type B (~80% of isolates)
- Penicillin: 100,000–200,000 U/kg/d divided q4h to q6h for streptococcal disease
- Oxacillin: 100–200 mg/kg/d for staphylococcal disease

ISSUES FOR REFERRAL
Airway should be secured by clinician most skilled in airway management (e.g., otolaryngologist, anesthesiologist) prior to any attempt to transport a child with expected epiglottitis

IN-PATIENT CONSIDERATIONS
Initial Stabilization
- Airway management: Maintain child upright, never supine. Personnel experienced in airway management should accompany the child at all times, including during transport and in radiology.
- Rapid assembly of a team, which should include an anesthesiologist, an otolaryngologist, and a pediatrician, if possible. In a recent review of almost 3 million pediatric discharges from 36 states, ~12% of cases of epiglottitis in children required an artificial airway, and 63% of the children were <2 years old.
- Allow the child to assume his or her most comfortable position (usually in the mother's arms/lap).
- Oxygen by mask or blown by face
- Transport to operating room as soon as possible for anesthesia and intubation, followed by positive pressure ventilation as necessary.
- Institute intravenous catheterization and blood collection, and culturing of epiglottis only after the airway is secured.
- Perform emergent cricothyrotomy if obstruction occurs prior to controlled airway management.
- Use fluid resuscitation in cases of septic shock.

Admission Criteria
Admit all children with suspicion of epiglottitis for airway management.

 ## ONGOING CARE

FOLLOW-UP RECOMMENDATIONS
Patient Monitoring
- Extubation is usually possible within 24–48 hours. Criteria include decreased erythema and edema of the epiglottis on direct inspection and development of an air leak around the endotracheal tube.
- Defervescence is usually prompt after initiation of appropriate antimicrobial therapy.

PROGNOSIS
- Mortality is estimated to be 8% in hospital series.
- Virtually all cases in which arrest occurred prior to transfer to tertiary center resulted in fatality.

COMPLICATIONS
- Without prompt medical intervention: Complete airway obstruction leading to respiratory arrest, hypoxia, and death
- Necrotizing cervical fasciitis (rarely)
- Therapeutic complications:
  – Aspiration
  – Endotracheal tube dislodgment and extubation
  – Tracheal erosion or irritation
  – Pneumomediastinum
  – Pneumothorax
  – Pulmonary edema
- Complications of *H. influenzae* type B bacteremia:
  – Septic shock
  – Pneumonia
  – Cervical lymphadenopathy
  – Rarely, arthritis and pericarditis

ADDITIONAL READING
- Guldfred LA, Lyhne D, Becker BC. Acute epiglottis: Epidemiology, clinical presentation, management and outcome. *J Laryngol Otol.* 2008;122(8):818–823.
- Heath PT, Booy R, Azzopardi HJ, et al. Non-type b *Haemophilus influenzae* disease: Clinical and epidemiologic characteristics in the *Haemophilus influenzae* type b vaccine era. *Pediatr Infect Dis J.* 2001;20:300–305.
- Midwinter KI, Hodgson D, Yardley M. Paediatric epiglottitis: The influence of the *Haemophilus influenzae* B vaccine, a ten-year review in the Sheffield region. *Clin Otolaryngol Allied Sci.* 1999;24:447–448.
- Rafei K, Lichenstein R. Airway infectious disease emergencies *Pediatr Clin North Am.* 2006;53(2):215–242.
- Shah RK, Stocks C. Epiglottitis in the United States: National trends, variances, prognosis, and management. *Laryngoscope.* 2010;120:1256–1262.
- Stroud RH, Friedman NR. An update on inflammatory disorders of the pediatric airway: Epiglottitis, croup, and tracheitis. *Am J Otolaryngol.* 2001;22:268–275.

 ## CODES

ICD9
- 464.30 Acute epiglottitis without mention of obstruction
- 464.31 Acute epiglottitis with obstruction

ICD10
- J05.10 Acute epiglottitis without obstruction
- J05.11 Acute epiglottitis with obstruction

FAQ
- Q: What is the incidence of epiglottitis since the introduction of conjugate vaccines against *H. influenzae* type B?
- A: Because *H. influenzae* type B caused 90% of epiglottitis and the incidence of all invasive disease due to *H. influenzae* type B has decreased by 99% in children <5 years of age, it is estimated that the incidence of epiglottitis has been reduced by more than 90%.
- Q: Have there been reports of epiglottitis caused by *H. influenzae* type B after complete vaccination?
- A: Yes. Several cases due to *H. influenzae* type B have been reported in the US and abroad after partial and complete vaccination. Therefore, even a history of having received a full vaccination series does not eliminate the possibility of HiB-associated epiglottitis.
- Q: How many cases of invasive disease due to *H. influenzae* type B occur in children with inadequate vaccination?
- A: During 1994 and 1995, 47% of children <4 years of age were too young (aged 5 months or younger) to have completed a primary series for HiB vaccine:
  – Among children old enough to have been fully vaccinated, 63% of those developing disease were undervaccinated, and the remainder (37%) had completed a primary series in which vaccine failed.
  – In a recent report from Australia, 34 of 412 cases (8%) of invasive HiB disease (including epiglottitis) were reported as vaccine failures.
  – Therefore, HiB cannot be ruled out as a cause of epiglottitis in a fully vaccinated child, although the overwhelming majority of cases occur in unvaccinated children.
  – An increase in cases of epiglottitis due to *H. influenzae* type B has been reported in relation to dropping immunization rates with a subsequent fall in cases resulting from improved vaccination rates.
- Q: Should a fully vaccinated child who develops invasive disease due to *H. influenzae* type B be tested for an underlying immunodeficiency?
- A: Probably. In one study, about 1/3 of children diagnosed with invasive disease due to *H. influenzae* type B were found to have a previously undiagnosed immunoglobulin deficiency.
- Q: Can epiglottitis recur?
- A: Yes, but rarely.
- Q: Are corticosteroids of any value in the management of epiglottitis?
- A: There appears to be no benefit.

EPSTEIN–BARR VIRUS (INFECTIOUS MONONUCLEOSIS)

Jessica Newman
Jason Newland
Kevin C. Osterhoudt (5th edition)

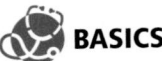 **BASICS**

DESCRIPTION
A double-stranded DNA virus implicated as the causative agent for infectious mononucleosis by an infected laboratory worker in 1968

GENERAL PREVENTION
- No vaccine is clinically available.
- Standard precautions should be utilized in the hospitalized patient.
- Restriction of intimate contact with immunosuppressed individuals may be advisable.
- Patients with recent Epstein–Barr virus (EBV) infection, either proven or suspected, should not donate blood or solid organs.

EPIDEMIOLOGY
- Worldwide distribution
- Humans are the only known reservoir.
- Transmission occurs through saliva and, occasionally, via blood transfusions
- Incubation period is 4–7 weeks.
- Antibodies to EBV are almost universally present in adult populations.
- Areas with a high population density or low socioeconomic status usually become primarily infected within the first 3 years of life.

Incidence
In developed countries, acquisition of EBV is biphasic:
- Initial peak in incidence occurs before the age of 5 years.
- Second peak occurs during adolescence, coinciding with an increased frequency of intimate oral contacts.

Prevalence
90–95% of adults have demonstrable EBV titers

PATHOPHYSIOLOGY
- Replicates initially in the oropharyngeal epithelium
- Selective infection of B lymphocytes occurs.
- The clinical syndrome of infectious mononucleosis results from proliferation of cells in the tonsils, lymph nodes, and spleen.
- Nonspecific humoral immune responses include the formation of heterophile antibodies and autoantibodies.
- Specific antibodies to EBV antigens are produced.
- Despite humoral responses, cellular immunity is responsible for controlling EBV infection.
- Latent, lifelong infection of B lymphocytes occurs.
- Latent virus may be reactivated during periods of immunosuppression.

COMMONLY ASSOCIATED CONDITIONS
- Subclinical infection:
  – Most EBV infections in children, and even in adolescents, are clinically inapparent.
  – Mild, nonspecific symptoms may include coryza, diarrhea, and/or fever.
  – Immunologic seroconversion does occur.
- Infectious mononucleosis ("glandular fever"): Most commonly observed with late primary acquisition of EBV. The classically defined illness is characterized by:
  – Fatigue
  – Malaise
  – Fever
  – Tonsillopharyngitis (often exudative)
  – Lymphadenopathy
  – Splenomegaly
  – Usually associated with increased numbers of atypical lymphocytes in the peripheral blood
- Rare illnesses of the nervous system have been reported including:
  – Guillain–Barré syndrome
  – Bell palsy
  – Aseptic meningitis
  – Meningoencephalitis
  – Peripheral and/or optic neuritis
- Hematologic complications have been reported in association with EBV:
  – Aplastic anemia
  – Hemolytic anemia
  – Agranulocytosis
  – Hemophagocytic syndrome
- Other illnesses associated with EBV in case reports include:
  – Hemolytic–uremic syndrome
  – Hepatitis
  – Pancreatitis
  – Myocarditis
  – Mesenteric adenitis
  – Orchitis
  – Genital ulcerative disease
- Lymphoproliferative disorders:
  – Burkitt lymphoma
  – Nasopharyngeal carcinoma
  – Lymphoma and non-Hodgkin lymphoma (in immunocompromised children)
  – Lymphomatoid granulomatosis
  – Posttransplant lymphoproliferative disorders (PTLD)
  – X-linked lymphoproliferative disease (Duncan disease)

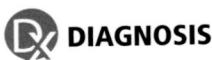 **DIAGNOSIS**

HISTORY
- A prodrome may occur:
  – Most often, lasts 3–5 days
  – Malaise, fatigue, with or without fever
- In the acute phase, the following features are common:
  – Fever: Begins abruptly, lasts 1–2 weeks
  – Fatigue
  – Malaise
  – Anorexia
  – Sore throat
  – "Swollen glands"
  – Rash; more common with ampicillin administration
- Young children are more likely to have rash or abdominal pain.

PHYSICAL EXAM
- Tonsillopharyngitis:
  – May be exudative and mimic streptococcal pharyngitis
  – Often accompanied by palatal petechiae
- Lymphadenopathy:
  – Occurs in 90%
  – Most prominent in cervical chains
  – May be diffuse
  – Usually nontender, nonerythematous, and discrete
- Hepatosplenomegaly:
  – Splenomegaly occurs in more than half the cases
  – Even if not palpable, splenomegaly may be demonstrated on ultrasound
  – Most prominent in 2nd to 4th week of illness
  – Hepatomegaly is less common

DIAGNOSTIC TESTS & INTERPRETATION
Lab
- Complete blood count with differential:
  – Leukocyte count up to 20,000/mm^3
  – Lymphocytosis
  – Atypical lymphocytes often constitute >10% of total leukocyte count.
  – Thrombocytopenia may occur.
  – False-positives: Atypical lymphocyte counts >10% of the total leukocyte count also occur with cytomegalovirus and toxoplasmosis infections.
- Liver enzymes:
  – Mild hepatitis is often found.
  – Jaundice is rare.
- "Monospot" (mononucleosis rapid slide agglutination test for heterophile antibodies):
  – Detects heterophile antibodies (nonspecific IgM antibodies to unrelated antigens)
  – Appears in first 2 weeks of illness, usually slow decline over 6 months
  – Often negative in children <4 years of age
  – Detects 85% of cases in adolescents and adults
  – False-positives: Infrequent; heterophile antibodies are also produced in serum sickness and neoplastic processes; heterophile antibodies may persist for months after acute infection and be indicative of past illness.

- EBV serology:
  - Usually reserved for heterophile-negative patients or children <4 years of age when strong clinical suspicion persists
  - Antibodies detected by indirect immunofluorescence or enzyme-linked immunosorbent assay techniques
  - Acute or past infection can usually be detected and differentiated.
- Other technology:
  - Tissue culture of EBV is difficult and, therefore, not clinically useful.
  - Polymerase chain reaction (PCR) may detect EBV genetic material.
  - Real-time PCR may quantify the amount of EBV genome present, which is useful in patients with PTLD.

ALERT
- Heterophile antibodies may not appear early in the illness.
- Up to 10% of patients with acute EBV infection may have no heterophile response 3 weeks into the illness.
- The heterophile response is less common in infants and children and should not be used in children <4 years of age.

DIFFERENTIAL DIAGNOSIS
- Infectious:
  - Group A streptococcus
  - Adenovirus
  - Cytomegalovirus
  - *Toxoplasma gondii*
  - Human herpes virus-6
  - *Mycoplasma pneumoniae*
  - Human immunodeficiency virus
  - Rubella
  - Diptheria
  - Viral hepatitis (A,B,C)
- Noninfectious:
  - Leukemia/Lymphoma

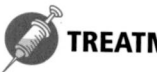 TREATMENT

MEDICATION (DRUGS)
- Acetaminophen or ibuprofen reduces fever and provides analgesia.
- Corticosteroids (prednisone 1 mg/kg/d—maximum of 20 mg/d) may reduce swelling of lymphoid tissues (see "FAQ"):
  - Indicated for patients with impending airway obstruction
  - May be considered for patients with severe tonsillopharyngitis requiring IV hydration
  - May be considered for patients with rare, life-threatening manifestations of EBV infection, such as hepatitis, aplastic anemia, and central nervous system dysfunction
  - 7-day treatment followed by tapering
- Acyclovir has not been shown to provide clinical benefit; sometimes, used in cases of active replicating EBV in posttransplant situations
- Patients with PTLD should have immunosuppression reduced
- Advise avoidance of contact sports until resolution of symptoms and no further splenomegaly

IN-PATIENT CONSIDERATIONS
Admission Criteria
- Respiratory distress secondary to airway obstruction
- Dehydration secondary to severe pharyngitis and poor oral intake

Discharge Criteria
- Resolved airway obstruction
- Good oral intake

ISSUES-FOR-REFERRAL
- PTLD
- EBV in immunocompromised host
- EBV associated lymphoproliferative disorders
- Considering steroid use as treatment

 ONGOING CARE

FOLLOW-UP RECOMMENDATIONS
Patient Monitoring
- Immunocompetent individuals usually recover uneventfully in 1–4 weeks.
- Recovery is often biphasic, with a worsening of symptoms after a period of improvement.
- Splenomegaly may persist for weeks after primary infection (see "FAQ").
- Fatigue may persist months after recovery.

PROGNOSIS
- Most patients with primary EBV infection will recover uneventfully in 1–4 weeks.
- Long-lasting immunity generally ensues.
- Prognosis of patients with unusual manifestations of EBV infection depends on the severity of the illness and the organ system involved.
- Patients with inherited or acquired immunodeficiency are at higher risk of complications and neoplasms.

COMPLICATIONS
- Dehydration:
  - Severe pharyngitis often limits fluid intake.
  - Most common problem requiring hospitalization
- Antibiotic-induced rash:
  - Morbilliform in appearance
  - Most common after administration of ampicillin or amoxicillin
  - Rare association with penicillin
  - Usually benign, resolves with discontinuation of the aminopenicillin
- Splenic rupture:
  - Incidence of ~1 in 1,000 patients
  - More common in males
  - 50% of the cases of splenic rupture are spontaneous; 50% follow blunt trauma,
- Airway obstruction: May result from massive lymphoid hyperplasia and mucosal edema

ADDITIONAL READING
- Bravender T. Epstein–Barr Virus, Cytomegalovirus and infectious mononucleosis. *Adolesc Med.* 2010;21:251–264.
- Hurt C, Tammaro D. Diagnostic evaluation of mononucleosis-like illness. *Am J Med.* 2007; 20(10):911.e1–e8.
- Jenson HB. Acute complications of Epstein–Barr virus infectious mononucleosis. *Curr Opin Pediatr.* 2000;12:263–268.
- Macsween KF, Crawford DH. Epstein–Barr virus—recent advances. *Lancet Infect Dis.* 2003;3:131–140.
- Okano M. Overview and problematic standpoints of severe chronic active Epstein–Barr virus infection syndrome. *Crit Rev Oncol Hematol.* 2002;44: 273–282.
- Putukian M, O'Connor FG, Stricker P, et al. Mononucleosis and athletic participation: An evidence-based subject review. *Clin J Sport Med.* 2008;18(4):309–315.

 CODES

ICD9
075 Infectious mononucleosis

ICD10
- B27.90 Infectious mononucleosis, unspecified without complication
- B27.92 Infectious mononucleosis, unspecified with meningitis
- B27.99 Infectious mononucleosis, unsp with other complication

FAQ
- Q: Should all patients with infectious mononucleosis be given corticosteroids?
- A: Although children may feel tired, weak, and ill, symptomatic EBV infection is most often self-limited and requires only symptomatic care.
- Long-term effects from the use of steroids to treat EBV are not known.
- EBV has been linked to certain lymphoproliferative disorders, and theoretic risks to modulating the host immune response with corticosteroids have been proposed.
- Q: How long after infectious mononucleosis may a patient return to athletic activity?
- A: More than half of patients with "mono" will have a boggy, enlarged spleen, which is prone to rupture even if it is not palpable.
- All athletic activity should be restricted until no evidence exists for a clinically enlarged or tender spleen. If this criterion is met, and the patient feels subjectively better, light (noncontact) activities may be resumed.
- Return to contact sports is not advised until at least 4–6 weeks after resolution of all signs and symptoms of illness.
- Some experts recommend ultrasound study of the spleen before a return to heavy contact sports such as rugby, football, lacrosse, and hockey.

ERYTHEMA MULTIFORME

James Treat
Albert C. Yan (5th edition)

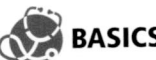 **BASICS**

DESCRIPTION

- An acute self-limited cutaneous eruption with many different or multiform lesions
- Characterized classically as a target or iris lesion but may appear as erythematous macules, papules, vesicles, and bullae and can be associated with mucosal involvement
- There are many triggers of erythema multiforme (EM), which is thought to encompass a spectrum of disease from relatively mild disease (EM minor) to severe forms with more severe mucosal surface involved (EM major).
- Although they can both present with targetoid skin lesions, many authors now feel Stevens Johnson Syndrome (SJS) and toxic epidermolysis (TEN) are separate entities from typical erythema multiforme. SJS and TEN involve ≥2 mucous membranes, and extensive skin blistering or sloughing (<10% is SJS, 10–30% is SJS-TEN overlap and >30% is TEN). SJS and TEN have significant morbidity and mortality, whereas EM is typically self-limited.

EPIDEMIOLOGY

- Believed by some to occur more frequently in spring and summer, with the more severe form of EM major occurring in winter
- Occurs predominantly in young adults

Incidence
Male = Female (some studies suggest a slightly higher incidence of EM minor in women)

Prevalence
Seen in ~1% of all dermatology patients

RISK FACTORS

Genetics
Emerging evidence shows strong genetic predisposition for EM in patients with certain HLA subtypes.

ETIOLOGY

- The major causes of EM, which is thought to be an immune-mediated reaction, include drugs such as sulfa, penicillin, and phenytoin and infections such as herpes simplex virus and *Mycoplasma*.
- There are a host of other etiologic factors, including exposure to various chemicals and tumors. The eruption usually occurs 1–2 weeks after initial exposure.
- Often the causative factor is not identified.
- Recurrent EM is generally secondary to herpes simplex virus.

DIAGNOSIS

HISTORY

- Cutaneous findings are sometimes preceded by a prodrome with fever and malaise.
- A careful drug and exposure history, as well as any signs or symptoms of infection or herpetic lesions, may reveal the cause.
- Inquire in detail about the patient's drug history, OTC preparations, and signs or symptoms of infection or herpetic lesions.

PHYSICAL EXAM

- EM classically appears as target lesions characterized by a dark, dusky center surrounded by a pale zone and then a zone of erythema:
  – The lesions are typically acrally distributed.
- Lesions occur in many forms and may appear as red macules, papules, urticarial lesions, or vesicles and bullae.
- Oral involvement is typically seen.
- Mucosal involvement with superficial denudation may also occur in the eyes, nasopharyngeal mucosal, or anogenital region.

DIAGNOSTIC TESTS & INTERPRETATION

No diagnostic laboratory tests; however, biopsy is often helpful, and other tests may help identify a cause.

Lab

- A WBC count with differential, looking for eosinophilia, may help identify a drug as causative.
- Direct fluorescent antibody testing, polymerase chain reaction, or cultures to evaluate for herpes or chest radiographic studies to evaluate for pneumonia or infectious cause of EM
- Cold agglutinins, serology, and polymerase chain reaction associated with *Mycoplasma*
- Erythrocyte sedimentation rate may be elevated, but is nonspecific.

Diagnostic Procedures/Other
Biopsy of lesion not usually needed

Pathological Findings

- Vary according to the lesion examined:
- Biopsy reveals necrosis of keratinocytes to varying degrees, depending on the clinical lesion biopsied
- Moderate to severe papillary dermal edema with mild to moderate perivascular dermal infiltrate composed predominantly of mononuclear cells and also some eosinophils (particularly if drug related)
- Subepidermal blistering may be seen.
- Extravasated blood cells are found, but there is no evidence of vasculitis.
- Hydropic degeneration of the basement membrane also may be seen, as may epidermal spongiosis.

DIFFERENTIAL DIAGNOSIS

Classic presentation with targetoid lesions and mucosal involvement is generally not a diagnostic challenge; however, given the many forms of presentation, the diagnosis of EM may be difficult. The differential diagnosis may be extensive depending on the presentation and includes:

- Viral exanthem
- Bullous impetigo
- Staphylococcal scalded-skin syndrome

- Bullous pemphigoid
- Urticaria
- Urticarial vasculitis
- Systemic lupus erythematosus
- Serum sickness
- Pemphigus vulgaris
- Secondary syphilis
- Chickenpox
- Rocky Mountain spotted fever
- Acute neutrophilic dermatosis
- Lyme disease
- Fixed drug eruption

 TREATMENT

ADDITIONAL TREATMENT
General Measures
- Mild forms:
  – Oral lesions are often painful, and oral preparations to swish and spit, made of diphenhydramine or viscous lidocaine, may provide relief.
  – Treatment of the underlying process is helpful (eg, acyclovir for herpes simplex virus–associated cases).
- EM major:
  – Supportive care, ophthalmology consultation, monitoring of fluid and electrolyte balance, local wound care, and vigilant observation for infection are necessary.
  – The use of systemic steroids is controversial, but when helpful, they are given early in the course of disease for ~2 weeks when there is no contraindication, such as infection.

IN-PATIENT CONSIDERATIONS
Initial Stabilization
- Mild EM: Resolves spontaneously without scarring and require only supportive therapy, including antihistamine or topical steroid for pruritus associated with the lesions
- EM major may be life-threatening and may require hospitalization.
- SJS/TEN: Higher associated mortality (than EM) is often secondary to infection given the larger body surface area involvement; care is ideally at a burn center, with careful attention to infection and to fluids and electrolytes.

Admission Criteria
Severe mucositis with inability to adequately hydrate.

 ONGOING CARE

PROGNOSIS
- Mild forms of EM are acute and self-limited, with lesions resolving in 2–4 weeks with postinflammatory hyperpigmentation or hypopigmentation.
- Sequelae owing to mucosal scarring may occur.
- When recurrent, EM is often associated with herpes simplex virus.

COMPLICATIONS
- EM minor is generally self-limited, with rare complications.
- In EM major, mucosal involvement may lead to stricture formation of the urethra, trachea, and esophagus, as well as conjunctivitis, corneal erosions, and rarely, blindness.

ADDITIONAL READING
- Ayangco L, Rogers RS 3rd. Oral manifestations of erythema multiforme. *Dermatol Clin.* 2003;21: 195–205.
- Duvic M. Erythema multiforme. *Dermatol Clin.* 1983;1:493–496.
- Huff JC, Weston WL, Tonnessen MG. Erythema multiforme: A critical review of characteristics, diagnostic criteria and causes. *J Am Acad Dermatol.* 1983;8:763–775.
- Metry D, Jung P, Levy ML. Use of IV immunoglobulin in children with Stevens-Johnson syndrome and toxic epidermal necrolysis: Seven cases and review of the literature. *Pediatrics.* 2003;112(6 pt 1):1430–1436.
- Riley M, Jenner R. Towards evidence based emergency medicine: Best BETs from the Manchester Royal Infirmary. Bet 2. Steroids in children with erythema multiforme. *Emerg Med J.* 2008;25(9):594–595.
- Schofield JK, et al. Recurrent erythema multiforme: tissue typing in a large series of patients. *Br J Dermatol.* 1994;131(4):532–535.
- Weston WL, Badgett JT. Urticaria. *Pediatr Rev.* 1998;19:240–244.

 CODES

ICD9
- 695.10 Erythema multiforme, unspecified
- 695.11 Erythema multiforme minor
- 695.19 Other erythema multiforme

ICD10
- L51.1 Stevens-Johnson syndrome
- L51.8 Other erythema multiforme
- L51.9 Erythema multiforme, unspecified

E

ERYTHEMA NODOSUM

James R. Treat
Albert C. Yan (5th edition)

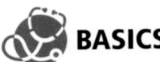 **BASICS**

DESCRIPTION
Delayed, cell-mediated hypersensitivity panniculitis characterized by red, tender, nodular lesions that are usually seen on the pretibial surface of the legs and occasionally on other areas of the skin where subcutaneous fat is present.

EPIDEMIOLOGY
- Girls are affected more often than boys.
- Most cases are seen in the 3rd decade, but not uncommon after age 10.

Incidence
Greatest seasonal incidence in spring and fall

PATHOPHYSIOLOGY
- Septal panniculitis: Lymphocytic perivascular infiltrate in the dermis; lymphocytes and neutrophils in the fibrous septa in the subcutaneous fat
- In older lesions, histiocytes, giant cells, and occasionally plasma cells are seen on histopathology.
- No fat cell destruction or vasculitis is present.

ETIOLOGY
- Thought to be a result of a host hypersensitivity immune response to circulating immune complexes secondary to infectious and/or inflammatory stimuli, which then results in chronic injury to the blood vessels of the reticular dermis and subcutaneous fat
- There are many associated triggering/underlying diseases:
- Infectious:
  - Bacterial: Streptococcal infection is the most common cause in children.
  - Other bacteria: Psittacosis, yersiniosis, lymphogranuloma venereum, cat-scratch disease, rickettsial diseases including conorii and tsutsugamushi.
  - Mycobacterial: Tuberculosis and atypical mycobacteria
  - Fungal: Histoplasmosis, coccidioidomycosis

- Systemic:
  - Sarcoidosis
  - Inflammatory bowel disease
  - Hodgkin disease
  - Behcet disease
- Pregnancy
- Medications: Oral contraceptives, sulfonamides, phenytoin, and halides

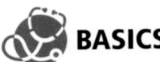 **DIAGNOSIS**

HISTORY
- In >50% of patients, a history of arthralgia is noted 2–8 weeks prior.
- Prodromal symptoms of fatigue/malaise or upper respiratory infection often proceed by 1–3 weeks.
- Patients often present with pain and tenderness of extremities, sometimes to the point of difficulty in ambulation.
- Special questions:
  - Recent streptococcal infection
  - Medication history (oral contraceptives, sulfonamides, iodides/bromides)
  - Last menses (erythema nodosum is seen in pregnancy)
  - History of diarrhea (inflammatory bowel disease or infectious diarrhea)
  - Tuberculosis exposure

PHYSICAL EXAM
- Red, often tender nodules on anterior lower legs, 2–6 cm in diameter, can also affect the extensor arms and face.
- Overlying skin is normal except for erythema.
- Initially, lesions are bright to deep red with palpable warmth.
- Later, lesions develop a brownish red or violaceous, bruise-like appearance.
- Smaller lesions are slope-shouldered nodules.
- Larger lesions are flat-topped plaques.

- Exam pearls:
  - Erythema nodosum never ulcerates or suppurates.
  - Palpation is very important to feel the painful nodules.
  - Usually, there are no more than 6 lesions at a time.
  - As a rule, both legs are affected.

DIAGNOSTIC TESTS & INTERPRETATION
Lab
- Throat culture
- Antistreptolysin-O titer
- Purified protein derivative
- CBC
- ESR
- Stool culture, if history of diarrhea
- Serologic testing, if yersiniosis, rickettsial disease, histoplasmosis, or coccidioidomycosis suspected

Imaging
Chest radiographic study, if diagnosis is in doubt

Diagnostic Procedures/Other
Excisional biopsy specimen for histopathology and bacterial, mycobacterial, and fungal cultures is helpful but not always needed.

Pathological Findings
False-positives: Bilateral hilar adenopathy may also be seen with sarcoidosis, coccidioidomycosis, histoplasmosis, tuberculosis, streptococcal infection, or lymphomatosis.

DIFFERENTIAL DIAGNOSIS
- Infection:
  - Erysipelas/cellulitis
  - Superficial or deep thrombophlebitis
  - Erythema induratum (nodular vasculitis)
  - Deep fungal infection
  - Angiitis
  - Leprosy

- Environmental (poisons)
- Tumors
- Trauma: Accidental or from child abuse
- Bruise
- Palmoplantar hidradenitis
- Metabolic:
  − Panniculitis secondary to pancreatic disease
  − Congenital
- Immunologic:
  − Major insect bite reaction
  − Psychosocial (self-injection with foreign material)
- Sarcoidosis
- Polyarteritis nodosa
- Granuloma annulare
- Miscellaneous
- Weber-Christian (thighs and trunk) lesions may suppurate and heal with atrophy/localized depression.

 TREATMENT

MEDICATION (DRUGS)
- Salicylates or other NSAIDs, such as ibuprofen, naproxen, or indomethacin
- Potassium iodide 300 mg PO t.i.d. for 3–4 weeks, especially for cases diagnosed early in course
- Corticosteroids are effective but rarely necessary:
  − Duration: 2–4 weeks

ADDITIONAL TREATMENT
General Measures
Bed rest and leg elevation

 ONGOING CARE

FOLLOW-UP RECOMMENDATIONS
Patient Monitoring
- When to expect improvement:
  − Within 2–3 days
  − Return visit in 1 week
- Signs to watch for: If lesions recur after cessation of treatment, underlying infection may worsen as well.
- If atypical locations or exuberant or suppurative nodules are present, a biopsy is warranted to rule out a disseminated infection.

PROGNOSIS
- Most individual lesions will completely resolve in 10–14 days.
- In general, erythema nodosum resolves in 3–6 weeks with or without treatment unless the underlying cause is a chronic infection or systemic disorder.
- Aching of legs and swelling of ankles may persist for weeks; rarely, symptoms may persist for up to 2 years.
- In children, the recurrence rate is 4–10% and is often associated with repeated streptococcal infection.

ADDITIONAL READING

- Chachkin S, Cheng JW, Yan AC. Erythema nodosum. In: Burg FD, Ingelfinger JR, Polin RA, et al., eds. *Current Pediatric Therapy.* 18th ed. Philadelphia: WB Saunders; 2006.
- Gonzalez-Gay MA, Garcia-Porrua C, Pujol RM, et al. Erythema nodosum: A clinical approach. *Clin Exp Rheumatol.* 2001;19:365–368.
- Hassink RI, Pasquinelli-Egli CE, Jacomella V, et al. Conditions currently associated with erythema nodosum in Swiss children. *Eur J Pediatr.* 1997;156(11):851–853.
- Pettersson T. Sarcoid and erythema nodosum arthropathies. *Best Pract Res Clin Rheumatol.* 2000;14:461–476.
- Premaratna R, Chandrasena TG, Rajapakse RP, et al. Rickettsioses presenting as major joint arthritis and erythema nodosum: Description of four patients. *Clin Rheumatol.* 2009;28:867–868.

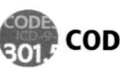 CODES

ICD9
695.2 Erythema nodosum

ICD10
L52 Erythema nodosum

FAQ
- Q: Will the lesions leave a scar?
- A: Erythema nodosum virtually always heals without scarring.

E

EWING SARCOMA
Edward F. Attiyeh

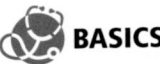 **BASICS**

DESCRIPTION
- Represents a family of tumors including:
  - Ewing sarcoma of bone
  - Extraosseous Ewing sarcoma (arises in soft tissue adjacent to bone)
  - Peripheral neuroectodermal tumor (PNET) of bone or soft tissue
- May develop in any bone of the body, with equal involvement of flat and long bones (unlike osteosarcoma, which arises more commonly in long bones):
  - ~25% have detectable metastases at diagnosis:
    - Lung
    - Bone
    - Bone marrow

EPIDEMIOLOGY
- 2nd most common malignant bone tumor of children and young adults
- More common in males than in females
- Associations (rare):
  - Skeletal anomalies (endochondroma, aneurysmal bone cyst)
  - Genitourinary anomalies (hypospadias, duplicated renal collecting system)

Incidence
- ~110 new cases are diagnosed in the US each year.
- Most (~65%) occur in the 2nd decade of life:
  - Rare under the age of 5 years
- 96% of cases occur in the white population:
  - Extremely rare in Asians and blacks

Prevalence
Accounts for ~2–5% of all childhood cancers

RISK FACTORS
Genetics
- Most cases occur sporadically.
- Not associated with familial cancer syndromes

PATHOPHYSIOLOGY
- One of the "small round blue cell" tumors of childhood
- Rearrangement of the EWS (EWing Sarcoma) gene is detected in >95% of cases.
  - Usually (85%) through a t(11;22) translocation resulting in a fusion EWS-FLI1 protein
  - Other translocation partners include other members of the ETS transcription factor family such as ERG (21q; 10% of cases).
- A large soft tissue component is often present.
- Necrosis and hemorrhage are common.
- The PNET variant has more neural differentiation.

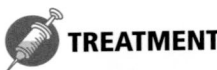 **DIAGNOSIS**

HISTORY
- Presenting symptoms and their frequency of occurrence:
  - Local pain (85%)
  - Local swelling (60%)
  - Fever (30%)
  - Paraplegia, back pain (2%)
- Systemic symptoms (fever, weight loss) are more common among patients with metastatic disease.
- Delay between 1st symptom and diagnosis is quite common; the duration of symptoms ranges from 4 weeks to 4 years, with an average of 9 months.

PHYSICAL EXAM
- Distribution of primary sites include the following:
  - Extremities (53%):
    - Usually begins in the midshaft
    - Lower extremities affected more than upper extremities
  - Central axis (47%):
    - Pelvis (45%)
    - Chest wall (34%)
    - Spine or paravertebral (12%)
    - Head or neck (9%)
- Extraskeletal Ewing sarcoma is rare; however, it may be found in most soft tissue regions of the body.

DIAGNOSTIC TESTS & INTERPRETATION
Lab
- CBC
- Serum lactate dehydrogenase (LDH) is often elevated at diagnosis.
- Electrolytes, liver function tests, and renal function tests in anticipation of starting chemotherapy

Imaging
- To evaluate primary site and confirm diagnosis:
  - Radiography:
    - Bony destruction with "onion skinning" appearance most often seen
    - Raising of the periosteum may result in a Codman triangle
    - Diaphyseal location
  - CT or preferably MRI scan
- To evaluate for evidence of distant metastases (present in 25% of patients at diagnosis):
  - Chest radiograph and CT scan
  - 99m-Tc-diphosphonate bone scan
  - PET scan

Diagnostic Procedures/Other
- Biopsy:
  - Should be performed by an experienced orthopedic surgeon:
    - Avoid contamination of surrounding tissues (use of a longitudinal incision is important).
    - Ensure adequate tissue sampling to make the diagnosis.
  - In addition to routine morphologic and immunohistochemical stain assessments, analysis of tumor genetics by traditional cytogenetics, fluorescent in situ hybridization, or reverse transcriptase PCR is helpful in making the diagnosis and may provide information regarding prognosis.
  - Because of the importance of these studies, consultation with a pediatric oncologist before the biopsy is essential.
- Bilateral bone marrow aspirates and biopsies

DIFFERENTIAL DIAGNOSIS
- Malignant:
  - Osteosarcoma
  - Neuroblastoma
  - Non-Hodgkin lymphoma
  - Rhabdomyosarcoma
- Nonmalignant:
  - Osteomyelitis
  - Tendonitis
  - Trauma/fracture
  - Langerhans cell histiocytosis (eosinophilic granuloma)
  - Benign bone tumor (giant cell tumor) or cyst

TREATMENT

MEDICATION (DRUGS)
- All patients with localized disease at diagnosis also have tumor cells outside the primary site that cannot be detected by standard measures; chemotherapy is therefore essential for cure.
- Common agents used include vincristine, dactinomycin, cyclophosphamide, doxorubicin, etoposide, and ifosfamide. Other agents, such as irinotecan, are being investigated.
- Most patients require placement of an indwelling central venous catheter for the duration of their therapy.

ADDITIONAL TREATMENT
General Measures
- Therapy is multimodal with chemotherapy, radiation therapy, and surgery. Typically structured as:
  - Neoadjuvant chemotherapy
  - Local control (surgery, radiation therapy)
  - Adjuvant chemotherapy
- Most children are treated according to large cooperative group protocols at pediatric oncology centers.
- Treatment is characterized by significant side effects, including increased susceptibility to infection, severe mucositis, and poor nutritional status.
- Experimental therapies such as immunotherapy (vaccination with fusion-gene peptide products) and antiangiogenic therapies are being investigated in clinical trials for patients with high-risk or relapsed disease.

Additional Therapies

Radiotherapy:

- Ewing sarcomas are generally radiosensitive.
- Radiation therapy can be used to aid in local control and for control of metastatic disease.

ISSUES FOR REFERRAL

Consultation with a pediatric oncologist is essential before any attempt is made at a diagnostic biopsy.

SURGERY/OTHER PROCEDURES

- Goal is to remove the entire tumor with adequate tissue margins.
- Surgical approach depends on the affected site.
- Limb salvage surgery is often possible but may not be best in some cases:
  - Amputation may be the only way to ensure complete resection and a chance for cure.
  - The morbidity associated with limb salvage is sometimes unacceptable, especially when combined with the effects of radiation therapy.
  - Limb salvage is often associated with longer recovery times and the need for more physical therapy.
  - Amputation with a mechanical prosthesis may provide more function (especially in the lower extremities).

 ONGOING CARE

PROGNOSIS

- Overall, 50–70% of patients will be disease free at 5 years from diagnosis.
- Unfavorable prognostic features:
  - Age >12 years
  - Primary tumor site: Pelvis
  - Larger primary tumor
  - Metastatic disease at diagnosis, especially involving bone or bone marrow (<30% disease-free survival)
  - Elevated LDH at diagnosis
  - Poor histologic response to chemotherapy:
    - Assessed at the time of surgical resection

COMPLICATIONS

- Cord compression secondary to vertebral involvement
- Metastatic spread is seen in 25% of cases at diagnosis. Sites include lung, bone, and bone marrow; liver and lymph nodes are less often involved.
- Acute effects of therapy:
  - Frequent admissions to the hospital for chemotherapy or complications of the therapy
  - Bone marrow suppression:
    - Transfusions are usually necessary.
    - Neutropenia: Increased risk of bacterial and fungal infections; granulocyte colony-stimulating factor is usually administered daily following chemotherapy to shorten the duration of neutropenia.

- Complications from the GI side effects of chemotherapy or radiotherapy:
  - Nausea and vomiting, relieved with ondansetron and other antiemetic agents
  - Malnutrition secondary to reduced appetite and mucosal ulcerations; nutritional supplements (oral, nasogastric, gastrostomy tube or parenteral) may be necessary.
  - Complications from radiotherapy
  - Skin erythema or breakdown
  - Pathologic fracture
- Late effects of therapy:
  - Cardiomyopathy:
    - Anthracyclines (doxorubicin) weaken cardiac muscle, leading to reduced left ventricular function many years after therapy.
    - ~5% of patients receiving cumulative doses of doxorubicin >500 mg/m^2 will develop CHF.
    - Radiation to the heart can lower the cumulative dose threshold to 300 mg/m^2.
    - Any patient who has received an anthracycline should be cautioned against initiating strenuous physical activity without adequate preparation. Pregnant women who have received anthracyclines in the past should inform their obstetrician so that appropriate cardiac assessment can be completed prior to vaginal delivery.
  - Kidney and bladder damage:
    - Urinalysis should be performed to detect hemorrhagic cystitis or tubular damage with spilling of sugar, protein, and phosphate into the urine.
    - BP should be monitored in patients who received irradiation to the kidneys; vascular damage and hypertension may develop many years after therapy.
  - Infertility and delayed puberty:
    - Reduced or absent gonadal function is related to high doses of alkylating agents (cyclophosphamide, ifosfamide): Males are at high risk of azoospermia; females may be fertile but are at risk for premature menopause.
    - Low-dose estrogen therapy with oral contraceptive medications may be necessary for amenorrheic women.
  - 2nd malignant neoplasms:
    - Sarcomas may occur within the radiation field.
    - Myelodysplastic syndromes and acute myeloid leukemia may occur secondary to chemotherapy.
  - Growth abnormalities/functional defects at the primary site:
    - Radiation doses >20 Gy will cause growth retardation in prepubertal children.
    - Scoliosis may occur if the vertebrae are involved in the radiation field.
    - Risk for pathologic fractures or aseptic necrosis of joints remains elevated.

ADDITIONAL READING

- Bacci G, Ferrari S, Bertoni F, et al. Prognostic factors in nonmetastatic Ewing's sarcoma of bone treated with adjuvant chemotherapy: Analysis of 359 patients at the Instituto Ortopedico Rizzoli. *J Clin Oncol*. 2000;18:4–11.
- Kennedy JG, Frelinghuysen P, Hoang BH. Ewing sarcoma: Current concepts in diagnosis and treatment. *Curr Opin Pediatr*. 2003;15:53–57.
- Kim SY, Tsokos M, Helman LJ. Dilemmas associated with congenital Ewing sarcoma family tumors. *J Pediatr Hematol Oncol*. 2008;30(1):4–7.
- Krasin MJ, Davidoff AM, Rodriguez-Galindo C, et al. Definitive surgery and multiagent systemic therapy for patients with localized Ewing sarcoma family of tumors: Local outcome and prognostic factors. *Cancer*. 2005;104(2):367–373.
- Rodriquez-Galindo C, Spunt SL, Pappo AS. Treatment of Ewing sarcoma family of tumors: Current status and outlook for the future. *Med Pediatr Oncol*. 2003;40:276–287.
- Spunt SL, Rodriguez-Galindo C, Fuller CE, et al. Ewing sarcoma-family tumors that arise after treatment of primary childhood cancer. *Cancer*. 2006;107(1):201–206.

 CODES

ICD9
170.9 Malignant neoplasm of bone and articular cartilage, site unspecified

ICD10
C41.9 Malignant neoplasm of bone and articular cartilage, unspecified

FAQ

- Q: At what time point is a child with Ewing sarcoma considered cured?
- A: Typically, cure is measured as 5-year survival without evidence of disease. However, late relapses or 2nd tumors do occur in children with Ewing sarcoma.
- Q: Should a Ewing sarcoma be completely resected at the time of diagnosis?
- A: Most times, this is not recommended as Ewing sarcoma is very sensitive to chemotherapy, facilitating an improved delayed surgical resection.
- Q: What factors determine whether to amputate or attempt a limb salvage procedure?
- A: In determining the best surgical approach, one must consider:
  - The chance of a complete resection with clean margins
  - Maximizing function
  - The effect of potential radiation therapy on the surgical site
  - Patient and family preferences

EXSTROPHY OF THE BLADDER, CLOACAL EXSTROPHY, AND EPISPADIAS

Matt Christman
Aseem Shukla
Douglas Canning

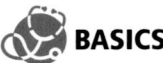 **BASICS**

DESCRIPTION
An anomaly in which the open bladder is part of the anterior abdominal wall. Presents as part of a complex of anomalies including male and female epispadias and wide separation of the pubis symphysis. The most severe variant of this complex is cloacal exstrophy, in which there is a large omphalocele, split bladder, imperforate anus, shortened colon, and multiple upper urinary tract and limb anomalies. Epispadias is less common than bladder exstrophy and presents with the urethral meatus at the penopubic junction, or rarely more distal on the dorsum of the penis.

EPIDEMIOLOGY
Incidence
- Estimated to be between 1/20,000 and 1/50,000 live births for classic bladder exstrophy
- Male:female ratio for classic bladder exstrophy is between 2:1 and 4:1.
- Cloacal exstrophy is exceedingly rare, with an incidence of 1/200,000 births (incidence continues to decrease because of prenatal diagnosis and termination).
- Male:female ratio for cloacal exstrophy is between 1:1 and 2:1
- Male epispadias: 1/117,000 male births
- Female epispadias: 1/484,000 female births
- Risk of bladder exstrophy in offspring of individuals with bladder exstrophy and epispadias is 1/70 births (500-fold greater than the general population).
- Risk of 2nd affected family member is 3.6%.

PATHOPHYSIOLOGY
Embryology:
- Normal development:
  - Cloacal membrane is located at the caudal end of the infraumbilical abdominal wall by 2 weeks' gestation.
  - Mesenchyme from the primitive streak migrates between the layers of the cloacal membrane to reinforce the abdominal wall as the cloacal membrane regresses.

- Bladder exstrophy:
  - Pathogenesis is still unclear, but represents an error in embryogenesis.
  - It is proposed that an abnormal overdevelopment of the cloacal membrane prevents medial migration of the mesenchymal tissue and normal lower abdominal wall development.
  - Because the membrane lacks reinforcement, it ruptures. The timing of this rupture determines the variant of the exstrophy–epispadias complex. In bladder exstrophy, rupture of the membrane occurs after the urorectal septum has descended.
- Cloacal exstrophy: Abnormally large cloacal membrane ruptures prior to division of the cloaca by the urorectal septum.

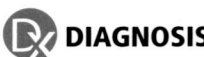 **DIAGNOSIS**

PHYSICAL EXAM
- Bladder exstrophy:
  - All cases have widening of the symphysis pubis caused by outward rotation of the innominate bones.
  - Triangular defect caused by premature rupture of the abnormal cloacal membrane is occupied by the exstrophied bladder and posterior urethra and bounded by the umbilicus superiorly, the 2 separated pubic bones laterally, and the anus inferiorly:
    ○ The distance between the umbilicus and anus is shortened in exstrophy.
  - Indirect inguinal hernia and incarceration are common in boys:
    ○ Perineum is short and broad with the compromised pelvic support structures.
  - Male genital anomalies:
    ○ Penis in boys with exstrophy is short and wide.
    ○ Corpora cavernosa are short and widely separated.
    ○ Marked dorsal chordee causes upward curvature of the penis with a short urethral plate.
    ○ Epispadias is nearly always present with the urethral meatus located on the dorsum at the penopubic junction.

  - Female genital anomalies:
    ○ Overall less complex
    ○ Mons pubis is displaced laterally, with bifid clitoris.
    ○ Vagina and introitus are displaced anteriorly.
    ○ Uterus and vagina may be duplicated. May be at risk of uterine prolapse if exstrophy closure fails
    ○ Epispadias may be less obvious.
  - Urinary defects:
    ○ Bladder mucosa at birth usually appears normal.
    ○ Ectopic bowel mucosa or polyp may be present in rare exstrophy variants.
    ○ Exstrophic bladder may exhibit maturational delay that improves following closure.
    ○ Upper urinary tract usually normal
    ○ Horseshoe, pelvic, hypoplastic, solitary, or dysplastic kidney occasionally occurs.
    ○ Most children with exstrophy have vesicoureteral reflux requiring correction.
- Cloacal exstrophy:
  - 2 halves of the exstrophied bladder separated by an exstrophied ileocecal bowel segment that represents the hindgut
  - Prolapsed ileum superiorly and blind-ending colon stump inferiorly
  - Imperforate anus
  - Penis may be duplicate or diminutive.
  - Bifid vagina and uterine abnormalities likely
  - Large omphalocele usually present
  - Upper urinary tract anomalies seen in up to 70% of children
  - Vertebral and neurologic abnormalities present in >50% of children

DIAGNOSTIC TESTS & INTERPRETATION
Imaging
- Prenatal sonographic findings by 20 weeks consistent with absence of a normal fluid-filled bladder, an anterior abdominal mass increasing in size, low-set umbilicus, and wide pubic ramus are suggestive of bladder exstrophy.
- A baseline renal ultrasound should be obtained after birth and a KUB will demonstrate the extent of pubic symphysis diastasis.

TREATMENT

SURGERY/OTHER PROCEDURES
Goals: Provide urinary continence and preserve renal function; surgically reconstruct the male penis to provide an erection straight enough for vaginal penetration and upright voiding:

- Complete primary repair of exstrophy (CPRE):
  - Bladder closure, bladder neck reconstruction, and epispadias repair completed in single procedure. May be performed with or without bilateral posterior iliac and anterior innominate osteotomy
  - May be postponed until 4–6 weeks of age to allow maternal bonding and to facilitate surgical planning to include orthopedic and pediatric urologic support
  - Regaining popularity as initial approach in neonates
  - Total penile disassembly involves total mobilization of the urethra to its ventral position without tension, and the bladder and urethra are closed in continuity.
  - Prophylactic antibiotic therapy should be continued in all children until antireflux procedure is completed or until vesicoureteral reflux resolves.
  - Practical advantage of allowing more normal bladder cycling that may facilitate bladder development
  - Results and complications: Daytime continence and volitional voiding in selected patients in up to 76% over 5 years of age; additional bladder neck surgery to gain continence is often required; >50% require subsequent hypospadias repair and bladder neck fistula rate is up to 40%.
- Staged closure of bladder exstrophy:
  - In the early neonatal period, bladder, posterior urethra, and abdominal wall closure is performed with or without osteotomy.
  - Results and complications: Daytime continence in 60–80% following bladder neck surgery, may require clean intermittent catheterization (long-term follow-up)—bladder capacity strong predictor of continence and previous failed bladder closure increases risk of incontinence; minimal risk for upper urinary tract changes or hydronephrosis

- Epispadias repair at 6 months to 1 year of age:
  - Bladder neck reconstruction with an antireflux procedure delayed until 3.5–4 years to facilitate adequate bladder growth and development
  - Results and complications: Cosmetic and functional success with a straight penis with erections ranges from 60–95%; urethral strictures and urethrocutaneous fistula are the most common complications of epispadias repair seen in ≤25% of patients.
- Complications for both types of closure:
  - Dehiscence, stone formation, and hydronephrosis requiring urethral dilation or vesicostomy may occur. Patients must be followed carefully.
  - Initial closure success very important for continence: 2nd attempt at closure delayed 6 months; expectation for continence decreases with each closure attempt.
  - Failed bladder neck repair in 20–50% may require further reconstruction.
  - Adenocarcinoma of the bladder occurs in patients with exstrophy 400 times more than in the normal population. This disease is not reported in adults who have had bladder closure after infancy.
- Fertility and pregnancy:
  - Sexual function and libido in exstrophy patients are normal following successful reconstruction.
  - Up to 87% of boys have erections following epispadias repair.
  - Retrograde and small-volume ejaculation should be expected.
  - Successful impregnation has been achieved with assisted reproductive techniques.
  - Pregnancy is commonly achieved in women with bladder exstrophy, but uterine and cervical prolapse are common following pregnancy. Cesarean section is recommended in females completing reconstruction.

IN-PATIENT CONSIDERATIONS
Initial Stabilization
Postnatal and nursery care:
- Tie umbilical cord with 2-0 silk to avoid traumatizing the bladder mucosa with an umbilical clamp.
- Cover bladder with a hydrated gel dressing or plastic wrap to prevent mucosa from sticking to clothing or diapers.
- Immediate transfer to an appropriate center for evaluation by a pediatric urologist and surgical correction.

ONGOING CARE

PROGNOSIS
Prospective parents of children with bladder exstrophy should be counseled as to excellent overall prognosis and favorable long-term outcome with early intervention by a pediatric urologist.

ADDITIONAL READING

- Gargollo PC, Borer JG, Diamond DA, et al. Prospective followup in patients after complete primary repair of bladder exstrophy. *J Urol*. 2008;180:1665–1670.
- Gearhart JP, Baird AD. The failed complete repair of bladder exstrophy: Insights and outcomes. *J Urol*. 2005;174(4 Pt 2):1669–1672; discussion 1672–1673.
- Kibar Y, Roth CC, Frimberger D, et al. Our initial experience with the technique of complete primary repair for bladder exstrophy. *J Pediatr Urol*. 2009;5:186–189.
- Kidoo DA, Carr MC, Dulczak S, et al. Initial management of complex urological disorders: Bladder exstrophy. *Urol Clin North Am*. 2004;31:417–426.
- MacLellan DL, Diamond DA. Recent advances in external genitalia. *Pediatr Clin North Am*. 2006;53(3):449–464, vii.
- Poli-Merol ML, Watson JA, Gearhart JP. New basic science concepts in the treatment of classic bladder exstrophy. *Urology*. 2002;60:749–755.
- Shnorhavorian M, Grady RW, Andersen A, et al. Long-term followup of complete primary repair of exstrophy: The Seattle experience. *J Urol*. 2008;180:1615–1620.
- Stein R, Thuroff JW. Hypospadias and bladder exstrophy. *Curr Opin Urol*. 2002;12:195–200.

CODES

ICD9
- 752.62 Epispadias
- 753.5 Exstrophy bladder (urinary)
- 753.6 Atresia and stenosis of urethra and bladder neck

ICD10
- Q64.0 Epispadias
- Q64.10 Exstrophy of urinary bladder, unspecified
- Q64.12 Cloacal extrophy of urinary bladder

E

FAILURE TO THRIVE

Michelle Terry

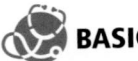 **BASICS**

DEFINITION

- Failure to thrive (FTT): Refers to a child whose physical growth is significantly less than that of peers.
- There is no official consensus on what constitutes FTT. Failure to thrive usually refers to a child whose growth is below the 5th percentile for their age or whose growth has fallen off precipitously and crossed 2 major growth percentiles (e.g., from above the 75th percentile to below the 25th percentile) as measured on standard growth charts, or if the child is 20% below the ideal weight for height. As defined, FTT is a sign of medical or environmental dysfunction vs. a definitive diagnosis or disease state.

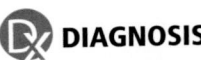 **DIAGNOSIS**

DIFFERENTIAL DIAGNOSIS

- **Inadequate caloric intake**
  - Incorrect preparation of formula
  - Inadequate breast milk supply or inefficient lactation techniques
  - Unsuitable feeding habits (i.e., food fads)
  - Disorganized mealtime routine
  - Behavior problems affecting eating
  - Poverty and food shortages
  - Disturbed parent–child or caregiver–child relationship
  - Mechanical feeding difficulties in the child (swallowing dysfunction, craniofacial anomalies, CNS injury, gastroesophageal reflux)
  - Voluntary restriction of intake/eating disorder
  - Child abuse and neglect
- **Inadequate caloric absorption**
  - Biliary atresia or liver disease
  - Celiac disease
  - Cystic fibrosis
  - Food allergies
  - Gastroesophageal reflux disease
  - Inflammatory bowel disease
  - Malrotation of the gut
  - Necrotizing enterocolitis or short-gut syndrome
  - Pyloric stenosis
  - Parasitic infection
  - Vitamin or mineral deficiencies

- **Increased metabolic expenditure**
  - Chromosomal abnormalities
  - Congenital or acquired heart disease
  - Cancer
  - Kidney disease
  - Chronic systemic disease (i.e., systemic lupus erythematosus [SLE], idiopathic juvenile arthritis, sickle cell disease, thalassemia)
  - Chronic or recurrent systemic infections (i.e., tuberculosis, hepatitis, AIDS and other immune deficiency syndromes, recurrent urinary tract infections, recurrent sinusitis)
  - Chronic respiratory insufficiency (i.e., obstructive sleep apnea, chronic lung disease)
  - Chronic metabolic disorders (i.e., aminoacidurias, organic acidurias, glycogen and lysosomal storage diseases, diabetes mellitus, adrenal insufficiency, pituitary disease, thyroid disease)

APPROACH TO THE PATIENT

General Goals

Determine if the child has growth failure and, if present, explore its etiology in order to provide the appropriate therapy.

- **Phase 1:** Is the malnutrition acute or chronic? With acute malnutrition, weight loss is evident first, and with chronic malnutrition, height and then head circumference are compromised. In order to thoroughly evaluate growth failure, the prenatal, developmental, feeding, and review of systems histories must be completely documented. The physical exam also provides clues as to the etiology of the growth failure in any of the following domains—general appearance, vital signs, head and neck, chest, abdomen, genitourinary, musculoskeletal, neurologic, and skin systems.
- **Phase 2:** If the medical database (history and physical exam) indicates a possible medical cause for FTT, then the appropriate diagnostic workup should be done in consultation with the relevant medical specialists.
- **Phase 3:** If no organic medical condition is identified as a reason for growth failure, then begin intensive nutritional and family support services.

HISTORY

Important aspects of the medical history include:

- **Question:** Pre- and perinatal history?
- *Significance:* Low birth weight, intrauterine growth restriction, perinatal illnesses, and prematurity are important predisposing factors to FTT. In addition prenatal exposures (e.g., alcohol, street drugs, and herbal supplements) may compromise growth and/or affect parent–child interactions.

- **Question:** Past medical history?
- *Significance:*
  - Presence of genetic or chronic diseases may hinder nutritional intake, nutrition absorption, or caloric expenditure; chronically malnourished children may be more susceptible to infection, and chronic infections may indicate immunodeficiency.
  - Family history should include the height and weight of parents and biologically related siblings and the constitutional rate of growth if known.
  - A careful review of systems history may give historical cues of potential significance.
- **Question:** Detailed information regarding diet and feeding?
- *Significance:*
  - Timing, location, and duration of mealtimes
  - Type of foods served
  - Quantity of food consumed
  - The dietary history should be as complete as possible with information, for example, regarding how a formula is mixed, or the volume of fruit juice consumed.
- Medical history symptoms that may be of particular significance:
  - Vomiting, diarrhea, and/or chronic constipation
  - Snoring or mouth breathing
  - Frequent infections
  - Frequent urination
  - Recent travel to a developing country
  - "Picky" eater preferences
  - Dietary restrictions because of food allergies
  - Child care attendance
  - Homelessness
- Psychosocial conditions that may be of particular significance:
  - Poverty
  - Parental depression
  - Parental substance abuse
  - Parental developmental delay
  - The psychosocial history should include an assessment of family composition, family stressors, and community supports.

PHYSICAL EXAM

A complete physical exam is necessary for the workup of FTT. A few examples of significant findings are as follows:

- **Finding:** Dysmorphic features (e.g., microcephaly, small palpebral fissures, flat philtrum, and thin upper lip)?
- *Significance:* Clinical or genetic syndrome associated (e.g., fetal alcohol syndrome or trisomy 21)

- **Finding:** Cataracts?
- *Significance*: Congenital infection, galactosemia
- **Finding:** Oropharyngeal lesions (e.g., dental caries, tongue enlargement, small jaw, tonsillar hypertrophy, defects in soft or hard palate)?
- *Significance*: May cause difficulties with suck and swallow
- **Finding:** Wheezing, crackles, prolonged expiratory phase, barrel-shaped chest?
- *Significance*: Diseases that contribute to chronic lung disease, e.g., asthma, cystic fibrosis.
- **Finding:** Cardiac murmur, rub, gallop?
- *Significance*: Congenital or acquired heart disease
- **Finding:** Abdominal distension, hepatosplenomegaly?
- *Significance*: Liver disease, glycogen storage disease, malignancy
- **Finding:** Bony deformities (abnormal skull shape, beading of the ribs, scoliosis, bowing of the legs or distal radius and ulna, enlargement of the wrist), scaling skin, spoon-shaped nails?
- *Significance*: Vitamin and mineral deficiencies (e.g., rickets, zinc deficiency, iron deficiency)
- **Finding:** Bruises and/or burns in characteristic object marks?
- *Significance*: Possible child physical abuse

DIAGNOSTIC TESTS & INTERPRETATION
Accurately measure the child:

- Measure the child' weight, length/height, and head circumference accurately using properly calibrated equipment and plot the measurements on a standard growth grid before tracking the data points over time.
- Perform a developmental screen: Assess the child's physical skills such as rolling over, sitting, standing, and walking. In older children it is important to assess the child's social, emotional, and cognitive skills as well.

    Order laboratory tests based on the data gathered in the history and physical exam.
- **Test:** CBC
- *Significance*: To identify anemia
- **Test:** Serum electrolytes, protein, albumin, calcium, magnesium, phosphorus, blood urea nitrogen, and creatinine
- *Significance*: To evaluate for potential metabolic problems and renal insufficiency; the values are useful to follow to prevent re-feeding syndrome in severe malnutrition. Re-feeding syndrome includes electrolyte and mineral disturbances in severely malnourished individuals who are provided with enteral nutrition too quickly.

- **Test:** Hemoglobin electrophoresis
- *Significance*: To determine the presence of conditions such as sickle cell disease
- **Test:** Hormone studies including thyroid function tests
- *Significance*: To evaluate for hormonal dysfunction
- **Test:** X-rays to determine bone age
- *Significance*: To determine stunting of growth by premature maturation of long bones
- **Test:** Urinalysis and urine culture
- *Significance*: To screen for urinary tract infection and renal tubular acidosis

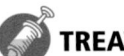 ## TREATMENT

EMERGENCY CARE
Children who meet criteria for severe malnutrition should be hospitalized, and a feeding plan should be determined in consultation with a registered dietician in order to avoid the risk of re-feeding syndrome. In addition children who are suspected to have growth failure as a result of child neglect or abuse should be hospitalized for their safety, and child welfare workers should be notified immediately.

ISSUES FOR REFERRAL
- Consider referring children with a specific organ disease or genetic syndrome to the appropriate pediatric medical specialty clinics.
- Physicians are considered "mandatory reporters" by every jurisdiction in the US, so if child abuse or neglect is suspected, the child's condition must be reported to the local version of child and family welfare protective services and/or law enforcement.
- In some medical centers, multidisciplinary teams consisting of physicians, nutritionists, occupational/speech therapists, social workers, psychologists, and clinical nurse practitioners work together to care for a child and the family.

ADDITIONAL READING
- Committee on Nutrition, American Academy of Pediatrics. Failure to thrive. In: Kleinman RE, ed. *Pediatric nutrition handbook*, 6th ed. Elk Grove Village, IL: American Academy of Pediatrics, 2009.
- Maggioni A, Lifshitz F. Nutritional management of failure to thrive. *Pediatr Clin North Am*. 1995;42: 791–810.

- MedlinePlus. Failure to thrive, August 2, 2009. Available at: http://www.nlm.nih.gov/medlineplus/ency/article/000991.
- Schmitt BD, Mauro RD. Nonorganic failure to thrive: An outpatient approach. *Child Abuse Negl*. 1989; 13:235–248.

 ## CODES

ICD9
- 779.34 Failure to thrive in newborn
- 783.41 Short stature

ICD10
- R62.51 Failure to thrive (child)
- P92.6 Failure to thrive in newborn

FAQ
- Q: What are the long-term effects of FTT?
- A: Poor physical growth can lead to multi-organ dysfunction as well as developmental delays.
- Q: What are the treatments for FTT?
- A: The treatment depends on the cause of the delayed growth and development. Delayed growth due to nutritional factors can be resolved by providing a well-balanced diet. Delayed growth due to medical disease can be addressed by treating the illness. Delayed growth due to psychological factors may improve by addressing family dynamics and improving living conditions.

CLINICAL PEARLS
- FTT may be due to inadequate caloric intake, inadequate caloric absorption, or excessive metabolic demand.
- Organic and environmental causes of FTT frequently co-exist.
- A medical reason for FTT is found <50% of the time.
- If the period of FTT has been short, and the cause is determined and can be corrected, normal growth and development will resume. If FTT is prolonged, the effects may be long-lasting, and normal growth and development may not be achieved.

FEEDING DISORDERS

Diane Barsky

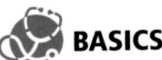 **BASICS**

DESCRIPTION
- Feeding disorder: Inability to consume by mouth in quantity or quality nutrition that is developmentally appropriate for that child
- Dysphagia: Disorder of swallowing characterized by difficulty in oral preparation for the swallow or in moving food or liquid from the mouth to the stomach
- Aspiration: Food or fluid falling below vocal cords proceeding to lungs
- Penetration: Food or fluid remaining above vocal cords and cleared by patient through coughing to prevent aspiration

RISK FACTORS
- Congenital heart disease
- Cystic fibrosis
- Metabolic disorders
- Autism spectrum disorder
- Developmental delay/Cerebral palsy
- Prolonged tube feeders (>4 weeks)
- Prematurity
- Neuromotor dysfunction
- Anatomic deformities (i.e., Pierre Robin sequence, laryngomalacia, tracheotomy)
- GI disorders: Gastroesophageal reflux
- Tachypnea (respiratory rate >40 breathes per minute)
- Oral motor disorder: Inability to manipulate age-appropriate diet; often related incoordination of facial muscles and/or tongue
- Pharyngeal dysphagia: Inability to protect airway during swallow; may be due to anatomic abnormality or neurological dysfunction
- Voluntary food or fluid refusal due to learned fear when caregiver pushes foods or textures before the child is developmentally or medically ready; may result in maladaptive interactions at meals

GENERAL PREVENTION
- Monitor weight, height, head circumference, weight for height, and BMI percentiles at regular interval office visits to identify changes in nutritional status early, especially in high-risk populations.
- Selective eater: Educate parents on age-appropriate portion sizes and foods.
- Provide vitamin and mineral supplementation or refer to nutritionist for complete assessment if patient is at risk for deficiencies.
- Developmental delay: Evaluate diet and feeding skills to manipulate nutrition provided.
- Ensure foods offered match developmental age if different than chronological age.

DIAGNOSIS

HISTORY
- Medical diagnoses past and present
- Treatments in past or present, especially those aversive to face and upper body and face (i.e., suctioning, tracheostomy, intubation)
- 24-hour diet: Recall food and fluid consumed over a 24-hour period
- Previous hospitalizations, especially respiratory illnesses
- Allergies or food intolerances
- Growth history
- Developmental history
- History of snoring or sleep apnea: May indicate adenoidal or tonsillar hypertrophy
- GI history: Stool pattern, vomiting, gagging, spitting up, pain
- Previous diagnostic testing
- Family history: GI disease, allergies, developmental delays, genetic abnormalities
- Failure to thrive:
  – Poor linear growth
  – Sucking and swallowing incoordination: Infant should demonstrate 1:1:1 suck, swallow, breathe pattern when sucking from breast or bottle.
  – Recurrent pneumonia
  – Coughing during or after feeding
  – Refractory asthma
  – Drooling
  – Refusal to drink or eat
  – Feeding selectivity
  – Difficulty with texture progression

PHYSICAL EXAM
- HEENT: Dysmorphic facial features, shape of head and sutures, facial tone, intact soft and hard palate, shape of mandible, tonsillar size, patency of nares, movement of lips and tongue, presence of stridor, mouth closure, dentition, drooling
- Pulmonary: Rate of breathing, use of accessory muscles for respiration, rales
- Cardiac: Murmur, rate and rhythm
- GI: Bowel sounds, masses, stool palpable, tenderness, distension
- Neurologic: Tone, positioning, cranial nerves, gait, affect, head control
- Extremities: Subcutaneous stores, muscle development, adipose tissue
- Skin: Rashes, alopecia

DIAGNOSTIC TESTS & INTERPRETATION
Perform feeding observation: Watch caregiver feed child, preferably thru 1-way observation mirror. Monitor child's behavioral response to placement in the feeding chair and presentation of bottle, breast, or cup and a variety of food types and textures; observe parental reaction to child's behaviors; child's ability to manipulate foods and fluids

Lab
- Based on nutritional and/or developmental concerns.
- Failure to thrive: Celiac panel, CBC, comprehensive metabolic panel, lead, urine analysis, thyroid function. Other tests if suspect vitamin or mineral deficiency (i.e., zinc, iron)
- Developmental and/or genetic concerns: Chromosomes, FISH test for 22Q11 deletion, FISH test for Prader-Willi syndrome, Fragile X (males), serum and urine organic acids, lactate, pyruvate, CPK
- Sweat test if suspected cystic fibrosis: Failure to thrive, diarrhea, and/or recurrent pulmonary infections

Imaging
- Tests indicated based on history and physical
- Suspected pharyngeal dysphagia: modified barium swallow study (MBSS) (also known as videofluoroscopic swallow study) evaluates swallow function and can visualize aspiration during swallow; usually performed by radiologist and speech therapist. Study visualizes function of pharyngeal muscles and structures. See below:
  – Upper GI series ensures normal anatomy of esophagus, stomach, and duodenum.
  – Chest x-ray: Determine if infiltrates or atelectasis is present; right upper and/or middle lobe changes indicative of potential aspiration.
  – Gastric emptying scan: Assess gastric emptying and assess if gastroparesis is present.
  – Salivagram: Radionucleotide study to evaluate if patient aspirating oral secretions
  – Chest CT scan: Allows detection of subtle changes from silent aspiration not detectable by pulmonary exam or chest x-ray.

Diagnostic Procedures/Other
- MBSS: Speech therapist feeds a variety of textures: Thin and thickened liquid of honey and nectar consistency, thin and thick purees and chewable foods to determine safety of oral feeding. Allows visualization of oral and pharyngeal phases of swallowing. Can determine appropriate positioning, type of infant bottles and cups to minimize the risk for aspiration.
  – Timing of aspiration is evaluated to determine if volume and fatigue result in aspiration, patient may be safe to drink or eat for short periods of time before the swallow becomes uncoordinated and leads to aspiration.
- Fiberoptic endoscopic evaluation of swallowing (FEES): Usually performed by ENT specialist. Direct visualization of airway structures and swallowing mechanism. Provides information on pharyngeal phase of swallowing but not oral phase. Best used if pharyngeal or laryngeal abnormality is suspected, tracheostomy in place, and there is difficulty managing secretions. Can observe food or fluid falling below vocal cords, resulting in aspiration
- Bronchoscopy: Visualizes tracheobronchial tree and lungs, sample for lipid-laden macrophages in lungs indicative of aspiration
- Endoscopy: To perform esophageal, gastric, and small bowel biopsies to determine presence of eosinophilic esophagitis, celiac disease (positive or inconclusive celiac panel), or presence of gastroesophageal reflux disease (GERD)

DIFFERENTIAL DIAGNOSIS

- Cardiorespiratory:
  - Congenital heart disease:
    ○ Infectious pneumonia
    ○ Bronchopulmonary dysplasia
- Neurological:
  - Diencephalic syndrome:
    ○ Congenital myopathy
    ○ Arnold-Chiari malformation
    ○ Hypoxic-ischemic encephalopathy
- GI/Nutritional:
  - GERD
  - Gastroparesis
  - Eosinophilic esophagitis
  - Failure to thrive
  - Celiac disease
- Metabolic syndromes
- Psychological disorders:
  - Behavioral refusal
  - Psychosocial deprivation
  - Anxiety disorder
- Food allergies
- Anatomic:
  - Laryngeal cleft
  - Tracheoesophageal fistula
- Genetic disorders
- Developmental disorders:
  - Autistic spectrum disorder
  - Sensory integration disorder

 TREATMENT

- Pharyngeal dysphagia: Pulmonary referral, oral stimulation program, NPO as indicated by clinical exam and studies, initiate tube feeds; monitoring by speech therapist
- Feeding disorders are complex and should be evaluated and managed by multidisciplinary team involving medical, nutrition, psychology, occupational therapy, and speech therapy.

MEDICATION (DRUGS)

- Appetite enhancing medications are not routinely recommended.
- Medications are administered to treat underlying medical condition (e.g., GERD); refer to specific sections for treatment of identified medical issues resulting in feeding disorder.

ADDITIONAL TREATMENT
General Measures
- Calorie counts
- Ensure adequate hydration

Additional Therapies
- Obtain a list of all supplemental vitamins, minerals, herbs, etc. that the parent may be providing to the patient.
- Investigate if parent is following any special diets (e.g., casein/gluten-free diet in autistic spectrum disorder).
- Note that the current literature does not support special diets or excessive dosing of vitamin and/or mineral supplements in developmental disorders unless indicated in treatment of a specific metabolic disorder.

COMPLEMENTARY & ALTERNATIVE THERAPIES

- Speech therapy: Evaluate oral motor skill and safety of swallowing mechanism; perform MBSS when indicated.
- Occupational therapy: Evaluate fine motor skills, sensory processing, and posture to support feeding.
- Psychology: May identify behaviors interfering with food acceptance and recommend strategies to improve oral acceptance
- Nutrition: Perform complete nutritional assessment, including evaluation of growth parameters, identifying patient's nutrition requirements, and adequacy of current diet. The nutritionist can develop a care plan to meet patient's nutritional requirements and monitor intake and weight gain during hospitalizations.

SURGERY/OTHER PROCEDURES

- Consider gastrostomy tube placement if tube feedings for >3 months are anticipated.
- For GERD not responding to medications, consider bypassing stomach and feeding into intestine with jejunostomy tube or Nissen fundoplication.

IN-PATIENT CONSIDERATIONS
Initial Stabilization
- Prior to initiation of behavioral program, ensure weight gain and growth are adequate.
- Evaluate and treat vitamin and mineral deficiencies.
- If weight-for-height or BMI is <5%, inappropriate weight gain crossing down 2 percentiles on growth chart occurs, or weight loss occurs, consider initiating supplemental nasogastric tube feeds.
- If aspiration pneumonia is suspected, obtain blood cultures, chest x-ray; keep NPO and start IV fluids and antibiotics. Measure oxygen saturation and initiate supplemental oxygen if <95%.

 ONGOING CARE

FOLLOW-UP RECOMMENDATIONS
Appointment with multidisciplinary feeding team, if available within reasonable geographic radius

Patient Monitoring
- Patient's weight should be checked within 2 weeks of discharge.
- Pediatrician should monitor patients with respiratory difficulties related to aspiration every 2 weeks until stable.

DIET
- Keep patient NPO if aspiration is suspected, until further evaluation (MBSS) can be performed.
- Order diet appropriate for child's current level of feeding skills (i.e., accepts baby food; may trial pureed diet).
- If nutritional intake is inadequate, offer nutritional supplements, monitor calorie counts, and initiate supplemental nasogastric tube feeds if unable to meet nutritional requirements.
- Caregiver education regarding administration of supplemental tube feeds

PROGNOSIS

- Nutritional rehabilitation can be achieved with tube feedings if patient is monitored closely.
- Patients with pharyngeal dysphagia resulting in aspiration may improve over time.
- Structural abnormalities, as seen with CHARGE association or subglottic stenosis, may improve over 1st 2–3 years of life or require surgical intervention prior to oral feeding.
- Static or degenerative neurological conditions resulting in aspiration generally do not resolve.
- Patient demonstrating dysphagia during illness may improve when healthy.

ADDITIONAL READING

- Rudolph CD, Thompson LD. Feeding disorders in infants and children. *Pediatr Clin North Am.* 2002;49(1):97–112.
- Tobin S, et al. Children's Hospital of Philadelphia's Pediatric and Swallowing Center: The role of our interdisciplinary feeding team in the assessment and treatment of feeding problems. Special Focus on Nutrition. *Building Block of Nutrition.* March 2006:1–34.
- Williams KE, Field DG, Seiverling L. Food Refusal in children: A review of the literature. *Res Develop Dis.* 2010;31:625–633.

 CODES

ICD9
- 307.59 Other disorders of eating
- 779.31 Feeding problems in newborn
- 787.21 Dysphagia, oral phase

ICD10
- F98.29 Other feeding disorders of infancy and early childhood
- P92.9 Feeding problem of newborn, unspecified
- R13.11 Dysphagia, oral phase

FAQ

- Q: What is the difference between aspiration and penetration in a swallowing disorder?
- A: Penetration occurs when food or fluid enter the trachea but remains above the vocal cords and is cleared by the patient. Aspiration occurs when the food or fluid falls below the vocal cords thus entering the lungs.
- Q: How is a modified barium swallow study used to evaluate dysphagia?
- A: A speech therapist in conjunction with the radiologist feeds the patient a variety of textures, including thin and thickened liquids, thin honey and nectar, thick purees, and chopped food if indicated, visualizing the pathway during swallowing to determine if it moves safely into the esophagus without entering the airway. The speech therapist also will engage in therapeutic endeavors, such as repositioning the patient, to determine if they can eliminate aspiration.

F

FETAL ALCOHOL SYNDROME

Michelle E. Melicosta
Janet M. Li-Tempest (5th edition)

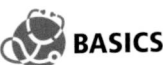 **BASICS**

DESCRIPTION
- Pattern of structural, behavioral, and neurocognitive abnormalities in individuals exposed to alcohol in utero.
- The four major features are:
  - Facial malformations
  - Growth abnormalities
  - Neurodevelopment symptoms
  - Maternal alcohol use during pregnancy.
- First described in 1973; has since been recognized that fetal alcohol syndrome (FAS) is the "tip of the iceberg" of a larger spectrum of disorders, from subtle to serious:
  - In 1996, the Institute of Medicine addressed this with a classification system which differentiated FAS from "partial FAS," alcohol-related birth defects (ARBD). and alcohol-related neurodevelopmental disorder (ARND).
  - Currently, the CDC, with the National Task Force on FAS/FAE, has developed a set of standardized diagnostic criteria for FAS; the other categories do not thus far have a uniformly accepted set of diagnostic criteria.

EPIDEMIOLOGY
Incidence
Ranges from 0.2–2.0 per 1,000 live births. Higher rates, up to 3–5 per 1,000, are found among selected subgroups (e.g., lower socioeconomic level, Native Americans).

RISK FACTORS
Genetics
- Maternal polymorphisms of the alcohol dehydrogenase gene (ADH): The presence of the ADH1B*3 allele appears to protect the fetus.
- Concordance of FAS is higher in monozygotic than in dizygotic twins; differential sensitivities to in utero alcohol exposure in different strains of mice.
- Other factors that contribute to variable susceptibility include older maternal age/parity, nutritional status, and concomitant use of other drugs.

GENERAL PREVENTION
- Studies have shown that up to 15% of women report alcohol use during pregnancy.
- The highest risk for FAS occurs in children whose mothers consume ≥5 drinks per occasion per week (peak blood alcohol level is more important than a lower sustained blood alcohol level).
- No minimum safe level of alcohol consumption has been determined.
- Recent FASD prevention research has focused on finding and treating women who drink alcohol during pregnancy (e.g., using a screening questionnaire to assess problem drinking in women, and then intervening at a level determined by the level of drinking).
- Good maternal nutritional status may be protective of the fetus in mothers who drink alcohol.

PATHOPHYSIOLOGY
- May involve increased susceptibility to cell damage by free radicals in the developing tissues, leading to cell death or decreased cellular proliferation
- Alcohol and its metabolite, acetaldehyde, are embryotoxic and teratogenic, capable of reducing fetal growth and inducing malformations during critical periods in the development of the fetus.
- Exposure in the 1st trimester affects organogenesis and craniofacial development, resulting in characteristic facial features and birth defects.
- Exposure at varying times can cause CNS neurodevelopmental effects, because brain formation and neuronal maturation occur throughout pregnancy.
- Exposure also causes prenatal and postnatal growth retardation, probably by inhibiting protein and DNA synthesis.

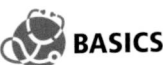 DIAGNOSIS

HISTORY
- Neurodevelopmental symptomatology is very age and development-dependent.
- Birth history, birth and subsequent growth parameters (weight, height, head circumference)
- Maternal history of alcohol use (binge drinking, average number of drinks per day, timing in pregnancy), and other drug use
- Family history: Neurobehavioral abnormalities should *not* be typical of other family members who were not exposed to ETOH prenatally.
- Learning/behavior problems, infancy:
  - May or may not have ethyl alcohol withdrawal as newborn
  - Irritability, irregular sleep, poor feeding, hypotonia, delayed motor function
- Learning/behavior problems, preschool and school age:
  - Hyperactivity
  - Slow verbal learning
  - Slow visual-spatial learning
  - Poor abstract thinking (planning and organizing)
  - Perseveration (inability to abandon ineffective strategies)
  - Attention problems
  - Difficulty with peer interactions
- Learning/behavior problems, adolescence and adulthood:
  - Substance abuse
  - Criminal behavior
  - Inability to work
  - Inability to live independently
  - Difficulty managing time and money
- Child in a high-risk living situation:
  - Keep in mind that external influences, such as poverty, unstable home environment, poor emotional support, and lack of educational resources, contribute to behavioral problems.

PHYSICAL EXAM
- Weight, height, head circumference
- Microcephaly persists throughout life.
- Weight can often be improved by interventions.
- History of growth deficits is required for diagnosis.
- Facial exam (short palpebral fissures, ptosis, flat midface, upturned nose, smooth philtrum, thin upper lip)
- Facial features become less prominent in adolescence and adulthood.

DIAGNOSTIC TESTS & INTERPRETATION
Neuropsychological testing:
- Simple IQ tests cannot distinguish children with FAS from those with other developmental disabilities.
- Tests of executive functioning most consistently show deficits; these include the WISC-III mazes and the Wisconsin category test.

Lab
No laboratory marker exists for FAS.

Diagnostic Procedures/Other
- FAS diagnosis requires all three of the following markers.
- I. Facial features:
  - Short palpebral fissures (≤10th percentile)
  - Thin vermilion border upper lip (score of 4 or 5 on the lip/philtrum guide [Astley, 2000])
  - Smooth philtrum (4 or 5 on lip/philtrum guide).
  - Other findings, such as ptosis, maxillary hypoplasia, and short, upturned nose are not diagnostic but are commonly seen in children with FAS.
- II. Documentation of growth deficits:
  - Height or weight ≤10th percentile at any time in patient's history.
- III. Documentation of CNS abnormality (any 1 below):
  - Structural:
    - Microcephaly at birth OFC <10th percentile, or disproportionate to height; or
    - Structural brain abnormalities (eg, agenesis of corpus callosum, cerebellar hypoplasia)
  - Neurological:
    - Seizures, poor coordination, impaired memory, or other soft neurological signs not attributable to postnatal insult or fever.
  - Functional: Performance substantially below that expected for an individual's age and circumstances, as evidenced by either:
    - Global cognitive deficits (IQ or developmental delays in multiple domains) >2 standard deviations below the mean, *OR*
    - Functional deficits 1 SD below the mean in at least 3 specific domains (e.g., attention, executive functioning, motor functioning, social skills, language, or specific learning disabilities)

- Maternal alcohol exposure:
  - Confirmed maternal exposure to alcohol is defined as substantial regular intake or heavy episodic drinking. Evidence may include self-report or that of a reliable informant; medical records showing an elevated blood alcohol level or alcohol-related medical problems (e.g., hepatic disease); legal problems related to drinking.
  - If there is no available history, or conflicting reports, then described as "Unknown maternal exposure."
  - If maternal alcohol abstinence can be confirmed (rare, for example, if mother incarcerated for entire pregnancy), then FAS is eliminated as a diagnosis.

DIFFERENTIAL DIAGNOSIS
- By physical features:
  - Aarskog syndrome
  - Williams syndrome
  - Noonan syndrome
  - Brachmann-De Lange syndrome
  - Dubowitz syndrome
  - Fetal valproate syndrome
  - Fetal hydantoin syndrome
  - Maternal phenylketonuria fetal effects
  - Toluene embryopathy
- By neurobehavioral features:
  - Fragile X syndrome
  - 22q11 deletion syndromes
  - Turner syndrome
  - Opitz syndrome

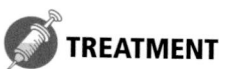

TREATMENT

ADDITIONAL TREATMENT
General Measures
- The role of the pediatrician is early identification (with help from specialists), appropriate referrals, and development of a multidisciplinary case plan, including the pediatrician, specialists, early intervention providers, psychologists, and social and educational resources in the community to support family and child.
- Specific medical referrals should include:
  - Comprehensive neuropsychologic evaluation (IQ, achievement, executive function, memory, adaptive function, language, reasoning and judgment, behavior)
  - Ophthalmologic exam (consider routine screening prior to school, then every 2 years)
  - Hearing test (consider brainstem auditory evoked response [BAER] at 6–12 months)

 ONGOING CARE

FOLLOW-UP RECOMMENDATIONS
Patient Monitoring
- Growth and nutrition in infancy: Failure to thrive is a common problem.
- Regular evaluations of vision and hearing: Problems occur at a high rate.
- As indicated by other medical/psychologic problems

PROGNOSIS
- 50% are mentally retarded (IQ <70). Average IQ in individuals with FAS is in the 60s (mild mental retardation); however, a wide range of IQ exists, from 16–115.
- 62% have severe behavioral problems, even if a normal IQ exists.
- The major disabilities of FAS caused by the neurocognitive/neurobehavioral effects leading to poor academic performance, legal problems, employment difficulties, and secondary mental health problems.
- Many are unable to live independently as adults.

ADDITIONAL READING
- American Academy of Pediatrics. Fetal alcohol syndrome and alcohol-related neurodevelopmental disorders. *Pediatrics*. 2000;106:358–361.
- Astley SJ. Diagnosing the full spectrum of fetal-alcohol exposed individuals. *Alcohol Alcohol*. 2000;35:400–410.
- Hoyme HE. A practical clinical approach to Diagnosis of fetal alcohol spectrum disorders: Clarification of the 1996 IOM Criteria. *Pediatrics*. 2005;115:39–47.
- National Center for Birth Defects and Developmental Disabilities, Centers for Disease Control, in coordination with the National Task Force on Fetal Alcohol Syndrome and Fetal Alcohol Effects. *Fetal alcohol syndrome*, 3rd revision, July 2005.
- National Institute on Alcohol Abuse and Alcoholism. *Fetal alcohol exposure and the brain*. Alcohol Alert no. 50. Bethesda, MD: National Institutes of Health; 2000.

 CODES

ICD9
760.71 Alcohol affecting fetus or newborn via placenta or breast milk

ICD10
Q86.0 Fetal alcohol syndrome (dysmorphic)

FAQ
- Q: What is FAE (fetal alcohol effect)?
- A: FAE originally described abnormalities seen in animal studies, then was adopted by clinicians, who widely used the term to refer to behavioral and cognitive problems in children exposed to alcohol in utero, but without the typical diagnostic features of FAS.
- Because of lack of diagnostic criteria for FAE and the imprecise use of this term, IOM replaced FAE with the terms ARND and ARBD.
  - Use of the terms ARND and ARBD remains controversial in that they imply that confirmed maternal alcohol exposure is causative of the associated abnormalities, which at present, is not proven.
  - In summarizing the problem list for an individual who may not meet the criteria for FAS or partial FAS, many leading dysmorphologists recommend listing the elements separately without attribution, rather than using the confusing terms FAE or ARND/ARBD. Example: Impression 1, prenatal alcohol exposure; 2, cleft lip and palate, complete bilateral; 3, cognitive deficit.
- Q: How much alcohol does it take to produce damage?
- A: The highest risk for FAS occurs in children whose mothers consume ≥5 drinks per occasion at least once per week. However, NO minimum safe level of alcohol consumption has been determined
- Q: Do most children with FAS have ADHD?
- A: Although hyperactivity appears to be common in FAS, many of these children are misdiagnosed as having ADHD. Instead of difficulty focusing and sustaining attention, children with FAS often have difficulty shifting attention from one task to another. Use of stimulant medication is not routinely supported, although a small proportion may respond to stimulant medication in educational settings.

F

FEVER AND PETECHIAE

Lisa Mcleod
Evaline A. Alessandrini (5th edition)

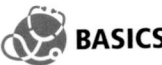 **BASICS**

DEFINITION
- Petechiae:
  - Small hemorrhages into the superficial layers of the skin
  - <3 mm in size
  - Manifest as a reddish purple, macular, nonblanching skin rash
- Purpura:
  - Larger skin hemorrhages
  - Purple
  - Often macular like petechiae but may be raised or tender

EPIDEMIOLOGY
- Although there are no strong epidemiologic data, the presentation of fever and petechiae is rare compared with the presentation of fever alone.
- A great majority of patients (70–80%) presenting with fever and petechiae have defined or presumed viral infections, which are most often caused by enterovirus or adenovirus.
- Several prospective studies have documented that 2–15% of children presenting with fever and petechiae will have an invasive bacterial disease, most commonly *Neisseria meningitidis*.
- Infants and toddlers are at greatest risk of having an invasive bacterial infection with fever and petechiae.
- Teenagers and young adults are most commonly affected by outbreaks of meningococcemia, presenting with fever and petechiae.
- Streptococcal pharyngitis may cause fever and petechiae in the well-appearing child.
- Recent epidemiologic investigations suggest that certain strains of Parvovirus B19 may be responsible for many cases of fever and generalized petechiae in children.
- Other etiologies, such as acute leukemia, idiopathic thrombocytopenic purpura (ITP), and Henoch–Schönlein purpura (HSP), are responsible for 5–10% of cases of fever and petechiae.

GENERAL PREVENTION
- Vaccine recommendations:
  - All children should complete the *Streptococcus pneumoniae* and *Haemophilus influenzae* type B immunization series that begins at 2 months of age.
  - Routine childhood immunization with meningococcal vaccine is now recommended for all children 11 years of age or older and for children ≥2 years who are at high risk, defined as asplenic, or with terminal complement deficiencies. A booster dose should be given 5 years later through age 21 years. Annual immunization against influenza viruses should be encouraged for all children >6 months of age.
- Chemoprophylaxis is recommended for close contacts of patients with meningococcal disease. Ideally, treatment with rifampin, ceftriaxone, or ciprofloxacin should begin within 24 hours.

PATHOPHYSIOLOGY
Petechiae may result from several different mechanisms:
- Disruption of vascular integrity—due to infections, vasculitis, or trauma
- Platelet deficiency or dysfunction—typically thrombocytopenia due to sepsis, disseminated intravascular coagulation (DIC), ITP, or leukemia
- Factor deficiencies (more likely to manifest as ecchymoses and deep bleeding)

DIAGNOSIS

DIFFERENTIAL DIAGNOSIS
- Viral infections (see "Etiology")
- Invasive bacterial infections:
  - Most commonly *N. meningitidis*
  - Less often *Staphylococcus aureus*, *Escherichia coli*, *S. pneumoniae*, and *H. influenzae* type B. *S. pneumoniae* and *H. influenzae* type B are less common because of widespread childhood immunization.
- Streptococcal pharyngitis—due to *Streptococcus pyogenes*
- Rickettsial infections: Diagnosis aided by season, history of tick bite accompanied by fever, petechiae, headache, and myalgias
- Stress petechiae in the distribution of the superior vena cava (SVC) after significant coughing or vomiting
- Coining or other traumatic causes
- Acute leukemias: Diagnosis aided by clinical findings of pallor, adenopathy, hepatosplenomegaly, and laboratory findings
- ITP: Diagnosis aided by findings of mucous membrane bleeding and isolated thrombocytopenia on laboratory testing
- HSP: Diagnosis aided by clinical findings consistent with HSP, including palpable purpura on the buttocks and lower extremities, usually in the absence of fever
- Endocarditis: Diagnosis aided by a history of congenital heart disease, cardiac surgery, or rheumatic fever

ETIOLOGY
Petechiae, when accompanied by fever, most often have an infectious cause. Multiple organisms are associated with fever and petechiae. Less commonly, fever and petechiae may be caused by other entities such as acute leukemia, ITP, and bacterial endocarditis.

- Bacterial:
  - *N. meningitidis*
  - *S. pneumoniae*
  - *H. influenzae* type B
  - *S. aureus*
  - *S. pyogenes*
  - *E. coli*

- Viral:
  - Enterovirus
  - Adenovirus
  - Influenza
  - Parainfluenza
  - Parvovirus B19
  - Epstein–Barr virus (EBV)
  - Rubella
  - Respiratory syncytial virus
  - Hepatitis viruses
- Rickettsial diseases:
  - Rickettsia rickettsii
  - Ehrlichiosis

HISTORY
Important historical factors to obtain include:
- Age of the child
- Any underlying immunodeficiency
- Immunizations received
- Exposure to infectious contacts, particularly *N. meningitidis*
- Duration and height of fever
- Duration and progression of rash
- Excessive coughing or vomiting
- Pallor or other bleeding
- Level of activity, excess fatigue
- Travel or history of tick bites
- History of trauma in location of rash

PHYSICAL EXAM
- Important components on which to concentrate:
  - Vital signs, particularly noting tachycardia or hypotension
  - Mental status
  - Meningismus/nuchal rigidity
  - Character of rash: Petechiae or purpura, body distribution, number of lesions, progression during exam
- Important findings suggesting specific diagnoses:
  - **Finding:** Pallor, adenopathy, organomegaly
  - *Significance:* Suggesting leukemia, EBV infection
  - **Finding:** Mucous membrane bleeding
  - *Significance:* Suggesting thrombocytopenia, such as that which occurs in ITP
  - **Finding:** Myalgias, centripetal rash distribution
  - *Significance:* Suggesting Rocky Mountain spotted fever

DIAGNOSTIC TESTS & INTERPRETATION

All children with fever and petechiae require laboratory testing. At a minimum, children should receive a CBC with differential, C-reactive protein (CRP), and a blood culture.

- Children >12–18 months with fever and petechiae should have a throat culture.
- Children who are ill-appearing may warrant coagulation studies including prothrombin time (PT), partial thromboplastin time (PTT), and DIC screen.
- Viral testing, including cultures, serology, and antibody immunofluorescence, is not routinely required and may be ordered at the discretion of the managing practitioner based on exposures, need for specific therapeutic interventions, admission to the hospital, and severity of illness.
- Nontoxic-appearing children >2 years of age with fever and petechiae should have a CBC with differential, CRP, blood culture, PT, and PTT.
- Although no one factor is 100% sensitive in identifying children with invasive bacterial disease, a constellation of factors is useful in identifying children with fever and petechiae in whom invasive bacterial disease is unlikely:
  - Multiple studies have demonstrated that well-appearing children with a normal WBC count (between 5,000 and 15,000), a normal absolute neutrophil count (between 1,500 and 9,000), an absolute band count <500, and petechiae limited to above the nipple line are exceedingly unlikely to have an invasive bacterial infection. In general a CRP <5 mg/L has been shown to have a high negative predictive value for ruling out invasive bacterial infection.

ALERT

Unsuspected invasive bacterial disease is the most common pitfall with fever and petechiae. A thorough history and physical exam, accompanied by laboratory testing and a period of close observation, may minimize missed serious diagnoses.

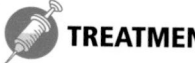 **TREATMENT**

ADDITIONAL TREATMENT
General Measures

- Prudent antibiotic choices are effective against meningococcal and streptococcal diseases, including third-generation cephalosporins such as cefotaxime and ceftriaxone.
- Doxycycline should be administered if rickettsial disease is considered.
- Vancomycin should be administered to children with suspected pneumococcal meningitis.
- Empiric antibiotic use should be decided on a case-by-case basis. There are no studies investigating the efficacy of antibiotic therapy in the outpatient management of patients with fever and petechiae. However, this author advocates use of parenteral ceftriaxone since *N. meningitidis*, the most likely bacterial pathogen in this circumstance, has a high morbidity and mortality.

IN-PATIENT CONSIDERATIONS
Initial Stabilization

- The management of children who are ill-appearing and have meningismus or purpura consists of a full sepsis evaluation, admission to the hospital with parenteral antibiotics, and fluids and vasoactive infusions to maintain normal hemodynamics.
- Because sporadic as opposed to epidemic cases of meningococcemia appear to occur in children in the first 2 years of life, and these children have less competent immune systems in fighting encapsulated organisms, full sepsis evaluation and admission for all children in this young age group are recommended.
- The well-appearing child with fever and petechiae and a positive streptococcal antigen test may be treated as an outpatient with antistreptococcal antibiotics.
- After a several-hour period of observation, children who remain well-appearing, are not tachycardic, have no progression of petechiae, and have normal lab studies may be considered for management as outpatients.

 ONGOING CARE

FOLLOW-UP RECOMMENDATIONS
Patient Monitoring

- Children managed as outpatients:
  - Give instructions to return immediately for progression of rash or worsening illness
  - Follow-up in 12–18 hours
  - Monitor cultures closely
- Most children with viral causes have little progression of their petechiae and are clinically better within several days with the resolution of fever.

PROGNOSIS

- Depends on the underlying cause
- Since most cases of fever and petechiae are caused by viral infections, particularly enteroviruses and adenoviruses, the prognosis is excellent.
- Studies demonstrate that the mortality rate of meningococcemia is 7–20%.

COMPLICATIONS

- Related to the underlying cause
- Most common complications of invasive bacterial disease causing fever and petechiae include sepsis and meningitis.
- Morbidity from *N. meningitidis* includes neurologic deficits, limb loss, and skin sloughing, necessitating skin grafts. Mortality is estimated to be 7–20%.

ADDITIONAL READING

- Mandl KD, Stack AM, Fleisher GR. Incidence of bacteremia in infants and children with fever and petechiae. *J Pediatr.* 1997;131:398–404.
- Neilsen HE, Andersen EA, Andersen J, et al. Diagnostic assessment of haemorrhagic rash and fever. *Arch Dis Child.* 2001;85:160–165.
- Wells LC, Smith JC, Weston VC, et al. The child with a non-blanching rash: How likely is meningococcal disease? *Arch Dis Child.* 2001;85:218–222.

 CODES

ICD9
- 772.6 Cutaneous hemorrhage of fetus or newborn
- 780.60 Fever, unspecified
- 782.7 Spontaneous ecchymoses

ICD10
- R23.3 Spontaneous ecchymoses
- R50.9 Fever, unspecified
- P54.5 Neonatal cutaneous hemorrhage

FAQ

- Q: What is the most common cause of fever and petechiae in children?
- A:
  - Viruses are the most common overall cause of fever and petechiae in children.
  - The most common invasive bacterial disease causing fever and petechiae in children in the 21st century is *N. meningitidis*.
- Q: Is there ever a role for outpatient management of children with fever and petechiae?
- A:
  - Practitioners may consider outpatient management in well-appearing children >2 years of age with all of the following criteria after a period of observation in which they have normal vital signs and no progression of petechiae:
    - A normal WBC count (between 5,000 and 15,000)
    - A normal absolute neutrophil count (between 1,500 and 9,000)
    - An absolute band count <500
    - Petechiae limited to above the nipple line

F

FEVER OF UNKNOWN CAUSE

Samir S. Shah

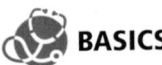

BASICS

DEFINITION
Fever of unknown origin (FUO) implies:
- A febrile illness (38.3°C on multiple occasions)
- Present for >14 days
- No apparent source despite careful history taking, physical exam, and preliminary lab studies

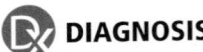

DIAGNOSIS

DIFFERENTIAL DIAGNOSIS
FUO is more often an unusual presentation of a common disease than a common presentation of an unusual disease. Possible causes include:

- **Common infectious causes**
  - Respiratory infections (otitis media, mastoiditis, sinusitis, pneumonia, pharyngitis, peritonsillar/retropharyngeal abscess)
  - Systemic viral syndrome
  - Urinary tract infection (UTI)
  - Bone or joint infection
  - Enteric infection (*Salmonella, Yersinia enterocolitica, Yersinia pseudotuberculosis, Campylobacter jejuni*)
  - Cat-scratch disease
- **Less common infectious causes**
  - Tuberculosis (TB)
  - Infectious mononucleosis (Epstein–Barr virus [EBV], cytomegalovirus [CMV])
  - Lyme disease
  - Rickettsial disease (Rocky Mountain spotted fever, ehrlichiosis)
  - Malaria
  - CNS infection (bacterial or viral meningoencephalitis, intracranial abscess)
  - Dental or periodontal abscess
  - Subacute bacterial endocarditis (SBE)
  - HIV infection
  - Acute rheumatic fever
- **Other infectious causes**
  - Q fever
  - Brucellosis
  - Toxoplasmosis
  - Syphilis
  - Parvovirus B19
  - Endemic fungi (histoplasmosis, blastomycosis, coccidioidomycosis)
  - Psittacosis
  - Chronic meningococcemia

- **Possible noninfectious causes**
  - Collagen-vascular disease (systemic juvenile idiopathic arthritis [JIA], systemic lupus erythematosus, dermatomyositis, sarcoidosis, vasculitis syndrome)
  - Malignancy
  - Kawasaki syndrome
  - Inflammatory bowel disease (IBD)
  - Drug fever
  - Hyperthyroidism
  - Factitious fever or Munchausen syndrome by proxy
  - Centrally mediated fever
  - Periodic fever syndrome
  - Kikuchi–Fujimoto disease (histiocytic necrotizing lymphadenitis)

ETIOLOGY
Etiology has changed as the use of more sensitive tests (e.g., MRI, PCR tests) permits earlier detection of many conditions that caused FUO in the past. Fever resolves in 40–60% of children without identification of a specific cause.

APPROACH TO THE PATIENT
Find the cause of the fever and begin treatment of the underlying illness.
- **Phase 1**
  - Document fever
  - Thorough history and physical exam
  - Determine whether constitutional symptoms (e.g., growth failure, developmental arrest) suggest a serious underlying disease.
  - Create broad differential diagnosis
  - Begin initial laboratory evaluation while tailoring the cadence of evaluation to patient's severity of illness.
- **Phase 2**
  - Begin invasive studies to seek rarer forms of fever, such as lymphoma, brucellosis, and SBE.
- **Phase 3**
  - Re-examine patient, consider additional testing, and reconsider causes such as systemic JIA, sarcoidosis, and factitious fever.

Repeat history and physical exam combined with the results of previous testing should guide the subsequent evaluation.

HISTORY
Initial studies should include a CBC, liver function tests, blood culture, urinalysis, urine culture, stool culture, and stool ova and parasite testing.

- **Question:** Temperatures and how they were measured (tympanic, oral, axillary, rectal)?
- *Significance:*
  - As many as 50% of children referred for evaluation of FUO have multiple unrelated infections, parental misinterpretation of normal temperature variation, or complete absence of fever at time of evaluation.
  - Parents are sometimes told to add a 1–2°F "correction" onto a temperature measured in the axilla to better approximate the core temperature. Such practices may further cloud the evaluation of the febrile child.
- **Question:** Exposure to animals?
- *Significance:*
  - Household exposures including pets and rodents
  - Recreational activities (e.g., hunting)
  - Household contacts with occupational exposure to animals
  - Consider cat-scratch disease, brucellosis, tularemia, leptospirosis, and lymphocytic choriomeningitis virus (from mice)
- **Question:** Ingestion of raw meat, fish, or unpasteurized milk?
- *Significance:* Trichinosis, brucellosis
- **Question:** Travel history, including past residence?
- *Significance:* Malaria, endemic fungi (e.g., coccidioidomycosis, blastomycosis), TB
- **Question:** Pica or dirt ingestion?
- *Significance: Toxocara canis* or *Toxoplasma gondii* infection
- **Question:** Change in behavior or activity?
- *Significance:* Brain tumor, TB, EBV, Rocky Mountain spotted fever
- **Question:** Pattern of fever?
- *Significance:* May correlate with underlying cause. A fever diary kept by the parent or caretaker may provide more objective documentation of the fever pattern than simple recall.
- **Question:** Medications (including OTC medications and eyedrops)?
- *Significance:* Drug fever, atropine-induced fever, methylphenidate, and antibiotics (especially penicillin, cephalosporins, and sulfonamides)
- **Question:** Well-water ingestion?
- *Significance:* Giardiasis

PHYSICAL EXAM

- **Finding:** Impaired weight gain or linear growth?
- *Significance:* Collagen-vascular disease, malignancy, IBD
- **Finding:** Toxic appearance?
- *Significance:* Kawasaki syndrome
- **Finding:** Conjunctivitis?
- *Significance:* Kawasaki syndrome, adenovirus, measles
- **Finding:** Ophthalmologic exam?
- *Significance:* Brain tumor, TB, systemic lupus erythematosus, Kawasaki syndrome (uveitis), sarcoidosis
- **Finding:** Sinus tenderness, nasal discharge, or halitosis?
- *Significance:* Sinusitis
- **Finding:** Pharyngitis?
- *Significance:* Kawasaki syndrome, EBV, SBE
- **Finding:** Tachypnea?
- *Significance:* SBE, pneumonia
- **Finding:** Rales?
- *Significance:* Histoplasmosis, sarcoidosis, coccidioidomycosis
- **Finding:** Cardiac murmur, gallop, or friction rub?
- *Significance:* SBE, acute rheumatic fever, pericarditis
- **Finding:** Hepatosplenomegaly?
- *Significance:* Hepatitis, EBV, CMV
- **Finding:** Rectal abnormalities?
- *Significance:* Pelvic abscess, IBD
- **Finding:** Arthritis?
- *Significance:* JIA, IBD
- **Finding:** Bony tenderness?
- *Significance:* Juvenile rheumatoid arthritis, leukemia, osteomyelitis

DIAGNOSTIC TESTS & INTERPRETATION

The laboratory evaluation for a child with FUO should be directed toward the most likely diagnostic possibilities. Consider the following initial studies:

- **Test:** CBC with differential and careful examination of WBC morphology
- *Significance:* Kawasaki syndrome, cyclic neutropenia, malignancy, ehrlichiosis, babesiosis
- **Test:** ESR, C-reactive protein, or procalcitonin
- *Significance:* Collagen-vascular disease, IBD, occult infection. Generally normal in drug fever and central fever.
- **Test:** Blood cultures
- *Significance:* Endocarditis, salmonellosis, other bloodstream infections
- **Test:** Urinalysis and urine culture
- *Significance:* UTI, Kawasaki syndrome (sterile pyuria)
- **Test:** Tuberculin skin test (by purified protein derivative)
- *Significance:* TB
- **Test:** Stool bacterial culture and examination for ova and parasites
- *Significance:* Salmonella, Giardia
- **Test:** Specific antibody testing
- *Significance:* Depending on clinical suspicion, consider:
- First line: Streptococcal enzyme titers (antistreptolysin O, anti-DNase B), EBV, CMV, cat-scratch disease, Lyme disease, HIV, hepatitis A, B, or C
- Second line: Rocky Mountain spotted fever; ehrlichiosis/anaplasmosis, toxoplasmosis, brucellosis, Q fever, leptospirosis, tularemia, dengue fever
- Viral testing of nasopharyngeal aspirates
- Evaluation for immune deficiency
- Bone marrow examination and culture: *Salmonella* infection, *Mycobacterium avium* complex, histoplasmosis, brucellosis, malignancy
- Lumbar puncture

Imaging

- Sinus CT: Sinusitis
- Chest radiograph: TB, endemic fungi, pneumonia
- Chest and/or abdominal CT scan: TB, liver abscess, hepatosplenic cat-scratch disease
- Pelvic or extremity MRI: Osteomyelitis, pyomyositis
- Gallium or bone scan: Osteomyelitis

ADDITIONAL READING

- Drenth JPH, Van Der Meer JWM. Hereditary periodic fever. *N Engl J Med.* 2001;345:1748–1757.
- Gattorno M, Caorsi R, Meini A, et al. Differenting PFAPA syndrome from monogenic periodic fevers. *Pediatrics.* 2009;124:e721–e728.
- Jacobs RF, Schutze GE. *Bartonella henselae* as a cause of prolonged fever and fever of unknown origin in children. *Clin Infect Dis.* 1998;26:80–84.
- McClung HJ. Prolonged fever of unknown origin in children. *Am J Dis Child.* 1972;124:544–550.
- Talano JM, Katz BZ. Long-term follow-up of children with fever of unknown origin. *Clin Pediatr.* 2000; 39:715–717.

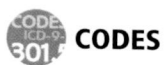 **CODES**

ICD9
780.60 Fever, unspecified

ICD10
R50.9 Fever, unspecified

FAQ

- Q: Do all of the above-mentioned tests need to be performed?
- A: A "shotgun" approach to testing is rarely useful in making the diagnosis.

F

FLOPPY INFANT SYNDROME

Garrick A. Applebee

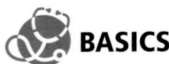 **BASICS**

DESCRIPTION
- "Floppy infant" implies generalized hypotonia presenting at birth or early in life with decreased movement, decreased resistance to movement, or increased joint laxity.
- Neuropathology includes CNS, lower motor neuron, peripheral nervous system (PNS), and primary muscle disease.
- Nonspecific transient hypotonia occurs in nonneurologic illnesses and may suggest endocrine, GI, or metabolic disease.

EPIDEMIOLOGY
Prevalence
No comprehensive prevalence known for this heterogeneous syndrome; overall, diseases affecting the CNS are more common than the PNS.

RISK FACTORS
Genetics
Many heritable disorders, including those with autosomal dominant, autosomal recessive, X-linked, and non-Mendelian inheritance patterns, feature infantile hypotonia.

PATHOPHYSIOLOGY
Neurologic causes may be divided into 2 major categories:
- Nonparalytic hypotonia: Hypotonia without weakness generally resulting from CNS or other organ system pathology
- Paralytic hypotonia: Hypotonia due to weakness from neuromuscular pathology

COMMONLY ASSOCIATED CONDITIONS
- Hip dislocation/contractures/joint laxity
- Feeding difficulties
- Seizure disorders
- Developmental/motor delay
- Apnea/hypoventilation
- Hypersomnolence

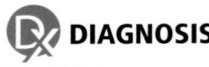 **DIAGNOSIS**

HISTORY
- Prenatal period and delivery:
  - Prenatal period:
    ○ Family history
    ○ Parental consanguinity
    ○ Maternal illness
    ○ Drug/teratogen exposure
    ○ Polyhydramnios (poor prenatal swallow)
    ○ Fetal movements
  - Delivery:
    ○ Birth trauma
    ○ Shortened umbilical cord
    ○ Apgar scores
- Neonatal period:
  - Maternal perinatal infection
  - Seizures
  - Apnea

- Later infancy:
  - Delayed motor milestones
  - Delayed social, fine motor, or language milestones point to CNS defect
  - Feeding difficulties

PHYSICAL EXAM
Exam findings will help determine if hypotonia is due to systemic or neurologic disease. If the latter is suspected, physical findings will help localize to specific region of nervous system (CNS vs. PNS). Perform:
- General physical exam
- Neurologic exam

FINDINGS/SIGNS AND SYMPTOMS
- General physical exam:
  - Look for dysmorphology.
  - Alertness: Infants with neuromuscular disease (unlike CNS disease) are typically alert.
  - Poor spontaneous movement
  - Abnormal head size and/or shape
  - High-arched palate (neuromuscular disorders)
  - Tongue fasciculations (anterior horn cell)
  - Large tongue (storage disorders)
  - Ophthalmologic exam: Cataracts, pigmentary retinopathy (peroxisomal disorders), cherry-red spot (storage disorders)
  - Visceral enlargement (storage disorders)
  - Arthrogryposis (central, neuromuscular, or connective tissue disorders)
  - Hip dislocation (intrauterine hypotonia)
  - Joint laxity (connective tissue disorders)
- Neurologic exam:
  - Muscle tone:
    ○ Infants exhibit abnormal resting posture (abducted, externally rotated legs, flaccid arms) and prominent head lag with pull-to-sit.
    ○ Fisting indicates spasticity.
    ○ Posture and tone in supine position, ventral and horizontal suspension, and traction abnormal. Elbow may extend beyond midsternum easily (scarf sign).
    ○ Generalized hypotonia with increased tone in thumb adductors, wrist pronators, and hip adductors often noted in early cerebral palsy
  - Strength:
    ○ Strength of cry
    ○ Decreased expression indicates facial weakness (myotonic dystrophy, congenital muscular dystrophy, congenital myopathies).
    ○ Ptosis and ophthalmoplegia (myasthenic syndromes, congenital myopathies, and congenital muscular dystrophies)
    ○ Regional strength differences may suggest certain disorders. Spinal muscular atrophy (SMA) spares diaphragm, face muscles, and pelvic sphincters. Neuropathies present with distal limb weakness and proximal sparing. Myasthenic syndromes affect bulbar and oculomotor muscles.
    ○ Fatigability is a cardinal feature of myasthenic syndromes and may occur in other neuromuscular diseases.

  - Reflexes:
    ○ Increased deep tendon reflexes (DTRs) imply central dysfunction.
    ○ In myopathic diseases, DTRs are diminished in proportion to degree of weakness.
    ○ Absent reflexes in setting of minimal weakness typical of neuropathic disease.

DIAGNOSTIC TESTS & INTERPRETATION
History and exam will guide both laboratory testing and imaging studies to establish a diagnosis.

Lab
- Initial tests may include:
  - Electrolytes (including Ca and Mg)
  - Thyroid function tests
  - Creatine kinase (CK)
  - Arterial blood gas
- Blood, urine, CSF cultures: Evaluate for infection.
- To identify an inborn error of metabolism:
  - Assays for uric acid, ammonia, and lactate (blood, urine, CSF)
  - Quantitative amino acid analysis (blood, urine)
  - Organic acid and acylcarnitine profiles (blood)
  - Assays of very-long-chain fatty acids (plasma)
- Molecular studies:
  - Karyotype: Chromosomal duplications, deletions, and trisomies
  - DNA microarray
  - DNA methylation, mutation analyses: A variety of diagnoses (Prader-Willi)
- Stool could be evaluated for *Clostridium* toxin when botulism suspected (endemic in Pennsylvania, some northwestern states).

Imaging
- MRI: Preferable to CT if CNS basis is suspected
- In some centers, muscle imaging is used to delineate a neuromuscular problem.

Diagnostic Procedures/Other
- Administration of an anticholinesterase in suspected myasthenia may be diagnostic.
- Electromyography (EMG) and nerve conduction velocity:
  - Useful tools in assessing the lower motor unit and localizing site of involvement

> **ALERT**
> Pitfalls:
> - EMG and nerve conduction velocity in young infants require expertise to perform and interpret. Values change with development.
> - Electroencephalogram, neuroimaging, if CNS abnormalities suspected
> - Muscle biopsy for specific biochemical and immunohistochemical tests may reveal specific diagnoses.
> - Electron microscopy may identify abnormal organelles, inclusions, or storage material.

Pathological Findings
Muscle biopsy: For suspected congenital myopathies, storage myopathies (acid maltase), muscular dystrophies (latter often feature high CK, and may be diagnosed via blood DNA testing)

DIFFERENTIAL DIAGNOSIS

Remember, many acute illnesses in infancy may present with decreased tone and/or weakness.

- Nonparalytic hypotonia:
  - Benign congenital hypotonia: Transient hypotonia without dysmorphology, weakness, or other neurologic, physical, or laboratory abnormalities
  - Connective tissue disorders:
    - Ehlers-Danlos syndrome
    - Marfan syndrome
    - Osteogenesis imperfecta
    - Chondrodysplasia
    - Benign joint laxity
  - Acute metabolic/systemic disorders:
    - Sepsis
    - Trauma
    - Malnutrition
    - Drug intoxication (maternal sedative, analgesic, and/or anesthetic exposure)
    - GI disease (obstruction, bleed)
  - Chronic metabolic/systemic disorders:
    - Congenital heart disease
    - Endocrinopathies (e.g., hypothyroidism)
    - Renal tubular acidosis
    - Rickets
    - Hypercalcemia
    - Cystic fibrosis, malabsorption
    - Organic acidemias
    - Glycogen storage disease
    - Mucopolysaccharidoses
    - Peroxisomal disorders (cerebrohepatorenal, neonatal adrenoleukodystrophy)
  - Disorders involving cerebral cortex, cerebellum, brainstem, cord:
    - Congenital malformations (lissencephaly, holoprosencephaly)
    - Hypoxic-ischemic encephalopathy
    - Intracranial hemorrhage
    - Infections (meningitis, encephalitis)
    - Trauma
    - Metabolic encephalopathies
    - Chromosomal disorders (Angelman, Prader-Willi, and Down syndromes)
    - Neuronal migration disorders
    - Sphingolipidoses
  - Disorders involving spinal cord:
    - Myelodysplasias (meningomyeloceles, diplomyelia, diastematomyelia)
    - Traumatic injury
- Paralytic hypotonia: Paralytic causes must be considered in floppy infants whose physical exam reveals significant weakness and decreased or absent DTRs. This category includes disorders of anterior horn cell, peripheral nerve, neuromuscular junction, and muscle:
  - Disorders of anterior horn cell:
    - Spinal muscular atrophy
    - Arthrogryposis multiplex congenita
    - Pompe (glycogen storage type II)
    - Neonatal poliomyelitis
  - Disorders of peripheral nerve:
    - Dejerine-Sottas disease
    - Guillain-Barré syndrome
    - Familial dysautonomia
    - Congenital hypomyelinating neuropathy
    - Leukodystrophies
    - Leigh/mitochondrial disease
  - Disorders of neuromuscular junction:
    - Myasthenia gravis (congenital, transient)
    - Toxic–metabolic defects (hypermagnesemia, antibiotics [especially aminoglycosides], nondepolarizing neuromuscular blockers)
    - Infantile botulism
  - Disorders of muscle:
    - Congenital structural myopathies: Central core, nemaline, centronuclear myopathy
    - Congenital myotonic dystrophy
    - Congenital muscular dystrophies
    - Metabolic myopathies (mitochondrial disorders, glycosylation disorders, lipid storage disease, others)

 TREATMENT

MEDICATION (DRUGS)

- Anticholinesterase medications may be required in treatment of myasthenic syndromes.
- IV immunoglobulin and plasmapheresis have been used in treatment of infants with Guillain-Barré syndrome

ADDITIONAL TREATMENT
General Measures

- Address apnea, hypoventilation, hypoxia:
  - Intubation or positive pressure devices may be required.
  - Chest physical therapy, antibiotics, bronchodilators, and oxygen may be needed.
  - Hypermagnesemia can cause apnea.
  - Weak infants in car seats may be at risk of acute respiratory problems.
- Underlying toxic or metabolic causes should be addressed and treated appropriately.

COMPLEMENTARY & ALTERNATIVE THERAPIES

- Physical therapy:
  - May help maintain maximum muscle function and reduce secondary deformities
  - Orthopedic consultation to evaluate hips and contractures should be obtained.

SURGERY/OTHER PROCEDURES

Surgical intervention in later childhood to correct primary as well as secondary deformities

IN-PATIENT CONSIDERATIONS
Admission Criteria

Respiratory insufficiency, feeding intolerance, failure to thrive, metabolic abnormality

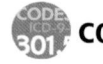 ONGOING CARE

FOLLOW-UP RECOMMENDATIONS

Individualized multidisciplinary care including specialists in neurology, pulmonary, orthopedics, development, physical therapy, and nutrition ensures optimal outcomes.

DIET

Feeding and swallowing difficulties may necessitate nutritional supplementation and/or feeding tube placement.

PROGNOSIS

Many of the paralytic hypotonias are quite variable in their clinical course. Severity of disease depends on underlying cause and associated respiratory and nutritional factors.

COMPLICATIONS

- Respiratory insufficiency/recurrent pneumonia
- Orthopedic deformities
- Poor nutritional status

ADDITIONAL READING

- Bodensteiner JB. The evaluation of the hypotonic infant. *Semin Pediatr Neurol.* 2008;15(1): 10–20.
- Harris SR. Congenital hypotonia: Clinical and developmental assessment. *Dev Med Child Neurol.* 2008;50:889–892.
- Johnston H. The floppy weak infant revisited. *Brain Dev.* 2003;25:155–158.
- Prasad A, Prasad C. The floppy infant: Contribution of genetic and metabolic disorders. *Brain Dev.* 2003;25:457–476.
- Riggs J, Bodensteiner J, Schochet S. Congenital myopathies/dystrophies. *Neurol Clin.* 2003;21: 779–794.

CODES

ICD9
- 358.8 Other specified myoneural disorders
- 779.89 Other specified conditions originating in the perinatal period

ICD10
P94.2 Congenital hypotonia

FAQ

- Q: By what age should one expect resolution of benign congenital hypotonia?
- A: Hypotonia typically resolves by the time the infant is walking, up to 18 months of age.
- Q: What clinical sign can help distinguish between SMA and infantile botulism?
- A: Tongue fasciculations are seen in SMA. Also, decreased pupillary light reflex is seen in botulism.

F

FOOD ALLERGY

Jackie P-D. Garrett
Terri Brown-Whitehorn
Stephen McGeady (5th edition)

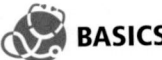 **BASICS**

DESCRIPTION

Food allergy has recently been defined as "an adverse health effect arising from a specific immune response that occurs reproducibly on exposure to a given food." Most commonly, the protein component of the food is responsible for the adverse immunologic response.

- Classifications of food allergies:
  - IgE-mediated, including:
    ○ Anaphylaxis
    ○ Acute urticaria
    ○ Oral allergy syndrome
  - Non-IgE-mediated (cell-mediated), including:
    ○ Food protein enterocolitis syndrome (FPIES)
    ○ Food protein-induced allergic proctocolitis
    ○ Celiac disease
  - Mixed IgE and non-IgE-mediated, including:
    ○ Atopic dermatitis
    ○ Eosinophilic gastroenteropathies (eosinophilic esophagitis, eosinophilic gastroenteritis)
- Most common IgE-mediated food allergies:
  - Children:
    ○ Milk
    ○ Egg
    ○ Soy
    ○ Peanut
    ○ Wheat
    ○ Fish
  - Adults:
    ○ Peanuts
    ○ Tree nuts
    ○ Fish
    ○ Shellfish

- Most common non-IgE-mediated food allergies associated with food protein enterocolitis and proctocolitis:
  - Milk
  - Soy
  - Wheat
  - Rice
  - Oat

EPIDEMIOLOGY

Food-induced anaphylaxis is the most common cause of anaphylactic reactions treated in emergency departments in the U.S. Many studies suggest that the prevalence of food allergy has increased over the past 10–20 years.

Prevalence

- 5–8% of children <3 years of age, 4% of teens and adults
- Nearly 2.5% of infants have hypersensitivity reactions to cow's milk during 1st year (thoughts are that 1/2 are GI diseases); outgrown by most (80%) by 5 years of age.
- 1.3% have egg allergy by 2.5 years (based on population-based studies); 66% of children outgrow egg allergy by 7 years of age.
- 0.6% of U.S. population have peanut allergy.
- 37% of children with moderate to severe atopic dermatitis have a food allergy.
- 34–49% of children with food allergy have asthma.
- 33–40% of children with food allergy have allergic rhinitis.
- Fatal and near-fatal reactions are associated with uncontrolled asthma.

RISK FACTORS

- Genetic
- Family history
- Presence of atopic dermatitis
- Other unknown factors suspected

ETIOLOGY

- Oral tolerance to food proteins believed to develop through T-cell anergy or induction of regulatory T cells. Food hypersensitivity develops when oral tolerance fails to develop or breaks down.
- IgE-mediated: T cells induce B cells to produce IgE antibodies that initially bind on the surface of mast cells and basophils; reexposure to the food protein binds to IgE antibodies, leading to degranulation of those cells, leading to release of histamine and other chemical mediators.
- Non–IgE-mediated (cell-mediated): T cells react to protein-inducing proinflammatory cytokines, leading to inflammatory cell infiltrates and increased vascular permeability. These factors lead to subacute and chronic responses primarily affecting the GI tract.
- Mixed IgE and non–IgE-mediated: Eosinophilic esophagitis and eosinophilic gastroenteropathy are characterized by eosinophilic infiltration of intestinal wall, occasionally reaching to serosa.

COMMONLY ASSOCIATED CONDITIONS

- Asthma (4-fold more likely)
- Allergic rhinitis (2.4-fold more likely)
- Other atopic diseases
- Dermatitis herpetiformis (celiac)

℞ DIAGNOSIS

Vary depending on the individual and the type of food hypersensitivity (see Table for symptoms of specific illnesses)

- IgE-mediated:
  - Urticaria
  - Angioedema
  - Immediate GI reactions (emesis, cramping, etc.)
  - Oral allergy syndrome
  - Rhinitis
  - Anaphylaxis (hypotension, dyspnea, dysphonia, wheezing, coughing, angioedema)
  - Nausea, abdominal pain, colic vomiting develop within 2 hours of ingesting offending foods
  - Diarrhea: Develops within 2–6 hours
- Mixed IgE- and non–IgE (cell-mediated):
  - Eosinophilic gastroenteropathy:
    ○ Weight loss (key feature), pain, emesis, failure to thrive (FTT), anorexia
    ○ Some infants have large protein-losing enteropathy component causing low serum albumin and hypogammaglobulinemia.
  - Eosinophilic esophagitis:
    ○ Dysphagia
    ○ Food impaction
    ○ Intermittent vomiting
    ○ Food refusal
    ○ Abdominal pain
    ○ Irritability
    ○ Failure to respond to reflux medication
    ○ Failure to thrive
    ○ Gastroesophageal reflux

- Non–IgE-mediated:
  - Food protein enterocolitis:
    ○ Severe vomiting 2 hours after ingestion; profuse diarrhea
    ○ Shock due to fluid/electrolyte loss
    ○ Very ill appearing
  - Food protein proctocolitis:
    ○ Blood in stool
  - Food protein-induced enteropathy:
    ○ Diarrhea, bloating, FTT, anemia

PHYSICAL EXAM

- IgE mediated:
  - Hives/angioedema (in 12% of patients with anaphylaxis, there are no skin findings and often these are most severe cases)
  - Wheezing/dyspnea
  - Hypotension/tachycardia
  - Vomiting, abdominal tenderness
  - Ill-appearing
- Mixed IgE-mediated, non–IgE-mediated:
  - Eosinophilic esophagitis: Abdominal tenderness (variable), growth concerns (in some)
  - Eosinophilic gastroenteropathy:
    ○ Abdominal tenderness
    ○ Weight loss
- Cell mediated:
  - Food protein–induced enterocolitis
    ○ Abdominal distension
    ○ FTT
    ○ Severe dehydration (may present in shock)
  - Celiac disease:
    ○ Abdominal distension
    ○ FTT

DIAGNOSTIC TESTS & INTERPRETATION
Lab
Initial lab tests
Depends on clinical presentation and patient symptoms; may include:

- CBC with differential:
  - Anemia in patients with enteropathy
  - Eosinophilia not consistently seen in patients with eosinophilic esophagitis, eosinophilic gastroenteritis, or enteropathy
- Serum IgE: May be elevated in:
  - IgE-mediated hypersensitivities
  - Eosinophilic esophagitis, eosinophilic gastroenteritis
- Albumin: Low with:
  - Protein-losing enteropathies
  - Non-IgE-mediated protein enterocolitis
  - Eosinophilic gastroenteritis
- Tryptase: May be elevated in anaphylaxis; obtain within 4 hours of initial reaction:
  - ImmunoCAP assay may be helpful in IgE-mediated illness
  - ImmunoCAP has many false-positives (do not send food allergy panels)

Diagnostic Procedures/Other
- Skin prick testing:
  - Used in conjunction with clinical history for IgE-mediated food allergies
  - 50% positive predictive value; 95% negative predictive value
  - Performed upon evaluation of patients with eosinophilic esophagitis
- Food challenges:
  - Gold standard for diagnosis of food allergy is double-blind placebo-controlled challenge but impractical in many clinical settings.
  - Most sites use single-blind or open food challenge.
  - Used to confirm food allergy in patients when unsure of diagnosis or to assess whether someone has outgrown food allergy (either IgE-mediated or food protein–induced enterocolitis)
  - Challenge must be performed in setting equipped to treat severe allergic reactions

F

- Endoscopy with biopsies of esophagus, stomach, and small bowel:
  – Patients should be on proton pump inhibitor prior to endoscopy if there are concerns of eosinophilic esophagitis as GERD may also lead to eosinophils in esophagus.
- Colonoscopy:
  – If lower GI symptoms present
- Patch skin testing:
  – May be used to evaluate for mixed (IgE/non–IgE-mediated) or cell-mediated sensitivities
  – Standards for interpretation and methods for reliability are under development.
- Elimination diets:
  – Should be conducted with care
  – May lack critical nutrients
  – Oral rechallenge should be carefully planned, because a more severe reaction may ensue after a food has been temporarily removed.

Pathological Findings
- Increased eosinophils in eosinophilic gastroenteropathy
- Presence of intraepithelial lymphocytes and variable villous damage in celiac disease

 TREATMENT

MEDICATION (DRUGS)
First Line
- Anaphylaxis:
  – Epinephrine for severe allergic reaction or anaphylaxis
  – H$_1$-antihistamines (diphenhydramine) may be given for milder symptoms.
  – H$_2$ antihistamines may be given in conjunction with H$_1$ antihistamines.
  – Systemic steroids
- Eosinophilic gastroenteritis:
  – Systemic steroids (briefly)
  – Swallowed steroids
  – Elemental formulas
  – Dietary restrictions

ADDITIONAL TREATMENT
General Measures
- Avoidance of food allergen
- Anaphylaxis:
  – Full monitoring of vital signs
  – Epinephrine for severe allergic reaction or anaphylaxis given intramuscularly: May be repeated
  – IV fluid bolus
  – Antihistamines may be given for hives or mild skin swelling.
  – Antihistamines (H$_1$ and H$_2$ blocker) and bronchodilators may be used as adjunct to epinephrine for severe reactions.
  – Glucocorticoids may prevent biphasic reaction.
- Nonanaphylactic food allergies: Eosinophilic esophagitis
- Systemic steroids for a brief course, swallowed steroids (NPO for 30 minutes after use)
- Hydrolyzed or elemental formulas: Patients may respond to hypoallergenic formulas.

ISSUES FOR REFERRAL
Allergy/Immunology and/or gastroenterology follow-up needed for most patients for diagnosis and long-term management

 ONGOING CARE

DIET
Nonanaphylactic and anaphylactic food allergies: Removal of the offending food agent from diet

PATIENT EDUCATION
- Epinephrine self-administration if anaphylaxis
- Anaphylaxis plan for families to know which medication to use when, along with education regarding emergency room avoidance
- Education regarding specific food avoidance and label reading

PROGNOSIS
- Generally good, after offending food antigens are removed from diet and adequate nutrients are ensured
- Tolerance to food allergens may develop over time.
- IgE-mediated disease may persist longer than non–IgE-mediated.
- Eosinophilic esophagitis and eosinophilic gastroenteritis are considered chronic illnesses.

COMPLICATIONS
- Food-protein allergy can be associated with:
  – Poor growth
  – Feeding disorder
  – Protein-losing enteropathy
  – Anemia
- Eosinophilic esophagitis:
  – Strictures
  – Hiatal hernia concerns
  – Poor growth
  – Feeding disorder
- Respiratory food-hypersensitivity reactions:
  – Heiner syndrome: Rare food-induced pulmonary hemosiderosis

Food Allergy/Hypersensitivity

Illness	Classification	Symptoms	Diagnosis
IgE mediated	Anaphylaxis	Rapid onset; nausea, vomiting; abdominal pain; hives, coughing, wheezing, involvement of other organ systems—skin, respiratory system	History + mediated skin-prick or ImmunoCAP test; oral challenge only in monitored setting with emergency access and anaphylaxis therapy
IgE mediated	Oral allergy syndrome (children and adults); due to cross-reactivity between food protein and pollen	Mild pruritus; angioedema of lips and oropharynx; sense of tightness in throat; rare systemic symptoms	History + skin-prick tests; oral challenge positive with fresh foods and negative with cooked foods
IgE and cell mediated	Allergic eosinophilic gastroenteritis	Failure to thrive; weight loss, abdominal pain, irritability, early satiety, vomiting, protein-losing enteropathy, edema, ascites	History + skin prick, endoscopy and colonoscopy with biopsy; elimination diet; monitor closely, may need immunosuppressants
IgE and cell mediated	Eosinophilic esophagitis	GERD with failure to respond to proton pump inhibitor; vomiting; FTT, dysphagia, intermittent abdominal pain; irritability	History, endoscopy with biopsy, elimination diet based on testing or history, elemental diet or swallowed steroids
Cell mediated	Allergic proctocolitis "breast-milk colitis" (infants)	Bloody stool, melena in first few months of life; no diarrhea or failure to thrive	Elimination of food (cow's milk or soy most commonly) clears bleeding in 72 hours; reexposure causes recurrence; RAST/skin prick not helpful; typically outgrown by 12–18 months of age
Cell mediated	Food protein induced enterocolitis syndrome (FPIES)	Severe symptoms; vomiting 2 hours after meal, severe vomiting; 6–8 hours later, diarrhea +/? blood, abdominal distention, failure to thrive dehydration, hypotension	Elimination of protein clears symptoms in 1–3 days ImmunoCAP/skin prick NOT helpful; patch testing may be helpful
Cell-mediated	Food protein enteropathy (infants)	Diarrhea, steatorrhea, abdominal distention, flatulence, failure to thrive or weight loss, nausea/vomiting oral ulcers	Endoscopy with biopsy; elimination diet resolves symptoms. Similar symptoms to celiac, but resolves by 2 years of age.
Celiac disease (infants to adults)	Diarrhea, steatorrhea, failure to thrive, abdominal distention, flatulence, weight loss, nausea/vomiting, oral ulcers	Endoscopic biopsy when patient is on gluten; gluten-free diet resolves symptoms. Anti-gliadin and TTG antibodies; HLA-DQ2 & DQ8 are often found.	

ADDITIONAL READING

- Bock SA. Pediatric food allergy: Diagnostic evaluation. *Pediatrics.* 2003;111:1638–1644.
- Burks W. Pediatric food allergy: Skin manifestations of food allergy. *Pediatrics.* 2003;111:1617–1624.
- Cianferoni A, Spergel JM. Food allergy: Review, classification and diagnosis. *Allergol Int.* 2009;58(4):457–466.
- Guidelines for the Diagnosis and Management of Food Allergy in the United States: Report of the NIAID-Sponsored Expert Panel. *J Allergy Clin Immunol.* 2010;126(6):S1–S58.
- John MJ. Pediatric food allergy: Respiratory manifestations of food allergy. *Pediatrics.* 2003;111:1625–1630.
- Sampson HA. Update on food allergy. *J Allergy Clin Immunol.* 2004;113:805–819.
- Sicherer SH, Sampson HA. Food allergy: Recent advances in pathophysiology and treatment. *Annual Rev Med.* 2009;60:261–277.

CODES

ICD9
- 530.13 Eosinophilic esophagitis
- 558.3 Allergic gastroenteritis and colitis
- 693.1 Dermatitis due to food taken internally

ICD10
- L27.2 Dermatitis due to ingested food
- T78.1XXA Other adverse food reactions, not elsewhere classified, initial encounter
- Z91.018 Allergy to other foods

FAQ

- Q: What are the most common food allergens leading to IgE mediated allergic reactions in childhood?
- A: The most common allergens to which children are sensitive are milk, egg, soy, wheat, fish, peanuts, and nuts.
- Q: Do you recommend elimination diets?
- A: Elimination diets are recommended when necessary to treat underlying disease. Nutrition evaluation is often necessary to avoid nutrient-deficient diets and malnutrition. They are used only in extreme circumstances because they can result in nutrient-deficient diets and malnutrition without identifying the offending allergen. Double-blinded food challenges are a better method for identifying the offending agent.

F

FOOD POISONING OR FOODBORNE ILLNESS

Christina B. Bales

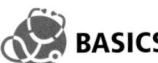 **BASICS**

DESCRIPTION
Any illness resulting from the ingestion of food or drink contaminated with an infectious organism or associated toxin

GENERAL PREVENTION
- Vaccination:
  - Oral rotavirus vaccine
  - Inactivated hepatitis A vaccine
- Preventive strategies:
  - Hand washing
  - Proper food handling (adequate cooking and refrigeration)
  - Avoidance of unpasteurized dairy products and juices
  - Avoidance of raw or undercooked eggs, meat, and shellfish
  - Avoidance of honey in children <1 year old
  - Avoidance of well water, which may contain nitrates, in preparing infant formulas

EPIDEMIOLOGY
Incidence (US Annual Estimates)
- 48 million illnesses
- 128,000 hospitalizations
- 3,000 deaths

PATHOPHYSIOLOGY
- Bacteria (often causes secretory diarrhea):
  - Invades intestinal epithelium
  - Elaborates toxin into the GI tract
  - Elaborates toxin into food (preformed toxin is ingested)
- Virus (often causes osmotic diarrhea): Invasion analysis of intestinal epithelial cells, leaving predominantly immature cells with inadequate disaccharidase activity

ETIOLOGY
- Viruses including calciviruses (noro and astro)
- Bacteria and/or associated toxins. Most common (in descending order):
  - *Salmonella* (nontyphoid)
  - *Clostridium perfringens*
  - *Campylobacter*
  - *Staphylococcus aureus*
- Parasites

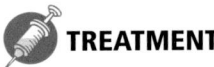 **DIAGNOSIS**

SIGN AND SYMPTOMS
- GI illness:
  - Nausea and vomiting
  - Diarrhea (watery vs. mucoid vs. bloody)
  - Abdominal pain or cramping
  - Constitutional symptoms (fever, malaise,)
  - Jaundice (may be present in hepatitis A)
- Botulism:
  - Impaired cranial nerve activity (sluggish or fixed pupils, ptosis, diminished corneal and oculovestibular reflexes, facial weakness, diminished gag, weak cry)
  - Constipation
  - Hypotonia with progressive symmetric descending paralysis
  - Absent deep tendon reflexes
  - Apnea

HISTORY
- Similarly exposed persons with related symptoms
- Timing of illness in relation to ingestion
- Duration of illness
- Type of food ingested

PHYSICAL EXAM
- Detailed neurologic examination
- Assessment of dehydration status (examination of mucous membranes, skin turgor)
- Assessment of potential liver involvement (hepatomegaly, jaundice, icterus)
- Careful abdominal examination

DIAGNOSTIC TESTS & INTERPRETATION
Lab
- Organism culture within:
  - Stool
  - Vomitus
  - Food (10^5 organisms/g)
  - Hand lesions of food handlers
  - Intestinal tissue
- Toxin identification in stool
- Serum antibody identification (e.g., HAV IgM in hepatitis A)
- Polymerase chain reaction (PCR) identification of viral RNA (e.g., norovirus) in stool or vomitus
- Virus identification via electron microscopy (e.g., norovirus)
- Latex agglutination tests (e.g., *Brucella*)

Diagnostic Procedures/Surgery
- Electrophysiology (botulism)
- Electroneurography (ENG): Normal
- Electromyography (EMG): Incremental response with repetitive stimulation

DIFFERENTIAL DIAGNOSIS
- Non-foodborne infection:
  - GI
  - Urinary tract
  - Upper respiratory (e.g., otitis media)
- Food intolerance or allergy:
  - Cow's milk (protein allergy)
  - Carbohydrate intolerance (e.g., lactose)
- Dietary manipulations:
  - Hyperosmolar formulas
  - Food additives (dyes, processing materials, coloring)
  - Caffeine
  - Overfeeding
  - Low fat intakes
  - Excessive fluids
- Miscellaneous:
  - Antibiotic induced
  - Malnutrition

TREATMENT

ADDITIONAL TREATMENT
General Measures
- Gastroenteritis:
  - Treat dehydration with oral rehydration solution (ORS):
    - Standard ORS contains 75–90 mEq of sodium and 74–111 mmol/L of glucose.
    - Alternative ORS, including rice-based carbohydrate or amylase-based solutions, may be more effective for *Vibrio cholerae* infections.
  - Transition rapidly (after 3–4 hours of ORS tolerance) to regular diet (see below).
  - Continue breastfeeding infants if possible.
- Botulism:
  - Continuous cardiac and respiratory monitoring
  - Endotracheal intubation and assisted ventilation in cases of respiratory insufficiency
  - Naso- or orogastric tube feeding

DIET
- BRATT diet (bananas, rice, apple sauce, toast, tea): Inappropriate due to low calorie, protein, and fat contents
- Balanced, varied diet, providing easily digestible, complex carbohydrates will promote improved stool consistency.

SPECIAL THERAPY
Botulism:
- Foodborne: Equine-derived immunoglobulin
- Infant: Human-derived immunoglobulin (BABY BIG) reduces hospital stay, duration of ventilation, duration of tube feeding, and cost.

IV Fluids
- If patient is unable to be rehydrated via oral route (because of ileus, circulatory failure, CNS complications) *or*
- If >10% dehydration

Complementary and Alternative Therapies

- Probiotics (especially lactobacillus) have been shown to reduce duration of less severe, nonrotavirus diarrhea and hospital stays.
- Zinc supplementation may be beneficial in malnourished children.

MEDICATION (DRUGS)

Use of antibiotics is:

- Always indicated:
  - *Shigella*
  - *Brucella*
  - *Listeria monocytogenes* (invasive disease)
  - *Salmonella typhi*
  - *Cyclospora cayetanensis*
  - *Trichinella*
  - *Entamoeba histolytica*
  - *Giardia lamblia*
- Sometimes indicated:
  - *Escherichia coli* (prolonged enterotoxigenic)
  - *Vibrio cholerae* (moderate to severe cases)
  - *Campylobacter* (Early treatment limits duration, prevents relapse, and shortens duration of shedding.)
  - Non-typhi *Salmonella* (Only patients who are <3 months old, are immunocompromised, have hemoglobinopathy, or have chronic GI conditions should be treated. Other patients should not be treated as antibiotics prolong organism shedding in the stool and promote disease spread.)
  - *Yersinia* pestis (sepsis)
  - *Toxoplasma gondii* (pregnant and immunocompromised patients)
  - Cryptosporidium (severe, <12 years of age)

  Contraindicated: *Clostridium* botulinum (aminoglycosides potentiate paralytic effects)

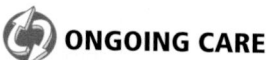

ONGOING CARE

PROGNOSIS

- Most gastroenteritis secondary to food poisoning is mild and self-limited.
- Recovery is complete in 2–5 days in most individuals.
- In the very young, prognosis is more guarded because these patients can become dehydrated quickly.
- After the patient has survived the paralytic phase of botulism, the outlook for complete recovery is excellent.

REPORTING REQUIREMENTS

- Foodborne diseases and conditions designated as notifiable at the national level include:
  - Notifiable bacterial foodborne diseases and conditions: Botulism, Brucellosis, Cholera, *Enterohemorrhagic E. Coli*, Hemolytic uremic syndrome, Listeriosis, Salmonellosis (other than *S. typhi*), Shigellosis, Typhoid fever (*S. typhi and S. paratyphi* infections).
  - Notifiable viral foodborne diseases and conditions: Hepatitis A.
  - Notifiable parasitic foodborne diseases and conditions: Cryptosporidiosis, Cyclosporiasis, Trichinellosis, Giardiasis.
- In the US, additional reporting requirements may be mandated by state and territorial laws and regulations. Details on specific state reporting requirements are available from state health departments and from the Council of State and Territorial Epidemiologists (http://www.cste.org/nndss/reportingrequirements.htm or phone 770-458-3811)

ADDITIONAL READING

- Centers for Disease Control and Prevention (CDC). Diagnosis and management of foodborne illnesses. *MMWR*. 2004;53(RR04):1–33.
- Davidson G, Barnes G, Bass D, et al. Infectious diarrhea in children: Working group report of the first world congress of pediatric gastroenterology, hepatology, and nutrition. *J Pediatr Gastroenterol Nutr*. 2002;25:143–150.
- Greer FR, Shannon M; American Academy of Pediatrics Committee on Nutrition; American Academy of Pediatrics Committee on Environmental Health. Infant methemoglobinemia: The role of dietary nitrate in food and water. *Pediatrics*. 2005;116(3):784–786.
- NASPGHAN Nutrition Committee report. Clinical efficacy of probiotics: Review of the evidence with a focus on children. *J Gastroenterol Hepatol Nutr*. 2006;43(43):550–557.
- Scallan E, Hoekstra RM, Angelo FJ et al. Foodborne illness acquired in the United States: Major pathogens. *Emerging Infect Dis*. 2011;17(1):1–15.

CODES

ICD9

- 003.9 Salmonella infection, unspecified
- 005.2 Food poisoning due to Clostridium perfringens (C. welchii)
- 005.9 Food poisoning, unspecified

ICD10

- A02.9 Salmonella infection, unspecified
- A05.2 Foodborne Clostridium perfringens intoxication
- T62.91XA Toxic effect of unsp noxious sub eaten as food, acc, init

FAQ

- Q: What are the most common causes of food poisoning?
- A: Viruses, particularly Norovirus, are the leading cause of forborne illnesses. The most common bacterial infections include *Salmonella*, *C. perfringens*, and *Campylobacter jejuni*.
- Q: How are the signs and symptoms of food poisoning different from those of a viral gastroenteritis?
- A: The signs and symptoms of food poisoning and gastroenteritis are similar in that the patient displays diarrhea, vomiting, and fever. Historically, food poisoning is distinguished by its association with a common food that affects multiple individuals who consumed it.
- Q: Which foods are most likely to be contaminated?
- A: Poorly cooked foods (eggs, meats, fish, shellfish), unpasteurized milk and juices, inadequately washed fresh produce, home canned goods, soft unpasteurized cheeses. Use of well water, which may be contaminated with nitrates, to prepare infant formula can result in infant methemoglobinemia

F

FRAGILE X SYNDROME

Chad R. Haldeman-Englert
Marni J. Falk

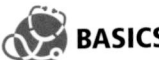 **BASICS**

DESCRIPTION
- Most common cause of inherited intellectual disability
- Caused by mutations in the *FMR1* gene on chromosome Xq27.3

EPIDEMIOLOGY
- Fragile X syndrome accounts for 1.2% of males with intellectual disability and 30% of X-linked intellectual disability cases
- Affects ~16–25/100,000 in males; prevalence in females is ~1/2 that in males.
- Carrier prevalence in females for *FMR1* premutation is 1:382 and for intermediate allele(s) is 1:143.

RISK FACTORS
Genetics
- Caused by loss-of-function mutations in the *FMR1* gene on chromosome Xp27.3
- >99% of affected individuals have a trinucleotide (CGG) repeat expansion (>200 repeats) within exon 1 of the *FMR1* gene
- Repeat size categories (based on guidelines from the American College of Medical Genetics):
  – Normal number of repeats: 5–44
  – Intermediate ("gray zone"): 45–54
  – Premutation: 55–200
  – Full mutation: >200
- Other *FMR1* gene mutations may rarely occur (<1% cases).
- Genetic counseling:
- Fragile X syndrome is inherited in an X-linked manner, but may not always follow typical inheritance patterns.
- Fragile X is a CGG trinucleotide repeat disorder that shows anticipation, in which the phenotype can be more severe in subsequent generations due to an expansion in the number of CGG repeats.
- Expansion only may occur in the germline of mothers who carry a premutation range repeat allele of *FMR1*.
  – Expansion does not always occur in offspring of female premutation carriers. In general, the larger the number of CGG repeats (>50), the higher the probability that expansion to a full mutation will occur.
- A male with a premutation will pass on the premutation to 100% of his daughters and none of his sons.
- Females with a full mutation are typically less severely affected than males because their 2nd *FMR1* allele is typically normal and, assuming random X-inactivation occurs, produces variable amounts of Fragile X mental retardation protein (FMRP).
- Males with mosaicism for the *FMR1* full mutation (some cells with the full-mutation and other cells with the premutation) are generally less severely affected (average IQ 60) relative to males with the full mutation in all of their cells.

- Males with the full mutation who have >50% of cells unmethylated have higher FMRP levels and are generally less severely affected (average IQ 88).
- Patients with larger chromosomal deletions involving *FMR1* and other nearby genes typically have a more severe phenotype.

GENERAL PREVENTION
- Prenatal diagnosis by chorionic villous sampling (~10–12 weeks' gestation) or amniocentesis (~16–20 weeks' gestation) is possible for at-risk pregnancies.
- Preimplantation genetic diagnosis in the setting of *in vitro* fertilization is possible for at-risk couples, but requires a familial *FMR1* mutation be known.

PATHOPHYSIOLOGY
Residual FMRP protein levels directly correlate with the severity of Fragile X syndrome manifestations:
- Absence of FMRP results in characteristic facial, neurologic, and connective tissue abnormalities.
- Decreased FMRP levels may also cause long-term depression of hippocampal synaptic transmission via specific glutamate receptors, with resulting behavioral and neuronal phenotypes.

COMMONLY ASSOCIATED CONDITIONS
Other *FMR1*-related disorders include Fragile X-associated tremor/ataxia syndrome (FXTAS) and premature ovarian failure (POF):
- FXTAS can be seen in older (>age 50 years) male and female premutation carriers. Clinical features include intention tremors, abnormal gait with frequent falling, cerebral atrophy, and memory deficits.
- POF can be seen in 20–25% of female premutation carriers, with menopause occurring prior to age 40.

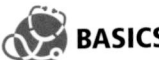 **DIAGNOSIS**

HISTORY
- Birth/Neonatal history:
  – Normal to increased birth weight
  – May have large head circumference at birth
  – Feeding problems and frequent emesis due to gastroesophageal reflux may occur, but improves with growth.
  – Irritability may result from sensory integration difficulties and tactile defensiveness.
- Past medical history:
  – Strabismus and hyperopia occur in 40%
  – Frequent ear infections in 60%: Conductive hearing loss is possible
  – Mitral valve prolapse and aortic root dilation can occur, typically in adults.
  – Seizures occur in ~20% of children and may resolve by adolescence.
  – Periventricular heterotopia seen on magnetic resonance imaging (MRI)
  – Pes planus
  – Scoliosis

- Developmental/Behavioral history:
  – Motor delay due to hypotonia
  – Speech may be absent to minimally affected.
  – Autism (60% of males with full mutation)
  – Intellectual disability
  – Severe intellectual disability in males (average IQ of males with the full mutation is 41, with range of 30–55)
  – Borderline or mild intellectual disability in 50% of females with the full mutation (IQ range 70–85)
  – Tantrums occur around age 2 years.
  – Hyperactivity can be severe during childhood.
  – Obsessive and compulsive behaviors also common
  – Often require a routine for daily activities
  – Social anxiety; patients are shy and easily overwhelmed by noisy environments
- Family history:
  – Fragile X syndrome
  – Intellectual disability or autism, especially in males related through the maternal side
  – Tremors or ataxia developing >50 years
  – Premature ovarian failure in females <40 years
  – No male–male transmission

PHYSICAL EXAM
- Growth parameters:
  – Height, weight, and head circumference
- Characteristic facial features:
  – Large head
  – Prominent forehead
  – Long face
  – Large and protruding ears
  – High palate
  – Prominent chin (after puberty)
- Murmur or midsystolic click (mitral valve prolapse)
- Large testicles (after puberty)
- Joint hypermobility, pes planus, scoliosis
- Skin often feels soft and smooth

DIAGNOSTIC TESTS & INTERPRETATION
Lab
Initial lab tests
- Consider *FMR1* mutation testing in:
  – Males or females with features of autism, developmental delays, or intellectual disability
  – Males or females with clinical findings consistent with Fragile X syndrome
  – Family history of Fragile X syndrome, recurrent intellectual disability or autism, especially through the maternal side
  – Males or females with tremor and/or ataxia developing >age 50
  – Females with premature ovarian failure <age 40
- Southern blot or PCR-based analyses are the first-line genetic tests to determine if there is a repeat expansion and define the number of CGG repeats within the *FMR1* gene.

Follow-Up & Special Considerations
- Methylation status can be determined by using a restriction enzyme that selectively cuts nonmethylated DNA or by methylation-sensitive PCR techniques. This study may be helpful in higher-functioning males who have a full mutation to establish their degree of *FMR1* methylation.

- Standard karyotype analysis will typically not be able to detect the repeat expansion.
- If the patient has many clinical features of Fragile X syndrome and the Southern blot is normal, consider further molecular techniques to detect point mutations or whole/partial *FMR1* gene deletions.

Diagnostic Procedures/Other
- Echocardiogram if cardiac exam is consistent with mitral valve prolapse (usually in adults)
- Aortic root dilation may be seen, but typically does not progress or require specific treatment.
- Evaluate for hypertension.
- Assess for seizure activity.
- Developmental evaluations
  - Feeding assessment in infants
  - Education planning:
    ○ Speech and language, including hearing assessment
    ○ Occupational and physical therapy
    ○ Behavioral and neuropsychological testing

DIFFERENTIAL DIAGNOSIS
- In early childhood, the symptoms of Fragile X syndrome are often nonspecific.
- Other genetic syndromes with overlapping features include:
  - Fragile XE syndrome (FRAXE): These patients have a milder degree of intellectual disability, as well as less specific physical characteristics compared to patients with typical Fragile X syndrome (FRAXA)
  - Mutations of the *FMR2* gene on chromosome Xq28 are associated with FRAXE
  - Sotos syndrome: Patients have overgrowth (macrocephaly), intellectual disability, behavioral abnormalities, and cardiac and renal defects. Mutations or deletions of the *NSD1* gene are causative of this syndrome.
  - Prader-Willi syndrome: A few patients with Fragile X syndrome have features that are similar to those in Prader-Willi syndrome, such as obesity and hyperphagia. Other features of Prader-Willi syndrome include hypotonia in infancy, developmental delay, cognitive deficits, and behavioral abnormalities. Abnormal parent-specific imprinting of chromosome 15q11-q13 causes this syndrome.
  - A range of other genes is now recognized to cause X-linked intellectual disability. Clinical diagnostic testing for many of these disorders is now available (www.genetests.org).

TREATMENT
MEDICATION (DRUGS)
- No specific medications are available.
- Some medications are used to treat specific symptoms in individual patients:
  - Stimulant medications (e.g., methylphenidate) or clonidine for hyperactivity
  - Selective serotonin reuptake inhibitors (e.g., fluoxetine) can be used for obsessive and compulsive behaviors, social phobia, anxiety, and depression.
  - Atypical psychotic medications (e.g., risperidone) if psychotic or paranoia symptoms
  - Valproic acid or carbamazepine for seizures or mood stabilization

ADDITIONAL TREATMENT
General Measures
- Treatment is aimed at supportive measures.
- Early developmental services:
  - Physical therapy
  - Occupational therapy
  - Speech and language therapy
  - Social integration therapy
  - Learning support classroom
- Some patients do well in a mainstream school with appropriate support, whereas others require a school for children with special needs.
- Behavioral therapies involve avoidance of overstimulation and providing positive reinforcement.

Additional Therapies
Experimental therapies:
- Fenobam, a glutamate receptor antagonist, was given to adults with Fragile X syndrome. The treated patients showed calmer behavior with reduced anxiety and hyperactivity.

SURGERY/OTHER PROCEDURES
- Myringotomy tubes if frequent ear infections and evidence of conductive hearing loss
- Inguinal hernia repair, if present
- Strabismus repair, if necessary
- Corrective lenses for refractive errors

ONGOING CARE
FOLLOW-UP RECOMMENDATIONS
Routine evaluation for strabismus, nystagmus, and ptosis. If abnormal, referral to an ophthalmologist is indicated.

Patient Monitoring
- Regular follow-up with a behavioral and developmental pediatrician, as well as a psychiatrist/psychologist is recommended for patients with significant behavioral abnormalities.
- Hypertension can occur in adults with Fragile X syndrome. Therefore, blood pressure and cardiac exam should be performed annually in these patients. Hypertension can be treated with typical medications used in the general population. If hypertension is refractory to treatment, evaluate for other causes of high blood pressure (e.g., renal).

DIET
No specific dietary requirements

PROGNOSIS
Most patients generally have a normal lifespan.

ADDITIONAL READING
- American Academy of Pediatrics. Health supervision for children with Fragile X syndrome. *Pediatrics.* 1996;98:297–300.
- Fragile X mental retardation syndrome. Online Mendelian inheritance in man. At: http://www.ncbi.nlm.nih.gov/omim/300624
- Fragile X syndrome. In: Firth HV, Hurst JA, Hall JG, eds. *Clinical genetics.* New York: Oxford; 2005: 324–326.
- Fragile X syndrome. In: Jones KL, ed. *Smith's recognizable patterns of human malformation.* Philadelphia: Elsevier; 2006:160–161.
- Hagerman RJ. Fragile X syndrome. In: Cassidy SB, Allanson JE, eds. *Management of genetic syndromes.* Hoboken, NJ: Wiley; 2005:251–253.
- Hagerman RJ, Berry-Kravis E, Kaufmann WE, et al. Advances in the treatment of fragile X syndrome. *Pediatrics.* 2009;123:378–390.
- Sherman S, Pletcher BA, Driscoll DA. Fragile X syndrome: Diagnostic and carrier testing. *Genet Med.* 2005;7:584–587.

See Also (Topic, Algorithm, Electronic Media Element)
- National Fragile X Foundation, www.fragilex.org
- FRAXA Research Foundation, www.fraxa.org

 ## CODES

ICD9
- 315.9 Unspecified delay in development
- 759.83 Fragile X syndrome

ICD10
- F89 Unspecified disorder of psychological development
- Q99.2 Fragile X chromosome

CLINICAL PEARLS
- Expansion of a CGG triplet repeat premutation *FMR1* allele can only occur in the offspring of female carriers. No expansion occurs in the germline of premutation carrying males, who will pass on the premutation size allele to each of their daughters and none of their sons.
- Fragile X syndrome cannot be diagnosed on routine karyotype. Specific genetic testing has to be requested to evaluate for this syndrome.

FAQ
- Q. Why is it called "Fragile X syndrome"?
- A. Early cytogenetic studies of male patients with intellectual disability identified a site on the X chromosome that would appear constricted when the patient's cells were grown with special culture techniques to induce "fragile" sites.
- Q. How many repeats are necessary to cause the full mutation that results in Fragile X syndrome?
- A. >200.
- Q. What are typical facial features seen in patients with Fragile X syndrome?
- A. Prominent forehead, long face, protruding ears, and a prominent chin.
- Q. When does the macroorchidism associated with Fragile X syndrome typically develop?
- A. After puberty.

F

FROSTBITE

Denise A. Salerno

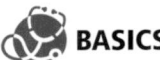 **BASICS**

DESCRIPTION
- Localized injury of epidermis and underlying tissue resulting from exposure to extreme cold or contact with extremely cold objects
- Distal extremities and unprotected areas (i.e., fingers, toes, ears, nose, and chin) most commonly affected
- Feet and hands account for 90% of frostbite injuries.
- Classified according to severity:
  - Superficial, 1st degree: Partial skin freezing
  - Superficial, 2nd degree: Full-thickness skin freezing
  - Deep, 3rd degree: Full-thickness skin and subcutaneous tissue freezing
  - Deep, 4th degree: Full-thickness skin, subcutaneous tissue, muscle, tendon, and bone freezing
- New classification of severity at day 0 has been proposed based on findings that correlate extent of frostbite with outcome of involved body part along with results of bone scans:
  - 1st degree: Leads to recovery
  - 2nd degree: Leads to soft-tissue amputation
  - 3rd degree: Leads to bone amputation
  - 4th degree: Leads to large amputation with systemic effects

RISK FACTORS
- Alcohol use
- Arthritis
- Atherosclerosis
- Constricting clothing
- Diabetes mellitus
- High altitude
- Hypothermia
- Immobilization
- Improper use of aerosol sprays
- Previous cold injury
- Smoking tobacco
- Trauma
- Vasoconstrictive drugs
- Body parts most affected:
  - Fingers
  - Toes
  - Nose
  - Cheeks
  - Ears
  - Male genitalia
- Groups at risk:
  - Mentally ill patients
  - Patients with impaired circulation
  - Winter sports enthusiasts and fans
  - Homeless persons
  - Very thin individuals
  - Malnourished people
  - Outdoor laborers
  - Military personnel, especially those of African American and Afro-Caribbean descent, exposed to cold, wet climates
  - Elderly people
  - Very young people

GENERAL PREVENTION
- Avoid prolonged cold exposure whenever possible.
- Maintain adequate nutrition and hydration when spending time in cold weather.
- Dress appropriately for cold weather:
  - Dress in layers: Clothing should be made of material that absorbs perspiration and prevents heat loss, and outerwear should be windproof and water repellent.
  - Cover head, ears, and neck.
  - Mittens help to conserve heat better than gloves do.
  - Footwear should be water-repellent and insulated.

PATHOPHYSIOLOGY
- Tissue damage and cell death result from initial freeze injury and inflammatory response that occurs with rewarming.
- Direct cellular damage can occur from frostbite. As temperature of freezing tissue approaches −2°C, extracellular ice crystals form and cause increased osmotic pressure in the interstitium, leading to cellular dehydration. As freezing continues, these shrinking, hyperosmolar cells die due to abnormal intracellular electrolyte concentrations. With rapid freezing, intracellular ice crystal formation occurs, resulting in immediate cell death.
- Indirect cellular damage results from progressive microvascular insult. Initial tissue response to extreme cold exposure is vasoconstriction. Blood flow to extremities is reduced as freezing continues. Ice crystals form in plasma, blood viscosity increases, and decreased circulation and formation of microthrombi occur in distal extremities, resulting in hypoxia, tissue damage, and ischemia.
- Oxygen free-radicals and inflammatory mediators, especially prostaglandin F2 and thromboxane A2, contribute to tissue injury following rewarming and reperfusion of damaged tissue.
- Most severe injuries are seen in tissues that freeze, thaw, and freeze again.

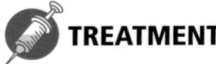 **DIAGNOSIS**

- Depends on severity
- Superficial, 1st degree: Transient tingling, stinging, and burning followed by throbbing and aching with possible hyperhidrosis (excess sweating)
- Superficial, 2nd degree: Numbness, with vasomotor disturbances in more severe cases
- Deep, 3rd degree: No sensation initially, followed by shooting pains, burning, throbbing, and aching
- Deep, 4th degree: Absence of sensation, presence of muscle function, pain, and joint discomfort

HISTORY
- Was there prolonged exposure to cold environment? In frostbite, history of prolonged cold exposure is typical.
- Was there contact with a cold object, especially metal? Metal will drain heat from skin through conduction and increase the risk of frostbite.
- What was the timing and duration of exposure?
- Was there any treatment prior to presentation?
- Does the patient have any underlying conditions or behaviors that put him or her at risk?
  - (Peripheral vascular disease, medications, smoking, etc.)

PHYSICAL EXAM
- Superficial, 1st degree: Waxy appearance, erythema, and edema of involved area without blister formation
- Superficial, 2nd degree:
  - Erythema, significant edema, blisters with clear fluid within 6–24 hours
  - Desquamation may occur with eschar formation 7–14 days after initial injury.

- Deep, 3rd degree: Hemorrhagic blisters, necrosis of skin and subcutaneous tissues, skin discoloration in 5–10 days
- Deep, 4th degree: Initially, little edema with cyanosis or mottling; eventually, complete necrosis, then becomes black, dry, and mummifies; occasionally results in self-amputation

DIAGNOSTIC TESTS & INTERPRETATION
Lab
Usually not necessary, but may be indicated when infection is suspected

Imaging
- No diagnostic studies done immediately after rewarming can accurately predict amount of nonviable tissue.
- Radionucleotide angiography with 99m-Tc-pertechnetate or triple-phase bone scanning with 99m-Tc-methylene diphosphonate 1–2 weeks after initial injury is advocated by some to assess tissue viability in cases of 3rd- and 4th-degree frostbite.
- MRI and MRA are being advocated by some as superior techniques for severe frostbite. They allow for direct visualization of occluded vessels and tissue, giving a more clear-cut demarcation of ischemic tissue injury, which may allow for earlier surgical intervention.

DIFFERENTIAL DIAGNOSIS
- Frostnip: Mild form of cold injury with pallor and painful, tingling sensation. Warming of cold tissue results in no tissue damage.
- Hypothermia
- Thermal injury: Easily excluded based on history, but can result from warming techniques.

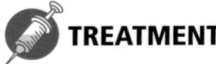 **TREATMENT**

MEDICATION (DRUGS)
- Tetanus prophylaxis: dT, dTap, or DT/DTaP, depending on age, and tetanus immunoglobulin if patient not fully immunized
- NSAIDs: Recommended by some to prevent prostaglandin-induced platelet aggregation and vasoconstriction
- Pentoxifylline (a phosphodiesterase inhibitor) should be considered with severe frostbite. It has been shown to enhance tissue viability by increasing blood flow and reducing platelet activity.
- Analgesics: As indicated
- Antibiotics: Given prophylactically by some; others recommend waiting for signs of infection or necrotic tissue.
- Tissue plasminogen activator (tPA) is being used by frostbite specialists within 24 hours of acute, severe frostbite. Studies have shown it can significantly reduce digital amputation rates.

ADDITIONAL TREATMENT
General Measures
- Check core temperature to rule out hypothermia, which would need to be addressed first.
- Rapid rewarming in warm water (40–42°C) for 15–45 minutes
  - Do not rewarm slowly.
  - Rewarming is complete when skin is soft and sensation returns.
  - Usually all that is needed for superficial, 1st-degree frostbite

- Apply dry, sterile dressings to affected areas and between frost-bitten toes and fingers.
- Intact nontense clear blisters should be left in place and wrapped with loosely applied dry gauze dressings. Rupturing may increase the risk of infection.
- Tense or hemorrhagic blister may be carefully aspirated but this increases the risk for infection
- Ruptured blisters should be debrided and covered with antibiotic ointment and nonadhesive dressings.
- Elevate affected parts to minimize edema.
- Daily hydrotherapy with hexachlorophene or povidone-iodine added to water
- Topical application of aloe vera (for its antiprostaglandin effect) to débrided blisters and intact hemorrhagic blisters, to minimize further thromboxane synthesis

ALERT
- Prohibit nicotine use because of its vasoconstrictive properties.
- Full extent of injury may not be apparent at presentation. Close observation is important

SURGERY/OTHER PROCEDURES
- Conservative surgical intervention: Recommended because it usually takes 6–8 weeks for injured tissue to declare viability
- Escharotomy: Performed on digits with impaired circulation or movement
- Fasciotomy: Performed if significant edema causes compartment syndrome
- Early amputation and debridement with closure of wound site: Necessary for uncontrolled infection
- Débridement of mummified tissue: Performed after 1–3 months

IN-PATIENT CONSIDERATIONS
Initial Stabilization
- Do not rub the area; may cause mechanical injury.
- Do not expose the area to direct heat; may cause burn injury.
- Refreezing after thawing leads to increased injury.
- Remove wet clothing and constricting jewelry.

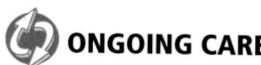 ONGOING CARE

PROGNOSIS
- Depends on degree of cold injury
- Superficial, 1st-degree frostbite heals in a few weeks.
- Favorable indicators: Sensation in affected area, healthy-looking skin color, blisters filled with clear fluid
- Unfavorable indicators: Cyanosis, blood-filled blisters, unhealthy-looking skin color

COMPLICATIONS
- Arthritis
- Changes in skin color
- Chronic numbness
- Chronic pain
- Cold hypersensitivity
- Digital deformities
- Gangrene
- Growth-plate abnormalities (only in children)
- Hyperesthesias
- Neuropathy
- Reduced sensitivity to touch
- Rhabdomyolysis
- Squamous cell carcinoma (rare)

- Tetanus
- Tissue loss
- Wound infection

ADDITIONAL READING

- Biem J, Koehncke N, Classen D, et al. Out of the cold: Management of hypothermia and frostbite. *Can Med Assoc J*. 2003;168:305–311.
- Hallam MJ, Cubison T, Dheansa B, et al. Managing frostbite. *BMJ*. 2010;341:1151–1156.
- Murphy J, Banwell PE, Roberts AH, et al. Frostbite: Pathogenesis and treatment. *J Trauma*. 2000;48:171–185.
- Simon TD, Soep JB, Hollister JR. Pernio in pediatrics. *Pediatrics*. 2005;116(3):e472–e475.
- Twomey JA, Peltier GL, Zera RT. An open-label study to evaluate the safety and efficacy of tissue plasminogen activator in treatment of frostbite. *J Trauma*. 2005;59:1350–1354.

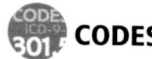 CODES

ICD9
- 991.0 Frostbite of face
- 991.1 Frostbite of hand
- 991.3 Frostbite of other and unspecified sites

ICD10
- T33.09XA Superficial frostbite of other part of head, initial encounter
- T33.529A Superficial frostbite of unspecified hand, initial encounter
- T33.90XA Superficial frostbite of unspecified sites, initial encounter

FAQ

- Q: What type of clothing can protect my child from getting frostbite?
- A: Dress your child in layers of clothes. Outer garments should be waterproof and windproof, and make sure your child is wearing a hat, scarf, and mittens. To protect their feet, they should wear thick socks and warm waterproof boots.
- Q: I've heard that your eyes can get frostbite. Is that true?
- A: Frozen corneas (the surface layer of the eye) have been reported in persons partaking in high wind-chill activities such as snowmobiling and skiing. Prevention is possible with the use of protective goggles/sunglasses.
- Q: My children's doctor recommended that we use sunscreen when we go skiing. Will the sunscreen help prevent frostbite?
- A: Although sunscreen is necessary to prevent getting sunburn that can occur from the sunlight's reflection off the snow, it will not decrease the risk for frostbite from the cold exposure.
- Q: I live in Buffalo, New York, where the winters are very cold and the wind-chill factor is often below zero. My children like playing outside, especially in the snow. How can I prevent them from getting frostbite?
- A: Because there is a risk of frostbite with a wind-chill factor of −25°C, try to encourage indoor play when the temperature dips this low. It is important to have the children come inside frequently to warm up, and for you to check for signs of cold injury.

- Q: My family members are avid skiers. While traveling in Europe last winter, I purchased a protective emollient that was sold there. Can protective emollients prevent frostbite if used on the face and exposed areas while skiing?
- A: No. Research has shown that the use of "protective" emollients and creams leads to a false sense of safety and leads to an increased risk of frostbite. This is thought to be due mostly to the failure to use more efficient protective measures when the emollients and creams are used.
- Q: If my child has had frostbite in the past, can she get it again?
- A: Yes. Children who have had a previous frostbite injury are at increased risk for repeat injury, especially in the location of previous damage. Appropriate clothing and limitation of cold exposure should be strictly enforced.
- Q: To prevent frostbite, is there a temperature below which I should not let my child go out to play?
- A: Although body tissue freezes more quickly at lower temperatures, the degree of damage from frostbite is related to the length of time tissue remains frozen. Therefore, the amount of time spent outside during cold weather should never be prolonged.
- Q: How can I tell if my child has frostbite or just cold fingers?
- A: Cold fingers are red and may be painful but do not become numb or white. Frostbitten fingers are painful, white, and waxy prior to rewarming and turn red with rewarming. The sequential development of digital blanching, occasional cyanosis, and erythema of the fingers or toes following cold exposure and subsequent rewarming is known as Raynaud phenomenon.
- Q: If I suspect frostbite in my child and we are outdoors without access to warm water, are there any options for treatment?
- A: If there is a delay in reaching shelter, you can start to thaw your child's body part by using your body as a warmer by placing the exposed body part under your armpit and keeping it there until further care can be initiated. Before starting the rewarming process you must be sure refreezing will not recur.
- Q: When should I call the doctor?
- A: The doctor should be called if, after rewarming, the skin is not soft and/or sensation does not return to normal. Call the doctor immediately if the skin is discolored and cold, blisters develop during rewarming, or there are signs of infection, such as the appearance of red streaks leading from the affected area, pus accumulation, or fever.
- Q: We are going on a winter vacation this year and expect to spend a lot of time outside skiing and sledding. What types of clothing should I pack for my 6-year-old son?
- A: It would be a good idea to pack a few pairs of waterproof mittens, a ski suit or ski pants, waterproof boots, thick cotton socks, and cotton thermal under garments. Try to make sure your son stays dry and warm. Take frequent breaks indoors to warm up and check your child for any early signs of cold injury.
- Q: Is frostnip the same thing as frostbite?
- A: No. Frostnip is the mildest form of cold injury, which commonly occurs on exposed parts of the body, such as the fingers, nose, and ears. The symptoms of frostnip are numbness and pallor of the involved body parts. Warming of these areas is the only treatment that is needed, and there is no associated tissue damage.

F

FUNCTIONAL DIARRHEA OF INFANCY OR TODDLER'S DIARRHEA

Vered Yehezkely Schildkraut
Raanan Shamir

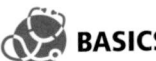

BASICS

DESCRIPTION
- Benign chronic diarrhea in a toddler or a preschool child who appears healthy and is normally active and growing without evidence of systemic illness, infection, malabsorption, or malnutrition.
- Also known as chronic nonspecific diarrhea of childhood, toddler's diarrhea, and irritable bowel of childhood

RISK FACTORS
Genetics
Family members often report nonspecific GI complaints or functional bowel disorders.

GENERAL PREVENTION
- Limit the consumption and delay the introduction of sorbitol or fructose-rich fruit juices to the infant diet.
- In the treatment of acute gastroenteritis, parents should be instructed to give an oral rehydration solution (ORS) and resume normal feeding early, avoiding diet restrictions.
- Avoid restrictive diets that may cause caloric deprivation.

PATHOPHYSIOLOGY
- Carbohydrate malabsorption:
  - Diarrhea is often preceded by acute gastroenteritis or other viral infection that results in dietary restrictions. Increased oral fluids, including juices, are used to compensate for stool losses and to prevent dehydration.
  - Capacity of the small intestine to absorb fructose is limited. Foods that contain equivalent amounts of fructose and glucose are more readily absorbed because of the additive effect of a glucose-dependent fructose co-transport mechanism. Excessive consumption of juices high in sorbitol (which inhibits fructose absorption) and those with a high fructose/glucose ratio (e.g., apple juice) result in fructose malabsorption and increased intraluminal gas caused by fermentation. The end result is abdominal distension, excessive flatulence, and diarrhea.
  - Colonic function: Possibly, disruption of colonic ability to ferment unabsorbed carbohydrates into short-chain fatty acids (SCFA), which maintain colonic function and prevent colon-based diarrhea
- Disturbed motility: Short mouth-to-anus transit time
  - Persistence of immature bowel motility pattern. Failure of initiation of normal postprandial delayed gastric emptying.
  - Low-fat meals. Meals with high dietary fat delay gastric emptying.
  - Excess fluid intake. Infant's colon already operates in high efficiency (in children, higher volume of fluids reach the caecum). Excessive fluids can lead to diarrhea.
  - Low-fiber diet. Dietary fiber serves as a bulking agent.
  - Excessive fecal bile acids. Rapid transit resulting in excess conjugated bile salt entering the colon. Bacterial degradation produces unconjugated bile salts, which decrease net water absorption in the colon.

ETIOLOGY
- Nutritional factors: Excessive consumption of fruit juice; high-carbohydrate, low-fat, and low-fiber diet
- Disordered intestinal motility (i.e., variant of irritable bowel syndrome of infancy) with rapid transit

DIAGNOSIS

- The typical age is 12 to 36 months, but range is 6 months to 5 years.
- Diagnostic criteria (Rome III):
  - Daily, painless, recurrent passage of ≥3 large unformed stools
  - Symptoms that last >4 weeks
  - Onset of symptoms that begins between 6 and 36 months of age
  - Passage of stools that occurs during waking hours
  - There is no FTT if caloric intake is adequate:
    ○ There is no definite diagnostic test. The diagnosis is primarily clinical based on age of onset, the history, symptoms, clinical course, and limited number of laboratory tests. Usually, it is an evident condition and not a diagnosis of exclusion.

HISTORY
- Nutritional history is essential, with attention to the 4 Fs (fiber, fluid, fat, and fruit juices) and dietary changes.
- Diarrhea:
  - For a toddler, it may not be abnormal to have >3 soft and occasionally loose stools a day with visible food remnants.
  - Children typically have intermittent symptoms and are often diagnosed with recurrent viral gastroenteritis
- Stool characteristics:
  - Stools that smell foul and contain undigested food particles. Presence of blood or mucus suggests another diagnosis.
- Timing of diarrhea:
  - No stools passed at night, and typically the 1st stool of the day is large and has firmer consistency than those occurring later on in the day.
- Recent enteric infection:
  - Presence of other affected family members, history of travel, day care, and infectious contacts suggests infectious cause.
- Signs and symptoms:
  - Thorough history is required because all illnesses in the differential diagnosis are associated with morbidity if diagnosis is delayed.

PHYSICAL EXAM
- Normal: Children look healthy, eat well, and are growing normally according to serial plots on the growth chart.
- There are no signs of malnutrition or malabsorption. Weight might be influenced by the dietary measures.
- Fecal matter found on abdominal palpation should alert for constipation.

DIAGNOSTIC TESTS & INTERPRETATION
- The following tests would be helpful only if indicated by history and physical exam:
  - Cystic fibrosis: Sweat test, stool for pancreatic enzymes, and genetic testing
  - Celiac disease is common and warrants a high level of suspicion: Serology (antiendomysial antibodies, tissue transglutaminase antibodies with IgA serum levels)
  - CBC, iron studies, vitamin levels, serum albumin
  - Inflammatory markers
- Diarrhea as the sole symptom of malabsorption in a normally thriving child is rare.

Lab
- Stool tests and culture: Negative for white blood cells, blood, fat, and pathogens including ova, parasites, and *Giardia* antigen.
- Celiac serology: Negative
- CBC normal: No anemia
- Serum electrolytes normal: No dehydration

Imaging
Usually unnecessary: Plain abdominal radiograph could demonstrate colonic fecal retention.

Diagnostic Procedures/Other
- A trial of lactose and fruit juice–free diet done separately is practical and diagnostic.
- Breath hydrogen test has limited benefit and is inferior to a trial of milk avoidance.
- Small bowel biopsy is rarely indicated unless strong evidence suggests another cause (e.g., positive celiac serology).

DIFFERENTIAL DIAGNOSIS
- All causes of chronic diarrhea should be considered.
- Infection: Bacterial, viral*, and parasite (giardiasis*, cryptosporidiosis)
- Celiac disease*
- Malabsorption: Carbohydrate: Postinfectious secondary lactose intolerance*, sucrase-isomaltase deficiency
- Pancreatic: Cystic fibrosis*, Shwachman-Diamond syndrome, Johannson-Blizzard syndrome, chronic pancreatitis
- Bile acid disorders: Chronic cholestasis, terminal ileum disease, bacterial overgrowth*
- Immunologic: Cow's milk and soy protein intolerance*, food allergy*, immunodeficiency
- Miscellaneous: Antibiotic-associated diarrhea, laxatives, fecal retention constipation*, UTI, abetalipoproteinemia, inflammatory bowel disease, short-bowel syndrome, hormone-secreting tumors, Munchausen by proxy
- Common conditions that may cause diarrhea without FTT: Constipation, lactose intolerance, and persistent infective diarrhea
- Constipation-related diarrhea is frequently overlooked. Consider it if diarrhea alternates with hard stools.

---

* More common conditions to be considered

TREATMENT

MEDICATION (DRUGS)
- Medications are unwarranted for a condition primarily caused by food that does not hamper growth.
- Metronidazole may be beneficial for patients with undetected giardiasis
- Loperamide is effective in normalizing bowel patterns, but only for duration of therapy.

ADDITIONAL TREATMENT
General Measures
Daily diet and defecation diary may document a specific food responsible for loose stools.

Additional Therapies
Reassure parents that there is no underlying GI disease, infection, or inflammation.

ISSUES FOR REFERRAL
- Failure of response to diet
- Weight loss despite adequate intake
- Presence of other symptoms (e.g., anorexia, irritability, fever, vomiting)
- Fat, blood, and mucus in the stool

ONGOING CARE

FOLLOW-UP RECOMMENDATIONS
- Improvement with dietary changes confirms the diagnosis and reassures the parents.
- Follow-up phone call to parents within a few days of instituting diet. If no improvement within 2 weeks despite good compliance with dietary recommendations, then reconsider diagnosis; consider more diagnostic tests and referral to a specialist.

Patient Monitoring
- Follow growth parameters.
- Monitor symptoms indicating nonfunctional illness.

DIET
- The child's feeding pattern should be normalized according to the 4 Fs:
  - Overconsumption of *fruit juices* should be discouraged, especially those that contain sorbitol and a high fructose/glucose ratio (e.g., apple juice, pear nectar).
    - Cloudy apple juice or white grape juice may be safe as alternatives.
  - *Fiber intake* should be normalized by introduction of whole-grain bread and fruits.
  - Increase *dietary fat* to at least 35–40% of total energy intake. Substitution of low-fat milk with whole milk may be sufficient.
  - Restrict *fluid intake* to <90 mL/kg/d if history is significant for fluid consumption >150 mL/kg/d.
- Improvement occurs within a few days to a couple of weeks after initiating the above therapy.

PROGNOSIS
- Good
- Symptoms resolve by school age.
- Long-term benefit of low-carbohydrate diet: contributes to balanced nutrition and the prevention of obesity.

COMPLICATIONS
Although children tend not to suffer from the symptoms, parents are often worried and frustrated and require frequent reassurance.

ADDITIONAL READING

- Hoekstra JH. Toddler diarrhoea: More a nutritional disorder than a disease. *Arch Dis Child*. 1998;79: 2–5.
- Huffman S. Toddler's diarrhea. *J Pediatr Health Care*. 1999;13:32–33.
- Hyman PE, et al. Childhood functional GI disorders: Neonate/toddler. *Gastroenterology*. 2006;130: 1519–1526.
- Judd RH. Chronic nonspecific diarrhea. *Pediatr Rev*. 1996;17:379–384.
- Kneepkens CM, Hoekstra JH. Chronic nonspecific diarrhea of childhood: Pathophysiology and management. *Pediatr Clin North Am*. 1996;43: 375–390.
- Moukarzel AA, Lesicka H, Ament ME. Irritable bowel syndrome and nonspecific diarrhea in infancy and childhood: Relationship with juice carbohydrate malabsorption. *Clin Pediatr (Phila)*. 2002;41:145–150.
- Vernacchio L, Vezina RM, Mitchell AA, et al. Characteristics of persistent diarrhea in a community-based cohort of young US children. *J Pediatr Gastroenterol Nutr*. 2006;43:52–58.

 CODES

ICD9
- 564.5 Functional diarrhea
- 787.91 Diarrhea

ICD10
- K59.1 Functional diarrhea
- R19.7 Diarrhea, unspecified

FAQ
- Q: How do I know that my toddler's diarrhea is not serious?
- A: Growth is usually normal and your child looks and feels well. His activity and development seem unaffected by the diarrhea. The change of diet results in improvement
- Q: What are the components of a successful treatment plan?
- A: Attention to the 4 Fs in the diet: Decreased fruit juice intake, increased fat intake, decreased fluid, and increased fiber intake.
- Q: Are probiotics useful in the treatment of toddler's diarrhea?
- A: There is no adequate data to support such a recommendation but evidence is emerging that probiotics are effective in IBS associated with diarrhea and bloating.
- Q: When should care by a pediatric gastroenterologist be sought?
- A: If no response after 2 weeks of compliance with dietary therapy, if growth is delayed, or if other GI or systemic complaints are present, seek a pediatric gastroenterologist's care.
- Q: Did my child get diarrhea because he goes to child care or because he is not clean?
- A. No. Functional diarrhea is not caused by infection.

F

FUNGAL SKIN INFECTIONS (DERMATOPHYTE INFECTIONS, CANDIDIASIS, AND TINEA VERSICOLOR)

William R. Graessle

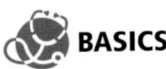 BASICS

DESCRIPTION
Superficial mycoses (fungal infection) involving skin, hair, or nails, usually characterized by scaling, erythema, and/or change in skin pigmentation

EPIDEMIOLOGY
- Dermatophyte infections:
  - Tinea capitis:
    ○ Most common in prepubertal and African American children
    ○ Peak age ~4 years
    ○ Incidence has increased over past decade.
  - Tinea corporis usually seen in younger children
  - Tinea cruris, tinea pedis, and onychomycosis uncommon in preadolescent children
- Candidiasis: Vast majority of infants colonized with *Candida albicans*
- Tinea versicolor (pityriasis versicolor): Usually seen in adolescents and young adults

GENERAL PREVENTION
- Children should be discouraged from sharing clothing, especially hats.
- Hair utensils and hats should be washed in hot, soapy water at onset of therapy.
- Pets should be watched and treated early for any suspicious lesions.
- Isolation of hospitalized patient is unnecessary.

PATHOPHYSIOLOGY
- Fungal elements penetrate skin, hair shaft, or nail.
- Predisposing factors may include moisture, macerated skin, and immunocompromise.
- Fungistatic fatty acids in sebum after puberty may offer protection against tinea capitis.
- Host immune response is usually able to contain infection.
- Inflammatory response is variable; highly inflammatory forms may lead to pustular lesions and kerion (large inflammatory mass) formation.

ETIOLOGY
- Varies by geographic region
- Dermatophyte infections:
  - Tinea capitis: >90% *Trichophyton tonsurans* in North America; *Microsporum canis* is a predominant organism in other geographic regions.
  - Nonhairy sites: *M. canis, T. tonsurans, T. rubrum, M. audouinii*
  - Fomites and pets may be a source of infection. Cats and dogs are major sources of *M. canis*.
- Candidiasis: Usually *Candida albicans*
- Tinea versicolor (pityriasis versicolor): *Malassezia furfur* (also called *Pityrosporum ovale*)

DIAGNOSIS

HISTORY
- Onset is usually gradual, except for candidal diaper rash, which is often abrupt.
- Usually pruritic
- Contacts, including exposure to pets
- Immunocompromised state
- Medications
- Signs and symptoms:
  - Dermatophyte infections:
    ○ Tinea capitis: May have various presentations ranging from round, distinct lesions to a diffusely dry scalp.
    ○ Tinea corporis: Lesions may occur anywhere on the body.
    ○ Onychomycosis: Patients present with thickened, discolored, and/or chipping nails.

PHYSICAL EXAM
- Dermatophyte infections:
  - Tinea capitis: May have various presentations:
    ○ Round to oval patches of alopecia with erythema
    ○ Diffusely dry scalp
    ○ Seborrheic dermatitis-like pattern with minimal or no alopecia
    ○ Follicular pustules with crusting, resembling bacterial folliculitis
    ○ Boggy, tender plaque with follicular pustules (kerion)
    ○ Presence of occipital lymphadenopathy may be more likely in tinea capitis.
  - Tinea corporis:
    ○ Skin lesions usually annular, hence the term ringworm; may be flesh-colored, erythematous, or violet to brown in color
    ○ Highly inflammatory forms may be frankly pustular.
    ○ Lesions may occur anywhere on the body.
  - Onychomycosis:
    ○ White, yellow, or silvery discoloration of lateral border or distal portion of nail
    ○ Nail eventually becomes discolored, thickened, and deformed.
    ○ Affects toenails more often than fingernails
- Candidiasis:
  - Diffuse erythema (often "beefy" red)
  - Raised edge with sharp margin
  - Pustulovesicular, satellite lesions
  - Prefers dark, warm, moist environments; favors skin folds/creases (axillae, groin, below breasts, and in infants, diaper area)
- Tinea versicolor (pityriasis versicolor):
  - Scaling, oval macular patches
  - Hypopigmented or hyperpigmented, depending on sunlight exposure and complexion
  - Distributed on upper trunk, neck, and proximal arms (high amount of sebum and free fatty acids, which organism requires); occasionally occurs on face

DIAGNOSTIC TESTS & INTERPRETATION
Lab
- KOH preparation:
  - Clean site with alcohol.
  - Scrape lesion along scaling edge with a scalpel blade; obtain material from hair follicles and crusts.
  - Place material on glass slide with 1 drop of 10% KOH.
  - Warm slide gently or let sit for 30 minutes.
  - Place cover slip on slide.
  - Examine slide under microscope at low power under low light. Look for:
    ○ Dermatophytes: Arthrospores around or within hair shaft; long, branching hyphae for skin infections
    ○ Candidiasis: Budding yeast, pseudohyphae
    ○ Tinea versicolor (pityriasis versicolor): Hyphae and spores ("spaghetti and meatballs")
- Fungal culture:
  - Obtain specimen with scalpel blade as described above or damp cotton swab for nonhairy sites.
  - For scalp, sample is obtained by rubbing toothbrush or cytology brush over dry scalp or area of concern; can be plated on appropriate media.
  - Results are available in several weeks.
  - Some laboratories provide drug susceptibility testing in addition to identification of fungus.
  - Distinguishing normal skin colonization from infection may be difficult.

Diagnostic Procedures/Other
Diagnosis usually made by characteristic lesions; if in doubt, may do:
- Potassium hydroxide (KOH) preparation
- Fungal culture
- Wood's lamp examination (short-wave ultraviolet light):
  - Examine in completely darkened room.
  - Dermatophytes: Hair infections caused by microsporum species will give a green fluorescence, but trichophyton does not fluoresce; not helpful for skin or nail infections.
  - Tinea versicolor: Yellow, coppery-orange, or bronze fluorescence

DIFFERENTIAL DIAGNOSIS
- Dermatophyte infections:
  - Dermatologic conditions:
    ○ Tinea capitis: Seborrheic dermatitis, psoriasis, alopecia areata, trichotillomania, folliculitis, impetigo, atopic dermatitis
    ○ Tinea corporis: Herald patch of pityriasis rosea, nummular eczema, psoriasis, contact dermatitis, tinea versicolor, granuloma annulare
  - Systemic diseases: Cutaneous T-cell lymphoma, histiocytosis, primary skin cancer, sarcoid
- Candidiasis:
  - Dermatologic conditions: Contact dermatitis, seborrheic dermatitis, atopic dermatitis, bacterial infection
  - Systemic diseases: Acrodermatitis enteropathica, histiocytosis
- Tinea versicolor (pityriasis versicolor): Dermatologic conditions: pityriasis alba, postinflammatory hypopigmentation, vitiligo, seborrheic dermatitis, pityriasis rosea

TREATMENT

MEDICATION (DRUGS)
First Line
- Dermatophyte infections:
  - Tinea capitis (requires systemic therapy):
    - Griseofulvin: 20–25 mg/kg once daily, taken with high-fat food (e.g., milk or ice cream) for 6–12 weeks. Side effects include vomiting, diarrhea, headache, hepatotoxicity, and photosensitivity. Concomitant therapy of 2.5% selenium sulfide or ketoconazole shampoo twice weekly will suppress viable spores and decrease spread. Laboratory monitoring is considered unnecessary.
  - Tinea capitis with kerion:
    - Treat as tinea capitis.
    - May require oral steroids if significant inflammation present alone
  - Tinea corporis:
    - Topical imidazole (1% clotrimazole, 2% ketoconazole) or 1% terbinafine cream applied twice daily for 2–4 weeks
  - Onychomycosis:
    - Terbinafine 3–6 mg/kg/d for 6–12 weeks. May be associated with hepatic failure; should not be used in patients with underlying liver disease. Strongly consider liver enzymes before and during treatment.
    - Itraconazole in weekly pulses for 3–4 months is effective; 200 mg twice daily for 7 days, then off for 3 weeks.
- Candidiasis: Topical nystatin cream or ointment 3–4 times daily for 7–10 days.
- Tinea versicolor (pityriasis versicolor):
- Selenium sulfide 2.5% applied to affected skin for 10 minutes. Wash off thoroughly. Apply daily for 7–10 days. Monthly applications may help prevent recurrences.

ALERT
- Topical steroids: Application will decrease inflammation and may mask infection ("tinea incognito").
- Systemic therapies are associated with elevated hepatic enzymes and hepatic failure.
- Possible interactions:
  - Many antifungals have drug interactions.
  - Consult a reference (e.g., *Physician's Desk Reference*) when prescribing them to a patient already on medication.

Second Line
- Dermatophyte infections:
  - Tinea capitis:
    - Itraconazole: 3–5 mg/kg once daily for 4–6 weeks. May also use terbinafine 3–6 mg/kg/d for 2–4 weeks or fluconazole 5 mg/kg/d for 4–6 weeks. All of these may be associated with hepatic failure and should not be used in patients with underlying liver disease. Liver enzymes before and during treatment are recommended.
  - Tinea corporis:
    - Oral griseofulvin 15–25 mg/kg/d for 4 weeks may be used for persistent or extensive involvement.

- Candidiasis:
  - Oral fluconazole:
    - 6 mg/kg on day 1, then 3 mg/kg/d for 2 weeks
    - May be used if poor response to topical therapy
- Tinea versicolor:
  - Topical imidazoles are effective but more expensive.
  - Oral ketoconazole 200–400 mg/d for 5–10 days, or itraconazole 200 mg/d for 5–7 days may be used if extensive, recurrent, or persistent.

 ## ONGOING CARE

FOLLOW-UP RECOMMENDATIONS
Patient Monitoring
- Watch for signs of secondary bacterial infection.
- Highly inflammatory lesions may require systemic steroids.
- Repeated infection may indicate a source that needs to be diagnosed and treated (e.g., family member or pet).

DIET
Griseofulvin is better absorbed with a fatty meal. It may be taken with foods such as milk, eggs, or ice cream.

PROGNOSIS
- Dermatophyte: Inflammation should improve within several days, but may take several weeks to resolve completely; nail infections may take 6–12 months to show improvement.
- Candidal skin lesions improve within 24–48 hours and resolve by 1 week.
- Tinea versicolor may take weeks to improve; repigmentation may take months and requires exposure to sunlight.
- Relapses and recurrences are not uncommon.
- Areas with significant inflammatory component may become scarred and permanently alopecic.

COMPLICATIONS
- Dermatophyte infections:
  - Secondary bacterial infection (which may obscure diagnosis of dermatophyte infection)
  - Kerion may lead to scarring alopecia.
- Candidiasis:
  - Scarring in severe disease
  - Fungemia in immunocompromised host

ADDITIONAL READING

- Elewski BE. Tinea capitis: A current perspective. *J Am Acad Dermatol*. 2000;42:1–20.
- González U, Seaton T, Bergus G, et al. Systemic antifungal therapy for tinea capitis in children. *Cochrane Database Syst Rev*. 2007;17:CD004685.
- Gupta AK, Cooper EA, Lynde CW. The efficacy and safety of terbinafine in children. *Dermatol Clin*. 2003;21:511–520.
- Gupta AK, Cooper EA, Montero-Gei F. The use of fluconazole to treat superficial fungal infections in children. *Dermatol Clin*. 2003;21:537–542.
- Shy R. Tinea corporis and tinea capitis. *Pediatr Rev*. 2007;28:164–174.

CODES

ICD9
- 110.9 Dermatophytosis of unspecified site
- 111.9 Dermatomycosis, unspecified
- 112.9 Candidiasis of unspecified site

ICD10
- B35.0 Tinea barbae and tinea capitis
- B37.9 Candidiasis, unspecified
- B49 Unspecified mycosis

FAQ

- Q: What is the role of topical and systemic steroids in the treatment of dermatophyte infections?
- A: Topical corticosteroids may be used in conjunction with antifungal therapy to reduce inflammation for fungal skin infections. Only mildly potent steroids should be used. Combination products containing a potent corticosteroid and an antifungal should be avoided, especially in the diaper area, where absorption may be increased. For tinea capitis, significant inflammation and kerion formation may benefit from a short course of systemic steroids. Reducing the inflammation with steroids may help prevent scarring alopecia.
- Q: What can be done to prevent recurrent tinea versicolor in an adolescent?
- A: *Malassezia furfur* is a ubiquitous organism and is present on the skin of postpubertal individuals. Humid environments, excessive sweating, and unclear genetic factors result in infection. Recurrences are common and can be prevented by monthly application of selenium sulfide 2.5%.
- Q: What is the role of the newer antifungal agents in the treatment of tinea capitis?
- A: Griseofulvin has long been considered the gold standard for the treatment of tinea capitis, because of its efficacy and safety profile. Development of resistance to griseofulvin has required the use of larger doses and longer courses, which increase the likelihood of noncompliance and treatment failures. In addition, longer courses increase the cost of griseofulvin therapy. The newer antifungals, terbinafine and itraconazole, offer some advantages over griseofulvin. Concentration of these drugs in nails and hair may allow for shorter courses of therapy, with improved compliance and lower cost than griseofulvin. Fluconazole has also been used for treatment of dermatophyte infections. It is available in a liquid formulation and is already FDA approved for treatment of candidal infections in children. Although still considered by many to be the preferred drug for tinea capitis, griseofulvin is likely to be replaced by these newer antifungals as experience with their use increases.

F

GASTRITIS

Janice A. Kelly

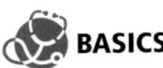 **BASICS**

DESCRIPTION
Microscopic inflammation of mucosa of stomach. Most common cause of upper GI tract hemorrhage in older children

EPIDEMIOLOGY
Prevalence
- 8 out of every 1,000 people
- >2% of ICU patients have heavy bleeding secondary to gastritis.

ETIOLOGY
- *Helicobacter pylori* (children more likely to have more severe gastritis, specifically located in antrum of stomach). Classified by WHO as a class I carcinogen in 1994.
- Physiologic stress (e.g., in CNS disease, overwhelming sepsis, ICU patients)
- Major surgery; severe burns; renal, liver, respiratory failure; severe trauma
- Idiopathic
- Caustic ingestions (e.g., lye, strong acids, pine oil)
- Celiac Disease: Lymphocytic gastritis
- Drug-induced (e.g., NSAIDs, steroids, valproate; more rarely, iron, calcium salts, potassium chloride, antibiotics)
- Ethanol
- Protein sensitivity (e.g., cow's milk-protein allergy), allergic enteropathy
- Eosinophilic gastroenteritis
- Crohn's Disease:
  - Up to 40% of Crohn patients have gastroduodenal involvement.
  - Gastric Crohn may manifest itself as highly focal, non- *H. pylori*, non-granulomatous gastritis.
- Infection (e.g., tuberculosis, *H. pylori*, cytomegalovirus, parasites)
- Less common causes:
  - Radiation
  - Hypertrophic gastritis (Ménétrier disease)
  - Autoimmune gastritis
  - Collagenous gastritis
  - Zollinger–Ellison syndrome
  - Vascular injury
- Direct trauma (nasogastric tubes)

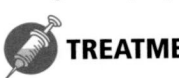 **DIAGNOSIS**

HISTORY
- Epigastric pain
- Abdominal indigestion
- Nausea
- Vomiting postprandially
- Vomiting blood or coffee ground-like material
- Diarrhea
- Dark or black stools (or bright red blood from rectum, if bleeding is brisk and intestinal transit time is short)
- Irritability
- Poor feeding and weight loss
- Less often: Chest pain, hematemesis, melena

PHYSICAL EXAM
- Epigastric tenderness is physical finding that most closely correlates with gastritis on endoscopy.
- Normal bowel sounds

DIAGNOSTIC TESTS & INTERPRETATION
Lab
- Heme-test all stools.
- CBC for anemia with other signs of chronic blood loss (e.g., microcytosis, low reticulocyte count)
- *H. pylori* identification:
  - Noninvasive *H. pylori* tests, including antibody (from serum, whole blood, saliva, or urine), antigen (from stool), or urea breath testing (UBT). UBT (using C_{13}) and stool antigen tests are more reliable and sensitive than antibody testing; serologic testing is not recommended. However, UBT is not widely available, and is used primarily in adults.
  - Rapid urease test from gastric biopsy specimen for *H. pylori*
  - Silver Warthin–Starry stain, Genta stain, modified Giemsa stain, or cresyl violet stain of gastric biopsy for *H. pylori*
  - Culture of homogenized gastric biopsy for *H. pylori* (difficult to perform outside of research setting)

Imaging
- Upper GI radiography when endoscopy not available
- Chest radiograph may detect free abdominal air secondary to perforation.

DIFFERENTIAL DIAGNOSIS
Of epigastric abdominal pain:
- Gastroesophageal reflux with esophagitis
- Peptic ulcer disease
- Biliary tract disorders
- Pancreatitis
- Inflammatory bowel disease
- Genitourinary pathology (renal stones, infection)
- Nonulcer dyspepsia
- Functional pain
- Allergic enteropathy

TREATMENT

MEDICATION (DRUGS)
- Proton pump inhibitors drug of choice as first-line therapy. Can also use antacids or H_2 blockers to maintain gastric pH >4–5:
  - Ranitidine: 2–3 mg/kg/dose b.i.d. to t.i.d. in children
  - Cimetidine: 10 mg/kg/dose q.i.d. (can be used prophylactically for hospitalized patients at risk for physiologic stress)
  - Famotidine: 0.5–2 mg/kg/d divided twice
  - Omeprazole, lansoprazole, rabeprazole, or esomeprazole: 1 mg/kg/d
- Misoprostol may reduce risk of progression of gastritis to ulcers in patients taking NSAIDs; concerns exist for increased cardiovascular events in adults when using misoprostol.
- Discontinue NSAIDs
- *H. pylori*:
  - Triple therapy with proton pump inhibitor and antibiotics, e.g., omeprazole, amoxicillin, and clarithromycin
  - If eradication unsuccessful, quadruple therapy is recommended for 7–14 days, including:
    - Bismuth (of note, may need to avoid bismuth subsalicylate and choose instead bismuth subcitrate)
    - Metronidazole
    - A proton pump inhibitor
    - Another antibiotic (either amoxicillin, clarithromycin, or tetracycline)
  - Drug regimens change frequently; clarithromycin resistance becoming increasingly problematic.

- Precautions:
  - Antacids are not palatable to children and can lead to diarrhea or constipation. Prolonged use of large doses of aluminum hydroxide-containing antacids may lead to phosphate depletion and aluminum-related CNS toxicity (particularly in patients with renal disease).
  - If *H. pylori* eradication is attempted, important to use a tested regimen. Untested substitutions in the triple or quadruple regimens should be avoided.
- Interactions: Ranitidine is less effective and can increase toxicity when given to patients receiving other medicines metabolized by cytochrome P-450 system (e.g., theophylline).

SURGERY/OTHER PROCEDURES

Upper endoscopy with biopsies:
- Sensitivity greatest
- Possible findings:
  - Edema around small ulcers
  - Thickened hyperemic mucosa
  - Atrophic mucosa
  - Antral micronodules (represent lymphoid follicles) commonly seen in children with *H. pylori* infection
  - Antral and prepyloric edema with retained gastric secretions

ONGOING CARE

FOLLOW-UP RECOMMENDATIONS
Patient Monitoring
- For stress gastritis with hemorrhage, provide vigilant supportive care with close monitoring of hemodynamics, fluids, and electrolytes.
- Monitor for hemoccult-positive stools
- Follow CBCs
- May elect to repeat endoscopy in severe cases

DIET
- Benefit of changes in diet is inconclusive.
- Eliminate alcohol, tobacco, and caffeine

PROGNOSIS
Significant gastritis relapse rates for children who remain infected with *H. pylori*

COMPLICATIONS
- Bleeding (from mild to hemorrhagic)
- When gastritis caused by acid/alkali ingestions, outlet obstruction may result from prepyloric strictures (4–8 weeks after ingestion)

ADDITIONAL READING

- Aannpreung P. Hematemesis in infants induced by cow's milk allergy. *Asian Pac J Allergy Immunol.* 2003;21(4):211–216.
- Drumm B, Koletzko S, Oderda G. *Helicobacter pylori* infection in children: A consensus statement. European Paediatric Task Force on Helicobacter pylori. *J Pediatr Gastroenterol Nutr.* 2000;30: 207–213.
- Hino B, Eliakim R, Levine A, et al. Comparison of invasive and non-invasive tests for diagnosis and monitoring of *Helicobacter Pylori* infection in children. *J Pediatr Gastroenterol Nutr.* 2004;39: 519–523.
- Pashankar DS, Bishop W, Mitros FA. Chemical gastropathy: A distinct histopathologic entity in children. *J Pediatr Gastroenterol Nutr.* 2002;35: 653–657.
- Vesoulis Z, Lozanski G, Ravichandran P, et al. Collagenous gastritis: A case report, morphologic evaluation, and review. *Mod Pathol.* 2000;13: 591–596.
- Weinstein WM. Emerging gastritides. *Curr Gastroenterol Rep.* 2001;3:523–527.
- Zheng P-Y, Jones NL. Recent advances in *Helicobacter pylori* infection in children: From the petri dish to the playground. *Can J Gastro.* 2003;17:448–454.
- Zimmermann AE, Walters JK, Katona BG, et al. A review of omeprazole use in the treatment of acid-related disorders in children. *Clin Ther.* 2001;23:660–679.

 CODES

ICD9
- 041.86 *Helicobacter pylori* [*H. pylori*]
- 535.50 Unspecified gastritis and gastroduodenitis, without mention of hemorrhage
- 535.51 Unspecified gastritis and gastroduodenitis, with hemorrhage

ICD10
- B96.81 Helicobacter pylori as the cause of diseases classd elswhr
- K29.70 Gastritis, unspecified, without bleeding
- K29.71 Gastritis, unspecified, with bleeding

FAQ

- Q: Will a bland diet help to resolve gastritis?
- A: Dietary changes have not been shown to affect the natural course of gastritis.
- Q: What is *Helicobacter pylori*?
- A: *H. pylori* is a bacterium frequently found in the gastric mucosa of patients with gastritis and peptic ulcer disease. It can be diagnosed by a variety of means, often including a combination of upper endoscopy and urea breath tests. Relapse rates for gastritis secondary to *H. pylori* are high when the infection is left untreated.
- Q: Is it appropriate to treat cases of gastritis, not proven by culture?
- A: No. It is important to treat only confirmed *H. pylori* infections, not to treat on suspicion of infection.
- Q: If a patient is treated for *H. pylori* and they still have symptoms and a positive stool *H. pylori* Ag, what would be the next course of action?
- A: Consider re-treating with a proton pump inhibitor, amoxicillin and flagyl, as clarithromycin resistance in *H. pylori* infection is an increasingly frequent cause for treatment failure.
- Q: What are newly recognized complications of treating patients with proton pump inhibitors?
- A: Some adult studies show hypomagnesemia, increased risk of pneumonia, hip fracture, and clostridium difficile infection are associated with proton pump inhibitor use.

G

GASTROESOPHAGEAL REFLUX

Jessica Hoseason
Yasemen Eroglu
Joel Friedlander

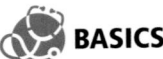 **BASICS**

DESCRIPTION

- Effortless regurgitation of gastric contents. Occurs physiologically at all ages, and most episodes are brief and asymptomatic. Important to identify the rare child with pathologic reflux, to perform appropriate diagnostic studies, and to start effective therapy.
- Divided into physiologic and pathologic processes:
  - Physiologic reflux (normal gastroesophageal reflux [GER] of infancy) is the more common form. Symptoms peak around 4 months of age in the majority of children. Most children outgrow their symptoms by 1 year of age. GER measured via pH probe is acceptable if it occurs ≤4–6% per 24 hours in children and adolescents and ≤11.6% per 24 hours in infants, if there are no more than 50 episodes in 24 hours, and if there are no prolonged episodes.
  - Pathologic reflux or gastroesophageal reflux disease (GERD) is defined by increased number of reflux episodes according to age-accepted norms with symptoms and/or complications of GER. Often includes complications such as esophagitis, bleeding, esophageal stricture, failure to thrive, or chronic/recurrent respiratory tract disease.

EPIDEMIOLOGY

Prevalence

- Pathologic GERD: 10% of adults, 2–8% of children, 7% of infants
- 80% of children with documented GERD at age 5 may have persistent symptoms as an adult.

RISK FACTORS

Neurologic disorders (cerebral palsy/quadriplegia), esophageal atresia, tracheoesophageal fistula, cystic fibrosis, asthma, gastroparesis, hiatal hernia

PATHOPHYSIOLOGY

Transient relaxation of the lower esophageal sphincter during episodes of increased abdominal pressure; multifactorial process involving number of reflux events, acidity, emptying, mucosal barriers, visceral hypersensitivity, and airway responsiveness.

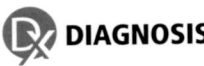 **DIAGNOSIS**

- Complicated GERD:
  - Vomiting
  - Irritability
  - Chest/abdominal pain
  - Heartburn
  - Hematemesis, melena
  - Blood loss
  - Dysphagia
  - Food refusal
  - Cough, wheezing
  - Obstructive apnea
  - Dysphonia
  - Aspiration pneumonia
  - Posturing (Sandifer syndrome)
- Other suspected complications include chronic or recurrent otitis media and sinusitis.
- GERD may be asymptomatic and still carry risk of complications.

HISTORY

- Infant:
  - Pay attention to feeding volume and frequency in addition to weight gain, failure to thrive, irritability.
  - Identify episodes of pneumonia, obstructive apnea, chronic cough, laryngitis, stridor, wheezing.
  - Identify additional signs/symptoms that suggest formula allergy (rash, diarrhea, hematochezia, irritability, failure to thrive).
  - Exclude evidence of bowel obstruction (emesis, polyhydramnios during pregnancy).
  - If vomiting is atypical or associated with other signs/symptoms, rule out infection, metabolic disease, anatomic abnormality, or neurologic disease.
  - Special questions:
    - Presence of polyhydramnios or bilious emesis?
    - Family history of metabolic disease?
    - Family history of allergies/atopy?
    - Perinatal asphyxia (and other neurologic disorders)?
    - History of prematurity?
- Older child:
  - Identify typical adult GERD complaints (chest pain, heartburn, regurgitation, dysphagia), but recognize that children describe discomfort poorly (isolated abdominal pain).
  - Identify episodes of pneumonia, choking, chronic cough, laryngitis, stridor, wheezing.
  - Consider evidence suggesting food allergy (rash, diarrhea, reactive airways disease).
  - Special questions:
    - Family history of GERD?
    - Family history of allergies/atopy?

PHYSICAL EXAM

- May be normal
- Growth failure
- Blood in stool
- Reactive airway disease and other manifestations of pulmonary complications
- Anemia
- Erosive dental (molar) disease
- Pharyngeal erythema/edema

DIAGNOSTIC TESTS & INTERPRETATION

Diagnosis of GERD is made clinically. Testing is only needed to identify questionable cases, potential causes, complications, or symptom-reflux correlations. Evaluation should include:

- Stool heme-occult
- Growth parameters

Imaging

- Barium swallow or upper GI series: Evaluate anatomy.
- Chest x-ray: Evaluate for recurrent pneumonia.
- Milk scan/gastric-emptying study: Evaluate gastric motility and/or pulmonary aspiration.
- Salivagram: Evaluate for aspiration.

Diagnostic Procedures/Other

- Medication trial
- pH probe:
  - Attempts to correlate acid GERD with symptoms over a 24-hour period
  - Simple (single-channel)
  - Double-channel
  - Combined pH/multichannel intraluminal impedance: New technology that allows detection of both acid and nonacid GERD events. Recent

studies suggest may be able to detect 45% additional pathologic refluxes than pH probe.
  - pH/thermistor (apnea) study
  - Wireless pH monitoring
- Esophagogastroduodenoscopy
- Laryngoscopy
- Bronchoscopy
- Manometric studies
- Esophageal manometry
- Antroduodenal manometry

Pathological Findings

Evidence of esophagitis, Barrett's esophagus, adenocarcinoma, stricture

DIFFERENTIAL DIAGNOSIS

Not all pediatric vomiting is reflux. Other causes of vomiting include:

- Cardiac: Congestive heart failure
- Toxin:
  - Lead
  - Fe
  - Medications
- Renal:
  - Obstructive uropathy
  - Uremia
- Infection:
  - Gastroenteritis
  - Urinary tract infection
  - Sepsis
  - Pneumonia
  - Hepatitis
  - Otitis media
  - Pancreatitis
  - Cholecystitis
- Neurologic:
  - Meningitis/Encephalitis: Intracranial injury
  - Brain tumor
  - Hydrocephalus
  - Subdural hematoma
- Metabolic:
  - Urea cycle defects
  - Aminoacidopathies (phenylketonuria, maple syrup urine disease)
  - Adrenal hyperplasia
  - Galactosemia, fructosemia
- Food intolerance:
  - Milk/Soy protein allergy
  - Eosinophilic esophagitis
  - Celiac disease
  - Hereditary fructose intolerance
- Anatomical malformation:
  - Diaphragmatic hernia
  - Gastric outlet obstruction
  - Esophageal atresia
  - Pyloric stenosis
  - Antral/Duodenal web
  - Volvulus/Malrotation
  - Meconium ileus
  - Enteral duplications
  - Intussusception
  - Trichobezoar
  - Foreign body
  - Incarcerated hernia
- Drugs that affect lower esophageal sphincter pressure:
  - Nitrates
  - Nicotine

- Narcotics
- Caffeine
- Theophylline
- Anticholinergic agents
- Estrogen
- Somatostatin
- Prostaglandins

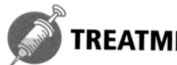 **TREATMENT**

Several modes of therapy are available, depending on severity, duration of reflux, and complications. Treatment should be individualized, and cost effectiveness should be considered.

MEDICATION (DRUGS)
First Line
H_2 blockers: For initial therapy of pain, esophagitis, or respiratory complications
- Ranitidine (Zantac):
  - 2–8 mg/kg/d split b.i.d. to t.i.d. *OR*
  - Adults 150 mg b.i.d. or 300 mg nightly
- Famotidine (Pepcid):
  - <3 months: 0.5 mg/kg daily
  - 3 months to 1 year: 0.5 mg/kg b.i.d.
  - 1–12 years: 1 mg/kg/d divided b.i.d. (max 80 mg/d)
  - 12 years–adults: 20 mg b.i.d.
- Side effects: Low incidence
- Medication interactions: Few

Second Line
- Proton pump inhibitors: For symptoms refractory to H_2 blockers or severe esophagitis:
  - Omeprazole (Prilosec):
    - <1 year: 1 mg/kg (daily or b.i.d.); studies demonstrate no clinical symptom (crying, irritability) improvement.
    - >1 year: 1 mg/kg (daily or b.i.d.) to adult dose range
    - >20 kg: 20–40 mg/d once daily or b.i.d.
    - Up to 3.5 mg/kg/d have been used
  - Lansoprazole (Prevacid):
    - <1 year: 0.4–1.8 mg/kg/d (daily or b.i.d.); studies demonstrate no clinical symptom (crying, irritability) improvement.
    - 1–11 years: <10 kg 7.5 mg/d
    - 10–30 kg: 15 mg/d or b.i.d.
    - >30 kg: 30 mg/d or b.i.d.
    - Up to 2.88 mg/kg/d have been used
  - Children often require a higher mg/kg. Side effects (uncommon) include headache, abdominal pain, and diarrhea.
  - Maximal effect not obtained until after 2 weeks of completed therapy
- Prokinetics: As adjunctive therapy for more severe GERD complications and hypomotility:
  - No single drug has optimal prokinetic effect and minimal side effects. There are many side effects associated with these medications, and they are not recommended as routine therapy.
  - Metoclopramide (Reglan):
    - 0.1 mg/kg q.i.d. 30 minutes before meals (0.3–0.8 mg/kg/d is acceptable)
    - Adults: 10–15 mg q.i.d. 30 minutes before meals
    - Side effects: May cause dystonia or oculogyric crisis
- Cisapride use has been withdrawn in the U.S., but a limited-access program is available for special situations.
- Calcium and aluminum/magnesium-containing antacids:
  - Require multiple dosing

- Side effects: Carry risk of diarrhea and aluminum toxicity
- Interactions: May lead to malabsorption of other medications
- Mucosal protective agents: Sucralfate (Carafate) for erosive esophagitis; maximally effective at pH 4 and on mucosal lesions

ADDITIONAL TREATMENT
General Measures
- Parental reassurance and education. Small, frequent feedings
- Thickening of feedings (~1 tablespoon cereal/ounce of formula): Helps with actual vomiting, not with stopping GER.
- Positioning: Prone positioning not recommended, keeping infant upright after feeds, head elevation in older children only (in infants, it increases GER)

SURGERY/OTHER PROCEDURES
- Fundoplication (open or laparoscopic)
  - To increase lower esophageal sphincter tone by wrapping portion of gastric fundus around lower esophagus to provide for a more effective barrier to GERD
  - Variations may include addition of a gastric emptying procedure (i.e., pyloroplasty) or gastrostomy placement.
  - Indications: Failure of aggressive medical management resulting in complications (i.e., esophageal stricture; high-grade intestinal metaplastic changes, as in Barrett esophagus), presence of large hiatal hernia, poor airway protection leading to aspiration of gastric contents (i.e., severe neurodevelopmental delay)
- Complications include:
  - Gas bloating syndrome
  - Intractable retching
  - Bowel obstruction
  - Dumping syndrome
  - Dysphagia
  - Paraesophageal hernia
  - Wrap failure with recurrent GERD (up to 6% failure at 48 months)
  - Limited long-term clinical effectiveness
- Greater morbidity associated with fundoplication in cohort of children with severe physical and mental disabilities

 ONGOING CARE

FOLLOW-UP RECOMMENDATIONS
Recurrent endoscopy for evidence of pathological changes of esophagus

DIET
- Consider use of hypoallergenic formula or eliminating milk/soy from mother's diet for patients with associated food allergy
- Dietary restrictions in older child: Caffeine, chocolate, acidic/spicy food, peppermint, but recent adult studies show this is on an individual basis only.

ADDITIONAL READING

- Colletti RB, Di Lorenzo C. Overview of pediatric gastroesophageal reflux disease and proton pump inhibitor therapy. *J Pediatr Gastroenterol Nutr.* 2003;37(Suppl 1):S7–S11.
- Craig WR, Hanlon-Dearman A, Sinclair C, et al. Metoclopramide, thickened feedings, and positioning for gastro-oesophageal reflux in children under two years. *Cochrane Database Syst Rev.* 2004;(4):CD003502.
- El-Serag HB, et al. Childhood GERD is a risk factor for GERD in adolescents and young adults. *Am J Gastroenterol.* 2004;99(5):806–812.
- Lobe TE. The current role of laparoscopic surgery for gastroesophageal reflux disease in infants and children. *Surg Endosc.* 2007;27:167–174.
- McGuirt WF Jr. Gastroesophageal reflux and the upper airway. *Pediatr Clin North Am.* 2003;50:487–502.
- Thakkar K, et al. Gastroesophageal reflux and asthma in children: A systematic review. *Pediatrics.* 2010;125(4):e925–e930.
- Vandenplas Y, et al. Pediatric gastroesophageal reflux clinical practice guidelines: Joint recommendations of the North American Society for Pediatric Gastroenterology, Hepatology, and Nutrition (NASPGHAN) and the European Society for Pediatric Gastroenterology, Hepatology, and Nutrition (ESPGHAN). *J Pediatr Gastroenterol Nutr.* 2009;49(4):498–547.

 CODES

ICD9
530.81 Esophageal reflux

ICD10
- K21.0 Gastro-esophageal reflux disease with esophagitis
- K21.9 Gastro-esophageal reflux disease without esophagitis

FAQ
- Q: How long will my baby suffer with GERD?
- A: Most infantile reflux resolves by 9–12 months of age, but symptoms may persist up to 24 months. If GERD continues after 2–3 years, it is more likely to behave clinically like adult GERD.
- Q: Should all babies with reflux be treated with medication?
- A: No. It is reasonable to 1st try conservative treatments such as thickened feedings and frequent small feedings.
- Q: Is there an association between asthma and GERD?
- A: The relationship between GERD and asthma is unclear based on recent studies and reviews.
- Q: What are the long-term effects of giving my child antacid medications?
- A: Although the effect of long-term acid suppression remains unknown, most medications used to treat GERD are quite safe. Although safe, some new adult research data suggest a possibility of osteoporosis and pneumonia after many years of treatment. Newer studies also demonstrate a very slight increased risk of *C. difficile* infection with their use. One must also recognize, however, that untreated reflux has the potential to lead to serious complications (Barrett esophagus, which can predispose patients to esophageal cancer). When considering safety, not treating reflux disease and esophagitis may be the more dangerous course of action.
- Q: Will the usage of PPI therapy stop my infant's crying and irritability from reflux?
- A: Recent studies demonstrate that although PPI therapy will decrease acid in the stomach and allow for mucosal healing of the esophagus, infants under 1 year had no significant change in the reported reflux symptoms of crying and irritability.

G

GERMAN MEASLES (THIRD DISEASE, RUBELLA)
Michael J. Smith

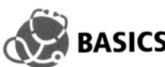 **BASICS**

DESCRIPTION
- *Rubella* derived from Latin, meaning "little red"
- Disease initially considered variant of measles
- Viral infection characterized by mild symptoms (often subclinical), with an erythematous rash progressing from head to toes
- Congenital rubella syndrome can be devastating.
- Rubella virus:
  - Classified as a Rubivirus in the Togaviridae family:
    - ○ RNA virus with single antigenic type
    - ○ 1st isolated in 1962 by Parkman and Weller

EPIDEMIOLOGY
- Spread person-to-person via airborne transmission; worldwide infection
- Infection most contagious when rash is erupting. However, virus may be shed beginning 7 days before rash to 14 days after
- Infants with congenital rubella syndrome may shed virus for up to 1 year

Incidence
- In temperate regions, peaks in late winter and early spring
- In prevaccine era, incidence of infection in U.S. was ~58 per 100,000 population
- From 2001–2004, nearly 1/2 of the 57 cases reported to the CDC occurred in persons born outside the U.S.
- 2004: No longer endemic in the U.S.
- Infection occurs equally in following age groups: <5 years, 5–19 years, and 20–39 years
- Congenital rubella syndrome:
  - 1964: 20,000 newborns
  - 1980s: Reported rarely, with <5 cases annually
  - 1990–1991: ~30 cases reported annually
  - 2001–2004: Total of 4 cases reported to CDC, only one with mother born in the U.S.

GENERAL PREVENTION
- Prevention of congenital rubella syndrome is main objective of vaccination programs
- Rubella vaccine:
  - Current strain of vaccine (RA 27/3, developed at the Wistar Institute in Philadelphia) was licensed in 1979 and has replaced all other strains
  - Given as part of MMR vaccine at 12–15 months and again at 4–6 years
  - Immunity occurs in 95% of vaccinees and is thought to be lifelong
  - Important to ensure full vaccination for preschool-aged children
  - Vaccine virus is not communicable: Pregnant women and persons who are immunodeficient (except asymptomatic HIV infection) should not receive vaccine, but household contacts should
- Isolation:
  - Pregnant women should avoid contact with source patient
  - Postnatal: Droplet precautions and/or school exclusion is indicated for 7 days after onset of rash
  - Congenital: Contact isolation until 1st birthday, or until 2 nasopharyngeal and urine cultures consecutively negative

PATHOPHYSIOLOGY
- Respiratory transmission
- Replication in nasopharynx and regional lymph nodes
- Viremia 5–7 days after exposure, with spread of virus throughout body
- In congenital rubella syndrome, transplacental infection of fetus occurs during viremia

ETIOLOGY
Rubella virus

COMMONLY ASSOCIATED CONDITIONS
Congenital rubella syndrome (see "Complications")

 DIAGNOSIS

If rubella is suspected, case should be reported to local public health authorities

HISTORY
- In children, prodrome is not often recognized
- In adults, a 1–5-day prodrome of low-grade fever, malaise, and cervical adenopathy may precede rash
- Inquire about immunizations and exposures

PHYSICAL EXAM
- Rash:
  - Begins on face, then progresses to trunk and extremities
  - Does not usually coalesce
  - Lasts for 3 days
- Adenopathies, especially postauricular, posterior cervical, and suboccipital, are commonly noted, along with conjunctivitis
- Arthralgia/arthritis may be seen in adolescents and adults

DIAGNOSTIC TESTS & INTERPRETATION
Lab
- Congenital infection:
  - Serologic testing should be performed on both mother and infant
  - Rubella-specific IgM in infant is highly suggestive
  - Viral isolation from throat or nasal specimen can confirm diagnosis. Blood, urine, and CSF samples may also be diagnostic
  - Diagnosis is difficult to verify after neonatal period
- Postnatally acquired:
  - Rubella-specific IgM or a ≥4-fold rise in rubella-specific IgG antibodies between acute and convalescent titers is diagnostic

worse the earlier in gestation

ffected if infection occurs in

ection occurs after 20th week
ongenital rubella

nmon defect
fects: Cataracts, glaucoma,

tent ductus, arteriosus,
efect, pulmonic stenosis,
a
  Mental retardation,

of congenital rubella
ellitus, progressive
be delayed for years

EADING

Pediatrics. Rubella. In:
 Long SS, et al., eds. *2009*
 e Committee on Infectious
 Grove Village, IL: American
 ; 2009:579–584.
 demiology and prevention of
 liseases, 2nd ed. Bethesda,
 ase Control and Prevention,

ontrol and Prevention.
 a and congenital rubella
 States, 1969–2004. *MMWR*
 ep. 2005;54:279–282.
 mphoid-nodular hyperplasia,
 and pervasive developmental
 . *Lancet.* 2010;375:445.

 CODES

ICD9
- 056.9 Rubella without mention of complication
- 771.0 Congenital rubella

ICD10
- B06.9 Rubella without complication
- P35.0 Congenital rubella syndrome

FAQ

- Q: While pregnancy is a contraindication to rubella vaccination, if a pregnant woman is inadvertently vaccinated, will there be harm to the fetus?
- A: Data collected since 1979 by the CDC show no evidence of congenital rubella syndrome in 321 susceptible women who were vaccinated while pregnant.
- Q: Is there any evidence that the MMR vaccine causes autism spectrum disorder?
- A: No. Multiple epidemiologic studies have shown no difference in the rates of autism spectrum disorder in children who received the MMR vaccine versus those who did not. The original paper that suggested a link between vaccines and autism was retracted in 2010.

G

GIARDIASIS

Lindsay Abenberg
Alan D. Baldridge (5th edition)

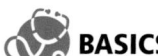 **BASICS**

DESCRIPTION
Infection of duodenum and jejunum with flagellated protozoan *Giardia lamblia*

EPIDEMIOLOGY
* Giardiasis has a worldwide distribution.
* Giardia lamblia is the most common intestinal parasite of humans identified in the U.S.
* Peaks at ages 1–9 years; 2nd peak at ages 35–44 years
* More common in summer and fall
* Water-dwelling mammals and household pets can become infected and may serve as reservoir of infection.

Incidence
U.S. average is 9.5 cases per 100,000.

Prevalence
* Direct person-to-person transmission accounts for the very high prevalence rates in institutions, daycare centers, and family contacts.
* High prevalence rates have been reported in patients with cystic fibrosis as well as Crohn disease.
* Waterborne transmission is an important source of endemic or epidemic spread, especially when water is supplied by surface source such as streams and reservoirs (outdoor recreation and international travel).
* Foodborne infection is uncommon and generally from uncooked or undercooked food or food contaminated after cooking by water source.

RISK FACTORS
* Daycare attendance
* International adoption
* Hypochlorhydria (previous gastric surgery)
* Hypogammaglobulinemia/immunodeficiency
* Blood group A
* Certain human leukocyte antigen alleles

GENERAL PREVENTION
* Maintenance of good sanitary conditions (strict handwashing and diaper disposal)
* Breastfeeding
* Family members and close contacts should be examined and treated if necessary.
* Examine water source in endemic areas.
* Boiling or iodine-based water treatment for camping and hiking

ETIOLOGY
* *G. lamblia:*
  – 2-form life cycle: Cyst (transmission) and trophozoite (infection):
    ○ Trophozoites adhere to duodenal mucosa with a ventral disk leading to mucosal damage and symptoms. Organism is noninvasive and does not lead to mucosal necrosis.
    ○ Cyst formation occurs in the colon and is passed into the environment. It can survive for a prolonged time if moist.
* Infection occurs after cyst ingestion from fecally contaminated water or by direct fecal–oral transmission in poor sanitary conditions; ingestion of between 10 and 100 cysts can produce infection.
* Anti-*Giardia* properties in breast milk may be related to free fatty acids cleaved from milk triglyceride by a bile salt-stimulated lipase present in human milk.
* *Giardia* also exhibits antigenic variation over the course of an infection.
* Mechanism of diarrhea is poorly understood but could include:
  – A glycoprotein located on the surface of *G. lamblia* trophozoites has been demonstrated to induce fluid accumulation in ligated ileal loops in rabbits.
  – Giardiasis results in decreased jejunal electrolyte, water, and 3-O-methyl-D-glucose absorption, thus leading to electrolyte, solute, and fluid malabsorption.
  – Damage to the intestinal brush border and the corresponding decrease in disaccharidase activity may lead to increased quantities of disaccharides in the intestinal lumen, which can result in osmotic diarrhea.
  – Giardia infection in gerbils accelerates intestinal transit time and increases smooth muscle contractility, both of which may play a role in giardial diarrhea.

 DIAGNOSIS

* Most (60%) infected individuals are asymptomatic.
* Common manifestations:
  – Sudden-onset watery, foul-smelling diarrhea without blood
  – Abdominal cramps
  – Bloating/flatulence
  – Anorexia
  – Dyspepsia
  – Nausea
  – Malaise
* Chronic course is associated with:
  – Weight loss
  – Loose, semiformed stool
  – Abdominal distention
  – Anorexia
  – Flatulence
  – Depression
* Malabsorption syndrome may include:
  – Steatorrhea
  – Secondary lactase deficiency
  – Deficiencies of iron, folic acid, vitamins A, B_{12}, and E
  – Protein-losing enteropathy

HISTORY
* Exposure to well water
* Habitation in endemic area
* Attendants of child care centers or inhabitants of institutions
* Asymptomatic infection can occur.
* Camping or hiking near fresh water
* Exposure to infected individual
* Immune function

PHYSICAL EXAM
* Abdominal distention
* Aphthous ulcers in oral mucosa
* Urticaria
* Arthralgia/Arthritis

DIAGNOSTIC TESTS & INTERPRETATION
Lab
Initial lab tests
- Identification of trophozoites or cysts in stool specimens, duodenal fluid, or small bowel tissue using staining methods
- Commercial ELISA test for detection of *G. lamblia* antigen in stool
- Empiric therapeutic trail of antiparasitic therapy in endemic area or populations
- If immunodeficiency is suspected, check immune function, especially IgA.

Diagnostic Procedures/Other
If strong suspicion of giardiasis, but 3 negative stool samples:
- Small intestinal aspirate sample may be obtained from duodenum.
- Duodenal biopsy specimen appears to be most sensitive.

Pathological Findings
Mucosal lesions vary from normal to subtotal villous atrophy, with crypt hyperplasia and proliferation of intraepithelial and lamina propria lymphocytes. Trophozoites may be seen on biopsies as an S-like curled shape on longitudinal sections.

DIFFERENTIAL DIAGNOSIS
- Celiac disease
- Cystic fibrosis
- Lactose intolerance
- Irritable bowel syndrome
- Inflammatory bowel disease
- Nonulcer dyspepsia

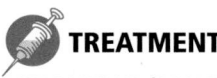 TREATMENT

MEDICATION (DRUGS)
- Metronidazole (not approved by FDA):
  – Most effective and best tolerated
  – Dose: 15 mg/kg/d divided t.i.d. for 5–7 days
- Tinidazole (approved for children ≥3 years)
  – 50 mg/kg to 2 g; single dose
  – Available in tablet form only
- Nitazoxanide (approved for ages 1–11 years)
- Furazolidone: Lower efficacy but better tolerated than metronidazole
- If therapy fails, a course can be repeated with the same drug.
- Asymptomatic giardiasis, in absence of risk factors, should not be treated.
- Treatment of patients with cystic fibrosis and household contacts of pregnant or immunocompromised persons may be considered.
- Repeat ova and parasite exam and antigen detection with recurrence of symptoms.
- May need to test for cure in patients with multiple organism infections

 ONGOING CARE

FOLLOW-UP RECOMMENDATIONS
Patient Monitoring
- Incubation period usually 1–4 weeks
- Reinfection common if source not eradicated
- If symptoms persist, with negative diagnostic studies, consider alternative etiology or another enteropathogen.

DIET
- High-fiber diet may aid in clearance.
- Low-lactose diet to prevent bloating and diarrhea for 1 month after treatment
- Probiotics may aid in prevention and clearance of infection.

PROGNOSIS
- Remains good for symptomatic patients
- Combination therapy with 2 medications has been successful when repeated courses of single drug have failed.

COMPLICATIONS
- Malabsorption syndrome
- Steatorrhea
- Lactose deficiency
- Deficiencies of iron, folic acid, and vitamins A, B_{12}, and E
- Protein-losing enteropathy
- Urticaria
- Arthralgia
- Growth retardation

ADDITIONAL READING
- Ali SA, Hill DR. Giardia intestinalis. *Curr Opin Infect Dis*. 2003;16:453–460.
- American Academy of Pediatrics (AAP). Giardia intestinalis infection (Giardiasis). *AAP Redbook*. 2009:303–305.
- Katz DE, Taylor DN. Parasitic infections of the gastrointestinal tract. *Gastroenterol Clin North Am*. 2001;30:797–815.

- Leitch GJ, et al. Dietary fiber and giardiasis: Dietary fiber reduces rate of intestinal infection by Giardia lamblia in the gerbil. *Am J Trop Med Hyg*. 1989; 41:512–520.
- Long KZ, et al. Impact of vitamin A on selected gastrointestinal pathogen infections and associated diarrheal episodes among children in Mexico City, Mexico. *J Infect Dis*. 2006;194(9):1217–1225. Epub 2006 Sep 26.
- Yoder JS, Harral C, Beach MJ. Giardiasis surveillance-United States, 2002–2006. *MMWR. Surveill Summ*. 2010;59(6):15–25.

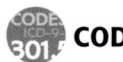 CODES

ICD9
007.1 Giardiasis

ICD10
A07.1 Giardiasis [lambliasis]

FAQ
- Q: Where is a likely place that *Giardia lamblia* occurs?
- A: Well water is a common place.
- Q: What do I do if I suspect *Giardia*, but the stool sample is negative?
- A: 3 samples are needed. If you are in an endemic area, you may choose to treat empirically.

G

GINGIVITIS
Daniel Walmsley

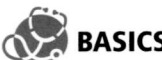 BASICS

DESCRIPTION
Gingivitis is a reversible dental plaque-induced inflammation of the gingival tissues. Symptoms may include bleeding, swelling, ulceration, and pain; although gingivitis is usually mild and asymptomatic.

EPIDEMIOLOGY
Incidence
- Affects >90% of children between the ages of 4 and 13 years. Most of these children have low-grade gingivitis.
- 13–40% of children aged 6–36 months have eruption gingivitis, which commonly resolves after teeth eruption.
- The prevalence of gingivitis increases with age; by puberty nearly 100% of all children are affected. This pubertal peak is likely due to hormonal influences and inconsistent dental hygiene.
- After puberty, the prevalence remains relatively constant at 50% of all adults.

RISK FACTORS
- Behavioral factors: Smoking, stress, alcohol consumption
- Medications: Antiepileptics, cyclosporine, calcium channel blockers
- Hormonal changes: Puberty, pregnancy
- Chronic illnesses: Diabetes mellitus, chronic renal failure, histiocytosis X, scleroderma, secondary hyperparathyroidism
- Immunologic deficiencies: HIV, Chediak–Higashi, cyclic neutropenia
- Neurologic problems: Cerebral palsy, mental retardation, seizures, and other conditions where routine dental care is difficult
- Miscellaneous: Chronic mouth breathing, malnutrition, viral illnesses

GENERAL PREVENTION
- Consistent daily oral hygiene described as the following by age:
  – Infants: Gum massage, washcloth to remove plaque; toothbrush using baby toothpaste (i.e., enzyme-based; no fluoride)
  – Young children: Assistance with brushing with a small amount of fluoridated toothpaste
  – School-aged children: Supervise brushing and assist if necessary
  – Older children and adolescents: Brush teeth twice a day with fluoridated toothpaste in addition to daily flossing. Some dentists recommended flossing as early as age 4 years.
  – Children with fixed orthodontics: Careful brushing and flossing is critical.

- Fluoride: Supplements are appropriate if the water supply is not fluoridated. It is important to be careful to treat with the appropriate amount of fluoride in order to prevent fluorosis.
- Sealants: Adherent plastic coating may be applied to the pits and fissures of the permanent teeth to provide a mechanical barrier.
- The AAP recommends that children at high risk for dental caries should establish routine dental care by their first birthday. Children should then continue routine dental checkups at a minimum of every 6 months.

ETIOLOGY
- Poor dental hygiene
- Bacterial plaque, calcified and noncalcified
- Caries
- Orthodontic appliances
- Malocclusion
- Crowded teeth
- Mouth breathing
- Erupting teeth margins
- Poor nutrition: Vitamin deficiencies (e.g., vitamin C deficiency), diet low in coarse detergent like foods (e.g., raw carrots, celery, apples), high prevalence of anaerobic microflora
- Infections: Herpes simplex virus (HSV) type I, *Candida albicans*, HIV, bacterial pathogens
- Drugs: Phenytoin, cyclosporine, nifedipine, oral contraceptive pills
- Trauma

 DIAGNOSIS

HISTORY
- Review the frequency of dental care visits and the home dental hygiene regimen.
- Review significant medical history, asking about chronic illnesses, bleeding disorders, and immunodeficiency.
- Review the diet of the child to assess for nutritional deficiencies.
- Dental appliances worn by patient:
  – Orthodontic equipment makes gingiva more difficult to clean, and reactive tissue growth is more common.
- Regular medications taken by patient:
  – Phenytoin may result in gingival hyperplasia, and chemotherapeutic agents, exogenous hormone therapy, and calcium channel blockers may result in gingivitis.
- Signs and symptoms:
  – Edema and erythema of the gingiva
  – Bleeding at gum line
  – Pain near the gingival margin

PHYSICAL EXAM
- Evaluate the gingival tissue for erythema, swelling, ulceration, fluctuance, or drainage. Erythema and edema are the most common findings in gingivitis.
- In severe cases, the gingival tissues may bleed spontaneously from ulcerations in the sulcus and there may be significant gingival hypertrophy.
- In herpetic gingivostomatitis, there is often significant ulceration and swelling of the gingiva associated with systemic symptoms such as fever, malaise.
- Evaluate the teeth for caries, fractures, looseness, malocclusion, pain, and plaque.
- Examine the face and neck for signs of swelling, erythema, warmth, or enlarged maxillary lymph nodes which may be signs of more extensive bacterial infection.
- Tanner staging: Normal pubertal changes seem to aggravate gingival inflammation so paying special attention to the gingiva of patients entering puberty is important.
- Assess the patient's oral hygiene technique in the office. This is the single largest contributor to gingivitis.

DIAGNOSTIC TESTS & INTERPRETATION
Lab
- Most patients will not need laboratory evaluation.
- If there is a concern for excessive bleeding, a CBC with differential, PT, PTT may be helpful to rule out thrombocytopenia, pancytopenia, or a clotting disorder.
- Blood culture: If there is concern for sepsis.
- Direct fluorescent antibody testing for HSV-1: If herpes is suspected (stomatitis is usually present), swab the base of a stoma/vesicle and smear on a slide. HSV culture is the gold standard.
- Biopsy is rarely necessary.

Imaging
Panoramic or individual tooth radiographic imaging is important to assess the bones for evidence of periodontal extension of the gingivitis in the more severe cases.

DIFFERENTIAL DIAGNOSIS
- Infectious:
  – Abscess
  – Herpetic gingivostomatitis—ulcerative lesions of the gingiva and mucous membranes of the mouth
- Traumatic:
  – Food impaction
  – Orthodontic appliances
  – Self-inflicted minor injury
- Hematologic:
  – Gingival bleeding due to hemophilia (factor VIII or IX deficiency)
  – Thrombocytopenia

- Immunologic:
  – Neutrophil disorders
  – Leukemia
  – HIV
  – Graft-versus-host disease (infiltrative gingivitis)
- Miscellaneous:
  – Gingival hyperplasia due to medications (i.e., phenytoin and nifedipine)
  – Periodontitis
  – Aphthous stomatitis
  – Vitamin C deficiency
  – Behçet's disease
  – Acute necrotizing ulcerative gingivitis (ANUG)—painful gingivitis associated with rapid onset and tissue ulceration and necrosis
    ○ Peaks in adolescence and young adulthood
    ○ Related to high oral concentrations of spirochetes and/or *Prevotella intermedia*

 TREATMENT

MEDICATION (DRUGS)
Mouth rinses for plaque inhibition can be used to augment daily oral care routine. The most commonly used rinses include 0.12% chlorhexidine and 0.075% or 0.1% cetylpyridinium chloride.

ADDITIONAL TREATMENT
General Measures
A daily oral care routine, including brushing and flossing, is essential to prevent gingivitis.
- Mild gingivitis:
  – Careful daily dental hygiene, including meticulous brushing and flossing
  – Mechanical plaque and calculus removal by scaling or root planing. This is then followed by frequent dental cleanings every 3–6 months to prevent recurrence.
- Moderate-to-severe gingivitis:
  – Care as outlined for mild gingivitis
  – Should be evaluated by a pedodontist in addition to a general dentist
  – Mouth rinses for plaque inhibition using either 0.12% chlorhexidine or 0.075% or 0.1% cetylpyridinium chloride
  – Irrigation devices
  – Sonic toothbrushes
  – Gingivectomies in cases of overgrowth to permit better cleaning
  – Antibiotics to cover mouth flora in more severe cases when bacterial superinfection is suspected

ISSUES FOR REFERRAL
- It is important for providers to evaluate the oral health of all children. When gingival inflammation is noted, the patient should be referred to a dentist.
- Routine dental care with professional cleaning and plaque removal is recommended for all children and adults.

- If the extent of involvement is great or the underlying disease of the patient requires more aggressive care, a periodontist should be consulted.
- The inability to resolve gingivitis by oral hygiene measures necessitates the consideration of other causes such as leukemia, vitamin C deficiency, or other chronic disease.

SURGERY/OTHER PROCEDURES
Only the most severe cases require gingivectomy.

 ONGOING CARE

FOLLOW-UP RECOMMENDATIONS
- Routine dental care with professional cleaning and plaque removal is recommended for all children and adults.
- Children with gingivitis should have frequent dental visits; most dentists recommend every 3 months.

Patient Monitoring
Routine dental exam and cleaning should be performed every 6 months to monitor for signs of inflammation.

DIET
- Avoid high sugar content food and beverages.
- Xylitol-containing chewing gum can improve oral hygiene by reducing plaque adherence to the gum line.

PATIENT EDUCATION
- Establish a daily mouth care routine.
- Brushing and flossing each morning and at bedtime will reduce plaque formation.
- Mouth rinses, if recommended by your dentist, can also reduce plaque formation.
- See the dental health professional every 6 months beginning at your child's first birthday for examination and cleaning.

PROGNOSIS
- Good oral hygiene may reverse mild-to-moderate gingivitis within several months.
- Periodontal disease is not reversible; therefore, prevention is essential.

COMPLICATIONS
- Periodontal disease
- Osteomyelitis
- Tooth decay

ADDITIONAL READING

- American Academy of Pediatric Dentistry. Guideline on periodicity of examination, preventive dental services, anticipatory guidance, and oral treatment for children. Available at: http://www.aapd.org/media/Policies_Guidelines/G_Periodicity.pdf
- Bacci C, Sivolella S, Pellegrini J, et al. A rare case of scurvy in an otherwise healthy child: Diagnosis through oral signs. *Pediatr Dent*. 2010;32(7):536–538.
- Califano JV, Research Science and Therapy Committee American Academy of Periodontology. Periodontal diseases of children and adolescents. *J Periodontol*. 2003;74(11):1696–1704.
- Kallio PJ. Health promotion and behavioral approaches in the prevention of periodontal disease in children and adolescents. *Periodontology*. 2001;26:135–145.
- Mankodi S, Bauroth K, Witt JJ, et al. A 6-month clinical trial to study the effects of a cetylpyridinium chloride mouth rinse on gingivitis and plaque. *Am J Dent*. 2005;18:9A–14A.

 CODES

ICD9
- 523.00 Acute gingivitis, plaque induced
- 523.10 Chronic gingivitis, plaque induced

ICD10
- K05.00 Acute gingivitis, plaque induced
- K05.5 Other periodontal diseases
- K05.10 Chronic gingivitis, plaque induced

FAQ

- Q: Are there differences among toothpastes and prevention of gingivitis?
- A: Yes. A study demonstrated that stabilized stannous fluoride toothpaste is effective in preventing gingivitis. When essential-oil mouthwashes (e.g., Listerine) are added, there is additional reduction in the amount of gingivitis noted.
- Q: What dietary changes may improve gingival health?
- A: Avoiding frequent carbohydrate intake may reduce gingivitis. Carbonated beverages, sugared chewing gum, and candy often adhere to teeth. When daily dental care is inconsistent, plaque formation is increased and gingivitis is much more likely.
- Q: Why do children generally not have the significant periodontal disease that adults get?
- A: No one knows for sure; however, it is known that the gingiva of the primary dentition is rounder and thicker and contains more blood vessels and less connective tissue than the gingival seen later in life. Whether these differences mask disease or are helpful is unclear.
- Q: How do intraoral piercings impact gum health?
- A: In addition to fractured teeth, gingival recession and gingivitis are complications of the trauma inflicted by a foreign body in the oral cavity.
- Q: Why is smoking associated with gingival disease?
- A: Nicotine inhibits phagocyte and neutrophil function, reduces bone mineralization, impairs vascularization, and reduces antibody production. Smokers do not respond as well as nonsmokers to surgical and nonsurgical treatments.

GLAUCOMA—CONGENITAL
Julie Y. Kwon
Graham E. Quinn

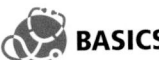 **BASICS**

DESCRIPTION
Improper development of drainage system for aqueous humor, leading to elevated intraocular pressure with enlargement of eye and damage to optic nerve

EPIDEMIOLOGY
- 1:10,000 births
- Male > Female (5:2)
- 70% bilaterally affected
- Primary congenital glaucoma accounts for ~1/2 of all cases of glaucoma in children.

PATHOPHYSIOLOGY
- Primary congenital glaucoma caused by structural abnormalities of aqueous outflow mechanism, which includes trabecular meshwork, iris, and cornea
- Secondary glaucoma may be associated with systemic abnormalities such as Lowe's syndrome, aniridia, rubella, and Sturge–Weber syndrome.
- Glaucoma may also be acquired from an ocular abnormality such as cataract, from trauma, or after intraocular surgery.
- Glaucoma may be caused by certain medications, most notably steroids. Angle closure glaucoma has been associated with Topiramate use.

ETIOLOGY
- Aqueous humor, a clear fluid produced by ciliary body at posterior base of iris, passes through pupil and exits through trabecular meshwork and Schlemm canal, which are located at the junction of the cornea and anterior iris
- Outflow blockage of aqueous may cause pressure to build in eye, resulting in enlargement of eye in younger children and destruction of fibers of the optic nerve in children with abnormally high intraocular pressures. The blockage may be microscopic (open-angle glaucoma) or due to obstruction of the outflow by iris (angle-closure glaucoma).

COMMONLY ASSOCIATED CONDITIONS
- Aniridia
- Axenfeld–Rieger's syndrome
- Sturge–Weber syndrome
- Neurofibromatosis Type 1
- Marfan syndrome
- Pierre Robin syndrome
- Homocystinuria
- Lowe (oculocerebrorenal) syndrome
- Rubella
- Chromosomal abnormalities
- Persistent fetal vasculature-type cataract
- Congenital cataract
- Ocular trauma or surgery
- Uveitis (juvenile rheumatoid arthritis)

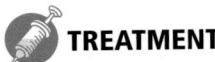 **DIAGNOSIS**

SIGNS AND SYMPTOMS
- Corneal enlargement (11 mm suspicious in patients younger than 1 year) or asymmetry.
- Corneal haze from edema and/or scarring, often seen with acute ruptures in Descemet's membrane
- Buphthalmos (ocular enlargement) due to stretching of immature collagen in infants
- Myopia, often extreme degrees
- Usually painless loss of vision without ocular inflammation
- Optic nerve cupping develops rapidly in infants but may be reversible with control of glaucoma in very young children.
- General signs of many systemic syndromes associated with glaucoma (neurofibromatosis, Sturge–Weber syndrome)
- Elevated intraocular pressure (IOP) > 21 mm Hg in one or both eyes in at least two occasions

HISTORY
- Epiphora (tearing), photophobia (light sensitivity), and blepharospasm (lid squeezing) may be present due to corneal edema from increased intraocular pressure.
- Acute pain, redness, and blurry vision in acute angle-closure glaucoma
- Loss of vision in advanced cases.

PHYSICAL EXAM
May have red eye or asymmetry of eye size, in particular the corneal size and clarity. Nystagmus may be noted if corneal haze is very severe

Imaging
Ultrasound: Axial length using A-scan:
- Eye usually abnormally long for age
- Longitudinal data very useful in determining progression of glaucoma

Genetics
- Primary congenital glaucoma is generally sporadic; an autosomal recessive form has been associated with P4501B1 (CYP1B1) gene

Diagnosis Procedures/Surgery
- Intraocular pressure measurement:
  - An awake child is ideal; use bottle or breast to quiet, along with low lighting
  - If examination under anesthesia is needed, check intraocular pressure as soon as possible after induction, as intraocular pressure drops with anesthetic agents

- Corneal inspection:
  - Diameter measured with calipers:
    - Normal newborn: 10–10.5 mm
    - >11.0 mm suspicious
    - Watch for asymmetry
  - Clarity: Haze may be due to edema or breaks in Descemet membrane (called Haab striae)
  - Refractive error:
    - High myopia common
    - Useful as office measure of change over time
  - Optic disc assessment
    - Cupping of nerve head is early sign
    - May reverse with good intraocular pressure control in the very young
- Gonioscopy: Evaluation of anterior chamber angle (between iris and cornea)
  - In trabeculodysgenesis, insertion of iris into corneoscleral angle often flat or concave
  - Iris defects may suggest type of abnormality causing glaucoma
  - Abnormal iris vessels may influence surgical plan
  - In angle-closure glaucoma: Diagnostic apposition of iris on cornea

DIFFERENTIAL DIAGNOSIS
- Excessive tearing, most commonly due to nasolacrimal duct obstruction
- Megalocornea:
  - May be associated with high myopia
  - Often familial
- Corneal haze
- Birth trauma, forceps
- Congenital corneal dystrophies
- Developmental anomalies
- Intrauterine inflammation (rubella, syphilis)
- Mucopolysaccharidoses
- Cystinosis

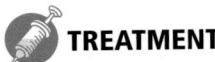 **TREATMENT**

ADDITIONAL TREATMENT
General Measures
Immediate:
- Medical treatment for glaucoma in children is usually a temporizing measure prior to surgical intervention.
- In other types of pediatric glaucoma, medical treatment involves use of the same medications as those used in adults, such as β-blockers, adrenergic agents, and carbonic anhydrase inhibitors. In general, miotics are not used because they may cause a paradoxical rise in intraocular pressure in children.

MEDICATION (DRUGS)
- Ensure that potential systemic medicines do not increase intraocular pressure
- Topical α-adrenergic agonists are associated with mental status changes, hypersomnolence, and apnea and are contraindicated in infants and children.

First Line
- Carbonic anhydrase inhibitors:
  - Systemic:
    - Acetazolamide
    - Methazolamide
  - Topical:
    - Brinzolamide
    - Dorzolamide
- β-Blockers, topical:
  - Timolol
  - Betaxolol
  - Levobunolol
  - Metipranolol
- Prostaglandins, topical:
  - Latanoprost
  - Bimatoprost
  - Travoprost

SURGERY/OTHER PROCEDURES
- Treatment of infantile glaucoma is typically surgical; medications usually not effective for long-term control
- Goniotomy/trabeculotomy: Both procedures open portions of Schlemm canal (goniotomy approaches Schlemm canal from inside eye and trabeculotomy from outside) into anterior chamber, allowing easier outflow of aqueous humor to subconjunctival space.
- Trabeculectomy: Similar to trabeculotomy but includes excision of a small portion of Schlemm canal and trabecular meshwork
- Seton procedures: Various devices inserted from subconjunctival space into anterior chamber, allowing free flow of aqueous humor from eye
- Cyclodestructive procedures: Procedures involving destruction of ciliary body (which produces aqueous humor) decrease production of aqueous humor.
- Iridectomy: If mechanism of glaucoma is angle closure (limited outflow of aqueous humor due to anatomic blockage with iris), then removal of portion of iris may eliminate obstruction

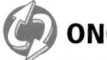 ONGOING CARE

FOLLOW-UP RECOMMENDATIONS
Early postoperative:
- Postoperative steroids and cycloplegic drops to decrease pain and prevent adhesions due to inflammation.
- Corneal edema clears slowly, but intraocular pressure falls quickly if surgery is successful.
- Examination under anesthesia may be required frequently during the first 3–4 years of life, to ensure adequate control of intraocular pressure.

Longer term:
- Follow-up needed throughout life
- Contact with social services for blind and visually handicapped individuals must be made for children even if the child is only suspected of being visually impaired. Encourage families to make contact even when child may be too young to provide objective data on extent of visual handicap.

PATIENT EDUCATION
Children and parents must understand that glaucoma may recur at any point, and that continued, long-term surveillance is essential.

PROGNOSIS
Guarded; even if pressure well controlled and amblyopia treatment undertaken vigorously, child still at high risk for visual impairment. Must be carefully followed for:
- Amblyopia
- Abnormal refractive errors
- Recurrence of glaucoma

COMPLICATIONS
- Severe visual impairment or blindness due to optic nerve damage, amblyopia, and corneal scarring likely if glaucoma is undetected or uncontrollable
- If glaucoma controlled, the following are relatively common:
  - Unrecognized and untreated amblyopia (most serious threat to child's vision)
  - High degrees of myopia
  - Anisometropia (difference in refractive error between fellow eyes)
  - Buphthalmos and corneal scarring

ADDITIONAL READING

- Beck AD. Diagnosis and management of pediatric glaucoma. *Ophthalmol Clin North Am.* 2001;14: 501–512.
- Bejjani B, Edward, D. Primary Congenital Glaucoma. *Gene Reviews [Internet].* Seattle (WA): University of Washington, Seattle. Last updated Dec. 3, 2007.
- Mandal AK, Gothwal VK, Bagga H, et al. Outcome of surgery on infants younger than 1 month with congenital glaucoma. *Ophthalmology.* 2003;110: 1909–1915.
- Mandal A, Netland P. *The Pediatric Glaucomas.* Butterworth-Heinemann, Burlington, MA, 2005.
- Nootheti S, Bielory L. Risk of cataracts and glaucoma with inhaled steroid use in children. *Compr Ophthalmol Update.* 2006;7(1):31–39.
- Papadopoulos M, Khaw PT. Advances in the management of paediatric glaucoma. *Eye.* 2007;21(10):1319–1325.

 CODES

ICD9
- 365.14 Glaucoma of childhood
- 365.31 Corticosteroid-induced glaucoma, glaucomatous stage
- 743.20 Buphthalmos, unspecified

ICD10
- H40.50X0 Glaucoma secondary to oth eye disord, unsp eye, stage unsp
- H40.60X0 Glaucoma secondary to drugs, unsp eye, stage unspecified
- Q15.0 Congenital glaucoma

FAQ
- Q: Can glaucoma be painful?
- A: If the ocular pressure rises quickly (hours), pain occurs frequently. Very high intraocular pressures may be present without pain if they occur slowly (months to years). However, most patients with glaucoma are asymptomatic until they have advanced vision loss.
- Q: Can glaucoma occur after eye trauma?
- A: Yes. This is a very common cause of glaucoma and may be asymptomatic, thus requiring periodic follow-up ophthalmic examinations for early detection and treatment.
- Q: Is infantile glaucoma heritable?
- A: Yes, both primary infantile glaucoma and glaucoma related to systemic or ocular syndromes may be inherited. Siblings and children of affected individuals should be examined for glaucoma.

G

GLOMERULONEPHRITIS

Christine B. Sethna
Kevin E.C. Meyers

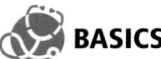 **BASICS**

DESCRIPTION
- Glomerulonephritis (GN) presents with nephritic syndrome: Hematuria with RBC casts, hypertension, azotemia and edema. Proteinuria and oliguria may also be present.
- Acute glomerulonephritis is associated with inflammation and proliferation of the glomerular tuft. It may be rapidly progressive.
- Chronic glomerulonephritis indicates permanent damage has occurred.

EPIDEMIOLOGY
Acute poststreptococcal glomerulonephritis can occur in anyone >2 years, but is most frequently found in boys 5–15 years old.

Incidence
- Incidence of acute poststreptococcal glomerulonephritis in the U.S. has declined over the last 2 decades.
- Chronic glomerulonephritis occurs more often at the end of the 1st decade of life and in adults.

Genetics
Genetic predisposition: Familial glomerulonephritis (e.g., Alport syndrome, X linked)

ETIOLOGY
- Low serum complement level: Systemic diseases:
  - Vasculitis and autoimmune disease (e.g., systemic lupus erythematosus [SLE])
  - Subacute bacterial endocarditis (SBE)
  - Shunt nephritis
  - Cryoglobulinemia
- Low serum complement level: Renal diseases:
  - Acute poststreptococcal glomerulonephritis
  - Membranoproliferative glomerulonephritis (types 1, 2, and 3)
- Normal serum complement level: Systemic diseases:
  - Microscopic Polyangiitis
  - Wegener vasculitis
  - Henoch-Schönlein purpura
  - Hypersensitivity vasculitis
  - Visceral abscess
- Normal serum complement level: Renal diseases:
  - IgA nephropathy
  - Idiopathic rapidly progressive glomerulonephritis
  - Immune-complex disease
- Pauci-immune glomerulonephritis

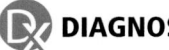 **DIAGNOSIS**

SIGNS AND SYMPTOMS
- Macroscopic hematuria (tea-colored urine)
- Sore throat
- Impetigo
- A prior upper respiratory infection in the previous 7–14 days or skin lesions in the preceding 14–21 days suggests acute poststreptococcal glomerulonephritis.
- An upper respiratory infection in the previous few days suggests IgA nephropathy.
- Reduced output of urine
- Dyspnea, fatigue, lethargy
- Headache
- Seizures (hypertensive encephalopathy)
- Symptoms of a systemic disease such as fever, rash (especially on the buttocks and legs, posteriorly), arthralgia, and weight loss
- Special questions:
  - Establish the time relationship between a sore throat and the acute glomerulonephritis. The onset of acute poststreptococcal glomerulonephritis is usually associated with a time delay of >1 week.

PHYSICAL EXAM
- Hypertension
- Pallor
- Signs of volume overload (e.g., edema, jugular venous distention, hepatomegaly, basal pulmonary crepitation, and a triple cardiac rhythm)
- Impetigo or ecthyma (pyoderma)
- Signs of vasculitis such as rash, loss of fingertip pulp space tissue, Raynaud phenomenon, and vascular thrombosis
- Signs of a systemic disorder (see comment on vasculitis)
- Signs of chronic kidney disease, such as short stature, pallor, sallow skin, edema, excoriations, pericardial friction rub, pulmonary rales and effusion, breath that smells of urine, asterixis, myoclonus, and neuropathy

DIAGNOSTIC TESTS & INTERPRETATION
Lab
Initial lab tests
- Urine:
  - Microscopy of the urine for crenated erythrocytes and erythrocyte casts—hallmark of nephritis
  - Proteinuria
- Evidence of previous strep infection:
  - Throat culture for beta-hemolytic *Streptococcus* (result is positive in 15–20% with acute poststreptococcal glomerulonephritis)
  - Antistreptolysin O titer: Positive result in 60% of patients with acute poststreptococcal glomerulonephritis
  - Streptozyme test: A mixed antigen test for β-hemolytic streptococcus. Together, the antistreptolysin O titer plus streptozyme tests have a >85% sensitivity.
  - Complement C3 serum level will be low in acute poststreptococcal glomerulonephritis and in other causes of acute glomerulonephritis as detailed herein.
- Blood chemistry:
  - Can be normal in acute glomerulonephritis
  - In chronic glomerulonephritis, serum chemistries will reflect the degree of chronic kidney disease (i.e., raised serum urea and creatinine). The serum potassium and phosphate levels will be elevated and the calcium level decreased.
  - With chronic kidney disease: Normocytic, normochromic, or hypochromic microcytic anemia

Imaging
- Chest radiograph to look for pulmonary edema and determine cardiac size
- Renal ultrasound if presentation or course not typical of acute poststreptococcal glomerulonephritis. The ultrasound is to assess the size and parenchymal texture.

Diagnostic Procedures/Other
Electrocardiogram to assess ventricular size and for hyperkalemia

Pathological Findings
In acute poststreptococcal glomerulonephritis, light microscopy reveals enlarged swollen glomerular tufts, mesangial and epithelial cell proliferation, with polymorphonuclear cell infiltration. There is granular deposition of C3 and IgG on immunofluorescence, and electron-dense subepithelial deposits or humps are seen on electron microscopy. The histology varies in chronic glomerulonephritis and depends on the cause. Rapidly progressive glomerulonephritis is associated with crescent formation.

DIFFERENTIAL DIAGNOSIS
- Acute postinfectious glomerulonephritis (Lancefield group A β-hemolytic streptococci, *Pneumococcus, Mycoplasma*, mumps, Epstein-Barr virus)
- Infection-related (hepatitis B and C, syphilis)
- IgA nephropathy
- Membranoproliferative glomerulonephritis
- Autoimmune glomerulonephritis (e.g., SLE)
- Familial glomerulonephritis
- Acute interstitial nephritis
- Hemolytic uremic syndrome
- Pyelonephritis

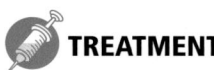 TREATMENT

MEDICATION (DRUGS)
- The following may be required:
  - Loop diuretics (furosemide) for volume, BP, and potassium control
  - Antihypertensive agents; vasodilators such as calcium channel blockers (e.g., nifedipine, isradipine, amlodipine), and loop diuretics are useful as first-line agents; IV hydralazine, labetalol, nicardipine, or nitroprusside may be required to treat severe refractory hypertension.
  - Serum potassium-lowering agents (sodium polystyrene sulfonate [Kayexalate], furosemide, bicarbonate, insulin/glucose, β-agonists). IV calcium is used to stabilize the myocardium in severe hyperkalemia.
  - Phosphate binders (calcium carbonate, sevelamer)
  - Immunosuppressive agents such as prednisone, cyclophosphamide, mycophenolate mofetil, and sometimes rituximab are used in the treatment of vasculitis-associated glomerulonephritis, membranoproliferative glomerulonephritis, and rapidly progressing glomerulonephritis. Plasmapheresis may be used to treat rapidly progressing glomerulonephritis. Penicillin is used in acute poststreptococcal glomerulonephritis to prevent rheumatic fever, but does not affect the course of the disease.

ADDITIONAL TREATMENT
General Measures
- Acute poststreptococcal glomerulonephritis is a self-limiting disease. Acute therapy is usually sufficient.
- The therapy of chronic glomerulonephritis depends on the underlying disease process; it may include immunosuppressives and, ultimately, the management of chronic kidney disease.

IN-PATIENT CONSIDERATIONS
Initial Stabilization
Treat hypertensive encephalopathy and life-threatening electrolyte disturbances immediately.

Admission Criteria
- Hypertension
- Edema
- Acute kidney injury

 ONGOING CARE

FOLLOW-UP RECOMMENDATIONS
In acute poststreptococcal glomerulonephritis, improvement usually occurs within 3–7 days, hypertension is not sustained, and macroscopic hematuria is transient. Watch for ongoing oliguria, unresolved hypertension, increasing proteinuria, or progressive azotemia. Complement levels return to normal within 6–8 weeks of the initial presentation.

> **ALERT**
> - Microscopic hematuria may be present up to 2 years after an episode of poststreptococcal glomerulonephritis.
> - If complement levels do not return to normal after presumed poststreptococcal glomerulonephritis, consider SLE and MPGN.

PATIENT MONITORING
- Look for and treat hyperkalemia.
- To control seizures, treat the hypertension; anticonvulsants play a secondary role.
- Monitor the degree of acute kidney injury.
- Home testing: BP monitoring may be required.
- Do not fail to check serum potassium levels.
- Be certain to recognize fluid overload.
- Be certain to recognize the severity and type of renal failure.

DIET
Restrictions of intake of fluid, sodium, potassium, and phosphate are initially required.

PROGNOSIS
- Prognosis is excellent in acute poststreptococcal glomerulonephritis and variable for other causes of glomerulonephritis in childhood.
- Acute poststreptococcal glomerulonephritis rarely recurs.

COMPLICATIONS
- Acute renal failure
- Hyperkalemia
- Hypertension
- Volume overload (e.g., congestive cardiac failure, pulmonary edema, hypertension)
- Chronic kidney disease

ADDITIONAL READING
- Ahn SY, Ingulli E. Acute poststreptococcal glomerulonephritis: An update. *Curr Opin Pediatr.* 2008;20(2):157–162.
- Madaio MP, Harrington JT. The diagnosis of acute glomerulonephritis. *N Engl J Med.* 1984;309: 1299–1302.
- Pan CG. Evaluation of gross hematuria. *Pediatr Clin North Am.* 2006;53(3):401–412.

 CODES

ICD9
- 580.9 Acute glomerulonephritis with unspecified pathological lesion in kidney
- 582.9 Chronic glomerulonephritis with unspecified pathological lesion in kidney
- 583.9 Nephritis and nephropathy, not specified as acute or chronic, with unspecified pathological lesion in kidney

ICD10
- N00.9 Acute nephritic syndrome with unspecified morphologic changes
- N03.9 Chronic nephritic syndrome with unspecified morphologic changes
- N05.9 Unspecified nephritic syndrome with unspecified morphologic changes

FAQ
- Q: When does the complement return to normal?
- A: Hemolytic complement levels (C3) return to normal within a 6–8-week period in acute poststreptococcal glomerulonephritis. Persistently low C3 levels suggest a cause other than acute poststreptococcal glomerulonephritis.
- Q: What are the indications for renal biopsy in acute glomerulonephritis?
- A: Patients in whom there is sustained hypertension, ongoing or progressive azotemia, or persistent proteinuria of >1.5 g/d should be biopsied.

G

GLUCOSE-6-PHOSPHATE DEHYDROGENASE DEFICIENCY

Michele P. Lambert

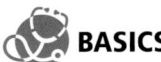 **BASICS**

DESCRIPTION
Deficiency of the enzyme glucose-6-phosphate dehydrogenase (G6PD) in the RBC, which may result in hemolytic anemia. Several types of genetic mutations result either in deficient enzyme production or in production of an enzyme with diminished activity:

- Although most patients with this deficiency are never anemic and have mild to no hemolysis, the classic manifestation is acute hemolytic anemia in response to oxidative stress.
- World Health Organization classification of G6PD:
  - Class 1: Congenital nonspherocytic hemolytic anemia: Rare. Chronic hemolysis without exposure to oxidative stressors—splenomegaly in 40%. Affected individuals tend to be white males of Northern European background.
  - Class 2: Severe deficiency (1–10% enzymatic activity): Oxidative stress–induced hemolysis. Prototype is G6PD-Mediterranean.
  - Class 3: Mild deficiency (10–60% enzymatic activity): Most common type. Acute hemolytic anemia uncommon, occurs only with stressors
  - Class 4: Nondeficient variant (60–100% enzymatic activity): No symptoms, even during oxidant stressors, e.g., G6PD A+(variant with normal activity); 20–40% allelic frequency in Africans
  - Class 5: >150% of normal activity
- Deficient neonates may have hyperbilirubinemia out of proportion to their anemia. May, in part, account for increased prevalence of African Americans among patients with bilirubin encephalopathy. Should be considered as cause of hyperbilirubinemia in neonates of appropriate racial background and may contribute to kernicterus

GENERAL PREVENTION
Avoid drugs and toxins known to cause hemolysis. Prompt follow-up with febrile illness and signs of hemolysis.

EPIDEMIOLOGY
Prevalence
- Most common of all clinically significant enzyme defects, affecting ~400 million people worldwide
- X linked (Xq28): Primarily affects males
- Almost 400 allelic variants
- Frequency of different mutations varies by population:
- Africans: 20–40% of X chromosomes are G6PD A+ (mutant enzyme with normal activity)
- Sardinians (some regions): 30% have G6PD-Mediterranean
- Saudi Arabians: 13% have G6PD deficiency
- African Americans: 10–15% have G6PD A− (mutant enzyme with decreased activity).
- High incidence of mutant genes in some regions may relate to survival advantage against malarial infection (*Plasmodium falciparum*).

Genetics
Gene is on the X chromosome (Xq28).

- Males express the enzyme (mutant or normal) from their single X chromosome (hemizygotes).
- Female homozygotes (rare) are more severely affected than female heterozygotes.
- Heterozygote females show variable intermediate expression because of random X inactivation.

PATHOPHYSIOLOGY
- RBCs lose G6PD activity throughout their life span; therefore, older cells are more prone to oxidative hemolysis.
- Normal RBC life span of ~120 days is unaffected in unstressed states, even with severe enzyme deficiency, but may be shortened during oxidant stress.
- Enzyme-deficient RBCs are destroyed by intravascular hemolysis on exposure to the oxidative stressor, and acute hemolytic anemia results.
- Oxidant stressors include infections and chemicals (mothballs, antimalarials, some sulfonamides, methylene blue).
- Hemolysis usually follows stressor by 1–3 days, and nadir occurs 8–10 days postexposure. Obtain hemoglobins for >1 week after the initial exposure.
- Favism: Severe hemolytic anemia in patients with more severe forms of G6PD deficiency after fava bean ingestion.
- Normal G6PD activity is 7–10 IU per gram of hemoglobin.

DIAGNOSIS

HISTORY
- Symptoms of anemia include fatigue, irritability, and malaise.
- Dark urine (cola or tea colored) may follow moderate-to-severe hemolysis. May develop jaundice (particularly scleral icterus).
- Patient may have required phototherapy in newborn period for hyperbilirubinemia.
- Recent drug, chemical, or food (fava bean) exposures may precipitate moderate-to-severe hemolysis.
- Family history of intermittent jaundice, splenectomy, cholecystectomy, or blood transfusion may indicate an inherited condition.
- Ethnicity may help determine type/severity of disease.

PHYSICAL EXAM
- Tachycardia, a flow murmur, or pallor: Signs of anemia
- Jaundice or scleral icterus: Signs of hemolysis

DIAGNOSTIC TESTS & INTERPRETATION
Lab
- CBC:
  - Usually reveals a normochromic normocytic anemia with appropriate reticulocytosis
  - Hemoglobin can drop precipitously; should be monitored closely until stable or trending upward; checking a single hemoglobin the day of exposure to the stressor is not sufficient.
- Peripheral blood smear:
  - Often shows bizarre RBC morphology with marked anisocytosis and poikilocytosis
  - Can see schistocytes, hemighost cells (uneven distribution of hemoglobin), bite cells, blister cells, and occasional Heinz bodies (on supravital staining)
- Hemoglobinemia: Seen as plasma (pinkish red supernatant) or measured as free serum hemoglobin
- Hemoglobinuria: Occurs when hemoglobin-binding sites in the plasma (haptoglobin and hemopexin) are saturated; may be visible as dark urine—heme positive on dipstick and no RBC on microscopy.
- Free haptoglobin levels decrease.
- Direct and indirect Coombs tests:
  - Must be done to exclude autoimmune hemolytic anemia
  - Should be negative in G6PD deficiency
- Other: Plasma indirect bilirubin, lactate dehydrogenase, and aspartate aminotransferase may be elevated; hemosiderin may be found in the urine several days after hemolysis. Liver function tests should be normal. Renal functions to rule out thrombotic thrombocytopenic purpura and hemolytic uremic syndrome:
  - Rapid screening tests for G6PD activity in RBCs are qualitative; will miss some female heterozygotes with measurable but low enzyme levels
  - Necessary to confirm a deficiency or to diagnose a suspected heterozygote with a test to quantify G6PD activity
  - Normal activity: 7–10 IU/g hemoglobin
    - Accurately detects deficiency in males and homozygous females with no recent hemolysis
    - Helpful with heterozygous women

- Newborn screening for G6PD deficiency
  - Included in some panels of genetic screening tests performed on newborns
  - Typically performed by DNA-based methods that detect a few of the most common variants in US populations. Does not screen for all G6PD variants and can miss severe but rare variants.
  - Results may be reported in terms of predicted enzyme levels but not a true measurement of enzymatic activity.

ALERT
Confirm with G6PD enzyme activity; measured enzyme levels will be higher immediately after an acute hemolytic event because younger RBCs (reticulocytes) with normal levels of enzyme will have replaced the older, more deficient population.
- Screening tests may be falsely negative during this time.
- Most cost-effective approach: Defer screening until 1–2 weeks after resolution of hemolysis.
- Heterozygote female detection:
  - 2 RBC populations exist because of mosaicism from random X inactivation.
  - On average, 50% are normal and 50% are deficient, but there may be variability.

DIFFERENTIAL DIAGNOSIS
Intravascular hemolysis is very rare in children, but other causes include:
- Acute hemolytic transfusion reactions (Coombs test is positive)
- Microangiopathic hemolytic disease, such as hemolytic uremic syndrome, thrombotic thrombocytopenic purpura, and prosthetic cardiac valves
- Physical trauma (e.g., March hemoglobinuria); severe burns (uncommon)
- Other inherited RBC enzyme deficiencies
- Paroxysmal nocturnal hemoglobinuria.

Extravascular hemolysis can also be confused with G6PD deficiency and includes: Hereditary spherocytosis (spherocytes on smear); autoimmune hemolysis and delayed hemolytic transfusion reactions (both Coombs positive); hemoglobinopathies; hypersplenism or severe liver disease; Gilbert disease

TREATMENT

General Measures
- Removal of the oxidant stressor is of primary importance:
  - Discontinue the suspected drug and/or treat the infection.
    - In class 3 and 4 patients, essential drug therapy may be continued while monitoring for signs of severe hemolysis.
    - Transfusion is may be necessary (esp. in some type 1 and 2 deficiencies), but any patient who is symptomatic with anemia or has a low hemoglobin and signs of ongoing brisk hemolysis should be transfused immediately with packed RBCs.

- Supportive care, evaluation of renal function (risk of acute tubular necrosis with brisk hemolysis), and monitoring degree of anemia and ongoing hemolysis are important.
- For the affected neonate:
  - Monitor the bilirubin closely and start phototherapy early.
    - If necessary, exchange transfusion should be carried out.
    - Phenobarbital may decrease bilirubin level.
    - Early discharge is not recommended in infants with jaundice and known risk for G6PD deficiency.

ONGOING CARE

FOLLOW-UP RECOMMENDATIONS
- Most deficient individuals remain asymptomatic.
- When hemolysis does occur, it tends to be self-limited and resolves spontaneously, with a return to normal hemoglobin levels in 2–6 weeks.
- Development of renal failure is extremely rare in children, even with massive hemolysis and hemoglobinuria.

DIET
- Avoid fava beans. Fava beans have a variety of names in different cultures.

PROGNOSIS
- For those with the milder forms, the prognosis is excellent.
- Can cause significant morbidity, but rarely mortality, in those with the more severe forms

COMPLICATIONS
Neonates can be at risk for hyperbilirubinemia requiring treatment. Kernicterus has been reported in infants with G6PD deficiency.

ADDITIONAL READING

- Cappellini MD, Fiorelli G. Glucose-6-phosphate dehydrogenase deficiency. *Lancet*. 2008;371: 64–74.
- Frank JE. Diagnosis and management of G6PD deficiency. *Am Fam Physician*. 2005;72(2): 1277–1282.
- Nkhoma ET, Poole C, Vannappagari V, et al. The global prevalence of glucose-6 phosphate dehydrogenase deficiency: A systematic review and meta-analysis. *Blood Cells Mol Dis*. 2009;42: 267–278.
- Watchko JF. Hyperbilirubinemia in African American neonates: Clinical issues and current challenges. *Sem Fet Neo Med*. 2010;15(3):176–182.

 CODES

ICD9
282.2 Anemias due to disorders of glutathione metabolism

ICD10
D55.0 Anemia due to glucose-6-phosphate dehydrogenase deficiency

FAQ

- Q: Do I need to follow a special diet or avoid medications if I have G6PD deficiency?
- A: Although most patients will have no symptoms of their disease, certain medications may cause transient hemolytic anemia, and these should be avoided. When prescribing medications, your physician and pharmacist should know about your G6PD, but most necessary medications are safe and well tolerated. People with severe variants of the deficiency should also avoid fava beans, but otherwise no dietary restrictions are necessary.
- Q: Do I need to know which variant of G6PD I have?
- A: It may be clear which variant you are likely to have based on your clinical symptoms and ethnic background.
- Q: Should my family be screened if someone has G6PD deficiency?
- A: In families of patients with G6PD, screening members may help provide meaningful genetic counseling to female carriers and affected but asymptomatic males.
- Q: How does G6PD affect sickle cell anemia and vice versa?
- A: Having sickle cell disease is somewhat protective in patients with G6PD A deficiency, because their RBC population is young and, therefore, has higher enzymatic activity. On the other hand, G6PD has no effect on the clinical characteristics of sickle cell disease.

G

GOITER

Adda Grimberg

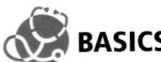

BASICS

DESCRIPTION
Goiter is enlargement of the thyroid gland.

EPIDEMIOLOGY
- The most common cause of pediatric goiter in the US is chronic lymphocytic thyroiditis.
- Prevalence of goiter in the US is 3–7%, although the incidence is much higher in regions of iodine deficiency.
- Thyroid cancers make up 0.5–1.5% of all malignancies in children and adolescents.
- Both thyroid tumors and autoimmune thyroid disease are more common in females than males.

Prevalence
World Health Organization (WHO) Global Database on Iodine Deficiency (1993–2003):
- Global goiter prevalence is 15.8% of the general population.
- Insufficient iodine intake among school-aged children ranged from 10.1% in the Americas to 59.9% in Europe.
- 54 countries had iodine deficiency, 29 countries had excessive iodine intake, and 43 countries achieved optimal iodine intake.

ETIOLOGY
- The multinodular goiter 1 (MNG1) locus has been identified on chromosome 14q and on chromosome Xp22.
- Germline mutations in DICER1 (chromosome 14q31) have been found in familial multinodular goiter, with and without ovarian Sertoli-Leydig cell tumors.
- Germline mutation in thyroid transcription factor-1 (TITF-1/NKX2.1) has been found in patients with papillary thyroid carcinoma and a history of multinodular goiter.
- Other genes implicated in simple goiter formation: Thyroglobulin, thyroid-stimulating hormone (TSH) receptor, and Na^+/I^- symporter.
- Thyroid peroxidase mutations lead to iodide organification defects and goitrous congenital hypothyroidism.
- Twin and family studies show a modest to major effect of environmental factors, especially iodine deficiency and cigarette smoking.
- Excessive maternal ingestion of iodine during pregnancy can lead to congenital goiter with increased iodine uptake on scan and in some babies, a transient hypothyroidism.
- Autoimmune goiters, such as chronic lymphocytic thyroiditis, occur in children with a genetic predisposition.
- Thyroid cancers are usually sporadic. Medullary carcinoma can be familial (autosomal dominant), as part of multiple endocrine neoplasia (MEN) type 2A and 2B, or as isolated malignancy.
- Pendred syndrome (autosomal recessive) causes congenital sensorineural deafness and an iodine organification defect that leads to goiter.

DIAGNOSIS

HISTORY
- Symptoms of hypothyroidism:
  - Increase in sedentary behavior
  - Lethargy
  - Weight gain
  - Constipation
  - Cold intolerance
  - Dry skin and/or hair
  - Hair loss
- Symptoms of hyperthyroidism:
  - Hyperactivity
  - Irritability
  - Difficulty concentrating or focusing in school
  - Hyperphagia
  - Weight loss
  - Diarrhea
  - Heat intolerance
- Careful dietary and medication history
- History of head, neck, or chest irradiation is associated with increased risk of carcinoma.
- Family history of thyroid carcinoma or MEN syndrome

PHYSICAL EXAM
Inspect, palpate, and auscultate the neck:
- Neck extension aids inspection.
- Palpation is best performed standing behind the child.
  - Determine if the thyroid is diffusely enlarged or asymmetric, evaluate gland firmness, and assess for any nodularity.
  - Check for cervical lymphadenopathy.
  - Pain on palpation suggests acute inflammation.
- Auscultate with the stethoscope diaphragm (while patient holds his or her breath) for a bruit, which indicates the hyperthyroidism-associated hypervascularity.
- Careful examination for signs of hypothyroidism or hyperthyroidism:
  - Pulse
  - Linear growth and weight pattern
  - Sexual development
  - Deep tendon reflexes
  - Skin
- Have patient drink water during inspection of gland.

DIAGNOSTIC TESTS & INTERPRETATION
- Thyroid function tests: Total T_4 and TSH are the best screens for hypothyroidism or hyperthyroidism.
- T_3 radioimmunoassay in cases of suspected hyperthyroidism (Note: Radioimmunoassay, which measures total T_3, and not resin uptake, which indirectly assesses thyroid hormone–binding capacity!)
- In cases of suspected chronic lymphocytic thyroiditis: Antithyroglobulin and antimicrosomal (antiperoxidase) antibodies
- In cases of suspected Graves disease: Thyroid-stimulating immunoglobulins (or TSH-receptor antibodies)
- Fine-needle aspiration biopsy in children should be considered only for evaluation of low-risk or purely cystic thyroid nodules. (A higher percentage of solitary thyroid nodules are malignant in children compared with adults.)
- Calcitonin levels: Elevated in 75% of patients with medullary carcinoma

Lab
Urinary iodine (UI) concentration is the best measure of the adequacy of iodine intake.

Imaging
- Ultrasound to determine the number, size, and nature (cystic, solid, or mixed) of nodules
- ^{123}I thyroid scans in cases of solitary nodules to establish whether the nodule concentrates iodide:
  - "Cold" nodules (no I uptake) suggest neoplasia and require immediate evaluation by a pediatric endocrinologist and surgeon.
- Barium swallow studies can reveal a fistulous tract between the left piriform sinus and the left thyroid lobe in children with recurrent acute suppurative thyroiditis. Such fistulas are amenable to surgical resection.

ALERT
False positives:
- Fat neck: Adipose tissue, large sternocleidomastoid muscles
- Thyroglossal duct cysts
- Nonthyroidal neoplasms: Lymphoma, teratoma, hygroma, ganglioneuroma

DIFFERENTIAL DIAGNOSIS
- Immunologic:
  - Chronic lymphocytic thyroiditis (often referred to as Hashimoto thyroiditis)
  - Graves disease
  - Amyloid deposition (familial Mediterranean fever, juvenile rheumatoid arthritis)
- Infectious:
  - Acute suppurative thyroiditis (most often *Streptococcus pyogenes*, *Staphylococcus aureus*, and *Streptococcus pneumoniae*)
  - Subacute thyroiditis (often viral)
- Environmental:
  - Goitrogens: Iodide, lithium, amiodarone, oral contraceptives, perchlorate, cabbage, soybeans, cassava, thiocyanate in tobacco smoke (smoking is especially goitrogenic in iodine-deficient areas)
  - Iodine deficiency (exacerbated by pregnancy)
- Neoplastic:
  - Thyroid adenoma/carcinoma
  - Follicular adenoma: Benign
  - Follicular, papillary, or mixed carcinoma: Well differentiated; follicular 90%
  - Medullary carcinoma: 4–10% as part of the MEN type 2 syndrome
  - TSH-secreting adenoma
  - Lymphoma
- Congenital:
  - Ectopic gland
  - Unilateral agenesis of gland
  - Dyshormonogenesis
  - Thyroxine resistance
- Miscellaneous:
  - Simple colloid goiter
  - Multinodular goiter

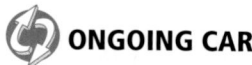
TREATMENT

ALERT
Possible conflicts: In manic depressive patients on lithium and cardiac patients on amiodarone, medication-induced thyroid abnormalities can be a significant problem that should be addressed by the endocrinologist and appropriate subspecialist.

MEDICATION (DRUGS)
- Goiters with hypothyroidism: L-thyroxine
- Goiter with hyperthyroidism: Treatment consists of antithyroid drugs (methimazole); if remission is not achieved after 1 or 2 years, radioactive iodine ablation [(131)I] or surgery (near-total or total thyroidectomy) may be considered.
- Duration depends on the cause of the goiter.

ALERT
FDA issued a black box warning (6/4/2009) against propylthiouracil (PTU) use in treating Graves disease owing to risk of severe liver injury including life-threatening acute liver failure.

ADDITIONAL TREATMENT
Additional Therapies
Intra-amniotic injections of L-thyroxine may treat fetal goitrous hypothyroidism. Large fetal goiters pose a risk of airway compromise at birth.

SURGERY/OTHER PROCEDURES
- Surgery solely to decrease the size of a goiter is indicated only if adjacent structures are compressed.
- Rates of complications after pediatric total thyroidectomy are similar for benign and malignant thyroid diseases; the most common is transient hypocalcemia.

Cancer:
- Surgery is recommended for a nonfunctioning nodule if there is:
  – A history of radiation
  – Rapid growth of a firm nodule
  – Evidence of satellite lymph nodes
  – Evidence of impingement on other neck structures
  – Evidence of distant metastases
- Following surgery, radioiodide therapy is administered if a follow-up iodine scan reveals any residual tissue or metastases.
- Suppressive doses of exogenous thyroid hormone are then given to maintain TSH levels <0.2 ulU/mL.
- Thyroglobulin levels are useful as markers of thyroid tissue; calcitonin level serves as tumor marker for medullary carcinoma.

ONGOING CARE

FOLLOW-UP RECOMMENDATIONS
- Potential for goiter regression depends on its cause. Goiters associated with chronic lymphocytic thyroiditis and Graves disease may or may not decrease in size with treatment.

- A goiter patient who is clinically and biochemically euthyroid still requires careful follow-up for the detection of the early signs of developing thyroid dysfunction.
- Potential complications of thyroid surgery include laryngeal nerve damage and hypoparathyroidism. Complication rates are lower in high-volume centers.

ALERT
Work up solitary thyroid nodules aggressively; remember, incidence of malignancy in these nodules in children is 15–40% (less in adults).
- Malignancy is more likely in euthyroid pediatric patients with nodules that have palpable lymph nodes, compressive signs, microcalcifications, intranodular vascularization, and lymph node alterations.
- Differentiated thyroid carcinoma in prepubertal children, compared to pubertal adolescents, has a more aggressive presentation and more frequently a family history of thyroid carcinoma.

DIET
- Depends on the cause of the goiter
- Incidence of iodine deficiency (endemic) goiter has greatly declined since the addition of potassium iodide to table salt.
- Iodide can also be added to communal drinking water or administered as iodized oil in isolated rural areas.

PROGNOSIS
- Depends on the cause of the goiter
- Thyroid cancers usually follow an indolent course with excellent prognosis, especially the well-differentiated follicular cell carcinoma. Mortality is most common in medullary and undifferentiated carcinomas, which are relatively rare in children.

COMPLICATIONS
- Depending on gland size, goiters can produce a mass effect on midline neck structures. If the goiter is intrathoracic, it may cause pleural effusions or chylothorax.
- Typically, the child is euthyroid, but clinical hypothyroidism or hyperthyroidism may result from certain types of goiters.
- Therapy for thyroid cancer may induce permanent hypothyroidism.

ADDITIONAL READING

- Andersson M, Takkouche B, Egli I, et al. Current global iodine status and progress over the last decade towards the elimination of iodine deficiency. *Bull World Health Organ.* 2005;83:518–525.
- Corrias A, Mussa A, Baronio F, et al. Diagnostic features of thyroid nodules in pediatrics. *Arch Pediatr Adolesc Med.* 2010;164:714–719.
- Hashimoto H, Hashimoto K, Suehara N. Successful in utero treatment of fetal goitrous hypothyroidism: Case report and review of the literature. *Fetal Diagn Ther.* 2006;21:360–365.
- Josefson J, Zimmerman D. Thyroid nodules and cancers in children. *Pediatr Endocrinol Rev.* 2008;6:14–23.
- Lazar L, Lebenthal Y, Steinmetz A, et al. Differentiated thyroid carcinoma in pediatric patients: Comparison of presentation and course between pre-pubertal children and adolescents. *J Pediatr.* 2009;154:708–714.
- Raval MV, Browne M, Chin AC, et al. Total thyroidectomy for benign disease in the pediatric patient—feasible and safe. *J Pediatr Surg.* 2009;44:1529–1533.
- Rivkees SA. Pediatric Graves' disease: Controversies in management. *Horm Res Paediatr.* 2010;74: 305–311.
- Stevens C, Lee JK, Sadatsafavi M, et al. Pediatric thyroid fine-needle aspiration cytology: A meta-analysis. *J Pediatr Surg.* 2009;44:2184–2191.
- Zimmermann MB, Hess SY, Molinari L, et al. New reference values for thyroid volume by ultrasound in iodine-sufficient schoolchildren: A World Health Organization/Nutrition for Health and Development Iodine Deficiency Study Group Report. *Am J Clin Nutr.* 2004;79:231–237.

CODES

ICD9
- 240.9 Goiter, unspecified
- 241.1 Nontoxic multinodular goiter
- 759.89 Other specified congenital anomalies

ICD10
- E00.9 Congenital iodine-deficiency syndrome, unspecified
- E04.2 Nontoxic multinodular goiter
- E04.9 Nontoxic goiter, unspecified

FAQ
- Q: Does a bigger thyroid gland mean increased thyroid functioning?
- A: Goiters can be euthyroid, hypothyroid, or hyperthyroid, depending on cause.
- Q: Will the goiter decrease in size with treatment?
- A: This depends on the cause of the goiter.
- Q: Does a bigger thyroid gland mean cancer?
- A: Most pediatric goiters are benign, and thyroid cancers often are detected as solitary nodules within an otherwise normal gland (in children with solitary nodules, up to 40% are carcinomas). Patients with a history of goiter or benign nodules/adenomas have an increased risk of developing thyroid cancer.
- Q: Does thyroid cancer usually present with hyperthyroidism?
- A: No. The usual chief complaint is a solitary, hard, painless nodule in a euthyroid patient.
- Q: Is there an increased risk of thyroid cancer from diagnostic radiographs (chest radiographs, lateral neck films)?
- A: Routine diagnostic radiographs should fall well below the levels of radiation thought to increase risk of thyroid neoplasia. During more prolonged radiologic procedures that might expose the thyroid to higher doses of radiation, a lead neck shield is used.
- Q: Should prophylactic thyroidectomy be performed in children identified genetically as having familial medullary carcinoma?
- A: Yes, because of the poorer prognosis associated with development of this cancer.

G

GONOCOCCAL INFECTIONS

Jane Nathanson
Samir S. Shah

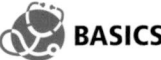 **BASICS**

DESCRIPTION
Neisseria gonorrhoeae, an aerobic gram-negative diplococcus, is the etiologic agent of gonorrhea.

EPIDEMIOLOGY
- Gonorrhea is the most common STD found in sexually abused children.
- Gonococcal conjunctivitis, although rare in adults, occurs by autoinoculation of infected secretions in patients with anogenital infection.

Prevalence
- In the U.S., there are >700,000 new infections each year. Rates are highest among 15–19-year-old women and 20–24-year-old men.
- Pelvic inflammatory disease occurs in 10–20% of women with endocervical gonococcal infection.
- The risk of male-to-female transmission is 50% per episode of vaginal intercourse; the risk of female-to-male transmission is ~20% per episode. Rectal intercourse is also a mode of transmission.
- Racial disparities include an incidence of infection in African Americans 18 times that of Caucasians.

GENERAL PREVENTION
- Neonatal ophthalmia: Prophylactic ophthalmic ointment is mandatory in the U.S. Instillation of either 1% tetracycline or 0.5% erythromycin ophthalmic ointment in both eyes occurs immediately (or within 1 hour) after birth.
- Maternal infection: Routine screening cervical cultures should be performed at the 1st prenatal visit; repeat at term if high risk.

PATHOPHYSIOLOGY
- Incubation period is 2–7 days.
- Transmission results from contact with infected mucous membranes and secretions, usually through sexual activity, parturition, and (rarely) household contact in prepubertal children.
- Immunity is not induced by infection.

ETIOLOGY
N. gonorrhoeae

COMMONLY ASSOCIATED CONDITIONS
Pediatric gonococcal infections can be categorized by age group: Neonates, prepubertal children, and sexually active adolescents.

- Neonatal gonococcal diseases include ophthalmia neonatorum, scalp abscess (complication of fetal scalp monitoring), and, rarely, vaginitis or systemic disease with arthritis, bacteremia, funisitis, or meningitis.
- Prepubertal gonococcal disease usually occurs in the genital tract. Vaginitis is the most common manifestation. Pelvic inflammatory disease (PID), perihepatitis (Fitz-Hugh-Curtis syndrome), urethritis, proctitis, and pharyngitis rarely occur. Sexual abuse must be considered when genital, rectal, or tonsillopharyngeal gonococcal infections occur in prepubertal children.

- Gonococcal diseases in sexually active adolescents resemble those found in adults and are mostly asymptomatic:
  - Both sexes: Pharyngitis or anorectal infection.
  - Females: Genital tract infection may cause urethritis, vaginitis, and endocervicitis. Ascending genital tract infection may lead to PID and perihepatitis.
  - Males: Acute urethritis is the predominant manifestation. Epididymitis also occurs.

DIAGNOSIS

HISTORY
- Premature or prolonged membrane rupture is a risk factor for conjunctivitis. Fetal scalp monitoring places the infant at risk for gonococcal scalp abscess.
- Vaginal itching and discharge indicate vaginitis. In prepubertal children, genital infection is mild; ascending or disseminated infection rarely occurs. In adolescents, estrogenization protects the vagina from infection and instead serves as a conduit for cervical exudate.
- Urethritis: Purulent urethral discharge and dysuria without urgency or frequency.
- Abdominal pain:
  - Ascending infection is characterized by diffuse lower quadrant abdominal pain, including discomfort with ambulation. Low back pain, dyspareunia, and abnormal vaginal bleeding occasionally occur. Fever, chills, nausea, and vomiting may be present. Acute perihepatitis causes right upper quadrant pain and results from direct extension of infection from the fallopian tube to the liver capsule.
- Symptoms of extragenitourinary disease including pharyngitis, arthritis, dermatitis, meningitis, or endocarditis.

PHYSICAL EXAM
- Neonatal ophthalmia:
  - Typical findings include bilateral eyelid edema, chemosis, and copious purulent discharge. Onset is usually between 2–5 days of age but ranges from the 1st day of life (with prolonged rupture of membranes) to several weeks of age.
- Neonatal scalp abscess
- Pelvic inflammatory disease:
  - Signs include cervical motion tenderness, pelvic adnexal tenderness (usually bilateral), and lower or right upper quadrant abdominal pain (with perihepatitis). Most females with PID also have either mucopurulent cervical discharge or WBCs on microscopic evaluation of a saline preparation of vaginal fluid.
- Cervicitis and urethritis:
  - Purulent vaginal discharge. Associated bacterial vaginosis may be noted.
- Bacteremia:
- Classically discrete, tender, necrotic pustules on distal extremities though macules, papules, and bullae occasionally occur; also tenosynovitis, migratory arthritis.

DIAGNOSTIC TESTS & INTERPRETATION
Lab
Initial lab tests
- Gram stain (low sensitivity) and culture of infected exudate or body fluid:
  - Intracellular gram-negative diplococci on gram stain. Confirmation depends on isolation of *N. gonorrhoeae* from culture. Specimens are immediately inoculated onto Thayer-Martin or chocolate-blood agar-based media at room temperature and incubated in an enriched CO_2 environment. In cases of suspected sexual abuse, genital, rectal, and pharyngeal cultures should be collected.
- STD panel:
  - Test for other STDs including *Chlamydia trachomatis*, *Treponema pallidum* (syphilis), *Trichomonas vaginalis*, hepatitis B, and HIV in the child in whom sexual abuse is suspected or when evaluating the sexually active adolescent.
- Nonculture gonococcal tests:
  - Nucleic acid amplification tests (NAAT) for urine specimens (freshly voided specimens), male urethral, female endocervical or vaginal (self-administered introital) swabs are highly sensitive and specific, but should not be used in investigations of possible sexual abuse (owing to the possibility of false-positive results). NAATs also cannot provide antimicrobial susceptibility test results.
- CBC, ESR, and C-reactive protein:
  - Leukocytosis and elevated ESR and C-reactive protein occur in 2/3 of patients with PID.
- Synovial fluid cell count and culture:
  - In septic gonococcal arthritis, synovial fluid has >50,000 leukocytes/mm^3 and the synovial fluid culture is positive, whereas the blood culture is usually negative. In arthritis-dermatitis syndrome, the synovial fluid contains <20,000 leukocytes/mm^3, and the synovial fluid culture is sterile, whereas the blood culture is positive.

Imaging
Pelvic ultrasound may detect ectopic pregnancy and in PID reveals thick, dilated fallopian tubes or tubo-ovarian abscess.

DIFFERENTIAL DIAGNOSIS
- Ophthalmia neonatorum: Other causes of neonatal conjunctivitis include infection with *C. trachomatis*, *S. aureus*, *S. pneumoniae*, *Haemophilus* species, and herpes simplex virus.
- Scalp infection: Gonococcal scalp abscesses may be difficult to distinguish from abscesses caused by staphylococcal species, group B *Streptococcus*, *H. influenzae*, Enterobacteriaceae, and herpes simplex virus.
- Vaginitis: In the prepubertal child, other causes include chemical or environmental irritants, pinworms, foreign body, and infections (i.e., streptococci, *T. vaginalis*). In cases of sexual abuse, *C. trachomatis* and syphilis may occur.
- Genitourinary tract infection: In adolescents, other causes include *C. trachomatis*, syphilis, and *T. vaginalis*.

- Arthritis: Other bacterial causes of septic arthritis, Reiter syndrome, and reactive arthritis.
- Abdominal pain: Ectopic pregnancy, appendicitis, cholecystitis, and UTI/pyelonephritis.

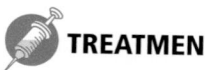 **TREATMENT**

MEDICATION (DRUGS)
First Line
- Increased fluoroquinolone resistance in the U.S. led to extended-spectrum cephalosporin as initial therapy.
- Neonates:
  - Ophthalmia neonatorum or mother known to have gonorrhea: Ceftriaxone, 25–50 mg/kg IV or IM (single dose; maximum, 125 mg); alternate agent for infants with hyperbilirubinemia is cefotaxime, 100 mg/kg IV or IM (single dose).
  - Neonates with gonococcal ophthalmia also require eye irrigation with sterile saline at presentation and at frequent intervals until the mucopurulent drainage has ceased.
  - Disseminated infection: Ceftriaxone daily or cefotaxime b.i.d. for 7 days; continue treatment for 10–14 days for meningitis.
- Older children and adolescents:
- Uncomplicated gonococcal infection (including epididymitis or pharyngeal infection): A single IM dose of ceftriaxone, 125 mg, or a single PO dose of cefixime, 8 mg/kg (max 400 mg, use 400 mg if >45 kg and >8 years). Follow with a treatment regimen for C. trachomatis.
- If allergic to cephalosporins, use single IM dose of spectinomycin, 40 mg/kg (max 2 g) or consider cephalosporin desensitization.
- Pelvic inflammatory disease: See Pediatric Red Book for treatment regimens.
- Complicated gonococcal infection: Ceftriaxone or cefotaxime for 7 days (arthritis and septicemia), 10–14 days (meningitis), or ≥28 days (endocarditis). Include concomitant C. trachomatis therapy: For arthritis, add erythromycin, azithromycin, or doxycycline for 7 days; for meningitis or endocarditis, add erythromycin for 7 days.

IN-PATIENT CONSIDERATIONS
Admission Criteria
Neonate: Hospitalize and obtain appropriate cultures (blood, CSF, conjunctival fluids, or those from any other site of infection).

 ONGOING CARE

FOLLOW-UP RECOMMENDATIONS
- Provide risk reduction education.
- Sexual contacts and mother and her partner(s) of patients with gonorrhea should be counseled and treated.
- Evaluate for concurrent infection with other sexually transmitted diseases, including syphilis, C. trachomatis, T. vaginalis, hepatitis B, and HIV. Patients whose age has progressed beyond the neonatal period should be treated presumptively for C. trachomatis infection.

- All cases of gonorrhea must be reported to public health officials.
- Contact isolation precautions recommended for all hospitalized patients with gonococcal disease in the neonatal and prepubescent age groups; no special policies are recommended for other patients.
- Consider and evaluate for abuse in prepubertal children.

ALERT
Pitfalls:
- Failure to consider the diagnosis of sexual abuse in a prepubertal child with a gonococcal infection. Cases of transmission via nonsexual contact have been reported (i.e., from freshly infected towels, or other fomites, or by digital transmission from an infected caregiver), but such mode cannot be assumed without first excluding sexual abuse.
- Failure to use culture to diagnose infection in cases of suspected abuse.
- Failure to differentiate N. gonorrhoeae by culture from other Neisseria species, especially in prepubertal children, given concern for sexual abuse.
- Failure to consider acute gonococcal perihepatitis/Fitz-Hugh-Curtis syndrome in females with right upper quadrant pain.
- Classic findings of fever, leukocytosis, and elevated erythrocyte sedimentation rate or C-reactive protein are not found in 1/3 of patients with laparoscopically diagnosed PID.

PROGNOSIS
Prognosis has been improved by treating all forms of infection with a 3rd-generation cephalosporin.

COMPLICATIONS
- Gonococcal infection during pregnancy is associated with spontaneous abortion, preterm labor, and perinatal infant mortality.
- Ophthalmia neonatorum of gonococcal origin may rapidly progress to corneal ulceration and perforation, with subsequent scarring and blindness.
- Pelvic inflammatory disease:
  - Endometritis, salpingitis, tubo-ovarian abscess, and pelvic peritonitis occur as a consequence of untreated vaginal disease.
  - Scarring secondary to salpingitis causes sterility in ≤20% of women with a single infection and ≤50% of women after 3 episodes of infection.
  - Risk of ectopic pregnancy increases sevenfold after 1 episode of PID.
- In males, rare complications include periurethral abscess, acute prostatitis, seminal vesiculitis, and urethral strictures.
- Disseminated disease:
  - Consider evaluation for complement deficiency in those with multiple episodes.
  - In neonates, arthritis is the most frequent systemic manifestation; symptoms develop 1–4 weeks after delivery. Involvement of multiple joints is typical, and most of these infants do not have ophthalmia neonatorum.

- In older children and adolescents, septic arthritis (1 joint) and a characteristic polyarthritis-dermatitis syndrome are predominant manifestations.
- Gonococcal meningitis, endocarditis, and osteomyelitis are rare in children.
- Gonococcal infection can serve as a cofactor in increasing HIV infection and transmission.

ADDITIONAL READING
- American Academy of Pediatrics. Pelvic inflammatory disease. In: Pickering LK, Baker CJ, Kimberlin DW, Long SS, eds. Report of the committee on infectious diseases, 28th ed. Elk Grove Village, IL: American Academy of Pediatrics; 2009:500–504.
- Bala M, Sood S. Cephalosporin resistance in Neisseria gonorrhoeae. J Global Infect Dis. 2010;2:284–290.
- Ingram DM, Miller WC, Schoenbach VJ, et al. Risk assessment for gonococcal and chlamydial infections in young children undergoing evaluation for sexual abuse. Pediatrics. 2001;107:e73.
- Ison C, Hughes G. Gonorrhoea themed issue. Sex Transm Infect. 2010;86:409–410.

 CODES

ICD9
- 098.7 Gonococcal infection of anus and rectum
- 098.49 Other gonococcal infection of eye
- 098.89 Gonococcal infection of other specified sites

ICD10
- A54.39 Other gonococcal eye infection
- A54.89 Other gonococcal infections
- P39.8 Other specified infections specific to the perinatal period

FAQ
- Q: What are the advantages of the nucleic amplification tests for making a diagnosis?
- A: The transcription mediated amplification (TMA) test of urine samples, approved by the FDA for women, can be used to simultaneously test for C. trachomatis and N. gonorrhea.
- Q: When is this test not approved?
- A: For rectal and pharyngeal swabs and for cases of suspected abuse.

GRAFT VERSUS HOST DISEASE

Valerie I. Brown

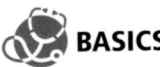 **BASICS**

DESCRIPTION
Multiorgan inflammatory process that develops when immunologically competent T lymphocytes from a histoincompatible donor are infused into an immunocompromised host unable to reject them.. Divided into acute and chronic, historically based on time of presentation, but best distinction based on clinicopathologic findings:
- Acute: Develops within 100 days after allogeneic stem cell transplant; with damage to skin, GI tract and/or liver
- Chronic: Develops 100–500 days after allogeneic stem cell transplant; with diverse features resembling autoimmune syndromes
- Chronic subtypes:
  - Progressive: Extension of acute GvHD
  - Quiescent: After resolution of acute GvHD
  - De novo: No prior acute GvHD

EPIDEMIOLOGY
- Acute GvHD (grades II–IV): 10–80% of patients receiving T-cell replete hematopoietic stem cell transplant (HSCT), 35–45% for human leukocyte antigen (HLA)–identical sibling donor bone marrow:
  - 60–80% if 1-antigen HLA-mismatched unrelated donor bone marrow or peripheral stem cells
  - 35–65% if 2-antigen HLA-mismatched unrelated umbilical cord blood
- Chronic GvHD: Most common late complication, cause of decreased quality of life, and late mortality of allogeneic HSCT
  - 15–25% if HLA-identical related marrow
  - 40–60% if HLA-matched unrelated marrow
  - 54–70% if HLA-matched unrelated peripheral stem cells
  - 20% if unrelated umbilical cord blood
- Flare-ups triggered by infection (usually viral)

RISK FACTORS
- HLA disparity (both major and minor antigens).
- Older donor or recipient age
- Stem cell source and dose: Highest with peripheral stem cells; lowest with umbilical cord
- Donor leukocyte infusions.
- Reactivation of viruses (e.g., HHV6, CMV)
- T-cell depletion decreases incidence.
- Acute disease specific:
  - Higher-intensity conditioning regimen
  - Prior pregnancies in female donors
  - Gender mismatch
- Chronic disease specific:
  - Severity of acute GvHD
  - Malignancy as indication for transplantation
  - Use of total-body irradiation
  - Type of immunosuppressive prophylaxis

Genetics
- HLA gene complex on chromosome 6; inherited as haplotype
- Full siblings: 25% chance HLA identical
- Minor histocompatibility antigen differences likely account for GvHD in HLA-identical sibling stem cell transplants.

GENERAL PREVENTION
- Transfusion: Irradiation of all cellular blood products for patients at risk
- Stem cell transplantation:
  - Selection of a histocompatible donor
  - Immunosuppression (gold standard): Cyclosporine or tacrolimus and a short course of methotrexate
  - Other options: Corticosteroids, usually with cyclosporine or tacrolimus, mycophenolate mofetil, sirolimus, and low-dose cyclophosphamide
  - Ex vivo depletion of donor T lymphocytes in graft and anti–T-cell antibodies to recipient

PATHOPHYSIOLOGY
- Acute GvHD: Interaction of donor and host innate and adaptive immune responses
  - Severity related to degree of HLA mismatch
  - 3 phases ending in "cytokine storm":
    - Tissue damage by conditioning regimen
    - Priming and activation of donor T cells: Infiltration of activated T cells into skin, GI tract, and liver resulting in apoptosis
- Chronic GvHD: Findings similar to autoimmune disorders: Donor T cell directed against host antigens, donor T-cell autoreactivity, B-cell dysregulation, regulatory T-cell deficiency. Marked collagen deposition in target organs and lack of T-cell infiltration

ETIOLOGY
- Hematopoietic stem cell transplantation
- Transfusion of nonirradiated blood products to immunodeficient hosts: Viable donor lymphocytes engraft in the recipient.
- Transfusion of nonirradiated blood from a donor homozygous for 1 of the recipient's HLA haplotypes (usually 1st- or 2nd-degree relative)
- Intrauterine maternal–fetal transfusions and exchange transfusions in neonates
- Solid organ grafts: Contain immunocompetent T cells into immune-suppressed recipient

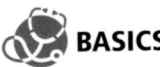 **DIAGNOSIS**

HISTORY
- Acute GvHD: Median onset: 19 days posttransplant:
  - Rash: Usually 1st manifestation; pruritus or burning sensation can precede rash.
  - Diarrhea, abdominal pain, and intestinal bleeding: Unusual to precede skin disease
  - Anorexia, nausea, vomiting, and dyspepsia
  - Jaundice (liver involvement)
- Chronic GvHD:
  - Dry eyes and/or dry mouth (sicca syndrome)
  - Blurry vision, eye irritation, photophobia, and eye pain (keratoconjunctivitis)
  - Difficulty swallowing or retrosternal pain (esophageal strictures)
  - Sensitivity to mint, spicy foods, or tomatoes
  - Weight loss, failure to thrive, diarrhea, anorexia, nausea, and vomiting
  - Dyspnea, wheezing, and cough (bronchiolitis obliterans)
  - Poor wound healing, especially after trauma
  - Joint stiffness
  - Muscle cramps
- Infections: Pneumococcal sepsis, *Pneumocystis carinii* pneumonia, invasive fungal infections

PHYSICAL EXAM
- Acute/transfusion-associated GvHD:
  - Skin (most common site): Erythema of palms, soles, ears, malar cheeks, nape of neck:
    - Can become confluent erythroderma
  - Severe form: Bullae formation, even full-thickness necrosis
  - GI tract: Diarrhea is profuse, watery, and often green and bloody.
  - Liver: Jaundice; atypical: Painful hepatomegaly, ascites, rapid weight gain
- Chronic GvHD:
  - Skin (involved in almost every patient):
    - Hyperpigmentation or hypopigmentation, xerosis (skin dryness), pruritus, patchy erythema, scaling, poikiloderma, skin atrophy; lichenoid, eczematous, and/or sclerodermatous changes
    - Advanced scleroderma: Thickened, tight, and fragile skin
  - Hair: Thin, fragile; premature graying
  - Scalp: Dry or seborrheic
  - Nails: Vertical ridging; dystrophic and fragile; entire nail can be lost.
  - Mouth: Mucositis, ulcers, pseudomembranes. Whitish lacey plaques or ulcers on tongue or buccal surfaces: May be painful
  - Cannot open mouth fully owing to sclerosis
  - Esophageal strictures, stenosis, or webs
  - Blood: Thrombocytopenia, anemia, eosinophilia, hypo- or hypergammaglobulinemia, autoantibodies
  - Joints: Stiffness and/or swelling. Contractures may occur without joint swelling.
  - Eosinophilic fasciitis, myositis
  - Lung: Bronchiolitis obliterans (obstructive), bronchiolitis obliterans organizing pneumonia (restrictive)
  - Other: Pericardial/pleural effusions, cardiomyopathy, nephritic syndrome, peripheral neuropathy, genital ulceration

DIAGNOSTIC TESTS & INTERPRETATION
Diagnosis is often made on clinical grounds.

Lab
- Complete blood count with differential and Coombs test: Autoimmune thrombocytopenia (most common), hemolytic anemia, and neutropenia. Eosinophilia: Resolves with treatment
- Howell-Jolly bodies on blood smear: Functional asplenia of chronic GvHD
- Elevated ALT/AST without hyperbilirubinemia
- Vitamin D: May be low; risk for osteoporosis
- Urinalysis: May show protein, glucose, blood
- Schirmer test: Decreased tear production
- Pulmonary function tests
- Echocardiogram/electrocardiogram
- Fluorescein biomicroscopy: Punctate keratopathy

Imaging
- High-resolution chest CT: Bronchiolitis obliterans
- Barium swallow: Strictures, webs

Diagnostic Procedures/Other
- Endoscopy with biopsy: Upper GI tract GvHD
- Skin biopsy: Localized epidermal atrophy
- Liver biopsy: Bile duct damage reminiscent of primary biliary cirrhosis
- Buccal/labial biopsy: Rule out viral/fungal infections
- Analysis of pleural, pericardial fluid

DIFFERENTIAL DIAGNOSIS
- Acute GvHD:
  - Skin: Drug reaction, chemoradiotherapy, viral exanthema, engraftment syndrome; TEN for grade IV skin GvHD
  - Liver: Hepatic veno-occlusive disease, side effect of total parenteral nutrition, drug toxicity, bacterial sepsis, or viral infection
  - GI: Diarrhea secondary to transplant conditioning regimen, infectious causes (e.g., *Clostridium difficile*, CMV), or opiate withdrawal
- Chronic GvHD:
  - Skin: Keratosis pilaris, eczema, psoriasis

ALERT
- Do not give live vaccine if chronic GvHD is present. May result in symptomatic infection
- Sudden high fevers may indicate bacterial sepsis that can be overwhelming. Chronic GvHD patients often functionally asplenic and have profound immune function impairment

 TREATMENT

MEDICATION (DRUGS)
- Treatment of acute GvHD (grades II–IV):
  - Systemic steroids (2 mg/kg/d) for 2 weeks, followed by a quick taper
  - Cyclosporine or tacrolimus if patient is not already receiving it as prophylaxis
  - Mycophenolate mofetil, sirolimus (rapamycin), antithymocyte globulin, and etanercept (experimental) as 2nd-line drugs
  - Infliximab (Remicade) for steroid-refractory GI tract disease
  - Other options: Extracorporeal photophoresis; mesenchymal stem cells (experimental)
  - Visceral organ involvement requires urgent start of 2nd-line therapy.
  - For isolated, mild skin GvHD, topical tacrolimus ointment and triamcinolone
- Treatment of chronic GvHD:
  - Steroids alone or with cyclosporine, sirolimus, tacrolimus, or mycophenolate mofetil
  - Goal: Steroids <0.5 mg/kg alternating days with cyclosporine or tacrolimus
- Steroid-refractory GvHD:
  - Mycophenolate mofetil, sirolimus, pentostatin (investigational)
  - Other options many off-label: Antithymocyte globulin; rituximab, especially for low platelets; low-dose methotrexate in liver GvHD; thalidomide; hydroxychloroquine; imatinib; low-dose cyclophosphamide; etanercept; alefacept alemtuzumab: High infection risk
- Extracorporeal photopheresis: Very effective for chronic skin GvHD; lower response rate if visceral organs involved
- Psoralen plus ultraviolet A is of some benefit in skin GvHD (lichenoid, not sclerotic).
- Oral rinses with dexamethasone: Oral GvHD
- Ursodeoxycholic acid: Hepatic GvHD

ADDITIONAL TREATMENT
General Measures
- Prophylaxis for *Pneumocystis carinii* pneumonia and pneumococcal infection
- Antifungal coverage if on multiple immunosuppressive agents
- IV immunoglobulin if low serum IgG levels
- Monitor closely for viral reactivation.
- Skin care: Lubricate dry skin with petroleum jelly. Protect skin from injury. Avoid sunburn.
- Artificial tears for sicca syndrome.
- Correct electrolyte imbalances for muscular aches and cramps.
- Physical therapy/range-of-motion exercises to prevent contractures
- Inhaled corticosteroids and azithromycin (experimental) for bronchiolitis obliterans
- Nutrition consults for malnutrition and wasting
- If chronic GvHD persists past 2–3 months or prednisone needed at 1 mg/kg/d, alternative therapy should be used.
- Hospitalization may be required for hydration, nutritional support, IV medications, monitoring, treatment of infections, and other supportive care.

 ONGOING CARE

FOLLOW-UP RECOMMENDATIONS
Patient Monitoring
- Steroids: Osteoporosis, diabetes
- Calcineurin inhibitors: Hypertension, renal dysfunction, hypomagnesemia
- Sirolimus: Hyperlipidemia, leucopenia, microangiopathic hemolytic anemia
- Mycophenolate mofetil: GI discomfort, diarrhea, leukopenia

PROGNOSIS
Prognosis of GvHD is based on severity:
- Acute GvHD: Graded from I to IV based on organ involvement, percent of body surface area involved (skin), volume of diarrhea (gut), and/or elevation of serum bilirubin (liver):
  - Grade I: One organ, usually skin; survival is the same as for patients without GvHD.
  - Grade II: >1 organ, with skin rash >50% body surface area, severe nausea/vomiting, diarrhea, and/or bilirubin elevation
  - Grade III: Severe multiorgan involvement, 25% long-term survival
  - Grade IV: Generalized erythroderma with bullae and desquamation; stage 4 liver. Survival is only 5–15%.
- Acute GvHD: 50–60% of patients respond to corticosteroids plus cyclosporine or tacrolimus.
- Poor prognosis for survival: Extensive skin involvement, progressive onset, GI involvement, thrombocytopenia, weight loss, and low Karnofsky performance status (40–60% survival)
- 50% of patients still require therapy 5 years after diagnosis of chronic GvHD.

COMPLICATIONS
- Mortality from GvHD after stem cell transplantation is usually related to infection.
- Rarely, patients die of hepatic failure or abdominal catastrophe.
- In transfusion-associated GvHD, death is usually from bone marrow aplasia with destruction of the host's marrow by donor lymphocytes.

ADDITIONAL READING
- Baird K, Cooke K, Schultz KR. Chronic graft-versus-host disease (GVHD) in children. *Pediatr Clin North Am.* 2010;57:297–322.
- Carpenter PA, MacMillan ML. Management of acute graft versus host disease in children. *Pediatr Clin North Am.* 2010;57:273–295.
- Jacobsohn DA. Optimal management of chronic graft-versus-host disease in children. *Br J Haematology.* 2010;150:278–292.
- Ram R, Gafter-Gvili A, Yeshurun M, et al. Prophylaxis regimens for GVHD: Systematic review and meta-analysis. *Bone Marrow Transplant.* 2009;43:643–653.
- Reddy P, Arora M, Guimond M, et al. GVHD: A continuing barrier to the safety of allogeneic transplantation. *Biol Blood Marrow Transplant.* 2009;15:162–168.
- Schlomchik WD. Graft-versus-host disease. *Nat Rev Immunol.* 2007;7:340–357.
- Wolff D, Schleuning M, von Harsdorf S, et al. Consensus Conference on Clinical Practice in Chronic GVHD: Second-line treatment of chronic graft-versus-host disease. *Biol Blood Marrow Transplant.* 2011;17:1–17.

 CODES

ICD9
996.85 Graft versus host disease

ICD10
- D89.810 Acute graft-versus-host disease
- D89.811 Chronic graft-versus-host disease
- D89.813 Graft-versus-host disease, unspecified

FAQ
- Q: If a child gets acute GvHD, does that mean that he will get chronic GvHD?
- A: No. ~30% of patients <10 years of age who receive HLA-identical sibling bone marrow transplantation will get acute GvHD, whereas only 13% will develop chronic GvHD. Of note, chronic GvHD can develop in a patient who did not have acute disease; the prognosis is much more favorable than for the progressive form.
- Q: Do patients with severe chronic graft versus host disease all die?
- A: No. Occasionally the graft versus host disease will "burn out." This is rare, and the process by which it happens is not understood.

G

GRAVES DISEASE
Adda Grimberg

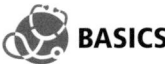 **BASICS**

DESCRIPTION
Multisystem autoimmune disorder that presents with the classic triad of hyperthyroidism (goiter), exophthalmos, and dermopathy (rare in children)

EPIDEMIOLOGY
Female > male (4–5:1)

Incidence
- 10–15% of all childhood thyroid disorders
- Incidence increases with age, peaking in adolescence and in the 3rd–4th decades.

RISK FACTORS
- No simple hereditary pattern (i.e., genetic susceptibility plus environmental factors):
  - Up to 60% of patients have a family history of autoimmune thyroid disease (hyperthyroidism or hypothyroidism).
  - Concordance rates of Graves disease: 17% in monozygotic twins (although another 17% had chronic lymphocytic thyroiditis and 10% had other nonthyroid autoimmune conditions); 2% in dizygotic twins; 4% of 1st-degree relatives
- Associated with higher frequency of HLA-DR3
- Increased incidence in genetic syndromes:
  - Down syndrome: Presents at a younger age, no female predominance as seen in the general population. Usually milder course
  - Turner syndrome

PATHOPHYSIOLOGY
- Autoimmune process that includes production of immunoglobulins against antigens in the thyroid, orbital tissue, and dermis
- IgG1 anti-TSH (thyroid-stimulating hormone receptor autoantibody, thyroid-stimulating immunoglobulin (Ig)) activates the receptor, causing constitutive stimulation; thyroid follicular cells increase production and release of thyroid hormone.

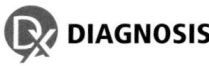 **DIAGNOSIS**

ALERT
Failure to recognize thyroid storm, which constitutes an endocrinologic medical emergency

HISTORY
- Growth acceleration also associated with precocious puberty
- Hyperthyroidism can accelerate the bone age (i.e., advance the developmental tempo).
- Declining school performance, mind racing, concentration difficulty. May be mistaken for ADHD
- Symptoms of hyperthyroidism and their duration (if child complains of these symptoms, evaluate for possible hyperthyroidism):
  - Restlessness, emotional lability, nervousness
  - Fine tremor
  - Insomnia and disturbed sleep pattern; may result in daytime fatigue
  - Weight loss, despite increased appetite
  - Palpitations or chest pain with minimal exertion or at rest; low exercise tolerance
  - Heat intolerance
  - Diarrhea and increased urination

- Muscle weakness (proximal)
- Plummer nails (separation of nail from bed)
- Menstrual irregularities
- Thyroid gland enlargement (duration and tenderness): Graves disease can present with goiter. Tenderness suggests an infectious cause.
- Bulging of the eyes, increased staring, change in vision or in facial appearance: Exophthalmos due to retro-orbital immune depositions is a hallmark of Graves disease.
- Familial history: Increased incidence of Graves disease in families with thyroid disease

PHYSICAL EXAM
- Accelerated growth, or height above expected genetic potential due to bone age advancement
- Symmetrically enlarged, smooth, nontender goiter in >95% of cases
- Auscultate the thyroid gland for bruit while patient holds his or her breath.
- Glandular hyperperfusion is associated with hyperthyroidism.
- Resting tachycardia with widened pulse pressure; hyperdynamic precordium: Cardiac effects of excessive thyroid hormone
- Slightly elevated temperature: Thyroid hormone controls basal metabolic rate and upregulates catecholamine-induced thermogenesis.
- Lid lag/stare; exophthalmos and proptosis: Severe ophthalmopathy is rare.
- Fine tremor especially visible in hands and tongue in ~60% of children with Graves disease.
- Proximal muscle weakness is common but seldom severe.
- Exaggerated deep tendon reflexes are variable.
- Skin warmth and moisture: Heat intolerance and excessive sweating in >30% of children

DIAGNOSTIC TESTS & INTERPRETATION
Lab
- Total or free thyroxine: Elevated
- Triiodothyronine assessment by radioimmunoassay: Elevated (triiodothyronine radioimmunoassay, as direct measurement of triiodothyronine, and not triiodothyronine resin uptake, which indirectly evaluates thyroid hormone–binding capacity)
- TSH: Significantly suppressed or undetectable
- TSI titer: Positive in 90% of children.

  False-positive test results: Elevated total thyroxine levels can also be caused by conditions involving increased protein binding, but they are not necessarily diagnostic for hyperthyroidism: Increased estrogen states (e.g., pregnancy and oral contraceptive use) lead to augmented hepatic thyroid-binding globulin (TBG) production. Familial dysalbuminemic hyperthyroxinemia: Mutation affecting the binding affinity leads to increased protein-bound pool.

Imaging
I^{123} scan: Not needed to diagnose Graves disease. Shows diffuse increased uptake at 6 and 24 hours. If palpation suggests a nodule, scan may reveal a hot nodule within a suppressed gland.

DIFFERENTIAL DIAGNOSIS
- Infectious:
  - Acute suppurative thyroiditis (i.e., transient thyroxine elevations)
  - Subacute thyroiditis after viral illness (also transient hyperthyroidism)

- Environmental:
  - Thyroid hormone ingestion
  - Ingestion of excess iodine (escape from Wolff-Chaikoff block due to impaired autoregulation)
- Tumors (all rare in childhood):
  - TSH-producing pituitary adenoma
  - Thyroid adenoma/hyperfunctioning autonomous thyroid nodule (most pediatric patients are euthyroid; incidence of nodule hyperfunctioning rises with patient age)
  - Thyroid carcinoma (rarely presents with hyperthyroidism)
- Congenital:
  - Neonatal Graves disease (transplacental antibody transfer from mothers with Graves disease or chronic thyroiditis)
- Genetic and developmental:
  - Pituitary resistance to thyroid hormones (dominant negative thyroid-receptor gene mutations causing loss of pituitary negative feedback loop and inappropriately elevated levels of TSH; can be isolated, with clinical hyperthyroidism, or associated with peripheral thyroid resistance and clinical euthyroidism or hypothyroidism)
  - TSH-receptor gene mutations (rare; germline activating TSH-receptor mutations cause autosomal dominant nonautoimmune hereditary hyperthyroidism)
  - McCune-Albright syndrome: Activating G-protein mutation can lead to indolent hyperthyroidism in addition to the classic features of this syndrome
  - Ectopic thyroid tissue
- Other causes of hyperthyroidism: See "Goiter."

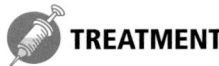 **TREATMENT**

Radiotherapy
I^{131} ablation therapy:
- 90–100% effective; safe and definitive, with predictable outcome
- Results in permanent hypothyroidism requiring lifelong thyroxine replacement
- Adequate dose should be used (>150 μCi/g of thyroid tissue) to prevent residual tissue that would be at risk of developing thyroid cancer.
- Current recommendations advise avoiding I^{131} ablation in children <5 years of age owing to theoretical concerns relating radiation exposure and cancer risks.
- Radioiodine ablation may exacerbate the ophthalmopathy, but this effect can be prevented with concomitant glucocorticoid administration.

MEDICATION (DRUGS)

ALERT
- Antihistamines and cold medications may worsen sympathetic nervous system symptoms.
- Stopping antithyroid drugs because of low thyroxine values where TSH is still suppressed, reflecting continued TSI activity, will likely result in relapse. Antithyroid medication dosage should be decreased, or L-thyroxine should be added.
- FDA issued a black box warning (6/4/2009) against propylthiouracil (PTU) use in treating Graves disease owing to risk of severe liver injury including life-threatening acute liver failure.

First Line
- Drug therapy is the 1st-line choice in children.
- Antithyroid medications (thiourea derivatives): 65–95% effective:
  - Medications block thyroid hormone synthesis but not the release of existing hormone.
  - Methimazole
  - Propylthiouracil (PTU): Note black box warning. Limited, short-term use of PTU may be considered for patients requiring antithyroid medication (neither I[131] ablation nor prompt surgery are options) or after a toxic reaction to methimazole. PTU is preferred during 1st trimester of pregnancy (teratogenic effects of methimazole).
- Propranolol and atenolol block adrenergic symptoms; should be used along with antithyroid medications at the start of treatment and whenever cardiac symptoms are prominent.
- Duration of treatment:
  - Antithyroid medications can be tapered and potentially discontinued after 2–3 years of therapy, depending on the patient's course.
  - β-Blockers: Continue until thyroxine and triiodothyronine are under control (~6 weeks).
  - If remission not achieved in 1–2 years, ablation with radioactive iodine [(131)I] or total or subtotal thyroidectomy may be considered.

SURGERY/OTHER PROCEDURES
Total or near-total thyroidectomy:
- Effective, rapid, and definitive (vs. 30% recurrence rate for subtotal thyroidectomy)
- Lifelong thyroxine replacement needed
- Surgical complication rates higher for children age 0–6 years and in lower-volume centers

ISSUES FOR REFERRAL
Treatment for severe ophthalmopathy: Must refer patient to an ophthalmologist:
- 3 options: High-dose glucocorticoids, orbital radiotherapy, or surgical orbital decompression
- Rehabilitative surgery for eye muscles or eyelids is often needed after the ophthalmopathy has been treated.

ONGOING CARE

PROGNOSIS
- Good, if compliant with treatment
- Mortality in severe thyrotoxicosis is possible from cardiac arrhythmias or cardiac failure.
- Spontaneous remission occurs in 20–30% of children after 1–2 years, but can relapse in 30%. Large thyroid gland size (by ultrasound) and high titers of TSH-receptor antibody (TRAb) predict lower chance of remission.
- Neonatal hyperthyroidism remits by 48 weeks and more commonly by 20 weeks.
- Propranolol or atenolol should result in rapid relief of symptoms of sympathetic hyperactivity.
- 4–6 weeks of medical treatment should result in normalization of levels of thyroxine and triiodothyronine, although TSH levels may remain suppressed owing to persistent underlying activity of the thyroid-stimulating Ig.

- Persistent suppression of TSH is associated with pretreatment presence of thyrotropin-binding inhibitory Ig, severity of thyrotoxicosis, and time to recovery of thyroid hormone levels.
- Duration and type of treatment depend on patient age and remission and relapse pattern.

COMPLICATIONS
- Endocrine disturbances: Delayed/early puberty, menstrual irregularity, hypercalcemia
- Ophthalmologic: 3–5% of patients develop severe ophthalmopathy, including eye muscle dysfunction and optic neuropathy, requiring specific treatment by an ophthalmologist. Pediatric ophthalmologic findings (lid lag, soft tissue involvement, and proptosis) are more common but usually less severe than in adults.
- Bone: Osteopenia common at diagnosis due to high bone turnover. Corrects with treatment of Graves disease and return to euthyroid status.
- Fetal/Neonatal: Intrauterine growth retardation (IUGR), nonimmune hydrops fetalis, craniosynostosis, intrauterine death, goiter that complicates labor and can cause life-threatening airway obstruction at delivery, hyperkinesis, failure to thrive, diarrhea, vomiting, cardiac failure and arrhythmias, systemic and pulmonary hypertension, hepatosplenomegaly, jaundice, hyperviscosity syndrome, thrombocytopenia.
- Medication side effects: Agranulocytosis (in 0.2–0.5% of patients), rash (most common side effect), gastrointestinal upset, headache, transient transaminitis/hepatitis and life-threatening liver failure with PTU, vasculitis with PTU (frequently associated with perinuclear antineutrophil cytoplasmic antibody [pANCA] titers)

ADDITIONAL READING

- De Luca F, Corrias A, Salerno M, et al. Peculiarities of Graves' disease in children and adolescents with Down's syndrome. *Eur J Endocrinol*. 2010;162: 591–595.
- Gogakos AI, Boboridis K, Krassas GE. Pediatric aspects in Graves' orbitopathy. *Pediatr Endocrinol Rev*. 2010;7(Suppl 2):234–244.
- Hemminki K, Li X, Sundquist J, et al. The epidemiology of Graves' disease: Evidence of a genetic and an environmental contribution. *J Autoimmun*. 2010;34:J307–J313.
- Langley RW, Burch HB. Perioperative management of the thyrotoxic patient. *Endocrinol Metab Clin North Am*. 2003;32:519–534.
- Manji N, Carr-Smith JD, Boelaert K, et al. Influences of age, gender, smoking, and family history on autoimmune thyroid disease phenotype. *J Clin Endocrinol Metab*. 2006;91:4873–4880.
- Papendieck P, Chiesa A, Prieto L, et al. Thyroid disorders of neonates born to mothers with Graves' disease. *J Pediatr Endocrinol Metab*. 2009;22: 547–553.
- Rahhal SN, Eugster EA. Thyroid stimulating immunoglobulin is often negative in children with Graves' disease. *J Pediatr Endocrinol Metab*. 2008;21:1085–1088.
- Rivkees SA. Pediatric Graves' disease: Controversies in management. *Horm Res Paediatr*. 2010;74: 305–311.
- Wilhelm SM, McHenry CR. Total thyroidectomy is superior to subtotal thyroidectomy for management of Graves' disease in the United States. *World J Surg*. 2010;34:1261–1264.

CODES

ICD9
- 242.00 Toxic diffuse goiter without mention of thyrotoxic crisis or storm
- 242.01 Toxic diffuse goiter with mention of thyrotoxic crisis or storm

ICD10
- E05.00 Thyrotoxicosis with diffuse goiter without thyrotoxic crisis or storm
- E05.01 Thyrotoxicosis with diffuse goiter with thyrotoxic crisis or storm

FAQ
- Q: Does Graves disease lead to thyroid cancer?
- A: No, although controversy surrounds the role of TSH and the closely related TSH-receptor antibodies of Graves disease in thyroid cancer's incidence and aggressiveness. There is an increased incidence of benign thyroid adenoma from 0.6–1.9% after therapy involving I[131] ablation.
- Q: Does hyperthyroidism affect long-term growth or final adult height?
- A: No. Hyperthyroidism can cause tall stature and acceleration of skeletal maturity, but does not typically affect final adult height.
- Q: Should WBC counts be monitored routinely while patients are on antithyroid medications?
- A: No. Routine monitoring is not cost effective because agranulocytosis is rare and sudden in onset. WBC counts should be checked when a patient on antithyroid medication develops fever.
- Q: Will the ophthalmopathy correct with antithyroid treatment?
- A: Not necessarily. It may require specific intervention by an ophthalmologist.
- Q: Can mothers breastfeed while they are being treated for Graves disease?
- A: Yes. PTU has a lower milk/serum concentration ratio than methimazole (0:1 and 1:0, respectively). In 1 study, 3 of 11 infants exclusively breastfed by women on 300–750 mg daily PTU had high levels of TSH; of these 3, 1 was just above the normal range and the other 2 completely corrected while the mother was still being medicated.

G

GROWTH HORMONE DEFICIENCY

Jeffrey D. Roizen
Craig A. Alter
Preneet Brar (5th edition)

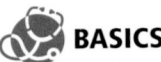

BASICS

DESCRIPTION
Growth hormone deficiency (GHD) is one of the rare causes of growth failure due to a lack of growth hormone action caused by a defect in GH synthesis (insufficient hormone), release or signalling (decreased responsiveness to normal or high levels of hormone).

EPIDEMIOLOGY
- Incidence in the USA is 1:4,000.
- Males are more commonly diagnosed than females.
- 2 peak ages of diagnosis:
  - infantile at—<1 year of age, usually because of associated hypoglycemia
  - childhood—>4 years of age, usually because of poor linear growth

Prevalence
~1:3,500 in school age children

Genetics
- Spontaneous
- Autosomal recessive
- Autosomal dominant
- X-linked forms

PATHOPHYSIOLOGY
Absence of GH action leads to decreased levels of insulin like growth factor I (IGF-I, formerly somatomedin-C), a protein that acts on cartilage at the growth plate to stimulate linear growth. GH has some direct effect on growth as well.

ETIOLOGY
- Idiopathic (the most common cause, a diagnosis of exclusion).
- Congenital idiopathic: Congenital malformation of the pituitary which can be associated with:
  - Holoprosencephaly
  - Septo-optic dysplasia
  - Midline defects: Cleft lip, cleft palate, central maxillary incisor
  - Ectopic posterior pituitary, small anterior pituitary, and/or hypoplastic infundibulum
  - Genetic mutations:
    o Familial multiple anterior pituitary hormone deficiency (Pit-1, Prop-1)
    o GH gene mutations (Type Ia, Ib, II, III)
  - GH insensitivity:
    o Laron dwarfism, which is an autosomal recessive disorder classically caused by mutation of the GH receptor, presents with the phenotype of severe GH deficiency (severe short stature, hypoplastic nasal bridge, sparse hair, high-pitched voice, and delayed bone age).
    o Postreceptor and second messenger defects such as IGF-I gene deletion, IGF-I receptor mutation, STAT5b mutation

- Acquired idiopathic (many likely due to hypophysitis):
  - Tumors: Craniopharyngioma, Germinoma, Medulloblastoma, Glioma, Pinealoma
  - Pituitary or hypothalamic irradiation
  - Trauma: Child abuse or closed head injury
  - Surgical resection/damage of the pituitary gland/stalk
  - Birth injury/Perinatal insult
  - Infection: Viral encephalitis, Bacterial or fungal infection, Tuberculosis,
  - Vascular: Pituitary infarction or aneurysm
  - Infiltration affecting pituitary gland or sella turcica: Histiocytosis, Sarcoidosis
  - Psychosocial deprivation.

DIAGNOSIS

HISTORY
- Family history:
  - Parents' height
  - Family history of short stature (women <4 feet 11 inches or men <5 feet 4 inches) indicates genetic shortness.
  - Family history of delayed puberty "late bloomer" (growth after high school, menarche at ≥14 years): Constitutional delay of growth and development tends to occur in family members.
- Birth history:
  - Babies born small for gestational age. 10–15% will not show "catch up growth," but are not typically GHD
  - Babies with congenital GHD may not be short at birth but will grow poorly over the next few years.
- Medication history: Look for overusage of corticosteroids, either systemic or inhaled. Ask about nonprescription drugs and health food store supplements.
- Dentition history: "Poor man's bone age," i.e., when first tooth was lost as an indicator of delay in skeletal maturation.
- Psychosocial history: Poor growth occurring at the time of a major stressful event may be due to psychosocial deprivation.
- Clues to etiology:
  - Hypopituitarism: Hypoglycemia, prolonged jaundice, micropenis
  - Increasing weight for height indicates an endocrinologic cause for the poor growth (GHD, hypothyroidism, hypercortisolism).
  - Hypothyroidism: Lethargy, weight gain, constipation, and dryness of skin
  - Turner syndrome: Wide-spaced nipples, marked short stature, cubitus valgus, scoliosis, and delayed puberty
  - Celiac disease or inflammatory bowel disease: Poor weight gain, vomiting, loose stools diarrhea, food-provoked GI distress

- Cardiac disease, renal tubular acidosis, chronic renal insufficiency, HIV, tuberculosis
- Prader–Willi or Down syndrome: Hypotonia and developmental delay
- Skeletal changes such as achondroplasia/hypochondroplasia; often have abnormal body proportions.

PHYSICAL EXAM
- Measure accurate weight and height with wall stadiometer.
- Neurologic examination, including visual fields and fundoscopic examination for evaluation of brain tumors
- Dental age, scoliosis, and proportionality of limbs relative to height are good skeletal indicators.
- Cubitus valgus and shortened 4th metacarpal for girls with Turner syndrome
- Midline facial defects such as submucous cleft, cleft lip and palate are associated with hypopituitarism.
- Tanner stage: Micropenis is associated with congenital hypopituitarism; delayed puberty suggests constitutional delay, but may also be indicative of panhypopituitarism
- Cherubic facies with frontal bossing, thin hair, high pitched voice, and relative truncal obesity with adiposity are seen in GHD.

DIAGNOSTIC TESTS & INTERPRETATION
Lab
- IGF-I and IGF binding protein-3 (IGFBP-3) production is regulated directly by GH. IGF-I values are low early in life and in conditions other than GHD such as hypothyroidism, diabetes, renal failure, and undernutrition.
- GH provocative testing: A random GH level is generally of little value to diagnose GHD beyond the neonatal period, after this time, GH is mostly secreted only in brief pulses during deep sleep (at night). Fully 20% of healthy GH-replete children can fail any provocative test. False-positive and negative results are common.
- CBC with differential: Anemia, malignancy, cell-based immunodeficiency and inflammatory processes
- Sedimentation rate and CRP: Inflammatory processes such as in Crohn disease
- Hepatic and renal function tests: Hepatic or renal disease
- Chromosomes in females (to exclude Turner syndrome)
- Thyroid function tests [thyroid-stimulating hormone (TSH) and either a T4 or a Free T4]

Imaging
- Bone age: Radiography of left hand and wrist
- If provocative testing shows GH deficiency an MRI with contrast of the pituitary and hypothalamus to look for central nervous system tumor or anomaly of the hypothalamus/pituitary

DIFFERENTIAL DIAGNOSIS
- Constitutional delay of growth and adolescence
- Familial short stature
- Malnutrition
- Intrauterine growth retardation
- Renal failure
- Inflammatory bowel disease
- Celiac sprue
- Hypochondroplasia, achondroplasia, or other skeletal dysplasia
- Turner syndrome
- Noonans syndrome
- Russell–Silver syndrome
- Prader–Willi syndrome
- Other genetic syndromes
- Congenital heart disease
- Hypothyroidism
- Hypercortisolism
- Metabolic disorders
- Rickets

ALERT
- Children with constitutional growth delay or pubertal delay show poor growth when peers are going through their pubertal growth spurts, and have a delayed bone age, mimicking GH deficiency.
- GH provocative testing may yield false-positive or false-negative results:
  - 20% of normal children will fail at least 1 GH provocative test.
  - Obese but otherwise normal children are more likely to fail provocative GH testing.
  - When GH testing is done in a child at high risk for GHD or if the growth pattern is concerning, the predictive value of GH testing is markedly improved.
- Malnutrition can cause low IGF-I.
- Psychosocial deprivation mimics GHD. Such deprived patients may have low growth factors and respond poorly to GH provocative testing.
- rhGH is associated with idiopathic intracranial hypertension (pseudotumor cerebri). This side effect is usually transient and often reverses without cessation of therapy.
- rhGH is usually not given in cancer patients until 1 year has elapsed without recurrence
- Carefully evaluate any limp, or hip or knee pain in patients on rhGH therapy because these symptoms may be associated with SCFE; SCFE necessitates orthopedic consultation.

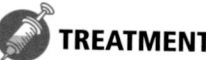 TREATMENT

MEDICATION (DRUGS)
- Recombinant human GH (rhGH) was approved by FDA) for use in 1985 by SQ injection daily.
- IGF-I therapy for the rare cases of GH insensitivity
- Duration of therapy (in children and adolescents):
  - Until growth velocity drops to 2.5 cm/year
  - When puberty is complete
  - GH-deficient adults may benefit from lifelong rhGH therapy due to its effects on body composition, lipids, bone density, and general sense of well being.
  - Adult patients should undergo repeat GH provocative testing (off rhGH therapy unless there is panhypopituitarism).

 ONGOING CARE

FOLLOW-UP RECOMMENDATIONS
Every 3 months by an endocrinologist:
- When to expect improvement:
  - Immediate effect on hypoglycemia
  - Growth velocity improves within 3–6 months
- Signs to watch for:
  - Pseudotumor cerebri (headache, vision problems)
  - Slipped capital femoral epiphysis
  - Theoretically, increased risk of leukemia (although most studies indicate no significant increased risk)
  - In adults, edema and carpal tunnel syndrome, but uncommon in children

PROGNOSIS
Excellent with treatment

COMPLICATIONS
- Short stature
- Lack of self-esteem because of short stature
- Delay in pubertal changes (sexual characteristics and growth spurt) due to delayed bone age
- Hypoglycemia (in the newborn period)
- Osteopenia

ADDITIONAL READING
- Camach-Hubner C, Rose S, Preece M, et al. Pharmacokinetic studies of recombinant human insulin-like growth factor-1 (rhIGF-I)/rhIGF-binding protein-3 complex administered to patients with growth hormone insensitivity syndrome. *J Clin Endocrinol Metab*. 2006;91:1246–1253.
- Clayton PE, Cohen P, Tanaka T, et al. Diagnosis of growth hormone deficiency in childhood. On behalf of the Growth Hormone Research Society. *Horm Res*. 2000;53(suppl 3):30.

- Clayton PE, Cowell CT. Safety issues in children and adolescents during growth hormone therapy—a review. *Growth Hormone IGF Res*. 2000;10:306–317.
- Cohen P, Bright G, Rogol A, et al. Effects of dose and gender on growth and growth factor response to GH in GH deficient children: Implications for efficacy and safety. *J Clin Endocrinol Metab*. 2001;87:90–98.
- Pitukcheewanont P, Desrosiers P, Steelman J, et al. Issues and trends in pediatric growth hormone therapy—an update from the GHMonitor observational registry. *Pediatr Endocrinol Rev*. 2008;5(Suppl 2):702–707.
- Richmond EJ, Rogol AD. Growth hormone deficiency in children. *Pituitary*. 2008;11(2):115–120
- Rosenfeld RG. Biochemical diagnostic strategies in the evaluation of short stature: The diagnosis of insulin-like growth factor deficiency. *Horm Res*. 1996;46:170.

 CODES

ICD9
253.3 Pituitary dwarfism

ICD10
E23.0 Hypopituitarism

FAQ

- Q: Does GH increase adult height in patients with familial short stature?
- A: Clinical studies have shown that rhGH may improve final adult height in some children; however, the results are unpredictable. The FDA recently added severe idiopathic short stature (predicted adult height <3rd percentile) as an approved indication for human GH therapy, but its use in this setting is not uncontroversial—with a treatment duration of 4–7 years, these children gain an average of roughly 3.5–7.5 cm in their adult height, but there is significant variation and many children have no final adult height gain..
- Q: Does GH cause tumors?
- A: Clinical studies have not confirmed an association.

G

GUILLAIN-BARRÉ SYNDROME

James Boyd

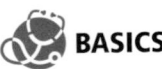

BASICS

DESCRIPTION
Guillain–Barré syndrome (GBS) is an acute disorder of the peripheral nerves—an inflammatory polyradiculoneuropathy. It causes progressive weakness in the limbs, face, and respiratory muscles. Autonomic and sensory disturbance occur with loss of sensation or pain. Neurologic deficits peak by 4 weeks or sooner.

EPIDEMIOLOGY
Incidence
Overall yearly incidence rate of 0.6–1.9 cases per 100,000. Of 95 reported pediatric GBS patients, 45 were aged 1–5 years, 36 were aged 6–10 years, and 14 were aged 11–15 years.

RISK FACTORS
Genetics
Particular subtypes of GBS are more common among certain human leukocyte antigen (HLA) types. No data indicate an increase in GBS among first-order relatives.

PATHOPHYSIOLOGY
Inflammatory cell-mediated and humoral-mediated immune mechanisms play a role in segmental demyelination on nerve biopsy; lymphocytes and macrophages participate in myelin destruction. Axonal variants of GBS feature axonal degeneration without demyelination. Circulating anti-ganglioside antibodies (e.g., GM1, GM2, GQ1B) found in particular subtypes suggest a molecular mimicry mechanism stimulated by infection.

ETIOLOGY
- Follows viral infection in >50% of cases. Cytomegalovirus, Epstein–Barr virus, varicella-zoster virus, acute HIV infection, others
- Also associated with bacterial infection (especially *Campylobacter jejuni*), surgery, and vaccination
- Tetanus toxoid is the only vaccination in common use with a clear link to GBS. Often, no precipitating event can be identified.

COMMONLY ASSOCIATED CONDITIONS
- GBS is seen in a higher-than-expected rate in patients with sarcoidosis, systemic lupus erythematosus, lymphoma, HIV infection, Lyme disease, and solid tumors.
- Muscle atrophy, joint contractures, pressure ulcers, chronic pain, hypertension, voiding difficulty

DIAGNOSIS

HISTORY
- GBS has a variety of clinical presentations so that index of suspicion is critical. Typical features are progressive motor weakness and areflexia, often following distal sensory changes. Common presentations include decreased ambulation (or crawling in toddlers), facial weakness, back pain, or sensory changes in the extremities.
- After respiratory status has been stabilized, address autonomic dysfunction and pain. Close monitoring required for dysautonomic symptoms: Arrhythmias, BP lability/orthostasis, ileus, urinary retention.
- Most patients first note leg weakness or gait instability that progresses over days to weeks.
- Paresthesias and pain typically occur in a stocking/glove distribution frequently early in the course.
- 2/3 of patients will report symptoms of an infection 2–3 weeks earlier. Consider polio if fever is present at symptom onset.
- Weakness may lead to respiratory paralysis in 20–30% of children with GBS.

PHYSICAL EXAM
- Weakness and sensory changes:
  - Typical signs of GBS, classically with distal greater than proximal involvement. A proximal predominance of symptoms does not preclude the diagnosis.
  - Typically, deep tendon reflexes are lost within 1 week.
- Respiratory difficulty-impaired upper airway or restrictive/neurogenic, with decreased vital capacity, maximum inspiratory (PiMax) and expiratory (PeMax) pressures:
  - Respiratory failure leads to intubation in up to 25% of patients. Bulbar weakness and poor airway protection can also necessitate intubation. Impending respiratory failure can often be unpredictable, and blood gas determination is not a useful indicator of neuromuscular respiratory failure until intubation is imminent. If close monitoring of vital capacity, inspiratory, or expiratory pressures suggests >30% decline in 24 hours, monitor patient in ICU.
- Bilateral facial weakness occurs in ≤50% of cases.
- Neonates and infants may (rarely) present as floppy infants.

DIAGNOSTIC TESTS & INTERPRETATION
Lab
- In atypical cases, consider heavy metal screen, HIV titer, Lyme titer, porphyria screen, acetylcholine receptor antibodies (myasthenia), conversion disorder:
  - See "Differential Diagnosis."
- IgA level should be considered if the child has a history of frequent pulmonary infections: IgA deficiency could contraindicate intravenous immunoglobulin (IVIg) therapy (risk of anaphylaxis).

Imaging
MRI of the spine (with gadolinium enhancement): Consider MRI for spinal cord compression syndrome in a child presenting with paraparesis. Spinal nerve root enhancement on MRI can support the diagnosis of GBS.

Diagnostic Procedures/Other
- Electrodiagnosis:
  - Nerve conduction studies (NCS) and electromyography (EMG) can confirm diagnosis of GBS and are helpful when clinical or CSF findings are ambiguous. NCS and EMG are abnormal in 50% of patients in the first 2 weeks and in 85% of patients afterwards.
  - Initially, needle EMG may be normal. Consider serial studies if initially nondiagnostic, high clinical suspicion.
- Lumbar puncture: Elevated levels of CSF protein after the 1st week of symptoms. Minimal pleocytosis (<20 leukocytes/mm^3), largely mononuclear leukocytes, may occur.

DIFFERENTIAL DIAGNOSIS
- Myasthenia gravis
- Botulism
- Intoxication (e.g., heavy metals, organophosphates)
- Myopathy/myositis
- Poliomyelitis and other acute (i.e., viral) motor neuron diseases
- Acute cerebellar ataxia (sometimes associated with neuroblastoma)
- Transverse myelitis

- Chronic inflammatory demyelinating polyneuropathy (CIDP)
- Vasculitic neuropathy
- Diphtheritic neuropathy (rare)
- Porphyric neuropathy
- Locked-in state
- Conversion, psychogenic weakness, astasia/abasia

ALERT
- Initially, gait instability may mistakenly be interpreted as having a psychogenic source.
- Reflexes may be preserved in early stages of illness.
- Proximal symptoms may predominate early on.
- Check for reflexes in patients with bilateral Bell palsy. Close observation for further development of symptoms or signs of GBS.

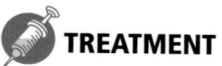 TREATMENT

ALERT
- Respiratory failure may occur quickly.
- Treat hypertension cautiously; catastrophic refractory hypotension may ensue.

ADDITIONAL TREATMENT
Additional Therapies
Physical therapy: Avoid contractures with lower extremity splinting and early passive range of motion. Aggressive physical and occupational therapy are essential for good outcomes.

COMPLEMENTARY & ALTERNATIVE THERAPIES
A combination of supportive therapy and immunotherapy is the mainstay of treatment for patients with GBS:

- Regular monitoring of vital capacity; strongly consider intubation if vital capacity reaches <50% of normal.
- IVIg and plasmapheresis have equivalent efficacy as first-line immunotherapy. Combination of the 2 therapies has not proven more effective than either monotherapy alone. Complications and discontinuation of therapy are less common with IVIg.
- Pediatric studies have shown IVIg and plasmapheresis to be well tolerated and efficacious.
- IVIg at 0.4 g/kg (body weight) for 5 consecutive days and initiated in ambulatory patients within 2–4 weeks of symptom onset

- Plasmapheresis requires placement of a central catheter. Total plasma exchange volume of 200–250 mL/kg divided in 3–5 treatments over 7–14 days. Therapy initiation is recommended within 4 weeks of symptom onset for patients who cannot walk and 2 weeks for patients who can.
- Corticosteroids have not been shown to be helpful and are not recommended.
- Pain from nerve root inflammation is common in GBS and should be treated aggressively.

IN-PATIENT CONSIDERATIONS
Initial Stabilization
Key elements center around respiratory management and deciding on hospitalization to monitor/treat progressive symptoms including heart block, hypotension, urinary retention, and neuropathic pain.

Admission Criteria
Admit patients with symptoms progressing over hours to days, with any respiratory or bulbar complaints, or who are nonambulatory.

Nursing
Particular attention to preventing skin breakdown, contractures, venous thrombosis, and secondary compressive neuropathies

Discharge Criteria
- Completion of immunotherapy
- Stabilization of symptoms
- Severity of bulbar, respiratory, and autonomic involvement dictates duration of hospital stay. Consider intensive inpatient rehabilitation.

 ONGOING CARE

FOLLOW-UP RECOMMENDATIONS
- Improvement typically begins 2–3 weeks after onset of symptoms, up to 2 months in some patients.
- Improvement continues for up to 2 years.

PATIENT EDUCATION
Parent Internet Information: Guillain–Barré Syndrome Foundation International. http://www.gbsfi.com

PROGNOSIS
- ~85% have a good recovery; ultimate functional recovery depends on the degree of axonal injury, which can be predicted from electrodiagnostic studies in adults.
- Early prognosticators include the severity of weakness at the disease nadir and fulminant onset.
- Overall prognosis in children is better than in adults.

COMPLICATIONS
- Complications include respiratory failure, BP dysregulation (hypotension and/or hypertension), urinary retention, aspiration, pain syndromes, deep venous thrombosis, and infection.
- Death from early respiratory failure, autonomic instability, or other complications occurs in 3–6%.

ADDITIONAL READING

- Hughes RA, Raphaël JC, Swan AV, et al. Intravenous immunoglobulin for Guillain-Barré syndrome. *Cochrane Database Syst Rev.* 2006;1:CD002063.
- Hughes RA, Swan AV, van Koningsveld R, et al. Corticosteroids for Guillain-Barré syndrome. *Cochrane Database Syst Rev.* 2006;2:CD001446.
- Hughes RA, Wijdicks EF, Barohn R, et al. Practice parameter: Immunotherapy for Guillain–Barré syndrome: Report of the Quality Standards Subcommittee of the American Academy of Neurology. *Neurology.* 2003;61:736–740.
- Lawn ND, Fletcher DD, Henderson RD. Anticipating mechanical ventilation in Guillain-Barré syndrome. *Arch Neurol.* 2001;58:893–898.
- Tekgul H, Serdaroglu G, Tutuncuoglu S. Outcome of axonal and demyelinating forms of Guillain-Barré syndrome in children. *Pediatr Neurol.* 2003;28:295–299.

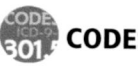 CODES

ICD9
357.0 Acute infective polyneuritis

ICD10
G61.0 Guillain-Barre syndrome

FAQ

- Q: Is GBS contagious?
- A: No.
- Q: Will I get GBS again?
- A: Acute relapses occur in 1–5% of patients in large series. Treatment-related fluctuations (worsening after completion of immunotherapy) can occur in CIDP and can be indistinguishable from GBS.
- Q: Do all cases require hospitalization and immunomodulatory treatment?
- A: Some youngsters with mild, nondisabling symptoms may be observed as outpatients (≤10%).

G

GYNECOMASTIA
Julie A. Boom

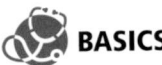

BASICS

DESCRIPTION
Any visible or palpable proliferation of breast glandular tissue, unilateral or bilateral, owing to an increase in estrogen action in relation to androgen action at the level of the breast

EPIDEMIOLOGY
2 peaks in age distribution occur in the pediatric population:
- Neonatal period
- Puberty

Incidence
Peak incidence for pubertal gynecomastia in males is 14 years of age (range: 10–16 years), usually during Tanner stage 3–4.

Prevalence
- Neonatal gynecomastia occurs in 60–90% of all newborns.
- ~40% of boys develop transient gynecomastia (measuring ≥0.5 cm) during puberty.

RISK FACTORS
Any situation that leads to an increase in the net effect of estrogen action relative to androgen action at the level of the breast may lead to gynecomastia. These situations could include:
- Increased estrogen concentration (endogenous or exogenous)
- Normal estrogen levels with decreased androgen concentrations
- Congenital reduction in estrogen receptors
- Pharmacologic blockade of androgen receptors
- Increased breast or peripheral tissue aromatase, which converts androgens to estrogens
- Elevated leptin levels, which may increase aromatase enzyme activity, stimulate growth of mammary cells or increase breast receptor sensitivity to estrogen
- Testicular dysfunction
- High levels of serum gonadotropins or increased sex hormone–binding globulin
- Elevated estrogen levels, which may lead to proliferation of the ducts and surrounding mesenchymal tissue, resulting in breast enlargement

ETIOLOGY
- Physiologic:
  - Neonatal: Transient palpable breast tissue developing in newborns owing to elevated estrogen levels in the fetoplacental unit. This condition resolves as estrogen levels decline.
  - Pubertal: Benign transient gynecomastia occurring in otherwise healthy adolescent males. Breast tissue in pubertal gynecomastia measuring <4 cm in diameter has a high likelihood of spontaneous regression.
  - Involutional: Breast enlargement occurs in elderly men.

- Pathologic:
  - Drug-induced:
    - Hormones: Estrogen, androgens, gonadotropins, anabolic steroids, growth hormone, antiandrogens, and cosmetics, foods, hair products, and herbal remedies that contain estrogenic or antiandrogenic compounds
    - Anti-infective agents: Ethionamide, isoniazid, ketoconazole, metronidazole, antiretrovirals
    - Antiulcer drugs: Cimetidine, ranitidine, omeprazole
    - Chemotherapeutic agents: Alkylating agents, methotrexate, vinca alkaloids
    - Cardiovascular agents: Amiodarone, captopril, digitoxin, diltiazem, enalapril, methyl-dopa, nifedipine, reserpine, spironolactone, verapamil
    - Psychotropic agents: Diazepam, haloperidol, phenothiazines, tricyclic antidepressants
    - Drugs of abuse: Alcohol, amphetamines, heroin, marijuana, methadone
    - Miscellaneous: Metoclopramide, phenytoin, penicillamine, theophylline, gabapentin, clonidine, pregabalin
  - Hypogonadism: Primary or secondary
  - Tumors: Testicular, adrenal, ectopic tumors that produce human chorionic gonadotropin
  - Chronic disease: Hyperthyroidism, renal failure, liver disease, malnutrition with refeeding, HIV infection
  - Congenital disorders: Klinefelter syndrome, vanishing testes syndrome (also known as anorchism, gonadal agenesis, or testicular regression), androgen resistance syndromes, true hermaphroditism, excessive peripheral tissue aromatase
  - Acquired testicular failure: Viral orchitis, trauma, granulomatous disease, or castration
  - Chest wall trauma or intercostal nerve damage following surgery or herpes zoster
  - Psychologic stress
  - Spinal cord injury

DIAGNOSIS

ALERT
- Do not mistake pseudogynecomastia (i.e., fatty enlargement of the breasts) for true gynecomastia.
- Do not overlook a potentially drug-related cause. Drug-related gynecomastia is usually reversible if diagnosed within 1 year of onset.

HISTORY
- Family history: 1/2 of adolescents with gynecomastia will have a positive family history.
- Time of onset relative to puberty:
  - Genital maturation develops at least 6 months before onset of breast development.
- Rate of progression:
  - Rapidly enlarging, painful gynecomastia with acute onset is of more concern than longstanding enlargement.
- Drug exposures, including alcohol and substance abuse:
  - Marijuana and heroin addiction may cause gynecomastia.
- Exposure to exogenous estrogen
- Symptoms suggestive of hyperthyroidism
- Symptoms suggestive of liver disease, such as cirrhosis:
  - Liver disease may alter the estrogen-to-androgen ratio and thus cause gynecomastia. Damaged hepatic cells may lose the ability to inactivate estrogens. Impaired hepatic removal of androstenedione from the bloodstream; provides more androstenedione for the peripheral conversion to estrogen. Liver disease may result in the elevation of sex-steroid binding globulin, which reduces circulating free testosterone.
- Symptoms suggestive of renal failure:
  - Renal disease may alter the estrogen-to-androgen ratio and thus cause gynecomastia. Chronic uremia can cause direct testicular damage resulting in decreased plasma testosterone levels. Renal disease may also result in an increased luteinizing hormone level.
- Symptoms suggestive of neoplastic disease:
  - In patients <10 years of age, consider pituitary, adrenal, or testicular tumor. Liver tumors may cause gynecomastia owing to increased aromatization of circulating adrenal androgens or by secretion of chorionic gonadotropins.
- Symptoms suggestive of hypogonadism, such as decreased libido, decreased erectile function, or infertility, may indicate an abnormal estrogen-to-androgen ratio.

PHYSICAL EXAM
- Assess height, weight, growth velocity, and BP.
- Assess for malnourishment: May result in hepatic dysfunction causing higher estrogen-to-androgen ratio.
- Perform a complete breast exam:
  - With patient in the supine position, grasp the breast between the thumb and forefinger and move digits toward the nipple: Look for a firm, rubbery, mobile, discoid mound of tissue arising concentrically below the nipple and areola. Measure the diameter of the disc of glandular tissue. Asymmetry and tenderness are common.
- Pseudogynecomastia:
  - If pseudogynecomastia (fatty enlargement of breasts) is present, no glandular disc will be palpable.
- Check for galactorrhea:
  - Seen in association with drug ingestion and pituitary tumor
- Determine whether macrogynecomastia (disc diameter >5 cm with a secondary mound above the level of the breast) is present:
  - Macrogynecomastia may be physiologic or pathologic and is unlikely to regress.
- Examine the thyroid gland for the presence of a goiter:
  - Gynecomastia may be seen in hyperthyroidism.
- Gynecomastia is a physiologic process found in many males during early puberty. Perform a careful testicular exam with measurement of size. Consider Klinefelter syndrome if testes <3 cm in length or 8 mL in volume. Check for the presence of a varicocele:
  - Boys 12–14 years of age with varicoceles are more likely to also have gynecomastia

DIAGNOSTIC TESTS & INTERPRETATION
Lab
- None indicated for pubertal and neonatal gynecomastia
- Karyotype: To rule out Klinefelter syndrome.
- Morning levels of luteinizing hormone (LH), follicle-stimulating hormone (FSH), estradiol, testosterone, dehydroepiandrosterone (DHEA), and human chorionic gonadotropin (hCG):
  - To determine whether hypogonadism, precocious puberty, testicular tumor, or adrenal tumor could be present. An isolated elevated estradiol level in an otherwise normal prepubertal boy may suggest direct or indirect exogenous estrogen exposure.
- Morning prolactin level

Imaging
- None indicated for pubertal and neonatal gynecomastia
- Bone age (radiograph of the left hand and wrist):
  - Elevated estrogen levels may accelerate skeletal maturation.
- Testicular ultrasound:
  - To rule out testicular tumor, or elevated levels of human chorionic gonadotropin and estradiol, or finding of asymmetric testes on physical exam
- Chest radiograph with abdominal CT
- Adrenal CT or MRI:
  - To rule out adrenal neoplasm, if estradiol elevated, DHEA elevated, LH level decreased or normal, and testicular ultrasound normal
- Skull radiograph, brain MRI or CT: If pituitary tumor is suspected

DIFFERENTIAL DIAGNOSIS
- Infectious:
  - Breast abscess
- Neoplastic:
  - Breast neoplasm
  - Neurofibroma
  - Lymphangioma
  - Lipoma
  - Neuroblastoma metastasis
- Trauma:
  - Hematoma
- Miscellaneous:
  - Pseudogynecomastia: Excessive adipose tissue only; no discrete subareolar tissue
  - Dermoid cyst

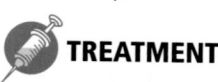 TREATMENT

MEDICATION (DRUGS)
- Generally, drug therapy should proceed under the guidance of an endocrinologist.
- Raloxifene and tamoxifen (as unlabeled or investigational use) and testolactone (an aromatase inhibitor for which safety and efficacy in pediatric patients has not been established) have shown some benefit in adolescents with benign pubertal gynecomastia.
- If gynecomastia has been present for >1 year, pharmacologic therapy is of little benefit. After 1 year, regardless of the cause of gynecomastia, epithelial growth becomes less prominent, whereas periductal fibrosis and hyalinization are more evident. Because of the increase in fibrosis, gynecomastia of longer duration is less amenable to medical treatment.

ADDITIONAL TREATMENT
Additional Therapies
- Reassurance for patients with pubertal gynecomastia measuring <4 cm. Treatment guidelines are variable for gynecomastia measuring 4–5 cm. Surgical consultation in these patients should be considered.
- Re-examine at 3–6 month intervals.
- Discontinue any drugs known to induce gynecomastia, and follow-up in 1 month.

ISSUES FOR REFERRAL
Consider surgical consultation in patients with >4 cm diameter of glandular tissue.

SURGERY/OTHER PROCEDURES
- Surgery is the therapy of choice for macrogynecomastia or persistent gynecomastia refractory to medical therapy.
- Obesity should not preclude surgical intervention.
- Obese adolescents may experience greater preoperative psychologic impact than nonobese adolescents.
- Surgical options include periareolar incision with adjunctive liposuction or glandular tissue removal through 2 incisions in the anterior axillary regions.
- Ultrasound-assisted liposuction has emerged as a new alternative surgical option.

 ONGOING CARE

FOLLOW-UP RECOMMENDATIONS
- Watch for signs of psychologic stress.
- Watch for symptoms of chronic disease and abnormal physical changes.

PROGNOSIS
- Overall, good
- Pubertal gynecomastia: 75% disappears spontaneously within 2 years, and 90% within 3 years.
- Neonatal gynecomastia usually resolves within the 1st year of life.

COMPLICATIONS
- Physical pain, which may interfere with sports
- Psychologic stress
- Embarrassment
- Skin erosion of the nipple owing to rubbing against clothing
- Breast cancer: Patients with Klinefelter syndrome have a 16-fold increased risk of breast cancer; other causes of gynecomastia are not associated with an increased risk of breast cancer.

ADDITIONAL READING

- Braunstein GD. Gynecomastia. *N Eng J Med.* 2007;357:1229–1237.
- Ma NS, Geffner ME. Gynecomastia in prepubertal and pubertal men. *Curr Opin Pediatr.* 2008:20(4): 465–470.
- Maidment SL. Question 2. Which medication effectively reduces pubertal gynecomastia? *Arch Dis Child.* 2010;95(3):237–239.
- Nordt CA, DiVasta AD. Gynecomastia in adolescents. *Curr Opin Pediatr.* 2008;20(4): 375–382.
- Rosen H, et al. Adolescent gynecomastia: Not only an obesity issue. *Ann Plast Surg.* 2010;64: 688–690.

 CODES

ICD9
- 611.1 Hypertrophy of breast
- 778.7 Breast engorgement in newborn

ICD10
- N62 Hypertrophy of breast
- P83.4 Breast engorgement of newborn

FAQ
- Q: When should a patient with gynecomastia be referred to a specialist?
- A: If macrogynecomastia is present, if there is an abnormal hormonal workup or an abnormal imaging study, or if there is an abnormal rate of progression.
- Q: For how long does neonatal gynecomastia persist?
- A: Studies of healthy term infants have shown that the diameter of the breast tissue may actually increase during the 1st 2 weeks of life. The breast tissue then decreases to an average diameter of 10 mm until about 4–6 months of age. The breast tissue of female infants is generally larger and may persist longer than in males. Occasionally, the breast tissue will fail to regress and remain after the 1st year of life.
- Q: Is it normal for a newborn baby's breasts to secrete milk?
- A: In the later stages of gestation, the developing breast undergoes a small amount of secretory activity. This produces the so-called "witch's milk" that is expressed from the breasts of many full-term infants from the day 5–7 of life. Witch's milk may persist for 1–7 weeks after birth. As fetal prolactin, placental estrogen, and progesterone decline, the breast tissue regresses.
- Q: How is gynecomastia distinguished from breast cancer?
- A: Breast cancer usually presents as a unilateral, eccentric hard or firm mass that is fixed to underlying tissues. Associated findings can include dimpling of the skin, retraction of the nipple, nipple discharge, or axillary lymphadenopathy. The incidence of breast cancer in the pediatric population is extremely low: <0.1% of all breast cancers occur in patients <20 years of age. Benign tumors, such as fibroadenomas, are much more common than malignant breast tumors.
- Q: Has the incidence of gynecomastia increased?
- A: As the prevalence of childhood and adolescent obesity has increased, the presence of pseudogynecomastia has also increased. If glandular tissue is not present, pseudogynecomastia should be treated with diet and exercise.

G

HAND, FOOT, AND MOUTH DISEASE

Ross Newman
Jason Newland

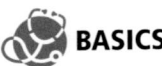 **BASICS**

DESCRIPTION
Hand, foot, and mouth disease is a viral illness with the characteristic clinical features of:
- Vesiculoulcerative stomatitis
- Papular or vesicular exanthem on the hands and/or the feet
- Mild constitutional symptoms such as fever and malaise

GENERAL PREVENTION
- Frequent hand washing, especially after changing diapers, and good personal hygiene are the most useful means to prevent spread of enteroviral illnesses.
- Contact precautions should be maintained with all hospitalized patients.
- The prodromal and enanthem periods appear to be the most contagious; however, some may shed virus in the stool 3 months after infection (see "FAQ").

EPIDEMIOLOGY
- In temperate climates, hand, foot, and mouth disease is most common in the summer and fall (a pattern common to many of the enterovirus infections).
- In tropical climates, disease is present year round
- Transmitted by oral–fecal route. Respiratory secretions may also transmit the virus.
- Incubation period is 3–6 days.
- Highly contagious, afflicting up to 50% of those exposed
- Close household contacts are particularly susceptible.
- Most common in children under 5 years, but may affect adults
- May occur as an isolated case or in an epidemic distribution

PATHOPHYSIOLOGY
- Enteroviruses are acquired primarily from oral-fecal contamination
- Lymphatic invasion leads to viremia and spread to secondary sites.
- Viremia ceases with antibody production.
- Direct inoculation of the extremities from oral lesions has been hypothesized with regard to hand, foot, and mouth disease.

ETIOLOGY
Coxsackie A16 virus is the most common causative agent. Other serotypes associated with HFMD:
- Coxsackieviruses A5, A7, A9, A10, A16, B1, and B3
- Enterovirus 71
- Echoviruses
- Other enteroviruses

DIAGNOSIS

HISTORY
- History of ill contacts:
  – Incubation period may be up to 1 week.
- Any fever, pain, or other symptoms:
  – A mild prodrome occasionally precedes the characteristic enanthem and exanthem by 1 or 2 days: Low-grade fever [usually near 101°F (38.3°C)], malaise, sore mouth, anorexia, coryza, diarrhea, abdominal pain.
- Bone pain:
  – Bone and joint aches infrequently accompany this illness.
- Lesions in mouth:
  – Oral lesions typically occur shortly before the hand and foot manifestations.
- Illness in family:
  – Family members or close contacts are often similarly affected.
- Hydration status:
  – Determine quality and amount of oral intake, quality and amount of urine output, recent weight loss, duration of symptoms.

PHYSICAL EXAM
- Enanthem:
  – Oral lesions begin as small, red papules.
  – Papules quickly evolve to small vesicles on an erythematous base.
  – Lesions progress to ulcerations.
  – Tongue, buccal mucosa, palate, gingiva, uvula, and/or tonsillar pillars may be involved.
  – Usually 2–10 lesions
  – Oral lesions may persist up to 1 week.
- Exanthem:
  – Less consistently present than oral lesions (occur in 1/4–2/3 of patients)
  – Maculopapular eruptions progress to vesicles.
  – Rarely tender or pruritic
  – Most frequent on the dorsal aspects of fingers and toes
  – May also occur on the palms, soles, arms, legs, buttocks, and face
- Adenopathy:
  – Enlarged anterior cervical, or submandibular nodes are present in one quarter of cases.
- Other:
  – Attention should be given to the patient's vital signs; general appearance; and respiratory, cardiac, and neurologic functioning to help identify the rare patient with a threatening complication of hand, foot, and mouth disease.

DIAGNOSTIC TESTS & INTERPRETATION
Lab
- Hand, foot, and mouth disease has unique clinical features and a relatively benign course. Laboratory confirmation of the diagnosis is seldom needed or indicated.
- Culture:
  – Causative viruses may be cultured from many sites:
    ○ Oral ulcers
    ○ Cutaneous vesicles
    ○ Nasopharyngeal swabs
    ○ Stool (Isolation of an enterovirus from the stool does not confirm it to be the cause of disease because the virus can be shed for many weeks after infection.)
    ○ Cerebrospinal fluid (in cases where meningoencephalitis is suspected). Reverse transcription-polymerase chain reaction (RT-PCR) can be used.

DIFFERENTIAL DIAGNOSIS
Few infectious diseases have such characteristic clinical findings. Oral ulcerations followed by lesions on the distal extremities are virtually pathognomonic. The most difficult diagnostic dilemmas may occur early in the disease course when isolated oral lesions predominate:
- Herpangina:
  – Also caused by Coxsackie A viruses
  – Associated with higher fever
  – Usually limited to the posterior oropharynx
- Herpetic gingivostomatitis:
  – Most common cause of stomatitis in children
  – Associated with higher fever
  – More frequently associated with lymphadenopathy
  – Gingival involvement severe
  – Aphthous ulcers
  – Generally occurs without fever or upper respiratory symptoms
  – Does not occur in outbreaks
- Stevens–Johnson syndrome:
  – Ulcerations frequently coalesce.
  – Usually affects other mucous membranes
  – Often appears with separate cutaneous manifestations
- The Boston exanthem:
  – Caused by echovirus 16
  – Mild febrile illness with a macular rash on the palms and soles occurring at time of or after defervescence
  – Oral lesions absent

TREATMENT

SUPPORTIVE CARE
No specific therapy is indicated or usually necessary. Most cases are mild and self-limiting and only require parental reassurance.

SPECIAL THERAPY
- Symptomatic relief from particularly painful oral ulcers may be accomplished by application of a topical antihistamine or anesthetic directly to the sores (see "FAQ").
- Dehydration should be treated when present. IV fluids may be required in the more severe cases, especially in infants and young children.
- Good supportive care is generally sufficient to treat most complications.

MEDICATION (DRUGS)
Acetaminophen may relieve malaise and minor discomfort associated with the oral ulcers. It also may be used as an antipyretic in those children with fever.

IN-PATIENT CONSIDERATIONS
Admission Criteria
Dehydration and inability to maintain adequate oral hydration

Discharge Criteria
Rehydrated and good oral intake

 ONGOING CARE

FOLLOW-UP RECOMMENDATIONS
Small children must be followed closely for signs of dehydration.

DIET
Dietary adjustments often improve oral intake from painful oral lesions and prevent or relieve dehydration:
- Avoid spicy or acidic foods.
- Provide cool or iced liquids in small quantities frequently.

PROGNOSIS
- Hand, foot, and mouth disease generally resolves spontaneously within 1 week after diagnosis.
- In nearly all instances, hand, foot, and mouth disease will resolve quickly, requiring only supportive care.
- Careful history and examination should distinguish those patients with the rare aforementioned complications.
- Rare cases may recur at intervals for up to 1 year.

COMPLICATIONS
- Hand, foot, and mouth disease is usually self-limited and uncomplicated, resolving within 7–10 days.
- Dehydration is the most frequent morbid complication:
  - Oral ulcerations are painful and interfere with feeding.
  - Infants and children are at highest risk.
- Rare reports of other complications include:
  - Neurologic complications such as aseptic meningitis, encephalitis, and acute flaccid paralysis
  - Pneumonia
  - Myocarditis
  - A possible association with first-trimester spontaneous abortions in previously infected women

ADDITIONAL READING

- American Academy of Pediatrics. Herpes simplex. In: Pickering LK, ed. *2009 Red Book: Report of the Committee on Infectious Diseases*. 27th ed. Elk Grove Village, IL: American Academy of Pediatrics; 2009.
- Robinson CR, Doane FW, Rhoades AJ. Report of an outbreak of febrile illness with pharyngeal lesions and exanthem: Toronto, 1957—isolation of Coxsackie virus. *Can Med Assoc J.* 1958;79:615–621.
- Scott LA, Stone MS. Viral exanthems. *Dermatol Online J.* 2003;9:4.
- Slavin KA, Frieden IJ. Picture of the month: Hand-foot-and-mouth disease. *Arch Pediatr Adolesc Med.* 1998;152:505–506.

CODES

ICD9
074.3 Hand, foot, and mouth disease

ICD10
B08.4 Enteroviral vesicular stomatitis with exanthem

FAQ
- Q: What is in the "magic mouthwash" often used to relieve the pain of stomatitis?
- A: Many health care providers will prescribe a "magic mouthwash" for symptomatic relief of oral ulcers, pharyngitis, and teething pain. The most common such treatment consists of an aluminum hydroxide/magnesium hydroxide gel suspension and diphenhydramine elixir (12.5 mg/5 mL) in a 1:1 formulation. It can be applied directly to the sores with a cotton swab or a small syringe before meals. Note: Some people will have a reaction to topical diphenhydramine.
- Q: Should lidocaine be used topically or in suspension with "magic mouthwash" for symptomatic relief of oral ulcers?
- A: The routine use of lidocaine in this situation is not recommended. Lidocaine is an effective topical anesthetic and comes in a 2% viscous suspension. In practice, the pain relief is short lived, which encourages frequent administration. Lidocaine is absorbed from the mucous membranes (bypassing first-pass liver metabolism) and has been frequently reported to cause poisoning of the cardiovascular and central nervous systems. Both pediatric and adult fatalities have occurred. Topical viscous lidocaine should be reserved for use by physicians knowledgeable about its proper dosage and potential side effects, and by educated, compliant parents or caregivers.
- Q: When may children with hand-foot-and-mouth disease return to school?
- A: Good hygiene will greatly reduce viral transmission. Isolation from school or day care contacts should occur while fever remains and/or while the enanthem persists. As mentioned, some patients may shed the virus in their stool for weeks after symptoms have resolved (again stressing the need for good personal hygiene).

H

HANTAVIRUS

Bruce Tempest

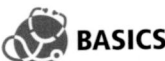 **BASICS**

DESCRIPTION
Hantavirus pulmonary syndrome (HPS) is a disease in humans caused by a Hantavirus; it is acquired from certain chronically infected rodent species. When acquired by humans, it results in a syndrome characterized by a flu-like illness, then by a rapidly progressive cardiac and respiratory failure with a high mortality.

EPIDEMIOLOGY
- The host rodent develops a chronic nonfatal infection and excretes virus in urine, feces, and saliva.
- Humans acquire the infection by inhaling virus-contaminated airborne particles from the dried rodent excreta. Typically, this occurs when sweeping or otherwise disturbing dusty areas in a rodent-infested building.
- Nosocomial transmission has been observed only with the Andes strain in Argentina, never in the US.
- In the US, HPS has occurred primarily in young healthy adults, although in South America a larger proportion of cases are in children.

Incidence
Human cases are more common in the spring and summer and also in years when the population of the rodent host has increased.

GENERAL PREVENTION
- Universal precautions are appropriate in caring for patients with HPS; person-to-person transmission has been demonstrated only with the Andes strain in the Southern Hemisphere, not in the US.
- Preventing infection depends on avoiding contact with airborne particles contaminated by rodent excreta.
- Eliminate rodents and seal off rodent access into the house.
- Reduce rodent shelter and food sources in the immediate vicinity of the home by cutting brush, removing trash, and storing grain and animal feed in rodent-proof containers.
- Wearing gloves, clean up rodent-contaminated areas by spraying nests and droppings with household disinfectants or dilute bleach, and seal material in bags for burning or burial.
- Ventilate closed areas before initiating cleanup.

PATHOPHYSIOLOGY
- The 2 most important pathophysiologic changes are:
  – Myocardial depression resulting in shock
  – Alveolar capillary leak pulmonary edema resulting in hypoxia
- The cardiac dysfunction is characterized by a falling cardiac output, increased systemic vascular resistance, and normal or low pulmonary artery wedge pressure.
  – Alveolar capillary leak pulmonary edema resulting in hypoxia
- The pulmonary alveoli are flooded with fluid devoid of erythrocytes but with a protein content similar to serum.

ETIOLOGY
The original human outbreak recognized in the southwestern US was caused by the Sin Nombre strain of Hantavirus transmitted from chronically infected deer mice (*Peromyscus maniculatus*). Subsequent cases were recognized throughout the seemingly ubiquitous distribution of the deer mouse. Since then, additional strains of Hantavirus have been recognized, each with a unique rodent host. The resulting human cases of HPS have now been identified from Canada to Argentina.

 DIAGNOSIS

Pitfalls:
- Recognizing the prodrome of HPS is difficult and requires a careful history, evaluation of the risk of exposure, and rapid access to testing:
  – The diagnosis depends on serologic testing, which can take some time.
  – Lacking serologic confirmation, one mostly depends on clinical history and serial hematologic tests.
  – In anticipation of the rapid progression of the cardiopulmonary phase, it is preferable to have the patient closely observed in the hospital.

HISTORY
- Clinical symptoms, physical findings, and laboratory findings progress in sequence. Early suspicion of the syndrome allows the clinician to prepare for that phase of the illness characterized by the rapid onset of respiratory failure and shock:
  – Fever and myalgia are usually severe and characterize the prodromal phase lasting 3–6 days.
  – GI complaints are frequently prominent, including combinations of nausea, vomiting, diarrhea, and abdominal pain.
  – Headache is present in >50% of patients.
  – Cough is uncommon at the onset of the prodrome, but heralds the onset of dyspnea and tachypnea, which is then followed by the rapid progression of cardiorespiratory failure.
  – Coryza and sore throat are rarely part of the prodrome.
  – A history of activities that might expose the patient to airborne virus-contaminated particles should be sought.
    ○ HPS is acquired by inhalation of airborne particles.

PHYSICAL EXAM
- Tachycardia and hypotension are late findings.
- During the prodromal phase, fever is the only finding.
- With the onset of the cardiopulmonary phase, cough and dyspnea are associated with the production of frequently copious amounts of nonpurulent material.

DIAGNOSTIC TESTS & INTERPRETATION
Lab
- Platelet count:
  – The platelet count falls on serial testing during the prodromal phase and may be the only abnormality measurable using laboratory methods.
- In addition to leukocytosis, myelocytes and immunoblasts appear in the peripheral blood.
- Hemoconcentration
- Liver function test results are only mildly abnormal.
- Hypoxemia accompanies the onset of the cardiopulmonary phase.
- Diagnostic serology demonstrates IgM antibody present at the time of clinical presentation.

Imaging

- Chest radiograph:
  - During the prodrome, chest radiography is normal. With the onset of cardiopulmonary symptoms, chest radiography will show evidence of interstitial fluid manifested by Kerley B lines, hilar indistinctness, and peribronchial cuffing. Alveolar flooding and pleural effusions develop in severe cases. Heart size remains normal.

DIFFERENTIAL DIAGNOSIS

- Septicemic plague
- Influenza
- Bacterial sepsis, especially that caused by *Pneumococcus* and other streptococci
- Other causes of shock and pneumonia or shock and pulmonary edema

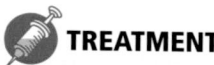 TREATMENT

ADDITIONAL TREATMENT

General Measures

- Because of the rapid progression of cardiorespiratory failure, all patients with HPS should be managed in an ICU setting with a pulmonary artery catheter to guide therapy.
  - Oxygen, intubation, and mechanical ventilation are frequently needed.
  - Use fluids cautiously in view of the capillary leak.
  - Extracorporeal membrane oxygenation has been used for patients who fail to respond to maximal inotropic and ventilatory support.
  - To date, antiviral agents have not been shown to be beneficial.

MEDICATION (DRUGS)

- If the patient develops hypotension, an inotropic agent such as dobutamine should be added; if the patient continues to be hypotensive on maximal doses of dobutamine, vasopressors can be added to maintain blood pressure.
- Use empiric antibiotics because serologic tests confirming HPS are usually delayed and the differential diagnosis includes sepsis from a variety of antibiotic-responsive organisms.

 ONGOING CARE

PROGNOSIS

- Patients who survive the shock phase typically then diurese fluid. Recovery is then generally rapid.
- Easy fatigability and mild pulmonary function abnormalities may persist.

ADDITIONAL READING

- Butler JC, Peters CJ. Hantaviruses and hantavirus pulmonary syndrome. *Clin Infect Dis*. 1994;19:387–395.
- Centers for Disease Control and Prevention. Hantavirus. Available at: http://www.cdc.gov/hantavirus/
- Duchin JS, Koster FT, Peters CJ, et al. Hantavirus pulmonary syndrome: A clinical description of 17 patients with a newly recognized disease. *N Engl J Med*. 1994;330:949–955.
- Graziano KL, Tempest B. Hantavirus pulmonary syndrome: A zebra worth knowing. *Am Fam Physician*. 2002;66:1015–1020.
- Hallin GW, Simpson SQ, Crowell RE, et al. Cardiopulmonary manifestations of hantavirus pulmonary syndrome. *Crit Care Med*. 1996;24:252–258.
- MacNeil A, Ksiazek TG, Rollin PE. Hantavirus Pulmonary Syndrome, United States, 1993–2009. *Emerg Inf Dis*. 2011;17:1195–1201.
- Ramos MM, Overturf GD, Crowley MR, et al. Infection with Sin Nombre hantavirus: Clinical presentation and outcome in children and adolesents. *Pediatrics*. 2001;108:E27.

 CODES

ICD9
079.81 Hantavirus infection

ICD10
B33.4 Hantavirus (cardio)-pulmonary syndrome [HPS] [HCPS]

FAQ

- Q: What should I do if I find a dead mouse indoors?
- A: Determine whether it is a house mouse or a species that could be infected with Hantavirus. If the latter, assume that it is infected and dispose of it as described previously and then seal off rodent access to the home and eliminate any individuals still left inside.
- Q: What should I do if I find what look like rodent droppings?
- A: Clean up with gloves and disinfectant as noted earlier. Then use traps to catch and identify the rodents involved and proceed as in the answer to the previous question.
- Q: Could a patient have hantavirus pulmonary syndrome without knowing it?
- A: In the US, asymptotic hantavirus pulmonary syndrome infections would appear to be uncommon based on serum screening of household contacts of cases and other populations at high risk, which show only infrequent evidence of prior infection.

H

HEAD BANGING

Ana Catarina Garnechor
Yvette E. Yatchmink

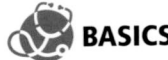

BASICS

DESCRIPTION
- Head banging (HB) is defined as the hitting of head on solid object such as a wall, side of crib, mattress or floor.
- Tend to hit the front or side of the head
- Usually last for 15 minutes but can go on for >1 hour
- Regular rhythm of 60–80 bpm
- Can be seen along with body rocking or head rolling

EPIDEMIOLOGY
- Average age on of onset is 9 months; usually extinguished by 3 years of age. Older patients with head-banging are more likely to have a developmental delay or other medical problems.
- More common in boys than girls (3:1)
- Occurs in 3–15% of typically developing children
- Estimated that 2–3% of kids with Intellectual disability have stereotypic movement disorder (SMD/HB) and 5% of kids with Tourette syndrome have SMD/HB)

ETIOLOGY
- Can be comforting and be a part of other self-soothing activities such as body rocking or head rolling
- Temper tantrum secondary to frustration or anger
- In typically developing children, as an expression of happiness or as a method of self-stimulation (sometimes secondary to sensory deprivation)

- Part of a sleep rhythmic disorder called *Jactatio capitis nocturna* (partial arousal during light, non-REM sleep); HB occurs when drowsy or falling asleep
- SMD is a repeated, rhythmic, purposeless movement or activity; these usually cause self-injury or severely interfere with normal activities. These are most prevalent in adolescence and tend to occur in clusters of symptoms. Diagnosis requires 4 weeks of duration.

COMMONLY ASSOCIATED CONDITIONS
- Medical causes: Teething (pain), ear infection, seizures, meningitis, headaches, drug use (cocaine, amphetamines)
- SMD is associated with: Cerebral palsy, Intellectual disability, schizophrenia, autism/PDD, Down syndrome, Lesch-Nyhan syndrome, blindness, deafness
- Tic disorder/Tourette syndrome
- Infantile spasms
- Rule out child abuse if significant scalp laceration, skull fracture, or intracerebral or subdural hemorrhage

DIAGNOSIS

- Determine factors associated with behavior, including age of child, degree of parental concern, location of behavior, associated behaviors, motivations of the child, benefits to the child.
- Determine if a medical cause exists, particularly if sudden onset.
- Determine if psychological factors are involved.

DIAGNOSTIC TESTS & INTERPRETATION
- Usually, no laboratory testing is needed for diagnosis.
- Physical exam to look for bruising, swelling, scratches, or minor lacerations
- If swelling or blood loss is involved, brain imaging may be necessary to rule out damage.
- If severe and persistent HB is reported, an ophthalmology exam is warranted to rule-out complications.
- Developmental screening to rule out possible developmental delay
- If developmental delay is suspected, formal psychoeducational testing can be recommended.

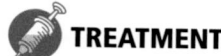 **TREATMENT**

- For patients with particularly violent movements of jactatio capitis nocturna, trials with clonazepam and citalopram have shown some success.
- For patients with SMD, medications may help, including: Antipsychotics, tricyclic antidepressants, SSRIs, and benzodiazepines. These should be closely monitored.

ISSUES FOR REFERRAL

- Referral to ophthalmologist is recommended, if vision disturbance appear. Such ophthalmologic complications include cataracts, glaucoma, or retinal detachment.
- Older children may need psychological/developmental follow-up to determine delay/cognition status and to determine if behavioral modification therapy could be beneficial in decreasing symptomatology

 ONGOING CARE

PROGNOSIS

- Normally disappears by age 3–4 years
- Jactatio capitis nocturna is usually benign and resolves by age 5 years.
- SMD usually peaks in adolescence and then declines.

ADDITIONAL READING

- Harris K, et al. Nonautistic motor stereotypies: Clinical features and longitudinal follow-up. *Pediatr Neurol*. 2008;38(4):267–72.
- Leekam S, et al. Repetitive behaviors in typically developing 2-year-olds. *J Child Psychol Psychiatry*. 2007;48(11):1131–1138.
- Miller J, et al. Behavioral therapy for treatment of stereotypic movements in nonautistic children. *J Child Neurol*. 2006;21(2):119–125.
- Sallustro F, Atwell C. Body rocking, head banging and head rolling in normal children. *J Pediatr*. 1978;93(4):704–708.
- Vinston R, Gelinas-Sorrell D. Head banging in young children. *Am Fam Phys*. 1991;43(5):1625–1628.

 CODES

ICD9
307.3 Stereotypic movement disorder

ICD10
F98.4 Stereotyped movement disorders

FAQ

- Q: Can head banging lead to serious head injury or neurological damage?
- A: Typically developing children rarely bang their heads hard enough to cause bleeding or fracture.
- Q: What can a parent do to prevent injury or diminish head banging behavior?
- A: Remove sharp or breakable objects from child's environment to avoid accidental injury.
- Place a rubber pad on the floor or a thick rug.
- Secure the crib to the wall to decrease noise and vestibular input to the child.
- If behavior occurs during tantrum, ignore the behavior once safety is established. Reward the child for appropriate behaviors.

H

HEADACHE AND MIGRAINE

Katherine A. Wayman
Brad C. Klein (5th edition)

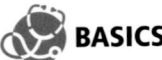

BASICS

DESCRIPTION
- Primary headache: No underlying condition (migraine, tension headache, cluster headache, autonomic cephalgias)
- Secondary headache: Symptomatic of a specific cranial, oral, dental, or cervical pathologic process (e.g., trauma or tumor)

EPIDEMIOLOGY
Prevalence
Headache prevalence approaches 60–80% by age 20. Migraines may start by age 3, but mean age of onset is 7 years for boys and 11 years for girls. About 7% of prepubertal children are affected; about 3% of younger school-age children and up to 20% of older adolescents are affected. Prevalence of chronic daily headache (a primary headache) in preadolescents is 4–5%.

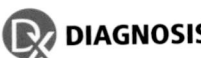

DIAGNOSIS

Migraine in children is classified into the following groups
- Migraine without aura: Most cases. Mood changes or withdrawal from activity, sensitivity to light and sound
- Migraine with aura: Aura lasts <60 minutes and usually precedes migraine. May be visual (spots, colors, image distortions, scintillating scotoma), sensory (paresthesias, hemisensory changes)
- Basilar-type migraine (13–19% childhood migraines): Vertigo, diplopia, ataxia, visual field deficits, often occipital headache
- Childhood periodic syndromes that may be precursors to migraine (sometimes called migraine equivalents): Benign paroxysmal vertigo of childhood, cyclic vomiting, abdominal migraine, benign paroxysmal torticollis
- Alice in Wonderland syndrome: Distortions of vision, space, and/or time (e.g., micropsia, metamorphopsia, sensory hallucinations)
- Confusional migraine: Impaired sensorium, agitation, and lethargy; may progress to stupor. Likely an overlap of hemiplegic migraine and basilar migraine

HISTORY
- Clarify temporal pattern, location, duration, and intensity. Also, time of onset, associated symptoms, precipitating and ameliorating factors, response to therapy, and family history
- The following questions should be asked:
  – Is there more than 1 type of headache? How are they different from each other?
  – Since they started, have headaches gotten worse or stayed the same?
  – How is the pain described (e.g., pounding, squeezing, stabbing, or some other description)?
  – Do the headaches occur at any special time of day?
  – Do they wake the patient up?
  – What does the patient do during the headaches?
  – Does the patient have ideas about what is causing the headaches?

- Migraine = acute recurrent headache. Nausea, vomiting, photophobia, phonophobia, and transitory neurologic disturbances suggest migraine.
- Agitation, pacing, and loud crying are atypical for migraine and more consistent with cluster headache.
- Tension-type headache (TTH) usually presents as a chronic or episodic nonprogressive headache pattern. Pain is often bilateral, bandlike, diffuse, dull, nonpulsatile, and of mild to moderate intensity.
- Mixed headache patterns: Migraine superimposed on tension headache
- Red flags: First or worst headache, occipital location, recent headache onset, increasing severity or frequency, headache in the morning associated with vomiting, headache causing awakening from sleep
- Ask about common comorbidities: Motion sickness, allergic rhinitis, depression
- 70% of those with migraine have a family history of migraine, especially those with migraine with aura.
- TTH is associated with higher rate of divorced parents and fewer close friends, unlike migraine.

PHYSICAL EXAM
- Vital signs: Especially blood pressure and height and weight
- Obesity: Consider pseudotumor or sleep apnea syndrome.
- Skin changes consistent with neurocutaneous syndrome: Patients with neurofibromatosis commonly experience headache.
- Auscultation for bruits over the supraclavicular areas, neck, and temporal and occipital areas: Arteritis, vascular malformation
- Examination for sinus tenderness, limitation of jaw excursion, or occipital trigger points
- Funduscopic exam: The presence of venous pulsations, best seen at the origin of branch points of the veins, decreases chance of intracranial hypertension.
- Visual acuity exam may reveal eye strain–related headache.
- Neurologic exam should be normal in primary headache syndromes (migraine, tension), except during a migraine with prolonged aura or migraine variant. Stiff neck, head tilt, decreased alertness, abnormal eye movements, asymmetric deep tendon reflexes, asymmetric motor weakness or sensory deficit, ataxia, and gait disturbance may signal infection, stroke, hemorrhage, tumor, or demyelination.
- Migraine without aura criteria: In children, 5 or more headache attacks that:
  – Last 1–72 hours
  – Have at least 2 of the following:
    ○ Bilateral or frontal (2/3 of cases) or unilateral, frontal/temporal location
    ○ Pulsating or throbbing quality
    ○ Moderate to severe intensity
    ○ Aggravated by routine physical activities
  – At least 1 of the following accompanies headache:
    ○ Nausea and/or vomiting
    ○ Photophobia and/or phonophobia (may be inferred from behavior)

DIAGNOSTIC TESTS & INTERPRETATION
Imaging
- Neuroimaging studies (CT or MRI): Emergency evaluation should focus on identifying acute processes that require urgent intervention. These include subarachnoid hemorrhage, meningitis, and mass lesions causing elevated intracranial pressure that may lead to herniation:
  – CT should be used if there is any suspicion for subarachnoid hemorrhage, but otherwise MRI is generally preferred.
  – Consider MR venogram if acute deficits/focal seizures present.
- Neuroimaging is not necessarily warranted in patients with acute recurrent or chronic nonprogressive headache who have normal findings on neurologic exam.
- Neuroimaging should be performed for:
  – Acute 1st episode of severe headache ("worst headache of my life")
  – Headaches or vomiting in the morning
  – Headache worse in supine position
  – Seizures
  – Cognitive decline
  – New, focal/persistent neurologic symptoms or findings (e.g., papilledema, hemiparesis, ataxia, abnormal eye movements, alteration of consciousness, nuchal rigidity)
  – Presence of ventriculoperitoneal shunt

Diagnostic Procedures/Other
- EEG: Although 10% of children with migraine may show nonspecific abnormalities, there is no role for EEG in routine testing of patients with headache.
- Other modalities:
  – Sinus films or CT if concern for sinusitis
  – Sphenoid sinusitis may produce unremitting chronic frontal headache.
  – Migraine may mimic sinusitis and vice versa.
- Lumbar puncture (LP):
  – In addition to meningitis, diagnostic considerations include subarachnoid hemorrhage, sinus thrombosis, pseudotumor cerebri, and low-pressure headache.
  – CT (prior to LP): Considered in chronic progressive headache in a nonfebrile patient, even when chronic migraine or tension headache is (statistically) more likely.
  – Measure opening pressure (abnormal if >20 cm) with patient recumbent to rule out pseudotumor cerebri (where result of cerebrospinal fluid analysis otherwise is normal).
  – Check urine drug screen in suspect cases.

DIFFERENTIAL DIAGNOSIS

The temporal pattern of headache can help clarify the differential. There are roughly 5 patterns:

- Acute, 1st severe headache:
  - Meningitis, encephalitis, cocaine or other substance abuse, medication (methylphenidate, steroids, psychotropic drugs, analgesics, cardiovascular agents), hypertension (usually secondary); hydrocephalus, pseudotumor cerebri (idiopathic intracranial hypertension), post-LP, subarachnoid hemorrhage, intracerebral hemorrhage, ventriculoperitoneal shunt malfunction, sinus thrombosis, migraine, upper respiratory tract infection, somatization
- Chronic progressive headache:
  - Brain tumor, abscess, hydrocephalus, vascular malformation, hematoma, chronic meningitis (e.g., Lyme disease), sinus thrombosis, idiopathic intracranial hypertension, depression, anemia, rheumatologic diseases
- Acute recurrent headache:
  - Migraine and variants, cluster, tension
- Chronic nonprogressive or daily headache:
  - Medication overuse, substance abuse, (rebound headache), caffeine, sinusitis, occipital neuralgia, temporomandibular joint syndrome, orthostatic headache, post-LP, other systemic disease, posttraumatic, sleep disorder, depression, anxiety, other psychiatric illness, tension headache, fibromyalgia
- Mixed headache = Migraine-superimposed tension headache

TREATMENT

MEDICATION (DRUGS)

- Acute treatment:
  - Abortives are generally most effective if given early in the acute migraine attack.
  - 1st line is ibuprofen (10 mg/kg).
  - Acetaminophen (10–15 mg/kg)
  - Naproxen sodium 2.5–5 mg/kg per dose
- Additional acute treatments for refractory patients:
  - Antiemetics (prochlorperazine, metoclopramide, ondansetron) also enhance effectiveness of analgesics and may abort migraines.
  - Sumatriptan (Imitrex), nasal in 5, 10, or 20 mg (Class 1 trials of 12–17-year-olds)
  - Sumatriptan, 25-mg oral tablets; rizatriptan (Maxalt, Maxalt-MLT) 5–10-mg tablets or oral dissolving wafers; and zolmitriptan (Zomig) 2.5–5-mg tablets or oral dissolving wafers may provide relief, although not proven statistically. An SC injection of sumatriptan may be necessary. SC dose is 0.06 mg/kg; 3 mg for children >6 years and weighing <30 kg; 6 mg for those >30 kg
  - Although safe, triptans are not currently FDA approved for use in children or adolescents.
  - Triptans/ergotamines not recommended in basilar, hemiplegic migraine, or with vascular risk factors
  - Drugs containing caffeine/isometheptene may cause rebound headaches.

- Status migrainosus:
  - Migraine lasting >72 hours
  - Hydrate patient with IV fluids: D5 1/2 NS or NS (dehydration exacerbates).
  - Raskin protocol: Dihydroergotamine: Not well studied in children and adolescents; use under guidance of neurologist.
  - IV valproate: Similar effectiveness to DHE-45 and metoclopramide for status migrainosus. Typical administration: 15 mg/kg at 3 mg/kg/min up to 1 g
  - Corticosteroids and IV ketorolac may be effective; remain controversial in children
  - Narcotics not recommended: Often lose efficacy, greater levels of sedation than pain relief. Addiction and rebound potential also of concern
- Prophylaxis:
  - >10 headache days/month or 3–4 severe attacks per month (i.e., leading to missed school or social activities, etc.) constitutes a relative indication for prophylaxis.
  - Start medication at a low dose; increase weekly toward maximum until headaches relent or adverse effects supervene. Choose a drug that may address other comorbidities.
  - Consider limited duration of treatment (i.e., through the calendar school year and then taper off in the summer).
  - Calcium channel blockers (e.g., verapamil)
  - β-Blockers (e.g., propranolol, nadolol) are discouraged in patients with asthma, depression, or diabetes.
  - Tricyclic agents (e.g., amitriptyline, nortriptyline) may provide relief from insomnia or depression.
  - Anticonvulsants: topiramate (evidence level A) and valproic acid (evidence level B) may have dual efficacy in patients with epilepsy. Emerging evidence for levetiracetam
  - Cyproheptadine, an antihistamine/antiserotonin agent = prophylactic therapy in younger children (i.e., 5–12 years old).

COMPLEMENTARY & ALTERNATIVE THERAPIES

- Relaxation techniques (meditation, progressive muscle relaxation, self-hypnosis)
- Stress management (cognitive behavioral therapy), biofeedback
- Some evidence for vitamins, supplements, and herbs such as riboflavin (300 mg/d), magnesium (200–300 mg/d), coenzyme q10, feverfew, and ginkgolide B

ADDITIONAL READING

- Abu-Arafeh I, Razak S, Sivaraman B, et al. Prevalence of headache and migraine in children and adolescents: A systematic review of population-based studies. *Dev Med Child Neurol.* 2010;52(12):1088–1097.
- Lewis D. Pediatric migraine. *Pediatr Rev.* 2007;28: 43–53.
- Lewis D, Ashwal S, Hershey A, et al. Practice parameter: Pharmacological treatment of migraine headache in children and adolescents. *Neurology.* 2004;63:2215–2224.
- Ozge A, Termine C, Antonaci F, et al. Overview of diagnosis and management of paediatric headache. Part I: Diagnosis. *J Headache Pain.* 2011;12:13–23.
- Papetti L, Spalice A, Nicita F, et al. Migraine treatment in developmental age: Guidelines update. *J Headache Pain.* 2010;11:267–276.
- Termine C, Ozge A, Antonaci F, et al. Overview of diagnosis and management of paediatric headache. Part II: Therapeutic management. *J Headache Pain.* 2011;12:25–34.

 CODES

ICD9
- 339.00 Cluster headache syndrome, unspecified
- 339.10 Tension type headache, unspecified
- 346.9 Migraine

ICD10
- G43.909 Migraine, unspecified, not intractable, without status migrainosus
- G44.009 Cluster headache syndrome, unspecified, not intractable
- G44.209 Tension-type headache, unspecified, not intractable

FAQ

- Q: What about allergy and headache?
- A: Many believe that headache may represent a symptom of hypersensitivity. Headache in the setting of allergic rhinitis/asthma may be a result of associated sinusitis/sinus congestion, a side effect of treatment (especially theophylline), or muscle tension.

H

HEAT STROKE AND RELATED ILLNESS

Patrick B. Solari
Paige L. Wright
George A. Woodward

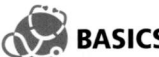 **BASICS**

DESCRIPTION
- Heat stroke results from imbalance in heat production, absorption, and dissipation. It can result from excessive body heat generation and storage without appropriate dissipation, high ambient temperature, low radiation or convective heat loss, decreased evaporation, or inadequate fluid/electrolyte replacement in response to ongoing losses through sweat or GI disturbance.
- 2 forms of heat stroke exist:
  - Exertional heat stroke (EHS), which occurs during periods of intense exertion
  - Nonexertional heat stroke (NEHS), in which the body is unable to compensate for an increase in ambient temperature; more common in very young and elderly, and during heat waves.

RISK FACTORS
- Environmental predisposition: Hot and humid without wind, heat wave, overheated indoor environment, lack of air conditioning. Social isolation, inability to care for self, or entrapment in closed space (e.g., car, trunk; internal automobile temperature in sunlight with poor ventilation can reach 131–172°F; the sharpest temperature increase occurs within 1st 15 minutes).
- Medical: Obesity, low fitness level, cardiac disease, diabetes mellitus and insipidus, diarrhea, hyperthyroidism, dehydration, vascular disease, sweat gland dysfunction, sunburn, viral illness
- Drugs/Medications:
  - Anticholinergics
  - Antihistamines
  - Beta-blockers
  - Diuretics
  - Psychiatric medications
  - Recreational drugs and alcohol
- Behaviors:
  - Lack of recognition of risk factors or warning signs
  - Overexertion or inadequate fluid intake
  - Inappropriate clothing; heavy, dark, tight-fitting, overbundling
  - Lack of acclimatization and conditioning
  - Children in enclosed space within vehicle

GENERAL PREVENTION
- Avoid enclosed spaces (e.g., children in closed cars).
- Reduce activity levels, keep cool, use shaded areas. Adaptation to warmer climates may take 8–10 exposures of 30–45 minutes each daily or every other day.
- Air conditioning or fans during hot weather
- Cool or tepid baths
- Increase fluid intake before, during, and after scheduled exercise or strenuous activity (up to 200–300 mL q10–20min); do not wait until thirsty. Cool water and large volumes increase gastric emptying (high osmolality and carbohydrate content decrease gastric emptying).
- Loose, light-colored clothing, protective hat

- Acclimatization via gradual conditioning over 10–14 days in hotter environment.
- Liberal dietary sodium:
  - Avoid NaCl tablets (possible hypernatremia, potassium depletion, gastric irritation, delayed gastric emptying)
- Frequently flex leg muscles when standing.
- Avoid prolonged standing in hot environments.
- Avoid caffeine and alcohol.

PATHOPHYSIOLOGY
- Heat production is increased 10–20 times by strenuous exercise.
- When environmental temperature is greater than body temperature, body gains heat by conduction and radiation and can lose heat by evaporation.
- Children have greater body surface-to-mass ratio, higher metabolic rate, inability to increase cardiac output, decreased sweat production, and inability to independently change environments, compared to adults:
  - Dehydration results in loss of sweating, hence decreased evaporation.
  - Above 40°C, cell volume, membrane integrity, metabolism, acid–base balance is affected.
  - Extreme core temperatures >42°C can uncouple oxidative phosphorylation and allow enzyme systems to cease functioning.

COMMONLY ASSOCIATED CONDITIONS
- Miliaria rubra (prickly heat): Heat rash, usually caused by obstruction of sweat glands by clothes or lotions, produces an erythematous papular rash; usually self-limited
- Heat cramps/Spasms: Related to physical exercise in people who have not trained or are poorly acclimatized with mild dehydration; thought to be related to water and sodium depletion
- Heat tetany: Paresthesias and carpopedal spasm help distinguish tetany from heat cramps.
- Heat syncope: Alteration of consciousness (i.e., dizziness, syncope) at end of strenuous or upright event
- Heat edema: Swollen feet and ankles (i.e., vascular leak, orthostatic pooling)
- Heat exhaustion: Relatively slow onset. Water and/or salt depletion. Clinically copious perspiration with headache, nausea, vomiting, malaise, myalgias, pallor, light-headedness, visual disturbances, syncope, temperature 38–40°C, dehydration, electrolyte imbalance, hemoconcentration; can evolve into heat stroke

- Heat stroke: Core body temperature exceeding 40°C with altered mental status ranging from confusion, disorientation, and incoherent speech to delirium, decerebrate posturing, seizure, and coma. May have acute, sudden onset (80%) or slower onset (minutes to hours, 20%). Classic heat stroke is associated with dry skin and prolonged exposure to elevated temperatures at rest. Exertional heat stroke may present with dry skin or profuse sweating.

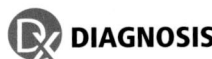 **DIAGNOSIS**

HISTORY
- Heat exhaustion:
  - Weakness, lethargy, thirst, malaise, diminished ability to work or play, headache, nausea, vomiting, myalgias, pale skin, dizziness
- Heat stroke:
  - History of CNS dysfunction in environment consistent with, or predisposing conditions conducive to, development of heat-related illness should suggest heat stroke.

PHYSICAL EXAM
- Heat exhaustion:
  - Visual disturbances, syncope, mild CNS dysfunction, impaired judgment, cramps, vertigo, hypotension, tachycardia, hyperventilation, paresthesias, agitation, ataxia, psychosis, temperature <40°C, sweating, environmental exposure, and activity; no coma or seizures
- Heat stroke:
  - Temperature >40°C (may be cooler owing to prehospital interventions and maneuvers)
  - Altered level of consciousness (confusion, drowsiness, irritability, neurologic deficits, euphoria, combativeness, obtundation), ataxia, posturing, incontinence, seizures, coma, purpura, or petechiae; 2/3 with constricted pupils; may have muscle rigidity with tonic contractions and dystonia that mimic seizures
  - Shock: Tachycardia, hypotension, widened pulse pressure, tachypnea
  - Hot, dry (classic), or clammy (exercise-induced) skin, pink or ashen color
  - Weakness, nausea, vomiting, anorexia, headache, dizziness
- Temperature measurement (continuous best):
  - Esophageal thermometry probably the best
  - Deep rectal thermometry a good approximation of core temperature
  - Tympanic, oral, axillary, temporal artery temperatures are less accurate measures of core temperature.

DIAGNOSTIC TESTS & INTERPRETATION
Lab
Initial lab tests
Tests only to confirm diagnosis, evaluate extent of injury, or rule out other processes because treatment should be empiric:

- Heat cramps: Decreased levels of serum and urine sodium and chloride; BUN level normal or slightly increased
- Heat exhaustion: May see hyponatremia or hypernatremia (free water loss), hypochloremia, low urine sodium, and chloride hemoconcentration; normal LFTs
- Heat stroke:
  - Electrolytes abnormalities: Sodium chloride level normal or high, hypokalemia, increased BUN/creatinine; Low K+, Ca, P; hypoglycemia
  - Hematologic: Hemoconcentration, leukocytosis, thrombocytopenia
  - Prerenal azotemia
  - Elevated AST/ALT
  - Metabolic acidosis: Lactate high, especially with exertional heat stroke
  - Coagulopathy
- Others: Creatine phosphokinase (rhabdomyolysis), arterial blood gases (classic heat stroke: Respiratory alkalosis and hypokalemia early; exertional heat stroke: lactic acidosis), urinalysis (casts, brownish color proteinuria, microscopic hematuria, myoglobinuria), CSF, EKG, chest radiograph

DIFFERENTIAL DIAGNOSIS
- Heat cramps: Rhabdomyolysis, tetany
- Heat edema: Thrombophlebitis, lymphedema, congestive heart failure
- Heat stroke: CNS process with fever (cerebrovascular stroke, meningitis, encephalitis), other infections, anticholinergic poisoning (dilated pupils), drug/medication-induced, temperature rise, severe dehydration. Chills suggest febrile illness, not heat stroke.
- Neuroleptic malignant syndrome
- Serotonin syndrome
- Malignant hyperthermia

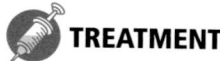

TREATMENT

MEDICATION (DRUGS)
- Antipyretics not useful because an intact hypothalamus is required for action.
- Avoid anticholinergic drugs (atropine), which can inhibit sweating.
- May require inotropic support
- Chlorpromazine may improve peripheral vasodilatation and prevent shivering.
- Benzodiazepine for sedation and/or seizures
- Dantrolene not shown to be effective

ADDITIONAL TREATMENT
General Measures
- Heat stroke: Treat empirically, then rule out other causes of presentation. Maintain airway, breathing, and circulation including securing airway as indicated, supplemental oxygen delivery:
  - Fluid replacement: IV 0.9% NS or LR solution. Rule out hypoglycemia.
  - Miscellaneous therapies:
    - Foley catheter to monitor urine output
    - Nasogastric tube
    - Myoglobinuria therapy (mannitol, bicarbonate, dialysis if necessary)
    - Electrolyte replacement if symptomatic from hypokalemia or hypocalcemia
    - Fresh frozen plasma for disseminated intravascular coagulation (DIC)

IN-PATIENT CONSIDERATIONS
Initial Stabilization
- Rapid recognition and cooling imperative
- Specific therapy:
  - Heat cramps: Rest, salt, and water replacement
  - Heat syncope: Self-limited as return to horizontal position is treatment; rest and fluids, salted liquids
  - Heat exhaustion: Clinical findings (heart rate, BP, orthostatic changes, urine output) should direct therapy. Most treated as outpatient with rapid rehydration, cooling; mild case: Oral electrolyte solution (0.1–2% saline = ~1/4–1/2 teaspoon table salt in 1 quart of water); if nausea, vomiting, inability to drink: IV (0.5% [similar to sweat losses] to 0.9% normal saline solution (NS); avoid rapid overcorrection of hypernatremia (treat as with hypernatremic dehydration); if hyponatremic seizures, treat with 3% saline at ~5 mL/kg
  - Heat stroke: Immediate cooling and support of cardiovascular system. Remove clothing, remove patient from hot environment; use air conditioning, open vehicle for transport if possible; esophageal or rectal temperature probe (continuous temperature measurements); cooling should exceed 0.1–0.2°C/min; slow cooling down at 38.5–39°C to avoid overshoot
  - Cooling options: Cold water immersion (15–16°C) has lowest morbidity and mortality for exertional heat stroke, is as effective as ice bath without discomfort, shivering, or vasoconstriction
    - Also: Ice packs to neck, groin, axillae, wet sheet over patient; moisten skin with water spray, convection increase (fan) to increase evaporative cooling; cooling blankets; cool/ice water lavage (peritoneum, rectum, gastric); cold to room temperature IV fluids; massage with ice (decreases shivering response)

Admission Criteria
- Patients with symptoms suggestive of heat stroke require immediate cooling and should be watched closely.
- Patients with evidence of multisystem disease (altered mental status, electrolyte imbalances, hematologic abnormalities) should be admitted until such issues are resolved.

ONGOING CARE

PROGNOSIS
- Heat-related illness (e.g., heat rash, edema, cramps, tetany, syncope, exhaustion): Rapid recovery with supportive care
- Heat stroke: Poor prognosis if not recognized and aggressively managed. Morbidity and mortality directly proportional to how rapidly core temperature is reduced.

ADDITIONAL READING
- Bouchama A, Knochel JP. Heat Stroke. *N Engl J Med.* 2002;346:1978–1988.
- Jardine DS. Heat illness and heat stroke. *Pediatr Rev.* 2007;28(7):249–258.
- MMWR. Heat illness among high school athletes–US, 2005–2009. *Morb Mortal Wkly Rep.* 2010;59(32):1009–1013.
- Tobin JR, Jason DR, Challa VR, et al. Malignant hyperthermia and apparent heat stroke. *JAMA.* 2001;286:168–169.

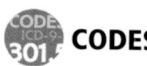

CODES

ICD9
992.0 Heat stroke and sunstroke

ICD10
- T67.0XXA Heatstroke and sunstroke, initial encounter
- T67.0XXD Heatstroke and sunstroke, subsequent encounter
- T67.0XXS Heatstroke and sunstroke, sequela

FAQ
- Q: How can one distinguish between heat exhaustion and heat stroke?
- A: Heat stroke involves temperature >40°C with CNS and LFT abnormalities, whereas heat exhaustion refers to inability to continue exercise.
- Q: When should heat stroke be suspected?
- A: Suspect heat stroke in a patient with or without sweating, who demonstrates alterations of CNS function.
- Q: Does the presence or absence of sweating help with the diagnosis of heat exhaustion versus heat stroke?
- A: No. Sweating will be present with heat exhaustion and may or may not be present with heat stroke.
- Q: Are children at increased risk of heat illness?
- A: Yes. They have a number of predisposing factors: Greater surface area-to-body mass ratio than adults, production of more metabolic heat/kg body weight, slower rate of sweating than adults, temperature when sweating starts is higher, lower cardiac output at a given metabolic rate than adults, rate of acclimatization is slower, thirst response is blunted, and access to fluids may be limited.

H

HEMANGIOMAS AND OTHER VASCULAR LESIONS

Carol A. Miller

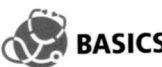 **BASICS**

DESCRIPTION
- Vascular tumors: Neoplasms of the vasculature:
  - Hemangioma of infancy
  - Diffuse hemangiomatosis
  - Tufted angioma
  - Kaposiform: Hemangioendothelioma
  - Pyogenic: Granuloma
  - Hemangiopericytoma
- Vascular malformations (VM); anomalous blood vessels without endothelial proliferation:
  - Capillary (salmon patch, port-wine stain/nevus flammeus)
  - Venous malformations
  - Arterial malformations (arteriovenous malformations [AVMs], complex/combined)
- Lymphatic malformations (macrocystic and microcystic)
- Vascular malformations
- Other types of VM may occur in any part of the body and may be associated with overgrowth of the involved part.

EPIDEMIOLOGY
Incidence
Hemangiomas:
- ~10% of infants by 12 months of age
- Increased incidence in low-birth-weight infants
- Increased incidence if chorionic villus sampling was performed during pregnancy
- Other demographic risk factors include white non-Hispanic race, female sex, born of multiple gestations, advanced maternal age, maternal history of miscarriage, and positive family history.

COMMONLY ASSOCIATED CONDITIONS
- Hemangiomas:
  - Lumbosacral; be aware an underlying spinal dysraphism may be present.
  - Segmental: Commonly located on the face and involving a developmental unit (segment) and frequently associated with complications
  - PHACES: Rarely occurring segmental hemangioma associated with other developmental anomalies (Posterior fossa malformations; Hemangioma; Arterial anomalies; Cardiac anomalies, including aortic coarctation; Eye abnormalities; Sternum defects)
  - Congenital hemangiomas: Noninvoluting congenital hemangioma (NICH) and rapidly involuting hemangioma (RICH)
- Vascular malformations:
  - Port-wine stains may be present as part of syndromes (e.g., Sturge-Weber, von Hippel-Landau, Rubinstein-Taybi, Beckwith-Wiedemann, Cobb syndrome)

DIAGNOSIS

HISTORY
- Onset of lesions and timing of changes
- Hemangiomas are often inapparent at birth or present with precursor lesions followed by a rapid growth phase.
- Vascular malformations are present at birth. Some may fade slowly over time (salmon patches) and others remain, sometimes becoming more obvious with overall growth, or slowly enlarge over time.
- PMHx: Low birth weight, twin or other multiple gestation, premature
- FHx: Familial hemangiomas or syndromes associated with port-wine stains
- ROS: Other developmental anomalies (e.g., PHACES)

PHYSICAL EXAM
- Hemangiomas:
  - Neonate: Flat pale lesion, superficial telangiectasia with halo border, pinkish ecchymotic lesion
  - Infant: Raised red rubbery nontender lesion with well-demarcated borders. Overlying skin is usually intact although sometimes ulceration may be present.
  - Deep layer lesion: Raised soft mass with bluish-purplish discoloration with smooth, intact, overlying skin
  - Complex/combined: Lesions will have both cutaneous and deep layer features.
  - Involuting lesion: Flat, atrophic pale or gray center with surrounding raised reddish border with stippled texture. Bleeding from ulceration may be present.
  - The presence of large numbers of small to moderate-sized cutaneous hemangiomas may indicate a rare condition called diffuse neonatal hemangiomatosis. Internal organ involvement (liver, lungs, GI tract, CNS) is likely to be present if this condition is diagnosed.
- Vascular malformations:
  - Salmon patches (nevus simplex): Most notable at birth as pinkish-red macules that often blanch and are most commonly found at the nape of the neck, glabella, and upper eyelids. Frequently all three locations are involved in an individual newborn.
  - Port-wine stains (nevus flammeus): Easily seen at birth and are deep red to purplish, nonblanching macules with well-demarcated borders. Most commonly located on the face and often cover a large area

  - Matured port-wine stains are deeper in color and frequently develop raised nodules or a bleblike appearance.
  - If an extremity is heavily involved, there may be underlying bony overgrowth and limb hypertrophy.
  - AVMs: Raised pulsating lesions with bruits audible by stethoscope if large in size. Smaller lesions may vary in appearance from macular erythema to thin vascular plaques. Some lesions may show elements similar to venous malformations.
  - Signs of cardiac compromise (i.e., tachycardia, gallop rhythm, shortness of breath, hepatomegaly) may be associated with very large AVMs.
  - Venous malformations: Deep blue to purplish, soft, fleshy nodules in the skin and may be surrounded by superficial venules. The drainage pattern is generally obvious upon inspection. Mature lesions may include small calcifications (phleboliths).
  - Lymphatic malformations: Present differently depending on size. Large lesions are rubbery, skin-colored, massive nodules with ill-defined borders, most often located in the head, neck, axilla, or chest (referred to as cystic hygromas). Lesions in the neck area may be associated with respiratory compromise if the airway is constricted. Microcystic lesions present as nodules or plaques, sometimes in clusters, with overlying skin changes such as discoloration. Complicated lesions may be hemorrhagic or leak translucent lymph fluid.

DIAGNOSTIC TESTS & INTERPRETATION
Diagnosis is usually made by recognition of the typical physical exam findings.

Imaging
- Occasionally helpful in distinguishing hemangiomas from vascular malformations
- May be necessary to determine the extent of internal or visceral lesions or characterize complex lesions
- Preoperative MRI, CT angiography, or venography aids in planning resection of large or invasive lesions such as cystic hygromas.

Diagnostic Procedures/Other
- Biopsy: Rarely required but may be helpful to differentiate lesions suspicious for malignancy. Should be avoided if lesion is highly suspected to be vascular as significant bleeding may ensue
- Other diagnostic tests should be considered if concerns for syndromes or other complications (e.g., cardiac or respiratory compromise) exist.

TREATMENT

ADDITIONAL TREATMENT
General Measures
- Hemangiomas:
  - Most patients will not need treatment as lesions will spontaneously involute without complications.
  - Consider treatment of lesions interfering with critical organ functions, such as vision or breathing, large lesions causing consumptive coagulopathy, or lesions significantly affecting appearance, such as on the face.
  - Timing of surgical treatment of hemangiomas should be carefully determined to minimize the risk of undesirable cosmetic outcome.
  - Intralesional and/or systemic steroids
  - Propranolol either systemically or topically has increased in popularity in recent years as an alternative to steroid therapy.
  - Interferon may be useful in refractory or severe lesions. The development of spastic diplegia has been reported as a complication of interferon therapy.
  - Apply compresses and topical dressings for ulcerations.
  - Topical or systemic antibiotics covering staphylococcal and streptococcal species for infected lesions
  - Laser therapy useful for superficial lesions
  - Liquid nitrogen has been used in selected situations
- Vascular malformations:
  - Pulsed dye laser is the treatment of choice for port-wine stains and other superficial vascular malformations. Serial applications over several years may be necessary. Large lesions may not completely respond. Better outcomes noted in children treated <1 year of age
  - Surgical resection, sclerotherapy, or embolization may be appropriate depending on the character of the malformation.

ISSUES FOR REFERRAL
Consider referral to specialty services if the following conditions are present:
- Lesions in locations where function may be impacted such as periorbital, ear canal, tip of nose, lips, or anogenital areas
- Lesions distributed in a "beardlike" format, which may constrict the airway

- Presence of numerous cutaneous lesions increasing the likelihood of visceral involvement (including the GI tract, liver, CNS, lungs)
- Lesions causing or likely to cause significant disfigurement
- Lesions located over the spine, which may be associated with spinal dysraphism
- Lesions located in a segmental distribution about the head and face
- Large AVMs impacting circulation and cardiac function (e.g., resulting in high output heart failure)
- Presence of dysmorphic features along with vascular lesions
- Lesions that are ulcerating or bleeding

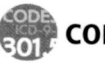
ONGOING CARE

PATIENT EDUCATION
Vascular Birthmarks Foundation (www.birthmark.org)

PROGNOSIS
- Hemangiomas:
  - All infantile hemangiomas undergo spontaneous involution. By 9–10 years of age, 90% will have completed involution. Greater than 85% will resolve without need for treatment.
  - Residual areas of skin atrophy and/or discoloration are common.
  - Complicated lesions marked by ulceration, bleeding, or infection may result in scarring or disfigurement.
- Vascular malformations:
  - VMs generally do not involute or resolve.
  - Salmon patches fade over time and generally are not a cosmetic problem.
  - Port-wine stains may darken and become nodular with age.
  - Larger lesions can be associated with excessive growth of the involved body area resulting in hypertrophy.
  - Malignant transformation is rare.

COMPLICATIONS
- Hemangiomas:
  - Bleeding, ulceration, superinfection
  - Iron deficiency anemia
  - Interference with function of important organs (including vision, airway, GI tract, CNS)
  - Disfigurement and cosmetic problems
  - Kasabach-Merritt phenomenon or syndrome; thrombocytopenia (due to platelet trapping, coagulopathy, and microangiopathic hemolytic anemia), usually associated with rapidly enlarging lesions, kaposiform hemangioendothelioma, or tufted angiomas
  - Hypothyroidism may occur with large hemangiomas that stimulate increased breakdown of thyroid hormone.

- Vascular malformations:
  - High-output cardiac failure due to circulatory "steal" associated with AVMs
  - Skeletal overgrowth of the involved limb can occur with disfigurement and emotional distress.
  - Limitation of movement and pain from localized ischemia
  - Problems associated with lymphedema, such as excessive leg and foot swelling
  - Airway compromise from constriction by large neck lesions

ADDITIONAL READING

- Chang LC, Haggstrom AN, Drolet BA, et al. Growth characteristics of infantile hemangiomas: Implications for management. *Pediatrics*. 2008; 112(2):360–367.
- Greene AK. Current Concepts of Vascular Anomalies. *J Craniofac Surg*. 2012;23:220–224.
- Haggstrom AN, Drolet BA, Baselga E, et al. Prospective study of infantile hemangiomas: Clinical characteristics predicting complications and treatment. *Pediatrics*. 2006;118(3):882–887.
- Kilcline C, Frieden IJ. Infantile hemangiomas: How common are they? A systematic review of the medical literature. *Pediatr Dermatol*. 2008;25(2): 168–173.

CODES

ICD9
- 228.01 Hemangioma of skin and subcutaneous tissue
- 228.09 Hemangioma of other sites
- 459.9 Unspecified circulatory system disorder

ICD10
- D18.00 Hemangioma unspecified site
- I99.9 Unspecified disorder of circulatory system
- Q28.8 Other specified congenital malformations of circulatory system

H

HEMATURIA

Ann Salerno

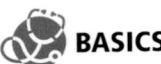

BASICS

DEFINITION
Hematuria is defined as ≥5 RBCs per high-power field (hpf), using a standard urinalysis technique on a centrifuged sample. This correlates with a urine dipstick reaction of ≥1+.

EPIDEMIOLOGY
- Asymptomatic microscopic hematuria (on >1 sample): 0.5–2% of school-aged children
- Gross hematuria: 0.13% children in walk-in clinic
- Gross hematuria is more commonly observed in boys.

RISK FACTORS
Hematuria, hypercalciuria, nephrolithiasis, and nephritis can be inherited.

PATHOPHYSIOLOGY
Bleeding can occur from anywhere along the urinary tract or kidney. In glomerular hematuria, RBCs cross the glomerular basement membrane (GBM) into the urinary space.

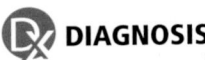

DIAGNOSIS

DIFFERENTIAL DIAGNOSIS
Hematuria may originate at any site along the urinary tract. Nonglomerular causes are more common than glomerular causes.

- **Factitious causes:** Urine appears bloody, but no RBCs are present.
  - Endogenous pigments:
    - Myoglobin (rhabdomyolysis)
    - Hemoglobin
    - Bile pigments
    - Urate crystals (pink diaper syndrome)
    - Beets, blackberries
  - Exogenous pigments:
    - Food and beverage dyes
    - Drugs that cause urinary discoloration:
      - Phenazopyridine (Pyridium)
      - Deferoxamine
      - Rifampin
      - Sulfa
      - Others
  - *Serratia marcescens*
- **Glomerular causes**
  - Common:
    - Strenuous exercise
    - Acute postinfectious glomerulonephritis (GN)
    - IgA nephropathy
    - Thin basement membrane disease (benign familial hematuria)
  - Uncommon:
    - Alport syndrome, hereditary nephritis
    - Membranoproliferative GN
    - Nephritis of systemic disease (Henoch–Schönlein purpura [HSP], systemic lupus or other vasculitis)

- **Nonglomerular (interstitial) renal causes**
  - Common:
    - Pyelonephritis
    - Hypercalciuria/nephrolithiasis/nephrocalcinosis
    - Renal trauma (contusion), particularly in hydronephrotic or cystic kidneys
    - Ureteropelvic junction obstruction
    - Hemoglobinopathies (sickle cell disease, sickle cell trait)
  - Uncommon:
    - Drug-induced interstitial nephritis (penicillins, cephalosporins, NSAIDs, phenytoin)
    - Cystic disease (simple cyst, polycystic kidney disease)
    - Neoplasm: Wilms tumor
    - Coagulopathy
    - Renal venous thrombosis, renal arterial thrombosis
    - "Nutcracker" phenomenon
- **Urinary tract causes**
  - Common:
    - Bladder catheterization, Foley catheter
    - Cystitis (bacterial, viral, occasionally chemical)
    - Perineal trauma or irritation
    - Urethrorrhagia
    - Meatal stenosis
    - Urethritis
    - "Terminal hematuria" syndrome (trigonitis)
    - Epididymitis
  - Uncommon:
    - Bladder tumor
    - Polyp
    - Urethral or bladder trauma
    - Foreign body in bladder or urethra
    - Schistosomiasis
- **External causes of "hematuria"**
  - Menstrual contamination
  - Diaper rash, perineal irritation
- No identifiable cause is found in the majority (up to 80%) of children with asymptomatic microscopic hematuria and in up to 30% of children with a single episode of gross hematuria.

APPROACH TO THE PATIENT
Evaluate all children with gross hematuria and those children with microscopic hematuria confirmed on 2 of 3 consecutive samples over several weeks:

- **Phase 1:** Determine if the pigment in urine is from blood or another source. Are RBCs present on microscopy?
- **Phase 2:** Determine the source of bleeding: Glomerular or nonglomerular, kidney or urinary tract?
- **Phase 3:** Select those who will require referral vs. those who will simply require follow-up.

HISTORY
- **Question:** Blood on voiding?
- *Significance*: Glomerular or renal source will be constantly bloody; urethral bleeding is more likely at initiation of stream.

- **Question:** Prior episodes of gross hematuria or abnormal urinalyses?
- *Significance*: Chronic vs. acute process
- **Question:** Antecedent infection, streptococcal pharyngitis, or impetigo?
- *Significance*: Suggests postinfectious GN
- **Question:** Concurrent upper respiratory infection (URI) or gastroenteritis?
- *Significance*: Suggests IgA nephropathy
- **Question:** Any precipitating factors (trauma, exercise)?
- *Significance*: Renal contusion, exercise hematuria, or myoglobinuria
- **Question:** Voiding symptoms, dysuria, urgency, frequency?
- *Significance*: Suggests bacterial or viral (adenovirus) hemorrhagic cystitis
- **Question:** Renal colic or other pain?
- *Significance*: Suggests stones
- **Question:** Drops of blood or spotting in underwear after or between voiding in prepubertal boys?
- *Significance*: Suggests urethrorrhagia
- **Question:** Fever, rash, arthritis?
- *Significance*: Signs or symptoms of systemic illness or immune-mediated process
- **Question:** Bleeding from any other source (i.e., gums, GI tract)?
- *Significance*: Suggests coagulopathy
- **Question:** Symptom-less "terminal" hematuria?
- *Significance*: Suggests trigonitis, hemorrhagic cystitis
- **Question:** Medications and diet?
- *Significance*: Food or drug pigment, drug nephrotoxicity
- **Question:** Family history?
- *Significance*:
  - Hematuria in family members: Familial hematuria, kidney failure, or premature deafness suggests Alport syndrome
  - Sickle cell disease or trait in child or family members: Suggests sickle nephropathy, papillary necrosis, or hemoglobinuria
  - Renal stone disease in family members: Suggests renal stones, hypercalciuria, or metabolic disease
  - Cystic kidney disease in family members: Autosomal-recessive or autosomal-dominant polycystic kidney disease
  - Kidney failure or identified kidney disease/nephritis in family members: Suggests hereditary nephritis, cystic disease

PHYSICAL EXAM
- **Finding:** Head, ears, eyes, nose, throat (HEENT) exam (periorbital edema)?
- *Significance*: GN, renal failure, volume overload
- **Finding:** Cardiovascular exam (hypertension, tachycardia, murmur, gallop)?
- *Significance*: GN, renal failure, volume overload
- **Finding:** Abdominal exam (ascites, organomegaly, tenderness, or masses)?
- *Significance*: Volume overload, tumor, polycystic kidneys, venous thrombosis

- **Finding:** Back exam (flank tenderness)?
- *Significance:* Pyelonephritis, renal calculi, large cysts
- **Finding:** Genital exam (blood at urethral meatus)?
- *Significance:* Urethral trauma
- **Finding:** Perineal exam (skin breakdown, irritation)?
- *Significance:* External source of bleeding or infection
- **Finding:** Extremities (pretibial edema, arthritis)?
- *Significance:* GN, volume overload, systemic illness
- **Finding:** Skin and mucosal exam (petechial, vasculitic rash, ulcerations)?
- *Significance:* Systemic illness (lupus, HSP)

DIAGNOSTIC TESTS & INTERPRETATION
Positive test for blood on urine dipstick may be myoglobin or hemoglobin. If the urinary sediment does not show RBCs, investigate for problems such as rhabdomyolysis (elevated creatinine phosphokinase [CPK]) or hemolysis.

- **Test:** Repeated urinalysis to confirm persistent microscopic hematuria
- *Significance:*
  - Patient should be told not to exercise before the urine collection.
  - 2 of 3 positive specimens over several weeks should be documented in an otherwise well child before diagnostic testing is initiated.
- **Test:** Gross and microscopic analyses of fresh urine specimen
- *Significance:*
  - Absence of RBCs suggests factitious hematuria.
  - Dimorphic RBCs suggest glomerular source.
  - Eumorphic RBCs suggest nonglomerular source/collecting system etiology.
  - RBC casts: Diagnostic for GN
  - WBCs suggest cystitis.
  - WBC casts suggest pyelonephritis.
- **Test:** Screening of the family members for occult hematuria
- *Significance:* Familial benign hematuria or Alport syndrome
- **Test:** Testing for hypercalciuria (random urine calcium/creatinine ratio >0.2 in children >6 years; >0.6 in children 6–12 months; >0.8 in children <6 months)
- *Significance:* If elevated, 24-hour urine calcium collection >4 mg/kg/d in children >2 years of age: Hypercalciuria
- **Test:** Culture
- *Significance:* Bacterial, viral—cystitis, *S. marcescens*, adenovirus
- **Test:** Serum electrolytes, BUN, and creatinine levels
- *Significance:* Impaired renal function suggests inflammation, infection, or obstruction.
- **Test:** Evaluation for GN
- *Significance:*
  - Hematuria with RBC casts in combination with proteinuria, edema, hypertension, and/or impaired renal function
  - Streptococcal serology (ASOT, streptozyme): Acute postinfectious GN
  - Complement studies (C3,C4): Hypocomplementemic GN—immune complex-mediated (lupus nephritis, postinfectious GN, membranoproliferative GN)
  - Antinuclear antibody (ANA) titer or anti-double-stranded DNA if hypocomplementemic: Vasculitis (lupus)
  - Quantitation of proteinuria and serum albumin concentration:

○ 3–4+ proteinuria, urine protein/creatinine ratio >2, and hypoalbuminemia suggest glomerular disease/nephrosis.
○ 24-hour urine protein ≥1 g/d
- **Test:** CBC with platelets, coagulation times
- *Significance:* May suggest hemolysis, clotting disorder, or systemic illness
- **Test:** Hemoglobin electrophoresis should be considered in black patients.
- *Significance:* Sickle cell disease or sickle trait may cause hematuria.
- Rarely, additional studies, such as cystourethrogram, renal angiography, cystoscopy, and renal biopsy, will be required with an appropriate referral to urology or nephrology.
- Audiometry may be indicated if hereditary (Alport) nephritis is suspected; should be performed on boys with familial hematuria.

Imaging
Every child with gross hematuria should have imaging of the kidneys and urinary tract. It may or may not be indicated in children with microscopic hematuria.

- Ultrasound of kidneys and bladder: Urinary tract obstruction, congenital malformation, cysts, stones, nephrocalcinosis, malignancy
- Abdominal CT scan: After trauma if there are >50 RBCs/hpf or if microscopic hematuria persists for several weeks
- Helical CT without contrast: Study of choice for the visualization of stones; however, must consider radiation exposure risk. Ultrasound is reasonable first test for stones.

 TREATMENT

ADDITIONAL TREATMENT
General Measures
- For children with microscopic hematuria, in the absence of other clinical, laboratory, or imaging findings, no specific treatment is indicated besides routine longitudinal follow-up.
- For children with glomerular hematuria, treatment depends on the histopathologic diagnosis, clinical features, renal function, and degree of proteinuria.
- For children with an anatomic/structural etiology, treatment is specific to abnormality.

ISSUES FOR REFERRAL
- Nephrology: Recurrent gross hematuria, proteinuria, RBC casts, nephrosis, edema, hypocomplementemia, hypertension, azotemia, cysts, hypercalciuria, family history of hereditary nephritis, deafness, or cystic kidney disease
- Urology: Congenital anomaly of urinary tract, uncontrollable bleeding after trauma, recurrent, painful or large stones, recurrent urinary infections
- Bleeding secondary to coagulopathy or sickle cell disease papillary necrosis

 ONGOING CARE

FOLLOW-UP RECOMMENDATIONS
Patient Monitoring
A healthy child with asymptomatic isolated hematuria and a negative workup should be reassessed annually with a complete physical exam, measurement of BP, and urinalysis. If hematuria is persistent, periodic assessment of renal function should also be performed. The development of significant proteinuria, hypertension, elevated creatinine, or other concerns should prompt evaluation by a pediatric nephrologist.

PROGNOSIS
- Most children with asymptomatic isolated microscopic hematuria detected on a well-child examination, without proteinuria, hypertension, or azotemia, will NOT be found to have serious underlying pathology and will simply require longitudinal follow-up.
- Many children with hematuria will not have an identifiable cause; however, long-term prognosis is still generally good.
- Children with asymptomatic microscopic or gross hematuria combined with proteinuria have a high likelihood of glomerular disease.
- Children with a history of stones or hypercalciuria are at increased risk of developing renal stones in the future.
- Familial hematuria secondary to thin GBM disease is a diagnosis of exclusion. Although it often has a benign prognosis, in some families it can progress to chronic kidney disease. Children should be examined yearly for the development of proteinuria or hypertension.

ADDITIONAL READING
- Bergstein JB, Leiser J, Andreoli S. The clinical significance of asymptomatic gross hematuria and microscopic hematuria in children. *Arch Pediatr Adolesc Med*. 2005;159(4):353–355.
- Carasi C, Van't Hoff WG, Rees L, et al. Childhood thin GBM disease: Review of 22 children with family studies and long-term follow-up. *Pediatr Nephrol*. 2005;20:1098–1105.
- Cohen RA, Brown RS. Clinical practice: Microscopic hematuria. *N Engl J Med*. 2003;348:2330–2338.
- Diven SC, Travis LB. A practical primary care approach to hematuria in children. *Pediatr Nephrol*. 2000;14:65–72.
- Feld LG, Meyers KE, Kaplan BS, et al. Limited evaluation of microscopic hematuria in pediatrics. *Pediatrics*. 1998;102:E42.
- Meglic A, Cavic M, Hren-Vencelj H, et al. Chlamydial infection of the urinary tract in children and adolescents with hematuria. *Pediatr Nephrol*. 2000;15:132–133.
- Patel HP, Bissler JJ. Hematuria in children. *Pediatr Clin North Am*. 2001;48:1519–1537.
- Quigley R. Evaluation of hematuria and proteinuria: how should a pediatrician proceed? *Curr Opin Pediatr*. 2008;20(2):140–144.
- Youn T, Trachtman H, Gauthier B. Clinical Spectrum of Gross Hematuria in Pediatric Patients. *Clin Pediatr*. 2006;45(2):135–141.

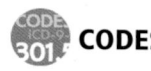 **CODES**

ICD9
- 599.70 Hematuria, unspecified
- 599.71 Gross hematuria
- 599.72 Microscopic hematuria

ICD10
- R31.0 Gross hematuria
- R31.1 Benign essential microscopic hematuria
- R31.9 Hematuria, unspecified

H

HEMOLYSIS
Julie W. Stern

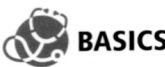 **BASICS**

DEFINITION
Premature destruction of RBCs, either intravascularly or extravascularly, leading to a shortened red cell survival time.

EPIDEMIOLOGY
Hereditary RBC membrane defects may be mild and may be diagnosed at an older age.

RISK FACTORS
Although many of these disorders are autosomal dominant, 20% of these patients represent new spontaneous mutations and have no affected family members.

GENERAL PREVENTION
Avoid glucose-6-phosphate dehydrogenase (G6PD) triggers such as fava beans, broad beans, and mothballs.

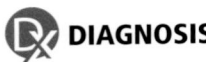 **DIAGNOSIS**

DIFFERENTIAL DIAGNOSIS
See Table 1.

- **Congenital/anatomic**
  - ABO blood type incompatibility and Rh incompatibility between infant and mother
  - Cardiac lesions with turbulent flow; left-sided more common than right-sided
  - Prosthetic heart valve (especially aortic)
  - Kasabach–Merritt syndrome
  - Hypersplenism
- **Infectious**
  - Congenital infections with syphilis, rubella, cytomegalovirus, and toxoplasmosis
  - Malaria
  - Bartonellosis
  - *Clostridium perfringens* (via a toxin)
  - *Mycoplasma pneumoniae*
  - HIV
  - Hemolytic uremic syndrome
- **Toxic, environmental, drugs**
  - Immune-complex "innocent bystander" mechanism:
    ○ Quinidine
    ○ Acetaminophen
    ○ Amoxicillin
    ○ Cephalosporins
    ○ Isoniazid
    ○ Rifampin
  - Immune-complex drug-adsorption mechanism:
    ○ Penicillin
    ○ Cephalosporins
    ○ Erythromycin
    ○ Tetracycline
    ○ Isoniazid
  - Drug-induced autoimmune hemolytic anemia: Alpha-methyldopa
  - Toxic drug-induced hemolysis: Ribavirin (generally mild and not clinically significant)
  - Snake and spider venoms
  - Extensive burns

- **Mechanical hemolysis**
  - Cardiac hemolysis
  - Abnormal microcirculation:
    ○ Thrombotic thrombocytopenic purpura (TTP)
    ○ Disseminated intravascular coagulopathy
    ○ Malignant hypertension
    ○ Eclampsia
    ○ Hemangiomas
    ○ Renal graft rejection
  - March hemoglobinuria (prolonged physical activity)
- **Tumor**
  - Lymphomas
  - Thymoma
  - Lymphoproliferative disorders
- **Genetic/metabolic**
  - RBC membrane defects:
    ○ Hereditary spherocytosis
    ○ Hereditary elliptocytosis
    ○ Pyropoikilocytosis
    ○ Paroxysmal nocturnal hemoglobinuria (can be acquired)
  - Enzyme defects:
    ○ PK deficiency
    ○ G6PD deficiency
  - Thalassemias (β-thalassemia major is the most severe)
  - Hemoglobinopathies:
    ○ Sickle cell anemia (Hgb SS and SC variants)
    ○ Unstable hemoglobins
- **Allergic/inflammatory/immune**
  - Autoimmune hemolytic anemia:
    ○ Warm antibody mediated
    ○ Cold antibody mediated
    ○ Hemolytic transfusion reaction

ALERT
Factors that constitute an emergency:
- Hemoglobin <5 g/dL, especially with signs of cardiovascular compromise
  - Attempts to stabilize cardiovascular compromise with volume should be undertaken with care since hemodilution may occur.
  - Transfusion may be riskier in autoimmune hemolysis because of potential problems with cross-matching.
- Renal failure may accompany severe hemolysis in TTP or hemolytic uremic syndrome.
- Hemolysis in the neonatal period secondary to ABO or Rh incompatibility may require exchange transfusion either for anemia or for hyperbilirubinemia.

ETIOLOGY

Table 1. Common mechanisms of hemolysis

Acquired disorders	Hereditary disorders
Infectious	Hemoglobinopathies
Drug induced	RBC membrane defects
Immune mediated	RBC enzyme defects
Microangiopathic	

APPROACH TO THE PATIENT
General goal is to establish existence of hemolysis rather than other causes of anemia, such as blood loss and hypoproduction.

- **Phase 1:** Determine acuity and severity of the anemia and hemolysis:
  - With acute onset, there will be evidence of unstable vital signs and possibly heart failure.
  - Parents may give a history of a rapid deterioration of the child's physical and/or mental state.
  - Patients with chronic anemia that has progressed slowly may have a low hemoglobin yet be well compensated with fairly normal vital signs (except for tachycardia).
  - CBC with a corrected reticulocyte count will help determine if there is an appropriate bone marrow response to the level of anemia and, therefore, whether the process is hypoproductive or hemolytic.
- **Phase 2:** Determine the cause of hemolysis. Treatment approaches will vary depending on the underlying etiology.

HISTORY
Hemoglobinuria is a sign of intravascular hemolysis, whereas pallor, fatigue, and jaundice may occur with either intravascular or extravascular hemolysis.

- **Question:** History of anemia, splenectomy, or early cholecystectomy in multiple family members?
- *Significance*:
  - Although hereditary membrane defects and enzyme deficiencies may be autosomal dominant, recessive, and X-linked disorders, a negative familial history does not always rule out these diagnoses.
  - In some cases, the diagnosis of hereditary spherocytosis has not been identified, yet multiple members of a family have had their gallbladders removed at an early age, which may indicate the presence of this defect.
  - Thalassemia (especially β-thalassemia) and sickle cell anemia may present in early childhood with chronic hemolysis with or without a familial history.
- **Question:** History of travel?
- *Significance*: Malaria is endemic to Africa, India, and parts of Central America.
- **Question:** Drugs and diet history?
- *Significance*: Specifically ask about exposure to fava beans, mothballs, and antibiotics. Drugs can themselves cause hemolysis or can induce hemolysis if there is an underlying disorder such as G6PD deficiency.
- **Question:** Age at first signs and symptoms of hemolysis (pallor or jaundice)?
- *Significance*:
  - Hereditary causes of hemolysis are most often chronic or recurrent, although the diagnosis may be delayed until the child is older if the process is mild.
  - Acute, acquired hemolytic disorders may also recur.

PHYSICAL EXAM

Hemolysis that is a secondary problem (e.g., related to infection, tumors) may be found incidentally during evaluation of the primary process.

- **Finding:** Acute processes such as autoimmune hemolytic anemia (both warm and cold antibody mediated) may present with a child in extremis.
- *Significance:*
  - Tachycardia is a common finding in nearly all cases of acute hemolysis.
  - BP instability is a late finding.
- **Finding:** More chronic processes, such as hereditary spherocytosis, G6PD, pyruvate kinase (PK) deficiencies, thalassemia intermedia, and sickle cell disease, may be picked up at well visits or by laboratory examination.
- *Significance:* These children often appear well (except for jaundice) but may become more anemic with an acute illness.
- **Finding:** Splenomegaly (often impressive) and hepatomegaly are common findings in extravascular hemolysis.
- *Significance:*
  - Hepatomegaly may be more pronounced if the child is in heart failure due to acute, severe anemia.
  - Splenomegaly may be either the cause of or, more frequently, a result of a hemolytic process.
  - If significant lymphadenopathy is present, look for an underlying cause such as lymphoproliferative disorders or other tumors.
- **Finding:** Skin?
- *Significance:*
  - Pallor is nearly a universal finding in acute hemolysis and in exacerbations of chronic hemolysis.
  - Jaundice is more common in intravascular hemolysis.
  - Presence of ecchymoses or petechiae suggests disseminated intravascular coagulopathy or thrombocytopenia.

DIAGNOSTIC TESTS & INTERPRETATION

- **Test:** CBC with differential and reticulocyte count
- *Significance:*
  - Level of anemia and the reticulocyte count must be interpreted together. Chronic hemolysis in hereditary spherocytosis, for example, may have a nearly normal hemoglobin count but usually has an increased reticulocyte count.
  - With a rapid fall in hemoglobin, as in acute autoimmune hemolytic anemia, the reticulocyte count may be low at the start, rise in response to anemia, and fall during recovery.
  - Thrombocytopenia should raise suspicions about TTP or hemolytic uremic syndrome.
- **Test:** Peripheral blood smear
- *Significance:*
  - Fragmented RBCs, schistocytes, and helmet cells are seen in disseminated intravascular coagulopathy, TTP, hemolytic uremic syndrome, and cardiac valve hemolysis.
  - Helmet or bite cells are nearly pathognomonic for G6PD deficiency.
  - Other findings on the smear that may be helpful in the diagnosis are spherocytes (hereditary spherocytosis and warm autoimmune hemolytic anemia), target cells (hemoglobin C and thalassemias), and acanthocytes (anorexia nervosa).

- **Test:** Bilirubin
- *Significance:* Total and unconjugated bilirubins are elevated in most cases.
- **Test:** Urinalysis
- *Significance:*
  - Hemoglobinuria is present in intravascular hemolysis; established by a urine dipstick positive for heme with no intact red cells microscopically.
  - Myoglobinuria can also give this picture.
- **Test:** Coombs test
- *Significance:*
  - Direct Coombs test (direct antiglobulin test) detects antibodies or complement fragments present on the patient's RBCs.
  - Indirect antiglobulin test detects antibodies in the patient's serum that can bind normal RBCs.
  - Direct antiglobulin test provides direct evidence of immune-mediated hemolysis.
  - Warm antibody autoimmune hemolytic anemia is caused by an IgG antibody that coats RBCs, which are subsequently removed by the spleen.
  - Cold antibody autoimmune hemolytic anemia is caused by an IgM antibody that binds RBCs, fixes complement, and can cause both extravascular and intravascular hemolysis.
- **Test:** Haptoglobin, hemopexin, and lactate dehydrogenase
- *Significance:*
  - In intravascular hemolysis, haptoglobin levels may be undetectable, hemopexin is reduced, and lactate dehydrogenase is significantly increased.
  - In extravascular hemolysis, haptoglobin is decreased (but detectable) and lactate dehydrogenase may be increased, but not to the level seen in intravascular hemolysis.
- **Test:** Bone marrow aspiration
- *Significance:* Rarely indicated, but if performed, erythroid hyperplasia should be present.
- Blood for diagnostic RBC enzyme or hemoglobinopathy studies must be drawn prior to transfusion.

 TREATMENT

ADDITIONAL TREATMENT
General Measures
- Red cell transfusion may be indicated for symptomatic anemia regardless of cause: Amount of rate will depend on severity of anemia and speed of onset (generally slower transfusion rate needed in chronic anemia).
- Plasmapheresis for TTP
- Withdrawal of inducing drug/agent (G6PD)

ISSUES FOR REFERRAL
- Most patients with severe, acute hemolysis or an underlying chronic hemolytic disorder will need to be evaluated by a hematologist.
- Suspected RBC membrane and enzyme defects, as well as hemoglobinopathies, should be referred for initial evaluation.

Admission Criteria
Unstable vital signs with acute hemolysis, significant exacerbation of chronic hemolysis

ADDITIONAL READING

- Gallagher PG. Update on the clinical spectrum and genetics of red blood cell membrane disorders. *Curr Hematol Rep.* 2004;3:85–91.
- Lo L, Singer ST. Thalassemia: Current approach to an old disease. *Pediatr Clin North Am.* 2002;49:1165–1191.
- Maisels MJ, Kring E. The contribution of hemolysis to early jaundice in normal newborns. *Pediatrics.* 2006;118(1):276–279.
- Old JM. Screening and genetic diagnosis of haemoglobin disorders. *Blood Rev.* 2003;17:43–53.
- Perkins SL. Pediatric red cell disorders and pure red cell aplasia. *Am J Clin Pathol.* 2004;122(Suppl 1):S70–S86.
- Shah S, Vega R. Hereditary spherocytosis. *Pediatr Rev.* 2004;25:168–172.

 CODES

ICD9
- 282.2 Anemias due to disorders of glutathione metabolism
- 282.7 Other hemoglobinopathies
- 773.1 Hemolytic disease of fetus or newborn due to ABO isoimmunization

ICD10
- D55.0 Anemia due to glucose-6-phosphate dehydrogenase deficiency
- P55.1 ABO isoimmunization of newborn
- D58.2 Other hemoglobinopathies

FAQ

- Q: When are blood transfusions indicated in patients with active hemolysis?
- A: Patients with severe, acute hemolysis that is causing cardiovascular compromise may require a transfusion if the process cannot be stopped with standard therapy (e.g., steroids for warm autoimmune hemolytic anemia, plasmapheresis for TTP). Transfusions must be given slowly if the hemolytic process has been chronic and the patient's blood volume is expanded.
- Q: Can hemolysis always be identified on a peripheral blood smear?
- A: No. Schistocytes, fragments, spherocytes, targets, and other morphology may provide clues to specific diagnoses but are not always present. The presence of a hemolytic process is inferred from a fall in hemoglobin, rise in the reticulocyte count, and elevation of the bilirubin and lactate dehydrogenase levels.

H

HEMOLYTIC DISEASE OF THE NEWBORN

Deborah A. Sesok-Pizzini

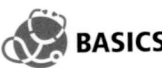 **BASICS**

DESCRIPTION
Hemolytic anemia occurring in the newborn owing to passive transfer of maternal RBC antibodies (IgG) against fetal RBCs

EPIDEMIOLOGY
- 15% of whites are Rh negative (dd)
- 48% are heterozygous (Dd)
- 35% are homozygous (DD)
- Prevalence of Rh-positive fetus in Rh-negative mother: 15%
- Incidence of Rh hemolytic disease: 6–7/1,000 live births
- Of all Rh-sensitized pregnancies:
  – 50% require no treatment.
  – 31% require treatment after a full-term delivery.
  – 10% are delivered early and require exchange transfusion.
  – 9% require intrauterine transfusion.
- Reasons for spectrum of clinical severity:
  – Rh immunization rarely occurs in 1st pregnancy.
  – Many subsequent infants may be Rh negative.
  – Only a fraction of women at risk develop antibodies.
- 50% of cases of ABO hemolytic disease of the newborn (HDN) occur in 1st pregnancy.

GENERAL PREVENTION
- Rh hemolytic disease can be prevented by administration of RhIG to an Rh-negative woman after any exposure to Rh-positive blood, prophylactically during pregnancy, and postpartum (within 72 hours) after birth of an Rh-positive newborn.
  – Standard dose of 300 mcg of RhIG given to unsensitized Rh(−) women at 28 weeks and at birth, or following an abortion or ruptured tubal pregnancy.
  – Calculate RhIG dose if fetal screen is positive and a Kleihauer-Betke or flow cytometry test is performed to determine the percentage of fetal cells in maternal circulation.
- Smaller doses of 50 mcg are indicated in the 1st trimester following sensitizing events.
- An Rh(−) woman known to be sensitized to Rh(D) (not due to antenatal RhIG administration) is not a candidate for RhIG.
- Severe HDN due to other RBC antibodies (i.e., Kell, Duffy) may be prevented by following maternal antibody titers and performing an analysis of amniotic fluid for bilirubin, ultrasound of the fetus, and Doppler ultrasonography of the middle cerebral artery.

PATHOPHYSIOLOGY
- Rh alloimmunization (or other antibody) results from passage of fetal RBCs that express surface Rh(D) antigen (or other RBC antigen) across the placenta into the circulation of an Rh-negative (or other antigen-negative) mother.
- The passage of fetal RBCs occurs as a result of transplacental hemorrhage.
- Initial exposure results in production of maternal IgM antibodies, which do not cross the placenta. This is followed by production of IgG antibodies, which can cross the placenta. On subsequent exposures, there is a rapid production of IgG antibodies.
- Mothers may have initial sensitization owing to transfusion or previous pregnancy.
- IgG produced in the maternal circulation crosses the placenta and coats fetal RBCs. These cells are then destroyed in the reticuloendothelial system, primarily the fetal spleen.
- Isoimmunization may lead to severe anemia, hydrops, and hyperbilirubinemia.
- Extramedullary hematopoiesis in the fetal liver and spleen occurs as a response to fetal anemia, leading to severe hepatosplenomegaly.
- ABO HDN occurs more frequently in type O mothers due to anti-A, B (IgG antibody) with type A or B fetus, and results in a clinically milder hemolysis and rarely requires intervention.
- HDN due to other RBC antibodies such as anti-Kell and anti-Ge may be a result of an additional mechanism that involves either suppression or destruction of RBC precursors.

ETIOLOGY
- Most common antigen system involved: ABO with mild HDN
- Failed or omitted anti-D prophylaxis
- 1% of cases involve other antigens.
- Other antigens include Kell*, Kidd, Duffy, MNS, C, E, c*, e, Ge, C^w, SARA, Jr^a (most severe HDN*)

DIAGNOSIS

HISTORY
- Previous stillbirths and/or abortions
- Neonatal hyperbilirubinemia requiring therapy in previous pregnancy
- Exposure of mother to blood products or previous pregnancy
- Father's ABO and Rh and other RBC antigen type
- RhIG not given after previous pregnancy or abortion

PHYSICAL EXAM
- Pallor, tachycardia, tachypnea due to CHF secondary to severe anemia
- Jaundice developing within 24 hours of birth
- Usually no jaundice at birth
- Generalized edema in cases with severe anemia and hydrops
- Massive hepatosplenomegaly in severe cases
- Milder cases manifest with neonatal hyperbilirubinemia only.
- ABO incompatibility usually manifests jaundice at 24 hours.

DIAGNOSTIC TESTS & INTERPRETATION
Lab
- Antenatal:
  – ABO and Rh type of all mothers at 1st prenatal visit
  – Zygosity of the father: If the father is Rh-positive homozygous, then all children will be Rh positive; if the father is heterozygous, then only 50% of children will be Rh positive.
  – Fetal blood group genotyping can be performed from a maternal blood sample during 2nd trimester.
  – Monitor antibody titer.
  – Spectrophotometric assessment of bilirubin concentration in amniotic fluid
  – Amniotic fluid values in Liley zone 3 and high zone 2 indicative of severe fetal disease (Liley test measures optical density in amniotic fluid as an indicator for bilirubin levels; do not use for Kell sensitization as it is not a reliable indicator of severity of disease in these patients)
  – Fetal blood sampling in severe cases to assess degree of anemia
- Neonatal:
  – Cord blood or neonate red blood cells for ABO and Rh types
  – Cord blood or neonate blood for hemoglobin (Hb), hematocrit (Hct), bilirubin (direct and indirect), reticulocyte count
  – Direct Coombs test on cord or neonate red blood cells will be positive in immune hemolytic disease.
  – Indirect Coombs test on neonate's serum for passively transferred antibody
  – Identification of antibody after elution from RBC
  – Administration of RhIG during pregnancy may result in a positive indirect Coombs result (antibody screen), but no risk to the fetus
  – Peripheral smear: Nucleated RBCs (spherocytes in ABO disease)

Imaging
- Fetal ultrasound (visualize fetal size and organomegaly)
- Doppler ultrasonography of fetal middle cerebral artery peak systolic velocity

Diagnostic Procedures/Other
- Fetal cordocentesis (for fetal anemia)
- Amniocentesis
- Intrauterine transfusion

Pathological Findings
- Kernicterus
- Extramedullary hematopoiesis
- Hepatosplenomegaly
- Edema

DIFFERENTIAL DIAGNOSIS
- Neonatal hyperbilirubinemia:
  – Galactosemia
  – Glucose-6-phosphate dehydrogenase (G6PD) deficiency
  – Hypothyroidism
  – Pyruvate kinase deficiency
  – Crigler-Najjar syndrome
  – α-Thalassemia
  – Gilbert syndrome
  – Spherocytosis
  – Breast milk jaundice

- Hydrops fetalis:
  - Hematologic: α-Thalassemia, severe G6PD deficiency, twin-to-twin transfusion
  - Cardiac: Hypoplastic left heart syndrome, myocarditis, endocardial fibroelastosis, heart block
  - Congenital infections: Parvovirus, syphilis, cytomegalovirus (CMV), rubella
  - Renal: Renal vein thrombosis, urinary tract obstruction, nephrosis
  - Placental: Umbilical vein thrombosis, true knot of umbilical cord
  - Miscellaneous: Trisomy 13, 18, 21; triploidy; aneuploidy; diaphragmatic hernia

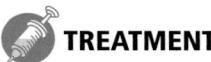 TREATMENT

ADDITIONAL TREATMENT
General Measures
- In severely affected fetuses (fetal Hct <25–30%) where early delivery is not possible owing to lung immaturity, intrauterine RBC transfusion is the therapy of choice. Usually not performed until after 20 weeks' gestation. Risks include fetal loss (2%), premature labor, rupture of membranes, chorioamnionitis, fetal bradycardia, cord laceration, and fetomaternal hemorrhage.
- Maternal plasma exchange and IVIG administration have been attempted as an alternative to intrauterine transfusion. Antibody titers are temporarily reduced.
- Early delivery and subsequent resuscitation may be required in severe HDN:
  - If there has been a previous stillbirth or hydrops and the fetus is high risk after amniocentesis, plan early delivery.
  - Careful fetal monitoring and induction of pulmonary maturation
  - After delivery, treatment depends on age, birth weight, severity, and other illness. Phototherapy starts as soon as possible.
- Exchange transfusion removes sensitized fetal RBCs and circulating bilirubin and also has the following benefits:
  - Corrects anemia in severely anemic infants
  - Prevents or corrects hyperbilirubinemia
  - Removes circulating antibodies
- Indications for early exchange transfusion:
  - Cord blood bilirubin >4.5 mg/dL and cord blood Hb <10 g/dL
  - Bilirubin rising at rate >1 mg/dL/hr despite optimal phototherapy
  - Indirect bilirubin ≥20 mg/dL or rising to reach that level
  - Lower indirect bilirubin triggers are used in preterm or high-risk infants.
  - Hb between 11 and 13 g/dL and bilirubin rising at rate >0.5 mg/dL/hr despite optimal phototherapy
- In hydropic infants, immediate partial exchange may be needed to correct anemia and CHF.
- Double-volume exchanges may be needed for hyperbilirubinemia.
- Selection of blood for exchange transfusion:
  - As fresh as possible or washed, CMV-safe, and irradiated, hemoglobin S negative

  - For Rh disease (if prepared before delivery): Type O Rh negative cross-matched against mother's blood
  - For ABO disease: Type O Rh negative or Rh compatible cross-matched against mother or infant's serum
  - For other antibodies: Antigen-negative RBCs selected to avoid the clinically significant antibody. ABO type-specific blood can be used if baby's type confirmed.
- Risks of exchange transfusion include prolonged neutropenia, thrombocytopenia, late anemia, metabolic abnormalities, arrhythmias, thrombosis, and death.
- Some studies indicate that administration of IVIG to the neonate diminishes hemolysis and may prevent the need for exchange transfusion.
- Most infants with ABO incompatibility require no treatment or phototherapy only.
- Some infants with milder Rh isoimmunization may have only exaggerated physiologic anemia at 12 weeks.
- Avoid drugs that interfere with bilirubin metabolism or its binding to albumin (sulfonamides, caffeine, and sodium benzoate).
- Infants who had HDN are at risk for late anemia owing to reticulocytopenia related to persistent high titers of circulating maternal antibody. They should have weekly Hct measured during the 1st few months of life. These infants may require small-volume transfusion.
- Erythropoietin and oral iron supplements may be used to avoid blood transfusion.

Additional Therapies
- Phototherapy
- Exchange transfusion

 ONGOING CARE

FOLLOW-UP RECOMMENDATIONS
Patient Monitoring
- Weekly Hct, especially for patients who had exchange transfusion
- Watch for exaggerated physiologic anemia at 12 weeks.
- Assess for neurologic damage.

PROGNOSIS
- ~50% of the infants have minimal anemia and hyperbilirubinemia and require either no treatment or phototherapy only.
- 1/4 will require exchange transfusions.
- Hydropic infants have high mortality.

COMPLICATIONS
- Hydrops fetalis
- Stillbirths
- Neonatal hyperbilirubinemia and kernicterus
- Fetal anemia

ADDITIONAL READING

- Chen WX, Wong VC, Wong KY. Neurodevelopmental outcome of severe neonatal hemolytic hyperbilirubinemia. *J Child Neurol*. 2006;21(6): 474–479.
- Dhodapkar KM, Blei F. Treatment of hemolytic disease of the newborn caused by anti-Kell antibody with recombinant erythropoietin. *J Pediatr Hematol Oncol*. 2001;23:69–70.
- Judd WJ. Practice guidelines for prenatal and perinatal immunohematology, revisited. *Transfusion*. 2001;41(11):1445–1452.
- Lee AI, Kaufman RM, Transfusion medicine and the pregnant patient. *Hematol Oncol Clin North Am*. 2011;25(2):393–413.
- Maisels MJ, Newman TB. Kernicterus, the Daubert decision, and evidence-based medicine. *Pediatrics*. 2007;119(5):1038; author reply 1038–1039.
- Moise KJ. Management of Rhesus alloimmunization in pregnancy. *Obstet Gynecol*. 2002;100:600–611.
- Oepkes D, Seaward G, Vandenbussche FP, et al. Doppler ultrasonography versus amniocentesis to predict fetal anemia. *N Engl J Med*. 2006;355: 156–154.
- Palfi M, Hilden J-O, Matthiesen L, et al. A case of severe Rh(D) alloimmunization treated by intensive plasma exchange and high-dose intravenous immunoglobulin. *Transfus Apher Sci*. 2006;35: 131–136.

 CODES

ICD9
773.2 Hemolytic disease of fetus or newborn due to other and unspecified isoimmunization

ICD10
P55.8 Other hemolytic diseases of newborn

FAQ
- Q: Does the condition become worse with each pregnancy?
- A: The fetus may be more affected in a 2nd or subsequent pregnancies with HDN due to Rh antibodies. Other antibodies, such as Kell, may result in severe HDN even in a 1st pregnancy.
- Q: Can maternal blood be used to transfuse the affected baby?
- A: Washed maternal blood may be used, but donor infectious disease testing protocols would need to be followed so it would not be routinely available in an emergency situation. However, for certain high-frequency antigens, such as Kp^b, maternal blood should be considered.
- Q: When are O red blood cells indicated for exchange transfusion?
- A: O red blood cells are indicated when the neonate's blood type is unknown or the reason for the HDN is ABO incompatibility between mom and neonate.

H

HEMOLYTIC UREMIC SYNDROME

Divya Moodalbail
Andres J. Greco (5th edition)

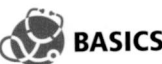 **BASICS**

DESCRIPTION
- HUS is a disease phenotype characterized by renal impairment, thrombocytopenia, and anemia with fragmentation of erythrocytes (schistocytes noted on peripheral smear).
- The kidney dysfunction may manifest as hematuria and/or proteinuria and/or azotemia.
- HUS is the leading cause of acute renal failure in infants and young children.
- ~90% of childhood cases follow a diarrheal prodrome (D+HUS or Stx HUS, or classic HUS).
- This syndrome can also be non–diarrhea-related (atypical) and represent a heterogeneous group of disorders: Hereditary (defects in complement proteins), *Streptococcus pneumoniae*–related HUS and HUS secondary to malignancies, bone marrow transplant, collagen-vascular disorder or drugs (calcineurin inhibitors).
- Non-Stx forms of HUS usually have a poor outcome.

EPIDEMIOLOGY
- Stx HUS (D+HUS):
  - Tends to occur in the summer months, and epidemics have been reported in daycare centers and nursing homes.
  - Occurs mainly in older infants and young children, between 6 months and 4 years of age.
- Atypical HUS (D-HUS):
  - Has no seasonal variation and can occur at any age; can occur sporadically or in families.

GENERAL PREVENTION
- Shiga toxin-producing *E. coli* (STEC) is found in the intestine of beef cattle. Ground beef may be contaminated throughout with Shiga toxin.
- For adequate prevention, it is imperative to wash hands and food well and to cook food, especially meat, thoroughly.

PATHOPHYSIOLOGY
- Vascular endothelial cell injury is central to the pathogenesis of all forms of HUS
- STEC colonize colonic mucosa, adhere to mucosal villi, and release Shiga toxin (Stx).
- Stx binds to cell surface receptors, translocates into the cell, interrupts protein synthesis, and causes cell death. This produces endothelial cell injury, exposing the thrombogenic basement membrane, and this causes platelet activation and local intravascular thrombosis.
- Recently, it has been shown that upregulation of chemokine and cytokine production occurs with Stx-1 and 2 and increased binding of the inflammatory cells to the endothelial cells.
- In vitro studies show that glomerular endothelial cells have receptors with very high affinity to the Stx.

ETIOLOGY
- Stx HUS: Most cases are caused by STEC, most often the O157:H7 subtype:
  - STEC most commonly infect children from 9 months to 4 years of age in the summer and the fall. The primary reservoir is cattle.
  - A negative stool culture in a patient who has HUS does not eliminate STEC as the cause.
- Atypical HUS: Mutations have been reported in the complement regulatory protein factor H in both sporadic and familial HUS, with mutations identified in 10–20% of cases.
- Mutations in other complement regulators (membrane cofactor protein CD46) have also been associated with familial HUS.
- One of the common causes of sporadic non–Stx-HUS is *S. pneumoniae* infection.

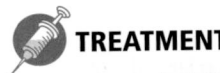 **DIAGNOSIS**

HISTORY
- GI prodrome: Stx HUS can develop 2–14 days after the onset of diarrhea (usually bloody). There can be associated vomiting and fever.
- Symptoms of pneumonia: *S. pneumoniae* associated HUS is associated with severe disease.
- Recent hamburger ingestion, consumption of unpasteurized milk, cheese, or apple cider
- Direct animal contact (petting zoos)
- Family history of HUS

PHYSICAL EXAM
- Pallor and petechiae
- Dehydration secondary to the gastroenteritis
- Edema
- Pulmonary edema (volume overload)
- Hypertension
- Irritability
- Behavioral changes

DIAGNOSTIC TESTS & INTERPRETATION
Lab
- CBC: Anemia, thrombocytopenia (usually <60,000/mm^3 in most of the cases), leukocytosis (often seen in typical HUS)
- Blood smear: Fragmented RBCs or schistocytes
- Markers of hemolysis: Elevated LDH, circulating free hemoglobin, decreased haptoglobin, elevated unconjugated bilirubin, increased reticulocyte count
- Renal function: Elevated BUN and serum creatinine
- Serum electrolytes: Hyperkalemia (hypokalemia can be observed in severe GI involvement), metabolic acidosis, hyponatremia, hypocalcemia, hyperphosphatemia
- Serum albumin: Usually low due to enteral losses and/or hypercatabolic state

- Amylase/Lipase: Elevated in pancreatic involvement.
- Stool culture: Should be screened for *E. coli* O157:H7 (>90% cases), preferably before 6 days after the onset of diarrhea. The local health department should be notified of any isolates.
- Identification of Shiga-toxin

Imaging
- Plain film of the abdomen often demonstrates colonic distension or evidence of bowel perforation.
- Barium enema may show "thumb-printing," secondary to bowel wall edema and submucosal bleeding.

Pathological Findings
The lesions are usually limited to the kidneys and involve the glomerular capillaries and the afferent arterioles. Renal biopsy findings usually comprise diffuse thickening of the glomerular capillary wall and swelling of endothelial cells. Thrombi containing platelets and small amounts of fibrin are visible in the capillary lumina.

DIFFERENTIAL DIAGNOSIS
- Severe hemolytic anemia
- Malaria

TREATMENT

MEDICATION (DRUGS)
- Antihypertensives: Vasodilators, such as calcium-channel blockers or hydralazine, are useful in the acute phase. After recovery, if a patient persists with hypertension and/or proteinuria, then ACE inhibitors are indicated.
- In patients with seizures, diazepam or lorazepam are of choice. In patients with recurrent seizures or cerebral infarcts, long-term anticonvulsant therapy is indicated.
- Treatment with insulin may be needed in patients with pancreatic necrosis.
- Patients with invasive bacterial infections or abscesses should be treated with appropriate antibiotic coverage.

ADDITIONAL TREATMENT
General Measures
- Treatment of HUS is generally supportive.
- The mainstay of therapy involves:
  - Strict fluid balance
  - Nutritional support
  - Control of hypertension
  - Treatment of seizures
- In patients with GI illness secondary to STEC, it's advisable to avoid administration of antibiotics unless there is sepsis, to prevent antibiotic-induced damage to the bacterial membranes, which can result in release of large amounts of toxin.

- Renal replacement therapy for severe acidosis, fluid overload, electrolyte imbalance or uremia
- Treatment of severe anemia: Packed RBCs are transfused slowly if the hemoglobin decreases below 6 g/dL (BP can increase during transfusion)
- Platelet transfusion: Indicated if there is active bleeding and severe thrombocytopenia, or the patient needs surgery or invasive procedure

Additional Therapies
- Renal replacement therapy:
  - Unless contraindicated, peritoneal dialysis is the treatment of choice.
  - It should be started in patients with anuria >24 hours.
  - Kidney transplant should be considered in patients who progress to end-stage renal disease.
- Plasmapheresis or fresh frozen plasma infusion may be beneficial in idiopathic (atypical) forms of HUS.

SURGERY/OTHER PROCEDURES
Some patients can have extensive bowel necrosis requiring resection.

IN-PATIENT CONSIDERATIONS
IV Fluids
Any fluid deficit should be corrected, and composition of additional fluid should be limited to ongoing losses (insensible water loss plus urine and/or GI losses).

 ## ONGOING CARE

FOLLOW-UP RECOMMENDATIONS
- Resolution is usually heralded by a rise in platelet count and a gradual decrease in the frequency of blood transfusions.
- Pancreatic insufficiency may persist, requiring long-term insulin therapy beyond resolution of acute illness.
- If a patient who attends a daycare center has Stx HUS, contacts should be informed that any episodes of gastroenteritis merit close follow-up for evidence of anemia, thrombocytopenia, and renal failure. No prophylaxis is indicated. Ill children should not be permitted to reenter the child care center until diarrhea has resolved and 2 stool cultures obtained 48 hours after antimicrobial therapy has been discontinued are negative for E. coli O157:H7.

DIET
- Aggressive nutritional support is important due to the hypercatabolic state of these patients.
- Enteral feeding can be tried if diarrhea is resolved.
- Total parenteral nutrition can be used in patients with severe GI involvement and dialysis.
- Avoid antiperistaltic agents for treatment of colitis.
- Some patients can have pancreatic involvement with subsequent exocrine or endocrine pancreatic insufficiency.

PROGNOSIS
- Factors associated with poor prognosis are:
  - Anuria lasting >2 weeks
  - WBC count >20,000/mm^3
  - Coma
  - Atypical HUS
  - Renal cortical necrosis
  - Prolonged diarrhea
- Patients with D+HUS can be mildly or severely affected. ~25% of survivors demonstrate long-term sequelae such as proteinuria and hypertension.
  - Mildly affected patients never develop anuria, almost never have seizures, are rarely hypertensive, do not require dialysis, and have an excellent outcome
  - Severely affected patients develop anuria and require dialysis, develop hypertension, and may have seizures. They can also progress to end-stage renal disease. Recurrence after renal transplantation is very uncommon.

COMPLICATIONS
- GI:
  - Acute colitis is usually transient.
  - Rectal prolapse, toxic megacolon, bowel wall necrosis, intussusception, perforation, and stricture
  - Pancreatic involvement may result in pancreatitis or insulin-dependent diabetes mellitus.
- CNS:
  - Most patients have mild CNS symptoms that include irritability, lethargy, and behavioral changes.
  - Major symptoms such as stupor, coma, seizures, cortical blindness, posturing, and hallucinations occur in 20–40% of patients.
  - Thrombotic or hemorrhagic stroke may occur.
  - The risk of seizures is associated with hyponatremia.

ADDITIONAL READING

- *Escherichia coli* diarrhea (including hemolytic-uremic syndrome). In: Pickering LK, ed., *Red Book: 2006 Report of the Committee on Infectious Diseases*, 27th ed. Elk Grove Village, IL: American Academy of Pediatrics, 2006:291–296.
- Fiorin EK, Raffaelli R. Hemolytic-uremic syndrome. *Pediatr Rev.* 2006;10:398–399.
- Kaplan BS, Meyers KE, Schulman SL. The pathogenesis and treatment of hemolytic uremic syndrome. *J Am Soc Nephrol.* 1998;9:1126–1133.

- Noris M, Remuzzi G. Hemolytic uremic syndrome, disease of the month. *J Am Soc Nephrol.* 2005; 16:1035–1050.
- Siegler RL. The hemolytic uremic syndrome. *Pediatr Clin North Am.* 1995;6:1505–1525.

 ## CODES

ICD9
283.11 Hemolytic uremic syndrome

ICD10
D59.3 Hemolytic-uremic syndrome

FAQ

- Q: What are some predictors of the severity of enteropathic HUS?
- A: Predictors include an elevated white cell count, a severe GI prodrome, anuria early in the course of illness, and age <2 years.
- Q: In a patient with nonenteropathic HUS, what is the chance other siblings will be affected?
- A: Familial HUS due to factor H deficiency may be autosomal dominant or recessive.
- Q: How many patients with gastroenteritis from *E. coli* 0157:H7 will develop HUS?
- A: 10–20%
- Q: What should the family tell the daycare staff and neighbors?
- A: If the patient has enteropathic HUS, contacts should be informed that any episodes of gastroenteritis merit close follow-up for evidence of anemia, thrombocytopenia, and renal insufficiency. No prophylaxis is indicated. Exclusion of infected children from daycare centers until 2 consecutive stool cultures are negative for *E. coli* 0157:H7 has been shown to prevent additional transmission.

H

HEMOPHILIA
Char Witmer

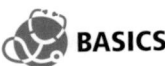 **BASICS**

DESCRIPTION
- Hemophilia A is factor VIII deficiency, and hemophilia B is factor IX deficiency. Both are inherited in an X-linked recessive manner.
- Deficiency or absence of FVIII or FIX leads to a delay and disruption of blood clotting that results in prolonged bleeding.
- The severity of bleeding depends on the percentage of clotting activity. No activity (<1%) results in severe disease; 1–5% is moderate, and 6–30% is mild hemophilia.

EPIDEMIOLOGY
- Most common severe inherited bleeding disorder
- Distribution:
  - Hemophilia A: 80–85%
  - Hemophilia B: 10–15%
- No geographic or ethnic associations
- 30% of cases are sporadic (no family history)

Incidence
- Hemophilia A: 1 per 5,000 male births
- Hemophilia B: 1 per 30,000 male births

RISK FACTORS
Genetics
- X-linked recessive disorder
- Daughters of fathers with hemophilia are obligate carriers for the hemophilia gene mutation. An obligate carrier has a 50% chance of passing the hemophilia gene mutations to her offspring.
- Carrier status and prenatal testing available
- Hemophilia A:
  - The intron 22 inversion mutation in the factor VIII gene is found in ~40–50% of patients with severe hemophilia A; detectable by direct gene mutation analysis.
- Hemophilia B:
  - Most factor IX gene defects are single–base pair changes that result in missense, frameshift, or nonsense mutations. Mutations have been detected in all regions of the factor IX gene.

GENERAL PREVENTION
- Prophylaxis: The regularly scheduled infusion of clotting factor concentrate with the goal of preventing bleeding episodes; primarily used in patients with severe disease.
  - Primary prophylaxis: Regularly scheduled infusion of clotting factor before joint bleeding is typically initiated before 1 year of age.
  - Secondary prophylaxis: Regularly scheduled infusion of clotting factor after joint bleeding has occurred
- Anticipatory guidance and prevention:
  - Good dental hygiene
  - Immunizations: No intramuscular injections; give subcutaneously with a small-gauge needle and apply direct pressure for several minutes.
  - Rapid treatment of hemarthrosis to avoid chronic joint damage
  - Avoidance of contact sports (e.g., football, hockey, rugby)
  - Encourage physical fitness to ensure strong muscles to maintain joint health and prevent joint bleeding. Some recommended activities include swimming, bicycle riding, and walking/hiking. Other sports that can be considered include soccer, tennis, and track.

- Home infusion therapy for prophylaxis as appropriate
- Self-infusion training: Usually starts in adolescence

PATHOPHYSIOLOGY
- Both factors VIII and IX are crucial for normal thrombin generation via the intrinsic pathway. The absence or decrease in activity of either protein severely impairs the ability to generate thrombin and fibrin.
- Hemophilia patients do not bleed more rapidly; rather, there is delayed formation of an abnormal clot resulting in prolonged bleeding.
- The friable clot formed has a tendency to ooze and rebleed.
- In closed spaces (e.g., joint), bleeding stops by tamponade; in open spaces (e.g., iliopsoas muscle, open wounds), significant amounts of blood may be lost.
- Repeated joint hemorrhages lead to synovial thickening and joint cartilage erosion. Joint space becomes narrowed and eventually fuses.

 DIAGNOSIS

HISTORY
- Family history:
  - Familial history of hemophilia in male offspring of female blood relatives is present in only 70% of cases. 30% of the time there is no family history of hemophilia.
- Excessive bleeding in a male neonate:
  - Excessive bleeding with circumcision may be an initial presentation of hemophilia, although only 50% of patients with hemophilia will have excessive bleeding with circumcision.
  - Muscle bleeding from intramuscular injections (e.g., vitamin K or immunizations); presents as increasing swelling at the site of injection
  - Prolonged oral bleeding from a torn frenulum or prolonged bleeding from venipuncture or heel puncture can be seen.
  - 3.5–4% of neonates with hemophilia may present with an intracranial hemorrhage.
- Pattern of bleeding in severe hemophilia:
  - Characterized by easy, excessive, and palpable bruising with normal activity, spontaneous joint and muscle hemorrhages, and prolonged and potentially fatal hemorrhage after trauma or surgery
- Age of onset of bleeding:
  - Bleeding events occur frequently when the child begins to crawl and walk or with the eruption of teeth.
  - Patients with mild hemophilia may not present until they are older.
- Location of hemarthroses:
  - Large weight-bearing joints are most often involved: Knees, ankles, and hips. Other nonweight-bearing joints can be involved including elbows and shoulders.
- Early symptoms of a hemarthroses:
  - Aura of tingling or warmth, visible swelling, followed by increasing pain and decreasing range of motion (ROM), and inability to bear weight

PHYSICAL EXAM
Joint exam:
- Acute hemarthrosis: Limitation and pain with ROM, warmth, swelling, tenderness
- Chronic joint changes: Crepitus, decreased ROM, synovial hypertrophy, boney abnormalities, and proximal muscle weakness
- Intramuscular hematomas: May not have external bruising; there will be pain with motion and swelling. With larger bleeds there will be a discrepancy in limb circumference.
- Distal extremity neurovascular compromise can be a sign of compartment syndrome from bleeding into the forearm.

DIAGNOSTIC TESTS & INTERPRETATION

ALERT
- Neonates have a normal physiologic reduction in the vitamin K–dependent factors, including factor IX, making a determination of the degree of factor IX deficiency difficult in the neonatal period. The factor IX level must be confirmed after 6 months of age.
- When interpreting coagulation testing in a neonate, neonatal normal values for the PT and aPTT are different from those in adults.

Lab
Patients with hemophilia either A or B will have a normal PT and a prolonged aPTT. Assay for factor VIII and factor IX levels:
- <1%: Severe hemophilia, characterized by spontaneous bleeding; hemarthroses and deep-tissue hemorrhages; will need frequent factor replacement therapy
- 1–5%: Moderate hemophilia. Bleeding following mild to moderate trauma; hemarthrosis and muscle bleeding, seldom spontaneous hemorrhage
- 5–30%: Mild hemophilia. Bleeding from trauma only, no spontaneous hemorrhages; patients require factor replacement only with significant trauma or prior to surgery or dental extraction

DIFFERENTIAL DIAGNOSIS
- Isolated prolonged aPTT associated with increased bleeding tendency:
  - von Willebrand disease
  - "Acquired hemophilia" owing to development of an inhibitory antibody to factor VIII or IX (extremely rare in children)
  - Hereditary factor deficiency of either VIII, IX, or XI
  - Afibrinogenemia
- Prolonged aPTT without increased bleeding tendency:
  - Factor XII deficiency
  - High-molecular-weight kininogen deficiency
  - Prekallikrein deficiency
  - Antiphospholipid antibody (lupus anticoagulant)
  - Heparin artifact
  - Underfilling of the specimen tube
  - Polycythemia

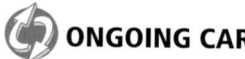 **TREATMENT**

MEDICATION (DRUGS)

Acute bleeding episodes:

- Factor replacement:
  - Factor VIII replacement products:
    ○ Recombinant, non–plasma-derived factor VIII
    ○ Plasma-derived, monoclonal antibody–purified factor VIII concentrate; heat or solvent detergent treated for viral inactivation
    ○ Cryoprecipitate (rarely used)
  - Factor IX replacement products:
    ○ Recombinant, non–plasma-derived factor IX
    ○ Plasma-derived, immunoaffinity-purified factor IX concentrate; heat or solvent detergent treated for viral inactivation
    ○ Prothrombin complex concentrate (PCC): Crude plasma fraction that contains variable amounts of activated factors II, VII, IX, and X; heat-treated for viral inactivation
    ○ Fresh frozen plasma (rarely used)
- Calculation of dose for pediatrics:
  - Recombinant factor VIII dosing (units) = % desired rise in plasma factor VIII × body weight (kg) × 0.5
  - Recombinant factor IX dosing (units) = % desired rise in plasma factor IX level × body weight (kg) × 1.4
- Target factor levels:
  - Joint bleed: 30–50% for 24–48 hours
  - Large muscle bleed: 70–100% repeated over 12–48 hours for large muscle bleeds
- CNS bleeding: 80–100% maintained for 10–14 days
- Desmopressin (DDAVP):
  - Synthetic vasopressin analog that stimulates release of endogenous factor VIII and von Willebrand factor
  - Only suitable for patients with mild or moderate factor VIII deficiency who have shown a response to DDAVP in a trial
  - Tachyphylaxis (unresponsiveness) may occur with repeated dosing.
  - Hyponatremia may also occur. Fluid restriction is recommended after each dose. Should not be used in neonates.
- Antifibrinolytic therapy:
  - Antifibrinolytic therapy is used to stabilize a clot by inhibiting the normal process of clot lysis by the fibrinolytic system.
  - Agents used for the treatment of oral hemorrhages and to minimize bleeding from dental and some surgical procedures: Aminocaproic acid, 100 mg/kg PO q6h (maximum, 6 g/dose), or tranexamic acid, 10 mg/kg PO q6–8h (maximum, 1.5 g/dose)

ADDITIONAL TREATMENT
General Measures

- Immobilization:
  - Splints, casts, crutches, and/or bed rest (24–48 hours)
  - Prolonged immobilization may reduce recovery of joint ROM
  - Initiation of physical therapy with factor coverage may be recommended, particularly after joint surgery.
- Special bleeding situations:
  - Intracranial hemorrhage:
    ○ Significant bleeding can occur despite a minor mechanism of head injury and the absence of external bruising. In severe hemophilia spontaneous intracranial bleeding can occur.

○ Factor replacement to 100% should be administered immediately followed by the diagnostic evaluation.
  - Major surgery:
    ○ Factor replacement to 100% preoperatively and postoperatively
    ○ Regular dosing of factor for a minimum of 1 week postoperatively, even in mild hemophilia
  - Compartment syndrome:
    ○ Bleeding within the fascial compartments of muscles
    ○ Most often occurs in the forearm
    ○ Neurovascular compromise can lead to Volkmann contracture.
  - Iliopsoas bleed:
    ○ Lower abdominal or upper thigh pain may be the 1st symptom.
    ○ Exam is notable for inability to extend hip with preservation of internal and external rotation (allows distinction from hemarthrosis of hip joint).
    ○ Diagnosis confirmed by ultrasound or CT scan
  - Oral bleeding/epistaxis:
    ○ Constant pressure for 15–20 minutes
    ○ Aminocaproic acid or tranexamic acid
    ○ Topical thrombin directly to the site of bleeding
  - Dental care:
    ○ Factor replacement is required for significant dental procedures like tooth extraction or procedures that require a mandibular block injection.
    ○ Preferably done in a hospital setting where hematology consultation is available.
    ○ Factor replacement is not required for routine teeth cleaning.
  - Lacerations:
    ○ Factor replacement is necessary at time of placement and removal of the sutures.
  - Hematuria:
    ○ Increased fluid intake and bed rest as initial treatment
    ○ If hematuria persists 24–48 hours, 30–40% factor replacement
    ○ Antifibrinolytics are contraindicated in the setting of hematuria because of the concern of obstructive uropathy from excessive clot formation.
- Patients should be followed regularly at a comprehensive hemophilia treatment center.

IN-PATIENT CONSIDERATIONS
Initial Stabilization

Life-threatening hemorrhages:
- CNS bleeding
- Bleeding into and around the airway
- Exsanguinating hemorrhage
- Prompt therapy with clotting factor concentrate should start immediately and prior to any diagnostic procedures.

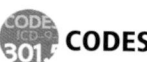 **ONGOING CARE**

COMPLICATIONS

- Complications of disease:
  - Hemophilic arthropathy: Joint contractures, limited ROM, and chronic pain
  - Intracranial bleeding (can occur without known trauma in severe hemophilia)
  - Compartment syndrome
  - Airway compromise owing to bleeds in the pharynx, tongue, or neck
  - Life-threatening hemorrhage owing to GI, posttraumatic, or perioperative bleeds

- Complications of therapy:
  - Inhibitors: Antibodies against factor VIII or IX, which can inactivate infused factor
  - Viral transmission (HIV, hepatitis B and C) through clotting factor concentrates derived from pooled plasma preparations. This risk is now minimized through the creation of recombinant factor products.
  - Anaphylaxis: Seen primarily with infusions of factor IX
- Thromboembolic disease: The use of central lines in pediatric patients with hemophilia for factor infusions has been associated with thrombotic complications. Bypassing agents including activated prothrombin complex concentrates or activated recombinant factor VIIa have also been linked with thrombosis.

ADDITIONAL READING

- Dunn AL, Abshire TC. Recent advances in the management of the child who has hemophilia. *Heme/Oncol Clin North Am.* 2004;18:1249–1276.
- Ljung R. Intracranial haemorrhage in haemophilia A and B. *Br J Haematol.* 2007;140:378–384.
- Mannucci PM, Tuddenham EGD. The hemophilias: From royal genes to therapy. *N Engl J Med.* 2001;344:1773–1779.
- Pipe SW, Valentino LA. Optimizing outcomes for patients with severe haemophilia A. *Haemophilia.* 2007;13(Suppl 4):1–16.
- Pruthi RK. Hemophilia: A practical approach to genetic testing. *Mayo Clin Proc.* 2005;80:1485–1499.
- Raffini L, Manno C. Modern management of haemophilic arthropathy. *Br J Haematol.* 2007;136:777–787.

CODES

ICD9
- 286.0 Congenital factor VIII disorder
- 286.1 Congenital factor IX disorder

ICD10
- D66 Hereditary factor VIII deficiency
- D67 Hereditary factor IX deficiency

FAQ

- Q: Are there any medications contraindicated in a child with hemophilia?
- A: Aspirin should not be given, as it interferes with platelet function. NSAIDs cause a milder effect on platelets and should also be avoided when possible. Patients with hemophilia should use acetaminophen for fever or pain.
- Q: Can immunizations be given to a child with hemophilia?
- A: To prevent bleeding from immunizations, they should be given SQ (instead of IM) with the smallest gauge needle available. Ice or cold packs should be applied to the area to minimize hematoma formation.

H

HEMOPTYSIS

Suzanne E. Beck

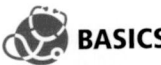 BASICS

DESCRIPTION
Hemoptysis is the coughing up of blood from the respiratory tract. The term comes from the Greek words *haima*, meaning blood, and *ptysis*, meaning spitting. The amount and nature of bleeding should be characterized by taking a careful history. Bleeding from the respiratory tract can range from blood-streaked sputum to massive hemoptysis from the lung. The source of bleeding can be anywhere in the respiratory tract, from the nose to the alveolus. Associated symptoms vary and may include cough, chest pain, rhinorrhea, or dyspnea, or there may be none. Consequences of hemoptysis may include exsanguination, hypoxemia, and anemia, or there may be none.

EPIDEMIOLOGY
Large series of pediatric patients with massive hemoptysis have not been described. Most instances of massive hemoptysis take place in older children, usually with underlying cardiac or pulmonary conditions.

PATHOPHYSIOLOGY
- Related to the underlying pulmonary or cardiac disease
- Vascular origin of hemoptysis is from 2 sites: Pulmonary arteries or bronchial arteries

ETIOLOGY
- Aspiration
- Bronchiectasis
- Bronchitis
- Cavitary infections (e.g., tuberculosis, abscess, histoplasmosis)
- Cystic fibrosis
- Congenital vascular or airway lesions (pulmonary arteriovenous malformation, hemangioma, bronchogenic cyst)
- Congenital heart disease with collateral vessels or pulmonary hypertension
- Factitious hemoptysis
- Foreign body aspiration
- Hemorrhagic diathesis, including anticoagulant therapy
- H-type tracheoesophageal fistula
- Pneumonia
- Pulmonary embolism
- Pulmonary hemosiderosis
- Tracheostomy-related complications
- Trauma (pulmonary contusion, bronchoscopy, airway manipulation)
- Tumors (lymphomas)

DIAGNOSIS

HISTORY
- Distinguish the source of bleeding: Nose, mouth, gastrointestinal (GI) tract versus lungs:
  - Bleeding from the nose and mouth may be associated with recurrent episodes, recent trauma, or pain at the site and is usually self-limited.
  - Bleeding from the GI tract may be associated with vomiting, history of gastritis, or abdominal pain.
  - Bleeding from the lungs may be associated with chest discomfort or sensations, shortness of breath, or coughing.
  - Blood from the GI tract is often darker and acidic, whereas blood from the airway tends to be bright red and alkaline, or pink and frothy.
- Determine amount of bleeding (>1 cup in 24 hours is considered massive).
- Determine associated symptoms/conditions:
  - Familial history of pulmonary disease or bleeding disorder
  - Systemic symptoms (weight loss, may indicate tumor)
  - Exposure to environmental toxins (mold or flood-damaged homes)
  - Exposure to tuberculosis
  - Medication/drug use: Cocaine, marijuana, propylthiouracil
  - Recurrent episodes of cough associated with blood-tinged sputum or hemoptysis suggests underlying bronchiectasis or chronic pulmonary infection.
  - Acute pleuritic chest pain raises the possibility of pulmonary embolism with infarction or other pleural lesion.

PHYSICAL EXAM
- Respiratory distress or hypoxemia: Indicates significant ventilation–perfusion mismatch due to airspace disease, shunt due to pulmonary embolism, or acidosis due to hypovolemia and blood loss
- Paleness: Indicates anemia or poor perfusion
- Pleural friction rub: May be associated with pulmonary embolism
- Loud 2nd heart sound: Suggests primary pulmonary hypertension, mitral stenosis, or Eisenmenger syndrome
- Localized wheeze over a major lobar airway: Suggests an intramural lesion such as hemangioma, foreign body, or carcinoma
- Presence of a murmur over the lung fields: May suggest pulmonary arteriovenous malformation
- Clubbing: Indicates the presence of underlying pulmonary disease such as cystic fibrosis, congenital cardiovascular disease, or liver disease

DIAGNOSTIC TESTS & INTERPRETATION
Lab
- CBC, reticulocyte count, erythrocyte sedimentation rate, and coagulation profile: May indicate the volume of blood loss, chronicity of blood loss, inflammatory conditions, and evidence of bleeding diathesis
- Comprehensive metabolic panel: To determine hepatic and renal function, acid-base status
- Sputum for bacterial culture, Gram stain, and acid-fast bacilli
- Purified protein derivative (PPD) testing
- Drug screen: If appropriate
- ECG: Determine presence of right ventricular hypertrophy.
- ESR, CRP, other rheumatologic studies if suspected

Imaging
- Chest radiograph, both anteroposterior and lateral: May reveal pleural effusion, bronchiectasis, foreign bodies, or consolidation. Fleeting alveolar infiltrates suggest pulmonary hemorrhage.
- CT: Useful when chest radiographs and fiberoptic bronchoscopy are normal. High-resolution CT may identify an area of bleeding, especially if bronchiectasis and arteriovenous malformation are suspected.
- Angiogram or CT angiograms: Used to detect bleeding from a vascular malformation or pulmonary embolism
- Ventilation–perfusion scans: Important studies in patients suspected of having hemoptysis from pulmonary embolism or infarct

Diagnostic Procedures/Other

- Flexible fiberoptic bronchoscopy:
  - Usually performed to localize the site of bleeding. Preferred if bleeding is distal or if alveolar bleeding is suspected, such as in alveolar hemorrhage due to capillaritis or pulmonary hemosiderosis
  - Fiberoptic bronchoscopy performed acutely (during hemoptysis or within 48 hours of event) is more likely than delayed bronchoscopy to visualize and stop active bleeding.
- Rigid bronchoscopy has the advantage of providing a means of airway stabilization, ventilation, and oxygenation while identifying and treating the source of bleeding or airway obstruction (clot, hemangioma) if the lesion is proximal, or to perform a therapeutic intervention (e.g., foreign body removal).

DIFFERENTIAL DIAGNOSIS

- Infections: Pneumonia, pulmonary abscess, tuberculosis, bronchitis
- Pulmonary disease: Cystic fibrosis, bronchiectasis, foreign body aspiration, arteriovenous malformation, congenital lung malformation, pulmonary emboli, pulmonary hemosiderosis, alveolar capillaritis, aspiration, isolated unilateral pulmonary agenesis
- Cardiovascular disease: Congenital heart malformations, pulmonary hypertension
- Collagen vascular disease: Systemic lupus erythematosus, vasculitis, Goodpasture disease, Wegener granulomatosis
- Trauma
- Coagulation disorder
- Munchausen syndrome
- Bronchogenic cysts, neoplasms, hemangiomas

 ## TREATMENT

ADDITIONAL TREATMENT
General Measures

- Initial management should follow the lines of basic life support.
- Support IV volume with packed RBCs or fresh frozen plasma.
- Methods used to stop localized bleeding include tamponade with balloon-tipped catheters, ice water lavage, local instillation of epinephrine, catheter-directed umbilication, IV vasopressin, and surgical resection. Surgical resection is usually reserved for the most difficult cases, such as extensive collateralization of bronchial arteries or arteriovenous malformations unresponsive to embolization. The most effective nonsurgical treatment is bronchial artery embolization. Some newer techniques include endoscopic instillation of fibrinogen/thrombin and endobronchial argon plasma coagulation.

 ## ONGOING CARE

PROGNOSIS

- Depends on the cause and nature of hemoptysis
- Immediate airway management decreases morbidity and mortality.

COMPLICATIONS

- Respiratory insufficiency
- Acute airway obstruction
- Hypovolemic shock
- Anemia
- Pneumonia
- Death

ADDITIONAL READING

- Batra PS, Holinger LD. Etiology and management of pediatric hemoptysis. *Arch Otolaryngol Head Neck Surg.* 2001;127:377–382.
- De Gracia J. Use of endoscopic fibrinogen-thrombin in the treatment of severe hemoptysis. *Respir Med.* 2003;97:790–795.
- Godfrey S. Pulmonary hemorrhage/hemoptysis in children. *Pediatr Pulmonol.* 2004;37(6):476–484.
- Jean-Baptiste E. Clinical assessment and management of massive hemoptysis. *Crit Care Med.* 2000;28:1642–1647.
- Lasso-Pirot A, Goldsmith D, Pascasio J, et al. Pulmonary hemorrhage in a child due to propylthiouracil. *Pediatr Pulmonol.* 2005;39(1):88–92.
- Salih ZN, Akhter A, Akhter J. Specificity and sensitivity of hemosiderin-laden macrophages in routine bronchoalveolar lavage in children. *Arch Pathol Lab Med.* 2006;130(11):1684–1686.

CODES

ICD9
786.30 Hemoptysis, unspecified

ICD10
R04.2 Hemoptysis

H

HENOCH-SCHÖNLEIN PURPURA

Blaze Robert Gusic

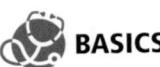 BASICS

DESCRIPTION
Henoch-Schönlein purpura (HSP) is an immunologically mediated, nonthrombocytopenic, purpuric, and systemic vasculitis involving the small blood vessels of the skin, gastrointestinal (GI) tract, joints, and kidneys.
- Defined by the presence of 2 of the following:
  - Palpable purpura
  - Age of onset <20 years
  - Abdominal pain
  - Granulocytic infiltration of vessel walls
- In children, only palpable purpura with normal platelet count needs be documented. Although most children do have purpura, colicky abdominal pain, and arthritis, up to 1/2 may present with symptoms other than purpura.

EPIDEMIOLOGY
Incidence
Incidence of 13.5 cases per 100,000 school-aged children per year (90% of patients are <10 years)

RISK FACTORS
Genetics
- There is only anecdotal evidence of genetic predisposition.
- Familial history of IgA-related disorders or inherited defects in complement (C2, C4 deficiency) may predispose to HSP.

PATHOPHYSIOLOGY
- Capillaries, arterioles, and venules are affected in HSP as opposed to polyarteritis nodosa, Wegener granulomatosis, and systemic lupus erythematosus (SLE), where small arteries are affected.
- Biopsy of the involved kidneys shows endocapillary proliferative glomerulonephritis involving endothelial and mesangial cells. Crescent formation may also be present. IgA, IgG, C3, and fibrin are commonly found in the mesangial regions.
- Considered to be an immune-mediated vasculitic disorder involving primarily IgA, specifically subclass IgA1. This is indirectly suggested by the elevation of serum IgA levels, circulating IgA immune complexes, IgA rheumatoid factor, IgA–fibronectin complexes, and immunoregulatory abnormalities involving IgA production.
- IgA from mucosal B cells interacts with IgG to form immune complexes that activate the alternate pathway of the complement system. Circulating IgA is deposited in the affected organs causing the inflammatory process.

ETIOLOGY
- No single etiologic agent has been identified.
- Most cases associated with preceding upper respiratory tract infections (URIs), usually group A β-hemolytic streptococci. A recent study shows a significant association with *Bartonella henselae*. Also reported following infections with parvovirus, adenovirus, hepatitis A virus, *Helicobacter pylori*, and *Mycoplasma pneumoniae*. Parvovirus B19 previously proposed, but evidence is inconclusive
- Also reported after drug ingestion (e.g., thiazides) and insect bites

DIAGNOSIS

HISTORY
- Previous disease: Especially infections such as hepatitis, URI, and streptococcal infections
- Abdominal pain: Pain is the most common GI tract symptom. 2/3 of children have GI tract symptoms. Emesis and melena are also reported.
- Transient, nondeforming, nonmigratory arthritis of knees, ankles, wrists, elbows, and digits is a frequent problem, and most common in knees and ankles.
- Presence of testicular pain or scrotal swelling, headache, cough, edema of the ankles or periorbital region, and hematuria suggests vasculitic lesions in the associated system.

PHYSICAL EXAM
- Particular attention to BP: Hypertension is common.
- Low-grade fever is present in 50% of the cases.
- Rash that is petechial or purpuric in a pressure-dependent, symmetric distribution, usually around the lateral malleoli of the ankles, on the ventral surfaces of the feet, and on the buttocks:
  - Purpura may be briefly preceded by maculopapular or urticarial lesions.
  - Lesions may ulcerate or present as hemorrhagic bullae.
- Joints should be examined for swelling and limitation of motion: Redness and warmth are not common. Symptoms precede the rash by up to 2 weeks in 25% of patients.
- Nonpitting subcutaneous edema of the scalp, periorbital region, hands, and feet is often noted:
  - Generalized edema is more common in children <3 years. The edema may lead to acute hemorrhagic edema, now considered to be a variant of HSP.
- Abdomen is often tender to palpation, but without rebound tenderness. Hepatosplenomegaly may be found. Because intussusception and appendicitis are possible complications, serial examinations may be necessary to determine if radiographic studies are indicated:
  - Abdominal symptoms may precede the rash by up to 2 weeks.
  - Symptoms of pancreatitis may appear after the onset of the rash, but pancreatitis has been reported as a rare presenting symptom.
- Orchitis, where affected testicle may be tender and swollen:
  - Swelling and bruising may be noted on the scrotum.
  - Testicular torsion has also been reported in HSP and may mimic orchitis.
- Neurologic changes:
  - CNS involvement may present with headaches, seizures, or behavioral changes.
  - Guillain-Barré syndrome has been reported.

DIAGNOSTIC TESTS & INTERPRETATION
There are no definitive diagnostic tests.
Lab
- CBC:
  - Normal platelet count differentiates from thrombocytopenic purpura. Hemoglobin is usually normal; leukocytosis; (especially eosinophilia), may be present.
- ESR: Normal or elevated
- Prothrombin (PT) and partial thromboplastin time (PTT): Normal
- IgA: Often elevated in the acute phase of illness, with normal or increased IgG and IgM
- C3: Normal (decreased in poststreptococcal glomerulonephritis and SLE)
- Antinuclear antibody: Negative (elevated in SLE)
- Von Willebrand factor antigen elevated with active HSP due to endothelial damage
- Throat swab for group A β-hemolytic streptococci: Positive in up to 75% of cases
- Serum basic/comprehensive chemistries: Elevated BUN and creatinine levels and decreased protein and albumin are seen with renal involvement.
- Urinalysis: Gross hematuria and proteinuria are present in many patients. Proteinuria alone is rare. Microscopic blood, RBCs, WBCs, and casts suggest glomerulonephritis.
- Stool guaiac: GI tract involvement may present as guaiac-positive stools, bloody stools, or melena. Important to have a low suspicion for intussusception, which is a known complication of HSP

Imaging
- Chest radiograph: May show interstitial lung disease
- Abdominal ultrasound: May be helpful if intussusception or appendicitis suspected
- Barium enemas are *not* indicated for suspected intussusception:
  - They will not reduce the ileoileal intussusception common to HSP (idiopathic intussusception is usually ileocolic in location) and may damage or perforate the inflamed bowel.
- Testicular ultrasound if torsion of the testes or appendix testes, known complications of HSP, suspected on clinical exam

Diagnostic Procedures/Other
- Renal biopsy: With severe renal failure, a biopsy should be performed to determine the extent of disease.
- Skin biopsy (optional): Direct immunofluorescence for IgA helpful in confirming the diagnosis

DIFFERENTIAL DIAGNOSIS
- Petechial and purpuric rashes seen in thrombocytopenia from:
  - Idiopathic thrombocytopenic purpura (ITP)
  - Sepsis/infection: Meningococcemia, Rocky Mountain spotted fever
  - Leukemia
  - Hemolytic uremic syndrome (HUS)
  - Coagulopathies

- Vasculitic rashes may result from primary and secondary vasculitides:
  - Polyarteritis nodosa
  - Wegener granulomatosis
  - Infection related
  - Connective tissue diseases (e.g., SLE), Berger disease (IgA nephropathy): Glomerulonephritis similar to HSP both clinically and immunologically, but not associated with the skin, GI tract, or joint manifestations of HSP streptococcal glomerulonephritis
  - Infantile acute hemorrhagic edema: Vasculitis that presents with urticarial or maculopapular rash, which then becomes purpuric. It is differentiated from HSP in that it usually affects children from 4 months to 2 years of age, is more common in the winter, and is not associated with systemic symptoms. On biopsy, IgA deposits are not as consistent a finding as they are with HSP.
  - Rheumatoid arthritis
  - Rheumatic fever

 TREATMENT

ADDITIONAL TREATMENT
General Measures
HSP usually resolves spontaneously without specific therapy:

- Analgesics and NSAIDs may be used for control of joint pain and inflammation, but salicylates and other agents that affect platelet function should be avoided if GI tract bleeding is present.
- Steroids are used for painful cutaneous edema, arthritis, and abdominal pain (2 mg/kg/d of prednisone until clinical resolution); however, steroids have not been shown to affect purpura or to decrease duration of disease or frequency of recurrences:
  - No consensus on management of GI and renal involvement. Oral prednisone at 2 mg/kg/d has shown faster resolution of abdominal pain, whereas other studies indicate that the symptoms will resolve similarly without intervention.
  - Steroids may mask associated problems such as intussusception and bowel perforation.
  - In nephritis, immediate treatment with steroids may prevent more serious renal disease; however, most will improve spontaneously. Treatment should be considered for children at high risk for chronic renal insufficiency or failure (those presenting with nephrotic syndrome or renal insufficiency).
- >50% crescentic glomerulonephritis on renal biopsy has a greater risk of future renal failure. Such cases should be considered for aggressive therapy with pulse or oral steroids and/or immunosuppressants (azathioprine, cyclophosphamide, cyclosporine) or plasmapheresis, intravenous immunoglobulin (IVIG), danazol, or fish oil.
- Treatment of hypertension may delay or prevent progression of renal disease in patients with glomerulonephritis.

 ONGOING CARE

FOLLOW-UP RECOMMENDATIONS
Patient Monitoring
- Patients should be seen weekly during the acute illness. Visits should include history and physical exam, along with BP measurement and urinalysis.
- All patients, even those who did not present with renal involvement, should have urine checked for blood weekly for 6 months and then monthly for 3 years because deterioration of renal function has been observed years after presentation in some patients.
- Women with a history of HSP should be monitored for proteinuria and hypertension during pregnancy.

PROGNOSIS
- Generally excellent: Most (>60%) children are better within 4 weeks of the onset.
- Better prognosis associated with younger age
- Recurrence within the 1st 6 weeks in up to 40%, usually as rash and abdominal pain
- No laboratory or clinical findings have been found to be predictive of recurrence.
- Most have only 1–3 episodes of purpura; however, a few will continue to experience symptoms for months or years. These patients have a poor prognosis and are more likely to develop severe nephritis.
- GI tract disease accounts for the most significant morbidity in the short term.
- Renal involvement is the cause of the most serious long-term morbidity. Microscopic hematuria alone or with mild proteinuria generally has a good outcome. A nephritic and nephrotic combination is more guarded, and those patients with a high percentage of crescent formation have worse outcomes.

COMPLICATIONS
- Persistent hypertension
- End-stage kidney disease (acute or as a late sequela)
- Intussusception (most common GI tract complication; affecting 1–5% of patients)
- Protein-losing enteropathy
- Hemorrhagic pancreatitis
- Hydrops of the gallbladder
- Strictures of the esophagus and ileus
- Bowel perforations, ischemia, and infarctions
- Pseudomembranous colitis
- Appendicitis
- Skin necrosis
- Subarachnoid, subdural, and cortical hemorrhage and infarction
- Peripheral mononeuropathies and polyneuropathies (Guillain-Barré syndrome)
- Pulmonary hemorrhage (uncommon, but may result in death)
- Torsion of the testis and appendix testes, and priapism
- Renal failure and hypertension, which can develop up to 10 years after onset of disease
- Scrotal swelling and pain

ADDITIONAL READING
- Davin JC, Weening JJ. Henoch Schönlein purpura nephritis: An update. *Eur J Pediatr.* 2001;160:689–695.
- Gedalia A, Cuchacovich R. Systemic vasculitis in childhood. *Curr Rheumatol Rep.* 2009;11:402–409.
- Peru H, Soylemezoglu O, Bakkaloglu SA, et al. Henoch Schönlein purpura in childhood: Clinical analysis of 254 cases over a 3-year period. *Clin Rheumatol.* 2008;9:1087–1092.
- Prais D, Amir J, Nussinovitch M. Recurrent Henoch-Schonlein purpura in children. *J Clin Rheumatol.* 2007;13(1):25–28.
- Saulsbury FT. Henoch-Schönlein purpura. *Curr Opin Rheumatol.* 2001;13:35–40.
- Soyer T, Egritas O, Atmaca E, et al. Acute pancreatitis: A rare presenting feature of Henoch Schonlein purpura. *J Paediatr Child Health.* 2008;3:152–153.
- Zaffanello M, Fanos V. Treatment-based literature of Henoch-Schönlein purpura nephritis in childhood. *Pediatr Nephrol.* 2009;24(10):1901–1911.

 CODES

ICD9
287.0 Allergic purpura

ICD10
D69.0 Allergic purpura

FAQ
- Q: When should I consider hospitalization for HSP?
- A: Often it is not necessary. Severe complications may require admission. These include GI hemorrhage, protein-losing enteropathy requiring total parenteral nutrition (TPN), decreased glomerular filtration rate (GFR) or hypertension, and pulmonary hemorrhage.
- Q: Is there a role for prophylactic penicillin?
- A: In patients with frequent relapses in whom group A β-hemolytic streptococci is often the inciting agent, administration of penicillin may be helpful.
- Q: Who are Henoch and Schönlein?
- A: The clinical finding of joint pain associated with purpura was named "purpura rheumatica" in 1837 by Schönlein. Henoch, a student of Schönlein's, later described the association of GI tract and renal involvement. However, the 1st report was by Heberden in 1801. Of note, it has been speculated that Mozart—whose symptoms included fever, vomiting, exanthem, arthritis, anasarca, and coma—died of HSP.

H

HEPATIC FAILURE

Charles Vanderpool
Lynette A. Gillis

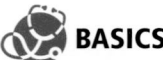 **BASICS**

DESCRIPTION
- A set of criteria has been proposed to diagnose acute hepatic failure in the pediatric population:
  - Biochemical evidence of liver injury
  - No previous history of chronic liver disease
  - Coagulopathy not responsive to vitamin K administration
  - International normalized ratio (INR) >1.5 in presence of encephalopathy or INR >2 without encephalopathy
- In older children and adolescents, in whom hepatic encephalopathy can be more easily assessed, acute hepatic failure may more simply be defined as:
  - Onset of encephalopathy <8 weeks after the onset of symptoms referable to liver dysfunction in a patient without preexisting liver disease

EPIDEMIOLOGY
- Prevalence of specific causes is often age-dependent and may vary based on geographic region.
- In infants and children <3 years of age, indeterminate and metabolic etiologies predominate.
- In older children and adolescents, drug-induced toxicity, especially acetaminophen, becomes more common.
- Infectious etiologies, especially viral hepatitis, vary in prevalence based on geographic region.

PATHOPHYSIOLOGY
Hepatocellular necrosis leads to release of growth factors that promote hepatic regeneration:
- Hepatic failure may become irreversible if:
  - The initial insult overcomes the liver's regenerative capacity.
  - The offending agent or derangement is not eliminated or corrected.
  - Secondary complications, such as shock or disseminated intravascular coagulation (DIC), lead to further injury.

ETIOLOGY
The major causes of acute liver failure can be grouped into the following broad categories:
- Indeterminate
- Drug Induced/Toxin: Acetaminophen, nonacetaminophen drug toxicity
- Metabolic/Genetic
- Infectious
- Vascular/Ischemic
- Malignancy
- Autoimmune

DIAGNOSIS

HISTORY
- Age: May suggest possible etiologic subgroup
- Toxin exposure: Prescription, over-the-counter, herbal, or supplemental medications
- Symptoms of viral prodrome
- Travel history, exposure history
- Length of symptoms, acuity of onset
- Associated symptoms/ROS:
  - Bleeding, bruising
  - Weakness, fatigue
  - Abdominal distension, pain, diarrhea
  - Pruritus secondary to cholestasis

PHYSICAL EXAM
- Skin: Jaundice, bruising
- Eyes: Scleral icterus
- Abdomen: Hepatomegaly, ascites with dullness to percussion or fluid wave, splenomegaly
- Neurologic:
  - Sequential mental status exams are paramount to monitor for change and should include age-appropriate questions.
  - Assess for presence of encephalopathy:
    - Grade I: Confused, altered sleep habits; reflexes normal, may have tremor or apraxia
    - Grade II: Drowsy, inappropriate behavior; hyperreflexic or asterixis; dysarthria or ataxia
    - Grade III: Stupor but may obey simple commands, sleepy; hyperreflexic, asterixis, Babinski positive; increased general tone
    - Grade IV: Comatose; reflexes absent; decerebrate or decorticate posturing

DIAGNOSTIC TESTS & INTERPRETATION
Imaging
- Abdominal ultrasound with Doppler: Visualization of both hepatic parenchyma and vasculature (direction of portal flow, presence of thrombosis)
- Abdomen/Pelvic CT with or without contrast depending on renal function
- Head CT scan without IV contrast in presence of encephalopathy or neurologic signs to rule out intracranial hemorrhage or cerebral edema

Diagnostic Procedures/Other
- Comprehensive metabolic panel:
  - Hepatocellular injury: Aminotransferases (AST, ALT) often are markedly elevated, degree of elevation may depend upon mechanism and time frame of injury
  - Biliary injury/obstruction: Elevated alkaline phosphatase, gamma glutamyl transpeptidase (GGT), total/direct bilirubin
- Assessment of hepatocellular synthetic function:
  - Prolonged PT/INR (with adequate supply of vitamin K)
  - Depressed factor V, VII levels
  - Hypoalbuminemia
  - Hypoglycemia: Frequent glucose measurements should be followed during initial evaluation and should be checked with any mental status or neurologic change.

- Encephalopathy: Ammonia level (has not been proven to correlate directly to presence or grade of encephalopathy)
- Tests to determine etiology:
  - Toxin: Urine or serum drug screen, serum acetaminophen and aspirin level
  - Infectious: Hepatitis virus serologic testing, comprehensive viral cultures; PCR testing for EBV, CMV, HSV and other viruses; antibody tests
  - Autoimmune hepatitis: Antinuclear, anti–smooth muscle, anti–f-actin and anti-LKM antibodies
  - Wilson disease: Decreased serum ceruloplasmin (may not be reliable in setting of acute liver failure), increased serum or urinary copper, evidence of hemolysis (oxidative stress from serum copper)
- Liver biopsy: Timing and approach depends on clinical stability, platelet level, presence of coagulopathy or ascites.

DIFFERENTIAL DIAGNOSIS
The cause of hepatic failure can be indeterminate in up to 50% of cases. Etiologic subgroups include:
- Drug-induced/Toxin:
  - Acetaminophen: Most common in older children and adolescents
  - Salicylates
  - Iron compounds
  - Anticonvulsants
  - Isoniazid
  - Ethanol
  - Antibiotics
  - *Amanita* species (mushrooms)
- Metabolic/Genetic/Miscellaneous: Early infancy:
  - Galactosemia
  - Tyrosinemia
  - Neonatal hemochromatosis
  - Storage diseases
  - Mitochondrial disorders
  - Fatty acid oxidation disorders
  - Hereditary fructose intolerance
- Metabolic/Genetic/Miscellaneous: Childhood/Adolescence:
  - Autoimmune hepatitis
  - Wilson disease
  - Pregnancy (HELLP syndrome, acute fatty liver)
  - Reye syndrome
- Infectious:
  - Hepatitis virus: A, B, E; less commonly C
  - Herpes Virus: HSV, EBV, CMV, VZV, HHV6
  - Echovirus, especially in neonates
  - Parvovirus
  - Adenovirus
- Vascular/Ischemic:
  - Congestive heart failure
  - Hypotensive shock
  - Budd-Chiari syndrome: Hepatic venous outflow obstruction
  - Veno-occlusive disease: Nonthrombotic occlusion of hepatic venules, typically occurs following stem cell transplantation
- Malignancy:
  - Primary: Hepatoblastoma, hepatocellular carcinoma
  - Other: Leukemia, lymphoma, hemophagocytic lymphohistiocytosis
- Heatstroke, hyperthermia, rhabdomyolysis

TREATMENT

MEDICATION (DRUGS)
- Medications should be mixed in fluids without sodium, such as D5 or D10W, whenever possible.
- Hematologic:
  - Coagulopathy should be corrected conservatively in the absence of active bleeding.
  - Vitamin K: Administer IV or SQ/IM for prolonged PT/INR and monitor response with repeat PT/INR 4–6 hours following vitamin K administration.
  - FFP and cryoprecipitate should be reserved for acute severe bleeding; their use prohibits subsequent monitoring of PT/INR or specific factor levels.
  - Recombinant factor VIIa can be used in cases of acute severe bleeding.
- Infectious disease:
  - Prophylactic antibiotics and antifungal medications if febrile, following obtaining cultures from any central venous access or catheterization.
- Renal:
  - Nephrotoxic drugs should be avoided when possible.
  - Renal dose medications if renal compromise present.
  - Renal replacement therapy as indicated, as per nephrology team.
- Neurologic/Hepatic encephalopathy:
  - Sedatives, especially benzodiazepines, should be avoided if possible as they may worsen encephalopathy.
  - Lactulose (oral, enema forms) should be used if encephalopathy present; goal is to acidify stool (pH <6) and increase frequency of stool, but not cause profuse diarrhea.
  - Oral or rectal administration of antibiotics (neomycin, rifaximin) may be effective in treatment of hepatic encephalopathy by reducing ammonia production in the gut. Antibiotic administration has also been studied in prevention of hepatic encephalopathy.
- Other:
  - N-acetylcysteine is the cornerstone of treatment for acetaminophen-induced hepatic toxicity.
  - IV acid suppression should be considered

ADDITIONAL TREATMENT
General Measures
- Patients with acute liver failure should be closely monitored, preferably in an ICU setting at a tertiary-care center with a liver transplant program.
- Therapy should be directed at the underlying cause if a cause can be determined.
- General supportive care:
  - Fluid restriction: Total fluids should remain at or just below maintenance requirements, including all drips, medications, blood products.
  - Sodium restriction: Patients should typically not receive >0.25 NS as maintenance fluids. A total sodium intake of 1.0 mEq/kg/d is usually adequate. Hyponatremia should not be corrected with hypertonic saline as this can worsen fluid overload and encephalopathy.
  - Glucose infusion: Maintenance fluid typically should include 10% dextrose; glucose infusion may need to be increased as patients are at risk for hypoglycemia

- General system-based care:
  - Hematologic: Blood products should be given slowly to avoid rapid expansion of intravascular space.
  - Infectious disease: Minimize invasive catheterization when possible due to infection risk.

SURGERY/OTHER PROCEDURES
- Those likely to require liver transplantation include children with acute liver failure secondary to indeterminate cause, idiosyncratic drug toxicity, or Wilson disease.
- Those likely to have spontaneous recovery include children with autoimmune hepatitis, acetaminophen toxicity without severe acidosis, or ischemic shock.
- 1-year patient and graft survival is excellent, often >90%. Long-term survival >1 year is also typically excellent, from 70–85% or higher 4-year survival.

IN-PATIENT CONSIDERATIONS
Initial Stabilization
- Initial evaluation should include assessment of neurologic status.
- Elective intubation should be considered in grades III or IV encephalopathy with somnolence.
- Aggressive initial fluid resuscitation should be avoided unless there is evidence of hemodynamic compromise.
- Secure venous access should be obtained immediately; central venous access should be considered to allow for higher glucose infusion rates if needed.

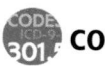 **ONGOING CARE**

PROGNOSIS
- King's College Criteria have been used to predict a poor prognosis in patients with acetaminophen-induced acute liver failure:
  - pH <7.3 regardless of encephalopathy grade OR
  - All of: PT >100 sec (INR >6.5), serum creatinine >3.4 g/dL, stage III or IV encephalopathy
- There is no consensus regarding prognostic criteria in patients in non–acetaminophen-induced liver failure. Factors associated with a poor prognosis include:
  - Factor V levels <10%
  - PT >50 sec (INR >3.5), especially if unresponsive to vitamin K
  - Grade III or IV encephalopathy
  - Duration of jaundice to encephalopathy >7 days
  - Ratio of total to direct bilirubin >2

COMPLICATIONS
- Complications are a direct consequence of loss of hepatic metabolic function:
  - Hepatic encephalopathy: Decreased elimination of neurotoxins or depressants
  - Cerebral edema: Pathogenesis incompletely understood
  - Coagulopathy: Failure of hepatic synthesis of clotting and fibrinolytic factors
  - Hypoglycemia: Impaired glucose synthesis and release, decreased degradation of insulin
  - Acidosis: Failure to eliminate lactic acid or free fatty acids

- In cases of suspected hepatic encephalopathy, consider other etiologies of neurologic change including hypoglycemia, intracranial hemorrhage, acute infection, or sepsis
- There is often rapid progression through the stages of encephalopathy. Increased intracranial pressure can develop quickly and can lead to irreversible neurologic sequelae.

ADDITIONAL READING
- Alonso EM, Squires RH, Whitington PF. Acute liver failure in children. In: Suchy FJ, Sokol RJ, Balistreri WF, eds. *Liver disease in children*, 3rd ed. New York: Cambridge University Press, 2007:71–96.
- Bass NM, Mullen KD, Sanyal A, et al. Rifaximin treatment in hepatic encephalopathy. *N Engl J Med*. 2010;362(12):1071–1081.
- Bucuvalas J, et al. Acute liver failure in children. *Clin Liver Dis*. 2006;10:149–168.
- Kortsalioudaki C, Taylor RM, Cheeseman P, et al. Safety and efficacy of n-acetylcysteine in children with non-acetaminophen-induced acute liver failure. *Liver Transplant*. 2008;12:25–30.
- Miyake Y, Sakaguchi K, Iwasaki Y, et al. New prognostic scoring model for liver transplantation in patients with non-acetaminophen-related fulminant hepatic failure. *Transplantation*. 2005;80:930–936.
- Squires RH, Shneider BL, Bucuvalas J, et al. Acute liver failure in children: The first 348 patients in the pediatric acute liver failure study group. *J Pediatr*. 2006;148:652–658.

CODES

ICD9
- 570 Acute and subacute necrosis of liver
- 572.8 Other sequelae of chronic liver disease

ICD10
- K72.00 Acute and subacute hepatic failure without coma
- K72.90 Hepatic failure, unspecified without coma
- K72.91 Hepatic failure, unspecified with coma

H

HEPATOMEGALY
John M. Good

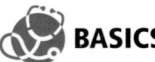

BASICS

DEFINITION
Liver enlargement beyond age-adjusted normal values; can be a common component of many diverse disease processes seen in infants and children.

- In children <2 years of age, the liver edge can extend 1–3 cm below the right costal margin in the midclavicular line.
- In older children, the liver edge rarely extends beyond 2 cm.

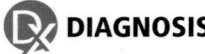

DIAGNOSIS

DIFFERENTIAL DIAGNOSIS
- **Congenital/anatomic**
  - Alagille syndrome
  - Biliary atresia
  - Choledochal cyst
  - Congenital hepatic fibrosis
  - Obstruction of the common bile duct due to stones, strictures, or tumors
- **Infections**
  - Viral infections:
    - Hepatitis types A–E
    - Cytomegalovirus
    - Epstein–Barr virus
    - Coxsackievirus
  - Congenital infections:
    - Toxoplasmosis
    - Rubella
    - Cytomegalovirus
    - Herpes
    - HIV
  - Parasitic infections:
    - Amebiasis
    - Flukes
    - Schistosomiasis
    - Malaria
  - Fungal diseases:
    - Candidiasis
    - Histoplasmosis
  - STDs:
    - Gonococcal perihepatitis
    - Syphilis
    - HIV
  - Zoonotic diseases: Brucellosis
  - Leptospirosis
  - Hepatic abscess
  - *Bartonella henselae*
  - *Pasteurella multocida*
  - Tuberculosis
  - Septicemia

- **Toxic, metabolic, drugs**
  - Drug-induced hepatitis:
    - Acetaminophen
    - Alcohol
    - Corticosteroids
    - Erythromycin
    - Hypervitaminosis A
    - Iron
    - Isoniazid
    - Nitrofurantoin
    - Oral contraceptives
    - Phenobarbital
    - Valproate
- **Trauma**
  - Hemorrhage
  - Subcapsular hematoma
  - Traumatic cyst
- **Tumor**
  - Benign tumors:
    - Hemangioma
    - Hemangioendothelioma
    - Mesenchymal hamartoma
    - Focal nodular hyperplasia
    - Adenoma
  - Malignant tumors:
    - Hepatoblastoma
    - Hepatocellular carcinoma
  - Metastatic tumors
  - Histiocytic disease
- **Genetic/metabolic**
  - α-1-Antitrypsin deficiency
  - Amyloidosis
  - Beckwith–Wiedemann syndrome
  - Chédiak–Higashi syndrome
  - Crigler–Najjar syndrome
  - Cystic fibrosis
  - Diabetes mellitus
  - Galactosemia
  - GM1 gangliosidoses
  - Glycogen storage diseases
  - Hemochromatosis
  - Hereditary fructose intolerance
  - Homocystinuria
  - Lipidoses
  - Mucopolysaccharidoses
  - Urea cycle defects
  - Wilson disease
  - Zellweger syndrome
- **Allergic/inflammatory**
  - Chronic active hepatitis
  - Sclerosing cholangitis
  - Sarcoidosis
  - Systemic inflammatory disease:
    - Juvenile rheumatoid arthritis
    - Systemic lupus erythematosus
    - Inflammatory bowel disease

- **Miscellaneous**
  - Congestive heart failure (CHF)
  - Extramedullary hematopoiesis
  - Pulmonary hyperinflation
  - Restrictive pericarditis
  - Veno-occlusive disease
  - Malnutrition
  - Reye syndrome
  - Total parenteral nutrition

ALERT
Indications for immediate hospitalization include:
- Persistent anorexia and vomiting
- Mental status changes
- Worsening jaundice
- Relapse of symptoms after initial improvement
- Known exposure to a liver toxin
- Rising PT
- Rising ammonia level
- Bilirubin >20 mg/dL
- Aspartate aminotransferase >2,000
- Development of new ascites
- Hypoglycemia
- Leukocytosis and thrombocytopenia

ETIOLOGY
- Most cases of hepatic failure in children are due to acute viral hepatitis.
- Toxic exposure accounts for 25% of cases, with the most common drug being acetaminophen.

HISTORY
A detailed history and physical exam will direct the practitioner to any additional laboratory testing or appropriate radiologic evaluation.

- **Question:** Prenatal history suggesting possible toxoplasmosis, other, rubella, cytomegalovirus, or herpes (TORCH) infection or HIV infection?
- *Significance:*
  - TORCH infections and HIV may cause hepatomegaly.
  - Liver involvement with HIV is usually secondary to disseminated opportunistic infections or neoplastic processes, rather than from the primary infection itself.
- **Question:** Any transfusions received before 1990?
- *Significance:* Hepatitis C is the most common cause of transfusion-associated hepatitis.
- **Question:** History of sexual activity or IV drug use?
- *Significance:* Consider not only hepatitis B and HIV, but also gonococcal perihepatitis (Fitz-Hugh–Curtis syndrome) and syphilis
- **Question:** Foreign travel?
- *Significance:* Suggests increased risk for parasitic infections or liver abscess
- **Question:** Contaminated shellfish?
- *Significance:* Has been the source of several large outbreaks of hepatitis A
- **Question:** Nonprescription and recreational drug use?
- *Significance:* Many pharmaceuticals have hepatotoxic side effects; ask about vitamin A, alcohol, and certain mushroom species, which can be hepatotoxic.

- **Question:** Other chronic illnesses?
- *Significance:*
  - Patients with heart disease may have liver enlargement due to CHF failure.
  - Patients with cystic fibrosis can have focal biliary cirrhosis.
  - Patients with diabetes mellitus often have hepatomegaly secondary to increased glycogen secretion.
  - Severely anemic patients have hepatomegaly because of extramedullary hematopoiesis.
- **Question:** Total parenteral nutrition?
- *Significance:* Cholestasis, bile duct proliferation, fatty infiltration, and early cirrhosis are all well-described complications.
- **Question:** Pruritus?
- *Significance:* Can be a subtle sign of cholestasis

PHYSICAL EXAM
- **Finding:** Liver edge?
- *Significance:*
  - In children <2 years of age, the liver edge can extend 1–3 cm below the right costal margin in the midclavicular line.
  - In older children, the liver edge rarely extends beyond 2 cm.
  - Verify all suspected cases of hepatomegaly by checking the liver span.
- **Finding:** Signs of chronic liver disease?
- *Significance:*
  - Liver is usually firm and enlarged, although actually may decrease in size eventually with advanced disease.
  - Splenomegaly, caput medusae, spider angiomas, esophageal varices, and hemorrhoids suggest portal hypertension.
  - Ascites may develop as a result of elevated hydrostatic pressures and decreased oncotic pressures secondary to hypoalbuminemia.
  - Also look for signs of occult bleeding or bruising due to impaired vitamin K production.
- **Finding:** Splenomegaly?
- *Significance:*
  - In the context of chronic liver disease, implies portal hypertension
  - In the context of other signs of viral illness, such as adenopathy, fever, malaise, and pharyngitis, suggests acute viral hepatitis
  - In the absence of these signs, suggests storage disease or hematologic malignancy
- **Finding:** Conditions that may mimic hepatomegaly by downwardly displacing a normal-sized liver?
- *Significance:*
  - Pulmonary hyperinflation
  - Subdiaphragmatic abscesses
  - Retroperitoneal mass lesions
  - Rib cage anomalies
- **Finding:** Clinical pearls?
- *Significance:*
  - Until age 2, girls have a slightly larger liver span than boys.
  - A Reidel lobe is a normal variant in which the right lobe of the liver appears elongated due to its adhesion to the mesocolon.
  - Administration of vitamin K in an attempt to correct PT can be a valuable assessment of the liver's synthetic function.
  - Fetor hepaticus is a sweetish odor that can be detected on the breath and urine of patients with liver failure.
  - Asterixis or liver flap is rare in children.

DIAGNOSTIC TESTS & INTERPRETATION
All patients with hepatomegaly should have a laboratory evaluation, including CBC with differential, comprehensive metabolic panel (including liver function tests, total protein and albumin, total and direct bilirubin, basic electrolytes and glucose), a PT, and a PPT.
- **Test:** CBC with differential
- **Test:** Aminotransferase and alanine aminotransferase
- *Significance:*
  - Elevations reflect the amount of damage to hepatocytes.
  - Elevations >1,000 indicate severe damage.
- **Test:** PT and PTT
- *Significance:*
  - Good indicators of the liver's synthetic function
  - Elevations can occur with an acute injury or illness.
  - Combined with albumin level, this test can be a sensitive indicator of chronic liver disease as well.
- **Test:** γ-Glutamyltransferase and alkaline phosphatase
- *Significance:*
  - Elevations of γ-glutamyltransferase out of proportion to elevations in aminotransferase and alanine aminotransferase can indicate an obstructive or infiltrative abnormality.
  - If an elevated γ-glutamyltransferase is associated with elevations in bilirubin, cholesterol, and alkaline phosphatase, an obstructive process is more likely.
- **Test:** Ammonia level
- *Significance:* Rising ammonia levels with a prolongation of the PT and PTT suggest liver failure.
- **Test:** Hepatitis profile
- *Significance:* Should be obtained in all patients with appropriate prodromal illness
- **Test:** Mono spot
- *Significance:*
  - Although this is a nonspecific heterophile antibody test for Epstein–Barr virus infection, it can be predictive in association with an elevation of the atypical lymphocyte count.
  - High false-negative rate in children <4 years of age
  - Epstein–Barr virus titer is the only confirmatory test.
- **Test:** α-Fetoprotein and carcinoembryonic antigen
- *Significance:* Tumor markers for hepatoblastoma and hepatocellular carcinoma, respectively
- **Test:** TORCH titers
- *Significance:* Consider in newborns with hepatomegaly
- **Test:** Serum immunoglobulins, antinuclear antibody, smooth muscle antibody, antimicrosomal antibody
- *Significance:* Additional autoimmune evaluation is indicated for those patients with chronic active hepatitis.
- **Test:** Serum ceruloplasmin level and urinary excretion of copper
- *Significance:*
  - Decreased ceruloplasmin levels and increased urinary excretion of copper characterize Wilson disease, especially after the administration of oral d-penicillamine.
  - Consider the diagnosis for patients with unexplained liver disease

Imaging
Abdominal ultrasound should be performed on all patients with acholic stools, asymmetric liver enlargement, or abdominal mass.

ADDITIONAL READING
- Clayton PT. Diagnosis of inherited disorders of liver metabolism. *J Inherit Metab Dis.* 2003;26(2–3): 135–146.
- Wolf AD, Lavine JE. Hepatomegaly in neonates and children. *Pediatr Rev.* 2000;21:303–310.

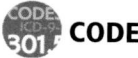 ## CODES

ICD9
- 751.69 Other anomalies of gallbladder, bile ducts, and liver
- 789.1 Hepatomegaly

ICD10
- R16.0 Hepatomegaly, not elsewhere classified
- Q44.7 Other congenital malformations of liver

FAQ
- Q: Why does cholestasis cause pruritus?
- A: This probably reflects an abnormal accumulation of bile acids in the skin.
- Q: Do patients with chronic liver disease have any different nutritional needs?
- A: Patients may have impaired fat absorption, and therefore may have deficiencies of fat-soluble vitamins A, D, E, and K, which may become evident as anemia, neuropathy, rickets, pathologic fractures, visual disturbances, or skin changes. Also consider supplementing the diet with medium-chain triglycerides, which are more easily absorbed. There may also be higher than normal requirements of trace minerals.
- Q: What is the etiology of cholestasis caused by total parenteral nutrition?
- A: Certain amino acids present in total parenteral nutrition have been shown to increase the serum levels of bile acids, which may in turn affect peristalsis in the gallbladder. Fasting may also decrease the normal hormonal stimulation of bile secretion.

H

HEREDITARY ANGIOEDEMA
Mathew Fogg

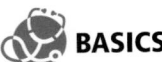 **BASICS**

DESCRIPTION
Hereditary angioedema is an autosomal-dominant disorder in which mutations in the *C1-INH* (C1 esterase inhibitor) gene results in a deficiency or an inactive form of plasma C1-INH. This permits unregulated activation of the complement and plasma kinin-forming pathways, leading to angioedema.

RISK FACTORS
Genetics
- Autosomal dominant
- Mutations may be present in either of 2 genes for C1-INH, located on chromosome 11.
- Acquired forms lack a genetic predisposition (there is no mutation in the *C1-INH* gene).

PATHOPHYSIOLOGY
- Deficiency of C1-INH leads to unopposed activation of the first complement component, resulting in the formation of bradykinin, which produces angioedema.
- Angioedema may occur in the upper airway, gastrointestinal tract, and extremities.
- Life-threatening upper airway obstruction may develop.

ETIOLOGY
- Classic hereditary form: Defect in 1 of 2 genes on chromosome 11 that code for C1-INH
- Acquired forms:
  - In 1 form, normal amount and functionally normal C1-INH is secreted into the plasma, but it is bound to circulating antibodies that inactivate it (associated with benign and malignant monoclonal B-cell lymphoproliferative disorders).
  - In the other form, an autoantibody not associated with lymphoproliferative disorders binds to C1-INH, resulting in increased degradation of C1-INH.
  - Third form (rare) found exclusively in women of childbearing age, may have normal plasma C1 inhibitor levels and function.

DIAGNOSIS

SIGNS AND SYMPTOMS
Decide if the patient's symptoms are consistent with hereditary angioedema (recurrent angioedema after minor trauma, family history, onset at puberty, lack of hives, poor response to epinephrine).

HISTORY
- Age at onset of recurrent episodes of subcutaneous and submucosal edema (recurrent episodes of angioedema usually begin at puberty)
- Characterize episodes of angioedema. Angioedema episodes are characterized by edema of the upper airway, extremities, or bowels (can cause severe abdominal pain).
- Determine whether angioedema episodes are associated with hives. Episodes of hereditary angioedema are not associated with hives; however, patients may have a nonpruritic erythema marginatum rash.
- Duration of angioedema episodes usually last 1–4 days.
- Triggers:
  - Emotional stress
  - Physical trauma such as surgery or dental procedures
  - Infection
  - Menstruation
  - Pregnancy
  - Estrogen-containing oral contraceptives
- Family history:
  - Angioedema can be inherited in an autosomal-dominant fashion.
  - There may be other affected family members.
- Response to epinephrine, antihistamines, or corticosteroids: Angioedema related to hereditary angioedema responds poorly to epinephrine, antihistamines, and corticosteroids.

PHYSICAL EXAM
Besides angioedema, the physical examination is normal. Erythema marginatum, a nonpruritic eruption, may also be present in patients with hereditary angioedema.

DIAGNOSTIC TESTS & INTERPRETATION
Lab
- C1 esterase inhibitor level and function:
  - If C1 esterase inhibitor level is normal and an acquired deficiency is suspected, order a functional assay of C1 esterase inhibitor.
  - Samples for complement assays must be placed on ice immediately; otherwise, the results may be falsely low.

- Direct measurement of C1-INH level and function (study of choice to identify the hereditary form of C1-INH deficiency):
  - This is an antigenic assay.
  - Affected patients may have a minimal quantity of C1-INH detected, and heterozygotes (carriers) have ~1/2 of normal levels detected.
  - Some patients may have normal levels of protein with reduced function.
- C1q level:
  - In acquired C1-INH deficiency, levels of C1q will be reduced.
  - In the hereditary form, C1q will be normal.
- CH50 level:
  - A general screen of the complement system
  - If abnormal, can indicate a deficiency of any of the complement components

DIFFERENTIAL DIAGNOSIS
- Toxic, environmental, drugs (patients on ACE inhibitors)
- Allergic inflammatory:
  - IgE-mediated allergic reactions: Drug, food, and contact allergies
  - Transfusion reaction
- Tumor (associated with neoplasms via unknown mechanism)
- Genetic/metabolic:
  - Urticaria pigmentosa/mastocytosis
  - Familial cold urticaria
  - C3b-inactivator deficiency
  - Amyloidosis with deafness and urticaria
  - Hereditary vibratory angioedema
- Physical/environmental
  - Urticarials: Cold urticaria, cholinergic urticaria, pressure urticaria (angioedema), vibratory angioedema, solar urticaria, aquagenic urticaria
  - Exercise-induced anaphylaxis
- Rheumatologic (collagen vascular disease)
- Psychologic:
  - Panic attacks
  - Globus hystericus
  - Vocal cord dysfunction
- Miscellaneous: Idiopathic angioedema

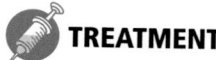 TREATMENT

ADDITIONAL TREATMENT
General Measures
- Prophylaxis:
  – Anabolic steroids (danazol or stanozolol) cause increased production of C1-INH, resulting in near-normal C2 and C4 levels (decreased degradation by activated C1) and a significantly decreased episode frequency. This therapy is indicated in patients with frequent or life-threatening episodes.
  – Plasmin inhibitors (β-aminocaproic acid or tranexamic acid) do not correct C2 and C4 levels, but are clinically effective.
  – Recombinant C1-INH concentrate is available outside the US and is highly effective. Prior to dental and surgical procedures, doses of androgen should be increased for 1–2 weeks. In addition, some experts recommend treatment with fresh frozen plasma shortly before and immediately after surgery, as this product contains C1-INH.
- Acute attacks:
  – Recombinant C1-INH concentrate is now available in the USA
  – Increase dose of androgen at first symptoms of an attack.
  – Immediately seek medical care; airway should be protected if any compromise is imminent.
  – Intermittent administration of subcutaneous epinephrine (This type of angioedema is usually poorly responsive, but in an emergency situation this may be considered.)
- Medical management: Treatment of the underlying condition often results in resolution of the angioedema.

ISSUES FOR REFERRAL
- Any patient with angioedema: An allergist/immunologist can help evaluate these patients for possible androgen prophylaxis therapy. In addition, they can assist in the creation of an emergency plan for management of acute attacks.
- Patients with difficult-to-control angioedema without an identified trigger: An allergist immunologist can assist with the appropriate evaluation.

 ONGOING CARE

FOLLOW-UP RECOMMENDATIONS
Patient Monitoring
- Patients should be seen at least annually.
- Follow-up should include the following:
  – Review of triggers
  – Prospective genetic counseling
  – Reinforcement of the need for prophylaxis
  – Review of attacks during the previous year
  – Creation of an emergency plan for the administration of recombinant C1 esterase inhibitor during severe attacks
- Regular follow-up with an endocrinologist is indicated for patients requiring androgen steroid therapy.

PATIENT EDUCATION
Education regarding:
- Role of triggers
- Prospective genetic counseling
- Need for prophylaxis
- Need for regular follow-up with an endocrinologist is indicated for patients who require androgen steroid therapy.

PROGNOSIS
Good with prophylactic and recombinant C1-INH therapies; recombinant C1-INH is not available in the US despite its proven clinical efficacy for treatment of acute attacks.

COMPLICATIONS
- Life-threatening upper airway obstruction
- Severe abdominal pain, often mistaken for a surgical abdomen

ADDITIONAL READING
- Bailey E, Shaker M. An update on childhood urticaria and angioedema. *Curr Opin Pediatr.* 2008;20(4):425–430.
- Frigas E, Nzeako UC. Angioedema: Pathogenesis, differential diagnosis, and treatment. *Clin Rev Allergy Immunol.* 2002;23:217–231.
- Gratten C, Powell S, Humphreys F. Management and diagnostic guidelines for urticaria and angio-edema. *Br J Dermatol.* 2001;144:708–714.
- Kaplan AP. Clinical practice: Chronic urticaria and angioedema. *N Engl J Med.* 2002;346:175–179.
- Kozel MM, Bossuyt PM, Mekkes JR, et al. Laboratory tests and identified diagnoses in patients with physical and chronic urticaria and angioedema: A systematic review. *J Am Acad Dermatol.* 2003;48:409–416.

 CODES

ICD9
- 277.6 Other deficiencies of circulating enzymes
- 279.8 Other specified disorders involving the immune mechanism

ICD10
D84.1 Defects in the complement system

FAQ
- Q: What is a good screening test for angioedema?
- A: C1 inhibitor functional and quantitative assays are readily available from commercial labs and are the test of choice for hereditary angioedema.
- Q: What are the side effects of prophylactic androgen therapy?
- A: Side effects include masculinization, menstrual irregularities, enhanced epiphyseal growth-plate closure, water retention, hypertension, cholestatic hepatitis, hepatic carcinoma, decreased spermatogenesis, and gynecomastia.

HEREDITARY SPHEROCYTOSIS

Michele P. Lambert

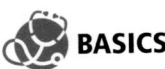 **BASICS**

DESCRIPTION

Hemolytic anemia with shortened RBC survival owing to selective destruction of RBCs in the spleen secondary to an inherent defect of the RBC membrane. Membrane loss is gradual; it results in spherocytosis, which results in increased osmotic fragility. Pathophysiologically related to Hereditary Elliptocytosis and hereitdary ovalocytosis)

EPIDEMIOLOGY

Most common in people of Northern European extraction (~1:3,000)

RISK FACTORS

Genetics

- ~75% of cases are inherited in an autosomal dominant pattern.
- The other 25% are autosomal recessive forms, dominant disease with reduced penetrance, or new mutations.
- Severity related to degree of membrane loss
  - Mild (20% of patients): Hemoglobin near normal, slight reticulocytosis (<6%), compensated hemolysis, mild splenomegaly. Often not diagnosed until adulthood due to gallstones
  - Moderate (60% of patients): hgb 8–10 mg/dL and reticulocytes generally >8%; >50% patients have splenomegaly
  - Moderately severe (10%): hemoglobin 6–8 mg/dL, retic >15%, intermittent transfusions
  - Severe (3–5%): life-threatening anemia requiring regular transfusions. Almost always recessive.

PATHOPHYSIOLOGY

The most common abnormality is a deficiency of ankyrin and subsequent decrease in spectrin, 2 major proteins of the erythrocyte membrane skeleton (50–60% Northern European decent; 5–10% Japan). Spectrin deficiency alone accounts for 20% of HS. Mutations in other erythrocyte surface proteins including beta-spectrin (typically mild to moderately severe), alpha-spectrin (sever HS), Band 3 (15–20% generally mild to moderately severe) and protein 4.2 (<5% HS, recessive and results in almost complete absence) and Rh antigen (<10% mild to moderate hemolytic anemia) also occur. The membrane skeletal defect causes RBC membrane fragility resulting in membrane loss. The sequelae are as follows:

- Loss of cell surface area relative to volume (spherocytosis) causes a decrease in cellular deformability.
- The spleen detains and "conditions" the nondeformable spherocytic RBC.
- Conditioning of cells involves depletion of adenosine 5'-triphosphate (ATP), increased glycolysis, increased influx and efflux of sodium, and loss of membrane lipid.
- Ultimately, these events lead to premature RBC destruction.

DIAGNOSIS

HISTORY

- Fatigue (a sign of anemia)
- Jaundice, scleral icterus, dark urine (signs of hemolysis)
- Phototherapy required in newborn period (50% of cases): Hyperbilirubinemia owing to hemolysis
- Positive familial history (for disease, gallstones, or splenectomy) is significant because of autosomal dominant inheritance.

PHYSICAL EXAM

- Splenomegaly is present in most older patients and may worsen with intercurrent illness.
- Icterus/Jaundice and pallor are present with increased hemolysis.
- Linear growth, weight gain, and sexual development may be delayed. Delayed growth is indication for splenectomy.

DIAGNOSTIC TESTS & INTERPRETATION

Lab

- CBC:
  - Mild to moderate anemia
  - Mean corpuscular volume usually normal
  - Mean corpuscular hemoglobin concentration (MCHC) elevated (useful screening test with high specificity)
  - Reticulocyte count: May be only slightly elevated
  - Often accompanied by elevated RBC distribution width
  - Indirect hyperbilirubinemia: Present in 50–60% of cases
  - Peripheral smear: Microspherocytes, polychromasia
- Coombs test: Negative
  - Important differential test in a patient with hemolytic anemia and spherocytes
- Urinalysis:
  - Hemoglobinuria
  - Increased urobilinogen

- Special tests:
  - Osmotic fragility (most useful test in diagnosis, but can be normal in 10–20% of patients):
    - Spherocytes are more fragile; less resistant to osmotic stress and therefore lyse in higher concentrations of saline than normal RBCs.
    - Test can result in a false-negative, especially in newborns whose RBCs may be more dehydrated and with high fetal hemoglobin
    - Important to use an age-matched control if possible
    - Any anemia that results in spherocytes will give increased osmotic fragility (especially autoimmune hemolytic anemia) and must be excluded.
  - Eosin-5-maleimide (EMA) binding: Flow cytometric analysis of RBCs with much higher sensitivity and specificity for HS, but not available at all centers.

DIFFERENTIAL DIAGNOSIS

- Hemolysis secondary to intrinsic RBC defects:
  - Membrane defects secondary to inherited disorders of membrane skeleton (HS and elliptocytosis) and RBC cation permeability and volume (stomatocytosis and xerocytosis)
  - Enzyme defects: Embden-Meyerhof pathway (i.e., pyruvate kinase deficiency) and hexose monophosphate pathway (i.e., glucose-6-phosphate dehydrogenase deficiency)
  - Hemoglobin defects:
    - Congenital erythropoietic porphyria;
    - Qualitative Hemoglobin S (Sickle cell), Hgb C, Hgb H, Hgb M
    - Quantitative: Thalassemias
  - Congenital dyserythropoietic anemias
- Hemolysis secondary to extracorpuscular RBC defects:
  - Immune-mediated (important in differential because spherocytes are present on smear and can give increased osmotic fragility if sent): isoimmune (e.g., hemolytic disease of the newborn, blood group incompatibility) and autoimmune (e.g., cold agglutinin disease, warm autoimmune hemolytic anemia)
  - Non–immune-mediated: Idiopathic and secondary to underlying disorder (e.g., hemolytic uremic syndrome, thrombotic thrombocytopenic purpura)

ALERT

- A patient with HS may become extremely anemic during an aplastic crisis, hyperhemolysis episode, or folic acid deficiency, requiring transfusion.
- False-negative osmotic fragility tests can occur in several situations; therefore, index of suspicion must be high to follow the clinical course and repeat test (e.g., in neonatal period, during megaloblastic crisis, and recovery from aplastic crisis after transfusion when cells are youngest and least spherocytic).
- 20–25% of HS patients have normal unincubated osmotic fragility (incubated test almost always positive; therefore, may need both)
- Spherocytes are often present in immune-mediated hemolysis.

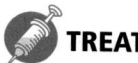 TREATMENT

ADDITIONAL TREATMENT

General Measures
- Folic acid supplement
- Penicillin prophylaxis (if splenectomized)
- Pneumococcal, meningococcal, and *Haemophilus influenza* B vaccines (prior to splenectomy)

SURGERY/OTHER PROCEDURES

Splenectomy: High response rate (most patients normalize their blood counts):

- Indications: Moderate-to-severe anemia with significant hemolysis resulting in transfusion dependence, decreased exercise tolerance, skeletal deformities, or delayed growth
- Complications: Risk of postsplenectomy sepsis, emerging data on increased risk of later pulmonary hypertension and increased risk of thrombosis
  - Cholecystectomy indications: Symptomatic gallbladder disease. Sometimes done simultaneously with splenectomy if gallstones evident by ultrasound
- Complications: Morbidity of surgical procedure and postoperative period

 ONGOING CARE

Physical exam: Splenomegaly, follow growth curves closely:

- CBC with reticulocyte count as needed: If patient develops fatigue, pallor, increased jaundice
- Penicillin prophylaxis after splenectomy

PROGNOSIS

Severity of disease is extremely variable, ranging from an incidental diagnosis in adulthood to severe anemia requiring transfusions.

COMPLICATIONS

- Gallstones: Most common complication of HS; pigment stones can lead to cholecystitis and/or biliary obstruction.
- Cholelithiasis in HS manifests in second and third decades of life.
- Aplastic crises: Can result in severe life-threatening anemia; often caused by parvovirus B_{19} infection. Epstein–Barr virus (EBV), influenza, cytomegalovirus (CMV) can also cause worsening anemia and reticulocytopenia
- Hyperhemolysis: Increased RBC destruction, often precipitated by infection
- Postsplenectomy sepsis: Lower risk of infection if postponed until 4–5 years of age and immunized with pneumococcal vaccine (50–70% sepsis caused by *Streptococcus pneumoniae*)
- Folate deficiency: Caused by insufficient dietary intake of folic acid for increased bone marrow requirement. Can result in megaloblastic crisis.
- Pulmonary hypertension: Long-term complication of splenectomy due to recurrent small vessel thrombosis in the lungs (either local clot or thromboembolic events). Long-term risk that weighs against splenectomy in patients with mild or well-compensated disease
- Other rare complications: Gout, indolent leg ulcers, or chronic erythematous dermatitis on legs

ADDITIONAL READING

- An X, Mohandas N. Disorders of red cell membrane; *BJH*. 2008;141;367–376.
- Bolton-Maggs PHB, Stevens RF, Dodd NJ, et al. Guidelines for the diagnosis and management of hereditary spherocytosis. *Br J Haematol*. 2004;126: 455–474.
- Delhommeau F, Cynober T, Schischmanoff P, et al. Natural history of hereditary spherocytosis during the first year of life. *Blood*. 2000;95:393–397.
- Gallagher P. Red cell membrane disorders. *Hematology Am Soc Hematol Educ Program*. 2005;13–18.
- Shah S, Vega R. Hereditary spherocytosis. *Pediatr Rev*. 2004;25:168–172.

 CODES

ICD9
282.0 Hereditary spherocytosis

ICD10
D58.0 Hereditary spherocytosis

FAQ

- Q: Will my child require blood transfusions?
- A: It depends on the clinical severity of your child's disease.
- Q: If a parent has HS, how should the newborn be followed?
- A: The infant has a 50% chance of having HS. In infants with HS, the CBC is usually normal in the first 72 hours of life, but then drops because of an inability to mount an appropriate erythropoietic response to increased destruction. Therefore, infants at risk should have a CBC with reticulocyte count after 72 hours. These infants also need to be monitored closely for hyperbilirubinemia.
- Q: What are the risks and benefits of splenectomy?
- A: Splenectomy is almost always successful in ameliorating anemia, but adds the risk of postsplenectomy infections and later risks for pulmonary hypertension and maybe increased risk of thrombosis and/or cardiovascular disease. The risks and benefits need to be carefully weighed and, in patients with mild, well-compensated hemolysis, splenectomy is not indicated.

H

HEROIN INTOXICATION

Fran Balamuth
Cynthia J. Mollen (5th edition)
Thomas J. Mollen (5th edition)

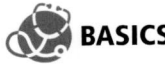 **BASICS**

DESCRIPTION
Heroin is a semisynthetic derivative of opium. The opioid family includes the following:
- Drugs that occur naturally in opium (from the poppy plant)
- Codeine
- Morphine
- Semisynthetic derivatives (e.g., hydromorphone, oxycodone)
- Synthetic compounds (e.g., meperidine, methadone)

EPIDEMIOLOGY
- Neonatal:
  - Fetal exposure commonly involves polysubstance abuse.
  - 60–80% of heroin-exposed infants develop withdrawal: Depends on maternal dosing and length of use.
- Adolescents:
  - Use peaked among U.S. adolescents in the 1970s and then declined.
  - Use is increasing again because a purer product allows for smoking or snorting as well as injecting.
  - Most use experimentally or intermittently; few become addicted and use daily.
  - There have been case reports of adolescents as heroin body packers.
  - Use of opioid analgesics has increased dramatically over the last 10 years, and has become more common than heroin use.
  - ED visits for opioid analgesics increased 111% from 2004–2008: Most common substances were oxycodone, hydrocodone, and methadone.
- Overdose:
  - Up to 1/3 of heroin users experience nonfatal overdose.
  - Most occur in the home and with other people present.
  - Risk factors include length of injecting history and concurrent use of CNS depressants.
- Deaths:
  - Most heroin deaths occur when drug is administered IV.
  - Most deaths occur in patients in their late 20s or 30s, with significant drug dependence.
  - Multiple drug use is common in heroin-related death.
  - Many deaths occur in people with a history of a nonfatal overdose.

Incidence
- Statistically significant increase in new heroin use since 1992
- 114,000 new users in 2008
- Mean age of 1st use in 2001 = 23.3

Prevalence
- Precise estimates of prevalence of use difficult
- ~2.9 million people used at least once
- ~213,000 used in 2008
- Prevalence of fetal exposure <1–3.7%
- Heroin users are more likely to visit EDs than users of other illicit substances.

PATHOPHYSIOLOGY
- Well-absorbed from GI tract, nasal mucosa, pulmonary capillaries, and SC and IM injection sites
- Oral dose less potent than parenteral because of 1st-pass hepatic metabolism
- IV heroin peaks in <1 minute; intranasal and IM heroin peak in 3–5 minutes.
- Very lipid soluble; crosses blood–brain barrier within 15–20 seconds
- Extensive distribution into skeletal muscle, kidneys, liver, intestine, lungs, spleen, brain, and placenta
- Rapidly crosses the placenta, entering fetal tissues within 1 hour
- Crosses into breast milk in quantities sufficient to cause addiction
- Excreted in urine as morphine
- Receptor types:
  - μ (mu or OP3):
    - Located in CNS, GI tract, and sensory nerve endings
    - Effect: Analgesia, euphoria, respiratory depression, physical dependence, GI dysmotility, miosis, pruritus, bradycardia
  - κ (kappa or OP2):
    - Located in CNS
    - Effect: Analgesia, miosis, diuresis, dysphoria
  - δ (delta or OP1):
    - Located in CNS
    - Effect: Spinal analgesia, modulation of mu receptors/dopaminergic neurons

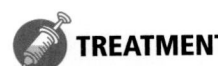 **DIAGNOSIS**

HISTORY
- Neonate:
  - Maternal history of heroin or other drug use
  - Extent of prenatal care
  - Time from most recent use to delivery
  - Breastfeeding
- Older child/Adolescent:
  - History of heroin use
  - Observed overdose
  - Found in setting consistent with possible drug use

PHYSICAL EXAM
- Neonate with in utero exposure:
  - Prematurity
  - Low birth weight
  - Perinatal depression with 5-minute Apgar <5
  - Hypotonia
- Intoxication/Overdose:
  - Classic toxidrome: Depressed level of consciousness, very decreased respiratory effort, miotic pupils, with or without diminished bowel sounds
  - More severe overdose: Bradycardia, hypotension, noncardiogenic pulmonary edema
- Withdrawal:
  - Early signs (8–24 hours): Anxiety, restlessness, insomnia, yawning, rhinorrhea, lacrimation, diaphoresis, stomach cramps, mydriasis
  - Late signs (up to 3 days): Tremor, muscle spasms, vomiting, diarrhea, hypertension, tachycardia, fever, chills, piloerection, seizures

- Additional neonatal withdrawal signs and symptoms:
- Hyperirritability
- Hypertonicity
- Posturing
- Exaggerated startle
- Tachypnea
- Hyperpyrexia
- Poor suck/swallow coordination
- High-pitched cry
- Poor weight gain
- Timing of neonatal symptoms depends on maternal substance used: Withdrawal from heroin within 48 hours, can be longer for methadone. Delayed withdrawal possible up to 4 weeks with both drugs

DIAGNOSTIC TESTS & INTERPRETATION
Diagnostic Procedures/Other
- Therapy should not be withheld pending laboratory results.
- Urine toxicology screen (heroin easily detected; synthetic opioids are not)
- Serum toxicology screen for acetaminophen level, etc., if suspect polydrug use
- Serum tests to rule out other causes, if needed (e.g., glucose)
- Meconium testing in neonates

DIFFERENTIAL DIAGNOSIS
- Neonatal exposure:
  - Sepsis
  - Hypoglycemia
  - CNS abnormality
  - Metabolic disorder
  - Withdrawal from other maternal drug use
- Intoxication/Overdose
- Other pharmacologic agents:
  - Clonidine, sedative hypnotics, barbiturates, antipsychotics, γ-hydroxy butyrate
- Hypoglycemia
- Hypothermia
- Hypoxia
- Heatstroke
- Pontine or subarachnoid hemorrhage

![syringe icon] **TREATMENT**

ADDITIONAL TREATMENT
General Measures
- Intoxication/Overdose:
  - Start with the ABCs (airway, breathing, circulation).
  - Antidote is naloxone (Narcan).
  - Assessment of respiratory status/adequacy of ventilation
  - If adequate respiratory effort, observe until normal level of consciousness:
    - Consider naloxone as diagnostic challenge.
  - If inadequate respiratory effort:
    - Bag-valve-mask ventilation
    - IV naloxone (or SC, IM, endotracheal)
    - If <20 kg, 0.1 mg/kg; 2 mg if >20 kg. Can repeat to 10 mg total dose

– If suspect dependence, start with lower dose (0.4 mg ampule)
– If no response to large dose, question diagnosis of heroin toxicity: Heroin is exquisitely sensitive to naloxone
– Naloxone loses efficacy in 20–40 minutes; may need repeat dosing
– Can give as continuous infusion if necessary; dosing recommendations vary
– One method: 2/3 of effective dose given over 1 hour with gradual wean
– Consider low-dose naloxone (0.01 mg/kg) in apneic infants exposed to opiates in utero
– Endotracheal intubation if no response to naloxone in 5–10 minutes, or other reason for invasive airway management
– Observe in ED for a minimum of 2–3 hours for respiratory status stabilization.
– Consider chest radiograph to evaluate for pulmonary edema.
– Consider glucose testing to evaluate for hypoglycemia.
– Consider whole bowel irrigation with Go-Lytely for symptomatic body packers, and consult local poison control center.
• Withdrawal:
– Standard treatment methadone maintenance (adolescents/adults):
  ○ Blocks euphoria and prevents withdrawal symptoms
  ○ Patients generally treated in established methadone maintenance programs
  ○ Buprenorphine is also an option.
  ○ Stabilize with 20–40 mg/d; wean by 2–5 mg/wk over several months.
  ○ Adjust wean if signs of withdrawal appear.
  ○ Some programs utilize heroin maintenance when methadone fails; research ongoing
– Clonidine (0.2 mg q4–6h for 7–10 days) can control acute withdrawal symptoms.
– Diazepam (10–15 mg q4–6h for 3–4 days), an alternative to clonidine
– Rapid and ultra-rapid detoxification (using opioid antagonist with or without general anesthesia) is a possibility in selected patients; recent review suggests high-rate adverse events:
  ○ Should be used only by experienced team with appropriate resources
– In neonates:
  ○ Paregoric (0.4 mg/mL) not recommended owing to high alcohol content (45%) and toxic compounds such as camphor, anise oil, benzoic acid, and glycerin
  ○ Tincture of opium (10 mg/mL) best diluted 25-fold to a concentration equal to paregoric (0.4 mg/mL)
  ○ 0.1 mL/kg (2 drops/kg) q4h; increase 0.1 mL/kg q4h as needed to control symptoms. After 3–5 days, wean dose by 0.1 mL/kg/d. Observe infant for 3–5 days after stopping therapy.
  ○ May need IV morphine in severe cases
  ○ Methadone and buprenorphine have also been shown to be effective
  ○ Clonidine gaining favor for use in infants; pharmacokinetic data not available; although use is currently recommended only in the context of a randomized clinical trial
  ○ Phenobarbital not a 1st-choice agent owing to long half-life, CNS depression, induction of drug metabolism, and rapid tolerance to sedative effect; however, has been shown to be effective in conjunction with diluted tincture of opium.

– Infants with opioid withdrawal have elevated metabolic demands: Consider higher-calorie (24 kcal/oz) feeds.
• Breastfeeding is not recommended in mothers using heroin, but can be considered for mothers on methadone treatment.

ISSUES FOR REFERRAL
• Social services and referral to substance abuse program
• Consider referral for testing for HIV and hepatitis B and C.

IN-PATIENT CONSIDERATIONS
Admission Criteria
Most patients with overdose warrant hospitalization.

 # ONGOING CARE

FOLLOW-UP RECOMMENDATIONS
Developmental follow-up for exposed neonates

PROGNOSIS
• Neonatal:
– Long-term morbidity from neonatal heroin dependence unclear owing to confounding variables (e.g., developmental environment)
• Intoxication/Overdose:
– With adequate early treatment, patients with uncomplicated overdoses do well: Key is to prevent respiratory arrest.
• Addiction:
– Dependent on involvement in other risky behaviors (polydrug use, high-risk sexual practices, school failure, delinquency, etc.)
– Longer treatment likely produces a better outcome.
– Most relapses require lifetime of therapy

COMPLICATIONS
• Intoxication/Overdose:
– Respiratory arrest
– Noncardiogenic pulmonary edema
– CNS depression/coma
– Hypotension
– Aspiration pneumonia
• Pregnancy:
– No known teratogenic effects
– Poor prenatal care
– Preterm labor
– Premature rupture of membranes
– Breech presentation
– Antepartum hemorrhage
– Toxemia
– Anemia
– Uterine irritability
– Infection (e.g., HIV, hepatitis B)
– Infantile dependence
• Naloxone use:
– May precipitate withdrawal syndrome in opioid-dependent patients
– Symptoms: Agitation, hypertension, tachycardia, emesis
– See dosing recommendations.
– May cause acute severe withdrawal in infants born to addicted mothers

ADDITIONAL READING
• Coyle MG, Ferguson A, LaGrasse L, et al. Neurobehavioral effects of treatment for opiate withdrawal. *Arch Dis Child Fetal Neonatal Ed.* 2005;90:F73–F74.
• Emergency department visits involving nonmedical use of selected prescription drugs—United States, 2004–2008. *MMWR.* 2010;59(23):705–709.
• Ferri M, Davoli M, Perucci CA. Heroin maintenance for chronic heroin dependents. *Cochrane Database Syst Rev.* 2005;2:CD003410.
• Gowing L, Ali R, White J. Opioid antagonists under heavy sedation or anaesthesia for opioid withdrawal. *Cochrane Database Syst Rev.* 2006;2:CD002022.
• http://www.oas.samhsa.gov/NHSDA/Treatan/treana11.htm.
• Jones HE, Kaltenbach K, Heil S, et al. Neonatal abstinence syndrome after methadone or buprenorphine exposure. *N Engl J Med.* 2010; 363:2320–2331.
• Osborn DA, Jeffery HE, Cole M. Opiate treatment for opiate withdrawal in newborn infants. *Cochrane Database Syst Rev.* 2010;10:CD002059.
• Osborn DA, Jeffery HE, Cole M. Sedatives for opiate withdrawal in newborn infants. *Cochrane Database Syst Rev.* 2010;10:CD002053.
• Peroon BE, Bohnert AS, Monsell SE. Patterns and correlates of drug-related ED visits: Results from a national survey. *Am J Emerg Med.* 2010;29(7): 704–710.

 # CODES

ICD9
• 304.00 Opioid type dependence, unspecified
• 779.5 Drug withdrawal syndrome in newborn
• E935.0 Heroin causing adverse effects in therapeutic use

ICD10
• F11.23 Opioid dependence with withdrawal
• F11.929 Opioid use, unspecified with intoxication, unspecified
• P96.1 Neonatal withdrawal symptoms from maternal use of drugs of addiction

FAQ
• Q: Is nalmefene an appropriate substitute for naloxone in a heroin overdose?
• A: Nalmefene, a long-acting specific narcotic antagonist, has not proved to be as effective as naloxone in a randomized, double-blind trial. It also may result in prolonged, dangerous withdrawal. It therefore has limited usefulness in this setting.

H

HERPES SIMPLEX VIRUS

Ross Newman
Jason Newland
Louis M. Bell (5th edition)

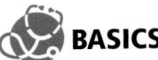 **BASICS**

DESCRIPTION

Herpes simplex virus (HSV) is a moderately large, double-stranded DNA virus. There are 2 serologically distinguishable subtypes: HSV-1 and HSV-2. HSV produces a wide spectrum of illness ranging from fever blisters to fatal viral encephalitis.

GENERAL PREVENTION

- Neonatal infection:
  - The risk of HSV infection in an infant born vaginally to a mother with a first-episode primary genital infection is high (25–60%). The risk to an infant born to a mother with recurrent HSV infection at delivery is much lower (2–5%).
  - Cesarean delivery in a mother with active genital herpes at the time of delivery is the main way to prevent neonatal infection. However, this does not prevent all cases because 60–80% of mothers of infected infants are asymptomatic or have unrecognized infection.
  - A cesearean delivery is not indicated for a mother with a history of genital HSV and absence of lesions at time of delivery
  - Fetal scalp monitors should be avoided in women suspected of genital HSV.
- Postnatal infection:
  - Universal body-substance precaution policies
  - Adults with oral herpes must be particularly careful to use appropriate hygiene.
  - Wrestlers with skin lesions suggestive of herpes
  - Patients with genital lesions from HSV should not have intercourse until the lesions heal.
  - Condoms can prevent the spread of virus.

EPIDEMIOLOGY

- Neonatal infection is usually acquired from the maternal genitourinary tract and causes serious disease with high mortality and morbidity.
- HSV-1 usually causes infections of the upper torso, head, and neck.
- HSV-2 usually causes genital infection. However, both forms can infect oral or genital cells, thus the virus type is not a reliable indicator of the anatomic site of infection.
- Route of spread is usually by close bodily contact or trauma such as teething or a break in the skin.
- Incubation period is 2–12 days (~6 days).
- Neonatal HSV infections are acquired from maternal strains, and 75–85% are caused by HSV-2.
- After the neonatal period, HSV-1 infections predominate, and 40–60% of children are seropositive for HSV-1 by the age of 5 years.

Prevalence

During puberty and early adolescence, the prevalence of HSV-2 increases, and 20–35% of adults are seropositive for HSV-2.

PATHOPHYSIOLOGY

- Initial viral replication occurs at the portal of entry.
- Vesicular fluid contains infected epithelial cells.
- After primary HSV infection, the virus remains latent in sensory neural ganglia innervating portions of the skin or mucous membranes originally involved. The virus can be reactivated by an appropriate stimulus such as sunlight or immune suppression.
- HSV can be replicated easily in the laboratory in tissue cultures.

COMMONLY ASSOCIATED CONDITIONS

- Gingivostomatitis is the most common form of HSV primary infection in children.
- Encephalitis due to HSV accounts for 2–5% of all encephalitis in the USA.

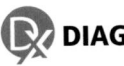 **DIAGNOSIS**

SIGNS AND SYMPTOMS

- Neonatal infection:
  - HSV-2, the most common cause of neonatal infection, is usually acquired from maternal labial lesions, but a history of previous or current genital HSV infection is present in only 20–30% of mothers who deliver infected infants. HSV-2 can be transmitted to the infant without rupture of the amniotic membranes or after delivery by cesarean section:
  - HSV-1 can be transmitted to a neonate by any adult with active herpes labialis.
  - Neonates can have nonspecific presentations with up to 75% presenting with fever alone.
  - A vesicular rash or bullae are clues to diagnosis and present in 60% of patients with disseminated infection and 80–85% of patients with skin, eye, or mouth disease. Diagnosis without skin lesions is challenging.
  - Disseminated infection (20% of cases) involves the liver, lungs, adrenals, and sometimes the CNS and classically presents in the first to second week of life.
  - Localized CNS infection (33% of cases) presents with irritability, bulging fontanelle, or seizures and classically presents in the second to third week of life.
  - Localized skin, eye, or mouth infection (40–45% of cases) presents with rash alone, keratitis, or chorioretinitis and classically presents in the first to second week of life.
- Gingivostomatitis:
  - Most common presentation during childhood.
  - Fever and irritability precede the development of vesicular lesions on the lips, gingiva, and tongue. The vesicles then break down and become gray ulcers that are friable and bleed easily.
  - Children refuse to drink because of the mouth pain and are at risk of dehydration.
  - The child usually starts to improve in 3–5 days and recovers in 14 days.
  - Latent virus causes recurrent stomatitis or labiitis.

- Encephalitis:
  - The illness begins with fever, malaise, and irritability that last 1–7 days and progress to mental status changes, seizures, and coma. Meningeal signs are not common.
  - Patients can develop hemiparesis, cranial nerve palsy, and visual field defects.
  - No presence of oral or genital lesions
  - It is the result of a primary infection in 30% of cases and recurrent in 70%.
- Vulvovaginitis:
  - 35–50% of patients with the 1st episode of genital herpes will be able to give a history of genital HSV infection in their contact.
  - The primary illness is characterized by fever, headache, malaise, and myalgias. Local genital symptoms include severe pain, itching, dysuria, vaginal or urethral discharge, and tender inguinal adenopathy. The genital lesions begin as vesicles and progress to ulcers before they crust over. Lesions last for 2–3 weeks.
  - An aseptic meningitis syndrome occurs in 1–35% of cases. Patients will have fever, headache, meningismus, and photophobia.
  - Latent virus causes recurrent episodes, which are painful but less severe than in primary infections.

HISTORY

- Neonatal period exposures:
  - History of herpes in mother
  - Active vulvar lesions at time of delivery
  - Skin lesions
  - Oral lesion
- General questions re: Contagious disease:
  - Contact with people with herpes
  - Unprotected sex
  - Drinking from common straws, glasses
  - Use of lipstick samples at cosmetic counters

PHYSICAL EXAM

See "Signs and Symptoms."

DIAGNOSTIC TESTS & INTERPRETATION

- Neonatal infection:
  - Samples for viral culture should be obtained from the eyes, oropharynx, and rectum.
  - Polymerase chain reaction (PCR) testing of the CSF is the test of choice for diagnosing CNS disease.
  - Cells from the base of freshly unroofed vesicles can be smeared on a slide for monoclonal antibody immunofluorescence.
  - Serologic tests are not useful for diagnosis of maternal or neonatal herpes during the acute phase of the disease.
- Encephalitis:
  - CSF reveals a pleocytosis with up to 2,000 WBCs/mm^3, and usually >60% of the cells are lymphocytes.
  - CSF protein is elevated (median, 80 mg/dL).
  - HSV PCR is the diagnostic test of choice.
  - EEG can reveal a typical pattern of unilateral or bilateral focal spikes.
  - CT or MRI may show enhancement in the temporal areas.

- Gingivostomatitis:
  - Physicians usually make this diagnosis clinically because it is so common in young children.
- Vulvovaginitis:
  - A viral culture of the vesicle is the gold standard. Sensitivity is 94% for early lesions and decreases to 27% for crusted lesions.
  - Immunofluorescence of infected cells is a more rapid diagnostic test and has a sensitivity of 78–88%.

DIFFERENTIAL DIAGNOSIS

- Neonatal HSV infection must be distinguished from severe neonatal enterovirus disease or bacterial sepsis, especially in the first 4 weeks of life.
- HSV infection should be considered in all neonates with vesicular rash, chorioretinitis, microcephaly, or hepatosplenomegaly. It must be distinguished from other congenital viral infections such as rubella or cytomegalovirus (CMV).
- Herpes gingivostomatitis must be distinguished from herpangina, an enteroviral infection usually presenting as posterior pharyngeal ulcers and, sometimes, as hand, foot, and mouth disease.
- HSV encephalitis must be distinguished from other viral encephalitis and from the HSV-induced aseptic meningitis syndrome, which is a complication of primary genital infection.
- HSV vulvovaginitis must be distinguished from chancroid and syphilis. Syphilis lesions are usually nonpainful, hard ulcers. Chancroid lesions are multiple purulent ulcers from which *Haemophilus ducreyi* can be cultured.

 TREATMENT

MEDICATION (DRUGS)

- Neonatal infection:
  - IV acyclovir (60 mg/kg/d in 3 divided doses) is the drug of choice. The recommended minimal duration of therapy is 14 days (if the disease is limited to the skin, eye, and mouth) and 21 days if disease is disseminated or involves the CNS. Infants with ocular involvement due to HSV infection should receive a topical ophthalmic drug (1–2% trifluridine, 1% iododeoxyuridine, or 3% vidarabine) in addition to parenteral antiviral therapy.
- Encephalitis:
  - IV acyclovir (30 mg/kg/d in 3 divided doses) for 21 days is appropriate therapy for HSV encephalitis beyond the neonatal period. In addition to parenteral antiviral therapy, appropriate management of fluids, intracranial pressure, and seizures is essential.
- Gingivostomatitis:
  - Most patients are managed with symptomatic therapy including antipyretics and oral fluids like popsicles. Oral anesthetics can be harmful and result in self-injury when children chew on anesthetized lips. Oral acyclovir has limited therapeutic benefit. If treatment is initiated, dosing is recommended at 80 mg/kg divided 4 times a day. Topical therapy is not recommended. Patients with frequent or severe recurrences may benefit from oral acyclovir at onset of symptoms.

- Vulvovaginitis:
  - Acyclovir (Zovirax) is the appropriate therapy for genital herpes infection. Oral acyclovir is used for patients with primary genital HSV infection and can decrease duration of illness and length of viral shedding. IV acyclovir is used for patients with severe local or systemic symptoms or complications like aseptic meningitis syndrome. Valacyclovir and famciclovir have not been shown to be more effective than acyclovir, however may lead to improved complicance with less frequent dosing. Topical therapy for primary genital lesions is not recommended.

 ONGOING CARE

PROGNOSIS

Neonatal infection:

- Overall mortality from untreated neonatal HSV infection is 50%, and only 26% of survivors are normal.
- Infants with disseminated disease or localized CNS disease have the worst prognosis with mortality up to 20% despite antiviral therapy.

COMPLICATIONS

The major sequelae in survivors are brain damage, seizures, and blindness.

ADDITIONAL READING

- American Academy of Pediatrics. Herpes simplex. In: Pickering LK, ed. *2009 Red Book: Report of the Committee on Infectious Diseases*. 27th ed. Elk Grove Village, IL: American Academy of Pediatrics; 2009:363–373.
- Hollier LM, Wendel GD. Third trimester antiviral prophylaxis for preventing maternal genital herpes simplex virus (HSV) recurrences and neonatal infection. *Cochrane Database Syst Rev.* 2008; 23;(1):CD004946.
- Kimberlin DW, Lin CY, Jacobs RF, et al. Safety and efficacy of high-dose intravenous acyclovir in the management of neonatal herpes simplex virus infections. *Pediatrics.* 2001;108:230–238.
- Long SS, Pool TE, Vodzak J, et al. Herpes simplex virus infection in young infants during 2 decades of empiric acyclovir therapy. *Ped Infect Dis J.* 2011; (30)7:1–5.
- Waggoner-Fountain LA, Grossman LB. Herpes simplex virus. *Pediatr Rev.* 2004;25:86–93.
- Whitley R. Neonatal herpes simplex virus infection. *Curr Opin Infect Dis.* 2004;17(3):243–246.

 CODES

ICD9

- 054.9 Herpes simplex without mention of complication
- 054.10 Genital herpes, unspecified
- 771.2 Other congenital infections specific to the perinatal period

ICD10

- A60.00 Herpesviral infection of urogenital system, unspecified
- B00.9 Herpesviral infection, unspecified
- P35.2 Congenital herpesviral [herpes simplex] infection

FAQ

- Q: What about recurrent cutaneous eruptions in a neonate? Should they be treated?
- A: The need for retreatment of infants with recurrent skin lesions is undetermined and under study. Because of concerns about silent CNS recurrent infection, some experts recommend acyclovir, 300 mg/m^2/dose in 3 doses for 6–12 months.
- Q: Is prophylactic therapy for recurrent herpes genitalia helpful? When is it indicated?
- A: Antiviral therapy has minimal effect on recurrent genital herpes. Oral acyclovir initiated within 2 days of onset of symptoms shortens the course. Topical acyclovir is not helpful.
- Q: What steps should be taken in the nursery for an infant born to an HSV-positive mother?
- A: Neonates with documented perinatal exposure to HSV may be in the incubation phase of infection and should be observed carefully. Infants of mothers with active HSV should be isolated if they have been delivered vaginally or by cesarean delivery after membranes were ruptured for more than 4–6 hours. The risk of HSV infection in possibly exposed infants (e.g., those born to a mother with a history of recurrent genital herpes) is low, and isolation is not necessary.
- Q: Is a repeated lumbar puncture necessary at the end of therapy for neonates or for children with HSV encephalitis?
- A: Experts recommend repeating the lumbar puncture at the end of the planned course of therapy to determine whether the virus is still present by PCR assay. If there is a positive test, therapy should be prolonged.

H

HICCUPS
Blaze Robert Gusic

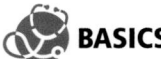 **BASICS**

DESCRIPTION
- Known medically as singultus, from the Latin *singult* (a sob or speech punctuated by sobs)
- Result of involuntary spasm of the diaphragm and intercostal muscles, leading to inspiration and abrupt closure of the glottis
- Affects nearly everyone at one time or another
- Hiccups serve no physiologic function and are often simply a benign affliction.

EPIDEMIOLOGY
- No male or female predominance for hiccup bouts; however, persistent and intractable hiccups are more frequent in males and are seen predominantly in adults.
- No racial, geographic, seasonal, or socioeconomic variability

Pregnancy Considerations
Fetal hiccups are common in the 3rd trimester of pregnancy.

GENERAL PREVENTION
Avoid precipitating factors.

PATHOPHYSIOLOGY
- A hiccup reflex arc has been postulated, although the exact anatomic mechanism remains unknown. The arc consists of:
  - The afferent limb: Phrenic and vagus nerves, the pharyngeal plexus from C2 to C4, and the thoracic sympathetic chain from T6 to T12
  - The efferent limb: Phrenic nerve to the diaphragm and the external intercostal nerves to the intercostal muscles
  - A central connection: A nonspecific location incorporating the medulla but independent of the respiratory center, the hypothalamus, and the phrenic nerve nuclei
- Hiccups have negligible effect on ventilation and usually involve only unilateral diaphragmatic contraction, most frequently on the left.
- Hiccups serve no respiratory function, despite activation of inspiratory musculature far more than during normal respiration.

ETIOLOGY
- Bouts may be precipitated by a number of benign causes including:
  - Gastric distention:
    - Aerophagia
    - Ingestion of excessive food, carbonated beverages, or alcohol
    - Gastric insufflation during endoscopy
  - Changes in the ambient or gastrointestinal temperature:
    - Cold showers
    - Ingestion of hot or cold beverages
    - Moving from cold to hot environment, or vice versa
  - Sudden excitement or stress
  - Tobacco use
- Persistent and intractable hiccups have many causes, which can be characterized as psychogenic, organic, or idiopathic:
  - Psychogenic:
    - Stress
    - Conversion reactions
    - Anorexia nervosa
    - Malingering
    - Personality disorders
  - Organic:
    - CNS disorders: Ventriculoperitoneal shunts, hydrocephalus, arteriovenous malformations, stroke, temporal arteritis, CNS trauma, encephalitis, meningitis, brain abscess
    - Peripheral nervous system disturbances: Irritation of the phrenic or vagus nerve from a variety of causes, including goiter, tumors or cysts of the neck, hiatal hernia, esophagitis, pneumonia, bronchitis, asthma, mediastinal lymphadenopathy, pericarditis, myocardial infarction, peptic ulcer disease, pancreatitis, inflammatory bowel disease, appendicitis, cholecystitis, and renal and hepatic disorders (stones or infections)
    - Infectious causes: Sepsis, influenza, herpes zoster, malaria, and tuberculosis
    - Metabolic or pharmacologic causes: Anesthesia, methylprednisolone, barbiturates, diazepam, methyldopa, uremia, hypocalcemia, and hyponatremia

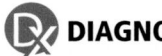 **DIAGNOSIS**

HISTORY
- Severity, duration, and characteristics of hiccups
- Medication and alcohol use
- Hiccups persisting during sleep suggest an organic cause.

PHYSICAL EXAM
- Head and neck exam may reveal evidence of trauma, foreign body in the ear, nuchal rigidity, masses, cervical lymphadenopathy, or an enlarged thyroid.
- Assess the chest for evidence of pneumonia, bronchitis, or pericarditis.
- Assess the abdomen for evidence of appendicitis, intestinal obstruction, ruptured viscus, pancreatitis, or hepatobiliary disease.
- Neurologic exam may provide evidence of trauma, meningitis, encephalitis, ventriculoperitoneal shunt malfunction, or neoplasm.

DIAGNOSTIC TESTS & INTERPRETATION
Lab
Tests should be chosen based on historic and physical findings:
- CBC
- Renal function and electrolytes
- Liver function tests and calcium
- Toxicology screen and blood gas

Imaging
Chest radiograph may rule out phrenic, vagal, and diaphragmatic irritation by pulmonary, cardiac, and mediastinal abnormalities.

DIFFERENTIAL DIAGNOSIS
Hiccups are not often mistaken for any other entity.

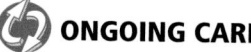 TREATMENT

MEDICATION (DRUGS)

- Studies confined to adult populations. Pharmaceuticals are rarely recommended for children.
- Chlorpromazine is widely used in adults in IV preparations. Intramuscular haloperidol has also been effective in adults.
- Anticonvulsants, including diphenylhydantoin, valproic acid, and carbamazepine, are reported effective.
- Combination of cisapride, omeprazole, and baclofen has been reported to be effective and is considered the mainstay for idiopathic chronic hiccups.
- Gabapentin has been shown to be effective as a substitute for baclofen or as an additional agent in the above regimen.
- Amantadine has been used with potential therapeutic response.

ADDITIONAL TREATMENT
General Measures
- Directed at the underlying disease
- If cause is unknown, empiric therapy may be necessary.
- Nonpharmacologic modalities:
  - Interruption of respiratory function: Sneezing, coughing, breath holding, hyperventilation, sudden pain or fright, and even positive airway pressure ventilation
  - Disruption of phrenic nerve transmission: Tapping over the 5th cervical vertebra, ice applied to the skin over the area of the phrenic nerve, and even transecting the phrenic nerve
  - Behavioral modification and hypnosis
  - Acupuncture: Reported to be successful in the treatment of persistent hiccups
  - Nasopharyngeal stimulation: Traction of the tongue, stimulation of the pharynx with a cotton swab, lifting the uvula with a spoon
  - Old-fashioned home remedies such as sipping ice water, swallowing granulated sugar, drinking water from the far side of a glass or through a paper towel, and biting on a lemon

SURGERY/OTHER PROCEDURES
Surgical treatment is rarely performed. Cases of phrenic nerve blockade, percutaneous phrenic nerve pacing, and crush injury have been cited, but mostly in adults and in those with underlying chronic illnesses.

 ONGOING CARE

FOLLOW-UP RECOMMENDATIONS
No specific follow-up is indicated unless a specific organic cause has been identified.

PROGNOSIS
- Self-limited and resolve without complications
- Usually terminate within hours
- Hiccup bouts may last up to 48 hours. Persistent hiccups last from 48 hours up to 1 month, and intractable hiccups last for >1 month.

COMPLICATIONS
- Adverse effects that have been associated with intractable hiccups:
  - Malnutrition and dehydration
  - Weight loss
  - Insomnia
  - Fatigue
  - Psychological stress
- Rare complications:
  - Cardiac dysrhythmia
  - Reflux esophagitis
  - Wound dehiscence
  - Pulmonary edema from the negative pressure
  - Death

ADDITIONAL READING

- Buyukhatipoglu H, Sezen Y, Yildiz A, et al. Hiccups as a sign of chronic myocardial ischemia. *South Med J.* 2010;103:1184–1185.
- Lierz P. Anesthesia as therapy for persistent hiccups. *Anesth Analg.* 2002;95:494–495.
- Payne BR. Vagus nerve stimulation for chronic intractable hiccups. Case report. *J Neurosurg.* 2005;102(5):935–937.
- Pearce JMS. A note on hiccups. *J Neurol Neurosurg Psychiatry.* 2003;74:1070.
- Petroianu G, Hein G, Stegmeier-Petroianu A, et al. Gabapentin "add-on therapy" for idiopathic chronic hiccup. *J Clin Gastroenterol.* 2000;30:321–324.
- Viera AJ, Sullivan SA. Remedies for prolonged hiccups. *Am Fam Physician.* 2001;63:1664–1668.
- Wilcox SK, Garry A, Johnson MJ. Novel use of amantadine: To treat hiccups. *J Pain Symptom Manage.* 2009;38(3):460–465.

CODES

ICD9
- 306.8 Other specified psychophysiological malfunction
- 786.8 Hiccough

ICD10
- F45.8 Other somatoform disorders
- R06.6 Hiccough

FAQ

- Q: Does rebreathing into a paper bag really work?
- A: As a fall in pCO_2 may increase the frequency of hiccups, rebreathing air will increase pCO_2 and thus terminate hiccups.
- Q: Will hiccups harm my baby?
- A: Hiccups alone are harmless. If they are truly persistent, are intractable, or disrupt sleep, they may have the side effects as mentioned. Premature babies have been observed to spend 2.5% of their time having hiccups.
- Q: Is there an association between gastroesophageal reflux and hiccups?
- A: Hiccups can be caused by esophageal irritation from gastroesophageal reflux disease, and chronic hiccups have been linked to reflux esophagitis.

H

HIRSCHSPRUNG DISEASE

Joy L. Collins

 BASICS

DESCRIPTION
- Characterized by aganglionosis of the distal bowel beginning at the anus and extending proximally for a variable distance, leading to abnormal intestinal motility and an abnormal or absent relaxation of the internal anal sphincter
- 1st description of congenital megacolon by Harald Hirschsprung in 1888
- May present as delayed passage of meconium, chronic constipation, partial or complete intestinal obstruction, or enterocolitis

EPIDEMIOLOGY
Incidence
- Most common cause of lower intestinal obstruction in neonates: 1 in 5,000 births
- Familial incidence in colonic aganglionosis: 75% of cases, rectosigmoid involved; 14%, descending colon involved; 8%, colon involved; 3%, small bowel affected

Prevalence
- Overall rate of male/female patients is 2.8:1; in long-segment disease, it is 2.8:1, and in total colonic aganglionosis, it is 2.2:1.
- Syndromic and nonsyndromic Hirschsprung disease: In the former there are other congenital anomalies (30% of cases), whereas in the latter it occurs as an isolated trait.

RISK FACTORS
Genetics
- Loci implicated include those at chromosomes 3p21, 10q11, 5p13, 22q13, 1p36, and 19q12
- Associated with mutations in the RET proto-oncogene
- ~5% of patients with Hirschsprung disease have mutations in the endothelin signaling pathway.

PATHOPHYSIOLOGY
- Basic histologic finding is the absence of Meissner and Auerbach plexuses and hypertrophied nerve bundles between the circular and the longitudinal muscles and in the submucosa.
- Defect is considered as a failure of caudal migration of the neural crest cells.

COMMONLY ASSOCIATED CONDITIONS
- In 3% of the patients, an association with Down syndrome, cardiac anomalies, and coexistent multiple neuroblastomas
- More recently, case reports of neurologic disorders associated in children with Hirschsprung disease
- May be familial and associated with disorders of the urogenital tract, cardiovascular defects, other GI system disorders, cleft palate, and extremity defects.
- Another study reveals upper gut dysmotility in patients with Hirschsprung disease and its allied disorders in adults.

 DIAGNOSIS

HISTORY
- 80% of patients present in the neonatal period.
- Typical symptoms: Failure to pass meconium by 48 hours of life; delayed passage of meconium after 24 hours of life; history of constipation; history of chronic laxative use, abdominal distention, bilious vomiting, diarrhea in 22% of patients
- Neonates usually have normal weight, but growth retardation may occur when the disease is severe.
- Children with Hirschsprung disease may have small-volume and small-diameter stools. Some may have overflow diarrhea as well.

PHYSICAL EXAM
- On rectal exam, the sphincter tone is usually normal or increased. Removal of the finger may be followed by explosive diarrhea. In most instances, especially in older children, the rectum is empty.
- Patients may be anemic owing to chronic blood loss from the large bowel secondary to infection.

DIAGNOSTIC TESTS & INTERPRETATION
Lab
CBC: Anemia, leukocytosis in the presence of enterocolitis

Imaging
- Plain film of abdomen:
  - May show distended intestinal loops
  - Diffuse intestinal pneumatosis has been reported as a rare presentation.
- Barium enema:
  - May be useful but not always diagnostic
  - Transition zone is a funnel-shaped area of intestine with normal distal area and dilated proximal area.
  - Reveals large intestinal mucosal pattern, prominently thickened folds, and irregular margins secondary to ulceration
  - Significant delay in excretion of barium should also raise one's suspicion for Hirschsprung disease.

Diagnostic Procedures/Other
- Anorectal manometry: May be diagnostic, but usually reserved for those cases causing diagnostic difficulties, as in the ultra–short-segment disease.
- Suction biopsy:
  - Should be done ~2–4 cm from the anal verge depending on the age of the patient
  - Biopsies must have adequate submucosa to demonstrate neurofibrils detected using acetylcholinesterase as a stain.
  - With the absence of ganglion cells, biopsy is diagnostic.
  - If the suction biopsies are not conclusive, a full-thickness biopsy is mandatory.

Pathological Findings
- Aganglionic segment
- Zone of hypoganglionosis proximal to the aganglionic segment
- Incomplete maturation of enteric nerve plexus
- Hypertrophy of nonmyelinated nerve fibers within bowel wall

DIFFERENTIAL DIAGNOSIS
- Mechanical obstruction
- Meconium ileus
- Meconium plug syndrome
- Neonatal small left colon syndrome
- Malrotation with volvulus
- Intestinal atresia
- Intussusception
- Necrotizing enterocolitis
- Functional obstruction
- Intestinal neuronal dysplasia
- Sepsis
- Metabolic disorders (e.g., uremia, hypothyroidism)
- Disorders of intrinsic enteric nerves (diabetes or dysautonomia)
- Disorders of smooth muscle function
- Electrolyte disturbances
- Chronic constipation

ALERT
Early recognition is of utmost importance in reducing the morbidity and mortality of Hirschsprung disease.

TREATMENT

MEDICATION (DRUGS)
- 1st line:
  - For constipation: Rhubarb, prune or pear juice, bran
  - For diarrhea: Bananas, carrots, blueberries
- 2nd line:
  - For constipation: Senna extract
- For diarrhea: Cholestyramine, loperamide (must make sure diarrhea is not due to enterocolitis or overflow)

ADDITIONAL TREATMENT
General Measures
Stabilizing treatment if child presents with suspected enterocolitis or obstruction:
- Fluid resuscitation
- Nasogastric decompression
- Broad-spectrum antibiotics
- Saline enemas for decompression

SURGERY/OTHER PROCEDURES

- Initial operation:
  - Defunctionalizing colostomy or ileostomy for total colonic aganglionosis or if child presents with obstruction not relieved by rectal irrigations:
    - Performed to avoid the hazards of enterocolitis
- Definitive surgery:
  - Performed 6 months to 1 year after the initial colostomy
  - May be performed as initial procedure in stable, nonobstructed child
- A multitude of surgical techniques have been described, including modifications on the traditional Swenson, Soave, and Duhamel procedures.
- Recent advances include:
  - The introduction of entirely transanal techniques
  - Increasing use of laparoscopic assistance with various procedures
  - Transition away from multistaged procedures to a variety of definitive single-stage operations
- In total colonic aganglionosis, the modified Lester Martin technique may be performed: Involves the anastomosis of the cecum and ascending colon as an onlay patch graft in the more distal normal small bowel, which is then pulled through the amputated rectum (which has been stripped of its mucosa), with a primary anastomosis.
- A Duhamel or modification thereof is also an option for total colonic aganglionosis; this involves total resection of the aganglionic colon with retrorectal pull-through of the ganglionated bowel and anastomosis in which a portion of aganglionic rectum is left in situ.

ALERT

- Clinicians must have *high* suspicion for enterocolitis both before and after definitive pull-through.
- Fecal incontinence could occur after surgery.

 ONGOING CARE

FOLLOW-UP RECOMMENDATIONS

Most children are followed on a regular basis for the 1st decade after surgery.

COMPLICATIONS

- Early (<4 weeks postoperation, usually related to technical issues):
  - Anastomotic leak
  - Cuff abscess and retraction of pull-through segment
  - Disturbance of micturition
  - Wound infection, intra-abdominal adhesions
- Late:
  - Chronic constipation
  - Long-term voiding dysfunction
  - Sexual dysfunction due to dissection around pelvic nerve plexus
  - Enterocolitis
- Enterocolitis is the most important complication:
  - Secondary to obstruction causing an increase in intraluminal pressure and decreased intramural capillary blood flow
  - Affects the protective mucosal barrier, enabling fecal breakdown products, bacteria, and toxins to enter the bloodstream
  - Usually presents with fever, diarrhea, and bilious vomiting
  - Can occur both before and after definitive pull-through
  - Clinicians must have *high* suspicion; can be rapidly progressive and FATAL

ADDITIONAL READING

- Dasgupta R, Langer JC. Evaluation and management of persistent problems after surgery for Hirschsprung disease in a child. *J Pediatr Gastroenterol Nutr.* 2008;46(1):13–19.
- de Lorijn F, Boeckxstaens GE, Benninga MA. Symptomatology, pathophysiology, diagnostic work-up, and treatment of Hirschsprung disease in infancy and childhood. *Curr Gastroenterol Rep.* 2007;9(3):245–253.

- Engum SA, Grosfeld JL. Long-term results of treatment of Hirschsprung's disease. *Semin Pediatr Surg.* 2004;13(4):273–285.
- Lyonnet S, Bolino A, Pelet A, et al. A gene for Hirschsprung disease maps to the proximal long arm of chromosome 10. *Nat Genet.* 1993;4:346–501.
- Rangel S, de Blaauw I. Advances in pediatric colorectal surgical techniques. *Semin Pediatr Surg.* 2010;19:86–95.
- Swenson O. Hirschsprung's disease: A review. *Pediatrics.* 2002;109:914–918.
- Teitelbaum DH, Coran AG. Primary pull-through for Hirschsprung's disease. *Semin Neonatol.* 2003; 8:233–241.
- Van der Zee DC, Bax KN. One-stage Duhamel-Martin procedure for Hirschsprung disease: A 5-year follow-up study. *J Pediatr Surg.* 2000;35: 1434–1436.

 CODES

ICD9

751.3 Hirschsprung's disease and other congenital functional disorders of colon

ICD10

Q43.1 Hirschsprung's disease

FAQ

- Q: Will the bowel movements be normal after surgery?
- A: Studies have shown that 83% of children have ≤3 stools per day at a mean follow-up of 4.1 ± 2.5 years.
- Q: Are laxatives required after surgery?
- A: In ~20% of children, some sort of laxative therapy or rectal irrigation may be required.

H

HISTIOCYTOSIS

Charles Bailey

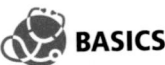 **BASICS**

DESCRIPTION
- Langerhans cell histiocytosis (LCH): Clinical condition associated with proliferation or inappropriate localization of Langerhans cells (dendritic cells, histiocytes, mononuclear phagocytes)
- Related disorders:
  - Macrophage hyperactivation syndromes (e.g., hemophagocytic lymphohistiocytosis [HLH], macrophage activation syndrome)
  - Malignant histiocytosis (lymphoma subtype)
- Disorder of unknown cause involving cells similar to Langerhans cells of the skin
- Other names include:
  - Histiocytosis X (superseded)
  - Eosinophilic granuloma: Refers to single lesion, usually of bone
  - Hand-Schüller-Christian syndrome: Chronic multifocal bone (especially cranial) and skin, diabetes insipidus, possibly with other organ involvement
  - Letterer-Siwe disease: Multisystem visceral LCH, often including hepatic and marrow involvement
  - Hashimoto-Pritzker syndrome: Infant dermatologic involvement, often self-limited

EPIDEMIOLOGY
- May occur at any age. Peak incidence in infancy, especially for multisystem disease
- Variable reports of mild male predominance

Incidence
2.5–9 cases per million

RISK FACTORS
Genetics
- Rare reports of recurrence within families
- Specific HLA alleles associated with disease phenotype in case series

PATHOPHYSIOLOGY
- Bone and skin lesions are most common in children, especially >1 year old
- Involvement of liver, spleen, marrow, and lung (rare in children) associated with more severe morbidity and mortality ("risk organs")
- Involvement of CNS, gut, other "nonrisk" organs less common than skin/bone, and not associated with mortality
- Clonal histiocytes have been detected in all forms of disease, but do not have malignant behavior, and may represent normal LC development.

ETIOLOGY
LCH cells differ structurally from normal Langerhans cells, but critical factors leading to disease remain largely uncharacterized.

DIAGNOSIS

HISTORY
- Swelling, pain, or pathologic fracture from soft tissue or bone lesion
- Erythematous or brown papular rash
- Persistent otorrhea
- Proptosis
- Gait disturbance
- Early loss of teeth
- Failure to thrive
- Diarrhea, possibly bloody
- Fever of unknown origin
- Headache
- Abdominal pain
- Jaundice
- Polydipsia or polyuria (diabetes insipidus)
- School/cognitive problems
- Dyspnea or persistent cough
- History of spontaneous pneumothorax
- Signs and symptoms:
  - Wide variation in presenting signs and symptoms depending on affected organ systems
  - Single-system skeletal disease may be asymptomatic, with incidental discovery of lesions on radiographs obtained for other reasons (e.g., trauma).

PHYSICAL EXAM
- Growth or pubertal delay
- Skin: Brownish-red papules often involving intertriginous areas, seborrheic dermatitis (cradle cap), purpura, petechial rash especially at areas of skin contact (e.g., top of diaper); rash may become ulcerated, crusted, or scaly.
- Ears: Otorrhea, hearing loss
- Skeleton: Swelling or mass; may be painless or very tender to palpation; skull, axial skeleton, long bones more often affected than hands or feet
- Teeth: Gingivitis, "floating teeth"
- Eyes: Orbital swelling, cranial nerve palsies
- Lungs: Tachypnea, intercostal retractions
- GI: Hepatosplenomegaly, ascites, edema, jaundice; stool with blood or mucus
- Neurologic: Ataxia, cognitive difficulties

DIAGNOSTIC TESTS & INTERPRETATION
Lab
- Routine diagnostic evaluation:
  - CBC with differential to evaluate for marrow involvement
  - Liver function tests (LFTs), prothrombin time (PT), partial thromboplastin time (PTT) to evaluate liver function
  - Morning urine specific gravity/osmolality
- Other investigations:
  - Pulmonary involvement: Pulmonary function tests
  - Polyuria/suspected diabetes insipidus: Endocrine evaluation including water deprivation test and evaluation of anterior pituitary hormone production
  - Auricular involvement: Audiogram; ear, nose, and throat evaluation
- Bone involvement: Biopsy of lesions unless diagnosis of LCH already established

Imaging
- Chest radiograph and skeletal survey (bone scan not as sensitive in most patients, but may be better for infants)
- Liver/spleen ultrasound
- High-resolution chest CT if pulmonary involvement suspected
- MRI of brain with contrast, including detailed evaluation of sella turcica, if neurologic involvement or signs of diabetes insipidus
- Dental radiographs if teeth are involved
- CT/MRI imaging of lytic-appearing lesions often obtained prior to diagnosis to evaluate potential malignancy; classic "punched out" lesions may not require imaging beyond plain films.

Diagnostic Procedures/Other
- Biopsy of lesion to establish diagnosis
- Cytopenias or other high-risk organ involvement: Bone marrow aspirate and biopsy
- Liver dysfunction: Liver biopsy to evaluate for sclerosing cholangitis
- GI involvement: Endoscopic biopsy of small and large intestine
- Pulmonary involvement: Consider bronchoalveolar lavage (BAL) or lung biopsy to evaluate for infection if diagnosis of LCH not already established from more accessible tissue or if appearance on CT is atypical.

Pathological Findings
- Lesions show proliferation of Langerhans-like cells in places where they are not typically found.
- Langerhans cells are characterized by the presence of tennis racquet–shaped inclusions (Birbeck granules) on electron microscopy or by staining with anti-CD1a or -CD207 (langerin).

DIFFERENTIAL DIAGNOSIS
- Broad differential, depending on constellation of presenting symptoms
- Bone/soft tissue lesions:
  - Sarcoma (especially osteogenic sarcoma, Ewing sarcoma, or rhabdomyosarcoma)
  - Benign bone lesion (e.g., osteoma, bone cyst)
  - Infection
  - Metastatic tumor (e.g., neuroblastoma, leukemia/lymphoma)
- Skin lesions:
  - Seborrheic dermatitis
  - Otitis externa
  - Tineal infection
  - Viral exanthem (especially herpes simplex virus [HSV] in neonates)
- CNS lesions:
  - Teratoma or malignant germ cell tumor
  - Craniopharyngioma
  - Primary CNS tumor
- Pulmonary involvement:
  - Infection
  - Emphysema (e.g., α_1-antitrypsin deficiency)

- Fever, lymphadenopathy (nontender, nonerythematous):
  – Lymphoma
  – Lymphadenitis (especially large DNA viruses)
  – Granulomatous (e.g., fungal, cat-scratch disease) infections
  – Rosai-Dorfman or Castleman disease
  – Rheumatologic disease
  – HLH
- Hepatic involvement:
  – Infections
  – Congenital hepatic and storage diseases
  – HLH
  – Tumor infiltration (e.g., leukemia)
  – Primary sclerosing cholangitis
- Cytopenias:
  – Leukemia or other tumor infiltration
  – Aplastic anemia
  – HLH
  – Myelofibrosis or storage diseases

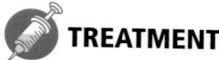 TREATMENT

MEDICATION (DRUGS)
First Line
- Corticosteroids
- Vinblastine
- Antimetabolites (6-mercaptopurine [6-MP], methotrexate)

Second Line
- 2-Chlorodeoxyadenosine ± cytarabine
- Etoposide also has activity; used in early LCH treatment trials
- Thalidomide has shown some efficacy for persistent disease not involving high-risk organs.
- Cyclosporin A or antithymocyte globulin used less often for immunomodulation in refractory disease

ADDITIONAL TREATMENT
General Measures
- Type of therapy depends primarily on:
  – Number of organ systems affected
  – Number of bone lesions, if sole system involved
  – Involvement of "risk organs" associated with morbidity or mortality: Liver, spleen, bone marrow, and possibly lung
- Single system (most often bone, skin):
  – Observation of isolated lesions; often remain stable or spontaneously resolve
  – Local therapy:
    ○ Excision or biopsy/disruption often curative for bone or lymph node lesion
    ○ Steroids for confirmed LCH of skin or multiple nodes
    ○ Topical nitrogen mustard or tacrolimus used for refractory skin lesions
    ○ Systemic therapy used for multiple/refractory lesions
  – Systemic therapy:
    ○ Low-dose chemotherapy for some multifocal bone disease or multiple recurrent single bone lesions; superior results with multiagent regimens
    ○ Reduces risk of later DI in patients with skull, vertebral, or CNS lesions
    ○ Cotrimoxazole effective for some patients with cutaneous involvement.

- Multisystem:
  – Chemotherapy:
    ○ Typically 6–12-month course
    ○ Steroid, vinblastine, plus antimetabolites depending on extent of disease and risk organ involvement
  – Limited response by 6 weeks merits intensification (e.g., 2-CdA + AraC)
  – Less common: Immunotherapy or radiation
  – Limited experience with allogeneic stem cell transplantation for very high-risk refractory disease
  – Most patients treated at pediatric oncology centers
  – International clinical trials in progress
- Treatment of disease-related morbidity:
  – Lifelong intranasal desmopressin acetate often needed for the management of diabetes insipidus; posterior pituitary dysfunction is rarely reversible.
  – Organ transplantation may be necessary for high-risk patients with organ dysfunction.

Additional Therapies
Radiotherapy
Rarely used; reserved for refractory or critical bone lesions (e.g., spinal cord compression)

ISSUES FOR REFERRAL
Multidisciplinary care involving several specialties may be required for management of orthopedic, endocrinologic, hepatic, hematologic, or pulmonary complications.

SURGERY/OTHER PROCEDURES
- Initial biopsy for diagnosis: Often curative for solitary bone lesions
- Excision of isolated bone or lymph node lesions

 ONGOING CARE

FOLLOW-UP RECOMMENDATIONS
- Evaluation at regular intervals for recurrence of lesions or new high-risk organ involvement, depending on extent of prior disease
- Because the course is quite variable, patients need to be followed closely at a center experienced in the management of histiocytosis.

Patient Monitoring
- Laboratory and imaging follow-up as described for initial evaluation, with focus on previously affected and high-risk organ systems
- Routine follow-up typically includes history, physical exam, CBC, LFTs, and skeletal imaging.

DIET
Maintain fluid and electrolyte intake if diabetes insipidus is present.

PROGNOSIS
- Single-system or bone/skin disease carries low risk of morbidity.
- <20% of patients with single-system disease, but up to 75% of patients with multifocal bone disease will have a remitting and relapsing course. Mortality is <5%.
- Often disease will "burn out" by the end of childhood. ~5% of patients will continue to have exacerbations as adults.

- 45% of patients with multisystem disease who reach CR will have reactivation; most do not involve risk organs.
- For patients with liver, spleen, bone marrow, or lung ("risk organ") involvement who have not responded to initial 6 weeks of therapy, the risk for mortality is >66%. For good responders, mortality is ~10%.

COMPLICATIONS
- Most common long-term morbidities include orthopedic problems, diabetes insipidus, and neurologic dysfunction.
- Some patients with single-system bone involvement will have a chronic remitting and relapsing course.
- Craniofacial and vertebral involvement is associated with a higher risk of diabetes insipidus; risk improves with multidrug therapy.
- Smoking strongly associated with development of pulmonary disease in LCH patients
- Chronic disabilities with multisystem disease include pulmonary fibrosis, hepatic fibrosis, deafness, orthopedic problems, short stature, permanent ataxia, neurocognitive deficits, and poor dentition.

ADDITIONAL READING

- Filipovich A, McClain K, Grom A. Histiocytic disorders: Recent insights into pathophysiology and practical guidelines. *Biol Blood Marrow Transplant.* 2010;16:S82–S89.
- Gadner H, Grois N, Pötschger U, et al. Improved outcome in multisystem Langerhans cell histiocytosis is associated with therapy intensification. *Blood.* 2008;111:2556–2562.
- Minkov M, Grois N, McClain K, et al. *Langerhans cell histiocytosis: Histiocyte Society evaluation and treatment guidelines.* 2009. Available at: http://www.histiocytesociety.org/site/c.mqISL2PIJrH/b.4442715/k.A339/Treatment_Plans.htm.
- Satter EK, High WA. Langerhans cell histiocytosis: A review of the current recommendations of the Histiocyte Society. *Pediatr Dermatol.* 2008;25:291–295.

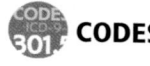 CODES

ICD9
- 202.5 Abt-Letterer-Siwe; acute histiocytosis X
- 277.89 Hand-Schüller-Christian; chronic histiocytosis X

ICD10
- C96.5 Multifocal and unisystemic Langerhans-cell histiocytosis
- C96.6 Unifocal Langerhans-cell histiocytosis
- C96.9 Malignant neoplasm of lymphoid, hematopoietic and related tissue, unspecified

H

HISTOPLASMOSIS

Marleine Ishak
Sumit Bhargava
Julian L. Allen (5th edition)

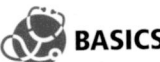

BASICS

DESCRIPTION
- Spectrum of illness, ranging from primary pulmonary to disseminated infection:
  - Pulmonary
  - Extrapulmonary
  - Disseminated
- Caused by the dimorphic fungus *Histoplasma capsulatum*
- Acute or chronic
- Primary or reactivation

EPIDEMIOLOGY
- Most common systemic fungal infection in U.S.
- Organism found in nitrogen-rich soil and high-carbon content, lower pH soil contaminated by animal droppings, especially those of bats and birds
- Outbreaks reported in pigeon breeders or cleaners of chicken coops, explorers of caves with bats, and populations living close to construction
- Endemic in eastern and central U.S., specifically in the St. Lawrence, Mississippi, and Ohio River valleys, the Rio Grande, Texas, Oklahoma, Kansas, Pennsylvania, Maryland, and Virginia
- No human-to-human or animal-to-human transmission
- Incubation period variable, 1–3 weeks

Incidence
Severity of symptoms depends on immunologic status of the host and size of inoculum:
- Asymptomatic in up to 95% of cases
- With heavy inoculum, 50–100% develop symptoms. Of these, 80% develop flu-like symptoms, lasting about a week; 10–20% develop pericarditis, arthritis, or erythema nodosum, resolving after a few weeks

Prevalence
80–90% of adults in endemic areas are skin-test positive.

RISK FACTORS
Risk factors for severe disease (progressive disseminated histoplasmosis) include very old and very young (<2 years) and cellular immunocompromise.

GENERAL PREVENTION
- Investigate common source of infection in outbreaks. Limit exposure to soil and dust from areas contaminated with bat and bird droppings.
- For occupational exposure to *H. capsulatum*-contaminated soil:
  - Wetting agents to prevent aerosolization of contaminated dust
  - National Institute for Occupational Safety and Health (NIOSH)-approved respirators; e.g., N95, gloves, and dispensable clothing (see NIOSH website in Bibliography)
- Isolation of the hospitalized patient: Standard precautions recommended

ETIOLOGY
- Inhalation of *H. capsulatum* spores
- The dimorphic fungus exists in mycelial form in the environment at 25°C and in yeast form in tissues at 37°C.

DIAGNOSIS

HISTORY
- Environmental exposures (pigeon breeding, construction, cave exploration, travel in endemic areas): Epidemiologically suggestive of histoplasmosis
- Upper respiratory symptoms, low-grade fever, cough, pleuritic chest pain: Suggestive of mild disease lasting 1–5 days
- Arthritis, more severe chest pain, skin lesions, pericarditis, or pleural effusion: Suggestive of moderate disease lasting ~15 days
- High fever, night sweats, weight loss, cough, chest pain, shortness of breath, hoarseness lasting >2–3 weeks: Suggestive of disseminated disease and underlying immune suppression
- Chronic cough, dyspnea, disabling respiratory dysfunction: Suggestive of chronic cavitary pulmonary disease

PHYSICAL EXAM
- Flu-like signs and symptoms are common in mild disease; physical exam may be normal.
- Less usual manifestations suggest moderate or disseminated disease:
  - Hepatosplenomegaly
  - Adenopathy
  - Pneumonitis
  - Skin lesions (erythema nodosum)
  - Pericardial friction rub
  - Pallor, petechiae
  - CNS findings
  - Severe disease can present as sepsis syndrome with hypotension, DIC, renal failure, and acute respiratory distress

DIAGNOSTIC TESTS & INTERPRETATION
Lab
- Culture of the organism in sputum, tissue specimens, peripheral blood, or bone marrow:
  - Definitive, but requires 2–6 weeks
  - Sputum cultures are negative in most patients with mild disease.
  - Cultures are positive in 2/3 of patients with cavitary disease and 1/3 of patients with noncavitary disease.
  - In progressive disseminated histoplasmosis in patients with AIDS, bone marrow, and blood cultures are positive in 80–90% of patients, and bronchoscopic cultures are positive in 80–90% of patients with abnormal chest radiographs.
- Identification of organism by microscopy:
  - Histologic identification in sputum, blood, bone marrow, biopsy specimens, and/or CSF
  - Staining methods: Hematoxylin and eosin, Wright, Giemsa, periodic acid-Schiff; Gomori methenamine silver more likely to detect sparse organisms
  - Histopathology is a valuable diagnostic tool and can demonstrate noncaseating granulomas in histoplasmosis.

- Radioimmune and hemagglutinin assays for *H. capsulatum* antigen:
  - Radioimmunoassay: Specific, sensitive, and rapid for diagnosing progressive disseminated histoplasmosis, but low sensitivity for acute pulmonary histoplasmosis in immunocompetent patients
  - May cross-react with coccidiomycosis and blastomycosis antigens
  - Hemagglutinin found in urine or blood in 50–90% of patients with progressive disseminated histoplasmosis (urine more sensitive) and in bronchoalveolar lavage fluid in 70% of AIDS patients with pulmonary histoplasmosis
  - Antigenuria is detected in 75% of patients with severe acute pulmonary histoplasmosis. Only 10–20% of patients with less severe acute pulmonary histoplasmosis or chronic cavitary pulmonary histoplasmosis will have antigenuria.
  - Antigen tests are generally useful only in 1st month of infection, but can persist for much longer in AIDS patients.
  - Antigen levels decrease with treatment and can increase again with relapse.
  - DNA probes increasingly used
- Serologic studies for antibodies:
  - Titers become positive 4–6 weeks after infection, peak at 2–3 months, and decline over a period of 2–5 years.
  - Positive titers in 90% of patients with symptomatic disease
  - False positives occur in patients with coccidiomycosis, blastomycosis, tuberculosis, or paracoccidiomycosis.
  - False negatives occur in immunocompromised patients with progressive disseminated histoplasmosis.
- Complement fixation:
  - Single titer 1:32 (1:8 in nonendemic areas) is diagnostic; 4-fold increase in titers is diagnostic.
  - More sensitive than immunodiffusion test, which is more specific
- Precipitating antibodies by immunodiffusion:
  - H band suggests active infection.
  - M band is less specific.
  - Presence of H and M bands is highly diagnostic.
- Evaluation for meningitis:
- Relative sensitivities:
  - Stain of CSF <10%
  - Culture CSF 20–60%
  - Antigen CSF 40–70%
  - Antibody CSF 60–80%
  - Meningeal or brain biopsy 50–80%

Imaging
Chest radiograph:
- Normal in 75% of patients with histoplasmosis, 25–50% of immunocompromised patients with disseminated disease
- Most common radiologic changes include:
  - Small 2–5-mm infiltrates in lung bases
  - Lobar or diffuse infiltrates
  - Enlarged or calcified hilar nodes
  - Buckshot calcifications seen in patients with large inoculum

- Cavitary lesions
- Pleural effusions in 10% of chest radiographs in adults
- Calcified nodules in liver and spleen

DIFFERENTIAL DIAGNOSIS
- Infections:
  - Pneumonia (viral, bacterial)
  - Influenza and other viral syndromes
  - Tuberculosis
  - Other fungal diseases:
    - Aspergillosis
    - Blastomycosis
    - Coccidiomycosis
  - Sarcoidosis
- Malignancy

ALERT
- Can be difficult to distinguish between active disease and previous exposure in patients from endemic regions
- May be confused with tuberculosis and other fungal diseases
- Isolated pulmonary nodule on chest radiograph may be difficult to distinguish from malignancy.

 TREATMENT

MEDICATION (DRUGS)
- Uncomplicated cases of primary histoplasmosis of the lungs may not require drug therapy.
- Treatment should be considered for patients with pulmonary symptoms lasting >4 weeks or with obstructing granulomatous disease.
- Patients with more severe or disseminated disease or the immunocompromised require treatment with antifungal agents. Treatment regimens vary. Amphotericin B, 0.5–1.0 mg/kg/d IV for 4–6 weeks (or 35 mg/kg total). Recommended for disseminated disease or patients with respiratory compromise and hypoxemia. Alternative treatment in children: Amphotericin B for 2–3 weeks, followed by oral itraconazole for 3–6 months.
- Milder disease: For the following drugs, interactions with other drugs are common; consult drug interaction database or reference before prescribing. Limited or no information about use in newborn infants, and, in the case of ketoconazole, children <2 years:
  - Ketoconazole:
    - 3.3–6.6 mg/kg/d PO (400 mg/d initially, then 200 mg/d is maximum dose) for 3–6 months
    - Should be used with caution in patients receiving H$_2$ blockers; absorption is decreased in achlorhydric state
    - Levels can also be reduced by rifampin and phenytoin.
    - Fluconazole or itraconazole are generally preferred due to fewer side effects (hepatotoxicity, anaphylaxis, thrombocytopenia, hemolytic anemia, other GI side effects).

- Fluconazole:
  - 6–12 mg/kg/d PO (400–800 mg/d is maximum dose) for 3–6 months
  - Reduced dose may also be given IV.
  - Achieves levels in CSF
- Itraconazole:
  - 5–10 mg/kg/d PO (400 mg/d is maximum dose) for 3–6 months
  - May also be given IV
  - Although not approved for use in children, effective in the treatment of HIV patients with histoplasmosis
  - Does not achieve levels in CSF
- In patients with AIDS, lifelong suppressive therapy is recommended.
- Adjunct therapy with corticosteroids may be added in patients with life-threatening airway obstruction secondary to hilar adenopathy.
- Prophylaxis: Considered for patients with AIDS, low CD4 counts, and who live in endemic areas
- Pericarditis and mediastinal fibrosis: Treat with indomethacin.

 ONGOING CARE

FOLLOW-UP RECOMMENDATIONS
When to expect improvement:
- In mild-to-moderate cases not requiring drug therapy, usually 1–2 weeks
- In cases requiring therapy, improvement usually noted within 2 weeks
- Response to therapy more variable in AIDS patients

PROGNOSIS
- In most cases, prognosis is excellent.
- 90% mortality within 3 months in patients with acute disseminated histoplasmosis if left untreated
- High relapse in AIDS patients if not treated with chronic suppressive therapy

COMPLICATIONS
- In general, complications rare; usually indicate disseminated disease
- Symptoms include:
  - Prolonged fever, malaise, cough, weight loss, hepatosplenomegaly, diarrhea
  - Patients may also develop disseminated intravascular coagulopathy, adult respiratory distress syndrome, renal failure, endocarditis, or Addison disease.
- Disseminated disease can involve:
  - Skin
  - Eyes (uveitis)
  - Liver
  - Spleen
  - Adrenal glands (adrenal insufficiency)
  - Bone marrow
  - Heart
  - CNS (meningitis)

- Other complications include:
  - Tracheobronchial compression
  - Mediastinal granuloma formation or fibrosing mediastinitis
  - Fistula formation
  - Pericarditis can be severe enough to cause cardiac tamponade.
  - Obstruction of superior vena cava, esophagus, or pulmonary arteries
- Chronic cavitary pulmonary disease very similar to tuberculosis

ADDITIONAL READING
- Kauffman CA. Histoplasmosis: A clinical and laboratory update. *Clin Microbiol Rev.* 2007;20: 115–132.
- Montenegro BL, Arnold JC. North American Dimorphic fungal infections in children. *Pediatr Rev.* 2010;31:40–48.
- National Institute for Occupational Safety and Health (NIOSH) Web site: http://www.cdc.gov/niosh/97–146.htm.
- Wheat LJ, Freifeld AG, Kleiman MB, et al. Clinical practice guidelines for the management of patients with histoplasmosis: 2007 update by the Infectious Disease Society of America. *Clin Infect Dis.* 2007; 45:807–825.

 CODES

ICD9
- 115.00 Infection by Histoplasma capsulatum, without mention of manifestation
- 115.05 Infection by Histoplasma capsulatum, pneumonia
- 115.90 Histoplasmosis, unspecified, without mention of manifestation

ICD10
- B39.2 Pulmonary histoplasmosis capsulati, unspecified
- B39.3 Disseminated histoplasmosis capsulati
- B39.9 Histoplasmosis, unspecified

FAQ
- Q: What are the most common clinical presentations of histoplasmosis?
- A: Asymptomatic, mild primary pulmonary (1–2 weeks), moderate (2–3 weeks), disseminated, and cavitary are common.
- Q: How is histoplasmosis best diagnosed?
- A: Skin test generally is not useful; culture and serologic testing is recommended.
- Q: Does histoplasmosis need to be treated with antifungal therapy?
- A: Mild primary disease—no; more severe or disseminated disease—yes.
- Q: How can histoplasmosis be prevented?
- A: Prevention can be achieved only by controlling the environmental factors in the affected areas; there are no vaccines for the prevention of histoplasmosis.
- Q: Do patients with histoplasmosis need to be isolated?
- A: No isolation of infected patients is required.

HODGKIN LYMPHOMA
Leslie S. Kersun

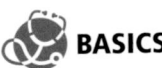

BASICS

DESCRIPTION
Malignant enlargement of lymph nodes characterized by a pleomorphic cellular infiltrate with multinucleated giant cells (Reed-Sternberg cells)

EPIDEMIOLOGY
Incidence
- Male > female
- Incidence shows bimodal age distribution:
  - Early peak, before adolescence in developing countries, mid- to late 20s in US
  - 2nd peak, late adulthood >50 years of age
  - Childhood cases rare before 5 years of age
    - Most common in whites >15 years of age

RISK FACTORS
Risk groups: Defintions vary in different countries and cooperative groups. For the largest cooperative group in the US:
- Low risk: IA–IIA, without bulk disease
- Intermediate risk:
  - IA–IIA with bulk disease (defined by nodal aggregate >6 cm or mediastinal mass >1/3 the thoracic diameter)
  - IAE, IIAE: IB–IIB
  - IIIA, IVA
- High risk: IIIB, IVB
- Prognostic factors:
  - Disease stage
  - Presence of "B symptoms" (see "History")
  - Bulk disease or mediastinal mass
  - Laboratory abnormalities including hemoglobin (Hb) <11 g/dL, WBC >13.5 thousand/uL, elevated ESR
  - Timing of response to treatment

Genetics
Familial clustering suggests both genetic and environmental factors in pathogenesis:
- 3–7-fold increased risk of disease among siblings in families where twins are concordant
- Reports of parent–child pairs

PATHOPHYSIOLOGY
Reed-Sternberg cells are the malignant cells of Hodgkin lymphoma. They are monoclonal and derived from germinal center B cells.
- WHO classification divides disease into histologic categories:
  - Nodular lymphocyte–predominant Hodgkin lymphoma
  - Classical Hodgkin lymphoma (90%)
    - Nodular sclerosis: Most common subtype in children
    - Mixed cellularity
    - Lymphocyte depletion
    - Lymphocyte rich

ETIOLOGY
- Exact cause unknown
- Infections with Epstein-Barr virus may play role in transmission of disease.

DIAGNOSIS

HISTORY
- Stage B symptoms occur in 20–30% and include 1 of the following:
  - Unexplained fever >38°C for ≥3 days
  - Unexplained weight loss > 10% of body weight in previous 6 months
  - Drenching night sweats
- Stage A disease signifies absence of B symptoms or asymptomatic.
- Other systemic symptoms can include fatigue, anorexia, pruritus, chest pain, and orthopnea
- History relative to possible immunodeficiency, Epstein-Barr virus, or HIV infection should be recorded.

PHYSICAL EXAM
Painless lymphadenopathy most common:
- Nodes usually firmer, rubbery in texture, and less mobile than inflammatory nodes. Cervical chain involved in 80% of patients
- Mediastinal mass in 2/3 of patients that may cause nonproductive cough or difficulty breathing
- Hepatosplenomegaly and bone tenderness in advanced stages
- If bone marrow involvement, can see pallor, bruising, or petechiae
- Rare cases present with autoimmune hemolytic anemia (AIHA) or idiopathic thrombocytopenic purpura (ITP) and can have jaundice, petechiae, or bleeding as a result.

DIAGNOSTIC TESTS & INTERPRETATION
Lab
- CBC, ESR
- Liver and renal function studies
- Baseline thyroid function (pre-radiotherapy)
- Baseline electrocardiogram, echocardiogram
- Baseline pulmonary function tests (pre-radiotherapy and/or bleomycin)
- Bone marrow biopsy in selected cases

Imaging
- Chest radiograph (posterior-anterior and lateral) for mediastinal mass
- CT scan (neck, chest, abdomen, pelvis) to rule out disseminated disease
- PET scan is now standard in children and young adults.

Diagnostic Procedures/Other
Excisional lymph node biopsy for definitive diagnosis
Ann Arbor Staging System:
- I: Involvement of a single lymph node region (I) or of a single extralymphatic organ or site (IE) by direct extension
- II: Involvement of 2 or more lymph node regions on the same side of the diaphragm (II) or localized involvement of an extralymphatic organ or site and 1 or more lymph node regions on the same side of the diaphragm (IIE)
- III: Involvement of lymph node regions on both sides of the diaphragm (III), which may be accompanied by involvement of the spleen (IIIS) or by localized involvement of an extralymphatic organ or site (IIIE) or both (IIIES)
- IV: Diffuse or disseminated involvement of 1 or more extralymphatic organs or tissues with or without associated lymph node involvement
- Staging further subclassified A or B according to absence or presence of symptoms (listed above), respectively

DIFFERENTIAL DIAGNOSIS
- Infection is most common cause for acute lymphadenopathy:
  - Bacterial (*Staphylococcus aureus*, hemolytic streptococcus, tuberculosis, atypical mycobacterium)
  - Other (Epstein-Barr virus, cytomegalovirus, cat-scratch disease, toxoplasmosis, HIV, histoplasmosis)
- Malignancy more common with chronic adenopathy:
  - Non-Hodgkin lymphoma
  - Neuroblastoma
  - Leukemia
  - Rhabdomyosarcoma
- Mediastinal masses divided anatomically:
  - Anterior: Lymphoid and thyroid tumors, bronchogenic cysts, aneurysms, lipomas
  - Middle: Lymphoid tumors, angiomas, pericardial cysts, teratomas, esophageal lesions, hernias
  - Posterior: Neurogenic tumors, cysts, thoracic meningocele, sarcomas

TREATMENT

MEDICATION (DRUGS)

Chemotherapy:

- Multiple agents allow different mechanisms of action (to circumvent resistance) and nonoverlapping toxicities so that full doses can be given. Some common combinations used in initial therapy include:
  - COPP: Cyclophosphamide, vincristine (Oncovin), procarbazine, prednisone. Often used in combination with ABV below.
  - ABV: Doxorubicin (Adriamycin), bleomycin, vinblastine
  - ABVD: ABV (as above) + dacarbazine
  - ABVE: Doxorubicin + bleomycin + vincristine + etoposide
  - ABVE-PC: ABVE (as above) + prednisone and cyclophosphamide
  - VAMP: Vinblastine, Adriamycin, methotrexate, prednisone
  - BEACOPP: Bleomycin, etoposide, Adriamycin, cyclophosphamide, vincristine, procarbazine, prednisone

ALERT

For patients with lymphocyte-predominant histology: Excision alone has been used for patients with low-stage disease.

ADDITIONAL TREATMENT

General Measures

Radiotherapy

Exquisitely responsive to radiotherapy: In pediatric setting, radiotherapy used in conjunction with chemotherapy and not used as sole treatment modality. Some combinations of chemotherapy have only been studied with radiation as additional treatment modality. Often recommended if patient has slow or incomplete response to chemotherapy. Some chemotherapy regimens have been used in the setting of a clinical trial without radiation therapy if rapid and complete response to chemotherapy alone.

ONGOING CARE

FOLLOW-UP RECOMMENDATIONS

Patient Monitoring

Once therapy is complete, office visits at decreasing frequency over time for:

- Laboratory evaluation including CBC, ESR
- Imaging of involved areas every 3 months for 1st year, every 3–4 months for years 2–3, then every 6 months for years 4–5 after therapy
- Relapse of disease usually occurs within 1st 3 years. Some may relapse as late as 10 years after initial diagnosis.
- Special studies as needed for toxicity-related complications. For example:
  - Yearly thyroid function tests if history of irradiation
  - Regular self-breast exam for females treated with chest radiation

  - Mammograms beginning by the age of 25 or 7 years post–chest radiation (whichever is later in females)
  - Periodic ECGs and Holter monitors if treated with radiation and/or anthracyclines
  - Periodic pulmonary function tests if treated with radiation and/or bleomycin
  - Refer to survivorship clinic at 5 years after completion of therapy
- Late effects secondary to chemotherapy and/or radiation
  - Pulmonary: Pneumonitis, pulmonary fibrosis, decreased pulmonary function, pneumothorax
  - Cardiac/vascular: Cardiomyopathy resulting in congestive heart failure, pericarditis, valvular damage, coronary heart disease, arrhythmias, myocardial infarction, and stroke
  - Gonadal dysfunction: Ovarian damage can be avoided by performing temporary oophoropexy prior to involved field radiotherapy (IFRT). Azoospermia secondary to alkylating agents is almost always permanent in postpubertal boys. Sperm banking recommended for boys with development of Tanner III or higher
  - Thyroid: Hypothyroidism, hyperthyroidism, thyroid nodules, thyroid cancer
  - Growth/musculoskeletal: Growth retardation more common in past when prepubertal patients received high doses of radiotherapy
  - Secondary malignant neoplasms: A major concern in selecting therapy:
    ○ Breast cancer most common solid tumor
    ○ Other secondary neoplasms: Thyroid and skin carcinomas, bone, colorectal, gastric, leukemia

PROGNOSIS

With current therapy including chemotherapy and/or radiation, 5-year disease-free survival:

- Low-risk disease: >90%
- Advanced disease: 60–95% depending on regimen used

COMPLICATIONS

Acute toxicity of treatment:

- Radiation: Include erythema, nausea, fatigue, possibly myelosuppression
- Chemotherapy: The general side effects include:
  - Hair loss
  - GI toxicity including nausea, vomiting, diarrhea, mucositis, risk for typhlitis
  - Myelosuppression (most common dose-limiting toxicity)
  - Transfusions may be required.
  - Febrile neutropenia and infection
  - All patients take prophylaxis for *Pneumocystis*.
  - Each chemotherapeutic agent has its own specific potential side effects, which are not reviewed here.

ADDITIONAL READING

- Bhatia S, Yasui Y, Robinson LL, et al. Late Effects Study Group. High risk of subsequent neoplasms continues with extended follow-up of childhood Hodgkin's disease: Report from the Late Effects Study Group. *J Clin Oncol.* 2003;21:4386–4394.
- Freed J, Kelly KM. Current approaches to the management of pediatric Hodgkin lymphoma. *Pediatr Drugs.* 2010;12(2):85–98.
- Olson MR, Donaldson SS. Treatment of pediatric Hodgkin lymphoma. *Curr Treat Options Oncol.* 2008;9(1):81–94.
- Smith RS, Chen Q, Hudson MM, et al. Prognostic factors for children with Hodgkin's disease treated with combined-modality therapy. *J Clin Oncol.* 2003;21:2026–2033.

 CODES

ICD9

- 201.50 Hodgkin's disease, nodular sclerosis, unspecified site, extranodal and solid organ sites
- 201.60 Hodgkin's disease, mixed cellularity, unspecified site, extranodal and solid organ sites
- 201.90 Hodgkin's disease, unspecified type, unspecified site, extranodal and solid organ sites

ICD10

- C81.10 Nodular sclerosis classical Hodgkin lymphoma, unspecified site
- C81.20 Mixed cellularity classical Hodgkin lymphoma, unspecified site
- C81.90 Hodgkin lymphoma, unspecified, unspecified site

FAQ

- Q: Is my child at risk for other cancers?
- A: Yes. Although the incidence is low, children with Hodgkin lymphoma are primarily at risk for cancers resulting from their treatment. Breast cancer is the most common solid tumor and can occur decades after therapy. Therefore, long-term follow-up is essential.
- Q: Will my child be infertile following treatment?
- A: It depends on the therapy received. Certain chemotherapy agents are associated with a higher risk of infertility (alkylating agents), and boys are more sensitive than girls. Radiation to the gonads is also associated with infertility.

H

HUMAN IMMUNODEFICIENCY VIRUS INFECTION

Richard M. Rutstein

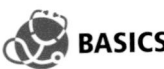 **BASICS**

DESCRIPTION
- HIV-1 and HIV-2 are the etiologic agents of HIV infection and AIDS.
- HIV infection is lifelong.
- For most infected individuals, a long clinically asymptomatic period (5–15 years in adults, frequently shorter in children) is followed by the development of generalized nonspecific signs and symptoms (weight loss, adenopathy, hepatosplenomegaly) and mild clinical immunodeficiency.
- Eventually, after progressive immunologic deterioration, patients are susceptible to a wide variety of opportunistic infections and cancers, which represent the clinical syndrome known as AIDS.

GENERAL PREVENTION
- HIV infection is almost completely preventable.
- It is now possible to significantly decrease the risk to newborns of HIV-infected women:
  - With prenatal 3-drug regimens, delivery via elective cesarean section for selected cases, and 6 weeks of postnatal zidovudine, perinatal transmission rates are now 2% or less in HIV specialty care sites.
  - All pregnant women should be offered HIV testing at the first prenatal visit. In areas of high incidence, repeat testing should be done at 36 weeks of gestation.

EPIDEMIOLOGY
HIV infection is transmitted via:
- Sexual contact:
  - Male-to-female transmission more efficient than female to male
  - Anal receptive sex more likely to transmit than vaginal sex
- Exposure to infected blood:
  - Almost always involves parenteral exposure to infected blood (via transfusions or sharing needles)
  - In occupational exposure, risk of transmission from percutaneous exposure to a needle contaminated with HIV-infected blood is 1/300.
- Breast milk:
  - Overall risk of breast-feeding is ~15%.
  - In countries where breast-feeding is the norm, up to 30% of perinatally acquired HIV infections occur through breast-feeding.
- Perinatally, either *in utero* or during labor and delivery:
  - Of perinatally infected infants, 5–10% are believed infected in utero; the rest acquire the infection around the time of birth.
  - Risk of an HIV-infected mother (not on treatment) giving birth to an infected infant is ~20%, (in the absence of breastfeeding) with increased rate of transmission for women with low CD4 counts or higher viral titers. Vaginal delivery, especially with rupture of membranes >8 hours, appears to increase the risk of infant infection.
  - Presence of untreated STDs, chorioamnionitis, and prematurity all increase the risk of mother-to-child transmission of HIV.

- HIV is not believed to be transmitted by:
  - Bites
  - Sharing utensils, bathrooms, bathtubs
  - Exposure to urine, feces, vomitus (except where these fluids may be grossly contaminated with blood, and even then transmission is rare, if it happens at all)
  - Casual contact in the home, school, or daycare center

DIAGNOSIS

SIGNS AND SYMPTOMS
Indications for HIV testing:
- Infants whose maternal HIV status is unknown
- Infants of HIV+ mothers
- IV drug use
- Noninjectable drug use
- STDs, especially syphilis
- All sexually active adolescents, at least annually
- Transfusions before 1986
- Frequent infections
- Sinopulmonary infections
- Recurrent pneumonia/invasive bacterial disease
- Severe acute pneumonia (*Pneumocystis*)
- Recurrent or resistant thrush, especially after 12 months of age
- Congenital syphilis
- Acquired microcephaly
- Progressive encephalopathy, loss of developmental milestones
- History of idiopathic thrombocytopenic purpura/thrombocytopenia
- Failure to thrive
- Recurrent/chronic diarrhea
- Recurrent/chronic enlargement of parotid gland

PHYSICAL EXAM
- May be entirely normal in the 1st few months of life
- 90% will have some physical findings by age 2 years
- Most common findings are:
  - Adenopathy, generalized
  - Hepatosplenomegaly
  - Failure to thrive
  - Recurrent/Resistant thrush, especially after 1 year of age
  - Recurrent or chronic parotitis

DIAGNOSTIC TESTS & INTERPRETATION
Lab
- Enzyme-linked immunosorbent assay (ELISA) antibody screen:
  - For children >18 months of age, repeatedly reactive ELISA antibody screen, followed by confirmation with Western blot analysis, is diagnostic of HIV infection.
  - Any positive test should always be repeated before a definitive diagnosis is discussed with family.
  - In first year of life, positive HIV ELISA and Western blot antibody tests simply confirm maternal infection, because the antibody test is IgG based and maternal anti-HIV antibodies readily cross placenta. Maternal antibodies may remain detectable in the infant until 15 months of age.

- HIV RNA or DNA polymerase chain reaction (PCR) DNA testing:
  - Most reliable way of diagnosing HIV infection in infancy
  - Both tests have sensitivities and specificities >95% when done after 2 weeks of age.
- Elevated IgG levels: First observed immune abnormality noted in HIV-infected infants, generally reaching twice the normal values by 9 months of age
- CD4 counts:
  - Obtained at diagnosis and every 1–3 months
  - Results need to be evaluated on the basis of age-adjusted normal values. Absolute CD4 counts are elevated in childhood, with normal median values >3,000/mm³ in the first year of life, which then gradually decline with age, reaching values comparable with adult levels (800–1,000/mm³) by age 7.
- Quantitative viral RNA PCR assays:
  - Termed "viral loads," results are reported in a range from undetectable, usually <50 copies/mL, to upper values of >10 million cpm
  - Long-term prognosis is closely related to viral loads.
  - Viral loads that remain >100,000 are associated with poor short-term (2- to 5-year) outcomes.
  - Also used as a marker of efficacy of treatment; goal is to suppress viral replication to the undetectable range for as long as possible. 50–65% of pediatric patients presently followed at tertiary sites have an undetectable viral load.
  - Test is done at time of diagnosis (twice) to establish baseline, 1 month after initiating or changing therapies, and every 1–3 months thereafter.
- Neurologic evaluation, with consideration of psychometric testing, at entry, and annually. Neuroimaging is indicated in those with abnormal results. Postimmunization antibody levels to assess B cell function
- Other frequent lab abnormalities include thrombocytopenia, anemia, and elevated liver enzymes.

DIFFERENTIAL DIAGNOSIS
- Neoplastic disease:
  - Lymphoma
  - Leukemia
  - Histiocytosis X
- Infectious:
  - Congenital/perinatal cytomegalovirus
  - Toxoplasmosis
  - Congenital syphilis
  - Acquired Epstein–Barr virus
- Congenital immunodeficiency syndromes:
  - Wiskott–Aldrich syndrome
  - Chronic granulomatous disease

ALERT
The result of failing to screen for HIV infection is the inability to offer antiretroviral therapy for pregnant women, therefore, possibly preventing infant infection, and also the inability to prescribe *Pneumocystis carinii* pneumonia prophylaxis to infected newborns.

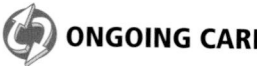 **TREATMENT**

ADDITIONAL TREATMENT
General Measures
- Immunizations:
  - All infected children receive standard childhood immunizations, including the recently approved pneumococcal conjugate vaccine.
  - Infected children should receive yearly influenza A/B immunizations and the 23 valent pneumococcal vaccine at age 2 years.
  - Symptomatic children should not receive the varicella vaccine, and those with severely low CD4 counts should not receive measles–mumps–rubella vaccination.
- Immune enhancement:
  - Passive: Studies done before the present era of antiretroviral therapy indicate that monthly gamma globulin infusions somewhat decreased febrile episodes and pneumococcal bacteremia. The children who benefit the most are those not on antibiotic prophylaxis for *P. carinii* pneumonia and/or who have had at least 2 episodes of invasive bacterial infections.
- Prophylaxis: One of the major advances in the care of HIV-infected children and adults has been the ability to offer prophylaxis against the most common opportunistic infections.

MEDICATION (DRUGS)
- Antiretroviral therapy:
  - Specific combination antiretroviral therapy prolongs life, delays progression of illness, promotes improved growth, and improves neurologic outcome.
  - Standard of care now involves the administration of combination therapy (usually 3 or more drugs), termed highly active antiretroviral therapy (HAART). There are now more than 25 approved antiretroviral agents, of 5 different drug classes.
  - Given the complexities of therapy, and the rapid changes in available therapies, antiretroviral therapy should always be prescribed in consultation with a specialist in pediatric/adolescent HIV infection.
  - Adherence to prescribed schedules is critical: When patients miss even 10–20% of doses, the durability of response is short.

ONGOING CARE

FOLLOW-UP RECOMMENDATIONS
- Psychosocial support for the family is critical.
- Because of the complex, rapidly changing therapies available to treat pediatric HIV infection, all infected patients should be co-managed with an HIV specialty care site.
- Patients should be seen every 1–3 months to monitor immune status (CD4 counts) and virologic suppression (quantitative plasma viral RNA).

PROGNOSIS
Because the use of HAART has become standard, morbidity and mortality have both greatly decreased:
- Median survival is now clearly into adulthood.
- Incidence of new opportunistic infections (AIDS signal illnesses) has decreased greatly, as have hospital admissions.

COMPLICATIONS
- *P. carinii* pneumonia:
  - Most common early fatal illness in HIV-infected children (peak age 3–9 months) mortality is 30–50%. A high index of suspicion is necessary for prompt diagnosis (by lavage) and initiation of therapy.
  - 40% of new cases of HIV-related pediatric *P. carinii* pneumonia involve infants not previously recognized as HIV infected.
- Lymphocytic interstitial pneumonitis:
  - Frequently asymptomatic; can lead to slow onset of chronic respiratory symptoms
  - Causes a distinctive diffuse reticulonodular pattern on chest radiographs
  - Usually diagnosed between 2 and 4 years of age; related to dysfunctional immune response to Epstein–Barr virus infection
  - Definitive diagnosis is made by lung biopsy.
  - For symptomatic patients, prednisone is effective.
- Recurrent invasive bacterial infections:
  - Prior to the use of pneumococcal conjugate vaccines and HAART, the risk of bacteremia/pneumonia was ~10%/year in HIV-infected children.
  - Pneumococcal bacteremia is the most common invasive bacterial disease.
  - Bacterial pneumonia, sinusitis, and otitis media are common among infected children.
- Progressive encephalopathy:
  - Diagnosed between 9 and 18 months of age, the hallmark is progressive loss of developmental milestones or neurologic dysfunction.
  - Cerebral atrophy, with or without basal ganglion calcifications, on neuroimaging
- Disseminated *Mycobacterium avium* intracellulare:
  - Older children, usually >5 years of age, with severe immunodeficiency (CD4 ≤100)
  - Symptoms include prolonged fevers, abdominal pain, anorexia, and diarrhea.
- *Candida* esophagitis: Older children with severe immunodeficiency usually present with dysphagia or chest pain and oral thrush. Diagnosis indicated by findings on barium swallow, but definitive diagnosis made by biopsy
- Disseminated cytomegalovirus disease:
  - Retinitis less common in HIV-infected children than in adults
  - Cytomegalovirus may also cause pulmonary disease, colitis, and hepatitis.

- HIV-related cancers: Non-Hodgkin lymphoma most common cancer, with primary site usually located in the CNS
- Other organ dysfunction associated with HIV-infection in children:
  - Cardiomyopathy
  - Hepatitis
  - Renal disease
  - Thrombocytopenia/Idiopathic thrombocytopenic purpura

ADDITIONAL READING
- Chen TK, Aldrovandi GM, Review of HIV antiretroviral drug resistance. *Pediatr Infect Dis J.* 2008;27(8):749–752.
- Perinatal HIV Guidelines Working Group. PHS Task Force recommendations for use of antiretroviral drugs in pregnant HIV-1 infected women for maternal health and interventions to reduce perinatal transmission in the United States. Revised February 2011. Available at: http://www.hivatis.org. Accessed March 2011.
- Working Group on Antiretroviral Therapy and Medical Management of HIV-1 Infected Children. Guidelines for the use of antiretroviral agents in pediatric HIV infection. Available at: http://www.hivatis.org. Accessed March 2011.

 CODES

ICD9
- 042 Human immunodeficiency virus [HIV] disease
- 795.71 Nonspecific serologic evidence of human immunodeficiency virus [HIV]
- V08 Asymptomatic human immunodeficiency virus [HIV] infection status

ICD10
- B20 Human immunodeficiency virus [HIV] disease
- R75 Inconclusive laboratory evidence of human immunodef virus
- Z21 Asymptomatic human immunodeficiency virus infection status

FAQ
- Q: When the HIV-exposed infant has seroreverted to antibody-negative status, how sure are we that he or she is uninfected?
- A: With today's technology, if the child has also been RNA or DNA PCR negative at least twice, and is clinically well, the chance that the child still harbors HIV is very low and appears to be <1/5,000. The CDC considers any child with 2 negative HIV PCRs as definitively uninfected, provided one of the PCRs was done after 4 months of age.

H

HUMAN PAPILLOMA VIRUS

Sarah E. Winters
Elizabeth M. Wallis
Kristen Feemster (5th edition)
Jane Lavelle (5th edition)

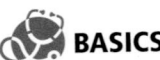 **BASICS**

DESCRIPTION
- Members of the Papovaviridae family, the human papillomaviruses (HPV) cause warts of the skin and mucous membranes. Exophytic venereal warts or condylomata acuminata are caused by HPV types 6 and 11.
- Warts can be found on the external genitalia and the urethra, vagina, cervix, anus, and mouth. HPV types 6 and 11 are also associated with squamous cell carcinoma of the external genitalia.
- Virus types 16, 18, 31, 33, and 35 typically cause subclinical infection in the anogenital region and have been associated with intraepithelial genital carcinomas.
- HPV can also cause recurrent respiratory papillomatosis (RRP) in infants and young children. RRP primarily impacts the larynx but can also cause lesions anywhere along the respiratory tract.

EPIDEMIOLOGY
- General:
  - HPV is the most common viral STI.
  - Genital warts and HPV infection are diseases of young adults 16–25 years of age.
  - Cervical cancer is the leading cause of female malignancy in the developing world.
- Genital HPV:
  - Peak prevalence among women 18–24 years
  - 40% of sexually active adolescents are infected with HPV
  - <1% of adolescents develop genital warts.
  - 21% of HPV positive women have low-grade squamous intraepithelial lesions (LSIL) on Pap smear.
  - 500,000 new cases of cervical cancer diagnosed each year internationally
- RRP:
  - RRP impacts 4.3 per 100,000 children, mostly those age 2–3 years.
  - 67% of children with RRP are born to mothers who had condyloma during pregnancy.

RISK FACTORS
- Infants:
  - Primarily vertical transmission at birth
- Adolescents:
  - Behavioral risks, including young age at 1st coitus, multiple partners, cigarette use, and having older male partners
  - Biologic risk in adolescent girls secondary to cervical anatomy

GENERAL PREVENTION
- Condom use may diminish transmission.
- Examine partners; treat those infected.
- Pap smear to assess for cervical dysplasia
- Vaccination to prevent HPV types 6, 11, 16, and 18. Vaccination is recommended for female and male patients starting at age 11 and is approved for use for persons aged 9–26
- HPV infection is not a reportable disease.

PATHOPHYSIOLOGY
- Transmission is primarily through sexual contact.
- It can also be acquired during the birth process.
- Transmission from nongenital sites occurs rarely.
- The incubation period is variable and ranges from 3 months to several years.
- The virus is trophic for epithelial cells and infects the basal layer of actively dividing cells.
- Infection results in koilocytosis and nuclear atypia. Genital infections may progress to severe dysplasia and carcinoma in situ (CIS).
- Spontaneous regression of clinical disease occurs in 90% of low-risk types and 75% of high-risk types
- Recurrence is common.

COMMONLY ASSOCIATED CONDITIONS
- Epidermodysplasia verruciformis
- Other STIs

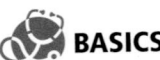 **DIAGNOSIS**

HISTORY
- Genital HPV:
  - Most patients have no symptoms.
  - Presence of warts, often painless
  - Vaginal, urethral, or anal discharge, bleeding, local pain
  - Dysuria
  - Pruritus
- RRP:
  - Infants have hoarse or weak cry, stridor, and failure to thrive.
  - Older children have hoarseness, stridor, dysphonia, and obstructive sleep apnea.

PHYSICAL EXAM
- Genital HPV:
  - Warts appear as soft, sessile tumors with surfaces ranging from smooth to rough with many fingerlike projections.
  - HPV may also cause flat keratotic plaques that project only slightly with a hyperpigmented surface and are difficult to identify without the addition of acetic acid.
  - Subclinical infection is common, causing many foci of epithelial hyperplasia invisible to the examiner.
  - In males, infection is found on the penis, urethra, scrotum, and perianal areas.
  - In females, infection involves the urethra, vagina, cervix, and perianal area.
  - Diagnosis is made by visual inspection of the anogenital region. Cervical dysplasia is clinically inapparent on exam.
- RRP:
  - Often normal exam, but may be evident on respiratory exam

DIAGNOSTIC TESTS & INTERPRETATION
Lab
- Application of 3–5% acetic acid for 5 minutes causes lesions to appear white and thus more readily apparent and can help with the detection of cervical disease.
- Tissue specimens may show koilocytosis typical for HPV infection.
- Pap smear with liquid cytology to assess for evidence of cervical dysplasia resulting from HPV infection
- Colposcopy aids the diagnosis of cervical lesions.
- Polymerase chain reaction is commercially available for HPV typing and is used in patients >21 with abnormal Pap smears.

Diagnostic Procedures/Other
- Genital HPV:
  - Pap smear or colposcopy to screen for cervical dysplasia
- RRP:
  - Direct visualization of the airway through laryngoscopy

DIFFERENTIAL DIAGNOSIS
- Genital HPV:
  - Condyloma lata
  - Molluscum contagiosum
  - Pink pearly papules or hypertrophic papillae of the penis
  - Lipomas
  - Fibromas
  - Adenomas
- RRP:
  - Croup
  - Vocal cord paralysis
  - Other forms of nasal, laryngeal, pharyngeal or tracheal obstruction

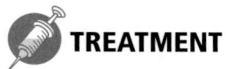

TREATMENT

MEDICATION (DRUGS)

Table 1. Treatment for external warts

Medication	Procedure	Side effect
Podofilox 0.5%	Patient applies medicine with a cotton swab b.i.d. for 3 days. After 4 days, it is repeated as necessary for 4 cycles. The area for treatment should not exceed 10 cm^2, and total drug should not exceed 0.5 mL/d.	Local
Imiquimod 5% cream	Patient applies cream at bedtime 3 times per week for up to 16 weeks. It is washed off after 6–10 hours.	Local
Podophyllin 10–25%	A practitioner applies a small amount to each wart and allows it to air dry. It is washed off 1–4 hours later. Dose is limited to 0.5 mL per treatment to avoid systemic toxicity.	Local
Trichloroacetic acid (TCA) 80–90%	The practitioner applies this sparingly to each wart directly. Talc is applied to remove unreacted acid. It is washed off after 4 hours.	Local
Laser surgical excision	Requires special equipment and training; often requires general anesthesia; controlled tissue destruction	Local
Cryotherapy	Liquid nitrogen or cryoprobe is used every 1–2 weeks by a specially trained provider.	Local

ADDITIONAL TREATMENT
General Measures
- To date, no therapy exists that eradicates the virus. Recurrences are likely due to reinfection.
- Most patients require a course of therapy rather than a single treatment.
- Genital HPV:
  – Lesions on mucosal surfaces respond better to topical treatments.
  – All available therapies have equal efficacy in eradicating warts, ranging from 22–94%, with the significant rate of relapse of 25% within 3 months (see table in "Medication"):
    ○ Consider size, location, number of warts, previous treatment, and patient preference.
    ○ Also consider patient preference, expense, and side effects.
    ○ Patients with extensive lesions should be referred to physicians who routinely treat these lesions.
  – Treatment:
    ○ External: See table in "Medication."
    ○ Meatal: Cryotherapy or podophyllin
    ○ Anal: Cryotherapy or trichloroacetic acid
    ○ Vaginal: Trichloroacetic acid
    ○ Cervical: Refer to an expert.
- RRP:
  – Surgical excision

ONGOING CARE

FOLLOW-UP RECOMMENDATIONS
Patient Monitoring
- Follow-up should continue until the warts have disappeared.
- Patients should return for recurrent disease.
- Latent infection and recurrent disease are common.
- USTPTF and American College of Obstetrics and Gynecology (ACOG) recommend initial Pap smear at age 21, while the American Cancer Society (ACS) recommends initial Pap smear after 3 years of initiating sexual activity, but no later than age 21.

PROGNOSIS
Therapy will not eradicate the virus; thus, HPV causes recurrent disease.

ADDITIONAL READING

- Brentjens MH, Yeung-YueK A, Lee PC, et al. Human papillomavirus: A review. *Dermatol Clin.* 2002;20: 315–331.
- Centers for Disease Control and Prevention. Sexually Transmitted Diseases Treatment Guidelines, 2010. *MMWR.* 2010;59(RR-12).
- Gunter J. Genital and perianal warts: New treatment opportunities for human papillomavirus infection. *Am J Obstet Gynecol.* 2003;189(3 Suppl): S3–S11.
- Kahn JA, Hillard PA. Human papillomavirus (HPV) In Children and Adolescents. In: Emans SJ, Goldstein DP, eds. *Pediatric and adolescent gynecology,* 5th ed. Boston: Lippincott Williams & Wilkins; 2005:649–684.
- Kliegman RM, Behrman RE, Jenson HB. *Nelson textbook of pediatrics,* 18th ed. Philadelphia: Elsevier; 2007.

CODES

ICD9
- 078.10 Viral warts, unspecified
- 079.4 Human papillomavirus in conditions classified elsewhere and of unspecified site
- 569.49 Other specified disorders of rectum and anus

ICD10
- B34.4 Papovavirus infection, unspecified
- B97.7 Papillomavirus as the cause of diseases classified elsewhere
- L08.9 Local infection of the skin and subcutaneous tissue, unspecified

FAQ
- Q: What treatment is indicated during pregnancy?
- A: Most experts recommend surgical removal if necessary. Podophyllin is absolutely contraindicated.
- Q: Should partners of patients with genital warts be referred for examination?
- A: Recurrence is due to reactivation of the virus; reinfection plays no role. Partner may benefit from an examination to evaluate for the presence of warts, and for education and counseling. There is no information regarding prophylaxis to prevent infection, so treatment for this is not indicated. Most partners have subclinical infection. Female partners/patients should follow the routine recommendations for Pap smear screening.
- Q: Are genital warts in children always indicative of sexual abuse?
- A: No. The HPV virus has an incubation period of many months. Thus, warts transmitted to infants at the time of birth may not become clinically apparent for 1–2 years. Whether the incubation period can be longer than this remains unknown. Thus, maternal history and, potentially, examination are both important factors. However, all children with anogenital warts should be carefully evaluated by experienced clinicians for child abuse. It is possible that caregivers may transmit the virus to children through close but nonsexual contact; thus, this history is also important in older children.
- Q: Will young women still need to get Pap smears if they have received the HPV vaccine?
- A: Yes. The vaccine does offer good protection against the strains most commonly associated with genital warts and cervical cancer, 6, 11, 16, and 18. However, these strains are not the only ones that can cause infection or lead to cervical cancer. It is important to continue regular screening to ensure that one has not been exposed to other strains that may cause cervical dysplasia.

H

HYDROCEPHALUS

Jennifer A. Markowitz

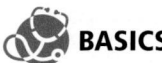 **BASICS**

DESCRIPTION
- Accumulation of CSF in the ventricles and subarachnoid spaces, leading to their enlargement
- Overall head size may enlarge in response, depending on age and cause.

PATHOPHYSIOLOGY
- Normal pathway of CSF: Choroid plexus and interstitial fluid (sources), lateral ventricles, foramina of Monro, 3rd ventricle, aqueduct of Sylvius, 4th ventricle, foramina of Luschka and Magendie, subarachnoid space, arachnoid villi, and venous circulation
- Hydrocephalus results from obstruction to CSF flow, impaired reabsorption, or overproduction of CSF.
- Noncommunicating (obstructive) hydrocephalus results from obstruction within the ventricular system.
- Communicating hydrocephalus usually results from impaired CSF reabsorption or (rarely) overproduction (e.g., due to a choroid plexus papilloma).
- The noncommunicating/communicating distinction has no prognostic significance, but has implications for etiology and choice of therapeutic intervention.

ETIOLOGY
- Intraventricular hemorrhage is most commonly due to prematurity, but may also occur with trauma. It results in impaired CSF absorption due to meningeal adhesions, granular ependymitis, and clots. Posthemorrhagic hydrocephalus (PHH) occurs in 35% of all neonates surviving intraventricular hemorrhage; its incidence increases with increasing severity of hemorrhage.
- Tumors or cysts near the foramina or the aqueduct, or within the ventricular system
- Infection (meningitis, intrauterine infection) can lead to leptomeningeal adhesions and granulations that block reabsorption of CSF.
- Developmental:
  - Chiari malformation, type II (associated with myelomeningocele, brain migrational disorders, small posterior fossa, inferior displacement of medulla and cerebellar vermis, kinking of the brainstem, aqueductal stenosis, beaking of the tectum)
  - Dandy-Walker malformation (absence of cerebellar vermis, small cerebellar hemispheres, enlarged posterior fossa, often with cystic 4th ventricle)
  - X-linked and autosomal dominant hydrocephalus; the former is often associated with aqueductal stenosis and mutations in L1CAM on Xq28.
  - Sporadic primary aqueductal stenosis
  - Dysmorphic syndromes (e.g., Apert syndrome, Cockayne syndrome, Crouzon syndrome, Pfeiffer syndrome, trisomy 13, trisomy 18, trisomy 21, triploidy)
  - Alexander disease
  - Mucopolysaccharidoses (e.g., type II [Hunter], type VI [Maroteaux-Lamy])
  - Migrational disorders/congenital muscular dystrophies (e.g., Miller-Dieker, muscle-eye-brain disease, Fukuyama congenital muscular dystrophy, Walker-Warburg syndrome)
  - Achondroplasia
  - Neurocutaneous syndromes (e.g., neurofibromatosis type 1, rare)
  - Idiopathic

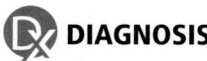 **DIAGNOSIS**

HISTORY
Presenting concerns:
- Infants: Enlarging head, irritability, vomiting, somnolence, poor feeding
- Older children: Headache, vomiting, double vision, somnolence

PHYSICAL EXAM
- Vital signs: In advanced acute hydrocephalus, Cushing triad (hypertension, reflex bradycardia, respiratory irregularities): This is not generally seen in infants prior to fusion of the sutures.
- Rapidly increasing head circumference in infants. Fullness of the anterior fontanelle neither sensitive nor specific, but should be noted. May observe splaying of the sutures
- Mental status: Irritability or somnolence in infants, behavioral changes in children (acute or chronic)
- Cranial nerves: "Setting sun" sign due to paralysis of upgaze, disconjugate gaze, papilledema, optic atrophy, and visual changes in the chronic setting
- Motor: Gait ataxia; spastic paraparesis in chronic hydrocephalus related to pressure on white matter tracts surrounding the ventricles
- Reflexes: Increased in chronic hydrocephalus

DIAGNOSTIC TESTS & INTERPRETATION
Imaging
- Head ultrasound:
  - Standard screening test for neonates with suspected hydrocephalus or intraventricular hemorrhage
  - Anterior fontanelle must be patent for this test.
  - Demonstrates ventricular size, presence or absence of blood, associated structures, and anomalies
- Unenhanced CT of the brain:
  - Mainly used in infants and children whose anterior fontanelles have closed and following shunt procedures
  - Better visualization of 4th ventricle/brainstem and calcifications than with ultrasound; standardized technique that is less operator dependent; better availability in the emergency room setting
- MRI:
  - Definitive test for analyzing brain anatomy
  - Can identify posterior fossa developmental malformations such as Chiari and Dandy-Walker
  - Not indicated in acute hydrocephalus, especially when patient is unstable

- Techniques such as diffusion tensor imaging may help to estimate local pressure on white matter adjacent to ventricles, as a correlate of increased intracranial pressure. This may help identify increased intracranial pressure in patients with unchanged ventricular size and aid in the assessment of postsurgical outcome.

Note: When imaging to diagnose shunt malfunction, it is important to consider the lifetime cumulative radiation exposure for each child; fast-sequence shunt MRI series may be able to replace CT for certain patients, if available.

> **ALERT**
> Head CT often will not show developmental malformations that may accompany hydrocephalus. MRI is the imaging procedure of choice for elective study.

DIFFERENTIAL DIAGNOSIS
- Other causes of macrocephaly:
  - Familial macrocephaly/" benign external hydrocephalus"
  - Pericerebral effusions
  - Congenital anomalies of intracerebral or extracerebral veins
  - Tumors, intracranial cysts
  - Primary megalencephaly, hemimegalencephaly
  - GM2 gangliosidosis
  - Some leukodystrophies (e.g., Alexander disease, Canavan disease)
  - Head-sparing intrauterine growth retardation (relative macrocephaly)
  - Rapid catch-up growth following prolonged malnutrition
- Other causes of ventriculomegaly, typically with normal head circumference: Brain atrophy and chronic ethanol or corticosteroid exposure (reversible)
- Enlargement of the subarachnoid spaces: Usually bifrontal, normal to mildly enlarged ventricles. May be seen in children with macrocephaly, who if otherwise normal are diagnosed with "benign external hydrocephalus." Recognize that metabolic and genetic disorders can also present with enlarged subarachnoid spaces (e.g., glutaric aciduria type I, others listed above).

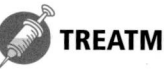 **TREATMENT**

SURGERY/OTHER PROCEDURES
Acute interventions:
- Ventricular shunt:
  - Indication: Progressive or acute symptomatic hydrocephalus
  - Contraindications: Active central nervous system infection, active intraventricular hemorrhage, and poor overall prognosis
  - Components: Ventricular catheter, reservoir (target of shunt taps), valve, distal catheter
  - Distal sites: Peritoneum is the most common choice; pleura, ureter, venous system, gallbladder, and right atrium are other options.
  - Approach: Usually performed as an open procedure; endoscopic procedures available in some centers

– Complications:
- ○ Shunt failure occurs in 40% of shunts within the 1st year after placement, and 50% within the 1st 2 years. Causes are obstruction, infection, disconnection, or fracture of components; migration of shunt components; overdrainage; erosion into an abdominal viscus. Presents with symptoms similar to those of acute hydrocephalus
- ○ Infections occur at a rate of ~8–10% per shunt manipulation, usually during the 1st 6 months after surgery. Present with low-grade persistent fever, and less commonly with erythema of overlying skin. Most common organism is *Staphylococcus epidermidis*; reinfection occurs in 30% of patients harboring this organism.
- ○ Siphon effect: Drop in ventricular pressure on sitting or standing causing headache; newer shunt systems with antisiphon mechanisms are available.
- ○ Newer shunts have programmable valve mechanisms; one must be cautious when obtaining an MRI in patients with this type of shunt in place as the magnet may affect valve settings.

ALERT
- Timing of shunt placement is critical and problematic: Sometimes watchful waiting can obviate the procedure, whereas waiting too long may result in brain damage.
- Don't assume hydrocephalus is "cured." Late shunt failure may occur years after placement, often due to fracture of tubing, and can result in death from acute hydrocephalus causing herniation.
- Posthemorrhagic hydrocephalus (PHH) in the neonate may be managed initially with serial lumbar puncture; this has been shown to improve cerebral perfusion in these patients. Most do not require shunt placement. Ultimately some may require ventriculosubgaleal or ventriculoperitoneal shunts.
- 3rd ventricle fenestration (endoscopic 3rd ventriculostomy):
  - Indications: Most effective for obstructive hydrocephalus due to aqueductal stenosis or space-occupying lesions
  - Complications: Overall rate of serious complications 9.4%; these include infection, CSF leak, neurologic deficits, extraparenchymal hemorrhage; rare risk of damage to the basilar artery

ONGOING CARE

FOLLOW-UP RECOMMENDATIONS
- When the etiology or need for shunt placement is unclear, it is important to follow clinical status, head circumference, and ventricular size (by head ultrasound or CT).
- Chronic hydrocephalus is often accompanied by spastic paraparesis, visual problems, and learning problems.

- Most interventions are supportive:
  - Physical therapy, occupational therapy, and orthopedic therapies for spasticity; interdisciplinary cerebral palsy clinics can be critical in providing easy access to these resources.
  - Special education programs may be appropriate for children with severe developmental delay.

ALERT
- It is important for long-term patients in intensive care nurseries to have head circumferences recorded at least twice weekly. Macrocephaly is not always obvious on visual inspection.
- Absence of papilledema does not exclude chronic increased intracranial pressure.

PATIENT EDUCATION
Parent Internet Information: National Hydrocephalus Foundation, http://www.nhfonline.org

PROGNOSIS
Depending on the severity and cause of hydrocephalus, efficacy of treatment, and presence or absence of concomitant neurologic disorders, outcome may vary widely from normal neurologic development to severe impairment or death.

COMPLICATIONS
- Acute hydrocephalus: Herniation syndromes may be fatal.
- Chronic hydrocephalus:
  - Macrocephaly
  - Spastic paraparesis may lead to gait and motor problems.
  - Vision loss
  - Developmental delay
  - Precocious puberty due to pressure on the hypothalamus

ADDITIONAL READING

- Air EL, Yuan W, Holland SK, et al. Longitudinal comparison of pre- and postoperative diffusion tensor imaging parameters in young children with hydrocephalus. *J Neurosurg Pediatr.* 2010;5: 385–391.
- Browd SR, Ragel BT, Gottfried ON, et al. Failure of cerebrospinal fluid shunts: Part I: Obstruction and mechanical failure. *Pediatr Neurol.* 2006;34:83–92.
- Browd SR, Ragel BT, Gottfried ON, et al. Failure of cerebrospinal fluid shunts: Part II: Overdrainage, loculation, and abdominal complications. *Pediatr Neurol.* 2006;34:171–176.
- Drake JM. The surgical management of pediatric hydrocephalus. *Neurosurgery.* 2008;62(Suppl 2): 633–640; discussion 640–642.
- Paciorkowski AR, Greenstein RM. When is enlargement of the subarachnoid spaces not benign? A genetic perspective. *Pediatr Neurol.* 2007;37:1–7.

- Partington MD. Congenital hydrocephalus. *Neurosurg Clin North Am.* 2001;12:737–742, ix.
- Smith MD, Narayan P, Tubbs RT, et al. Cumulative diagnostic radiation exposure in children with ventriculoperitoneal shunts: A review. *Childs Nerv Syst.* 2008;24:493–497.
- Soul JS, Eichenwald E, Watter G, et al. CSF removal in infantile posthemorrhagic hydrocephalus results in significant improvement in cerebral hemodynamics. *Pediatric Res.* 2004;55:872–876.

 CODES

ICD9
- 331.3 Communicating hydrocephalus
- 331.4 Obstructive hydrocephalus
- 742.3 Congenital hydrocephalus

ICD10
- G91.0 Communicating hydrocephalus
- G91.1 Obstructive hydrocephalus
- G91.9 Hydrocephalus, unspecified

FAQ

- Q: When does an infant need a head ultrasound?
- A: Any infant whose head circumference increases by more than a quartile on the growth chart needs a head ultrasound. Preterm infants below a certain gestational age or birth weight (varies from hospital to hospital) should all receive screening head ultrasounds while in the intensive care nursery.
- Q: When should an infant or child receive an MRI rather than an ultrasound or CT?
- A: Although MRI may be superior in many cases, the logistics of ordering the proper sequences and the need for sedation or anesthesia for long studies must be strongly considered. Consultation with a neurologist or neurosurgeon is generally advised.
- Q: What is the workup for shunt obstruction and shunt infection?
- A: Symptoms and signs of increased intracranial pressure should lead to a neurosurgical evaluation; the most useful studies include head CT (to assess ventricular size and placement of ventricular catheter) and shunt series (plain films of the entire shunt system to check for disruptions). "Pumping" the shunt reservoir is a procedure with a low positive predictive value for shunt failure. Tapping the shunt to assess pressure must be done with discretion, as repeated taps may disrupt the valve mechanism. Fever is the most important indication for a shunt infection evaluation (shunt tap with CSF cell count, protein, glucose, Gram stain, and culture). Often patients will be evaluated for both complications.

H

HYDRONEPHROSIS

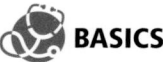

J. Christopher Austin
Michael C. Carr

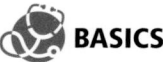 BASICS

DESCRIPTION
- Hydronephrosis: Dilation of the renal pelvis (pelviectasis) and calyces (caliectasis) due to excess urine in the collecting system of the kidney
- Hydroureteronephrosis: Dilation of the renal collecting system and the ureter to the level of the bladder

EPIDEMIOLOGY
- Incidence of genitourinary abnormalities noted on routine prenatal ultrasound is 0.2%.
- 87% of these are antenatally detected hydronephrosis/hydroureteronephrosis.
- 5% of fetuses with hydronephrosis are due to ureteropelvic junction obstruction.
- Perinatal mortality associated with hydronephrosis has ranged from 13–72%, but is most strongly correlated with the presence of chromosomal abnormalities, multiple system abnormalities, detection earlier in gestation, oligohydramnios, and evidence of infravesical obstruction.
- Posterior urethral valves and triad syndrome account for 6% of cases.

ETIOLOGY
- Ureteropelvic junction obstruction:
  – Intrinsic narrowing or an aperistaltic segment of distal ureter. These are also called megaureters.
- Vesicoureteral reflux:
  – In primary reflux (grades I to V depending on the severity), it is due to an insufficient flap valve–type mechanism at the ureterovesical junction.
  – Hydroureteronephrosis is usually seen only with higher grades of reflux (grades III to V) or secondary reflux (reflux in the presence of an abnormal bladder, in which the reflux is often due to high storage or voiding pressures within the bladder). Secondary reflux is not graded.
- Ureterocele:
  – Hydroureteronephrosis secondary to obstruction of the ureter from a cystic dilation of the intravesical portion of the distal ureter
  – Most often associated with the upper pole ureter in a duplicated collecting system; less frequently associated with a single system
  – Ureterocele is further classified as intravesical (contained completely within the bladder) or ectopic (extending down the bladder neck and often into the urethra).
- Ectopic ureter:
  – A ureter that drains into an abnormal location away from the trigone
  – The hydroureteronephrosis can be the upper pole ureter of a duplicated collecting system or a single system.
  – Ectopic ureters can drain at various sites along the lower urinary tract depending on the sex of the child. In boys, they can drain into the bladder neck, prostatic urethra, vas deferens, seminal vesicle, or epididymis. In girls, they can drain into the bladder neck, urethra, introitus, and vagina.
  – The ectopic locations often require passage through the bladder neck or urogenital diaphragm, which produces obstruction of the distal ureter.

- Urolithiasis:
  – Obstructing calculi often produce dilation of the urinary tract proximal to its location.
  – Stone disease is rare in infancy except in preterm infants who receive furosemide.
  – The hydronephrosis is usually associated with renal colic.
- Posterior urethral valves:
  – Hydroureteronephrosis, nearly always bilateral, produced by outflow obstruction of the bladder from valve leaflets in the prostatic urethra
  – Because both kidneys are affected, there is a significant risk of chronic renal insufficiency and development of end-stage renal disease.
- Triad syndrome:
  – Hydroureteronephrosis, often with massively dilated ureters, and a large bladder
  – Also known as prune belly syndrome or Eagle–Barrett syndrome
  – These boys have a triad of hypoplastic abdominal wall musculature (leading to a prunelike appearance), bilateral undescended testes, and a dilated urinary tract.
  – Many have associated urethral atresia, which imparts a worse prognosis for renal function.
  – Exact cause of triad syndrome remains elusive.
  – Significant risk of renal insufficiency in these patients
  – A similar syndrome may occur in girls with a prunelike appearance to the abdomen and anomalies of the urogenital tract; however, it is very rare.

DIAGNOSIS

HISTORY
- Newborns:
  – Antenatal hydronephrosis: Presence of hydronephrosis or hydroureteronephrosis
  – If unilateral, severity of hydronephrosis and the status of contralateral kidney
  – If bilateral, presence of bladder wall thickening, bladder enlargement, bladder emptying, or a dilated posterior urethra (keyhole sign) may indicate posterior urethral valves or triad syndrome.
  – If oligohydramnios is present, pulmonary hypoplasia is a concern. The presence of oligohydramnios, increased renal echogenicity, and cystic changes in the kidneys are indicators of poor renal function and dysplasia.
- Older children:
  – History of urinary tract infections or gross hematuria
  – General health and growth (poor growth with chronic renal insufficiency or acidosis)
  – Daytime incontinence, poor urinary stream, or symptoms of voiding dysfunction may be an indicator of bladder dysfunction due to posterior urethral valves.
  – History of episodic abdominal (which may not lateralize well), flank, or back pain in the presence of hydronephrosis is often due to symptomatic ureteropelvic junction obstruction (see topic "Ureteropelvic Junction Obstruction").

PHYSICAL EXAM
- Neonate:
  – Signs of oligohydramnios (Potter facies, lateral patellar dimples, clubfeet, and other limb deformities) and respiratory distress
  – Palpable abdominal mass
  – Palpable walnut-sized bladder (posterior urethral valves)
  – Patent urachus
  – Ascites
  – Development of abdominal wall musculature (wrinkled prunelike appearance in triad syndrome)
- Older children:
  – Presence of abdominal mass
  – Abdominal or flank tenderness

DIAGNOSTIC TESTS & INTERPRETATION
Lab
- Newborn:
  – Hydronephrosis or hydroureteronephrosis with a normal contralateral kidney does not require any immediate laboratory testing.
  – If both kidneys are affected or a solitary kidney is affected, there is a need for serial assessments of renal function (serum electrolytes and creatinine).
- Older children:
  – Urinalysis to detect hematuria or pyuria. Culture if infection suspected
  – In cases where both kidneys are affected or there is a solitary kidney, renal function should be evaluated.

Imaging
- Infants with antenatally detected hydronephrosis typically are evaluated with 3 imaging studies:
  – Renal/bladder ultrasound
  – Voiding cystourethrogram
  – Renal scan
- The timing can be elective for a unilateral lesion with a normal contralateral kidney, but if both kidneys are affected or a solitary kidney is involved, prompt evaluation of the newborn should be undertaken.
- Renal/bladder ultrasound:
  – Because of a period of relative oliguria of a newborn in the first 24–48 hours of life, an ultrasound may underestimate the degree of hydronephrosis during this time and thus should be postponed until the infant is at least 48 hours old.
  – This should not preclude evaluating an infant during this time as long as a study is repeated in 4–6 weeks.
  – In cases where both kidneys were affected or there is a solitary affected kidney, the evaluation should not be delayed.
  – Ultrasound of the kidneys should reveal the severity of dilation of the renal pelvis and calyces, changes in the amount and echogenicity of the parenchyma, and presence of cortical cysts.
  – Evaluation of the full bladder is important as well. It will show dilated distal ureters, which may indicate a ureterovesical junction obstruction, vesicoureteral reflux, or hydroureteronephrosis from posterior urethral valves or triad syndrome.

- Voiding cystourethrogram:
  - Evaluates for the presence of vesicoureteral reflux
  - Allows for the grading of the severity of reflux as well
  - The shape of the bladder, presence of diverticulum, and trabeculations may indicate hypertrophy from posterior urethral valves, neurogenic bladder dysfunction, or voiding dysfunction (in older children)
  - Test can be delayed until after discharge from the nursery unless there is concern about posterior urethral valves, in which case it should be done in the early postnatal period.
- Renal scan:
  - Can quantify the differential renal function or the amount each kidney contributes to overall renal function (the normal differential function is 50% ± 5% for each kidney)
  - The 2 most commonly used radionuclides are 3-mercaptoacetyl triglycine (MAG-3) and diethylenetriamine penta-acetic acid (DTPA). MAG-3 is the best choice for infants and babies.
  - In addition to the ability to detect diminished function, if there is poor drainage of the affected kidney, furosemide is given to wash out the radiotracer. The duration for washing out 1/2 of the accumulated radiotracer ($T_{1/2}$) is often given in the report. A prompt $T_{1/2}$ (<10 min) is indicative of a nonobstructed kidney. A slower $T_{1/2}$ may be indicative of obstruction when it is >20 minutes. An intermediate $T_{1/2}$ (10–20 minutes) is indeterminate for obstruction. Many factors affect the $T_{1/2}$ making it less reliable for indicating obstruction. These factors include the hydration status, presence of vesicoureteral reflux, and the overall function of the kidney (very poorly functioning kidneys have a poor response to diuretics).
- IV pyelogram:
  - Most useful for evaluating the anatomy of the kidney and the ureters
  - Also a useful test for evaluating an older child with intermittent symptoms of abdominal or flank pain
  - Can be diagnostic of an intermittent ureteropelvic junction obstruction as the cause of the child's pain
- CT scan:
  - Most commonly done in cases where the hydronephrosis is symptomatic
  - Noncontrast spiral CT is the most sensitive way to detect stones, as even stones radiolucent on plain films (uric acid) will be detected by CT.
- MRI: Currently has a limited role in evaluating hydronephrosis, but contrast-enhanced MRI is currently being studied as an alternative to renal scans and ultrasound in the evaluation of hydronephrosis.

DIFFERENTIAL DIAGNOSIS

- Cystic renal tumor:
  - Most commonly Wilms tumor
  - Should be distinguished from hydronephrosis by ultrasound or CT scanning
- Multicystic dysplastic kidney:
  - Can be difficult to distinguish from severe hydronephrosis with marked parenchymal thinning
  - Renal scan will show no function or perfusion with a multicystic dysplastic kidney

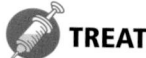 **TREATMENT**

ADDITIONAL TREATMENT
General Measures
Neonates with hydronephrosis are started on prophylactic antibiotics (1/4 the therapeutic dose given once a day) of amoxicillin. When the baby is 2 months old, the antibiotic can be changed to trimethoprim, trimethoprim/sulfamethoxazole or nitrofurantoin.

 ONGOING CARE

FOLLOW-UP RECOMMENDATIONS
- Ureteropelvic junction obstruction:
  - After initial evaluation, the infants are usually followed with serial studies, either ultrasound or renal scans, depending on the degree of functional impairment, the severity of the hydronephrosis, and the pattern of drainage on the renal scan.
  - From more information, see topic "Ureteropelvic Junction Obstruction."
- Ureterovesical junction obstruction:
  - After initial evaluation, these children are followed with serial studies as with ureteropelvic junction obstruction.
  - These lesions are much less common than ureteropelvic junction obstruction, and most of the time, the affected kidneys have normal function and can be followed conservatively.
  - If the function of the kidney is significantly diminished (differential function of 35–40%), surgical treatment of the obstruction is indicated.
- Vesicoureteral reflux:
  - Infants with reflux are kept on prophylactic antibiotics.
  - In the absence of breakthrough infections, they are re-evaluated annually.
  - If persistent high-grade reflux continues or breakthrough infections are a problem, surgical correction is carried out.
  - For more information, see topic "Vesicoureteral Reflux."
- Ureterocele/ectopic ureter: Because these are obstructive lesions, they are generally treated surgically early in life at the time of diagnosis.

- Posterior urethral valves:
  - Full-term infants undergo cystoscopic valve ablation, whereas preterm infants may require a temporary vesicostomy until endoscopic treatment is feasible.
  - These boys require careful follow-up from a pediatric urologist and nephrologist as they grow up.
  - For more information, see topic "Posterior Urethral Valves."
- Triad syndrome: Typically these boys will undergo bilateral orchiopexy with or without an abdominoplasty depending on the severity of the hypoplasia of the abdominal wall during the first 6–12 months of life.

ADDITIONAL READING

- Cooper CS, Andrews JI, Hansen WF, et al. Antenatal hydronephrosis: Evaluation and outcome. *Curr Urol Rep.* 2002;3:131–138.
- Estrada CR Jr. Prenatal hydronephrosis: Early evaluation. *Curr Opin Urol.* 2008;18(4):401–403.

CODES

ICD9
- 591 Hydronephrosis
- 753.21 Congenital obstruction of ureteropelvic junction

ICD10
- N13.1 Hydronephrosis w ureteral stricture, NEC
- N13.30 Unspecified hydronephrosis

FAQ

- Q: If my baby has hydronephrosis affecting only 1 kidney, will he need a kidney transplant?
- A: In the absence of oligohydramnios and bilateral hydroureteronephrosis, it would be a very rare event that a child would develop renal failure requiring transplantation.
- Q: My unborn baby has hydronephrosis in only one kidney, and the other kidney is normal. What are the chances that it is a ureteropelvic junction obstruction?
- A: The chances are ~45% that isolated hydronephrosis will be due to a ureteropelvic junction obstruction.
- Q: My male unborn baby has bilateral hydronephrosis but a "normal" bladder. Is there still a chance that he has posterior urethral valves?
- A: Yes. Although it is less likely to be due to posterior urethral valves than if a thick-walled, enlarged, poorly emptying bladder were seen, prenatal ultrasonography is operator dependent and can miss dilated ureters or bladder abnormalities.

H

HYPERIMMUNOGLOBULINEMIA E SYNDROME

Erin E. McGintee

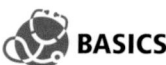 **BASICS**

DEFINITION
Rare disorder characterized by markedly elevated serum IgE levels, chronic eczematoid dermatitis, skeletal abnormalities, and recurrent staphylococcal infections

RISK FACTORS
Genetics
- Most cases sporadic, but both autosomal-dominant (AD-HIES) and autosomal-recessive forms (AR-HIES) have been reported.
- AD-HIES is caused by mutations in STAT3, a transcriptional regulator.
- Mutations in DOCK8 and Tyk2 have been identified in AR-HIES.

PATHOPHYSIOLOGY
- Impaired cytokine signaling (IFN-γ, IL-6, and IL-10 defects have been identified) leads to a variety of immunologic impairments.
- Phagocytic: Impaired chemotaxis
- T cell: Impaired proliferative response to antigens
- B cell: Variable heterogeneity of ability to form antibodies to antigens

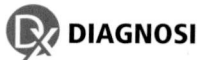 **DIAGNOSIS**

HISTORY
- Recurrent infection: "Cold" abscesses, pneumonia, pneumatoceles, otitis media, sinusitis
- Organisms that cause infection: *Staphylococcus aureus, Candida, Haemophilus influenzae, Streptococcus pneumoniae*, group A *Streptococcus*
- Superinfection with fungal and opportunistic organisms.
- AR-HIES may present with severe viral infection or molluscum.
- Severe eczematoid dermatitis as early as 1 week of age.
- Delayed shedding of primary teeth (AD-HIES)

PHYSICAL EXAM
- Coarse facial features, prominent forehead, broad nasal bridge, prominent nose
- Growth retardation can occur with recurrent illnesses.
- Osteoporosis complicated by recurrent fractures
- Eczematoid dermatitis
- Hyperextensible joints

DIAGNOSTIC TESTS & INTERPRETATION
Diagnostic Procedures/Other
- Eosinophilia: Peripheral eosinophils, >700 cells/mL
- Quantitative immunoglobulins: IgG, IgA, IgM usually normal, but IgE elevated, usually >10,000 IU/mL
- IgE antibodies against *S. aureus*
- Functional antibodies to diphtheria, tetanus, *Haemophilus influenzae* Type b, and *Pneumococcus* results are variable, but there is a subgroup of patients who are unable to mount an appropriate antibody response to these antigens.
- Some patients demonstrate impaired polymorphonucleocyte (PMN) chemotaxis.
- Pulmonary function tests to evaluate extent of lung disease from infections such as pneumatoceles

DIFFERENTIAL DIAGNOSIS
- Atopic dermatitis
- Wiskott-Aldrich syndrome
- Omenn syndrome
- IPEX
- Chronic granulomatous disease

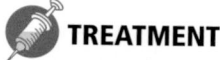
TREATMENT

ADDITIONAL TREATMENT
General Measures
- Supportive, based on clinical and laboratory findings
- Lifelong use of antistaphylococcal therapy: Dicloxacillin or amoxicillin/clavulanate potassium (Augmentin) at therapeutic doses
- Surgical intervention for management of pneumatoceles for drainage or secondary to compression of nearby parenchyma
- IV immunoglobulin as replacement therapy for abnormal functional antibodies is usually given at starting dose of 400 mg/kg monthly.

ONGOING CARE

FOLLOW-UP RECOMMENDATIONS
- Long-term outcome is unknown; it depends on a timely diagnosis that allows for close monitoring and aggressive treatment of infections.
- Sequelae from recurrent infections, such as pneumonias and pneumatoceles, can result in a debilitating course.
- Increased chance of malignancy has been reported in some cases.

ADDITIONAL READING

- Buckley RH. The hyper-IgE syndrome. *Clin Rev Allergy Immunol*. 2001;20:139–154.
- Erlewyn-Lajeunesse MDS. Hyperimmunoglobulin-E syndrome with recurrent infection: A review of current opinion and treatment. *Pediatr Allergy Immunol*. 2000;11:133–141.
- Lavoie A, Rottem M, Grodofsky MD, et al. Anti-Staphylococcus aureus IgE antibodies for diagnosis of hyperimmunoglobulinemia E—recurrent infection syndrome in infancy. *Am J Dis Child*.1989;143:38–104.
- Leung DYM, Geha RS. Clinical and immunologic aspects of the hyperimmunoglobulin E syndrome. *Hematol Oncol Clin North Am*. 1988;2:81–97.
- Marone G, Florio G, Triggiani M, et al. Mechanisms of IgE elevation in HIV-1 infection. *Crit Rev Immunol*. 2000;20:477–496.
- Ozcan E, Notarangelo LD, Geha RS. Primary immune deficiencies with aberrant IgE production. *J Allergy Clin Immunol*. 2008;122:1054–1062.
- Saini SS, MacGlashan D. How IgE upregulates the allergic response. *Curr Opin Immunol*. 2002;14:694–697.
- Sheerin KA, Buckley RH. Antibody response to protein, polysaccharide, and Ox174 antigens of the hyperimmunoglobulinemia E syndrome. *J Allergy Clin Immunol*. 1991;87:803–811.

CODES

ICD9
- 279.3 Unspecified immunity deficiency
- 288.1 Functional disorders of polymorphonuclear neutrophils

ICD10
D82.4 Hyperimmunoglobulin E [IgE] syndrome

FAQ

- Q: Is this disease also referred to as Job syndrome?
- A: Yes, because Job suffered from difficulties with boils and other skin manifestations.

H

HYPERINSULINISM

Vaneeta Bamba
Diva D. De León

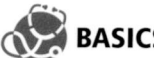

BASICS

DESCRIPTION
Hyperinsulinism (HI) is a disorder of dysregulated insulin secretion characterized by excessive and/or inappropriate insulin secretion resulting in severe hypoglycemia. Hyperinsulinism can occur transiently but congenital HI refers to a permanent inborn condition.

EPIDEMIOLOGY
Most common cause of persistent or recurrent hypoglycemia in children beyond the immediate neonatal period.

Incidence
- Annual incidence estimated at ~1:40,000–50,000 live births in the USA.
- May be as high as 1:2,500 in select populations (Saudi Arabians, Ashkenazi Jews)

Prevalence
- Estimated prevalence of hypoglycemia due to hyperinsulinism in the USA is 0.0008%.

Genetics
- Autosomal recessive mutations of K_{ATP} channel genes (*ABCC8* and *KCNJ11*) at chromosomal locus 11p14-15.1 resulting in diffuse involvement throughout the pancreas (diffuse HI)
- Autosomal dominant mutations of K_{ATP} channel genes
- A nonmendelian mode of inheritance with reduction to homozygosity (or hemizygosity) of paternally inherited mutation of K_{ATP} channel gene, and a specific loss of maternal alleles of the imprinted chromosome region 11p15 (focal HI).
- Autosomal dominant mutations of glucokinase (*GCK*): Activating mutations in the glucokinase gene
- Autosomal dominant mutations of glutamate dehydrogenase (*GLUD-1*): Known as hyperinsulinism/hyperammonemia syndrome due to activating mutations of glutamate dehydrogenase (GDH) enzyme
- Autosomal recessive mutations of the mitochondrial enzyme short-chain-3-dydroxyacyl-CoA dehydrogenase (SCHAD; encoded by *HADHSC*)
- Autosomal dominant mutations in *HNF4A*, mutations known to cause a familial form of monogenic diabetes can present with neonatal hyperinsulinism
- Autosomal dominant promoter activating mutations in *SLC16A1* encoding monocarboxylate transporter 1 (MCT1): Causes exercise-induced HI

PATHOPHYSIOLOGY
- These mutations result in uncoupling of insulin secretion from the glucose-sensing machinery of the pancreatic β-cell and inappropriate insulin secretion even in the face of low blood glucose.
- The most common and severe forms of HI arise from mutations in the K_{ATP} channel, which can manifest in focal or diffuse disease.
- In the focal form of the disease, only a cluster of pancreatic β-cells are affected, whereas in diffuse disease, all pancreatic β-cells are abnormal.
- In hyperinsulinism/hyperammonemia syndrome, activating mutations of glutamate dehydrogenase result in protein-induced insulin secretion and cause persistently elevated ammonia level.
- *HNF4A* mutations known to cause a familial form of monogenic diabetes, can present with neonatal hypoglycemia due to HI.
- In the case of exercise-induced HI, ectopic expression of MCT1, allows transport of lactate and pyruvate across the β-cell membrane, particularly during anaerobic exercise. Pyruvate is metabolized and there is an increase in ATP to ADP ratio, thus stimulating insulin secretion. Hypoglycemia occurs 30–45 minutes after intensive anaerobic exercise.

ETIOLOGY
- Mutations in 7 genes have been associated with congenital HI: Genes coding for either of the two subunits of the beta cell K_{ATP} channel [SUR1, sulfonylurea receptor (*ABCC8*); Kir6.2, inwardly rectifying potassium channel (*KCNJ11*)], glucokinase (*GCK*), glutamate dehydrogenase (GLUD-1), SCHAD (*HADHSC*), monocarboxylate transporter-1 (*SLC16A1*), and *HNF4A*.
- A transient form of HI has been associated with perinatal stress [small for gestational age (SGA) birth weight, maternal hypertension, precipitous delivery, or hypoxia], but the mechanism has not been elucidated.

COMMONLY ASSOCIATED CONDITIONS
Hyperinsulinism can be associated with Beckwith–Wiedemann syndrome and congenital disorders of glycosylation. The underlying mechanism of hyperinsulinism in these disorders is not clear.

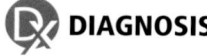

DIAGNOSIS

HISTORY
Symptoms of hypoglycemia in the infant:
- Poor feeding
- Hypotonia
- Lethargy
- Cyanosis
- Tachypnea
- Tremors
- Seizures
- Early-morning irritability that responds to feeding

PHYSICAL EXAM
- Macrosomia:
  - Indicates congenital HI due to mutations in the K_{ATP} channel
- Small for gestational age:
  - Indicates transient HI
- Macroglossia, umbilical hernia, visceromegaly:
  - Indicates Beckwith Wiedeman syndrome
- No midline defects, including normal palate and genitalia
  - Midline defects indicate hypopituitarism.

DIAGNOSTIC TESTS & INTERPRETATION
Lab
- Plasma insulin levels are rarely dramatically elevated in HI; rather there is inadequate suppression of insulin (>2 μU/mL) at time of hypoglycemia.
- Suppressed levels of plasma free fatty acids (<1.5 mmol/L) and ketones (β-hydroxybutyrate level <2.0 mmol/L) at time of hypoglycemia
  - Indirect signs of excessive insulin action
- Glycemic response to glucagon (blood sugar rise >30 mg/dL) at time of hypoglycemia:
  - Indicates inappropriately stored glycogen at time of hypoglycemia (sign of excessive insulin action)
- Suppressed insulin-like growth factor binding protein-1 (IGFBP-1) level:
  - IGFBP-1 production is inhibited by insulin (sign of excessive insulin action).
- Elevated plasma ammonia levels:
  - Indicate hyperinsulinism/hyperammonemia syndrome
- Elevated plasma 3-hydroxybutyryl-carnitine and urinary 3-hydroxyglutarate
  - Indicates SCHAD
- Normal growth hormone, cortisol, and thyroxine levels:
  - Exclude hypopituitarism

Imaging
- PET scans at specialized hyperinsulinism centers using 18-fluoro-DOPA may identify and localize focal lesions.
- Traditional imaging studies such as ultrasound, CT scan and MRI are not helpful in identifying focal HI lesions.

Pathological Findings
- Pancreatic histology in children with HI due to K_{ATP} channel mutations can be subdivided into 2 major forms:
  - Diffuse HI: Abnormally enlarged islet cell nuclei found diffusely throughout the pancreas
  - Focal HI (40–60% of cases): Discrete region of adenomatous hyperplasia surrounded by normal-appearing pancreas
- Normal histology can also be seen in HI.

DIFFERENTIAL DIAGNOSIS
- Sepsis
- Congenital heart disease
- Infant of diabetic mother (IDM)
- Beckwith–Wiedemann syndrome (BWS)
- Panhypopituitarism
- Congenital disorders of glycosylation
- Respiratory distress syndrome
- Erythroblastosis fetalis
- Other inborn errors of metabolism
- Children with dumping syndrome after fundoplasty can have severe post-meal hypoglycemia due to excessive insulin secretion after a meal.

 ## TREATMENT

ADDITIONAL TREATMENT
General Measures
The major goal is prevention of brain damage by controlling blood glucose:
- Parenteral dextrose infusions to stabilize blood sugar acutely: For an acute hypoglycemic event, give a bolus of 2–3 mL/Kg of 10% dextrose (0.2–0.3g/kg). For maintenance, use glucose infusion rates of 8–10 mg/kg/min to maintain BG >70 mg/dL (some HI patients may need up to 25 mg/kg/min).
- Supplemental oral or nasogastric/G tube feeds

MEDICATION (DRUGS)
- Diazoxide, a suppressant of insulin secretion, at 5–15 mg/kg/d divided q12h (most patients with KATP HI do not respond to diazoxide). Most patients with transient HI who require medical therapy respond well to diazoxide and resolve spontaneously.
- Octreotide, a long-acting somatostatin analog, at 5–20 μg/kg/d divided q6h or given by continuous SQ infusion. Octreotide may increase the risk of necrotizing enterocolitis in neonates.
- Glucagon, at 1 mg/d by continuous intravenous infusion, may stabilize blood glucose levels in preparation for surgery.

SURGERY/OTHER PROCEDURES
- Subtotal pancreatectomy in children refractory to medical therapy or in those with focal lesions
- For focal HI, surgery can be curative.

 ## ONGOING CARE

FOLLOW-UP RECOMMENDATIONS
- Up to 30–44% of patients can have neurodevelopmental retardation due to hypoglycemia
- Diabetes may develop later in life, especially after pancreatectomy

Patient Monitoring
- Home blood glucose monitoring, especially with longer fasts or intercurrent illnesses
- Hospitalizations for IV glucose infusions may be necessary during intercurrent illnesses with vomiting.
- Follow-up fasting studies may be needed to evaluate safety and/or disease regression.
- Diazoxide may cause fluid retention and hypertrichosis.
- Neonates treated with octreotide should be closely monitoring for evidence of necrotizing enterocolitis.
- Tachyphylaxis and hyperglycemia may occur with octreotide.
- Close observation of linear growth is necessary, because octreotide can suppress GH secretion.

DIET
- Frequent feedings and avoidance of long fasts
- Avoidance of protein loads in those with hyperinsulinism/hyperammonemia, as high-protein diets may stimulate insulin secretion

COMPLICATIONS
- Severe refractory hypoglycemia
- Cognitive deficits, especially of short-term memory, visual–motor integration, and arithmetic skills
- Seizures
- Coma
- Permanent brain damage
- Glucose intolerance or frank diabetes mellitus

ADDITIONAL READING

- De León DD, Stanley CA. Mechanisms of disease: advances in diagnosis and treatment of hyperinsulinism in neonates. *Nat Clin Prac Endocrinol Metab*. 2007;3(1):57–68.
- Dunne MJ, Cosgrove KE, Sheperd RM, et al. Hyperinsulinism in infancy: From basic science to clinical disease. *Physiol Rev*. 2004;84:239–275.
- Hoe FM, Thornton PS, Wanner LA, et al. Clinical features and insulin regulation in infants with syndrome of prolonged neonatal hyperinsulinism. *J Pediatr*. 2006;148:207–212.
- James C, Kapoor RR, Ismail D, et al. The genetic basis of congenital hyperinsulinism. *J Med Genet*. 2009;46(5):289–299.
- Marquard J, Palladino AA, Stanley CA, et al. Rare forms of congenital hyperinsulinism. *Semin Pediatr Surg*. 2011;20(1):38–44.
- Meissner T, Wendel U, Burgard P, et al. Long-term follow-up of 114 patients with congenital hyperinsulinism. *Eur J Endocrinol*. 2003;149:43–51.
- Otonkoski T, Jiao H, Kaminen-Ahola N, et al. Physical exercise-induced hypoglycemia caused by failed silencing of monocarboxylate transporter 1 in pancreatic beta cells. *Am J Hum Genet*. 2007; 81(3):467–474.
- Palladino AA, Stanley CA. A specialized team approach to diagnosis and medical versus surgical treatment of infants with congenital hyperinsulinism. *Semin Pediatr Surg*. 2011;20(1):32–37.
- Pearson ER, Boj SF, Steele AM, et al. Macrosomia and hyperinsulinaemic hypoglycaemia in patients with heterozygous mutations in the HNF4A gene. *PLoS Med*. 2007;4(4):e118.

 ## CODES

ICD9
251.1 Other specified hypoglycemia

ICD10
E16.1 Other hypoglycemia

FAQ
- Q: What is the chance of hyperinsulinism in the sibling of an affected child?
- A: 25% in the autosomal-recessive type; 50% in the autosomal-dominant type; <1% for siblings of children with focal hyperinsulinism
- Q: How low and for how long can glucose go before brain damage occurs?
- A: The definition of hypoglycemia has been the subject of controversy in pediatrics, but activation of glucose counterregulatory systems occurs when blood glucose levels reach the 65–70 mg/dL range; symptoms of hypoglycemia present at the 50–55 mg/dL level, and cognitive dysfunction occurs when blood glucose levels are in the 45–50 mg/dL range. Taking these data into account, blood glucose concentration should be maintained >70 mg/dL. The duration of hypoglycemia necessary for brain damage to occur is unknown.
- Q: What is the chance that HI will eventually resolve without surgery?
- A: Only ~40–50% of cases are controlled with medication alone. Patients with mutations in KATP channel may be more likely to require surgery, and in those patients with focal disease, surgery may be curative. Perinatal-stress induced hyperinsulinism usually resolves within the first 3 months of life.

H

HYPERLIPIDEMIA

Dale Y. Lee
Ruben W. Cerri (5th edition)

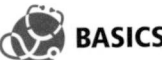 **BASICS**

DESCRIPTION

Hyperlipidemia is an elevation of serum lipids. These lipids include cholesterol, cholesterol esters (compounds), phospholipids, and triglycerides. Lipids are transported as part of large molecules called lipoproteins.

- 5 major families of lipoproteins:
  - Chylomicrons
  - Very low-density lipoproteins (VLDL)
  - Intermediate-density lipoproteins (IDL)
  - Low-density lipoproteins (LDL)
  - High-density lipoproteins (HDL)
  - Normal serum lipid concentrations: Total cholesterol: 170 mg/dL (borderline, 170–199 mg/dL)
  - LDL cholesterol: <110 mg/dL (borderline, 110–129 mg/dL)
  - HDL cholesterol: ≥35 mg/dL
  - Total triglycerides: 100 mg/dL (borderline, 100–140 mg/dL)
  - More detailed age and gender specific values are available (refer to Table 2 of 2008 *Clinical Report: Lipid Screening and Cardiovascular Health in Childhood*)
- Primary hypercholesterolemia or hypertriglyceridemia (hyperlipidemia): Elevation in serum cholesterol as a result of an inherited disorder of lipid metabolism (i.e., familial hypercholesterolemia)
- Secondary hypercholesterolemia or hypertriglyceridemia: Elevation in serum cholesterol as a result of another disease process (e.g., nephrotic syndrome)

EPIDEMIOLOGY
Incidence
The incidence of homozygous familial hypercholesterolemia is 1 in 1,000,000; the incidence of the heterozygous state is 1 in 500. Unknown causes result in hypercholesterolemia and/or hypertriglyceridemia occurring in 2% of the population.

Prevalence
- National Health and Nutrition Exam Surveys (NHANES I-III) have provided information about the serum cholesterol levels in children.
- For all children 4–17 years, the 95th percentile for serum total cholesterol is 216 mg/dL and the 75th percentile is 181 mg/dL.
- The average total and LDL cholesterol levels are, before puberty, significantly higher in girls than they are in boys.
- The mean total cholesterol level for all children from 4–11 years old peaks at age 9–11 and then gradually decreases until mid to late adolescence.

RISK FACTORS
Genetics
- Familial hypertriglyceridemia (FHTG): Dominantly inherited disorder
- Familial hypercholesterolemia (FH): Dominantly inherited defect of LDL receptor
- Familial combined hyperlipidemia (FCHL): Dominantly inherited lipid disorder

GENERAL PREVENTION
- Fat intake is generally unrestricted prior to 2 years of age. After age 2, 2 complementary approaches are recommended.
- Diet and lifestyle guidelines are to promote:
- Consumption of an overall healthy diet
- A healthy body weight (BMI: 18.5–24.9 kg/m^2)
- Recommended lipid levels:
  - LDL cholesterol <110 mg/dL
  - HDL cholesterol >50 mg/dL in women, >40 mg/dL in men
  - Triglycerides <150 mg/dL
- Normal BP (age appropriate)
- Normal blood glucose level (fasting blood glucose ≤100 mg/dL)
- Being physically active
- Avoiding use of and exposure to tobacco products
- Screen children and adolescents who have:
  - Positive family history of dyslipidemia or premature CVD (≤55 years old for men, ≤65 years old for women), such as coronary atherosclerosis, documented MI.
  - Unknown family history
  - Obesity (BMI ≥95th percentile), or are overweight (BMI ≥85th–<95th percentile)
  - Cigarette smoking exposure
  - Diabetes mellitus

DIAGNOSIS

HISTORY
- Family history of premature heart disease or dyslipidemia:
  - Almost all cases of primary hyperlipidemia are of dominant inheritance.
- Smoking:
  - Smoking reduces HDL cholesterol levels and increases the risk of vascular disease.
- Use of oral contraceptives:
  - Birth control pills have been shown to cause elevations in lipoprotein levels and, when coupled with already elevated lipid levels, can increase the risk of atherosclerosis.
- Regular exercise
- Diet:
  - Children with increased intake of fat, carbohydrates, sugar added drinks, and fast foods are likely to be overweight/obese
- Obesity:
  - Obese children are more likely to have abnormal serum lipids.

PHYSICAL EXAM
- Eye exam:
  - Arcus corneae: Deposits of cholesterol, resulting in a thin, white circular ring located on the outer edge of the iris
- Skin exam:
  - Tendon xanthomas: Thickened tissue surrounding the Achilles and extensor tendons
  - Xanthelasma: Yellowish deposits of cholesterol surrounding the eye
  - Palmar xanthomas: Pale lines in creases of palms
  - Eruptive xanthomas: Characteristic of hypertriglyceridemia; papular yellowish lesions with a red base that occur on the buttocks, elbows, and knees
  - Enlarged tender liver may present in association with fatty liver.

DIAGNOSTIC TESTS & INTERPRETATION
Lab
- Screening for patients with:
  - A parental history of elevated total cholesterol levels (>240 mg/dL) or other dyslipidemia
  - A family history of premature coronary heart disease
  - Incomplete or unavailable family histories
  - Other risk factors for CVD (obese or overweight, cigarette smoking, hypertension, diabetes, inactivity)
- Fasting lipid profile: Total cholesterol, HDL cholesterol, LDL cholesterol, and triglycerides:
  - Determine the type of hyperlipidemia.
- First screening should take place after 2 years of age, but no later than 10 years of age
- If fasting lipid profile is within normal range, repeat test in 3–5 years
- Chemistry panel (ALT, AST, bilirubin, BUN, creatinine, urinalysis):
  - Screening test for liver and kidney disease
- Thyroid evaluation (thyroxine, thyroid stimulating hormone):
  - Determines the presence of hypothyroidism

ALERT
- Serum total cholesterol is inaccurate when serum triglycerides are >400 mg/dL.
- Hypertriglyceridemia is associated with falsely lowered serum Na.

DIFFERENTIAL DIAGNOSIS
- Hypercholesterolemia:
  - Primary hypercholesterolemia (see above)
  - Hypothyroidism
  - Nephrotic syndrome
  - Liver disease (cholestatic)
  - Renal failure
  - Anorexia nervosa
  - Acute porphyria
  - Medications (antihypertensives, estrogens, steroids, microsomal enzyme inducers, cyclosporine, diuretics)
  - Pregnancy
  - Dietary: Excessive dietary intake of fat, cholesterol, and/or calories

- Hypertriglyceridemia:
  – Primary hypertriglyceridemia (see above)
  – Acute hepatitis
  – Nephrotic syndrome
  – Chronic renal failure
  – Medications (diuretics, retinoids, oral contraceptives)
  – Diabetes mellitus
  – Alcohol abuse
  – Lipodystrophy
  – Myelomatosis
  – Glycogen storage disease
  – Dietary: Excessive dietary intake of fat and/or calories

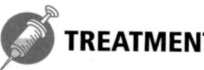 TREATMENT

MEDICATION (DRUGS)
- Drug therapy should be considered only for children ≥8 years of age after an adequate trial of diet therapy (for 6–12 months) and if they have one of the following:
  – LDL cholesterol level remains >190 mg/dL
  – LDL cholesterol level remains >160 mg/dL and there is a family history of premature cardiovascular disease (≤55 years of age for men, ≤65 for women) or ≥2 other risk factors are present (obesity, hypertension, cigarette smoking).
  – LDL ≥130 mg/dL and have diabetes mellitus
- Physicians caring for overweight and obese children who have lipid disorders should emphasize the importance of diet and exercise rather than drug therapy for most of their patients.
- Statins (1st-line drug therapy): Decrease endogenous synthesis of cholesterol and increase clearance of LDL from circulation
  – Similar safety and efficacy in the treatment of lipid disorders in children as in adults
  – Side effects include hepatitis and myositis
- Bile-acid-binding resins: Bind cholesterol in bile acids in intestine and prevent reuptake into enterohepatic circulation
  – Associated with GI discomfort
  – Very poor compliance in children
- Niacin: Lowers LDL and triglycerides while increasing HDL; however, poorly tolerated in children due to side effects occur in >50%, including flushing, itching, and elevated hepatic transaminases
  – Drugs needing further pediatric studies: Cholesterol absorption inhibitors and fibrates

ADDITIONAL TREATMENT
General Measures
- Outpatient management unless secondary hyperlipidemia caused by liver or renal failure, which would necessitate inpatient management of primary illness. Note: The cause of secondary hyperlipidemia should be treated with disease-specific therapy to reduce elevated lipid levels.
- For primary hyperlipidemia: It is recommended that once a lipoprotein analysis is obtained, it should be repeated so that an average LDL cholesterol level can be calculated.

- Risk assessment and treatment:
  – Population approach: General emphasis on healthy lifestyle to prevent development of dyslipidemias. Recommendations include increasing intake of fruits, vegetables, fish, whole grains, and low-fat dairy products; reducing intake of fruit juice, sugar-sweetened beverages and food.
  – Individual approach: Focuses on patients who are high risk. Initial intervention is focused on changing diet, but patients often require pharmacologic intervention.

Additional Therapies
Activity:
- 60 minutes of moderate to vigorous play or physical activity daily
- Reduce sedentary behaviors (e.g., watching TV, playing videogames, using computers)
- Participation in organized sports.

 ONGOING CARE

FOLLOW-UP RECOMMENDATIONS
Patient Monitoring
- For patients with primary hyperlipidemia who are off medication, follow-up should be performed every 1–2 years with lipoprotein profile evaluation. For those patients on medication, follow-up should be conducted every 3–6 months.
- For all other patients with risks factors and normal lipid profile a monitored lifestyle and diet changes should be strongly recommended at every office visit.

DIET
- Dietary modification is safe in the treatment of hyperlipidemia in children >2 years of age:
  – Restrict saturated fat to <7% daily calories
  – Restrict dietary cholesterol to 200 mg/d
  – Limit trans fatty acids to <1% daily calories
  – Supplemental fiber at goal dose of child's age + 5 g/d (up to 20 g/d)
- For children between 12 months and 2 years who are overweight, obese, or have a family history of dyslipidemia or CVD, the use of reduced fat milk can be considered.

PROGNOSIS
- Familial hypercholesterolemia:
  – Homozygotes: Coronary artery disease in 1st or 2nd decade of life
  – Heterozygotes: 50% of males develop premature heart disease by age 50 (females, age 60)
- Familial combined hyperlipidemia: Occurs in 1–2% of the population and accounts for 10% of all premature heart disease. A reduction of LDL cholesterol by 1% reduces risk by 2%.
- Children and adolescents with high cholesterol levels are more likely than the general population to have high levels as adults.

COMPLICATIONS
- Hypercholesterolemia has been linked to premature coronary artery disease and vascular disease.
- Severe hypertriglyceridemia can cause pancreatitis.
- Hypercholesterolemia:
  – Premature heart disease
  – Stroke
  – Carotid artery disease
- Hypertriglyceridemia:
  – Pancreatitis

ADDITIONAL READING
- Daniels SR, Greer FR, Committee on Nutrition. Clinical report: Lipid screening and cardiovascular health in childhood. *Pediatrics*. 2008;122: 198–208.
- Gidding SS, Dennison BA, Birch LL, et al. American Heart Association; American Academy of Pediatrics. Dietary recommendations for children and adolescents: A guide for practitioners: Consensus statement from the American Heart Association. *Circulation*. 2005;112:2061–2075.
- Kavey RW, Allada V, Daniels SR, et al. Cardiovascular Risk Reduction in high-risk pediatric patients. A scientific statement from the American Heart Association. *Circulation*. 2006;114: 2710–2738.
- Lichtenstein AH, Appel LJ, Brands M, et al. Diet and lifestyle recommendations revision 2006. A scientific statement from the American Heart Association Nutrition Committee. *Circulation*. 2006;114:82–96.
- McCrindLe BW, Urbina EM, Dennison BA, et al. Drug therapy of high-risk lipid abnormalities in children and adolescents. A scientific statement from the American Heart Association. *Circulation*. 2007;1115:1948–1967.

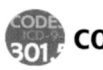 CODES

ICD9
- 272.0 Pure hypercholesterolemia
- 272.1 Pure hyperglyceridemia
- 272.4 Other and unspecified hyperlipidemia

ICD10
- E78.0 Pure hypercholesterolemia
- E78.1 Pure hyperglyceridemia
- E78.5 Hyperlipidemia, unspecified

H

HYPERTENSION

Christine B. Sethna
Kevin E. C. Meyers

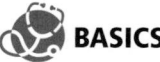 **BASICS**

DESCRIPTION

- Hypertension: Average systolic and/or diastolic BPs above the 95th percentile for age, gender, and height percentile on at least 3 separate occasions as defined by the Fourth Report on the Diagnosis, Evaluation, and Treatment of High Blood Pressure in Children and Adolescents.
- Prehypertension: BP between the 90th percentile and 95th percentile or BP >120/80 in adolescents.
- Stage 1 hypertension: BP 95–99% plus 5 mm Hg.
- Stage 2 hypertension: BP >99th% plus 5 mm Hg.
- Primary (essential) hypertension: Hypertension for which there is no underlying cause
- Secondary hypertension: Hypertension for which an underlying cause can be identified
- White coat hypertension: Elevated BP readings in a medical setting with normal actual blood pressures
- Masked hypertension: Normal BP readings in a medical setting with elevated actual blood pressures

EPIDEMIOLOGY

- Secondary hypertension is more common in children than in adults.
- Primary hypertension is now identifiable in children and adolescents, and is associated with overweight, the metabolic syndrome, and family history of hypertension.

Prevalence

- The prevalence of hypertension is increasing due to the epidemic of youth obesity and the metabolic syndrome.
- Hypertension in the pediatric population is estimated between 1% and 23%.
- 30% of children with BMI >95% have hypertension.
- Primary hypertension in blacks is twice that of whites.

RISK FACTORS

- Primary hypertension: Obesity, sedentary lifestyle, low birth weight, smoking, alcohol use, hyperlipidemia, family history, stress, sodium intake, sleep apnea
- Secondary hypertension: Umbilical artery catheterization, UTI, genetic disease
- The younger the child and the more elevated BP, the greater likelihood of a secondary cause.

Genetics

- The genetic basis of primary hypertension is polygenic, but more likely to develop in individuals when there is a strong family history.
- The genetics of secondary causes depend on the condition:
  - Polycystic kidney disease: Autosomal dominant, autosomal recessive
  - Neurofibromatosis: Autosomal dominant
  - Glucocorticoid-remediable aldosteronism: Autosomal dominant

GENERAL PREVENTION

Avoidance of excess weight gain and regular physical activity can prevent obesity-related hypertension.

PATHOPHYSIOLOGY

- Many different mechanisms play a role in primary hypertension: Volume overload (sodium retention, excess sodium intake), volume distribution (sympathetic and renin overactivity, stress), and increased peripheral resistance (renin and sympathetic activity, insulin, endothelin)
- Secondary causes, with examples, include:
  - Renal: Acute glomerulonephritis, chronic renal failure, polycystic kidney disease, reflux nephropathy
  - Renovascular: Fibromuscular dysplasia, neurofibromatosis, vasculitis
  - Cardiac: Coarctation of the aorta
  - Endocrine: Pheochromocytoma, hypo/hyperthyroid, neuroblastoma, glucocorticoid-remediable aldosteronism, Conn syndrome, apparent mineralocorticoid excess, congenital adrenal hyperplasia, Liddle syndrome, Gordon syndrome
  - Neurologic: Increased intracranial pressure
  - Drugs: Corticosteroids, oral contraceptives, sympathomimetics, illicit drugs (cocaine, phencyclidine)
  - Other: Pain, burns, traction

DIAGNOSIS

- Hypertensive emergency: Severely elevated BP with evidence of target organ injury (encephalopathy, seizures, renal damage)
- Hypertensive urgency: Severely elevated BP with no evidence of secondary organ damage

HISTORY

- Headache, blurry vision, epistaxis, unusual weight gain or loss, chest pain, flushing, fatigue
- UTIs can be associated with reflux nephropathy and hypertension.
- Gross hematuria, edema, fatigue may suggest renal disease.
- Birth history: Umbilical artery catheterization
- Medications: Corticosteroids, cold preparations, oral contraceptives, illicit drugs
- Family history: Hypertension, diabetes, obesity, familial endocrinopathies, renal disease
- Trauma: Arteriovenous (AV) fistula, traction
- Review of symptoms: Sleep apnea, obesity

PHYSICAL EXAM

- BP:
  - Children >3 years should have their BP measured during a health care episode
  - Child should be seated quietly for 5 minutes, feet on the floor with the right arm supported at the level of the heart. Routine BPs pressures are measured in the arm.
  - Use the proper cuff size. The inflatable bladder should completely encircle the arm and cover ~80–100% of the upper arm. A cuff that is inappropriately small will artificially increase the measurement.
  - Elevated BPs obtained by oscillometric devices should be repeated by auscultation.
  - When hypertension is confirmed, BP should be measured in both arms and in a leg. Normally, BP is 10–20 mm Hg higher in the legs. If leg BP is lower than arm, consider coarctation of the aorta.
- Tachycardia in hyperthyroidism, pheochromocytoma
- Body habitus: Thin, obese, growth failure, virilized, stigmata of Turner or Williams syndromes
- Skin: Café au lait spots, neurofibromas, rashes, acanthosis, malar rash
- Head/Neck: Moon facies, thyromegaly
- Eyes: Funduscopic changes, proptosis
- Lungs: Rales
- Heart: Rub, gallop, murmur
- Abdomen: Mass, hepatosplenomegaly, bruit
- Genitalia: Ambiguous, virilized, femoral pulses
- Neurologic: Bell's palsy

DIAGNOSTIC TESTS & INTERPRETATION

Lab

- The laboratory evaluation to determine the cause of hypertension should proceed in a stepwise fashion.
- Patients should have the following: Urinalysis, urine culture; serum electrolytes, blood urea nitrogen, creatinine, calcium, cholesterol; CBC; ECG, echocardiogram (the most sensitive study to monitor end-organ changes); renal ultrasound; retinal exam
- Further evaluation is based on history, physical exam, and/or to prove secondary causes: Voiding cystourethrogram, DMSA renal scan, 3D CT angiogram, MRA, urine or plasma for catecholamines and metanephrines, plasma renin activity, aldosterone levels
- More invasive studies include renal angiogram; renal vein renin concentrations; MIBG scan; renal biopsy; genetic studies to identify rare causes of hypertension

Diagnostic Procedures/Other

Ambulatory BP monitoring refers to a procedure in which a portable BP device, worn by the patient, records BP over a specified period, usually 24 hours. Ambulatory BP monitoring may be helpful in cases assessing in which the diagnosis of hypertension is uncertain (white coat hypertension and masked hypertension, labile hypertension, effectiveness of antihypertensive agents and children at high risk of cardiovascular disease; e.g., diabetes mellitus, chronic kidney disease, labile hypertension).

DIFFERENTIAL DIAGNOSIS

The initial objective after diagnosing hypertension in children is distinguishing primary from secondary causes. Generally, the younger the child and more elevated the BP measurements, the more likely the cause of hypertension is secondary.

TREATMENT

MEDICATION (DRUGS)

- Classes of antihypertensive agents include α- and β-blockers, diuretics, vasodilators (direct and calcium channel blockers), ACE inhibitors, and angiotensin receptor blockers (ARB).
- Therapy should be initiated with a single drug.
- Avoid multiple medications with the same mechanism of action.
- Elicit a history of adverse effects and adjust medications accordingly.
- Specific classes should be used with concurrent medical conditions: ACE inhibitors or ARBs in children with diabetes and microalbuminuria or proteinuric renal diseases; β-blockers or calcium channel blockers with migraine headaches.
- Certain classes of medication should be avoided in patients with specific conditions, such as asthma and diabetes (β-blockers) and bilateral renal artery stenosis (ACE inhibitors).
- ACE inhibitors are associated with congenital malformations and are contraindicated during pregnancy; calcium channel blockers and β-blockers are alternatives.

ADDITIONAL TREATMENT
General Measures

- If BP is >95th percentile, it should be repeated on 2 more occasions.
- If BP is >99th percentile plus 5 mm Hg, prompt referral for evaluation and therapy should be made.
- If the patient is symptomatic, immediate referral and treatment are indicated.
- Mild primary hypertension may be managed with nonpharmacologic treatment: Weight reduction, exercise, sodium restriction, avoidance of certain medications such as pseudoephedrine.
- Pharmacologic therapy should be directed to the cause of secondary hypertension when this is known or for severe, sustained hypertension.
- Medications may be needed in children with mild-to-moderate hypertension if nonpharmacologic therapy has failed, or if end-organ changes are present or diabetes is present.

Additional Therapies
- Regular aerobic physical activity (30–60 minutes several days a week)
- Limitation of sedentary activities to <2 hours per day
- Patients with uncontrolled stage 2 hypertension should be restricted from high-static competitive sports until the BP is in normal range.

COMPLEMENTARY & ALTERNATIVE THERAPIES
Dialysis may be needed for hypertension in chronic renal failure.

SURGERY/OTHER PROCEDURES
Surgical correction of renovascular hypertension and coarctation of the aorta. Percutaneous transluminal angioplasty has been used for renal artery stenosis.

IN-PATIENT CONSIDERATIONS
Initial Stabilization
- Hypertensive emergencies should be treated with IV blood pressure medications, aiming to decrease the BP by 25% over the 1st 8 hours and gradually normalizing BP over 24–48 hours.
- Hypertensive urgencies can be treated by either IV or PO antihypertensives depending on symptomatology.

Admission Criteria
- Hypertensive emergencies should be admitted to the ICU if indicated.
- Hypertensive urgencies should be admitted to the hospital.

ONGOING CARE

FOLLOW-UP RECOMMENDATIONS
Patient Monitoring
The reduction of BP with medication should be gradual to avoid side effects. The medications themselves cause adverse effects, such as exercise intolerance (β-blockers), headaches (vasodilators), renal insufficiency or hyperkalemia (ACE inhibitors), or hypokalemia (diuretics).

DIET
- Dietary increase in fresh vegetables, fresh fruits, potassium, fiber, and nonfat dairy
- Restriction of sodium, calories, saturated fat, and refined sugar

PATIENT EDUCATION
- Diet:
  - Increase in fresh vegetables, fresh fruits, fiber, and nonfat dairy
  - Restriction of sodium and calories
- Activity:
  - Regular aerobic physical activity (30–60 minutes several days a week)
  - Limitation of sedentary activities to <2 hours per day
- Prevention:
  - Avoidance of excess weight gain, smoking, and alcohol use; regular physical activity

PROGNOSIS
The patient's prognosis depends on the underlying cause of the hypertension. It is excellent if the BP is well controlled.

COMPLICATIONS
- CHF
- Renal failure
- Encephalopathy
- Retinopathy

ADDITIONAL READING

- Demorest, et al. Athletic participation by children and adolescents who have systemic hypertension. *Pediatrics*. 2010;125:1287–1294.
- Feld LG, Corey H. Hypertension in childhood. *Pediatr Rev*. 2007;28(8):283–298.
- Flynn JT. Pediatric hypertension: Recent trends and accomplishments, future challenges. *Am J Hypertens*. 2008;21(6):605–612.

- McCrindle B. Assessment and management of hypertension in children and adolescents. *Nat Rev Cardiol*. 2010;7:155–163.
- National Heart, Lung, and Blood Institute. The fourth report on the diagnosis, evaluation and treatment of high blood pressure in children and adolescents. *Pediatrics*. 2004;114(2):S555–S576.
- Portman R, Sorof J, Ingelfinger J, eds. *Pediatric hypertension*. New Jersey: Humana Press Inc., 2004.
- Suresh S, Mahajan P, Kamat D. Emergency management of pediatric hypertension. *Clin Pediatr*. 2005;44:739–745.
- Varda N, Gregoric A. A diagnostic approach for the child with hypertension. *Pediatr Nephrol*. 2005; 20:499–506.

CODES

ICD9
- 401.9 Essential hypertension (unspecified)
- 405.99 Other unspecified secondary hypertension

ICD10
- I10 Essential (primary) hypertension
- I15.9 Secondary hypertension, unspecified

FAQ

- Q: What is the value of ambulatory BP monitoring?
- A: This device is similar to a Holter monitor and measures BPs over a 24-hour period while the patient is awake and asleep. By reviewing the BPs, one can determine if a significant proportion of readings are elevated and whether or not the normal dip in pressures during sleep is seen. Thus, conditions such as white coat hypertension can be verified or discounted.
- Q: What are the indications for invasive studies, such as angiography?
- A: This decision should be individualized and based on the severity of the hypertension, response to medication, the clinical presentation (e.g., neurofibromatosis), and results of other studies. In general, young children and all children with severe, unexplained hypertension should be completely evaluated.
- Q: Can adolescents with elevated BP compete in sports?
- A: Adolescents with hypertension should be encouraged to participate in athletics if their BP is well controlled. The use of stress testing in this population is controversial.
- Q: Do I need to worry about isolated systolic hypertension?
- A: Studies in adults have shown that sustained systolic hypertension may be just as important as diastolic hypertension.

H

HYPOGAMMAGLOBULINEMIA

Timothy Andrews

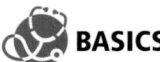 **BASICS**

DEFINITION
Humoral immunodeficiency signified by low or absent immunoglobulin levels, as compared with age-matched controls, and defective specific antibody production

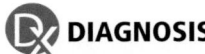 **DIAGNOSIS**

DIFFERENTIAL DIAGNOSIS
- **Selective IgA deficiency**
  - For details, refer to the topics "Common Variable Immunodeficiency (CVID)" and "Immunoglobulin A Deficiency."
- **X-linked agammaglobulinemia (Bruton agammaglobulinemia)**
  - Intrinsic defect in B-cell maturation due to mutations in the gene on the X chromosome encoding a B-cell-associated tyrosine kinase is involved in cytoplasmic signal transduction.
  - All immunoglobulin isotypes significantly decreased or absent
  - Significant reduction or absence of B cells
  - Bacterial infections caused by pyogenic encapsulated organisms such as *Staphylococcus aureus*, *Streptococcus pneumoniae*, *Haemophilus influenzae*, and *Pseudomonas* species
  - Recurrent respiratory tract infections including otitis, sinusitis, bronchitis, and pneumonia
  - Associated complications include arthritis of the large joints, chronic meningoencephalitis due to echoviruses, chronic diarrhea due to *Giardia lamblia*, inflammatory bowel disease, neutropenia, autoimmune hemolytic anemia, dermatomyositis, and an increased incidence of lymphoreticular malignancies.
  - Patients are also susceptible to viral infections, particularly enterovirus; live viral vaccines are contraindicated in these patients because some patients have vaccine-associated poliomyelitis.
  - Autosomal recessive agammaglobulinemia
  - Similar phenotype to X-linked agammaglobulinemia
  - Hyper-IgM syndrome
- **X-linked hyper IgM: Hyper IgM syndrome type**
  - Defect is caused by mutations in the gene encoding the CD40 ligand surface molecule on T cells. This leads to defective T-cell signaling for B-cell immunoglobulin class switching.
  - Normal to elevated IgM levels with low to absent IgG, IgA, and IgE
  - Recurrent upper respiratory tract infections, otitis, pneumonia, sinusitis
  - Associated complications include autoimmune hemolytic anemia/thrombocytopenia/neutropenia, opportunistic infections with *Pneumocystis carinii*, and lymphoproliferative disease.
- **CD40 mutation: Hyper IgM syndrome type 3**
  - Type I integral membrane glycoprotein encoded by gene chromosome 20 defect results in defective B-cell class switching.
  - Autosomal recessive form of hyper IgM clinically similar to X-linked hyper IgM

- **Activation-dependent cytidine deaminase mutation: Hyper IgM syndrome type 2**
  - Activation-dependent cytidine deaminase is an RNA-editing enzyme encoded by a gene on chromosome 12p13 expressed in germinal center B cells.
  - Deficiency causes impaired terminal differentiation of B cells and failure of isotype switching.
  - Extreme elevation of IgM with low to absent IgG, IgA, and IgE
  - Lymphoid hyperplasia, unlike X-linked hyper IgM in which there is minimal lymphoid tissue
  - Older at age of onset
  - No susceptibility to *P. carinii*
- **Transient hypogammaglobulinemia of infancy**
  - Difficult to differentiate this from the normal physiologic nadir of IgG that occurs between 3 and 6 months of age owing to the loss of maternally derived immunoglobulin. This nadir is normally short-lived.
  - Affected infants have abnormally prolonged delay in the onset of their own immunoglobulin production to compensate for this nadir.
  - Cause is unknown.
  - Self-limited; most infants recover by 18–36 months
  - Clinical course is typically benign. Therapy with IV immunoglobulin should be considered only in infants with severe recurrent infections.
  - This syndrome is frequently seen in infants with a familial history of severe combined immunodeficiency or other immunodeficiencies.
- **Selective IgG subclass deficiency (the 4 subclasses of IgG, in decreasing order of serum levels: IgG1, IgG2, IgG3, and IgG4)**
  - Total serum IgG levels can be normal even when 1 subclass is low or absent.
  - Deficiency of IgG3 is most common in adults, whereas deficiency of IgG2 is seen more frequently in children.
  - IgG2 deficiency has been associated with an inability to respond to polysaccharide antigens.
  - Clinical significance of IgG subclass deficiency has not been fully defined. Many patients have an increased frequency of upper and lower respiratory tract infections, whereas others are asymptomatic.
  - No consensus on standard therapy for these patients in regard to replacement IV immunoglobulin
- **Kappa-chain deficiency**
  - Absence of the kappa subtype of light chains in immunoglobulin molecules
  - Described in 2 families
  - Associated with variable defects in specific antibody formation
- **Immunodeficiency with thymoma**
  - Seen in adults, typically between 40 and 70 years
  - Associated with significantly decreased to absent IgG, IgA, and IgM
  - Secondary causes of hypogammaglobulinemia

- **Viruses**
  - Epstein–Barr virus
  - Cytomegalovirus
  - Congenital rubella
  - Mechanism by which antibody responses and immunoglobulin production are altered in infected patients is not clearly defined.
- **Infectious mononucleosis**
  - Has been associated with defective specific antibody responses to neoantigens and impaired in vitro B-cell function in normal individuals. These defects are transient and resolve within 6–8 weeks after the onset of the disease.
  - A disastrous response to Epstein–Barr virus infection is seen in X-linked lymphoproliferative syndrome. These patients develop fatal infectious mononucleosis, marrow aplasia, B-cell lymphoma, and agammaglobulinemia.
  - HIV, cytomegalovirus, and rubella infections have been associated with abnormal specific antibody responses.
- **Drugs**
  - Immunosuppressive/chemotherapeutic agents, phenytoin-associated defects in immune function and antibody production usually resolve after therapy is discontinued.
- **Other**
  - Protein-losing enteropathy
  - Intestinal lymphangiectasia
  - Nephrotic syndrome
  - The hypogammaglobulinemia is due to direct loss through the GI tract or kidneys.
  - Lymphoreticular malignancies have been associated with various immune defects and decreased immunoglobulin production.

HISTORY
Detailed history for recurrent infection is key to evaluating suspected humoral immunodeficiency.
- **Question:** Humoral immunodeficiencies?
- *Significance*: Usually present with recurrent infections caused by encapsulated bacteria such as *H. influenzae* type B and *S. pneumoniae*
- **Question:** It is important to rule out hypogammaglobulinemia in patients with recurrent infections because replacement therapy with IV IgG is readily available.
- *Significance*:
  - Patients with hypogammaglobulinemia usually present after 3–6 months of age.
  - Late onset of infections may be more consistent with common variable immunodeficiency.
- **Question:** Recurrent severe infections such as meningitis, sepsis, and osteomyelitis?
- *Significance*: Some of the congenital immunodeficiency syndromes are signified by specific infections such as chronic meningoencephalitis with echoviruses, vaccine-associated poliomyelitis, and *P. carinii* pneumonia.
- **Question:** Familial history of immunodeficiencies?
- *Significance*: Previously affected males suggest an X-linked inheritance pattern.

- **Question:** Early infant deaths due to overwhelming infection?
- *Significance:* May indicate a previously undiagnosed congenital immunodeficiency. Many of the congenital immunodeficiencies have associated arthritis, autoimmune disease, chronic lung disease, and GI manifestations.

PHYSICAL EXAM
Patients should be examined for signs of acute and chronic infections.
- **Finding:** Growth parameters?
- *Significance:* Children with significant, recurrent infections and GI disease related to immunodeficiency may present with failure to thrive.
- **Finding:** Signs of chronic otitis media or conjunctival recurrent disease?
- *Significance:* Patients with X-linked agammaglobulinemia frequently have signs of chronic conjunctivitis.
- **Finding:** Gingivitis and stomatitis?
- *Significance:* May occur with the neutropenia-associated hypogammaglobulinemia syndromes
- **Finding:** Lymphoid tissue?
- *Significance:* Absence of tonsillar tissue and palpable lymph nodes is suggestive of X-linked agammaglobulinemia.
- **Finding:** Lymphadenopathy and tonsillar hypertrophy?
- *Significance:*
  – Can be seen in hyper-IgM syndrome and common variable immunodeficiency
  – Persistently enlarged nodes should be investigated.
- **Finding:** Wheezes, rales?
- *Significance:* May signify acute pneumonia or chronic lung disease
- **Finding:** Hepatosplenomegaly or masses?
- *Significance:*
  – May be seen in hyper-IgM syndrome and common variable immunodeficiency
  – Abdominal masses should be investigated promptly to rule out malignancy.
- **Finding:** Arthritis, clubbing?
- *Significance:*
  – Arthritis can be seen in patients with X-linked agammaglobulinemia and common variable immunodeficiency.
  – Clubbing can be seen in the presence of chronic lung disease or bronchiectasis.

DIAGNOSTIC TESTS & INTERPRETATION
- **Test:** CBC with differential
- *Significance:* Autoimmune hemolytic anemia, neutropenia, and thrombocytopenia can be seen in X-linked agammaglobulinemia, hyper-IgM, and common variable immunodeficiency.
- **Test:** Quantitative immunoglobulin levels
- *Significance:*
  – Each isotype should be measured (IgG, IgA, IgM, IgE).
  – Normal or elevated IgM level in face of low to absent IgG, IgA is characteristic of hyper-IgM syndrome.

- **Test:** Serial testing of immunoglobulins
- *Significance:* Should be done in infants suspected of transient hypogammaglobulinemia to document subsequent normalization of immunoglobulin levels
- **Test:** Qualitative antibody levels
- *Significance:*
  – Isohemagglutinins are primarily IgM antibodies to the main blood groups.
  – Should be present in normal patients, but will be absent in patients with AB blood type
  – Presence is inconstant in children <1 year of age.
- **Test:** Antibody titers to tetanus, diphtheria, *S. pneumoniae*, and *H. influenzae* type B measured postvaccination
- *Significance:* Ability to mount a protective antibody response to childhood vaccinations may indicate a less severe clinical course in hypogammaglobulinemia.
- **Test:** B-cell enumeration
- *Significance:*
  – Number of peripheral B cells will be decreased to absent in X-linked agammaglobulinemia and in autosomal-recessive agammaglobulinemia.
  – Usually normal in other hypogammaglobulinemia syndromes
- **Test:** Total lymphocyte count
- *Significance:* T-lymphocyte number and function are normal.

Imaging
Chest and sinus radiography and CT scans:
- May be helpful in evaluating for acute and chronic disease
- Bronchiectasis can be a long-term sequela of chronic pulmonary infection.

 # TREATMENT

ADDITIONAL TREATMENT
General Measures
- Prompt and appropriate antibiotic therapy is an important part of routine treatment.
- May be a role for prophylactic antibiotics in patients with persistent recurrent infections
- Replacement therapy with IV immunoglobulin is the primary therapeutic modality for X-linked agammaglobulinemia, hyper-IgM syndrome, and common variable immunodeficiency.
  – Usual initiating doses are 200–400 mg/kg every 3–4 weeks.
  – Nadir IgG levels should be >300 mg/dL.

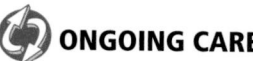 # ONGOING CARE

PROGNOSIS
Therapy is usually lifelong in patients with documented humoral immunodeficiency.

> **ALERT**
> Patients receiving IV immunoglobulin therapy should not receive routine vaccinations; they are passively immunized with the therapy.

ADDITIONAL READING
- Chinen J, Shearer WT. Advances in basic and clinical immunology in 2009. *J Allergy Clin Immunol.* 2010;125:563–568.
- Conley ME, Rohrer J, Minegishi Y. X-linked agammaglobulinemia. *Clin Rev Allergy Immunol.* 2000;19:183–204.
- Huston DP, Kavanaugh AF, Rohane PW, et al. Immunoglobulin deficiency syndromes and therapy. *J Allergy Clin Immunol.* 1991;87:1–17.
- Ochs HD, Smith CI. X-linked agammaglobinemia: A clinical and molecular analysis. *Medicine.* 1996; 75:287–299.
- Schaffer FM, Ballow M. Immunodeficiency: The office work-up. *J Respir Dis.* 1995;16:523–541.
- Skull S, Kemp A. Treatment of hypogammaglobulinemia with intravenous immunoglobulin, 1973–93. *Arch Dis Child.* 1996;74:527–530.
- Vale AM, Schroeder HW. Clinical consequences of defects in b-cell development. *J Allergy Clin Immunol.* 2010;125:778–787.
- Woroniecka M, Ballow M. Office evaluation of children with recurrent infection. *Pediatr Clin North Am.* 2000;47:1211–1224.

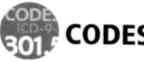 ## CODES

ICD9
- 279.00 Hypogammaglobulinemia, unspecified
- 279.01 Selective IgA immunodeficiency
- 279.06 Common variable immunodeficiency

ICD10
- D80.0 Hereditary hypogammaglobulinemia
- D80.1 Nonfamilial hypogammaglobulinemia
- D80.2 Selective deficiency of immunoglobulin A [IgA]

FAQ
- Q: When should I make a referral?
- A: Refer any patient suspected of having a primary humoral immunodeficiency to a specialist in allergy and immunology. These are patients with chronic disease who require prolonged follow-up and good communication between the referring physician and specialist.

H

HYPOPARATHYROIDISM

Adda Grimberg

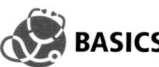 **BASICS**

DESCRIPTION
Hypoparathyroidism is decreased parathyroid hormone (PTH) effect.

EPIDEMIOLOGY
- Many normal neonates can have hypocalcemia (serum calcium >8 mg/dL) during the 1st 3 weeks of life owing to physiologic transient hypoparathyroidism.
- Parathyroid gland immaturity can lead to deficient PTH release and exaggerated normal fall in serum calcium concentration during the 1st 3 days of life.
- Relative immaturity of renal phosphorus handling and response to PTH can lead to late neonatal hypocalcemia precipitated by a high-phosphate diet (cow's milk-based formulas).
- Following total thyroidectomy, 10% of patients develop transient hypoparathyroidism, and of these, less than half remain with permanent hypoparathyroidism.

RISK FACTORS
Genetics
- X-linked recessive: Neonatal onset
- Autosomal dominant and autosomal recessive forms:
  - Chromosome 3q13: Activating mutations in the calcium-sensing receptor (CaSR) gene
  - Chromosome 6p23-24: Homozygous loss of function of GCMB gene (transcription factor required for parathyroid gland embryology)
  - Chromosome 10p15: GATA3 gene mutations cause dominantly inherited familial hypoparathyroidism, sensorineural deafness, and renal anomaly ([HDR] syndrome).
  - Chromosome 11p: Mutations in the PTH gene
  - Chromosome 22q11: DiGeorge syndrome
  - Chromosome 21q22 (AIRE gene): Type 1 polyglandular autoimmune disease; some cases of chronic hypoparathyroidism without associated Addison disease or chronic candidiasis
  - Chromosome 20q13: Albright hereditary osteodystrophy
- Mitochondria diseases: Kearns-Sayre syndrome (progressive external ophthalmoplegia before age 20 years and pigmentary retinal degeneration, frequently with other organ system involvement including cardiac, neurologic, and hypoparathyroidism)

PATHOPHYSIOLOGY
Diminished or absent PTH activity results in:
- Hypocalcemia and hyperphosphatemia
- Reduced vitamin D activation to 1,25(OH)2-vitamin D
- Hypocalcemia leads to increased neural excitability.

COMMONLY ASSOCIATED CONDITIONS
- Transient:
  - Fetal parathyroid suppression: Maternal hypercalcemia, diabetic mother
  - Hypomagnesemia: Direct effects (suppressed PTH secretion, increased PTH resistance)
  - Alcohol intoxication
  - Congenital
  - Familial: X-linked recessive, autosomal dominant, autosomal recessive
  - Sporadic and isolated
  - DiGeorge syndrome: Parathyroid gland hypoplasia, thymic hypoplasia/aplasia, facial abnormalities, aortic arch and cardiac defects, and neuropsychiatric disorders including speech difficulties, learning disabilities, and high risk for developing psychotic disorders including schizophrenia
- Acquired:
  - Postsurgical
  - Postirradiation
  - Following severe burns
  - Type 1 polyglandular autoimmune disease (Blizzard syndrome): Hypoparathyroidism associated with chronic mucocutaneous candidiasis and autoimmune adrenal insufficiency; can also have diabetes mellitus, lymphocytic thyroiditis, hypogonadism, pernicious anemia, chronic hepatitis
  - Iron deposition: Thalassemia, hemochromatosis
  - Copper deposition: Wilson disease
  - Metastatic carcinoma
  - Miliary tuberculosis
- Pseudohypoparathyroidism: Resistance to PTH:
  - Albright hereditary osteodystrophy: G-protein mutation

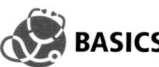 **DIAGNOSIS**

HISTORY
- In neonates: Maternal calcium and magnesium abnormalities, maternal diabetes
- Family history of calcium disorders
- Medications
- Recurrent infections
- Recurrent muscle cramps
- Paresthesias

PHYSICAL EXAM
- Chvostek sign: Facial nerve stimulation (tapping anterior of external auditory meatus) causes contraction of orbicularis oris, producing upper lip or mouth twitch.
- Trousseau sign: Inflation of BP cuff reduces the blood flow to peripheral motor nerves and thereby can elicit carpopedal spasm in latent tetany.
- Carpopedal spasm
- Laryngeal stridor
- Mental status changes
- Irritability
- Papilledema

- Cataracts
- Bradycardia, hypotension
- Dry skin, coarse hair, brittle nails
- Albright hereditary osteodystrophy (pseudohypoparathyroidism type Ia): Short stature, round face, thick neck, barrel chest, obesity, subcutaneous calcifications, brachydactyly (short 4th metacarpal bones)

DIAGNOSTIC TESTS & INTERPRETATION
Lab
- Total and ionized serum calcium concentrations: Low
  - False positives: Hypomagnesemia
- Serum phosphorus concentration: Elevated in hypoparathyroidism; low in rickets
- Serum magnesium concentration: Rule out hypomagnesemia.
- Albumin: Assess calcium binding (if cannot get ionized calcium).
- Intact PTH levels
- 25-OH- and 1,25(OH)2-vitamin D levels: Distinguish hypoparathyroidism from rickets.
- Urinary calcium/creatinine ratio: Low in idiopathic hypoparathyroidism, higher (almost equal to normocalcemic controls) in calcium ion-sensing receptor gain-of-function mutations
- Urinary cyclic AMP response to PTH: Diagnostic test if concerned about pseudohypoparathyroidism; otherwise, not routinely done

Imaging
- Chest radiograph: Rachitic rosary (rickets), absence of thymus (DiGeorge syndrome)
- Head CT: Intracranial calcifications are associated with chronic hypoparathyroidism and pseudohypoparathyroidism.

DIFFERENTIAL DIAGNOSIS
Hypocalcemia:
- Vitamin D deficiency
- Vitamin D-dependent rickets type I and II
- Hyperphosphatemia
- Prematurity
- Acute pancreatitis
- Malignancy: Osteoblastic metastases, tumor lysis syndrome
- Medication: Citrated blood products, phenobarbital, Dilantin, phosphate

TREATMENT

MEDICATION (DRUGS)

- Titer therapy to maintain serum calcium concentrations >8.0 mg/dL. In cases requiring lifelong therapy, compromise for serum calciums in the 8–9-mg/dL range to decrease the long-term risk for developing nephrocalcinosis:
  - 1,25(OH)2-vitamin D: <1 year: 0.04–0.08 mcg/kg/d; 1–5 years: 0.25–0.75 mcg/d; >6 years and adults: 0.5–2 mcg/d
  - Calcium: Dose depends on preparation and on patient needs.
  - A recent 3-year randomized trial comparing twice-daily calcitriol (plus calcium and cholecalciferol in four daily doses) versus subcutaneous synthetic human PTH-(1–34) treatment in 12 children with chronic hypoparathyroidism (and without severe renal or hepatic insufficiency) showed stable calcium homeostasis and normal bone mineral accrual, linear growth, and weight gain with both treatments.
  - Duration: For life
- Activating mutations in the calcium sensor are treated with thiazide diuretics and hydration.

ONGOING CARE

FOLLOW-UP RECOMMENDATIONS
Patient Monitoring
- Regularly with the endocrinologist
- When to expect improvement: Immediately
- Signs to watch for:
  - Patients with acute, severe hypocalcemia should be placed on telemetry to monitor for cardiac arrhythmias (especially prolonged QTc)
  - Muscle cramps
  - Carpedal spasms
  - Seizures

DIET
Unrestricted

PROGNOSIS
Fair; long-term outcome: Development of nephrocalcinosis resulting in renal insufficiency

COMPLICATIONS
- Hypocalcemia can cause tetany, arrhythmias, seizures, and respiratory arrest.
- Long-standing untreated hypoparathyroidism and pseudohypoparathyroidism can lead to intracranial calcifications, especially in the basal ganglia. These may cause extrapyramidal signs (e.g., choreoathetosis, dystonic spasms, parkinsonism). Cognitive impairment and psychiatric disturbances can also be seen.
- Untreated hypoparathyroidism can also lead to dilated cardiomyopathy, which improves with restoration of normocalcemia.

ADDITIONAL READING

- Cervato S, Morlin L, Albergoni MP, et al. AIRE gene mutations and autoantibodies to interferon omega in patients with chronic hypoparathyroidism without APECED. *Clin Endocrinol (Oxf)*. 2010;73:630–636.
- Gelfand IM, Eugster EA, DiMeglio LA. Presentation and clinical progression of pseudohypoparathyroidism with multi-hormone resistance and Albright hereditary osteodystrophy: A case series. *J Pediatr*. 2006;149:877–880.
- Herwadkar A, Gennery AR, Moran AS, et al. Association between hypoparathyroidism and defective T cell immunity in 22q11.2 deletion syndrome. *J Clin Pathol*. 2010;63:151–155.
- Hieronimus S, Bec-Roche M, Pedeutour F, et al. The spectrum of parathyroid gland dysfunction associated with the microdeletion 22q11. *Eur J Endocrinol*. 2006;155:47–52.
- Kemp EH, Gavalas NG, Krohn KJ, et al. Activating autoantibodies against the calcium-sensing receptor detected in two patients with autoimmune polyendocrine syndrome type 1. *J Clin Endocrinol Metab*. 2009;94:4749–4756.
- Klein GL, Langman CB, Herndon DN. Persistent hypoparathyroidism following magnesium repletion in burn-injured children. *Pediatr Nephrol*. 2000;14:301–304.
- Lima K, Følling I, Eiklid KL, et al. Age-dependent clinical problems in a Norwegian national survey of patients with the 22q11.2 deletion syndrome. *Eur J Pediatr*. 2010;169(8):983–989.
- Marx SJ. Hyperparathyroid and hypoparathyroid disorders. *N Engl J Med*. 2000;343:1863–1875.
- McKay CP, Portale A. Emerging topics in pediatric bone and mineral disorders 2008. *Semin Nephrol*. 2009;29:370–378.
- Perheentupa J. Autoimmune polyendocrinopathy-candidiasis-ectodermal dystrophy. *J Clin Endocrinol Metab*. 2006;91:2843–2850.
- Safford SD, Skinner MA. Thyroid and parathyroid disease in children. *Semin Pediatr Surg*. 2006;15:85–91.
- Shaw N. A practical approach to hypocalcaemia in children. *Endocr Dev*. 2009;16:73–92.
- Thakker RV. Genetic developments in hypoparathyroidism. *Lancet*. 2001;357:974–976.
- Winer KK, Sinaii N, Reynolds J, et al. Long-term treatment of 12 children with chronic hypoparathyroidism: A randomized trial comparing synthetic human parathyroid hormone 1–34 versus calcitriol and calcium. *J Clin Endocrinol Metab*. 2010;95:2680–2688.

CODES

ICD9
- 252.1 Hypoparathyroidism
- 775.4 Hypocalcemia and hypomagnesemia of newborn

ICD10
- E20.9 Hypoparathyroidism, unspecified
- E89.2 Postprocedural hypoparathyroidism
- P71.4 Transitory neonatal hypoparathyroidism

FAQ

- Q: Is the thyroid also involved?
- A: No
- Q: Are seizures common?
- A: Yes. Seizures are a common presentation of hypoparathyroidism in childhood, and physiologic transient hypoparathyroidism is the most common cause of neonatal seizures.
- Q: Can hypoparathyroidism be associated with other abnormalities?
- A: Yes. Investigate neonates at the time of diagnosis for cardiac defects and thymic aplasia (DiGeorge syndrome), and monitor patients with hypoparathyroidism for development of other autoimmune endocrinopathies and chronic mucocutaneous candidiasis (type 1 polyglandular autoimmune disease).
- Q: When should IV versus oral calcium supplementation be used?
- A: IV calcium supplementation provides the quickest correction of hypocalcemia and is therefore useful in severe cases (seizures, stridor, tetany, cardiac arrhythmias) or in the initiation of therapy (as you await establishment of adequate vitamin D levels, which are necessary for enteral calcium absorption). Switch to oral calcium supplementation as soon as possible to reduce the risk of potential IV calcium-mediated venous sclerosis and tissue extravasation.

H

HYPOPLASTIC LEFT HEART SYNDROME

Javier J. Lasa (5th edition)
Laura Mercer-Rosa

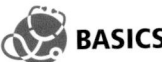 **BASICS**

DESCRIPTION
Hypoplastic left heart syndrome (HLHS) is a continuum of congenital cardiac defects resulting from severe underdevelopment of the structures on the left side of the heart (left atrium, mitral valve, left ventricle, aortic valve, and ascending aorta).

EPIDEMIOLOGY
Incidence
- 0.16–0.36 per 1,000 live births
- 8% of congenital heart disease (CHD); third most common cause of critical CHD in the newborn
- 23% of all neonatal mortality from CHD
- Familial inheritance: Sibling recurrence risk ranges from 8% to 21% with higher recurrence observed when cardiovascular malformations are present in either parent. In addition, rare kinships have a frequency approaching autosomal-dominant transmission.
- Comorbid forms of CHD (13.5%)
- Male predominance (67%)
- Increased mortality when associated with definable genetic disorders, which comprise 10–28% of HLHS patients:
  - Turner syndrome, Noonan syndrome, Smith-Lemli-Opitz syndrome, Holt-Oram syndrome
  - Trisomy 13, 18, 21, or other microdeletion syndromes
- Major extracardiac anomalies (diaphragmatic hernia, omphalocele)

PATHOPHYSIOLOGY
- The etiology of HLHS appears multifactorial, most likely resulting from an in utero reduction of left ventricular inflow or outflow (mechanisms postulated include premature closure of the foramen ovale and fetal cardiomyopathy).
- As a result, the right ventricle (RV) must supply both the pulmonary and systemic circulations (via the ductus arteriosus) before and after birth.
- The reduction in pulmonary vascular resistance that occurs with lung expansion at birth reduces the proportion of RV output to the systemic circulation. If the ductus arteriosus closes, shock occurs.

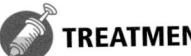 **DIAGNOSIS**

HISTORY
- Respiratory distress (tachypnea, grunting, flaring, retractions)
- Cyanosis
- Cardiovascular collapse and profound metabolic acidosis when the ductus arteriosus closes

PHYSICAL EXAM
- CHF secondary to pulmonary overcirculation (e.g., tachycardia, hepatomegaly, gallop)
- Normal S1 and single S2 (A2 absent); a murmur of tricuspid regurgitation may be auscultated.
- Varying degrees of cyanosis
- Decreased perfusion and weak peripheral pulses

DIAGNOSTIC TESTS & INTERPRETATION
Lab
- Chest radiograph: Varying degree of cardiomegaly with increased pulmonary vascular markings (if the atrial septum is intact or highly restrictive, lungs will appear hazy with a pulmonary venous obstructive pattern)
- EKG: Right axis deviation (+90 to +210 degrees), RV hypertrophy with a qR pattern in the right precordial leads, decreased left ventricular forces with an rS pattern in the left precordial leads
- Echocardiogram: Varying degrees of hypoplasia or atresia of the mitral valve, left ventricle, aortic valve, ascending aorta, and aortic arch; patent ductus arteriosus with right-to-left shunt in systole and diastolic flow reversal; atrial septal defect with left-to-right flow
- Cardiac catheterization: No longer routinely performed; similar findings as with echocardiography

DIFFERENTIAL DIAGNOSIS
- Cardiac: Other causes of circulatory collapse in the neonate include critical aortic stenosis and coarctation of the aorta, cardiomyopathy (infectious, metabolic, or hypoxic), persistent supraventricular tachycardia, obstructive cardiac neoplasms, and large arteriovenous fistulae.
- Noncardiac: Neonatal septicemia, respiratory distress syndrome, inborn errors of metabolism

TREATMENT

ADDITIONAL TREATMENT
General Measures
Supportive:
- Although surgical intervention has become the medical standard, supportive measures are sometimes offered, especially when multiple noncardiac congenital anomalies exist or when severe multiorgan system damage is present.
- The preoperative goal is to balance the systemic and pulmonary circulations provided by the RV to a Qp/Qs (ratio of pulmonary to systemic blood flow) of ~1:1, usually achieved with a pulse oximetry measurement of 75%.
- Prostaglandin E1 infusion: 0.05–0.1 mcg/kg/min.
- Aggressive treatment of metabolic acidosis with fluid boluses, bicarbonate, and/or tromethamine (THAM)
- 0.21 FiO_2, goal PaO_2 of 35–40 mm Hg.
- Careful use of small amounts of inotropic agents (in cases of sepsis or RV failure). Aggressive use of inotropic agents (alpha effect) may worsen systemic perfusion.

SURGERY/OTHER PROCEDURES
- Palliative surgery is generally performed in 3 stages:
  - Stage I (Norwood) palliation (performed in the first few days of life or soon after presentation): Involves transection of the main pulmonary artery with anastomosis of the augmented aortic arch to the pulmonary valve stump to form a neoaortic valve and arch, placement of an aorta-to-pulmonary artery shunt (modified Blalock-Taussig shunt), and often an atrial septectomy. The RV provides both systemic and pulmonary blood flows with post-operative saturations of ~75%.
  - Stage I Sano modification: Developed in 2003 as an alternative to the Norwood procedure, the Sano modification replaces the modified Blalock-Taussig shunt with an RV to pulmonary artery conduit with the RV continuing to supply both pulmonary and systemic circulations.
  - Hybrid Procedure: This recent alternative to the Norwood procedure utilizes both median sternotomy (pulmonary artery banding) and interventional cardiac catheterization (PDA stenting) to provide both systemic and pulmonary blood flow while avoiding cardiopulmonary bypass.
  - Stage II/Hemi-Fontan or bidirectional Glenn procedure: Involves anastomosis of the superior vena cava to the pulmonary artery, resulting in volume unloading of the RV. All prior shunts are usually removed. The oxygen saturations after this procedure are usually 85–90%.
  - Stage III/Modified Fontan procedure: Baffling the inferior vena cava to the pulmonary artery with placement of a small fenestration in the baffle, permitting a small residual right-to-left shunt. The RV is now supplying only systemic blood flow. The oxygen saturations after this procedure are usually 90–95%.

- There are many surgical modifications to these 3 procedures. In addition, these procedures may be performed at different ages based on an institution's experience. Our approach has been to perform the hemi-Fontan operation at 4–6 months of age and the Fontan operation at 18 months to 2 years of age.
- Orthotopic heart transplantation may be performed either as an initial approach or after a stage I palliation.

IN-PATIENT CONSIDERATIONS
Initial Stabilization
During initial resuscitation and stabilization of a newly diagnosed infant:

- Prostaglandin E1 therapy should be initiated as soon as possible to maintain ductal patency.
- Avoid using oxygen despite low pulse oximetry saturation. Increasing FiO_2 will lower pulmonary vascular resistance preferentially shunting cardiac output away from the systemic circulation towards the lungs, thereby worsening systemic perfusion.
- Should invasive ventilation be required, avoid hyper-ventilation. Permissive hypercapnia is preferred due to the secondary increase in pulmonary vascular resistance, and subsequent improvement in systemic perfusion. Maintain mildly elevated $PaCO_2$ levels (40–50 mm Hg).

Admission Criteria
The admission for the first operation usually lasts for about 3–4 weeks after birth. Patients are watched to ensure stable oxygen saturation and weight gain. Nutritional needs often require nasogastric tube feed supplementation.

 ## ONGOING CARE

FOLLOW-UP RECOMMENDATIONS
Patient Monitoring
Interval pediatric evaluations should include careful consideration of growth parameters, cardiovascular symptoms, and developmental milestones. Examinations should focus on the presence or absence of cyanosis, edema, pleural effusions, diarrhea, ascites, and arrhythmias.

- For patients after staged palliation, frequent echocardiograms and intermittent cardiac catheterizations may be needed to assess for:
  – RV dysfunction
  – Residual or recurrent aortic arch obstruction
  – Branch pulmonary artery narrowing
  – Venous collateral formation causing increased cyanosis
  – Protein-losing enteropathy
  – Sinus node dysfunction
  – Atrial arrhythmias
- For patients treated alternatively with heart transplantation, other lifelong issues should be addressed:
  – Graft rejection and/or coronary vasculopathy
  – Infection
  – Hypertension
  – Lymphoproliferative disease

- Follow-up medications:
  – Lifelong subacute bacterial endocarditis (SBE) prophylaxis (high-risk category)
  – Furosemide is generally administered until the hemi-Fontan.
  – Afterload reduction (i.e., angiotensin-converting enzyme inhibitors) may be used to reduce the workload on the heart at any stage.
  – Antiplatelet (aspirin) and anticoagulant (Coumadin) therapies are used by most physicians after stage I and later in the setting of the low-flow state of the cavopulmonary connection.
- For transplant patients, immunosuppressive regimens are managed differently according to institution preferences.

PROGNOSIS
- Fatal if untreated (95% mortality within the 1st month of life)
- In the current era, HLHS is often diagnosed prenatally, and improved outcomes may result from early diagnosis and prevention of the presentation as neonatal shock.
- 90% early survival after stage I palliation if treated in a timely fashion at experienced institutions
- 5% mortality at stage II hemi-Fontan (bidirectional cavopulmonary anastomosis) procedure
- Recently, 1% mortality at Fontan operation (with the addition of a fenestration to allow right-to-left shunting)
- Excluding infants who die waiting for a donor organ, the 5-year actuarial survival for either staged palliation (Fontan) or heart transplantation is similar, ~75%.

COMPLICATIONS
Neonatal presentation:

- Circulatory collapse with resultant metabolic acidosis
- Multiorgan system failure (i.e., necrotizing enterocolitis, renal failure, liver failure, CNS injury)

ADDITIONAL READING

- Alsoufi B, Bennetts J, Verma S, et al. New developments in the treatment of hypoplastic left heart syndrome. *Pediatrics.* 2007;119(1):109–117.
- Grossfeld P. Hypoplastic left heart syndrome: New insights. *Circ Res.* 2007;100(9):1246–1248.
- Mahle WT, Clancy RR, McGaurn SP, et al. Impact of prenatal diagnosis on survival and early neurologic morbidity in neonates with the hypoplastic left heart syndrome. *Pediatrics.* 2001;107:1277–1282.
- McClure CD, Johnston JK, Fitts JA, et al. Postmortem intracranial neuropathology in children following cardiac transplantation. *Pediatr Neurol.* 2006;35(2):107–113.
- Pigula FA, Vida V, Del Nido P, et al. Contemporary results and current strategies in the management of hypoplastic left heart syndrome. *Semin Thorac Cardiovasc Surg.* 2007;19(3):238–244.
- Stamm C, Friehs I, Duebenew L, et al. Long-term results of the lateral tunnel Fontan operation. *J Thorac Cardiovasc Surg.* 2001;121:28–41.
- Tabbutt S, Dominguez T, Ravishankar C, et al. Outcomes after the stage I reconstruction comparing the right ventricular to pulmonary artery conduit with the modified Blalock Taussig shunt. *Ann Thorac Surg.* 2005;80(5):1582–1590.
- Tworetzky W, McElhinney DB, Reddy VM, et al. Improved surgical outcome after fetal diagnosis of hypoplastic left heart syndrome. *Circulation.* 2001;103:1269–1273.
- Wernovsky G, Ghanayem N, Ohye RG, et al. Hypoplastic left heart syndrome: Consensus and controversies in 2007. *Cardiol Young.* 2007;17(Suppl 2):75–86.

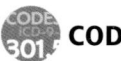 ## CODES

ICD9
746.7 Hypoplastic left heart syndrome

ICD10
Q23.4 Hypoplastic left heart syndrome

FAQ

- Q: What should the differential diagnosis include when an infant with hypoplastic left heart syndrome (HLHS) who has undergone stage I palliation presents with cyanosis and respiratory distress?
- A: Modified Blalock-Taussig shunt thrombosis, anemia, intercurrent lower respiratory tract infection leading to V/Q mismatch, low cardiac output state, sepsis.

  Infants with HLHS status post stage I palliation are solely dependent on the modified Blalock-Taussig shunt for pulmonary blood flow. This synthetic tube graft ranges from 3.5 to 4 mm in diameter and is prone to thrombosis, especially during periods of illness, which leads to dehydration (gastroenteritis), poor nutrition, or systemic inflammation.
- Q: Should there be a specific concern if a patient with HLHS who has completed the 3-stage palliation with Fontan procedure presents with complaints of unremitting diarrhea, crampy abdominal pain, ascites, and peripheral edema?
- A: Yes, protein-losing enteropathy (PLE) is a poorly understood disease process affecting patients with single ventricle after Fontan operation associated with significant morbidity and mortality. PLE is defined as the abnormal loss of serum proteins into the lumen of the GI tract and occurs in up to 11% of patients after Fontan palliation. Diuretic therapy and nutritional supplementation are often insufficient management strategies, frequently requiring the addition of somatostatic analogs (octreotide), sildenafil, and/or the creation of a fenestration in the Fontan circuit to palliate potentially elevated Fontan pressures.

H

HYPOSPADIAS

Douglas Canning
Matt Christman

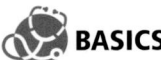 **BASICS**

DESCRIPTION
Hypospadias is the incomplete development of the anterior urethra due to the failure of the urethral folds to unite over and cover the urethral groove. Minor glanular hypospadias form from abnormal ingrowth of ectoderm from the glans to the corona.

EPIDEMIOLOGY
Incidence
- 1/250–1/300 live male births
- With affected father: 8%
- With affected brother: 14%
- With 2 or more affected family members: 21%
- Unexplained increase in incidence since the 1970s may be due to more diagnostic precision and awareness

RISK FACTORS
Genetics
- Increased incidence in monozygotic twins (8.5-fold greater than in singletons)
- Reported mutations include defects in the androgen receptor, 5α-reductase enzyme defects, alterations in homeobox genes, and variants of fibroblast growth factor, although these are found only in a minority of patients.

ETIOLOGY
- Polygenic/multifactorial
- Higher familial incidence
- Proposed theories include:
  - Estrogenic environmental contamination
  - Pressure of the fetal limbs on developing penis
  - Insufficient human chorionic gonadotropin (HCG) in placenta
  - Abnormality in androgen metabolism as a local manifestation of a systemic endocrinopathy

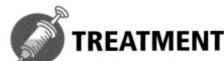 **DIAGNOSIS**

HISTORY
- Important to inquire about:
  - Other affected family members
  - Other congenital anomalies
- Increased incidence of cryptorchidism
- Consider workup for disorders of sexual differentiation (DSD) if cryptorchidism is found along with severe hypospadias
  - May be associated with an enlarged utricle, complicating urethral catheter placement
  - Severe hypospadias (perineal and penoscrotal) may have associated vesicoureteral reflux (VUR). No need to screen for VUR even in severe hypospadias.

PHYSICAL EXAM
- Incomplete foreskin
- Distal urethral pit on glans
- Ventral curvature of penis:
  - Localize meatal position by pulling outward on ventral penile shaft skin
  - Record position as glanular; coronal; distal, middle, or proximal shaft; penoscrotal; or perineal
  - Important to document position of testes
  - If testes impalpable, consider workup for disorder of sexual differentiation

DIAGNOSTIC TESTS & INTERPRETATION
Lab
Karyotype in patients with bilateral undescended testes and hypospadias; may also be obtained in cases of unilateral undescended testis and hypospadias.

Imaging
- If there is a question of ambiguous genitalia, pelvic ultrasound or cystography may be indicated.
- There is no need for imaging in cases of routine, isolated hypospadias.

DIFFERENTIAL DIAGNOSIS
Ambiguous genitalia, namely, XX disorder of sexual differentiation

TREATMENT

ADDITIONAL TREATMENT
General Measures
If the patient has a very small penis, he may benefit from hormonal stimulation with testosterone preoperatively.

> **ALERT**
> - Newborn circumcision is absolutely contraindicated.
> - Bilateral impalpable testes and hypospadias must be worked up to rule out salt-losing adrenogenital syndrome.

SURGERY/OTHER PROCEDURES

- Surgical repair:
  - Surgical repair is usually performed in the first 3–6 months of life.
  - Mild glanular hypospadias may not need surgery.
- Type of repair depends on position of meatus and degree of chordee:
  - Tubularized incised plate
  - Meatal advancement
  - Onlay island flap
  - Tubularized island flap
  - 90% success rate for distal repairs
  - Success rate may be less for proximal repairs.
- Potential complications include:
  - Urethrocutaneous fistula
  - Urethral diverticulum
  - Urethral stricture
  - Unacceptable cosmetic outcome

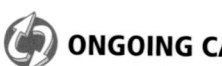 **ONGOING CARE**

FOLLOW-UP RECOMMENDATIONS

Patient Monitoring

- Compressive dressing for 2 days, removed by parents at home
- Indwelling urethral catheter/stent remains for about 2 weeks
- Postoperative visit at 2 weeks to remove catheter
- Longer term follow-up includes witness of urinary stream as toddler to identify fistula or recurrent curvature if present.

ADDITIONAL READING

- Baskin L. Hypospadias and urethra development. *J Urol.* 2000;163:951–956.
- Baskin LS, Ebbers MB. Hypospadias: Anatomy, etiology, and technique. *J Pediatr Surg.* 2006;41:463–472.
- Dolk H. Rise in prevalence of hypospadias. *Lancet.* 1998;351:770.
- Fisch M. Urethral reconstruction in children. *Curr Opin Urol.* 2001;11(3):253–255.
- Kalfa N, Sultan C, Baskin L. Hypospadias: Etiology and current research. *Urol Clin N Am.* 2010; 37:159–166.
- Kraft KH, Shukla AR, Canning DA. *Hypospadias. Urol Clin N Am.* 2010;37:167–181.
- Lambert SM, Snyder HM 3rd, Canning DA. The history of hypospadias and hypospadias repairs. *Urology.* 2011;77:1277–1283.
- Liu G, Yuan J, Feng J, et al. Factors affecting the long-term results of hypospadias repairs. *J Pediatr Surg.* 2006;41(3):554–559.
- Moriya K, Kakizaki H, Tanaka H, et al. Long-term cosmetic and sexual outcome of hypospadias surgery: Norm related study in adolescence. *J Urol.* 2006;176(4 Pt 2):1889–1892; discussion 1892–1893.
- Snodgrass WT, Shukla AR, Canning DA. Hypospadias. In: Docimo SG, Canning DA, Khoury AE, eds. The Kelalis-King-Belman textbook of clinical pediatric urology. London: Informa, 2007: 1205–1238.

 CODES

ICD9

752.61 Hypospadias

ICD10

- Q54.8 Other hypospadias
- Q54.9 Hypospadias, unspecified

FAQ

- Q: Does the patient with hypospadias routinely have other anatomic problems?
- A: No. The majority of patients with hypospadias have no other problems.
- Q: Why is there no need for routine imaging?
- A: Studies have been done and show that without symptoms or problems, patients with hypospadias have no other congenital problems.

H

IDIOPATHIC INTRACRANIAL HYPERTENSION (PSEUDOTUMOR CEREBRI)

Sabrina E. Smith
Dennis J. Dlugos

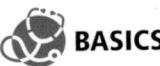 BASICS

DESCRIPTION
Diagnostic criteria of idiopathic intracranial hypertension (IIH) include:
- Signs and symptoms of increased intracranial pressure (e.g., headache, vomiting, ocular manifestations, and papilledema)
- Elevated cerebrocranial fluid pressure but otherwise normal CSF
- Normal neurologic exam except for papilledema (occasional abducens or other motor cranial neuropathy)
- Normal neuroimaging study (or incidental findings only)

EPIDEMIOLOGY
- Boys and girls are affected equally in childhood; in adulthood, more women than men are affected.
- IIH has been reported in patients as young as 4 months of age, with a median age of 9 years.

Incidence
Incidence in children is unknown.

RISK FACTORS
Genetics
Sporadic, no clear genetic predisposition, unless related to an underlying hormonal, toxic, or inflammatory condition; no data are available in children.

PATHOPHYSIOLOGY
Pathogenesis unknown, but may involve decreased CSF absorption owing to arachnoid villi dysfunction or elevated intracranial venous pressure. For example, obesity may lead to increased intra-abdominal, intrathoracic, and cardiac filling pressure, leading to elevated intracranial venous pressure.

ETIOLOGY
- Numerous precipitants of IIH have been reported. In adolescents, it is clearly associated with obesity and weight gain, but not clearly linked to obesity in children <11 years. Many weaker associations may be due to chance.
- IIH is often linked to minocycline, tetracycline, sulfonamides, isotretinoin, and thyroid replacements, and to corticosteroid withdrawal. It is also linked to vitamin A deficiency or intoxication, chronic anemia, and hypothyroidism.

COMMONLY ASSOCIATED CONDITIONS
- Visual loss due to optic nerve pressure
- Endocrinopathies, exogenous steroids, lead exposure, and therapy involving tetracycline and several other antibiotics may be associated with IIH.

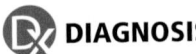 DIAGNOSIS

HISTORY
- Headache
- Blurred vision
- Transient visual darkening
- Stiff neck
- Pulsatile tinnitus
- Dizziness
- Infants and young children may present with irritability, somnolence, or ataxia.
- IIH should be considered in any child with chronic headache or unexplained visual changes.
- Directed history for signs of associated endocrinopathy, exposure to antibiotics or steroids, sinus infection, abnormal clotting, or familial tendency to thrombosis or visual disturbance

PHYSICAL EXAM
- Examination of the fundi is essential.
- Recording baseline visual acuity and visual fields in older children is essential.
- Papilledema is almost always present in older children with IIH.
- Most infants have some degree of papilledema, even with open fontanelles and split sutures.
- 6th cranial nerve (abducens) palsies are common in children with IIH; they were found in 29 of 68 patients in 1 series.
- Facial or other cranial nerve deficits rare

DIAGNOSTIC TESTS & INTERPRETATION
Lab
- CSF exam including opening pressure; cell count, glucose, and protein are essential and should be normal in IIH.
- CBC and thyroid function tests should be obtained because anemia, hypothyroidism, and hyperthyroidism have rarely been associated with IIH.
- The following may be useful in selected cases:
  - ANA test
  - ESR
  - Urine cortisol
  - Serum lead level
  - Serologic testing for Lyme disease

Imaging
Cranial CT or MRI should be normal. MRI is recommended because of superior imaging of brainstem, posterior fossa, and venous sinuses. Magnetic resonance venography is strongly suggested to evaluate for venous sinus thrombosis, which can be difficult to distinguish from IIH.

Diagnostic Procedures/Other
- Lumbar puncture manometry, with the patient in a relaxed lateral decubitus position, should show an opening pressure >280 mm H_2O.
- Goldmann perimeter visual field testing or computerized visual fields are useful in children >5 years to document field deficits and monitor response to therapy.

DIFFERENTIAL DIAGNOSIS
Some conditions may be confused with IIH, but the clinical picture and CSF analysis usually permit their distinction:
- Chronic meningitis (e.g., CNS, Lyme disease), encephalitis, or cerebral edema (may show minimal changes on neuroimaging with elevated CSF protein levels and little evidence of pleocytosis)
- Cerebral venous sinus thrombosis
- Chronic headache (common) with pseudopapilledema (optic nerve disc drusen)

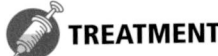 TREATMENT

MEDICATION (DRUGS)
First Line
- For patients with mild to moderate visual loss, acetazolamide, a carbonic anhydrase inhibitor that decreases CSF production, is the drug of choice:
  - The pediatric dosage is 60 mg/kg/d divided q.i.d. for the standard form and b.i.d. for the long-acting form (Diamox sequels).
  - The initial adult dose is 250 mg q.i.d. or 500 mg b.i.d., increased to 750 mg q.i.d. or 1,500 mg b.i.d. if tolerated.
- If visual loss, papilledema, and symptoms of pressure resolve, acetazolamide dosage can be tapered after 2 months of therapy.

Second Line
Furosemide can be used if acetazolamide is ineffective or has intolerable adverse effects.

ISSUES FOR REFERRAL
Follow-up and tapering of acetazolamide should be done in conjunction with a neurologist or neuro-ophthalmologist.

SURGERY/OTHER PROCEDURES
- Serial lumbar punctures are not recommended as standard therapy, although the initial puncture can be useful to relieve symptoms quickly.
- Surgical therapy (e.g., optic nerve sheath fenestration, lumboperitoneal shunt) is indicated for progressive visual loss despite medical therapy and may also be considered as an urgent intervention at presentation depending on degree of visual loss. Optic nerve sheath fenestration may be the preferred surgical treatment, especially in children, because of the high failure rates of lumboperitoneal shunting. High-dose IV steroids and acetazolamide therapy may be used while awaiting surgical therapy.

IN-PATIENT CONSIDERATIONS
Initial Stabilization
- The urgency of diagnosis and treatment depends on the severity of visual loss. Recent reports suggest that severe visual loss may progress rapidly, warranting close initial (weekly) tracking of vision and prompt consideration of surgical treatment (see below).
- For patients with no visual loss, removal of possible causative agents may be the only intervention needed, along with treatment of associated conditions (e.g., obesity, anemia, thyroid disease). Consider treatment with acetazolamide (Diamox; see later comment). Headache can be treated symptomatically if needed.

 ONGOING CARE

FOLLOW-UP RECOMMENDATIONS
Patient Monitoring
- Initially, patients should have visual acuity, visual fields, and fundi evaluated weekly or biweekly.
- If vision is stable, monthly visits may be adequate for 3–6 months.
- More frequent follow-up is required for any signs of progressive visual loss.
- IIH can recur. In one pediatric series, nearly 1/4 of patients had recurrence.
- Pitfalls: Children are not exempt from permanent visual loss as a consequence of IIH. Ophthalmologic follow-up is important. Occasional patients, especially adolescents, may experience headache weeks or months after resolution of objective signs of IIH (i.e., even though intracranial pressure has returned to normal).
- IIH may be diagnosed erroneously if:
  - Pseudopapilledema is mistaken for papilledema. (Pseudopapilledema is apparent optic disc swelling that simulates papilledema, but is usually secondary to an underlying benign process. It can be differentiated by an experienced ophthalmologist or neurologist.)
  - CSF abnormalities (i.e., isolated increase in protein) are overlooked.
  - Clinician fails to identify underlying cerebral venous sinus thrombosis.

ADDITIONAL READING
- Avery RA, Licht DJ, Shah SS, et al. CSF opening pressure in children with optic nerve head edema. *Neurology.* 2011;76(19):1658–1661.
- Friedman DI, Jacobson DM. Diagnostic criteria for idiopathic intracranial hypertension. *Neurology.* 2002;59:1492–1495.
- Lim M, Kurian M, Penn A, et al. Visual failure without headache in idiopathic intracranial hypertension. *Arch Dis Child.* 2005;90:206–210.
- Kesler A, Bassan H. Pseudotumor cerebri - idiopathic intracranial hypertension in the pediatric population. *Pediatr Endocrinol Rev.* 2006;3(4):387–392.
- Soiberman U, Stolovitch C, Balcer LJ, et al. Idiopathic intracranial hypertension in children: Visual outcome and recurrence risk. *Childs Nerv Syst.* 2011. Epub ahead of print.

 CODES

ICD9
348.2 Benign intracranial hypertension

ICD10
G93.2 Benign intracranial hypertension

FAQ
- Q: What are the side effects of acetazolamide?
- A: Side effects of acetazolamide include GI upset, paresthesias, loss of appetite, drowsiness, metabolic acidosis, and renal stones. An alternative is furosemide.
- Q: If IIH occurs on tetracycline, can the patient take penicillin?
- A: Penicillins/cephalosporins have not been reported as a significant cause of IIH.
- Q: Are there any limitations on physical activity?
- A: Activity can be graded entirely according to the child's symptoms.

I

IDIOPATHIC THROMBOCYTOPENIC PURPURA

Charles Bailey

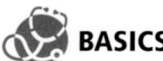 **BASICS**

DESCRIPTION
- Idiopathic thrombocytopenic purpura (ITP) is an autoimmune syndrome characterized by:
  - Isolated thrombocytopenia (platelet count <100,000/mm^3)
  - Shortened platelet survival
  - Presence of circulating platelet autoantibodies
  - Increased number of megakaryocytes in the bone marrow
- There are 3 types of ITP:
  - Acute ITP resolves (platelet count normal) within 6 months after diagnosis, without relapse.
  - Chronic ITP is defined by persistent thrombocytopenia >6 months after initial presentation.
  - Recurrent ITP exhibits an intermittent pattern of thrombocytopenia after an initial recovery to normal count.

EPIDEMIOLOGY
- Most common acquired platelet disorder in childhood
- Males and females are equally affected in childhood ITP (mild male predominance in younger children; female/male ratio is 3:1 in adult and chronic ITP).
- Median age at diagnosis is 4 years. Children <1 year or >10 years more likely to develop chronic ITP
- >70% of childhood ITP is acute (i.e., resolves within 6–12 months).
- Risk of severe bleeding is <5%.

Incidence
Incidence is 2–5/100,000 children per year (<15 years of age).

PATHOPHYSIOLOGY
- Thrombocytopenia results from increased destruction of antibody-coated platelets by phagocytic cells in the reticuloendothelial system, particularly the spleen.
- It is hypothesized that antibodies generated in response to foreign antigen or drug cross-react with platelet membrane glycoproteins (most commonly IIb/IIIa and Ib/IX). Multiple mechanisms of immune dysregulation have been implicated.
- Typical bone marrow aspirate shows increased numbers of immature megakaryocytes. However, some studies suggest that inhibition of thrombocytopoiesis limits ability to compensate for destruction.

COMMONLY ASSOCIATED CONDITIONS
- Autoimmune disorders (e.g., systemic lupus erythematosus [SLE], autoimmune lymphoproliferative syndrome [ALPS])
- HIV

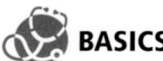 **DIAGNOSIS**

HISTORY
- Unusual bruising (with minor or no trauma, or in uncommon locations such as torso, neck, face), petechiae, epistaxis, or prolonged bleeding with minor trauma, gingival bleeding, hematuria, or hematochezia
- Ask about headache, abdominal or back pain, and any change in neurologic status.
- Onset is acute in an otherwise well child.
- Not associated with pallor, fatigue, weight loss, or persistent fevers
- 50% of cases are preceded by a viral infection 1–3 weeks before onset (particularly varicella; also Epstein-Barr virus, cytomegalovirus).
- Recent vaccination, especially live virus
- Drug history, focusing on drugs with antiplatelet effects (e.g., aspirin, seizure medications, heparin)
- Evidence of other autoimmune diseases (e.g., rheumatoid or collagen vascular symptoms, thyroid disease, hemolytic anemia)
- Family history is usually negative for bleeding disorders. Ask about family autoimmune disease.
- Risk factors for HIV should be elicited, because ITP-like thrombocytopenia may be a presentation of HIV in children.

PHYSICAL EXAM
- Clusters of petechiae or large or purple bruises readily apparent on skin or oropharynx
- Dried blood or clots in the nares
- Persistent slow bleeding from nares, gums, or wounds
- A funduscopic exam should be performed on all patients (retinal hemorrhage).

DIAGNOSTIC TESTS & INTERPRETATION
Lab
- Thrombocytopenia (typically <20,000/mm^3) with a normal WBC count and hemoglobin (mild anemia in proportion to amount of blood loss)
- Mean platelet volume may be increased.
- Peripheral blood smear should always be reviewed to differentiate platelet clumps from true thrombocytopenia. Smear will be otherwise normal, with no red cell fragmentation, no spherocytes, and no blasts.
- Prothrombin time and partial thromboplastin time are normal. Bleeding time will be prolonged, but testing is unnecessary.
- Direct antiglobulin test to exclude coexisting autoimmune RBC hemolysis (Evans syndrome)
- Antinuclear antibody (ANA) in subset of patients for whom causes of thrombocytopenia other than acute childhood ITP must be ruled out, including adolescents, especially girls, patients with chronic ITP, and those with suspicion of autoimmune disease

- HIV testing if risk factors are identified
- Bone marrow aspirate if anemia, abnormal WBC, leukemic blasts on peripheral smear, organomegaly, jaundice, or lymphadenopathy is present; otherwise controversial. It is safe to perform with a low platelet count.
- Most hematologists examine bone marrow before initiating corticosteroids.
- Marrow shows normal to increased numbers of megakaryocytes with otherwise normal morphology and cellularity.
- Assays for platelet-associated antibodies (either direct or indirect) are not routinely indicated.
- Demonstration of platelet-associated IgG may be useful in more complicated patients in whom chronic ITP is a possible diagnosis.
- *Helicobacter pylori* testing and treatment of infection may improve platelet recovery.

Imaging
As indicated by symptoms, particularly abdominal pain, headache, vision or focal neurologic change

DIFFERENTIAL DIAGNOSIS
- Consider other diagnoses if there is pallor, jaundice, adenopathy, bone pain, arthritis, or organomegaly (mild splenomegaly may occur in 5–10%).
- Destructive thrombocytopenias (normal or increased megakaryocytes in marrow):
  - Immunologic: ITP, infection (HIV, cytomegalovirus, Epstein-Barr virus, varicella zoster virus, parvovirus B19), drug induced, posttransfusion purpura, autoimmune hemolytic anemia (Evans syndrome), lymphoproliferative disorders, SLE, hyperthyroidism
  - Nonimmunologic: Microangiopathic hemolytic anemia, hemolytic uremic syndrome, disseminated intravascular coagulopathy (DIC), thrombotic thrombocytopenic purpura, Kasabach-Merritt syndrome (giant hemangioma), cardiac defects (left ventricular outflow obstruction, prosthetic heart valves, repaired intracardiac defects), malignant hypertension
- Impaired or ineffective production (decreased or absent megakaryocytes in marrow):
  - Marrow-infiltrative processes (leukemias, myelofibrosis, lymphomas, neuroblastoma, other solid tumor metastases, osteopetrosis, storage diseases)
  - Drug- or radiation-induced aplastic anemia, nutritional deficiency states (iron, folate, vitamin B$_{12}$)
  - Infection-associated suppression: Typically viral (e.g., hepatitis, Epstein-Barr virus, HIV, parvovirus B19), also severe or neonatal sepsis
  - Congenital disorders: Thrombocytopenia absent radii (TAR) syndrome, Fanconi anemia, trisomy 13 and 18, Bernard-Soulier syndrome, Wiskott-Aldrich syndrome, May-Hegglin anomaly, other inherited thrombocytopenias (X linked or autosomal dominant), metabolic disorders (e.g., methylmalonic acidemia)

TREATMENT

MEDICATION (DRUGS)

First Line

- IVIG: 94–97% will have an increase in platelet count >20,000/mm³ by 72 hours. The usual dose is 0.8–1 g/kg over 6–8 hours. Response typically peaks after 1 week and lasts 3–4 weeks:
  - Advantages: Faster time to platelet count >20,000/mm³ (24 hours), marrow aspirate may be deferred, helps confirm diagnosis
  - Disadvantages: High cost, long infusion time, allergic reactions, 10–30% have evidence of aseptic meningitis with severe headache and stiff neck, 50–75% have headache, nausea, vomiting, or fever
  - Routine acetaminophen and diphenhydramine prior to and for 24 hours after infusion may reduce acute side effects.
  - Subcutaneous administration has been used successfully as an alternative to IV infusion.
- Corticosteroids: 80% respond with platelet counts >20,000/mm³ by 72 hours (faster with high-dose pulse therapy). Oral prednisone at 2 mg/kg/d tapered over 2–4 weeks is typical:
  - Advantages: Ease of dosing (oral, outpatient), low cost, often longer duration of response
  - Disadvantages: Most pediatric hematologists require a bone marrow aspirate before steroid therapy is begun, to exclude leukemia. Short-term side effects: Mood changes, increased appetite and weight gain, hypertension, insulin resistance. Long-term side effects with chronic use: Adrenal suppression, osteopenia, growth delay
- Anti-Rh D immunoglobulin (patient must be Rh[+] and nonsplenectomized): 80% respond with platelet counts >20,000/mm³ after 72 hours. Dose is 50–75 mcg/kg IV over 3–5 minutes. Response lasts ~5 weeks:
  - Advantages: Less expensive than IVIG but more costly than steroids. Lower rate of allergic side effects (10%) than with IVIG and does not cause aseptic meningitis. Amenable to outpatient administration.
  - Disadvantages: Fever/chills, mild hemolysis (Hb decrease of 1–3 g/dL) in all patients. Rare reports of catastrophic hemolysis; subcutaneous route may ameliorate risk.
- Any of these therapies may be repeated if responsive patient later develops recurrent thrombocytopenia.

Second Line

- Rituximab (anti-CD20 monoclonal antibody) induces response in many refractory patients (after median 5 weeks), but duration is often limited (median <12 months).
- Thrombopoietin receptor agonists (e.g., eltrombopag, romiplostim) have been shown in trials to improve platelet counts and bleeding risk in patients with chronic ITP. Cost, concerns about adverse effects including myelofibrosis and thrombosis, and paucity of long-term follow-up data limit use of these agents.
- Cytotoxic chemotherapy (vincristine or low-dose cyclophosphamide) or immunosuppression (CsA or MMF) is effective in some patients refractory to other therapy and splenectomy.

ADDITIONAL TREATMENT

General Measures

- Platelet transfusions are generally ineffective, because transfused platelets are rapidly destroyed. Role is limited to emergent support for critical hemorrhage.
- Medical treatment slows antibody-mediated platelet clearance and raises platelet counts acutely, but does not alter the long-term course.
- Because severe hemorrhage is rare and ITP resolves spontaneously in 90% of pediatric cases, most patients will not require treatment.
- Guidelines put forth by the American Society of Hematology recommend treatment for:
  - Patients with severe or life-threatening bleeding
  - Patients with moderate bleeding, overt mucosal bleeding, or developmental or psychosocial risk for injury
  - Patients with a platelet count <10,000/mm³ are at higher risk for bleeding, but platelet count alone is not an indication for treatment.
- Active toddlers or children at risk for trauma may require treatment when platelet count is <20,000–30,000/mm³.
- Observation alone is acceptable for older children without serious bleeding, and with adequate supervision and assured follow-up. May be preferable to repeated courses of treatment in clinically well children with chronic ITP
- Avoid medications that affect platelet function, such as aspirin, ibuprofen, most other NSAIDs, and anticoagulants.
- Educate parents about signs and symptoms of intracranial hemorrhage (ICH), elevated intracranial pressure (ICP), and GI bleeding.
- Avoid activities with significant fall, collision, or other trauma risk while thrombocytopenic.

SURGERY/OTHER PROCEDURES

Splenectomy: 60–80% respond with complete remission. No reliable presurgical predictors of response have been found.

- Advantages: Response in patients refractory to medical therapy
- Disadvantages: Surgical morbidity; risk of sepsis with encapsulated organisms (Immunize preoperatively against *Haemophilus influenzae*, pneumococcus, and meningococcus, and consider lifelong penicillin prophylaxis.)

IN-PATIENT CONSIDERATIONS

Initial Stabilization

Life-threatening hemorrhage: The goal is to stop bleeding rapidly. Platelet transfusion, IVIG, and steroids (after emergent marrow exam, if possible) should be given concomitantly. Emergent splenectomy is necessary in rare cases.

ONGOING CARE

FOLLOW-UP RECOMMENDATIONS

Patient Monitoring

- Platelet count biweekly when <20,000/mm³, weekly when <50,000/mm³ or after treatment, except in stable chronic ITP. Increase interval if no symptoms and platelet count >50,000/mm³.
- Platelet counts may fall transiently with intercurrent illnesses prior to resolution of ITP.
- Discontinue monitoring when no symptoms and normal platelet count for >3 months.

PROGNOSIS

- Acute ITP: In 3 months, 60% of children will have a normal platelet count; at 1 year from diagnosis, 90%. Recurrence with future infections/illnesses is rare.
- Chronic ITP: Platelet count tends to be higher, at 40,000–80,000/mm³. Remissions can occur many years after diagnosis (predicted spontaneous remission rate 61% after 15 years).
- Not yet possible to prospectively distinguish patients with acute ITP from those who will persist with chronic ITP
- Patients with chronic ITP should be periodically re-evaluated for secondary ITP associated with underlying diseases such as systemic lupus erythematosus, HIV infection, ALPS, or Evans syndrome.
- Of patients with chronic ITP, 50–60% eventually stabilize without need for ongoing therapy or need for splenectomy.
- Spontaneous resolution of thrombocytopenia can occur as long as 10–20 years after diagnosis.

COMPLICATIONS

- The incidence of significant bleeding-related morbidity and mortality is low (<5%):
  - ICH is a rare (0.1%) but potentially fatal event in acute ITP.
  - Platelet count always <20,000/mm³ in published literature (80% of cases <10,000/mm³)
  - May occur any time and without prior trauma
- Mucosal bleeding from nose, gums, lower GI tract, or kidneys is not uncommon. Hematemesis and melena are rare.
- Menorrhagia may be severe.
- Retinal hemorrhage is rare.

ADDITIONAL READING

- Bennet CM, Tarantino M. Chronic immune thrombocytopenia in children: Epidemiology and clinical presentation. *Hematol Oncol Clin North Am.* 2009;23(6):1223–1238.
- Blanchette V, Bolton-Maggs P. Childhood immune thrombocytopenic purpura: Diagnosis and management. *Hematol Oncol Clin North Am.* 2010;24(1):249–273.
- Provan D, Atasi R, Newland AC, et al. International consensus report on the investigation and management of primary immune thrombocytopenia. *Blood.* 2010;115(2):168–186.

CODES

ICD9
287.31 Immune thrombocytopenic purpura

ICD10
D69.3 Immune thrombocytopenic purpura

IMMUNE DEFICIENCY
Kathleen E. Sullivan

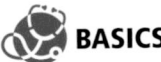 **BASICS**

DEFINITION
Immunodeficiencies generally represent a defect in host defense.
- Congenital and acquired forms exist.
- Defects in antibody production: Most often characterized by frequent sinopulmonary infections with typical organisms
  - X-linked agammaglobulinemia: Onset of symptoms after 6 months of age; sinopulmonary infections with typical bacterial pathogens. Markedly decreased immunoglobulins and B cells are characteristic. Tonsils are absent.
  - Hyper-IgM syndromes: Several forms. Usually present with recurrent bacterial infections in infancy; *Pneumocystis jiroveci* is seen; intermittent neutropenia is common. Decreased IgG, IgE, IgA with normal or increased IgM.
  - Common variable immunodeficiency: Usually presents with recurrent bacterial infections; most commonly arises in the 2nd or 3rd decade of life (but is seen in all ages). Immunoglobulin levels and function gradually decline; autoimmunity is common.
  - IgG subclass deficiency: IgG2 subclass deficiency is seen as a transient developmental delay in the acquisition of humoral immunity. May also precede the development of common variable immunodeficiency and can rarely be seen as an isolated defect.
  - IgA deficiency: The most common congenital immunodeficiency (1:500); most are asymptomatic. Symptoms can be seen at any age; typically sinopulmonary infections; increased risk of allergy, autoimmune disease, and anaphylaxis from blood products.
  - Transient hypogammaglobulinemia of infancy: A developmental delay of immunoglobulin production; function is intact; typically resolves between 9 and 15 months of age.
- T-cell defects: Most often characterized by persistent viral infections or opportunistic infections.
  - Severe combined immunodeficiency (SCID): Most common presentation is a respiratory virus that fails to clear or chronic diarrhea. Failure to thrive, thrush, and *P. jiroveci* pneumonia are also common; see "Failure to Thrive" and "Pneumocystis Pneumonia."
  - Chromosome 22q11.2 deletion syndrome (DiGeorge syndrome/velocardiofacial syndrome): See "DiGeorge Syndrome."
  - Chronic mucocutaneous candidiasis: There are multiple forms of this disorder. One form is also called autoimmune polyendocrinopathy candidiasis ectodermal dystrophy (APECED) and has a very strong association with polyendocrinopathies and ectodermal dysplasia. The other types are more likely to have an associated T-cell defect. Infants have extensive or recurrent *Candida*; predisposition to other infections is modest.
  - IPEX (immunodeficiency, polyendocrinopathy, enteropathy, X-linked syndrome): Diarrhea associated with villous atrophy and a T-cell infiltrate, progressive autoimmune destruction of endocrine organs. Infections can be severe but the autoimmune manifestations predominate.

- Neutrophil defects: *Staphylococcus*, *Pseudomonas*, unusual bacterial or fungal infections are characteristic.
  - Autoimmune neutropenia of infancy: Most common neutrophil defect of childhood; usually detected at ~6–12 months of age; often resolves by 2 years of age.
  - Congenital neutropenia: Infections may be skin infections or sinopulmonary; patients have either persistently absent or markedly low neutrophil counts. Some patients will have 21-day cycles of neutropenia—cyclic neutropenia.
  - Leukocyte adhesion deficiency: ~10% have delayed separation of the umbilical cord; most common presentations are recurrent skin ulcers and periodontitis. Spontaneous peritonitis occurs.
  - Chronic granulomatous disease: Recurrent skin abscesses common, deep hepatic abscesses, and pulmonary infections. Typical organisms are *Staphylococcus aureus*, *Burkholderia*, *Serratia*, *Nocardia*, mycobacteria, *Aspergillus*, and *Candida*; age of onset is usually 1–3 years.
- Innate defects in signaling: Typically present with severe bacterial or viral infections in early infancy
  - IRAK4 and MyD88 deficiencies are associated with staphylococcal, streptococcal, or pseudomonal sepsis/meningitis.
  - Unc93 and other defects are associated with neonatal herpes encephalitis.
- Macrophage activation defects: Universally associated with atypical mycobacteria. *Salmonella* is also seen. Biopsies may reveal poorly formed granulomas.
- Multiple genetic types have a broad range of severity: IFNGR1, IFNGR2, STAT1, IL12P40, IL12RB1.
  - Complement deficiency: Deficiencies of C5–C9 are associated with *Neisseria* infections; deficiencies of C1, C2, and C4 are associated with lupus and recurrent bacterial infections. C3 deficiency is associated with glomerulonephritis and severe recurrent infections. Defects in complement regulatory proteins are associated with atypical hemolytic uremic syndrome (HUS).
  - Immunodeficiency syndromes
    - Ataxia telangiectasia: Progressive cerebellar ataxia beginning at ~2 years of age; ocular telangiectasias beginning at about 5–15 years of age; recurrent sinopulmonary infections; α-fetoprotein is elevated, IgA and IgG2 are diminished.
    - Wiskott–Aldrich syndrome: Clinical triad of eczema, thrombocytopenia, and recurrent infections. Immunoglobulin levels are variable but responses to vaccines are often poor; platelets range from 20,000 to 90,000 and are small.
    - Hyper-IgE syndrome: Recurrent infections of the skin and lungs; *S. aureus* is a major cause of infection, and pulmonary infections typically heal with pneumatoceles.
    - X-linked lymphoproliferative syndrome: 4 main types of presentation and 2 genetic types: Acute Epstein–Barr virus infection with hemophagocytosis, lymphoma, hypogammaglobulinemia, and aplastic anemia. Family history is key to diagnosis.

    - Chédiak–Higashi syndrome: Pigmentary dilution, progressive neuropathy, and frequent infections; associated with a hemophagocytic process. Neutrophil counts are low and neutrophils have giant inclusions.
    - Familial hemophagocytic lymphohistiocytosis: A defect in cytotoxic function; presents with fever, pancytopenia, and hepatosplenomegaly; usually <5 years of age.
    - Ectodermal dysplasia with immune deficiency also known as NEMO (NFκB essential modulator) deficiency: Variable ectodermal dysplasia and variable immune deficiency. Immunoglobulin levels are variable as are responses to vaccines. Susceptibility to mycobacteria, *Pneumocystis*, and common bacterial pathogens.
  - Secondary immunodeficiencies include:
    - HIV infection
    - Malignancy
    - Viral suppression
    - Nephrotic syndrome
    - Protein-losing enteropathy
    - Malnutrition
    - Medications
    - Splenectomy

EPIDEMIOLOGY
Primary immune deficiencies range from the common (1:600) to the very rare (1:1,000,000)
- 1:600 for IgA deficiency in Caucasians
- 1:3,000 for chromosome 22q11.2 deletion syndrome (DiGeorge syndrome)
- 1:20,000 for common variable immune deficiency
- 1:50,000 for SCID
- 1:200,000 for chronic granulomatous disease
- 1:1,000,000 for NEMO deficiency

RISK FACTORS
- The immunodeficiencies are generally autosomal recessive, although there are several important exceptions.
- X-linked (Properdin deficiency, X-linked agammaglobulinemia, X-linked hyper-IgM, X-linked SCID, X-linked chronic granulomatous disease, X-linked lymphoproliferative syndrome [2 types], IPEX, Wiskott–Aldrich syndrome, NEMO deficiency). All of these have autosomal-recessive phenocopies or may be seen in females with altered X inactivation.
- Autosomal dominant: Hyper-IgE syndrome, chromosome 22q11.2 deletion syndrome, some macrophage activation defects
- Polygenic: IgA deficiency and common variable immunodeficiency

DIAGNOSIS

DIFFERENTIAL DIAGNOSIS
- Chronic inflammation of mucous membranes such as that due to reflux or allergies can lead to recurrent infections.
- Immunocompromise due to chemotherapy and immunosuppressive drugs
- Malnutrition
- Intercurrent viral infections such as Epstein–Barr virus and cytomegalovirus

- Medications such as Dilantin and gold can cause IgA deficiency or hypogammaglobulinemia
- Inborn errors of metabolism
- Chromosomal syndromes
- Protein loss can be associated with hypogammaglobulinemia.
- HIV infection

HISTORY
- **Question:** Family history?
- *Significance:* X-linked disorders are common.
- **Question:** Number and duration of infections?
- *Significance:* To determine whether the problem is one of clearance, or frequency
- **Question:** Types of infections?
- *Significance:* Infections of skin are frequently due to neutrophil problems, whereas recurrent infections of a single site imply an anatomic problem. Opportunistic infections are associated with both neutrophil defects (unusual bacteria and fungi) and T-cell defects (opportunistic viruses).
- HIV risk factors

PHYSICAL EXAM
The physical exam should be directed at defining organ damage as a result of infection, the presence of any current infections, the presence of any syndromic features, the presence of signs of autoimmune disease, and the characterization of accessible lymphoid organs.
- **Finding:** Examination of lymph nodes, tonsils, liver, and spleen?
- *Significance:* Hypoplasia or expansion

DIAGNOSTIC TESTS & INTERPRETATION
- **Test:** Laboratory evaluations should focus on the quantity and function of antibodies: IgG, IgA, IgM, IgE levels, and responses to vaccines such as diphtheria and tetanus.
- *Significance:* A patient with recurrent sinopulmonary infections with typical organisms could have a defect in antibody production.
- **Test:** Evaluation of T-cell production and function—T-cell enumeration and lymphocyte proliferation studies
- *Significance:* Chronic viral infections or opportunistic infections suggest a T-cell defect.
- **Test:** Evaluation of neutrophil numbers and function—a CBC with differential, morphologic examination of neutrophils, and a measure of respiratory burst
- *Significance:* Neutrophil disorders typically present with skin abscesses or ulcers or deep infections with *Staphylococcus* or fungi.
- **Test:** Special studies designed to test the function of the toll-like receptor signaling complex
- *Significance:* Innate defects, such as IRAK4, MyD88, and NEMO deficiencies, can be detected.
- **Test:** A CH50
- *Significance:* Complement deficiencies—a CH50 will detect most of the structural component deficiencies. Special studies are needed for defects of the alternative pathway and the regulatory proteins.
- **Test:** CBC with differential, IgG, IgA, IgM levels, and diphtheria and tetanus titers
- *Significance:* In certain patients it may be difficult to differentiate between viral processes and bacterial processes. In these cases, a CBC with differential, IgG, IgA, IgM levels, and diphtheria and tetanus titers are a useful screen to evaluate for the most common immunodeficiencies.

TREATMENT
- Prophylactic antimicrobials:
  - IgG subclass deficiency
  - Chronic mucocutaneous candidiasis
  - Ataxia telangiectasia
  - Hyper-IgE syndrome
  - Chronic granulomatous disease

ADDITIONAL TREATMENT
General Measures
- Suspected SCID requires isolation, cytomegalovirus negative/irradiated blood products, and a prompt evaluation for hematopoietic stem cell transplant.
- Immunoglobulin replacement (either IV or SC)
  - X-linked agammaglobulinemia
  - Hyper-IgM
  - Common variable immunodeficiency
  - IgG subclass deficiency (infrequently)
- Probiotics can be useful for patients exposed to frequent antibiotics.
- Hand washing and topical measures to prevent infections

SURGERY/OTHER PROCEDURES
- Hematopoietic stem cell transplantation:
  - SCID
  - Wiskott–Aldrich syndrome
  - X-linked lymphoproliferative syndrome
  - Chédiak–Higashi syndrome
  - Familial hemophagocytic lymphohistiocytosis
  - Selected cases of hyper-IgM, chronic granulomatous disease, macrophage activation defects, NEMO deficiency
- Thymus transplantation:
  - Severe chromosome 22q11.2 deletion syndrome (DiGeorge syndrome)

ONGOING CARE

PROGNOSIS
- Most antibody deficiencies have an excellent prognosis. Transient or developmental deficiencies of IgG or IgG subclasses typically resolve by 2 years of age.
- Some patients with common variable immunodeficiency can develop malignancy or autoimmune disease is this defines the prognosis.
- The treatment of neutrophil disorders remains problematic, and most children with chronic granulomatous disease will not have a full life expectancy.
- Patients with T-cell disorders for whom bone marrow transplantation is not performed can do well if the defect is mild and if they do not suffer from autoimmune disease, malignancy, or recurrent infections.

COMPLICATIONS
- Bronchiectasis
- Deafness
- Autoimmune disease
- Lymphoreticular malignancies occur in patients with T-cell disorders.
- Live viral vaccines administered to patients with significant T-cell dysfunction can result in unchecked viremia.
- Oral polio vaccine administered to patients with agammaglobulinemia can cause meningoencephalitis.

ADDITIONAL READING
- Ballow M. Approach to the patient with recurrent infections. *Clin Rev Allergy Immunol.* 2008;34: 129–140.
- Fischer A. Human primary immunodeficiency diseases. *Immunity.* 2007;27:835–845.
- International Union of Immunological Societies. Primary immunodeficiencies: 2009 update. *J Allergy Clin Immunol.* 2009;124:1161–1178.
- Slatter MA, Gennery AR. Primary immunodeficiency syndromes. *Adv Exp Med Biol.* 2010;685:146–165.
- www.immunodeficeincysearch.com

CODES

ICD9
- 279.3 Unspecified immunity deficiency
- 279.04 Congenital hypogammaglobulinemia
- 279.06 Common variable immunodeficiency

ICD10
- D80.0 Hereditary hypogammaglobulinemia
- D83.9 Common variable immunodeficiency, unspecified
- D84.9 Immunodeficiency, unspecified

FAQ
- Q: I have many patients with recurrent episodes of green rhinorrhea. Do these episodes all need to be treated with antibiotics, and should the child have an immunologic evaluation?
- A: Many viral infections cause green rhinorrhea and thus do not require antibiotics. Children with no other infections may be safely observed.
- Q: Does a child with thrush require evaluation?
- A: A child with severe thrush in the absence of risk factors should have an evaluation for T-cell dysfunction, HIV, and the possibility of chronic mucocutaneous candidiasis of childhood. Moderate thrush or recurrent simple thrush does not require evaluation unless it is occurring in an older child.
- Q: A newborn in my practice still has his umbilical cord attached at 6 weeks of age. Is that abnormal, and does it require an evaluation for leukocyte adhesion deficiency?
- A: A completely healthy-appearing cord at 6 weeks of age does not require any evaluation. If there is clinical suspicion of leukocyte adhesion deficiency, a CBC can be performed to identify neutrophilia.

CLINICAL PEARLS
- Boys with X-linked agammaglobulinemia and X-linked hyper-IgM do not have tonsils and adenoids.
- Children and adults with hyper-IgE syndrome develop abscesses that are not painful.
- Infections in patients with IRAK4 or MyD88 deficiency may not be accompanied by fever.

I

IMMUNOGLOBULIN A DEFICIENCY

Mathew Fogg

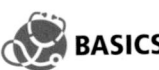 **BASICS**

DESCRIPTION

Serum IgA <5 mg/dL and a normal serum IgG and IgM, in patients >1 year

RISK FACTORS

Genetics

Most common autosomal dominant mode of inheritance with variable expressivity, but the following rare associations also occur:

- 18q syndrome
- Partial deletions in the long or short arm, and ring forms of chromosome 18
- Also associated with HLA-A1, HLA-A2, B8, and Dw3

PATHOPHYSIOLOGY

Increased incidence of the following:

- Atopy
- Sinopulmonary infections
- GI infections (especially *Giardia lamblia*)
- Crohn disease
- Ulcerative colitis
- Celiac disease
- Autoimmune illnesses:
  - Arthritis
  - Lupus
  - Immune endocrinopathies
  - Autoimmune hematologic conditions
  - Chronic active hepatitis

 DIAGNOSIS

HISTORY

- Patients with IgA deficiency:
  - Can have frequent sinopulmonary infections
  - Can have frequent GI infections
  - Tend to be allergic
  - Have an increased incidence of autoimmune diseases
- ~30% of patients with IgA deficiency are completely healthy.

PHYSICAL EXAM

- Look for signs of recurrent infection and atopy.
- Allergies are associated with IgA deficiency. Signs include:
  - Cobblestoning of the conjunctiva caused by allergic inflammation in the eyes
  - Allergic shiners
- Serous otitis media may be the result of recurrent ear infections:
  - Increased ear infections can be seen in IgA deficiency.
  - Serous otitis media can be secondary to allergies, also associated with IgA deficiency.
- Pain on palpation of the sinuses: Recurrent sinus infections are associated with IgA deficiency.
- An increased frequency of pneumonia is associated with IgA deficiency.
- Swollen joints: An increased frequency of autoimmune diseases is associated with IgA deficiency.

DIAGNOSTIC TESTS & INTERPRETATION

Diagnostic Procedures/Other

The general goal is to decide whether the patient's complaints are consistent with IgA deficiency (frequent upper respiratory and GI infections, or allergies).

- Measure serum IgA level:
  - If the patient is IgA deficient, exclude other conditions associated with IgA deficiency.
  - Serum IgA level: Patient is considered deficient if the serum IgA level is <5 mg/dL.
- Total immunoglobulins: If normal, helps rule out X-linked agammaglobulinemia (Bruton), common variable immunodeficiency, and severe combined immunodeficiency
- IgG subclasses: Study helps rule out an associated IgG2 subclass deficiency; clinical significance of IgG2 subclass deficiency is controversial.
- Lymphocyte mitogens:
  - A functional lymphocyte study
  - If normal, helps rule out common variable immunodeficiency, severe combined immunodeficiency, ataxia telangiectasia, DiGeorge syndrome, and Nezelof syndrome
- Lymphocyte *Candida* antigen stimulation: No response to *Candida* in vivo is consistent with chronic mucocutaneous candidiasis.

DIFFERENTIAL DIAGNOSIS

- Toxic, environmental, drugs: Penicillamine and anticonvulsants can induce IgA deficiency.
- Genetic/Metabolic:
  - X-linked agammaglobulinemia (Bruton)
  - Common variable immunodeficiency
  - Severe combined immunodeficiency
  - Ataxia telangiectasia
  - DiGeorge syndrome
  - Chronic mucocutaneous candidiasis
  - Nezelof syndrome
  - Selective IgG2 deficiency

- Miscellaneous: Patients may be completely healthy, and IgA deficiency may be an incidental finding.
- Common causes: May be the result of decreased synthesis or impaired differentiation of IgA B lymphocytes into IgA plasma cells

ALERT
Factors that may help alert you to make a referral include:
- Suggestion that IgA deficiency may be part of a more complex immune deficiency: An allergist/immunologist can assist with an appropriate immunologic evaluation.
- IgA deficiency associated with autoimmune disease: Evaluation and treatment by a rheumatologist would be indicated.
- Patient likely to need a blood transfusion: IgA-deficient patients show an increased incidence of anaphylaxis to IgA-containing blood products. The allergist can help select appropriate blood products for these patients.

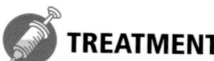 **TREATMENT**

ADDITIONAL TREATMENT
General Measures
- There is no specific drug therapy.
- Recurrent infections should be treated aggressively with broad-spectrum antibiotics.
- Antibiotic prophylaxis to prevent recurrent sinopulmonary infections is often indicated.
- IV γ-globulin is not indicated.

ALERT
Patients with IgA deficiency may develop antibodies against IgA in transfused blood products. These patients are at risk for anaphylactic (or anaphylactoid) transfusion reactions. To avoid these reactions, these patients may receive:
- Packed RBCs (only if these cells have been washed 3 times)
- Plasma products from IgA-deficient donors
- Autologous banked blood

 ONGOING CARE

FOLLOW-UP RECOMMENDATIONS
- Patients should be observed for:
  - Sinopulmonary infections
  - GI infections
  - Autoimmune diseases
  - Inflammatory bowel disease
- It is important to manage infectious complications aggressively and to intervene promptly when the associated conditions present.

PATIENT EDUCATION
- Recurrence risk for a couple with an affected child depends on the mode of inheritance.
  - Most commonly, the mode of inheritance is autosomal dominant and the risk would be 50%.
  - However, expressivity is variable, and the patient's phenotype may not be that of an IgA-deficient person.
- IgA deficiency can be induced by some anticonvulsants and by penicillamine.
- IgA-deficient patients should wear medical alert bracelets. These patients can have anaphylaxis if administered blood products containing IgA. In an emergency situation, this is important information for the caregivers to have.

PROGNOSIS
Survival into the 7th decade is common.

COMPLICATIONS
Increased incidence of the following:
- Respiratory tract infections
- GI tract infections
- Atopy

ADDITIONAL READING
- Burrows PD, Cooper MD. IgA deficiency. *Adv Immunol*.1997;65:245–276.
- Janzi M, et al. Selective IgA deficiency in early life: Association to infections and allergic diseases during childhood. *Clin Immunol*. 2009;133(1): 78–85.
- Smith CA, et al. Increased prevalence of immunoglobulin A deficiency in patients with the chromosome 22q11.2 deletion syndrome (DiGeorge syndrome/velocardiofacial syndrome). *Clin Diagn Lab Immunol*.1998;5:415–417.
- Stiehm RE. The four most common pediatric immunodeficiencies. *Adv Exp Med Biol*. 2007; 601:15–26. Review.
- Yel L. Selective IgA deficiency. *J Clin Immunol*. 2010;30(1):10–16.

 CODES

ICD9
279.01 Selective IgA immunodeficiency

ICD10
D80.2 Selective deficiency of immunoglobulin A [IgA]

FAQ
- Q: What is the recurrence risk for a couple with an affected child?
- A: It depends on the mode of inheritance. Most commonly, the mode of inheritance is autosomal dominant and the risk would be 50%. However, the expressivity is variable, and the patient's phenotype may not be that of an IgA-deficient person.
- Q: Does the patient take any medications?
- A: The IgA deficiency can be induced by some anticonvulsants and by penicillamine.
- Q: Should IgA-deficient patients wear medical alert bracelets?
- A: Yes. These patients can have anaphylaxis if they are given blood products containing IgA. In an emergency situation, this is important information for the caregivers to have.

I

IMPERFORATE ANUS

Judith Kelsen

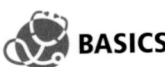 **BASICS**

DESCRIPTION
Congenital abnormality in which the bowel fails to perforate or only partially perforates the pelvic muscular floor and/or the epidermal covering

EPIDEMIOLOGY
- Incidence is estimated to be in the range of 1:3,000–1:9,000.
- High lesions are more common in males (2:1).
- Low lesions occur with equal frequency in both sexes.

RISK FACTORS
Genetics
- Can be an isolated defect or part of a syndrome or association
- Can be part of omphalocele-exstrophy of the bladder-imperforate anus-spinal defects (OEIS) complex or cloacal exstrophy (EC)
- Syndromic disorders that contain imperforate anus are associated with defects on chromosomes 6, 7, 10, and 16.
- Can be associated with Trisomy 21

PATHOPHYSIOLOGY
- The hindgut comes in contact with the cloacal membrane during the 6th week of fetal development. At this time, the hindgut is divided into a ventral urogenital and dorsal rectal component. By the 8th week, the dorsal 1/2 perforates to the exterior. In imperforate anus, the process is arrested during this critical period.
- There are many anatomic variants of imperforate anus. From the prognostic point of view, the most important is classification and distinguishing the main types: Supralevator (high) and translevator (low). In the low variant, the rectal termination is above the anal pit and not related to the urethra.
- A separate group is of cloacal malformation, in which the urinary genital and digestive systems drain to a common channel that communicates with the perineum.

- A fistula communicating from the gut to the urogenital system or to the external opening is present in 90% of cases. In females, most commonly the fistula leads to the opening in the posterior fourchette of the vagina (in low lesions) or to the upper vagina (in high lesions). In males, the fistula leads to the raphe of the scrotum (in low lesions) or to the urethra (in high lesions).

COMMONLY ASSOCIATED CONDITIONS
- Other anomalies are present in 1/3 of patients with an imperforated anus.
- Imperforate anus can be associated with vertebral and cardiac anomalies, tracheoesophageal fistula, and renal and limb anomalies (VACTERL).
- Other anomalies associated with imperforate anus include intestinal atresia, malrotation, omphalocele, annular pancreas, urologic anomalies, spinal anomalies, duplicate uterus, septate vagina, vaginal atresia, and absence of rectal muscles.

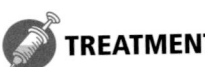 **DIAGNOSIS**

HISTORY
- Most children are diagnosed in the 1st days of life by abnormal findings on physical exam.
- Failure to pass meconium, a history of constipation, and signs of low intestinal obstruction (abdominal distention and vomiting) should mandate re-exam of perianal area.

PHYSICAL EXAM
- Lesion presents as no opening, an inadequate caliber of anus, or an anterior malposition of the opening.
- Attempt to localize the opening of the fistula and look for associated anomalies.
- Evaluate for lumbosacral neurologic function. Anal wink can usually be elicited, because a vertiginous external anal sphincter is present in most cases.

DIAGNOSTIC TESTS & INTERPRETATION
Imaging
- Invertogram: After sufficient time for a transit of gas (>12 hours after birth), the child is placed in an upside-down position for 3 minutes, after which a lateral view of the pelvis is obtained.
- Lumbosacral films to evaluate for vertebral anomalies
- MRI of the spine should be considered to look for a tethered cord.
- Renal ultrasound, voiding cystoureterogram, and IV pyelogram can be used to evaluate for urinary tract anomalies.

DIFFERENTIAL DIAGNOSIS
- No disorders can mimic imperforate anus
- Task is to define the location of the termination of the bowel and the opening of the fistula.

TREATMENT

SURGERY/OTHER PROCEDURES
- Surgery should be performed by an experienced surgeon.
- High lesions require an emergent diverting colostomy and pull-through procedure with a Pena midsagittal anorectoplasty at 3–9 months of age. The colostomy is closed after the anoplasty has healed and any necessary secondary dilations have been completed.
- New techniques: While the above procedure has been the gold standard, a significant percentage of patients continue to have fecal disorders postoperativerly.

- The use of the laparoscopically assisted anorectal pull-through using laparoscopy and muscle electrostimulation (LAARP) has been developed.
- Transanal anorectoplasty was recently shown to have sphincter sparing and results in accurate placement of anus in external canal with good neurological function.
- After surgery, follow-up with anal dilatation helps minimize the risk of stricture formation and helps the newly constructed canal to become functional.
- Complications of surgery include stricture of the anocutaneous anastomosis, rectourinary fistula, mucosal prolapse, constipation, and incontinence.

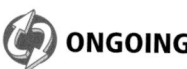 ONGOING CARE

PATIENT EDUCATION
- Imperforate anus can be associated with multiple other anomalies and not necessarily isolated.
- Renal and vertebral anomalies must be excluded.
- Genetic basis: Imperforate anus can be associated with chromosomal anomalies or can be an isolated problem.

PROGNOSIS
- Continence can be attained in 90% if patients have low lesions.
- <50% of patients with high lesions are continent before school age, but most continue to improve and achieve continence by adolescence.
- Highest incidence of incontinence occurs in males with rectobladder fistulae.

COMPLICATIONS
- Constipation is the most common problem following repair.
- A significant percentage will have incontinence.
- Many patients will need regular enemas for years to prevent or reduce constipation and fecal incontinence.
- Although some patients experience significant problems early in school years, overall studies have shown patients with imperforate anus did not experience psychosocial impairment despite significant functional problems.

ADDITIONAL READING

- Arbell D, Gross E, Orkin B. Imperforate anus, malrotation and Hirschsprung's disease, a rare and important association. *J Pediatr Surg.* 2006;41(7): 1335–1337.
- Chen CJ. The treatment of imperforate anus: Experience with 108 patients. *J Pediatr Surg.* 1999;34:1728–1732.
- Javid PJ, et al. Immediate and long-term results of surgical management of low imperforate anus in girls. *J Pediatr Surg.* 1998;33:198–203.
- Keppler-Noreuil K, et al. Ascertainment of OEIS complex/cloacal exstrophy: 15 new cases and literature review. *Am J Med Genet A.* 2007; 143A(18):2122–2128.
- Khalil BA, Morabito A, Bianchi A. Transanoproctoplasty: A 21 year review. *J Pediatr Surg.* 2010;45(9): 1915–1919.
- Lima M, Tursini S, Ruggeri G. Laparoscopically assisted anorectal pull-through for high imperforate anus: Three years' experience. *J Lapaoroendos Adv Surg Tech A.* 2006;16(1):63–69.
- Pakarinen M, Rintala R. Management and outcome of low anorectal malformations. *Pediatr Surg Int.* 2010;26:1057–1063.
- Pena A, Hong A. Advances in the management of anorectal malformations. *Am J Surg.* 2000;180: 370–376.
- Rintala RJ, Pakarinen MP. Imperforate anus: I: Long- and short-term outcome. *Semin Pediatr Surg.* 2008;17(2):79–89.

 CODES

ICD9
- 565.1 Anal fistula
- 751.2 Imperforate anus

ICD10
- Q42.2 Congenital absence, atresia and stenosis of anus with fistula
- Q42.3 Congenital absence, atresia and stenosis of anus without fistula

FAQ

- Q: Is this an isolated defect in my child?
- A: Often, imperforate anus can be associated with multiple other anomalies and not necessarily isolated. Renal and vertebral anomalies must be excluded.
- Q: What is the genetic basis for this defect?
- A: Imperforate anus can be associated with chromosomal anomalies or can be an isolated problem.

I

IMPETIGO
Michelle Terry

 BASICS

DESCRIPTION
Impetigo is a superficial skin infection characterized by the eruption of shallow pustules that rupture and form thick yellow crusts.

- Impetigo occurs most commonly in children and is contagious.
- Pyoderma and impetigo contagiosa are synonyms for impetigo.

CLASSIFICATION:
- Primary impetigo is defined as direct bacterial invasion of previously normal skin.
- Secondary impetigo is defined as infection at sites of minor skin trauma such as abrasions, insect bites, or underlying conditions such as eczema.

TYPES OF IMPETIGO
- Non-bullous impetigo—the most common form of impetigo. Lesions begin as papules that progress to vesicles surrounded by erythema. Over the course of a week, they become pustules that enlarge and break down to form thick, adherent yellow crusts.
- Bullous impetigo—characterized by vesicles containing clear yellow fluid, that then becomes darker and more turbid; ruptured bullae leave a "honey"-colored crust.
- Ecthyma—an ulcerative form of impetigo in which the lesions extend through the epidermis and deep into the dermis.

MICROBIOLOGY
The predominant bacteria are:

Non-bullous impetigo
- Group A beta-hemolytic streptococcus (GABHS)
- *Staphylococcus aureus*
- Miscellaneous gram-negative and anerobic bacteria have also been isolated from lesions.

Bullous impetigo
- *Staphylococcus aureus*

Ecthyma
- Group A beta-hemolytic streptococcus (GABHS)
- *Staphylococcus aureus*
- Miscellaneous gram-negative and anerobic bacteria (including *Pseudomonas aeruginosa* in ecthyma gangrenosum)

EPIDEMIOLOGY
- Frequency: Impetigo accounts for approximately 10% of skin problems observed in pediatric clinics and is one of the more common dermatologic infections.
- Location: Impetigo occurs more frequently in warm, humid environments.
- Age: Impetigo is found most commonly in preschool-aged children and can spread rapidly through child care centers and schools.

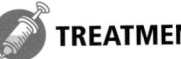 DIAGNOSIS

DIFFERENTIAL DIAGNOSIS
- Varicella
- Staph scalded skin syndrome
- Erythema multiforme
- Herpes simplex virus infection
- Burns (thermal and chemical)
- Nummular eczema
- Tinea corporis
- Insect bites
- Scabies
- Lice

HISTORY
- Patients with impetigo may report a history of minor trauma, insect bites, scabies, herpes simplex virus infection, varicella infection, or eczema before the development of the infection. Impetigo lesions are usually present for a few days to weeks before the patient seeks medical attention.
- Impetigo is usually painless, although patients may complain of that the lesions are itchy. Additional symptoms such as fever, respiratory distress, vomiting, or diarrhea are rare and perhaps indicative of another diagnosis besides impetigo.
- Outbreaks commonly occur in families and child care centers, as well as among sports team members.

PHYSICAL EXAM
- Nonbullous impetigo
  - Lesions first begin as thin-walled vesicles or pustules on an erythematous base. The lesions promptly rupture, releasing their serum, which dries and forms a light brown, "honey-colored" crust.
  - Multiple lesions generally occur at the same site, often coalescing.
  - As the lesions resolve with treatment, the crusts slough from the affected areas and usually heal without scarring.
- Bullous impetigo
  - Lesions may form on grossly normal or previously traumatized skin.
  - The vesicles do not rupture as easily or quickly as in nonbullous lesions, but they do enlarge into bullae that are usually 1–2 cm in diameter. The bullae initially contain a clear yellow fluid that subsequently turns cloudy and dark yellow.
  - After the lesions rupture, a thin, light brown, crust remains.

- Ecthyma
  - The lesion is a vesicle or pustule overlying an inflamed area of skin that deepens into a dermal ulceration with overlying crust.
  - The crust of ecthyma lesions is gray-yellow and is thicker and harder than the crust of impetigo.
  - A shallow, punched-out ulceration is apparent when adherent crust is removed and the deep dermal ulcer has a raised and indurated surrounding margin.
  - Ecthyma heals slowly and commonly produces a scar.
  - Regional lymphadenopathy is common in ecthyma, even with solitary lesions. Lymphadenopathy is less common in bullous impetigo and is rare in nonbullous impetigo.

Lab
- Usually, no lab evaluation is required, impetigo is a clinical diagnosis.
- Gram stain and wound culture is helpful, especially if MRSA is suspected.
- CBC with differential and blood cultures are helpful if systemic symptoms are present.
- A skin biopsy may be useful if the diagnosis is uncertain.

TREATMENT

Supportive
- Clipping the patient's fingernails short to discourage scratching of the lesions is recommended.
- Cleansing and debriding the lesions are unnecessary.

MEDICATION (DRUGS)
Topical therapy:
- The preferred treatment when there are a limited number of lesions without bullae. Topical therapy has fewer side effects and lower risk for contributing to bacterial resistance compared with oral therapy.
- Mupirocin 2% ointment or cream, children >2 months old: Applied to affected areas three times daily for 5 days
- Retapamulin 1% ointment, children >9 months old: applied to affected area (up to 2% BSA) twice daily for 5 days
- Although the components of over-the-counter triple antibiotic ointments (consisting of bacitracin–neomycin–polymyxin B) do have some activity against the organisms causing impetigo, they are not considered effective for treatment.

Oral therapy

- Oral antibiotic therapy should be used for impetigo when the lesions are bullous, and when it is impractical to use topical therapy either due to the extent or location of lesions:
- Amoxicillin/clavulanic acid 40mg/kg/d in 2 divided doses × 10 days
- Cephalexin 25 mg/kg/d in 4 divided doses × 10 days
- Clindamycin 15–25 mg/kg/d in 3 divided doses × 10 days
- Erythromycin 40 mg/kg/d in 4 divided doses × 10 days
- When MRSA is suspected:
  - Please become familiar with resistance patterns in the community.
  - Clindamycin 15–25 mg/kg/d in 3 divided doses × 10 days
  - Trimethoprim–sulfamethoxazole: Trimethoprim 8 mg/kg and sulfamethoxazole 40 mg/kg daily in 2 divided doses × 10 days

 ONGOING CARE

FOLLOW-UP RECOMMENDATIONS
Duration of Therapy:
The duration of antimicrobial therapy should be tailored to clinical improvement; 7–10 days of treatment is usually appropriate. The skin covered with the crusted lesions can be cleansed gently with soap and water. In addition, regular hand washing is important for reducing spread among children.

Signs of Incomplete Therapy:
- Recurrent infection may indicate incomplete therapy, reinfection, or an *S. aureus* carrier state.
- Development of fever is unusual, and may indicate a more serious infection and/or the presence of cellulitis or an abscess.

Pitfalls:
- Impetigo frequently spreads among close contacts and family members. Patients and family members should wash their hands frequently, keep clothes and bedding clean, and not share towels and other personal care items.
- Underlying skin conditions (e.g., eczema) and infestations (e.g., scabies) should be treated appropriately to decrease the likelihood of the development of impetigo.

COMPLICATIONS
Cellulitis, lymphangitis, suppurative lymphadenitis, and staphylococcal scalded skin syndrome occur in as many as 10% of patients with impetigo. In addition, acute post streptococcal glomerulonephritis, scarlet fever, osteomyelitis, septic arthritis, pneumonia, septicemia, and rheumatic fever have also been observed in patients with impetigo.

PROGNOSIS
The sores of impetigo usually heal; although there may be some post-inflammatory hyperpigmentation. Overall, the infection is highly curable, but the condition often recurs in young children.

ADDITIONAL READING

- Bass JW, Chan DS, Creamer KM, et al. Comparison of oral cephalexin, topical mupirocin and topical bacitracin for treatment of impetigo. *Pediatr Infect Dis J*. 1997;16:708–710.
- Darmstadt GL, Lane AT. Impetigo: An overview. *Pediatr Dermatol*. 1994;11(4):293–303.
- George A, Rubin G. A systematic review and meta-analysis of treatments for impetigo. *Br J Gen Pract*. 2003;53:480–487.
- Stevens DL, Bisno AL, Chambers HF, et al. Practice guidelines for the diagnosis and management of skin and soft-tissue infections. *Clin Infect Dis*. 2005; 41:1373–1406.

 CODES

ICD9
684 Impetigo

ICD10
- L01.00 Impetigo, unspecified
- L01.01 Non-bullous impetigo
- L01.03 Bullous impetigo

FAQ

- Q: Which is the more effective treatment for impetigo—oral or topical antibiotics?
- A: In general, if there are a few localized lesions, topical therapy with mupirocin is preferred. If there is more diffuse involvement, or systemic symptoms, a course of oral antibiotics is recommended.
- Q: Can a child with impetigo attend school or child care?
- A: After a child begins antibiotic therapy and the lesions begin to improve, the child may resume his or her activities without restrictions.
- Q: How does one help prevent impetigo from spreading?
- A: Gently wash the affected areas with mild soap and running water, use the antibiotics (topical or oral) as directed, and then cover lesions with bandages. Wear gloves when applying any antibiotic ointment to the patient's lesions and endorse thorough hand washing afterwards. Do not share clothes, linens, or towels used by the affected individual until the infection has cleared.

I

INAPPROPRIATE ANTIDIURETIC HORMONE SECRETION

Sogol Mostoufi-Moab
Sheela N. Magge
Paul S. Thornton (5th edition)

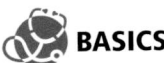

BASICS

DESCRIPTION
Inappropriate secretion of antidiuretic hormone (ADH) or ADH-like peptide in the presence of low serum sodium, low serum osmolality, and high urine osmolality, and in the absence of renal, adrenal, or thyroid pathology

EPIDEMIOLOGY
Incidence
The syndrome of inappropriate antidiuretic hormone (SIADH) can occur at any age. Its incidence depends on the various possible etiologies.

RISK FACTORS
Genetics
Genetic causes of SIADH are exceedingly rare. However, 2 cases have been described with gain-of-function mutation in the vasopressin-2 receptor contributing to SIADH and undetectable serum ADH levels.

PATHOPHYSIOLOGY
- ADH is synthesized within the neurons of the hypothalamus, transported in conjunction with neurophysin down the supraopticohypophyseal tract, and stored in the posterior pituitary.
- ADH acts on the renal collecting ducts.
- Interaction of ADH with its receptors forms intracellular cyclic AMP (cAMP), which increases water permeability through insertion of aquaporins (water channels) in renal collecting ducts and consequently enhances reabsorption of free water.
- SIADH results when elevated levels of ADH or ADH-like peptides cause free water retention and hypervolemia leading to hyponatremia. Three possible mechanisms include:
  – Increased hypothalamic production of ADH (e.g., CNS disorders such as stroke or meningitis)
  – Independent production of ADH or ADH-like substances from ectopic sources (e.g., lung oat cell carcinoma or olfactory neuroblastoma)
  – Decreased venous return that stimulates atrial volume receptors and thereby leads to ADH release (e.g., heart failure, cirrhosis, pulmonary and intrathoracic diseases, such as tuberculosis)

ETIOLOGY
- Idiopathic
- CNS pathology, causing increased secretion of ADH or ADH-like peptides: Meningitis, head trauma, neurosurgical procedures, encephalitis, Guillain-Barré syndrome, brain tumor, brain abscess, hydrocephalus, hypoxia, subarachnoid hemorrhage, cerebral venous thrombosis
- Ectopic production of ADH or ADH-like peptides: Oat cell carcinoma of the lung, bronchogenic carcinoma, olfactory neuroblastoma, and pancreatic carcinoma
- Pulmonary disease (leading to secondary elevation in ADH secretion or ADH-like peptides): Tuberculosis, viral or bacterial pneumonia, asthma, cystic fibrosis, pneumothorax, positive pressure ventilation

- Drugs (which mimic ADH or stimulate its release): Vincristine, cyclophosphamide, carbamazepine, chlorpropamide, phenothiazines, clofibrate, nicotine, fluoxetine, sertraline
- Iatrogenic exogenous administration of ADH: Vasopressin infusion for treatment of diabetes insipidus, excess desmopressin (DDAVP) in conjunction with fluid intake
- Severe, prolonged nausea
- Postoperative patient (e.g., as part of triple-phase response after hypothalamic–pituitary surgery, after transsphenoidal pituitary surgery)
- Rocky Mountain spotted fever

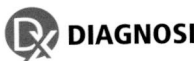

DIAGNOSIS

HISTORY
- Unusual water intake (suspicious for psychogenic polydipsia)
- Review of intake and output for inpatients
- Decreased urine output
- Anorexia, lethargy
- Weight gain or weight loss
- Renal disease
- Vomiting
- Diarrhea
- Use of diuretics
- Burns
- Heart disease
- Liver disease
- Brain injury: Trauma, surgery, hypoxia, toxin

PHYSICAL EXAM
- A complete neurologic and physical exam must be performed. Classically, patients with SIADH manifest subtle signs of hypervolemia but without increased urine output.
- With or without edema
- No signs of dehydration
- Signs of fluid overload
- Absent hyperpigmentation of skin creases/gums (presence suggests Addison disease)
- Hyponatremia, may cause lethargy or irritability, and muscle cramps. In severe cases, patients may lose deep tendon reflexes, seize, or be comatose.

ALERT
- Pitfall: Failure to distinguish SIADH from other causes of hyponatremia such as adrenal insufficiency, hypothyroidism, or cerebral salt wasting (CSW) can result in erroneous medical management and lead to worsening hyponatremia.
- Patients with SIADH are still capable of making urine; basing the diagnosis on urine volume alone can be misleading.

DIAGNOSTIC TESTS & INTERPRETATION
Lab
- Specific tests:
  – Simultaneous urinary osmolality, serum osmolality, and serum sodium (order a basic metabolic panel)
  – Urine sodium: Usually >30 mmol/L
  – Serum uric acid: Usually low in SIADH
  – Presence of hyponatremia (serum sodium <130 mEq/L), decreased serum osmolality (<260 mOsm/kg), with an inappropriately elevated urinary osmolality (>260 mOsm/L)
  – Plasma ADH concentration: Diagnostic but not helpful for rapid diagnosis
- Nonspecific tests:
  – Fractional renal excretion of sodium: Net sodium loss is normal or elevated and is dependent on sodium intake.
  – Urinary specific gravity: Helpful but not as specific as urine osmolality
  – Blood glucose: Hyperglycemia results in pseudohyponatremia.
  – Triglycerides: Hyperlipidemia causes pseudohyponatremia.

Imaging
Head MRI with special cuts of the pituitary and hypothalamus if indicated

DIFFERENTIAL DIAGNOSIS
- Hypovolemic hyponatremia (e.g., hyponatremic dehydration, seen after running a marathon)
- Euvolemic hyponatremia (e.g., hypothyroidism, adrenal insufficiency)
- Hypervolemic hyponatremia (e.g., CHF, cirrhosis, nephrotic syndrome)
- Diuretics
- Total body sodium loss through vomiting, nasogastric suction, diarrhea, or increased intestinal secretions
- Renal failure
- Severe potassium depletion
- Water intoxication
- Cerebral salt wasting: Excess production or effects of atrial and/or brain natriuretic peptide hormones
- Reset hypothalamic osmostat
- Rocky Mountain spotted fever
- Pseudohyponatremia with hyperglycemia (diabetic ketoacidosis), severe hyperlipidemia, or after administration of mannitol

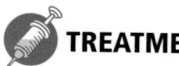 ## TREATMENT

MEDICATION (DRUGS)

- For emergency use only: Hypertonic saline (1.5–3% NaCl)
- Diuretics should be avoided because they worsen hyponatremia.
- ADH antagonists, such as tolvaptan, have been shown to be effective for treatment of SIADH in research trials for adults.
- Demeclocycline (for chronic SIADH)

ADDITIONAL TREATMENT
General Measures
- The most important aspects of therapy for SIADH are diagnosis and treatment of the underlying cause.
- Hyponatremia may result in seizures, which will require immediate treatment with 3% hypertonic saline until the seizure activity stabilizes. Despite the urgent need for correction of hyponatremia to address the severe neurologic symptoms, the rate of sodium correction should not exceed 12 mEq/L in 24 hours.

IN-PATIENT CONSIDERATIONS
Admission Criteria
Patients with severe hyponatremia and/or neurologic manifestations will need to be admitted for correction of hyponatremia under close medical supervision.

IV Fluids
- Fluid restriction is essential to treat and prevent worsening hyponatremia. Thus, IV fluid, in general, is not recommended for patients with SIADH. If IVF is clinically necessary, a rate comparable to insensible losses (1/3 daily maintenance) is recommended with close attention to the serum sodium levels.
- The hyponatremia in SIADH is due to free water retention and not due to decreased total body sodium content. For this reason, changing IV fluid from hypotonic solutions to hypertonic (normal saline) without restriction of rate will still result in worsening hyponatremia.

Discharge Criteria
- Depends on the primary etiology causing SIADH
- Generally, when the serum sodium is stabilized and the patient is neurologically stable

 ## ONGOING CARE

FOLLOW-UP RECOMMENDATIONS
Patient Monitoring
- When to expect improvement: Usually during the 1st 48–72 hours
- Signs to watch for: Changes in neurologic status

DIET
Fluid restriction is the most important aspect in the treatment of SIADH. Generally, only fluids for insensible losses (1/3 daily maintenance) are recommended.

PROGNOSIS
Based on the primary cause

COMPLICATIONS
- Severe hyponatremia can cause seizures and, rarely, brain damage. Correcting hyponatremia too quickly can lead to central pontine myelinolysis (CPM), a devastating demyelinating disease, which impairs vital functions such as breathing.
- Susceptibility to CPM due to correction of hyponatremia is strongly influenced by the severity and preexisting duration of hyponatremia in the patient.
- Serum sodium should not be increased >12 mEq/L in 24 hours.

ADDITIONAL READING

- Ellison DH, Berl T. The Syndrome of Inappropriate Antidiuresis. *N Engl J Med*. 2007;356(20): 2064–2072.
- Feldman BJ, Rosenthal SM, Vargas GA, et al. Nephrogenic syndrome of inappropriate antidiuresis. *N Engl J Med*. 2005;352:1884.
- Fenske W, Allolio B. The syndrome of inappropriate secretion of antidiuretic hormone: Diagnostic and therapeutic advances. *Horm Metab Res*. 2010; 42(10):691–702.
- Schrier RW, Gross P, Gheorghiade M, et al. Tolvaptan, a selective oral vasopressin V2-receptor antagonist, for hyponatremia. *N Engl J Med*. 2006;355:2099–2112.
- Singh S, Bohn D, Carlotti AP, et al. Cerebral salt wasting: Truths, fallacies, theories, and challenges. *Crit Care Med*. 2002;30(11):2575–2579.

 ## CODES

ICD9
253.6 Other disorders of neurohypophysis

ICD10
E22.2 Syndrome of inappropriate secretion of antidiuretic hormone

FAQ

- Q: Is the use of diuretics beneficial in treating SIADH?
- A: No. Although diuretics may relieve the effects of volume overloading, they also worsen hyponatremia. Overall, diuretics usually cause more detriment than benefit.
- Q: What distinguishes SIADH from cerebral salt wasting?
- A: CSW occurs because of increased natriuresis from increased plasma and CSF levels of atrial natriuretic peptide (ANP) after neurologic insults (e.g., subarachnoid hemorrhage). Owing to the natriuresis, these patients become dehydrated with notable decreased plasma volume and elevated BUN. In contrast, patients with SIADH have free water overload, causing hyponatremia. CSW is associated with very high urine output, in contrast to SIADH, which has low urine output. However, patients with SIADH who are treated with excess solute (3% saline) may exhibit a natural natriuresis and a high urine output. Thus, polyuria alone should never be used to distinguish between CSW and SIADH. Net sodium loss is very high in CSW, but SIADH has normal to slightly elevated net sodium loss; thus, urinary sodium levels are often not very helpful in distinguishing CSW from SIADH. Laboratory features of CSW include suppressed plasma aldosterone and normal serum uric acid concentration. Note that plasma ADH concentration is high in SIADH, and initially in CSW as well. However, in CSW, after the intravascular volume has been restored, the ADH will decrease again, and patients may not exhibit elevated urine osmolality. In these patients, persistent hyponatremia with elevated urine osmolality is more suggestive of SIADH, which is far more common than CSW.
- Q: Why is it important to distinguish SIADH from CSW?
- A: Therapies differ dramatically for these conditions. Unlike the water restriction used to treat SIADH, treatment of dehydration, such as that seen in CSW, requires replacement of ongoing salt and water losses. However, CSW is much less common than SIADH and appropriate diagnosis of each condition is necessary to avoid worsening of hyponatremia by the treatment regimen.

I

INFANTILE SPASMS

Juliann Paolicchi
Amy R. Brooks-Kayal (5th edition)
Eric Marsh (5th edition)

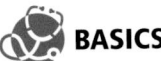 **BASICS**

DESCRIPTION
- An epileptic encephalopathy of infancy or early childhood consisting of myoclonic seizures and electroencephalographic pattern: High-voltage slowing, asynchrony, disorganization, and multifocal spikes (hypsarrhythmia)
- Seizures can be flexor, extensor, mixed flexor/extensor, or arrest/akinetic. They occur in clusters, typically upon awakening or drowsiness, and can have focal features.
- The combination of infantile spasms, hypsarrhythmia, and developmental arrest is known as West syndrome.
- Infantile spasms (ISs) are symptomatic if the child has a coexistent neurologic condition or developmental delay at presentation, or if a specific etiology can be identified. They are cryptogenic if no underlying cause is found.

EPIDEMIOLOGY
90% have onset <1 year of age, with the majority between 3 and 7 months. Onset after 18 months is rare.

Incidence
Incidence is 0.16–0.42/10,000 live births. In patients with tuberous sclerosis complex the incidence is 68%.

RISK FACTORS
Genetics
- Most cases are sporadic with a positive family history of IS present in 3–6%.
- Tuberous sclerosis complex may be sporadic or autosomal dominant.
- X-linked infantile spasm syndromes (ARX, CDKL-5), and chromosomal (STXBP-1) show variable penetrance.

ETIOLOGY
- Genetic syndromes:
  – Neurocutaneous disorders: Tuberous sclerosis complex, incontinentia pigmenti, neurofibromatosis type I (NF1)
  – Down syndrome
  – X-linked infantile spasm syndromes: ARX, CDKL5, Aicardi syndrome
  – Autosomal infantile spasm syndromes: Miller-Dieker syndrome (17p13.3), 18q and 7q duplication, partial 2p trisomy, and STXBP1 and MAGI2 deletions
- Metabolic disorders:
  – Congenital lactic acidoses and mitochondrial disorders
  – Phenylketonuria
  – Nonketotic hyperglycinemia
  – Pyridoxine and folinic acid deficiency syndromes
- Malformations of cortical development
- Almost any cause of prenatal, perinatal, or early infant brain injury may lead to infantile spasms, including meningitis, encephalitis, hypoxic-ischemic injury, abusive head trauma, stroke, and congenital infection.
- ~40% of infantile spasms are cryptogenic, but that percentage may decrease with recent genetic discoveries.

COMMONLY ASSOCIATED CONDITIONS
- Intrauterine infection, CNS infections
- Cerebral malformations: Malformation of cortical development
- Hypoxic-ischemic encephalopathy, perinatal asphyxia, prenatal/perinatal stroke
- Abusive head trauma
- Intraventricular hemorrhage
- Kernicterus
- Genetic and neurocutaneous conditions noted above

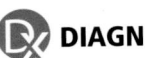 **DIAGNOSIS**

HISTORY
- Prenatal and perinatal history, including maternal age, pregnancy complications, perinatal difficulties
- Family history of tuberous sclerosis, epilepsy, or previous children with infantile spasms or early infant demise
- Developmental history to establish any preexisting developmental delay
- Description of spells to differentiate spasms from nonepileptic seizures

PHYSICAL EXAM
- Check general growth parameters, especially head circumference.
- Microcephaly suggests preexisting brain abnormality, poorer prognosis.
- Dysmorphism (Down stigmata)
- Retinal defects as in Aicardi syndrome or metabolic diseases
- Hepatomegaly, suggesting inborn errors of metabolism or congenital infection
- Careful skin exam, including Wood lamp exam, should be performed for evidence of neurocutaneous disorders, especially the hypopigmented macules associated with tuberous sclerosis.
- Neurologic exam: Particular attention should be paid to level of alertness (visual attentiveness often impaired at presentation), developmental milestones, and motor tone.

DIAGNOSTIC TESTS & INTERPRETATION
- EEG: High-voltage, disorganized, multifocal spikes; asynchronous, hypsarrhythmia
- Infants with cutaneous signs of tuberous sclerosis should undergo cardiologic and ophthalmologic evaluation and renal ultrasound; genetic counseling for family; other family members should be evaluated.
- Pyridoxine or folinic acid challenge during electroencephalogram: Infantile spasms can present as pyridoxine or folinic acid–dependent seizures.

Lab
- Routine blood studies:
  – Electrolytes
  – Calcium
  – Glucose (although generally unrevealing)
- Chromosomal analysis:
  – Karyotype for Down phenotype
  – Tuberous sclerosis complex screening for clinical or radiologic evidence of tuberous sclerosis. Genetic testing available for other neurocutaneous disorders, if suspected
  – Chromosome microarray for suspected genetic or cryptogenic cases
  – Specific genetic panels available for infantile spasm–associated syndromes
- Metabolic screening, including blood lactate, pyruvate, and ammonia. Serum amino acids, cholesterol panel (pyridoxine disorders), urine organic acids. Review neonatal metabolic screening for phenylketonuria and biotinidase.
- TORCH titers, depending on level of suspicion for congenital infection or microcephaly

Imaging
- MRI is the single most useful laboratory test; intracranial calcifications associated with intrauterine infections and tuberous sclerosis are more apparent on CT, but CT rarely needed
- PET imaging for refractory infantile spasms and suspected cortical malformations

Diagnostic Procedures/Other
If no cause is found using other diagnostic modalities, consider lumbar puncture for lactic acid, amino acids, folate metabolites, glucose, glycine, and abnormalities of neurotransmitter levels.

Pathological Findings
Depends on etiology: May include gliosis, atrophy, remote stroke, malformation of cortical development, tubers, etc.

DIFFERENTIAL DIAGNOSIS
- Nonepileptic disorders:
  – Benign myoclonus
  – Benign sleep myoclonus
  – Paroxysmal torticollis
  – Posturing related to gastroesophageal reflux (Sandifer syndrome)
  – Shuddering spells
  – Exaggerated startle in children with cerebral palsy
- Myoclonic epilepsies of infancy:
  – Benign myoclonic epilepsy of infancy
  – Severe myoclonic epilepsy (early infantile epileptic encephalopathy)

 TREATMENT

MEDICATION (DRUGS)
First Line
- Adrenocorticotropic hormone (ACTH) is the historical treatment option, and many different protocols are in use with variability between high- and low-dose protocols.
- Treatment is often initiated at 150 U/m^2/d IM) (high dose) or 20–30 U/d (low dose) for 1–2 weeks. If the low-dose protocol is not effective after 2 weeks, the patient receives high dose at 40 U/d. The dose in either case is gradually tapered over 1–3 months. A recent study showed no difference in the high- and low-dose protocols in terms of efficacy (50–58%), but the high-dose group had greater side effects. A recent consensus study recommended high dose for 2 weeks, followed by a taper.

- Side effects: Weight gain, irritability, sleep disturbance, hyperglycemia, hypertension, electrolyte abnormalities, cardiomyopathy, immunosuppression, gastritis/GI bleeding, osteoporosis, growth failure
- ACTH therapy has not been proven to affect outcome in infants whose spasms are caused by prenatal or perinatal brain abnormalities (symptomatic infantile spasms).
- Patients are typically admitted for initiation and education of ACTH therapy, and weekly monitoring of BP, glucose, electrolytes, BUN/creatinine, stool guaiac, and signs of infection is recommended. Stopping ACTH resolves its side effects.
- Vigabatrin is considered the 1st-line agent for infantile spasms secondary to tuberous sclerosis complex. Dosing is initiated at 50 mg/kg/d and increased to 100–200 mg/kg/d for efficacy. The duration of therapy is not established owing to potential visual field constriction that may be related to duration of therapy. Other side effects include hypotonia, drowsiness, irritability, and reversible MRI abnormalities. Comparison trials with ACTH suggest better tolerance, similar long-term outcomes in the symptomatic group, and potentially less short-term efficacy.

Second Line
- A trial of pyridoxine (100 mg IV) and folinic acid (2.5 mg IV) should be considered to rule out pyridoxine and folinic acid deficiency or dependency. Reports (primarily from Japan) exist of successful treatment of infantile spasms with daily high-dose pyridoxine (200–300 mg/d).
- Topiramate (at dosages up to 20–60 mg/kg/d)
- Zonisamide (5–15 mg/kg/d)
- Clonazepam (0.1–0.15 mg/kg/d) or nitrazepam (0.5–3.5 mg/kg/d)
- Ketogenic diet
- Prednisone (2 mg/kg/d)
- Less used alternatives:
  – Tiagabine (0.3–1.3 mg/kg/d)
  – Valproate used cautiously because of the increased rate of fatal hepatotoxicity in this age group

SURGERY/OTHER PROCEDURES
May be indicated in malformations of cortical development, particularly hemimegalencephaly and treatment-refractory infantile spasms, especially due to tuberous sclerosis. Referral to a pediatric epilepsy center is recommended.

IN-PATIENT CONSIDERATIONS
Initial Stabilization
- If patient appears ill (possible with metabolic disorders) tend to ABCs before treatment of spasms. (Infantile spasms themselves rarely threaten vital functions.)
- General:
  – The goal of treatment is cessation of spasms and resolution of electroencephalogram.
  – The primary options for treatment are ACTH and vigabatrin, approved for the treatment of IS; however, owing to the difficulty of placebo-controlled trials for IS and the variability of the many treatment protocols, a clear consensus on treatment has not been reached.

 ONGOING CARE

PROGNOSIS
- Developmental retardation occurs in 85% of patients, and long-term outcome is dependent on underlying etiology. Patients with cryptogenic IS have an overall better prognosis than symptomatic IS.
- 10% of patients achieve normal cognitive, physical, and educational development.
- 50–90% of children develop other seizure types, most commonly in the symptomatic group. 27–50% develop severe epileptic encephalopathy (Lennox-Gastaut syndrome).

COMPLICATIONS
- Hypertension and hemorrhagic gastritis may occur during ACTH therapy and must be anticipated by weekly follow-up visits. Parents need to be educated about immunosuppression during therapy, and vaccinations are typically held for 3 months.
- Infantile spasm recurrence is common, as is the development of secondary epilepsy syndromes, and requires additional treatment.

ADDITIONAL READING
- Darle K, Edwards SW, Hancock E, et al. Developmental and epilepsy outcomes at age 4 years in the UKISS trial comparing hormonal treatments to vigabatrin for infantile spasms: A multi-centre randomized trial. *Arch Dis Child.* 2010;95:382.
- Elterman RD, Shields WD, Bittman RM, et al. Vigabatrin for the treatment of infantile spasms: Final report of a randomized trail. *J Child Neurol.* 2010;25:1340.

- Epilepsy Foundation. *Patient information.* Available at: http://www.epilepsyfoundation.org.
- Goh S, Kwiatkowski DJ, Dorer DJ, et al. Infantile spasms and intellectual outcomes in children with tuberous sclerosis complex. *Neurology.* 2005;65:235.
- Holland KD, Hallinan BE. What causes epileptic encephalopathy in infancy? The answer may lie in our genes. *Neurology.* 2010;75(13):1132.
- McKay MT, Weiss SK, Adams-Webber T, et al. Practice parameter: Medical treatment of infantile spasms: Report of the American Academy of Neurology and the Child Neurology Society. *Neurology.* 2004;62:1668.
- The National Institute of Neurological Disorders and Stroke. *NINDS infantile spasms information page.* Available at: http://www.ninds.nih.gov/disorders/infantilespasms/infantilespasms.htm.
- Pellock JM, Hrachovy R, Shinnar S, et al. Infantile spasms: A US consensus report. *Epilepsia.* 2010;51:2175.

CODES

ICD9
- 345.60 Infantile spasms, without mention of intractable epilepsy
- 345.61 Infantile spasms, with intractable epilepsy

ICD10
- G40.401 Other generalized epilepsy and epileptic syndromes, not intractable, with status epilepticus
- G40.409 Other generalized epilepsy and epileptic syndromes, not intractable, without status epilepticus

FAQ
- Q: Do infantile spasms ever remit spontaneously?
- A: Spontaneous remission of infantile spasms has been reported but appears to be rare.
- Q: What is the developmental prognosis in idiopathic infantile spasms?
- A: Guarded; periodic evaluation by a child neurologist or developmental pediatrician helps to detect delays in motor or cognitive development and involvement of early intervention services is recommended. Cessation of spasms and resolution of electroencephalogram are associated with the best outcome.

I

INFLUENZA

Kristen A. Feemster
Joel A. Fein (5th edition)

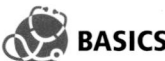 **BASICS**

DESCRIPTION
An acute febrile illness characterized by fever, malaise, and respiratory symptoms

EPIDEMIOLOGY
- Although influenza affects people of all ages, the highest morbidity and mortality occur in young children <2 years old and the geriatric population.
- Attack rates are highest among school-aged children and range from 10–40%. ~1% of infections result in hospitalization but infection and hospitalization rates vary significantly across seasons.
- 20% of hospitalized children develop severe outcomes, and complication rates increase in children <2 years and those with high-risk conditions (see "Complications"). Epidemics of influenza occur almost exclusively during winter months, peak ~2 weeks after the index case, and last 4–8 weeks. Up to 75% of school children in the epidemic region may be affected.
- Transmission of influenza virus occurs by aerosol droplets, as well as by direct or indirect contact.
- Viral shedding starts 24 hours before symptoms onset and usually continues for 7 days:
  - Prolonged shedding may occur in young children, immunocompromised individuals

RISK FACTORS
High-risk conditions for severe disease include: Chronic pulmonary disease (i.e., asthma), hemodynamically significant cardiac disease, HIV and other immunodeficiencies, chronic immunosuppressive therapy, hemoglobinopathies (i.e., sickle cell disease), long-term salicylate use, chronic renal dysfunction, chronic metabolic disease, morbid obesity, and neuromuscular disorders.

General Prevention
- Vaccination:
  - American Academy of Pediatrics recommends influenza vaccination for:
    ○ All children ≥6 months during influenza season (October–March)
    ○ Health care professionals
    ○ Out-of-home caregivers and household contacts of all children <5 years old OR children 5–18 years old who are at high risk for complications from influenza infection (see Risk Factors)
    ○ Pregnant women
  - Vaccine types:
    ○ Trivalent inactivated influenza vaccine (TIV) approved for children ≥6 months; administered as an intradermal injection.
    ○ Live-attenuated influenza vaccine (LAIV) approved for healthy nonpregnant 2- to 49-year-olds; administered as an intranasal spray; not recommended for high-risk persons, contacts of severely immunocompromised persons, or children receiving chronic aspirin therapy (because of the association between aspirin use, influenza infection, and Reye syndrome.)
  - Children <10 years old receiving seasonal influenza vaccination for the 1st time should receive 2 doses of vaccine administered at least 1 month apart.

- LAIV can be given simultaneously with both live and inactivated vaccines. However, after administration of any live vaccine, a minimum of 4 weeks should pass before administering another live vaccine.
- People with a known anaphylactic hypersensitivity to eggs or a history of Guillain-Barré syndrome within 6 weeks of previous influenza vaccination should consult a physician before receiving the vaccine.
- Postexposure chemoprophylaxis:
  - Prophylactic administration of antiviral medications is indicated for: High-risk children who are unvaccinated or were vaccinated within 2 weeks of exposure, immunocompromised patients who have a poor response to vaccine, and high-risk patients who cannot receive the vaccine (anaphylactic reaction to chicken or eggs); also for control of outbreaks in institutions housing high-risk people
  - Chemoprophylaxis should begin within 48 hours of exposure to be most effective
  - The neuraminidase inhibitors zanamivir and oseltamivir are now approved for prophylaxis. Amantadine and rimantadine should not be used due to widespread resistance.

ETIOLOGY
- The orthomyxoviruses influenza types A, B, and C; influenza C virus has not been reported as a cause of influenza epidemics.
- Influenza A has subtypes defined by 2 surface antigens: Hemagglutinin and neuraminidase:
  - Currently circulating subtypes include novel 2009 H1N1 and H3N2
- Mild variation, or antigenic drift, for both A and B viruses results in seasonal epidemics; antigenic shift occurs only with A viruses and results in pandemics.

COMMONLY ASSOCIATED CONDITIONS
- Pharyngitis
- Laryngotracheitis (croup)
- Bronchitis/bronchiolitis
- Pneumonia
- Gastroenteritis
- Conjunctivitis
- Otitis media

DIAGNOSIS

- Illness is marked by acute onset of constitutional and respiratory symptoms.
- Infection with influenza causes distinct clinical pictures based on the affected individual's age:
  - Infants and young children are less likely to present with typical symptoms but may suffer higher fevers and more severe respiratory symptoms.
  - Many older children and adults infected with influenza are diagnosed with a "viral respiratory infection," without specific reference to the viral etiologic agent.
- The diagnosis of influenza infection is more commonly made in light of previously identified index cases or specific findings, such as myositis.

HISTORY
- Abrupt onset of illness, beginning with chills, headache, malaise, and dry cough
- Subsequent increase in respiratory tract symptoms that can range from mild cough to severe respiratory distress (infants)
- Other symptoms: Fever, anorexia, myalgias, sore throat, irritability
- GI complaints in younger children may include vomiting, diarrhea, and severe abdominal pain.
- Children may also commonly present with otitis media.

PHYSICAL EXAM
- Cough is the predominant respiratory sign. Infants and small children may exhibit a "barky" cough (croup).
- Nasal congestion and conjunctival and pharyngeal infections are common.
- Cervical adenopathy is more common in children than in adults.
- Neonates may appear septic with apnea, circulatory collapse, or petechiae.
- A generalized macular or maculopapular rash is sometimes observed.

DIAGNOSTIC TESTS & INTERPRETATION
Lab
- Culture is the traditional gold standard for diagnosis of influenza. Viral culture from nasopharyngeal secretions will be positive within 2–6 days:
  - Only culture isolates can be used to measure subtype and antiviral resistance of circulating strains.
- Direct immunofluorescent antibody (DFA) and indirect immunofluorescence antibody (IFA) tests have moderate sensitivity (6–70%) and excellent specificity (>95%), and are completed within 2–4 hours.
- Rapid antigen testing is available for diagnosing influenza A and influenza B. The tests can be completed within 10–15 minutes but have a wide range of sensitivities (22–77% in community settings), which may limit their usefulness. A negative test result should not guide management, especially when community prevalence is high.
- Reverse transcriptase-polymerase chain reaction (RT-PCR) is now the most accurate and sensitive testing modality. These tests are increasingly available but labor intensive.
- False positives:
  - The false-positive rate of DFA, IFA, and rapid antigen testing may be as high as 20% for influenza A and 40% for influenza B.
  - The use of nasopharyngeal aspirates rather than nasopharyngeal swabs may reduce this false-positive rate by 5–10%.

Imaging
Chest x-ray:
- May be normal despite significant respiratory involvement
- X-rays of patients with lower airway involvement are indistinguishable from those in patients with other viral lower respiratory infections.

DIFFERENTIAL DIAGNOSIS
- Viral infections including but not limited to respiratory syncytial virus, parainfluenza, adenovirus:
  - Difficult to distinguish infection from other respiratory pathogens based upon clinical presentation alone
- *Streptococcus pyogenes* infection
- Bacterial sepsis in young infants

 TREATMENT

MEDICATION (DRUGS)
- Neuraminidase inhibitors (oseltamivir and zanamivir) are the recommended antiviral medications for both treatment of and chemoprophylaxis against influenza A and B:
  - Although amantadine hydrochloride and rimantadine are approved for treatment of influenza A in children >1 year of age, the CDC has recommended against their use for both treatment and prophylaxis due to increasing resistance. Neither is effective against influenza B.
- Early treatment decreases duration of illness and can decrease symptom severity among patients at high risk of complications
- Antiviral treatment is recommended for any patient who is:
  - Hospitalized
  - Has severe or progressive illness
  - At high risk for complications
- Treatment is most effective when initiated <2 days after symptom onset but may still reduce morbidity and mortality for hospitalized patients or patients with severe disease if started after >2 days of symptoms.
- Treatment of healthy children with suspected or confirmed influenza in the outpatient setting is at the clinician's discretion but should be initiated <2 days after symptom onset
- Dosage recommendations:
  - Zanamivir is approved for treatment in children ≥7 years and prophylaxis in children ≥5 years of age.
    - Treatment: Two 10 mg inhalations b.i.d. × 5 days
    - Prophylaxis: Two 10 mg inhalations once per day × 10 days
    - Can cause bronchospasm, so should not be used in patients with history of chronic pulmonary diseases such as asthma

- Oseltamivir is approved for treatment and prophylaxis in children ≥1 year of age:
  - Dose depends upon weight (<15 kg: 30 mg, 15–23 kg: 45 mg, >23–40 kg: 60 mg, >40 kg: 75 mg), b.i.d. × 5 days for treatment and once daily x 10 days for prophylaxis
  - Treatment guidelines for infants <1 year were developed for 2009 pandemic influenza A (H1N1) under an Emergency Use Authorization (now expired)
  - May cause nausea and vomiting
- Investigational parenteral medications (peramivir and zanamivir):
  - For severely ill high risk patients with suspected or confirmed oseltamivir-resistant infection
  - Available through emergency Investigational New Drug protocol only
- Longer courses of therapy can be administered if patients remain severely ill after 5 days.
- Recommended duration of chemoprophylaxis is 10 days for household contacts and 7 days in other settings
- Preexposure prophylaxis can be considered for very-high-risk patients who cannot otherwise be protected against infection (i.e., cannot receive the vaccine) when there is high risk of exposure to influenza cases:
  - Duration depends upon expected duration of exposure, but 4–6 weeks has been well tolerated.
- Chemoprophylaxis should not be given within 14 days after LAIV receipt as the vaccine strains are susceptible to the antiviral medications.

ADDITIONAL TREATMENT
General Measures
Most patients with influenza infection require supportive oral hydration, antipyresis, and routine decongestant therapy.

 ONGOING CARE

FOLLOW-UP RECOMMENDATIONS
When to expect improvement:
- Fever associated with influenza infection usually lasts up to 5 days. Recrudescence of fever does not necessarily signify the onset of a secondary bacterial infection.
- Cough may last up to 2 weeks.
- Lethargy or malaise may persist for up to 2 weeks.
- Influenza A infection usually lasts longer than influenza B or influenza C infection.'

ADDITIONAL READING

- Cooper NJ, Sutton AJ, Abrams KR, et al. Effectiveness of neuraminidase inhibitors in treatment and prevention of influenza A and B: Systematic review and meta-analyses of randomized controlled trials. *Brit Med J.* 2003;326:1235–1241.
- Fiore AE, Fry A, Shay D, et al. Advisory Committee on Immunization Practices. Antiviral agents for the treatment and chemoprophylaxis of influenza: r: Recommendations of the Advisory Committee on Immunization Practices (ACIP). *MMWR Recomm Rep.* 2011;60(1):1–25.
- Glezen WP. Clinical practice. Prevention and treatment of seasonal influenza. *N Engl J Med.* 2008;359(24):2579–2585.
- Rouleau I, Charest H, Douville-Fradet M, et al. Field performance of a rapid diagnostic test for influenza in an ambulatory setting. *J Clin Microbiol.* 2009; 47(9):2699–2703.
- Stebbins S, Stark JH, Prasad R, et al. Sensitivity and specificity of rapid influenza testing of children in a community setting. *Influenza Other Respi Viruses.* 2011;5(2):104–109.

 CODES

ICD9
- 487.1 Influenza with other respiratory manifestations
- 487.8 Influenza with other manifestations
- 488.12 Influenza due to identified 2009 H1N1 influenza virus with other respiratory manifestations

ICD10
- J10.1 Influenza due to other identified influenza virus with other respiratory manifestations
- J11.1 Influenza due to unidentified influenza virus with other respiratory manifestations
- J11.89 Influenza due to unidentified influenza virus with other manifestations

FAQ
- Q: When is it safe for a child with influenza to return to daycare or school?
- A: Older children with influenza may shed the virus in nasal secretions for up to 7 days from onset of symptoms, and younger children even longer. Therefore, older children with influenza may return to school 1 week after the onset of symptoms, and infants and toddlers should remain home for 10–14 days.
- Q: Can a child on chronic steroid therapy be immunized against influenza?
- A: In general, children who require maintenance steroid therapy for their underlying illness should still receive influenza immunization. If possible, immunize while the child is on the lowest possible dose of steroids and not during a period of high-dose therapy.
- Q: What are the chances of acquiring influenza despite annual vaccination?
- A: Vaccination against influenza is >70–90% effective in preventing disease and >90% effective in preventing death from the infection.
- Q: Is chemoprophylaxis an acceptable alternative for protecting children against influenza?
- A: In general, chemoprophylaxis should not be used as a substitute for vaccination; specific recommendations and indications for chemoprophylaxis can be found at: www.aapredbook.org/flu

INGUINAL HERNIA

Joy Collins
Eugene Schneider (5th edition)

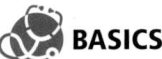 **BASICS**

DESCRIPTION
A hernia is defined as the protrusion of an organ or its portion through the wall that normally contains it. Inguinal hernia is a protrusion of abdominal contents (intestine, omentum) through the inguinal canal outside the peritoneal cavity.

EPIDEMIOLOGY
- Extremely common; represents the most frequent problem requiring surgical intervention in the pediatric age group
- Much more common in boys (90% of cases) than girls, has a definite familial tendency, and presents more frequently on the right side, possibly as a result of later descent of the right testis and delayed obliteration of the right processus vaginalis
- Clinical presentation is on the right side in 60% of cases, on the left side in 30%, and bilateral in 10%.
- Incidence varies with age and ranges from 3–5% in full-term babies to 7–30% in preterm infants.

RISK FACTORS
- Prematurity
- Urologic conditions: Cryptorchidism, hypospadias, epispadias, bladder exstrophy
- Abdominal wall defects: Gastroschisis, omphalocele
- Conditions that increase intra-abdominal pressure: Ascites, peritoneal dialysis, ventriculoperitoneal shunt
- Meconium peritonitis
- Cystic fibrosis
- Congenital dislocation of the hip
- Connective tissue disease: Marfan syndrome, Ehlers-Danlos syndrome
- Mucopolysaccharidoses
- Family history

PATHOPHYSIOLOGY
- In boys, during the 7th month of gestation, the testes begin their descent from the peritoneal cavity, where they developed, through the inguinal canal and down into the scrotum.
- Between the 7th and 9th months of gestation, the testes reach the scrotum, at which point the processus vaginalis—an outpouching of the peritoneum attached to the testes—begins to obliterate spontaneously, leaving a small potential space adjacent to the testes, called tunica vaginalis.

- In girls, although the ovaries do not leave the abdomen, the round ligament (part of the gubernaculum) travels through the inguinal ring into labium majus. When the processus vaginalis remains open, it is called the canal of Nuck.
- Incomplete obliteration of the processus vaginalis leaves a sac of peritoneum extending all the way from the internal inguinal ring to the scrotum or labium majus, from which an inguinal hernia may develop.

DIAGNOSIS

HISTORY
- Location of the bulge:
  - Swelling or bulge in the inguinal area is the most common presenting sign of inguinal hernia.
- Does the bulge change in size, and if so, what activities bring about these changes? The usual history is of an intermittently appearing bulge, especially noted at times of increased intra-abdominal pressure, such as during crying or straining.
- Does the child appear to be bothered by the swelling (extreme fussiness during diaper changes in babies or complaints of pain/discomfort in older children)? Hernias are usually asymptomatic. The parents may perceive the bulge as being painful to the baby because it often is more pronounced when the baby is crying. However, if the parents provide definitive history of a painful bulge in the inguinal region, incarcerated inguinal hernia must be suspected.

PHYSICAL EXAM
- Examine the child in the supine and standing positions. Reduction of hernia contents through the inguinal ring is confirmatory.
- If the bulge is apparent in the standing position but disappears when the child is supine, presence of a hernia is strongly suggested.
- If the bulge is not readily apparent, perform maneuvers that increase intra-abdominal pressure (have the patient blow up balloons, gently press on his or her abdomen, or have him or her cough or strain).
- Transillumination of the scrotum may help in differentiating hernias, which usually do not transilluminate, from hydroceles, which typically do (unreliable sign).

- When the empty hernia sac is palpated over the cord structures, the sensation may be similar to that of rubbing 2 layers of silk together. This finding is known as "the silk sign" and when detected by an experienced practitioner is highly suggestive of an inguinal hernia.
- Always consider an incarcerated hernia, testicular torsion, epididymitis, orchitis, or trauma when exam reveals a tender scrotal mass.
- Try to reduce the hernia with the child in the supine or head-down position so that gravity assists the maneuver. Use a pacifier to calm the infant. Do not force a difficult incarcerated hernia.
- Sliding hernia occurs when 1 wall of the hernia is composed of viscera.
- Richter hernia results from the herniation of only a part of the bowel wall, which results in bowel ischemia without bowel obstruction (very rare).
- Hernia of Littre has Meckel diverticulum in the hernia sac.

DIAGNOSTIC TESTS & INTERPRETATION
Karyotyping should be considered when a testis is palpable in the inguinal canal or found at herniorrhaphy in phenotypic females, because there is an association between androgen insensitivity and inguinal hernia.

Imaging
The diagnosis of an inguinal hernia can usually be made on the basis of the clinical history and exam. However, in some cases, use of scrotal or inguinal ultrasonography may be indicated:
- Suggestion of torsion (use duplex ultrasound to evaluate blood flow)
- Suggestion of the spermatic cord or testicular tumor
- Scrotal trauma and concern about testicular rupture

Diagnostic Procedures/Other

Consult a pediatric surgeon when a diagnosis of inguinal hernia or hydrocele is suspected. In the event of incarceration and/or strangulation, request an urgent consultation.

DIFFERENTIAL DIAGNOSIS

- Lymphadenopathy
- Hydrocele
- Retractile testis
- Undescended testis
- Varicocele
- Testicular tumor

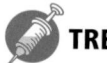 TREATMENT

SURGERY/OTHER PROCEDURES

Herniorrhaphy:

- Complication rate after an elective repair is low (1–2%) but increases dramatically (~20%) if the hernia becomes incarcerated. This excessive morbidity, along with a fairly high rate of incarceration in the 1st year of life, is responsible for the recommendation to repair pediatric inguinal hernias soon after they are diagnosed.
- ~10% of patients develop a contralateral hernia after a unilateral repair. Routine contralateral inguinal exploration in children with unilateral hernia has been a topic of debate for more than 50 years.
- Some surgeons perform diagnostic laparoscopy to evaluate for a contralateral patent processus vaginalis at the time of unilateral herniorrhaphy.
- Laparoscopic inguinal hernia repair has been performed in children of all ages, with a variety of techniques described in the literature. Currently, open repair remains the standard of care, but further study of laparoscopic repair is ongoing.

IN-PATIENT CONSIDERATIONS

Initial Stabilization

An inguinal hernia will not resolve spontaneously; herniorrhaphy (an outpatient procedure) is accepted universally as the treatment of choice.

 ONGOING CARE

PATIENT EDUCATION

Following operative repair, avoidance of major physical activity for 1 week is recommended.

COMPLICATIONS

- Incarceration (>50% of cases occur within the 1st 6 months of life)
- Strangulation
- Intestinal infarction leading to perforation and peritonitis
- Testicular/ovarian ischemia or infarction

ADDITIONAL READING

- Brandt ML. Pediatric hernias. *Surg Clin North Am.* 2008;88(1):27–43, vii–viii.
- Erez I, Rathause V, Vacian I, et al. Preoperative ultrasound and intraoperative findings of inguinal hernias in children: A prospective study of 642 children. *J Pediatr Surg.* 2002;37:865–868.
- Kapur P, Caty MG, Glick PL. Pediatric surgery for the primary care pediatrician, part I. *Pediatr Clin North Am.* 1998;45:773–789.
- Lee SL, Sydorak RM, Iau ST. Laparoscopic contralateral groin exploration: Is it cost-effective? *J Pediatr Surg.* 2010;45:793–795.
- Niyogi A, Tahim AS, Sherwood WJ, et al. A comparative study examining open inguinal herniotomy with and without hernioscopy to laparoscopic inguinal hernia repair in a pediatric population. *Pediatr Surg Int.* 2010;26:387–392.
- Parelkar SV, Oak S, Gupta R, et al. Laparoscopic inguinal hernia repair in the pediatric age group—experience with 437 children. *J Pediatr Surg.* 2010;45:789–792.

- Sheldon CA. The pediatric genitourinary examination: Inguinal, urethral, and genital diseases. *Pediatr Clin North Am.* 2001;48: 1339–1380.
- Tackett LD, Breuer CK, Luks FI, et al. Incidence of contralateral inguinal hernia: A prospective analysis. *J Pediatr Surg.* 1999;34:684–688.
- Toki A, Watanabe Y, Sasaki K, et al. Ultrasonographic diagnosis for potential contralateral inguinal hernia in children. *J Pediatr Surg.* 2003;38:224–226.
- Zendejas B, Zarroug A, Erben YA, et al. Impact of childhood inguinal hernia repair in adulthood: 50-years follow-up. *J Am Coll Surg.* 2010;211: 762–768.

 CODES

ICD9

- 550.90 Inguinal hernia, without mention of obstruction or gangrene, unilateral or unspecified (not specified as recurrent)
- 550.91 Inguinal hernia, without mention of obstruction or gangrene, unilateral or unspecified, recurrent

ICD10

- K40.90 Unilateral inguinal hernia, without obstruction or gangrene, not specified as recurrent
- K40.91 Unilateral inguinal hernia, without obstruction or gangrene, recurrent

FAQ

- Q: Are trusses helpful to keep the hernia from incarcerating?
- A: No. Surgery is the accepted treatment.

INTESTINAL OBSTRUCTION

Vered Yehezkely Schildkraut
Raanan Shamir

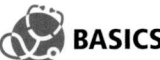 **BASICS**

DESCRIPTION

- Pathologic blockage of progression of intestinal contents:
  - May be partial or complete
  - May arise from **intrinsic abnormalities** (e.g., meconium ileus, intestinal atresia or **extrinsic abnormalities** (e.g., adhesions, bands or volvulus). May be of small bowel origin (most cases) or colon.
  - May be simple or strangulation obstruction (i.e., associated with bowel ischemia).
- May be mechanical or functional: **Paralytic ileus:** Failure of intestinal motor function without mechanical obstruction:
  - Common after abdominal operations.
  - Causes:
    ○ Infection (pneumonia, gastroenteritis, peritonitis, systemic sepsis).
    ○ Drugs (e.g., opiates, loperamide, vincristine).
    ○ Metabolic abnormalities (hypokalemia, uremia, myxedema, and diabetic ketoacidosis).
- **Chronic intestinal pseudo-obstruction (CIPO):** A severe intestinal motility disorder described in diverse conditions, including muscular, endocrine, metabolic and autoimmune disorders. CIPO is characterized by episodes of continuous symptoms and signs of bowel obstruction in the absence of a fixed lumen-occluding lesion. It may be congenital or acquired, primary or secondary. Examples include mitochondrial diseases (primary), fetal alcohol syndrome (intrauterine exposure) and post viral dysmotility (e.g., secondary to Epsten-Barr virus).

PATHOPHYSIOLOGY

- Mechanical obstruction:
  - Intestinal contents accumulate proximal to the site of obstruction.
  - The bowel distends with swallowed air, ingested food, secretions, and gases from intestinal reactions and bacterial fermentation.
  - Retrograde flow of intestinal contents and reflex gut distention results in vomiting.
  - Internal and external losses result in hypovolemia, oliguria, and azotemia.
  - Bacteria proliferate in the small bowel and its contents become feculent.
- Strangulation obstruction: Impaired blood flow to the intestine in addition to intestinal content obstruction
  - Loss of plasma into the bowel, leading to shock.
  - When strangulation progresses, gangrene, peritonitis, and perforation may ensue.
  - Damage to the normal gut barrier may enable bacteria, bacterial toxins, and inflammatory mediators to enter the circulation causing sepsis.

ETIOLOGY

May be **congenital** (e.g., atresia, duplication), **acquired** (e.g., neoplastic, inflammatory), or **iatrogenic** (e.g., adhesions, radiation stricture). Etiology varies according to age group:

- **Neonates:**
  - Intestinal atresia (the most common cause in the neonate, approximately one third of cases).
  - Meconium ileus primarily in cystic fibrosis) and meconium plug.
  - Duodenal atresia (associated with Down syndrome).
  - Anorectal malformation: Anal atresia and stenosis.
  - Necrotizing enterocolitis.
- Hirschsprung disease.
- **Infants:**
  - Pyloric stenosis (the most common cause).
  - Intussusception (the most common cause between 3 months and 6 years of age.
  - Postoperative adhesions.
  - Incarcerated inguinal hernia.
  - Hirschsprung disease.
  - Duplications.
  - Meckel diverticulum.
- **Older children:**
  - Postoperative or postinfectious intestinal adhesions.
  - Inflammatory bowel disease.
  - Cancer-related intestinal obstruction and radiotherapy-induced adhesions.
  - Malrotation.
  - Annular pancreas.
  - Meckel diverticulum.
  - Superior mesenteric artery syndrome.
  - Esophageal injury, corrosive injury, or foreign body ingestion.
  - Juvenile polyposis and related syndromes.
  - Distal intestinal obstruction syndrome (in cystic fibrosis).
  - Roundworm (*A. lumbricoides*).
  - Gastric and intestinal bezoars.
  - Colonic volvulus secondary to aerophagia and constipation in children with intellectual disability.

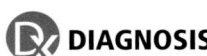 **DIAGNOSIS**

ALERT
There is no spontaneous resolution of inguinal hernia. Surgery should be scheduled before incarceration occurs. Inguinal hernias have 10–28% risk for incarceration.

SIGNS AND SYMPTOMS

- Presentation may be acute and obvious or chronic and subtle. The latter and partial obstruction could be difficult to diagnose.
- Careful history, physical examination, and consideration of age-related etiology most often will identify the specific cause.

HISTORY

- The classic symptoms of intestinal obstruction include vomiting (often bile stained), abdominal distention, colicky abdominal pain, and failure to pass stool.
- In neonates:
  - History of maternal polyhydramnios and aspiration of >20 mL gastric fluid after birth are suggestive of high intestinal obstruction.
  - Failure to pass meconium within 48 hours of birth.

- Older children:
  - Pain is one of the cardinal manifestations. It can be poorly localized, colicky visceral pain or sharp peritoneal pain.
  - Nausea and vomiting: High obstruction causes bilious emesis; distal obstruction may lead feculent emesis; in colonic obstruction, vomiting may be absent or late.
  - No passage of stool in low obstruction or bloody stool with mucus in strangulation (e.g., intussusception and volvulus).

ALERT
Neonates, more so than older children, with unrecognized intestinal obstruction deteriorate rapidly, with increased morbidity, mortality, and surgical complications.

PHYSICAL EXAM

- General assessment and vital signs, signs of dehydration, sepsis, or malnutrition.
- Palpation may reveal the presence of a hernia, a mass suggestive of intussusception. Tenderness and rigidity result from peritonitis.
- Bowel sounds may be initially increased, but later become decreased, occasional, or absent.
- Anal inspection excludes anal atresia and stenosis. Rectal examination reveals, at times, a palpable polyp or intussusceptum and blood (overt, occult, or "currant jelly", typical of intussusception).
- Strangulation is suspected when there is fever, tachycardia, signs of peritonitis, and severe pain that persists after nasogastric decompression.

DIAGNOSTIC TESTS & INTERPRETATION
Lab
- No laboratory studies are diagnostic.
- Full blood count, electrolytes, and blood gas should be taken.
- High obstruction may lead to hypochloremic hyperkalemic metabolic alkalosis.
- Bowel infarction may lead to marked leukocytosis, thrombocytopenia, and metabolic acidosis.
- Serum amylase and lipase should be determined to rule out pancreatitis, but they might be mildly elevated in intestinal obstruction.

Imaging
- **Plain abdominal X-rays** in the supine and erect or decubitus views will identify the classic features: Gasless abdomen, air–fluid levels and distended loops of intestine. High small bowel obstruction or strangulation obstruction may present with normal or nearly normal X-rays.
  - In small bowel obstruction: Dilated bowel, air-fluid levels without gas in the colon.
  - Paralytic ileus: Distended loops of bowel.
  - Duodenal obstruction: "Double-bubble" sign.

- Pneumoperitoneum in perforation.
- Peritoneal calcifications in meconium peritonitis.
- Right lower quadrant ground-glass appearance in meconium ileus.
- Obstruction with intraluminal calcifications in rectourinary fistula, colonic aganglionosis, or intestinal atresia.
- **Ultrasonography:** May identify a mass (e.g., perforated appendix), pyloric stenosis, malrotation, volvulus, intussusception ("target sign" or "Doughnut sign") or pelvic pathology in adolescents.
- **CT or MRI:** Localize the obstruction, diagnosis of strangulation; helpful in postoperative obstruction, Crohn disease, and neoplasms.
- **Barium enema** to confirm intussusception or Hirschsprung disease and "microcolon" in neonatal small bowel obstruction.
  - Upper GI series for malrotation or volvulus.
  - Water-soluble, low osmolarity materials should be preferred (risk of perforation). Effort should be made to minimize radiation exposure.

ALERT
- Evaluation for associated congenital anomalies is mandatory, as some are life threatening. The most frequent are cardiac and renal abnormalities.
- **Manometry** in is used in CIPO to assess neuromuscular function and can distinguish myopathy from neuropathy.

DIFFERENTIAL DIAGNOSIS
Other causes of abdominal pain and vomiting should be considered and ruled out by history and physical examination:
- Appendicitis.
- Torsion of testis or ovary.
- Lower lobe pneumonia.
- Pancreatitis.
- Sickle cell crisis.
- Henoch–Schönlein purpura.
- Biliary colic.
- Lead poisoning.
- Acute adrenal insufficiency.
- Diabetic ketoacidosis.
- Acute intermittent porphyria.

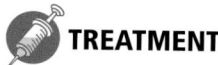 **TREATMENT**

Initial Stabilization
- Hold oral intake.
- Decompress the stomach by nasogastric tube.
- Administer IV fluids, correct electrolyte imbalance, and ensure adequate urine output.
- Identify etiology of obstruction and establish definitive repair.
- Cultures and broad-spectrum antibiotics (covering Gram-negative aerobes and anerobes) according to patient's age and status.

General Measures
- In intussusception, hydrostatic or air reduction is successful in 90% of cases.
- Nasogastric decompression or anti-inflammatory medication for adhesions or inflammatory strictures.

- Contrast-material enemas, manipulation, and direct enteral irrigation with *N*-acetylcysteine for uncomplicated meconium ileus.
- Manual reduction of incarcerated inguinal hernia.
- Colonic volvulus may be treated with endoscopic decompression followed by elective surgery.
- Endoscopic removal of foreign bodies.
- Paralytic ileus is usually self-limiting and resolves with supportive treatment.

SPECIAL THERAPY
- Conservative management with decompression by nasogastric tube and IV fluids is the first-line approach in:
  - Early postoperative, partial, and recurrent adhesive obstructions.
  - Necrotizing enterocolitis.
  - Meconium ileus.
  - Duodenal hematomas.
  - Superior mesenteric artery syndrome.
  - Crohn's disease.

SURGERY/OTHER PROCEDURES
- Definitive treatment requires an urgent operation.
- Exceptions to this rule include the above mentioned conditions managed conservatively.
- In all situations: if no improvement within 12–24 hours, surgery is advisable.
- The surgical procedure is individualized according to the specific type, site, anatomy of the obstruction, and associated conditions.
- **Laparoscopy-assisted surgery** can be used for the diagnosis and repair of small bowel obstruction and for adhesiolysis.

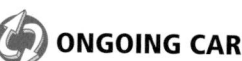 **ONGOING CARE**

PROGNOSIS
- Varies with different causes of intestinal obstruction, age of the patient, presence of prematurity, and associated anomalies.
- Short bowel syndrome continues to be a major impediment to improved survival rate; permanent parenteral nutrition is associated with morbidity and mortality.

COMPLICATIONS
May result from delayed operation:
- Dehydration.
- Intestinal ischemia with sepsis and shock.
- Bowel perforation and peritonitis.
- Short-gut syndrome.

ADDITIONAL READING
- Connor FL, Di Lorenzo C. Chronic intestinal pseudo-obstruction: Assessment and management. *Gastroenterology.* 2006;130:S29–S36.
- Hajivassiliou CA. Intestinal obstruction in neonatal/pediatric surgery. *Semin Pediatr Surg.* 2003;12:241–253.
- Lampl B, Levin TL, Berdon WE, et al. Malrotation and midgut volvulus: A historical review and current controversies in diagnosis and management. *Pediatr Radiol.* 2009;39:359–366.
- Liakakos T, Thomakos N, Fine PM, et al. Peritoneal adhesions: Etiology, pathophysiology, and clinical significance. Recent advances in prevention and management. *Dig Surg.* 2001;18:260–273.
- Nicolaou S, Kai B, Ho S, et al. Imaging of acute small-bowel obstruction. *AJR Am J Roentgenol.* 2005;185:1036–1044.
- Stollman TH, de Blaauw I, Wijnen MH, et al. Decreased mortality but increased morbidity in neonates with jejunoileal atresia; a study of 114 cases over a 34-year period. *J Pediatr Surg.* 2009;44:217–221.

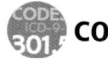 **CODES**

ICD9
- 751.1 Atresia and stenosis of small intestine
- 560.9 Unspecified intestinal obstruction
- 777.1 Meconium obstruction in fetus or newborn

ICD10
- K56.60 Unspecified intestinal obstruction
- P76.0 Meconium plug syndrome
- Q41.9 Congen absence, atresia and stenosis of sm int, part unsp

FAQ
- Q: Will my child need surgery for this problem?
- A: Most likely; It depends on the cause. Surgical treatment is necessary to correct intestinal obstruction, except in a few cases, such as intussusception, pseudo-obstruction, and paralytic ileus.
- Q: What is the most common cause of this problem in my 3-day-old son?
- A: In an infant, the most common causes are atresias of the intestine, which are absences of the normal amount of large or small intestine in the abdomen.
- Q: Is my child likely to have recurrent episodes of intestinal obstruction?
- A: It depends on the cause for the obstruction. Conditions associated with recurrence include intussusception, inflammatory conditions (e.g., Crohn's disease) and postoperative adhesions.

INTOEING–TIBIAL TORSION

Ali Al-omari
John P. Dormans

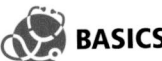 **BASICS**

DESCRIPTION
- Tibial torsion: Twisting (internal or external) of the tibia (may be associated with femoral torsion)
- Medial or internal tibial torsion associated with intoeing (most common)
- Lateral or external tibial torsion associated with outtoeing
- Normal defined as within 2 standard deviations of mean

EPIDEMIOLOGY
- Common and usually normal (i.e., within 2 standard deviations of the mean).
- It is often associated with physiologic bowleg.

RISK FACTORS
Genetics
No strong evidence to suggest that this is an inherited condition (heredity-familial tendency)

PATHOPHYSIOLOGY
- Tibial torsion: Twisting the tibia; usually medial or internal; associated with intoeing
- If associated with increased femoral anteversion, may be associated with patellofemoral malalignment (kneecap subluxation)

ETIOLOGY
- Normal fetal development
- Intrauterine position
- Heredity-familial tendency
- Posturing (sitting position): Cause or effect?
- Associated pathology (e.g., spasticity, fracture malunion, or developmental dislocation of the hip [DDH])

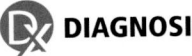 **DIAGNOSIS**

HISTORY
- Birth history: Common in 1st-borns
- Pain or limping may indicate other diagnosis.
- Metatarsus adductus, torticollis, and DDH may be associated with other conditions that result from immobility in uterus.
- Functional limitations (i.e., child trips and falls frequently) may suggest other diagnosis, such as mild cerebral palsy, especially if abnormal birth history, abnormalities in developmental milestones, and physical findings consistent with cerebral palsy.

PHYSICAL EXAM
- If child is ambulatory, watch gait and assess for foot progression angle: The angle formed between the axis of the foot and the axis of forward progression of gait.
- Also assess other aspects of gait: Stride, heel–toe gait, cadence, limping, other abnormalities. Unilateral or bilateral torsion
- Leg-length discrepancy, hip abnormalities, contractures, spasticity, thigh–foot axis (TFA)
  - With the child prone, the knee flexed to 90°, and the ankle at neutral, measure the difference between the axis of the foot and the axis of the femur.
    ○ If the TFA is internal, this suggests internal tibial torsion; If external, external tibial torsion.
- Transmalleolar axis: With the child seated and the knee flexed to 90°, assess the malleolar axis in reference to the coronal plane (less reliable than TFA).

- Look for abnormalities of the feet: Metatarsus adductus or clubfoot may be a primary cause of intoeing. Significant calcaneovalgus may be a component of outtoeing.
- Careful neurologic exam: To see if intoeing is related to a mild neurologic abnormality, such as mild spastic diplegic cerebral palsy
- Physical exam tricks:
  - "Torsional profile" consists of foot-progression angle, medial hip rotation in extension (to assess femoral torsion), lateral hip rotation in extension (to assess femoral torsion), thigh–foot angle (to assess tibial torsion), transmalleolar axis (to assess tibial torsion), and configuration of the foot.
  - "Kissing patellae": Occurs when bilateral increased femoral anteversion causes the patellae to face one another, giving the appearance of kissing patellae

DIAGNOSTIC TESTS & INTERPRETATION
Lab
Usually not helpful (i.e., normal with tibial torsion)

Imaging
- Usually not needed; physical exam gives information needed.
- Hip radiograph: May be indicated if hip pathology (i.e., DDH) is suspected

- CT: An accurate way to measure tibial and femoral torsion, but there is radiation exposure. An occasional indication may be a patient who is being evaluated for surgery.
- MRI and ultrasound: Have been described to quantify torsion, but generally are less accurate than CT

DIFFERENTIAL DIAGNOSIS

Look for DDH, spasticity (e.g., mild cerebral palsy), metatarsus adductus, femoral anteversion

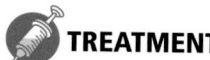 **TREATMENT**

ADDITIONAL TREATMENT
General Measures
- Observation
- Activity: No restrictions

Additional Therapies
- Physical therapy
  – Will not change natural history (it may help with associated patellofemoral malalignment pain)
  – Devices (casts, shoe wedges, twister cables, splints, Denis-Brown bars): No proven benefit

SURGERY/OTHER PROCEDURES
- Rarely needed
- Tibial osteotomy is seldom, if ever, needed.

IN-PATIENT CONSIDERATIONS
Initial Stabilization
- Observation and familial and patient reassurance (almost always the treatment of choice)
- Devices such as casts, shoe wedges, twister cables, splints, and Denis-Brown bars have no proven benefit (i.e., they will not change the natural history). Some of these may in fact cause problems such as ligamentous damage to hip, knee, ankle, and foot.
- Reassurance is usually enough. The condition improves spontaneously. Usually corrects enough by 8 years of age
- Surgery seldom needed
- Tibial osteotomy: When done, is usually a distal supramalleolar osteotomy

 ONGOING CARE

PROGNOSIS
- Good; usually not painful, cosmetically unattractive, or dysfunctional
- Usually corrects enough by 8 years of age
- Should improve with growth and development. There is no substantial evidence that increased femoral anteversion will cause arthritis of the hip or knee.
- Overall, good prognosis for the majority of patients

COMPLICATIONS
Functional if severe; no long-term complications (osteoarthritis) proven. However, most of the complications are related to operative treatment.

ADDITIONAL READING

- Craig CL, Goldberg MJ. Foot and leg problems. *Pediatr Rev*. 1993;14:395–400.
- Schoenecker PL, Rich MM. The lower extremity. In: Morrissy RT, Weinstein SL, eds. *Lovell and Winter's pediatric orthopaedics*, 6th ed. Philadelphia: Lippincott Williams & Wilkins; 2005:1157–1212.
- Staheli LT. Lower positional deformity in infants and children: A review. *J Pediatr Orthop*. 1990;10:559–563.

 CODES

ICD9
754.43 Congenital bowing of tibia and fibula
ICD10
Q68.4 Congenital bowing of tibia and fibula

FAQ

- Q: When are special shoes or braces indicated for tibial torsion?
- A: Almost never. The situation will improve without treatment in most patients. There is no convincing evidence that any of these treatments truly alter the natural history of the condition.
- Q: Why do patients with torsional pathology occasionally have knee pain?
- A: Children may have increased femoral anteversion with associated external tibial torsion (i.e., an external rotation of the tibia that matches and, in effect, balances the internal rotation of the femur). This can be diagnosed by observing the above rotational profile and by noting increased Q-angle. This situation is sometimes a "setup" for patellofemoral pain.

INTRACRANIAL HEMORRHAGE

Irfan Jafree
Peter Binghan (5th edition)

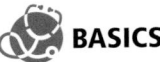

BASICS

DESCRIPTION
Extravasation of blood from intracranial vessels to the epidural, subdural, intraparenchymal (intracerebral), or intraventricular space within the cranial vault

EPIDEMIOLOGY
- Germinal matrix hemorrhage is the most common intracranial hemorrhage (ICH) in premature infants.
- Trauma: Common cause of ICH in children
- Arteriovenous malformations (AVMs): Most common cause of nontraumatic ICH in children
- Children with change in mental status or seizure at presentation have worse outcome.

Incidence
Stroke in children (birth to 14 years of age): 2.5–2.7 cases per 100,000 children; 55% are believed to be ischemic, others represent ICH.

RISK FACTORS
Genetics
Increased frequency with hereditary disorders of coagulation, congenital heart disease, and polycystic kidney disease associated with intracranial aneurysms

GENERAL PREVENTION
- Automobile seat belts
- Bicycle, skating, and skateboarding helmets
- Child abuse prevention
- Diving safety practices
- Preventing falls
- Maintaining safe driving speeds
- Keeping children away from firearms
- Hematologic monitoring for those at risk for hemorrhage due to blood disorders

PATHOPHYSIOLOGY
- Epidural hematoma (blood between the dura mater and the skull) is frequently arterial, related to skull fracture; typically middle meningeal artery bleeding following temporal bone fracture. 1/4 epidural hematomas in children are from dural venous laceration.
- Subdural hematoma (blood between the dura mater and the arachnoid membrane) is frequently venous from trauma causing stretching and tearing of bridging cortical veins or coagulopathy.
- Subarachnoid hemorrhage (blood between the arachnoid membrane and brain): Ruptured intracranial aneurysm, AVM, or trauma
- Blood within the brain parenchyma may be the result of trauma, hypertension, infections such as herpes simplex encephalitis, brain tumor, venous sinus thrombosis, or cerebral infarction (occurs mostly with rupture of medium or smaller branches of major cerebral arteries).
- Subependymal germinal matrix hemorrhage: Especially in premature infants born <34 weeks' gestation

- Intraventricular hemorrhage commonly with intraparenchymal or subependymal germinal matrix (in the subependymal layer of the lateral ventricle) hemorrhage extends into the ventricular system. 4 grades:
  – Grade I: Isolated to 1 or both germinal matrices
  – Grade II: Intraventricular hemorrhage without ventricular dilatation
  – Grade III: Intraventricular hemorrhage with ventricular dilatation (hydrocephalus)
  – Grade IV: Intraventricular hemorrhage with ventricular dilatation and extension into the adjacent hemispheric white matter

ETIOLOGY
- Vascular:
  – Congenital vascular anomalies: AVM, venous angioma, cavernous malformation, hereditary hemorrhagic telangiectasia, aneurysm, coarctation with intracranial aneurysm, vein of Galen malformation
  – Developmental/acquired vasculopathy: Ehlers-Danlos syndrome type IV, Moyamoya syndrome, pseudoxanthoma elasticum, sickle cell disease, hypertension, mycotic aneurysm, vasculitis (cocaine, inflammatory diseases)
- Trauma:
  – Child abuse
  – Angioplasty
  – Trauma (subdural, epidural, subarachnoid)
- Other contexts of ICH:
  – Prematurity
  – Neonatal asphyxia
  – Sinovenous thrombosis
  – Cerebral infarction, especially resulting from venous thrombosis
- Alcohol, cocaine, and other sympathomimetics are associated with ICH
- Hematologic disorders:
  – Immune thrombocytopenic purpura
  – Thrombotic thrombocytopenia
  – Purpura
  – Autosomal recessive afibrinogenemia
  – Disseminated intravascular coagulation
  – Hemolytic uremic syndrome
  – Iatrogenic (chemotherapy) thrombocytopenia
  – Congenital serum C2 deficiency
  – Kidney or liver dysfunction
  – Vitamin K deficiency
  – Factor deficiency (factor V, protein C, or S deficiency)
  – Leukemia, lymphoma

DIAGNOSIS

HISTORY
- Head trauma
- Delivery, circumstances during
- Headache severity, quality
- Abrupt, severe headache and stiff neck may suggest a "warning leak" from aneurysm.
- Change in level of consciousness, "lucid interval" with epidural hematoma

- Seizures, especially new onset
- Visual problems
- Focal neurologic deficits
- Epistaxis (may occur with leakage of cerebrospinal fluid if skull fracture is present)
- Meningeal symptoms
- Patient or family history of coagulopathy
- Risk factors for cerebral venous sinus thrombosis: Dehydration, coagulopathy, polycythemia, sepsis, and asphyxia (especially in newborns)
- Risk factors for arterial aneurysms: Polycystic kidney disease, coarctation of the aorta
- Failure to thrive, hydrocephalus with vein of Galen malformation
- Signs and symptoms:
  – Presentation may include change or decrease in consciousness, seizure, severe headaches, meningismus (because blood is an irritant), or sudden focal neurologic deficit.
  – With posterior fossa bleed: Disconjugate gaze, ataxia, and rapid deterioration to coma
  – Expeditious history, exam, and emergency CT
  – Increasing intracranial pressure from hemorrhage or hydrocephalus is life threatening.

PHYSICAL EXAM
- Signs of increased intracranial pressure or herniation, such as Cushing triad (hypertension, bradycardia, abnormal respiratory pattern), papilledema, pupils that do not constrict to light, ophthalmoparesis, decorticate or decerebrate posturing. Intraventricular blood may present with signs of increased intracranial pressure caused by communicating hydrocephalus. Increased intracranial pressure may result in a bulging fontanel and splayed sutures.
- Meningeal signs, low-grade fever
- In setting of trauma:
  – Leakage of CSF from the ear or nose
  – Battle sign: Bruising over the mastoid process suggestive of basilar skull fracture
  – Raccoon eyes: Periorbital ecchymosis suggestive of basilar skull fracture
  – Subhyaline retinal hemorrhages
- Herpes simplex type 1 encephalitis: Frequently presents with fever, cognitive impairment, seizures
- Germinal matrix hemorrhages often clinically silent but may present with apnea in the newborn
- ICH should be suspected in the septic-appearing neonate, especially if there are no obvious risk factors for sepsis.
- Subarachnoid hemorrhage frequently presents as worst headache ever experienced, subhyaloid hemorrhages, signs of meningeal irritation
- Unexplained subdural hemorrhage in infants, particularly bilateral: Inflicted trauma until proven otherwise

DIAGNOSTIC TESTS & INTERPRETATION
Immediate stroke evaluation (1st 24 hours): Consider:
- Head CT
- Chest radiograph
- Electrocardiogram (ECG for evaluation of acute cardiac ischemia or old infarction)
- Urine toxicology screen
- CBC
- Metabolic profile (high creatinine and glucose associated with hematoma expansion)

- Prothrombin time/partial thromboplastin time (PT/PTT), international normalized ratio
- ESR/ANA
- Lumbar puncture: Lumbar puncture will show RBCs, reduced glucose, xanthochromia (best detected by spectrophotometry), and bloody CSF. Consider spinal fluid evaluation if CT negative.
- MRI/magnetic resonance angiogram/venography
- Transcranial/carotid ultrasound (for vasospasm)

Imaging

- CT of the head:
  - The most important study to obtain when considering ICH in the differential diagnosis, because of its relative convenience, speed, and low false-negative rate
- CT angiography and contrast-enhanced CT, based on the presence of contrast extravasation within the hematoma, may identify patients at high risk of ICH expansion:
  - Fresh intracerebral blood increased density; between 1 and 6 weeks, becomes isodense with adjacent brain parenchyma. Acute ICH may appear isodense if hemoglobin <8–10 g/dL.
  - "Biconvex and displacing gray–white interface": Extradural hemorrhage
  - "Crescent shaped": Subdural hemorrhage; bilateral subdural hemorrhage frequent in intentional injury
- MRI gradient echo and T2 susceptibility weighted MRI are helpful not only for acute hemorrhage, but also for old hemorrhage such as seen with amyloid angiopathy.
- CTA, CT venography, MRA/MRV: Helpful for evaluation of structural lesions, including vascular malformations, dissection, tumors, venous sinus thrombosis, etc.
- Head ultrasound: Hemorrhages in infants with gestational age of <32 weeks with birth weight <1,800 g; serial ultrasound exams are warranted.

DIFFERENTIAL DIAGNOSIS

- Stroke
- Brain tumor
- Migraine headache

ALERT

- Early subarachnoid hemorrhage may not be apparent on CT and may require lumbar puncture (if safe to perform) or serial CT evaluation while the patient is under clinical observation.
- ICH, especially in young infants and children without an obvious etiology, should raise the suspicion of nonaccidental trauma.
- Patients with concussion without ICH may still develop cerebral edema; observe for signs of increasing intracranial pressure.

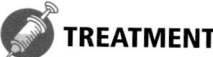 TREATMENT

IN-PATIENT CONSIDERATIONS

Initial Stabilization

- Admission to neuro-ICU
- Institute acyclovir therapy if herpes simplex type 1 encephalitis is considered.
- Blood pressure management. Definite optimal values have not been established, but systolic BP <160 mm Hg are probably best, while avoiding compromised cerebral blood flow. This can be achieved by using IV agents including nicardipine (5 mg/hr with titration 2.5 mg/hr every 5 minutes up to maximum of 15 mg/hr), labetalol (10–20 mg IV over 2 minutes, then 40–80 mg IV every 10 minutes until either BP goal achieved or 300 mg has been given, then repeat effective every 6–8 hours), enalaprilat (0.625–1.2 mg every 6 hours).
- Glucose monitoring to achieve normoglycemia
- DVT prophylaxis: ICH is associated with a high risk of thromboembolic disease. Use combination of intermittent pneumatic compression and elastic stockings.
- Temperature management: Fever associated with worse neurologic outcome; maintain normothermia.
- Correction of coagulopathies (suggested by PT, PTT, platelet abnormalities), should be done promptly, may require hematology evaluation and include various therapies such as vitamin K, fresh frozen plasma, prothrombin complex concentrate, recombinant factor VII, or platelet infusion.
- ICP monitoring when elevated ICP is suspected
- Antiepileptic drugs: Only for clinical seizures or electrograph seizures (suspected when change in mental status is disproportionate to ICH or subtle signs including intermittent nystagmus, myoclonus, or marked blood pressure fluctuations and confirmed by continuous EEG monitoring)
- Neurosurgical intervention is frequently necessary for subdural and epidural hematomas. Serial neurologic exams on patients treated for ICH. Surgical treatment is suggested for cerebellar hemorrhage with brainstem compression or hydrocephalus from ventricular obstruction. It can also be considered for lobar clots >30 mL and within 1 cm of the surface.
- Intracranial aneurysms: Frequently amenable to neurosurgical intervention to decrease the likelihood of rebleeding. In addition, careful control of intracranial pressure and prompt attention to hydrocephalus may be necessary.
- Definitive treatment of AVMs consists of surgical resection or interventional neuroradiologic techniques, or proton beam irradiation.

 ONGOING CARE

FOLLOW-UP RECOMMENDATIONS

Patient Monitoring

Long-term observation for signs of injury: Cognitive deficits, focal weakness, seizures

PROGNOSIS

Often, good neurologic recovery is possible.

COMPLICATIONS

- Increased intracranial pressure and brain herniation syndromes
- Hydrocephalus: Communicating/noncommunicating
- Vasospasm secondary to blood and breakdown products of erythrocytes
- Seizures, death
- Motor, visual, and cognitive deficits secondary to ischemic infarction

ADDITIONAL READING

- Bonnier C, Nassogne MC, Saint-Martin C, et al. Neuroimaging of intraparenchymal lesions predicts outcome in shaken baby syndrome. *Pediatrics.* 2003;112:808–814.
- Hintz SR, Slovis T, Bulas D, et al. NICHD Neonatal Research Network. Interobserver reliability and accuracy of cranial ultrasound scanning interpretation in premature infants. *J Pediatr.* 2007;150(6):592–596, 596.e1–5.
- Morgenstern LB, Hemphill JC, Anderson C, et al. Guidelines for the management of spontaneous ICH. *Stroke.* 2010;41;2108–2129.
- National Stroke Association. *Stroke information.* Available at: http://www.stroke.org
- Nelson KB, Lynch JK. Stroke in newborn infants. *Lancet Neurol.* 2004;3:150–158.
- Proust F, Toussaint P, Garnieri J, et al. Pediatric cerebral aneurysms. *J Neurosurg.* 2001;94: 733–739.
- Squier W. Shaken baby syndrome: The quest for evidence. *Dev Med Child Neurol.* 2008;50(1):10–14.

 CODES

ICD9

- 432.9 Unspecified intracranial hemorrhage
- 853.00 Other and unspecified intracranial hemorrhage following injury without mention of open intracranial wound, unspecified state of consciousness

ICD10

- I62.9 Nontraumatic intracranial hemorrhage, unspecified
- S06.330A Contusion and laceration of cerebrum, unspecified, without loss of consciousness, initial encounter

FAQ

- Q: What is a lucid interval and how long will it last?
- A: Epidural hematoma may present in a delayed fashion after head trauma, may last 24 hours before change in consciousness, or other signs appear.
- Q: What is the role of CT in the diagnosis of subarachnoid bleeding?
- A: Early subarachnoid hemorrhage may not be apparent on CT initially but may require either a lumbar puncture or follow-up CT studies.

I

INTUSSUSCEPTION

Andrew B. Grossman

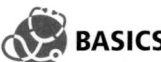 **BASICS**

DESCRIPTION

- The most common abdominal emergency of early childhood
- The telescoping of one part of the bowel into itself or adjacent bowel, causing abdominal pain, vomiting, and eventually bloody stools and lethargy
- Telescoping of the bowel causes diminished venous blood flow and bowel wall edema, which can result in ischemia and obstruction. Eventually, arterial blood flow is inhibited and infarction of the bowel wall occurs, which results in hemorrhage and, if untreated, possible perforation.
- Strangulation of the bowel rarely occurs in the first 24 hours but evolves afterward.
- Ileocolic type accounts for 80–90% of intussusceptions; ileoileal and colocolic types also occur.
- Typical triad of acute onset of colicky abdominal pain, right upper quadrant (RUQ) mass, and "currant jelly" stools, although clinical presentation can vary
- Increased incidence in children who received the RotaShield rotavirus vaccine. The currently available vaccine (RotaTeq) has not been shown to increase the risk.

EPIDEMIOLOGY

- Male/Female ratio: 3:2
- Generally occurs in patients 6 months to 3 years of age
- Peak age from 6–12 months

Incidence
1–4/1,000 live births

ETIOLOGY

- Children <3 years: Usually idiopathic or enlarged Peyer patch from viral infection
- Children ≥3 years: Often a pathologic lead point: Meckel diverticulum, hematoma from Henoch-Schönlein purpura or bleeding diatheses, tumors (polyps, lymphoma, sarcoma, lipoma, neurofibroma), adhesions, duplication, postsurgical anastomotic sutures or staples, cystic fibrosis

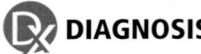 **DIAGNOSIS**

HISTORY

- The typical presentation is the sudden onset of severe intermittent (colicky) abdominal pain, with the child often drawing the legs up to the abdomen and crying. Can be asymptomatic between paroxysms of pain
- Lethargy out of proportion to the severity of dehydration
- Nonbilious emesis initially, becomes bilious with progressive obstruction
- "Currant-jelly" stools (sloughed mucosa, blood, and mucous) appear in 50% of cases: A sign of a longer course

PHYSICAL EXAM

- Lethargic with colicky pattern of abdominal pain
- Mass in the RUQ may be palpated ("RUQ sausage")
- Absence of bowel contents in right lower quadrant (Dance sign)
- Abdominal distention
- Rectal exam: Blood-tinged mucous or currant jelly stool; occasionally the intussusception can be felt
- Peritoneal signs if intestinal perforation has occurred

DIAGNOSTIC TESTS & INTERPRETATION
Lab
CBC, electrolytes

Imaging
- Abdominal x-ray: Not sensitive or specific. Normal in early stages, later can have absence of gas in right lower quadrant (RLQ) and RUQ, as well as RUQ soft tissue mass; with obstruction, will have air-fluid levels, paucity of distal gas
- Abdominal ultrasound: If performed by experienced radiologist, highly sensitive and specific; "doughnut sign" with presence of several concentric rings

- Contrast enema: Diagnostic and therapeutic with reduction often achieved; air enema preferred because less perforation risk than barium; can miss a lead point

ALERT
- Only 30% present with the classical triad of abdominal pain, palpable abdominal mass, and currant-jelly stool, so high clinical suspicion is necessary
- Clinical status of hypovolemic patients may worsen with high-osmotic contrast agents.

DIFFERENTIAL DIAGNOSIS
- Infection: Gastroenteritis, enterocolitis, parasites
- Immunologic: Henoch-Schönlein purpura
- Miscellaneous:
  - Appendicitis
  - Meckel diverticulum: May act as a lead point in the absence of bleeding
  - Incarcerated hernia
  - Crohn disease
  - Celiac disease
  - Henoch Schönlein purpura
- Obstruction: Adhesions, hernia, volvulus, stricture, bezoar, foreign body, polyp, tumor

TREATMENT

ADDITIONAL TREATMENT
General Measures
- Prompt reduction is imperative.
- Spontaneous reduction occurs in 5%.
- Obtain surgical consultation before contrast enema reduction attempt secondary to risk of perforation; failed reduction requires surgical correction.
- Absolute contraindications to reduction by enema: Peritonitis, shock, and perforation
- Relative contraindications to reduction by enema: Symptoms >24 hours, evidence of obstruction (i.e., air fluid levels), sonographic evidence of ischemia
- Perforation during reduction occurs in 1% of cases, mostly in the transverse colon.

SURGERY/OTHER PROCEDURES
If perforation/peritonitis exists, patient is unstable, nonoperative reduction is unsuccessful, or lead point is identified, proceed to surgical reduction.

IN-PATIENT CONSIDERATIONS
Initial Stabilization
- Nasogastric tube placement: Bowel decompression
- IV line placement: Correction of fluid and electrolyte losses

ONGOING CARE

FOLLOW-UP RECOMMENDATIONS
Recurrence after nonoperative reduction has been reported in up to 10% of cases and usually is seen within 24 hours of the reduction.

PROGNOSIS
- Timely diagnosis results in a highly favorable prognosis.
- Hydrostatic reduction by contrast enema is therapeutic in 50–90% of cases.
- Risk of recurrence is ~10% after contrast enema reduction, 1% after manual reduction, and not reported after intestinal resection; the greatest risk is in the 24–72 hours after reduction.

COMPLICATIONS
- Bowel necrosis secondary to local ischemia
- GI bleeding
- Bowel perforation
- Sepsis, shock

ADDITIONAL READING

- Byrne A, Goeghegan T, Govender P, et al. The imaging of intussusception. *Clin Radiol.* 2005;60:39–46.
- Daneman A, Navarro O. Intussusception. Part 1: A review of diagnostic approaches. *Pediatr Radiol.* 2003;33:79–85.
- Daneman A, Navarro O. Intussusception. Part 2: An update on the evolution of management. *Pediatr Radiol.* 2004;34:97–108.
- Davis CF, McCabe AJ, Raine PA. The ins and outs of intussusception: History and management over the past fifty years. *J Pediatr Surg.* 2003;38(Suppl 7): 60–64.
- Fishman D, Chumpitazi BP, Ngo PD, et al. Small bowel intussusception in celiac disease: Revisiting a classic association. *J Pediatr Gastroenterol Nutr.* 2010;50:237.
- McCollough M, Sharieff GQ. Abdominal surgical emergencies in infants and young children. *Emerg Med Clin North Am.* 2003;21:909–935.
- Vesikari T, et al. Safety and efficacy of a pentavalent human-bovine (WC3) reassortant rotavirus vaccine. *N Engl J Med.* 2006;354:23–33.

CODES

ICD9
560.0 Intussusception

ICD10
- K38.8 Other specified diseases of appendix
- K56.1 Intussusception
- Q43.8 Other specified congenital malformations of intestine

FAQ

- Q: Can my child have a recurrent intussusception?
- A: Yes. The risk is very low, probably <10% if the child has had a nonsurgical reduction. If the lead point is removed surgically, recurrence is very unlikely. The greatest risk is in the 1st 72 hours after reduction.
- Q: What are the common ages for presentation?
- A: 6 months to 3 years is the age range associated with the greatest risk of intussusception, but it may occur at any age. The prevalence of pathologic conditions rises with the age of a child diagnosed with intussusception.

I

IRON DEFICIENCY ANEMIA

Peter de Blank
Janel L. Kwiatkowski (5th edition)

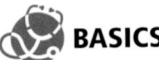 BASICS

DESCRIPTION
A reduction in hemoglobin production due to an insufficient supply of iron that results in a microcytic, hypochromic anemia

EPIDEMIOLOGY
- Iron deficiency is the most common nutritional deficiency of children
- Leading cause of anemia among infants and children in the US
- Most commonly seen in children ages 9 months to 3 years and in teenage girls

Prevalence
- Prevalence is variable depending on socioeconomic status, availability of iron-fortified formulas, prevalence and duration of breastfeeding, and the way that iron deficiency is defined.
- Prevalence of iron deficiency anemia in US is generally between 1% and 5% of children.

RISK FACTORS
- Low socioeconomic status
- Certain ethnic groups (e.g., Southeast Asian) may be at increased risk owing to dietary practices.

GENERAL PREVENTION
- Maintain breastfeeding for the 1st 5–6 months of life if possible. The iron concentration is lower in breast milk than formula, but iron in breast milk is more bioavailable (50% vs. 10%).
- Iron supplementation (1 mg/kg/d) for infants who are exclusively breastfed beyond 6 months
- Iron-fortified formula for the 1st 12 months of life for infants who are not breastfed
- Iron supplementation after 2 months of life for low-birth-weight and premature infants because of decreased iron stores and increased growth rate
- Encourage iron-enriched cereal when infants are started on solid food.
- Avoid whole cow's milk during the 1st year of life, to prevent occult GI bleeding.
- Screen hemoglobin level at periodic intervals. The American Academy of Pediatrics recommends 9 months, 5 years, and 14 years.

PATHOPHYSIOLOGY
- Iron is required for oxygen transport by hemoglobin.
- Iron absorption and distribution regulated by hepcidin, a peptide hormone secreted by liver, macrophages, and adipocytes
- Iron is absorbed primarily in the duodenum.
- Iron deficiency develops because of an inadequate supply or increased demand for iron, or a combination of these.
- Sequential stages of iron deficiency:
  - Depletion of iron stores: Reflected by low serum ferritin and absent bone marrow stores (Prussian blue staining)
  - Iron-deficient erythropoiesis: Near-normal number of red blood cells produced, but they have abnormal hemoglobin synthesis with wide distribution in RBC size
  - Iron deficiency anemia: Microcytosis evident

ETIOLOGY
- Causes of inadequate supply include dietary deficiency and malabsorption:
  - Dietary deficiency in infants and young children results from introduction of cow's milk prior to age 12 months, exclusive breastfeeding beyond age 6 months without iron supplementation, and excessive cow's milk intake (>24 oz/d).
  - Malabsorption results from surgical resection of intestine, celiac disease.
  - Certain foods impair iron absorption (tannins in tea and coffee, phytates).
- Causes of increased demand include rapid growth and blood loss:
  - Periods of rapid growth include infancy (especially low-birth-weight and premature infants) and adolescence.
  - GI blood loss is most common and includes cow's milk enteropathy (seen in infants), inflammatory bowel disease (IBD), and bleeding from Meckel diverticulum.
- Other etiologies of blood loss include perinatal loss, menorrhagia, pulmonary hemosiderosis, and hematuria.

 DIAGNOSIS

HISTORY
- Evaluate dietary intake of iron, including breast- or formula feeding and type of formula (iron fortified or low iron).
- Age at introduction of cow's milk
- Daily intake of cow's milk
- Birth history for prematurity or blood loss
- Pica
- Lead exposure
- Blood loss from urine, stool, menorrhagia
- Iron deficiency anemia often develops slowly, and no symptoms may be present. When present, signs and symptoms include:
  - Irritability and behavioral disturbances
  - Fatigue, exercise intolerance
  - Pallor
  - Headache
  - Pica or pagophagia (chewing ice)

PHYSICAL EXAM
- Often normal
- Pallor, irritability
- Tachycardia, flow murmur if anemia is more severe
- Koilonychia (spoon nails)
- Glossitis or stomatitis

DIAGNOSTIC TESTS & INTERPRETATION
Lab
- Hemoglobin level <2 standard deviations below the age-specific mean defines anemia.
- Low MCV (red cell volume) and MCH (hemoglobin concentration) for age

- High RDW (red cell distribution width):
  - Measures the variation in red cell size
  - Normal is <14.5%.
  - Often increased before anemia is present
- Low serum ferritin (≤12 ng/mL) reflects reduced tissue iron stores:
  - Earliest laboratory abnormality
  - May be normal or increased with concurrent infection or inflammation
  - Higher cutoff improves sensitivity of the test: Ferritin ≤30 ng/mL has sensitivity of 92% and PPV of 83% for iron deficiency anemia, vs. sensitivity of 25% for ferritin ≤12 ng/mL.
- Low serum iron
- Increased total iron-binding capacity
- Low transferrin saturation; measures the iron available for hemoglobin synthesis
- Increased soluble transferrin receptor (sTfR):
  - Indicator of increased tissue iron demand
  - Also increased in thalassemia syndromes but not in anemia of chronic inflammation (ACI)
  - sTfR/log(ferritin) <1 suggests anemia of chronic inflammation.
  - sTfR/log(ferritin) >2 suggests iron deficiency anemia.
- Decreased reticulocyte hemoglobin content: This test is an early indicator of iron deficiency because reticulocytes have a short (1–2-day) life span before becoming mature red cells.
- Increased free erythrocyte protoporphyrin, a precursor molecule in hemoglobin synthesis. Also high in lead poisoning and chronic inflammation
- Thrombocytosis (can approach 1 million/dL)
- Peripheral blood smear with microcytosis, hypochromia, poikilocytosis (varying shapes), pencil forms, and anisocytosis (varying sizes)
- Test for occult blood in stool often positive with gastrointestinal blood loss:
  - However, the test can be positive with oral iron supplementation.
- Iron absorption test can assess adequacy of PO iron supplementation. 3 mg/kg elemental iron should increase serum iron more than 100 mcg/dL within 4 hours of ingestion.

Diagnostic Procedures/Other
Bone marrow examination: Shows decreased iron stores by Prussian blue staining; rarely needed to establish diagnosis

DIFFERENTIAL DIAGNOSIS
- Recent infection
- Lead poisoning
- Thalassemia trait
- Anemia of chronic inflammation (e.g., juvenile rheumatoid arthritis, IBD)
- Sideroblastic anemias

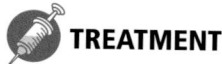 **TREATMENT**

- Iron supplementation (see below)
- Family education regarding age-appropriate diet and iron-containing foods
- Specific treatment if underlying condition causing blood loss is found (e.g., hormonal therapy for menorrhagia, medications for IBD)
- May require initial inpatient observation in cases of severe anemia
- Red cell transfusion only if evidence of cardiovascular compromise (rarely indicated)

MEDICATION (DRUGS)
First Line
Oral replacement with ferrous iron, 3–6 mg/kg/d of elemental iron divided into 2 or 3 doses.

- Iron should be given on an empty stomach or with a vitamin C–containing juice to increase absorption. Ascorbic acid increases oral absorption of iron by ~30%.
- Side effects (in 10–20%) include nausea, constipation, GI upset, and vomiting. Iron suspensions can stain teeth temporarily.

Second Line
Parenteral (IM or IV) iron formulations indicated only for severe noncompliance or malabsorption, or if ongoing loss exceeds absorption capacity. Administration may be associated with pain at injection site or anaphylaxis.

ISSUES FOR REFERRAL
- Evaluation for source of GI blood loss
- Unexplained recurrence after treatment
- Failure to improve with iron supplementation

IN-PATIENT CONSIDERATIONS
Admission Criteria
- Active bleeding
- Severe anemia (hemoglobin level <6 g/dL) especially if symptoms or ongoing blood loss
- Tachycardia, S_3 gallop, or other signs of CHF

Nursing
Family education: Teaching administration of iron and dietary counseling

Discharge Criteria
- No signs of CHF
- If blood loss, bleeding is controlled
- Stable hemoglobin level
- Parent demonstrates ability to administer oral iron therapy to young children and demonstrates adequate knowledge about dietary modifications.
- Adequate follow-up ensured

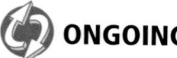 **ONGOING CARE**

FOLLOW-UP RECOMMENDATIONS
Patient Monitoring
- Reticulocyte count increases in 3–4 days.
- Hemoglobin concentration should rise by at least 1 g/dL in 2–3 weeks.
- Continue iron for 2 months beyond correction of anemia to replenish body stores.
- Causes of poor response to oral iron supplementation include:
  - Noncompliance (most common)
  - Ongoing blood loss
  - Insufficient duration of therapy
  - High gastric pH
  - Concurrent lead intoxication
  - Other diagnosis: Thalassemia trait and anemia of chronic disease are not iron responsive

DIET
- Milk should be restricted to <24 oz daily or eliminated in those with milk protein enteropathy.
- Bottle should be discontinued after 12 months.
- Diet should include foods rich in iron: Meats, beans, iron-fortified cereal, strawberries, spinach

PATIENT EDUCATION
- Activity: Usually, no activity restriction is needed. Those with severe anemia resulting in CHF should have limited activity until the anemia is corrected.
- Diet: A diet containing iron-rich foods should be encouraged. Limit milk intake to <24 oz daily.
- Prevention: Prevention of iron deficiency is preferable. Anticipatory guidance about diet, prolonged bottle use, etc., should be given, and government-sponsored programs such as the Special Supplemental Nutrition Program for Women, Infants and Children (WIC) should be used.

PROGNOSIS
- Anemia is readily corrected with iron replacement.
- Developmental delay may be long lasting or irreversible.

COMPLICATIONS
- Impaired cognitive and motor development in infants and toddlers
- Impaired immunity
- Short-term memory impairment and poor exercise performance in adolescents

ADDITIONAL READING

- Goodnough LT, Nemeth E, Ganz T. Detection, evaluation, and management of iron-restricted erythropoiesis. *Blood.* 2010;116(23):4754–4761.
- Griffin IJ, Abrams SA. Iron and breastfeeding. *Pediatr Clin North Am.* 2001;48:401–413.
- Konofal E, Lecendreux M, Deron J, et al. Effects of iron supplementation on attention deficit hyperactivity disorder in children. *Pediatr Neurol.* 2008;38(1):20–26.
- Looker AC. Iron deficiency–United States 1999–2000. *Morb Mortal Wkly Rep.* 2002;51:897–899.
- McCann JC, Ames BN. An overview of evidence for a causal relation between iron deficiency during development and deficits in cognitive or behavioral function. *Am J Clin Nutr.* 2007;85:931–945.
- Pappas DE. Iron deficiency anemia. *Pediatr Rev.* 1998;19:321–322.
- Wharton BA. Iron deficiency in children: Detection and prevention. *Br J Haematol.* 1999;106:270–280.
- Wu AC, Lesperance L, Bernstein H. Screening for iron deficiency. *Pediatr Rev.* 2002;23:171–177.

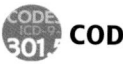 **CODES**

ICD9
280.9 Iron deficiency anemia, unspecified

ICD10
D50.9 Iron deficiency anemia, unspecified

FAQ

- Q: What dietary changes can help prevent the recurrence of iron deficiency?
- A: Limit milk to 24 oz/day so that your child has a better appetite for iron-containing foods. Heme iron, found in meats, fish, and poultry, is absorbed better than nonheme iron and also enhances absorption of nonheme iron. Other foods that have iron are raisins, dried fruit, sweet potatoes, lima beans, chili peppers, green peas, peanut butter, and enriched foods. Give iron on an empty stomach along with an ascorbic acid–containing juice to increase absorption. Foods that decrease absorption include bran, vegetable fiber, tannins found in tea, and phosphates. Antacids may also decrease iron absorption.
- Q: What are the side effects of iron therapy?
- A: Iron may cause temporary staining of the teeth, which can be decreased by diluting the iron with a small amount of juice. Iron will also change the color of bowel movements to greenish black and may be associated with constipation.
- Q: What are the most important tests to do to establish the diagnosis of iron deficiency?
- A: For patients with a history of dietary deficiency or known blood loss, a CBC that shows a low hemoglobin and MCV and an elevated RDW is very suggestive of iron deficiency. A therapeutic trial of iron without further laboratory testing is an appropriate next step. A rise in the hemoglobin concentration of ≥1 g/dL after 1 month of therapy confirms the diagnosis. If this does not occur, further laboratory testing is necessary and other diagnoses should be considered.
- Q: How does a concurrent infection affect the diagnosis of iron deficiency?
- A: Common childhood infections may be associated with a mild microcytic anemia that resembles iron deficiency. Laboratory tests to diagnose iron deficiency may be misleading while a child is acutely ill. Acute infection is associated with a shift of iron from serum to storage sites, causing a decrease in serum iron and an increase in ferritin. It is more helpful to test a child for iron deficiency 3–4 weeks after an acute infection.

IRON POISONING

Carla Campbell
Carl Tapia

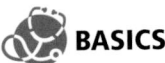 **BASICS**

DESCRIPTION
- The nontherapeutic ingestion of an iron-containing preparation, which may be available in a number of iron salts
- Ingested doses of <20 mg/kg of elemental iron are generally nontoxic; of 20–60 mg/kg lead to moderate toxicity; and of >60 mg/kg lead to severe toxicity and can be potentially fatal

EPIDEMIOLOGY
- Most frequent cause of pediatric unintentional ingestion fatalities in the 1980–1990s, accounting for ~30% of fatalities in 1 series; incidence of fatalities and poison control center calls has been declining in recent years, perhaps due to changes in package labels
- Almost all iron-related injuries are in children <4 years of age, and are usually due to ingestion of adult iron formulations.
- Risk factors for iron poisoning include ready availability of iron preparations in homes with pregnant women and young children, and the similarity in appearance of some iron pills and vitamins to candy.

PATHOPHYSIOLOGY
- Direct corrosive effects of iron on GI mucosa may lead to abdominal pain, vomiting, hematemesis, diarrhea, hematochezia, and melena. These effects may cause intestinal ulceration, edema, and inflammation.
- Hepatotoxicity from free iron accumulation can lead to periportal necrosis and hepatic failure, as well as coagulopathy.
- GI fluid losses can lead to hypotension and tissue hypoperfusion.
- Decreased cardiac output from decreased venous filling pressures, decreased preload, relative bradycardia, and a possible direct negative inotropic effect of iron on the myocardium can lead to shock.
- Metabolic acidosis results from tissue hypoperfusion with lactate formation, unbuffered hydrogen ion as absorbed ferrous iron is converted to ferric iron, disruption of oxidative phosphorylation, and lipid peroxidation of mitochondrial membranes.
- Acute respiratory distress syndrome (ARDS) may present in severe cases, and may be caused by iron-induced alveolar membrane damage.

- Stages of the clinical effects of iron poisoning: Stage I (early acute): 0–6 hours postingestion: Characterized by GI, CNS, and cardiovascular (CV) signs and symptoms. Stage II (quiescent): 6–24 hours: Characterized by decrease in GI symptoms and relative improvement in overall clinical condition. Stage III (recurrent): 12–48 hours: Characterized by cyanosis, profound metabolic acidosis, shock, evidence of hepatic and renal failure, bowel ischemia, myocardial depression, and cerebral dysfunction sometimes causing seizures and coma. Stage IV (late): 2–8 weeks postingestion: Characterized by gastric scarring and pyloric stenosis, sometimes leading to obstruction

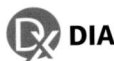 **DIAGNOSIS**

HISTORY
- Discovery of iron-containing pills, pill fragments, or other preparations in a young child's mouth or in opened containers in the home
- Detailed information on iron compound ingested such as iron salt type (determines percentage of elemental iron potentially ingested), number of pills ingested, and approximate ingestion time can be used to calculate estimated ingested iron dose in mg/kg of elemental iron.
- As a reference, the percentage of elemental iron in ferrous fumarate is 33%; in ferrous chloride is 28%; in ferrous sulfate is 20%; and in ferrous gluconate is 12%.

PHYSICAL EXAM
- A lethargic, hypotensive, vomiting toddler: The diagnosis of iron poisoning should be strongly considered for this scenario.
- Hypotension, decreased capillary refill, pallor, tachycardia, and CNS depression (lethargy or coma) suggest hypovolemic and/or hemorrhagic shock.
- Abdominal tenderness, vomiting, diarrhea, and occult or apparent GI bleeding may be seen as the direct corrosive effects of iron on gastric mucosa.

DIAGNOSTIC TESTS & INTERPRETATION
Diagnostic Procedures/Other
- Iron level:
  - The serum iron level at 4–6 hours postingestion is most predictive of the clinical course, and is used in conjunction with the clinical assessment.
  - Iron levels 300–500 mcg/dL are usually associated with GI toxicity and moderate systemic toxicity.
  - Iron levels 500–1,000 mcg/dL are usually associated with significant systemic toxicity and shock.
  - Iron levels >1,000 mcg/dL are usually associated with significant morbidity and mortality:
    - Chemistries including hepatic profile: To assess for hepatic injury and/or metabolic acidosis (positive anion-gap acidosis)
    - CBC: To determine degree of anemia from blood loss
    - Coagulation studies: To monitor for coagulopathy
    - ABG: To monitor metabolic acidosis

- Pitfalls:
  - Total iron-binding capacity (TIBC) not recommended to assess degree of toxicity.
  - Lower iron levels do not necessarily preclude the possibility of serious iron toxicity.
  - Radiographic studies: Abdominal radiograph: May reveal iron pills, which can then guide approach to GI decontamination. Liquid iron preparations and multivitamins with iron are typically not radiopaque. Absence of pills on x-ray does not exclude potential iron ingestion and toxicity.

DIFFERENTIAL DIAGNOSIS
- Ingestions: Methanol, paraldehyde, ethanol, ethylene glycol, salicylate, theophylline, or digoxin ingestions.
- GI:
  - GI hemorrhage
  - GI trauma with perforation
  - Appendicitis with rupture
  - Intussusception
  - Hemolytic uremic syndrome
  - Gastritis
  - Esophagitis
  - Mallory-Weiss tear
  - Vascular malformation
- Other:
  - Reye syndrome
  - Fulminant sepsis
  - Meningitis
  - Diabetic ketoacidosis

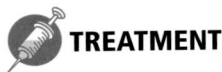 **TREATMENT**

General Measures
- Asymptomatic patients with minimal or no GI involvement can be observed in the emergency department for a 6-hour period and discharged home.
- Symptomatic patients with GI or mild symptoms should be admitted for inpatient management.
- Symptomatic patients with significant toxicity should be treated in an intensive care setting by specialists skilled in management of this ingestion. Metabolic acidosis and radiopaque material on abdominal radiograph predict significant iron absorption and toxicity.

SPECIAL THERAPIES

- GI decontamination:
  - Goal is to decrease iron absorption and break up pill concretions, which may directly damage the GI mucosa.
  - Whole-bowel irrigation with a polyethylene glycol electrolyte solution until all pill remnants have passed in the stool is recommended for most cases.
  - Gastric lavage with normal saline or tap water may be attempted, but iron tablets are often too large to pass through nasogastric tube.
  - Activated charcoal: Iron does not bind well to it, so this method of decontamination is not effective.
  - Syrup of ipecac is not recommended.
  - Rarely, endoscopy or gastrotomy may need to be performed to remove embedded pills.
- Chelation with deferoxamine (DFO):
  - Given parenterally via continuous IV infusion at 5–15 mg/kg/h. (Consult specialist or guidelines for specific dosing instructions.) This is recommended for symptomatic or ill patients, patients with a positive abdominal radiograph or significant exposure history, and all patients with levels of ≥500 mcg/dL.
  - Chelation can be discontinued with clinical improvement, resolution of metabolic acidosis, resolution of radiograph radiopacities, and urine color normalization.
  - If renal failure develops, chelation can be continued and dialysis performed (the iron–DFO complex is dialyzable).
  - The most common side effect of chelation is hypotension; therefore, adequate fluid resuscitation is imperative.

IN-PATIENT CONSIDERATIONS

Initial Stabilization

- Evaluate for presence of GI or systemic involvement, including acidosis, shock, or lethargy.
- Supportive care should include assessment of airway, supplemental oxygen, establishing IV access, and supporting BP with normal saline or Ringer's lactate.
- Endotracheal intubation and oro- or nasogastric tube placement should be considered in a lethargic patient to facilitate GI decontamination.

 ONGOING CARE

FOLLOW-UP RECOMMENDATIONS

- Abdominal x-ray should be followed until complete decontamination is documented.
- Patients should be monitored for possible late complications, such as strictures of the GI tract.

PATIENT EDUCATION

- Strategies include parental education, package-labeling warning of the potential pediatric ingestion hazard, regulatory change to require prescription status for preparations containing iron, and improved packaging of iron preparations.
- The Consumer Product Safety Commission (CPSC) requires child-resistant packaging for packages containing ≥250 mg of elemental iron. The FDA regulation that required individually packaged units for products containing ≥30 mg of elemental iron per dosage unit was repealed in 2003; still, most children's multivitamin preparations only contain up to 18 mg of elemental iron per tablet.

PROGNOSIS

- Manifestations of iron ingestion can range from asymptomatic to severe systemic toxicity and death.
- Prognosis can be estimated based on factors such as estimated ingestion dosage, serum iron level, clinical course, and presence of complications.

COMPLICATIONS

- Small bowel infarction and necrosis
- Gastric or intestinal scarring and strictures, which may present as gastric outlet or intestinal obstruction
- Hepatic failure
- Metabolic acidosis
- Hypovolemic and hemorrhagic shock
- Coagulopathy
- ARDS
- CNS effects including lethargy, seizures, and coma
- *Yersinia enterocolitica* infection or sepsis
- Death

ADDITIONAL READING

- Fine JS. Iron poisoning. *Curr Probl Pediatr*. 2000; 30(3):71–90.
- Henretig FMI. Acute iron poisoning. In: Shaw LM, Kwong TC, eds. *The Clinical Toxicology Laboratory: Contemporary Practice of Poisoning Evaluation*. Washington, DC: AACC Press; 2001:401–409.
- Madiwale T, Liebelt E. Iron: Not a benign drug. *Curr Opin Pediatr*. 2006;18:174–179.
- Manoguerra AS, Erdman AR, Booze LL, et al. Iron ingestion: An evidence-based consensus guideline for out-of-hospital management. *Clin Toxicol*. 2005;42:553–570.
- Mills KC, Curry SC. Acute iron poisoning. *Emerg Med Clin North Am*. 1994;12:397–413.
- Tenenbein M. Unit-dose packaging of iron supplements and reduction of iron poisoning in young children. *Arch Pediatr Adolesc Med*. 2005;159:557–560.

 CODES

ICD9

964.0 Poisoning by iron and its compounds

ICD10

- T45.4X4A Poisoning by iron and its compounds, undetermined, initial encounter
- T45.4X4D Poisoning by iron and its compounds, undetermined, subsequent encounter
- T45.4X4S Poisoning by iron and its compounds, undetermined, sequela

FAQ

- Q: Why isn't syrup of ipecac recommended to induce vomiting?
- A: Because the major early signs and symptoms involving the GI tract include vomiting, inducing vomiting may interfere with the clinical assessment. There is also the risk of aspiration in the patient with severe poisoning.
- Q: What is the recommendation regarding observation of a patient for development of symptoms with iron ingestion of an unknown quantity?
- A: Observe for 6 hours. Those who are asymptomatic 6 hours after ingestion are not likely to exhibit systemic illness.
- Q: What is the recommendation regarding nonintentional ingestion of children's vitamins with iron, carbonyl iron formulations, or polysaccharide iron complex formulations?
- A: These ingestions are generally deemed to contain low levels of iron, and the American Association of Poison Control Centers recommends against emergency room referral for nonacute patients with adequate home supervision. Even patients with mild diarrhea and emesis can be safely observed in the home following these ingestions, although consultation with a physician and Poison Control hotline is still advised.

I

IRRITABLE BOWEL SYNDROME

Edisio Semeao

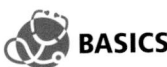 **BASICS**

DESCRIPTION

- Irritable bowel syndrome (IBS) is the best known and one of the most common functional GI tract disorders.
- These disorders are characterized by chronic and/or recurrent GI tract symptoms not explained by structural abnormalities, infection, or neoplastic or metabolic changes on routine testing.
- Terms such as *spastic colon*, *nervous colon*, and *spastic colitis* have also been used to describe IBS. Spastic colitis, however, is inaccurate because these patients do not have evidence of inflammation of their colon (colitis) at colonoscopy.
- Patients with IBS have a constellation of symptoms that include:
  - Chronic abdominal pain, usually lower abdomen
  - Altered bowel pattern:
    - Constipation
    - Diarrhea
  - Alternating constipation and diarrhea

EPIDEMIOLOGY

- 60–70% of patients with IBS are women.
- More common in adolescents in the pediatric population
- Poses a significant health care burden, with a total cost of $30 billion annually
- There is no known genetic predisposition for developing IBS.
- Women are 2 times more likely to be diagnosed with IBS than men.

Prevalence

- IBS is a prevalent disorder that occurs in 10–20% of the US population.
- It is more prevalent than hypertension, asthma, diabetes, and ischemic heart disease.
- Up to 28% of referrals for gastroenterology consults are for IBS.
- In adults, IBS is the 7th most common cause of visits to primary care physicians.
- 50% of patients present with symptoms before age 35, and 33% can trace their symptoms back into childhood.

PATHOPHYSIOLOGY

- Most commonly, IBS is thought to be a disorder of GI function relating to motility, sensation, and/or perception.
- The pathogenesis of IBS is believed to be multifactorial, with a variety of factors influencing the gut–brain axis at various levels.
- These factors interact to cause the symptoms of IBS and include:
  - Predisposing factors (social, cultural, environmental) include genetics, early life experiences, gender, and intergenerational illness behavior.
  - Precipitating factors (physiologic) may be associated with IBS but not directly a cause: Stress, infection/inflammation, bacterial flora, intestinal motility, and hormonal dysregulation.
  - Perpetuating factors (behavioral) further amplify the GI dysfunction in patients with IBS and include depression, anxiety, panic disorder, somatization, poor social support, and maladaptive behavior.
- There are no actual histologic, microbiologic, or biochemical abnormalities noted in patients with IBS.

DIAGNOSIS

- There are no specific diagnostic tests or pathognomonic signs or symptoms for the diagnosis of IBS.
- Over the past several years investigators have developed symptom-based, consensus diagnostic criteria for IBS, and the latest version (Rome III) has allowed for a confident diagnosis of this disorder based on a cluster of symptoms, minimal diagnostic evaluation, and the absence of "red flags."
- Rome III criteria: The signs and symptoms for the diagnosis of IBS may occur on a recurrent basis and need not be continuous. At least 3 months, with onset at least 6 months previously of recurrent abdominal pain or discomfort associated with 2 or more of the following:
  - Improvement in the abdominal pain after a bowel movement
  - An increasing number of stools with the start of the pain
  - Change in the form and appearance of the stool with the onset of pain:
    - Based on type of symptoms, IBS can be further classified into 1 of 3 subtypes:
      1. Diarrhea predominant
      2. Constipation predominant
      3. Mixed
    - Female IBS patients are more likely to have constipation-predominant disease.

HISTORY

- Evaluation of these patients needs to include a careful and detailed history, including a description of the symptoms, with assessment if they recur on a regular basis.
- Detailed diet and travel history
- Inciting and exacerbating factors
- Characteristics of abdominal pain:
  - Sharp, dull, crampy, or burning
  - Usually periumbilical or lower abdominal in nature, but not necessarily
  - Starts after a meal and rarely awakens a patient from sleep
- Patients, especially children, describe associated symptoms, such as pallor, nausea, anorexia, and fatigue with the abdominal pain.
- Presence or absence of abdominal distention
- Presence of increased belching and/or flatulence
- Change in bowel habits: Presence of alternating diarrhea and constipation:
  - Patients tend to have one predominant form.
  - Most patients experience relief of pain after a bowel movement.
  - Patients with constipation may go several days to a week without any stool passage.
  - In some instances, mucus may be described in this group of patients. However, blood is a rare finding and is usually associated with local/anal irritation or fissure secondary to diarrhea or constipation.

- Red flags:
  - Prolonged, unexplained fevers
  - Significant, unexplained weight loss, anorexia
  - Family history of colorectal cancer or GI disorders
  - Onset in older patients
  - Joint complaints
  - Nocturnal symptoms that awaken a patient
  - Recent major change in the nature or severity of the symptoms

PHYSICAL EXAM

- Findings, including those from rectal exam, are usually completely normal.
- There is usually no evidence of weight loss or growth failure.
- Red flags: Abdominal mass or other abnormal finding

DIAGNOSTIC TESTS & INTERPRETATION

- There are no specific tests for the diagnosis of IBS. The use of various tests may be indicated to evaluate for organic disease based on the presence of "red flags" in the history or the physical exam.
- Confine testing to basic screening tests so that patients are not left with the impression that there is a significant organic disease present.
- Tests may include:
  - Lactose breath test: Presence of lactose intolerance
  - Stool cultures for routine specimen, *Clostridium difficile*, and ova and parasites: Exclude infectious etiologies for symptoms.
  - Gastric emptying, antral-duodenal, and anal-rectal manometry are special tests.

Lab

There are no laboratory tests that are diagnostic for IBS. Routine CBC, ESR, urinalysis, electrolytes, liver function tests, albumin, amylase, lipase, celiac antibodies, and thyroid studies are performed to exclude other diseases.

Imaging

Abdominal radiograph or CT scan may exclude an intra-abdominal process.

Diagnostic Procedures/Other

Upper endoscopy and/or colonoscopy: Indications include:

- Bleeding
- Profuse diarrhea
- Weight loss
- Iron deficiency anemia
- Abnormal laboratory or radiographic studies
- Extraintestinal manifestations of inflammatory bowel disease

Pathological Findings

Red flags from testing that would raise concern about the diagnosis of IBS include:

- Anemia
- Leukocytosis
- Elevated ESR or C-reactive protein
- Positive fecal occult blood
- Positive stool cultures
- Positive serology for celiac disease
- Abnormal histology on endoscopy/colonoscopy

DIFFERENTIAL DIAGNOSIS

- Common disorders that need to be considered are those that may present with recurrent abdominal pain and altered bowel patterns, including:
  - Chronic inflammatory conditions of the bowel (Crohn disease, ulcerative colitis, indeterminate colitis, celiac disease)
  - Infectious disorders (parasites, bacterial)
  - Lactose intolerance
  - Complications of constipation (megacolon, encopresis, intermittent sigmoid volvulus)
  - Drug-induced diarrhea or constipation
  - Gynecologic disorders
  - Neoplasms
  - Psychiatric disorders
- Patients fulfilling Rome III criteria for IBS rarely (<1% probability) have an underlying illness. In contrast, IBS is so prevalent that there may be a co-occurrence with other disorders that can modify and/or amplify the clinical features of IBS. Common disorders include celiac disease and lactose intolerance.

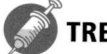 TREATMENT

MEDICATION (DRUGS)
First Line
Limited by marginal therapeutic benefits, side effects, and potential exacerbation of IBS

- Bulking agents: Fiber supplementation in the diet is a usual 1st step in therapy that prolongs stool transit time and absorption.
- Laxatives: Unproven benefits, no real trials, and frequent complications
- Antispasmodics: Dicyclomine (Bentyl) and hyoscyamine (Levsin) may aid in pain relief, but overall efficacy in global symptom control is not proven.
- Antidiarrheal agents: Unproven benefits and associated with some risks.

Antidepressants

- Tricyclic antidepressants: Play a role in pain relief. They have also been shown to decrease symptoms independent of their effect on anxiety and depression. May have unwanted side effects
- Selective serotonin reuptake inhibitors: Improvement in symptoms independent of their effect on anxiety and depression. The mechanism of action may be related to the effect of serotonin's role in motility, sensation, and secretion in the GI tract
  - Serotonin receptor medications
    - 5-HT$_3$ antagonist: Alosetron (Lotronex) inhibits cholinergic neurons and visceral sensory mechanisms. Presently, it is only available in limited, restricted use in females with severe diarrhea-predominant IBS who have failed other therapies. Complications of ischemic colitis (3:1,000) and severe constipation have been reported. A few cases of ischemic colitis resulted in either death or need for surgical resection.

- Probiotics
  - 25% of patients with IBS report start of symptoms after a GI intestinal infection. Recent studies have concluded that probiotics may be useful; however, dose, formulation, and type greatly affect the results.
- Antibiotics: Neomycin and rifaximin. Can be used to treat for possible bacterial overgrowth
- Dietary restrictions: Can be used as adjuvant therapy; however, have not been shown to be beneficial as a primary therapy
- Herbal medications
  - St John's wort: Has not been shown to have any positive effect in the treatment of IBS
  - Peppermint: Studies have shown that its use can decrease the symptoms of IBS. It is accepted as an adjunct therapy.
- Psychotherapy: Patients are taught a variety of techniques and exercises to use during the episodes of pain that allow them to focus on other subjects, not on the pain.
- Future therapies: Tachykinins—biologically active peptides that affect bowel function. They include substance P and neurokinin A and their clinical significance is unclear.
- Overall, the most effective intervention may be to combine therapies that will target specific symptoms and arms of the gut–brain axis to globally control the symptoms from IBS.

COMPLICATIONS

- A large number of the complications that arise from IBS include depression and anxiety, causing a decreased quality of life.
- Patients with IBS show a significant amount of absenteeism from both school and work.

ADDITIONAL TREATMENT
General Measures

- For patients with mild symptoms of IBS, reassurance, education, and lifestyle changes such as avoiding identified triggers may be adequate for management.
- In patients with more severe or complex symptoms, a multidisciplinary approach including pharmacotherapy and psychosocial intervention may be needed.

 ONGOING CARE

FOLLOW-UP RECOMMENDATIONS
Patient Monitoring
There is no standard or specific follow-up needed for patients with IBS. They should continue with routine care, and one should ensure effective communication between the patient and physician to review the clinical symptoms and evaluate for any changes in the symptoms that may indicate another underlying problem.

ADDITIONAL READING

- Camilleri M. Treating irritable bowel syndrome: Overview, perspective and future therapies. *Br J Pharmacol*. 2004;141:1237–1248.
- Chiou E, Nurko S. Management of functional abdominal pain and irritable bowel syndrome in children and adolescents. *Expert Rev Gastroenterol Hepatol*. 2010;4(3):293–304.
- Cremonini F, Talley N. Irritable bowel syndrome: Epidemiology, natural history, health care seeking and emerging risk factors. *Gastroenterol Clin North Am*. 2005;34:189–204.
- Drossman D. The functional gastrointestinal disorders and the Rome III process. *Gastroenterology*. 2006;130:1377–1390.
- Huertas-Ceballos A, Logan S, Bennett C, et al. Dietary interventions for recurrent abdominal pain (RAP) and irritable bowel syndrome (IBS) in childhood. *Cochrane Database Syst Rev*. 2008;(1): CD003019.
- Katiraei P, Bultron G. Need for a comprehensive medical approach to the neuro-immuno gastroenterology of irritable bowel syndrome. *World J Gastroenterol*. 2011;17(23):2791–2800.

 CODES

ICD9
564.1 Irritable bowel syndrome

ICD10
- K58.0 Irritable bowel syndrome with diarrhea
- K58.9 Irritable bowel syndrome without diarrhea

FAQ

- Q: Is evidence of microscopic colitis consistent with the diagnosis of IBS?
- A: There should be no histologic or laboratory abnormalities.
- Q: Will patients with IBS have a coexisting GI disorder?
- A: Frequently, patients may be diagnosed with lactose intolerance or celiac disease. In these instances, both disorders need to be treated to alleviate the symptoms.

JAUNDICE

Kathleen M. Loomes

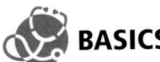 **BASICS**

DEFINITION
- Jaundice is derived from the French word jaune, which means "yellow."
- Jaundice: A yellow or green/yellow hue to the skin, sclerae, and mucous membranes which can be appreciated at serum bilirubin levels >2 mg/dL. Intensity of color is directly related to the serum bilirubin level.
- Unconjugated bilirubin: 80% is due to hemoglobin turnover and 20% is from degradation of hepatic and renal heme proteins. It is a hydrophobic compound that must be carried to the liver by albumin for processing.
- Conjugated bilirubin: Conjugated to glucuronic acid in the liver, a water-soluble derivative that helps lipid emulsification and absorption
- Conjugated hyperbilirubinemia (direct hyperbilirubinemia): A conjugated bilirubin of >2 mg/dL or >20% of the total bilirubin

EPIDEMIOLOGY
The most common causes of pathologic jaundice:
- Newborn period: Biliary atresia, idiopathic neonatal hepatitis, α-1-antitrypsin deficiency, infection
- Older child: Autoimmune hepatitis, viral hepatitis, Wilson disease, biliary obstruction

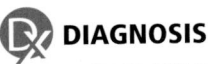 **DIAGNOSIS**

DIFFERENTIAL DIAGNOSIS
- **Unconjugated hyperbilirubinemia**
  - Congenital/anatomic:
    - Placental dysfunction/insufficiency resulting in polycythemia (e.g., infants of diabetic mothers)
    - Upper GI tract obstruction (e.g., pyloric stenosis, duodenal web, atresia)
    - Congenital hypothyroidism
  - Infectious:
    - Sepsis
  - Trauma/delivery complications:
    - Cephalohematoma/bruising
    - Delayed cord clamping, twin–twin transfusion, maternal–fetal transfusion leading to polycythemia
    - Intrauterine hypoxia (secondary to cocaine abuse, high altitude) resulting in polycythemia
    - Induction of labor with oxytocin
    - Prematurity
  - Genetic/metabolic:
    - Inherited red cell enzyme, membrane defects (e.g., spherocytosis, glucose 6-phosphate-dehydrogenase deficiency, phosphokinase deficiency, elliptocytosis)
    - Red cell abnormalities (sickle cell anemia, thalassemia)
    - Defect in hepatic bilirubin conjugation (e.g., Crigler–Najjar types I and II, Gilbert)
    - Inborn errors of metabolism
  - Allergic/inflammatory/immunologic:
    - Isoimmunization (ABO, Rh, Kell, other incompatibility)
  - Functional:
    - Physiologic jaundice—peaks during the day
    - Breastfeeding-associated jaundice
    - Swallowed maternal blood
    - Increased bilirubin load due to infant bleeding from a clotting disorder
    - Familial benign unconjugated hyperbilirubinemia in mother and neonate (Lucey–Driscoll syndrome)
- **Conjugated hyperbilirubinemia**
  - Extrahepatic:
    - Extrahepatic biliary atresia
    - Choledochal cysts and other abnormalities of the choledochopancreatic ductal junction
    - Spontaneous perforation of the bile duct
    - Bile or mucous plug or biliary sludge
    - Gallstones
  - Infectious etiologies:
    - Bacterial: Gram-negative sepsis, urinary tract infection
    - Viral: Cytomegalovirus; echovirus; herpes simplex virus; rubella; Epstein–Barr virus; HIV, hepatitis A, B, C, D, and E
    - Toxoplasmosis
    - *Pneumocystis carinii*
    - *Entamoeba histolytica*
    - *Mycobacterium tuberculosis*
    - Mycobacterium avium-intracellulare
    - Syphilis
  - Toxic, environmental, drugs:
    - Post-shock or post-asphyxia (ischemic injury to liver)
    - Drugs: Acetaminophen, valproate, chlorpromazine, Amanita toxin and others
    - Hyperalimentation (total parenteral nutrition)
  - Tumor:
    - Neuroblastoma, hepatic, biliary, pancreatic, duodenal, peritoneal
    - Portal hepatis nodes
  - Genetic/metabolic:
    - Arteriohepatic dysplasia (Alagille syndrome)
    - Progressive familial intrahepatic cholestasis (including FIC1, BSEP, and MDR3 deficiency)
    - Benign recurrent intrahepatic cholestasis
    - Defects in bile acid metabolism
    - Defects in amino acid metabolism
    - Defects in lipid metabolism: Wolman disease, Niemann–Pick disease, Gaucher disease
    - Defects in carbohydrate metabolism: Galactosemia, hereditary fructose intolerance, glycogenosis type IV
    - Defects in fatty acid oxidation
    - Defects in mitochondrial DNA and respiratory chain defects
    - α-1-antitrypsin deficiency
    - Cystic fibrosis
    - Wilson disease (older children)
    - Inherited noncholestatic conjugated jaundice syndromes (e.g., Dubin–Johnson and Rotor syndrome)
    - Hereditary cholestasis with lymphedema (Aagenaes syndrome)
  - Inflammatory/immunologic/endocrine:
    - Idiopathic neonatal hepatitis
    - Neonatal iron storage disease
    - Idiopathic panhypopituitarism
    - Autoimmune hepatitis (children and adolescents)
    - Sclerosing cholangitis (children and adolescents, unless neonatal form)

APPROACH TO THE PATIENT
- **Phase 1:** Determine if hyperbilirubinemia is unconjugated or conjugated.
- **Phase 2:** If unconjugated hyperbilirubinemia
  - Obtain CBC and indices
  - Reticulocyte count
  - Coombs test: If test is positive, the diagnosis is isoimmune; if test is negative, then consider polycythemia, extravascular bleed, or RBC structural or enzyme defects.
- **Phase 3:** If conjugated hyperbilirubinemia
  - Alanine aminotransferase (ALT), aspartate aminotransferase (AST), γ-glutamyltranspeptidase (GGT)
    - PT/PTT/international normalized ratio (INR)
  - Ultrasound of the liver/pancreas/gallbladder and biliary tree
  - Rule out those etiologies of conjugated hyperbilirubinemia that may adversely affect the outcome if diagnosis is delayed (biliary atresia, tyrosinemia, galactosemia, inborn error of bile acid synthesis, hereditary fructose intolerance, panhypopituitarism and others).

HISTORY
- **Question:** Unexplained itching?
- *Significance*: Cholestatic liver disease (conjugated hyperbilirubinemia)
- **Question:** History of poor school performance, change in mental status, handwriting?
- *Significance*: Wilson disease
- **Question:** History of other family members having prolonged jaundice, hepatic failure, or sudden death in infancy?
- *Significance*: Suggests an underlying inborn error of metabolism such as tyrosinemia, galactosemia, or a fatty acid oxidation defect
- **Question:** History of IV drug abuse or exposure to blood or blood products, especially prior to 1992?
- *Significance*: The patient may have transfusion-associated hepatitis (e.g., hepatitis C).

PHYSICAL EXAM
- **Finding:** Scratch marks?
- *Significance*: Pruritus secondary to cholestasis
- **Finding:** Spider angioma, palmar erythema?
- *Significance*: Chronic liver disease
- **Finding:** Petechiae, purpura, microcephaly, thrombocytopenia?
- *Significance*: Congenital TORCH infection
- **Finding:** Heart murmur?
- *Significance*: Alagille syndrome (peripheral pulmonic stenosis)
- **Finding:** Splenomegaly?
- *Significance*: Suggests acute hemolysis (in unconjugated hyperbilirubinemia) or chronic liver disease and portal hypertension (conjugated hyperbilirubinemia)
- **Finding:** Ascites?
- *Significance*: Suggests portal hypertension
- **Finding:** Acholic stool?
- *Significance*: Severe cholestasis or biliary obstruction

DIAGNOSTIC TESTS & INTERPRETATION

- Percutaneous liver biopsies: Liver pathology—in infants with cholestasis, the most common patterns are giant cell hepatitis, bile duct proliferation, and bile duct paucity. A pattern of duct proliferation, bile plugs, portal expansion, and fibrosis suggests biliary obstruction.
- Intraoperative cholangiogram is indicated for infants with a liver biopsy suggestive of biliary obstruction and possible biliary atresia. If the cholangiogram is consistent with biliary atresia, the surgeon will perform the Kasai portoenterostomy.
- **Test:** Total bilirubin with fractionation into unconjugated, conjugated, and delta fractions
- *Significance*: Direct vs. indirect hyperbilirubinemia

If unconjugated hyperbilirubinemia, investigation is initiated with:

- **Test:** CBC with indices, reticulocyte count, and peripheral blood smear for RBC morphology
- *Significance*: Polycythemia in neonate, hemolysis, or other conditions associated with increased destruction of red cells
- **Test:** Coombs test
- *Significance*: Isoimmune and autoimmune hemolytic anemia
- **Test:** PT/PTT/INR, platelet count
- *Significance*: Coagulopathy associated with hemorrhage that causes an increased bilirubin load

If neonatal conjugated hyperbilirubinemia, investigation is initiated with:

- **Test:** Serum aminotransferases (ALT, AST)
- *Significance*: Ongoing liver inflammation
- **Test:** Alkaline phosphatase and GGT
- *Significance*: Biliary tree obstruction, bile duct injury, or cholestasis
- **Test:** PT/INR, PTT, serum albumin, fibrinogen
- *Significance*: Liver synthetic function
- **Test:** Sepsis evaluation (blood and urine, and spinal fluid)
- *Significance*: Sepsis can impair conjugation and excretion of bilirubin; results in poor feeding with bile sludging and subsequent formation of gallstones.
- **Test:** Free T3, T4, and thyroid-stimulating hormone
- *Significance*: Congenital hypothyroidism
- **Test:** α-1-antitrypsin serum levels and PI phenotype
- *Significance*: Serum α-1-antitrypsin levels will be low in inherited protease inhibitor deficiency. Levels can be falsely elevated due to the fact that α-1-antitrypsin is an acute-phase reactant.
- **Test:** Urine dipstick for glucose and reducing substances
- *Significance*: Positive reducing substances seen in galactosemia and hereditary fructose intolerance.

- **Test:** Urine for bile acid analysis
- *Significance*: Inborn error of bile acid metabolism
- Metabolic workup may be performed depending on clinical setting, including plasma amino acids, urine organic acids, succinylacetone, lactate, pyruvate, and other tests as indicated.
- In an older child presenting with conjugated hyperbilirubinemia, the most common causes are biliary obstruction due to gallstones, viral hepatitis, and autoimmune hepatitis.

Imaging

- Ultrasound:
  - A noninvasive method to examine the overall liver appearance, size, and density
  - Allows for examination of the biliary tree and gallbladder to rule out choledochal cysts, sludge/stones, and ductal dilatation indicating possible obstruction
  - Infants with biliary atresia/splenic malformation syndrome may have other findings including polysplenia, asplenia and pre-duodenal portal vein with azygous continuation.
- Hepatobiliary scintigraphy (HIDA scan): Tracer secretion into the duodenum excludes biliary atresia or extrahepatic biliary obstruction.

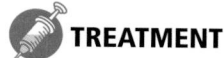 TREATMENT

ADDITIONAL TREATMENT
General Measures
- Treat Crigler–Najjar syndrome promptly with phototherapy and phenobarbital to prevent kernicterus
- Older children with Wilson disease may present with profound hemolysis and may have predominantly unconjugated hyperbilirubinemia with severe parenchymal liver disease and fulminant liver failure.

ISSUES FOR REFERRAL
- Any infant with jaundice beyond 10–14 days of age should have a fractionated bilirubin sent.
- Any infant with conjugated hyperbilirubinemia should be referred immediately to a pediatric gastroenterologist for further workup.

ADDITIONAL READING

- Cappellini MD, Fiorelli G. Glucose-6-phosphate dehydrogenase deficiency. *Lancet*. 2008; 371(9606):64–74.
- Cohen RS, Wong RJ, Stevenson DK. Understanding neonatal jaundice: A perspective on causation. *Pediatr Neonatol*. 2010;51(3):143–148.
- Davenport M, Betalli P, D'Antiga L, et al. The spectrum of surgical jaundice in infancy. *J Pediatr Surg*. 2003;38:1471–1479.
- Kelly DA, Davenport M. Current management of biliary atresia. *Arch Dis Child*. 2007;92(12): 1132–1135.
- Maisels MJ, McDonagh AF. Phototherapy for neonatal jaundice. *N Engl J Med*. 2008;358(9): 920–928.
- Subcommittee on Hyperbilirubinemia. Management of hyperbilirubinemia in the newborn infant 35 or more weeks of gestation. *Pediatrics*. 2004;114(1): 297–316.
- Takaya J, Muneyuki M, Tokuhara D, et al. Congenital dilation of the bile duct: Changes in diagnostic tools over the past 20 years. *Pediatr Int*. 2003;45: 383–387.

 CODES

ICD9
- 774.6 Unspecified fetal and neonatal jaundice
- 782.4 Jaundice, unspecified, not of newborn

ICD10
- P59.9 Neonatal jaundice, unspecified
- R17 Unspecified jaundice

FAQ

- Q: Are there any characteristic findings in neonatal jaundice that are specifically concerning?
- A: These findings are concerning until proven otherwise:
  - Development of jaundice before 36 hours of life
  - Persistent jaundice beyond 10 days of life
  - Serum bilirubin concentration >12 mg/dL
  - Elevation of direct bilirubin >2 mg/dL or 20% of total bilirubin at any time
- Q: Are there any ethnic/social factors associated with higher bilirubin levels?
- A: Factors that have been associated with high serum bilirubin levels are low birth weight, certain ethnic groups (Asian, Native American, Greek), delayed meconium passage after birth, and breastfeeding. Factors that have been associated with lower serum levels in neonates include maternal smoking, black race, and certain drugs such as phenobarbital.

J

KAWASAKI DISEASE

Jeffrey S. Gerber

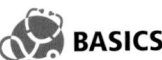

BASICS

DESCRIPTION
An idiopathic, multisystem disease of young children characterized by vasculitis of the small- and medium-sized blood vessels. The acute phase is self-limited; signs and symptoms evolve over the 1st 10 days, then resolve spontaneously. However, 20–25% of untreated patients will develop coronary artery aneurysms.

EPIDEMIOLOGY
Kawasaki disease (KD) has surpassed rheumatic fever as the leading cause of acquired heart disease in children in the U.S.

Incidence
- The annual U.S. hospitalization rate for children <5 years of age with KD is estimated at 20.815 per 100,000 children.
- Rates were highest among Asian and Pacific Islander children (30.3 per 100,000), followed by African American children.
- Kawasaki disease accounted for >4,200 hospitalizations in the U.S. in 2000, with hospital charges of ~$35 million. No deaths were reported among hospitalized patients during the acute phase of illness.
- Median age of cases is 3 years. 76.82% of cases occurred in children <5; 95% in children <10. Slightly higher incidence in boys.
- Recurrence rate is <1–31%

ETIOLOGY
- Etiology is uncertain.
- Epidemiologic and clinical features (seasonal peak in winter/spring, peak in toddler age group, with sparing of young infants, and low recurrence rate) suggest an infectious cause trigger in a genetically susceptible child, although there is no convincing evidence linking a particular pathogen with KD.
- Controversial evidence suggests that KD may be associated with infection with superantigen-producing bacteria (either *Staphylococcus aureus* or group A streptococci).
- Association with recent carpet cleaning, humidifier use, or residence near water has not been substantiated.

COMMONLY ASSOCIATED CONDITIONS
- Diarrhea and abdominal pain may be seen.
- Patients may develop arthralgias or even frank arthritis.
- Pancarditis may present as myocardial dysfunction early in the course of disease, with signs of CHF.
- Infantile periarteritis nodosa:
  - A previously described entity in which the pathologic findings of coronary artery aneurysms are indistinguishable from those seen in KD.
  - Most patients with periarteritis nodosa do not have the other findings of KD.

DIAGNOSIS

- Diagnosis of KD requires fever for ≥45 days and ≥4 of the following criteria, which are not required to be present simultaneously:
  - Bilateral nonexudative conjunctival injection
  - Polymorphous, nonvesicular rash
  - Mucosal involvement of the upper respiratory tract that may include erythema, fissured lips, crusting of the lips and mouth, strawberry tongue, or injected, nonexudative pharyngitis.
  - Edema or erythema of the hands and feet
  - Cervical adenopathy (>1.5 cm diameter), which is often unilateral
- Incomplete KD:
  - Patients may present with fever and <4 of the 5 diagnostic criteria and still develop aneurysms
  - Children with KD at the extremes of age (>9 or <1) are more likely to have incomplete disease, and coronary aneurysm is more common in children <1.

HISTORY
- Typical presentation proceeds through 3 recognizable phases:
  - Acute phase (1–2 weeks from onset):
    - Highly febrile (generally >39°C), irritable, toxic appearing
    - Occasionally toxic; rarely hypotensive
    - Fever generally >39°C
    - Oral changes usually quickly follow and also may last 1–2 weeks.
    - Rash prone to occur in perineal area
    - Edema and erythema of the feet are usually painful and limit ambulation.
  - Subacute phase (from 2–8 weeks after onset):
    - Without treatment, gradual improvement occurs; fever decreases and there is desquamation of the perineal area, palms, soles, and/or periungual areas.
    - Coronary artery aneurysms often appear during the early portion of this phase, and acute myocardial infarction (MI) may be seen rarely.
    - May have persistent arthritis or arthralgias
  - Convalescent phase (from months to years after):
    - Resolution of remaining symptoms
    - Laboratory values return to normal
    - Aneurysms may resolve or patients may have persistent aneurysms, persistent cardiac dysfunction, or even MI.

PHYSICAL EXAM
- High, unremitting fevers that last 1–2 weeks
- Rash is erythematous and polymorphous; not vesicular or bullous:
  - Often prominent on trunk, perineum; usually maculopapular, may coalesce and may be petechial
- Conjunctivitis: Bilateral and nonexudative
- Oral changes may be erythema, fissures, and crusting of lips, diffuse oropharyngeal erythema, or the presence of a strawberry tongue or any combination of these findings. Not exudative.

- Extremity changes may include erythema of the palms and soles and/or induration of the hands and feet:
  - Desquamation, especially periungual, usually occurs in the subacute phase.
  - Transverse grooves across the fingernails (Beau lines) may be seen 2–3 months after onset.
- Adenopathy is usually cervical and often unilateral:
  - Least often seen of the major criteria
  - May be fleeting and easily missed
- Aseptic meningitis: Common; patients are extremely irritable and may show signs of encephalopathy or ataxia.
- Pancarditis during the acute phase: May present with tachycardia, gallop rhythms, muffled heart sounds, signs of CHF, and murmurs consistent with aortic or mitral insufficiency
- Abdominal exam GI: Patients may have a right upper quadrant mass abdominal pain, diarrhea, (hydrops of gallbladder [<10%]), diarrhea, hepatosplenomegaly, or jaundice.
- Meatitis and vulvitis: May be seen in association with urethritis and sterile pyuria (70%)
- Arthralgias are common; frank arthritis is seen in up to 20% of patients.
- May involve large and small joints
- Is nondeforming
- Onset may be as late as 2nd or 3rd week
- Usually resolves in <1 month
- Uveitis (25–50%): During acute phase, slit-lamp exam may reveal anterior uveitis.

DIAGNOSTIC TESTS & INTERPRETATION
There is no diagnostic test for KD. However, a constellation of laboratory tests provides support for the diagnosis within the appropriate clinical context. Such data become most helpful in less definitive clinical scenarios, and most useful for aiding the diagnosis of incomplete KD. Exclusion of other diseases (adenovirus, scarlet fever, toxic shock syndrome, roseola, enterovirus, EBV) is paramount.

Lab
- CBC:
  - WBC usually increased with a left shift; >15,000 in 50% of cases
  - Anemia for age
  - Elevated ESR and C-reactive protein
- Platelet count:
  - Platelets may be low, normal, or high at presentation but increase rapidly after the 2nd week of illness; may be >1 million/mm³
  - During subacute phase, platelet counts may increase to $1–2 \times 10^6$.
- Other laboratory abnormalities include:
  - Sterile pyuria (70%)
  - Mild increases in hepatic transaminases
  - A CSF pleocytosis with a normal protein and glucose
  - Mild hypoalbuminemia

Imaging
- Chest x-ray: May show dilated heart during acute phase
- Echocardiography:
  - During acute phase can show a decreased shortening fraction and effusion
  - Coronary ectasia, dilation, or aneurysms may be detected as early as 6 days into the illness; peak onset is between 3 and 4 weeks.

Diagnostic Procedures/Other
ECG: During acute phase may show prolonged PR interval, decreased QRS voltage, flat T waves, and ST changes

DIFFERENTIAL DIAGNOSIS
- Infections:
  - In 1 series, measles and group A -β-hemolytic streptococcal infections most closely resembled KD and accounted for 83% of patients referred who did not have KD.
  - Severe staphylococcal infections with toxin release (e.g., toxic shock syndrome) may also resemble KD, although there is usually renal involvement (extremely rare in KD) and low platelets.
  - Other infections that must be considered include adenovirus, Epstein-Barr virus EBV, roseola, enterovirus, Rocky Mountain spotted fever, and leptospirosis.
- Immunologic:
  - Juvenile idiopathic arthritis and unusual variants of acute rheumatic fever
  - Hypersensitivity reactions and Stevens-Johnson syndrome (SJS)
  - In SJS the conjunctivitis is more likely to be exudative, the rash is more likely to be vesicular with crusting, and there is often a history of drug ingestion.

 TREATMENT

MEDICATION (DRUGS)
- IV immunoglobulin (IVIG):
  - Usual dose is 2 g/kg as a 1-time dose
  - Efficacy of IVIG after the 10th day of illness is unclear.
  - Patients who fail to respond to an initial dose of IVIG or who have a recrudescence of their symptoms should be retreated with IVIG (up to 2/3 may have a good response to repeat doses).
  - Side effects: Patients may develop signs of fluid overload and CHF. Aseptic meningitis may also be seen. This may be difficult to differentiate from the aseptic meningitis seen in patients as part of their KD.
- Aspirin:
  - High-dose aspirin (was the mainstay of therapy; still used in conjunction with IVIG, although no data look at IVIG with aspirin versus IVIG alone has been evaluated)
  - Usual initial dose is 80–100 mg/kg/d in divided doses.
- Corticosteroids:
  - A randomized controlled trial did not support the addition of steroids to IVIG for primary treatment.
  - The role of steroids for refractory disease remains unclear.
  - Cyclophosphamide, plasma exchange, TNF-α antagonists biologics (e.g., infliximab), and other salvage therapies have also been reported useful in patients who do not respond to repeated doses of IVIG.

- Duration:
  - Aspirin is continued at high dose until day 14 of the illness or when the child has been afebrile for 48 hours.
  - Aspirin dose is then decreased to 3–5 mg/kg/d for 6 weeks or until platelet count returns to normal.
  - If there are coronary artery abnormalities, additional antiplatelet/anticoagulation drugs therapy should be considered depending upon the severity of structural and clinical disease.

ADDITIONAL TREATMENT
General Measures
- The acute treatment of KD is aimed at reducing the inflammation of the coronary arteries to inhibit the development of aneurysm formation.
- If aneurysms are present, chronic imaging and therapy is directed at inhibiting coronary thrombosis and resultant MI.

 ONGOING CARE

FOLLOW-UP RECOMMENDATIONS
- The natural course is a gradual improvement during the subacute phase.
- With IVIG, children usually defervesce and show significant resolution of clinical symptoms within 2–3 days of treatment (70–80%).
- 2/3 of patients who receive a repeat dose of IVIG will respond to this dose.

Patient Monitoring
- WBC count, platelet count, and ESR should be followed weekly to biweekly until they return to normal.
- ECG and echo should be done performed to rule out the development of coronary artery aneurysms at diagnosis, at 2 weeks, and at 6–8 weeks from disease onset; more frequent imaging is recommended in patients with coronary abnormalities.
- If aneurysms are present, cardiology follow-up should include coronary artery catheterization and imaging at some time (usually 8–12 weeks after onset of illness).
- Symptoms of cardiac insufficiency (fatigue, chest pain, dyspnea on exertion) should be respected and an evaluation for myocardial dysfunction undertaken when these are present.

PROGNOSIS
- Without treatment with IVIG, 15–25% of patients develop coronary aneurysms.
- Use of IVIG decreases the incidence of coronary artery aneurysms to 4–8<5%.
- Death occurs secondary to cardiac disease in 0.13–0.2% of cases; ~10% is related to early myocarditis, and the remainder is due to MIs.
- MI can occur several years after the initial illness.
- Patients who are <1 year old, >98 years old, male, and whose fevers persist for >14 days are more likely to develop aneurysms.
- Mortality rates are much higher in males and patients who develop giant coronary artery aneurysms (diameter of >8 mm).
- Patients with a history of KD may have a worse cardiovascular risk profile in later life, indicative of an increased risk of atherosclerotic heart disease compared to the general population.

COMPLICATIONS
- Aneurysms are usually 1st noted 12–28 days after onset of the disease. They rarely appear >28 days after onset.
- Aneurysms may thrombose, leading to MI and death.
- Rarely, aneurysms may rupture acutely.
- A pancarditis is often present in the 1st 10 days of the illness. Pericardial effusions may accompany this.

ADDITIONAL READING
- Baumer JH, Love SJ, Gupta A, et al. Salicylate for the treatment of Kawasaki disease in children. *Cochrane Database Syst Rev.* 2006;(4):CD004175.
- Burns JC, Glode MP. Kawasaki syndrome. *Lancet.* 2004;364:533–44.
- Freeman AF, Shulman ST. Refractory Kawasaki disease. *Pediatr Infec Dis J.* 2004;23:463–4.
- Holman RC, et al. Hospitalizations for Kawasaki syndrome among children in the U.S., 1997–2007. *Pediatr Infect Dis J.* 2010;29: 483–8.
- Manlhiot C, Yeung RS, Clarizia NA, et al. Kawasaki disease at the extremes of the age spectrum. *Pediatrics.* 2009;124;e410–e405.
- Newburger JW, Sleeper LA, McCrindle BW, et al. Randomized trial of pulsed corticosteroid therapy for primary treatment of Kawasaki disease. *Pediatric Heart Network Investigations. N Engl J Med.* 2007; 356(7):663–675.
- Newburger JW, Takahashi M, Gerber MA, et al. Diagnosis, treatment, and long-term management of patients with Kawasaki disease: A statement for health professionals from the committee on rheumatic fever, endocarditis, and Kawasaki disease, Council on Cardiovascular Disease in the Young, American Heart Association. *Pediatrics.* 2004;114: 1708–1733.
- Pinna GS, Kafetzis DA, Tselkas OI, et al. Kawasaki disease: An overview. *Curr Opin Infect Dis.* 2008;21(3):263–270.
- Baumer JH, et al. Salicylate for the treatment of Kawasaki disease in children. *Cochrane Database Syst Rev.* 2006;4:CD004175.
- Silva AA, et al. Cardiovascular risk factors after Kawasaki disease: A case-control study. *J Pediatr.* 2001;138:400–405.

 CODES

ICD9
446.1 Acute febrile mucocutaneous lymph node syndrome [MCLS]

ICD10
M30.3 Mucocutaneous lymph node syndrome [Kawasaki]

FAQ
- Q: Do coronary artery aneurysms associated with KD ever resolve?
- A: Most coronary artery aneurysms do resolve. Even some giant aneurysms (those >8 mm in diameter) will resolve; there is concern, however, that even if aneurysms resolve, these patients may be at risk for the early development of atherosclerosis.

K

KNEE PAIN, ANTERIOR/PATELLOFEMORAL MALALIGNMENT SYNDROME

Theodore J. Ganley

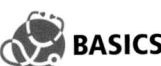 **BASICS**

DESCRIPTION
- Condition characterized by discomfort at the anterior aspect of the knee that is generally associated with activities, especially those that involve running, jumping, and climbing stairs
- Has also been called "miserable malalignment syndrome"

PATHOPHYSIOLOGY
- Predisposing factors for patellofemoral malalignment syndrome include:
  – Femoral anteversion
  – Genu valgus
  – Pes planus
- These 3 anatomic features have been commonly referred to as a terrible triad contributing to anterior knee pain. Because the entire kinetic chain is linked in function, malalignment at 1 area can lead to secondary stresses at a distant location.
- Excess femoral anteversion, as well as marked pes planus, can contribute to the increase lateral pull on the patella and subsequent patellofemoral pain.
- Further contributing factors include a wider pelvis and more laterally positioned tibial tubercle, both of which also contribute to altered biomechanics at the knee.
- Tight hamstrings, heel cords, and quadriceps, as well as diminished quadriceps tone, can lead to increased forces across the patellofemoral joint.

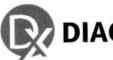 **DIAGNOSIS**

HISTORY
- Pain under and around the kneecap with activities including squatting, sitting for prolonged periods with the knees bent, and going up or down stairs or hills: These activities increase patellofemoral contact stress.
- Recent history of direct trauma to the kneecap: A blunt trauma to the kneecap can cause soft tissue or subchondral contusion that may exacerbate this condition.

PHYSICAL EXAM
- Cracking noises from the front of the knee with flexion and extension:
  – Cracking can be a sign of softening of the undersurface of the patella
  – Chondromalacia is patellar articular cartilage pathologic changes, which range from mild cracking attributed to softening to locking and catching attributed to cartilage disruption.
- There is no single angulation or rotation profile that is universal for all anterior knee pain patients. Those with anterior knee pain however more commonly have femoral anteversion, genu valgus and pes planus. Low quadriceps tone and hamstring as well as quadriceps tightness may also be found.

DIAGNOSTIC TESTS & INTERPRETATION
Imaging
- Anterior and posterior, lateral, Merchant plain radiographs of the knee:
  – The Merchant kneecap view shows the shape of the patella within the trochlea.
  – Patients will frequently be found to have lateral patellar tilt, as well as an abnormally shaped patella with excessive elongation of the lateral portion of the patella/lateral patellar facet.
- MRI: Not a 1st-line study for patellofemoral syndrome; however, it may be performed to rule out associated pathology in patients with recalcitrant pain and unusual clinical presentations.

DIFFERENTIAL DIAGNOSIS
- Osgood-Schlatter disease:
  – Tenderness not at the patella but at the anterior tibial tubercle
  – A self-limiting inflammation of the apophysis that tends to occur in growing teenagers and pre-teens
  – Irregularity and fragmentation of the apophysis are seen on lateral radiographs.
- Meniscus tear:
  – Disruption of the crescent-shaped fibrocartilaginous tissue adjacent to the tibial and femoral articular surfaces
  – Most commonly presents as posteromedial or posterolateral hemijoint tenderness with knee hyperflexion and rotation

- Prepatellar bursitis:
  - An inflammation of the fluid-filled bursal sac beneath the SC tissue and immediately anterior to the patella
  - More common in patients who kneel for extended periods of time and has been called "carpet layer's knee"
  - Swelling and tenderness immediately anterior to the patella; does not primarily present with deeper tenderness in the medial and lateral parapatellar regions found in patellofemoral syndrome

ALERT
Patients with a traumatic effusion, locking, catching, instability to ligamentous stress testing, multiple joint effusions, or night waking should be evaluated for other traumatic or medical conditions.

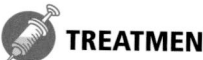

TREATMENT

ADDITIONAL TREATMENT
General Measures
- A progressive exercise program is the main focus of treatment.
- Strength and flexibility exercises are needed to increase the strength and control the quadriceps muscle, as well as to stretch the quadriceps, hamstrings, and tendoachilles complex.
- Straight-leg-raising program can help to strengthen the quadriceps:
  - This can be performed several times each day as a home exercise program or formally with physical therapy in more recalcitrant cases.
  - Quadriceps, hamstrings, and tendoachilles stretches can be performed at the same time intervals as the strengthening program.

- Patients can be advanced from low-resistance exercises such as swimming, stationary bike, and elliptical trainers to higher-level running activities.
- Activity restriction in the initial acutely symptomatic stage is instituted to eliminate high-impact sports, including especially those that involve running and jumping.

ADDITIONAL READING

- Flynn J, Lou J, Ganley T. Prevention of sports injuries in children. *Curr Opin Pediatr*. 2002;14:719–722.
- Ganley TJ, et al. Pediatric sports medicine. *Curr Opin Orthopaed*. 2001;12:456-61.
- Hamer AJ. Pain in the hip and knee. *BMJ*. 2004; 328(7447):1067–1069.
- Hart L. Supervised exercise versus usual care for patellofemoral pain syndrome. *Clin J Sport Med*. 2010;20(2):133.
- Murray KJ. Hypermobility disorders in children and adolescents. *Best Pract Res Clin Rheumatol*. 2006; 20(2):329–351.
- Saperstein AL, Nicholas SJ. Pediatric and adolescent sports medicine. *Pediatr Clin North Am*. 1996;43:1013–1033.

 ## CODES

ICD9
- 719.46 Knee pain
- 733.92 Chondromalacia

ICD10
- M22.40 Chondromalacia patellae, unspecified knee
- M25.569 Pain in unspecified knee
- M94.269 Chondromalacia, unspecified knee

FAQ

- Q: Is it acceptable to play sports, or is this condition too dangerous?
- A: Patients with a history of patellofemoral syndrome who have regained their strength and flexibility are permitted to return to their activities, provided that they do not have pain and limping during their activities. A history of catching, locking, or knee effusions may be a sign of further biomechanical intraarticular pathology that should be addressed.
- Q: Is bracing indicated?
- A: Some patients with anterior knee pain respond to neoprene sleeves, and those with a component of increased lateral translation may benefit from neoprene sleeves with lateral patellar supports. Bracing, however, is not a substitute for a strength and conditioning program.
- Q: Is chondromalacia patella the same as patellofemoral syndrome?
- A: No. Chondromalacia is a classification of the anatomic pathologic changes of the undersurface of the patella. Patellofemoral syndrome is the clinical condition encompassing the patient's history, physical, and radiographic elements of anterior knee pain.

K

LACRIMAL DUCT OBSTRUCTION

Scott M. Goldstein
Femida Kherani (5th edition)

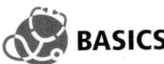 **BASICS**

DESCRIPTION
Congenital or acquired blockage of the distal portion of the tear drainage system extending from the lacrimal sac to the opening of the nasolacrimal duct in the inferior meatus in the nose. This results in chronic tearing.

EPIDEMIOLOGY
Incidence
~6% of newborns, most of which resolves spontaneously

PATHOPHYSIOLOGY
• Congenital obstruction occurs from incomplete canalization of the nasolacrimal duct during embryogenesis.
• Acquired obstructions result from scar tissue occluding the duct. This usually results secondarily from infection, inflammation, or trauma.

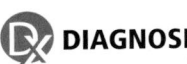 **DIAGNOSIS**

HISTORY
• Determine when the symptoms began.
• Clarify which eye is more symptomatic and whether frank epiphora is present.
• Congenital obstruction usually manifests itself within the 1st few months of life.
• Patients with acquired obstruction usually have a history of eye infection, dacryocystitis, or trauma to the drain system.
• Both present with symptoms including tearing, crusting of eyelashes particularly on awakening, and discharge from eye.

PHYSICAL EXAM
• Common symptoms:
  – Increased tear meniscus
  – Maceration of eyelid skin
  – Mucopurulent discharge
  – Crusted debris on the eyelashes
  – Occasionally conjunctival hyperemia
• Palpation of lacrimal sac with expression of mucoid discharge: Distal obstruction in the lacrimal system allowing accumulation of mucopurulent material in the sac, which can be expressed through the puncta with pressure on the lacrimal sac

DIAGNOSTIC TESTS & INTERPRETATION
Imaging
• Lacrimal scintigraphy can be performed on occasion to evaluate drainage from the eye into the nose, but is rarely done in children.
• CT scan be obtained if there is concern of a nasolacrimal cyst or dacryocele.

Diagnostic Procedures/Other
• Dye disappearance test:
  – Fluorescein is applied to the conjunctival cul-de-sac, and the patient is observed for 5 minutes.
  – In a negative test (normal), the tear meniscus will become relatively unstained as the tears naturally flow down through the drainage system. Dye can sometimes be found in the nose.
  – In a positive test (abnormal), the height of the stained tear meniscus will either increase or fail to decrease owing to the obstructed lacrimal system.
• In teenagers and adults, in-office irrigation of lacrimal system at the level of the canaliculus can be used diagnostically to evaluate for obstruction.

DIFFERENTIAL DIAGNOSIS
• Causes of increased tear production:
  – Congenital glaucoma
  – Reflex tearing secondary to dry eye
  – 7th nerve palsies
  – Trichiasis
  – Entropion
  – Corneal abrasion
• Causes of decreased drainage:
  – Imperforate puncta or canaliculi
  – Ectropion
  – Lateral canthus dystopia
  – Traumatic injury to the nasolacrimal drainage system

 TREATMENT

ADDITIONAL TREATMENT
General Measures
• Initially, in congenital obstruction lacrimal sac, massage and either ophthalmic antibiotic drops or ointment is applied when ocular discharge increases. Polysporin or erythromycin ophthalmic is typically recommended for coverage of the eyelid normal flora. This conservative approach is applied for the 1st year of life.
• If symptoms persist after 12 months of age, probing and irrigation of the nasolacrimal system are is performed. An inferior turbinate infracture is performed in cases of distal obstruction to increase the space in the inferior meatus and facilitate outflow.

- If the initial probing and irrigation procedure fails, which it does in about 10% of cases, the procedure is repeated with placement of silastic intubation and/or stretching of the lacrimal duct via balloon dacryoplasty. Silastic intubation can be monocanalicular or bicanalicular and is typically maintained for 3–6 months.
- If all else fails, a dacryocystorhinostomy, a permanent surgical connection between the lacrimal sac and the nose, is created to prevent recurrent infections (dacryocystitis).
- Patients with acquired obstructions typically require surgery. Probing and irrigation are performed to determine the location of the obstruction. These patients may also require silastic intubation, balloon dacryoplasty, and/or dacryocystorhinostomy surgery.

IN-PATIENT CONSIDERATIONS
Admission Criteria
Infants with an acute dacryocystitis associated with a lacrimal obstruction should be admitted for IV antibiotic therapy and surgery to drain the collection.

 # ONGOING CARE

FOLLOW-UP RECOMMENDATIONS
Patient Monitoring
- Children with congenital obstruction should be re-evaluated at 9–12 months of age and referred for probing and irrigation if still symptomatic.
- Children with acquired obstruction should be referred to an ophthalmologist for surgical treatment.
- Referral for probing and irrigation is delayed until the patient is ~12 months of age; the probing and irrigation should be performed in a timely fashion to ensure a good outcome.

PROGNOSIS
- Spontaneous resolution in ~90% of children by 12 months of age with congenital obstruction. If no spontaneous resolution, surgical intervention involving a probing and irrigation is recommended.
- Acquired obstruction requires surgical intervention.

COMPLICATIONS
- Acute dacryocystitis (acute infection and inflammation of the lacrimal sac), which rapidly appears as an erythematous nodule and surrounding cellulitis in the inferior medial canthal area and medial lower eyelid
- Chronic low-grade dacryocystitis manifested by subtle mucopurulent discharge from the eye that may be intermittently symptomatic

ADDITIONAL READING
- Casady DR, Meyer DR, Simon JW, et al. Stepwise treatment paradigm for congenital nasolacrimal duct obstruction. *Ophthal Plast Reconstr Surg*. 2006;22:243–247.
- Granet DB, Olitsky S, Burke MJ. Nasolacrimal duct obstruction. *J Pediatr Ophthalmol Strabismus*. 2000;37:103–106.
- Mandeville JT, Woog JJ. Obstruction of the lacrimal drainage system. *Curr Opin Ophthalmol*. 2002;13:303–309.
- Pediatric Eye Disease Investigator Group, Repka MX, Chandler DL, Beck RW, et al. Primary treatment of nasolacrimal duct obstruction with probing in children younger than 4 years. *Ophthalmology*. 2008;115(3):577–584.
- Robb RM. Congenital nasolacrimal duct obstruction. *Ophthalmol Clin North Am*. 2001;14:443–446, viii.

 # CODES

ICD9
- 375.55 Obstruction of nasolacrimal duct, neonatal
- 375.56 Stenosis of nasolacrimal duct, acquired
- 743.65 Specified congenital anomalies of lacrimal passages

ICD10
- H04.539 Neonatal obstruction of unspecified nasolacrimal duct
- H04.559 Acquired stenosis of unspecified nasolacrimal duct
- Q10.4 Absence and agenesis of lacrimal apparatus

FAQ
- Q: Is my child in any danger while the nasolacrimal duct remains obstructed?
- A: Not usually. The obstruction presents more of a nuisance. However, occasionally the contents of the sac can become infected and will require oral or parenteral antibiotics.
- Q: Why not wait longer to do the probing and irrigation in congenital nasolacrimal duct obstruction?
- A: The failure rate of the initial procedure increases with age: If performed before 13 months of age, 96% success rate; between 13 and 18 months of age, 77% success rate; and between 18 and 24 months, 54% success rate.

L

LACTOSE INTOLERANCE

Kathleen M. Loomes
Vera de Matos (5th edition)

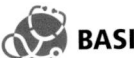 **BASICS**

DESCRIPTION
- Lactose is a disaccharide built from glucose and galactose and is the major carbohydrate in infants' food (breast milk or milk-based formula).
- Lactose is important as a source of energy; it promotes the absorption of calcium, phosphorus, and iron and has a probiotic effect on the gut flora.
- Lactose intolerance is defined as the inability to digest the disaccharide lactose secondary to deficiency of the enzyme lactase, resulting in clinical symptoms.
- Four types of lactase deficiency:
  - Congenital lactase deficiency:
    - Extremely rare
    - Presents during the newborn period, often with the 1st feeding of lactose-containing formula
    - Will cause severe diarrhea and failure to thrive and risk the newborn's life
  - Primary lactase deficiency or adult-type hypolactasia is due to relative or absolute absence of lactase:
    - Develops during childhood at different ages in different racial groups
    - Most common cause of lactose intolerance
  - Secondary lactase deficiency results from small bowel injury (acute gastroenteritis, persistent diarrhea, small bowel bacterial overgrowth, chemotherapy). Can present at any age, but is more common in infancy
  - Developmental lactase deficiency is the relative lactase deficiency observed in premature infants of <34 weeks' gestation.

EPIDEMIOLOGY
Prevalence
- ~70% of the world's population has primary lactase deficiency.
- The prevalence of primary lactase deficiency in Northern Europeans, who have a diet rich in dairy, is 2%.
- In Hispanic people, the prevalence of primary lactase deficiency is 50–80%.

- In Ashkenazi Jewish people as well as in African Americans the prevalence is 60–80%.
- In the Asian population, the prevalence of primary lactase deficiency is almost 100%.
- Nearly 20% of children <5 years from Hispanic, Asian, or African American descent have lactase deficiency and lactose malabsorption.
- Caucasian children usually do not develop symptoms until after 5 years of age.

RISK FACTORS
Genetics
- Posttranslational regulatory mechanisms in primary lactase deficiency or adult-type hypolactasia
- Correlation between the genetic polymorphism of mRNA and persistence of lactase activity with early loss at 1–2 years in Thai children and late loss at 10–20 years in Finnish children

PATHOPHYSIOLOGY
- The symptoms depend on the amount of lactose ingested.
- Malabsorbed lactose creates an osmotic load that draws fluid and electrolytes into the bowel lumen, leading to diarrhea.
- Nonabsorbed lactose is the substrate for intestinal bacteria. In the colon, bacteria metabolize lactose, producing volatile fatty acids and gases leading to flatulence, bowel distension, pain, and low pH.

 DIAGNOSIS

HISTORY
- Classic symptoms include bloating, gaseousness, colicky abdominal pain, and diarrhea after digestion of lactose-containing meal.
- Diet history provides important information.
- Detailed history of symptoms: Blood or mucus in the stools, failure to thrive, fat malabsorption, or any extraintestinal symptoms strongly suggest different causes.
- Symptoms vary in severity with dose of lactose ingested.
- Association with milk ingestion may not be evident.

PHYSICAL EXAM
- Height and weight should be measured and plotted against age-appropriate norms; any deviation should not be attributed to lactose intolerance alone.
- Abdomen percussion: Abdomen may be distended and tympanitic.
- Blood in the stool must be further evaluated, because lactose intolerance does not cause bleeding.

DIAGNOSTIC TESTS & INTERPRETATION
Lab
- Stool-reducing substances and fecal acidity:
  - A positive result indicates malabsorption of carbohydrates.
  - A pH <6.0 or reducing substances >0.5% are interpreted as a positive result.
- Lactose hydrogen breath test:
  - Noninvasive and highly sensitive
  - The only source of hydrogen is fermented unabsorbed carbohydrates. A rise of breath H_2 concentration of ≥ 20 ppm over baseline appears to correlate with enzyme deficiency.
  - However, the frequently poor association between symptoms of lactose intolerance and breath H_2 excretion suggests caution in the interpretation of the clinical significance of the breath hydrogen test.
  - False-positive test results occur owing to inadequate fasting before the test, rapid intestinal transit, toothpaste, smoking, and bacterial overgrowth.
  - False-negative results occur owing to diarrhea, hyperventilation, recent antibiotic exposure, and delayed gastric emptying. Up to 10% of the population is colonized with bacteria unable to produce hydrogen and will give a negative result.
- Lactase activity measurement in duodenal (invasive and expensive): Reserved for patients undergoing upper endoscopy to exclude celiac disease

Pathological Findings
- Disaccharidase activity can be measured in biopsy specimens of the small bowel and compared with normal values.
- The small bowel intestinal histology will often be normal in primary lactase deficiency (unless the reason is insult/damage to the small bowel mucosa).

DIFFERENTIAL DIAGNOSIS
Lactose intolerance may be secondary to a generalized small bowel mucosal dysfunction; the presence of other symptoms should prompt an evaluation. The differential diagnosis includes:
- Infection:
  - Viral and bacterial infections can cause secondary lactose intolerance due to villous injury. Most common pathogen is rotavirus.
  - Parasitic infections can mimic lactose intolerance (giardiasis).
- Inflammatory: Small intestinal Crohn disease can have associated lactose intolerance.
- Congenital:
  - Other carbohydrate enzyme deficiencies can mimic lactose intolerance. These include sucrase–isomaltase or glucose–galactose malabsorption.
  - Cystic fibrosis
  - Shwachman-Diamond syndrome (SDS): Primary features include:
    o Bone marrow insufficiency
    o Pancreatic insufficiency
    o Skeletal abnormalities
    o Short stature
- Allergic/Immune:
  - Celiac disease often is associated with lactose intolerance due to small intestinal damage.
  - Protein allergy can cause secondary lactose intolerance.

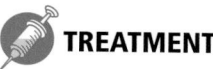 ## TREATMENT

MEDICATION (DRUGS)
- Oral lactase replacement capsules
- Calcium supplements to meet daily recommended intake levels if dairy-free diets are used

ADDITIONAL TREATMENT
General Measures
- Removal of lactose from the diet is effective in eliminating symptoms. However, a milk-free diet may result in calcium deficiency.
- Predigestion of lactose can be done by the addition of commercially available enzyme supplementation. Multiple products are available over the counter. Liquid preparations, capsules, and chewable tablets can be obtained.
- Acquired deficiencies, particularly those associated with infection, may resolve over time or with specific treatment. Most patients with lactose intolerance will not recover the ability to digest lactose.
- Supplemental probiotics may improve symptoms of lactose intolerance.

 ## ONGOING CARE
DIET
- Lactose-free formula, lactase-containing milk
- Substitutes for cow's milk based on rice or soy
- Yogurt and aged cheeses have a smaller content of lactose.

PROGNOSIS
- Prognosis of lactase deficiency and clinical intolerance is excellent as elimination and enzyme replacements are possible. With lactose avoidance or with enzyme supplementation, the child can control and eliminate symptoms.
- However, lactose intolerance may be secondary to disease processes that should be treated promptly.

ADDITIONAL READING
- de Vrese M, Stegelmann A, Richter B, et al. Probiotics—compensation for lactase insufficiency. *Am J Clin Nutr*. 2001;73(2 Suppl):421S–429S.
- Heyman MB. Lactose intolerance in infants, children, and adolescents. *Pediatrics*. 2006;118:1279–1286.
- Kokkonen J, Tikkanen S, Savilahti E. Residual intestinal disease after milk allergy in infancy. *J Pediatr Gastroenterol Nutr*. 2001;32:156–161.
- Krawczyk M, Wolska M, Schwartz S, et al. Concordance of genetic and breath tests for lactose intolerance in a tertiary referral centre. *J Gastrointestin Liver Dis*. 2008;17(2):135–139.
- Law D, Conklin J, Pimentel M. Lactose intolerance and the role of the lactose breath test. *Am J Gastroenterol*. 2010;105(8):1726–1728.
- Usai Satta P, Congia M, Schirru E, et al. Genetic testing is ready to change the diagnostic scenario of lactose malabsorption. *Gut*. 2008;57(1):137–138.

 ## CODES

ICD9
271.3 Intestinal disaccharidase deficiencies and disaccharide malabsorption

ICD10
- E73.0 Congenital lactase deficiency
- E73.1 Secondary lactase deficiency
- E73.9 Lactose intolerance, unspecified

FAQ
- Q: When is the usual time for presentation of lactose intolerance?
- A: In whites, the age of presentation is after 5 years of age. In blacks, 2–3-year-old children may present with clinical signs and symptoms. The differential diagnosis must distinguish primary from secondary causes.
- Q: Does lactose intolerance prevent the child from ever eating lactose?
- A: No. The patient can take smaller amounts of lactose in the diet or have the enzyme supplemented.
- Q: Does this problem ever get better?
- A: No. It is a lifelong problem, but seems to become less symptomatic for adults, in light of their individual desire to tolerate symptoms. Secondary lactose intolerance may improve with time or treatment of the primary disorder.

LEAD POISONING

Carla Campbell

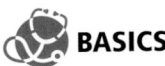 BASICS

DESCRIPTION
- One of the most common pediatric environmental health problems, involving a systemic intoxication by the heavy metal lead; most commonly this is with inorganic lead.
- The Centers for Disease Control and Prevention (CDC) considers a blood lead level (BLL) of $\geq$10 mcg/dL to represent undue lead exposure and absorption, and to be elevated:
  - The CDC has recently reported on adverse health effects at lower BLLs, with no clear threshold.
  - *Lead poisoning* is an older term that is less specific than an actual BLL.
- CDC classification, by BLL in mcg/dL:
  - Class I (0–9); Class IIa (10–14)
  - Class IIb (15–19); Class III (20–44)
  - Class IV (45–69); Class V ($\geq$70)

EPIDEMIOLOGY
- ~83% of American pre-1978 privately owned units contain some lead-based paint.
- A recent national survey estimates that 38 million housing units have lead-based paint and 24 million housing units have hazards from lead-based paint.

Prevalence
- Prevalence of elevated BLLs and geometric mean BLLs have decreased significantly in the past 20 years.
- ~310,000 American children aged 1–5 years (1.6% of a representative national sample) are estimated to have BLLs of $\geq$10 mcg/dL.

RISK FACTORS
- Young children with more oral behaviors are at greatest risk for lead poisoning.
- Children with developmental delays/mental retardation are at greater risk for elevated BLLs.
- Individuals with pica are at higher risk for lead ingestion and poisoning.

GENERAL PREVENTION
- Primary prevention: Removal of potential environmental lead hazards prior to exposure:
  - The CDC recommends that states and cities include primary prevention activities to reach the Healthy People 2020 goals of eliminating elevated BLLs in children.
  - Provide anticipatory guidance to all parents about lead exposure pathways and the prevention of these exposures.
  - Follow CDC guidelines for screening pregnant and lactating women.
- Secondary prevention as screening for elevated BLLs:
  - Minimum screening recommendations: Blood lead test for children at 1 and 2 years and for those 36–72 months old who have not had previous screening.
- Tertiary prevention: Case management and environmental remediation for children with lead poisoning

- Control measures:
  - Abatement of building-based (residential) lead hazards by removal, encapsulation, or enclosure of lead-containing structures
  - Control of environmental lead dust exposure and ingestion by good housekeeping (wet dusting and mopping of household dust) and personal hygiene (cleaning of child's hands, toys, personal items)
  - Removal of any other known lead source from the child's environment

PATHOPHYSIOLOGY
- Lead adversely affects many organ systems including neurologic, hematologic, GI, renal, and reproductive. Many toxic effects result from inhibition of enzymes involved in heme biosynthesis, as the electropositive metal binds to negatively charged sulfhydryl groups on active sites of δ-aminolevulinic acid dehydratase (ALA-D), ferrochelatase, porphobilinogen synthase, co-proporphyrinogen oxidase, and other enzymes.
- Divalent lead also acts competitively with calcium in various biologic systems.
- Children absorb lead more efficiently from the GI tract and are more likely than adults to ingest lead through hand-to-mouth activities.
- Because the developing, immature CNS is susceptible to toxic effects of lead, the neuropsychologic effects of lead poisoning on fetuses/young children are of particular concern.

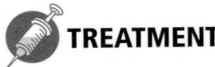 DIAGNOSIS

HISTORY
- Etiology/common sources of lead:
  - Ingestion of lead-based paint or contaminated dust or soil through residence in or visitation of older (pre-1980), deteriorated housing
  - A parental occupation or hobby involving lead exposure (e.g., construction or battery plant work, stained glass window or pottery making)
  - Use of remedies, cosmetics, pottery, toys or consumer products containing lead
  - Ingestion of contaminated water, food, or beverages
- Typical symptoms:
  - Most children asymptomatic
  - Although many of the clinical manifestations of symptomatic lead poisoning are nonspecific, a cluster of complaints including anorexia, intermittent abdominal pain, constipation, sporadic vomiting, change in mental status (such as irritability or lethargy), decreased play activity, and change in developmental status (particularly with regression of developmental milestones) may herald this condition.
- Lead encephalopathy:
  - Can present with change in consciousness, ataxia, persistent vomiting, seizures, coma
  - Often presents after a prodrome of symptoms mentioned above.

PHYSICAL EXAM
- Not generally helpful at lower lead levels. Symptomatic and/or encephalopathic patients may have acute GI, neurologic, hematologic, and systemic manifestations.
- Assess for developmental delay.

DIAGNOSTIC TESTS & INTERPRETATION
Lab
- Blood lead test, either venous or capillary:
  - Results may be reportable to local health authorities.
  - The test result is a measure only of recent lead exposure and does not indicate total body burden of lead.
  - Capillary testing is associated with more false-positive results. If abnormal, a venous lead should be sent.
- CBC: To assess for anemia:
  - Iron deficiency anemia is often seen concomitantly.
  - Anemia related to lead toxicity is typically normocytic and normochromic; a microcytic, hypochromic anemia may be seen with a mixed etiology.
  - Basophilic stippling is sometimes seen on peripheral blood smear.
- Free erythrocyte protoporphyrin:
  - Marker of lead-induced inhibition of heme synthesis
  - Can be useful clinically to follow the recovery from heme synthesis inhibition during management

Imaging
- Abdominal radiograph: Look for radiopaque foreign material suggestive of ingestion of lead paint chips or other lead-containing foreign body, when ingestion of such is suspected in the history.
- Long-bone radiographs, not recommended for routine use:
  - Look for lead lines or metaphyseal sclerosis, characterized by increased density along transverse lines in the metaphyses of growing long bones, representing increased mineralization owing to interference with the metabolism of the boney matrix. If present, lead lines imply chronic lead exposure.

DIFFERENTIAL DIAGNOSIS
- Consider lead poisoning as the etiology for the following diagnoses:
  - Seizures, altered mental status, and/or coma
  - Anemia

ALERT
Failure to diagnose results from:
- Delay in checking a blood lead test in the presence of clinical signs, symptoms of lead poisoning, or neuropsychologic disorders
- Failure to inquire about lead exposure possibilities

TREATMENT

MEDICATION (DRUGS)
- Chelation therapy:
  - Should complement environmental management in all children with venous levels of $\geq$45 mcg/dL (CDC class IV), using parenteral calcium disodium ethylenediamine tetra-acetate (EDTA; also calcium disodium versenate) or oral agents such as meso 2,3-dimercaptosuccinic acid (DMSA, succimer, Chemet)
  - Chelation of children with levels <45 mcg/dL is not recommended, as evidence suggests it does not reverse or diminish neuropsychological effects of lead.

– Outpatient therapy can take place if a lead-safe environment has been identified and compliance is expected.

– Succimer is given at 10 mg/kg (or 350 mg/m^2) q8h for 5 days, then q12h for 14 more days. Weekly monitoring for neutropenia, platelet abnormality, and increased liver enzymes is recommended. Succimer is more lead-specific than other chelators and causes less mineral depletion.

– Children with symptomatic lead poisoning or with levels of ≥70 mcg/dL (CDC class V) should be admitted immediately to a hospital for parenteral chelation with both intramuscular dimercaprol (British antilewisite, BAL) and IV or IM calcium disodium EDTA. Because there are many issues involved with administration of both chelating agents, consultation of appropriate guidelines and pharmacologic information is recommended.

• Children with encephalopathy constitute a medical emergency and should receive the preceding treatment in an intensive care setting with attentive neurosurgical support. Consultation with a clinician experienced in lead toxicity treatment is advised for these patients.

• Ingested lead-containing foreign bodies should be evacuated with whole-bowel irrigation using a high-molecular-weight glycol solution.

ADDITIONAL TREATMENT
General Measures
• Environmental management:
 – Includes removing children from the lead source(s)
 – Should occur when venous lead levels are recurrently 10 mcg/dL (CDC class IIA) and higher. Could be done for lower BLLs as resources allow.
• Reduction of lead:
 – Wet mopping and dusting with all-purpose household detergents is recommended to reduce lead dust exposure.

ISSUES FOR REFERRAL
• Close communication with the local health department is essential before, during, and after admission.
• Referral may be made to early intervention or development assessment programs, social workers, therapists, neurologists or other specialists, as needed.

IN-PATIENT CONSIDERATIONS
Admission Criteria
Admit all symptomatic children, those with BLLs ≥70, and those with BLLs ≥45 for which one cannot ensure a lead-safe environment and/or compliance with oral medication.

Discharge Criteria
Consider discharge when symptoms have resolved, BLL has significantly declined, and a lead-safe discharge environment has been identified.

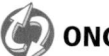 ONGOING CARE

FOLLOW-UP RECOMMENDATIONS
Patient Monitoring
• Prompt environmental follow-up of current lead exposure situations and investigation for additional exposure (e.g., with family moves, visitation of new residences) should occur.
• Follow-up venous lead levels should be performed for those with levels from 10–19 mcg/dL (CDC class IIA, IIB) about every 1–3 months, with less frequent follow-up after levels decline.
• Follow-up venous levels should be performed for those with levels of ≥20 mcg/dL at 1–2-month intervals until no additional lead exposure is present and levels have decreased.
• Follow-up venous levels should be performed 1–3 weeks following chelation therapy, with frequent monitoring thereafter.

DIET
• Nutritional support with calcium and iron supplementation should be given if intake is inadequate; deficiencies of these increase lead absorption from the GI tract.
• Iron supplementation should be withheld during chelation therapy.

PROGNOSIS
• In general, there is an increased risk for long-term neuropsychological sequelae, which increases with lead exposure and absorption that is more intense, of longer duration, and begins at an early age when the CNS is still developing.
• Recurrent episodes of symptomatic lead poisoning increase the risk for permanent sequelae.
• More subtle effects may not be detected until school entry.

COMPLICATIONS
• Acute encephalopathy
• Seizures
• Coma
• Death (predominantly owing to cerebral edema)
• Mental retardation
• Cognitive, behavioral, attentional, and neurodevelopmental impairment
• Anemia
• Fanconi syndrome
• Abdominal colic
• Adverse reproductive outcomes

ADDITIONAL READING

• American Academy of Pediatrics Committee on Environmental Health. Lead exposure in children: Prevention, detection and management. *Pediatrics.* 2005;116:1036–1046.
• Bellinger DC. Very low lead exposures and children's neurodevelopment. *Curr Opin Pediatr.* 2008;20(2):172–173.
• Binns, HJ, Campbell C, Brown MJ. Interpreting and managing blood lead levels of less than <10 μg/dL in children and reducing childhood exposure to lead: Recommendations of the Centers for Disease Control and Prevention Advisory Committee on Childhood Lead Poisoning Prevention. *Pediatrics.* 2007;120:e1285–e1298.
• Centers for Disease Control and Prevention. *Guidelines for the identification and management of lead exposure in pregnant and lactating women.* Atlanta: CDC, 2010.
• Centers for Disease Control and Prevention. *Preventing lead poisoning in young children.* Atlanta: CDC, 2005.
• Lanphear BP, Matte TD, Rogers J, et al. The contribution of lead-contaminated house dust and residential soil to children's blood lead levels. *Environ Res.* 1998;79:51–68.

CODES

ICD9
984.9 Toxic effect of unspecified lead compound

ICD10
• T56.0X4A Toxic effect of lead and its compounds, undetermined, initial encounter
• T56.0X4D Toxic effect of lead and its compounds, undetermined, subsequent encounter
• T56.0X4S Toxic effect of lead and its compounds, undetermined, sequela

FAQ

• Q: What is lead abatement?
• A: Lead abatement is removal of a lead hazard from the environment either by replacing it (e.g., installing a new window), enclosing the area with the lead source (e.g., installing paneling), removing the lead-based paint from a surface (burning or dry sanding methods should never be used), or encapsulating the area (placement of a specific coating over the lead-containing surface, which prevents access to the lead hazard).
• Q: Is lead abatement permanent?
• A: Often lead paint that is chipping or peeling is removed from a home. Any areas with intact lead-based paint may become deteriorated with aging, leading to new lead hazards, although ongoing maintenance and repair may prevent this.
• Q: Why didn't my child's brother and sister get lead poisoning at the same age since they lived in the same house?
• A: Children are different; some do much more hand-to-mouth activity than others, which is the main way that children get lead into their bodies. Also, your home may not have had the same lead dangers (hazards) when the siblings were younger.

L

LEARNING DISABILITIES

Monica Dowling
Jeffrey P. Brosco
Chloe Brittan (5th edition)

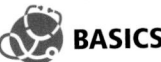 **BASICS**

DEFINITION

Learning problems may be caused by many factors besides specific learning disabilities (e.g., failure to attend school or significant behavioral problems).

- Learning disorders, or learning disabilities (LD), are defined in the *Diagnostic and Statistical Manual of Mental Disorders*, 4th edition (DSM-IV) as academic achievement that is substantially below the level expected for age, schooling, and general intellectual ability, that cannot be accounted for by psychosocial factors, economic disadvantage, or major sensory problems.
- Learning disabilities have neurobiologic and genetic roots. Symptoms are lifelong but can improve with early intervention. LD may affect reading, writing, spelling, or math. Any given child may have >1 learning disability.
- Learning disabilities are not comorbid with intellectual disability, but often coexist with coordination, speech-language, and auditory processing disorders as well as disorders involving executive functions (ADHD).
- Reading disorder (dyslexia) is the most frequently diagnosed type of learning disability, and is typically characterized by impairments in phonologic processing. Phonologic deficits have also been implicated in writing disorder along with motor problems, but further research is needed to identify core deficits. Children with math disorder show procedural and fact fluency deficits.

EPIDEMIOLOGY

- Estimated incidence is 5–10% in school-aged children: 2.7 million public school students in the US have identified LD (2007).
- Learning disabilities are typically not evident until academic demands are placed on affected children.

GENERAL PREVENTION

- High-quality preschool experiences that are developmentally appropriate
- Early literacy initiatives (e.g., Reach Out and Read)
- Early intervention for speech, language, motor difficulties
- Ongoing academic progress monitoring beginning in kindergarten
- Early intervention programs for reading and math skills in children who show early signs of learning problems

DIAGNOSIS

DIFFERENTIAL DIAGNOSIS

- **Academic problems:** May stem from a learning disability or other factors, including sensory impairments, intellectual disability, attention disorders, neurologic disorders, poor school attendance, or psychosocial problems
- **ADHD:** May present as a learning problem, especially when the inattentive and distractible symptoms of the diagnosis are greater than the hyperactive symptoms.
  - May be difficult to distinguish from a learning disability, and the 2 occur together in approximately half of diagnosed cases of learning disabilities
  - Careful psychoeducational assessment may be needed to clarify these diagnoses.
- **Sensory impairments**
  - Hearing or vision impairments may cause learning problems.
  - School screening results should be confirmed in children with learning problems.
- **Neurologic**
  - Absence seizures and other nonconvulsive epileptic disorders are much less common than ADHD but may mimic its symptoms.
  - Neurodegenerative disorders such as Niemann–Pick disease, adrenoleukodystrophy, ceroid lipofuscinosis, and subacute sclerosing panencephalitis may rarely present as school-age learning problems.
  - Intellectual disability (mental retardation): Borderline and mild ID are sometimes not recognized until school entrance.
- **Genetics**
  - Some genetic syndromes may show subtle dysmorphology that is not noted until learning problems arise. Examples include:
    ○ Sex chromosome aneuploidies
    ○ Fragile X syndrome in both boys and girls
    ○ Neurofibromatosis
    ○ Tuberous sclerosis
    ○ Velocardiofacial/DiGeorge syndrome
- **Nutritional, toxicologic, infections**
  - Lead intoxication, chronic malnutrition, iron deficiency, hypothyroidism, and HIV infection may have insidious effects on cognitive function.
- **Iatrogenic interventions**
  - Some medications (e.g., antiepileptic drugs) affect cognition.
- **Psychosocial**
  - Issues related to family stress, peer relationships, illness, or adolescence may present as academic difficulty.
  - Conversely, behavior problems at home or at school always should prompt evaluation of school functioning.

- **Psychiatric comorbidity occurs commonly**
  - Adjustment disorders, mood disorders, oppositional defiant disorder, conduct disorder, tic disorders, substance abuse, and other behavior problems may precede or follow the presentation of learning problems.
  - Less commonly, psychotic disorders, personality disorders, and obsessive-compulsive disorder may underlie learning problems.

APPROACH TO THE PATIENT

- Learning problems in general arise from a complex interplay of genetic and environmental factors.
- Many learning problems respond to appropriate educational interventions, regardless of specific etiology, and failure to respond to intervention is part of the diagnostic process for specific learning disabilities.
- It is the role of the educator to (a) monitor the academic progress of all students; (b) provide early educational intervention and frequent progress monitoring to struggling students; and (c) conduct a psychoeducational assessment of students who do not respond to initial intervention.
- Once a child presents with learning problems, it is the role of the physician to:
  - **Phase 1:** Help the family obtain timely educational interventions
  - **Phase 2:** Educate the family and communicate with the educators regarding the above process
  - **Phase 3:** Identify and treat underlying medical problems:
    ○ Sensory impairments, lead or other intoxication, absence seizures, medication side effects
    ○ Consider genetic syndromes that may cause learning problems, especially subtle ones such as Fragile X syndrome in girls
  - **Phase 4:** Identify and help treat underlying psychosocial issues:
    ○ Psychosocial stresses may exacerbate learning difficulties or be a primary etiologic factor.
    ○ School attendance is a particularly important factor in learning.
  - **Phase 5:** Identify and treat comorbid conditions
    ○ ADHD, depression, and anxiety may lead to learning problems or comorbid conditions with specific learning disabilities.

HISTORY

- **Question:** When and how does the child fail in his/her daily academic pursuits?
- *Significance*:
  - Learning disabilities typically impact only school activities and are often limited to one skill area such as reading or math.
  - Children with attention disorders typically show problems in multiple settings (school, home, extracurricular, peers).
  - Children with borderline intellectual disability (mental retardation) usually have a long history of developmental concerns.
- **Question:** Is decline in school performance recent and/or abrupt?
- *Significance*: Consider new pathophysiologic processes such as new vision or hearing impairment, side effect from new medication, or neurodegenerative disorders (rare)

- **Question:** Past medical history, medications, review of systems, psychosocial stresses?
- *Significance*:
  – School attendance
  – Early development and behavior
  – Family history of learning problems
  – Sleep patterns

PHYSICAL EXAM
- **Finding:** Subtle dysmorphology?
- *Significance*: May suggest the presence of a genetic syndrome or a pattern of malformation resulting from teratogenic fetal exposures (e.g., alcohol, phenytoin)
- **Finding:** Skin lesions?
- *Significance*: May suggest underlying genetic syndromes such as tuberous sclerosis
- **Finding:** Abnormal neurologic examination?
- *Significance*:
  – Any focal signs demand additional evaluation.
  – Soft signs such as slow rapid alternating finger movements (neuromaturational signs) are often present in children with learning problems, but are generally not helpful in diagnosis or treatment.

DIAGNOSTIC TESTS & INTERPRETATION
- Physician
  – Audiology and vision screening
  – Standardized behavior questionnaires (e.g., Teachers and Parent Vanderbilt: for evaluation of ADHD)
  – Consider other screening tools for depression, anxiety, family dysfunction, parental depression, and substance abuse
  – Genetic, neurologic evaluation if indicated by history or physical exam
- Educator
  – Teachers typically use a variety of screening measures (e.g., DIEBELS) or computer-administered tests to frequently monitor progress. Standardized achievement tests can be administered yearly and are used to measure current functioning and review progress.
- Psychologist
  – Testing must be performed individually and should include general intelligence and academic achievement testing as a minimum.
  – Federal law requires schools to provide comprehensive evaluations on written request by the parents to the school. Specific information for each state can be obtained from the National Dissemination Center for Children with Disabilities (800-695-0285; www.nichcy.org).
  – Many centers outside the school system (e.g., hospital-based centers) also conduct evaluations of children with learning disabilities.
  – For children who do not respond to educational interventions, or if the psychoeducational evaluation is inconclusive, more extensive neuropsychological testing may elucidate specific cognitive strengths and weaknesses that may help in developing an effective educational plan.

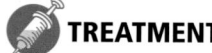

TREATMENT

ADDITIONAL TREATMENT
General Measures
- Physician
  – Responsible for treatment of underlying medical diagnoses
  – Ensure appropriate treatment of psychosocial problems with pharmacological therapy and behavioral therapy (family therapy, social skills training, cognitive-behavioral therapy) as needed
- Educator
  – Educational treatment varies with the age and educational level of the child and should follow an approach of increasing intensity as needed (academic improvement plan to 504 plan to IEP).
    ○ Tier 1: For patients displaying poor academic achievement, begin with extra support (e.g., homework clinic, tutoring) in the regular educational program (assuming culturally and linguistically appropriate instruction).
    ○ Tier 2: If academic problems disrupt classroom participation and impede progress as measured by universal screening, refer to school-based child study team and provide intensive assistance as part of general curriculum, such as summer school or specialized materials.
    ○ Tier 3: If child is >1 year behind or has shown minimal response to Tier 2 interventions, refer for a comprehensive psychoeducational evaluation to identify specialized interventions, typically provided under the umbrella of special education
  – Specialized instruction is at the center of treatment, often within the context of a regular classroom (inclusion) with supplemental instruction through either a consultant special teacher or resource room.
  – Children may also benefit from classroom accommodations such as preferential seating, extra time for test taking, electronic word processors and computer applications, recorded books, calculators, note-takers, and modified instructions (oral or written).
  – Treatment is most effective when it uses a team approach, including parents, teachers, and other therapists.
  – Grade retention, which provides only a repeat of the same educational approaches that have already failed the child, will not be helpful.

ONGOING CARE

Children with learning disabilities require continued monitoring of academic progress. Even when the initial learning problems are resolved, later difficulties may arise in writing, note-taking, composition, or organization, and with more abstract academic subjects.

PROGNOSIS
- In most cases, prognosis is quite good with treatment, although learning disabilities never go away.
- Prognosis varies with intensity, timing, and appropriateness of intervention.

- Early diagnosis and treatment is essential for minimizing impact and to take advantage of typical developmental progression.
- Current brain imaging research shows remedial reading instruction alters brain functioning if provided during critical window of development (before age 8–10 years).

ADDITIONAL READING
- AAP. Learning disabilities, dyslexia and vision. *Pediatrics*. 2009;124:837–844.
- Gabrieli JD. Dyslexia: A new synergy between education and cognitive neuroscience. *Science*. 2009;325:280–283.
- Glascher J, Tranel D, Paul L, et al. Lesion mapping of cognitive abilities. *Neuron*. 2009;61:681–691.
- Meyler A, Keller T, Cherkassky V, et al. Modifying the brain activation of poor readers during sentence comprehension with extended remedial instruction. *Neuropsychologia*. 2008;46:2580–2592.
- National Center for Learning Disabilities. The state of learning disabilities 2009. Available at: www.ncld.org
- Shaywitz SE, Gruen JR, Shaywitz BA. Management of dyslexia: Its rationale, and underlying neurobiology. *Pediatr Clin North Am*. 2007;54:609–623.

 CODES

ICD9
- 315.00 Developmental reading disorder, unspecified
- 315.02 Developmental dyslexia
- 315.2 Other specific developmental learning difficulties

ICD10
- F81.0 Specific reading disorder
- F81.2 Mathematics disorder
- F81.9 Developmental disorder of scholastic skills, unspecified

FAQ
- Q: What is the evidence that dietary restriction will help control hyperactivity?
- A: Despite the many anecdotal reports of value, random controlled studies have not shown that dietary restriction has value when the patients are followed for long term. There is a new study to take another look at food dyes.

CLINICAL PEARLS
- Discourage a "wait and see" approach to decision-making: Early intervention improves outcomes.
- Begin educational interventions as soon as possible (e.g., evidence-based reading intervention); children who do not respond require more thorough etiological workup.
- Academic or attention difficulties may lead to spiraling psychological problems, from depression or damaged self-esteem to conduct disorder and school dropout.

L

LEUKOCYTOSIS
Susan R. Rheingold

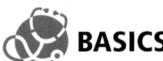 **BASICS**

DEFINITION
An increase in WBC count above normal for age

RISK FACTORS
- Allergic disorders
- Hematologic disorders
- Immunodeficiencies
- Inflammatory disorders
- Malignancy
- Rheumatologic diagnoses
- No specific genetic abnormality is associated with leukocytosis.

PATHOPHYSIOLOGY
Most frequent cause is an increase in the total neutrophil count, but leukocytosis may result from other type of conditions where WBC count is elevated, such as lymphocytosis, monocytosis, eosinophilia, and basophilia.

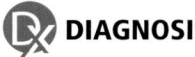 **DIAGNOSIS**

DIFFERENTIAL DIAGNOSIS
- **Infectious**
  - Bacterial:
    - *Streptococcus* (especially *S. pneumoniae*)
    - *Staphylococcus aureus*
    - *Haemophilus*
    - *Neisseria*
    - *Brucella*
    - *Bartonella* (cat-scratch disease)
    - *Clostridium difficile*
    - Pertussis
  - Viral:
    - Infectious mononucleosis
    - Cytomegalovirus
    - Rubella
    - Mumps
    - Hepatitis
  - Fungal:
    - *Aspergillus*
  - Parasitic:
    - *Toxocara*
    - *Toxoplasma*
    - *Trichinella*
    - Tapeworms
    - *Strongyloides*
    - Coccidioidomycosis
  - Tuberculosis
  - Syphilis
  - Acute infectious lymphocytosis
    - Benign viral mediated lymphocytosis (often >25,000/mm³)
  - Kawasaki disease

- **Congenital/Genetic**
  - Down syndrome
  - Sickle cell disease
  - Fanconi anemia
  - Thrombocytopenia with absent radii
  - Leukocyte adhesion deficiency
- **Drugs**
  - Corticosteroids
  - Epinephrine and beta-agonists
  - Lithium
  - Granulocyte colony-stimulating factor
  - Granulocyte–macrophage colony-stimulating factor
- **Trauma**
  - Acute hemorrhage
  - Severe burns
  - Splenectomy
- **Tumor**
  - Leukemia or lymphoma
  - Myeloproliferative disorders
- **Metabolic**
  - Hyperthyroidism
  - Acidosis
- **Inflammatory**
  - Juvenile idiopathic arthritis
  - Rheumatoid arthritis
  - Vasculitis
  - Inflammatory bowel disease
  - Chronic granulomatous disease
  - Pulmonary eosinophilic syndromes: Transient infiltrates with a peripheral eosinophilia
- **Allergic**
  - Asthma
  - Seasonal or drug allergies
  - Eczema
  - Psoriasis
- **Hematologic**
  - Severe hemolysis
- **Stress**
  - Anxiety
  - Overexertion/exercise
  - Seizures
  - Anesthesia
- **Artifactual**
  - Nucleated RBCs

ALERT
Beware of any differential that has a high percentage of monocytes or atypical lymphocytes, whether machine generated or manual. Leukemic blasts can be mistaken for these cell types.

APPROACH TO THE PATIENT
- **Phase 1:** Which WBC line is elevated?
  - Elevated neutrophil count is more likely with bacterial infections; lymphocytosis is usually associated with viral infections.
  - Eosinophilia: Possible allergic disorder
- **Phase 2:** Degree of elevation can be indicative of the diagnosis:
  - Most elevations of WBC count are in the 15,000–20,000/mm³ range.
  - WBC count in the 30,000/mm³ range is more consistent with pertussis, pneumococcal infection, or acute infectious lymphocytosis.
  - Higher counts are worrisome for acute or chronic leukemia or leukemoid reactions.
- **Phase 3:** Other signs/symptoms present?
  - Is there an obvious infectious source?
  - Fever, rash, and mild anemia are nonspecific and associated with infection, rheumatologic process, or malignancy.
  - Pallor or petechiae should make one think of hematologic or oncologic process.
- **Phase 4:** Is the WBC count dangerously elevated?
  - WBC count of 100,000/mm³ can increase viscosity, causing neurologic or respiratory distress.
  - WBC counts this high almost always indicate malignant bone marrow processes (leukemia, myeloproliferative disorder) and should be referred immediately to a hospital with a pediatric oncologist.
  - Children with elevated WBC counts with anemia and/or thrombocytopenia should be referred to a pediatric hematologist or oncologist to evaluate for malignancy.

ALERT
Many laboratories provide only machine-generated differentials. If there are any abnormalities, a manual differential must be obtained. It may be necessary to review the smear with a hematologist or pathologist.

HISTORY
- **Question:** Evidence for infection—fever, rash, or swelling?
- *Significance*:
  - Acute infection is the most common cause for leukocytosis.
  - Thorough history should be taken for apparent or occult infections.
  - Fever can also be a symptom of inflammatory diseases.
- **Question:** Other complaints?
- *Significance*: Chronic cough may point to tuberculosis; a whooping cough may indicate pertussis. Intermittent joint pain, rash, and/or fevers may point to a rheumatologic diagnosis.

- **Question:** Other medical problems?
- *Significance:*
  – Sickle cell disease: Elevated WBC count probably secondary to chronic inflammation or marrow expansion
  – Down syndrome: Transient myeloproliferative disease (especially in the first few months of life) that resolves spontaneously
- **Question:** Medications?
- *Significance:*
  – Corticosteroids will increase the neutrophil precursors.
  – Epinephrine can cause a transitory increase in neutrophil count.
- **Question:** Familial history of inflammatory diseases?
- *Significance:* Rheumatoid arthritis, thyroiditis, Crohn disease
- **Question:** Weight loss, chronic fatigue, night sweats, or pallor?
- *Significance:* Malignancy must be ruled out.

PHYSICAL EXAM
- **Finding:** Foci of infection?
- *Significance:*
  – Look for cellulitis, otitis, pharyngitis, or abscesses on examination
  – A careful lung examination is necessary since pneumonia can cause a WBC count as high as 30,000–40,000/mm³.
  – A murmur or gallop may be a sign of bacterial endocarditis.
  – Urinary tract infections (UTIs) present with dysuria and cloudy urine, vasculitis with bloody urine or stool.
- **Finding:** Lymphadenopathy or hepatosplenomegaly?
- *Significance:* Points toward a possible viral etiology but is also of concern for malignancy
- **Finding:** Tender or swollen joints or nonspecific bone pain?
- *Significance:* May indicate juvenile idiopathic arthritis, septic arthritis, or systemic lupus erythematosus
- **Finding:** Stigmata of Down syndrome?
- *Significance:* Transient Myeloproliferative Disease of infant

DIAGNOSTIC TESTS & INTERPRETATION
- **Test:** WBC count including manual differential
- *Significance:*
  – If neutrophilia is present, think of bacterial infections.
  – Pneumonia, UTIs, and soft-tissue infections are the most likely to cause leukocytosis.
  – May see Döhle bodies, toxic granulations, or vacuolization in WBCs in bacteremia
  – Recovering or stressed marrow may have an increase in monocytes or eosinophils.
  – Look for leukemic blasts
- **Test:** Hemoglobin/platelet count
- *Significance:* If either is low, consider a marrow-infiltrative process or a marrow that is hyperstimulated and overproducing WBCs as part of a response to a low hemoglobin or platelet count.
- **Test:** Chemistry panel
- *Significance:*
  – Liver function tests: Possible viral etiology
  – Uric acid and lactate dehydrogenase are elevated in leukemia and lymphoma.

- **Test:** Cultures
- *Significance:* Blood, urine, stool, throat, and others
- **Test:** Screen for infectious mononucleosis
- *Significance:* Mono spot, heterophil antibodies
- **Test:** EBV titers
- *Significance:* Mono spot can be falsely negative in younger children.
- **Test:** Leukocyte alkaline phosphatase
- *Significance:*
  – Elevated in infection but not in leukemia
  – Helps to differentiate chronic myelogenous leukemia from a leukemoid reaction
- **Test:** Antinuclear antibody/rheumatoid factor/anti-neutrophil cytoplasmic antibodies
- *Significance:* Nonspecific screen for rheumatologic etiology
- **Test:** Bone marrow biopsy and aspirate
- *Significance:*
  – Necessary if any other blood cell line is abnormally low or if the WBCs appear dysmorphic
  – Need to rule out malignancy, myelodysplasia, or other marrow processes. Should be performed at a pediatric oncology center.

Imaging
Chest radiograph for pneumonia, tuberculosis

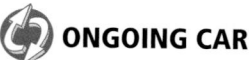 TREATMENT

ADDITIONAL TREATMENT
General Measures
- Antibiotics immediately if a child appears septic, otherwise tailor antibiotics to the underlying infectious etiology
- If an underlying rheumatologic, hematologic, or genetic cause is suspected, refer to the appropriate specialist.
- If leukemia is suspected, start hydration with fluids containing bicarbonate and no potassium, and administer oral allopurinol or urate oxidase.
- If the leukocytosis is >100,000/mm³ and the patient has symptoms of end-organ failure, emergent leukapheresis should be considered.

ISSUES FOR REFERRAL
- WBC counts >50,000/mm³
- Associated thrombocytopenia or anemia
- Any indication of malignancy
- Any indication of a rheumatologic etiology
- Inability to find an etiology with a persistent leukocytosis

 ONGOING CARE

Following appropriate treatment the WBC should return to normal. If it remains elevated or other symptoms persist the differential should be expanded to include noninfectious etiologies.

ADDITIONAL READING
- Abramson N, Melton B. Leukocytosis: Basis of clinical assessment. *Am Fam Physician*. 2000; 62:2053–2060.
- Lowe EJ, Pui CH, Hancock ML, et al. Early complications in children with acute lymphoblastic leukemia presenting with hyperleukocytosis. *Pediatr Blood Cancer*. 2005;45(1):10–15.
- Peterson L, Hrisinko MA. Benign lymphocytosis and reactive neutrophilia. *Clin Lab Med*. 1993;13: 863–877.
- Shah SS, Shofer FS, Seidel JS, et al. Significance of extreme leukocytosis in the evaluation of febrile children. *Pediatr Infect Dis J*. 2005;24(7):627–630.

 CODES

ICD9
- 288.3 Eosinophilia
- 288.8 Other specified disease of white blood cells
- 288.60 Leukocytosis, unspecified

ICD10
- D72.1 Eosinophilia
- D72.828 Other elevated white blood cell count
- D72.829 Elevated white blood cell count, unspecified

FAQ

- Q: What does "left-shifted" mean?
- A: Increased numbers of early granulocyte precursors (metamyelocytes, myelocytes, bands) are seen in the peripheral smear with a bandemia and neutrophilia. They are often seen with bacterial infections or marrow recovery from a suppressing drug/virus.
- Q: Infectious mononucleosis and acute lymphoblastic leukemia have many similar signs and symptoms. How can I differentiate them?
- A: Both can present with fever, malaise, headache, prominent lymphadenopathy, organomegaly, and suppressed hemoglobin and platelet counts. Infectious mononucleosis is associated with a sore throat, and acute lymphocytic leukemia with bone pain. The best test to differentiate between the two is the peripheral smear morphology. A heterophil AB or mono spot, if positive, helps with the diagnosis of infectious mononucleosis.
- Q: Is the degree of elevation of WBC significant?
- A: For most bacterial infections the WBC has not been found to be a sensitive or specific indicator of the seriousness of the infection. Leukocytosis has been found to be a predictor for the development of hemolytic uremic syndrome in patients with *Escherichia coli* O157:H7 infection. Higher presenting WBC count in leukemia has been associated with higher risk and worse outcomes.

L

LICE (PEDICULOSIS)

Alyssa Siegel
J. Nadine Gracia (5th edition)

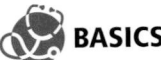 **BASICS**

DESCRIPTION
Infestation of the head, body, or anogenital region

EPIDEMIOLOGY
- Head lice:
  - Common in children 3–12 years of age, especially in daycare settings and school-age children
  - Affects all socioeconomic groups
  - Less common in African American children
  - Not indicative of poor hygiene
  - Not influenced by hair length, or frequency of brushing/shampooing
- Body lice:
  - Found on persons with poor hygiene
  - More common in extreme conditions such as crowding, homelessness
- Pubic lice:
  - Most common in adolescents and young adults

Incidence
Estimated 6–12 million cases per year in US.

GENERAL PREVENTION
- Examine household members and treat those who are infested.
- Prophylactically treat bed mates.
- Environmental cleaning is controversial and may not be necessary. Only items in contact with the infested person within 24–48 hours need to be considered:
  - Wash bedding, clothes, and cloth toys in hot water (>128°F).
  - Treat combs and hairbrushes by washing in hot water and soaking in pediculicide.
  - Seal anything not washable in plastic bags for 14 days.
  - Environmental insecticide is not helpful in the control of head lice.
  - Treatment of pets is not necessary.
- School attendance: "No-nit" school policies do not control head lice transmission and are not recommended. Children who have been treated with appropriate pediculicide should be allowed to return to school.

PATHOPHYSIOLOGY
- Head lice:
  - Female, adult louse survives for 3–4 weeks on scalp, laying up to 10 eggs per day
  - Eggs attach to base of hair, close to the scalp, camouflaged with pigment to match hair color
  - Eggs incubate by body heat, hatch within 7–12 days, leaving white empty shell (nit) on hair
  - Nymph emerges, passing through 3 stages in 9–12 days, reaching the adult stage capable of mating and laying viable eggs
  - Nymphs and adult lice feed on scalp blood, inject saliva, causing sensitization and associated pruritus

- Body lice:
  - 10–20% larger than head lice
  - Prefer to live on clothing, visiting human only to feed
  - Lay eggs along seams of clothing, which hatch when warmed by wear
  - Incubation period 6–10 days
  - Transmitted through contact with infested clothing or bedding
- Pubic lice:
  - Crab-like appearance with predilection for pubic hair
  - May also infest axillary hair, perineal area, eyelashes, eyebrows, and rarely scalp
  - Transmitted almost exclusively by sexual contact
  - Uncommonly spread by fomites (e.g., towels, bedding)
  - May infest eyebrows/lashes (pediculosis palpebrarum) in young children (associated with maternal infestation, but must consider possible sexual abuse)

ETIOLOGY
- 3 species of ectoparasites (6-legged, wingless, 1–4 mm insects that live on humans, feeding on human blood):
  - *Pediculus humanus capitis*: Head louse
  - *P. humanus corporis*: Body louse
  - *Phthirus pubis*: Pubic or crab louse
- Transmission:
  - Direct contact with hair or skin of an infested individual
  - Indirect spread of head lice via personal belongings (i.e., combs, brushes, hats) occurs rarely in head lice, more often in body lice; head lice only survive for 1–2 days away from the scalp, body lice 5–7 days.

COMMONLY ASSOCIATED CONDITIONS
- Head lice: Do not transmit disease. Rarely secondary scalp impetigo, cervical and occipital lymphadenopathy may develop.
- Body lice: Can act as vector for transmission of *Rickettsia prowazekii*, *Bartonella quintana*, and *Borrelia recurrentis* (causing endemic typhus, trench fever, relapsing fever); secondary bacterial skin infections due to pruritus.
- Pubic lice: Up to 50% of patients have another STD, particularly gonorrhea or syphilis.

 DIAGNOSIS

HISTORY
- Pruritus is the most common symptom, although some patients are asymptomatic.
- Intense nighttime pruritus is common with body lice.
- Special questions:
  - Ask about possible infested contacts (home, school, or sexual).
  - Ask about special living circumstances such as crowding or institutionalization.

PHYSICAL EXAM
- Direct visualization of live lice provides definitive diagnosis of active infestation:
  - Head lice may be difficult to identify as lice crawl quickly in response to a perceived threat, including light. Body lice sequester in clothing.
  - Wet combing with conditioner, oil, or water has been suggested to slow the movement of lice prior to inspection.
- Nits, empty egg cases attached to base of hair shaft, may indicate historic infestation, but suggest active infestation if within 1 cm of scalp.
  - Often clustered in parietal and occipital regions, in the perianal region (for pubic lice), or in the seams of clothing (for body lice)
  - Difficult to dislodge (unlike dandruff, hair casts, or debris)
- Bites from body lice result in pinpoint, erythematous macules, papules, wheals, or excoriation
- Other findings:
  - Secondary skin lesions (e.g., impetigo, excoriation); dermatitis of the neck, shoulder area
  - Cervical or occipital lymphadenopathy with head lice
  - Secondary infestation in eyebrows and/or eyelashes
  - Post-inflammatory hyperpigmentation with body lice
  - Maculae cerulea (sign of heavy pubic infestation): Bluish/slate macules, 0.5–1-mm diameter, usually on lower abdomen, thighs, buttocks

DIAGNOSTIC TESTS & INTERPRETATION
Diagnostic Procedures/Other
Tests are rarely necessary. Can examine louse or nit using hand lens or under microscope.

DIFFERENTIAL DIAGNOSIS
- Seborrheic dermatitis
- Contact dermatitis
- Eczema
- Impetigo
- Scabies

TREATMENT

MEDICATION (DRUGS)
Head and pubic lice:
- Permethrin (Nix) 1% cream rinse:
  - Neurotoxic to lice, ovicidal, residue on hair kills newly hatching nymphs as they emerge
  - Generally used as first-line therapy
  - High cure rate; resistance reported, but prevalence unknown
  - 10-minute application to damp hair, followed by optional 2nd application 7–10 days later
  - OTC preparation, low toxicity
- Pyrethrins (Rid, A-200):
  - Neurotoxic to lice, low ovicidal activity
  - Efficacy substantially reduced due to resistance, although highly variable among communities; not effective if resistant to permethrin.
  - 10-minute application to dry hair, 2nd application 7–10 days later to kill newly hatched
  - OTC preparation
  - Contraindicated in persons allergic to chrysanthemums or ragweed

- Malathion (Ovide) 0.5%:
  - True ovicidal activity; highly effective, although countries with long-term use now showing resistance
  - Requires 8–12-hour application to dry hair; 2nd application 7–10 days later only if live lice are present
  - Safety concerns: Theoretical risk of respiratory distress if ingested; flammability (due to alcohol base). Patients should be warned not to use external heat sources including hair dryers during treatment.
  - Not for use in children <24 months due to increased absorption through the scalp (safety not established for children <6 years)
- Benzyl alcohol 5%:
  - Kills lice by asphyxiation; no ovicidal activity
  - For use in children >6 months
  - Apply for 10 minutes, repeat in 7–9 days
  - Common adverse reactions include pruritus, erythema, pyoderma, ocular irritation
- Lindane (Kwell) 1% lotion:
  - No longer recommended due to human neurotoxicity, reports of severe seizure and death in children, high resistance/lack of efficacy
- Controversial treatments:
  - Sulfamethoxazole–trimethoprim (Bactrim): Not FDA approved as a pediculicide. Used with topical permethrin, may improve cure rate for treatment failures; 10-day course advised
  - Ivermectin: Not FDA approved as a pediculicide. For cases resistant to topical treatment, can be given as a single oral dose of 200 mcg/kg followed by 2nd dose 7–10 days later. Blocks neural transmission if it crosses blood–brain barrier (younger children at higher risk). Not for use in children <15 kg.
  - Essential oils such as lavender, peppermint, eucalyptus, coconut, anise, ylang-ylang, and tea tree oil may have some activity against lice and eggs, but preparations are unregulated, and some have potential for contact allergy and prepubertal gynecomastia.
  - A mechanical device delivering hot air to the scalp has shown successful desiccation of lice, but is expensive and requires training for use.
- Other considerations:
  - Topical corticosteroids and oral antihistamines for pruritus and inflammation
  - Antibiotics for impetiginized lesions

ALERT

Pediculosis palpebrarum: Pediculicides are oculotoxic and must be avoided.

ADDITIONAL TREATMENT

General Measures

- Head lice:
  - Wash hair with nonconditioning shampoo and towel dry.
  - Apply pediculicide (See "Medication")
  - If nit removal desired, comb through with a fine-tooth nit comb.
  - No clinical benefit of vinegar-based products for nit removal has been demonstrated and may interfere with pediculicide use.
  - No data to determine whether suffocation of lice by application of petroleum jelly, olive oil, or mayonnaise is effective.
- Body lice:
  - Pediculicide usually not necessary (insects live in clothing)
  - Improve hygiene.
  - Wash clothing and bedding in hot water at least weekly.
  - Dry cleaning is effective, as is hot ironing (particularly along seams of clothing).
- Pubic lice:
  - Apply pediculicide and retreat 7–10 days later with pediculicide.
  - Treat sexual contact to prevent reinfestation.
  - Removal of nits from pubic hair with fine-tooth comb is helpful.
- *P. palpebrarum*:
  - Petrolatum ointment applied to lashes 2–4 per day for 8–10 days
  - Remove nits by hand from the eyelashes.

ONGOING CARE

FOLLOW-UP RECOMMENDATIONS

- Itching or mild burning of scalp is common up to 2 weeks after use of topical agents.
- Risk of transmission is promptly reduced after a single application of pediculicide. Child may return to school or day care immediately after treatment.
- Recurrence of symptoms represents improper use of the treating agent, reinfestation, resistance, failure to recognize and treat other sites of infestation, such as perianal hair, axillary hair, or sexual contacts (in *P. pubis*.)

ADDITIONAL READING

- Burgess I. Current treatments for pediculosis capitis. *Curr Opin Infect Dis*. 2009;22:131–136.
- Diamantis S, Morrell D. Treatment of head lice. *Dermatol Ther*. 2009;22:273–278.
- Fournier PE, Ndihokubwayo JB, Guidran J, et al. Human pathogens in body and head lice. *Emerg Infect Dis*. 2002;8(12):1515–1518.
- Goates BM, Atkin JS, Wilding KG, et al. An effective nonchemical treatment for head lice: A lot of hot air. *Pediatrics*. 2006;118:1962–1970.
- Meinking TL, Serrano L, Hard B, et al. Comparative in vitro pediculicidal efficacy of treatments in a resistant head lice population in the United States. *Arch Dermatol*. 2002;138:220–4.
- Roberts R. Head lice. *N Engl J Med*. 2002;345:1645–1650.
- Wolf R, Davidovici B. Treatment of scabies and pediculosis: Facts and controversies. *Clin Dermatol*. 2010;28:511–518.

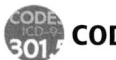 CODES

ICD9
- 132.2 Phthirus pubis [pubic louse]
- 132.3 Mixed pediculosis infestation
- 132.9 Pediculosis, unspecified

ICD10
- B85.2 Pediculosis, unspecified
- B85.3 Phthiriasis
- B85.4 Mixed pediculosis and phthiriasis

FAQ

- Q: Did my child get head lice because my house or my child is not clean enough?
- A: No. Head lice are unrelated to personal hygiene.
- Q: Should I cut my child's long hair to get the lice out?
- A: No. Meticulous application of the pediculicide to the entire scalp and pulling through all hair shafts is adequate treatment. Head lice infestation is not influenced by hair length.
- Q: Can infants become infested with pubic lice (*P. pubis*)?
- A: Yes. Although the primary mode of transmission of the crab louse is via sexual contact, it can be transmitted through close personal contact with an infested individual. Small children become infested on the eyebrows or lashes with crab lice.
- Q: If children are infested with the head lice, how can items such as stuffed animals or other cloth toys be decontaminated?
- A: Machine washable items can be washed in hot water at temperatures >128°F. An alternative method of decontamination is sealing the items in a plastic bag for 10–14 days.
- Q: Is removal of nits necessary to prevent spread?
- A: No. They can be removed for cosmetic reasons by using a fine-tooth comb.
- Q: What is appropriate treatment of infestation of the eyelashes?
- A: A petroleum ointment should be applied 2–4 times daily for 8–10 days. Nits should be removed mechanically from the lashes.

L

LOWER GI BLEEDING

Kristin N. Fiorino
Maria R. Mascarenhas

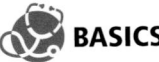 **BASICS**

DEFINITION
Lower GI bleeding refers to bleeding from the lower GI tract, distal to the ligament of Treitz

ETIOLOGY
Reasons for lower GI bleeding at different ages:
- Neonatal period (birth to 1 month):
  - Anorectal fissure
  - Necrotizing enterocolitis
  - Enteric infections
  - Allergic colitis
  - Upper GI source
  - Duplication cyst
  - Hirschsprung disease enterocolitis
  - Meckel diverticulum
  - Malrotation with volvulus
  - Hemorrhagic disease of the newborn
- Infancy (1 month to 2 years):
  - Anorectal fissure
  - Enteric infections
  - Allergic colitis
  - Intussusception
  - Meckel diverticulum
  - Malrotation with volvulus
  - Lymphonodular hyperplasia
  - Upper GI source
  - Duplication cyst
  - Enterocolitis with Hirschsprung disease
  - Vascular malformation
- Preschool age (2–5 years):
  - Anorectal fissure
  - Enteric infections
  - Polyps
  - Parasites
  - Meckel diverticulum
  - Intussusception
  - Lymphonodular hyperplasia
  - Inflammatory bowel disease
  - Hirschsprung disease enterocolitis
  - Hemolytic uremic syndrome
  - Henoch-Schönlein purpura
  - Vascular malformation
  - Volvulus
  - Rectal prolapse/rectal ulcer
  - Child abuse
  - Perianal streptococcal cellulitis
- School age (5–13 years):
  - Anorectal fissure
  - Enteric infections
  - Inflammatory bowel disease
  - Intussusception
  - Meckel diverticulum
  - Polyps
  - Henoch-Schönlein purpura
  - Hemolytic uremic syndrome
  - Intestinal ischemia
  - Neutropenic colitis (typhlitis)
  - Parasites
  - Child abuse
  - Vascular malformations
  - Perianal streptococcal cellulitis

- Adolescent (>13 years):
  - Anorectal fissure
  - Enteric infections
  - Inflammatory bowel disease
  - Hemolytic uremic syndrome
  - Intussusception
  - Midgut volvulus
  - Intestinal ischemia
  - Neutropenic colitis (typhlitis)
  - Polyps
  - Vascular malformations
  - Lymphonodular hyperplasia
  - Parasites
  - Hemorrhoids

 DIAGNOSIS

- General goals: Determine location of the bleeding and cause, and begin stabilization and treatment.
  - Phase 1: Determine if there is blood or other cause of bright red or black stools.
  - Phase 2: Assess patient to determine etiology; follow history, physical, and laboratory.
  - Phase 3: Stabilize patient, decide if emergency treatment or referral is needed. (See "Emergency Care" under "Treatment.")
- Hints for screening problem:
  - The more rapid the rate, the larger the volume of lower GI bleeding, and greater the drop in hemoglobin and change in pulse and BP.
  - Any significant blood loss will lead to pallor, tachycardia, orthostasis, poor capillary refill, CNS changes (restlessness, confusion), and hypotension.
  - Hypotension may not be seen even in the face of significant blood loss, because vasoconstriction will occur to maintain BP until decompensation.
  - Initial hemoglobin values may be unreliable, because a delay in hemodilution may falsely result in near-normal values.
  - In newborn, determine if this is swallowed maternal blood by the Apt–Downey test.

HISTORY
- Obtain a detailed history and note if any recently ingested foods resemble blood.
- Color of blood:
  - If bright red, then site of bleeding is probably in left colon, rectosigmoid, or anal canal
  - If darker red, then from right colon
  - If melena or tarry, then bleeding is proximal to ileocecal valve
- Location of blood in relation to the stool:
  - In colitis, the blood will be mixed with stool
  - With a fissure/constipation, it will be in streaks on the outer aspect of the stool
- Consistency of the stool:
  - If diarrhea, more likely to be colitis
  - If hard, then more likely to be a fissure/constipation
- Painful stools suggest anal fissure, local proctitis, or ischemic bowel.

- Painless rectal bleeding is associated with polyps, Meckel diverticulum, nodular lymphoid hyperplasia of colon, intestinal duplication, intestinal submucosal mass (GIST), or vascular anomaly.
- Abdominal pain can be seen with colitis, inflammatory bowel disease, or surgical abdomen.
- Any underlying known GI disease, previous GI surgery: Past history of colitis, Hirschsprung disease, necrotizing enterocolitis
- Any history of jaundice, hepatitis, liver disease, neonatal history: Suggestive of portal vein thrombosis (sepsis, shock, exchange transfusion, omphalitis, IV catheters), portal hypertension, and variceal bleeding
- Any familial history of bleeding diathesis: von Willebrand disease, hemophilia
- Medications: Heparin, warfarin
- Associated symptoms:
  - Mouth ulcers
  - Weight loss
  - Joint pains as in inflammatory bowel disease
  - Petechiae
  - Renal insufficiency
  - History of ingestion of uncooked meat as in hemolytic uremic syndrome
  - Purpuric rash as in Henoch-Schönlein purpura
  - Severe abdominal pain and vomiting as in a surgical abdomen

PHYSICAL EXAM
- Skin:
  - Petechiae or purpura
  - Ecchymosis
  - Hemangiomas
  - Evidence of chronic liver disease (spider angiomata, palmar erythema)
  - Jaundice
- HEENT:
  - Freckles on buccal mucosa: Peutz-Jeghers syndrome
  - Mouth ulcers: Crohn disease
  - Icteric sclera: Portal hypertension
- Abdomen:
  - Hepatosplenomegaly, ascites: Portal hypertension
  - Isolated splenomegaly: Cavernous transformation of the portal vein
- Rectal examination:
  - Evidence of any perianal disease: Inflammatory bowel disease
  - Polyps: Bright red blood in stool
  - Hemorrhoids: Portal hypertension

DIAGNOSTIC TESTS & INTERPRETATION
Lab
- CBC: Iron-deficiency anemia:
  - Leukopenia, anemia, and thrombocytopenia: Consider chronic liver disease and portal hypertension
  - Anemia with normal RBC indices: Truly an acute cause for bleeding
  - RBC indices indicate iron-deficiency anemia: Consider varices or a mucosal lesion, i.e., chronic blood loss
  - Thrombocytopenia: Consider hemolytic uremic syndrome

- Coagulation profile:
  - If PT and PTT are abnormal, consider liver disease or disseminated intravascular coagulation with sepsis.
- Liver function tests: Abnormal in chronic liver disease
- Renal function tests (BUN, creatinine, urine analysis): Abnormal in hemolytic uremic syndrome, Henoch-Schönlein purpura, acute bleed
- ESR or C-reactive protein (CRP): Abnormal in inflammatory disorders or infectious colitis
- Stool tests:
  - Stool culture (Salmonella, Shigella, Campylobacter, Yersinia, Aeromonas, Escherichia coli), Klebsiella
  - Stool for Clostridium difficile toxin A and B
  - 3 stool samples for ova and parasites (Amebae)
  - Stool smears for WBCs (not always positive in colitis) and eosinophils (not always positive in allergic colitis)
  - Stool CMV: Consider in immunocompromised

Imaging
- Abdominal x-ray helpful in surgical abdomen (dilated bowel, air–fluid levels, perforation), constipation (presence of excessive stool), colitis (edematous bowel, thumb-printing, pneumatosis intestinalis, and toxic megacolon
- Ultrasound can show bowel wall thickening and Meckel diverticulum and is diagnostic of intussusception.

Diagnostic Procedures/Other
- Lower and upper endoscopy:
  - Full colonoscopy to the terminal ileum helpful in diagnosing inflammatory bowel disease
  - Upper endoscopy diagnostic in massive upper GI bleeds presenting with hematochezia or melena
  - Push enteroscopy involves the passage of a special endoscope further in the small bowel, identifying rare lesions in the proximal 60–120 cm of the jejunum.
  - Double balloon enteroscopy: assists in further evaluating the entire GI tract
- Barium tests:
  - Air-contrast enema is diagnostic and therapeutic in intussusception and diagnostic in mucosal lesions (polyps).
  - Upper GI series with small-bowel follow-through is helpful in evaluating anatomy and Crohn disease and its complications (fistula, sometimes ulcer may be identified).
  - Enteroclysis or small bowel enema provides good mucosal detail.
- Meckel scan:
  - Diagnostic for Meckel diverticulum that secretes acid (can use H2-receptor antagonist to enhance uptake)
  - There may be false negatives if the Meckel diverticulum has different tissue expression.
- Bleeding scan:
  - Useful when endoscopy is not diagnostic
  - Technetium sulfur colloids versus tagged RBC scan: The former detects rapid bleeding but can miss small bleeds, especially if the patient is not bleeding during the scan. The latter can detect small bleeds, especially if intermittent.
- Angiography:
  - Useful in detecting vascular causes for GI bleeding >0.5 mL/min
  - Can also be therapeutic

- Video capsule endoscopy:
  - Useful in detecting distal small bowel hemorrhage
  - Approved for ages >2 years

DIFFERENTIAL DIAGNOSIS
- The majority of patients with lower GI bleeding have a fissure or infection.
- Mucosal lesions are more likely to be associated with antecedent occult bleeding.
- In most, the bleeding stops spontaneously.
- Pitfalls:
  - Make sure red substance in stool is really blood.
  - Initial hemoglobin, if normal, may be misleading.

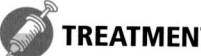
TREATMENT

ADDITIONAL TREATMENT
General Measures
- Anal fissure: Treat the underlying constipation (mineral oil, lactulose, MiraLax, high-fiber diet, increased water intake). Local therapy consists of sitz baths, local emollient creams, and steroid suppositories.
- Polyp: Colonoscopy and polypectomy
- Intussusception: Ultrasound is diagnostic. Air-contrast enema permits confirmation and hydrostatic reduction.
- Parasites: Antiparasitic drugs

ISSUES FOR REFERRAL
Refer the following patients to a specialist:
- Any patient with significant acute lower GI bleeding after initial stabilization
- Patients with less acute bleeding for whom an easily identifiable cause has not been found or patients with chronic or recurrent lower GI bleeding

SURGERY/OTHER PROCEDURES
In cases of massive or persistent bleeding with no identifiable site, exploratory laparotomy with intraoperative endoscopic evaluation of the entire bowel to identify mucosal lesions may be required.

IN-PATIENT CONSIDERATIONS
Initial Stabilization
Emergency care:
- If patient is critical, stabilize with IV fluids and blood products.
- Order laboratory tests: CBC, PT/PTT, disseminated intravascular coagulation screen, liver function tests, blood type, and cross-match
- Insert a nasogastric tube and lavage with saline to distinguish massive bleeding from an upper GI tract source.
- Monitor patient's vital signs and hemoglobin.
- Make appropriate diagnosis and institute appropriate therapy, i.e., abdominal x-ray, colonoscopy, bleeding scans.

ONGOING CARE

DIET
Introduce hydrolyzed protein formula in infants with cow's milk protein allergy.

ADDITIONAL READING

- Antao B, Bishop J, Shawis R, et al. Clinical application and diagnostic yield of wireless capsule endoscopy in children. *J Laparoendosc Adv Surg Tech A.* 2007;17(3):364–370.
- Boyle JT. Gastrointestinal bleeding in infants and children. *Pediatric Rev.* 2008;29(2):39–52.
- Fox V. Gastrointestinal bleeding in infancy and childhood. *Gastroenterol Clin North Am.* 2000;29:37–66.
- Lin TK, Erdman, SH. Double-balloon enteroscopy: Pediatric experience. *J Pediatr Gastroenterol Nutr.* 2010;51(4):429–432.
- Ross A. Editorial: Push-and-pull enteroscopy: One balloon or two? *Am J Gastroenterol.* 2010;105: 582–584.
- Turk D, Michaud L. Lower gastrointestinal bleeding. In: Walker WA, et al. *Pediatric Gastrointestinal Disease,* 4th ed. Philadelphia: BC Decker; 2004: 266–280.

CODES

ICD9
- 565.0 Anal fissure
- 578.9 Hemorrhage of gastrointestinal tract, unspecified
- 777.50 Necrotizing enterocolitis in newborn, unspecified

ICD10
- K60.2 Anal fissure, unspecified
- K92.2 Gastrointestinal hemorrhage, unspecified
- P77.9 Necrotizing enterocolitis in newborn, unspecified

FAQ

- Q: What is the most common cause of lower GI bleeding?
- A: In all age groups, fissures are the leading cause, followed by infections. However, in infancy, the most common cause is a fissure; in toddlers and young children, polyps; and in older children, inflammatory bowel disease.
- Q: What common foods cause stools to be red? Black?
- A: Red: Raspberries, cranberries, Kool-aid, artificial coloring in cereal. Black: Bismuth, spinach, blueberries, licorice.

L

LUPUS ERYTHEMATOSUS

Elizabeth Candell Chalom

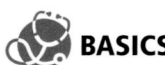 **BASICS**

DESCRIPTION
Multisystem, autoimmune disease characterized by production of antibodies to various components of cell nucleus, in conjunction with variety of clinical manifestations

EPIDEMIOLOGY
- Age: 20% of lupus begins in childhood, but it is very rare under 5 years old
- Female:Male ratio: Between 3–5:1 (prepubertal) and 9–10:1 (postpubertal)
- SLE occurs about 3 times more often in African Americans than Caucasians. It is also more common in Hispanic, Asian, and Native Americans.

Incidence
- Peak incidence: Between ages 15 and 40 years
- Incidence in children is from 10-20/100,000

Prevalence
- U.S. estimate: 5,000–10,000 children

RISK FACTORS
Genetics
- Increased frequency in 1st-degree family members of patients with SLE
- 10% of patients have ≥1 affected relative.
- Concordance rate of 25–50% in monozygotic twins and 5% in dizygotic twins
- Some major histocompatibility antigens are associated with increased incidences of lupus, such as HLA-DR2 and DR3 in whites and DR2 and DR7 in blacks.

ETIOLOGY
Although exact etiology is unknown, lupus is an autoimmune disease, with genetic, environmental, and hormonal factors playing a role.

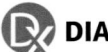 **DIAGNOSIS**

Diagnostic criteria: 4 of following 11 criteria, developed by the American College of Rheumatology, must be met to classify a patient as having SLE:
- Malar (butterfly) rash,
- Discoid rash,
- Photosensitivity,
- Oral or nasal ulcers,
- Arthritis,
- Cytopenia: Anemia, leukopenia ($<4,000/mm^3$), lymphopenia ($<1,500/mm^3$), or thrombocytopenia ($<100,000/mm^3$),
- Neurologic disease: Seizures or psychosis
- Nephritis: >0.5 g/d proteinuria or cellular casts
- Serositis: Pleuritis or pericarditis
- Positive immunoserology (revised 1997): Antibodies to double-stranded DNA or Smith nuclear antigen, false-positive serologic test for syphilis, lupus anticoagulant, or antiphospholipid antibodies
- Positive ANA

HISTORY
- History of photosensitivity or malar rash common but not necessary
- Many patients have systemic complaints, such as fevers, fatigue, and malaise.
- Many patients complain of joint pain, Raynaud's phenomenon, or alopecia.
- Chest pain from pericarditis or pleural effusions may be present.
- Signs and symptoms:
  - Immune complex–mediated vasculitis, which can occur in almost any organ system
  - Cutaneous lesions: Very variable. Include:
    - Erythematous malar or "butterfly" rash
    - Maculopapular rashes (which can occur anywhere on body)
    - Periungual erythema
    - Mucosal membrane vasculitis
  - Arthritis: Can affect large and small joints; usually symmetric and nonerosive
  - Hematologic pathology: Includes:
    - Hemolytic anemia
    - Anemia of chronic disease
    - Leukopenia
    - Lymphopenia
    - Thrombocytopenia

- Neurologic symptoms include:
  - Headaches
  - Psychosis
  - Depression
  - Seizures
  - Organic brain syndromes
  - Peripheral neuropathies
- Renal pathology (present in up to 75% children with SLE):
  - Includes mesangial changes and glomerulonephritis (focal, diffuse, proliferative, or membranous)
  - 1st signs of renal disease in lupus patient are often proteinuria and active urinary sediment.
  - Hypertension, nephrotic syndrome, and renal failure can also occur.
- Serositis: Usually seen as pericarditis or pleuritis, but peritonitis can also occur.
- Constitutional symptoms are very common: Fatigue, weight loss, fever

PHYSICAL EXAM
- Rash: May be malar, discoid, or vasculitic. Periungual erythema may also be seen.
- Oral or nasal ulcers (usually on hard or soft palate) that are painless and often go unnoticed by patients
- Arthritis of large and small joints
- Pericardial friction rub if patient has pericarditis
- Edema may be present secondary to renal disease.
- CNS changes such as personality changes, psychosis, or seizures

DIAGNOSTIC TESTS & INTERPRETATION
Lab
- ANA:
  - Found in >95% patients with SLE, but a positive ANA can occur in many diseases and in up to 20% of normal population
- Anti–double-stranded DNA and anti–Smith nuclear antigen:
  - Very specific to lupus, but not all patients with lupus have these autoantibodies. In many patients, anti-DNA levels vary with activity of disease.
- CBC:
  - Anemia, leukopenia, lymphopenia, and/or thrombocytopenia may be seen.

- Urinalysis:
  - May show proteinuria or active urinary sediment if there is renal dysfunction
- Complement levels:
  - Can fall very low during a lupus flare (C3 and C4)
- PTT:
  - Patients may also have prolonged PTT, as result of antiphospholipid (APL) antibodies, often seen in SLE. Patients with APL antibodies at increased risk for thrombotic events, such as deep venous thromboses, strokes, and fetal losses during pregnancies.

DIFFERENTIAL DIAGNOSIS
- Systemic juvenile-onset rheumatoid arthritis
- Oncologic disease (leukemia, lymphoma)
- Viral or other infectious illness
- Other vasculitic disorders
- Dermatomyositis
- Fibromyalgia
- Drug-induced lupus
- Pitfalls:
  - Avoid overdiagnosis; positive ANA in the absence of clinical signs or symptoms of SLE is not lupus.

 TREATMENT

MEDICATION (DRUGS)
- NSAIDs may be used for musculoskeletal and mild systemic complaints, although ibuprofen has been noted to cause aseptic meningitis in a small number of patients with SLE. NSAIDs can also exacerbate renal disease in lupus.
- Hydroxychloroquine often used to help control cutaneous manifestations and to help minimize the chance of lupus flares.
- Steroids often necessary to control systemic and renal manifestations
- Patients with renal disease often need immunosuppressive agents, such as cyclophosphamide (usually given as monthly IV boluses). Mycophenolate mofetil, cyclosporin, or azathioprine may also be used.
- Patients with mainly arthritic symptoms may be treated with weekly methotrexate, PO or SC
- Patients with antiphospholipid antibodies are often treated with a baby aspirin daily. If they have already had a significant clotting event, they need stronger anticoagulation.
- Angiotensin-converting enzyme (ACE) inhibitors are often used to help prevent renal damage from proteinuria.

- Patients with abnormal lipid profiles that do not respond to diet may need statins.
- Rituximab (anti-CD20 antibody) causes B-cell depletion and is used in SLE, especially for thrombocytopenia.
- Other biologic agents also being tested in lupus. A BLyS (B lymphocyte stimulator) inhibitor has been approved in adults but has not yet been tested in children. Antibodies to CD40 and C5 are also being studied.
- Plasmapheresis and IVIG have been used as well.

ADDITIONAL TREATMENT
General Measures
Avoid excessive sun exposure and use sunscreen liberally.

Additional Therapies
For very severe lupus, bone marrow immunoablation or transplantation are options.

 ONGOING CARE

PROGNOSIS
- Extremely variable. Renal disease and CNS involvement are poor prognostic signs, whereas systemic complaints and joint findings are not.
- 10-year survival in children presenting with SLE is >90%

COMPLICATIONS
- End-stage renal disease
- Infections secondary to treatments used to control disease
- Atherosclerosis and myocardial infarctions at a young age
- Libman-Sacks endocarditis, which increases risk of subacute bacterial endocarditis.
- Neonatal lupus:
  - Neonatal lupus (NLE) is due to maternal autoantibodies (usually SS-A or SS-B antibodies) that cross the placenta and can cause rashes, congenital heart block, cytopenias, and/or hepatitis in the newborn baby.
  - Most symptoms of NLE resolve by 6 months of age, but the heart block, if it occurs, is permanent.
  - Many mothers of babies with NLE are asymptomatic and unaware that they have these autoantibodies.
  - The rash, erythema annulare, can begin a few days after delivery or within the 1st few weeks of life.
  - Topical steroids can minimize the lesions. Congenital heart block is due to damage of the conducting system of the developing fetal heart.
  - Bradycardia may be noted by 22 weeks' gestation, and CHF with nonimmune hydrops fetalis may ensue.

ADDITIONAL READING
- Godfrey T, Khamashta MA, Hughes GR. Therapeutic advances in systemic lupus erythematosus. *Curr Opin Rheumatol.* 1998;10:435–441.
- Gottlieb BS, Ilowite NT. Systemic lupus erythematosus in children and adolescents. *Pediatr Rev.* 2006;27(9):323–330.
- Macdermott EJ, Adams A, Lehman TJ. Systemic lupus erythematosus in children: Current and emerging therapies. *Lupus.* 2007;16(8):677–683.
- Petty RE, Laxer RM. Systemic lupus erythematosus. In: Cassidy JT, Petty RE, Laxer RM, Lindsley CB, eds. *Textbook of pediatric rheumatology.* Philadelphia: Saunders, 2005:342–391.

 CODES

ICD9
- 695.4 Lupus erythematosus
- 710.0 Systemic lupus erythematosus

ICD10
- L93.0 Discoid lupus erythematosus
- M32.9 Systemic lupus erythematosus, unspecified

FAQ
- Q: If a patient has a positive ANA but no clinical signs of SLE, how often should the ANA be followed?
- A: A positive ANA will usually remain positive indefinitely, but it has no real significance in the absence of clinical or other laboratory disturbances. Up to 20% of the normal population may have a positive ANA, so there is no need to repeat the test.
- Q: Can SLE patients with end-stage renal disease obtain renal transplants?
- A: Yes, and SLE usually does not recur in the new kidney.

L

LYME DISEASE

Elizabeth Candell Chalom

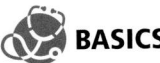 **BASICS**

DESCRIPTION

Multisystemic illness caused by the spirochete *Borrelia burgdorferi*, carried by the deer tick

EPIDEMIOLOGY

- Can affect people of all ages, but 1/3–1/2 of all cases occur in children and adolescents
- Male/Female ratio: 1:1–2:1
- Onset most often in summer months
- Endemic areas in northeast, north central, and Pacific Coast states

Prevalence

Has now become most common tick-borne disease in the U.S., with 29,595 confirmed cases reported in 2009. Although Lyme disease can be found anywhere, the majority of the cases in the U.S. are found in southern New England and the mid-Atlantic States. It is also seen frequently in California, Minnesota, and Wisconsin.

RISK FACTORS

Genetics

Chronic Lyme arthritis seems to be associated with increased incidence of HLA-DR4 and less so with HLA-DR2.

PATHOPHYSIOLOGY

B. burgdorferi is injected into skin with saliva of Ixodes tick. Spirochetes 1st migrate within skin, forming the typical rash, erythema migrans. Spirochetes then spread hematogenously to other organs, including heart, joints, and nervous system.

ETIOLOGY

The tick-borne spirochete *B. burgdorferi*

COMMONLY ASSOCIATED CONDITIONS

The same ticks that transmit Lyme disease can also transmit *Ehrlichia* and *Babesia*, so infections with those spirochetes can occur simultaneously.

DIAGNOSIS

HISTORY

- Tick bite:
  - History of tick bite can only be elicited in 1/3 of patients with Lyme disease, and most people with tick bites do not develop Lyme disease. Even in endemic areas, risk of developing Lyme disease after tick bite is <5%.
- Rash:
  - 50–80% will have or will recall the typical rash, which is not painful or pruritic, but does feel warm.
- Other symptoms:
  - Many patients will complain of fatigue, headaches, fevers, chills, myalgias, conjunctivitis, and arthralgias early on.
- Joint pain:
  - Many patients will complain of painful joints early on, and later will develop joint swelling.
- Signs and symptoms:
  - Skin: Erythema migrans (typical rash); starts as red macule or papule and then expands to annular lesion up to 30 cm in diameter with partial central clearing. The lesion is usually painless and lasts 4–7 days.
  - Musculoskeletal:
    ○ Early on, patient may experience fevers, myalgias, migratory joint pain (often without frank arthritis), and painful tendons and bursae.
    ○ Weeks to months later, 60% of untreated patients will develop monoarticular or pauciarticular arthritis of large joints, especially knees.
    ○ Joint fluid can have WBC count anywhere from 500–110,000 cells/mm^3, and cells are mostly neutrophils.
  - Neurologic:
    ○ Several weeks after initial rash, 14% of untreated patients will develop neurologic symptoms including aseptic meningitis, cranial nerve palsies (especially facial nerve palsies), mononeuritis, plexitis, or myelitis.
    ○ Months to years later, chronic neurologic symptoms may occur, including a subtle encephalopathy: Memory, mood, and sleep disturbances.
    ○ Significant fatigue can occur early or late in the course of Lyme disease.
  - Cardiac:
    ○ Several weeks after initial rash, ~5% of untreated patients develop cardiac disease.
    ○ Most common cardiac lesion is atrioventricular block (primary, secondary, or complete)
  - Pericarditis, myocarditis, or pancarditis can also develop.

PHYSICAL EXAM

- May be completely normal early in course of disease
- Rash of erythema migrans, if seen, is virtually pathognomonic for Lyme disease. If patient does not have the rash, no physical finding exists that gives definitive diagnosis of Lyme.
- Patient may have arthritis, Bell palsy, a cranial nerve palsy, conjunctivitis, or an irregular heartbeat.

DIAGNOSTIC TESTS & INTERPRETATION

Lab

Initial lab tests

- ELISA:
  - Can detect antibodies to *B. burgdorferi* several weeks after tick bite. However, has relatively high false-positive rate and occasionally false-negative results. Remains positive for years after treatment
- Western blot analysis:
  - Much more specific. After 4–8 weeks of infection, ≥5 of the following IgG bands must be present for test to be positive: 18, 21, 28, 30, 34, 39, 41, 45, 58, 66, and 93 kd. During 1st 2–4 weeks of infection, 2 IgM bands may establish diagnosis but false positive IgM blots are common.
- Positive ELISA with negative Western blot:
  - Usually means patient does not have Lyme disease and ELISA was a false-positive but false positive IgM blots are common.
- Polymerase chain reaction (PCR):
  - PCR testing may be done with synovial tissue or fluid, or with CSF. Positive PCR indicates active disease, but negative result does not rule out Lyme.
  - Urine tests for Lyme disease have been shown to be very inaccurate and should not be used.

DIFFERENTIAL DIAGNOSIS

- Viral arthritis/arthralgias
- Septic arthritis
- Juvenile rheumatoid arthritis
- Postinfectious arthritis
- Fibromyalgia syndrome
- SLE
- Pitfalls:
  - Incorrect diagnosis: Many patients with vague systemic complaints (fatigue, headaches, arthralgias) are incorrectly diagnosed with Lyme disease, even though their Lyme tests are negative (or ELISA mildly positive and Western blot negative).
  - These patients are then treated with multiple courses of oral antibiotics; if they do not respond, they are often treated with IV antibiotics, sometimes for prolonged periods.
  - This situation delays diagnosing true problem and subjects patients to unnecessary risks of long-term antibiotic use and occasionally of central venous lines.

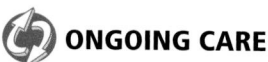 **TREATMENT**

MEDICATION (DRUGS)

- Oral antibiotics:
  - Initial therapy for early Lyme disease
  - Specific therapies:
    - Patients >8 years old: Doxycycline is drug of choice.
    - Younger children or people who do not tolerate tetracyclines: Amoxicillin or cefuroxime preferred, but penicillin V is also acceptable.
    - Penicillin-allergic patients: Erythromycin may be used, but is less effective.
  - Duration of therapy:
    - Patients with only skin rash: 14–21 days of oral antibiotics usually sufficient
    - If other symptoms present: 21–28 days recommended
- IV antibiotics:
  - Become necessary for:
    - Persistent arthritis unresponsive to oral medications
    - Severe carditis
    - Neurologic disease (other than an isolated 7th-nerve palsy)
  - Specific IV therapies
    - Ceftriaxone: Drug of choice
    - Penicillin V: May also be used
  - Duration of therapy: 14–21 days
- Prevention:
  - Some studies suggest that a single dose of doxycycline after tick bite will prevent Lyme disease.
  - Protective clothing, tick repellants, and checking daily for ticks are good preventive measures.

ONGOING CARE

PROGNOSIS

- In general, much better for children than for adults. Only 2% of children have chronic arthritis at 6 months.
- Most of the cardiac manifestations will disappear with or without treatment in a short time (3–4 weeks), but may later recur. Severe cardiac involvement rarely may be fatal.

COMPLICATIONS

- Chronic arthritis occurs in ∼2% of children.
- Other complications arise from treatment, such as:
  - Cholecystitis secondary to treatment with ceftriaxone
  - Infections from indwelling catheters used for IV antibiotics
  - Some patients develop what is thought to be a post-Lyme disease syndrome. This is not well defined and is very controversial. It often consists of arthralgias and fatigue, but may include paresthesias and cognitive complaints. Prolonged antibiotics have not been shown to be helpful. Some of these patients present with a fibromyalgia-like syndrome and improve with physical therapy.

ADDITIONAL READING

- Bunikis J, Barbour AG. Laboratory testing for suspected Lyme disease. *Med Clin North Amer*. 2002;86:311–340.
- Feder HM Jr. Lyme disease in children. *Infect Dis Clin North Am*. 2008;22(2):315–326, vii.
- Hayes E. Lyme disease. *Clin Evid*. 2002:652–664.
- Huppertz HI. Lyme disease in children. *Curr Opin Rheumatol*. 2001;13:434–440.
- Nachman SA, Pontrelli L. Central nervous system Lyme disease. *Semin Pediatr Infect Dis*. 2003; 14:123–130.
- Shapiro ED, Gerber MA. Lyme disease: Fact versus fiction. *Pediatr Ann*. 2002;31:170–177.
- Steere AC. Lyme disease. *N Engl J Med*. 2001;345:115–125.
- Weinstein A, Britchkov M. Lyme arthritis and post-Lyme disease syndrome. *Curr Opin Rheumatol*. 2002;14:383–387.

 CODES

ICD9
088.81 Lyme disease

ICD10
A69.20 Lyme disease, unspecified

FAQ

- Q: What does the deer tick look like?
- A: The deer tick is flat, very small (about the size of a pin head), and has 8 legs. The adult male is black, and the female is red and black. They can grow to 3 times their normal size when they are engorged with blood.
- Q: Do all bites from infected deer ticks cause Lyme disease?
- A: No. Even infected ticks will not cause Lyme disease if they are attached to the skin for a short period of time. If the tick is attached for <24 hours, the chances of transmitting the disease are exceedingly low. The longer the tick is attached, the higher the probability of disease transmission.
- Q: Should all patients be retested for Lyme disease after a full course of treatment?
- A: No. Lyme titers and the Western blot will remain positive for years after adequate treatment for Lyme disease. If the patient's symptoms have resolved, there is no point in rechecking the titer. If the patient is still symptomatic, titers and a Western blot may be checked before starting IV antibiotic therapy to look for a rising titer and to be sure the patient truly has Lyme disease. If symptoms remain after IV therapy, other diagnoses should be considered.
- Q: Should patients with nontraumatic Bell's palsy be tested for Lyme disease?
- A: Bell's palsy is seen in association with Lyme disease infections, so testing for Lyme disease is a good idea.

L

LYMPHADENOPATHY

Hans B. Kersten

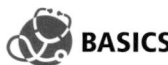 BASICS

DESCRIPTION
- Term used to describe ≥1 enlarged lymph nodes >10 mm in diameter (for inguinal nodes, >15 mm; for epitrochlear nodes, >5 mm)
- Any palpable supraclavicular, popliteal, or iliac lymph node considered abnormal
- Normal lymph nodes: Generally <10 mm
- Lymph nodes often palpable in normal, healthy children. They are present from birth, peak in size between 8 and 12 years of age, and then regress during adolescence.
- Lymph nodes drain contiguous areas:
  – Cervical nodes drain head and neck area.
  – Axillary nodes drain arm, thorax, and breast.
  – Epitrochlear nodes drain forearm and hand.
  – Inguinal nodes drain leg and groin.
  – Supraclavicular nodes drain thorax and abdomen.

EPIDEMIOLOGY
Incidence
Difficult to determine because it depends on the underlying process that causes lymph node enlargement.

Prevalence
Palpable nodes are present in 5–25% of newborns (cervical, axillary, inguinal) and in >50% of older children (all areas except epitrochlear, supraclavicular, and popliteal).

PATHOPHYSIOLOGY
- Lymphatic flow from adjacent nodes or inoculation site brings microorganisms to lymph nodes.
- Lymph node enlargement may occur via any of the following mechanisms:
  – Nodal cells may replicate in response to antigenic stimulation (e.g., Kawasaki disease) or malignant transformation (e.g., lymphoma).
  – Large number of reactive cells from outside node (e.g., neutrophils or metastatic cells) may enter node.
  – Foreign material may be deposited into node by lipid-laden histiocytes (e.g., lipid storage diseases).
  – Vascular engorgement and edema may occur secondary to local cytokine release.
  – Suppuration secondary to tissue necrosis (e.g., *Mycobacterium tuberculosis*)
- Many systemic infections (e.g., HIV) cause hepatic or splenic enlargement in addition to generalized lymphadenopathy.

ETIOLOGY
Usually determined by performing a thorough history and physical exam

COMMONLY ASSOCIATED CONDITIONS
Many systemic infections (e.g., HIV) cause hepatic or splenic enlargement in addition to generalized lymphadenopathy.

DIAGNOSIS

HISTORY
- Preceding symptoms (e.g., upper respiratory symptoms preceding cervical lymphadenopathy)
- Localizing signs or symptoms (e.g., stomatitis may be associated with submandibular lymphadenopathy)
- Duration: Days or weeks
- Constitutional or associated symptoms (e.g., fever, weight loss, or night sweats)
- Exposures: Cat exposure (cat scratch disease), uncooked meat (Toxoplasmosis), tick bite (Lyme disease)
- Medications (e.g., Phenytoin or Isoniazid)
- Travel to or residence in an endemic area should raise suspicion for Tuberculosis, Lyme disease.
- Signs and symptoms:
  – Localized lymphadenopathy: Involves enlarged nodes in any 1 region
  – Generalized lymphadenopathy: Involves ≥2 noncontiguous regions secondary to a systemic process, such as EBV infection.
  – Supraclavicular nodes seen with malignancy: Right-sided supraclavicular node is associated with mediastinal malignancy; left-sided node suggests abdominal malignancy.

PHYSICAL EXAM
- Complete physical exam is imperative to look for signs of systemic disease such as skin, oropharyngeal, or ocular findings; or hepatosplenomegaly.
- The child's weight should also be checked to be sure there has been no weight loss.
- If localized lymphadenopathy is suspected, examine the area that the lymph node drains for pathology. For example, an arm papule may be associated with axillary lymphadenopathy in cat scratch disease.
- Cervical, axillary, and inguinal nodes, as well as liver and spleen, must be palpated to help determine if signs of systemic disease or infection are present.
- Characterize nodes. Be sure to note:
  – Location: Be as exact as possible (see above).
  – Size: Specify dimensions.
  – Consistency: Soft, firm, solid, cystic, fluctuant, rubbery. Firm, rubbery nodes may be associated with lymphomas, while soft nodes are generally palpated with reactive lymphadenopathy.
  – Fixation: Normally freely mobile; infection or malignancy may cause adherence to surrounding tissues or nodes.
  – Tenderness: Suggests inflammation

DIAGNOSTIC TESTS & INTERPRETATION
Lab
Consider the following tests if ≥1 nodes is persistently enlarged, has increased in size, has changed in consistency or mobility, or if systemic symptoms are present:
- CBC: Consider with generalized lymphadenopathy, or if malignancy is in differential diagnosis.
- Purified protein derivative (PPD) testing: Consider with persistently enlarged node (2– 4 weeks) or travel to areas where tuberculosis is endemic.
- ESR or CRP: Increased with infection or inflammation
- Throat culture: If concern for group A β–hemolytic streptococcal (GAS) pharyngitis
- EBV/Cytomegalovirus (CMV) titers: Consider with persistent generalized adenopathy.
- *Bartonella henselae* titers: Consider with persistently enlarged unilateral node and/or history of cat exposure.
- *Toxoplasma gondii* titers: Consider with generalized lymphadenopathy and exposure to undercooked or raw meat.
- HIV testing: Consider with persistent generalized lymphadenopathy and failure to thrive.
- Lactate dehydrogenase (LDH), uric acid, and liver enzymes: Consider if history and physical exam raise concern for malignancy.
- Rapid plasma reagin (RPR): Consider with rash and generalized lymphadenopathy or other signs of syphilis.
- Antinuclear antibody (ANA): If persistent generalized lymphadenopathy and other signs of systemic disease, to rule out systemic lupus erythematosus (SLE)

Imaging
- Chest radiograph: Helpful with supraclavicular nodes, systemic symptoms, or if positive PPD
- US: May help differentiate cystic from solid masses
- CT: May help delineate anatomy or extent of the lesion

Diagnostic Procedures/Other
- Biopsy should be considered if:
  – Nodes are persistently enlarged, especially if accompanied by signs of systemic disease such as hepatosplenomegaly, weight loss, and exanthema.
  – Nodes are fixed to underlying skin.
  – Ulceration is present.
  – Node is supraclavicular, nontender, or increasing in size or firmness.
- Fine-needle aspiration: Cost-effective, but sometimes nondiagnostic; may result in fistulous tract
- Open biopsy: Often diagnostic, but requires general anesthesia

DIFFERENTIAL DIAGNOSIS
Must be carefully differentiated from lymphadenitis, defined as lymph node enlargement with signs of inflammation (including erythema, tenderness, induration, warmth); often treated with antibiotics.

- Localized lymphadenopathy:
  – Generally occurs as reactive adenopathy in response to local infection
  – Differential diagnosis for localized adenopathy varies depending on affected site:
    ○ Cervical adenopathy: Includes cystic hygroma, branchial cleft cyst, and thyroglossal duct cyst
    ○ Inguinal adenopathy: Includes inguinal hernia or other mass

- Generalized lymphadenopathy: May be seen in many systemic illnesses:
  - Miscellaneous: Kawasaki disease, Castleman disease, Rosai-Dorfman disease (sinus histiocytosis with massive lymphadenopathy), Kikuchi-Fujimoto disease (histiocytic necrotizing lymphadenitis), Churg-Strauss syndrome, infection-associated hemophagocytic syndrome, Gianotti-Crosti syndrome (papular acrodermatitis), sarcoidosis, lipid storage diseases (Niemann-Pick, Gaucher, Wolman, Faber diseases), hyperthyroidism
  - Viral infections: Adenovirus, rubella, enterovirus, herpes simplex virus, measles virus, varicella virus, EBV, cytomegalovirus, HIV, hepatitis A or B viruses
  - Bacterial infections: *Staphylococcus aureus*, *Bartonella henselae*, GAS, salmonella, yersinia, brucellosis, tularemia, *Mycobacterium tuberculosis*, *Mycoplasma pneumonia*, rickettsiae
  - Parasitic infections: Chagas disease, Schistosomiasis
  - Autoimmune disorders: SLE, juvenile rheumatoid arthritis, serum sickness
  - Malignancy: Lymphoma (Hodgkin and non-Hodgkin), histiocytosis, neuroblastoma, leukemia
  - Medications: Phenytoin, isoniazid, pyrimethamine, antileprosy drugs, antithyroid drugs, aspirin, barbiturates, penicillin, tetracycline, iodides, sulfonamides, allopurinol, phenylbutazone
  - Lymphoproliferative disorders: Wiskott-Aldrich syndrome, ataxia-telangiectasia syndrome, combined immunodeficiency syndrome, x-linked lymphoproliferative syndrome

 TREATMENT

MEDICATION (DRUGS)
Acute lymphadenitis should be treated with antibiotics directed against *Streptococcus* and *Staphylococcus*:

- Cephalexin 50 mg/kg/d in 4 divided doses OR
- Cefadroxil 30 mg/kg/d in 2 divided doses OR
- Dicloxacillin 50–100 mg/kg/d in 4 divided doses. Max 4 g/d.
- Consider using clindamycin 20–30 mg/kg/d in 4 divided doses OR trimethoprim-sulfamethoxazole (TMP–SMX) 8–10 mg/kg/d PO/IV in 2 divided doses in areas with a high prevalence of methicillin-resistant *Staphylococcus aureus* (MRSA)
- Penicillin-allergic patients: Erythromycin 50 mg/kg/d in 4 divided doses

First Line
Empiric treatment with antibiotics: 1st- or 2nd-generation cephalosporin to cover group A *Streptococcus* and *S. aureus* if meticulous history and physical exam are not revealing. Consider empiric treatment with clindamycin or trimethoprim-sulfamethoxazole if there is a high incidence of MRSA in the community.

Second Line
Consider broader antibiotic coverage for *B. henselae* and atypical mycobacterium: Azithromycin 10 mg/kg dose on day 1, followed by 5 mg/kg divided once for 4 more days

ADDITIONAL TREATMENT
General Measures
- Treat underlying disease.
- Close observation, unless history and physical suggest malignancy or lymphadenitis

ISSUES FOR REFERRAL
Refer to surgery or otolaryngology if biopsy or excision required.

SURGERY/OTHER PROCEDURES
Excision for special, prolonged cases

 ONGOING CARE

FOLLOW-UP RECOMMENDATIONS
Patient Monitoring
- Localized lymphadenopathy: Observe for several weeks or treat with antibiotics if indicated.
- Serial observation if nodes are persistently enlarged

PROGNOSIS
- Depends on underlying diagnosis
- Excellent for reactive lymphadenopathy

COMPLICATIONS
- Lymphadenitis
- Local infection (e.g., cellulitis)
- Lymph node abscess
- Sepsis via hematogenous spread of inadequately contained infection
- Fistula (e.g., with atypical mycobacteria)
- Fibrosis secondary to purulence or lymphadenitis
- Stridor secondary to enlarged cervical lymph nodes
- Wheezing secondary to enlarged parabronchial mediastinal lymph nodes

ADDITIONAL READING

- Albright JT, Pransky SM. Nontuberculous mycobacterial infections of the head and neck. *Pediatr Clin North Am*. 2003;50:503–514.
- Bamji M, Stone RK, Kaul A, et al. Palpable lymph nodes in healthy newborns and infants. *Pediatrics*. 1986;78:573–575.
- Friedmann AM. Evaluation and management of lymphadenopathy in children. *Pediatr Rev*. 2008;29(2):53–60.
- Jackson MA, Chesney PJ. Lymphatic system and generalized lymphadenopathy. In: Long SS, Pickering LK, Prober CG, eds., *Principles and practice of pediatric infectious diseases*, 3rd ed. New York: Churchill Livingstone; 2008:135–143.
- McClain KL, Fletcher RH. Approach to the child with peripheral lymphadenopathy. In: Bascow DS, ed., *UpToDate*. Waltham MA: UpToDate, 2010.
- Nield LS, Kamat D. Lymphadenopathy in children: When and how to evaluate. *Clin Pediatr*. 2004;43:25–33.
- Nizet N, Jackson MA. Localized lymphadenitis, lymphadenopathy, and lymphangitis. In: Long SS, Pickering LK, Prober CG, eds., *Principles and practice of pediatric infectious diseases*, 3rd ed. New York: Churchill Livingstone; 2008:165–168.
- Twist CJ, Link MP. Assessment of lymphadenopathy in children. *Pediatr Clin North Am*. 2002;49: 1009–1025.

 CODES

ICD9
- 785.6 Enlargement of lymph nodes

ICD10
- R59.0 Localized enlarged lymph nodes
- R59.1 Generalized enlarged lymph nodes

FAQ
- Q: When should there be concern about malignancy in a child with lymphadenopathy?
- A: Malignancy should be considered in any child who has lymphadenopathy that does not improve in spite of antibiotic therapy, that has a location of concern (e.g., supraclavicular) or physical exam features of concern (hard, large size [>2 cm]) that persistently enlarges, or if the child shows signs of systemic disease.
- Q: How much of a workup does a well child with localized lymphadenopathy need?
- A: As long as the lymph nodes are soft, mobile, and nontender, the lymphadenopathy is likely to be self-limited. If the cause is unclear, then children should be observed for a couple of weeks. Further workup is needed if the nodes persist or enlarge, or if there are signs of systemic disease (e.g., hepatomegaly or weight loss).
- Q: When should a child with lymphadenopathy be referred to a specialist?
- A: Most cases of lymphadenopathy in children are self-limited and can be observed for a few weeks and/or treated with antibiotics, if appropriate. Referral to a surgeon should be considered in any child with persistently enlarged lymphadenopathy (>4 weeks) or immediately if there are signs of malignancy.

L

LYMPHEDEMA

Robert K. Noll

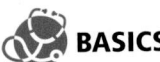 **BASICS**

DESCRIPTION
- Lymphedema is a chronic swelling, typically in an extremity or the genitals, which is caused by abnormal accumulation of interstitial fluid. It can be of primary or secondary origin.
- Primary lymphedema has 3 forms, all of which stem from a developmental abnormality of lymphatic flow. Not all primary lymphedemas are clinically evident at birth.
  - Congenital lymphedema
    ○ Present at birth
    ○ Female-to-male ratio: 2:1
    ○ Lower to upper extremity ratio: 3:1
    ○ 2/3 cases are bilateral
    ○ May improve with age
  - Lymphedema praecox (65–80% of primary lymphedema)
    ○ Usually becomes evident at puberty, but may appear between infancy to age 35
    ○ Female-to-male ratio: 4:1
    ○ 70% unilateral lower extremity (L>R)
  - Lymphedema tarda: Presents at age 35 or older
- Secondary lymphedema is from an acquired abnormality of lymphatic flow.
  - Common causes in children include:
    ○ Postsurgical obstruction
    ○ Burns
    ○ Insect bites
    ○ Infection
    ○ Surgery
    ○ Neoplasm
    ○ Trauma

EPIDEMIOLOGY
- Most lymphedemas in childhood are primary (or idiopathic) lymphedema (96%).
- Congenital lymphedema comprises 10–25% of primary lymphedema cases; lymphedema praecox, 65–80%; and lymphedema tarda, 10%.
- Female-to-male ratio in congenital lymphedema is 2:1; in lymphedema praecox the female-to-male ratio is 4:1.
- Affected males—most likely congenital and bilateral; affected females—most likely unilateral lymphedema praecox
- Secondary lymphedema is more common in adults, and rare in children. In the US, commonly from breast cancer; worldwide, due to filariasis.

Incidence
Incidence of 1.15/100,000 in children <20 years

RISK FACTORS
Genetics
- Chromosomal defect in Milroy disease mapped to long arm of 5q35
- Specific genes implicated in lymphedema are VEGFR3, FOXC2, and SOX18
- Genetic disorders are associated with lymphedema: Fabry disease, Milroy disease (congenital familial lymphedema with ocular findings), Meige disease (familial lymphedema praecox), and Down, Turner, Noonan, yellow nail, Klippel–Trenaunay–Weber, pes cavus, and other syndromes.
- Inheritance can be autosomal dominant, recessive, or sex-linked.

PATHOPHYSIOLOGY
- Abnormal accumulation of interstitial fluid due to impaired uptake by lymphatic vessels or excessive production of lymph due to venous obstruction and increased capillary pressure
- Initially edema is pitting, whereas chronic edema is generally non-pitting as a result of fibrosis.

 DIAGNOSIS

HISTORY
- Unilateral, painless lower extremity edema in healthy pubertal female strongly suggests lymphedema praecox.
- Painless swelling distal to site of extremity surgery or trauma suggests secondary lymphedema.
- Sites of previous cellulitis, infection, or insect bites can be associated with secondary lymphedema.

PHYSICAL EXAM
- Painless, pitting edema in unilateral limb is strongly suggestive of lymphedema, though nearly half of cases are bilateral.
- Most commonly affected sites: Extremities, usually legs, followed by genitalia
- Chronic inflammation leads to fibrosis and non-pitting or "woody" edema with induration.
- Hair loss and hyperkeratosis of the affected limb develop over time.
- Pain in affected limb uncommon and suggests secondary lymphedema due to thrombophlebitis, cellulitis, or reflex sympathetic dystrophy.
- Global edema suggests other disease states.
- Red streaking of extremity, fever, chills, or nodal enlargement suggests development of cellulitis or lymphangitis.

DIAGNOSTIC TESTS & INTERPRETATION
Lab
Not usually necessary but may be useful to rule out other causes of edema
- Urinalysis for proteinuria as seen with glomerulonephrosis
- Serum total protein and albumin to rule out hypoproteinemia
- Liver function tests to assess functional status
- Pregnancy test

Imaging
Usually unnecessary to make diagnosis, but may help to plan or evaluate therapy
- Lymphangiography is no longer used since related dyes caused inflammation and worsening of lymphatic obstruction.
- Radionuclide lymphoscintigraphy, when indicated, is the preferred method of imaging to define anatomy and to evaluate lymph flow and obstruction
- CT and MRI may be valuable if a malignancy is suspected.
- Doppler ultrasound may be helpful if deep vein thrombosis is suspected.

DIFFERENTIAL DIAGNOSIS
- Infection
  - Cellulitis
  - Lymphangitis
  - Herpes simplex virus type 2
- Tumors
  - Pelvic mass
  - Multiple enchondromatosis
- Metabolic
  - Cushing disease
  - Hyperthyroidism
  - Lipedema
- Anatomic
  - Venous stasis
  - Deep vein thrombosis
  - Hemihypertrophy
  - Arteriovenous fistula
  - Popliteal arterial aneurysm
  - Popliteal cyst (Baker cyst)
- Miscellaneous
  - Heart failure
  - Glomerulonephrosis
  - Cirrhosis
  - Hypoproteinemia
  - Reflex sympathetic dystrophy
  - Pregnancy

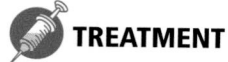 TREATMENT

General Measures
- Therapy should be instituted as soon as possible and before fibrosis develops.
- Goals of therapy are to minimize or decrease edema, and to prevent infection, fibrosis, and skin changes.
- Compression garments (e.g., Jobst stockings or elastic wraps) recommended long term, but compliance can be a challenge
- Extremity elevation, especially at night
- Exercise, swimming, or walking may be beneficial.
- Diligent skin care and appropriately fitting shoes to avoid infection
- Manual massage decompression can be helpful for digital edema and for infants who may not tolerate compression garments
- Automated intermittent pneumatic compression machines shown to facilitate home regimen compliance
- Published series reports 73% treated with compression stockings, 18% with pneumatic compression, and 13% required surgery
- Psychological effects of cosmesis should not be overlooked.

Diet
In children with chylous reflux syndromes, a diet low in long-chain triglycerides may be of benefit.

SPECIAL THERAPY
Complex or complete decongestive physiotherapy is part of a specialized treatment program offered at a few select centers. It may be more effective than massage or compression garments alone in reducing swelling and maintaining reduction in fluid accumulation.

MEDICATION (DRUGS)
- Diuretics: Not used in children and adolescents; efficacy for adults is debated.
- Prophylactic antibiotic use is indicated for patients with recurrent cellulitis or lymphangitis.

SURGERY
- Microsurgical treatment has been proven to show excellent outcomes in carefully selected patient populations via lymphatic-venous anastomoses or lymphatic-venous-lymphatic anastomoses.
- Traditional surgery has 1 of 2 goals: Removal of excess edematous tissue or attempts to restore lymph drainage
  - Both may decrease the rate of infections but have poor cosmetic results.
  - Recommended only for those with uncontrolled swelling with significant disability

 ONGOING CARE

PROGNOSIS
- Edema persists throughout life.
- Natural history: Plateau in severity of edema after an initial few years of progression in 50%, slow constant progression in 50%

COMPLICATIONS
- Cellulitis and lymphangitis are the most common complications and are treated with antibiotics; published series showed 24% of cases developed infection and half of these required hospitalization.
- Poor long-term compliance with compression garments due to uncomfortable nature of therapy
- Lymphangiosarcoma (rare)
- Psychological problems
- Physical limitations
- Chronic inflammation and edema ultimately lead to fibrosis and induration of the involved area.

ADDITIONAL READING
- Campisi C, Da Rin E, Bellini C, et al. Pediatric lymphedema and correlated syndromes: Role of microsurgery. *Microsurgery*. 2008;28:138–142.
- Mayrovitz HN. The standard of care for lymphedema: Current concepts and physiological considerations. *Lymph Res Biol*. 2009;7(2):101–108.
- Schnook CC, Fishman SJ, Mulliken JB, et al. Pediatric lymphedema: Clinical features in 136 children. *Plast Reconstr Surg*. 2010;125(6):88.
- Smeltzer DM, Stickler GB, Schirger A. Primary lymphedema in children and adolescents: A follow-up study and review. *Pediatrics*. 1985;76:206–218.
- Zuther JE. Lymphedema management: The comprehensive guide for practitioners, 2nd ed. New York, NY: Thieme, 2009.

 CODES

ICD9
- 457.1 Other lymphedema
- 757.0 Hereditary edema of legs

ICD10
- I89.0 Lymphedema, not elsewhere classified
- Q82.0 Hereditary lymphedema

FAQ
- Q: Is the swelling going to go away?
- A: No, this is a lifelong disorder in most cases.
- Q: Could this have been prevented?
- A: No, primary lymphedema is typically due to abnormal embryologic development.
- Q: If the lymph channels have been abnormal since birth, why does the swelling present during adolescence?
- A: No one really knows; hormones may play a role in lymphedema.

L

LYMPHOPROLIFERATIVE DISORDERS

David T. Teachey

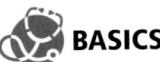 **BASICS**

DESCRIPTION
- Lymphoproliferative disorders are a class of nonmalignant diseases characterized by uncontrolled growth of lymphoid tissues (spleen, bone marrow, liver, lymph nodes)
- Can be congenital or acquired
- Most common in children include:
  – Autoimmune lymphoproliferative syndrome (ALPS)
  – Castleman's Disease (CD)
  – Rosai–Dorfman's Disease (RD)
  – EBV-associated lymphoproliferative disorder (ELD)
  – X-linked lymphoproliferative syndrome (XLP)
- Rarer disorders (not discussed in detail)
  – Angioimmunoblastic lymphadenopathy
  – Caspase eight deficiency syndrome
  – Dianzani autoimmune lymphoproliferative disease
  – Kikuchi–Fujimoto syndrome
  – Lymphomatoid granulomatosis
  – Lymphomatoid papulosis
  – Occular adnexal lymphoid proliferation
  – Ras-associated leukoproliferative disorder

EPIDEMIOLOGY
Incidence and Prevalence
All uncommon

RISK FACTORS
Often multifactorial with inherited genetic defect and acquired infection

Genetics
- ALPS (80% of patients have identifiable mutation)
  – 60–70% germline mutation in FAS (TNFRSF6)
  – 10% somatic mutation in FAS
  – 2% germline mutation in CASP10
  – <1% germline mutation in FASL
- XLP
  – Majority of cases mutation in SH2DIA
  – XLP-like syndrome caused by XIAP mutations

PATHOPHYSIOLOGY
- ALPS
  – Defective Fas-mediated apoptosis leads to abnormal lymphocyte survival with subsequent lymphoproliferation, autoimmunity, and cancer
- Castleman's Disease (CD)
  – Largely unknown but can be triggered by HHV8 infection, especially in immunocompromised patients
- EBV-associated lymphoproliferative disorder
  – EBV triggered lymphoproliferative disorder found in patients on chronic immune suppression typically after organ or bone marrow transplant (PTLD) or with inherited immune deficiency
- X-linked lymphoproliferative syndrome (XLP)
  – Mutation in SH2D1A leads to abnormal production of SAP protein in NK and T cells, leading to defective SAP-SLAM signaling and inability to appropriately respond to EBV infection.

DIAGNOSIS

HISTORY
- ALPS
  – Typically presents at young age (average 18 months) with massive lymphadenopathy and splenomegaly.
  – Many patients develop secondary autoimmune disease.
  – Most often, autoimmune destruction of blood cells (80% of patients). Can be mild to severe
  – Destruction of platelets: See chapter on Idiopathic thrombocytopenic purpura
  – Destruction of erythrocytes: See chapter on autoimmune hemolytic anemia
  – Destruction of neutrophils: See chapter on neutropenia
  – Can have autoimmune involvement of any organ system, similar to systemic lupus erythematosis
  – In young adult years, 10–20% develop lymphoma
  – Lymphoproliferation can improve or worsen with infection. Often progresses through teenage years and improves in adulthood
  – Autoimmune disease less likely to improve with older age
- Castleman's Disease (CD)
  – 2 variants:
  – Hyaline vascular: presents with enlarged single lymph node or chain of nodes. >90% with no other symptoms. Rarely can have fever, weight loss, fatigue
  – Plasma cell: presents with enlarged single lymph node or chain (unicentric) or diffuse adenopathy (multicentric). Often with constitutional symptoms (fever, sweats, lethargy, rashes, neuropathy, arthritis)
- Rosai–Dorfman's Disease (RDD)
  – Massive painless bilateral cervical lymphadenopathy with or without other involved nodal groups
  – Fever
  – Snoring common
  – Can have extranodal invasion of almost any organ (25% of patients have extranodal disease) and signs and symptoms depend on involved organ
- ELD/PTLD
  – Can be mild, with lymphadenopathy, fever, and/or diarrhea, or severe, with massive lymphadenopathy, high fever, night sweats, rash, and pruritus, and organ compression from involved nodes
- XLP
  – Can present as fulminant infectious mononucleosis or aplastic anemia or lymphoma or hematophagocytic syndrome
  – Often critically ill in the setting of EBV infection

PHYSICAL EXAM
- ALPS
  – Massive lymphadenopathy (90% of patients): Rarely can compress vital organs including trachea. Most common site of adenopathy is anterior cervical. Nodes hard but mobile
  – Splenomegaly (90% of patients)
  – Hepatomegaly (50% of patients)
  – Other physical exam findings as expected with autoimmune destruction of blood cells and/or end organ autoimmune disease.

- CD
  – Hyaline vascular: single enlarged lymph node or chain. Most often, cervical or mediastinal. May have shotty diffuse nonpathologic adenopathy
  – Plasma cell. Single or multiple pathologically enlarged lymph nodes. Abdominal nodes most common. Hepatosplenomegaly common. Peripheral edema, ascites, and pleural effusions may be present
- RDD
  – Massive bilateral anterior cervical lymphadenopathy (90% of patients). Other physical exam findings can vary based on extranodal disease
  – Hepatosplenomegaly (10% of patients)
- ELD/PTLD
  – Similar to other lymphoproliferative disorders (see Epstein–Barr virus chapter)
- XLP
  – Similar to other lymphoproliferative disorders; however, far more acutely ill (see also Epstein–Barr virus chapter and aplastic anemia chapter)

DIAGNOSTIC TESTS & INTERPRETATION
Lab
General
- Complete blood and reticulocyte count for anemia, thrombocytopenia, and neutropenia
- Direct antiglobin test (DAT) to check for autoimmune destruction of red blood cells
- Serum chemistries, uric acid, phosphorus to look for cell turnover (usually normal in lymphoproliferative disorders)
- Liver function tests, PT, PTT, and fibrinogen to measure liver function and for coagulopathy
- EBV PCR and titers, CMV PCR
- If acutely ill, consider ESR or CRP and ferritin
- Quantitative immunoglobulins. Often elevated in lymphoproliferative disorders

Diagnostic Tests for ALPS
- Mandatory criteria:
  – (1) chronic (>6 months) nonmalignant lymphoproliferation (lymphadenopathy and/or splenomegaly
  – (2) Elevated peripheral blood double negative T cells (DNTs); T cells that are CD3+, TCRalpha/beta+, CD4–, CD8–). DNTs are usually rare in peripheral blood (<1% of total lymphocytes or <2.5% of total T cells). DNTs are elevated and often markedly elevated in ALPS. Slight elevation in DNTs can be found in other autoimmune disorders
- Major (primary) criteria:
  – (1) Genetic mutation in ALPS causative gene (germline or somatic) in FAS, FASL or CASP10
  – (2) In vitro evidence of defective Fas mediated apoptosis. This assay requires growing blood cells from patient in culture for weeks and exposing to anti-Fas monoclonal antibody to see if T-cells are resistant to death. Only performed in a few labs

LYMPHOPROLIFERATIVE DISORDERS

- Minor (secondary) criteria
  - (1) Elevated vitamin B12 (>1500 ng/L)
  - (2) Elevated IL-10 (>20 pg/mL)
  - (3) Elevated IL-18 (>500 pg/mL)
  - (4) Elevated sFASL (>200 pg/mL)
  - (5) Classic histopathologic findings on lymph nodes or spleen biopsy
  - (6) Autoimmune cytopenias AND elevated serum IgG
  - (7) Positive family history
- Diagnosis
  - Definitive: Both mandatory and one major criteria
  - Probable: Both mandatory and one minor criteria (Probable ALPS should be treated the same as definitive ALPS)

Diagnostic Tests for CD
- Castleman syndrome diagnosed by histopathology
- Hypergammaglobulinemia, anemia, high ESR, high IL-6, HHV8 PCR+

Diagnostic Tests for RD
- Rosai–Dorfman's diagnosed by Histopathology
- Hypergammaglobulinemia, anemia, high ESR, leukocytosis with neutropenia, hematologic autoantiboides

Diagnostic Tests for EPD/PTLD
- Posttransplant lymphoproliferative diisorder after bone marrow graft
- Persistent EBV infection (positive EBV PCR or abnormal seroconversion by titers) in setting of immune suppression or immune compromise
- Diagnosis confirmed with imaging and/or histopathology

Diagnostic Tests for XLP
- Persistent EBV infection (positive EBV PCR or abnormal seroconversion on titers)
- Inverted CD4/8 ratio
- High IgM and IgA, Low IgG
- Defective NK activity
- Secondary hematophagocytic syndrome (Elevated ferritin, high triglycerides, low fibrinogen, cytopenias, high fever, splenomegaly, poor NK function, elevated s-IL-2R-alpha, and hematophagocytosis on marrow or node biopsy)
- Diagnosis confirmed by genetic testing for mutations in SH2D1A and XIAP genes, and/or SAP protein quantification

Imaging
- CT scans of head, neck, chest, abdomen and pelvis with IV contrast important for all lymphoproliferative disorders at initial diagnosis to define extent of disease
- IMPORTANT to obtain plain chest X-ray on initial presentation in patient with diffuse lymphadenopathy before CT scan to ensure a large mediastinal mass is not present. If present, it may be unsafe to lie patient flat and/or sedate for CT scan.
- Most lymphoproliferative disorders are very PET-avid

Diagnostic Procedures/Other
- ALPS and PTLD can be diagnosed without histopathology; however, most patients have a lymph node biopsy
- Other lymphoproliferative disorders typically require tissue for diagnosis (Biopsy, not fine needle aspirate)
- Consider bone marrow aspirate and/or biopsy to rule out marrow disease or other disease processes

Pathological Findings
- ALPS: DNTs in lymph node and spleen
- CD: Hyaline vascular (shrunken germinal centers with eosinophilic expansion of mantle zones with and vessel hyalinization); Plasma cell (extensive plasma cell infiltrate in interfollicular regions)
- RD: Emperipoiesis (lymphophagocytosis) hallmark of disease on biopsy. Presence of histiocytes
- XLP/PTLD/EPD: EBER+

DIFFERENTIAL DIAGNOSIS
- Other lymphoproliferative disorders
- Lymphoma
- Infection: EBV, CMV, Toxoplasmosis, HIV, TB
- Evans syndrome
- Rheumatologic disease

 # TREATMENT

ALPS
First Line
- Corticosteroids or IVIG for acute flares

Second Line
- Sirolimus or mycophenolate mofetil for chronic disease
- Sirolimus (rapamycin): Pros: Improves autoimmune disease and lymphoproliferation and eliminates DNTs. Cons: Drug–Drug interactions; requires therapeutic drug monitoring; 10% of patients develop mouth sores (most common in first month)
- Cellcept (mycophenolate): Pros: No drug–drug interactions, no mouth sores, no therapeutic drug monitoring. Cons: Not as effective. Does not help lymphoproliferation or lower DNTs. GI upset.
- Recommended treatment: Mild to moderate autoimmune disease start with cellcept and transition to sirolimus if poor response or side effects. More severe autoimmune disease or clinically significant lymphoproliferation start with sirolimus

Third Line
- Combination therapy. Stem cell transplant

Relative Contraindications (AVOID, if possible)
- Splenectomy: High incidence of pneumococcal sepsis even with antibiotic prophlylaxis and immunization
- Rituxiamb: Can lead to life-long hypogammaglobulinemia (5–10% of patients)

CD
Localized Disease
- Surgical resection or focal radiation. Steroids may be used to shrink lesions prior to surgery

Multicentric Disease
- Multiagent therapy (vincristine, prednisone, rituximab, cyclophosphamide, doxorubicin)

RD
- May self-resolve (20% of patients)
- If not consider, prednisone, or vinblastine plus prednisone, or mercaptopurine plus methotrexate, or 2CdA.

EPD/PTLD
- Reduce immune suppression or convert immune suppression to sirolimus if possible
- Consider rituximab, adoptive transfer of EBV-specific cytotoxic T cells
- If fails or generalized disease consider multi-agent chemotherapy similar to RD

XLP
- If hematophagocytosis or aplasia: Rituximab, etoposide, steroids, and cyclosporine
- Hematopoietic stem cell transplant is the only cure

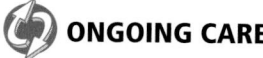 # ONGOING CARE

FOLLOW-UP RECOMMENDATIONS
- Recommended follow-up imaging varies among institutions. Most physicians will repeat imaging if patient's history changes OR to determine response to therapy.

PROGNOSIS
- Prognosis is good to fair for most lymphoproliferative disorders
- Prognosis is poor in XLP and advanced CD

ADDITIONAL READING

- Blaes AH, Morrison VA. Post-transplant lymphoproliferative disorders following solid-organ transplantation. *Expert Rev Hematol.* 2010;3(1): 35–44.
- Fleisher TA, Jaffe ES, Lenardo MJ, et al. Revised diagnostic criteria and classification for the autoimmune lymphoproliferative syndrome (ALPS): Report from the 2009 NIH International Workshop. *Blood.* 2010;7;116(14):e35–e40.
- Rezaei N, Mahmoudi E, Aghamohammadi A, et al. X-linked lymphoproliferative syndrome: A genetic condition typified by the triad of infection, immunodeficiency and lymphoma. *Br J Haematol.* 2011;152(1):13–30.
- Schulte KM, Talat N. Castleman's disease—a two compartment model of HHV8 infection. *Nat Rev Clin Oncol.* 2010;7(9):533–543. Epub 2010 Jul 6.
- Teachey DT, Seif AE, Grupp SA. Advances in the management and understanding of autoimmune lymphoproliferative syndrome (ALPS). *Br J Haematol.* 2010;148(2):205–216.

 # CODES

ICD9
- 238.77 Post-transplant lymphoproliferative disorder (PTLD)
- 238.79 Other lymphatic and hematopoietic tissues
- 279.41 Autoimmune lymphoproliferative syndrome

ICD10
- D47.Z1 Post-transplant lymphoproliferative disorder (PTLD)
- D89.82 Autoimmune lymphoproliferative syndrome [ALPS]

L

MALABSORPTION

Teena Sebastian
Maria R. Mascarenhas
Gabriel Arancibia (5th edition)

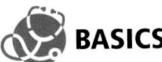 **BASICS**

DESCRIPTION
Malabsorption is characterized as a syndrome, as opposed to a disease entity, and is defined as any state in which there is a disturbance of digestion and/or absorption of nutrients across the intestinal mucosa. Additionally, there seems to be an association of chronic diarrhea with abdominal distention and failure to thrive in malabsorptive states.

EPIDEMIOLOGY
Depends on the underlying disease causing malabsorption

PATHOPHYSIOLOGY
- According to the nutrient affected:
  - Carbohydrate:
    - Monosaccharide: Congenital glucose-galactose deficiency, fructose intolerance
    - Disaccharide: Lactase deficiency (congenital or acquired), sucrase-isomaltase deficiency
    - Polysaccharide: Amylase deficiency (congenital or acquired)
  - Fat:
    - Bile salt deficiency: Cholestasis, resection of terminal ileum
    - Exocrine pancreatic insufficiency: Cystic fibrosis, chronic pancreatitis
    - Inadequate surface area: Celiac disease, flat villous lesions
  - Protein:
    - Protein-losing enteropathy: Intestinal lymphangiectasia, congenital heart failure
    - Exocrine pancreatic insufficiency: Cystic fibrosis, Shwachman syndrome
    - Inadequate surface area: Celiac disease
- According to the place where the alteration occurs:
  - Mucosal abnormality:
    - Anatomical: Post-enteritis syndrome, celiac disease, Inflammatory bowel disease (IBD)
    - Functional: Disaccharidase deficiencies
  - Luminal abnormality:
    - Exocrine pancreatic insufficiency: Cystic fibrosis, Shwachman-Diamond syndrome
    - Bile salt insufficiency: Biliary cholestatic liver disease, ileal resection
  - Anatomical abnormality:
    - Short gut: Surgical resection
    - Motility disturbance: Intestinal pseudo-obstruction

ETIOLOGY
The most common causes of malabsorption in developed countries are:
- Postenteritis syndrome
- Cow's milk protein intolerance
- Giardiasis
- Celiac disease
- Cystic fibrosis
- IBD

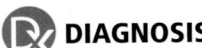 **DIAGNOSIS**

HISTORY
- GI symptoms:
  - Common in patients with malabsorption syndromes and range from mild abdominal gaseous distention to severe abdominal pain and vomiting. Chronic or recurrent diarrhea is by far the most common symptom.
  - Abdominal distention and watery diarrhea, with or without mild abdominal pain associated with skin irritation in the perianal area due to acidic stools, are characteristic of carbohydrate malabsorption syndromes.
  - Fat malabsorption can present with bulky, foul-smelling stools that are oily and thus float in water. Abdominal distension, increased gas, weight loss, and increased appetite are also seen.
  - Periodic nausea, abdominal distention and pain, and diarrhea are common in patients with chronic *Giardia* infections.
  - Vomiting, with moderate-to-severe abdominal pain and bloody stools, is characteristic of protein sensitivity syndromes.
  - Malabsorption syndromes can definitely cause abdominal pain or irritability (particularly seen in celiac disease).
- Stool characteristics:
  - Frequent loose watery stools may indicate carbohydrate intolerance.
  - Bulky, greasy, or loose foul-smelling stools indicate fat malabsorption.
  - In protein malabsorption, stools may be normal or loose.
  - Bloody stools are seen in patients with cow's milk protein allergy, infection, and inflammatory bowel disease.

- Other symptoms:
  - Malabsorption of carbohydrates, fats, or proteins can cause failure to thrive.
  - Anemia, with weakness and fatigue due to inadequate absorption of vitamin B_{12}, iron, and folic acid
  - Edema due to decreased protein absorption and hypoalbuminemia
  - Muscle cramping due to decreased vitamin D causing hypocalcemia, and decreased potassium levels
  - Failure to maintain growth velocity on standard charts

PHYSICAL EXAM
- In the absence of GI tract symptoms, malabsorption syndromes should be considered during the workup for failure to thrive, malnutrition, poor weight gain, or delayed puberty.
- Malabsorption syndromes should be suspected in infants with weight loss or little weight gain since birth and in infants with low weight and weight-for-height percentiles.
- Malnutrition symptoms may be present, as reduced SC fat, paleness, angular cheilosis, and muscle weakness. Abdominal distension, increased bowel sounds, rash around mouth and/or anus are commonly seen.

DIAGNOSTIC TESTS & INTERPRETATION
Lab
- Stool analysis:
  - The presence of reducing substances and pH <5.5 indicates that carbohydrates have not been properly absorbed.
  - The level of quantitative stool fat and the amount of fat intake in the diet should be measured and monitored for 3 days; a coefficient of fat absorption is calculated thus:

$$\frac{\text{Ingested fat (g)} - \text{fat in stool (g)}}{\text{Ingested fat (g)}} \times 100$$

  - Special stains are used for identification of fat. Normal values for the coefficient of fat absorption: $>93\%$ in children and adults, $>85\%$ in infants, $>67\%$ in premature infants. Moderate fat malabsorption ranges from 60–80%. Fat absorption of $<50\%$ indicates severe malabsorption.
  - The presence of large serum proteins in the stool, such as α_1-antitrypsin, indicates leakage of serum protein. A 24-hour stool collection for α_1-antitrypsin (along with a serum level) serves as a screening test for protein-losing enteropathy.

- Exam of the stool for ova and parasites or testing for the stool antigen may reveal the presence of *Giardia* species.
- Normally, stool bile acids should not be detected. If bile acid malabsorption is suspected, quantitative conjugated and unconjugated bile acids may be measured in stool, although this test is not commonly available and thus, not used in routine clinical practice.
- Other laboratory studies:
  - CBC may reveal anemia in patients with iron, folate and vitamin B_{12} malabsorption, and neutropenia is seen in patients with Shwachman-Diamond syndrome.
  - Total serum protein and albumin levels may be lower than reference range in syndromes in which protein is lost or not absorbed, particularly in protein-losing enteropathy and pancreatic insufficiency.
  - With fat malabsorption or ileal resection, fat-soluble vitamin levels in the serum are low.
  - With bile acid malabsorption, levels of LDL cholesterol may be low.
  - Serum calcium may be low due to vitamin D and amino acid malabsorption
  - Serum vitamin A, E, and carotene may be low due to bile salt deficiency and impaired fat absorption.
  - Other studies must be performed when a specific disease is suspected (e.g., mucosal biopsy for celiac disease, sweat test for cystic fibrosis, or appropriate workup for IBD).
  - Urine analysis should be done to rule out proteinuria in patients with low albumin levels.
  - An upper GI radiographic series is helpful for identification of segmental dilatation or stenosis secondary to bacterial overgrowth.
  - Genetic testing may be performed for identification of inherited malabsorption syndromes.
  - If tissue samples are acquired through a biopsy, ultrastructural analysis may be performed using electron microscopy.

DIFFERENTIAL DIAGNOSIS

- Pancreatic disorders:
  - Cystic fibrosis
  - Shwachman syndrome
  - Johanson-Blizzard syndrome
- Chronic cholestasis:
  - Biliary atresia
  - Vitamin E deficiency
  - Alagille syndrome

- Infectious diarrhea:
  - Giardiasis
  - Cryptosporidiosis
- Mucosal defect:
  - Celiac disease
  - Crohn disease
  - Postinfectious diarrhea
- Congenital brush border enzyme deficiencies:
  - Glucose-galactose transporter deficiency
  - Sucrase-isomaltase deficiency
  - Microvillus inclusion disease
- Abnormal intestinal lymphatic drainage:
  - Primary intestinal lymphangiectasia
  - Secondary intestinal lymphangiectasia

 TREATMENT

- The treatment depends on the underlying disease causing malabsorption. Appropriate nutritional support is of paramount importance.
- Specific treatment depends on etiology, for example, gluten-free diet for celiac disease, metronidazole for *Giardia* infection, or removal of the offending agent in a case of food intolerance.

ONGOING CARE

COMPLICATIONS

- Complications vary according to the underlying disease, but malnutrition and its consequences may worsen progressively if the cause is not determined and appropriate treatment prescribed.
- Some of the most frequent complications of malabsorption and malnutrition are: Growth failure, vitamins and micronutrient deficiency (zinc, magnesium, calcium), bone disease, hypoproteinemia and edema, essential fatty acid deficiency, perianal dermatitis, immune dysfunction and anemia.

ADDITIONAL READING

- Ali SA, Hill DR. Giardia intestinalis. *Curr Opin Infect Dis.* 2003;16:453–460.
- Crittenden RG, Bennett LE. Cow's milk allergy: A complex disorder. *J Am Coll Nutr.* 2005;24: 582S–591S.
- Dodge JA, Turck D. Cystic fibrosis: Nutritional consequences and management. *Best Pract Res Clin Gastroenterol.* 2006;20:531–546.

- Fasano A, Catassi C. Coeliac disease in children. *Best Pract Res Clin Gastroenterol.* 2005;19: 467–478.
- Pietzak MM, Thomas DW. Childhood malabsorption. *Pediatr Rev.* 2003;24:195–206.

 CODES

ICD9
- 271.3 Intestinal disaccharidase deficiencies and disaccharide malabsorption
- 579.8 Other specified intestinal malabsorption
- 579.9 Unspecified intestinal malabsorption

ICD10
- E74.39 Other disorders of intestinal carbohydrate absorption
- K90.4 Malabsorption due to intolerance, not elsewhere classified
- K90.9 Intestinal malabsorption, unspecified

FAQ

- Q: When should a patient with malabsorption be referred?
- A: Children with growth failure in whom malabsorption is suspected should be referred to a pediatric gastroenterologist because of the associated high morbidity.
- Q: What is the prognosis of malabsorption?
- A: Some malabsorption syndromes are transient, while others simply require a change in diet. Most disorders that cause secondary malabsorption are progressive and result in significant morbidity due to systemic complications.

M

MALARIA

Rakesh D. Mistry

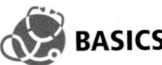 **BASICS**

DESCRIPTION
- Malaria is a febrile illness due to the *Plasmodium* species of protozoan parasites. *P. falciparum* and *P. vivax* most commonly infect humans, although *P. malariae* and *P. ovale* may also produce infection. The *Anopheles* mosquito serves as the vector for *Plasmodium* transmission.
- Malaria was described by the earliest medical writers in China, Assyria, and India, and by the 5th century B.C. Hippocrates was able to describe the characteristic fever patterns and clinical manifestations of the disease.

EPIDEMIOLOGY
- High-risk areas of endemic malaria include parts of Central and South America, Africa, and tropical regions of Asia.
- Malaria is a major cause of infant death in the tropical regions of the world.
- Malaria is the most common cause of fever in travelers returning from foreign countries.
- Risk of malaria infection is highest among travelers to Sub-Saharan Africa and Oceania.

Incidence
- Worldwide, an estimated 300–500 million cases of malaria occur annually.
- ~1,500 cases of malaria are imported into the U.S. each year.

RISK FACTORS
Genetics
- Sickle cell disease and trait confer protection against malaria by 2 postulated mechanisms:
  - Release of a toxic form of heme that possess antimalarial properties
  - The hemoglobin S erythrocyte tends to lose potassium required for adenosine triphosphatase (ATPase) activation, thereby depriving the parasites of nutrients.
- Thalassemia and G6PD deficiency may also provide innate resistance to malaria.

GENERAL PREVENTION
- In the hospital setting, universal precautions should be followed.
- Personal protective measures against *Anopheles* mosquito bites are extremely important:
  - Remain in well-screened areas.
  - Protective clothing is advised, including pants and long-sleeved shirts.
  - Insect repellents, such as DEET, are recommended. However, in children <2 years, concentrations of <10% are recommended; concentrations <35% may be used in older child.
- Chemoprophylaxis is strongly advised for travelers in endemic areas:
  - Chloroquine is the drug of choice in resistant areas (500 mg once a week or 5 mg/kg once a week)
  - Mefloquine is recommended in chloroquine-resistant areas (250 mg once a week; if weight is <15 kg, 5 mg/kg; if weight is 15–19 kg, 1/4 tablet; if weight is 20–30 kg, 1/2 tablet; if weight is 31–45 kg, 3/4 tablet).

- Contraindications include patients taking β blockers or other drugs that alter cardiac conduction, patients with seizure disorders or psychosis, and patients requiring fine-motor skill performance.
  - Atovaquone-proguanil (Malarone) is equally effective, with fewer side effects than mefloquine.
  - Doxycycline or chloroquine plus proguanil are also alternatives to mefloquine.
- Chloroquine and mefloquine should begin 1 week before travel, continued during the period of exposure, and 4 weeks after leaving the endemic region. Atovaquone-proguanil is started 2 days prior to travel, and continued 1 week after return.
- Travelers should use pyrimethamine-sulfadoxine (Fansidar) if a febrile illness occurs while on chloroquine and access to medical care is not readily available.

ETIOLOGY
- Infection may be acquired throughout the life of the female *Anopheles* mosquito but can also occur through contaminated blood transfusions or needles, or through congenital acquisition.
- The most common infecting species are *P. falciparum* and *P. vivax*.
  - *P. vivax* and *P. ovale* are associated with relapsing disease because of the persistent hepatic stage of the infection.

COMMONLY ASSOCIATED CONDITIONS
- Severe malaria is usually caused by P. falciparum.
- Defined as parasitemia >5% with CNS and other end-organ dysfunctions (shock, acidosis, renal failure, and/or hypoglycemia).
- Cerebral malaria is the most serious consequence of malaria infection. Prognosis depends on the management of other complications (e.g., acidosis, renal failure).
- Hemolytic anemia, the most common disease finding, can be severe, especially in *P. falciparum*; the predominant mechanism is due to IV hemolysis from fragile erythrocytes rather than solely rupture from infected cells.
- Tropical splenomegaly syndrome seen in chronic infections caused by *P. malariae* produces splenomegaly, hepatomegaly, portal hypertension, and pancytopenia. In *P. vivax* malaria, acute splenomegaly can induce rupture.
- Blackwater fever is due to acute renal failure caused by accumulation of hemoglobin in the renal tubules resulting in hemoglobinuria with dark urine. This often occurs after repeated attacks of *P. falciparum*.
- Pulmonary edema, distributive shock, dysentery, and nephrotic syndrome have been described.

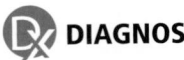 **DIAGNOSIS**

HISTORY
- Travel to malaria endemic region
- Pattern of fevers
- Poor compliance with malaria prophylaxis
- Signs and symptoms:
  - Upon return from a malaria endemic zone, presenting findings often include high fevers, headache, chills, sweating, and rigors.
  - Periodicity of fever is dependent on the *Plasmodium* species and is less commonly seen in young children and travelers.
  - Cough, irritability, anorexia, vomiting, abdominal pain, back pain, and arthralgias may be present.
  - Dark urine
  - Cerebral malaria will manifest with signs of increased intracranial pressure, encephalopathy, and seizures.

ALERT
- Failure to obtain a thorough travel history to determine exposure risk to developing malaria can delay the diagnosis and appropriate therapy.
- Delay in the diagnosis of malaria has been shown to increase the morbidity and mortality up to 20-fold compared with diagnosis and treatment within 24 hours of presentation.

PHYSICAL EXAM
- Ill-appearance during fever, with relatively well appearance in between
- Jaundice or pallor
- Hepatosplenomegaly may be present and is more likely observed in chronic infections due to *P. falciparum*.
- There is no rash present in malaria; presence of rash should elicit consideration of alternative diagnoses.

DIAGNOSTIC TESTS & INTERPRETATION
Lab
- Hemoglobin:
  - Hemolytic anemia is present initially as mild then more severe, depending on the *Plasmodium* species.
- WBC:
  - Leukocyte counts are usually normal or low; there is no eosinophilia.
  - Thrombocytopenia due to liver and splenic sequestration occurs in the more severe cases.
- Peripheral smear:
  - Thick and thin peripheral blood smears are required for definitive diagnosis (thick smears enable better sensitivity if the parasitemia is low; thin smears provide for species identification).
  - If initial smears are negative, repeated specimens should be obtained q8–12h during a 72-hour period to confirm a truly negative result.
  - The percent of red cells involved is an important risk factor for severe disease.
  - A parasitemia >5% of red cells, signs of CNS (mental status changes), or other organ involvement are indications for more intensive therapy.

- Rapid diagnostic tests:
  - Newly developed techniques exhibit excellent sensitivity for *Plasmodium* spp., require a small amount of blood for testing, and provide results in <20 minutes
  - Detection of parasitemia levels as low as 0.002%
  - Rapid testing is particularly useful in highly endemic areas; negative results may allow for expectant management and avoid unnecessary empiric therapy.
- Serologic tests:
  - Using indirect immunofluorescent assays may be helpful, but they have a low sensitivity in the early phases of acute infections.

DIFFERENTIAL DIAGNOSIS
- Because of its potential for severe disease, malaria must be ruled out in any febrile traveler returning from an endemic zone.
- Other causes of fever in travelers should be considered, based on the region of travel:
  - Typhoid fever
  - Dengue fever
  - Yellow fever
  - Hepatitis
  - Hemolytic-uremic syndrome
  - Leptospirosis
- Common etiologies of fever, such as sinusitis, pneumonia, and influenza should also be considered.

ALERT
Consider malaria when a patient with unexplained fever has a history of travel.

 TREATMENT

MEDICATION (DRUGS)
- Chloroquine phosphate is recommended at a dose of 10 mg/kg PO (maximum, 600 mg), then 5 mg/kg PO in 6 hours (maximum, 300 mg), then 5 mg/kg PO at 24 and 48 hours (maximum, 300 mg) For all *Plasmodium* species except chloroquine-resistant *P. falciparum* and chloroquine-resistant *P. vivax*
- If parenteral therapy is necessary, treatment with quinidine gluconate, 10 mg/kg IV initial dose (maximum, 600 mg) over 2 hours followed by 0.02-mg/kg/min infusion until PO therapy can be started.
- For chloroquine-resistant *P. falciparum* or chloroquine-resistant *P. vivax*; quinine sulfate, 25 mg/kg/d PO in 3 doses for 3–7 days plus doxycycline, 2 mg/kg/d PO b.i.d. for 7 days (maximum, 1 g/d) is recommended.
  - Instead of doxycycline, clindamycin 20–40 mg/kg/d PO in 3 doses for 5 days.
- A safe alternative for children is mefloquine, 15 mg/kg PO followed by 10 mg/kg PO 8–12 hours later.
- Other alternatives include pyrimethamine–sulfadoxine (Fansidar), quinine sulfate plus doxycycline, or atovaquone plus proguanil.

- Primaquine phosphate is used for the prevention of *P. vivax* and *P. ovale* relapses, but should not be used in patients with G6PD deficiency or in pregnancy.
- Artemisinin-based compounds such as artesunate are effective but are not currently licensed in the U.S. or United Kingdom.
- Artemisinin-based combinations are often used in 2nd and 3rd trimester of pregnancy in developing countries.

IN-PATIENT CONSIDERATIONS
Admission Criteria
Travelers diagnosed with malaria infection should be managed as inpatients.

 ONGOING CARE

PATIENT EDUCATION
- Consultation with a travel clinic is advisable when traveling into a malaria endemic zone.
- Chemoprophylaxis is not 100% effective; therefore, prevention measures against mosquito bites are equally important.

PROGNOSIS
- The prognosis depends on the *Plasmodium* species, relapsing nature of the disease, chloroquine resistance, and age of the patient.
- Infants with *P. falciparum* infection account for most of the mortality due to malaria, with case-fatality rates between 0.6–3.8%.
- If treated promptly, even *P. falciparum* malaria will respond well to current treatment options.

COMPLICATIONS
- *P. falciparum* tends to cause more severe disease, and morbidity is significantly increased due to multiorgan system involvement.
- Chronic relapses occur from *P. vivax* and *P. ovale* infections, and can occur during periods ranging from every few weeks to a few months.
- Pregnant women remain at higher risk for complication from malaria infection and should strongly be encouraged to refrain from travel to malaria endemic areas.
- Additionally, for semi-immune or nonimmune mothers, transplacental antibodies may be lacking, and the risk of congenital infection may be higher in this subgroup; fortunately, in pregnant patient, increased perinatal mortality has not been reported with malaria in stable, endemic regions.

ADDITIONAL READING
- Agarwal D, Teach SJ. Evaluation and management of a child with suspected malaria. *Pediatr Emerg Care*. 2006;22(2):127–133.
- d'Acremont V, Malila A, Swai N, et al. Withholding antimalarials in febrile children who have a negative result for a rapid diagnostic test. *Clin Infect Dis*. 2010;51(5):506–511.
- Freedman DO. Clinical practice. Malaria prevention in short-term travelers. *N Engl J Med*. 2008;359(6):603–612.

- Maitland K, Bejon P, Newton CR. Malaria. *Curr Opin Infect Dis*. 2003;16:389–395.
- Meremikwu MM, Donegan S, Esu E. Chemoprophylaxis and intermittent treatment for preventing malaria in children. *Cochrane Database Syst Rev*. 2008;(2):CD003756.
- White NJ. Antimalarial drug resistance. *J Clin Invest*. 2004;113:1084–1092.

 CODES

ICD9
- 084.1 Vivax malaria [benign tertian]
- 084.6 Malaria, unspecified
- 084.9 Other pernicious complications of malaria

ICD10
- B50.0 Plasmodium falciparum malaria with cerebral complications
- B51.9 Plasmodium vivax malaria without complication
- B54 Unspecified malaria

FAQ
- Q: What is the optimal drug regimen for the young infant or child or the lactating or pregnant female?
- A: The only drug not contraindicated in any of these patients is chloroquine. In chloroquine-resistant areas, mefloquine has been shown to be safe in the 2nd and 3rd trimesters. Limited data suggest safety in the 1st trimester also. Mefloquine is excreted in breast milk; however, limited data suggest safety for young infants. Atovaquone-proguanil is not recommended in pregnant or breastfeeding women, or in children <11 kg.
- Q: Is there a vaccine available to prevent malaria?
- A: No adequate vaccination is currently available; however, recent advances in the technology for introducing malarial DNA coding into bacteria may lead to an effective vaccine in the future.
- Q: How can I determine if the area my patient is traveling to has chloroquine-resistant malaria?
- A: The CDC has an automated traveler's hotline accessible from a touch-tone phone 24 hours a day, 7 days a week: (404) 332-4559. Questions can also be faxed to (404) 332-4565. The Internet address for information is www.cdc.gov.

M

MAMMALIAN BITES
Margaret Wolff
Jill C. Posner

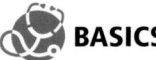 **BASICS**

DESCRIPTION
Injury to the human skin and/or subcutaneous tissues caused by bite, causing local, and in some cases systemic, effects

EPIDEMIOLOGY
- Animal bites:
  - Dogs are responsible for 90–95%, cats, 3–8%; rodents or rabbits, 1%; and raccoons and other animals, 1%.
  - 90% of the offending animals are well known to the victim.
  - Children are the most common victims:
    ○ Boys are twice as likely as girls to be bitten by dogs; girls are more likely to be bitten by cats.
- Human bites:
  - Incidence is unknown, due to lack of reporting.
  - Most common in children ages 2–5 years.
  - In older children, bites may occur accidentally during sports activities or intentionally during altercations or abusive situations.

Incidence
An estimated 4.5 million dog bites, 400,000 cat bites, and 250,000 human bites occur annually in the U.S.

GENERAL PREVENTION
Ensure that children receive routine immunizations against tetanus and hepatitis and that family pets are immunized against rabies. Encourage children to avoid contact with wild animals and dead animals.

PATHOPHYSIOLOGY
- Animal bites:
  - Dog: Crush and tear injuries, may involve bone
  - Cat: Puncture-type wounds, penetrate deeper and carry a higher risk of infection
  - Human: Generally only violate skin, although penetration into joint and tendon sheath spaces may occur (especially bites overlying the metacarpal-phalangeal areas).
- Infection:
  - Rate of infection:
    ○ Dog bites:3–18%
    ○ Cat bites:28–80%
    ○ Human bites: 15–20%
  - More recent studies have suggested an incidence of infection after dog and cat bites to be closer to 2–3%.

- Infections are most commonly polymicrobial with both aerobic and anaerobic organisms.
- Infected dog and cat bites:
  ○ *Pasteurella* species are the most frequent isolates.
  ○ Dog: *P. canis*
  ○ Cat: *P. multocida* and *P. septica*
  ○ Common anaerobes include *Fusobacterium*, bacterioids, *Porphyromonas*, and *Prevotella*.
- Infected human bites:
  ○ *Streptococcus anginosus*
  ○ *Staphylococcus aureus*
  ○ *Eikenella corrodens*
  ○ *Fusobacterium* species
  ○ *Prevotella* species

ETIOLOGY
- Animal bites:
  - Dogs
  - Cats
  - Rodents
  - Wild animals
- Human bites

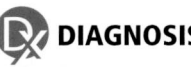 **DIAGNOSIS**

HISTORY
Animal bites:
- Type of animal
- Apparent health of the animal
- Provocation for the attack
- Location of the bite or bites
- Availability of animal for undergoing observation (i.e., is it a known animal as opposed to a stray or wild animal?)
- Rabies immunization status of the animal
- Tetanus immunization status of the child
- Hepatitis B immunization status of child
- PMH of patient: Is patient immunocompromised or asplenic?

PHYSICAL EXAM
- Carefully assess neurovascular integrity.
- Location of bite:
  - If bite is located over a joint, assess for violation of joint capsule.
- Examine entire patient to ensure that all wounds are identified and treated.
- Older wounds:
  - Assess for signs of infection such as erythema, induration, purulence, regional adenopathy, and elevated temperature.

DIAGNOSTIC TESTS & INTERPRETATION
Lab
- Blood culture if fever or systemic toxicity
- Aerobic and anaerobic cultures from infected wounds

Imaging
In penetrating injuries overlying bones or joints, consider radiography to evaluate for presence of fracture, foreign body (e.g., tooth), and air within joint.

Diagnostic Procedures/Other
No tests routinely done

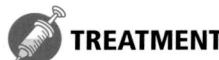 **TREATMENT**

MEDICATION (DRUGS)
- Antibiotics: Data are often contradictory. In general:
  - All cat bites should be treated with prophylactic antibiotics, due to high risk of infection with *P. multocida*.
  - Amoxicillin–clavulanic acid is drug of choice (50 mg/kg/d divided b.i.d. or t.i.d. for 5 days).
  - All human bites should be treated with antibiotic prophylaxis. Amoxicillin–clavulanic acid is drug of choice (50 mg/kg/d divided b.i.d. or t.i.d. for 5 days).
  - An alternative antibiotic regimen for penicillin-allergic patients is trimethoprim-sulfamethoxazole*plus*clindamycin.
  - Bites to the hand, face, deep puncture wounds, and wounds in immunocompromised patients may be treated empirically.
  - Skin and soft-tissue infections requiring hospitalization: Ampicillin/sulbactam 150 mg/kg/d in 4 divided doses. For penicillin-allergic patients, 3rd-generation cephalosporin. Antibiotics with poor activity against *Pasteurella* include penicillinase-resistant penicillins, clindamycin, and aminoglycosides.
- Tetanus prophylaxis if indicated

- Rabies prophylaxis if indicated:
  - Unknown dog or cat; dogs or cats with unknown immunization status that cannot be observed for 10 days
  - Bites from wild animals, including raccoons, bats, skunks, foxes, coyotes
  - Because bat bites may go undetected, especially by a sleeping child, rabies prophylaxis is now recommended after exposure to bats in a confined setting.
  - Rabies is unlikely if the child was bitten by an immunized dog, cat, or other pet (e.g., hamsters, guinea pigs, gerbils).
  - Rabies is unlikely if the child was bitten by a small rodent (squirrels, mice, or rats) or rabbit.
  - The regimen for patients who have not been vaccinated previously should include both human rabies vaccine (a series of 4 doses administered IM on days 0, 3, 7, and 14) and rabies immune globulin (20 IU/kg) administered as much as possible into the wound, the remainder given IM at a site distant from the site used for vaccine administration.
- HIV postexposure prophylaxis (PEP):
  - There are case reports describing transmission of HIV by human bites; however, the risk of transmission due to biting is unknown. It is estimated to be extremely small. Bites with saliva containing no visible blood have no associated risk for transmission and, therefore, are not considered exposures.
  - HIV PEP requires a multidrug regimen administered over 28 days that can be associated with significant toxicity.
  - Decisions to initiate PEP might best be made in consultation with local experts or by contacting the National Clinicians Post-Exposure Prophylaxis Hotline at 888-448-4911.
  - Hepatitis B has been transmitted from nonbloody saliva. Check the vaccination status of the bitten (or biter if necessary) to consider PEP. Unvaccinated children should begin the hepatitis B vaccine series.
  - The transmission rate of hepatitis C via human bites is unknown and no regimen for PEP currently exists.

ALERT

A bite with a break in the skin is considered low risk, and a bite with intact skin is felt to pose no risk.

ADDITIONAL TREATMENT
General Measures
- Wound care:
  - Copious irrigation with normal saline or tap water to remove visible debris
  - Do not use antimicrobial solutions to irrigate.
  - Cleanse but do not irrigate puncture wounds.
- Human bites over metacarpals (clenched-fist injuries) require orthopedic evaluation for possible surgical exploration and irrigation.
- Débride devitalized tissue.
- The increased risk of infection associated with suturing a potentially contaminated wound must be weighed against the cosmetic effect due to nonclosure:
  - Primary closure of larger wounds or significant facial wounds may be indicated unless wound is old or has evidence of infection.
- Hand wounds may be an exception, due to high propensity for infection.

ISSUES FOR REFERRAL
Local regulations dictate the reporting of animal bites to health departments.

 ONGOING CARE

FOLLOW-UP RECOMMENDATIONS
Patient Monitoring
- Signs and symptoms of infection
- All patients with significant bites should receive follow-up 48 hours after bite.

PROGNOSIS
Most injury from animal bites is trivial, but infections, and rarely deaths, do occur.

COMPLICATIONS
Human bites over metacarpals (clenched fist) can penetrate tendon sheaths, become infected, and result in a tenosynovitis.

ADDITIONAL READING

- Havens PL and the Committee on Pediatric AIDS. Postexposure prophylaxis in children and adolescents for nonoccupational exposure to human immunodeficiency virus. *Pediatrics*. 2003;111: 1475–1489.
- Medeiros IM, Saconato H. Antibiotic prophylaxis for mammalian bites. *Cochrane Database of Syst Rev*. 2008, Issue 3.
- Rupprecht CE, Briggs D, Brown CM, et al. Use of a reduced vaccine schedule for postexposure prophylaxis to prevent human rabies: Recommendations of the advisory committee on immunization practices. *MMWR Recomm Rep*. 2010;59(RR–2):1–9.
- Talan DA, Abrahamian FM, Moran GJ, et al. Clinical presentation and bacteriologic analysis of infected human bites in patients presenting to the emergency departments. *Clin Infect Dis*. 2003; 37:1481–1489.

CODES

ICD9
879.8 Open wound(s) (multiple) of unspecified site(s), without mention of complication

ICD10
- W55.81XA Bitten by other mammals, initial encounter
- W55.81XD Bitten by other mammals, subsequent encounter
- W55.81XS Bitten by other mammals, sequela

MASTOIDITIS

Sadiqa Edmonds
Frances M. Nadel
Oluwakemi Badaki (5th edition)

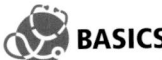 **BASICS**

DESCRIPTION
Infection of the mastoid air cells, characterized clinically by protrusion of the pinna and erythema/tenderness over the mastoid process; can range from an asymptomatic illness to a severe life-threatening disease.

EPIDEMIOLOGY
- Most patients are between 6–24 months old.
- Males more than females, ratio of 2:1
- It is unusual to see mastoiditis in the very young, because of incomplete pneumatization of the mastoid air cells.

Incidence
- At the start of the 20th century, 20–50% of cases of otitis media developed into coalescent mastoiditis. The routine use of antibiotics for otitis media and aggressive management of treatment failures has decreased incidence to 0.2–0.4%.
- Although some single-site reports have suggested that mastoiditis is on the rise, larger population-based studies demonstrate a stable incidence.

RISK FACTORS
- Age <2 years of age
- Acute otitis media

GENERAL PREVENTION
- Appropriate early treatment of otitis media and timely follow-up to identify treatment failures
- Avoid factors that predispose to otitis media, including caretaker smoking and bottle-feeding.
- Early recognition of mastoiditis decreases the risk of intracranial complications.
- Streptococcal vaccination may help decrease the occurrence of otitis media.

PATHOPHYSIOLOGY
- The mastoid process is the posterior portion of the temporal bone and consists of interconnecting air cells that drain superiorly into the middle ear. Because these mastoid air cells connect with the middle ear, all cases of acute otitis media are associated with some mastoid inflammation.
- Acute mastoiditis develops when the accumulation of purulent exudate in the middle ear does not drain through the eustachian tube or through a perforated tympanic membrane but spreads to the mastoid.
- Acute mastoiditis can progress to a coalescent phase after the bony air cells are destroyed and may then progress to subperiosteal abscess or to chronic mastoiditis.

ETIOLOGY
- Acute mastoiditis is generally caused by an extension of the inflammation and infection of acute otitis media into the mastoid air cells. However, up to 50% of patients present without evidence of preceding otitis media.
- The bacteria isolated from middle ear drainage or from the mastoid are usually *Streptococcus pneumoniae*, *Streptococcus pyogenes*, *Haemophilus influenzae*, or *Staphylococcus aureus*. However, many patients' cultures are sterile:
  – *S. pneumoniae* is the most frequently isolated cause of mastoiditis in pediatric patients. *S. pneumoniae* resistance to penicillin may be as high as 30%, with the 19A serotype being the most common. With the advent of the new 13 valent pneumococcal vaccine (which contains the 19A serotype), the epidemiology may change in the coming years.
- Chronic mastoiditis is usually caused by *S. aureus*, anaerobic bacteria, enteric bacteria, and *Pseudomonas aeruginosa*:
  – Chronic mastoiditis is often a multiple-organism infection.
- Unusual agents of chronic mastoiditis include *Mycobacterium tuberculosis*, atypical mycobacteria, *Nocardia asteroides*, and *Histoplasma capsulatum*.
- Cholesteatomas may contribute to the development of mastoiditis by impeding mastoid drainage or erosion of underlying bone.

DIAGNOSIS

HISTORY
- Usually includes a recent or a chronic history of treatment for otitis media
- Sign and symptoms:
  – May include fever, otalgia, otorrhea, and postauricular swelling:
    ○ Children who are already on antibiotics may present with more subtle findings.
  – Intracranial extension should be suspected if there is lethargy, a stiff neck, headache, focal neurologic symptoms, seizures, visual changes, or persistent fevers despite appropriate antibiotic treatment.
  – Labyrinthitis initially presents with tinnitus and nausea, which can progress to vomiting, vertigo, nystagmus, and loss of balance.

PHYSICAL EXAM
- The ear may protrude away from the scalp:
  – In infants, the ear protrudes out and is displaced down.
- The tympanic membrane often is hyperemic, with decreased mobility:
  – The tympanic membranes of children on antibiotics may have a normal appearance.
- The mastoid process is tender, with soft-tissue swelling:
  – The overlying skin may be warm and erythematous, with posterior auricular fluctuance.
- In chronic mastoiditis, the fever and posterior auricular swelling are often not present, and the patient presents with ear pain, persistent drainage, or hearing loss.

DIAGNOSTIC TESTS & INTERPRETATION
Lab
- CBC with differential:
  – May show a leukocytosis with a neutrophil predominance
- ESR/CRP:
  – May be elevated in acute mastoiditis but is usually normal in the chronic stage; more often seen elevated in complicated mastoiditis
- Purified protein derivative (PPD):
  – Should be done if tuberculosis is suspected
- Middle-ear aspirate obtained by myringotomy:
  – Gram stain and cultures for aerobic and anaerobic bacteria
  – There is some correlation between middle-ear bacterial cultures and mastoid cultures.

Imaging
- X-rays:
  – Reveal haziness of the mastoid air cells and can show bony destruction in more advanced disease
  – Are unreliable and can be falsely normal, as well as falsely abnormal
- Temporal bone and cranial CT:
  – Helpful in the confirmation of the diagnosis, identification of coalescence or a subperiosteal abscess, and evaluation for concomitant intracranial complications
  – Intracranial complications are best seen with MRI.

Diagnostic Procedures/Other
Lumbar puncture must be performed in any child with symptoms of meningitis.

DIFFERENTIAL DIAGNOSIS
- Parotitis
- Posterior auricular lymphadenopathy or cellulitis
- Otitis externa or an ear canal furuncle
- Neoplastic disease:
  – Leukemia
  – Lymphoma
  – Rhabdomyosarcoma
  – Histiocytosis X
- Branchial cleft anomaly
- Tuberculosis

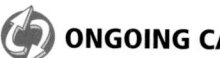 TREATMENT

MEDICATION (DRUGS)
- Parenteral antibiotics are chosen on the basis of the most likely organisms and regional bacterial resistance patterns.
- In acute mastoiditis, broad-spectrum antibiotics such as ampicillin-sulbactam, ceftriaxone, or clindamycin can be used. If pseudomonas is suspected, antibiotic coverage should be expanded to cover this organism.
- Broad-spectrum coverage, such as oxacillin and gentamicin is recommended for chronic mastoiditis.
- If *M. tuberculosis* is suspected, then antituberculosis therapy should be started.

ADDITIONAL TREATMENT
General Measures
Middle-ear drainage is essential; therefore, a myringotomy with or without tube placement should be performed early.

SURGERY/OTHER PROCEDURES
- Indications for surgical intervention include:
  – Subperiosteal abscess
  – Coalescence
  – Facial nerve palsy
  – Meningitis
  – Intracranial abscess
  – Venous thrombosis
  – Persistent symptoms despite adequate antibiotic treatment
- In the preantibiotic era, mastoidectomy was the treatment of choice for mastoiditis. Currently, this therapy is generally reserved for cases complicated by the indications above.

IN-PATIENT CONSIDERATIONS
Admission Criteria
Admit for IV antibiotics, and for ear, nose, and throat (ENT) evaluation to ensure response to antibiotics and to rule out complications.

ONGOING CARE

FOLLOW-UP RECOMMENDATIONS
Patient Monitoring
- If patients respond quickly to parenteral therapy, they can complete a 3-week course with oral antibiotics and weekly follow-up visits.
- Audiograms should be performed later to screen for hearing loss.

PROGNOSIS
- Mastoiditis has a good prognosis if treated early. However, intracranial extension of mastoiditis can lead to permanent neurologic deficits and death.
- Chronic mastoiditis can lead to irreversible hearing loss.

COMPLICATIONS
- The mastoid's proximity to many important structures can result in serious complications from extension of infection or as a response to the inflammatory process.
- Complication rates may be as high as 16%.
- Intracranial complications include meningitis and extradural, subdural, or brain parenchymal abscesses.
- Venous sinus thrombophlebitis results from extension of disease to the sigmoid or lateral sinus:
  – Sepsis, increased intracranial pressure, or septic emboli may result.
- Facial nerve palsy is usually unilateral and can be permanent.
- Labyrinthitis, petrositis, or osteomyelitis may result from extension of the infection into adjacent bones.
- Subperiosteal abscess
- Hearing loss can occur from destruction of the ossicles or from labyrinthine damage.
- Bezold abscess is a deep neck abscess along the medial sternocleidomastoid muscle that develops when the infection erodes through the tip of the mastoid bone and dissects down tissue planes.
- Gradenigo syndrome:
  – Triad of 6th nerve palsy, retro-orbital pain and otorrhea

ADDITIONAL READING

- Agrawal S, Husein M, MacRae D. Complications of otitis media: An evolving state. *J Otolaryngol*. 2005;34(Suppl 1):S33–S39.
- Anderson K, Adam H. Mastoiditis. *Pediatr Rev*. 2009;30:233–234.
- Bilavsky E, Yarden-Bilavsky H, Samra Z, et al. Clinical, laboratory, and microbiological differences between children with simple or complicated mastoiditis. *Int J Pediatr Otorhinolaryngol*. 2009;73:1270–1273.
- Kaplan SL, Mason EO Jr., Wald ER, et al. Pneumococcal mastoiditis in children. *Pediatrics*. 2000;106(4):695–699.
- Pang L, Barakete M, Havas T. Mastoiditis in a pediatric population: A review of 11 years of experience in management. *Int J Pediatr Otorhinolaryngol*. 2009;73:1520–1524.
- Smith JA, Danner CJ. Complications of chronic otitis media and cholesteatoma. *Otolaryngol Clin North Am*. 2006;39(6):1237–1255.
- Zanetti D, Nassif N. Indications for surgery in acute mastoiditis and their complications in children. *Int J Pediatr Otorhinolaryngol*. 2006;70(7):1175–1182.

 CODES

ICD9
- 383.00 Acute mastoiditis without complications
- 383.02 Acute mastoiditis with other complications
- 383.9 Unspecified mastoiditis

ICD10
- H70.009 Acute mastoiditis without complications, unspecified ear
- H70.099 Acute mastoiditis with other complications, unspecified ear
- H70.90 Unspecified mastoiditis, unspecified ear

FAQ
- Q: Do all children with mastoiditis need a CT scan of the head if mastoiditis is suspected?
- A: No. In general, if the child with mastoiditis has mild swelling, no fluctuance of the mastoid, and responds to therapy, no CT scan is needed. A patient who appears toxic or fails to respond to appropriate antibiotic therapy, or one who may be a surgical candidate, should undergo additional imaging studies.
- Q: Should all children with mastoiditis be admitted to the hospital?
- A: Yes. In general, admission with IV antibiotics and ENT evaluation is warranted to ensure response to antibiotics and rule out complications.

M

MEASLES (RUBEOLA, FIRST DISEASE)

Jeffrey S. Gerber

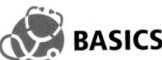 **BASICS**

DESCRIPTION

- An exanthematous disease that has a relatively predictable course, making clinical diagnosis possible.
- Misdiagnosis is common. Because it is rare and may occur in outbreaks, cases are often initially misdiagnosed as Kawasaki disease or Stevens-Johnson syndrome.
- Patients are contagious from 1–2 days before onset of symptoms (3–5 days before rash) until 5 days after the appearance of the rash. The incubation period is generally 8–12 days from exposure to onset of symptoms and ~14 days until the appearance of rash.
- Types of measles include the following:
  – Typical measles
  – Modified measles: Occurs in children with partial antibody protection (after post-exposure administration of immunoglobulin or in infants <9 months old with transplacental antibodies).
    ○ Clinically similar to typical measles but is generally mild
    ○ The patient may be afebrile and the rash may last only 1–2 days.
  – Atypical measles: Caused by a hypersensitivity reaction to measles infection in those who received killed virus vaccine between 1963 and 1967 and are subsequently exposed to wild-type virus.

EPIDEMIOLOGY

- Measles is one of the most highly contagious of all infectious diseases.
- Hospital or clinic waiting rooms (especially pediatric emergency department waiting rooms) have been identified as a major risk, accounting for up to 45% of the known exposures. With adequate immunization (2 doses = 99% effective), measles could be eliminated as a disease.
- Although no longer endemic in the U.S., networks of intentionally unvaccinated children have led to several recent U.S. outbreaks originating from measles virus imported from abroad.
- Since 20 million cases of measles occur globally per year (>150,000 deaths), it is critical to maintain high levels of vaccination coverage.

Incidence

- Before the 1963 licensure of vaccine, an estimated 3–4 million people acquired measles in the U.S. each year; by 1983, there were only 0.7 cases per 100,000 population.
- Delays in immunization facilitated large outbreaks in the U.S. from 1989–1991, peaking in 1990 when 27,672 cases were reported, 89 of which were fatal.
- From 2001–2008, 557 cases of measles and 38 outbreaks were reported in the U.S.; 42% were known to be imported from 44 countries.

GENERAL PREVENTION

- Vaccine recommendations:
  – Routine vaccination against measles, mumps, and rubella (MMR) for children begins at 12–15 months of age, with a second MMR vaccination at age 4–6 years.
  – With the recent resurgence of measles, aggressive employee immunization programs should be pursued for all health care workers.
  – Health care workers born after 1956 who have no documentation of vaccination or evidence of measles immunity should be vaccinated at the time of employment and revaccinated ≥28 days later.
- Infection control measures:
  – Any inpatient suspected of having measles should be in a negative-pressure respiratory isolation room; health care workers must wear masks, gloves, and gowns (airborne and contact precautions).
  – Isolation is required for 4 days after the 1st appearance of the rash; immune-compromised patients require isolation for the course of the illness.
  – All suspected cases of measles should be reported immediately to the local health department.

PATHOPHYSIOLOGY

Transmission of measles occurs through direct contact with infectious droplets; less commonly by airborne spread.

ETIOLOGY

Measles is an RNA virus (paramyxovirus, genus *Morbillivirus*) with only 1 serotype.

DIAGNOSIS

- The disease involves fever, cough, conjunctivitis, and coryza with an erythematous rash, which has a characteristic progression:
  – The rash appears on the face (often the nape of the neck, initially) and abdomen 14 days after exposure. The rash is erythematous and maculopapular and spreads from the head to the feet, often becoming confluent at more proximal sites.
- Pharyngitis, cervical lymphadenopathy, and splenomegaly may accompany the rash.

- Atypical measles:
  – This group of young adults (2nd and 3rd decades of life) may become quite ill, with sudden onset of fever from 103–105°F and headache. The rash, unlike typical measles, appears initially on the distal extremities, progressing cephalad.
  – Most patients with atypical measles have pneumonia, often with pleural effusions.
  – Diagnosis depends on clinical recognition and by serologic and molecular (RNA) testing.

HISTORY

- Case definition from the CDC includes:
  – Generalized rash lasting ≥3 days; and
  – A temperature of ≥38.3°C (101°F); and
  – Cough, coryza, or conjunctivitis; and
  – Positive testing or epidemiologic linkage to known case
- The mean incubation period is 10 days (range: 8–21 days).
- The prodrome of measles lasts 2–4 days and begins with symptoms of upper respiratory infection, fever up to 104°F, malaise, conjunctivitis, photophobia, and increasing cough.
- During the prodrome, Koplik spots (white spots on the buccal mucosa) appear on most people.
- Following this prodrome, the rash appears on the face (often initially at the hairline) and abdomen (14 days after exposure). The rash is erythematous and maculopapular and spreads from the head to the feet.
- After 3–4 days, the rash begins to clear, leaving a brownish discoloration and fine scaling.
- Fever usually resolves by the 4th day of rash.

DIAGNOSTIC TESTS & INTERPRETATION

- The course of typical measles follows a predictable pattern; therefore, laboratory studies to confirm infection are rarely indicated.
- At the beginning of a suspected case, confirmation of the index cases is important.

Lab

- Serum measles-specific IgM titer (simplest):
  – Sensitivity may be diminished if assay performed <72 hours from onset of rash; repeat if negative. IgM detectable for at least 1 month from onset of rash.
  – A comparison of IgG titers obtained during the acute and convalescent stages can be done. Blood samples must be taken at least 7–10 days apart.
  – Culture or RNA (RT-PCR) testing of nasopharyngeal, throat, blood, or urine.

DIFFERENTIAL DIAGNOSIS

With a careful history and physical exam, it is usually possible to diagnose measles. The differential diagnosis includes:

- Steven-Johnson syndrome
- Kawasaki disease
- Other viral exanthem
- Meningococcemia
- Rocky Mountain spotted fever (RMSF)
- Toxic shock syndrome

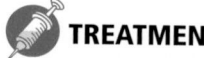 **TREATMENT**

ADDITIONAL TREATMENT
General Measures
- No specific therapy; supportive care.
- Ribavirin active in vitro, but not approved by FDA for treatment of measles.
- Antipyretics, oral fluids, and room humidification to help reduce cough are usually sufficient.
- Vitamin A treatment of children with measles in developing countries has been associated with decreases in both morbidity and mortality.
  - The World Health Organization recommends vitamin A for all children with measles worldwide.
  - Vitamin A is given once daily for 2 days:
    ○ 200,000 IU for children ≥12 months of age.
    ○ 100,000 IU for infants 6–11 months of age.
    ○ 50,000 IU for infants <6 months of age.
  - The higher dose may be associated with vomiting and headache for a few hours.
  - For children with ophthalmologic evidence of vitamin A deficiency, a 3rd dose at 4 weeks is indicated.
  - Vitamin A is available in 50,000 IU/mL solution and may be given orally.

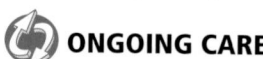 **ONGOING CARE**

FOLLOW-UP RECOMMENDATIONS
In uncomplicated measles infection, clinical improvement and fading of rash typically occur on the 3rd or 4th day.

PROGNOSIS
- Mortality in the modern outbreak of 1989–1990 occurred in 3 of every 1,000 cases in the U.S.
- Case fatality rates are increased in immunocompromised children.

COMPLICATIONS
- Complication rate in 1989–1990 outbreaks that occurred throughout the country was 23% and included diarrhea (9%), otitis media (7%), pneumonia (6%), and encephalitis (0.1%):
  - Encephalitis, which can lead to permanent neurologic sequelae, occurs in 1 of every 1,000 cases reported in the U.S.
  - Croup, myocarditis, pericarditis, and disseminated intravascular coagulation (black measles) can also occur.
- In 1990, ~18–20% of patients required hospitalization, many for either dehydration or pneumonia.
- In patients with poor nutrition, most common in developing countries, mortality is higher.
- Subacute sclerosis panencephalitis (SSPE) occurs in 1 per 100,000 children with naturally occurring measles:
  - After an incubation period of several years (mean 10.8), a progressive, usually fatal, encephalopathy develops among unvaccinated children.
  - Patients with SSPE are not infectious.

ADDITIONAL READING
- American Academy of Pediatrics. Measles. In: Pickering LK, Baker CJ, Kimberlin DW, Long SS. *Red Book: 2009 Report of the Committee on Infectious Diseases*, 28th ed. Elk Grove Village, IL: American Academy of Pediatrics; 2009:444–455.
- Duke T, Mgone CS. Measles: Not just another viral exanthema. *Lancet*. 2003;361:763–773.
- Farizo KM, Stehr-Green PA, Simpsons DM, et al. Pediatric emergency room visits: A risk factor for acquiring measles. *Pediatrics*. 1991;98:74.
- Global Measles Mortality, 2000–2008. *MMWR*. December 4, 2009;58(47):1321–1326.
- Huiming Y, Chaomin W, Meng M. Vitamin A for treating measles in children. *Cochrane Database System Rev*. 2005:CD001479.
- Parker Fiebelkorn A, Redd SB, Gallagher K, et al. Measles in the U.S. during the Postelimination Era. *J Infect Dis*. 2010;202(10):1520–1528.
- Perry RT, Halsey NA. The clinical significance of measles: A review. *J Infect Dis*. 2004;189(Suppl 1):S4–S16.
- Rall GF. Measles virus 1998–2002: Progress and controversy. *Annu Rev Microbiol*. 2003;57:343–367.
- Sugerman DE, Barskey AE, Delea MG, et al. Measles outbreak in a highly vaccinated population, San Diego, 2008: Role of the intentionally undervaccinated. *Pediatrics*. 2010;125;747–755.

 CODES

ICD9
055.9 Measles without mention of complication
ICD10
- B05.89 Other measles complications
- B05.9 Measles without complication

FAQ
- Q: If a health care worker has had a natural measles infection or measles immunization, should one be concerned about infection following exposure?
- A: Those persons born before 1957 who had wildtype measles virus infection are usually immune from reinfection. However, in a report in 1993, 4 health care workers who were previously vaccinated with positive preillness measles antibody levels developed modified measles following exposure to infected patients. Therefore, all health care workers should observe respiratory precautions in caring for patients with measles.
- Q: During an outbreak of measles, should children <12 months of age be vaccinated?
- A: In an outbreak of measles, public health officials may recommend vaccination of infants ages 6–11 months with a single-antigen measles vaccine; children initially vaccinated before their 1st birthday should be revaccinated at 12–15 months of age. A 2nd dose should be administered during the early school years.

MECKEL DIVERTICULUM

Edisio Semeao

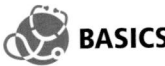 **BASICS**

DESCRIPTION
- Meckel diverticulum is the most common congenital abnormality of the GI tract.
- A congenital anomaly that is part of the group known as the omphalomesenteric duct remnants
- In pediatric patients, the most common clinical presentation is with painless rectal bleeding.
- Other symptoms that may also be described include recurrent abdominal pain, abdominal distention, nausea, and/or vomiting.

EPIDEMIOLOGY
- Meckel diverticulum was 1st described by Johann Meckel in 1809.
- A remnant of the embryonic yolk sac found in ~2% of all infants
- Although the presence of Meckel diverticulum is 2% in the population, the rarity of this anomaly in clinical practice is that only 4–6.5% of patients are symptomatic.
- The development of symptoms seems to be age related, with the peak incidence being early childhood (2 years).
- 80% of all patients requiring surgery were <10 years of age, and nearly 50% were <2 years of age.

Incidence
- Meckel diverticulum tends to be more common in males, with a male/female ratio of 3:2, and also with males having more symptomatic diverticula.
- These have also been associated with several other congenital anomalies that include:
  – Anorectal atresia (11%)
  – Esophageal atresia (12%)
  – Minor omphalocele (25%)
  – Cardiac malformations
  – Exophthalmos
  – Cleft palate
  – Annular pancreas
  – Some central nervous system malformations

PATHOPHYSIOLOGY
- Meckel diverticulum is a true diverticulum containing all 3 layers of the bowel wall, and its vascular supply comes from a remnant of the vitelline artery.
- Most of these diverticula are lined with ileal mucosa, but ectopic tissue is often present.
- ~50% of diverticula contain ectopic tissue.
  – Gastric tissue accounts for 60–85%.
  – Pancreatic tissue accounts for 5–16%.
  – Other less common tissue types include colonic and duodenal.
- Of the symptomatic cases of Meckel diverticulum, 40–80% have some type of ectopic tissue, with the most common being gastric or pancreatic type.

ETIOLOGY
- This abnormality results from the incomplete obliteration of the fetal omphalomesenteric (vitelline) duct between the 7th and 8th weeks of gestation.
- The vitelline duct communicates with the yolk sac and involutes as the placenta replaces the yolk sac as the source of fetal nutrition. Failure of this process results in various anomalies; Meckel diverticulum accounts for 90% of the vitelline duct anomalies.
- This diverticulum originates from the antimesenteric border of the bowel in the region of the terminal ileum and proximal to the ileocecal valve. It can be between 3 and 6 cm in length.
- Other intestinal diverticula are more common in the jejunum and on the mesenteric border of the bowel.

COMMONLY ASSOCIATED CONDITIONS
Malignancies have also been reported in association with Meckel diverticulum. These are present within the diverticulum and can cause obstructive symptoms or can be found incidentally. Sarcomas are most common, followed by carcinoids and adenocarcinomas.

DIAGNOSIS

HISTORY
- Bleeding:
  – In children, the most common presentation is with painless rectal bleeding, which may range from occult blood to frank bright red blood and hemodynamic instability.
  – Bleeding is thought to occur owing to the highly acidic secretions of the gastric tissue on the adjacent tissues, which may cause ulcerations that lead to bleeding. Similarly, the alkaline secretions of the pancreatic tissue may also cause ulcerations and lead to bleeding.
  – The bleeding, even in the most severe cases, tends to be self-limiting, because of constriction of the splanchnic vessels secondary to hypovolemia.
  – Bleeding is most commonly seen in children <5 years of age. In diverticula that bleed, 90% have ectopic gastric mucosa.
- Obstruction:
  – Partial or complete small bowel obstruction
  – The clinical symptoms in this setting include recurrent abdominal pain, abdominal distention, nausea, and vomiting.
  – This is the most common type of presentation in adults and can also occur in up to 40% of pediatric patients. It results from intussusception, in which the Meckel diverticulum serves as a lead point.
  – Intraperitoneal bands, volvulus, or internal herniation may also lead to an obstructive presentation.

- Inflammation/fever:
  – Another common presentation for symptomatic Meckel diverticulum is inflammation/diverticulitis, which can occur in 12–40% of cases.
  – Patients often present with signs and symptoms consistent with appendicitis, and the diagnosis is made at the time of surgical exploration.
  – In a subset of this group (~1/3), the diverticulum may perforate from infarction or ulceration and lead to a more acute and toxic presentation.
  – The rule of 2s: 2% of the population, 2 inches in length, 2 feet from the ileal cecal valve, 2 types of tissue, 2% are symptomatic, 2 times more boys affected than girls.

PHYSICAL EXAM
- Physical exam findings are variable and are dependent upon the type of presenting complications.
- In children with rectal bleeding, the exam is usually benign except for a positive rectal exam and usually low BP and tachycardia.
- Patients with obstructive symptoms may have abdominal distention and tenderness and hyperactive bowel sounds.
- Patients with an inflammatory (diverticulitis) type of presentation will have findings similar to those in appendicitis, with the possibility of peritoneal signs in cases of perforation.
- Signs and symptoms:
  – Rectal bleeding
  – Obstruction: Abdominal pain/vomiting
  – Inflammation: Fever

DIAGNOSTIC TESTS & INTERPRETATION
- The diagnosis of symptomatic Meckel diverticulum is difficult to make and requires a high index of suspicion.
- This diagnosis should be considered in any patient with recurrent unexplained abdominal pain, nausea and vomiting, or rectal bleeding.

Lab
- The diagnosis cannot be made with laboratory evaluation or plain radiography.
- Laboratory analysis may be helpful to determine the degree of bleeding with a hemoglobin count and a coagulation profile to rule out an underlying bleeding disorder.
- Plain radiographs may show evidence of obstruction, but are not diagnostic of Meckel diverticulum.

Imaging
- Contrast studies such as upper gastrointestinal series with small bowel follow-through or enteroclysis studies are limited in value because the layers of barium in the bowel can obscure the diverticulum.
- CT scan and ultrasound are often nonspecific in diagnosis but can be helpful in looking for other causes of presenting symptoms.

- Endoscopy and colonoscopy are not sensitive for the diagnosis but can be helpful in identifying other causes that may explain symptoms.
- Angiography may not be helpful because the vascular supply is usually normal.
- Red cell–tagged scans are not specific for Meckel diverticulum, but may be useful in localizing the site of bleeding.

Diagnostic Procedures/Other
- The most useful method of diagnosis of Meckel diverticulum is with a Meckel scan (technetium-99m pertechnetate scan):
  - This technique, however, depends on the presence of ectopic gastric mucosa within the diverticulum to have uptake of the isotope by the gastric mucosa. Because not all diverticula contain gastric mucosa, this scan may not be of value in all situations.
  - However, because complications such as bleeding are usually (90%) associated with ectopic gastric tissue, this test may be diagnostic in many symptomatic cases.
  - In children, the scan has a sensitivity and specificity of 85% and 95%, respectively, but in adults these values fall to 62.5% and 9%, respectively.
  - Technetium-99m pertechnetate is taken up by the ectopic gastric tissue (mucous neck secreting cells). Certain substances enhance the detection of the ectopic gastric tissue, including cimetidine, glucagon, and pentagastrin.
- False results can occur in 20% of the scans.
  - False-positive results with bleeding: Intussusception, hemangioma, arteriovenous malformation (AVM), inflammatory lesion, Crohn disease, peptic ulcer, carcinoid and uterine fibroids
  - False-positive results without bleeding: Ureteral obstruction, sacral meningomyelocele
  - False-negative results: Barium, bladder overdistention, no gastric mucosa present
- Surgery: In situations in which the Meckel scan is nondiagnostic or in patients with nonbleeding symptoms (but when there is a high index of suspicion for Meckel diverticulum), laparoscopy has been shown to be effective and have less morbidity than an exploratory laparotomy.

DIFFERENTIAL DIAGNOSIS
Based on the 2 main clinical symptoms:
- Bleeding:
  - Rectal fissure
  - Polyps
  - Allergic proctitis
  - Infectious colitis
  - Lymphonodular hyperplasia
  - AVM
  - Hirschsprung enterocolitis
  - Peptic ulcer disease
  - Inflammatory bowel disease
  - Hemolytic uremic syndrome
  - Henoch-Schönlein purpura

- Obstruction:
  - Appendicitis
  - Intussusception
  - Malrotation/volvulus
  - Intestinal duplication
  - Colonic diverticulitis
  - Adhesions/strictures

 TREATMENT

ADDITIONAL TREATMENT
General Measures
The treatment for Meckel diverticula that are symptomatic and identified is surgical removal.

SURGERY/OTHER PROCEDURES
- Surgical resection can be done with simple diverticulectomy, but in cases in which the adjunct ileum is damaged or there is further evidence of ectopic tissue, a limited resection may be required.
- The bigger dilemma is what should be the approach when a Meckel diverticulum is found incidentally and the patient is asymptomatic:
  - Previous research had indicated that the morbidity for diverticulectomy is ~9% and that, because the risk of developing symptoms in a lifetime was 4%, these diverticula should be left in place. More recent work has shown a much lower morbidity (2%) associated with the removal of the diverticulum; thus, some researchers have advocated removal of the diverticulum that is found incidentally.
  - The development of new techniques such as laparoscopy and stapling devices has aided in decreasing the morbidity and mortality in this procedure.
- There have been several series that have compared features of symptomatic versus asymptomatic diverticula to see if there are characteristics that would help in deciding the approach to asymptomatic diverticulum. If these features are noted, the risk of developing symptoms later in life if the diverticulum is not removed is significantly increased. These include:
  - Age, younger patients (<8–10 years of age)
  - Longer diverticulum (≥2 cm)
  - Narrower base (≤2 cm in diameter)

IN-PATIENT CONSIDERATIONS
Initial Stabilization
- Bleeding: Address issues of anemia and volume status based on vital signs and blood tests.
- Obstruction: Evaluate the need for acute management (surgical) and decompression.

ADDITIONAL READING

- McCollough M, Sharieff G. Abdominal surgical emergencies in infants and young children. Emerg Med Clin N Am. 2003;21(4):909–935.
- Mendelson K, Bailey B, Balint T, et al. Meckel diverticulum: Review and surgical management. Curr Surg. 2001;58(5):455–457.
- Ruscher KA, Fisher JN, Hughes CD, et al. National trends in the surgical management of Meckel diverticulum. J Pediatr Surg. 2011;46(5):893–896.
- Shalabi R, Soliman S, Fawy M, et al. Laparoscopic management of Meckel diverticulum in children. J Pediatr Surg. 2005;40(3):562–567.
- Snyder CL. Current management of umbilical abnormalities and related anomalies. Semin Pediatr Surg. 2007;16(1):41–49.
- Uppal K, ShaneTubbs R, Matusz P, et al. Meckel diverticulum: A review. Clin Anat. 2011;24(4): 416–422.

 CODES

ICD9
751.0 Meckel's diverticulum

ICD10
Q43.0 Meckel's diverticulum (displaced) (hypertrophic)

FAQ

- Q: What are the reasons for resection of a Meckel diverticulum?
- A: Narrowing at base of diverticulum or presence of ectopic tissue resulting in bleeding
- Q: What is the most common ectopic tissue present in Meckel diverticulum?
- A: Gastric
- Q: What is the most common presentation of a Meckel diverticulum?
- A: Intermittent, painless rectal bleeding

M

MEDIASTINAL MASS

Charles Bailey

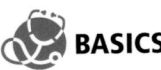 **BASICS**

DEFINITION
Space-occupying lesion of the mediastinum:
- Anterior mediastinum includes the thymus and other structures anterior to the pericardium.
- Middle mediastinum contains the heart, great vessels, ascending aorta, and aortic arch, as well as lymph nodes.
- Posterior mediastinum contains the tracheobronchial tree, esophagus, descending aorta, and neural structures.

PATHOPHYSIOLOGY
Morbidity is due to compression of adjacent normal structures, particularly large airways, heart, and great vessels.

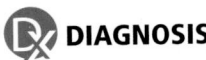 **DIAGNOSIS**

DIFFERENTIAL DIAGNOSIS
- Congenital/anatomic:
  - Thoracic meningocele (posterior)
  - Large normal thymus in neonate (anterior)
  - Bronchogenic, pericardial, or foregut cyst (middle)
  - Aortic aneurysm and other vascular anomalies (middle)
- Infectious (may cause mediastinal adenopathy and/or pulmonary nodules) (middle/posterior):
  - Tuberculosis
  - Histoplasmosis
  - Aspergillosis
  - Coccidioidomycosis
  - Blastomycosis
- Foreign body in the trachea or esophagus
- Sarcoidosis
- Tumor:
  - Benign:
    - Thymoma (anterior)
    - Teratoma/Dermoid cyst (anterior)
    - Lymphangioma/Cystic hygroma (middle/posterior)
    - Hemangioma (posterior/middle)
    - Ganglioneuroma (posterior)
    - Neurofibroma (posterior)
  - Malignant:
    - Hodgkin's lymphoma (anterior/middle)
    - Non-Hodgkin's lymphoma or leukemia (anterior/middle)
    - Neuroblastoma (posterior)
    - Ganglioneuroblastoma (posterior)
    - Ewing sarcoma or osteogenic sarcoma (anterior/posterior)
    - Malignant germ cell tumor (anterior)
    - Pheochromocytoma (posterior)
    - Rhabdomyosarcoma or pleuropulmonary blastoma (any)
    - Neurofibrosarcoma (posterior)

APPROACH TO THE PATIENT
Goal is to establish diagnosis promptly and begin treatment as indicated, because condition may progress rapidly and become life threatening. If you suspect a malignancy, the child should be immediately referred to an oncologist.

HISTORY
- **Question:** Systemic symptoms (fever, weight loss, night sweats, fatigue)?
- *Significance:* May be associated with infection or malignancy.
- **Question:** Cough, wheeze, dyspnea on exertion, orthopnea?
- *Significance:* May indicate early airway compromise.
- **Question:** Face/neck swelling?
- *Significance:* Suggests superior vena cava syndrome.

PHYSICAL EXAM
- Pulse oximetry
- Check for signs and symptoms noted below
- **Finding:** Edema/suffusion of face and neck, jugular venous distension, conjunctival injection, headache, altered mental status?
- *Significance:* Superior vena cava syndrome.
- **Finding:** Cough (nonproductive), orthopnea or dyspnea, stridor or wheezing?
- *Significance:* Airway compression.
- **Finding:** Quiet heart sounds, hypotension, narrowed pulse pressure, or pulsus paradoxus?
- *Significance:* Cardiac tamponade/diastolic dysfunction.
- **Finding:** Lymphadenopathy or hepatosplenomegaly?
- *Significance:* Suggests malignancy or infection. Low cervical, posterior, or supraclavicular adenopathy particularly concerning for malignancy.
- **Finding:** Ecchymoses, petechiae, and mucosal bleeding?
- *Significance:* Suggest thrombocytopenia, which can be seen in leukemia.
- **Finding:** Horner syndrome.
- *Significance:* Posterior mediastinal mass, most commonly a neuroblastoma in a young child?

DIAGNOSTIC TESTS & INTERPRETATION
Consider pulmonary function tests if respiratory reserve is in question.
- **Test:** CBC with differential.
- *Significance:* Anemia, thrombocytopenia, neutropenia, or circulating blasts frequently noted in leukemia or lymphoma; leukocytosis in infection.
- **Test:** Lactate dehydrogenase, uric acid, electrolytes, phosphate, creatinine.
- *Significance:* Tumor lysis screen.
- **Test:** Purified protein derivative (PPD) skin test.
- *Significance:* Tuberculosis.

- **Test:** Other assays for specific pathogens based on history of exposure.
- *Significance:* For a patient with a large mass or potential cardiopulmonary compromise, goal is rapid diagnosis using least invasive/painful procedure, to minimize need for sedation/anesthesia.
- **Test:** Bone marrow aspiration/biopsy.
- *Significance:* Simplest procedure if CBC is suspicious.
- **Test:** Lymph node biopsy.
- *Significance:* If adenopathy at easily accessible site.
- **Test:** Biopsy of mass.
- *Significance:* Consider radiologically guided needle biopsy.
- **Test:** Pleurocentesis, pericardiocentesis, or excision of isolated mass.
- *Significance:* May have both diagnostic and therapeutic roles.
- **Test:** Lumbar puncture.
- *Significance:* May be combined with other procedures if meningitis or hematologic malignancy is suspected.

ALERT
Recumbent positioning, sedation, or positive pressure ventilation may lead to catastrophic respiratory or cardiovascular collapse in patients with partial compromise. Procedures may need to be done with local anesthesia or minimal sedation in these patients.

Imaging
- Chest radiograph (lateral film required) to establish size and location of mass
- CT of the chest (if patient can tolerate semirecumbent positioning) to define size, location, and consistency of mass, and to assess large blood vessels and airways
- Echocardiogram to assess diastolic filling and vascular patency

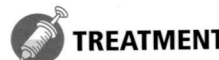 **TREATMENT**

- First Line
  - Steroids may be given after diagnosis is obtained to treat hematologic malignancies or decrease edema/inflammation.
  - Additional therapy depends on diagnosis (e.g., chemotherapy, antibiotics).

SPECIAL THERAPY
- Radiotherapy
  - May be indicated for emergent management of malignancies

ADDITIONAL TREATMENT
General Measures
- Close monitoring of cardiorespiratory status
- With cardiorespiratory compromise, attempt to avoid positive-pressure ventilation, if feasible
- Definitive therapy will be based on the diagnosis.

ALERT
- Do not treat a patient with wheezing who has no history of asthma with steroids without obtaining a chest radiograph to confirm that there is no mediastinal mass.
- If symptoms are progressing rapidly or there is evidence of superior vena cava syndrome, tracheal compression, or spinal cord compression, emergent steroids or radiation may be required, following rapid diagnostic procedures if possible.

SURGERY/OTHER PROCEDURES
- May be required for diagnostic biopsy
- Excision may relieve acute compression, and may be primary therapy for isolated benign mass.

 ## ONGOING CARE

DISPOSITION
Admission Criteria
- All patients with significant mass, until cardiopulmonary risk defined
- All patients with evidence of significant airway or vascular compression

Discharge Criteria
- Resolution/resection of mass, or clear evidence of cardiopulmonary stability through all activities of daily living (ADLs), including sleep.

COMPLICATIONS
- Superior vena cava syndrome
- Tracheal compression
- Spinal cord compression

- Pleural and pericardial effusions
- Secondary infection
- Horner syndrome: Ptosis, miosis, and anhydrosis resulting from compression of the cervical sympathetic nerve trunk
- Esophageal narrowing or erosion: May result in feeding difficulty or bleeding

ADDITIONAL READING
- Franco A, Mody NS, Meza MP. Imaging evaluation of pediatric mediastinal masses. *Radiol Clin North Am*. 2005;43:325–353.
- Gothard JW. Anesthetic considerations for patients with anterior mediastinal mass. *Anesthesiol Clin*. 2008;26:305–314.
- Jaggers J, Balsara K. Mediastinal masses in children. *Semin Thorac Cardiovasc Surg*. 2004;16:201–208.
- Pizzo PA, Poplack DG, eds. *Principles and Practice of Pediatric Oncology*, 6th ed. Lippincott, Williams, and Wilkins; 2010.

 ## CODES

ICD9
786.6 Swelling, mass, or lump in chest

ICD10
- D38.3 Neoplasm of uncertain behavior of mediastinum
- R22.2 Localized swelling, mass and lump, trunk

FAQ
- Q: What should be done if the child is asymptomatic and a mediastinal mass is an incidental finding on chest x-ray?
- A: Careful history and physical with specific attention to pulmonary, cardiac, and hematologic systems.
  - Vital signs to include temperature and pulse oximetry
  - CBC, differential, ESR, tumor lysis labs
  - PPD, anergy panel if high risk for tuberculosis or initial evaluation negative
  - CT of chest
  - Referral to oncologist, surgeon, or infectious disease specialist pending above results
- Q: When should an oncologist be consulted?
- A: With any of the following:
  - Rapidly enlarging mass
  - Signs and symptoms of tracheal compression, superior vena cava syndrome, or spinal cord compression
  - Hepatomegaly, lymphadenopathy, bruises, or petechiae on physical examination
  - Anemia, thrombocytopenia, or leukocytosis suggesting bone marrow involvement
  - Malignant histology demonstrated with biopsy
  - When help is needed in establishing diagnosis

M

MEGALOBLASTIC ANEMIA

Kim Smith-Whitley

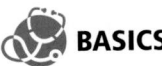 **BASICS**

DESCRIPTION
Anemia characterized by megaloblastic RBCs (large cells with abundant cytoplasm) in the bone marrow and hypersegmented neutrophils on peripheral blood smears.

EPIDEMIOLOGY
Exact incidence and prevalence figures in American children are unknown, but overall the disease is rare.

PATHOPHYSIOLOGY
- Abnormal DNA synthesis in hematopoietic precursors
- Anemia is due to ineffective hematopoiesis and hemolysis.

ETIOLOGY
Overall causes are numerous, but the following are the most common general etiologic categories:
- Vitamin B_{12} (cobalamin) deficiency
- Folate (folic acid) deficiency
- Refractory dyserythropoietic anemias—rare in children
- In adults, pernicious anemia is a common cause.

DIAGNOSIS

HISTORY
Insidious onset of anemia and associated symptoms such as pallor, fatigue, poor appetite, irritability. GI history may include:
- Malabsorption/diarrhea
- Special diets: Particularly strict vegan diets
- Prior gastrointestinal surgery
- Medications such as anticonvulsants and chemotherapeutic agents that interfere with folate metabolism
- Neurologic symptoms are commonly associated with vitamin B_{12} deficiency; symptoms may include:
  - Difficulty walking
  - Numbness/tingling in hands and/or feet

PHYSICAL EXAM
- Pallor and other associated signs of anemia:
  - Smooth and sometimes tender tongue
- Neurologic findings:
  - Abnormal position and vibratory sensation
  - Ataxia
  - Muscular weakness
  - Peripheral neuropathy
  - Positive *Babinski* sign

DIAGNOSTIC TESTS & INTERPRETATION
Lab
- CBC:
  - Decreased hemoglobin
  - Increased mean corpuscular volume
  - Increased red cell distribution width
  - Normal to decreased WBC count and platelets
- Peripheral blood smear:
  - Macro-ovalocytes
  - Hypersegmented neutrophils
  - Increased anisocytosis (variation in RBC size)
  - Increased poikilocytosis (variation in RBC shape)
- Reticulocyte count: Low
- Serum B_{12}: Low
- Folate: Low in serum and RBCs
- Serum methylmalonic acid (MMA) and homocysteine levels: May help to distinguish vitamin B_{12} deficiency and folate deficiency

Imaging
Barium studies may be needed to evaluate gastric, small bowel, and large bowel anomalies.

Diagnostic Procedures/Other
- Bone marrow aspirate and biopsy examination:
  - Large RBC, WBC, and platelet precursors with nuclear-to-cytoplasmic dissociation prominent in red cell line
  - Increased iron stores
  - Multiple binucleate and trinucleate RBC precursors
  - Multiple mitotic figures
- Schilling test assesses B_{12} absorption:
  - Part 1 evaluates vitamin B_{12} absorption by measuring urine radioactivity after oral radioactive vitamin B_{12}.
  - This test may be performed after the patient has been treated, but the test involves administration of vitamin B_{12}; therefore, all other tests, particularly bone marrow examination, should be performed beforehand or shortly thereafter.
  - If the urinary excretion is lower than expected, abnormal absorption is present, from either malabsorption or intrinsic factor disorders.
  - Part 2 should be performed if part 1 is abnormal; this involves oral intrinsic factor.
  - If part 2 is normal and part 1 is abnormal, pernicious anemia is highly likely.
  - If part 2 remains abnormal, a malabsorption syndrome is the most likely diagnosis.

DIFFERENTIAL DIAGNOSIS
- Macrocytic anemias must be differentiated from megaloblastic anemias. In macrocytic anemias, the mean corpuscular volume is increased but without megaloblastic bone marrow changes. Macrocytic red cells may be seen in aplastic anemia, liver disease, pregnancy and hypothyroidism.
- Diets deficient in vitamin B_{12} or folate
- Pernicious anemia: B_{12} deficiency due to loss of intrinsic factor normally produced in the stomach and necessary for B_{12} absorption in the terminal ileum. Caused by autoimmune disease affecting gastric parietal cells.

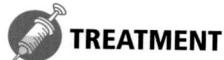 **TREATMENT**

MEDICATION (DRUGS)

ALERT

Treating undiagnosed vitamin B_{12} deficiency with high doses of folate may worsen neurologic complications, although a hematologic response may occur.

First Line
- Folic acid deficiency:
  - Folic acid at 1–5 mg PO daily for $\geq$2–3 months
  - Parenteral preparation also available if needed
- Vitamin B_{12} deficiency:
  - Acutely, daily doses of 25–100 mg IM
  - Long term, 200–1,000 mg monthly IM
  - Most patients with vitamin B_{12} deficiency require lifelong treatment because the underlying cause is abnormal absorption.

ADDITIONAL TREATMENT
General Measures
General considerations: The following 3 categories should be addressed for all patients:
- Replacement of deficient substance, vitamin B_{12}, or folate at adequate doses for an adequate duration
- Treatment/management of underlying disorder, such as malabsorption syndromes, chronic hemolytic anemias
- Monitoring response to therapy

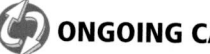 **ONGOING CARE**

FOLLOW-UP RECOMMENDATIONS
- The reticulocyte count should increase within the 1st 2 weeks of therapy, whereas the hemoglobin will take longer, in some cases months, to increase.
- If the hemoglobin fails to rise in 2 months, then other causes of anemia including iron deficiency and anemia of chronic disease should be considered.

PROGNOSIS
- Depends on cause of megaloblastic anemia; usually good if dietary deficiency
- Poor prognoses may be associated with inborn errors of metabolism that sometimes present with megaloblastic anemia.

COMPLICATIONS
- Mild congestive heart failure may develop as a result of anemia, but this is uncommon because of the insidious onset of megaloblastic anemia in general.
- Neurologic complications from vitamin B_{12} deficiency
- Folate deficiency may complicate vitamin B_{12} deficiency.

ALERT
- Microcytic anemias such as iron deficiency, thalassemia, and anemia of chronic disease may obscure the diagnosis of a megaloblastic anemia by falsely lowering the mean corpuscular volume; however, hypersegmented neutrophils should be present to aid in the correct diagnosis.
- Serum B_{12} and folate rise rapidly after beginning supplements; therefore, diagnostic levels must be drawn prior to administration of supplements or normal diets.

ADDITIONAL READING

- Dror DK, Allen LH. Effect of vitamin B_{12} deficiency on neurodevelopment in infants: Current knowledge and possible mechanisms. *Nutr Rev.* 2008;66(5):250–255.
- Oh RC, Brown DL. Vitamin B_{12} deficiency. *Am Fam Physician.* 2003;67:979–986, 993–994.
- Snow C. Laboratory diagnosis of vitamin B_{12} and folate deficiency: A guide for the primary care physician. *Arch Intern Med.* 1999;159:1289–1298.
- Weiss R, Fogelman Y, Bennett M. Severe vitamin B_{12} deficiency in an infant associated with a maternal deficiency and a strict vegetarian diet. *J Pediatr Hematol Oncol.* 2004;26(4):270–271.
- Whitehead VM. Acquired and inherited disorders of cobalamin and folate in children. *Br J Haematol.* 2006;34:125–136.

 CODES

ICD9
281.3 Other specified megaloblastic anemias not elsewhere classified

ICD10
D53.1 Other megaloblastic anemias, not elsewhere classified

FAQ
- Q: What are common dietary sources of vitamin B_{12}?
- A: Meat, eggs, and milk; liver contains the greatest amount of vitamin B_{12}.
- Q: What are common dietary sources of folate?
- A: Vegetables (primarily green, leafy vegetables), citrus fruits and berries, liver
- Q: Can food preparation destroy vitamin B_{12} and folate?
- A: Food preparation cannot destroy vitamin B_{12}, but excessive heating can destroy folate.

M

MENINGITIS

Ross Newman
Jason Newland
Louis M. Bell (5th edition)

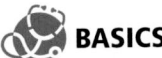 **BASICS**

DESCRIPTION
Inflammation of the membranes of the brain or spinal cord, usually caused by bacteria or viruses, and rarely fungi or parasites

EPIDEMIOLOGY
- Bacterial meningitis:
  - Most common agents in children of all ages include: *Streptococcus pneumoniae* and *Neisseria meningitidis*.
  - Underlying host factors, age, exposure, and geographic location alter incidence.
  - *S. pneumoniae* isolates are becoming more resistant to penicillin. Up to 50% of isolates causing invasive disease are resistant to penicillin.
- Viral meningitis:
  - Most commonly from enteroviruses that tend to occur in outbreaks in summer and early fall.
- Fungal meningitis:
  - *Cryptococcus neoformans* is a budding encapsulated yeast-like organism found in soil and avian excreta. Although associated with meningitis in immunocompromised adults (especially those with AIDS), this is rare in children with AIDS. 30% of patients with cryptococcal meningitis have no underlying immunodeficiency.
  - Meningitis caused by *Candida* species occurs in ill premature infants and other immunocompromised individuals.
- Tuberculous meningitis:
  - The incidence of disease due to *Mycobacterium tuberculosis* (TB) is on the rise throughout the world.
  - TB meningitis occurs in 0.5% of untreated primary TB infections.
  - Most common in children aged 6 months to 4 years
  - In ~50% of cases miliary TB is accompanied by meningitis.
  - Increasing number of patients suffer from multidrug-resistant TB.

GENERAL PREVENTION
- *Haemophilus influenzae* type b (HIB) vaccine has significantly reduced the incidence of meningitis and other invasive HIB infections by up to 99%.
- A 13-valent *S. pneumoniae* protein conjugate vaccine (PCV 13) has replaced the 7-valent vaccine (PCV 7) for use in all infants given at 2, 4, 6, and 12–15 months of age.
- A tetravalent meningococcal vaccine (MCV4) is recommended for all patients ≥11 years of age and select at-risk populations <11 years. A booster dose is recommended for all patient who receive the first dose of the vaccine between 11 and 15 years of age.

ETIOLOGY
- Bacterial:
  - Cause differs depending on age:
    - <1 month old: Group B streptococcus, *Escherichia coli*, other enteric bacteria, *Listeria monocytogenes*, *S. pneumoniae*
    - 1–3 months old: Group B streptococcus, *E. coli*, *S. pneumoniae*, HIB (almost disappearing secondary to immunization)
    - 3 months to 5 years old: *S. pneumoniae*, *N. meningitidis*
    - >5 years old: *S. pneumoniae*, *N. meningitis*
- Viral:
  - Herpes simplex virus (HSV) in the neonatal population
  - Enteroviruses: ~70 different strains that include polioviruses, Coxsackie A, Coxsackie B, and echoviruses. Recently discovered enteroviruses are not placed in these 4 groups, but are numbered (e.g., enterovirus 68).
  - Other, less common: Arboviruses (e.g., West Nile virus), mumps
- Fungal:
  - Fungi most commonly isolated include *Candida* species, *Coccidioides immitis*, *C. neoformans*, *Aspergillus* species
- Aseptic meningitis:
  - Agents not easily cultured in the viral or microbiology laboratory can cause meningitis and include *Borrelia burgdorferi* (Lyme disease), *Treponema pallidum* (syphilis)
- Tuberculous meningitis
- Unusual pathogens more likely in immunocompromised patients

 DIAGNOSIS

- Age specific
- Pain
- Fever
- Nausea and/or vomiting

HISTORY
- Bacterial meningitis:
  - Children >12 months old will often complain of classic meningeal inflammation signs including neck pain, headache, or back pain as well as photophobia, anorexia, and myalgias.
  - Nausea and vomiting are common.
  - In children <12 months old, symptoms are often nonspecific, including fever, hypothermia, irritability, and poor feeding as well as signs of increased intracranial pressure, including seizures and apnea.
  - Attention should be noted to the patient's immunization status, birth history, travel history, trauma, health status, geographic location, and exposure to high-risk contacts.
  - Common chief complaints by the infants' caregivers include the following:
    - Irritable or "sleeping all the time"
    - "Won't take to bottle"
    - "Not acting right"
    - "Cries when moved or picked up"
    - "Won't stop crying"
    - "Soft spot bulging out"
- Recurrent meningitis:
  - Recurrent meningitis with *S. pneumoniae* or *Enterococcus* may indicate a history of trauma causing a skull fracture or cribriform plate fracture with contamination of the CSF by nasopharyngeal secretions.
- Viral meningitis:
  - Headache and fever may precede signs of meningitis, such as stiff neck, vomiting, and photophobia.
  - Duration 2–6 days
- Fungal meningitis:
  - Cryptococcal meningitis is often indolent, with complaints of worsening headaches and vomiting for days to weeks.

- Exposure to pigeon droppings or other bird droppings can be a valuable clue to etiology if present.
- Tuberculous meningitis:
  - Symptoms are often nonspecific initially, with personality changes, fever, nausea, and vomiting progressing to anorexia, irritability, and lethargy (stage I disease).
  - Stage II disease is characterized by focal neurologic signs (most often involving the cranial nerves III, VI, and VII).
  - Stage III disease is characterized by coma and papilledema.

PHYSICAL EXAM
- Stiff neck in older children. Infants have poor neck muscle tone and this finding may be absent.
- Brudzinski and Kernig signs may be present.
  - Brudzinski sign: With the patient supine, flexion of the neck elicits involuntary flexion of the hips or knees.
  - Kernig sign: With the patient supine, the legs are flexed 90 degrees at the hip, extensions of the lower legs are unable to be accomplished beyond 135 degrees.
  - Negative Brudzinski or Kernig sign does not rule out meningitis.
- Children <12 months old may not have nuchal rigidity, Kernig, and/or Brudzinski signs.
- Classically, there may be "paradoxical" crying— crying that increases when child is picked up.
- Signs of increased intracranial pressure, including papilledema, asymmetric pupils, bulging fontanelle, diplopia.
- Skin exam for exanthems consistent with enterovirus infection, erythema migrans from borreliosis (Lyme disease), petechiae or purpura with invasive meningococcal disease, or vesicles in an infant <6 weeks old with HSV.

DIAGNOSTIC TESTS & INTERPRETATION
Lab
- CBC, platelet count, prothrombin time (PT), partial thromboplastin time (PTT), electrolytes, BUN, creatinine, glucose, liver function tests, arterial blood gas
- CSF analysis
- Blood culture

Diagnostic Procedures/Surgery
- Lumbar puncture with analysis of the CSF:
  - Contraindicated with cardiopulmonary compromise, uncorrected coagulopathy, and signs of increased intracranial pressure or focal neurologic findings until head imaging can be obtained
- If no etiology is discovered after the first lumbar puncture and the child is not responding to therapy, repeated lumbar puncture at 36–48 hours.
- Opening pressure: Normal is <200 mm H$_2$O in lateral recumbent position.
- Depending on the presentation, age, history, and physical exam findings, some or all of the following tests should be requested for CSF analysis:
  - Cell count with differential and gram stain
    - Bacterial meningitis is characterized by CSF pleocytosis ($>1.0 \times 10^3/\mu$L) with predominance of neutrophils. Culture is the gold standard for diagnosis.

○ Viral meningitis typically has a lower CSF cell count ($0.05–0.5 \times 10^3/\mu L$) compared to bacterial meningitis with a predominance of lymphocytes.
- Glucose: Compare with serum glucose; normal is >40 mg/dL or 1/2–2/3 of the serum glucose.
- Protein: Normal 5–40 mg/dL except in newborns, who may have protein levels of 150–200 mg/dL
  ○ >1.0 g/dL in bacterial meningitis and normal to slightly elevated in viral meningitis
- Cultures for bacteria, fungi, virus, and mycobacteria
  ○ 80% of blood cultures are positive in children with bacterial meningitis.
- Polymerase chain reaction (PCR) analysis for enterovirus, TB, HSV, Epstein–Barr virus
  ○ *Borrelia burgdorferi* PCR for CSF samples has a diagnostic yield as low as 17%. Antibody studies for neuroborreliosis are recommended.

DIFFERENTIAL DIAGNOSIS
- Encephalitis
- Toxic encephalopathy
- Epidural abscess
- Cerebral abscess

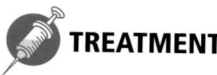 TREATMENT

ADDITIONAL TREATMENT
General Measures
- Assure adequate ventilation and cardiac function
  - *A*irway, *b*reathing, *c*irculation (ABCs)
- Initiate hemodynamic monitoring and support by achieving venous access and treat shock syndrome, if present
- Prompt initiation of appropriate antimicrobials
  - If a lumbar puncture cannot be obtained or is contraindicated a blood culture should be obtained and antimicrobials initiated.
- Monitor serum sodium concentrations because syndrome of inappropriate ADH secretion (SIADH) is a frequent complication during the first 3 days of treatment.
- Glucose should be given IV if <50 mg/dL at a dose of 0.25–1 g/kg.
- If pH is <7.2, acidosis should be corrected with 1–2 mEq/kg of sodium bicarbonate.
- Coagulopathy should be treated with platelet concentrates (0.2 U/kg) if platelets are <50,000/mm^3 and with fresh frozen plasma (10 mL/kg) if PT/PTT is prolonged.
- Steroids should be used in the initial therapy of TB meningitis along with anti-tuberculosis medication.
- Steroids indicated for HIB meningitis are controversial but can be considered in *S. pneumoniae* meningitis. Consult ID expert for use.
  - If giving steroids, use dexamethasone 0.6 mg/kg/d divided into 4 doses and given for 4 days. The first dose should be given before or with the first dose of antibiotic.

MEDICATION (DRUGS)
- Antimicrobial agents:
  - <1 month of age: Ampicillin IV 200–300 mg/kg/d divided q6–12h based on postnatal age and weight. If <7 days of age 200 mg/kg/d divided q8h; if >7 days of age, ampicillin 300 mg/kg/d divided q6h and cefotaxime IV 200 mg/kg/d divided q6h
  - >1 month of age: Vancomycin IV 60 mg/kg/d divided q6h; cefotaxime IV 300 mg/kg/d divided q6h or ceftriaxone 100 mg/kg/d divided q12h (should not be used in infants <2 months of age)

- Vancomycin IV 60 mg/kg/d divided q6h should be considered in a patient of any age suspected of *S. pneumoniae*.
- Alternative therapy for penicillin or cephalosporin allergic patients can include carbapenem or a quinolone in addition to vancomycin. Infectious disease specialist input should be considered in these patients.
- Fungal meningitis:
  - Amphotericin B with or without 5-flucytosine, depending on the type of fungi isolated
- Tuberculous meningitis:
  - Treatment is generally with 4 drugs for 2 months followed by 2 drugs for 10 months.
  - Initially, treat with isoniazid, rifampin, pyrazinamide, and streptomycin.
- Viral meningitis:
  - Enterovirus: No specific therapy other than supportive
  - HSV: Acyclovir 60 mg/kg/d divided q8h

ALERT
- Remember that in tuberculous meningitis, up to 50% of children will not react to the 5-tuberculin unit Mantoux tests. Therapy should be started if suspicious; do not rely on the skin testing.
- Be aware that the isolation of resistant strains of *S. pneumoniae* is increasing; therefore, antibiotics such as vancomycin and cefotaxime or ceftriaxone should be used until antibiotic sensitivity data are available.

 ONGOING CARE

FOLLOW-UP RECOMMENDATIONS
- Neonatal HSV meningitis should be evaluated with a repeat CSF HSV DNA PCR at day 21 and therapy extended if the PCR remains positive.
- Prophylaxis in HIB:
  - Rifampin (20 mg/kg/dose, maximum 600 mg/d for 4 days) should be given to all household contacts if 1 member is <4 years of age and is unvaccinated.
- Prophylaxis in *N. meningitidis*:
  - Rifampin (10 mg/kg/dose, maximum 600 mg b.i.d. for 2 days) for all household contacts, daycare contacts, and other persons with close contact 7 days prior to onset of illness.
- Note: If cefotaxime or ceftriaxone was used for treatment, the patient with *N. meningitidis* or HIB meningitis does not need to receive prophylaxis.

PATIENT MONITORING
- Most children with bacterial meningitis become afebrile by 7–10 days after starting therapy, with gradual improvement in activity with less irritability.
- Evaluation for neurologic sequelae, such as hearing and vision testing, is essential.

PROGNOSIS
- Bacterial meningitis:
  - Fatality approaches 100% if untreated.
  - ~500–1,000 deaths each year, or 5–10% of cases
  - Hearing deficits and neurologic damage may occur in up to 30% of children.
- Viral meningitis:
  - Prognosis for enteroviral meningitis is quite good.
- Aseptic meningitis:
  - Lyme disease: Prognosis with diagnosis and treatment is quite good (see "Lyme Disease").
- Tuberculous meningitis:

- The long-term prognosis in children with tuberculous meningitis depends on the stage of disease in which treatment is begun.
- Complete recovery occurs in 94% of those whose treatment was started in stage I, but only 51% and 18% for those whose treatment began in stage II or stage III, respectively.

COMPLICATIONS
- Bacterial meningitis:
  - Acute complications: SIADH, seizures occur in up to 1/3 of patients, focal neurologic signs occur in 10–15%.
  - Long-term complications: Mental retardation, hearing defects
- Viral meningitis:
  - Acute complications: SIADH in 10%
  - Long-term complications: Complications from viral meningitis are rare. However, neonates (<1 month of age) may develop severe EV disease and older agammaglobulinemic children may develop chronic EV meningoencephalitis.
- Tuberculous meningitis:
  - Acute complications: Most common are cranial nerve findings, especially 6th cranial nerve palsy affecting the eyes; hydrocephalus
  - Long-term complications: Many, including blindness, deafness, and mental retardation

ADDITIONAL READING

- El Bashir H, Laundy M, Booy R. Diagnosis and treatment of bacterial meningitis. *Arch Dis Child*. 2003;88:615–620.
- Hoffman JA, Mason EO, Schutze GE, et al. *Streptococcus pneumoniae* infections in the neonate. *Pediatrics*. 2003;112:1095–1102.
- Maconochie I, Baumer H, Stewart ME. Fluid therapy for acute bacterial meningitis. *Cochrane Database Syst Rev*. 2008;23(1):CD004786.
- Mann K, Jackson MA. Meningitis. *Pediatr Rev*. 2008;29:417–430.
- Saez-Llorens X, McCracken GH. Bacterial meningitis in children. *Lancet*. 2003;361:2139–2148.
- van de Beek D, de Gans J, McIntyre P, et al. Corticosteroids in acute bacterial meningitis. *Cochrane Database Syst Rev*. 2003;3:CD004305.

 CODES

ICD9
- 047.9 Unspecified viral meningitis
- 320.9 Meningitis due to unspecified bacterium
- 322.9 Meningitis

ICD10
- A87.9 Viral meningitis, unspecified
- G00.9 Bacterial meningitis, unspecified
- G03.9 Meningitis, unspecified

FAQ

- Q: Is a lumbar puncture required before starting antibiotics in the patient with suspected meningitis with unstable vital signs requiring resuscitation?
- A: No. In the unstable patient, it is contraindicated to perform a lumbar puncture. Appropriate IV antibiotics should be started. When resuscitated, a lumbar puncture should be performed.

M

MENINGOCOCCEMIA

Andrew P. Steenhoff

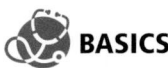 **BASICS**

DESCRIPTION
- A systemic infection with the bacterium *Neisseria meningitidis*, a Gram-negative diplococcus that is relatively fastidious. Despite treatment with appropriate antibiotics, this disease may have a fulminant course with a high likelihood of mortality.
- 13 serogroups have been described on the basis of capsular polysaccharide antigens; serotypes B, C, and Y account for most of the cases in the US. Serogroup Y accounted for 30% of cases between 1996 and 1998.

GENERAL PREVENTION
- Isolation of the hospitalized patient.

  Hospitalized patients require respiratory isolation until 24 hours after initiation of appropriate antibiotic therapy.
- Exposed contacts, including household, day care, and nursery school, should receive rifampin, 10 mg/kg (maximum 600 mg) q12h for 4 doses. Contacts younger than 1 month of age should receive 5 mg/kg PO q12h for 4 doses.

  Ceftriaxone is effective prophylaxis for contacts ≤15 years of age; a single dose of 125 mg IM is recommended. For contacts >15 years old, 250 mg IM is recommended. Its safety profile is preferred for pregnant women.
- Medical personnel should receive prophylaxis only if they had close contact with respiratory secretions.
- Vaccines for types A, C, Y, and W-135 are available and produce an immune response in 10–14 days.
- A tetravalent conjugate meningococcal vaccine, MCV4, is licensed for use in people in the age range of 2–55 years. It is recommended in all unimmunized 11- to 12-year-old adolescents with a booster dose at age 16 years.
- By February 2008, 26 cases of Guillain–Barre syndrome (GBS) had been reported in children within 6 weeks after receiving MCV4 vaccination. The currently available data cannot determine with certainty whether MCV4 increases the risk for GBS and the Centers for Disease Control (CDC) continues to recommend routine adolescent immunization with the exception of persons with a history of GBS who are not in a high-risk group for invasive meningococcal disease. An updated fact sheet on GBS and MCV4 is available at http://www.cdc.gov/vaccinesafety/Concerns/gbsfactsheet.html

EPIDEMIOLOGY
- The rates of meningococcal disease in the US have remained stable at 0.9–1.5 cases per 100,000 population per year.
- Children <5 years of age are most often affected, with peak incidence between 3 and 5 months of age.
- During epidemics, more school-aged children may be affected.
- The disease occurs most commonly in winter and spring months.
- Increased disease activity may follow an influenza A outbreak.

RISK FACTORS
- Patients with asplenia, deficiencies of properdin C3, or a terminal complement component (C5-9), and HIV are at increased risk for invasive and recurrent disease.
- Organism virulence factors, such as differences in the bacterial cell wall lipopolysaccharide, play a role in disease severity. Less virulent organisms are more likely in chronic meningococcemia which has a favorable prognosis.

Genetics
Inherited deficiency of terminal complement may be found in 5–10% of patients during epidemics. The frequency increases to 30% in patients with recurrent disease.

PATHOPHYSIOLOGY
- Fulminant disease is signified by diffuse microvascular damage and disseminated intravascular coagulation (DIC; see "Septic Shock").
- Death results from effects of endotoxic shock, including circulatory collapse and myocardial dysfunction.

ETIOLOGY
- Colonization and infection of the upper respiratory tract occurs after inhalation of, or direct contact with, the organism, usually in oral secretions.
- Disseminated disease occurs when the organism penetrates the nasal mucosa and enters the bloodstream, where it replicates.

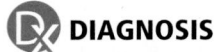 **DIAGNOSIS**

SIGNS AND SYMPTOMS
- Fever
- Malaise
- Rash
- Petechiae
- Tachycardia
- Delayed capillary fill
- Abnormal mental status
- Bacteremia without sepsis presents with fever, malaise, myalgias, and headache. Patients may clear the infection spontaneously, or it may invade meninges, joints, lungs, and so forth.
- Meningococcemia without meningitis occurs after initial bacteremia with systemic sepsis. A rash erupts, which may be nonspecific maculopapular, morbilliform, or urticarial. Progression to petechiae or purpura signifies evolution of disease.
- Fulminant disease is signified by hypotension, oliguria, DIC, myocardial dysfunction, and vascular collapse. Death occurs in ~20% of these patients.

HISTORY
Time of onset of fever, malaise, and rash

PHYSICAL EXAM
- Physical examination of a child with fever should include careful evaluation of the skin for petechiae and signs of early shock (tachycardia, delayed capillary refill, abnormal mental status, etc.).
- Recognition of abnormal vital signs and lethargy is necessary.
- Nuchal rigidity, lethargy, and irritability should be carefully evaluated.

DIAGNOSTIC TESTS & INTERPRETATION
The organism can be cultured from blood, CSF, and skin lesions.

Lab
- Gram stain of CSF or scraped petechial lesion (pressed against a glass slide):
  - Revealing Gram-negative diplococci will give a presumptive diagnosis.
- Rapid test for antigen detection: Supports diagnosis if found in CSF but not sensitive for serogroup B

Diagnostic Procedures/Other
Lumbar puncture: Antigen detection although culture remains the gold standard

DIFFERENTIAL DIAGNOSIS
- Meningitis due to *N. meningitidis* is indistinguishable from that of other causes, except for 1/3 of children who have a petechial rash.
- Sepsis from other microbial causes may appear identically, including the petechiae or purpuric rash.

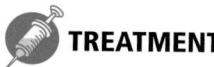

TREATMENT

ADDITIONAL TREATMENT
General Measures
- Patients with acute onset of petechial rash and fever should receive a prompt initial dose of antibiotics (preferably after blood culture)
- Close monitoring of vital signs and clinical status should follow, preferably in an ICU setting.

MEDICATION (DRUGS)
- Cefotaxime or ceftriaxone can be initiated as presumptive therapy. After sensitivity is confirmed, penicillin is preferred.
- After isolate is proven sensitive to penicillin, treatment of choice is aqueous penicillin G IV at a dose of 300,000 IU/kg/d q4–6h (maximum 12 million U/d) for 5–7 days.
- In penicillin-allergic patients, 3rd-generation cephalosporins or chloramphenicols are acceptable alternatives.

ISSUES FOR REFERRAL
Public health officials should be notified of *N. meningitidis* cases.

ONGOING CARE

FOLLOW-UP RECOMMENDATIONS
Patient Monitoring
Patients with bacterial meningitis should have hearing test as a follow-up.

PROGNOSIS
- Fatality rate of meningococcemia is 20%, even when recognized and treated.
- Fatality rate of meningococcal meningitis is 5%. The most severe cases often have a rapid progression from onset of symptoms to death over a matter of hours. At the time of hospital admission, the following signs predict poor survival:
  – Lack of meningitis
  – Shock
  – Coma
  – Purpura
  – Neutropenia
  – Thrombocytopenia
  – DIC
  – Myocarditis

COMPLICATIONS
- Complications may result directly from the infection or be classified as allergic immune complex mediated.
- Meningococcemia may be complicated by myocarditis, arthritis, hemorrhage, and pneumonia, digit or limb amputation and skin scarring.
- Meningococcal meningitis is most commonly complicated by deafness in 5–10% of survivors.
- Other complications of meningitis include seizures, subdural effusions, and cranial nerve palsies.
- Allergic complications include arthritis, vasculitis, pericarditis, and episcleritis.

ADDITIONAL READING
- Brouwer MC, Spanjaard L, Prins JM, et al. Association of chronic meningococcemia with infection by meningococci with underacylated lipopolysaccharide. *J Infection*. 2011;62:479–483.
- CDC Update: Guillain–Barre syndrome among recipients of Menactra® Meningococcal conjugate vaccine – United States, June 2005–September 2006. *MMWR*. 2006;55:1120–1124.
- Pathan N, Faust SN, Levin M. Pathophysiology of meningococcal meningitis and septicaemia. *Arch Dis Child*. 2003;88:601–607.
- Rosenstein NE, Perkins BA, Stephens DS, et al. Medical progress: Meningococcal disease. *N Engl J Med*. 2001;344:1378–1388.
- Welch SB, Nadel S. Treatment of meningococcal infection. *Arch Dis Child*. 2003;88:608–614.

CODES

ICD9
036.2 Meningococcemia

ICD10
- A39.2 Acute meningococcemia
- A39.3 Chronic meningococcemia
- A39.4 Meningococcemia, unspecified

FAQ
- Q: How long should antibiotic therapy be given to a patient with septic shock?
- A: 7 days.
- Q: Is MCV4 meningococcal vaccine indicated for all adolescents?
- A: Yes, MCV4 is now recommended in all previously unimmunized adolescents at the doctor visit from 11 to 12 year or at high school entry, whichever comes first. A booster dose is recommended at age 16 years.
- Q: How does one approach MCV4 immunization of adolescents who previously received MPSV4?
- A: If 3–5 years have elapsed since their MPSV4 vaccination, then MCV4 immunization is indicated.
- Q: When should one test for complement deficiency?
- A: In patients with recurrent disease.
- Q: Which hospital personnel should receive prophylaxis?
- A: Only those with direct exposure to index patient's secretions.

M

MENTAL RETARDATION

Rita Panoscha

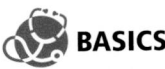

BASICS

DESCRIPTION

- Mental retardation or intellectual disability essentially means slow rate of learning or slow cognitive processing abilities. By definition, there are significant cognitive and adaptive delays 1st evident in childhood. Significant cognitive delays are defined as 2 standard deviations below the population mean on a standard cognitive or IQ test.
  - Usually indicates an IQ score of <70–75
- Adaptive skills are the functional skills of everyday life, including communication, social skills, daily living/self-care skills, and the ability to safely move about the home and community.
- Mental retardation is typically subdivided into mild, moderate, severe, and profound categories, depending on the severity of the delays. A more recent definition by the American Association on Mental Retardation (AAMR) puts more emphasis on the level of functioning and the amount of support required by an individual.

ALERT

- Children with behavioral problems may also be masking cognitive delays.
- Hearing impairment may present as a delay in development.
- Children with mild mental retardation may not be diagnosed as having a problem until they are having difficulties keeping up in elementary school.

EPIDEMIOLOGY

Found in both sexes and all racial and socioeconomic groups

Prevalence

- Prevalence of mental retardation is generally listed as 2–3% of the population.
- Of the different subcategories of mental retardation, the mild form is the most prevalent, at 85% of those with mental retardation:
  - Profound mental retardation is least prevalent, at ~1% of this group.

GENERAL PREVENTION

- There is no specific prevention, but prevention of some underlying causes may be possible.
- Immunization programs, early detection of metabolic disorders, and education programs for head injury/asphyxia prevention may be useful in some cases.
- Avoidance of alcohol and some drugs during pregnancy may also decrease some brain insults.

ETIOLOGY

- The cause of the mental retardation is usually an insult to the brain or abnormal development of the CNS but is not evident in many cases. The following represent potential causes.
- Genetic/Familial/Metabolic:
  - Fragile X syndrome
  - Trisomy 21 (Down syndrome) and other chromosomal abnormalities
  - Tuberous sclerosis
  - Neurofibromatosis
  - Phenylketonuria (PKU)
  - Other inborn errors of metabolism

- Nervous system anomalies:
  - Hydrocephalus
  - Lissencephaly
  - Seizures
- Endocrinologic:
  - Congenital hypothyroidism
- Infectious:
  - Prenatal cytomegalovirus, rubella, toxoplasmosis, HIV
  - Postnatal bacterial meningitis, neonatal herpes simplex
- Environmental toxins:
  - Heavy-metal poisoning such as lead
  - In utero drug or alcohol exposure, including fetal alcohol syndrome
- Traumatic:
  - Closed-head trauma
  - Asphyxia

COMMONLY ASSOCIATED CONDITIONS

- Associated findings are more common in the more severe forms of mental retardation.
- Mental retardation has many associated findings, including seizures, autism, cerebral palsy, communication disorders, failure to thrive, sensory impairments, and psychiatric disorders.
- Behavioral disorders can be seen, including attention deficit hyperactivity disorder, self-injurious and self-stimulating behaviors.
- Families often face additional stressors when caring for a child with mental retardation.

DIAGNOSIS

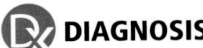

HISTORY

Complete information regarding the following:

- Pregnancy history:
  - Maternal age and parity
  - Maternal complications (including infections and exposures)
  - Medications/Drugs used
  - Tobacco or alcohol used, along with quantities
  - Fetal activity
- Birth history:
  - Gestational age
  - Birth weight
  - Route of delivery
  - Maternal or fetal complications/distress
  - Apgar scores
- General health:
  - Significant illnesses, hospitalizations, or surgeries
  - Accidents or injuries
  - Hearing and vision status
  - Medications used
  - Known exposures to toxins
  - Any new or unusual symptoms
- Developmental history:
  - Current developmental achievement in each stream of development
  - Age when developmental milestones were achieved
  - Any loss of skills
  - Where parents think their child is functioning developmentally

- Educational history:
  - Type of schooling and services received, if any
  - Any previous educational/developmental testing
- Behavioral history:
  - Any perseverative or stereotypical behaviors
  - Interaction skills
  - Attention and activity levels
- Family history:
  - Family members with developmental delays, neurologic disorders, syndromes, inherited disorders, or consanguinity
- Signs and symptoms are dependent on etiology:
  - Developmental delays
  - Slow learning behavior

PHYSICAL EXAM

A complete physical exam including growth parameters is needed looking for etiology. Key features to include are the following:

- Observation of interactions and behavior:
  - Atypical behaviors and general impressions
- Head circumference:
  - Macro- or microcephaly
- Skin exam:
  - Neurocutaneous lesions
- Major or minor dysmorphic features:
  - Indication of a syndrome or anatomic malformation
- Neurologic exam:
  - Assess for cranial nerve deficits, neuromuscular status, reflexes, balance and coordination, and any soft signs.

DIAGNOSTIC TESTS & INTERPRETATION

Lab
Initial lab tests

- There is no specific laboratory test battery for mental retardation. Testing must be tailored to the individual situation based on history and physical exam. A high index of suspicion should be maintained for any associated findings and delays in the other streams of development. Listed below are some of the more common studies.
- Genetic testing:
  - For any dysmorphic features, or a family history of delays or genetic disorder
  - A karyotype and fragile X DNA should be considered, particularly for significant cognitive delays, although the comparative genomic hybridization (CGH) microarray is increasingly recommended as a first line genetic test.
- Metabolic tests:
  - Quantitative plasma amino acid, quantitative urine organic acid, lactate, pyruvate, or ammonia levels should be considered if there is any loss of skills or indication of a metabolic disorder.
  - Additional metabolic tests may be indicated depending on symptoms.
- Thyroid function tests:
  - Most infants will have had screening for hypothyroidism shortly after birth. This should be rechecked if symptoms indicate.

Imaging
Head MRI: Consider for head abnormalities, significant neurologic findings, loss of skills, or for workup of a specific disorder, such as trauma or leukodystrophy.

Diagnostic Procedures/Other
- When developmental delays are present and mental retardation is suspected, more formal developmental screening or testing should be done.
- Possible tests for the pediatrician are the Denver-II Developmental Screening Test or the Cognitive Adaptive Test/Clinical Linguistic & Auditory Milestone (CAT/CLAMS).
- Diagnosis needs to be made based on standardized tests, usually done by a clinical psychologist. Such standardized testing might involve the Stanford Binet Intelligence Scale, the Wechsler Scales, and the Vineland Adaptive Behavior Scales.
- Audiological testing:
  – For any child with speech and language and/or cognitive delays
- EEG:
  – An EEG should be considered if there is any concern about seizures.

DIFFERENTIAL DIAGNOSIS
The differential can include several other developmental diagnoses, including the following:
- Borderline cognitive abilities
- Developmental language disorder
- Autism
- Learning disability
- Cerebral palsy
- Significant visual or hearing impairment
- Degenerative disorders

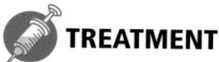 TREATMENT

ADDITIONAL TREATMENT
General Measures
- There is no specific cure for mental retardation. The ultimate goal of all therapies is to help the child reach his or her full potential.
- Therapy should consist of appropriate treatment for any underlying or associated medical condition.
- Early intervention and special education programs are available for an individualized education program based on the child's needs and abilities.
- Behavior management programs or selected use of medications is available for patients with severe behavioral problems.

ISSUES FOR REFERRAL
- A referral is made to a clinical psychologist for the formal diagnosis.
- Subspecialists:
  – Referral to other medical specialists may also be indicated.
  – These specialists may include developmental pediatrics, neurology, genetics, or ophthalmology.

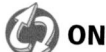 ONGOING CARE

FOLLOW-UP RECOMMENDATIONS
Patient Monitoring
- Children with mental retardation will need regular pediatric preventative care in addition to management of any underlying medical conditions.
- Ongoing monitoring of the educational programs, to ensure that it is still meeting the child's needs, is important.
- The family will also need ongoing counseling and support in dealing with a child having special needs.

PROGNOSIS
- The prognosis for longevity varies with the associated findings and overall health, but individuals with mental retardation can live to adulthood and old age.
- An individual's level of functioning is variable depending on the level of retardation, special individual skills, and family or community supports. In general, the following applies:
  – Mild mental retardation (IQ 55–70): Formerly called educable. May be in school with extra help and may achieve roughly a 4th–6th grade level in reading and math. May be employed in an unskilled to semiskilled job. May live in a group home or independently. Some marry.
  – Moderate mental retardation (IQ 40–54): May learn to recognize basic words and learn basic skills. May work in a sheltered workshop or with supported employment in an unskilled job. May live with family or in a group home doing much of their own care.
  – Severe mental retardation (IQ 25–39): May live with family, or in a group home or institution. Some may be in a sheltered workshop. May be able to do some daily self-care or chores with supervision.
  – Profound mental retardation (IQ <25): Live with family, in group home, or in institution. Usually require full-time care

ADDITIONAL READING
- Battaglia A. Neuroimaging studies in the evaluation of developmental delay/mental retardation. *Amer J Med Genet.* 2003;117C:25–30.
- Battaglia A, Carey JC. Diagnostic evaluation of developmental delay/mental retardation: An overview. *Am J Med Genet.* 2003;117C:3–14.
- Gilbride KE. Developmental testing. *Pediatr Rev.* 1995;16:338–345.
- Gropman AL, Batshaw ML. Epigenetics, copy number variation, and other molecular mechanisms underlying neurodevelopmental disabilities: New insights and diagnostic approaches. *J Dev Behav Pediatr.* 2010;31:582–591.

- Moeschler JB, Shevell M, Committee on Genetics. Clinical genetic evaluation of the child with mental retardation or developmental delays. *Pediatrics.* 2006;117:2304–2316.
- Shevell M. Global developmental delay and mental retardation or intellectual disability: Conceptualization, evaluation and etiology. *Pediatr Clin N Am.* 2008;55:1071–1084
- Stankiewicz P, Beaudet AL. Use of array CGH in the evaluation of dysmorphology, malformations, developmental delay, and idiopathic mental retardation. *Curr Opin Genet Develop.* 2007;17: 182–192.
- Walker WO, Johnson CP. Mental retardation: Overview and diagnosis. *Pediatr Rev.* 2006;27(6): 204–211.

 CODES

ICD9
- 315.9 Unspecified delay in development
- 317 Mild intellectual disabilities
- 319 Unspecified intellectual disabilities

ICD10
- F70 Mild mental retardation
- F79 Unspecified mental retardation
- F81.9 Developmental disorder of scholastic skills, unspecified

FAQ
- Q: Will my child be "normal" by adulthood?
- A: Generally, mental retardation is considered a life-long condition. Some individuals, usually with the milder form of mental retardation, can function well in the community, especially when given added supports.
- Q: Can my child learn?
- A: Except for the most severe forms of mental retardation, children do learn. This learning may not be as rapid or as extensive as that of a typically developing child.
- Q: But my child looks fine and has had appropriate motor development. How can he be mentally retarded?
- A: Mental retardation is a slowed rate of cognitive development. Many children with mental retardation do not have obvious dysmorphic features. Other streams of development, such as gross motor skills, may be reached on time or nearly so, yet the cognitive developmental streams can be significantly delayed.

M

MESENTERIC ADENITIS

Michelle Rook
Vera de Matos (5th edition)

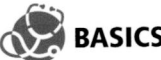 **BASICS**

DESCRIPTION
Mesenteric adenitis is defined as inflammation of the mesenteric lymph nodes. The inflamed nodes are usually clustered in the right lower quadrant (RLQ) small bowel mesentery or ventral to the psoas muscle.

EPIDEMIOLOGY
- Age related, most common in patients <15 years of age
- Affects males and females equally
- History of recent sore throat or upper respiratory tract infection found in 20–30% of subjects
- Most common cause of acute abdominal pain in young adults and children
- Self-limiting condition
- Most common cause of inflammatory adenopathy, more common than tuberculosis
- Acute RLQ pain; can mimic acute appendicitis
- Mesenteric adenitis in childhood is related to a decreased risk of ulcerative colitis in adulthood.

PATHOPHYSIOLOGY
- Lymph nodes involved are those draining the ileocecal area. Lymph nodes absorb toxic products or bacterial products secondary to stasis.
- Nodes are enlarged up to 10 mm, discrete, soft, and pink, and with time become firm. Calcification and suppuration are rare.
- Cultures of the nodes are negative.
- Reactive hyperplasia: Adenitis results from a reaction to some material absorbed from the small intestine, reaching the intestine from the blood or lymphatic system.
- Hypersensitivity reaction to a foreign protein

ETIOLOGY
- Viral: Adenovirus, echovirus 1 and 14, coxsackie viruses, Epstein-Barr virus (EBV), cytomegalovirus (CMV), (HIV)
- Bacterial: Tuberculosis, *Streptococcus* species, *Staphylococcus* species, *Escherichia coli*, *Yersinia enterocolitica*, *Bartonella henselae* (cat-scratch disease)

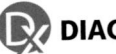 **DIAGNOSIS**

Can be difficult to differentiate from acute appendicitis clinically, and many patients may have a laparotomy before the right diagnosis is made

HISTORY
- Abdominal pain:
  - Ache to severe colic is the 1st symptom, due to stretch on the mesentery.
  - May initially be in the upper abdomen/RLQ or generalized
  - If generalized, eventually becomes localized to RLQ
  - An important point is that the patient cannot localize the exact point of the most intense pain, unlike appendicitis.
- Spasms: Between spasms, the patient feels well and can walk without any difficulty.
- Signs and symptoms:
  - Abdominal pain (RLQ)
  - Anorexia and fatigue are common.
  - Nausea and vomiting usually precede abdominal pain.
  - Fever
  - Diarrhea

PHYSICAL EXAM
- Patient flushed: Early in the attack, fever may be 38°C (100.4°F) to 38.5°C (101.3°F).
- May have associated upper respiratory tract infection symptoms, such as rhinorrhea or hyperemic pharynx
- Peripheral lymphadenopathy
- Abdominal examination shows tenderness of the RLQ: May be a little higher, more medial, and less severe than acute appendicitis
- Point of maximal tenderness may vary from one examination to the next.
- Voluntary guarding with or without rebound tenderness, and without rigidity
- Rectal tenderness

DIAGNOSTIC TESTS & INTERPRETATION
- Mesenteric adenitis is a diagnosis of exclusion. It can only be diagnosed accurately at laparoscopy or laparotomy. Ultrasound or CT scan may demonstrate enlarged mesenteric lymph nodes.
- See "Differential Diagnosis."

Lab
Complete blood count and C-reactive protein can be increased but are not specific.

Imaging
- Abdominal ultrasound: Differentiates among acute appendicitis, pelvic inflammatory disease, ovarian pathology, and mesenteric adenitis
- Contrast-enhanced CT scan of the abdomen and pelvis shows enlarged mesenteric lymph nodes, with possible ileal or ileocecal wall thickening, normal appendix
- MRI

Diagnostic Procedures/Other
- Laparoscopic surgery
- Laparotomy

DIFFERENTIAL DIAGNOSIS
- Infection:
  - Acute appendicitis: 20% of patients treated for possible acute appendicitis had mesenteric adenitis.
  - Infectious mononucleosis: Associated lymphadenopathy more generalized
  - Associated splenomegaly: Can screen for positive EBV titers
  - Tuberculosis: Associated intestinal involvement, positive purified protein derivative (PPD) test, elevated erythrocyte sedimentation rate (ESR)
  - Pelvic inflammatory disease: A consideration in sexually active adolescents; pelvic examination useful
  - Urinary tract infections/pyelonephritis: Urinalysis and urine culture are helpful.
  - Abscess: Related to missed acute appendicitis or inflammatory bowel disease (IBD)
  - *Y. enterocolitica* infection: Bloody diarrhea, arthropathy present; stool culture is diagnostic.
  - Typhlitis: Transmural inflammation of the cecum seen in patients with neutropenia
- Tumors:
  - Lymphoma: Adenopathy can be more generalized
  - CT scan of the abdomen and/or laparotomy to confirm the diagnosis
- Trauma:
  - Hematomas of the abdominal wall and intestines
  - History of trauma

- Metabolic:
  - Acute intermittent porphyria
  - Cyclic episodes of acute abdominal pain and vomiting
  - Appropriate metabolic workup diagnostic
- Congenital:
  - Duplication cysts: May present with abdominal pain due to rupture, bleeding, intussusception, or volvulus
  - Meckel diverticulum: May present with diverticulitis or act as a lead point for intussusception
- Miscellaneous:
  - Crohn disease: Associated mesenteric adenitis and intestinal involvement
  - Intussusception: Acute abdominal pain with "currant jelly" stools; barium/air enema is diagnostic and therapeutic.
  - Ovarian cysts: May need abdominal/pelvic ultrasound to differentiate between the two
  - Chronic mesenteric ischemia

 TREATMENT

Most patients recover completely without any specific treatment.

 ONGOING CARE

FOLLOW-UP RECOMMENDATIONS
Patient Monitoring
Watch for:
- Increasing abdominal pain
- Vomiting
- Fevers
- Toxic appearance
- Severe tenderness that is persistent
- Guarding
- Rigidity
- Decreasing bowel sounds

PROGNOSIS
- Most patients recover completely without any specific treatment.
- Death is very unusual and may occur only when secondary specific bacterial infection occurs with suppuration and rupture of the nodes with resulting abscess and peritonitis.
- When to expect improvement: Acute symptoms may take days to resolve and generally last a few days after the associated viral symptoms have resolved.

COMPLICATIONS
- Suppuration
- Intussusception (enlarged lymph nodes can be a lead point for intussusception)
- Rupture of lymph nodes
- Peritonitis
- Abscess formation

ADDITIONAL READING

- Carty HM. Paedtric emergencies: Non-traumatic abdominal emergencies. *Eur Radiol*. 2002; 12(12):2835–2848.
- Frisch M, Pedersen BV, Andersson RE. Appendicitis, mesenteric lymphadenitis, and subsequent risk of ulcerative colitis: Cohort studies in Sweden and Denmark. *BMJ*. 2009;338:b716.
- Karmazyn B, Werner EA, Rejaie B. Mesenteric lymph nodes in children: what is normal? *Pediatr Radiol*. 2005;35(8):774–777.
- Lucey BC, Stuhlfaut JW, Soto JA. Mesenteric lymph nodes seen at imaging: Causes and significance. *Radiographics*. 2005;25(2):351–365.
- Macari M, Balthazar EJ. The acute right lower quadrant: CT evaluation. *Radiol Clin North Am*. 2003;41:1117–1136.
- Macari M, Hines J, Balthazar E, et al. Mesenteric adenitis: CT diagnosis of primary versus secondary causes, incidence, and clinical significance in pediatric and adult patients. *AJR Am J Roentgenol*. 2002;178(4):853–858.
- Toorenvliet B, Vellekoop A, Bakker R, et al. Clinical differentiation between acute appendicitis and acute mesenteric adenitis in children. *Eur J Pediatr Surg*. 2011;21(2):120–123.
- Zeiter DK, Hyams JS. Recurrent abdominal pain in children. *Pediatr Clin North Am*. 2002;49:53–71.

 CODES

ICD9
- 014.80 Other tuberculosis of intestines, peritoneum, and mesenteric glands, unspecified
- 289.2 Nonspecific mesenteric lymphadenitis

ICD10
- I88.0 Nonspecific mesenteric lymphadenitis
- A18.39 Retroperitoneal tuberculosis

FAQ

- Q: Can one differentiate clinically between acute appendicitis and nonspecific mesenteric adenitis?
- A: Patients with nonspecific mesenteric adenitis cannot localize the exact point of the most intense pain, unlike those with appendicitis. Between spasms, patients with nonspecific mesenteric adenitis feel well and can walk without any difficulty. Abdominal examination shows tenderness of the RLQ that is a little higher, more medial, and less severe than that in acute appendicitis. Point of maximal tenderness may vary between examinations in patients with nonspecific mesenteric adenitis. There is no rigidity on abdominal examination in patients with nonspecific mesenteric adenitis. However, it is clinically difficult to differentiate the two entities.
- Q: Which investigations can be diagnostic for RLQ pain?
- A: An ultrasound or CT scan of the RLQ can differentiate between acute appendicitis, ovarian pathology, and lymphadenopathy. An upper gastrointestinal series with small bowel follow-through or a magnetic resonance enterography study can be diagnostic for IBD.

METABOLIC DISEASES IN HYPOGLYCEMIC NEWBORNS

Kristin E. D'Aco
Samantha A. Schrier
Ralph J. DeBerardinis (5th edition)
Sulagna C. Saitta (5th edition)

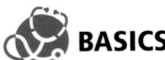 **BASICS**

DESCRIPTION

Inborn errors of metabolism are inherited defects in biochemical pathways affecting metabolism of fats, amino acids, or carbohydrates. Some inborn errors of metabolism predispose newborns to hypoglycemia. Because these conditions are life- threatening if not treated promptly, maintaining a high degree of clinical suspicion in sick neonates is essential. In the newborn period, the immediate goals should be to:

- Establish a tentative diagnosis.
- Initiate presumptive management.
- Send confirmatory studies.
- Involve a team trained in treating patients with inborn errors of metabolism.

RISK FACTORS
Genetics
Almost all inborn errors of metabolism causing hypoglycemia are autosomal recessive. One form of hyperinsulinism is autosomal dominant.

PATHOPHYSIOLOGY
- Through glycolysis and oxidative phosphorylation, glucose is a major source of cellular energy (ATP). Failure to produce ATP is probably the main source of hypoglycemia-associated tissue dysfunction.
- The brain preferentially uses glucose metabolism to produce energy and is particularly sensitive to hypoglycemia.
- A long list of metabolic disturbances in a variety of pathways can result in hypoglycemia.
- Neonates are at particular risk for hypoglycemia because they use glucose more rapidly than adults and have immature ability to obtain energy from other sources (glycogen, muscle protein, adipose tissue).

ETIOLOGY
Inherited defects in biochemical pathways affecting metabolism of fats, amino acids, or carbohydrates

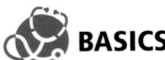 **DIAGNOSIS**

HISTORY
- Family history: Because inborn errors of metabolism are genetic disorders, patients may have a family history of poorly explained pediatric death. Diagnoses to ask about include:
  - Sepsis (was an organism identified?)
  - Sudden infant death syndrome
  - Cardiomyopathy
  - Uncontrollable seizures
  - Coma
  - Liver failure
- Unexplained developmental delay or hypoglycemia in older siblings
- Complications with the pregnancy:
  - Maternal diabetes
  - Certain disorders of fatty acid oxidation are associated with fatty liver of pregnancy or the HELLP (hypertension, elevated liver enzymes, low platelets) syndrome.
- Results of newborn screen: Children are tested for a variety of inborn errors of metabolism through newborn screening programs. Some of these disorders predispose to hypoglycemia and have specific therapies.
- Current diet and feeding schedule: Timing of hypoglycemia helps form differential diagnosis:
  - Hypoglycemia occurring shortly after feeding (0–4 hours) is suggestive of hyperinsulinism or inability to process carbohydrates.
  - Hypoglycemia between 2 and 10 hours after feeding is concerning for glycogen storage diseases or counter-regulatory hormone deficiencies.
  - Hypoglycemia after a prolonged fast (>6 hours) is suggestive of ketotic hypoglycemia, defects in gluconeogenesis, or fatty acid oxidation defects.

PHYSICAL EXAM
- ABCs and vital signs: Tachycardia and hypotension are commonly seen in hypoglycemia.
- Facies: Decreased interpupillary diameter or other midline anomalies occur in association with abnormalities of the pituitary.
- Skin: Diaphoresis is an effect of the catecholamine surge that accompanies hypoglycemia.

- Respiratory: Tachypnea may be the result of either respiratory compensation of metabolic acidosis or hyperammonemia.
- GI: Hepatomegaly occurs in many inborn errors of metabolism causing hypoglycemia and is a key feature in differentiating possible diagnoses. It can be a result of abnormal accumulation of lipid (e.g., in fatty acid oxidation defects) or glycogen (e.g., glycogen storage disease).
- Neurologic: Every neonate with a suspected inborn error of metabolism needs a complete neurologic exam to evaluate level of consciousness, tone, unusual movements, reflexes:
  - Tremulousness is a common early sign of hypoglycemia.
  - Stupor and coma occur if hypoglycemia is not reversed.
- Growth parameters: Infants of diabetic mothers may be large for gestational age. Beckwith-Wiedemann syndrome presents with an infant that is large for gestational age, hyperinsulinism, and physical stigmata (hemihypertrophy, macroglossia, abdominal wall defects).

DIAGNOSTIC TESTS & INTERPRETATION
Lab
The goal of the lab evaluation is to make a presumptive diagnosis as soon as possible. In many cases, definitive diagnosis requires specialized and time-consuming tests. Critical management points:

- Presumptive treatment should not await a definitive diagnosis, but should be based on clinical suspicion and initial labs. Delays in treatment can be fatal.
- Involvement of a biochemical genetics team is invaluable in directing the workup of suspected inborn errors of metabolism.
- In a neonate with a hypoglycemic dextrose stick, obtain the following critical labs as soon as possible:
  - Basic metabolic profile including glucose
  - Urinalysis for ketones: Inappropriately low or absent in hyperinsulinism and fatty acid oxidation defects
  - Arterial blood gas with lactate: Lactic acidosis occurs in gluconeogenic defects and in glycogen storage disease type I.
  - Insulin: Inappropriately high in hyperinsulinemic states
  - Cortisol, growth hormone levels: Inappropriately low in deficiency states
  - Plasma acylcarnitine profile: Diagnostic for fatty acid oxidation defects, some organic acidemias
  - Urine organic acids: Helps quantify accumulation of ketones and intermediates of amino acid and lipid metabolism
  - Review of the state newborn screen

DIFFERENTIAL DIAGNOSIS

Hypoglycemia is caused by increased glucose use or decreased glucose availability. Examples of disorders causing each:

- Increased glucose use:
  - Sepsis increases metabolic demand and is a leading cause of neonatal hypoglycemia.
  - Hyperinsulinemia
  - Decreased insulin counter-regulatory hormones (glucagon, cortisol, growth hormone)
- Decreased glucose availability/production:
  - Infants of diabetic mothers
  - From ingested carbohydrate: Galactosemia, hereditary fructose intolerance
  - Glycogen storage diseases
  - Decreased gluconeogenesis: Phosphoenolpyruvate carboxykinase deficiency, fructose-1,6-diphosphatase deficiency, pyruvate carboxylase deficiency
  - From decreased efficiency of pathways providing alternate energy sources: Organic acidemias, fatty acid oxidation defects
- Various toxins or medications interfere with pathways needed to maintain glucose homeostasis, including salicylates, valproate, β blockers, ethanol, and exogenous insulin.

 TREATMENT

ADDITIONAL TREATMENT
General Measures
- A well-appearing neonate with a low dextrose stick should be fed immediately. If feeds are contraindicated or not tolerated, obtain IV access.
- In children with associated physical or laboratory findings consistent with an inborn error of metabolism or other serious illness (e.g., vital sign instability, lethargy, acidosis), IV access should be obtained.
- A dextrose bolus (e.g., 5 cc/kg D10) and infusion rapidly corrects hypoglycemia in most cases. Infants requiring high glucose infusion rates are suspicious for hyperinsulinism.

Additional Therapies
Specific therapies vary according to the diagnosis and are best carried out with the help of a specialist familiar with each disease. Examples include:

- Hyperinsulinism:
  - May require continuous glucose administration (IV or via continuous gastric feeds)
  - Medical therapies including diazoxide and octreotide
  - Pancreatectomy
- Deficiencies in counter-regulatory hormones: Hormone supplementation
- Galactosemia, hereditary fructose intolerance: Eliminate offending agent from diet.
- Fatty acid oxidation disorders, glycogen storage disease type I, defects in gluconeogenesis: Frequent feeds, fasting avoidance, increase caloric intake during stress. Some children may benefit from cornstarch supplementation before bedtime to prevent nocturnal hypoglycemia.

 ONGOING CARE

COMPLICATIONS
- Hypoglycemic episodes must be recognized and treated promptly or permanent CNS injury ("hypoglycemic stroke") may occur.
- For many inborn errors of metabolism, episodes of hypoglycemia may recur. These are avoided by specific dietary measures during times of stress.

ADDITIONAL READING

- Hoe FM. Hypoglycemia in infants and children. *Adv Pediatr*. 2008;55:367–84.
- Saudubray JM, de Lonlay P, Touati G, et al. Genetic hypoglycaemia in infancy and childhood: Pathophysiology and diagnosis. *J Inherited Metab Dis*. 2000;23:197.
- Stanley CA. Hypoglycemia in the neonate. *Pediatr Endocrinol Rev*. 2006;4(Suppl 1):76–81.

 CODES

ICD9
- 775.6 Neonatal hypoglycemia
- 277.9 Unspecified disorder of metabolism

ICD10
- E88.9 Metabolic disorder, unspecified
- P70.4 Other neonatal hypoglycemia

FAQ

- Q: Why is hypoglycemia dangerous?
- A: Glucose is a crucial source of rapidly available energy for many tissues, especially the brain. Prolonged hypoglycemia causes CNS damage.
- Q: Why are the critical labs so important?
- A: In some metabolic disorders, the biochemical disturbance is apparent only during hypoglycemic episodes. Collecting this panel of informative labs during an episode greatly increases the chance of making a diagnosis.
- Q: If an infant dies before a diagnosis is made, what can be done to provide information for family members regarding future pregnancies?
- A: A postmortem exam and biochemical tests performed on various tissues obtained immediately after death can establish the diagnosis. A skin biopsy (obtained premortem or postmortem) yields fibroblasts for a variety of biochemical assays, including enzyme defects in fatty acid oxidation disorders and organic acidemias. Workup of primary lactic acidosis syndromes requires electron transport chain analysis of muscle, which must be harvested immediately (within 30 minutes) after death.

M

METABOLIC DISEASES IN ACIDOTIC NEWBORNS

Kristin E. D'Aco
Samantha A. Schrier
Ralph J. DeBerardinis (5th edition)
Sulagna C. Saitta (5th edition)

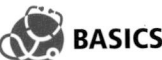 BASICS

DESCRIPTION

- Inborn errors of metabolism are inherited defects in biochemical pathways affecting fats, amino acids, or carbohydrates. Many affect the conversion of fuel to energy. Some present with catastrophic neonatal metabolic acidosis.
- Because these conditions are life-threatening if not treated promptly, a high degree of suspicion is essential. In the newborn period, the immediate goals should be to:
  – Establish a tentative diagnosis.
  – Initiate presumptive management.
  – Send confirmatory studies.
  – Involve a team trained in treating patients with inborn errors of metabolism.

RISK FACTORS
Genetics
Generally autosomal recessive. Exceptions include pyruvate dehydrogenase deficiency (a form of lactic acidosis, usually X-linked) and diseases of the mitochondrial genome (maternally inherited).

PATHOPHYSIOLOGY

- Inborn errors of metabolism presenting with metabolic acidosis usually produce an elevated anion gap owing to accumulation of an acidic intermediate. *Identification of this acid is the 1st step in establishing the diagnosis.*
- Tissue dysfunction results from toxicity of the accumulated byproduct and/or failure to produce sufficient energy to meet cellular needs.
- CNS toxicity results in increased intracranial pressure, emesis, lethargy, coma, seizures, abnormalities in muscle tone.
- Hepatic toxicity causes jaundice, failure to thrive, hypoglycemia, hyperammonemia, coagulopathy.
- Other organ systems may be involved, depending on the disease. These include the heart, the proximal renal tubule, the pancreas, and the bone marrow (see below).

ETIOLOGY
Inherited defects in biochemical pathways affecting fats, amino acids, or carbohydrates.

DIAGNOSIS

HISTORY

- Complications with the pregnancy: Some inborn errors of metabolism, particularly certain disorders of fatty acid oxidation, are associated with fatty liver of pregnancy or the HELLP (*h*ypertension, *e*levated *l*iver enzymes, *l*ow *p*latelets) syndrome.
- Current diet and feeding schedule (does baby wake spontaneously to feed?): Acidotic episodes may be triggered by specific food exposures or by prolonged fasting, including relatively short delays. In addition, diets low in protein content may delay the onset of symptoms in disorders of amino acid metabolism.
- Unusual odors to the urine or secretions: Some organic acids are associated with specific odors.

- Family history: Because inborn errors of metabolism are genetic disorders, there may be a family history of poorly explained pediatric death. Diagnoses to inquire about include:
  – Sepsis (was an organism identified?)
  – Sudden infant death syndrome
  – Cardiomyopathy
  – Uncontrollable seizures
  – Coma
  – Liver failure
  – Unexplained developmental delay or hypoglycemia in older siblings

PHYSICAL EXAM

- ABCs and vital signs: Cushing's triad (apnea, bradycardia, hypertension) should prompt immediate evaluation for elevated intracranial pressure. Are there signs of dehydration?
- Skin: Jaundice owing to liver toxicity occurs in many neonates with inborn errors of metabolism. Rashes are associated with biotinidase deficiency.
- Head, eyes, ears, nose, throat: Bulging fontanelle suggests elevated intracranial pressure. Minor dysmorphic features (e.g., frontal bossing, short/upturned nose, long philtrum, low-set ears) are sometimes seen in pyruvate dehydrogenase deficiency and severe disorders of fatty acid oxidation.
- Respiratory: Tachypnea may result from either respiratory compensation of metabolic acidosis or from hyperammonemia.
- Cardiovascular: Arrhythmias or signs of heart failure may signal a cardiomyopathy.
- GI: Hepatomegaly occurs in many inborn errors of metabolism that also cause acidosis. It can be the result of abnormal accumulation of lipid or glycogen. Abdominal pain and emesis can be caused by ketosis.
- Neurologic: Inborn errors of metabolism presenting with acidosis are often associated with neuronal toxicity. Every neonate with a suspected inborn error of metabolism must have a complete neurologic exam.
- Assessment for odors:
  – Burnt sugar: Maple syrup urine disease
  – Fruity: Ketosis
  – Sweaty feet: Isovaleric acidemia
- Growth parameters: Normal at birth for most inborn errors of metabolism

DIAGNOSTIC TESTS & INTERPRETATION
Lab

- The goal of the lab evaluation is to make a presumptive diagnosis as soon as possible. In most cases, definitive diagnosis requires specialized and time-consuming tests. Critical management points:
  – Presumptive treatment should not await definitive testing, but should be based on clinical suspicion and initial testing. Delays in treatment can be fatal.
  – Involvement of a biochemical genetics team is invaluable in directing the workup of suspected inborn errors of metabolism.
- A rational approach for acidotic neonates is to determine the inborn error of metabolism category using the tests below, then to send metabolic follow-up studies as indicated:
  – Initial tests:
    ○ Urinalysis for ketones. Can be bagged urine, but obtain by catheterization if necessary.
    ○ Dextrose stick
    ○ Basic metabolic profile
    ○ Arterial blood gas
    ○ Blood lactate*
    ○ Ammonia*
    ○ Liver function tests
    ○ Review of the state newborn screen

  *must be collected without tourniquet, from free flowing blood, and delivered to laboratory on ice

- Patterns and follow-up testing: These studies establish a presumptive diagnosis in most inborn errors of metabolism presenting with acidosis:
  – If elevated ketones, consider:
    ○ Branched-chain and other organic acidemias (methylmalonic acidemia, propionic acidemia, isovaleric acidemia, others): Ketoacidosis, hyperammonemia, with or without hypoglycemia. Obtain plasma amino acids, urine organic acids, plasma acylcarnitine profile with total/free carnitine.
    ○ Primary lactic acidosis syndromes (below)
  – If elevated blood lactate, consider:
    ○ Primary lactic acidosis syndromes: May be associated with ketosis (oxidative phosphorylation deficiency) and/or hypoglycemia (gluconeogenesis defects). Obtain lactate/pyruvate ratio, urine organic acids, creatine phosphokinase and biotinidase quantitation. Consider brain MRI and MR spectroscopy if CNS symptoms present.
    ○ Fatty acid oxidation defects: Hypoketotic hypoglycemia with or without hyperammonemia and lactic acidosis: Obtain creatine phosphokinase, plasma acylcarnitine profile with total/free carnitine, urine organic acids. Perform ECG/echo for signs of cardiac failure.
  – If anion is not identified on initial tests, consider branched-chain and other organic acidemias.
- Other tests: Consider organic acid, amino acid, and lactate/pyruvate analysis of the CSF in neonates with neurologic dysfunction.
- Definitive diagnosis may require enzyme testing or mutation analysis.

DIFFERENTIAL DIAGNOSIS

In neonates, many different inborn errors of metabolism present with similar symptoms, which can easily be confused with other serious diseases.

- Differential diagnosis in sick, acidotic neonate:
  - Sepsis
  - Congenital heart disease
  - Toxin/Drug exposure
  - Perinatal depression
  - Inborn error of metabolism
- Categories of inborn error of metabolism presenting with neonatal acidosis:
  - Lactic acidosis:
    - ○ Pyruvate dehydrogenase deficiency
    - ○ Pyruvate carboxylase deficiency
    - ○ Phosphoenolpyruvate carboxykinase deficiency
    - ○ Defects in tricarboxylic acid cycle enzymes
    - ○ Mitochondrial diseases or other conditions affecting oxidative phosphorylation
    - ○ Severe disorders of gluconeogenesis (e.g., glucose-6-phosphatase deficiency)
    - ○ Multiple carboxylase deficiency, biotinidase deficiency
    - ○ Disorders of fatty acid oxidation
  - Ketoacidosis:
    - ○ Disorders of ketone utilization (e.g., β-ketothiolase deficiency)
    - ○ Ketosis can also occur in lactic acidosis syndromes (above) and organic acidemias (below)
  - Other organic acids:
    - ○ Maple syrup urine disease
    - ○ Branched chain organic acidurias (methylmalonic acidemia, propionic acidemia, isovaleric acidemia)
    - ○ Many others. Note that in some cases, other abnormalities (e.g., lethargy, hyperammonemia) may occur prior to severe acidosis.

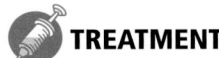

TREATMENT

ADDITIONAL TREATMENT
General Measures
Metabolic derangement usually worsens during times of stress (e.g., perinatal period, infection, fasting) and accompanying catabolism. Provide sufficient calories to reverse the catabolic state. Considerations include:

- IV access
- Many decompensated patients will have altered mental status and dehydration. Consider intubation if obtunded.
- Bicarbonate boluses and infusions may be necessary, especially if pH <7.22 or bicarb <14. Monitor sodium carefully in patients receiving NaHCO₃.
- In most cases, a high glucose infusion rate (e.g., with D10-based fluid) speeds stabilization. One important exception is pyruvate dehydrogenase deficiency, a primary lactic acidosis syndrome, in which rapid glucose infusion can worsen the lactic acidosis. These children should receive D5.
- Specific dietary measures require a presumptive diagnosis.

- Total parenteral nutrition is a useful option when a presumptive diagnosis has been made. Note that special amino acid mixtures are available for particular disorders (e.g., maple syrup urine disease).
- Insulin can be used to reverse states of severe catabolism.
- Nasogastric feeding using appropriate formulas is useful.
- In patients with large acid load and/or concomitant hyperammonemia, hemodialysis may be indicated.

Additional Therapies
Specific therapies are best carried out with the help of a biochemical geneticist or other specialist with experience treating inborn errors of metabolism, and a clinical nutritionist.

- Organic acidemias:
  - Protein restriction, protein elimination during times of stress, and avoidance of fasting
  - High glucose infusion rates during decompensation
- Primary lactic acidosis syndromes: Therapy is supportive and involves avoidance of stresses such as fasting.
- In pyruvate dehydrogenase deficiency, a ketogenic diet may improve chronic acidosis.
- Fatty acid oxidation disorders:
  - Low-fat, high-carbohydrate diets with frequent feeds

 ONGOING CARE

FOLLOW-UP RECOMMENDATIONS
Patient Monitoring
Should be determined with the input of a metabolic specialist, but may include:

- Serial ABG or basic metabolic profile to trend pH and bicarbonate levels
- Serial blood lactates
- Cardiorespiratory monitoring
- Frequent assessment of patient's mental status and peripheral perfusion

COMPLICATIONS
- Failure to treat patients promptly can be fatal or result in severe CNS insult and developmental disability. The basal ganglia are particularly susceptible to a variety of metabolic disturbances, and damage to these structures can cause "metabolic stroke."
- For many inborn errors of metabolism, recurrent episodes of acidosis, triggered by stress, intercurrent illness, or dietary noncompliance, are a major source of morbidity.
- Long-term effects may include progressive tissue dysfunction (e.g., liver or renal failure, cardiomyopathy) or failure to thrive.

ADDITIONAL READING

- Burton BK. Inborn errors of metabolism in infancy: A guide to diagnosis. *Pediatrics*. 1998;102: E69–E77.
- Dionisi-Vici C, Deodato F, Röschinger W, et al. Classical organic acidurias, propionic aciduria, methylmalonic aciduria and isovaleric aciduria: Long-term outcome and effects of expanded newborn screening using tandem mass spectrometry. *J Inherit Metab Dis*. 2006;29(2–3): 383–389.
- Ozand PT, Gascon GG. Organic acidurias: A review. Part 1. *J Child Neurol*. 1991;6:196–219.
- Ozand PT, Gascon GG. Organic acidurias: A review. Part 2. *J Child Neurol*. 1991;6:288–303.

 CODES

ICD9
- 775.7 Late metabolic acidosis of newborn
- 276.2 Acidosis
- 277.9 Unspecified disorder of metabolism

ICD10
- E87.2 Acidosis
- E88.9 Metabolic disorder, unspecified
- P74.0 Late metabolic acidosis of newborn

FAQ

- Q: If an infant dies before a diagnosis is made, what can be done to provide information for family members regarding future pregnancies?
- A: Postmortem exam and biochemical tests on tissues obtained immediately after death can establish the diagnosis. Skin biopsy (obtained premortem or postmortem) yields fibroblasts for a variety of biochemical assays. Workup of primary lactic acidosis syndromes requires electron transport chain analysis of muscle, which must be harvested within 30 minutes after death.
- Q: What determines developmental outcome in children with inborn errors of metabolism?
- A: Disease severity depends in part on the specific mutations in each patient. However, prompt initiation of appropriate therapy in the newborn period, as well as compliance with chronic management and avoidance of decompensation periods, all contribute to developmental outcome.

M

METABOLIC DISEASES IN HYPERAMMONEMIC NEWBORNS

Kristin E. D'Aco
Samantha A. Schrier
Ralph J. DeBerardinis (5th edition)
Sulagna C. Saitta (5th edition)

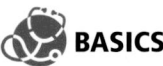 BASICS

DESCRIPTION
- Inborn errors of metabolism are inherited defects in biochemical pathways affecting metabolism of fats, amino acids, or carbohydrates.
- Some inborn errors of metabolism present with elevated ammonia in newborns (>100 micromolar). Because these conditions are life-threatening if not treated promptly, maintaining a high degree of clinical suspicion in sick neonates is essential. In the newborn period, the immediate goals include:
  – Establish a tentative diagnosis.
  – Initiate presumptive management.
  – Send confirmatory studies.
  – Involve a team trained in treating patients with inborn errors of metabolism.

RISK FACTORS
Genetics
Generally autosomal recessive. Ornithine transcarbamylase deficiency (the most common urea cycle defect) is X-linked. Incidence of urea cycle defects is ~1 in 45,000 births.

PATHOPHYSIOLOGY
The urea cycle coverts ammonia (NH3) to water-soluble urea in the liver and is the major mechanism for ammonia disposal. Inborn errors of metabolism causing hyperammonemia interfere with urea cycle function, either directly or indirectly, including the following mechanisms:
- Genetic defects in a urea cycle enzyme *per se*
- Decreased production, increased use, or defective transport of a urea cycle intermediate. Examples:
  – Hyperornithinemia, hyperammonemia, homocitrullinemia (HHH) syndrome
  – Lysinuric protein intolerance
  – Fatty acid oxidation defects
  – Hyperammonemia/Hyperinsulinemia syndrome
  – Organic acidemias
  – Pyruvate carboxylase deficiency
- Hepatotoxicity (galactosemia, hereditary fructose intolerance)

DIAGNOSIS

HISTORY
- Evidence of systemic disease: A variety of systemic newborn illnesses, including sepsis, can be complicated by a secondary hyperammonemia.
- Family history of poorly explained pediatric death or developmental disability raises suspicion for a genetic disorder, such as an inborn error of metabolism. Diagnoses to ask about:
  – Sepsis (was an organism identified?)
  – Sudden infant death syndrome
  – Cardiomyopathy
  – Uncontrollable seizures
  – Coma
  – Liver failure
- Current diet and feeding schedule: In urea cycle defects, hyperammonemia is exacerbated by protein intake.
- Failure to wake and feed spontaneously is a sign of CNS dysfunction in neonates.
- Perinatal hypoxia can cause temporary liver dysfunction and reduced urea cycle capacity. Relative immaturity of the urea cycle can cause hyperammonemia in premature infants.

PHYSICAL EXAM
- ABCs and vital signs: Cushing's triad (apnea, bradycardia, hypertension) should prompt immediate evaluation for elevated intracranial pressure, a complication of hyperammonemia.
- Skin: Jaundice is not typical in urea cycle defects, but occurs in other inborn errors of metabolism associated with hepatotoxicity.
- Head, eyes, ears, nose, and throat: Bulging fontanelle suggests elevated intracranial pressure.
- Respiratory: Effects of hyperammonemia on the brainstem respiratory center may cause tachypnea, leading to respiratory alkalosis.
- GI: Hepatomegaly occurs in some of these disorders (fatty acid oxidation, galactosemia).
- Neurologic: Hyperammonemia causes a variety of neurologic abnormalities, including abnormal tone, obtundation, and coma.

DIAGNOSTIC TESTS & INTERPRETATION
Lab
The goal of lab testing is to make a presumptive diagnosis as soon as possible. In many cases, definitive diagnosis requires specialized tests. Critical management points:
- Presumptive treatment should not await a definitive diagnosis, but should be based on clinical suspicion and initial labs. Delays in treatment can be fatal.
- Involvement of a biochemical genetics team is invaluable in directing the workup of suspected inborn errors of metabolism.
- Initial labs to evaluate neonatal hyperammonemia:
  – Dextrose stick
  – Electrolytes, BUN, creatinine
  – CBC, blood culture
  – Blood gas with lactate
  – Liver function tests and PT/PTT
  – Urinalysis for ketones, reducing substances
  – Frequent ammonia levels (q3–12 hours depending on level of elevation). These should be obtained as free-flowing samples without tourniquets and placed on ice.
  – Review state newborn screen
- Suspected disorders and follow-up testing:
  – Urea cycle defects: Plasma amino acids and urine orotic acid
  – Organic acidemias: Urine organic acids, plasma amino acids, and acylcarnitine profile
  – Fatty acid oxidation defects: Creatine phosphokinase, urine organic acids, plasma acylcarnitine profile
  – Galactosemia: Urine galactitol, red blood cell galactose-1-phosphate uridyltransferase (GALT) activity, and total galactose from blood
  – Definitive diagnosis may require enzyme testing or mutation analysis.

DIFFERENTIAL DIAGNOSIS
- Neonatal hyperammonemia not caused by inborn errors of metabolism:
  – Sepsis or other severe illness
  – Liver failure (any cause)
  – Transient neonatal hyperammonemia
  – Perinatal depression/hypoxia
  – Iatrogenic (valproic acid, asparaginase)

- Inborn errors of metabolism:
  - Urea cycle defects (N-acetylglutamate synthetase deficiency, carbamoyl phosphate synthase deficiency, ornithine transcarbamylase deficiency, argininosuccinate synthetase deficiency (citrullinemia), argininosuccinate lyase deficiency)
  - Organic acidemias (isovaleric acidemia, propionic acidemia, methylmalonic acidemia, multiple carboxylase deficiencies, others)
  - Fatty acid oxidation defects (medium-chain acyl-CoA dehydrogenase deficiency, multiple acyl-CoA dehydrogenase deficiency, others)
  - Hyperornithinemia, hyperammonemia, homocitrullinemia (HHH) syndrome
  - Pyruvate carboxylase deficiency
  - Hyperammonemia/Hyperinsulinemia syndrome
  - Galactosemia
  - Hereditary fructose intolerance

 TREATMENT

ADDITIONAL TREATMENT
General Measures
- Discontinue protein intake, which exacerbates ammonia production. Protein/Amino acid–free formula or parenteral nutrition should be used.
- Obtain IV access.
- Many patients will require intensive care transfer. Hyperammonemia interferes with normal CNS and respiratory function, so hyperammonemic neonates often require intubation.
- Nitrogen scavenging agents (e.g., sodium benzoate, sodium phenylacetate, sodium phenylbutyrate) are used in some settings. They improve hyperammonemia by combining with amino acids to yield products that can be excreted into the urine.
- Arginine or citrulline therapy may be used to supplement the residual function of the urea cycle. Use should be only under the supervision of a metabolic specialist.
- In severe hyperammonemia, dialysis may be indicated.
- In many disorders, catabolism and associated breakdown of endogenous protein exacerbates the nitrogen load. This can be treated with calories from high-rate dextrose infusion with insulin, if indicated, to enhance anabolism.
- Administration of N-carbamyl-L-glutamic acid (Carbaglu) has been shown to reduce ammonia levels in NAG synthetase deficiency, CPS1 deficiency, and the organic acidemias. Use should only be under the supervision of a metabolic specialist.

Additional Therapies
Specific therapies are best carried out with the help of a specialist experienced in treating inborn errors of metabolism, and a clinical nutritionist. Examples include:
- Urea cycle defects:
  - Protein-restricted diet, with protein elimination during illness/stress
  - Chronic therapy with nitrogen scavenging agents
  - Amino acid supplements when indicated (e.g., citrulline in ornithine transcarbamylase deficiency; arginine in citrullinemia, argininosuccinate lyase deficiency)
  - Long-term therapy may involve an orthotopic liver transplant.
- Fatty acid oxidation disorders:
  - Low-fat, high-carbohydrate diets with frequent feeds
- Organic acidemias:
- Protein restriction, protein elimination during times of stress, and avoidance of fasting

 ONGOING CARE

COMPLICATIONS
- Recurrent episodes of hyperammonemia
- Elevated intracranial pressure
- Developmental disability
- Coma
- Death

ADDITIONAL READING

- Batshaw ML, MacArthur RB, Tuchman M. Alternative pathway therapy for urea cycle disorders: Twenty years later. *J Pediatr*. 2001;38:S46–S55.
- Burton BK. Inborn errors of metabolism in infancy: A guide to diagnosis. *Pediatrics*. 1998;102: E69–E77.
- Haeberly J. Clinical practice: The management of hyperammonemia. *Eur J Pediatr*. 2011;170:21–34.
- Kasapkara C, Ezgu F, Okur U, et al. N-carbamylglutamate treatment for acute neonatal hyperammonemia in isovaleric academia. *Eur J Pediatr*. 2011; Epub ahead of print.
- Singh RH. Nutritional management of patients with urea cycle disorders. *J Inherit Metab Dis*. 2007; 30(6):880–887.
- Summar M, Tuchman M. Proceedings of a consensus conference for the management of patients with urea cycle disorders. *J Pediatr*. 2001;138(suppl 1): S6–S10.
- Summar M. Current strategies for the management of neonatal urea cycle disorders. *J Pediatr*. 2001; 138(Suppl 1):S30–S39.
- Walker V. Ammonia toxicity and its prevention in inherited defects of the urea cycle. *Diabetes Obesity Metabol*. 2009;11:823–835.

 CODES

ICD9
- 270.6 Disorders of urea cycle metabolism
- 277.9 Unspecified disorder of metabolism

ICD10
- E72.4 Disorders of ornithine metabolism
- E88.9 Metabolic disorder, unspecified

FAQ

- Q: Can females have ornithine transcarbamylase deficiency?
- A: Because ornithine transcarbamylase is an X-linked gene, females are generally asymptomatic carriers. However, "skewed" X inactivation, in which the normal ornithine transcarbamylase gene is inactive in a large majority of hepatocytes, has caused symptomatic disease in a number of females. Affected carrier females may exhibit protein intolerance, migraines, and personality changes. They are treated similarly to affected males.
- Q: Can any of these disorders present outside of the newborn period?
- A: Disease severity depends in large part on a patient's enzyme activity. In some patients, there is enough activity so that hyperammonemia does not occur until later in life during a period of illness, stress, or high protein intake.
- Q: What determines developmental outcome in children with inborn errors of metabolism?
- A: In most inborn errors of metabolism, severe mutations cause very low enzyme activity and a greater disease severity. However, prompt initiation of appropriate therapy in the newborn period, as well as compliance with chronic management, contributes to developmental outcome.

M

METABOLIC SYNDROME

George A. Datto, III
Sandra Gibson Hassink

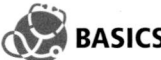 **BASICS**

DESCRIPTION
- A cluster of metabolic disorders that is the antecedent to cardiovascular disease and type 2 diabetes in adults
- The presence of 3 or more of the following metabolic abnormalities is required to meet the diagnosis:
  - Obesity:
    - BMI >97% (BMI Z score >2)
  - Low HDL cholesterol:
    - <5% for age and gender
  - Elevated triglycerides:
    - >95% for age and gender
  - Hypertension:
    - Systolic and/or diastolic BP >95% for age and gender
  - Impaired fasting blood sugar/impaired glucose tolerance:
    - Fasting blood sugar >100 mg/dL
    - 2-hour glucose tolerance test >140 mg/dL

EPIDEMIOLOGY
Prevalence
- Uncommon in children of normal weight
- 30% of obese children meet criteria for the metabolic syndrome.
- Rates increase with higher BMI.
- Highest rates in Mexican Americans > whites > African Americans
- More prevalent in males than females

RISK FACTORS
- Obesity
- Family history of cardiovascular disease
- Family history of type 2 diabetes mellitus

Genetics
Strong family history of early coronary heart disease and type 2 diabetes supports genetic component.

PATHOPHYSIOLOGY
- Visceral fat:
  - Deposition of fat centrally, which can be influenced by diet and genetics
- Adipocytes:
  - Adipocytes produce proinflammatory mediators (adiponectin, resistin, and tumor necrosis factor-α).
- Insulin resistance:
  - Inflammatory mediators affect cell's ability to respond to insulin.

ETIOLOGY
- Obesity
- Physical inactivity
- Insulin resistance
- Aging
- Genetics

COMMONLY ASSOCIATED CONDITIONS
- Polycystic ovarian syndrome
- Nonalcoholic steatohepatitis (NASH)
- Sleep apnea

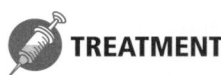 **DIAGNOSIS**

HISTORY
- Obesity trigger:
  - Age at which weight gain started
  - Family or patient stress
  - Life events
- Parents'/patient's beliefs:
  - Level of concern and motivation
  - Self-assessed reasons for weight gain
  - Previous attempts at weight control
- Family history:
  - Early coronary heart disease and diabetes mellitus
- Lifestyles:
  - Eating behavior
    - Sugared beverage consumption
    - Snacks: Frequency and content
    - Eating structure
  - Physical activity
    - Hours of screen time
    - Sports and activity participation
    - Time outdoors
- Parenting skills
  - Assessing the environment
  - Ability to set boundaries
  - Role modeling
  - Anger management
  - Hunger management
- Signs and symptoms:
  - Obese patients with the metabolic syndrome usually lack any symptoms, but may complain of:
    - Easy and rapid weight gain
    - Excessive hunger
    - Tiredness
    - Headaches
    - Darkening of neck and axillae (findings suggestive of acanthosis nigricans)
    - Nocturia

PHYSICAL EXAM
A complete physical should be done on all patients. Special attention should be paid to the following:
- Weight, height, and BMI
- Waist circumference
- Blood pressure
- Acanthosis nigricans
- Abdominal striae
- Hepatomegaly
- Tanner stage
- Affect

DIAGNOSTIC TESTS & INTERPRETATION
Lab
Metabolic screening (fasting specimens) should be done on all obese patients:
- Lipid profile: Cholesterol, HDL, and triglycerides
- Glucose
- Hemoglobin A1c
- Liver function tests: ALT and AST
- Thyroid function tests: Free T_4 and TSH
- A 2-hour glucose tolerance test should be considered in patients with a fasting blood sugar >100 mg/dL or a hemoglobin A1c >6% to document either impaired glucose tolerance or type 2 diabetes.
- Abnormal lab tests should be repeated after a trial of weight management.
- Normal lab studies should be repeated yearly with significant weight gain.

Imaging
All patients with hypertension (BP >95th percentile × 3) should have an ECG to evaluate for left ventricular hypertrophy.

DIFFERENTIAL DIAGNOSIS
- Hereditary dyslipidemia
- Essential hypertension
- Hypertriglyceridemia
- Diabetes mellitus
- Secondary hypertension

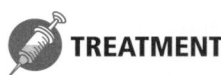 **TREATMENT**

MEDICATION (DRUGS)
Medications may be appropriate in certain clinical situations to treat the components of the metabolic syndrome when lifestyle interventions fail to show clinical improvement.
- Dyslipidemia
  - Statin therapy to treat hypercholesterolemia should be considered in adolescent patients with the following problems:
    - LDL >190 mg/dL
    - LDL >160 mg/dL with strong family history of early coronary artery disease (1st-degree relatives with coronary artery disease at age <55)
    - Patients with type 2 diabetes with dyslipidemia
  - Atorvastatin: 10 mg PO daily to max of 40
  - Treatment goal: LDL <130 mg/dL
  - Side effects: Elevation of liver function tests
- Hypertension (see "Hypertension" chapter)
  - Antihypertensive drug therapy should be considered in the following patients:
    - Stage 2 hypertension (99% + 5 mm Hg)
    - Hypertensive patients with insufficient clinical response to lifestyle modification
    - Patients with evidence of left ventricular hypertrophy on echocardiogram
    - Patients with type 2 diabetes

- ACE inhibitors or angiotensin-receptor blockers may have renal protective effects in diabetic patients.
- Impaired fasting blood sugar/impaired glucose tolerance; type 2 diabetes mellitus (see "Diabetes" chapter)
  - Drug therapy should be considered in all patients with a fasting blood sugar >126 mg/dL or a hemoglobin A1c >7.0%.

ADDITIONAL TREATMENT
General Measures
In the adults, lifestyle intervention has been more effective than metformin in decreasing the incidence of diabetes mellitus in patients who have the metabolic syndrome. Modest decreases in BMI by incorporating lifestyle interventions will decrease risk factors of the metabolic syndrome. Effective pediatric obesity management incorporates the following principles:

- Effective communication with patient and family:
  - Nonblaming approach
  - Be positive that change can occur.
- Assessing family's understanding of problem and readiness to make lifestyle change(s)
  - Incorporate motivational interviewing to help families with their stage of change.
- Identifying energy balance abnormalities
- Providing options for change
- Supporting families in planning and making lifestyle change
  - Goal setting
  - Parenting skills
  - Controlling the environment
  - Ongoing evaluation of treatment efficacy

Additional Therapies
- Activity: Increased physical activity has been shown to reduce insulin resistance and lower inflammatory markers associated with the metabolic syndrome.
- When possible, add structured physical activity into daily routine.
- Incorporate both resistance and aerobic activities.
- Non-weight-bearing activities such as swimming and stationary bike riding may be easier for the morbidly obese deconditioned patient.
- Limit sedentary activity to no more than 2 hours per day.
- Home monitoring:
  - Food and activity record logs may increase awareness and importance of healthy lifestyles.
- At home or in school, blood pressure monitoring may rule out white coat hypertension.
- Preprandial and 2-hour postprandial blood sugars are helpful in monitoring impairments in glucose metabolism:
  - Preprandial blood sugar <100 mg/dL
  - Postprandial blood sugar <140 mg/dL

ISSUES FOR REFERRAL
Refer for components of the metabolic syndrome that do not improve with reductions in BMI or treatment of complications (i.e., dyslipidemia, hypertension, diabetes).

SURGERY/OTHER PROCEDURES
Gastric bypass surgery should be considered for morbidly obese adolescent patients (BMI >40) who have severe comorbid conditions, including the following:

- Diabetes mellitus
- Sleep apnea
- Disabling orthopedic complications
- NASH with fibrosis

 ONGOING CARE

FOLLOW-UP RECOMMENDATIONS
Patient Monitoring
- Patients should be followed frequently, every 1–2 months, when they are implementing lifestyle changes.
- Therapy should be intensified (lifestyle and/or pharmacologic) if components of the metabolic syndrome are not clinically improving or worsening.

DIET
- Limiting intake of simple sugars has been shown to improve insulin resistance.
- Eliminate sugared beverages from the diet
- Increase amount of fruits, vegetables, whole grains, and protein in diet.
- Portion control junk food.
- Portion control carbohydrates.
- Family eats healthy together.
- Parents monitor child's food intake.

PROGNOSIS
Improvement in the components of the metabolic syndrome depends on the ability to implement lifestyle changes and achieve modest weight loss.

COMPLICATIONS
- Short term:
  - Increased risk of progression to type 2 diabetes mellitus with weight gain
- Long term:
  - Metabolic syndrome in adults increases risk of coronary heart disease:
    - 2–4-fold depending on population studied
    - 3.5-fold increase in cardiovascular mortality

ADDITIONAL READING

- Gungor N, Hannon T, Libman I, et al. Type 2 diabetes in youth: The complete picture to date. *Pediatr Clin North Am.* 2005;52(6):1579–1609.
- Knowler WC, Barret-Coonor E, Hamman RF, et al. Reduction in the incidence of type 2 diabetes with lifestyle intervention or metformin. *N Engl J Med.* 2002;246(6):393–403.
- Morrison JA, Friedman LA, Gray-McGuie C. Metabolic syndrome in childhood predicts adult cardiovascular disease 25 years later. The Princeton Lipids Research Clinics Follow-up Study. *Pediatrics.* 2007;120(2):340–345.
- Weiss R, Dziura J, Burquet TS, et al. Obesity and the metabolic syndrome in children and adolescents. *N Engl J Med.* 2004;350:2362–2374.
- Zimmet P, Ablerti K, George MM. The metabolic syndrome in children and adolescents – an IDY consensus report. *Pediatr Diabetes.* 2007;8: 299–306.

 CODES

ICD9
- 277.7 Dysmetabolic syndrome X
- 278.00 Obesity, unspecified

ICD10
- E66.9 Obesity, unspecified
- E88.81 Metabolic syndrome

FAQ

- Q: Why is it important to diagnose the metabolic syndrome in children?
- A: Making the diagnosis can help clinicians to educate patients and families that the metabolic syndrome is the antecedent to type 2 diabetes mellitus and increases risk of premature cardiovascular disease.
- Q: What is the 1st-line therapy for the metabolic syndrome?
- A: Weight loss, as modest as 5% reductions in body mass index, can improve the components of the metabolic syndrome.
- Q: How early can the metabolic syndrome be diagnosed?
- A: Prepubertal children can be diagnosed with the metabolic syndrome.

M

METHEMOGLOBINEMIA

Kevin C. Osterhoudt

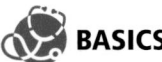 **BASICS**

DESCRIPTION
- Methemoglobin is dysfunctional hemoglobin in which the deoxygenated heme moiety has been oxidized from the ferrous (Fe^{2+}) to the ferric (Fe^{3+}) state.
- Methemoglobinemia is an undue accumulation of methemoglobin within the blood.

EPIDEMIOLOGY
- Toxic methemoglobinemia, resulting from exposure to oxidant chemicals or drugs, is the most common cause of methemoglobinemia among children older than 6 months.
- Enteritis-associated methemoglobinemia is the most common cause among children younger than 6 months:
  - As many as 2/3 of infants with severe diarrhea have methemoglobinemia.

PATHOPHYSIOLOGY
- Hemoglobin in the allosteric configuration of methemoglobin cannot carry oxygen.
- Methemoglobin increases the oxygen affinity of normal heme moieties in the blood and results in impaired oxygen delivery to tissues.
- NADH-dependent cytochrome b5 methemoglobin reductase is the major source of physiologic reduction of methemoglobin.
- A normally dormant NADPH-dependent methemoglobin reductase is the site of action for antidotal methylene blue therapy.

ETIOLOGY
- Toxic methemoglobinemia:
  - Dietary or environmental chemicals: Chlorates, chromates, copper sulfate fungicides, naphthalene, nitrates, and nitrites
  - Industrial chemicals: Aniline and other nitrogenated organic compounds
  - Drugs: Amyl nitrite, benzocaine, dapsone, lidocaine, metoclopramide, nitric oxide, nitroprusside, phenazopyridine, prilocaine, many others
  - Methemoglobinemia is a common iatrogenic complication of drug therapy.
- Enteritis-associated methemoglobinemia is multifactorial in origin:
  - Intestinal nitrate and nitric oxide promotes methemoglobin formation.
  - Innate enzymatic methemoglobin reduction systems may be underdeveloped during infancy.
  - Acidemia further inhibits enzymatic methemoglobin reduction systems.
  - Methemoglobinemia is also reported with nitrite-producing bacterial infections of the intestines or urinary tract.

- Congenital methemoglobinemia (rare):
  - Hemoglobin M: Heterozygotes for autosomal dominant hemoglobin M will exhibit lifelong cyanosis.
  - NADH-dependent methemoglobin reductase deficiency: Homozygotes for this autosomal recessive enzyme will have lifelong cyanosis; heterozygotes may have increased susceptibility to oxidative hemoglobin injury.

COMMONLY ASSOCIATED CONDITIONS
- Heinz body hemolytic anemia
- Oxidant stress on the globin protein may cause hemolysis.
- Sulfhemoglobinemia
- Oxidant stress on the hemoglobin porphyrin ring may cause sulfhemoglobinemia.

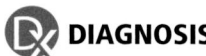 **DIAGNOSIS**

HISTORY
- Age of onset:
  - New onset of cyanosis in children older than 6 months is unlikely to be due to congenital or enteritis-associated methemoglobinemia.
- Source of water:
  - Well water may be contaminated with nitrates.
- Drug or chemical exposure:
  - May suggest a source of toxic methemoglobinemia
- Diarrhea:
  - May suggest enteritis-associated methemoglobinemia

PHYSICAL EXAM
- Cyanosis:
  - Cyanosis becomes apparent in the presence of 1.5 g/dL of methemoglobin (in contrast to 4–5 g/dL of deoxyhemoglobin).
- Heart murmur:
  - May suggest right-to-left intracardiac shunting, rather than methemoglobinemia
- Abnormal lung auscultation:
  - May suggest cyanosis due to pulmonary disorder
- Signs and Symptoms:
  - Malaise
  - Fatigue
  - Dyspnea
  - Tachycardia
  - Cyanosis

DIAGNOSTIC TESTS & INTERPRETATION
Lab
- Oxygen saturation:
  - Oxygen saturation measured by pulse oximetry is artificially low, but oxygen saturation calculated from arterial blood gas is normal (a "saturation gap").
- Co-oximetry:
  - Multiple-wavelength co-oximetry is the standard for quantifying methemoglobin in the blood.
- Hemoglobin quantitation:
  - The percent methemoglobin concentration must be considered in relation to the total hemoglobin.
  - Anemia may suggest concurrent hemolysis.
- Serum bicarbonate:
  - Metabolic acidosis is relatively mild in cases of <40% toxic methemoglobinemia.
  - Metabolic acidosis is typically profound in cases of enteritis-associated methemoglobinemia.
- Glucose-6-phosphate dehydrogenase (G6PD) assay:
  - G6PD deficiency does not predispose to methemoglobinemia and should not be routinely ordered.
- Hemoglobin electrophoresis:
  - Hemoglobin M is rare and does not respond to therapy.
  - This test should not be routinely ordered.

Diagnostic Procedures/Other
- Pulse oximetry may be inaccurate in the setting of methemoglobinemia or methylene blue therapy.
- Blood may have a "chocolate brown" appearance despite exposure to air.

DIFFERENTIAL DIAGNOSIS
- Environmental hypoxia
- Cardiovascular disease
- Pulmonary disease
- Sulfhemoglobinemia
- Factitious skin discoloration

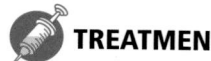 **TREATMENT**

MEDICATION (DRUGS)

- Consider administration of 1% methylene blue.
  - Dose: 1–2 mg/kg IV over 5 minutes, repeated as necessary (caution above 4–7 mg/kg total)
  - Indications: Signs of tissue hypoxia, CNS depression, >30% methemoglobinemia
  - Contraindications (relative): Known, severe G6PD deficiency
- Methylene blue therapy may be ineffective if:
  - Patient is G6PD deficient.
  - Ongoing drug or chemical absorption or biotransformation leads to continuing methemoglobin formation.
  - Sulfhemoglobin is present.
  - Hemoglobin M is present.
  - High doses of methylene blue add to, rather than ameliorate, the oxidant stress.

ADDITIONAL TREATMENT

General Measures

- Acquired methemoglobinemia:
  - Administer 100% oxygen.
  - Decontaminate or remove from toxic source of oxidative stress.
  - Alleviate enteritis with IV fluids or elemental formulas.
  - Treat identified bacterial infections.
  - Exchange transfusion is a consideration of last resort.
- Congenital methemoglobinemia:
  - No beneficial therapy exists for hemoglobin M.
  - Oral methylene blue or ascorbic acid may provide alternative reduction pathways for patients with NADH-dependent reductase deficiencies.

 ONGOING CARE

FOLLOW-UP RECOMMENDATIONS

- Toxic methemoglobinemia:
  - Consider consultation with a medical toxicologist.
  - May require environmental investigation
- Enteritis-associated methemoglobinemia:
  - Careful formula rechallenge warranted if possibility exists for milk protein allergy or other dietary intolerance
- Congenital methemoglobinemia:
  - Consider consultation with a hematologist.

PROGNOSIS

- Toxic methemoglobinemia:
  - Full recovery with recognition, removal of oxidant stress, and appropriate therapy
- Enteritis-associated methemoglobinemia:
  - Methemoglobinemia may be prolonged and relapsing until enteritis healed
- Congenital methemoglobinemia:
  - Lifelong cyanosis expected

COMPLICATIONS

- >10% methemoglobinemia:
  - Cyanosis
- >30% methemoglobinemia:
  - Malaise, fatigue, dyspnea, tachycardia
- >50% methemoglobinemia:
  - Somnolence, tissue ischemia
- 60% methemoglobinemia:
  - Potential lethality

ADDITIONAL READING

- Avner JR, Henretig FM, McAnaney CM. Acquired methemoglobinemia: The relationship of cause to course of illness. *Am J Dis Child*. 1990;144: 1229–1230.
- Osterhoudt KC. Methemoglobinemia. In: Erickson TB, Ahrens WR, Aks SE, eds. *Pediatric Toxicology*. New York: McGraw Hill; 2005:492–500.
- Pollack ES, Pollack CV. Incidence of subclinical methemoglobinemia in infants with diarrhea. *Ann Emerg Med*. 1994;24:652–656.
- Shihana F, Dissanayake DM, Buckley NA, et al. A simple quantitative bedside test to determine methemoglobinemia. *Ann Emerg Med*. 2010;55: 184–189.
- Wright RO, Lewander WJ, Woolf AD. Methemoglobinemia: Etiology, pharmacology, and clinical management. *Ann Emerg Med*. 1999;34:646–656.

 CODES

ICD9
289.7 Methemoglobinemia

ICD10
- D74.0 Congenital methemoglobinemia
- D74.8 Other methemoglobinemias
- D74.9 Methemoglobinemia, unspecified

FAQ

- Q: Can methemoglobinemia be diagnosed by the color of the blood?
- A: The "chocolate brown" blood of methemoglobinemia is most easily noted when compared to "control" blood on a white filter paper background. In contrast to deoxygenated blood from patients with cardiopulmonary disease, methemoglobin-darkened blood does not redden on exposure to room air.
- Q: Is methemoglobin responsible for the profound metabolic acidosis often found in diarrheal infants?
- A: Benzocaine-induced methemoglobinemia rarely causes acidosis in infants. In contrast, infants with enteritis-associated methemoglobinemia often have a profound acidemia with a relatively narrow anion gap. Acidosis should be considered a contributing or coexisting factor, rather than a result, of methemoglobinemia among infants with diarrhea.

M

MICROCYTIC ANEMIA

Alexis Teplick
Janel L. Kwiatkowski (5th edition)

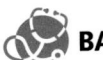 **BASICS**

DEFINITION
Low hemoglobin level and reduced red cell size:
- Mean corpuscular volume (red cell size) varies with age. Adult normal values cannot be applied to young children. Newborns have larger red cells with an average mean corpuscular volume of 108 fL and a lower limit of normal of 98 fL. The mean corpuscular volume then gradually declines. Lower limit of normal:
  – At 2 weeks: 86 fL
  – 2 months: 77 fL
  – 6 months to 2 years: 70 fL
  – 2–5 years: 75 fL
  – 6–12 years: 77 fL
  – 13–18 years: 78 fL
- A quick estimate of the lower limit of normal for mean corpuscular volume for children >1 year old can be made with the following formula:
  – Lower limit of normal mean corpuscular volume = 70 + age (years)

EPIDEMIOLOGY
- Iron deficiency anemia occurs with a prevalence of 1–5% in the US:
  – Young children and adolescent females are at greatest risk.
- β-Thalassemia mutations are common in Mediterranean countries, Southeast Asia, China, Africa, and India.
- Hemoglobin E mutations are common in certain Southeast Asian countries, particularly Cambodia, Laos, and Thailand.
- α-Thalassemia mutations occur in the Chinese subcontinent, Malaysia, Indochina, and Africa.

PATHOPHYSIOLOGY
- Disorders of globin chain synthesis include the thalassemias and hemoglobin E disease.
- β-E mutation leads to decreased production of functional β-globin messenger RNA (mRNA):
  – In the heterozygous form, there is usually mild microcytosis with minimal or no anemia and no clinical symptoms.
  – Homozygous E disease is also asymptomatic, but there is marked microcytosis and a mild anemia (hemoglobin is usually ≥10 g/dL).
- Combination of hemoglobin E and β-thalassemia often results in more severe anemia, similar to β-thalassemia intermedia or major.

ETIOLOGY
- Limited number of causes of microcytic anemia
- Hemoglobin molecule is made up of heme and globin components. Disorders of the production of either of these components may result in a microcytic anemia:
  – Heme production requires iron and is affected by iron deficiency or inadequate iron utilization as is seen in the anemia of chronic inflammation.
  – Inadequate production of porphyrin component can also impair heme synthesis; such disorders are known as sideroblastic anemias. Sideroblastic anemias can be inherited or acquired.
  – Disorders of globin production, the thalassemias, also cause microcytosis.

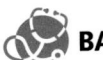 **DIAGNOSIS**

HISTORY
- Child's age:
  – Microcytic anemia in children age 9 months to 3 years and in adolescence is most commonly iron deficiency:
    ○ Term infants are born with adequate iron stores for 6 months and therefore should not have nutritional iron deficiency causing anemia.
    ○ β-Thalassemia major often presents in 1st year of life as fetal hemoglobin production declines.
- Child's diet:
  – Evaluate dietary iron intake as appropriate for age:
    ○ Iron in breast milk is more bioavailable (50% vs. 10%) than iron in formula.
    ○ Infants who are exclusively breastfed after 6 months are at an increased risk for iron deficiency if they do not receive supplements.
    ○ Infant formulas and cereals should be iron fortified. In preschool children and adolescents, assess intake of high iron-containing foods including red meats, fish, poultry, beans, and peanut butter.
  – Introduction of whole cow's milk at age <1 year provides little dietary iron and can cause occult intestinal bleeding leading to iron loss.
    ○ High intake of milk also causes a decreased appetite for other foods with a higher iron content.
    ○ Cow's milk intake >24 ounces daily is a risk factor for iron deficiency.
  – History of pica suggests iron deficiency and/or lead intoxication.

- Other factors:
  – History of blood loss:
    ○ Decreases iron stores
    ○ Ask about loss from stool, urine, chronic nosebleeds, and menorrhagia.
  – Premature birth or blood loss at birth:
    ○ Premature infants have lower total body iron stores and an increased growth rate that leads to increased iron requirements.
    ○ Significant blood loss at birth can deplete iron stores.
  – Child's ethnic background and familial history of anemia:
    ○ α-Thalassemia is most common among children of African or Asian descent.
    ○ β-Thalassemia is most common in children of Mediterranean, Asian, or African descent.
    ○ Hemoglobin E occurs most commonly in children of Southeast Asian descent.
  – Symptoms suggestive of a chronic disease such as joint pain/swelling or abdominal pain

PHYSICAL EXAM
- Child's general appearance: Most children with mild to moderate microcytic anemia are well appearing with a normal physical exam.
- Irritability or pallor:
  – Anemia is likely more severe.
  – Irritability is a common finding with iron deficiency.
- Cardiovascular examination:
  – Check for instability including tachycardia, hypotension, and presence of a gallop.
  – Flow murmurs are common with chronic anemia.
- Abnormal sclerae:
  – Blue sclera is associated with iron deficiency (very rare).
  – Icterus is seen with severe thalassemia syndromes and hemolytic anemias.
- Mouth lesions: Glossitis and stomatitis are signs of iron deficiency.
- Splenic enlargement: May be seen with thalassemia syndromes depending on the severity. The spleen is a site of extramedullary hematopoiesis and clears abnormal red cells.

DIAGNOSTIC TESTS & INTERPRETATION
- In the patient:
  – CBC: Low hemoglobin level and low mean corpuscular volume for age
  – Red cell distribution width:
    ○ Measures variation in red cell size
    ○ Elevated in iron deficiency
    ○ Normal in thalassemia trait, infection, and lead poisoning

- Reticulocyte count: Decreased in iron deficiency anemia and increased in moderate and severe thalassemia syndromes
- Peripheral blood smear:
  ○ Microcytosis and hypochromia
  ○ Marked poikilocytosis and anisocytosis with iron deficiency and thalassemia syndromes
  ○ Basophilic stippling with lead poisoning
  ○ Target cells are found with heterozygous or homozygous hemoglobin E.
- Ferritin:
  ○ Serum ferritin reflects tissue iron stores. It is reduced in iron deficiency.
  ○ Ferritin is an acute-phase reactant and is increased with infection, inflammation, and liver disease.
  ○ Normal or increased in thalassemia
- Serum iron:
  ○ Reduced in iron deficiency
  ○ Normal in thalassemia (unless chronically transfused, which leads to increased iron levels)
  ○ Normal or reduced in infection or inflammatory states
  ○ Can rise within hours of single oral dose
- Transferrin saturation:
  ○ Measures iron available for hemoglobin synthesis
  ○ Low in iron deficiency and chronic infection
  ○ Normal in thalassemia
- Lead level: Increased in lead intoxication
- Hemoglobin electrophoresis with quantitation:
  ○ Increased hemoglobin A2 in β-thalassemia trait and normal in α-thalassemia trait and other microcytic anemias
  ○ Iron deficiency anemia may cause a reduction in hemoglobin A2 production.
  ○ If microcytosis persists after iron is replenished, hemoglobin electrophoresis should be repeated.
- Soluble transferrin receptor:
  ○ Indicator of increased tissue iron demand
  ○ Increased in iron deficiency anemia and also in thalassemia syndromes, but not with the anemia of chronic inflammation
- Bone marrow aspirate:
  ○ Rarely needed to establish diagnosis
  ○ Iron stores can be assessed by hemosiderin staining.
  ○ In sideroblastic anemias, >10% of the nucleated red cell precursors are ringed sideroblasts.
- Family studies:
  - CBC
  - Peripheral blood smear
  - Hemoglobin electrophoresis

Diagnostic Procedures/Other
- Most commonly identified in children through routine screening
- Often the result of a chronic condition that does not require immediate intervention
- Review of the child's history, red cell indices, and peripheral blood smear should guide further laboratory evaluation.
- General guidelines for evaluation:
  - Initially identify severe anemia that requires inpatient observation and possible blood transfusion.

- Consider chronic lead intoxication early. If history is suspicious (e.g., peeling paint, pica), draw lead level.
- Iron deficiency is the most common cause of microcytic anemia. Screen by history. If history is suspicious, consider therapeutic iron trial prior to additional workup.
- If suspicious of a thalassemia syndrome, send hemoglobin electrophoresis with hemoglobin A2 quantification. CBCs and hemoglobin electrophoresis from parents may also be helpful.

DIFFERENTIAL DIAGNOSIS
- Metabolic: Iron deficiency (most common)
- Environmental: Chronic lead poisoning
- Congenital:
  - Thalassemia syndromes
  - Hemoglobin E trait (single gene affected) or disease (2 genes affected)
  - Selected congenital hemolytic anemias with unstable hemoglobin
- Inflammatory:
  - Recent inflammation or infection
  - Anemia of chronic inflammation (also known as anemia of chronic disease) may cause a microcytic anemia or normocytic anemia. Common causes of anemia of chronic inflammation include:
    ○ Chronic infection
    ○ Rheumatoid arthritis
    ○ Systemic lupus erythematosus
    ○ Inflammatory bowel disease (may also be a component of iron deficiency due to gastrointestinal blood loss)
    ○ Malignancy
- Miscellaneous: Sideroblastic anemia (rare in children)

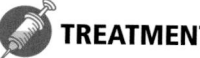 TREATMENT

ADDITIONAL TREATMENT
General Measures
- Consider therapeutic trial of iron supplementation if history is suspicious.
- May require initial inpatient observation in cases of severe anemia
- Red cell transfusion only if evidence of cardiovascular compromise (rarely indicated)
- Removal of environmental exposure and possible chelation for lead poisoning to prevent CNS toxicity
- No treatment needed for α- or β-thalassemia trait or hemoglobin E heterozygous or homozygous conditions:
  - Iron therapy is not indicated.
  - If concomitant iron deficiency is suspected, iron studies should be sent and treatment commenced if iron deficiency is documented.

 ONGOING CARE

FOLLOW-UP RECOMMENDATIONS
- In iron deficiency, reticulocyte count begins to increase in 3–4 days, and hemoglobin concentration should rise by $\geq$1 g/dL in 2–3 weeks following iron supplementation.
- Children with thalassemia trait have a persistent mild, microcytic anemia that is not clinically significant, but they require genetic counseling as they become older.
- Children with other thalassemia syndromes (β-thalassemia major, hemoglobin H disease) should be referred to a hematologist.

ALERT
Lead poisoning and iron deficiency can occur concurrently because iron deficiency causes increased lead absorption. If history is concerning for increased lead exposure in cases of documented iron deficiency, send lead levels.

ADDITIONAL READING
- Grantham-McGregor S, Ani CA. Review of studies on the effect of iron deficiency on cognitive development in children. *J Nutr.* 2001;131(2S-2): 649S–666S; discussion 666S–668S.
- McCann JC, Ames BN. An overview of evidence for a causal relation between iron deficiency during development and deficits in cognitive or behavioral function. *Am J Clin Nutr.* 2007;85(4):931–945.
- Pappas DE. Iron deficiency anemia. *Pediatr Rev.* 1998;19:321–322.
- Richardson M. Microcytic anemia. *Pediatr Rev.* 2007;28(1):5–14.
- Suskind DL. Nutritional deficiencies during normal growth. *Pediatr Clin North Am.* 2009;56(5): 1035–1053.
- Walters MC, Abelson HT. Interpretation of the complete blood count. *Pediatr Clin North Am.* 1996;43:599–622.
- Wharton BA. Iron deficiency in children: Detection and prevention. *Br J Hematol.* 1999;106:270–280.

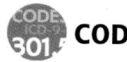 CODES

ICD9
280.9 Iron deficiency anemia, unspecified

ICD10
D50.8 Other iron deficiency anemias

M

MILIA

Albert C. Yan

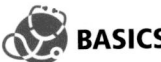 **BASICS**

DESCRIPTION
White papules that occur commonly and spontaneously on the face and frequently elsewhere; after healing of blisters when present on mucous membranes; referred to as *Epstein pearls*

EPIDEMIOLOGY
- Common in all age groups
- Up to 40% of newborns have milia on the skin.
- In older patients, most often related to trauma, sites of irradiation, or re-epithelializing blisters

PATHOPHYSIOLOGY
- Retention of keratin and sebaceous material within the pilosebaceous duct, eccrine sweat duct, or sebaceous collar surrounding vellus hair
- Lamellated keratin deposits are found in the superficial papillary dermis.

ETIOLOGY
Spontaneous, or related to trauma or healing blisters in older patients

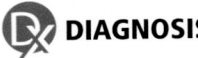 **DIAGNOSIS**

HISTORY
- Asymptomatic
- Recent trauma
- History of blistering diseases
- Special question:
  - If present periocularly, ask about history of atopy/allergic conjunctivitis.

PHYSICAL EXAM
- 1–2 mm bright white papules with smooth surface
- Most often found on cheeks, nose, chin, forehead, but occasionally on dorsal surface of hands and over knees, especially if related to trauma
- Occasionally, lesions may be seen on upper trunk, extremities, penis, or mucous membranes. Epstein pearls represent milia on the palate (often seen at the junction of the soft and hard palates).
- Distinguish from pustules by palpation.

DIAGNOSTIC TESTS & INTERPRETATION
Diagnostic Procedures/Other
Milia are firm and, when incised, reveal solid keratin rather than liquid contents.

DIFFERENTIAL DIAGNOSIS
- Infection:
  - Molluscum contagiosum
  - Impetigo (pustules)
  - Herpes simplex (clouded vesicles)
  - Environmental (poisons)
- Tumors:
  - Sebaceous gland hyperplasia.
- Miscellaneous:
  - Neonatal acne
  - Keratosis pilaris

TREATMENT

ADDITIONAL TREATMENT
General Measures
- No need for treatment in infants because milia are benign, asymptomatic, and often resolve on their own.
- Alternatively, cyst contents may be expressed by squeezing or with a comedone extractor, or after incision of the overlying epidermis with a needle or no. 11 scalpel blade.

ONGOING CARE

FOLLOW-UP RECOMMENDATIONS
Without treatment, most lesions resolve in 1–2 weeks in infants.

PROGNOSIS
- Spontaneous regression of milia occurs in infants.
- In older individuals, the lesions are usually chronic unless treated.
- Lesions uncommonly recur.

COMPLICATIONS
- Primarily of cosmetic concern
- Rare potential for foreign body reaction to occur
- If persistent milia in an unusual or widespread distribution when seen with other defects: Hereditary trichodysplasia (Marie Unna hypotrichosis), oral-facial-digital syndrome type I, absence of fingerprints (dermatoglyphs) associated with fragile skin (Baird or Basan or Rombo syndrome), or Loeys-Dietz syndrome (periocular milia, arachnodactyly, craniofacial and cardiovascular anomalies). Often seen in healed areas of dystrophic forms of epidermolysis bullosa

ADDITIONAL READING

- Baird HW, III. Kindred showing congenital absence of the dermal ridges (fingerprints) and associated anomalies. *J Pediat*. 1964;64:621–631.
- Berk DR, Bayliss SJ. Milia: A review and classification. *J Am Acad Dermatol*. 2008;59(6):1050–1063.
- Hurwitz S. *Clinical pediatric dermatology: A textbook of skin disorders of childhood and adolescence*, 2nd ed. Philadelphia: WB Saunders, 1993.
- Lloyd BM, Braverman AC, Anadkat MJ. Multiple facial milia in patients with Loeys-Dietz syndrome. *Arch Dermatol*. 2011;147(2):223–226.

 CODES

ICD9
- 528.4 Cysts of oral soft tissues
- 701.1 Keratoderma, acquired
- 706.2 Sebaceous cyst

ICD10
- K09.8 Other cysts of oral region, not elsewhere classified
- L72.0 Epidermal cyst
- L85.8 Other specified epidermal thickening

FAQ
- Q: Will the lesions get bigger before they go away?
- A: No. There is no tendency to enlarge with time.

M

MILK PROTEIN INTOLERANCE

Rosalyn Diaz

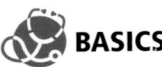 BASICS

DESCRIPTION
- A condition in which symptoms affecting the GI tract, skin, and respiratory tract result from ingestion of cow's milk protein
- Currently no distinction is being made between cow's milk protein allergy and intolerance since both seem to have similar pathogenesis and clinical presentation.

EPIDEMIOLOGY
Prevalence has been estimated at 2–7.5% of otherwise normal infants. The condition usually presents in the 1st 3 months of life. It may rarely present for the 1st time in older children (0.4%) and recur in adults.

PATHOPHYSIOLOGY
- Unprocessed cow's milk protein is 80% casein and 20% whey. The whey fraction contains >20 types of antigenic proteins, including α-lactoglobulin (the most allergenic of all), α-lactalbumin, bovine serum albumin, α_2-microglobulin, transferrin, and lactoferrin. Casein is thought to be weakly allergenic.
- Exclusively breastfed infants may also develop milk protein intolerance through exposure to allergens that appear in breast milk. Nevertheless, breastfeeding is protective in decreasing food allergies.
- Although α-lactoglobulin is suspected to be an antigen, no single protein fraction has been proven. Most children appear to be allergic to multiple cow's milk proteins; rarely are patients allergic to only 1 fraction.
- There is 25–30% cross-reactivity between milk proteins and soy proteins.

ETIOLOGY
Predisposing factors include:
- Age (diagnosis usually <2 years)
- Immune deficiency (immaturity of the mucosal immune system, immaturity or damage of mucosal barrier function, low IgA levels)
- History or presence of atopy
- Early milk protein–based formula feeding
- Allergenic formula
- GI infection
- Positive family history

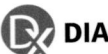 DIAGNOSIS

HISTORY
- Diagnosis is implied if clinical symptoms resolve upon removal of cow's milk protein–containing products.
- In some cases, no resolution is seen on soy-based formula, and hydrolyzed formula and even crystalline amino acid–based formulas are needed.
- Signs and symptoms:
  - GI manifestations such as blood and mucus in the stool in a normal-appearing infant are the most common presentation.
  - GI: Diarrhea, bloody stools, vomiting, feeding problems, constipation, GERD
  - Dermatologic: Atopic dermatitis, urticaria, angioedema, eczema
  - Respiratory: Allergic rhinitis, coughing, wheezing
  - General: Anaphylaxis, failure to thrive (FTT), hypoproteinemia

PHYSICAL EXAM
- Usually healthy-appearing child with normal physical exam
- Most patients will present in the 1st few months of life with:
  - Occult blood loss (without anemia in most cases)
  - Hematochezia
  - Emesis/reflux symptoms
- Some patients may present with:
  - Profuse watery diarrhea with signs of dehydration
  - Malabsorption (edema due to hypoalbuminemia, FTT, hemorrhage, rickets)
  - Abdominal distention

DIAGNOSTIC TESTS & INTERPRETATION
Diagnostic Procedures/Other
- Clinical diagnosis
- No single laboratory test appears to have significant sensitivity for detecting this syndrome.
- Radioallergosorbent testing (RAST) and skin testing may be used with positive predictive value of only 50%.
- Occasionally, peripheral blood and stool eosinophilia may be documented.
- Infectious causes of enteropathy may mimic the disorder; therefore, infection should be ruled out with stool cultures and duodenal fluid cultures, if available.

- Rectosigmoid biopsies are not routinely performed.
- Histologic changes in bowel mucosa tend to be nonspecific.
- Grossly, the mucosa appears friable and inflamed, rarely with erosions or gross ulcerations.
- Pathologic findings may include:
  - Partial villous atrophy with reduction in villous height on upper endoscopy
  - Moderate increase in intraepithelial lymphocytes
  - Prominent eosinophilic infiltrate

ALERT
In the rare situation of severe food allergy with shocklike picture and acidosis, fluid resuscitation and refeeding should be done in the hospital.

DIFFERENTIAL DIAGNOSIS
- GERD and colic are most often misdiagnosed in these infants.
- Diseases characterized by watery diarrhea, abdominal pain, and blood and mucus in the stool should be considered.
- Infectious causes (dysentery, *Clostridium*) should be excluded.
- Inflammatory bowel disease (IBD), celiac disease, autoimmune enteropathy, toddler diarrhea, anal fissures, and Meckel diverticulum (among others) should be considered, depending on the presentation.

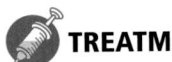 TREATMENT

ADDITIONAL TREATMENT
General Measures
- Removal of cow's milk protein–containing products from the diet is the cornerstone of treatment.
- ~10–30% of children with cow's milk protein intolerance will also be intolerant to soy protein. For this reason, soy-based formulas are rarely recommended.
- Casein hydrolysate formulas (Pregestimil, Nutramigen, Alimentum) are the formulas of choice for infants with cow's milk protein intolerance. Whey hydrolysate formula is not usually recommended for these patients.
- Resolution of grossly bloody stools usually occurs within 24–72 hours, but stool occult blood testing may continue to be positive for 2–6 weeks.

- Neocate, Nutramigen AA, and EleCare formulas are amino acid–, simple carbohydrate–, and fat-based formulas that have been more effective in recalcitrant cases of intolerance.
- If no clinical response is seen after 2–3 weeks of diet restriction, then other diagnoses should be considered.
- Epinephrine may be needed in cases of severe milk protein allergy and anaphylaxis.
- Corticosteroids are sometimes used to treat skin and respiratory manifestations.

 ONGOING CARE

FOLLOW-UP RECOMMENDATIONS

- It is important to restrict the diet completely for milk and soy protein during the 1st year of life.
- With the introduction of solids, it is important to read labels carefully for the presence of any milk or soy proteins.
- In most cases, tolerance to cow's milk protein develops at age 1–2 years, and a normal diet can be safely reintroduced.
- Occasionally, symptoms of intolerance may persist past the 3rd year of life; ~10% will have symptoms that persist at 6 years of age.
- Cow's milk protein challenge with RAST, skin testing, and possible GI biopsies can help to monitor the degree of allergic response in these older children.
- In cases of severe anaphylactic reactions or acute urticaria, the cow's milk challenge should be performed in a hospital under medical supervision.
- GI intolerance seems to persist in a certain proportion of subjects, with intestinal symptoms and increased prevalence of lactose intolerance.

ADDITIONAL READING

- Boyce JA, Assa'ad AH, Burks AW, et al. *Guidelines for the diagnosis and management of food allergy in the United States. 2010.* Available at: http://www.niaid.nih.gov/topics/foodAllergy/clinical/Pages/default.aspx. Accessed May 23, 2011.
- Branum AM, Lukacs SL. Food allergy among U.S. children: Trends in prevalence and hospitalizations. *NCHS Data Brief.* 2008;(10):1–8.
- Crittenden RG, Bennett LE. Cow's milk allergy: A complex disorder. *J Am Coll Nutr.* 2005;24(6 Suppl):582S–591S.
- Host A. Frequency of cow's milk allergy in childhood. *Ann Allergy Asthma Immunol.* 2002;89(6 Suppl 1):33–37.
- Kattan JD, Cocco RR, Järvinen KM. Milk and soy allergy. *Pediatr Clin North Am.* 2011;58(2):407–426.
- Kokkonen J, Tikkanen S, Savilahti E. Residual intestinal disease after milk allergy in infancy. *J Pediatr Gastroenterol Nutr.* 2001;32:156–161.
- Sampson HA, Anderson JA. Summary and recommendation: Classification of gastrointestinal manifestations due to immunologic reactions to foods in infants and young children. *J Pediatr Gastroenterol Nutr.* 2000;30:S87–S94.
- Vanto T, Helppila S, Juntunen-Backman K, et al. Prediction of the development of tolerance to milk in children with cow's milk hypersensitivity. *J Pediatr.* 2004;144(2):218–222.
- Walker-Smith J. Cow's milk allergy: A new understanding from immunology. *Ann Allergy Asthma Immunol.* 2003;90(6 Suppl 3):81–83.
- Walker-Smith J. Hypoallergenic formulas: Are they really hypoallergenic? *Ann Allergy Asthma Immunol.* 2003;90(6 Suppl 3):112–114.

 CODES

ICD9
- V15.02 Allergy to milk products
- 558.3 Allergic gastroenteritis and colitis

ICD10
- T78.1XXA Other adverse food reactions, not elsewhere classified, initial encounter
- Z91.011 Allergy to milk products

FAQ

- Q: Can a fully breastfed infant develop milk protein intolerance?
- A: Fully breastfed infants rarely develop milk protein intolerance because there are fewer cow's milk protein antigens in breast milk, but it may still occur. To continue to nurse, the mother needs to follow a strict elimination diet for milk and soy protein, and sometimes even fish, eggs, and other common allergens.
- Q: When does this problem usually resolve?
- A: In most infants who develop minimal symptoms, the problem will resolve by the 1st year of life, but the range can be several years. Some reports of residual GI disease exist.
- Q: When should a patient be referred to an allergist?
- A: Infants with severe symptoms, persistence of symptoms despite a strict elimination diet, and/or those >12 months of age should be referred to an allergist.

M

MUMPS/PAROTITIS

Nicholas Tsarouhas

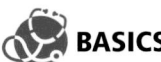 **BASICS**

DESCRIPTION
CDC clinical case definition: Illness with acute onset of unilateral or bilateral, tender, self-limited swelling of the parotid or other salivary gland, lasting ≥2 days, without other apparent cause

EPIDEMIOLOGY

Incidence
- In the prevaccine era, 90% of all children contracted mumps virus infection by 14 years of age.
- Incidence of this once very common disease has declined dramatically since the advent of universal childhood immunization.
- Outbreaks, however, continue to occur.
- Since 2001, 200–300 cases per year reported in the US
- In early 2006, a large epidemic broke out in Iowa and neighboring states:
  - 11 states reported >2,500 cases.
  - Largest epidemic since 1988
  - Median age of patient was 21 years (mostly college students).
  - Led CDC and American College Health Association to recommend 2 doses of MMR be a requirement for college entry.
- In 2006, 81–100% of children entering US schools had received 2 doses of mumps vaccine.
- Seroprevalence of antibody to mumps virus in the US population (1999–2004) estimated at 90%

GENERAL PREVENTION
- 2 combination mumps vaccine are used:
  - MMR: Measles, mumps, rubella
  - MMRV: Measles, mumps, rubella, varicella
- A single 0.5-mL SC injection of live mumps vaccine (MMR or MMRV) is recommended at 12–15 months.
- A 2nd vaccination is recommended between 4 and 6 years of age.
- Primary vaccine failure and waning vaccine-induced immunity have been reported.
- Some have suggested the need for a 3rd vaccination to mitigate waning immunity.
- The 1st dose of MMR vaccine sometimes causes fever and rash:
  - This occurs 7–10 days after immunization.
  - Measles component is usually the culprit.
- Both MMRV and MMR vaccines, but not varicella vaccine alone, are associated with increased outpatient fever visits and seizures 7–10 days after vaccination in 12–23-month-olds, with MMRV vaccine increasing fever and seizure twice as much as the MMR + varicella vaccine.
- Vaccine should not be administered to children who are immunocompromised by disease or pharmacotherapy, or to pregnant women.
- Children with HIV infection who are not severely immunocompromised should be immunized with the MMR vaccine.
- 1 attack of mumps (clinical or subclinical) usually confers lifelong immunity.
- Links of the MMR vaccine to autism by Dr. Andrew Wakefield in a 1998 *Lancet* publication have now been completely exposed as fraudulent and false.

PATHOPHYSIOLOGY
- The virus is spread by contact with respiratory secretions.
- The mumps virus enters via the respiratory tract, and a viremia ultimately ensues.
- The viremia spreads to many organs, including the salivary glands, gonads, pancreas, and meninges.
- Period of communicability: 7 days before to 9 days after onset of parotid swelling
- Most communicable period: 1–2 days before to 5 days after onset of parotid swelling
- Incubation period: 12–25 days after exposure
- Humans are the only known host for mumps.

ETIOLOGY
- Parotitis is usually caused by mumps, a Rubulavirus in the paramyxovirus family.
- Other viral causes of parotitis include cytomegaloviruses, influenza, parainfluenza, and enteroviruses.
- Bacterial cases are usually secondary to *Staphylococcus aureus* (suppurative parotitis).
- Streptococci, gram-negative bacilli, and anaerobic infections are also possible.
- Rare childhood cases may be secondary to an obstructing calculus, foreign body (sesame seed), or various drugs (antihistamines, phenothiazines, iodine-containing drugs/contrast media).

COMMONLY ASSOCIATED CONDITIONS
- Salivary adenitis:
  - Most common manifestation of mumps
  - 1/3 of cases occur subclinically
- Epididymoorchitis:
  - Up to 35% of adolescent mumps cases are complicated by orchitis.
  - Orchitis develops within 4–10 days of the onset of the parotid swelling.
  - Sterility is uncommon.
- Pancreatitis:
  - Mild inflammation is common.
  - Serious involvement is rare.

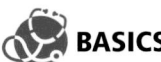 **DIAGNOSIS**

HISTORY
- Prodromal symptoms uncommon, but may include the following:
  - Fever
  - Anorexia
  - Myalgia
  - Headache
- Onset usually pain and swelling in front of and below ear
- Swelling:
  - Usually starts on one side of the face, then progresses to the other
- Mild fever:
  - Usually accompanies parotid swelling
- Dysphagia and dysphonia are common.
- Testicular pain and swelling, along with constitutional symptoms, usually begin ~1 week after the parotid swelling of mumps.
- Epigastric pain and constitutional symptoms with pancreatic involvement

- Fever, headache, and stiff neck with meningitis
- Behavioral changes, seizures, and other neurologic abnormalities are rare.
- Other symptoms are analogous to the particular organ involved.
- Parotid enlargement can be an initial sign in HIV-infected children.

PHYSICAL EXAM
- Nonerythematous, tender parotid swelling (erythema seen with suppurative parotitis)
- Swelling ultimately obscures the mandibular ramus.
- The ear is displaced upward and outward.
- Importantly, up to 30% of symptomatic cases of mumps are not associated with parotitis.
- Submaxillary and sublingual glands also may be swollen.
- Inflammation may be noted intraorally at the orifice of Stensen duct.
- Presternal edema is occasionally noted.
- Mumps are infrequently associated with truncal rash.
- Tender, edematous testicle in mumps orchitis (usually unilateral)
- Ask the patient if the pain (at the parotid) intensifies with the tasting of sour liquids:
  - Have the patient suck on a lemon drop or lemon juice, and note any discharge from Stensen duct.

DIAGNOSTIC TESTS & INTERPRETATION

ALERT
Skin tests should not be used for test of immunity; serologic studies are more reliable.

Lab
- Uncomplicated parotitis:
  - Mild leukopenia with lymphocytosis
- Suppurative parotitis and mumps orchitis:
  - Leukocytosis
- Pancreatic involvement:
  - Hyperamylasemia and elevated serum lipase
- Salivary adenitis without pancreatic involvement:
  - Isolated hyperamylasemia
- Gram stain and culture of pus expressed from Stensen duct is diagnostic in suppurative parotitis.
- CDC lab criteria for mumps diagnosis:
  - Isolation of mumps virus from clinical specimens: Blood, urine, buccal swab (Stensen duct exudates), throat washing, saliva, or CSF
  - Detection of mumps virus nucleic acid by reverse transcriptase PCR
  - Positive serologic test for mumps IgM
  - Significant rise between acute and convalescent titers in mumps IgG levels by any standard assay (complement fixation, neutralization, hemagglutination inhibition, or enzyme immunoassays)

Imaging
Sialography is useful to evaluate for stones or strictures but is contraindicated in acute infection.

Diagnostic Procedures/Other
Lumbar puncture if meningitis is suspected: CSF pleocytosis (predominately mononuclear)

DIFFERENTIAL DIAGNOSIS

- Mumps parotitis can be distinguished from the other viral causes by clinical presentation along with specialized laboratory studies.
- Cases of tuberculous and nontuberculous (atypical) mycobacterial parotitis are rare but have been reported.
- Salivary calculus can be diagnosed by sialogram.
- Recurrent childhood parotitis, aka juvenile recurrent parotitis:
  - Rare, recurrent swelling of parotids
  - Seen in children 3–6 years old
  - Not associated with suppuration or external inflammatory changes
  - Largely a diagnosis of exclusion
- Cervical or preauricular adenitis:
  - May simulate parotitis
  - Close anatomic localization should be diagnostic
- Infectious mononucleosis and cat-scratch disease are other considerations.
- Drug-induced parotid enlargement occasionally occurs.
- Malignancies of the parotid are extremely rare.
- Pneumoparotitis is seen in those with a history of playing a wind instrument, glass blowing, scuba diving, and even general anesthesia.

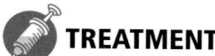

TREATMENT

ADDITIONAL TREATMENT
General Measures
- Supportive therapy is all that is required in mumps parotitis.
- Antibiotics directed against *S. aureus* should be used in cases of suppurative parotitis.

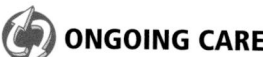

ONGOING CARE

FOLLOW-UP RECOMMENDATIONS
- Most children have resolution of glandular swelling by ~1 week.
- Disappearance of testicular pain and swelling can be expected 4–6 days after onset.
- Testicular atrophy is common, although infertility is rare.
- Markedly elevated pancreatic enzymes should be monitored until they improve.
- Children should not return to school until at least 9 days after the onset of parotid swelling.

PROGNOSIS
Complete recovery in 1–2 weeks is the rule.

COMPLICATIONS
- Meningitis:
  - >50% have a CSF pleocytosis.
  - This "aseptic meningitis" is usually benign.
- Encephalitis: Rarely causes permanent sequelae
- Cerebellitis
- Facial nerve palsy
- Oophoritis, nephritis, thyroiditis, myocarditis, mastitis, arthritis, transient ocular involvement, deafness, and sterility (all rare)

ADDITIONAL READING

- American Academy of Pediatrics. Mumps. In: Pickering LK, ed. *2009 Red Book: Report of the Committee on Infectious Diseases*, 28th ed. Elk Grove Village, IL: American Academy of Pediatrics; 2009:468–472.
- Brauser D. Autism and MMR vaccine study: An 'elaborate fraud,' charges BMJ. *Medscape Medical News*. January 6, 2011. Available at: http://www.medscape.com/viewarticle/735354.
- CDC. Update: Multistate outbreak of mumps—United States, Jan 1–May 2, 2006. *MMWR*. 2006;55:559–563.
- Deer B. How the case against the MMR vaccine was fixed. *BMJ*. 2011;342:c5347. Available at: http://www.bmj.com/content/342/bmj.c5347.full?sid=cd35b6db-3b0e-4e33-9393-fe1f08d424e8. Accessed January 10, 2011.
- Karmody KA. Mumps in emergency medicine. *Medscape Medical News*. January 31, 2011. Available at: http://emedicine.medscape.com/article/784603-overview.
- Klein NP, Fireman B, Yih WK, et al. Measles-mumps-rubella-varicella combination vaccine and the risk of febrile seizures. *Pediatrics*. 2010;126(1):e1–8. Epub 2010 Jun 29.
- Kutty PK, Kruszon-Moran DM, Dayan GH, et al. Seroprevalence of antibody to mumps virus in the US population, 1999–2004. *J Infect Dis*. 2010; 202(5):667–674.
- Offit PA. Autism and the MMR vaccine, revisited. *Medscape Infectious Diseases*. January 7, 2011. Available at: http://www.medscape.com/viewarticle/735439?src=ptalk.
- Quinlisk MP. Mumps control today. *J Infect Dis*. 2010;202(5):655–656. doi:10.1086/655395
- Senanayake SN. Mumps in the United States. *N Engl J Med*. 2008;359(6):654.
- Shacham R, Droma EB, London D, et al. Long-term experience with endoscopic diagnosis and treatment of juvenile recurrent parotitis. *J Oral Maxillofac Surg*. 2009;67(1):162–167.
- Virtanen M, Peltola H, Paunio M, et al. Day to day reactogenicity and the healthy vaccinee effect of measles-mumps-rubella vaccination. *Pediatrics*. 2000;106:5.

 CODES

ICD9
072.9 Mumps without mention of complication

ICD10
B26.9 Mumps without complication

FAQ

- Q: Should immunization be deferred in children with intercurrent illness?
- A: No. Children with minor illnesses, even with fever, should be vaccinated.
- Q: Should vaccination be withheld in children living with immunocompromised hosts?
- A: No. Vaccinated children do not transmit mumps vaccine virus.

M

MUNCHAUSEN SYNDROME BY PROXY

Cheryl L. Hausman

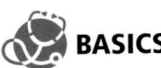 **BASICS**

DESCRIPTION
- Illness in a child that is fabricated by someone else (usually the parent)
- May also be known as "pediatric condition falsification" (PCF)
- Results in repeated interactions with the medical care system, often leading to multiple medical procedures
- Perpetrator denies the cause of the child's illnesses.
- Symptoms decrease when the child is separated from the perpetrator.

EPIDEMIOLOGY
- Typical victims are <4 years of age, equally divided between males and females. However, there have been case reports of older children.
- Victims average 21.8 months from onset of symptoms to diagnosis.
- Varies with presentation
- Of infants monitored in apnea programs, 0.27% are believed to be secondary to Munchausen syndrome by proxy.
- 5% of allergy patients in some clinic settings are estimated to be secondary to Munchausen syndrome by proxy.
- Mortality is ~6–9%.

ETIOLOGY
- The parent, commonly the mother, fabricates the illnesses.
- Little is known about the etiology in the parent:
  – Parent may have Munchausen syndrome.
  – Parent may be seeking secondary gain from the attention of medical staff or financial gain by having the child be disabled.

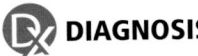 **DIAGNOSIS**

HISTORY
- Unexplained or unusual illness, symptoms, and signs that are incongruous or present only when the perpetrator is present
- Usual medical treatment is ineffective in treating the presenting symptom.
- Perpetrator may not be concerned about the patient, may be constantly present while the patient is in the hospital, or may form unusually close relationships with the hospital staff.
- Special questions:
  – History of frequent moves, or of other siblings who have either died or had unusual medical illnesses, may suggest Munchausen syndrome by proxy.
  – In the context of divorce, repeated allegations of sexual abuse may represent Munchausen syndrome by proxy.

PHYSICAL EXAM
- Examination of the patient with apnea presentation may indicate evidence of intentional suffocation.
- Patients who present with unusual bleeding may have lacerations on other parts of the body.
- Perpetrator also may have lacerations.
- Note the presence of indwelling IV, CSF, or bladder catheters.
- Patient may have evidence of old fractures.

DIAGNOSTIC TESTS & INTERPRETATION
Diagnostic Procedures/Other
Workup is dictated by presentation:
- Pneumogram to rule out apnea
- If bleeding is the major presentation, identify the blood as the patient's (as opposed to that of the perpetrator or an animal).
- A toxicology screen may be helpful for unusual presentations of poisoning.
- Separating the perpetrator from the patient, with resultant decrease in symptoms, may suggest the diagnosis.
- Suspect Munchausen syndrome by proxy when there is blood or urine culture with many organisms.
- If GI bleeding is the presenting symptom, use endoscopy or a Meckel scan to rule out anatomic causes of bleeding.
- Video monitoring of a patient's room may demonstrate the perpetrator harming the child.
- Ensure that the perpetrator cannot tamper with testing.

DIFFERENTIAL DIAGNOSIS

Diagnosis depends on presentation. Munchausen syndrome by proxy should be considered in unusual presentations of:

- GI bleeding
- Apnea/apparent life-threatening event
- Asthma
- Seizures
- Genitourinary bleeding
- Unexplained abnormalities in electrolytes
- Chronic diarrhea or vomiting
- Infections with multiple organisms found in blood or urine culture

ALERT

- Diagnosis is often delayed: Mean length of time to diagnosis is 21.8 months.
- Physicians and nursing personnel may be reluctant to suspect the parent because of their own involvement with the family.

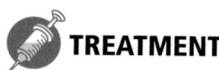

TREATMENT

ADDITIONAL TREATMENT
General Measures

- If Munchausen syndrome by proxy is documented, the patient must be separated from the perpetrator. Psychotherapy for the perpetrator is warranted.
- As long as the perpetrator is in need of intensive psychotherapy, the patient should be protected.

ONGOING CARE

FOLLOW-UP RECOMMENDATIONS

- If the perpetrator agrees to seek help, improvement usually occurs, but long-term follow-up is necessary.
- Watch for recurrence of original presentation, unusual new symptoms.

PROGNOSIS

- If undiagnosed, mortality has been estimated at 6–9%.
- Some children go on to develop Munchausen syndrome themselves.
- Long-term consequences to the child are unknown.

ADDITIONAL READING

- Carter KE, Izsak E, Marlos J. Munchausen syndrome by proxy caused by ipecac poisoning. *Pediatr Emerg Care*. 2006;9:655–656.
- Galvin HK, Newton AW, Vandeven AM. Update on Munchausen syndrome by proxy. *Opin Pediatr*. 2005;17(2):252–257.
- Giurgea I, Ulinski T, Touati G, et al. Factitious hyperinsulinism leading to pancreatectomy: Severe forms of Munchausen syndrome by proxy. *Pediatrics*. 2005;116(19):e145–e148.
- Hall DE, Eubanks L, Meyyazhagan LS, et al. Evaluation of covert video surveillance in the diagnosis of Munchausen syndrome by proxy: Lessons from 41 cases. *Pediatrics*. 2000;105: 1305–1312.
- Kamerling LB, Black XA, Riser RT. Munchausen syndrome by proxy in the pediatric intensive care unit: An unusual mechanism. *Pediatr Crit Care Med*. 2002;3:305–307.
- Pankratz L. Persistent problems with the Munchausen syndrome by proxy label. *J Am Acad Psychiatry*. 2006;34(1):90–95.
- Schreier H. Munchausen by proxy defined. *Pediatrics*. 2002;110:985–988.
- Sheridan MS. The deceit continues: An updated literature review of Munchausen syndrome by proxy. *Child Abuse Negl*. 2003;27:431–451.

CODES

ICD9
301.51 Chronic factitious illness with physical symptoms—Munchausen syndrome

ICD10
F68.13 Factitious disorder with combined psychological and physical signs and symptoms

FAQ

- Q: Is it legal to use video surveillance or to separate the parent from the patient?
- A: If suspicions of Munchausen syndrome by proxy are high and other laboratory tests are negative, it is important to make the diagnosis. Hospital administration and/or risk management should be consulted on how to proceed.
- Q: Should this be reported to child abuse authorities?
- A: If documented, this should be reported to protect the child.

M

MUSCULAR DYSTROPHIES

Hugh J. McMillan
Molly E. Rideout (5th edition)

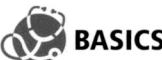 BASICS

DESCRIPTION
- Muscular dystrophies (MDs) are a heterogeneous group of disorders characterized by progressive skeletal muscle weakness. Cardiac muscle can be involved in some forms.
- Muscular dystrophies with childhood onset can be divided into 5 groups:
  - Dystrophinopathies (i.e., Duchenne MD [DMD], Becker MD [BMD])
  - Limb girdle MDs (LGMDs)
  - Congenital MD (CMD)
  - Facioscapulohumeral MD (FSH-MD)
  - Emery-Dreifuss MD (EDMD)
- Types of MDs can be differentiated by their clinical features (i.e., pattern of muscle weakness, joint contractures), age of onset, genetic test results, and/or muscle biopsy.

EPIDEMIOLOGY
Incidence
- Dystrophinopathies:
  - DMD: 1 per 3,500 boys (most common)
  - BMD: 1 per 30,000 boys
- LGMD (childhood onset): 5–10 per million
- CMD (all types): 1–10 per 100,000
- FSH-MD: 1 per 20,000
- EDMD: 1 per 300,000

RISK FACTORS
Genetics
Genetic testing is clinically available for most MDs:
- Dystrophinopathies (DMD/BMD): X linked:
  - DMD exon duplication/deletion in 70% cases
  - DMD point mutation in almost 30% cases
- LGMD: Most childhood-onset LGMDs are autosomal recessive.
  - Sarcoglycanopathies (LGMD2C–F) make up roughly 70% of childhood-onset LGMDs.
  - LGMD2I (FKRP): 5% childhood-onset LGMDs
- CMD: Most autosomal recessive (12 genes)
  - Nonsyndromic (LAMA2, COL6A1–COL6A3)
  - Syndromic (e.g., POMT1, POMGT1, FKRP)
- FSH-MD: Autosomal dominant (D4Z4 deletion)
- EDMD: X linked (EMD or FHL1 mutations) or autosomal dominant (LMNA mutation)

PATHOPHYSIOLOGY
- Deficient or defective muscle fiber proteins causing fiber dysfunction and/or increased membrane fragility
- Muscle biopsy: Increased variability in muscle fiber size (i.e., degenerating, regenerating, and necrotic fibers); split muscle fibers and increased internal nuclei; fibrosis. Immunohistochemistry may note decreased/absent sarcolemma proteins (e.g., DMD, LGMDs, CMDs).

DIAGNOSIS

HISTORY
- Neonatal hypotonia, feeding difficulty (CMD)
- Gross motor delay/regression
- Global developmental delay (syndromic CMD) or learning disorders (DMD)
- Exercise intolerance/cramping
- Myalgia (BMD, DMD)
- Seizures: Merosin-negative and syndromic CMD
- **DMD:** Onset typically <5 years old with gross motor delays, increasing falls, toe walking, and proximal muscle weakness (e.g., difficulty climbing stairs, rising from floor). Calf pseudohypertrophy is common. Serum creatine kinase (CK) levels are markedly elevated (often >50× normal). Serum transaminases may be elevated (muscle origin). Higher incidence of learning difficulties, ADHD, autism, OCD. Loss of ambulation occurs around 13–16 years old. Incidence of cardiomyopathy increases with age, although respiratory muscle weakness (e.g., ineffective cough, hypoventilation, and eventual respiratory failure) is the cause of death in about 75% of DMD boys.
- **BMD:** Milder version of DMD phenotype. Onset typically >8 years old. Boys remain ambulatory into their 20s. Higher incidence of myalgia, cramps, and myoglobinuria in BMD (vs. DMD). Rarely, cardiomyopathy may be sole or presenting feature.
- **LGMD:** Proximal muscle weakness (neck flexors, hip flexors, shoulder girdle). Disease onset and progression highly variable. Sarcoglycanopathies (LGMD2C–F) can mimic DMD (including calf pseudohypertrophy). Patients are cognitively normal.
- **CMD:** Hypotonia, gross motor delay, weakness, and feeding difficulty typically noted from birth. Two main groups of CMDs: (1) **nonsyndromic** CMD due to defective structural proteins (e.g., merosin-negative CMD, Ullrich/Bethlem MD) and (2) **syndromic** CMD due to defective glycosylation (e.g., Fukayama MD, muscle-eye-brain disease, Walker-Warburg syndrome):
  - Most children with nonsyndromic CMD are cognitively normal. Seizures may occur in merosin-negative CMD (20–30%). Ullrich MD shows characteristic proximal contractures and distal joint hyperlaxity (fingers, toes). Bethlem MD shows proximal muscle weakness and distal contractures.
  - Syndromic CMDs show variable severity, often associated with intellectual disability, eye manifestations, and brain anomalies (e.g., neuronal migration disorders, seizures, hydrocephalus).

- **FSH-MD:** Onset typically <20 years old with facial weakness, scapular winging, and humeral (biceps, triceps) weakness. Relative sparing of deltoid strength is seen. Rare infantile-onset cases have been reported. Retinal vasculopathy (Coates disease) can occur. Cardiac arrhythmia is occasionally noted (<10%), while cardiomyopathy is exceedingly rare.
- **EDMD:** Onset typically in 1st decade. Patients initially present with joint contractures (neck, elbow, and ankles) disproportionate to degree of weakness. Muscle weakness and wasting develop in biceps, triceps, spinates muscles, and (later) tibialis anterior and peroneal muscles. Cardiac arrhythmias are common by 2nd decade. Pseudohypertrophy is not seen.

PHYSICAL EXAM
- Facial weakness (FSH-MD)
- Pattern of muscle weakness and atrophy
- Scapular winging (FSH-MD)
- Pattern of joint contractures (EDMD) or joint hypermobility (Ullrich MD)
- Pattern of muscle pseudohypertrophy (e.g., calf muscles in DMD, BMD, LGMD)
- Reflexes normal to mildly decreased (except for joints with contractures). Reflexes are not lost until late in disease course.
- Normal sensory exam
- Scoliosis: Rapid progression if nonambulatory
- Gower maneuver (when arising from sitting to standing position patient must put his hand on his knees and "climb up himself")
- Gait abnormalities (e.g., toe walking, exaggerated lumbar lordosis, Trendelenburg gait)
- Cardiomyopathy (tachycardia, hypotension)
- Respiratory weakness (weak cough)

DIAGNOSTIC TESTS & INTERPRETATION
Lab
Serum CK: Markedly elevated in DMD, BMD, some LGMD and CMDs (e.g., Fukayama MD). CK may be normal late in disease owing to severe muscle atrophy. CK is typically normal in FSH-MD and some CMDs (e.g., Ullrich MD). Normal to mild CK elevation is seen in EDMD.

Diagnostic Procedures/Other
- Nerve conduction study: Merosin-negative CMD may show mild conduction velocity slowing.
- EMG: Nonspecific myopathic changes
- MRI muscle: Signal change noted reflecting muscle atrophy and fatty infiltration (may guide site of muscle biopsy but is not valuable for diagnostic purposes)

- MRI brain: Merosin-negative CMD show diffuse white matter signal abnormalities (typically visible by 6 months old)
- Muscle biopsy can be used to confirm dystrophy (see "Differential Diagnosis"), while immunohistochemistry can help in diagnosis of nondystrophic MDs (e.g., LGMD) if DMD genetic testing is normal.

DIFFERENTIAL DIAGNOSIS
- Inflammatory myopathy (e.g., dermatomyositis)
- Metabolic myopathy
- Congenital myopathy
- Anterior horn cell disease (e.g., SMA)
- Polyneuropathy (e.g., CIDP)
- Myotonic dystrophy (different pathology)

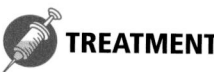 TREATMENT

MEDICATION (DRUGS)
- For DMD: Corticosteroids (prednisone [0.75 mg/kg/day] or deflazacort) 0.9 mg/kg/day: Improve muscle strength, prolong independent ambulation (mean = 2.5 years), delay onset of cardiomyopathy and scoliosis, and improve pulmonary function testing. Patients must be monitored for adverse effects of steroid therapy (weight gain, bone demineralization, behavior issues).
- All other MDs: No treatment

ADDITIONAL TREATMENT
General Measures
- Supportive care (e.g., routine immunizations)
- Psychological and/or school support
- Night splinting (DMD, LGMD) to prevent progression of joint contractures
- Physiotherapy: Passive stretching
- Orthopedic evaluation: Scoliosis surveillance and/or management of joint contractures
- Genetic counseling
- Ophthalmology (retinal) evaluation (FSH-MD); cataract surveillance (DMD patients on steroids)

Additional Therapies
Several potential therapies for DMD are being studied (e.g., antisense oligonucleotide therapy, DMD nonsense mutation read-through therapy, myostatin inhibitor therapy, stem cell therapy). These therapies remain experimental and are not commercially available in North America or Europe.

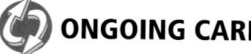 ONGOING CARE

FOLLOW-UP RECOMMENDATIONS
Patient Monitoring
- Respiratory surveillance:
  - Baseline respirology evaluation (DMD, CMD) with periodic PFT surveillance, incentive spirometry, and/or cough assist devices
  - Monitor for decline in PFT scores (especially FVC) and/or clinical evidence of nocturnal hypoventilation (e.g., morning headache/nausea, daytime somnolence, orthopnea). If noted, obtain sleep study to evaluate for potential need for nocturnal bilevel positive airway pressure (BiPAP).
  - Monitor kyphoscoliosis.
- Cardiology surveillance:
  - Cardiomyopathy is well documented for many MDs, necessitating periodic echocardiogram and ECG surveillance studies for DMD, BMD, LGMD1B, LGMD2C–F (20–30% risk), LGMD2I (30–60% risk), merosin-negative CMD, and EDMD.
  - American Academy of Pediatrics (AAP) guidelines recommend DMD patients receive complete cardiac evaluation every 2 years (until age 10 years) and annually thereafter.
  - Cardiac arrhythmia surveillance is required for EDMD, LGMD1B, and FSH-MD (<10% risk); also consider for any MD patient showing echocardiogram evidence of a cardiomyopathy.
  - Cardiac transplantation should be considered for BMD patients with severe cardiomyopathy, particularly if they have relatively minor skeletal muscle involvement.

PROGNOSIS
- DMD: Life expectancy into late 20s, death typically from respiratory failure
- BMD: Life expectancy into mid-40s, death typically due to cardiomyopathy
- LGMD: Variable. Sarcoglycanopathies may show a DMD-like progression. Autosomal dominant LGMD later onset with slow progression

ADDITIONAL READING
- American Academy of Pediatrics. Cardiovascular health supervision for individuals affected by Duchenne or Becker muscular dystrophy. *Pediatrics.* 2005;166:1569–1573.
- Bonnemann CG. Limb-girdle muscular dystrophy in childhood. *Pediatr Ann.* 2005;34:569–577.
- Bushby K, Finkel R, Birnkrant DJ, et al. Diagnosis and management of Duchenne muscular dystrophy, part 1: Diagnosis, pharmacological and psychosocial management. *Lancet Neurol.* 2010;9:77–93.

- Bushby K, Finkel R, Birnkrant DJ, et al. Diagnosis and management of Duchenne muscular dystrophy, part 2: Implementation of multidisciplinary care. *Lancet Neurol.* 2010;9:177–189.
- El-Bohy A, Wong B. Muscular dystrophies. *Pediatr Ann.* 2005;34:525–530.
- Guglieri M, Straub V, Bushby K, et al. Limb–girdle muscular dystrophies. *Curr Opin Neurol.* 2008;21:576–584.
- Hermans MCE, Pinto YM, Merkies IS, et al. Hereditary muscular dystrophies and the heart. *Neuromuscular Disord.* 2010;20:479–492.
- Kirschner J, Bonnemann C. The congenital and limb-girdle muscular dystrophies. *Arch Neurol.* 2004;61:189–197.
- Tawil R, Van Der Maarel SM. Facioscapulohumeral muscular dystrophy. *Muscle Nerve.* 2006;34:1–15.

 CODES

ICD9
- 359.0 Congenital hereditary muscular dystrophy
- 359.1 Hereditary progressive muscular dystrophy

ICD10
- G71.0 Muscular dystrophy
- G71.2 Congenital myopathies

FAQ
- Q: What test should be ordered 1st in a boy with suspected DMD?
- A: After confirmation that CK is elevated, 1st-line testing is *DMD* duplication/deletion analysis (detects 70% cases). If negative, *DMD* gene should be sequenced. Muscle biopsy is typically reserved for patients with negative genetic testing (i.e., LGMD) or if there is clinical suspicion for inflammatory myopathy (e.g., dermatomyositis). Nerve conduction studies can help differentiate neurogenic disorders (i.e., SMA, polyneuropathy) but show nonspecific myopathic changes in MDs.
- Q: What is the recurrence risk in DMD?
- A: About 2/3 of mothers of males with DMD are carriers. If a female DMD carrier has a son, that boy has a 50% chance of having DMD. If she has a daughter, that girl has a 50% chance of becoming a DMD carrier. Males with DMD or BMD will transmit the mutated gene to all daughters (who become carriers). The sons of DMD males will not be affected (X linked).
- Q: Can female DMD carriers be symptomatic?
- A: Yes. Owing to the random nature of X-chromosome inactivation, roughly 10% of female DMD heterozygotes may develop cardiomyopathy and/or proximal muscle weakness. The American Academy of Pediatrics recommends female carriers receive a cardiac evaluation in early adulthood and every 5 years after 25–30 years old.

M

MYASTHENIA GRAVIS

Diana X. Bharucha-Goebel
Brenda E. Porter (5th edition)
Grant T. Liu (5th edition)

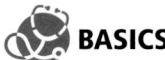 BASICS

DESCRIPTION
A neuromuscular (NM) disease presenting with varying weakness that worsens with exercise and improves with rest.
- Rare—Incidence 4–6 per million per year
- Prevalence of 40–80 per million
- Children account for 10–15% of cases of myasthenia gravis annually.
- 3 types of myasthenia gravis seen in childhood:
  - Neonatal transient: 10–20% of infants born to mothers with autoimmune myasthenia
  - Congenital myasthenia: Rare; <10% of all childhood myasthenia. Weakness usually starts in the 1st year of life and is caused by an inherited disorder in NM transmission. Can be classified by the site of mutation (e.g., presynaptic/postsynaptic) or by molecular genetics.
  - Juvenile myasthenia: Autoimmune disorder similar to adult-onset, autoimmune myasthenia gravis. Caused by aberrant production of antibodies against the acetylcholine receptor (AChR). Relatively rare: 1 new diagnosis per million per year. The average age of onset is 10–13 years, with a female predominance of 2:1 or 4:1.

RISK FACTORS
Genetics
- Congenital type: Generally autosomal-recessive (check consanguinity)
- Occasional family history

PATHOPHYSIOLOGY
- Caused by a disruption in signal transmission from the motor neuron to the muscle. Sensory or cognitive symptoms are absent.
  - The motor nerve terminal lies in close proximity to the end plate, a region of the muscle cell membrane with a high concentration of AChR.
  - Normally, when stimulated, the motor nerve terminal releases acetylcholine that binds receptors, causing contraction of the muscle. The cleft contains acetylcholinesterase (AChE), an enzyme that breaks down acetylcholine and helps terminate the muscle contractions.
- Autoimmune form (Juvenile)
  - Autoantibody blocks AChR activity → increased rate of receptor breakdown → fewer receptors are present → leads to decreased muscle contraction.
  - Thymic pathology is believed to be central to the pathogenesis of autoimmune myasthenia; hyperplasia is present in most children who undergo thymectomy.

- Neonatal (transient) myasthenia: Infants are born with weakness and hypotonia.
  - Due to maternal–fetal transmission of antibodies against the AChR
  - The severity of maternal symptoms does NOT predict the likelihood that the infant will be affected. Occasional arthrogryposis (joint contractures) reflects decreased fetal movement in utero.
  - High levels of maternal antibodies against the fetal form of AChR pose an increased risk of disease.
  - A previous pregnancy with an affected infant places future pregnancies at much higher risk. In rare cases, the mother is asymptomatic, despite presence of a (placentally transmitted) antibody.
- Congenital myasthenic syndromes—group of genetic disorders of NM junction; classified by site of NM transmission defect and more recently by molecular genetics
  - Includes presynaptic defects, synaptic defect (due to end-plate AChE deficiency); postsynaptic defects (primary AChR deficiency; primary AChR kinetic abnormality; OR perijunctional skeletal muscle sodium channel mutation)

COMMONLY ASSOCIATED CONDITIONS
- In juvenile myasthenia, other autoimmune disorders may occur:
  - Hyperthyroidism is present in 3–9% of patients.
  - Small increase in the incidence of rheumatoid arthritis and diabetes
- Some reports suggest an increased incidence of seizures in autoimmune myasthenia.
- Screening for thymoma at initial diagnosis is appropriate (by chest CT scan):
  - Children appear to have a lower incidence of thymic tumor than adults with autoimmune myasthenia.

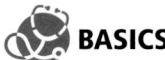 DIAGNOSIS

Most patients present with ptosis and diplopia alone or in combination with swallowing difficulties, dysphonia, and generalized weakness.

HISTORY
- Neonatal transient: Mother with known autoimmune myasthenia or a history of weakness, ptosis, or dysphagia
- Congenital myasthenia:
  - Usually presents in the 1st year of life (rarely later) with hypotonia, poor feeding, ptosis, and delayed motor milestones
  - Possible family history of similar weakness
  - No response to thymectomy or immunosuppressant medications

- Juvenile myasthenia:
  - Gradual onset of weakness over weeks, months, or even years
  - Symptoms are worse after prolonged activity or late in the day.
  - Intermittent ptosis, diplopia, dysphagia, and dysphonia are common.
  - Ocular myasthenia gravis: A subset of 10–15% of patients with myasthenia who have isolated ptosis and ophthalmoplegia (weakness in extraocular muscles) in absence of systemic or bulbar symptoms

PHYSICAL EXAM
- Neonatal transient: From birth, the infant is hypotonic, with a weak suck, a weak cry, and ptosis.
- Congenital and juvenile myasthenia:
  - Weakness of neck flexion
  - Reflexes often preserved
  - Ptosis, ophthalmoplegia, and variable-feeding problems are often the earliest findings.
  - Generalized weakness may be asymmetric in the limbs. The weakness is more pronounced with endurance tasks.
  - Shallow, rapid respirations suggest impending ventilatory failure. Vital capacity of <50% of predicted (in older children) suggests impending respiratory failure.
  - Check for scoliosis (anti-MuSK variant)

DIAGNOSTIC TESTS & INTERPRETATION
- Juvenile myasthenia:
  - Nerve conduction and electromyography studies: Repetitive stimulation of a nerve shows a diagnostic decremental response due to decreased AChR.
  - Single-fiber electromyography measures the variability in firing rates of 2 muscle fibers innervated by different branches of the same motor neuron. A large variability suggests a higher threshold for activation.
  - Edrophonium chloride (Tensilon) is a fast-acting AChE-blocking agent (no longer widely available in the US).
    - Patients with myasthenia often show an immediate, transient improvement in muscle strength after IV infusion of this drug.
    - A measurable weakness should be present prior to testing, and a placebo dose of saline should be given initially.
    - Although the risk of a hyperreactive cholinergic response with muscle weakness and bradycardia is low, atropine should always be available, and the patient's vital signs should be closely monitored during the test (contraindicated in patients with heart disease).
    - Measurable cranial nerve dysfunction, such as ptosis, is often responsive to edrophonium.
    - Children receive 20% of 0.2 mg/kg dose of Tensilon over 1 minute; if there is no response after 45 seconds, the rest of the dose is then given, up to a maximum of 10 mg. Have atropine and epinephrine readily available.

Lab
- AChR antibody levels (most specific): Elevated in ~80% of patients with generalized myasthenia and about 50% of patients with isolated ocular myasthenia
- Second most common—serum antibody to muscle-specific receptor tyrosine kinase (MuSK-Ab)

DIFFERENTIAL DIAGNOSIS
- Generalized botulism:
  - In endemic areas, may cause generalized weakness in infants; caused by *Clostridium* toxin that blocks the release of acetylcholine from nerve terminal.
- Guillain–Barré syndrome or acute inflammatory demyelinating polyneuropathy:
  - A frequent cause of rapidly progressive generalized weakness
  - Unlike myasthenia, there are often sensory symptoms, and areflexia occurs even with minimal weakness.
- Acute spinal cord compression:
  - Can present as generalized (but not variable) weakness of the extremities
  - Look for sparing of facial and extraocular muscles; a sensory level, bowel, or bladder dysfunction; and hyperactive reflexes
- Organophosphate ingestion: Pyridostigmine bromide (Mestinon)
  - Can cause profound weakness
  - Symptoms of parasympathetic hyperactivity, such as hypersalivation, miosis, diarrhea, and bradycardia, will usually be present.
- Penicillamine used for the treatment of autoimmune disorders can induce autoantibodies that bind the AChR, causing myasthenia gravis.

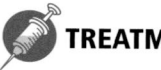 TREATMENT

INITIAL STABILIZATION
Treat respiratory failure, a rare but serious complication of juvenile myasthenia gravis:
- Shallow breathing, a vital capacity of <50% predicted, or a rapidly worsening vital capacity suggests impending respiratory failure.

General Measures
- Neonatal myasthenia:
  - Severity of disability should be used to guide the aggressiveness of therapy.
  - Respiratory or swallowing impairment: Pyridostigmine syrup, 60 mg/5 mL, 7 mg/kg, 30 minutes before feeds; 1 mg IM = 30 mg PO dose
- Juvenile myasthenia:
  - Most patients benefit from pyridostigmine bromide (Mestinon) given 3–4× per day. A long-acting formulation prior to bedtime may alleviate obstructive hypoventilation during sleep.
  - Pyridostigmine → blocks AChE activity → results in increased acetylcholine
  - A normal starting dosage is approximately 7 mg/kg/d. The dosage is slowly titrated upward, following symptoms, at several-day intervals. Common side effects are hypersalivation, blurry vision, and diarrhea.

- Glycopyrrolate (1 mg PO) may decrease diarrhea.
- Prednisone
  - Consider in patients with disabling symptoms and inadequate response to pyridostigmine
  - Watch for transient worsening within weeks in up to 50% of patients
  - Start daily dose at 2 mg/kg, watch for improvement in 3–6 weeks, taper toward 1.5 mg/kg/d on alternate-day schedule for 4 months. Taper slowly thereafter by 5 mg/wk.
  - Monitor for side effects, including growth stunting
  - Calcium and every-other-day dosing may limit the bone deterioration from chronic steroids.
- Azathioprine
  - Induces remission in 30% of patients and significant improvement in another 25–60%
  - Useful adjunctive to steroids and thymectomy; however, it takes 3–12 months for benefits to occur
- Juvenile myasthenics with profound weakness and respiratory failure (myasthenic crisis) should undergo immediate therapy to decrease the number of circulating antibodies:
  - Plasmapheresis or IV immunoglobulin can help within days by decreasing AChR antibodies.
  - Steroids diminish antibody production over weeks to months.
  - Newer immunosuppressants reported effective in small series (mycophenolate mofetil and anti-CD20)

SURGERY
Thymectomy:
- 20–60% remission; another 15–30% show marked improvement
- Thymectomy earlier in the course of illness appears to produce a higher rate of remission.

 ONGOING CARE

- The following medications can exacerbate myasthenia gravis:
  - Corticosteroids may worsen symptoms.
  - Aminoglycosides
  - Ciprofloxacin
  - β-Adrenergic blocking agents, including eye drops
  - Lithium
  - Procainamide
  - Quinidine
  - Phenytoin
- Prolonged recovery after exposure to nondepolarizing NM blocking agents
- Always start new medications cautiously

PROGNOSIS
- Neonatal transient:
  - A self-limited disorder that resolves spontaneously over weeks or months of life as maternal antibodies disappear
  - The infant may require ventilatory and nutritional support during the first few months of life.
  - Infants with arthrogryposis multiplex congenita (born to mothers with antibodies against the fetal form of AChR) may gain mobility over time and with passive range-of-motion therapy.

- Congenital myasthenia:
  - Prognosis varies, depending on the specific defect
  - Autosomal-recessive disorders tend to be more severe than the dominant disorders. Weakness shows variable response to cholinesterase inhibitors.
  - Immunosuppressants are not helpful. In general, these are indolent disorders.
  - Ptosis and fatigability resemble the juvenile type, but are more stable over time.
- Juvenile myasthenia:
  - Most patients do extremely well with treatment; patient selection for early surgery requires experience and may improve outcome.
  - Longitudinal studies suggest that the rate of spontaneous remission is ~2% per year.
  - Patients with generalized weakness are slightly less likely to experience remission.
  - The mortality rate from myasthenia is near that of the general population in patients <50 years.

PATIENT MONITORING
- Watch for transient worsening of symptoms
- Monitor for side effects of corticosteroids, including growth stunting
- Medication effects: GI upset due to AChE inhibitors

COMPLICATIONS
Respiratory failure, nocturnal hypoventilation, visual disturbance, thymic cancer, other autoimmune disorders

ADDITIONAL READING
- Harper CM. Congenital myasthenic syndromes. *Semin Neurol.* 2004;24:111–123.
- Lindner A, Schalke B, Toyka VK. Outcome in juvenile-onset myasthenia gravis: A retrospective study with long-term follow up. *J Neurol.* 1997;244:515–520.
- Newsom-Davis J. Therapy in myasthenia gravis and Lambert-Eaton myasthenic syndrome. *Semin Neurol.* 2003;23:191–198.
- Parent internet information: http://www.myasthenia.org
- Pineles SL, Avery RA, Moss HE, et al. Visual and systematic outcomes in pediatric ocular myasthenia gravis. *Am J Ophthalmol.* 2010;150:453–457.

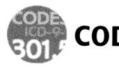 CODES

ICD9
- 358.0 Myasthenia gravis
- 358.01 Myasthenia gravis with (acute) exacerbation
- 775.2 Neonatal myasthenia gravis

ICD10
- G70.00 Myasthenia gravis without (acute) exacerbation
- G70.01 Myasthenia gravis with (acute) exacerbation
- P94.0 Transient neonatal myasthenia gravis

M

MYOCARDITIS

Bradley S. Marino
John L. Jefferies

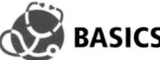 **BASICS**

DESCRIPTION
Myocarditis is defined as inflammation of the myocardium on histologic examination.

EPIDEMIOLOGY
Cardiovascular complications may be significant including myocardial dysfunction, arrhythmias, conduction abnormalities, and cardiac arrest.

Incidence
- True incidence of acute myocarditis is difficult to estimate because of the wide range in clinical severity, various etiologies, and under-diagnosis.
- Estimates of incidence from autopsy range from ~0.1% to 12%.
- More than 50% of pediatric cases seen are in infants <1 year of age.

Prevalence
Viral myocarditis has a seasonal distribution, which varies according to the viral species.

RISK FACTORS
- Exposure to infectious agents, drugs, toxins, and systemic diseases
- Drug exposure
- Autoimmune disease
- Systemic disease

PATHOPHYSIOLOGY
- Pathophysiology of myocarditis may vary based on cause (See Etiology)
- Viral myocarditis is best characterized and involves a complex interaction among the virus, host immune response, and environmental factors. 3 stages include: 1) Viral injury and innate immune response; 2) Acquired host immune response; and 3) Recovery or chronic cardiomyopathy.
- Inflammatory response from innate and acquired immune response may result in significant damage to the myocardium and conduction system
- Development of autoantibodies may also play a key role in acute and chronic myocardial damage.
- Virus may cause direct damage to the myocardium independent of inflammation secondary to cleavage of structural proteins.
- Pathogenesis of nonviral myocarditis is poorly understood.
- Regardless of the cause, symptom severity increases with worsening ventricular function and/or with worsening arrhythmias.
- Fulminant myocarditis may be characterized by both severe systolic and diastolic dysfunction.
- Progressive left ventricular systolic dysfunction may lead to hypotension, acidosis, and end-organ dysfunction.
- Left ventricular diastolic dysfunction may result in elevated left ventricular end diastolic pressures, leading to pulmonary venous and arterial hypertension, with concomitant pulmonary edema and right-sided heart failure.

ETIOLOGY
- Causes include infection, toxins, drugs, autoimmune disease, and systemic disease
- Infectious causes include: Viral, bacterial, rickettsial, fungal, helminthic, spirochetal, and protozoal infections
- Viral infection is the most common in developed countries. Both RNA and DNA viruses have been implicated. Previously, the enteroviruses, specifically Coxsackie B, were commonly seen. However, there has been a recent shift in the spectrum. Currently, parvovirus B19 is most commonly seen. There are growing reports of certain herpes viruses, specifically HHV6, becoming more prevalent.
- Nonviral infectious causes are far less common but must be considered especially in endemic areas, such as Central and South America where Chagas disease is prevalent.
- Nonviral myocarditis may be secondary to exposure to toxins, drug hypersensitivity, autoimmune disease such as SLE, or systemic disease such as Churg–Strauss or sarcoidosis.
- Giant cell myocarditis (GCM) is a very rare form of myocarditis in children that is associated with autoimmune disease and drug hypersensitivity. These patients respond poorly to typical care and frequently require cardiac transplantation.

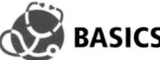 **DIAGNOSIS**

SIGNS AND SYMPTOMS
- Prodromal:
  - Antecedent flu-like illness
  - Gastroenteritis
  - Rheumatologic symptoms
  - Fever
- Left-sided heart failure:
  - Exercise intolerance
  - Easy fatigability
  - Dyspnea
  - Orthopnea
  - Anorexia, loss of appetite/poor feeding, early satiety
  - Emesis (especially in children)
- Right-sided heart failure:
  - Abdominal pain/cramping
  - Swelling of abdomen/lower extremities
  - Loose stools

HISTORY
- Duration of symptoms
- Travel history
- Family history

PHYSICAL EXAM
Any of the following may be present:
- Pulmonary:
  - Rales
  - Tachypnea
  - Retractions

- Cardiovascular:
  - Jugular venous distention
  - Normal to hyperdynamic precordium with or without right ventricular heave
  - Lateral displacement of the point of maximal impulse (PMI)
  - Tachycardia: Arrhythmia (atrial and/or ventricular ectopy may be present)
  - Heart sounds: Accentuation of second heart sound (secondary to pulmonary artery hypertension), murmur (mitral and/or tricuspid insufficiency), gallop, and/or rub.
- Abdomen: Hepatomegaly, splenomegaly, ascites
- Extremities:
  - Weak pulses
  - Poor capillary refill
  - Cool extremities

DIAGNOSTIC TESTS & INTERPRETATION
- Despite limited sensitivity and specificity, endomyocardial biopsy (EMB), using the Dallas criteria for histopathologic classification, remains the gold standard for confirming the diagnosis of acute myocarditis.
  - These criteria are limited in that they provide information with regard to inflammation but do not assess for the presence of viral pathogens.
  - Current approaches indicate benefit in analyzing the tissue for viral DNA by polymerase chain reaction.
  - EMB has inherent problems, including sample selection bias, as tissue is only obtained from the right ventricular endocardium, and possible morbidity and mortality associated with an invasive procedure.
- Other studies supportive of the diagnosis may include: EKG:
  - Highly variable findings may include sinus tachycardia, low voltage QRS, ST segment depression/elevation, flattening or inversion of the T wave, conduction system disease including complete heart block, prolongation of the QT interval, and arrhythmias (premature atrial contractions/supraventricular tachycardia, or premature ventricular contractions/ventricular tachycardia).

Lab
- ESR and C-reactive protein level may be elevated.
- Creatinine kinase MB fraction and troponin T and I levels may be elevated.
- Cultures (bacterial, viral, fungal) of blood, urine, stool, and nasopharyngeal swabs may be considered.
- Viral PCR analysis of tissue including myocardium, blood, or sputum may be considered.
- Acute and convalescent serologic studies may be considered for selected antibody studies.

Imaging
- Chest radiograph:
  - Cardiomegaly and varying degrees of pulmonary edema
  - Possible pleural effusions
- Echocardiography:
  - Depressed systolic function (may biventricular with normal to mildly dilated chamber sizes)
  - Depressed diastolic function
  - Focal wall motion abnormalities
  - Valvular insufficiency
  - Pericardial effusion
- Cardiac MRI
- Assessment of chamber size and systolic function
- Fibrosis by delayed enhancement
- Abnormal delayed enhancement and edema as seen by T_2 weighting

DIFFERENTIAL DIAGNOSIS
- Severe left-sided obstructive heart lesions:
  - Mitral stenosis
  - Valvular aortic stenosis
  - Coarctation of the aorta
- Congenital coronary artery anomalies:
  - Anomalous left coronary artery from the pulmonary artery and other coronary variants
- Incessant arrhythmias:
  - Incessant supraventricular tachycardia
  - Ventricular tachycardia
- Metabolic disorders including mitochondrial disease
- Drug use
  - Cocaine or other stimulants
- Acquired disease
  - Kawasaki disease
  - Coronary artery disease
- Genetic syndromes:
  - Neuromuscular disease
  - Genetically mediated cardiomyopathies

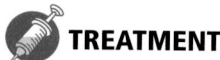 TREATMENT

ADDITIONAL TREATMENT
General Measures
- Initial management should be based on the clinical presentation. These include the following: Bed rest and limited activity (during acute phase).
- Standard medical regimens for acute care should be based on appropriate heart failure therapies and may include (a more complete list of recommendations for the management of acute and chronic heart failure may be found elsewhere; Jessup M et al.):
  - Inotropic support should be considered for patients with evidence of low cardiac output. Medication infusions may include milrinone, dopamine, dobutamine. If epinephrine is required, mechanical support should be considered.
  - Diuretics: Afterload reduction may be considered if volume overload exists with preserved cardiac output (e.g., nitroglycerin and nitroprusside)
  - Anti-arrhythmics may be used in cases of hemodynamically significant arrhythmias.

- Standard medical regimens for chronic care should be based upon appropriate heart failure therapies and may include:
  - Angiotensin converting inhibitors (ACEi)
  - β-blockers
  - Angiotensin receptor blockers
  - Diuretics (e.g., spironolactone for ventricular remodeling)
  - Immunosuppression/immunomodulation may be considered in the form of intravenous immunoglobulin
  - Steroids may also be considered in patients with evidence of myocardial necrosis or refractory arrhythmias
  - Anticoagulation with unfractionated or low molecular weight heparin acutely and aspirin and/or coumadin chronically for patients with severe myocardial depression and ventricular dilation
  - Implantable devices may be considered for patients with conduction system disease or those at risk for sudden cardiac death
  - Permanent pacemaker
  - Implantable cardioverter–defibrillator
  - Mechanical ventilation in patients with respiratory failure secondary to myocardial failure
  - Mechanical support (in patients with rapidly progressing, severe heart failure; used as a bridge to transplantation): Left ventricular or biventricular assist devices, extracorporeal membrane oxygenation (ECMO)
  - Rescue therapy: Cardiac transplantation

MEDICATION (DRUGS)
- Immunosuppression: High-dose gamma globulin (2 g/kg IV immunoglobulin [Ig] over 24 hours) during the acute phase has been associated with improved recovery of left ventricular function and with a tendency for better survival during the first year after presentation.
- Steroids, azathioprine, calcineurin inhibitors, cyclosporine, cyclophosphamide, and other immunosuppressive medications have all been proposed as effective agents, although insufficient evidence of therapeutic benefit is currently available to recommend routine use.
- Antiviral therapy does not currently have an accepted role in myocarditis management. Use of interferon therapy is being widely studied but there continues to be a lack of demonstrable benefit.

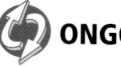 ONGOING CARE

FOLLOW-UP RECOMMENDATIONS
Patient Monitoring
- Clinical changes in systolic and diastolic function
- Observation for life-threatening arrhythmias
- Effects of the illness on other systems:
  - Nutritional status
  - Growth
  - Development
  - Comorbid illnesses

PROGNOSIS
- Statistics are hampered by the lack of complete ascertainment of all cases of acute myocarditis, with many patients likely exhibiting only mild symptoms, which spontaneously resolve.

- Prognosis is often dictated by clinical presentation. However, if treated appropriately early in the course, outcome can be quite favorable. Prognosis is poor in patients with fulminant lymphocytic myocarditis with significant hemodynamic compromise with a mortality of >40% in adults and ~75% in children without aggressive management strategies. Mortality is higher in children presenting in the neonatal period. Giant cell myocarditis represents a unique subgroup with a particularly poor prognosis unless transplanted.

COMPLICATIONS
- Acidosis
- End-organ hypoperfusion
- Pulmonary venous and arterial hypertension
- Pulmonary edema
- Unfavorable ventricular remodeling
- Conduction system disease including heart block
- Arrhythmias

ADDITIONAL READING
- Bowles NE, Ni J, Kearney DL, et al. Detection of viruses in myocardial tissues by polymerase chain reaction: Evidence of adenovirus as a common cause of myocarditis in children and adults. *J Am Coll Cardiol*. 2003;42:473–476.
- Blauwet LA, Cooper LT. Myocarditis. *Prog Cardiovasc Dis*. 2010;52(4):274–288.
- Foerster SR, Canter CE, Cinar A, et al. Ventricular remodeling and survival are more favorable for myocarditis than for idiopathic dilated cardiomyopathy in childhood: An outcomes study from the Pediatric Cardiomyopathy Registry. *Circ Heart Fail*. 2010;3(6):689–697.
- Jefferies JL, Price JF, Morales DLS. Mechanical circulatory support in childhood heart failure. *Heart Fail Clin*. 2010;6(4):559–573.
- Kühl U, Schultheiss HP. Myocarditis in children. *Heart Fail Clin*. 2010;6(4):483–496.
- Moulik M, Breinholt JP, Dreyer WJ, et al. Viral endomyocardial infection is an independent predictor and potentially treatable risk factor for graft loss and coronary vasculopathy in pediatric cardiac transplant patients. *J Am Coll Cardiol*. 2010;56(7):582–592.

 CODES

ICD9
- 422.90 Acute myocarditis, unspecified
- 422.91 Idiopathic myocarditis
- 429.0 Myocarditis, unspecified

ICD10
- I40.0 Infective myocarditis
- I40.9 Acute myocarditis, unspecified
- I51.4 Myocarditis, unspecified

M

NARCOLEPSY

Kiran P. Maski
Sanjeev V. Kothare

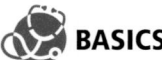 **BASICS**

DESCRIPTION
- Lifelong neurologic disorder that, often, initially manifests in childhood or adolescence and can cause significant functional impairment and disability
- Excessive daytime somnolence and inappropriate transition from wakefulness into REM sleep
- Principal features include uncontrollable and overwhelming daytime sleep attacks, cataplexy, hyponogogic hallucinations, and sleep paralysis.

GENERAL PREVENTION
- Narcolepsy is not preventable.
- Narcolepsy is an under-recognized disease, especially in children.
- Physicians should screen for sleep dysfunction and excessive sleepiness in anticipatory guidance.

EPIDEMIOLOGY
- Prevalence in the USA is reported to range from 3 to 16 per 10,000; prevalence may be higher in the Japanese population
- An estimated 200,000 Americans have narcolepsy, but fewer than 50,000 of these individuals have been diagnosed with the disorder
- Most often diagnosed in the third and fourth decade, but 34% of patient have symptoms before age 15
- Cataplexy is present in 50–70% of adult patients but is correctly identified in only 15% of children with a diagnosis of narcolepsy

RISK FACTORS
- First-degree relatives of patients with narcolepsy have a 1–2% risk (which is 10- to 40-fold more than the general population) of developing narcolepsy.
- Both genetic and environmental factors may be involved in the development of narcolepsy
- There is an association between narcolepsy and histocompatibility leukocyte antigens (HLA) sub-types DQ (specifically DQB1 0602 and DQA1 0102) and DR2 antigens.

PATHOPHYSIOLOGY
- Hypocretin/orexin is a neuropeptide produced by neurons in the periforniceal area of the posterior and lateral hypothalamus that is supplied to several areas of the brain that promote wakefulness, and it possibly also inhibits REM sleep
- Idiopathic narcolepsy is caused by selective loss of the hypocretin/orexin-producing neurons in the hypothalamic region
- The association between narcolepsy and specific HLA antigens may indicate immunologic pathogenesis; however, this is yet to be established.

COMMONLY ASSOCIATED CONDITIONS
- Secondary narcolepsy may be seen with CNS trauma, strokes, brain tumors, and demyelinating diseases, particularly involving the lateral and posterior hypothalamus, midbrain, and the pons.
- Genetic syndromes such as Prader–Willi syndrome, Myotonic dystrophy, and Niemann–Pick type C syndrome may be associated with secondary narcolepsy

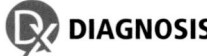 **DIAGNOSIS**

HISTORY
- Excess daytime sleepiness with irresistible urge to fall asleep and unintentional naps may be early signs of disease.
- In adults, naps tend to be restorative, but are more likely to be described as "unrefreshing" in children.
- Cataplexy, the abrupt loss of muscle tone provoked by strong emotions such as surprise, sadness, laughter, or anger, is the second most common symptom in narcolepsy. Loss of muscle tone can range from sagging of face, eyelids or jaw, blurred vision, knee buckling, to complete collapse, but with preservation of consciousness.
- Hypnagogic (on sleep onset)/hypnopompic (on awakening) hallucinations involve vivid auditory or visual hallucinations during transitions between sleep and wakefulness. Such hallucinations are also experienced infrequently by normal individuals.
- Sleep paralysis is the inability to move or speak for a few seconds or minutes at sleep onset or offset. Normal individuals can also occasionally experience sleep paralysis.

PHYSICAL EXAM
- Normal in most idiopathic cases; children with narcolepsy are often overweight/obese.
- Vertical gaze palsy, confusion, poor memory, developmental regression, impaired thermoregulation, and signs of endocrine dysfunction may be present in cases of secondary narcolepsy

DIAGNOSTIC TESTS & INTERPRETATION
Lab
- Levels of CSF hypocretin <100 pg/ml are strongly indicative of narcolepsy with cataplexy in children (range in healthy controls are reported as 280.3 ± 33 pg/mL).
- HLA antigen typing with HLA DQB1 0602 and DQA1 0102 and DR2 are strongly associated with idiopathic narcolepsy with cataplexy, but also present in 12–38% of the normal population.

Imaging
MRI brain is indicated with sudden onset of sleepiness, recent head injury, or an abnormal neurological exam

Diagnostic Procedures/Other
- Overnight polysomnography (PSG) and multiple sleep latency test (MSLT) are essential components of diagnosis
- MSLT is a series of four or five 20-minute naps, 2 hours apart after an overnight PSG to determine mean sleep latency (MSL) and sleep onset REM (SOREM) within 15 minutes of falling asleep. MSL <8 minutes and ≥2 SOREMs during the MSLT are diagnostic of narcolepsy

DIFFERENTIAL DIAGNOSIS
- Chronic sleep deprivation with erratic sleep–wake schedule
- Idiopathic CNS hypersomnia (without cataplexy or REM intrusion in wakefulness or sleep)
- Primary sleep disorders such as obstructive sleep apnea, restless leg syndrome, periodic limb movement disorder
- Klein–Levin syndrome (cyclical episodes of hypersomnolence, overeating, and hypersexuality lasting days to weeks with normal intervals in between)
- Psychiatric disorder/depression
- Medication side effects, drug/alcohol abuse
- Atonic drip attacks associated with childhood epilepsy syndromes such as Lennox Gastaut syndrome

 TREATMENT
MEDICATION (DRUGS)
- Daytime sleepiness
  - Modafinil Provigil, 100–400 mg/day
  - Methylphenidate, 10–30 mg (max. 60 mg/d). Consider other long-acting formulations such as Concerta, Ritalin SR, Metadate CD, Focalin XR, etc.
  - Dextroamphetamine (Dexedrine) 20–25 mg/d
  - Methamphetamine (Desoxyn) 10–40 mg/d
  - Amphetamine/dextroamphetamine mixture (Adderall XR) 10–30 mg/d
- Cataplexy
  - Clomipramine (Anafranil) 3 mg/kg/d in divided doses
  - Imipramine 1.5–5 mg/kg/d
  - Protriptyline (Vivactil) 2.5–10 mg/d in divided doses
  - Selective serotonin reuptake inhibitors. Fluoxetine (Prozac) 5–30 mg/d or sertraline (Zoloft) 25–100 mg/d
  - Sodium oxybate (Xyrem): A new drug that recently became available to treat hypersomnia and cataplexy in refractory cases of narcolepsy. Dose is given at 10 pm and 2 am.

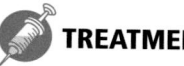 **ONGOING CARE**
PROGNOSIS
With proper sleep hygiene, including regular sleep hours and scheduled daytime short naps, and medications to reduce sleepiness and cataplexy, the prognosis is good, with normal life expectancy, and normal intellectual functioning.

ADDITIONAL READING
- Challamel MJ, Mazzola ME, Nevsimalova S, et al. Narcolepsy in children. *Sleep.* 1994;17(suppl): S17–20.
- Kotagal, S. Narcolepsy in Children. In Sheldon S, Kryger M, Ferber R (eds): *Principles and Practices of Pediatric Sleep.* Philadelphia; Elsevier Inc., 2005, pp. 171–179.
- Scammell T. The neurobiology, diagnosis, and treatment of narcolepsy. *Ann Neurol.* 2003;53: 154–166.
- Vendrame M, Havaligi N, Ali-Matadeen C, et al. Narcolepsy in children: A single-center clinical experience. *Ped Neuro.* 2008;38:314–320.

 CODES
ICD9
- 347.00 Narcolepsy, without cataplexy
- 347.01 Narcolepsy, with cataplexy
ICD10
- G47.411 Narcolepsy with cataplexy
- G47.419 Narcolepsy without cataplexy

FAQ
- Q: What is the chance that a sibling of the patient may develop narcolepsy
- A: There is a 1% possibility that siblings and offspring could be affected.
- Q: Will a patient with narcolepsy be able to drive a car?
- A: Narcolepsy patient can legally drive, provided they are on the appropriate medications to keep them from falling asleep at the wheel.

NECK MASSES

Nicholas Tsarouhas

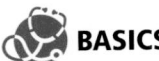

BASICS

DESCRIPTION
Any mass in the tissues of the neck; cervical adenopathy is usually defined as a neck node >1 cm.

ETIOLOGY
Varies depending on underlying condition

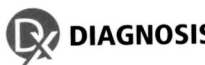

DIAGNOSIS

To diagnose and appropriately manage neck masses, one must combine the history with a careful examination of the mass. The major task of the differential diagnosis is to distinguish infections from congenital and malignant causes.

HISTORY
- Fever: Infection, Kawasaki disease, malignancy, "PFAPA" syndrome (periodic fever, aphthous stomatitis, pharyngitis, and cervical adenitis)
- Noticed with intercurrent infection: Reactive hyperplasia, mononucleosis, adenitis, abscess, congenital cyst
- Subacute or chronic cervical lymphadenitis: Cat-scratch disease, toxoplasmosis, Epstein–Barr virus (EBV), and mycobacterial infection
- Increasing size: Infection, congenital lesion newly infected, malignancy
- Sore throat: Mononucleosis, peritonsillar or retropharyngeal abscess
- Swallowing problems: Retropharyngeal or peritonsillar abscess, thyroglossal duct cyst
- Contact with cats: Cat-scratch disease, toxoplasmosis
- History of scratch or papule on face: Cat-scratch disease
- Recurrently infected neck mass: Infected congenital cyst (thyroglossal duct, branchial cleft)
- Mass noticed at or shortly after birth: Cystic hygroma, hemangioma, sternocleidomastoid tumor of infancy
- Weight loss, cough, or other chronic constitutional symptoms: Malignancy, tuberculosis
- Hypothyroid or hyperthyroid symptoms: Thyroglossal duct cyst, thyroidal diseases

PHYSICAL EXAM
- Tender, erythematous, indurated mass may indicate cervical adenitis, infected congenital lesion, or cat-scratch disease.
- Nontender, enlarged lymph nodes(s) suggest reactive hyperplasia or malignancy.
- Fluctuant mass may indicate adenitis with abscess or cystic hygroma.
- Drainage suggests adenitis with abscess, atypical mycobacterial disease, infected thyroglossal duct, or branchial cleft cyst.
- Regional adenopathy suggests reactive hyperplasia or cat-scratch disease.
- Exudative pharyngitis may be a sign of mononucleosis.
- Asymmetric soft palate with uvular deviation suggests peritonsillar abscess.
- Pulmonary findings may indicate tuberculosis or malignancy.
- Midline mass suggests thyroglossal duct or dermoid cyst, or thyroidal disease.

- If mass moves with tongue protrusion, thyroglossal duct cyst may be present.
- Sinus opening may indicate thyroglossal duct, branchial cleft, or dermoid cyst.
- Multiloculated mass which transilluminates suggests cystic hygroma.
- Matted-down mass may indicate malignancy.
- Mass posterior to sternocleidomastoid muscle may be malignancy or infection.
- Inferior deep cervical nodes (scalene and supraclavicular) suggest malignancy.
- Generalized adenopathy suggests malignancy.
- Hepatosplenomegaly may indicate malignancy or infectious mononucleosis.
- Skin discoloration suggests trauma, abscess, or atypical mycobacterial disease.
- A skin papule is a clue to cat-scratch disease.
- Conjunctivitis, oral involvement, extremity changes, rash, and adenopathy, in the context of fever, are the key diagnostic criteria in Kawasaki disease.
- Torticollis in a neonate suggests sternocleidomastoid (pseudo) tumor of infancy.

DIAGNOSTIC TESTS & INTERPRETATION
- CBC:
  - Leukocytosis in infections
  - Atypical lymphocytosis in mononucleosis
  - Thrombocytosis after 1st week in Kawasaki disease
  - Most patients with neck malignancies initially have a normal CBC.
- EBV titers, mononucleosis spot test: "Mono spot" test less reliable in children <4 years old; therefore, titers more useful
- Indirect fluorescent antibody titers for *Bartonella*: Reliable test to confirm clinical suspicion of cat-scratch disease
- Purified protein derivative: Negative or only weakly positive in atypical mycobacterial infections
- Chest radiograph: Cavitary lesions and infiltrates in tuberculosis; adenopathy in malignancies and tuberculosis
- Lateral neck radiograph: Prevertebral soft-tissue space at C2–C3 abnormally wide (>1/2 adjacent vertebral body diameter) in cases of retropharyngeal abscess
- Ultrasound:
  - Often the first imaging modality for neck masses
  - Provides immediate, noninvasive information on location, size, and composition of mass (cystic vs. solid)
  - Doppler adds information about vascularity.
- CT or MRI scan: Useful in evaluating deep neck infections and complex or extensive neck masses
- Thyroid scintigraphy: Useful in evaluating thyroid lesions, especially when malignancy is a concern
- Gram stain and culture of specimen after needle aspiration or incision and drainage: Diagnostic as well as therapeutic procedure when infection suspected
- Histologic evaluation of specimen after fine-needle aspiration or biopsy: Diagnostic to distinguish malignant causes from congenital and infectious ones

DIFFERENTIAL DIAGNOSIS
- **Infectious**
  - Reactive hyperplasia: Self-limited, usually viral enlargement of bilateral minimally tender nodes
  - Bacterial lymphadenitis:
    ○ Usually staphylococcal or streptococcal infection of unilateral, tender, swollen, warm, erythematous node
    ○ In neonates, a cellulitis–adenitis syndrome is usually caused by group B *Streptococcus*.
  - Cat-scratch disease:
    ○ A usually self-limited, though sometimes protracted, illness (2–4 months)
    ○ Caused by the Gram-negative bacillus *Bartonella henselae*
    ○ Starts as a papule at a cat-scratch site and then progresses to tender, regional adenopathy, 5–50 days later (median, 12 days)
    ○ Cervical nodes are second most commonly involved; axillary adenopathy is most common.
    ○ Nodes stay enlarged several weeks to several months.
  - Tuberculosis: Acute or insidious onset of fever and firm, nontender adenopathy in children exposed to adult infected with the acid-fast bacillus *Mycobacterium tuberculosis*
  - Atypical mycobacterial disease:
    ○ Infection usually caused by *Mycobacterium avium* complex or *Mycobacterium scrofulaceum* (ubiquitous agents found in the soil)
    ○ Rapidly enlarging mass of firm, nontender nodes in young children with no known exposure to tuberculosis
    ○ Nodes often occur with overlying skin discoloration and thinning; some spontaneously drain.
  - Infectious mononucleosis: EBV infection most commonly seen in older children who present with fever, exudative pharyngitis, adenopathy, and hepatosplenomegaly
  - Toxoplasmosis:
    ○ Parasitic disease caused by *Toxoplasma gondii* which presents with cervical adenopathy, rash, fever, malaise, and hepatosplenomegaly
    ○ Acquired from contact with cat feces or inadequately cooked meat
  - Retropharyngeal abscess:
    ○ Suppurative adenitis of the retropharyngeal nodes that presents in children <5 years of age
    ○ These children often have fever, neck stiffness, dysphagia, respiratory distress, drooling, and stridor.
  - Peritonsillar abscess: Suppurative sequela of a severe tonsillopharyngitis, usually caused by group A β-hemolytic *Streptococcus* (GABHS), which commonly presents in older children and adolescents with trismus, "hot potato" voice, and uvular deviation from a bulging palatal abscess.
  - Ludwig angina:
    ○ Rapidly expanding, diffuse inflammation of the submandibular and sublingual spaces
    ○ May compromise the airway
    ○ Often occurs with dental infections

- **Congenital**
  - Thyroglossal duct cyst: Most common congenital neck mass; a remnant of the embryonic thyroglossal sinus, which presents as a nontender (unless infected) mobile, anterior midline mass near the hyoid bone
  - Branchial cleft cyst: Remnant of the 2nd branchial cleft, which presents as a nontender (unless infected) cyst at the anterior border of the sternocleidomastoid
  - Cystic hygroma (lymphangioma): Complex, multiloculated mass of lymphatic tissue, which presents in the 1st year of life as a large, soft, compressible neck structure
  - Dermoid cyst: Small, firm, nontender mass, usually high in the midline
  - Hemangioma: Bluish purple, blanching mass appearing in 1st year of life
  - Sternocleidomastoid (pseudo) tumor of infancy (congenital muscular torticollis): Benign perinatal fibromatosis, often associated with difficult deliveries or abnormal uterine positioning, that results in a hard, immobile, fusiform mass in the sternocleidomastoid
  - Cervical wattle: Benign pedunculated congenital anomaly on lateral neck with a core of elastic cartilage
  - Cervical bronchogenic cyst: Cervical neck mass in the anteromedial neck (superior to the sternal notch), resulting from abnormal development of the tracheobronchial tree
  - Ectopic cervical thymus: Rare neck mass resulting from abnormal development of pharyngeal pouches and branchial clefts
- **Malignant**
  - Hodgkin lymphoma: Slowly enlarging, unilateral, firm, nontender neck malignancy, which usually presents in previously well adolescents
  - Non-Hodgkin lymphoma: Presents in young adolescents as a painless, rapidly growing, firm collection of lymph nodes
  - Leukemia: Most common tumor associated with cervical lymphadenitis in first 6 years of life
  - Neuroblastoma: Most commonly presents in toddlers as a large, nontender, abdominal mass, often associated with a myriad of signs and symptoms as a result of its propensity for metastasis
  - Rhabdomyosarcoma: Head and neck malignancy that usually presents as a rapidly enlarging mass
- **Thyroid**
  - Chronic lymphocytic thyroiditis (Hashimoto thyroiditis): Autoimmune childhood goiter that may be euthyroid, hypothyroid, or hyperthyroid
  - Thyrotoxicosis (Graves disease): Clinically hyperfunctioning thyroid caused by circulating thyroid cell-stimulating antibodies
  - Thyroiditis: Painful bacterial infection of the thyroid caused by *Staphylococcus* or *Streptococcus*

- **Miscellaneous**
  - Kawasaki disease:
    - Idiopathic vasculitis distinguished by prolonged fever, conjunctivitis, oral involvement, extremity changes, rash, and adenopathy
    - Cervical node: Least common clinical feature
    - Unilateral cervical node should be >1.5 cm.
  - PFAPA syndrome:
    - Periodic fever, aphthous stomatitis, pharyngitis, and cervical adenitis
    - Idiopathic, periodic, febrile syndrome most commonly described in young children
  - Sinus histiocytosis with massive lymphadenopathy (Rosai–Dorfman disease): Benign form of histiocytosis that presents as massive, painless enlargement of cervical nodes
  - Hematoma: Secondary to trauma
  - Hypersensitivity reaction: Secondary to bites, stings, or other allergens
  - Drugs: Notably phenytoin and isoniazid, may be associated with lymphadenopathy
  - Immunization: Lymphadenopathy has been reported following immunization with diphtheria–pertussis–tetanus and poliomyelitis.

TREATMENT

GENERAL MEASURES

- Infectious: Antibiotics; drainage for abscesses
- Community-acquired methicillin-resistant *Staphylococcus aureus* (CA-MRSA) infections continue to rise, especially in purulent abscesses.
- The mainstay of therapy for abscesses is I&D; if antibiotics are used adjunctively, clindamycin or trimethoprim–sulfamethoxazole should be used to cover *S. aureus.*
- Congenital: Antibiotics if infected; ENT referral for surgical excision
- Malignancy: Oncology referral for chemotherapy/radiation/excision
- Thyroidal: Endocrine referral for pharmacotherapy
- Miscellaneous:
  - Kawasaki disease: IV immunoglobulin (IVIG) and aspirin therapy to prevent coronary artery aneurysms; cardiology referral for echocardiography
  - PFAPA syndrome: Steroids (a single dose) are efficacious in aborting fever attacks.
  - Sternocleidomastoid tumor of infancy: Massage, range of motion, and stretching exercises

ONGOING CARE

Close follow-up is essential for all neck masses; consider referral for biopsy in the following cases:

- Nodes not responding to antibiotics
- Toxic illness/systemic symptoms
- Clinical signs of malignancy (weight loss, peripheral adenopathy, hepatosplenomegaly)
- Firm, nontender nodes fixed to deep tissues

- Nodes located posterior to the sternocleidomastoid or in the lower cervical/supraclavicular regions
- Bilateral nodes >2 cm
- Increasing size after 2 weeks
- No decrease in size after 4–6 weeks
- Not back to normal size after 8–12 weeks

ADDITIONAL READING

- Al-Khateeb TH, Al Zoubi F. Congenital neck masses: A descriptive retrospective study of 252 cases. *J Oral Maxillofac Surg.* 2007;65(11):2242–2247.
- Caorsi R, Pelagatti MA, Federici S, et al. Periodic fever, apthous stomatitis, pharyngitis and adenitis syndrome. *Curr Opin Rheumatol.* 2010;22(5):579–584.
- Dulin MF, Kennard TP, Leach L, et al. Management of cervical lymphadenitis in children. *Am Fam Physician.* 2008;78(9):1097–1098.
- Klotz SA, Ianas V, Elliott SP. Cat-scratch disease. *Am Fam Physician.* 2011;83(2):152–155.
- Niedzielska G, Kotowski M, Niedzielski A, et al. Cervical lymphadenopathy in children—incidence and diagnostic management. *Int J Pediatr Otorhinolaryngol.* 2007;71(1):51–56.
- Odell CA. Community-associated methicillin-resistant *Staphylococcus aureus* (CA-MRSA) skin infections. *Curr Opin Pediatr.* 2010;22(3):273–277.
- Rosenberg HK. Sonography of pediatric neck masses. *Ultrasound Q.* 2009;25(3):111–127.
- Sidell DR, Shapiro NL. Diagnostic accuracy of ultrasonography for midline neck masses in children. *Otolaryngol Head Neck Surg.* 2011;144(3):431–434.
- Tracy TF Jr, Muratore CS. Management of common head and neck masses. *Semin Pediatr Surg.* 2007;16(1):3–13.
- Wood LE, Tulloh RM. Kawasaki disease in children. *Heart.* 2009;95(10):787–792.

CODES

ICD9
784.2 Swelling, mass, or lump in head and neck

ICD10
R22.1 Localized swelling, mass and lump, neck

NECROTIZING ENTEROCOLITIS
Edisio Semeao

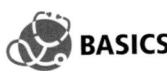 **BASICS**

DESCRIPTION
- Necrotizing enterocolitis (NEC) is an acquired condition of diffuse necrotic injury to the mucosal and submucosal layers of the bowel. It is the most common and serious GI disorder that occurs during the neonatal period. The entire GI tract, from the stomach to the anus, is susceptible, but the distal small bowel and proximal colon are involved most frequently. The lesions may be diffuse and contiguous or patchy and more focal in nature. Systemic signs and symptoms accompany GI injury.
- NEC affects mostly premature infants, but up to 10% of cases occur in term infants.

EPIDEMIOLOGY
- NEC usually has an onset within the 1st 2–3 weeks of life (3–20 days) and after enteral feedings have been initiated. The more premature the infant, the longer the child is at risk for developing NEC, and cases have been reported 3 months after birth.
- Mean gestational age is 31 weeks.

Incidence
- The incidence of NEC varies. It is stated most often as 1–7% of all neonatal intensive care unit (NICU) admissions, or 1–3 per 1,000 live births.
- Preterm infants account for 70–90% of total NEC cases; the more preterm the infant the higher the risk. By 36 weeks of gestation, there is a sharp decrease in incidence.
- Highest in infants with birth weights between 500 and 750 g (15%)
- Prevalence in infants weighing between 500 and 1,500 g is 7%.

RISK FACTORS
- The risk of NEC in full-term infants is ~10% of all cases. Risk factors include:
  - Cyanotic heart disease
  - Polycythemia
  - Exchange transfusions
  - Other coexisting conditions including hypothyroidism, Down syndrome, small bowel atresia, or gastroschisis
  - Perinatal asphyxia
  - Small size for gestational age
  - Umbilical catheters
  - Maternal preeclampsia
  - Antenatal cocaine abuse
  - Use of IV antibiotics

GENERAL PREVENTION
- Modifying the feeding regimen, especially with using maternal breast milk exclusively, has been advocated.
- Also using a low-osmolar protein hydrolysate, high medium-chain triglyceride (MCT) fat formula has been reported to reduce the risk of developing NEC.
- The rate of feeding advancement and the timing of initiation of feedings has been explored and does not seem to consistently contribute to the development of NEC.
- Interventions to prevent bacterial proliferation (formula supplemented with IgA–IgG preparation, use of probiotics) and enhancing the intestinal maturity of the neonate have been used with some success.

- The use of probiotics has been shown to be effective in decreasing incidence for very-low-birth-weight (VLBW) infants. However, 1 recent multicenter trial has shown no change in overall mortality. Some studies have also raised concern of an increased risk of sepsis when using probiotics.
- There are some suggestions that the use of various growth factors, anticytokine agents, and glucocorticoids may have some benefit.

PATHOPHYSIOLOGY
- Varying degrees of inflammation early in the course cause superficial mucosal ulcerations and submucosal edema and hemorrhage, leading to transmural coagulation necrosis and perforation.
- NEC can be transmural in nature in the most severe cases.
- The most common sites for NEC include the terminal ileum, ileocecal region, and ascending colon.
- 50% of infants have both colonic and small intestine disease, whereas the other 50% is divided fairly equally between isolated ileal and colonic involvement.

ETIOLOGY
- The etiology of NEC is unknown but thought to be a multifactorial process.
- Various factors causing direct and indirect mucosal disruption, which in turn may lead to an increased permeability in the gut of agents that lead to injury, include the following:
  - Hypoxia/ischemia leading to mucosal injury
  - GI immaturity, immature host defense
  - Enteral feedings
  - Patent ductus arteriosus (PDA), indomethacin therapy
  - Bacteria within the GI lumen
- Enteral alimentation:
  - Because 95% of infants who develop NEC have been enterally fed, the act of initiation of feedings has been implicated as a possible cause of NEC.
  - The composition of the formula (osmolarity), the rate of volume increase, and the immaturity of the mucosa have all been implicated as factors that may increase the risk of NEC.
- Because of the frequent report of epidemic, cluster-type episodes, a variety of microorganisms has been implicated in the development of NEC:
  - In most cases, no identifiable organism is recovered, but at times, certain microbes, such as *Escherichia coli*, *Klebsiella*, *Salmonella*, and *Staphylococcus epidermidis*, have been recovered.
  - Blood cultures may be positive in 20–30% of cases.
- Immaturity of the GI mucosal defense system against invading organisms has been noted in NEC.
- PDA, indomethacin therapy:
  - Both the left-to-right shunt and mesenteric steal associated with PDA and the acute decreased blood flow associated with indomethacin therapy increase the preterm infant's risk for NEC.

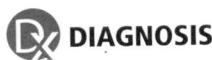 **DIAGNOSIS**

ALERT
The major pitfall occurs when there is a delay in making the correct diagnosis and instituting appropriate therapy. This delay leads to a rapid progression of symptoms and usually a worse outcome.

PHYSICAL EXAM
- The triad of abdominal distention, heme-positive stools, and bilious emesis is frequently seen shortly after initiating enteral feedings.
- Perforation in the setting of other clinical symptoms is also indicative of NEC.
- The clinical spectrum varies dramatically from nonspecific symptoms of feeding intolerance and sepsis to severe abdominal distention and shock. An organized staging system that ranks the disease into 3 categories based on severity of the clinical signs and symptoms has been developed. The staging criteria can be used to formulate individual treatment plans according to the specific stage of NEC:
  - Stage I (suspected NEC):
    ○ Temperature instability
    ○ Apnea
    ○ Bradycardia
    ○ Lethargy
    ○ Cyanosis
    ○ Glucose instability
    ○ Increased gastric residuals
    ○ Emesis (may be bilious)
    ○ Abdominal distention
    ○ Heme-positive stools
  - Stage II (definitive NEC): Stage I plus:
    ○ Mild metabolic acidosis
    ○ Mild thrombocytopenia
    ○ Poor perfusion
    ○ Severe abdominal distention
    ○ Absent bowel sounds
    ○ Abdominal tenderness
    ○ Grossly bloody stools
    ○ Possible abdominal wall cellulitis, fullness/mass
    ○ Ascites
  - Stage III (advanced NEC): Stage I and II plus:
    ○ Shock/deterioration of vital signs
    ○ Metabolic acidosis
    ○ Thrombocytopenia
    ○ Disseminated intravascular coagulation (DIC)
    ○ Significant abdominal tenderness/peritonitis
    ○ Respiratory compromise
    ○ Neutropenia

DIAGNOSTIC TESTS & INTERPRETATION
Lab
No single laboratory feature is diagnostic of NEC. Some laboratory findings that are important if present include:
- Thrombocytopenia
- Acidosis, metabolic
- Anemia
- Neutropenia
- DIC

Imaging
Abdominal radiographs will vary based on the stage of NEC:
- Stage I: Normal or possible mild dilatation of bowel loops
- Stage II:
  - Dilated loops
  - Loops may be fixed.
  - Pneumatosis intestinalis (presence of submucosal or subserosal air in the intestinal wall)
  - Possible portal venous gas
- Stage III: Likely pneumoperitoneum, free air

DIFFERENTIAL DIAGNOSIS
- Systemic:
  - Sepsis with ileus
  - Pneumothorax causing a pneumoperitoneum
  - Hemorrhagic disease of the newborn
  - Swallowed maternal blood
  - Postasphyxial bowel necrosis
- GI tract:
  - Volvulus
  - Malrotation
  - Pseudomembranous colitis
  - Hirschsprung colitis
  - Intussusception
  - Spontaneous bowel perforation
  - Stress ulcer
  - Meconium ileus
  - Milk protein allergy
  - Umbilical arterial thromboembolism

 TREATMENT

Early recognition of the disease and rapid medical management of infants with NEC are critical to minimize the progression of this aggressive disease.

ADDITIONAL TREATMENT
General Measures
- Length of therapy and reinstitution of feedings tend to be based on the severity of the episode and on clinical, laboratory, and radiologic abnormalities.
- If the infant responds immediately to therapy and there are no laboratory or radiographic abnormalities, feedings may be started as early as 72 hours after the episode.
- If mild abnormalities arise and the patient remains only mildly ill, a 10-day course of therapy is considered.
- In cases in which laboratory and radiologic abnormalities include pneumatosis intestinalis, acidosis, and/or thrombocytopenia, a 14-day course is indicated.
- Overall, the best therapy for NEC is prevention.

SURGERY/OTHER PROCEDURES
- NEC is medically managed in 50–75% of infants.
- Surgical intervention is required in 25–50% of all cases.
- Indications include:
  - Pneumoperitoneum
  - Cellulitis of the anterior abdominal wall, abdominal mass
  - Suspicion of intestinal infarction with a fixed loop of dilated bowel over 24 hours on radiography
  - Metabolic acidosis unresponsive to medical therapy
  - Progressive respiratory failure

- The goal of any surgical procedure for the treatment of NEC is to remove all necrotic bowel and to preserve as much bowel length as possible. Different surgical approaches have been adopted with varying degrees of success and complications:
  - The most widely accepted procedure is laparotomy with resection of gangrenous intestine and exteriorization of all viable ends as stomas.
  - Primary anastomosis prevents the necessity of a 2nd procedure to reconnect the gut and establish intestinal continuity.
  - Patch, drain, and wait technique: The infant undergoes a laparotomy, and the major perforations are patched without resection.
  - Clip and drop-back technique can be used if there is extensive intestinal necrosis. Areas of obvious necrosis with perforation are resected, and the ends of the bowel are clipped or stapled closed.
  - Peritoneal drains at the bedside: Developed as a palliative procedure to decrease surgical morbidity and mortality in infants weighing <1,000 g. The purpose of peritoneal drains is to decompress the peritoneal cavity of gas, necrotic debris, and stool. Recent studies have shown that this approach has a higher overall mortality rate than initial laparotomy.

IN-PATIENT CONSIDERATIONS
Initial Stabilization
- For patients who develop NEC, therapy is based on the severity and progression of the symptoms.
- Initial management of all patients with suspected or proven NEC:
  - NPO status
  - IV fluids
  - Nasogastric (NG) tube placement for decompression
  - IV antibiotics: Broad spectrum
  - Total parenteral nutrition (TPN) to ensure adequate nutrition and growth
  - Severely ill patients may require hemodynamic support, acid-base regulation, and respiratory support.
- Evaluate every 6 hours to once a day, depending on the severity of the episode:
  - Blood and stool cultures
  - CBC, electrolytes, DIC screen
  - Fluid status
  - Abdominal radiograph

 ONGOING CARE

FOLLOW-UP RECOMMENDATIONS
Despite early recognition and intervention, NEC is associated with a significantly high morbidity and mortality.

DIET
- NPO
- TPN

PROGNOSIS
- Overall mortality for infants with NEC is between 20% and 40% but can be as high as 60% in patients with stage III NEC:
  - Related to the presence of bacteremia, low birth weight, and low gestational age
  - Results from perforation, sepsis, shock, and DIC
- Prognosis for infants surviving the acute stage of NEC is very good: 80–95% of infants who are discharged from their 1st hospitalization have a good long-term survival.

- Morbidity may be related to anemia, IV access difficulties, and the risk for infection: The other most common long-term sequelae seen in 15–35% of infants with NEC are intestinal strictures and short gut syndrome if the patient undergoes a lengthy surgical resection of bowel.
- Recent studies are showing some long term neuro developmental concerns. Infants recovering form NEC have a 25% risk of microcephaly and serious neuro developmental delays.

COMPLICATIONS
- A variety of complications may occur in infants with this disease process. In the acute setting, these include GI perforation, DIC, sepsis and shock, fluid and electrolyte imbalance, and respiratory failure.
- Complications related to long-term effects on the GI tract occur in 10–30%. These include the following:
  - Intestinal strictures
  - Acquired short bowel syndrome
  - Enterocolic fistulas
  - Malabsorption
  - Cholestasis
  - Anastomotic leaks
- Most common complication (10–35%) is intestinal stricture: Occurs mainly in the left colon

ADDITIONAL READING
- Choo S, Papandria D, Zhang Y, et al. Outcomes analysis after percutaneous abdominal drainage and exploratory laparotomy for necrotizing enterocolitis in 4657 infants. *Pediatr Surg Int*. 2011;27(7): 747–753.
- Deshpande G, Rao S, Patole S. Progress in the field of probiotics: Year 2011. *Curr Opin Gastroenterol*. 2011;27(1):13–18.
- Lee JS, Polin RA. Treatment and prevention of necrotizing enterocolitis. *Semin Neonatol*. 2003;8:449–459.
- Lin P, Stoll B. Necrotising enterocolitis. *Lancet*. 2006;386:1271–1283.
- Neu J, Walker WA. Necrotizing enterocolitis. *N Engl J Med*. 2011;364:255–264.

CODES

ICD9
777.50 Necrotizing enterocolitis in newborn, unspecified

ICD10
P77.9 Necrotizing enterocolitis in newborn, unspecified

FAQ
- Q: What is the most common complication of NEC?
- A: Not recognizing the problem and the development of intestinal strictures
- Q: Is this preventable?
- A: The development of NEC is not clearly preventable, but clinicians should be careful to start feedings in extremely premature infants and use preferably breast milk or low-osmolar protein hydrolysate, medium-chain triacylglycerol (MCT) formulas.
- Q: Is NEC exclusively a process that occurs in the premature infant?
- A: ~10% of cases occur in full-term infants.

N

NEONATAL ALLOIMMUNE THROMBOCYTOPENIA

Kim Smith-Whitley

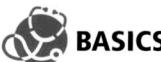 ## BASICS

DESCRIPTION
Neonatal alloimmune thrombocytopenia is analogous to hemolytic disease of the newborn.

EPIDEMIOLOGY
Incidence
- Occurs in 1 in every 1,000–5,000 live births, including 1st-born offspring
- Severe thrombocytopenia (platelet counts $<50,000/\mu L$) caused by human platelet antigen (HPA)-1a antibodies occurs in 1 in 1,100 births.

GENERAL PREVENTION
Although the disease cannot be prevented, mothers of infants with neonatal alloimmune thrombocytopenia can be monitored and possibly treated during subsequent pregnancies. Recent studies support the use of intravenous γ-globulin with or without steroids for fetal alloimmune thrombocytopenia.

PATHOPHYSIOLOGY
Antibody-coated platelets in the fetus or newborn are destroyed at an increased rate.

ETIOLOGY
Caused by maternal antibodies directed against fetal platelet antigens, inherited from the father. IgG antibodies cross the placenta and enter the fetal circulation:

- The most common antigens responsible are HPA-1a (formerly PLA1), in >75% of cases, HPA-5b (formerly Bra), and HPA-3 (formerly Bak); however, many other antigens can be responsible and vary in frequency according to ethnic group.
- Mothers who are HPA-1a negative and human leukocyte antigen (HLA)-DR3, -B8, or -DR52a positive form platelet antibodies at increased rates and are more likely to have severely affected neonates.
- Less commonly, maternal antibodies directed against fetal histocompatibility antigens may cause thrombocytopenia or neutropenia.

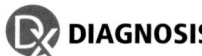 ## DIAGNOSIS

HISTORY
- Family history of bleeding disorders, particularly a history of thrombocytopenia or idiopathic thrombocytopenic purpura in the mother
- Medications used during pregnancy or in the newborn
- Infectious diseases in mother and/or newborn
- Affirmative answers to the following questions increase the likelihood of neonatal alloimmune thrombocytopenia in the thrombocytopenic newborn:
  – Is the mother's platelet count presently normal?
  – Has the mother had prior newborns with thrombocytopenia, neonatal alloimmune thrombocytopenia, or in utero intracranial hemorrhage?
  – Has the mother ever been told that she was HPA-1a or PLA1 negative?

PHYSICAL EXAM
- Most neonates with neonatal alloimmune thrombocytopenia are well appearing unless they have already experienced an intracranial hemorrhage.
- Skin and mucous membrane bleeding, petechiae, and ecchymoses are common findings.
- Less commonly, if significant hemorrhaging occurs, the following signs may be noted:
  – Irritability
  – Pallor
  – Lethargy
  – Focal neurologic deficits
  – Seizure
- If congenital anomalies, hepatosplenomegaly, or masses are present, causes of thrombocytopenia, other than immune mediated, should be investigated.

ALERT
Neonatal alloimmune thrombocytopenia is a difficult diagnosis to confirm and often requires expensive tests, the results of which are often not available to guide the acute management of the newborn; however, a complete workup is necessary for management of future pregnancies in the affected neonate's mother.

DIAGNOSTIC TESTS & INTERPRETATION
Lab
- Low platelet count: $<150,000/\mu L$, often $<50,000/\mu L$ at birth
- Hemoglobin and hematocrit should be normal. Infants with low values may have experienced perinatal blood loss or could have active bleeding.
- WBC count should be normal in uncomplicated neonatal alloimmune thrombocytopenia.
- PT/PTT should be considered to evaluate for disseminated intravascular coagulation, particularly if the infant is ill-appearing or has a complicated prenatal and/or perinatal history.
- Maternal platelet count: Usually normal in neonatal alloimmune thrombocytopenia, but a normal maternal platelet count does not rule out autoimmune thrombocytopenia.
- Maternal serum for antiplatelet antibody analysis: To confirm the diagnosis of neonatal alloimmune thrombocytopenia, the antibody detected should be specific for a known platelet antigen.
- Maternal and paternal platelet antigen typing: Crucial for counseling regarding future pregnancies
- Newborn platelet antigen typing: Use only when absolutely necessary to make the diagnosis, as large amounts of blood may be required for this test. Molecular diagnostic methods require less sample.
- Consider urine and stool for detection of occult blood.

Imaging
Head ultrasound to rule out intracranial hemorrhages

DIFFERENTIAL DIAGNOSIS
- Infection: Primarily related to disseminated intravascular coagulation:
  – Bacterial: Sepsis
  – Viral: Congenital rubella or cytomegalovirus
  – Spirochetal: Syphilis
  – Protozoal: Toxoplasmosis
- Tumor/malignancy: Marrow disease (congenital leukemia, neuroblastoma)
- Metabolic: Methylmalonic or isovaleric acidemia
- Congenital:
  – Thrombocytopenia with absent radii syndrome
  – Wiskott-Aldrich syndrome
  – May-Hegglin anomaly
  – Hemangiomata with Kasabach-Merritt syndrome
- Immunologic:
  – Autoimmune neonatal thrombocytopenia: Primarily seen in infants of mothers with a history of idiopathic thrombocytopenia purpura
  – Infants of mothers with systemic lupus erythematosus
- Miscellaneous:
  – Catheter-associated thrombosis with increased platelet consumption
  – Renal vein and other large-vessel thromboses
  – Disseminated intravascular coagulation
  – Necrotizing enterocolitis

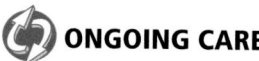

TREATMENT

General Measures
- Therapy primarily involves close monitoring for severe bleeding, including intracranial hemorrhage:
  – Daily platelet counts at minimum during the 1st several days of life
  – If significant bleeding occurs, the neonate should receive a platelet transfusion with the 1st available product, in order of preference:
    ○ Washed, irradiated maternal platelets
    ○ Irradiated platelets selected by cross-match with maternal serum
    ○ Irradiated PLA1-negative platelets
    ○ Irradiated random donor platelets: Often very limited success in increasing platelet count, as 98% of the US population is PLA1 positive
- Platelet transfusions, when needed, are usually required only once:
  – The treatment of severely thrombocytopenic neonates without evidence of significant bleeding is controversial because of the small but real risk of intracranial hemorrhages.
  – Often transfusions are performed at platelet counts of 20,000–30,000.
  – Other therapies have been reported with limited success, such as steroids, IV γ-globulin, and exchange transfusions.
  – Isolation of hospitalized patients is not required.
  – Head ultrasound to detect recent intracranial hemorrhage.
  – General avoidance of arterial and lumbar punctures.

ONGOING CARE

FOLLOW-UP RECOMMENDATIONS
- The thrombocytopenia of neonatal alloimmune thrombocytopenia usually resolves within 3–4 weeks, but can be present for up to 12 weeks.
- Family counseling regarding management of future pregnancies after a thorough diagnostic evaluation is strongly recommended.

Patient Monitoring
If the thrombocytopenia persists after 3 months, other causes of thrombocytopenia should be investigated.

PROGNOSIS
- Overall prognosis is fair, as most patients will experience little morbidity or mortality associated with bleeding; however, the risk of bleeding is higher than in infants of mothers with idiopathic thrombocytopenic purpura, and reported mortality is 10% in some series.
- Most future pregnancies are equally or more severely affected, but this is controversial.

COMPLICATIONS
Abnormal bleeding: Primarily skin and mucous membrane bleeding, including but not limited to:
- Petechiae and ecchymoses: These lesions are progressive and not confined to areas of birth trauma, such as the head and shoulders.
- Prolonged bleeding from the umbilical stump, from phlebotomy sites, and/or at circumcision
- Cephalohematoma
- Hematuria
- GI bleeding
- Intracranial hemorrhages: Reported in 2–20% of cases; 50% of these occur in utero.

ADDITIONAL READING
- Bussell J. Diagnosis and management of the fetus and neonate with alloimmune thrombocytopenia. *J Thromb Haemost.* 2009;7:253–257.
- Bussel JB. Identifying babies with neonatal alloimmune thrombocytopenia and the responsible antigens. *Transfusion.* 2007;47(1):6–7.
- Noninvasive antenatal management of the fetal and neonatal alloimmune thrombocytopenia: Safe and effective. *BJOG.* 2007;114:469–473.
- Roberts I, Murray NA. Neonatal thrombocytopenia: Causes and management. *Arch Dis Child Neonatal Ed.* 2003;88:F359–F364.

 # CODES

ICD9
776.1 Transient neonatal thrombocytopenia

ICD10
P61.0 Transient neonatal thrombocytopenia

FAQ
- Q: What is the HPA-1a- or PLA1-negative mother's risk of having other affected newborns?
- A: This depends on the genotype of the father:
  – If the father is homozygous for HPA-1a or PLA1, all offspring will be heterozygous PLA1 positive and at great risk for developing neonatal alloimmune thrombocytopenia.
  – If the father is heterozygous for HPA-1a or PLA1, 50% of offspring will be at risk for developing neonatal alloimmune thrombocytopenia.
- Q: What is the management of future pregnancies in mothers known to be HPA-1a or PLA1 negative?
- A: This depends on the risk of having an affected child and the clinical course of past affected children. Some perinatal monitoring and therapeutic techniques have shown limited success but not without risks. However, if the risk of having an affected child is high and the clinical course of prior affected newborns was associated with significant morbidity and/or mortality, consider the following perinatal management:
  – Percutaneous umbilical blood sampling for a platelet count
  – Maternal IV γ-globulin therapy
  – Maternal steroid therapy
  – Weekly intrauterine platelet transfusions
  – Early elective cesarean section to avoid birth trauma
- Q: Will the affected neonate be at increased risk for other bleeding problems later in life?
- A: If the neonate has confirmed neonatal alloimmune thrombocytopenia, there is no increased risk for bleeding problems later in life relative to the general population.

NEONATAL APNEA

Carl Tapia

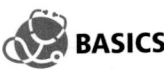

BASICS

DESCRIPTION
- Apnea of infancy is the unexplained cessation of breathing for ≥20 seconds—or a shorter pause associated with cyanosis, pallor, bradycardia, hypoxia, or hypotonia—with an onset after 37 weeks' gestational age.
- Apnea of prematurity is an abrupt respiratory pause for ≥20 seconds, accompanied by desaturation and bradycardia, in an infant <37 weeks' gestational age.
- Apnea has been traditionally classified into 3 categories:
  - Central: No evidence of upper airway obstruction
  - Obstructive: Obstructed upper airway, typically with respiratory effort, but no airflow
  - Mixed: Obstructed respiratory efforts, usually heralded by central pauses
- Periodic breathing is a normal neonatal breathing pattern, defined by ≥3 pauses, each ≥3 seconds, with <20 seconds of regular respiration between pauses.
- Apparent life-threatening event (ALTE) is a sudden event that is frightening to the observer, and characterized by apnea, color change, change in tone, and/or gagging.

EPIDEMIOLOGY
- Apnea and bradycardia occur in ~2% of all healthy term infants.
- Apnea of prematurity is inversely correlated to gestational age. It occurs in <10% of neonates 34–35 weeks' gestational age and in almost all neonates <28 weeks' gestational age at birth.
- ALTE occurs in 2.4 per 1,000 live births.

RISK FACTORS
- Prematurity
- Respiratory syncytial virus (RSV) infection
- Sepsis
- Following pertussis vaccine administration
- Gastroesophageal reflux
- Fluctuating incubator temperatures
- Large patent ductus arteriosus
- CNS insult, such as hemorrhage, hypoxia, or seizures
- Head flexion during holding or sleeping
- Maternal medications, such as magnesium sulfate, prostaglandins, or narcotics
- Anemia

PATHOPHYSIOLOGY
- Immature chemoreceptors in the brainstem may be responsible for the decrease in respiratory drive, especially in response to hypoxia.
- Hypercapnia leading to decreased muscle tone and uncoordination of respiratory muscles may result in mixed apnea.
- Activation of laryngeal afferent nerves, as with gastroesophageal reflux, may result in glottal closure.
- Vagally mediated responses to hypoventilation have been suggested as the cause of bradycardia.

DIAGNOSIS

HISTORY
- Review the prenatal history for prematurity, birth weight, maternal tobacco or other substance use, and the immediate postpartum course. In breastfeeding infants, ask about maternal medications that might cause drowsiness, such as pain or anxiety medications.
- Relevant factors in the past medical history include prior ALTE, feeding and respiratory patterns, and history of seizure, breath-holding spells, reflux, foreign-body aspiration, cardiac disease, metabolic or endocrine disease, or food allergy.
- Evaluate for recent illness, fever, poor feeding, irritability, weight trends, recent vaccine administration, and sick contacts.
- Probe for evidence or suspicion of child maltreatment.
- Pertinent family history includes sudden infant death syndrome (SIDS), home tobacco use, previous infant deaths, congenital problems, and cardiac disease.
- The event should be reviewed in detail for location, timing and duration, associated respiratory effort, color change, infant position and tone, relation to feeding, and resuscitative measures used.

PHYSICAL EXAM
- Monitor vital signs for fever, respiratory effort, arrhythmia, and oxygen saturation.
- Evaluate for dysmorphic features, abnormal growth parameters, and distress.
- Cardiac exam for evidence of arrhythmia or heart failure
- Respiratory evaluation for cyanosis, breathing pattern and effort, wheezing, rales, and absent air sounds
- Complete neurological exam, with emphasis on abnormalities in tone or development
- Examine for signs of child abuse, including bruises, loop marks, belt marks, and other suspicious lesions.

DIAGNOSTIC TESTS & INTERPRETATION
Lab
- CBC with differential to look for infection or anemia
- Electrolytes, glucose, calcium, magnesium to evaluate for acidosis, dehydration, or metabolic disease
- Lactate level to evaluate for hypoxia, toxic ingestions which cause acidosis, or inborn errors of metabolism
- Liver function tests when hepatic dysfunction or severe hypoxia is a consideration
- Ammonia when an inborn error of metabolism or a liver disorder is suspected
- Arterial blood gas when acidosis is considered
- Blood culture if sepsis is suspected
- Urinalysis to evaluate for infection
- Urine drug screen when ingestion or overdose is a concern

Imaging
- Chest x-ray to evaluate for infection or cardiac disease
- Head CT or head ultrasound (if <6 months old) to look for evidence of acute bleed if trauma or elevated intracranial pressure is suspected
- Head MRI, if indicated, to evaluate for congenital malformations
- Skeletal survey if child abuse is suspected

Diagnostic Procedures/Other
- EKG to evaluate arrhythmias or conduction problems
- Lumbar puncture if sepsis/meningitis is in the differential diagnosis
- Nasal aspirate for RSV if respiratory infections are considered
- Pertussis PCR, culture, and serology if suspected contact with pertussis, or a prolonged or paroxysmal cough
- Modified barium swallow if aspiration is suspected or if concerning event is associated with feeding
- Pneumography may be used when the diagnosis of apnea is uncertain. A 5-channel pneumogram records chest wall excursion, heart rate, EKG, pulse oximetry, and nasal airflow. A pH probe for gastroesophageal reflux or end-tidal CO_2 monitor may provide further information.

DIFFERENTIAL DIAGNOSIS
Although apnea of prematurity is very common, careful attention should be made for underlying illness or medical conditions. Apnea of infancy is uncommon and should warrant a thorough evaluation.

- Infections:
  - Respiratory illness, particularly due to RSV, pertussis, or pneumonia
  - Sepsis, urinary tract infection, necrotizing enterocolitis, or CNS infection
- Environmental:
  - Suffocation
  - Head injury
  - Child abuse
  - Hypothermia or hyperthermia
- Tumors:
  - CNS tumors, metastasis, or chest mass
- Neurologic:
  - Seizure
  - CNS bleeding
  - Brainstem malformation
  - Hydrocephalus
- Pulmonary/Airways:
  - Obstruction: Obstructive sleep apnea, nasal obstruction, airway obstruction, foreign-body aspiration
  - Breath-holding spells
  - Vocal cord abnormality
  - Laryngotracheomalacia
- Metabolic:
  - Inborn errors
  - Neuromuscular disease
  - Hypoglycemia or electrolyte disturbance

- Cardiovascular:
  - Congenital heart disease
  - Arrhythmia: Long QT syndrome, Wolff-Parkinson-White syndrome
  - Cardiomyopathy
  - Myocarditis
- GI:
  - Gastroesophageal reflux
  - Dysphagia or swallowing disorder
  - Intussusception
- Toxin/Drugs:
  - Overdose: Sedatives, seizure medications, pain medications

ALERT
Exclusion of specific causes should be performed before specific treatment for apnea is undertaken.

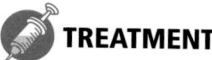

TREATMENT

MEDICATION (DRUGS)
- Theophylline and caffeine citrate have been the mainstays of treatment, but should be undertaken in consultation with a pulmonary or neonatal specialist. Caffeine has the advantage of a higher therapeutic index, lower toxicity, and once-daily dosing.
- Caffeine citrate is commonly administered as a 20 mg/kg bolus (IV or PO), followed by a once-daily dose of 5 mg/kg. The therapeutic range of caffeine is 5–25 mg/L. The alternative salt, caffeine benzoate, is not commonly used, as there is a theoretical risk of bilirubin displacement from albumin.
- Common side effects of theophylline and caffeine include tachycardia, arrhythmia, feeding intolerance, seizures, and diuresis.

ADDITIONAL TREATMENT
General Measures
- Appropriate resuscitation and supportive care directed at underlying disease and presenting signs/symptoms
- Continuous positive airway pressure may decrease airway obstruction and improve oxygenation. Positive-pressure ventilation may be needed for severe or persistent apnea.
- Gastroesophageal reflux and apnea frequently coexist; however, there is little evidence that treatment of reflux has a beneficial effect on apnea of prematurity.
- Aggressively treating anemia does not seem to reduce the incidence of apnea of prematurity.

ONGOING CARE

FOLLOW-UP RECOMMENDATIONS
- A car seat challenge test should be considered for preterm infants with respiratory problems and all infants born at <37 weeks. Parents should be advised to use car seats only for travel and with careful supervision during the 1st few months of life.
- Home cardiorespiratory monitoring may be considered for premature infants at high risk for recurrent apnea, particularly infants with frequent bradycardia and short, but not apneic, respiratory pauses. Monitoring of these infants should be discontinued at 43 weeks' corrected gestational age or when episodes cease.
- Infants who are technology-dependent, have unstable airways, symptomatic chronic lung disease, and medical conditions affecting the regulation of breathing may also be candidates for home monitoring.

PROGNOSIS
- Most apnea of prematurity resolves by 36–40 weeks' corrected gestational age, although infants born at <28 weeks gestation often continue with apnea until 40 weeks' corrected gestational age. After 43–44 weeks' corrected gestational age, the rate of apnea for preterm infants is the same as for term infants.
- Large studies have not found apnea of prematurity to be a precursor or predictor of SIDS.
- The mortality rate for ALTE is between 0–4%. There may be an increased risk of SIDS in infants with apnea of infancy and ALTE.
- There is mixed evidence regarding the occurrence of neurodevelopment delay or behavioral disorders in infants with ALTE. One study found that ≥5 apneic events in infants who were home monitored were associated with lower developmental achievement at 1 year.

ADDITIONAL READING

- American Academy of Pediatrics Committee on Fetus and Newborn. Policy statement: Apnea, sudden infant death syndrome, and home monitoring. *Pediatrics.* 2003;111:914–917.
- Abu-Shaweesh JM, Martin RJ. Neonatal apnea: What's new? *Pediatr Pulmonol.* 2008;43:937–944.
- DeWolfe CC. Apparent life-threatening event: A review. *Pediatr Clin N Am.* 2005;52:1127–1146.
- Hall KL, Zalman B. Evaluation and management of apparent life-threatening events in children. *Am Fam Physician.* 2005;71:2301–2308.
- Martin RJ, Abu-Shaweesh JM, Baird TM. Apnoea of prematurity. *Paediatr Respir Rev.* 2004;5(Suppl A): S377–S382.

- Shah S, Sharieff GQ. An update on the approach to apparent life-threatening events. *Curr Opin Pediatr.* 2007;19:288–294.
- Silvestri JM. Indications for home apnea monitoring (or not). *Clin Perinatol.* 2009;36:87–89.
- Winckworth LC, Powell E. Does caffeine treatment for apnea of prematurity improve neurodevelopmental outcome in later life? *Arch Dis Child.* 2010;95:757–759.

CODES

ICD9
- 770.82 Other apnea of newborn
- 786.03 Apnea
- 798.0 Sudden infant death syndrome

ICD10
- P28.2 Cyanotic attacks of newborn
- P28.3 Primary sleep apnea of newborn
- P28.4 Other apnea of newborn

FAQ

- Q: What recommendations should be given at discharge for neonates with apnea?
- A: Appropriate instruction in the supine sleeping position, a safe sleeping environment (adequate mattress size and removal of pillows and toys that represent a suffocation hazard), and tobacco cessation should be provided. Training in CPR/basic life support and monitor training should be provided.
- Q: What should be included in home monitoring training?
- A: When home monitoring is prescribed, families should be provided with realistic expectations (i.e., lack of efficacy regarding the prevention of SIDS), anticipated cessation of the monitor, and guidelines for intervention when the monitor alarms.
- Q: Should caffeine be given to prevent apnea?
- A: Caffeine is an effective treatment for apnea of prematurity, and recent evidence suggests its use may be beneficial in decreasing outcomes such as developmental delay and cerebral palsy. However, prophylactic caffeine in infants without apnea has not been well-studied, and the side effects likely outweigh any potential benefits.

N

NEONATAL CHOLESTASIS
Binita M. Kamath

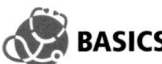 **BASICS**

DESCRIPTION
- Neonatal cholestasis presents at or shortly after birth with the accumulation of bilirubin, bile acids, and cholesterol in blood and extrahepatic tissues. Neonatal cholestasis most often manifests with conjugated hyperbilirubinemia and jaundice. Any infant who is jaundiced beyond 2 weeks of life warrants further evaluation for neonatal cholestasis.
- Biochemical definition: Serum conjugated bilirubin >2 mg/dL or >15% of the total bilirubin concentration

EPIDEMIOLOGY
Estimated frequency of causes of neonatal cholestasis:
- Biliary atresia: 25–30%
- Idiopathic neonatal hepatitis: 15%
- α_1-Antitrypsin deficiency: 7–10%
- Intrahepatic cholestasis syndromes (e.g., Alagille syndrome): 20%
- Infection: 3–8%
- Metabolic/Endocrine: 2–7%

Incidence
Overall incidence of neonatal liver disease is 1 in 2,500 live births

RISK FACTORS
Genetics
Genetics of biliary atresia, neonatal hepatitis, and most causes of neonatal cholestasis are unknown.
- α_1-Antitrypsin deficiency:
  - Autosomal recessive
  - 10–15% of individuals with at risk genotypes (e.g., PIZZ) develop liver disease
- Alagille syndrome:
  - Autosomal dominant, variable expressivity
  - Caused by mutations in Jagged1 and Notch2
- Progressive familial intrahepatic cholestasis:
  - Autosomal recessive
  - Caused by mutations in FIC1, BSEP, and MDR3

PATHOPHYSIOLOGY
Cholestasis is defined physiologically as a reduction in bile flow. In infancy, bile flow is primarily dependent on the secretion of bile acids by hepatocytes. The hepatobiliary excretory system is functionally and structurally immature at birth, leaving the neonate vulnerable to cholestasis. In neonates, bile acid synthesis and secretion are impaired; in addition, there is inefficient enterohepatic bile acid cycling due to reduced expression of bile acid transport proteins.

ETIOLOGY
- Idiopathic neonatal hepatitis
- Cholestasis associated with infection:
  - Sepsis (especially urinary tract infection)
  - Congenital viral infections (cytomegalovirus, adenovirus, herpesvirus, coxsackievirus, echovirus, rubella, hepatitis B, HIV, parvovirus B19)
  - Toxoplasmosis
  - Listeriosis
  - Syphilis
  - Tuberculosis
- Biliary obstruction:
  - Biliary atresia
  - Choledochal cyst
  - Inspissated bile
- Other biliary disorders:
  - Neonatal sclerosing cholangitis
  - Alagille syndrome
  - Caroli disease
  - Congenital hepatic fibrosis
- Metabolic and genetic disorders:
  - α_1-Antitrypsin deficiency
  - Cystic fibrosis
  - Tyrosinemia
  - Galactosemia
  - Neonatal hemochromatosis
  - Niemann-Pick disease
  - Gaucher disease
  - Bile acid synthetic defects
  - Progressive familial intrahepatic cholestasis
- Endocrine disorders:
  - Hypothyroidism
  - Panhypopituitarism
- Toxic:
  - Drugs
  - Total parenteral nutrition
- Vascular disorders:
  - Budd-Chiari syndrome
  - Perinatal asphyxia (shock)

COMMONLY ASSOCIATED CONDITIONS
- Biliary atresia (syndromic form):
  - Heterotaxy
  - Polysplenia
  - Malrotation
  - Congenital heart disease
- Alagille syndrome:
  - Cardiac lesions, typically peripheral pulmonary stenosis
  - Butterfly vertebrae
  - Posterior embryotoxon in the eye
  - Characteristic facies

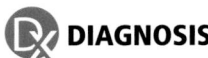 **DIAGNOSIS**

HISTORY
- Pregnancy and birth history
- Family history
- Presence of extrahepatic anomalies
- Stool color
- Signs and symptoms:
  - Jaundice
  - Hepatomegaly
  - Splenomegaly
  - Rickets
  - For specific diagnoses:
    ○ Acholic stools in biliary obstruction (usually biliary atresia)
    ○ Characteristic facies, heart murmur in Alagille syndrome
    ○ Low birth weight, microcephaly, purpura, chorioretinitis in congenital infections
    ○ Irritability, poor feeding, lethargy in metabolic disorders

PHYSICAL EXAM
- Dysmorphic facial features
- Cardiac exam
- Hepatomegaly
- Splenomegaly

DIAGNOSTIC TESTS & INTERPRETATION
- Ophthalmologic evaluation (for chorioretinitis, posterior embryotoxon)
- Sweat chloride/cystic fibrosis mutation analysis

Lab
- Fractionated serum bilirubin (total and conjugated)
- Serum transaminases (alanine transferase, aspartate transferase)
- Alkaline phosphatase, gamma glutamyl transpeptidase
- Serum albumin
- Prothrombin time, partial thromboplastin time, INR
- Serum cholesterol and triglycerides
- CBC
- Bacterial blood culture
- Urine culture
- Serologies for infectious serologies (hepatitis B surface antigen [HepBsAg], TORCH [toxoplasmosis rubella cytomegalovirus herpes], Venereal Disease Research Laboratory [VDRL], HIV, other)

- Serum α_1-antitrypsin level and PI type
- Metabolic screen (plasma and urine amino acids, urine organic acids, lactate/pyruvate)
- Red cell galactose-1-phosphate uridyl transferase (galactosemia)
- Urine succinylacetone (tyrosinemia)
- Thyroid function tests
- Serum iron and ferritin
- Serum and urine bile acids
- Genetic testing for Alagille syndrome
- Genetic testing for progressive familial intrahepatic cholestasis

Imaging
- Abdominal US
- Hepatobiliary scintigraphy
- X-rays of spine (for butterfly vertebrae)
- X-rays of skull and long bones (for congenital infections)

Diagnostic Procedures/Other
- Liver biopsy
- Percutaneous transhepatic cholangiogram
- Intraoperative cholangiogram
- Consider bone marrow exam (for storage disorders)

DIFFERENTIAL DIAGNOSIS
See "Etiology." Conjugated hyperbilirubinemia must be distinguished from physiologic or breast milk jaundice. Any infant who is jaundiced for >14 days should have a total and conjugated hyperbilirubinemia measured to identify neonatal cholestasis.

ALERT
Certain causes of neonatal cholestasis require expedited management (potentially life-threatening if not treated quickly):
- Sepsis
- Biliary atresia
- Galactosemia
- Tyrosinemia
- Hypothyroidism

TREATMENT

MEDICATION (DRUGS)
- Ursodeoxycholic acid (choleretic)
- Vitamin E (antioxidant)
- Antihistamines, rifampin, cholestyramine (pruritus)
- Antibiotics or antivirals (congenital infections)

ISSUES FOR REFERRAL
All neonates with conjugated hyperbilirubinemia should be referred to a pediatric gastroenterologist. In cases of suspected biliary atresia, sepsis, or metabolic disease, referral should be prompt.

COMPLEMENTARY & ALTERNATIVE THERAPIES
- Fat-soluble vitamin supplementation
- Water-soluble vitamin supplementation
- Milk thistle has been used in cholestasis, but its use is not validated.

SURGERY/OTHER PROCEDURES
- Kasai procedure (hepatoportoenterostomy) for biliary atresia
- Surgical drainage (choledochoenterostomy) for choledochal cyst
- Biliary diversion for Alagille syndrome and PFIC

IN-PATIENT CONSIDERATIONS
Initial Stabilization
- Identify and treat coagulopathy with parenteral vitamin K.
- Identify and treat sepsis.

IV Fluids
Limit sodium intake in children with liver disease. Use D10 1/2 normal saline.

ONGOING CARE

DIET
- Aggressive nutritional support is vital. A hydrolysate formula with a high content of medium-chain triglycerides is better absorbed in cholestasis.
- Special diets:
  - Galactose-free (galactosemia)
  - Low tyrosine/phenylalanine (tyrosinemia)

PROGNOSIS
Dependent on etiology. Biliary atresia is the most common indication for pediatric liver transplantation.

COMPLICATIONS
- Growth failure
- End-stage liver disease (ascites, coagulopathy) and portal hypertension
- Fractures

ADDITIONAL READING

- Emerick KM, Whitington PF. Neonatal liver disease. *Pediatr Ann.* 2006;35(4):280–286.
- Hartley JL, Davenport M, Kelly DA. Biliary atresia. *Lancet.* 2009;374(9702):1704–1713.
- Moerschel SK, Cianciaruso LB, Tracy LR. A practical approach to neonatal jaundice. *Am Fam Phys.* 2008;77(9):1255–1262.
- Moyer V, Freese DK, Whitington PF, et al. Guideline for the evaluation of cholestatic jaundice in infants: Recommendations of the North American Society for Pediatric Gastroenterology, Hepatology and Nutrition. *J Pediatr Gastroenterol Nutr.* 2004;39(2):115–128.

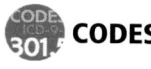

CODES

ICD9
- 774.4 Perinatal jaundice due to hepatocellular damage
- 751.61 Biliary atresia
- 751.69 Other anomalies of gallbladder, bile ducts, and liver

ICD10
- E80.6 Other disorders of bilirubin metabolism
- K83.1 Obstruction of bile duct
- P78.89 Other specified perinatal digestive system disorders

NEPHROTIC SYNDROME

Rebecca Ruebner
Lawrence Copelovitch

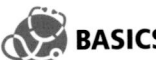 **BASICS**

DESCRIPTION
Nephrotic syndrome (NS) applies to any glomerular disorder associated with nephrotic-range proteinuria, hypoalbuminemia, edema, and hypercholesterolemia. Nephrotic-range proteinuria is found when there is 3–4+ protein on the urine dipstick, which usually correlates with proteinuria of >40 mg/m^2/hr or 50 mg/kg/d, or a spot protein-to-creatinine ratio >2 mg protein/mg creatinine.

EPIDEMIOLOGY
- Minimal change nephrotic syndrome (MCNS) is the most frequent cause of nephrotic syndrome in younger children:
  - Occurs mainly between 2–8 years, with a peak at 3 years.
  - Boys are more commonly affected than girls (3:2).
  - Atopy and minimal change nephrotic syndrome have an association.
- Focal segmental glomerulosclerosis (FSGS) is the 2nd most frequent cause of nephrotic syndrome in childhood:
  - Children with FSGS are more likely than children with MCNS to have steroid-resistant nephrotic syndrome (SRNS).
- Less common than MCNS and FSGS are congenital NS (<3 months) and infantile NS (<1 year).

Incidence
- 2–7 per 100,000 in children <16 years
- Black and Hispanic children have a higher incidence of FSGS than do white and Asian children.

Prevalence
16 per 100,000 in children <16 years

RISK FACTORS
- Risk factors for hypovolemia in NS:
  - Severe relapse, GI illness, diuretic use, or sepsis
- Risk factors for immunologic abnormalities that predispose to infection in patients with NS:
  - Defective opsonization, decreased serum levels of complement factors D and B, abnormal humoral immunity, decreased delayed hypersensitivity and proliferative responses, and increased suppressor-cell activity and suppressor lymphokine levels.
- Risk factors for thrombosis in patients with NS:
  - Hypovolemia, immobilization, thrombocytosis, increased platelet aggregability, urinary losses of protein C, protein S, and antithrombin III
- Risk factors for acute renal failure in patients with NS:
  - Hypovolemia, bilateral renal vein thrombosis, diuretics, or ACE inhibitors

Genetics
A positive family history is present in 3.5% of patients.

PATHOPHYSIOLOGY
- Disruption of podocyte architecture composing the glomerular filtration barrier leads to proteinuria, hypoalbuminemia, and subsequently edema.
- Hypercholesteremia occurs due to increased liver production of cholesterol in response to hypoalbuminemia, as well as to loss of lipoprotein lipase in urine.
- Pathology MCNS:
  - The glomerular tuft and size are normal.
  - Mesangial expansion is absent or minimal.
  - Immunofluorescence is usually negative, although scanty staining for C3, IgM, and IgA may occasionally be found; these patients are usually steroid-dependent.
  - Electron microscopy reveals effacement of the visceral (podocyte) epithelial foot processes, which is reversible.

ETIOLOGY
- Most pediatric cases are primary; 5–10% are secondary to other diseases.
- The most common primary cause of NS in childhood is MCNS. It is characterized by minimal histologic changes on light microscopy and is usually a steroid-sensitive nephrotic syndrome (SSNS).
- Other causes of primary nephrotic syndrome include FSGS, membranous, and membranoproliferative glomerulonephritis (GN).
- Secondary causes of NS include infections, vasculitis, diabetes, drugs (e.g., NSAIDs), and hereditary disorders.
- Examples of congenital NS include Finnish type, diffuse mesangial sclerosis (DMS), and syphilitic nephrosis.
- NS can also be caused by inherited mutations in proteins involved in the podocyte cytoskeleton, which often results in steroid-resistant NS and FSGS.

DIAGNOSIS

HISTORY
- Inquire about known atopy or food intolerance.
- Inquire about drug exposure (especially NSAID agents).
- Inquire about any infections or hernias.
- Signs and symptoms:
  - Fatigue and general malaise
  - Reduced appetite
  - Weight gain and facial swelling
  - Puffy eyes
  - Abdominal swelling or pain
  - Foamy urine
  - Atopy
  - Pitting-dependent edema
  - Fluid accumulation in body spaces (ascites, pleural effusions, scrotal swelling)
  - White nails, lusterless hair, soft ear cartilage
  - Mild hypertension (10–20% of patients)

PHYSICAL EXAM
Look for edema in the most dependent area of the child:
- Legs
- Lumbar spine
- Scalp
- Soft ear cartilage
- Scrotum/labia

DIAGNOSTIC TESTS & INTERPRETATION
Lab
Initial lab tests
- The urine dipstick usually shows 2,000 mg/dL (4+) of protein:
  - In small children with NS, the urine dipstick may show $<4+$.
- Timed or spot urine protein collection:
  - 24-hour urine shows >50 mg/kg/d.
  - Spot urine protein/creatinine ratio is >2.
- Microscopic hematuria in 10–20% of cases, but the presence of RBC casts more suggestive of glomerulonephritis
- Serum creatinine usually normal
- Serum albumin usually <2.5 g/dL
- Total cholesterol elevated, usually >200 mg/dL but can be as high as 500 mg/dL
- Home testing:
  - The 1st morning urine is tested for protein with urine dipsticks.

Imaging
In complicated cases, renal US to evaluate kidney size, parenchymal architecture, and renal venous thrombosis.

DIFFERENTIAL DIAGNOSIS
- Edema:
  - CHF
  - Liver failure
  - Protein-losing enteropathy
  - Protein energy malnutrition (Kwashiorkor)
- Minimal change nephrotic syndrome:
  - Focal glomerulosclerosis (FSGS)
  - Membranous GN
  - Membranoproliferative GN
  - Diffuse mesangioproliferative GN

TREATMENT

MEDICATION (DRUGS)
First Line
- Corticosteroids used as first-line therapy. There are a number of similar regimens:
  - On presentation: Daily corticosteroids for 4 weeks, followed by alternate-day therapy for 4 weeks, then taper over 3–6 months.
  - On relapse: Daily corticosteroids until in remission, followed by alternate-day therapy for 8–12 weeks

Second Line
- Alkylating agents (cyclophosphamide, chlorambucil)
- Mycophenolate mofetil (MMF)
- Calcineurin inhibitors (cyclosporine A, tacrolimus)
- Diuretics
- Albumin
- Rituximab

ALERT
- Live vaccines are contraindicated while daily corticosteroids or alkylating agents are being given.
- Children in relapse, on corticosteroids, or on alkylating agents and who are nonimmune and exposed to varicella should receive VZIG.
- Albumin and/or Lasix must be used cautiously to prevent fluid overload or intravascular dehydration.

ADDITIONAL TREATMENT
General Measures
- Influenza vaccination yearly
- Pneumococcal vaccination according to the "high-risk" schedule (23 valent pneumococcal vaccine)

 ONGOING CARE

FOLLOW-UP RECOMMENDATIONS
- When to expect improvement:
  - Remission occurs 2–4 weeks after starting corticosteroids in MCNS.
- Signs to watch for:
  - Fever, abdominal pain, oliguria
- Pitfalls:
  - Recognize situations in which hypovolemia may occur.
- Monitor complications of glucocorticoid therapy:
  - Growth failure
  - Cataracts
  - Hypertension
  - Osteopenia
  - Steroid-induced gastritis

DIET
Restrict salt intake while in relapse or on daily corticosteroids.

PATIENT EDUCATION
Educate the family about urine testing, complications, diet, and therapy.

PROGNOSIS
- The prognosis for MCNS is excellent, with a mortality rate of <1%:
  - 90% of MCNS are steroid-sensitive.
  - 20–30% of MCNS never have relapse.
  - 40% of MCNS become steroid-dependent or frequent relapsers.
  - Remaining 30–40% MCNS have infrequent relapses.
- Patients with FSGS, genetic forms of NS, or other secondary causes are more likely to be steroid-resistant and may progress to develop chronic kidney disease.

COMPLICATIONS
- Most complications are secondary to steroid therapy and include growth retardation, glaucoma, posterior lens cataracts, obesity, mood changes, hirsutism, osteoporosis, and infection.
- Primary peritonitis and cellulitis may occur de novo or with steroid therapy.
- Diarrhea and vomiting may result in rapid, severe hypovolemia.
- Vascular thromboses are found with NS in relapse, especially if hypovolemia is present.
  - Sites of thrombosis include lower extremities, IVC, renal veins, cerebral sinuses, and pulmonary emboli.
- Viral infections (measles, varicella) may be life-threatening in immunocompromised patients.
- Acute reversible renal failure is an uncommon complication of NS of childhood.

ADDITIONAL READING

- Chesney RW. The idiopathic nephrotic syndrome. *Curr Opin Pediatr*. 1999;11:158–161.
- Eddy AA, Symons JM. Nephrotic syndrome in childhood. *Lancet*. 2003;362:629–639.
- Gipson DS, Massengill SF, Yao L, et al. Management of childhood onset nephrotic syndrome. *Pediatrics*. 2009;124(2):747–757.
- Hodson EM, Knight JF, Willis NS, et al. Corticosteroid therapy for nephrotic syndrome in children. *Cochrane Database Syst Rev*. 2000;(4):CD001533.
- Hodson EM, Knight JF, Willis NS, et al. Corticosteroid therapy for nephrotic syndrome in children [update of *Cochrane Database Syst Rev*. 2001;(2):CD001533]. *Cochrane Database Syst Rev*. 2003;CD001533.
- Robson WLM, Leung AKC. Nephrotic syndrome in childhood. *Adv Pediatr*. 1993;40:287–323.

 CODES

ICD9
- 582.1 Chronic glomerulonephritis with lesion of membranous glomerulonephritis
- 581.3 Nephrotic syndrome with lesion of minimal change glomerulonephritis
- 581.9 Nephrotic syndrome with unspecified pathological lesion in kidney

ICD10
- N04.0 Nephrotic syndrome with minor glomerular abnormality
- N04.9 Nephrotic syndrome with unspecified morphologic changes
- N05.1 Unspecified nephritic syndrome with focal and segmental glomerular lesions

FAQ
- Q: Will the MCNS recur?
- A: The clinical course tends to be one of multiple remissions and relapses. Relapses usually stop about the time of puberty.
- Q: Can the NS return in adult life?
- A: Yes. This does occur.
- Q: Is macroscopic hematuria ever found with MCNS?
- A: Gross hematuria suggests a renovascular event or a diagnosis other than MCNS. Microscopic hematuria occurs in ~10–20% of cases.
- Q: What other agents are used to treat NS?
- A: Cyclosporin A, tacrolimus, mycophenolate mofetil (MMF), cyclophosphamide, and ACE inhibitors/angiotensin receptor blockers are used in children with steroid-dependent or -resistant NS.

N

NEURAL TUBE DEFECTS

Sabrina E. Smith
Dennis J. Dlugos

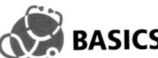 **BASICS**

DESCRIPTION
Neural tube defects (NTD) include clinical and subclinical defects resulting from failure of neural tube closure between the 3rd and 4th weeks of gestation. NTDs include anencephaly, encephalocele, myelomeningocele, meningocele, and occult spinal dysraphism. The latter 3 are different types of spina bifida.

GENERAL PREVENTION
- Folic acid supplementation in early pregnancy can reduce the incidence of NTDs by 50% in the general population and by 70% in women with a history of NTD in a previous pregnancy.
- Because many pregnancies are not discovered until after the 4th week of gestation, when neural tube closure occurs, the Centers for Disease Control and Prevention (CDC) recommend that all women of childbearing age receive a minimum of 0.4 mg of folic acid daily.
- The American Academy of Pediatrics recommends that women with a history of NTD in a previous pregnancy receive 4 mg of folic acid daily, starting 1 month before and through the first 3 months of pregnancy.
- Women on anticonvulsants and other medications linked to NTDs may benefit from receiving 4 mg (high-risk dose = 4,000 mcg) of folic acid daily.

EPIDEMIOLOGY
Prevalence
- 1 in 1,000 live births in the US (not including occult defects, for which no accurate epidemiologic data are available)
- Anencephaly: 3.7 in 10,000
- Encephalocele: 1.4 in 10,000
- Spina bifida: 5.5 in 10,000
- Myelomeningocele: 2–4 in 10,000

RISK FACTORS
Genetics
- Most cases are due to a combination of genetic, environmental, and dietary factors. Numerous candidate genes have been studied with mixed results. A chromosomal or gene abnormality can be identified in ~10% of children with NTDs, and this number increases if there are multiple congenital anomalies.
- Some recent studies suggest that the 677C >T mutation in the methylenetetrahydrofolate reductase gene in mother or child is associated with increased risk of NTDs, though other studies have not confirmed this association.
- 5% of patients are born to a couple with a family history of NTD.
- After 1 child with NTD, the recurrence rate is 2–4% for subsequent pregnancies.

PATHOPHYSIOLOGY
- Neural tube closure begins midway along the neural axis, spreads like a zipper in both rostral and caudal directions, and is completed in a few days.
- Failure of neural tube closure most often occurs in the lumbosacral region.

ETIOLOGY
- Genetic
- Maternal folic acid deficiency
- Gestational diabetes
- Maternal obesity
- Maternal hyperthermia during days 20–28 of gestation
- Use of valproic acid, carbamazepine, or alcohol during pregnancy

COMMONLY ASSOCIATED CONDITIONS
The defect itself may be only the tip of the iceberg, because the malformation may involve the entire central nervous system:
- Disorganized brain stem nuclei or brain stem herniation (Chiari II malformation) occurs.

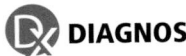 **DIAGNOSIS**

HISTORY
- Thorough health history: NTDs are associated with maternal folic acid deficiency, gestational diabetes, maternal obesity, maternal hyperthermia during days 20–28 of gestation, and use of valproic acid, carbamazepine, or alcohol during pregnancy.
- Activity and development:
  - Occult frontal encephaloceles may come to attention because of a history of developmental delay, seizures, or focal neurologic signs.
  - Occult spinal dysraphism presents with lower extremity weakness or sensory loss, gait abnormalities, bowel and bladder dysfunction, foot deformities, and (rarely) recurrent meningitis.

PHYSICAL EXAM
- Plot head circumference as a marker of developing hydrocephalus.
- Look for evidence of dysmorphic features: May indicate a syndrome.
- Check for integrity of the skin covering the defect, because this affects the timing of surgical intervention. A bony defect or sinus may be palpable in occult cases.
- Neurologic exam of the lower extremities in a myelomeningocele outlines the functional level of the lesion and can indicate ambulatory potential: Intact hip flexion (L1–L2) and knee extension (L3–L4) are favorable signs for future ambulation.
- Flaccid paralysis is present below the level of the lesion, and limb growth may be asymmetric:
  - Sensory level may not correspond to motor level.
  - Cranial neuropathies, such as strabismus, laryngeal paresis, and stridor, may be present at birth or may develop in the first months of life.
- Local signs of occult spinal dysraphism include a dimple, sinus, lipoma, skin pigment change, or tuft of hair in the lumbosacral area.
- Examination may show foot deformities, tight heel cords, unequal leg or foot length, decreased sphincter tone, lower extremity weakness, or sensory changes.

DIAGNOSTIC TESTS & INTERPRETATION
Lab
Maternal serum alpha fetoprotein (MSAFP) testing, done at 16–18 weeks' gestation, can identify 88% of cases of anencephaly and 79% of cases of myelomeningocele.

Imaging
- Ultrasonography:
  - Reveals >99% of cases of anencephaly and 90% of cases of myelomeningocele
- Encephalocele is more likely to be detected by ultrasound than by MSAFP testing.
- Serial cranial ultrasounds or CT scans can evaluate hydrocephalus, which can occur without rapid head growth in patients with NTDs.
- MRI for other brain anomalies, including areas of cortical dysplasia, found in 92% of patients in one neuropathologic study
- Suspected occult spinal dysraphism (often asymptomatic):
  - Incidentally noted on spine radiographs
  - Ultrasound (in the newborn period)
  - CT scan provides more detail of bony anatomy and MRI more detail of spinal cord anatomy.

Diagnostic Procedures/Surgery
- EEG for suspected seizures
- Urodynamic evaluation should be performed in all children with myelomeningocele to anticipate/prevent renal damage owing to reflux.

DIFFERENTIAL DIAGNOSIS
Diagnosis reflects the embryogenesis and anatomy of each defect:
- Anencephaly results from failure of anterior neural tube closure:
  - The diagnosis is obvious at birth.
  - The cerebral hemispheres, basal ganglia, and variable amounts of the upper brain stem are absent.
  - 75% are stillborn; the remainder die in the neonatal period.
- Encephalocele reflects partial failure of anterior neural tube closure:
  - Abnormal brain tissue protrudes through a skull defect usually covered by skin.
  - 70–80% are occipital, 20% are frontal.
  - 10–20% of occipital defects are meningoceles and contain no brain tissue.
  - Frontal encephaloceles, unless accompanied by craniofacial abnormalities, may not be identified unless a neuroimaging study is performed for an associated symptom (such as developmental delay or seizures).
- Myelomeningocele is a failure of posterior neural tube closure:
  - Abnormal neural tissue protrudes through a vertebral column defect.
  - 80% are thoracolumbar, lumbar, or lumbosacral.
  - By definition, this is an open defect, and the diagnosis is obvious at birth.

- Occult spinal dysraphism: Intact skin over the defect:
  - Wide spectrum of defects includes dermal sinus tracts, cysts, lipomas, other tumors, diastematomyelia (bifid spinal cord), and tethered spinal cord.
- Non-neural congenital defects suggest syndromic basis (e.g., telecanthus [Waardenburg syndrome]; heart defect [chromosome 22q11 deletion]).

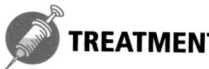 **TREATMENT**

ADDITIONAL TREATMENT
Initial Stabilization
- Acute hydrocephalus from shunt failure or tethered spinal cord from occult spinal dysraphism may arise later in life.

General Measures
- Route of delivery:
  - For most patients with NTDs who do not undergo fetal surgery and have vertex presentation, no clear benefit of cesarean delivery
  - One study demonstrated improved neurologic outcome in patients delivered via cesarean.
  - Infants who undergo fetal surgery must be born via cesarean delivery.
- Infants with high bladder pressure may be treated with anticholinergics and clean intermittent catheterization.

SURGERY/OTHER PROCEDURES
- Fetal closure of a myelomeningocele has been associated with reduced risk of hydrocephalus and improved mental development and motor outcomes in one prospective randomized trial.
- Fetal surgery should be considered in selected patients prior to 26 weeks' gestational age. In patients for whom fetal surgery is not an option, urgent stabilization in the newborn period should be provided, followed by prompt neurosurgical closure:
- Neurosurgical closure of a myelomeningocele is indicated within the first few days of life to prevent infection. Closure of the defect in the first hours of life is not necessary; keep defect clean and moist:
  - An encephalocele with adequate skin covering can be repaired less urgently.
- Ventriculoperitoneal shunts should be placed in infants with hydrocephalus; early shunting may improve cognitive outcome.

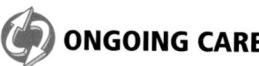 **ONGOING CARE**

- Multidisciplinary approach may include primary pediatrician, neurosurgeon, urologist, orthopedist, neurologist, physiatrist, and others.
- Anticipation of skin breakdown, decubitus ulcers, and leg injuries is important.
- Loss of motor or bladder function, pain, spasticity, or scoliosis may indicate tethered cord.

ISSUES FOR REFERRAL
Occult spinal dysraphism is most often benign/asymptomatic, but if there are possible neurologic signs or symptoms patient should be referred to neurosurgery for evaluation.

PROGNOSIS
- Anencephaly is uniformly fatal.
- Encephalocele: Prognosis is largely dependent on the size of the defect, the amount of brain tissue contained within the sac, and any associated brain malformations.
- Myelomeningocele:
  - Prognosis for ambulation depends on the location of the lesion: The lower the lesion, the more likely the patient will ambulate:
    ○ Most with sacral lesions can ambulate; 95% of adolescents and 40% of younger children with low lumbar lesions will ambulate; 30% of adolescents with high lumbar or thoracic lesions will ambulate.
  - ~80% of children with myelomeningocele will have a neurogenic bladder (urodynamic testing). The goal of therapy is urinary continence and control of high bladder pressure.
- Bowel programs involve high-fiber, low-fat foods; enemas; stool softeners; and biofeedback.
- ~60% of children with encephalocele and 80–85% with myelomeningocele are of normal intelligence.
- Risk of epilepsy corresponds to degree of mental retardation; high with frontal encephaloceles.

COMPLICATIONS
- Encephalocele:
  - Hydrocephalus (50%)
  - Intellectual deficits (40%)
  - Motor and cognitive deficits
  - Seizures likely owing to dysplastic cortex surrounding the encephalocele
- Myelomeningocele:
  - Hydrocephalus (80% with postnatal treatment vs. 40% with fetal surgery)
  - Chiari II malformation (80%), potential feeding difficulties, stridor, and apnea due to lower cranial nerve dysfunction
  - Neurogenic bladder (80%): Risk of renal damage
  - Orthopedic deformities; seizures (25%)
  - Below-average intelligence (15–20%)
  - Tethered spinal cord later in childhood
- Occult dysraphism:
  - Progressive lower extremity motor or sensory deficit
  - Sphincter dysfunction
  - Foot deformities
  - Scoliosis

Patient Monitoring
- The neurologic status of a patient with a repaired NTD should remain stable. Have a high index of suspicion for worsening hydrocephalus, syringomyelia, and tethered spinal cord.
- Tethered cord may accompany occult dysraphism and is a surgically treatable cause of cauda equina syndrome in young children.
- Vocal cord paralysis may appear episodically, resembling croup, in children with myelomeningocele.

ADDITIONAL READING
- Adzick NS. Fetal myelomeningocele: Natural history, pathophysiology and in-utero intervention. *Semin Fetal Neonatal Med.* 2010;15:9–14.
- Rowland CA, Correa A, Cragan JD, et al. Are encephaloceles neural tube defects? *Pediatrics.* 2006;118(3):916–923.
- Nicholas DE, Stanier P, Copp AJ. Genetics of human neural tube defects. *Hum Mol Genet.* 2009;18(R2): R113–R129.
- Liptak GS, Dosa NP. Myelomeningocele. *Pediatr Rev.* 2010;31(11):443–450.
- Adzick NS, Thom EA, Spong CY, et al. A randomized trial of prenatal versus postnatal repair of myelomeningocele. *NEJM.* 2011;364(11): 993–1004.

OTHER
Patient Information:
Spina Bifida Association of America Web site:
http://www.sbaa.org

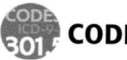 **CODES**

ICD9
- 740.0 Anencephalus
- 742.0 Encephalocele
- 742.8 Other specified congenital anomalies of nervous system

ICD10
- Q00.0 Anencephaly
- Q01.9 Encephalocele, unspecified
- Q07.9 Congenital malformation of nervous system, unspecified

FAQ
- Q: Will my child have learning problems?
- A: At least 80% of those with myelomeningocele have normal intelligence. Cognitive outcome appears improved with early shunting of hydrocephalus.
- Q: Could my baby have other problems besides neurologic problems?
- A: Infants with NTDs need to be checked periodically for signs of bladder problems. Some develop problems with control of eye movements (strabismus), but this is often correctable.
- Q: Should I stop taking anticonvulsants during pregnancy to reduce my risk of NTDs?
- A: Not unless your doctor recommends doing so. In general, continuing the lowest dose of the medicine that best controls your seizures is recommended during pregnancy. There are risks to the fetus from poorly controlled seizures during pregnancy. The overall risks and benefits of medications must be weighed. Any woman of childbearing age who is taking anticonvulsants should receive folic acid supplementation.

N

NEUROBLASTOMA

Edward F. Attiyeh

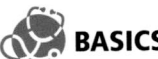 **BASICS**

DESCRIPTION
- Neuroblastoma is the most common extracranial solid tumor of childhood and the most common malignancy of infancy.
- It is derived from neural crest cells and can arise anywhere along the sympathetic chain of the peripheral nervous system, most commonly in the adrenal medulla.
- Neuroblastoma has the highest rate of spontaneous regression of any human malignancy; however, in most cases, it is one of the most aggressive cancers of childhood.
- Neuroblastoma should be distinguished from ganglioneuroma and ganglioneuroblastoma, which show features of differentiation or maturation.
- The International Neuroblastoma Staging System (INSS) is the current staging system:
  - Describes localized tumors (stages 1 and 2), more extensive primary tumors (stage 3), and metastatic tumors (stage 4)
  - Stage 4S ("Special") describes a distinct group of infants <365 days old who have a small primary mass with dissemination limited to the liver, skin, and/or <10% of the bone marrow.
- Risk grouping relies on patient age, tumor stage, MYCN amplification status, Shimada histopathology status, and tumor ploidy. In general:
  - Low-risk groups have localized disease and do not have MYCN amplification.
  - High-risk groups have disseminated disease (often involving the bones, bone marrow, liver, and/or skin) as well as unfavorable biologic characteristics (e.g., MYCN amplification).

EPIDEMIOLOGY
- Most children are <5 years of age at diagnosis.
- ~50% of children have disseminated disease at diagnosis.
- Male:female ratio 1.1:1
- More common in whites
- Most primary tumors are in the abdomen.

Incidence
About 800 new cases per year in the US (10 per million children per year)

Prevalence
Neuroblastoma accounts for ~7–10% of all childhood cancers.

RISK FACTORS
Genetics
- Neuroblastoma can rarely (~1%) show a genetic predisposition (autosomal dominant with variable penetrance).
- Most are due to inherited mutations of the *ALK* tyrosine kinase.
- Also associated with congenital central hypoventilation syndrome and *PHOX2B* mutations

PATHOPHYSIOLOGY
- One of the "small round blue cell" tumors of childhood
- Tumor growth causes mass effect:
  - Nerve/cord compression
  - Renal artery stenosis
- Bone metastases cause pain. Characteristic involvement of the bony orbit
- Bone marrow metastases may cause cytopenias.
- Amplification of the MYCN protooncogene is present in ~20% of tumors.
- There has not been a tumor suppressor gene identified: Many candidate tumor suppressor genes may lie in genomic regions frequently lost in neuroblastomas (e.g., 1p, 3p, and 11q).

ETIOLOGY
No known etiology or causative environmental exposures

COMMONLY ASSOCIATED CONDITIONS
- Neuroblastoma has been found to occur along with:
  - Neurofibromatosis type I
  - Hirschsprung disease
  - Central congenital hypoventilation syndrome
- This suggests that a dysregulated development of the peripheral nervous system may play a role in neuroblastoma initiation.

 DIAGNOSIS

HISTORY
- General appearance, activity level, appetite:
  - Patients with localized, low-risk disease may be very well-appearing (i.e., tumor is an incidental finding on imaging study).
  - Patients with disseminated, high-risk disease typically appear ill.
- Based on tumor location:
  - Thoracic:
    - Chest pain
    - Cough
    - Respiratory distress
  - Abdominal:
    - Pain
    - Swelling
  - Bone marrow:
    - Fatigue (anemia)

PHYSICAL EXAM
- Presenting signs and symptoms depend on the primary site of the tumor and the degree of dissemination.
- Abdomen:
  - Abdominal mass is usually firm, fixed, and irregular and often crosses the midline.
  - Abdominal distention with or without tenderness
  - Signs of bowel obstruction: Anorexia, vomiting, low stool output
  - Hypertension (renal artery compression)
  - Genital and lower extremity edema from obstruction of venous and lymphatic drainage

- Cervical/thoracic mass (posterior mediastinal):
  - Respiratory distress or stridor with thoracic masses
  - Horner syndrome with cervical or high thoracic masses: Ptosis, myosis, and anhydrosis
  - Superior vena cava syndrome with large mediastinal tumors
- Paraspinal mass:
  - Vertebral body involvement and nerve root compression
  - Bladder and bowel dysfunction, paraplegia, and back pain secondary to spinal cord compression
- Metastatic disease:
  - Liver: Hepatomegaly
  - Bone:
    - With or without bony pain
    - Periorbital ecchymoses
    - Proptosis
  - Bone marrow:
    - Cytopenias
    - Pain from marrow expansion
  - Lymph nodes: Adenopathy
  - General:
    - Fever
    - Irritability
    - Failure to thrive

DIAGNOSTIC TESTS & INTERPRETATION
Lab
- CBC: Decreased hemoglobin, platelets, and/or WBC counts may indicate bone marrow involvement.
- Electrolytes, liver function tests, and renal function tests in anticipation of starting chemotherapy
- Urine catecholamine metabolites are typically elevated: Homovanillic acid (HVA) and vanillylmandelic acid (VMA).

Imaging
- Generally an ultrasound or CT scan of the suspected primary tumor site (MRI may be necessary for paraspinal tumors): Calcification suggests neuroblastoma.
- Metaiodobenzylguanidine (MIBG) scan:
  - MIBG is taken up by 90% of neuroblastomas.
  - Radioisotope-labeled MIBG can detect both bone and soft tissue involvement.
- Bone scan to evaluate for bony metastasis: Only necessary if the tumor is not MIBG avid

Diagnostic Procedures/Other
- Tumor biopsy
- Bilateral bone marrow aspirates and biopsies

DIFFERENTIAL DIAGNOSIS
- Abdominal masses:
  - Wilms tumor
  - Lymphoma
  - Germ cell tumor
  - Hepatoblastoma
  - Pancreaticoblastoma

- Thoracic masses:
  - Lymphoma (usually non-Hodgkin)
  - Leukemia with bulky disease
  - Germ cell tumors
- "Small round blue cell tumors":
  - Non-Hodgkin lymphoma
  - Ewing sarcoma
  - Peripheral primitive neuroectodermal tumors (PNETs)
  - Rhabdomyosarcoma

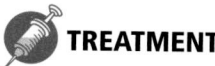 TREATMENT

MEDICATION (DRUGS)

- Multiagent chemotherapy typically includes a combination of vincristine, doxorubicin, cyclophosphamide, cisplatin, carboplatin, etoposide (VP-16), and/or topotecan.
- High-dose myeloablative chemotherapy is followed by autologous stem cell transplant.
- 13-cis-Retinoic acid induces differentiation of neuroblastoma cells and improves patient survival following stem cell transplant.
- Immunotherapy with antibodies directed against GD2, which is present on most neuroblastoma cells

ADDITIONAL TREATMENT
General Measures
Treatment protocols are based on risk classification:

- Patients with low-risk disease, such as stage 1 or 4S with favorable biologic features, may undergo spontaneous regression or only require surgery.
- Patients with intermediate-risk disease receive 2–8 cycles of outpatient chemotherapy.
- Patients with high-risk disease, such as stage 4 or MYCN amplified, receive a combination of surgery, high-dose chemotherapy requiring stem cell rescue, radiation therapy, and biologic response modification therapy.

Additional Therapies
Radiotherapy

- Radiation therapy is used for control of local disease or for palliation.
- Total-body irradiation may be part of high-dose therapy prior to stem cell transplant.

SURGERY/OTHER PROCEDURES

- Total surgical resection at the time of diagnosis may be attempted but not if it would involve significant morbidity.
- Neoadjuvant chemotherapy results in smaller tumors that make a future resection attempt more straightforward.

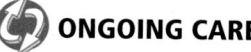 ONGOING CARE

FOLLOW-UP RECOMMENDATIONS
Referral to a pediatric oncologist is essential before any diagnostic procedures or therapeutic interventions.

Patient Monitoring

- On therapy:
  - Frequent laboratory evaluations to monitor for effects of chemotherapy:
    - Marrow suppression
    - Organ toxicity
  - Disease re-evaluation prior to surgery or stem cell transplant:
    - Imaging
    - Bone marrow evaluation
- Off therapy:
  - Close follow-up for disease recurrence for 2–3 years after completion of therapy:
    - Imaging of site of primary tumor
    - Urine catecholamine metabolites
    - Late effects of chemotherapy and radiation therapy require close monitoring.

PROGNOSIS

- Adverse prognostic factors:
  - Age >18 months
  - Advanced stage (especially stage 4 metastatic disease)
  - MYCN amplification (very powerful marker of poor outcome)
  - Unfavorable histology
  - Diploid tumor genome (primarily infants)
  - Loss of heterozygosity at chromosome arms 1p or 11q
- These factors stratify children at diagnosis as low, intermediate, or high risk of relapse. These risk groups predict survival:
  - Low- and intermediate-risk patients have excellent outcomes (>80–90% survival).
  - High-risk patients have poorer outcomes (30–50% survival) despite aggressive therapy.

COMPLICATIONS
Paraneoplastic syndromes:

- Vasoactive intestinal peptide (VIP) syndrome:
  - Neuroblastoma may secrete VIP, which causes watery diarrhea, abdominal distention, and electrolyte imbalances.
  - Usually resolves with removal of tumor
- Opsoclonus-myoclonus-ataxia (2–4%):
  - Chaotic eye movements (dancing eyes) and myoclonic jerks (dancing feet) with or without cerebellar ataxia
  - Up to 80% of patients have long-term neurologic deficits.
  - Likely due to autoimmune effect of antineural antibodies
  - Specific therapies: High-dose steroids and intravenous immunoglobulin (IVIG).
- Symptoms of catecholamine excess are rare.

ADDITIONAL READING

- Attiyeh EF, London WB, Mosse YP, et al. Chromosome 1p and 11q deletions and outcome in neuro-blastoma. N Engl J Med. 2005;353: 2243–2253.
- Kuroda T, Saeki M, Honna T, et al. Late complications after surgery in patients with neuroblastoma. J Pediatr Surg. 2006;41(12): 2037–2040.
- Lee KL, Ma JF, Shortliffe LD. Neuroblastoma: Management, recurrence, and follow-up. Urol Clin North Am. 2003;30:881–890.
- Moroz V, Machin D, Faldum A, et al. Changes over three decades in outcome and the prognostic influence of age-at-diagnosis in young patients with neuroblastoma: A report from the International Neuroblastoma Risk Group Project. Eur J Cancer. 2011;47(4):561–571.
- Maris JM. Recent advances in neuroblastoma. N Engl J Med. 2010;362(23):2202–2211.
- Mosse YP, Laudenslager M, Longo L, et al. Identification of ALK as a major familial neuroblastoma predisposition gene. Nature. 2008;455:930–935.

 CODES

ICD9
- 194.0 Malignant neoplasm of adrenal gland
- 195.1 Malignant neoplasm of thorax

ICD10
- C74.90 Malignant neoplasm of unspecified part of unspecified adrenal gland
- C74.91 Malignant neoplasm of unspecified part of right adrenal gland
- C74.92 Malignant neoplasm of unspecified part of left adrenal gland

FAQ

- Q: Are siblings of children with neuroblastoma at increased risk for neuroblastoma compared with the general population?
- A: No, except in rare families with a known history of neuroblastoma (<1%).
- Q: Can neuroblastoma spontaneously regress?
- A: Yes, but this is usually seen only in children <1 year of age with lower-stage disease or in infants with stage 4S disease.
- Q: What are the biggest risks during therapy?
- A: As with all intensive chemotherapy regimens, the risk of infection is high. This is especially true during the autologous stem cell transplant phase.
- Q: What therapy is available to patients who either fail to go into remission or relapse following aggressive therapy?
- A: There is no curative therapy after disease recurrence in high-risk neuroblastoma. However, the disease can be controlled with phase 1 or 2 therapies for many years, which allows patients to maintain a good quality of life.

N

NEUROFIBROMATOSIS

Leah Burke
Sunil Thummala

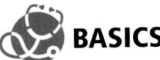

BASICS

DESCRIPTION
- Neurofibromatosis (NF) types 1 and 2 are multisystem neurocutaneous autosomal dominant genetic conditions. NF1 (Von Recklinghausen disease) is diagnosed based on the presence of any 2 of the following from National Institutes of Health (NIH) diagnostic criteria:
  - 2 or more cutaneous neurofibromas or 1 plexiform neurofibroma
  - 2 or more Lisch nodules
  - Inguinal or axillary freckling
  - 6 or more (smooth-edged) café au lait spots, at least 1.5 cm in diameter in postpubertal individuals or 0.5 cm in diameter in prepubertal individuals
  - Optic nerve glioma
  - Osseous lesions, including sphenoid wing dysplasia, pseudoarthrosis
  - A 1st-degree relative (parent, sibling, or offspring) with NF
- Approximately half of sporadic NF1 patients fail to meet NIH criteria by 1 year of age
- Tumors may be cosmetically disfiguring and physically limiting; 5–13% of plexiform neurofibromas undergo sarcomatous transformation.
- NF2 is 10 times less common than NF1 and is characterized by bilateral vestibular schwannomas, intracranial and spinal meningiomas, and cutaneous schwannomas.

EPIDEMIOLOGY
Incidence
- NF1: 1 in 2,700 live births
- NF2: 1 in 33,000 live births

Prevalence
- NF1: 1 in 4,560
- NF2: 1 in 56,161

RISK FACTORS
Genetics
- 50% of the cases are inherited; others occur as sporadic (new) mutations.
- One of the most commonly inherited autosomal dominant disorders, with no known gender or ethnic predisposition
- Penetrance is complete; however, expression is variable.
- *NF1* gene, which codes for neurofibromin, is located on chromosome 17q11.2.
- Expression varies widely within and among families, from mildly affected to severely impaired.
- Course impossible to predict; relative's disease cannot predict disease course in a patient.

COMMONLY ASSOCIATED CONDITIONS
- Hypertension
- Headache, brain tumor, cerebrovascular dysplasia
- Sarcoma, CML, Wilms tumor, pheochromocytoma
- Short stature, scoliosis, osteoporosis, thin long bones

DIAGNOSIS

HISTORY
- "Positive family history": Affecting a 1st-degree relative, mother, or father of the proband: 100% penetrance
- Vision: Optic pathway tumors (OPTs) generally occur between the ages of 2 and 6 years.
- Development: Speech delay, motor incoordination, learning problems and attention deficit hyperactivity disorder (ADHD), >50%
- Seizures: Twice as common in NF1 than in general population
- Joint/extremity pain: Neuropathic pain or abrasion due to neurofibroma
- Back pain: Could signal potentially serious cord or root compression
- Headache: Hydrocephalus; migraine also common in NF
- Neurofibromas may encroach on the airway
- Aberrant sexual development, abnormalities due to hypothalamic disease, psychiatric/behavioral symptoms, and depression are common.
- NF2 patients: Hearing loss, visual impairment, skin lesions

PHYSICAL EXAM
- Macrocephaly
- Café au lait spots are noted at birth or within the 1st year of life:
  - Macules are generally flush and circular, although they may have jagged edges or areas of hypertrichosis.
  - Café au lait spots result from a collection of heavily pigmented melanocytes of neural crest origin in the epidermis.
  - The macules will appear for the 1st 5 years of life and then slow or stop, although they will grow with the child.
- Axillary and inguinal freckling is generally seen by puberty. The freckling is a cluster often seen in the skinfolds.
- Lisch nodules are best assessed by slit-lamp examination:
  - Small bumps on the iris that do not interfere with vision
  - They are uncommon during infancy, but by age 20, 99% of patients with NF1 have Lisch nodules.
- OPTs are present in 20% of patients with NF1, although only ~20% of those will require intervention:
  - Funduscopy and acuity check for evidence of OPT
  - Treatment should be limited to those patients who have uncorrectable visual acuity, a change in visual fields, and/or endocrine abnormalities, or to those lesions that extend to the hypothalamus.

- Bony dysplasias occur in ~3% of patients with NF1:
  - Dysplasias especially affecting the tibia or the sphenoid wing
  - A pseudoarthrosis: Due to thinning of the long bone and its inability to heal after it breaks
- Hypertension
- Review of palpable tumors for extension or "stony" feel that could signal cancerous change
- Abdominal exam for masses
- Neck and spine palpation/mobility
- Reflexes for evidence of nerve root tumor
- Growth parameters (including head circumference) for evidence of hydrocephalus, hypothalamic disturbance
- Scoliosis

DIAGNOSTIC TESTS & INTERPRETATION
Lab
Urine catecholamines for pheochromocytoma

Imaging
- MRI brain:
  - Bright areas in cerebral white matter on T2-weighted MRI images are common in NF1, and their clinical significance is uncertain.
  - Indications for neuroimaging depend on findings such as progressive macrocephaly, sensory deficits (especially visual), new-onset seizure, chronic headaches, and hearing deficit (NF2).
- Renal studies may be indicated for persistent hypertension or difficulty with urine flow.

Diagnostic Procedures/Other
In most cases, the diagnosis of NF1 remains a clinical diagnosis. Radiologic tests to identify complications (see below)
- DNA testing has become more available and therefore may be useful in atypical cases or in making reproductive choices:
  - DNA-based testing of the NF1 gene is undertaken in a stepwise approach using a cascade of complementary tests that are able to detect a mutation in the NF1 gene in 95% of patients who meet the NIH criteria.

Pathological Findings
Biopsy of tumors that are enlarging, as this may be evidence of sarcomatous change

DIFFERENTIAL DIAGNOSIS
- Café au lait spots are most often benign findings unrelated to NF.
- NF2 may resemble NF1:
  - NF2 is also known as central bilateral acoustic NF, a rare disorder characterized by multiple tumors on the cranial and spinal nerves and by other lesions of the brain and spinal cord.
  - NF2 is genetically and clinically distinct from NF1. The NF2 gene, which codes for merlin protein, is located on chromosome 22.
  - The diagnosis of NF2 is made if the individual has the following: Bilateral acoustic neuromas or a 1st-degree relative with NF2 and either a unilateral acoustic neuroma or 2 of the following: Meningioma, glioma, schwannoma, or juvenile posterior subcapsular lenticular opacity.

- Soto syndrome features macrosomia, hypertelorism, ventriculomegaly, and cognitive difficulties.
- McCune-Albright syndrome has large café au lait spots with irregular margins and polyostotic fibrous dysplasia.
- Tuberous sclerosis (TS) may share autosomal dominant transmission and café au lait lesions in common with NF:
  - Features distinctive for TS include adenomal sebaceum, cardiac and renal tumors, and prominent epilepsy.
  - Genetic testing for TS is now available.

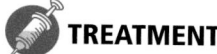 TREATMENT

ADDITIONAL TREATMENT
General Measures
- Treatment of NF is multidisciplinary.
- There is no treatment for tumor growth except surgical intervention, if symptomatic.
- Interventions are palliative and supportive.

ISSUES FOR REFERRAL
Orthopedic, oncology, ophthalmology, endocrine, surgery, and plastic surgery consultants may be helpful, depending on individual issues.

SURGERY/OTHER PROCEDURES
Surgical intervention is performed on those tumors that are compressive, painful, or cosmetically disfiguring:
- Subcutaneous nodules are flesh colored, raised, pealike nodules that may be present during childhood.
- These commonly appear and grow during puberty or pregnancy and do not grow into plexiform tumors.
- Resection of vestibular schwannomas, if symptomatic

 ONGOING CARE

FOLLOW-UP RECOMMENDATIONS
- Longitudinal care is essential for early detection and management of complications.
- Optimism: Natural history studies indicate that people with NF1 can live long, full lives.
- Pitfalls:
  - Macrocephaly is a common feature of NF, but growth curve for the head is necessary to determine whether it signifies a concern.
  - Regrowth of plexiform neurofibromas: Even after apparent total resection, regrowth is common and should be discussed before surgery.
  - The possibility of nerve injury after surgery on plexiform neurofibromas should also be discussed with the family/individual before surgery.

Patient Monitoring
- Vigilance/anticipatory care regarding common psychological and developmental issues, such as speech delay, incoordination, ADHD, and learning disabilities
- Early educational assessment and interventions may improve developmental outcome.

- Continuous yearly ophthalmologic examinations:
  - Goldman visual field perimetry is suggested in those with any question of an optic nerve tumor.
  - Some practitioners use yearly visual field testing (by an ophthalmologist) in addition to or as prescreen to MRI scanning.
- BP checks are increasingly important in adolescents and adults with NF.
- Monitoring for the development of tumors, hypertension, and psychological and developmental disabilities

PATIENT EDUCATION
- Family counseling regarding genetic implications, possible genetic testing using linkage, or, in some cases, mutation testing of the gene neurofibromin
- The children's tumor foundation: http://www.nfnetwork.org/
- NIH information page: http://www.ninds.nih.gov/disorders/neurofibromatosis/neurofibromatosis.htm

PROGNOSIS
- Deaths have been associated with cancer, heart disease, and strokes, similar to the general population.
- Tumors cannot be predicted on the basis of their occurrence in another member of the family with NF.

COMPLICATIONS
- Skeletal: Pseudoarthrosis, scoliosis, osteoporosis
- Oncologic: Overall risk of malignancy in NF1 is 2.7 times that of general population:
  - Neurofibromas are benign tumors of Schwann cells, nerve fibers, and fibroblasts that arise along the nerves.
  - Plexiform neurofibromas occur in ~15% of patients with NF1; these are extensive tumors that grow along the nerve root and may invade adjacent structures, threatening vital structures (especially in the neck and throat), or cause gross disfigurement. ~10% of these tumors undergo sarcomatous degeneration.
  - CNS tumors include optic nerve/pathway gliomas or gliomas elsewhere in the brain.
- Neurologic: Learning disability, language disorders, incoordination, autism, seizures, retardation, and attention deficit occur with higher-than-background frequency in NF.
- Renal: Hypertension
- Circulatory: Moyamoya disease, stroke
- Endocrine: Pheochromocytoma
- Hematologic: Leukemia

ADDITIONAL READING
- American Academy of Pediatrics Committee on Genetics. Health supervision for children with neurofibromatosis. *Pediatrics.* 1995;96:368–372.
- Evans DG, Howard E, Giblin C, et al. Birth incidence and prevalence of tumor-prone syndromes: Estimates from a UK family genetic register service. *Am J Med Genet A.* 2010;152A(2):327.

- Ferner RE. The neurofibromatoses. *Pract Neurol.* 2010;10:82–93.
- Gutman DH, Aylsworth A, Carey JC, et al. The diagnostic evaluation and multidisciplinary management of neurofibromatosis 1 and neurofibromatosis 2. *JAMA.* 1997;278:51–57.
- North KN, Riccardi V, Samango-Sprouse C, et al. Cognitive function and academic performance in neurofibromatosis 1: Consensus statement from the NF1 Cognitive Disorders Task Force. *Neurology.* 1997;48:1121–1127.
- Reynolds RM, Browning GG, Nawroz I, et al. Von Recklinghausen's neurofibromatosis: Neurofibromatosis type 1. *Lancet.* 2003;361:1552–1554.
- Rosser T, Packer RJ. Intracranial neoplasms in children with neurofibromatosis 1. *J Child Neurol.* 2002;17:630–637, 646–651.
- Walker L, Thompson D, Easton D, et al. A prospective study of neurofibromatosis type 1 cancer incidence in the UK. *Br J Cancer.* 2006;95(2):233.
- Williams VC, Lucas J, Babcock MA, et al. Neurofibromatosis type 1 revisited. *Pediatrics.* 2009;123(1):124–133.

 CODES

ICD9
- 237.70 Neurofibromatosis, unspecified
- 237.71 Neurofibromatosis, type 1 [von recklinghausen's disease]
- 237.72 Neurofibromatosis, type 2 [acoustic neurofibromatosis]

ICD10
- Q85.00 Neurofibromatosis, unspecified
- Q85.01 Neurofibromatosis, type 1
- Q85.02 Neurofibromatosis, type 2

FAQ

- Q: Can NF develop into cancer?
- A: Most tumors caused by NF are benign and remain benign (even large tumors). In rare cases, they may become malignant.
- Q: My child has NF1. What specialists must he see?
- A: Your child should have yearly checkups with a physician familiar with the issues of NF (could be a family physician, pediatrician, child neurologist, or geneticist) who will know when to refer to other specialists. Otherwise, periodic visits to an ophthalmologist with experience in NF are the only routine recommendation.

N

NEUTROPENIA
Cynthia F. Norris

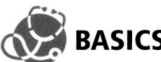 **BASICS**

DESCRIPTION
A decrease in the number of circulating neutrophils (both segmented and band forms), strictly defined as an absolute total neutrophil count (ANC) of $<1,500/mm^3$

- To calculate ANC, multiply the total WBC count by the percentage of segmented neutrophils and band forms.
- For example: WBC count 5,200 with 15% segs/polys, 4% bands, 76% lymphocytes, 5% monocytes: $ANC = 5,200 \times (0.15 + 0.04) = 988$.

EPIDEMIOLOGY
- Normal values for total WBC counts and ANC vary with age and race.
- Black children have lower total WBC counts and lower ANCs than do white children.
- Infants have a higher total WBC count and a higher percentage of lymphocytes in their differential counts.

RISK FACTORS
Genetics
- Some neutropenia syndromes can be inherited: Kostmann syndrome = SCN: severe congenital neutropenia: Autosomal recessive.
- Cyclic neutropenia: Autosomal dominant

ETIOLOGY
- Decreased production of neutrophils:
  - Marrow failure syndromes
  - Marrow suppression by drugs, chemotherapy, or radiation
  - Nutritional deficiencies
- Increased destruction of neutrophils:
  - Immune-mediated destruction
  - Increased utilization (usually with overwhelming infection)
  - Sequestration in the spleen
- Factitious causes of a low WBC count:
  - Long time period between when blood sample is drawn and when it is tested
  - Excessive leukocyte clumping (in presence of certain paraproteins)
  - Leukocyte fragility secondary to leukemia or medication use

DIAGNOSIS

HISTORY
- Current or recurrent fever, skin abscesses, infection, or oral ulceration helps establish pattern and duration of neutropenia.
- Medication use: Many can cause neutropenia.
- Results of prior CBC with differential: Prior normal WBC count and ANC essentially rule out Kostmann syndrome.
- Diet: Evidence of nutritional deficiency
- Family history of neutropenia, recurrent infection, or early death suggests an inherited condition.

PHYSICAL EXAM
- Fever (temperature should not be taken rectally), tachycardia, and hypotension may indicate systemic infection.
- Oral ulceration, gingival irritation, pharyngitis, thrush
- Cellulitis, perirectal, or labial abscesses
- Hepatomegaly or splenomegaly
- Bruises, petechiae, pallor (other cell lines may be involved)
- Phenotypic abnormalities (thumb anomalies, dwarfism, joint findings)
- Systemic infection: Fever, rash, upper respiratory symptoms, jaundice

DIAGNOSTIC TESTS & INTERPRETATION
Lab
- CBC with differential
- Antineutrophil antibodies: Present in autoimmune and isoimmune neutropenia on the neutrophils (direct) and in the serum (indirect)
- Cultures
- Genetic testing for Kostmann syndrome (HAX1) and cyclic neutropenia (ELA2)
- ELA2 mutations may also account for some cases of Kostmann syndrome.

Diagnostic Procedures/Other
Bone marrow aspirate and biopsy may be normal or may reveal a decrease in the number of myeloid precursors or a maturational arrest of the myeloid line (usually in the later stages), depending on the cause of neutropenia.

DIFFERENTIAL DIAGNOSIS
- Neutropenia associated with infection:
  - Bacterial: Group B streptococcal disease, tuberculosis, brucellosis, tularemia, typhoid, paratyphoid
  - Viral: Hepatitis A and B, parvovirus B19, respiratory syncytial virus (RSV), influenza A and B, rubeola, rubella, varicella, cytomegalovirus (CMV), Epstein-Barr virus (EBV), HIV
  - Other: Malaria, visceral leishmaniasis, scrub typhus, sandfly fever

- Drug induced:
  - Antibiotics: Sulfonamides (trimethoprim/sulfamethoxazole is a common offender), penicillin, chloramphenicol (may be irreversible)
  - Chemotherapy agents: Alkylating agents, antimetabolites, anthracyclines
  - Antipyretics: Aspirin, acetaminophen (uncommon)
  - Sedatives: Barbiturates, benzodiazepines
  - Phenothiazines: Chlorpromazine, promethazine
  - Antirheumatic agents: Gold, penicillamine, phenylbutazone
- Tumors:
  - Leukemia
  - Solid tumors that invade bone marrow
- Metabolic:
  - Nutritional: Malnutrition, copper deficiency, megaloblastic anemia secondary to folate or vitamin B_{12} deficiency
  - Inborn errors of metabolism: Hyperglycinemia, isovaleric acidemia, propionic acidemia, methylmalonic acidemia
- Congenital:
  - Kostmann syndrome: Severe congenital neutropenia
  - Cyclic neutropenia: Regular oscillations in the number of circulating neutrophils (periodicity every 7–36 days; duration of neutropenia, 3–10 days)
- Chronic benign neutropenia of childhood: This is a diagnosis of exclusion.
- Shwachman-Diamond syndrome: Neutropenia and exocrine pancreatic insufficiency
- Cartilage/hair hypoplasia: Neutropenia, dwarfism, abnormal cellular immunity
- Reticular dysgenesis
- Immunologic:
  - Neutropenia associated with primary immunodeficiencies: Abnormalities in T and B lymphocytes
  - Autoimmune neutropenia: Idiopathic (common in childhood; onset usually <2 years of age; diagnosis established by demonstrating antineutrophil antibodies; typically a benign course with resolution within several years; steroids may help in severe cases)
  - Felty syndrome (neutropenia, splenomegaly, and rheumatoid arthritis)
  - Secondary to drugs, infection, or rheumatologic process
  - Isoimmune neonatal neutropenia

- Miscellaneous:
  - Hypersplenism
  - Part of evolving aplastic anemia: Idiopathic, Fanconi anemia, familial aplastic anemia, dyskeratosis congenita
  - Bone marrow infiltration: Tumor, osteopetrosis, Gaucher disease
  - Radiation injury

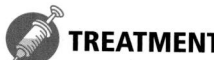 TREATMENT

MEDICATION (DRUGS)

- Hematopoietic growth factors:
  - Granulocyte colony-stimulating factor (G-CSF): Drug of choice for Kostmann syndrome
  - Granulocyte-macrophage colony-stimulating factor (GM-CSF)
- Corticosteroids and/or plasmapheresis: Most helpful in immune-mediated neutropenia
- IVIG may also be used in autoimmune neutropenia.

ADDITIONAL TREATMENT

General Measures

- Isolation of hospitalized patient: Prudent until the cause of the neutropenia is identified
- Correction of underlying cause of neutropenia (discontinue drug, treat infection, correct nutritional deficiency)
- Treatment of fever and suspected infection when neutropenic: Initially, broad-spectrum antibiotics are indicated; after the diagnosis has been established, this may not always be necessary (i.e., individuals with chronic benign neutropenia).
- Prophylactic antibiotics are not usually beneficial and may predispose to systemic fungal infection.
- Stool softeners may be helpful in the profoundly neutropenic patient at risk for constipation to prevent development of a perirectal abscess.
- No therapy may be required if neutropenia is not severe and there are no serious or recurrent infections (often the case in autoimmune neutropenia and chronic benign neutropenia).

Additional Therapies

Granulocyte transfusions: Rarely indicated for severe or refractory infections

ISSUES FOR REFERRAL

- Chronic or profound neutropenia
- History of recurrent skin infections
- When bone marrow examination is indicated
- When hematopoietic growth factors, plasmapheresis, or granulocyte transfusion is being considered

 ONGOING CARE

FOLLOW-UP RECOMMENDATIONS

Management of febrile episodes:

- Prompt evaluation by a physician
- Obtain CBC with differential.
- Obtain blood culture.
- Hospitalize.
- Treat with IV antibiotics.
- Monitor daily CBC with differential.

Patient Monitoring

CBCs and physical exams at regular intervals while the patient is neutropenic

PROGNOSIS

- Death from overwhelming infection does occur.
- Outcome varies according to diagnosis
  - Neutropenia resulting from infection or drug-related marrow suppression is usually short lived.
  - Congenital neutropenia syndromes may result in chronic lifelong neutropenia.
  - Immune-mediated neutropenia frequently improves with age.

COMPLICATIONS

- Systemic bacterial infection
- Localized infections such as cellulitis, labial abscesses, perirectal abscesses, oral mucosal ulceration, thrush

ADDITIONAL READING

- Alexander SW, Pizzo PA. Current considerations in the management of fever and neutropenia. *Curr Clin Topics Infect Dis*. 1999;19:160–180.
- Boxer LA. Neutrophil abnormalities. *Pediatr Rev*. 2003;24:52–62.
- Boxer L, Dale DC. Neutropenia: Causes and consequences. *Semin Hematol*. 2002;39:75–81.
- Christensen RD, Calhoun DA, Rimsza LM. A practical approach to evaluating and treating neutropenia in the neonatal intensive care unit. *Clin Perinatol*. 2000;27:577–601.
- James RM, Kinsey SE. The investigation and management of chronic neutropenia in children. *Arch Dis Child*. 2006;91(10):852–858.
- Kyono W, Coates TD. A practical approach to neutrophil disorders. *Pediatr Clin North Am*. 2002;49:929–971.

 CODES

ICD9

- 288.00 Neutropenia, unspecified
- 288.01 Congenital neutropenia
- 288.02 Cyclic neutropenia

ICD10

- D70.0 Congenital agranulocytosis
- D70.4 Cyclic neutropenia
- D70.9 Neutropenia, unspecified

FAQ

- Q: Do all episodes of fever and neutropenia require antibiotics?
- A: In severe neutropenia syndromes (i.e., Kostmann syndrome) or when the cause of the neutropenia is unclear, it is prudent to evaluate the child promptly, draw a blood culture, and administer IV broad-spectrum antibiotics. Certain neutropenia syndromes are not associated with an increased risk of infection (i.e., chronic benign neutropenia of childhood); children with these syndromes should be evaluated when they have fever, but probably do not require IV antibiotics if they look well.
- Q: Should a child with neutropenia be allowed to go to school?
- A: Yes
- Q: Does he or she need to wear a mask?
- A: No

N

NON-HODGKIN LYMPHOMA

Anne F. Reilly

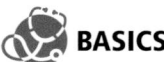 **BASICS**

DESCRIPTION

- Non-Hodgkin lymphoma (NHL) is a malignant proliferation of cells of lymphocytic or histiocytic lineage that spread in a pattern similar to the migration of normal lymphoid cells.
- No uniform staging system exists for childhood NHL. The commonly used Murphy's staging system is as follows:
  - Stage I: Single tumor (extranodal) or single nodal area, excluding mediastinum or abdomen
  - Stage II: Single tumor with regional nodal involvement, 2 or more tumors or nodal areas on the same side of the diaphragm, or a primary GI tract tumor (resected) with or without regional node involvement
  - Stage III: Tumors or lymph node areas on both sides of the diaphragm, any primary intrathoracic or extensive intra-abdominal disease (unresectable), or any paraspinal or epidural tumors
  - Stage IV: Bone marrow or CNS disease regardless of other sites; marrow involvement defined as 0.5–25% of malignant cells

EPIDEMIOLOGY

- 3rd most common childhood malignancy (~12% cancers in individuals <20 years of age in developed countries)
- Male/female ratio: 3:1

Incidence

- 1–1.5 per 100,000
- Higher frequency of endemic Burkitt-type in equatorial African countries (10–15 per 100,000 children younger than age 5–10)
- Incidence increases steadily with age; in children, usually seen in 2nd decade of life (unusual in those <3 years of age)

RISK FACTORS

Environmental factors:

- Drugs: Immunosuppressive therapy and diphenylhydantoin
- Radiation: Atomic bomb survivors and ionizing radiation
- Viruses: Epstein-Barr virus (EBV), HIV; EBV present in >95% of cases of endemic Burkitt versus <20% cases of sporadic

Genetics

Genetic predisposition: Increased risk in patients with immunologic defects (e.g., Bruton agammaglobulinemia, ataxia–telangiectasia, Wiskott-Aldrich, severe combined immunodeficiency)

PATHOPHYSIOLOGY

- In contrast to adult lymphomas, childhood NHL is almost never nodular alone and rarely occurs in peripheral nodal areas.
- Pediatric NHL can be divided into 3 major categories according to the National Cancer Institute (NCI) formulation:
  - Small noncleaved cell lymphomas (B cell):
    - 40% of childhood NHL
    - Subdivided into Burkitt and non-Burkitt based on the degree of pleomorphism

- A variety of B-cell markers are usually present (e.g., CALLA, CD20).
  - Expresses surface immunoglobulins (Ig), most bearing IgM of either κ or λ light-chain subtype
  - Terminal deoxyribonucleotidyl transferase (TdT) is negative.
  - Characteristic chromosomal translocation, usually t(8;14), rarely t(8;22) or t(2;8); all translocations involve the c-myc protooncogene.
- Lymphoblastic lymphomas (LL):
  - Make up 30% of childhood NHL
  - In children, 90% T-cell and 10% B-cell origin
  - Predominantly of thymocyte (T-cell) origin: Morphologically identical to acute leukemia T lymphoblasts. Bone marrow involvement of >25% blasts is considered leukemia.
  - T-cell lymphomas are positive for TdT and have a T-cell immunophenotype (e.g., CD7).
  - Most lack chromosomal translocations and seldom involve T-cell receptor genes on chromosomes 7 and 14q.
- Large cell lymphomas:
  - 30% of childhood NHL
  - 2/3 are a large noncleaved or cleaved type of B-cell origin; these can be diffuse large B-cell lymphoma (DLBCL) or mediastinal large cell lymphoma (LCLM).
  - 1/3 are anaplastic large cell lymphoma (ALCL) and are positive for CD30 (Ki-1).
  - ALK (anaplastic lymphoma kinase) positivity seen in systemic ALCL disease; ALK-negative ALCLs are more often localized/cutaneous. ALK-negative disease is rare in children.

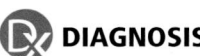 **DIAGNOSIS**

A diagnosis needs to be made expeditiously, as pediatric lymphomas generally have a rapid growth rate.

HISTORY

- B-cell lymphomas:
  - Systemic manifestation (e.g., fever, weight loss, anorexia, fatigue) if disseminated; less likely if tumor localized
  - Lump in neck unresponsive to antibiotics
  - Abdominal mass with pain, swelling, change in bowel habits, nausea, or vomiting
- T-cell lymphomas:
  - Mediastinal tumor symptoms include cough, hoarseness, dyspnea, orthopnea and chest pain, anxiety, confusion, lethargy, headache, distorted vision, syncope, and a sense of fullness in the ears.
  - Marrow involvement: Bleeding and/or bruising, bone pain, pallor, fatigue

PHYSICAL EXAM

- Small noncleaved cell lymphomas:
  - Intra-abdominal mass (up to 90%):
    - Involving ileocecal region, appendix, ascending colon, or a combination
    - Lymphadenopathy may be present in inguinal or iliac region.
    - Hepatosplenomegaly may be present.
    - Acute abdomen with intussusception, peritonitis, ascites, and acute GI bleeding
    - Lymphoma is the most frequent cause of intussusception in children >6 years.

- In endemic Burkitt lymphoma, jaw tumors are the most frequent; orbital involvement in infants; abdominal masses in 50%
  - Other sites: Testis, unilateral tonsil hypertrophy, peripheral lymph nodes, parotid gland, skin, bone, CNS, and marrow
- Lymphoblastic lymphoma:
  - Mediastinal mass (50–70%), possibly pleural effusion present with decreased breath sounds, rales, and cough with or without superior vena cava (SVC) syndrome or superior mediastinum syndrome (SMS):
    - Signs include swelling, plethora, and cyanosis of the face, neck, and upper extremities; diaphoresis; stridor; and wheezing.
  - Lymphadenopathy (50–80%); primarily above diaphragm
  - Abdominal involvement uncommon: Likely to involve only liver and spleen
  - Cranial nerve involvement: Rarely
- Large cell lymphomas:
  - Sites: Mediastinum, bone, inguinal nodes, skin
  - Bone marrow and CNS involvement: Rare at diagnosis

DIAGNOSTIC TESTS & INTERPRETATION

- Establish diagnosis with least invasive method.
- Bone marrow aspirate and biopsy may establish the diagnosis without further testing.
- Fluid from ascites in patients with abdominal disease or pleural fluid should be obtained for cytology, immunophenotyping, and cytogenetics.
- Take a biopsy of an enlarged lymph node.

Lab

- CBC
- Liver and renal function studies
- Serum lactate dehydrogenase (LDH) and uric acid levels
- Ascitic, CSF, or pleural fluid:
  - Cytology
  - Immunophenotyping
  - Cytogenetics

Imaging

- Abdominal ultrasound
- Chest radiographs: Posteroanterior and lateral
- CT scan of chest, abdomen, and pelvis
- PET/CT scan
- MRI (especially for bone involvement)

Diagnostic Procedures/Other

- Adequate surgical biopsy
- Bone marrow aspiration and biopsy
- Lumbar puncture with CSF cytology

DIFFERENTIAL DIAGNOSIS

- Abdominal mass:
  - Newborn: Hydronephrosis, renal cysts, Wilms tumor, or neuroblastoma
  - Older children: Constipation, full bladder, hamartoma, hemangioma, cysts, leukemic or lymphomatous involvement of the liver and/or spleen, Wilms tumor, or neuroblastoma

- Mediastinal mass:
  - Anterior: Masses of thymic origin, teratomas, angiomas, lipomas, or thyroid tumors
  - Middle: Metastatic or infectious lesions involving the lymph nodes, pericardial or bronchogenic cysts, esophageal lesions, or hernias
  - Posterior: Neurogenic tumors (e.g., neuroblastoma, ganglioneuroma, neurofibroma), enterogenous cysts, thoracic meningocele, or hernias

 **TREATMENT**

MEDICATION (DRUGS)

- Chemotherapy:
  - Histology and stage determine choice of a particular protocol.
  - Because of a high conversion rate of lymphomas to leukemias, prophylactic CNS treatment is given (except in patients with totally excised intra-abdominal tumor).
  - Duration: 1–8 months; lymphoblastic lymphomas longer, up to 24 months
  - Drugs: Cyclophosphamide, vincristine, methotrexate (IV and intrathecal [IT]), prednisone, daunorubicin, asparaginase, cytarabine, thioguanine, carmustine, hydroxyurea, hydrocortisone, doxorubicin, mercaptopurine, etoposide
  - Common side effects: Hair loss, myelosuppression with transfusions required, nausea/vomiting
- Immunotherapy: Rituximab:
  - A chimeric monoclonal antibody directed against the CD20 antigen, which is almost universally expressed on tumor cells in pediatric B-cell NHL
  - A new active agent for lymphoma
  - Has been used successfully in patients with relapsed/refractory B-cell NHL
  - Few overlapping side effects with the combination of rituximab and conventional chemotherapeutic agents

ADDITIONAL TREATMENT
General Measures
A multidisciplinary approach is imperative to ensure the best therapy.
- Prechemotherapy management:
  - Allopurinol, hydration, and alkalinization of urine to promote uric acid excretion; may use rasburicase for uric acid >8 mg/dL
  - Vigorous hydration with maintenance of brisk urine flow to prevent tumor lysis syndrome
  - Monitor uric acid, BUN, calcium, creatinine, potassium, and phosphate levels closely.
- Management of relapse:
  - Relapse indicates extremely poor prognosis.
  - No uniform approach to rescue therapy; different chemotherapy combinations may induce a new response.
  - For patients with chemosensitive relapse, salvage therapy followed by high-dose therapy with stem cell support is recommended, because this may result in prolonged survival.

Additional Therapies
Radiotherapy
- Adds no therapeutic benefit in children with limited disease. May be indicated in mediastinal DLBCL
- Used occasionally as emergent treatment for SVC obstruction or CNS or testicular involvement
- Cranial radiotherapy given for CNS-positive children with lymphoblastic lymphoma
- Increases short- and long-term toxicity

SURGERY/OTHER PROCEDURES
- Performed if total resection can be achieved
- Additional indications: Intussusception, intestinal perforation, suspected appendicitis, or serious GI bleeding
- Avoid extensive surgery in patients with NHL

 ONGOING CARE

FOLLOW-UP RECOMMENDATIONS
- Patient monitoring weekly to monthly with CBC and physical examination
- Radiologic imaging at intervals during and off therapy
- Monitor for toxicity-related complications:
  - Cardiac
  - Gonadal function
  - Second malignancies

Patient Monitoring
Late effects from therapy:
- Cardiomyopathy from anthracyclines
- Impaired reproductive function or infertility from alkylating agents or radiation
- Second malignant neoplasms from etoposide and alkylators
- Psychological consequences of severe illness

PROGNOSIS
- Important prognostic factors for outcome include tumor burden at presentation.
- Favorable:
  - Stages II and I with primary site head and neck (nonparameningeal), peripheral nodes, or abdomen (≥90% 2-year survival)
  - Burkitt: Most >90% 2-year survival
- Less favorable:
  - Stage III or IV ALCL, LL
  - Parameningeal stage II
  - Stage IV with CNS involvement (worst)
  - Incomplete initial remission within 2 months (50–80% 2-year survival)

COMPLICATIONS
- Tumor lysis syndrome:
  - Combination of hyperuricemia, hyperkalemia, and hyperphosphatemia with hypocalcemia, resulting in uric acid nephropathy that leads to renal failure
  - Correct before starting chemotherapy.
- GI obstruction, perforation, bleeding, intussusception
- Inferior vena cava obstruction and venous thromboembolism
- Neurologic (e.g., paraplegia, increased intracranial pressure)

- SVC syndrome and SMS: Associated with lymphoblastic lymphomas that invade the thymus and nodes surrounding the vena cava and airways
- Massive pleural effusion
- Cardiac tamponade or arrhythmia

ADDITIONAL READING

- Abramson SJ, Price AP. Imaging of pediatric lymphomas. *Radiol Clin North Am.* 2008;46: 313–338.
- Hochberg J, Waxman IM, Kelly KM, et.al. Adolescent non-Hodgkin lymphoma and Hodgkin lymphoma: State of the science. *Br J Haematol.* 2009;144(1): 24–40.
- Kjeldsberg CR, Meadows A, Siege IS, et al. Chromosome abnormalities may correlate with prognosis in Burkitt/Burkitt-like lymphomas of children and adolescents: A report from Children's Cancer Group Study CCG-E08. *J Pediatr Hematol Oncol.* 2004;26:169–178.
- Pinkerton CR. Continuing challenges in childhood non-Hodgkin's lymphoma. *Br J Haematol.* 2005; 130:480–488.
- Pulte D, Gondos A, Brenner H. Trends in 5- and 10-year survival after diagnosis with childhood hematologic malignancies in the United States. 1990–2004. *J Natl Cancer Inst.* 2008;100(18): 1301–1309.

CODES

ICD9
- 200.10 Lymphosarcoma, unspecified site, extranodal and solid organ sites
- 202.70 Peripheral T cell lymphoma, unspecified site, extranodal and solid organ sites
- 202.80 Other malignant lymphomas, unspecified site, extranodal and solid organ sites

ICD10
- C83.50 Lymphoblastic (diffuse) lymphoma, unspecified site
- C83.70 Burkitt lymphoma, unspecified site
- C85.90 Non-Hodgkin lymphoma, unspecified, unspecified site

FAQ

- Q: Did I do something to cause this?
- A: No. Most cases are sporadic and not associated with diet, underlying immune dysfunction, or viral illness.
- Q: When will my child be "cured"?
- A: For patients with small or large cell lymphomas, relapse most commonly occurs in the 1st year after therapy finishes. Therefore, a child may be considered cured if he or she remains in remission after the 1st year off therapy. A patient with lymphoblastic lymphoma is considered cured if he or she remains in remission after ~3 years from onset of therapy.
- Q: Is this contagious?
- A: No. Siblings may have slightly higher inherent risk than the general population, but they are not at risk from the affected child.

N

NOSEBLEEDS (EPISTAXIS)

Sheila M. Nolan

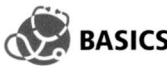

BASICS

DESCRIPTION
- Epistaxis: Bleeding from the nose
- Bleeding may be evident anteriorly through the nares or posteriorly through the nasopharynx.

EPIDEMIOLOGY
- Nosebleeds occur in all ages throughout the year.
- Children aged 2–10 years are most commonly affected.
- Nosebleeds are more common in the winter.

GENERAL PREVENTION
- Vaporizers, humidifiers, or saline sprays prevent desiccation of the nasal mucosa.
- Petroleum jelly applied to the anterior nasal septum aids healing of inflamed nasal mucosa.
- Antigen avoidance and medical therapy should be used to reduce allergic symptoms.
- Fingernails should be cut short, and nose-picking behavior should be discouraged.
- Protective athletic equipment should be worn.

PATHOPHYSIOLOGY
- The nasal mucosa has a rich blood supply originating from both the internal and external carotid arteries.
- Blood vessels of the nasal septum and lateral nasal walls have little anatomic support or protection. The thin mucosal surface is prone to drying.
- Blood vessels of the nose form many plexiform networks. Especially important is Kiesselbach plexus in the anterior nasal septum, the most common site of nosebleeds in children.
- The nose is subject, by position, to traumatic injury.

ETIOLOGY
- Inflammation of, or trauma to, the nasal passages accounts for most nosebleeds:
  - Viral upper respiratory infections, allergic rhinitis, bacterial rhinitis
  - Nose picking, external trauma, foreign bodies, postsurgical bleeding, chemical or caustic agents/inhalants

- Local structural abnormalities may predispose to epistaxis:
  - Rhinitis sicca, or environmental drying of the nasal mucosa, commonly promotes epistaxis.
  - Nasal polyps, telangiectasias, meningoceles, angiofibromas, vascular malformations, septal deviations or spurs
- Less commonly, nosebleeds may herald, or accompany, systemic illnesses:
  - Hematologic diseases such as leukemias, thrombocytopenias, hemophilias (and von Willebrand disease), and hemoglobinopathies
  - Clotting disorders owing to infection, hepatic failure, or poisoning/envenomation
  - Hypertension (usually not the cause, but can make hemostasis difficult)
- Pseudoepistaxes from pulmonary hemoptysis, bleeding esophageal varices, or pharyngeal/laryngeal tumors that bleed can be mistaken for epistaxis.

COMMONLY ASSOCIATED CONDITIONS
Hemoptysis, hematemesis, or melena may be the presenting concerns in individuals with bleeding from the nasopharynx.

DIAGNOSIS

HISTORY
- Frequency of occurrence
- Persistence of bleeding
- Nose-picking behavior/traumatic injury
- Nasal congestion, discharge, obstruction
- Allergies
- Medications or drugs of abuse (especially cocaine)
- Previous or concurrent bruising or bleeding
- Menstrual history
- Family history of systemic disease or hemorrhagic disorder

PHYSICAL EXAM
- Vital signs with blood pressure determination
- Inspection of nose, nasopharynx, and oropharynx
- General exam with attention to lymph nodes, liver and spleen size, rashes, icterus, pallor
- Procedure:
  - Exam of the nose may be facilitated by application of a topical vasoconstricting agent and/or anesthetic agent.
  - Anxiety may interfere with exam and treatment of children. Sedation and analgesia may be beneficial in some circumstances.

DIAGNOSTIC TESTS & INTERPRETATION
Lab
- Laboratory evaluation is not indicated in healthy children with readily controlled epistaxis from an anterior site.
- Recurrent or refractory nosebleeds or suspicious findings from the history and physical exam may warrant a directed laboratory evaluation (such as platelet count, PT and PTT, CBC, and/or bleeding time) and/or consultation.

DIFFERENTIAL DIAGNOSIS
Epistaxis is a common event in normal children. A careful history and physical exam should identify those children with unusual predisposing causes for nosebleeds.

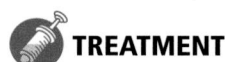

TREATMENT

ADDITIONAL TREATMENT
General Measures
- Elevate the head of the bed.
- Direct pressure, applied by gently squeezing the nostrils, is usually sufficient to stop most nosebleeds.
- Ice or cold packs to the neck or nasal dorsum appear not to have a significant benefit, but may be combined with application of pressure.
- A cotton pledget beneath the upper lip may aid hemostasis by compressing the labial artery.

- Vasoconstricting agents (0.25% phenylephrine, 0.05% oxymetazoline, 1:1,000 epinephrine, or 1–5% cocaine) will help reduce bleeding, as well as improve visualization.
- Application of topical thrombin or fibrin glue may be used when direct visualization of the bleeding site is achieved.
- Once identified, an offending vessel may be cauterized with a silver nitrate stick or a swab dipped in trichloroacetic acid:
  - For recurrent nosebleeds silver nitrate cauterization with antiseptic cream may have a slight advantage over the use of antiseptic cream alone.
  - Cautery should only be applied to one side of nasal septum to avoid the risk of septal perforation, as the septal cartilage receives its blood supply from the overlying mucous membrane.
- Anterior nasal packing with oxycellulose or petroleum jelly gauze may be required to control refractory epistaxis when the site of bleeding cannot be precisely identified.
- Parental reassurance is an important, but often neglected, aspect of therapy.

ISSUES FOR REFERRAL
Otorhinolaryngologic consultation may be needed for severe nosebleeds or when posterior nasal packing, fracture reduction, surgery, or embolization is required. Nasal endoscopy is now routinely used.

 ## ONGOING CARE

FOLLOW-UP RECOMMENDATIONS
- Nosebleeds are easily controlled and self-limited in most instances.
- Postsurgical nosebleeds can be particularly problematic.
- Referral to an otorhinolaryngologist is indicated for patients with specific local abnormalities, such as polyps, tumors, or vascular malformations, or severe nosebleeds, recurrent nosebleeds, and/or posteriorly located nosebleeds.
- Identification of systemic illness may require referral to the appropriate specialist.

PATIENT MONITORING
- Blood clots in the nasopharynx should be removed because they may obscure engorged, bleeding vessels.
- Failure to detect a posterior location within the nasal cavity as the source of bleeding may interfere with measures to control bleeding.
- After nasal packing, it is essential to examine the oropharynx to confirm adequate hemostasis.
- Absorbable-type packings should be used, if required, in patients with bleeding disorders. Standard packings are prone to rebleeding on removal.
- Impregnation of nasal packings with antibiotic ointment reduces the risk of toxic shock syndrome.

PATIENT EDUCATION
Families should be given instructions in basic first aid for nosebleeds, because minor insults, such as sneezing or excessive manipulation, may cause nosebleeds to recur.

PROGNOSIS
- Uncomplicated epistaxis is most often self-limited or resolves with simple first-aid techniques.
- Refractory or recurrent epistaxis may require more specialized techniques, surgical intervention, and/or otorhinolaryngologic intervention.

COMPLICATIONS
- Usually uncomplicated
- Rare complications: Significant blood loss, airway obstruction, aspiration, and vomiting

ADDITIONAL READING

- Calder N, Kang S, Fraser L, et al. A double-blind randomized controlled trial of management of recurrent nosebleeds in children. *Otolaryngol Head Neck Surg.* 2009;140(5):670–674.
- Mahmood S, Lowe T. Management of epistaxis in the oral and maxillofacial surgery setting: An update on current practice. *Oral Surg Oral Med Oral Pathol Oral Radiol Endod.* 2003;95:23–29.
- Tan LS, Calhoun KH. Epistaxis. *Med Clin North Am.* 1999;83:43–56.
- Viehweg TL, Roberson JB, Hudson JW. Epistaxis: Diagnosis and treatment. *J Oral Maxillofac Surg.* 2006;64(3):511–518.

 ## CODES

ICD9
784.7 Epistaxis

ICD10
R04.0 Epistaxis

FAQ

- Q: How should the patient with nosebleeds be positioned?
- A: When possible, patients with nosebleeds should be kept erect. The upright position decreases vascular congestion. Recumbent patients may appear to have less bleeding, but this is owing to redirection of blood flow through the posterior pharynx.
- Q: How does rhinitis sicca contribute to epistaxis, and why does it occur?
- A: The nose warms, humidifies, and filters inspired air. Many modern heating systems and air-conditioning units reduce household humidity to unnaturally low levels. Rhinitis sicca is the direct result of inhaling dry air and results in friable nasal mucosa. Turbulent airflow from a septal deformity also promotes drying.

N

OBESITY

George A. Datto
Sandra Gibson Hassink

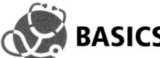 **BASICS**

DESCRIPTION
A chronic disease defined as having an excess of body fat. Body mass index (BMI), which is defined as weight in kilograms divided by height in meters squared, is accepted as a proxy measurement of adiposity in children.

- Children <2 years of age:
  - Weight for length >95% for age: Obese
- Children ≥2 years of age:
  - BMI <5%: Underweight
  - BMI 5–84%: Normal weight
  - BMI 85–94%: Overweight
  - BMI 95–99%: Obese
  - BMI >99%: Morbid obesity

EPIDEMIOLOGY
Prevalence
2007 data:
- 2–5 years of age: 10.4%
- 6–11 years of age: 19.6%
- 12–19 years of age: 19.1%
- Highest rates in Native American and Hispanic children
- 61% of overweight children have at least 1 additional risk factor for heart disease.

RISK FACTORS
- Intrauterine environment:
  - Gestational diabetes
  - Intrauterine growth retardation
- Obese parents:
  - 1 obese parent: 40% chance of having an obese child. 2 obese parents: 70% chance of having an obese child
- Low socioeconomic status/minority ethnic groups
- Limited intake of fruits and vegetables
- Postnatal environment:
  - Television viewing >2 hr/d
  - Consumption of sugared beverages
  - Inadequate sleep

GENERAL PREVENTION
- Prevention of gestational diabetes: Children of diabetic pregnancies have a greater risk of obesity and diabetes.
- Prevention of intrauterine growth retardation: Infants with intrauterine growth retardation are at increased risk of later obesity and cardiovascular disease; this risk is enhanced in infants and children who have had rapid weight gain or "catch-up growth."
- Encourage breastfeeding: There is a response effect on reduction of risk of obesity in children who have been breastfed.
- Early preventive counseling in patients with obese parents
- Early preventive counseling in children crossing BMI percentiles
- Promotion of nutrition guidelines, free play, and limited screen time in the general population

PATHOPHYSIOLOGY
Complex gene–environment–behavior interaction:
- Hypothalamus: Appetite regulation. Energy balance is regulated at the hypothalamic level. Neuropeptide regulation of hunger and satiety with input from cortical stimuli and gut hormone secretion. Energy stores and energy expenditure are regulated with input from leptin on energy stores and regulation of energy expenditure via the sympathetic nervous system.
- Adipose cells: Cytokines. Adipose tissue produces leptin (energy regulation) and adiponectin (cardiovascular risk).
- Tumor necrosis factor-α (inflammation)
- Psychobehavioral

ETIOLOGY
Energy imbalance:
- Excessive caloric intake: High caloric foods readily available in large portions and often preferred by children
- Inadequate caloric expenditure: Television, video games, and computers part of child's daily activities

COMMONLY ASSOCIATED CONDITIONS
- Type 2 diabetes mellitus
- Hypertension
- Dyslipidemia
- Metabolic syndrome
- Sleep apnea
- Asthma
- Polycystic ovarian syndrome
- Nonalcoholic steatohepatitis
- Slipped capital femoral epiphysis (SCFE)
- Blount disease (tibial bowing)
- Binge-eating disorder
- Mood disorder: Anxiety and depression
- Low self-esteem

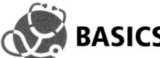 **DIAGNOSIS**

HISTORY
- Obesity trigger:
  - Age at which weight gain started
  - Family or patient stress
  - Life events
- Parents'/patient's beliefs:
  - Level of concern and motivation
  - Self-assessed reasons for weight gain
  - Previous attempts at weight control
- Family history:
  - Weight of parents
  - Obesity comorbidities in family
- Lifestyles:
  - Eating behaviors:
    ○ Age-appropriate meal structure
    ○ Sugared beverage (including juice, soda, sports drink) consumption
    ○ Snacks: frequency and content
  - Physical activity:
    ○ Hours of screen time from TVs, handheld devices, game stations, computers
    ○ Sports participation
    ○ Time outdoors

- Parenting skills:
  - Hunger management
  - Role modeling
  - Ability to set boundaries
- Obesity review of symptoms:
  - CNS: Pseudotumor
  - Respiratory: Sleep apnea, asthma
  - GI: Reflux
  - Orthopedics: SCFE/Blount disease
  - Psychology: Depression, attention deficit hyperactivity disorder (ADHD), anxiety, school difficulties
  - Skin: Acanthosis nigricans
- Prior interventions:
  - Ask about prior use of diet pills, laxatives.
  - Ask family about previous or current complementary and alternative medicine (CAM) weight loss products they have tried.

PHYSICAL EXAM
- Anthropometrics:
  - Weight, height
  - BMI
  - Blood pressure
- General:
  - Short stature
  - Dysmorphic features
  - Developmental delay
- Head, eyes, ears, nose, and throat (HEENT):
  - Papilledema
  - Tonsillar hypertrophy
- Cardiopulmonary:
  - Breath sounds
  - Heart murmur
- Abdomen: Hepatomegaly
- Genitourinary: Tanner stage
- Musculoskeletal:
  - Joint range of motion
  - Limp
  - Flat feet
- Skin:
  - Acanthosis nigricans
  - Hirsutism
  - Striae
- Psychological:
  - Mood: Assess for evidence of depression.
  - Affect

DIAGNOSTIC TESTS & INTERPRETATION
Lab
Metabolic screening (fasting specimens) should be done on all obese patients:
- Lipid profile: Cholesterol, HDL, and triglycerides
- Glucose or hemoglobin A1c
- Liver function tests to assess for liver disease
- Thyroid tests, cortisol, insulin, androgens (as indicated)

Diagnostic Procedures/Other
- Body composition: Excessive fat confirmation
  - Skinfold measurement
  - Bioelectric impedance analysis: Clinical estimate of basal metabolic rate and lean body mass
  - Indirect calorimetry: Clinical use in determining dietary requirements; calculates basal metabolic rate
- Comorbidity confirmation:
  - Sleep study: Assess for sleep apnea.
  - Hip radiographs: Rule out SCFE.
  - Knee and lower extremity radiographs: Rule out Blount disease.
  - Echocardiogram (echo): If hypertension present
  - Liver ultrasound: Nonalcoholic steatohepatitis (NASH)
  - Chromosomes: If dysmorphic features are present on examination
- DNA methylation study: Prader-Willi syndrome

DIFFERENTIAL DIAGNOSIS
Diseases in which obesity may be a component:
- Hypothalamic obesity
- Cushing syndrome
- Hypothyroidism
- Growth hormone deficiency
- Down syndrome

 TREATMENT

MEDICATION (DRUGS)
- Appetite suppressant:
  - Sibutramine (Meridia): Currently not marketed in US because of concerns about a 16% increase risk of cardiovascular disease as compared to patients taking placebo
- Lipase inhibitor:
  - Orlistat (Xenical):
    - Side effects: Abdominal pain, oily stools, flatulence
    - Minimal weight loss as compared to placebo
    - Not recommended for routine use

ADDITIONAL TREATMENT
General Measures
Early obesity recognition and treatment to prevent further excessive weight gain and obesity complications. Weight loss (initial goal of 5–10% reduction in BMI) and comorbidity treatment when clinically appropriate:
- Effective communication with patient and family:
  - Nonblaming
  - Using growth charts as visual aids
  - Being positive that change can occur
- Identify energy balance abnormalities.
- Supply developmentally appropriate nutrition and activity information.
- Support parents in planning and in making lifestyle changes:
  - Set goals.
  - Enhance parenting skills related to developing structure, setting boundaries, maintaining consistency, communication, and knowledge of child development.

Additional Therapies
Improve/change activity habits:
- Limit total screen time (television, video games, and computer) to a maximum of 2 hr/d.
- When possible, add structured physical activity into daily routine.
- Encourage non-weight-bearing activities, such as swimming or stationary bike riding, which may be easier for the severely deconditioned patient.
- Help family find opportunities for increased activity in both the child's school and community.

SURGERY/OTHER PROCEDURES
Gastric bypass or gastric banding (Lap-Band is not currently approved by the FDA in children) surgery may be appropriate for some adolescent patients with BMI >40 and severe comorbid conditions, including the following:
- Diabetes mellitus
- Sleep apnea
- Disabling orthopedic complications

 ONGOING CARE

FOLLOW-UP RECOMMENDATIONS
- Initially monthly to assess weight and behavioral change:
  - Intensify follow-up with weight gain
  - Spread out visits when efficacy of treatment has been established.
- Comorbidities that do not improve with reductions in BMI, or complications beyond a provider's expertise: Refer to appropriate specialist/pediatric obesity center.

DIET
Improve/change dietary habits:
- Encourage age-appropriate eating:
  - Review frequency of eating.
  - Review portion sizes.
- Discuss access to food.
- Discuss family meals.
- Limit sugared beverage consumption.
- Limit amount of junk food in house.
- Increase fruit and vegetable intake.
- Have parents model healthy eating habits.
- Encourage parents to work with child care, school, and extended family on supporting dietary changes.

PROGNOSIS
- Better prognosis in younger and less obese patients
- Better prognosis in patients and families who maintain ability to self-monitor health habits and maintain physical activity
- Long-term prognosis is guarded in morbidly obese patients.

COMPLICATIONS
- Medical emergencies:
  - Pseudotumor cerebri
  - SCFE
  - Nonketotic hyperosmolar hyperglycemia
  - Diabetic ketoacidosis
  - Pulmonary emboli

- Acute but generally nonemergent:
  - Hypertension
  - Sleep apnea
  - Gallstones
  - Type 2 diabetes
  - Polycystic ovarian syndrome
  - Gastroesophageal reflux
  - Asthma
  - Blount disease
- Chronic:
  - Dyslipidemia
  - Psychosocial issues
  - Increased risk of cardiovascular disease
  - Increased mortality of all causes in adulthood

ADDITIONAL READING

- CHS Health E stats. Available at: http://www.cdc.gov/nchs/data/hestat/obesity_child_07_08/obesity_child_07_08.htm.
- Inge TH, Krebs NF, Garcia VF, et al. Bariatric surgery for severely overweight adolescents: Concerns and recommendations. *Pediatrics*. 2004;114(1):217–223.
- Khan UI, Collier M. Medical interventions in adolescent obesity. *Adolesc Med State Art Rev*. 2008;19(3):406–420.
- Murray PJ. Bariatric surgery in adolescents: Mechanics, metabolism, and medical care. *Adolesc Med State Art Rev*. 2008;19(3):450–474.
- Van Cleave J, Gortmaker SL, Perrin JM. Dynamics of obesity and chronic health condition among children and youth. *JAMA*. 2010;303(7):623–630.

 CODES

ICD9
- 278.00 Obesity, unspecified
- 278.01 Morbid obesity

ICD10
- E66.01 Morbid (severe) obesity due to excess calories
- E66.3 Overweight
- E66.9 Obesity, unspecified

FAQ

- Q: How do I start addressing a child's weight?
- A: Review the height, weight, and BMI charts as part of the visit routine. Discuss family history in light of obesity and comorbidities, and link to the child's risk. Make obesity risk assessment part of the visit.
- Q: What do I do if family is not interested in addressing the child's weight?
- A: Introduce your concern about the child's health, ask the family to think about their priorities for the child and family, and help make links to good nutrition and activity habits (motivational interviewing).
- Q: How early can I start managing a child's weight?
- A: Attention to good nutrition and activity starts even before birth, at the prenatal visit. Parents need to see this as part of every interaction with their child's pediatrician.

OBSESSIVE COMPULSIVE DISORDER

C. Pace Duckett

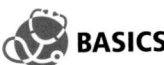 **BASICS**

DESCRIPTION

- Obsessive compulsive disorder (OCD), is a psychiatric illness manifested by repetitive obsessions and compulsions.
- Obsessions are defined as unwanted thoughts, images, or impulses that the patient recognizes as unwanted and intrusive.
- Compulsions are repetitive actions that are frequently in response to an obsession and are often preceded by an internal urge:
  - Compulsions are frequently performed according to a set of rules and often to prevent something from happening in the future.
- DSM-IV criteria:
  - Either obsessions or compulsions:
    - Obsessions: Recurrent or persistent ideas, thoughts, impulses, or images that are recognized as a product of one's own mind.
    - Compulsions: Repetitive behaviors or mental acts that a person feels driven to perform in response to an obsession, or according to rules that must be applied rigidly. These behaviors are aimed at reducing distress or preventing a feared event or situation.
    - It is not necessary that children recognize these thoughts or behaviors to be excessive or unreasonable.
    - The obsessions or compulsions cause marked distress, are time consuming (>1 hour daily), and cause impairment in daily functioning.

EPIDEMIOLOGY
Incidence
From 0.5–3%:
- The variability in these rates is understood in the context of the high prevalence of subclinical obsessions and compulsions in the population.

RISK FACTORS
- Acute streptococcal infection
- Familial heritability pattern
- Moderate genetic component based on twin studies

COMMONLY ASSOCIATED CONDITIONS
- Depression
- Anxiety disorders
- Tourette syndrome
- Trichotillomania

 DIAGNOSIS

HISTORY
- The diagnostic evaluation should entail gathering data through separate interviews with the child/adolescent and the parents.
- Current symptoms should be elicited within attention to severity, duration, and level of functional impairment.
- Core symptoms should be elicited concerning the content of obsessions and the nature of compulsions. These are most frequently checking behaviors, repetition rituals, or a focus on symmetry and organization.
- Sensitivity in assessing violent or sexually intrusive thoughts is necessary, as children may be uncomfortable disclosing these.
- Compulsions may manifest in physical action or in mental repetition.
- Assess the amount of functional impairment by estimating the time spent occupied by obsession and compulsions and how it interferes with their daily lives.
- Explore their level of insight into the irrationality of the symptoms. Diagnostically, children do not have to recognize the symptoms to be excessive. However, poor insight in an adult may represent a delusional disorder.
- Assess any parental accommodation of the ritualized behaviors, such as excessive cleaning.
- Determine if the onset was acute, severe, and temporally associated with symptoms of a streptococcal infection.

PHYSICAL EXAM
No pertinent findings

DIAGNOSTIC TESTS & INTERPRETATION
Lab
- No pathognomonic laboratory findings
- If onset is acute, severe, and associated with symptoms of a streptococcal infection, it may be reasonable to obtain an ASO titer.

Diagnostic Procedures/Other
Diagnostic scales:
- Children's Yale-Brown Obsessive Compulsive Scale (CY-BOCS)

DIFFERENTIAL DIAGNOSIS
- Anorexia nervosa
- Body dysmorphic disorder
- Delusional disorder
- Obsessive-compulsive personality disorder
- Pervasive developmental disorders
- Trichotillomania
- Tourette syndrome
- Schizophrenia
- Sydenham's chorea
- Pediatric autoimmune neuropsychiatric disorders associated with Strep infections (PANDA)

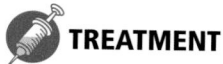 TREATMENT

General Measures
There are 2 types of treatment for OCD, psychosocial treatment and pharmacotherapy.

- Cognitive behavioral therapy (CBT) is most effective and well-studied psychosocial treatment:
  – SSRIs are the 1st-line agents for medication management.
  – Start intervention with CBT alone and add medication if treatment response limited.
- Emphasis is placed on graduated exposure with response prevention.
- Parental education is an important aspect of treatment adherence.

MEDICATION (DRUGS)
- SSRIs (1st-line) initiate 1/2 the starting dose for children with anxiety disorders:
  – Side effects include GI upset, headaches, dizziness, and agitation.
  – A black box warning by the FDA indicates that all antidepressants may increase suicidal thinking and behavior in children and adolescents.
  – Close monitoring is recommended following initiation.
  – Fluoxetine (Prozac) (10–60 mg)
  – Sertraline (Zoloft) (25–200 mg)
  – Fluvoxamine (Luvox) (25–200 mg)
- TCAs (2nd line):
  – Side effects include dizziness, xerostomia, blurred vision, postural hypotension, tachycardia, sedation, and constipation.
  – Clomipramine (Anafranil) (25–250 mg)

 ONGOING CARE

FOLLOW-UP RECOMMENDATIONS
Patient Monitoring
- Monitoring of response to psychosocial treatment should be performed routinely every 2–3 months.
- If medication is initiated, close monitoring on a weekly basis is recommended for the 1st 4 weeks, followed by monthly monitoring.
- CBT is performed on a weekly or twice weekly regimen.
- Monitoring of any emerging comorbidities is suggested.

PROGNOSIS
- OCD is a chronic condition. Treatments have been demonstrated to show significant response, but remission of symptoms is rare.
- Childhood onset is a poor prognostic indicator.

ADDITIONAL READING

- Martin A, Volkmar F. Obsessive-compulsive disorder. In: *Lewis's child and adolescent psychiatry*. Philadelphia: Lippincott Williams & Wilkins, 2007.
- March JS; Pediatric Obsessive-Compulsive Treatment Study Group. Cognitive-behavior therapy, sertraline, and their combination for children and adolescents with obsessive-compulsive disorder: The Pediatric OCD Treatment Study (POTS) randomized controlled trial. *JAMA*. 2004;292(16):1969–1976.

 CODES

ICD9
- 300.3 Obsessive-compulsive disorders
- 312.39 Other disorders of impulse control
- 315.9 Unspecified delay in development

ICD10
- F42 Obsessive-compulsive disorder
- F63.3 Trichotillomania
- F84.9 Pervasive developmental disorder, unspecified

CLINICAL PEARLS

Pitfalls include:
- Failing to utilize appropriate psychosocial treatments
- Not identifying the extent of the functional impairment

FAQ
- Q: Is OCD inherited?
- A: While no specific genes for OCD have been identified, there appears to be familial relationship to its inheritance.
- Q: What causes OCD?
- A: There is no proven cause of OCD. Research suggests that OCD involves problems in communication between the front part of the brain (the orbital cortex) and deeper structures (the basal ganglia).
- Q: Is there a cure?
- A: OCD is a chronic condition, but effective treatments are available.

OBSTETRIC BRACHIAL PLEXUS (ERB) PALSY

Richard S. Finkel

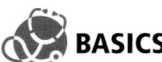

BASICS

DESCRIPTION
- The brachial plexus is a network of nerves in the neck and shoulder usually derived from the 5th cervical through the 1st thoracic nerve roots, consisting of anatomic structures termed trunks, divisions, and cords, terminating in specific nerves to individual muscles of the shoulder girdle, arm, and hand.
- Lesions of the brachial plexus can result in motor impairment—weakness, atrophy, and secondary joint contracture; sensory impairment—dermatomal or peripheral nerve distribution; functional and cosmetic impairment; limb length discrepancy; and chronic pain.
- Clinical and anatomic relationships:
  - 5th and 6th cervical (C5, C6) nerve roots fuse to form the upper trunk of the plexus:
    - C5 root impairment causes weakness of arm elevation to the front and side (flexion and abduction, due to deltoid and supraspinatus impairment).
    - C6 root compromise causes weakness of external rotation of the arm at the shoulder (infraspinatus), elbow flexion (mainly biceps), and partial supination (supinator) weakness.
    - If the lesion is at the C5, C6 root level or very proximal upper trunk, then winging of the scapula (serratus anterior) occurs. The biceps and brachioradialis deep tendon reflexes (DTRs) are depressed or absent.
  - 7th cervical (C7) nerve root alone forms the middle trunk of the plexus and is largely responsible for weakness in extension of the elbow (triceps), wrist (extensor carpi ulnaris), and fingers (extensor digitorum) and of wrist flexion (flexor carpi radialis).
  - 8th cervical (C8) and 1st thoracic (T1) nerve roots fuse to form the lower trunk of the plexus and innervate the intrinsic hand muscles responsible for grip and thumb opposition/abduction. The triceps DTR reflects the C7, C8 roots, but is difficult to obtain in newborns. The pectoralis DTR has the same distribution and is easier to elicit.

EPIDEMIOLOGY
- Erb palsy is the most commonly encountered partial lesion of the plexus seen in children, accounting for ~73–90% of all newborn cases, and occurs in ~1–4 per 1,000 live births. It involves the C5–6 and sometimes the C7 nerve roots and/or upper-middle trunks of the plexus:
  - Risk factors: Mainly large for gestational age (gestational diabetes), shoulder dystocia during vaginal delivery, and having a prior infant with Erb palsy
  - Antepartum compressive causes are well described in a minority of cases.
- Klumpke palsy in ~2% of neonatal cases, and is due to C8–T1 nerve root avulsion:
  - Risk factors: Breech delivery and face presentation

DIAGNOSIS

HISTORY, FOR BRACHIAL PLEXUS LESIONS IN OLDER CHILDREN
- Pregnancy and birth history, birth weight
- Trauma
- Recent viral infection
- Recent tetanus injection
- Family history, prior similar episodes that have resolved

PHYSICAL EXAM
- Testing of limb tone, strength, muscle bulk, joint range of motion, sensation, muscle stretch reflexes (DTRs) and elicited infant reflexes (Moro, asymmetric tonic neck response), diaphragm excursion, pupil size, pulses, and perfusion of the affected limb. Compare to the other side and the legs as well. Acute lesions often have severe pain, accentuated by movement of the arm.
- Sensory loss is difficult to assess because of overlap of dermatomes.
- Upper plexus lesion, such as Erb palsy (C5–6):
  - Arm hangs limply at the shoulder, adducted and internally rotated, the elbow extended and the forearm pronated, wrist and fingers flexed ("waiter's tip posture").
  - Hand grip is preserved.
  - Sensory impairment is often present over the lateral deltoid.
  - The biceps and brachioradialis muscle stretch reflexes (DTRs) are unelicitable; the triceps is present but often difficult to elicit in normal newborns.
  - The Moro reflex is asymmetric.
- Lower plexus lesion, such as Klumpke palsy (C8, T1):
  - Elbow flexion, supination of the forearm, wrist and finger extension, and an odd cupped-hand position
  - Triceps jerk is often absent.
  - Sensation may be impaired in the C8–T1 dermatomes.
  - An ipsilateral Horner sign (ptosis and miosis) indicates T1 involvement.
- Complete plexus lesion:
  - The entire upper limb and shoulder girdle is flaccid, anesthetic, and areflexic.

DIAGNOSTIC TESTS & INTERPRETATION
Imaging
- Chest and arm radiograph: Identifies subluxation of the spine or shoulder, fracture of the humerus or clavicle, and diaphragmatic palsy
- MRI has now largely replaced CT: Myelogram imaging of the cervical spinal cord, nerve roots, and plexus. There are occasional false-positive and false-negative findings for root avulsion, and many plexus lesions are not apparent on MRI.

Diagnostic Procedures/Other
Electrophysiologic testing: Electromyography (EMG) and nerve conduction velocity studies (NCV) can confirm the localization of the lesion, determine whether there has been axonal damage, and estimate timing of the lesion and the extent of reinnervation. Somatosensory and motor evoked potentials are not commonly done outside of the OR but can demonstrate conduction through a lesion in the plexus or nerve root. Usually the physical exam can give much the same information, reducing the need for EMG to selected settings.

DIFFERENTIAL DIAGNOSIS
- Lesions of the brain and spinal cord can produce focal weakness in mainly 1 limb. Usually the ipsilateral leg will have at least mild findings to indicate a hemiparesis.
- The pattern of weakness and hyperreflexia distinguish a central brain or spinal cord lesion from a peripheral nerve, root, or plexus lesion. A "congenital hemiparesis" presenting in early infancy, usually due to an antenatal stroke, often presents with arm and leg involvement and can mimic a brachial plexus lesion.
- Congenital malformations (Sprengel deformity) and contractures may mimic a brachial plexus palsy.
- Acute orthopedic problems such as a fracture or subluxation of the radial head
- Fascioscapulohumeral dystrophy has scapular winging and proximal arm weakness as main features, and when asymmetric can be similar to a brachial plexus lesion.

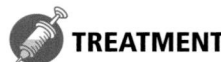

TREATMENT

ADDITIONAL TREATMENT
General Measures
- Mild weakness will recover in most cases without special treatment.
- For severe injury, with flaccid shoulder girdle and arm:
  - Immobilization: Babies with a fracture or who have significant pain with shoulder movement should have the limb partly immobilized for 2–3 weeks, to allow for rest during the acute phase of pain.
  - Cuff of the jersey can be pinned to the midline of the garment at the umbilicus level.
  - Caregivers should be instructed in proper lifting and positioning techniques to avoid pressure at the axilla.
  - Passive range-of-motion stretching: After 3 weeks, immobilization should be discontinued and gentle passive range of motion (PROM) should be initiated under the supervision of a therapist.
  - Fracture or shoulder subluxation needs to be excluded on radiography before starting PROM.
  - Regular visits to a pediatric occupational or physical therapist are necessary.
  - Electrical muscle stimulation: The data to support this therapy are limited, and there is no consensus at present regarding selection of patients for this treatment. It is not used routinely.

SURGERY/OTHER PROCEDURES

- Surgical issues: The critical window of time to consider surgical intervention is at 3–6 months if the deltoid/biceps remain flaccid and between 6 and 12 months when at least some early and steady recovery of strength is seen within the 1st 3 months but with later plateau. Primary repair of the nerve never results in full functional recovery.
- Surgical outcome is best if performed by 6–12 months and probably not useful if done after 24 months. Secondary surgery, usually after age 2 years, is often needed to address release of contractures, tendon transfers, and glenohumeral dysplasia.
- When an EMG at 1 month demonstrates no reinnervation in a flaccid deltoid or biceps, the prognosis for functional recovery is poor.
- There are no data to support the conjecture that repair at 4 months is more effective than later in the 1st year in the severely affected group.

 ## ONGOING CARE

FOLLOW-UP RECOMMENDATIONS

- The newborn with brachial plexus palsy should be re-evaluated at 2 weeks and if not nearly back to normal, then referred for weekly occupational or physical therapy and seen again at 2 to 3 months.
- When there is persisting weakness but steady improvement between 2 and 12 weeks, focus on therapy to prevent contractures.
- If elbow flexion against gravity has not evolved by 3 months of age, then referral to a surgical center with expertise in the management of Erb palsy should be considered.

PROGNOSIS

- ~75–85% of all patients regain very good to full strength and function, with 1/2 doing so rapidly (the mild group) and 1/2 more slowly (the moderate group).

Clinical Spectrum of Erb Palsy and Natural History

- For typical Erb palsy, return of elbow flexion (biceps) is the single most important prognostic factor in predicting functional recovery. Return of external rotation of the shoulder and forearm supination best predicts full recovery of function. Full recovery has been reported in 69–95% of patients. An estimated 1/4 of Erb palsy patients have some degree of permanent functional impairment.
- Pure C5, C6 Erb palsy patients do the best as a group.
- Prognosis is more guarded when C7 is involved.
- Involvement of the whole plexus or C8, T1 (Klumpke palsy) distribution fares least well.

- Mild: ~1/2 of patients have a mild injury due to stretching of the myelin sheath of the nerve fibers:
  - Initially there can be weakness limited to elevation of the arm and elbow flexion, or there can be full flaccidity of the arm and hand. Recovery of at least antigravity power in all muscle groups is seen by 2 weeks, and full strength returns by 3 weeks of age.
- Moderate: Another 1/4 of babies are very weak to fully flaccid at birth. This group appears initially like the mild one, but has slower recovery:
  - Those infants likely to recover fully develop at least antigravity strength in shoulder abduction and elbow flexion/extension by 3 months of age and recover full functional strength at a mean age of 6.5 months (range of 1.5–16 months). External rotation of the shoulder and forearm supination are the last motor functions to return. Mild weakness, contractures, and motor deficits may persist.
- Severe: If the arm remains flaccid at 3 months, the prognosis for spontaneous recovery of functional strength in the arm is guarded and with a high likelihood of developing shoulder and elbow joint contractures. When some improvement is seen at 3 months but is still less than antigravity, it is not possible to predict if a specific patient will be in the moderate or severe group. By 5–6 months, the group destined to recover functional strength will usually have developed antigravity strength in elbow flexion. If severe wrist and finger extensor weakness is still present at 6 months, there is little chance that a good functional recovery will occur.

COMPLICATIONS

- Ipsilateral diaphragm weakness is seen in about 5%, due to phrenic nerve (C4, C5) compromise.
- Bilateral arm weakness, typically asymmetric in degree, is noted in ~10%.
- Torticollis is frequent, and facial palsy is seen in ~10%. These do not carry an added unfavorable prognosis.
- Associated subluxation of the cervical spine and related spinal cord injury is identified in up to 5% and requires urgent neurosurgical attention.

ADDITIONAL READING

- Grossman JA. Early operative intervention for selected cases of brachial plexus birth injury. *Arch Neurol.* 2006;63:1031–1035.
- Hoeksma AF, ter Steeg AM, Nelissen RGHH, et al. Neurological recovery in obstetric brachial plexus injuries: An historical cohort study. *Dev Med Child Neurol.* 2004;46:76–83.
- Joyner B, Soto MA, Adam HM. Brachial plexus injury. *Pediatr Rev.* 2006;27(6):238–239.
- Lagerkvist A-L, Johansson U, Hohansson A, et al. Obstetric brachial plexus palsy: A prospective, population-based study of incidence, recovery, and residual impairment at 18 months of age. *Dev Med Child Neurol.* 2010;52:529–535.
- Pondaag W, Malessy MJA, van Dijk JG, et al. Natural history of obstetric brachial plexus palsy: A systematic review. *Dev Med Child Neurol.* 2004;46:138.
- *Semin Pediatr Neurol.* 2000;7(1). This entire issue is devoted to the evaluation and management of brachial plexus injuries in the newborn and child.

 ## CODES

ICD9
- 767.6 Injury to brachial plexus due to birth trauma
- 767.7 Other cranial and peripheral nerve injuries due to birth trauma

ICD10
- P14.0 Erb's paralysis due to birth injury
- P14.3 Other brachial plexus birth injuries

FAQ

- Q: What if my baby does not get better?
- A: About 1 in 4 babies have poor or limited recovery within the 1st few months, in which case it is advised to consult with a surgeon expert in this area and address whether an operation to fix the nerve injury will enhance the recovery. In the older child with some functional use of the arm, there may be a role for latter soft tissue surgery, to release contractures, transfer tendons, or stabilize the shoulder joint. Occupational therapy is important for infants and children with residual deficits in function.
- Q: When should an EMG be performed?
- A: If a baby with Erb palsy has no sign of recovery of biceps function at 1 month of age, then a EMG is helpful in establishing the prognosis. Lack of reinnervation features suggests a poor chance spontaneously gaining functional recovery, and surgical referral should be considered.

OMPHALITIS

Samir S. Shah

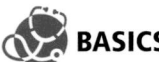 **BASICS**

DESCRIPTION
Omphalitis, an infection of the umbilical stump, begins in the neonatal period as a superficial cellulitis, but may progress to necrotizing fasciitis, myonecrosis, or systemic disease.

EPIDEMIOLOGY
- Episodes of omphalitis are usually sporadic, but rare epidemics occur.
- Mean age of onset is 5–9 days in term infants and 3–5 days in preterm infants.

Incidence
- Incidence varies from 0.2–0.7% in industrialized countries.
- Incidence is higher in hospitalized preterm infants compared with term infants.

RISK FACTORS
- Low birth weight
- Prior umbilical catheterization
- Septic delivery
- Prolonged rupture of membranes

GENERAL PREVENTION
- Antimicrobial agents applied to the umbilicus decrease bacterial colonization and prevent omphalitis.
- Effective methods of umbilical cord care include:
  – Triple dye daily until cord separation
  – Triple dye once and then alcohol daily until cord separation
  – Triple dye once and no further treatment
  – Povidone-iodine daily until cord separation
  – Silver sulfadiazine daily until cord separation
  – Bacitracin daily until cord separation
  – Chlorhexidine (4%) daily for 7 days
- There are no significant differences in the incidence of omphalitis with these regimens. However, the duration of umbilical cord attachment is significantly longer with triple dye daily compared with the other regimens (17 days vs. 6–12 days).
- Dry cord care: Spot cleaning of soiled skin in periumbilical area without application of any antibacterial agents is acceptable, but requires extreme vigilance for signs of infection. Infants treated with dry cord care as opposed to any of the above regimens are more likely to experience foul-smelling umbilical exudates (7% vs. <1%), bacterial colonization of umbilical stump, and omphalitis.

PATHOPHYSIOLOGY
- Potential bacterial pathogens normally colonize the umbilical stump after birth.
- These bacteria invade the umbilical stump, leading to omphalitis.
- Established aerobic bacterial infection, necrotic tissue, and poor blood supply facilitate the growth of anaerobic organisms.
- Infection may also extend beyond the subcutaneous tissues to involve fascial planes (fasciitis), abdominal wall musculature (myonecrosis), and the umbilical and portal veins (phlebitis).

ETIOLOGY
- Most (85%) cases of omphalitis are polymicrobial.
- The most common organisms include gram-positive cocci (*Staphylococcus aureus*, group A streptococci) and gram-negative enteric bacilli (*Escherichia coli*, *Klebsiella pneumoniae*, and *Proteus mirabilis*).
- Gram-positive organisms predominated in the past; however, the introduction of antistaphylococcal cord care (triple dye) has led to an increase in colonization and infection with gram-negative organisms.
- Anaerobic bacteria, including *Bacteroides fragilis* and *Clostridium perfringens*, are isolated in 1/3 of infections.
- Anaerobic organisms are more likely in cases complicated by necrotizing fasciitis or myonecrosis than in cases of superficial abdominal wall cellulitis.
- *Clostridium tetani* and *Clostridium sordellii* have been reported when deliveries have occurred outside a medical facility and when the cultural practice of placing cow dung on the umbilical stump after delivery was observed.

COMMONLY ASSOCIATED CONDITIONS
- Omphalitis may be the initial manifestation of an underlying disorder of neutrophil migration such as leukocyte adhesion deficiency, a rare immunologic disorder with an autosomal-recessive pattern of inheritance. These infants present with leukocytosis, delayed separation of the umbilical cord, and recurrent infections.
- Omphalitis may also be a manifestation of neutropenia in the neonate:
  – In neonatal alloimmune neutropenia, maternal IgG antibodies cross the placenta and result in an immune-mediated destruction of fetal neutrophils bearing antigens that differ from the mother's. The resultant neutropenia can last for several weeks to as long as 6 months. Antineutrophil antibodies are found in the serum of the mother and the infant. Affected infants may also present with other cutaneous bacterial infections, pneumonia, sepsis, and meningitis.
  – Causes of neutropenia associated with immune dysfunction include autoimmune neutropenias, X-linked agammaglobulinemia, hyper-IgM immunodeficiency syndromes, and HIV.
  – Other causes of neutropenia include metabolic disorders such as hyperglycinemia, isovaleric acidemia, propionic acidemia, methylmalonic acidemia, tyrosinemia, and glycogen storage disease type IB.
- Omphalitis complicated by sepsis can also be associated with neutropenia. Therefore, the underlying disease process producing neutropenia may not be immediately appreciated in affected newborns.
- Rarely, an anatomic abnormality such as a patent urachus or patent omphalomesenteric duct may be present.

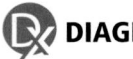 **DIAGNOSIS**

HISTORY
- Identify risk factors such as prolonged membrane rupture, septic or home delivery, and dry cord care.
- A history of change in mental status such as irritability, lethargy, somnolence, or decreased level of activity may indicate systemic dissemination of the infection.
- A history of urine or stool discharge from the umbilicus suggests an underlying anatomic abnormality.
- Family history may reveal individuals with metabolic disorders or recurrent infections.

PHYSICAL EXAM
- Varies with the extent of disease
- Localized infection:
  – Abdominal tenderness
  – Periumbilical edema and erythema
  – Purulent or malodorous discharge from the umbilical stump
- Indications of more extensive local disease, such as necrotizing fasciitis or myonecrosis:
  – Periumbilical ecchymoses or gangrene
  – Abdominal wall crepitus
  – Progression of cellulitis despite antimicrobial therapy
- Signs of systemic disease are nonspecific and include thermo dysregulation and evidence of multiorgan dysfunction:
  – Fever or temperature instability
  – Tachycardia, hypotension, delayed capillary refill
  – Apnea, tachypnea, flaring of the alae nasi, grunting, intercostal/subcostal retractions, hypoxemia
  – Abdominal distention, diminished bowel sounds
  – Cyanosis, petechiae, jaundice
  – Lethargy, hypotonia

DIAGNOSTIC TESTS & INTERPRETATION
Lab
- Umbilical stump Gram stain and culture for aerobic and anaerobic organisms:
  – Identify potential organisms and antimicrobial susceptibility patterns. Although suggestive, cultures of umbilical discharge may reflect only colonization of the stump and are not proof of an etiologic role in the underlying process. Therefore, if myonecrosis is suspected, specimens of muscle should be sent for culture.
- Blood culture:
  – Risks systemic dissemination of infection in the neonate.

- CBC:
  - Neutropenia or neutrophilia may be present.
  - An immature-to-total neutrophils ratio >0.2 is suggestive of systemic infection.
  - Thrombocytopenia may be present.
- D-dimers or prothrombin time, partial thromboplastin time, fibrinogen, and fibrinogen split products:
  - Indicated for sepsis or disseminated intravascular coagulation

Imaging
Radiographs (case dependent):
- Abdominal radiographs:
  - Portal venous or intramural air requires immediate surgical consultation.
- Abdominal CT:
  - Confirms involvement of fascia and muscle and delineates the extent of infection
- Voiding cystourethrogram:
  - Reveals patent urachus

Diagnostic Procedures/Other
Lumbar puncture is indicated in any neonate with a focal bacterial infection

DIFFERENTIAL DIAGNOSIS
- The characteristic clinical picture of omphalitis allows diagnosis on clinical grounds.
- Determine the presence of associated complications, such as necrotizing fasciitis, myonecrosis, or systemic infection.
- Consider an underlying immunologic or metabolic disorder.

 TREATMENT

MEDICATION (DRUGS)
Empiric coverage:
- Antistaphylococcal agent (e.g., oxacillin, vancomycin) plus an aminoglycoside (e.g., gentamicin, amikacin, tobramycin) or cefepime
- Add anaerobic coverage (e.g., metronidazole) in cases complicated by necrotizing fasciitis or myonecrosis. Clindamycin also provides anaerobic coverage and may be substituted for the antistaphylococcal penicillin.
- As with antimicrobial therapy for other infections, consider local antibiotic susceptibility patterns.
- Duration of therapy is typically 10–14 days; 7 days may be adequate for uncomplicated cases

ADDITIONAL TREATMENT
General Measures
Antibiotics and supportive care

Additional Therapies
The use of hyperbaric oxygen to treat anaerobic necrotizing fasciitis and myonecrosis is controversial:
- No prospective data are available.
- The delivery of high concentrations of oxygen to marginally perfused tissues may have a detrimental effect on the growth of anaerobic organisms and improve phagocyte function.
- Surgical therapy remains the highest priority.

SURGERY/OTHER PROCEDURES
- Early and complete surgical débridement of affected tissue and muscle is important.
- Delay in diagnosis or surgical intervention allows local progression of infection and worsening systemic toxicity.

IN-PATIENT CONSIDERATIONS
Initial Stabilization
Emergency care: Immediate evaluation, antimicrobial therapy, and supportive care are essential to survival.

 ONGOING CARE

FOLLOW-UP RECOMMENDATIONS
Infants developing associated portal vein thrombosis require follow-up for complications owing to portal hypertension.

PROGNOSIS
- The outcome of infants with uncomplicated omphalitis is generally good.
- The mortality rate among all infants with omphalitis, including those who develop complications, is 7–15%.
- The mortality rate is significantly higher (38–87%) with necrotizing fasciitis or myonecrosis.
- Risk factors for poor prognosis include male gender, prematurity, low birth weight, and septic delivery, including delivery outside a medical facility.

COMPLICATIONS
- Necrotizing fasciitis, a bacterial infection of the subcutaneous fat, and superficial and deep fascia, complicates 8–16% of cases of omphalitis. It is characterized by rapidly spreading infection, often with systemic toxicity.
- Myonecrosis refers to infectious involvement of the muscle. The rapid development of edema may constrict the muscle within its fascia and cause a superimposed ischemic myonecrosis. Extensive areas of necrotic tissue facilitate the growth of anaerobic organisms.
- Portal vein thrombosis and septic embolization follow infection of the umbilical vessels.
- Sepsis complicates omphalitis in 13% of cases.

ADDITIONAL READING
- Cushing AH. Omphalitis: A review. *Pediatr Infect Dis J.* 1985;4:282–285.
- Fraser N, Davies BW, Cusack J. Neonatal omphalitis: A review of its serious complications. *Acta Paediatr.* 2006;95:519–522.
- Mullany LC, Darmstadt DL, Khatry DK, et al. *Lancet.* 2006;367:10–18.
- Samuel M, Freeman N, Vaishnav A, et al. Necrotizing fasciitis: A serious complication of omphalitis in neonates. *J Pediatr Surg.* 1994;29:1414–1416.

 CODES

ICD9
- 041.00 Streptococcus infection in conditions classified elsewhere and of unspecified site, streptococcus, unspecified
- 041.10 Staphylococcus infection in conditions classified elsewhere and of unspecified site, staphylococcus, unspecified
- 771.4 Omphalitis of the newborn

ICD10
- B95.0 Streptococcus, group A, as the cause of diseases classified elsewhere
- P38.1 Omphalitis with mild hemorrhage
- P38.9 Omphalitis without hemorrhage

FAQ
- Q: Do all infants who develop omphalitis require evaluation for immunologic disorders?
- A: No, particularly if predisposing factors such as an umbilical catheter are present. Infants requiring further evaluation include those with persistent neutropenia, recurrent infections, delayed separation of the umbilical cord, or a family history of immunologic disorders.
- Q: Is surgical consultation required for all infants with omphalitis?
- A: No. Surgical consultation is not required for uncomplicated omphalitis. However, a high degree of suspicion should exist for associated complications. The presence of necrotizing fasciitis or myonecrosis requires immediate surgical consultation.

OSTEOGENESIS IMPERFECTA

Vikas Trivedi
John P. Dormans

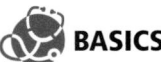 **BASICS**

DESCRIPTION
Osteogenesis imperfecta (OI) is a group of genetically and clinically heterogeneous connective tissue disorders affecting bone and soft tissue, causing abnormal fragility of bone, resulting in recurring fractures and deformity.

EPIDEMIOLOGY
Incidence
1 in 30,000 births

Prevalence
~20,000–50,000 cases in U.S.

RISK FACTORS
Genetics
- Majority of OI cases are caused by dominant mutations in type1 collagen: *COL1A1* and *COL1A2*, and by recessive mutations in recently identified *CRTAP* (cartilage-associated protein gene) and *LEPRE1*.
- Sillence classification:
  - Type I (mild, nondeforming): Autosomal dominant *COL1A1*, blue sclera, onset preschool:
    - A: Teeth involved
    - B: Teeth not involved
  - Type II (perinatal, lethal): Autosomal recessive, *CRTAP* and *LEPRE1*, lethal, blue sclera
  - Type III (severely deforming): Autosomal recessive, *CRTAP* and *LEPRE1*, severe, normal sclera
  - Type IV (moderately deforming): Autosomal dominant, *COL1A2*, normal sclera, mild form:
    - A: Teeth involved
    - B: Teeth not involved
- New descriptive phenotypic classification (type I–VIII) has been proposed that incorporates traditional Sillence classification with new genetic mutations as described above.

PATHOPHYSIOLOGY
- In general, both enchondral and intramembranous bone formation are disturbed:
  - Osteoid seams are wide and crowded by osteoblasts (woven bone).
  - Osteoclasts are normal.
  - Collagen fibrils are disorganized (by electron microscope).
- Physis broad and irregular:
  - Osteopenia
  - Long bones are slender and smaller.
  - Fractures (recent or healed)
  - Deformities:
    - Spine: Scoliosis, compression fractures, kyphosis, upper cervical spine instability
    - Skull: Multiple centers of ossification, wormian bones, basilar invagination/platybasia

ETIOLOGY
- Abnormality of collagen production and organization
- Failure of maturation of procollagen to type 1 collagen and failure of normal collagen cross-linking

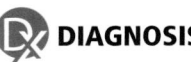 **DIAGNOSIS**

HISTORY
- Variable
- Family history

PHYSICAL EXAM
- Severe congenital forms:
  - Multiple fractures
  - Limbs deformed and short
  - Skull soft
- Mild and moderate forms:
  - General: Short stature, hernias
  - Extremities: Bowing, coxa vara deformity, cubitus varus, hypermobility of joints: Subluxations and dislocations
  - Pelvis: Trefoil pelvis, protrusio acetabuli

- Spine (cause: osteoporosis, compression fractures, and ligamentous laxity): Kyphoscoliosis (30–40%), platybasia
- Skin: Thin skin, subcutaneous hemorrhages, wide surgical scars
- Eyes: Blue sclera caused by thin collagen layer, Saturn ring (white sclera immediately) hyperopia, embryotoxon or arcus juvenilis occasionally, retinal detachment occasionally
- Teeth: Dentinogenesis imperfecta, enamel normal, both deciduous and permanent teeth affected, teeth easily broken, discoloration
- Deafness: Either conduction or nerve type

DIAGNOSTIC TESTS & INTERPRETATION
Lab
- Serum calcium and phosphorus levels:
  - Normal
- Alkaline phosphatase:
  - May be elevated
- No widely available specific diagnostic laboratory test
- Dermal biopsy involving collagen testing
- Current evidence favors DNA analysis over dermal biopsy

Imaging
- Osteopenia
- Fractures:
  - New, healing, or healed
  - Malunions
- Deformity
- Metaphyseal ends of long bones:
  - Honeycomb appearance of ends of long bones, popcorn calcifications, Erlenmeyer flask appearance, acetabular protrusion
- Spine:
  - Atlantoaxial subluxation, spondylolisthesis, scoliosis, compression fractures

DIFFERENTIAL DIAGNOSIS
- Severe:
  - Congenital hypophosphatasia
  - Achondroplasia
  - Camptomelic dwarfism
- Mild:
  - Cystinosis
  - Pyknodysostosis
  - Child abuse
  - Leukemia
  - Idiopathic juvenile osteoporosis
  - Steroid treatment
  - Rickets in very-low-weight infants
  - Menkes kinky hair syndrome (newborn male [X-linked recessive] with failure to thrive)
  - Metaphyseal corner fractures
  - Abnormal hair
- Hyperplastic callus formation may be confused with osteogenic sarcoma.

 TREATMENT

MEDICATION (DRUGS)
- Bisphosphonates are being used currently in clinical trials for children with severe involvement (gene therapy possibly in future).
- Sex hormones, fluoride, magnesium oxide, and calcitonin

ADDITIONAL TREATMENT
General Measures
- Fracture treatment:
  - Fractures heal at a normal rate; splinting, orthoses, casting, operations (intramedullary rod)
- Scoliosis:
  - Seen in ~50%
  - Orthoses usually ineffective
  - Spinal fusion for curves >50 degrees after the onset of puberty
- Correction of deformities (e.g., realignment osteotomies with intramedullary fixation most common for long-bone deformity)

IN-PATIENT CONSIDERATIONS
Initial Stabilization
Emergency care:
- For unstable fractures, such as femur fractures, spine instability
- Depends on location of fracture and details of individual situation
- Multidisciplinary approach:

Team member	Care problem
Pediatric Endocrinologist	Maintenance of bone mass
Pediatric orthopaedic surgeon	Fracture repair, rodding, scoliosis correction
Dentist	Dentinogenesis imperfecta: capping, orthodontics
Physiotherapist	Post operative
	Rehabilitation of all joints and spine, muscle strength and gait training
Psychologist/Social worker	School adjustment from kindergarten to college, work guidance

 ONGOING CARE

FOLLOW-UP RECOMMENDATIONS
- Techniques for safe handling, protective positioning, and safe movement are taught to parents.
- Children and youth learn which activities to avoid and how to practice energy conservation.
- Following a healthy lifestyle including not smoking, and maintaining a healthy weight is beneficial.

PATIENT EDUCATION
Education and fracture and injury prevention are important.

PROGNOSIS
- In general, the earlier the fractures occur, the more severe the disease.
- For moderate and mild types, there is a gradual tendency to improvement, with the incidence of fractures decreasing after puberty.
- Depends on severity of OI
- Moderate and mild types:
  - Gradual tendency to improvement, with incidence of fractures decreasing after puberty

COMPLICATIONS
- Pathological fractures
- Scoliosis
- Cardiorespiratory problems (aortic dilatation, mitral valve prolapse, and aortic regurgitation)
- Otosclerosis and hearing loss
- Dwarfism
- Skull fractures
- Intracranial bleeding and brain damage

ADDITIONAL READING
- Antoniazzi F, Zamboni G, Lauriola S, et al. Early bisphosphonate treatment in infants with severe osteogenesis imperfecta. *J Pediatr.* 2006;149(2): 174–179.
- Bachrach LK. Consensus and controversy regarding osteoporosis in the pediatric population. *Endocr Pract.* 2007;13(5):513–520.
- Dormans JP, Flynn JM. Pathologic fractures associated with tumors and unique conditions of the musculoskeletal system. In Beaty J, Kasser JR, eds., *Rockwood and Wilkins fractures in children.* Philadelphia: Lippincott Williams & Wilkins, 2007.
- Dormans JP. *Pediatric orthopaedics: Core knowledge in orthopaedics.* Philadelphia: Elsevier Mosby, 2005:393–394.
- Gertner JM, Root L. Osteogenesis imperfecta. *Orthop Clin North Am.* 1990;21:151–162.
- Hackley L, Merritt L. Osteogenesis imperfecta in the neonate. *Adv Neonatal Care.* 2008;8(1):21–30.
- Kamboj MK. Metabolic bone disease in adolescents: Recognition, evaluation, treatment, and prevention. *Adolesc Med State Art Rev.* 2007;18(1):24–46.
- Minch CM, Kruse RW. Osteogenesis imperfecta: A review of basic science and diagnosis. *Orthopedics.* 1998;21:558–567, 568–569 (quiz).
- Sillence DO. Osteogenesis imperfecta: An expanded panorama of variants. *Clin Orthop.* 1981;159:11.
- Shapiro JR, Sponseller PD. Osteogensis Imperfecta: Questions and answers. *Curr Opin Pediatr.* 2009;21: 709–716.
- Tosi LL. Osteogenesis imperfecta. *Curr Opin Pediatr.* 1997;9:94–99.
- Zaleske DJ. Metabolic and endocrine abnormalities. In Morrissy RT, Weinstein SL, eds., *Lovell and Winter's pediatric orthopaedics,* 5th ed. Philadelphia: Lippincott Williams & Wilkins, 2001:177–242.

 CODES

ICD9
756.51 Osteogenesis imperfecta

ICD10
Q78.0 Osteogenesis imperfecta

OSTEOSARCOMA

Naomi J. Balamuth
Susan R. Rheingold (5th edition)

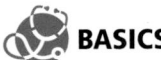 **BASICS**

DESCRIPTION
A tumor of the bone composed of spindle cells that produce malignant osteoid

EPIDEMIOLOGY
- Osteosarcoma is the most common malignant bone tumor of childhood and adolescence, representing 60% of all bone tumors in the pediatric age group.
- Overall, it accounts for <1% of all malignant neoplasms.
- ~90% of tumors occur at the metaphyseal ends of long tubular bones, but any portion of the skeleton may be involved.
- The most frequent site is the distal femur, followed by the proximal tibia and the proximal humerus.

Incidence
- Peak incidence is in adolescence and early adulthood, with a median age of 18 at diagnosis.
- Thought to begin during the adolescent growth spurt

RISK FACTORS
- Radiation exposure
- Paget disease of the bone
- Rothman–Thompson syndrome
- Enchondromatosis
- Hereditary multiple exostoses
- Fibrous dysplasia
- Hereditary retinoblastoma

Pathophysiology
- Osteosarcoma most often involves the medullary region of bone.
- Rarely, osteosarcoma occurs in soft tissue separate from underlying bone.
- Classic or conventional osteosarcoma, the largest group of osteosarcomas, is composed of connective tissue stroma containing highly malignant spindle-shaped cells as well as areas of osteoid production and calcification.
- 4 microscopic subtypes are osteoblastic, chondroblastic, fibroblastic, and telangiectatic. These variants are rare in the pediatric population and lack prognostic significance at present.
- 2 rare clinical subtypes, periosteal and parosteal osteosarcomas, rarely metastasize and carry a better prognosis.

ETIOLOGY
- The etiology of most cases is unknown.
- There is an association of osteosarcoma with exposure to ionizing radiation:
  - Secondary osteosarcoma is seen in up to 5% of patients who received radiation therapy for an initial malignancy.
- Children with hereditary retinoblastoma are at increased risk of developing osteosarcoma with and without prior exposure to radiation.

DIAGNOSIS

SIGNS AND SYMPTOMS
- A tender, soft-tissue mass and increased warmth may be present in the involved area.
- Localized erythema is uncommon.
- Unless there exists an underlying fracture, range of motion of the limb is normal and there is no difficulty weight bearing.
- Regional lymphadenopathy is rare.

HISTORY
- Pain at the site of the tumor is the most common presentation.
- Swelling over the involved area is also reported.
- The duration of symptoms varies.
- A history of recent trauma is common but unrelated. trauma often brings the affected area to the patient's or parents' attention, but does not actually cause osteosarcoma.
- Weight loss is rare, but may occur in advanced disease.
- If fever is present, it may indicate an infectious cause (osteomyelitis) rather than osteosarcoma.

DIAGNOSTIC TESTS & INTERPRETATION
Lab
- Laboratory tests are not generally helpful in osteosarcoma.
- Serum lactate dehydrogenase (LDH) and alkaline phosphatase may be elevated: The prognostic significance is controversial.
- An elevated WBC count, C-reactive protein, or sedimentation rate may suggest osteomyelitis.

Imaging
- A plain radiograph of the involved area always reveals some abnormality. Radiographic examination should include the primary tumor site as well as areas of potential metastases:
  - Most commonly, one sees a lytic or blastic region of the bone with ill-defined borders.
  - Other findings may include periosteal elevation adjacent to the primary lesion, a sunburst appearance of the primary lesion caused by neoplastic spicules adjacent to the bony cortex, or a pathologic fracture.
- A chest CT and bone scan should be done to assess for pulmonary and bone metastases.
- An MRI should be done to better evaluate the extent of the tumor:
  - Include the joint above and below the involved bony area.
  - MRI can delineate the intraosseous and extraosseous extent of the tumor as well as evaluate the neurovascular structures involved.

Diagnostic Procedures/Surgery
The diagnosis of osteosarcoma can be confirmed only by a biopsy, which should be done by an experienced pediatric orthopedic surgeon in conjunction with a pediatric oncologist and pediatric pathologist

DIFFERENTIAL DIAGNOSIS
- Infection:
  - Osteomyelitis
  - Septic arthritis
- Trauma: Stress fracture
- Benign tumors:
  - Unicameral bone cyst
  - Osteoblastoma
  - Eosinophilic granuloma
  - Giant-cell tumor
  - Aneurysmal bone cyst
  - Osteochondroma
  - Fibrous dysplasia
- Malignant tumors:
  - Ewing sarcoma
  - Chondrosarcoma
  - Fibrosarcoma
  - Leukemia
  - Metastatic lesions of other primary tumors

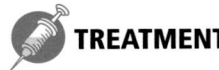 **TREATMENT**

RADIOTHERAPY
Osteosarcoma is not a radiation sensitive tumor. Radiation may be used in cases that are not surgically accessible.

Physical Therapy
- All patients need to work with specialists to learn how to adapt to their surgically induced disability.
- The duration of physical therapy and rehabilitation is dependent on the disability and the individual patient's needs.

MEDICATION (DRUGS)
- The goals of adjuvant chemotherapy are treatment of micrometastases and shrinkage of the primary tumor mass, particularly when limb-salvage procedures are surgical options. Response to adjuvant chemotherapy (degree of necrosis at the time of complete resection) is an important prognostic factor.
- Groups such as the Children's Oncology Group (COG) have developed chemotherapy protocols for osteosarcoma. Most children and adolescents with osteosarcoma are treated on these chemotherapy protocols. Many protocols are open to young adults up to the age of 30.

- The mainstays of treatment are cisplatin, high-dose methotrexate and doxorubicin, with many protocols adding ifosfamide and etoposide:
  - The duration of chemotherapy varies from 8–12 months according to the extent of the tumor at diagnosis, tumor response to therapy, and the individual protocol.

SURGERY/OTHER PROCEDURES

- In the past, when osteosarcoma was managed by surgery alone, most patients subsequently developed pulmonary metastases and died of progressive disease.
- Surgical options depend on the primary site of the tumor and the extent of tumor involvement.
- Complete surgical resection with wide margins is necessary for cure. Surgical options for osteosarcomas of the extremities include:
  - Amputation
  - Limb salvage with allograft or prosthetic reconstruction
  - Rotationplasty
- Macroscopic pulmonary metastases should be resected at the time of surgery if still visible by radiographic examination:
  - Localized pulmonary recurrences that develop after treatment also should be resected, as this can result in long-term cure or a prolonged symptom-free period.

 ONGOING CARE

ISSUES FOR REFERRAL

When a malignant bone tumor is suspected, the patient should be referred immediately to a pediatric cancer center:

- Children's cancer centers can provide the multidisciplinary team needed to diagnose, biopsy, treat, and rehabilitate children with bone tumors.

PROGNOSIS

- Most patients with osteosarcoma involving an extremity without pulmonary metastases can be cured.
- 5-year survival for nonmetastatic disease ranges from 60–70%. The following have been associated with a poorer prognosis:
  - Pulmonary metastases
  - Disseminated bone metastases
  - Poor response of the tumor to preoperative chemotherapy with tumor necrosis <95%
  - Inability to achieve a total surgical excision of the tumor

COMPLICATIONS

- 10–20% of patients have pulmonary metastases at the time of diagnosis; a smaller proportion has metastases to other bones
- Wound infections may develop in surgical sites in the initial postoperative period. Significant pain, fever, swelling, discharge, and foul odor from the surgical site should be evaluated, preferably by the surgeon.
- Poor healing of the surgical site may be a problem, particularly in patients receiving chemotherapy or in those with poor nutrition. Patients may require IV antibiotics, supplemental feeding, and/or surgical revision of the wound.

Patient Monitoring

- If prostheses are required, skin breakdown and fitting difficulties with prosthetic devices, such as adjustments for changes in height and weight, should be diagnosed and corrected. Scoliosis and back pain may develop in patients using improperly adjusted crutches and/or prosthetic devices after lower extremity or pelvic procedures. This requires expertise in prosthetic devices for children.
- Phantom pain is a normal phenomenon after amputation. Patients and their families should be reassured if this occurs. Sometimes medication can reduce the pain.
- All children need to be followed by an oncologist regularly after treatment is completed to monitor for recurrence as well as long-term side effects of the chemotherapy, such as cardiac toxicity, infertility, or secondary malignancy.

ADDITIONAL READING

- Arndt CAS, Crist WM. Medical progress: Common musculoskeletal tumors of childhood and adolescence. *N Engl J Med*. 1999;341:342–352.
- Bielack SS, Carrle D, Hardes J, et al. Bone tumors in adolescents and young adults. *Curr Treat Options Oncol*. 2008;9(1):67–80.
- Ferguson WS, Goorin AM. Current treatment of osteosarcoma. *Cancer Invest*. 2001;19:292–315.
- Grimer RJ. Surgical options for children with osteosarcoma. *Lancet Oncol*. 2005;6(2):85–92.
- Harting MT, Blakely ML. Management of osteosarcoma pulmonary metastases. *Semin Pediatr Surg*. 2006;15(1):25–29.
- Longhi A, Errani C, De Paolis M, et al. Primary bone osteosarcoma in the pediatric age: State of the art. *Cancer Treat Rev*. 2006;32(6):423–436.
- Miller SL, Hoffer FA. Malignant and benign bone lesions. *Radiol Clin North Am*. 2001;39:673–699.

 CODES

ICD9

170.9 Malignant neoplasm of bone and articular cartilage, site unspecified

ICD10

C41.9 Malignant neoplasm of bone and articular cartilage, unsp

FAQ

- Q: How does one differentiate osteosarcoma from Ewing sarcoma, the second most common bone tumor of childhood?
- A: Ultimately, only a biopsy can differentiate the two. In general, Ewing sarcoma is seen in younger children and tends to affect the axial bones, such as the pelvis. When found in the long bones, it is usually in the diaphyseal regions. Symptomatology does not differ, but Ewing sarcoma can be metastatic to the bone marrow, as well as the bone and lung.
- Q: How does one differentiate osteosarcoma from a benign bone lesion?
- A: Ultimately, only a biopsy can differentiate the two. Benign lesions tend to be very well circumscribed with smooth edges on radiograph. They are generally not associated with soft tissue masses, swelling, or fever. Fractures are just as likely through benign bone lesions as malignant ones. Only in very rare situations should bony lesions be presumed to be benign and observed without biopsy.
- Q: Is there an increased risk of osteosarcoma in the contralateral limb?
- A: No.
- Q: Does limb salvage incur a greater risk of recurrence than does amputation?
- A: Recent studies have shown that there is no increase in recurrence if wide margins are achieved at the time of surgery.

OSTEOMYELITIS

Virginia M. Pierce
Mitchell R. M. Schwartz (5th edition)

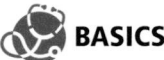 **BASICS**

DESCRIPTION
- Infection of the bone
- Any bone can be involved, but most commonly occurs in the metaphysis of a long bone (especially the femur or tibia)

EPIDEMIOLOGY
- One of the most common invasive bacterial infections in children, accounting for 1% of all pediatric hospitalizations
- ~50% of cases occur in children ≤5 years of age
- A history of minor trauma to the affected site is common, but of unclear significance.

RISK FACTORS
- Sickle hemoglobinopathy
- Primary or acquired immunodeficiency
- Bone trauma (open fractures, puncture wounds, bites, surgical manipulation)
- Implanted orthopedic devices
- Pressure ulcers

PATHOPHYSIOLOGY
- Usually, osteomyelitis is of hematogenous origin in children (inoculation of bone during an episode of bacteremia). The infecting organism enters the bone via a nutrient artery and then is deposited in the metaphysis due to its rich vascular supply. The organism replicates in metaphyseal capillary loops, causes local inflammation, spreads through vascular tunnels, and adheres to the bone matrix. Increased pressure in the metaphysis allows pus to perforate through the cortex and lift the periosteum.
- Local spread from a contiguous focus of infection and direct inoculation (e.g., penetrating injury) are less common mechanisms of infection.

ETIOLOGY
- *Staphylococcus aureus* is responsible for 70–90% of osteomyelitis in all age groups, with MRSA an increasingly common problem.
- *Streptococcus pyogenes, Streptococcus pneumoniae*, and *Kingella kingae* are the next most common pathogens in infants and children.

- Group B *Streptococcus* and gram-negative enterics are important causative organisms in neonates.
- *Salmonella* spp. can be the cause in children with sickle cell disease.
- *Pseudomonas aeruginosa* can be found after puncture wounds to the foot.
- There has been a significant decline in the incidence of *Haemophilus influenzae* type b (Hib) osteomyelitis since immunization with the Hib conjugate vaccine became widespread.
- Other, more unusual pathogens may be seen in patients with specific risk factors (e.g., coagulase-negative staphylococci in the presence of prosthetic material, anaerobes after animal or human bites).
- In a significant percentage of cases, a definitive causative microorganism is not identified.

DIAGNOSIS

HISTORY
- Persistent, increasing pain and tenderness over the affected bone
- Restricted use of the involved limb, refusal to bear weight, or limp
- Fever, malaise, anorexia
- Swelling, warmth, and erythema of the soft tissues over the affected bone may be noted.
- Exaggerated immobility/pain with micromotion of an adjacent joint suggests pyogenic arthritis (alternatively, or in addition to osteomyelitis).

DIAGNOSTIC TESTS & INTERPRETATION
Lab
Initial lab tests
- The white blood cell count may be normal or elevated.
- The erythrocyte sedimentation rate (ESR) and C-reactive protein (CRP) levels are usually elevated.
- Blood cultures are positive in ~50% of patients.

Imaging
- Plain radiographs may show deep soft-tissue swelling early in the course of infection and may help to suggest or exclude alternative diagnoses. Evidence of bone destruction and periosteal elevation are not typically seen until 10–14 days after the onset of symptoms.
- Bone scans are sensitive and are especially useful if the site of infection is poorly localized or if there is concern for multifocal osteomyelitis. However, they may be positive in other illnesses that cause osteoblastic activity.
- MRI is sensitive and offers superior anatomic resolution, making it a more useful modality for surgical planning and for identification of intraosseous, subperiosteal, and soft tissue abscesses.

Diagnostic Procedures/Other
- Biopsy or aspiration of the infected bone (or an associated abscess) for Gram stain and culture is useful for determining the etiologic organism. Inoculating a portion of an aspirated sample into a blood culture bottle enhances yield for *Kingella kingae*.
- If a plan is in place to rapidly obtain a bone culture in a clinically stable patient, it is reasonable to defer initiation of antibiotic therapy until after the culture specimen is secured.
- Biopsy may also help differentiate osteomyelitis from noninfectious bone pathology.

DIFFERENTIAL DIAGNOSIS
- Trauma
- Cellulitis
- Abscess
- Pyomyositis or fasciitis
- Septic arthritis
- Aseptic bone necrosis or bone infarction (sickle cell disease)
- Tumor (e.g., Ewing sarcoma, osteoid osteoma, eosinophilic granuloma)
- Acute leukemia, neuroblastoma with bone invasion
- Chronic recurrent multifocal osteomyelitis (CRMO)
- Inflammatory arthritis or juvenile idiopathic arthritis
- Transient synovitis

TREATMENT

MEDICATION (DRUGS)

- Empiric antibiotics should cover the most likely pathogens considering patient age, history of presentation, physical findings, and underlying medical conditions.
- Empiric therapy should always include an agent directed against *S. aureus*. In the past, oxacillin or nafcillin was the standard agent, but the increasing prevalence of MRSA has altered this approach. In areas where the rate of methicillin resistance among community *S. aureus* isolates exceeds 10%, an antibiotic effective against community-acquired MRSA should be selected (i.e., clindamycin or vancomycin).
- Clindamycin and vancomycin are also usually effective against *S. pneumoniae* and *S. pyogenes*, but are not effective in vitro against *K. kingae*.
- *Salmonella* spp. coverage is needed in patients with sickle cell disease.
- Gram-negative coverage should also be added to the empiric regimen for neonates.
- If the patient recently had a foot puncture wound, coverage for *P. aeruginosa* should be considered.
- If an organism is isolated and susceptibilities determined, antibiotic therapy should be modified based on the susceptibility profile.
- When clindamycin is considered for treatment of an identified MRSA isolate, the D-test (to exclude inducible macrolide, lincosamide, and streptogramin B resistance) should be performed by the clinical microbiology laboratory.

ADDITIONAL TREATMENT

General Measures

- Antibiotic therapy for 4–6 weeks is generally provided.
- Total treatment duration is individualized based on the extent of infection, the promptness and completeness of surgical débridement (when indicated), the rate of clinical response, the presence or absence of distant foci of infection, and the patient's underlying risk factors and comorbid conditions.
- If an intraosseous, subperiosteal, or soft tissue abscess is present, surgical débridement may be necessary in addition to antibiotic therapy.
- After an initial period of parenteral antibiotic administration, many patients can be transitioned to an oral regimen to complete therapy (assuming the availability of an oral antibiotic with an appropriate spectrum of activity and adequate bone penetration, as well as patient ability to adhere to and absorb an oral regimen). This sequential IV–oral approach reduces the risk of complications (e.g., catheter associated bloodstream infection, catheter malfunction, and thrombosis) associated with the prolonged presence of a central venous catheter.

 ONGOING CARE

FOLLOW-UP RECOMMENDATIONS

- Most children who receive appropriate treatment have no long-term sequelae.
- Inflammatory markers (ESR and CRP) are typically measured serially until they normalize during the course of antibiotic therapy.
- Patients should be followed to ensure medication compliance, adequacy of treatment, side effects of therapy, and continued growth of the involved extremity.

COMPLICATIONS

- Septic arthritis
- Recurrence or progression to chronic osteomyelitis in ~5% of patients
- Disturbances of bone growth, limb length discrepancy
- Arthritis
- Pathologic fractures

ADDITIONAL READING

- Gerber JS, Coffin SE, Smathers SA, et al. Trends in the incidence of methicillin-resistant *Staphylococcus aureus* infection in children's hospitals in the United States. *Clin Infect Dis*. 2009;49:65–71.
- Gutierrez K. Bone and joint infections in children. *Pediatr Clin N Am*. 2005;52:779–794.
- Harik NS, Smeltzer MS. Management of acute hematogenous osteomyelitis in children. *Expert Rev Anti Infect Ther*. 2010;8:175–181.
- Kaplan SL. Osteomyelitis in children. *Infect Dis Clin N Am*. 2005;19:787–797.
- Santiago Restrepo C, Gimenez CR, McCarthy K. Imaging of osteomyelitis and musculoskeletal soft tissue infections: Current concepts. *Rheum Dis Clin N Am*. 2003;29:89–109.
- Yagupsky P. *Kingella kingae*: From medical rarity to an emerging paediatric pathogen. *Lancet Infect Dis*. 2004;4:358–367.
- Zaoutis T, Localio AR, Leckerman K, et al. Prolonged intravenous therapy versus early transition to oral antimicrobial therapy for acute osteomyelitis in children. *Pediatrics*. 2009;123:636–642.

CODES

ICD9

- 730.20 Unspecified osteomyelitis, site unspecified
- 730.25 Unspecified osteomyelitis, pelvic region and thigh
- 730.26 Unspecified osteomyelitis, lower leg

ICD10

- M86.259 Subacute osteomyelitis, unspecified femur
- M86.659 Other chronic osteomyelitis, unspecified thigh
- M86.9 Osteomyelitis, unspecified

OTITIS EXTERNA

Lee R. Atkinson-McEvoy

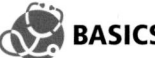 **BASICS**

DESCRIPTION
- Inflammation or infection of the external auditory canal and/or the auricle
- May be categorized as follows:
  - Acute: Also known as "swimmer's ear," usually an acute bacterial infection of the external auditory canal
  - Chronic: Persistent, low-grade infection and inflammation of the external ear
  - Atopic: Encompasses otitis externa due to atopic dermatitis, seborrheic dermatitis, psoriasis, and other inflammatory conditions
  - Fungal: Occurs more commonly in patients with diabetes mellitus or an immunodeficiency
  - Malignant or necrotizing: Severe otitis externa with invasive disease into the surrounding soft tissue, cartilage and bone; seen more commonly in patients with diabetes mellitus or immunodeficiency; may progress to invasive disease of the surrounding structures

EPIDEMIOLOGY
- Occurs more commonly in summer months
- 90% of cases are unilateral.
- Uncommon before 2 years of age

Incidence
1:100–250 annually in the general population

Prevalence
10% of the population is diagnosed with acute otitis externa at some point in their lives.

RISK FACTORS
- Increased environmental temperature
- High humidity
- Local trauma
- Exposure to water with high bacterial counts.

GENERAL PREVENTION
- Earplugs that prevent water from entering the ear canal should be used when swimming or participating in other water sports.
- Acetic acid drops (which can be made at home with 1 part vinegar to 2 parts rubbing alcohol) followed by wicking away moisture with cotton; can be used to restore the acidic pH of the ear canal and decrease moisture to prevent otitis externa after swimming.
- Discourage removal of cerumen with vigorous ear cleaning, especially by using cotton swabs in the ear. Remove impacted cerumen with cerumenolytics.
- Avoid known allergens.

PATHOPHYSIOLOGY
- Cerumen provides an acidic layer that prevents infection of the external auditory canal. Warm, humid air (i.e., in summer) can disrupt the integrity of cerumen.
- Trauma to the squamous epithelium of the external auditory canal or an increase in the pH of the external auditory canal increases the risk of inflammation and infection.

- Cleaning or removal of cerumen or introduction of water into the canal (i.e., from swimming, playing water sports) can lead to maceration of the canal and the onset of infection.
- Other factors such as sweating, allergy, stress, and alkaline eardrops have been implicated in disturbing the normal acidic pH of the external auditory canal, leading to infection.

ETIOLOGY
- Bacteria: Most commonly *Pseudomonas aeruginosa* 20–60% (particularly in malignant otitis externa) and *Staphylococcus aureus* 10% to 70%, *Staphylococcus epidermidis*. Other organisms make up ~2–3% of cases and usually are other staphylococcal species *Microbacterium* spp., *Streptococcus pyogenes*, *Streptococcus pneumoniae*, *Escherichia coli*, *Haemophilus influenzae*, *Klebsiella*, and other gram-negative bacteria.
- Fungal: More common in chronic otitis externa or acute otitis externa after treatment with topical antibiotics; *Candida albicans*, *Aspergillus niger*, *Aspergillus versicolor*
- Viral: Herpes simplex virus (acute infection and herpes zoster) and varicella

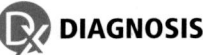 **DIAGNOSIS**

HISTORY
- Known risk factors:
  - Host: Excess wax leading to moisture retention, chronic skin conditions, immunocompromise
  - Environment: Excess moisture (i.e., swimming, high humidity), trauma, heat
- Hearing loss (associated with involvement of the tympanic membrane), pain that is worse with chewing or activities that result in motion of the ear, pruritus (associated with inflammation of the external auditory canal), and/or ear discharge
- Fever may suggest a more severe infection.
- Earrings or other ear jewelry:
  - Associated with atopic dermatitis as the etiology of the otitis externa
- Use of topical treatments for the ear or canal (including tattooing, permanent or nonpermanent), which is also associated with atopic dermatitis as the cause of the otitis externa
- Pain in jaw, particularly in temporomandibular joint area (referred pain).

PHYSICAL EXAM
- Rapid onset
- Pain with pressure applied to tragus and with traction on the pinna
- Canal appears macerated with erythema, purulent discharge, and/or edema.
- Look for the presence of foreign bodies, including pieces of cotton from cleaning with cotton swabs.
- Tympanic membrane should appear intact with normal landmarks. If not, there may be a concurrent otitis media.

- In cases of fungal infection, "mold" or black or white fungal hyphae with spores may be seen.
- In viral infections, vesicles may be present.
- In eczematous otitis externa, the skin is dry and flaky with crust. Excoriation may be visible as well.
- A somewhat fruity smell suggests infection due to *Pseudomonas*.

DIAGNOSTIC TESTS & INTERPRETATION
Diagnostic Procedures/Other
- In simple, uncomplicated otitis externa, testing is generally not indicated.
- If there is concern for concurrent acute otitis media, pneumatic otoscopy or tympanometry can be performed. These are normal in acute otitis externa, and show limited or absent mobility with pneumatic otoscopy or a flat tracing with tympanometry in acute otitis media.
- In more severe infections, recalcitrant infections, or immunocompromised patients, bacterial culture with Gram stain and fungal cultures should be obtained. *P. aeruginosa* is a frequent pathogen in malignant otitis externa
- Herpes has been described as an etiologic agent; therefore, direct fluorescence antibody (DFA) testing for herpes may be helpful. Viral cultures should be considered when there is a vesicular component to the otitis externa.

DIFFERENTIAL DIAGNOSIS
- Infectious:
  - Acute otitis media
  - Mastoiditis
  - Furunculosis
- Tumors:
  - Squamous cell carcinoma
  - Basal cell carcinoma
  - Acoustic neuroma
  - Other metastatic tumors
- Miscellaneous:
  - Foreign body
  - Cerumen impaction
  - Cholesteatoma
  - Atopic dermatitis

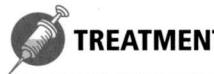 **TREATMENT**

MEDICATION (DRUGS)
- Topical antibiotics are the treatment of choice. They have been shown to be efficacious and to deliver a higher concentration of medication than can be achieved with systemic therapy.
- Ototopical drops should be placed with the patient lying down with the affected ear up. Drops should fill the canal. Gentle tugging on the pinna allows expulsion of ear and introduction of the drops. The patient should remain in this position for 5 minutes.
- In cases of severe canal edema, clinicians may place a wick, made of compressed cellulose that expands, or ribbon gauze to assist in medication delivery.
- Acetic acid drops are available, with similar efficacy to other antibiotic drops. These are least expensive.

- Polymyxin B, neomycin, and hydrocortisone combination otic solution or suspension can be used to treat a simple infection.
- In some cases, the neomycin component may cause allergy, leading to exacerbation of the otitis externa. If there is a suspected perforation of the tympanic membrane, neomycin is an ototoxic medication and should not be used.
- Fluoroquinolones, such as ofloxacin and ciprofloxacin (available only as a combination with hydrocortisone), have also shown high cure rates.
- Antibiotic–steroid combination drugs have not been shown to have greater clinical or bacteriologic cure than antibiotics alone. However, newer studies suggest that they result in rapid treatment response and symptom resolution.
- Topical ophthalmic antimicrobial/steroid drops, such as Cortisporin ophthalmic solution, may be tolerated better if there is severe maceration of the canal, since they are less acidic.

ADDITIONAL TREATMENT
General Measures
- Hydrogen peroxide or 3% hypertonic saline may be used to clean the ear:
  – Use a cotton swab to dry the canal after cleansing.
- Pain management is an important factor. Pain can usually be managed with mild analgesics, such as acetaminophen or NSAIDs. Benzocaine otic solution with or without antipyrine has not been evaluated for efficacy in clinical trials in acute otitis externa. This type of solution can mask progression of the disease and lead to a contact dermatitis.
- If there is significant edema of the canal, using ophthalmic drops (which tend to be less viscous than otic drops) in combination with a wick to facilitate introduction of medication into the ear canal may be useful. However, if there is concern about a concomitant acute otitis media with perforation, caution must be used with the introduction of any topical treatment to the external auditory canal.
- Specific therapies, depending on the presentation:
  – Remove foreign body if present.
  – For acute localized otitis externa with abscess, incision and drainage of the abscess in combination with antistaphylococcal penicillins or 1st-generation cephalosporins
  – For fungal otitis externa, antifungal drops such as clotrimazole 1% solution are used.
  – For atopic otitis externa, management of the underlying dermatologic condition is appropriate, along with the topical application of corticosteroid to the affected parts of the ear. Skin testing for specific allergies should be considered if atopic otitis externa is severe or recalcitrant.
  – For cellulitis, lymphadenitis, or otitis media, oral antimicrobials are used.
  – When pseudomonal infection is suspected, an antipseudomonal agent, such as a 3rd-generation cephalosporin (e.g., ceftriaxone sodium) or a fluoroquinolone (ofloxacin) should be used.

Additional Therapies
- No data are available regarding efficacy of these therapies.
- Isopropyl alcohol alone, isopropyl alcohol with equal part 5% acetic acid (white vinegar), and 5% acetic acid with an equal part water are common home remedies.
- Tea tree oil is effective in vitro against many bacteria associated with acute otitis externa, but *Pseudomonas* is commonly resistant to this and no controlled efficacy trials have been described.
- Ear candles should not be used to treat acute otitis externa; they have not been shown to be efficacious but they have been shown to cause ear obstruction from the wax, tympanic membrane perforation, and hearing loss.

ISSUES FOR REFERRAL
- Ear, nose, and throat specialist (ENT) referral when indicated:
  – Malignant otitis media (often caused by *P. aeruginosa* and found in immunocompromised individuals) and/or mastoiditis
  – Cases of chronic otitis externa with failure of long-term medical therapy: Refer for débridement and further evaluation.

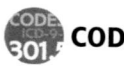 ## ONGOING CARE

FOLLOW-UP RECOMMENDATIONS
- Re-evaluate if there is no symptomatic improvement 24–48 hours after starting treatment.
- Fever or progression of symptoms in spite of treatment warrants more aggressive or broader therapy.
- Immunocompromised patients, including those with diabetes mellitus, should be followed closely depending on severity, to ensure improvement.

PROGNOSIS
Very good, with rapid response to treatment

COMPLICATIONS
- Cellulitis of adjacent tissues (facial or auricular), including facial nerve paralysis, mastoiditis, and osteomyelitis of the skull base.
- Lymphadenitis of upper neck or parotid lymph nodes
- Acute otitis media and rarely mastoiditis
- Facial nerve neuritis
- Canal stenosis (usually in chronic otitis externa that results in hypertrophy of the canal walls)
- Hearing loss, if there is significant edema of the canal walls

ADDITIONAL READING
- Bellez WG, Kalman S. Otolaryngologic emergencies in the outpatient setting. *Med Clin North Amer.* 2006;90:329–353.
- Dohar JE. Evolution of management approaches for otitis externa. *Pediatr Infect Dis J.* 2003;22: 299–308.
- Kaushik V, Malik T, Saeed SR. Interventions for Acute Otitis Externa. *Cochrane Database Syst Rev.* 2010;1:CD004740. DOI: 10.1002/14651858. CD004740.pub2
- Sander R. Otitis externa: A practical guide to treatment and prevention. *Am Fam Phys.* 2001;63:927–936.
- Stone KE. Otitis externa. *Pediatr Rev.* 2007;28(2): 77–78.

CODES

ICD9
- 380.10 Otitis externa
- 380.22 Other acute otitis externa
- 380.23 Other chronic otitis externa

ICD10
- H60.90 Unspecified otitis externa, unspecified ear
- H60.91 Unspecified otitis externa, right ear
- H60.92 Unspecified otitis externa, left ear

FAQ

- Q: How should I clean my child's ear?
- A: Only the external tragus, pinna, and visible parts of the ear should be cleaned with a cotton ball or washcloth. No foreign object should be placed in the canal. Ear cerumen is a normal protective substance to maintain protection of the fragile tympanic membrane. If impaction is suspected, use a cerumen-loosening agent such as carbamide peroxide. Although there is still common use of ear candles (small narrow candles that are placed at the opening of the external auditory canal and then lit with the goal of the heat causing the cerumen to loosen and exit the ear), this method has not been shown to remove significant impacted cerumen and can leave candle wax in the ear canal.
- Q: When can my child return to swimming after an episode of otitis externa?
- A: After completion of the prescribed therapy, your child may resume water sports. He or she should use waterproof earplugs and acetic acid drops to prevent another infection.
- Q: When should otitis externa be referred to an otolaryngologist?
- A: In refractory cases, chronic otitis externa, or persistent hearing loss after treatment, and when there are severe complications (e.g., malignant otitis externa, mastoiditis).

OTITIS MEDIA

William R. Graessle

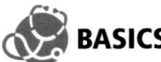 BASICS

DESCRIPTION
Otitis media refers to inflammation of the middle ear. A distinction is usually made between otitis media with effusion (OME) and acute otitis media (AOM). AOM implies that infection is present.

EPIDEMIOLOGY
- More common in fall and winter, and less common in spring and summer
- Inverse relationship with breastfeeding duration

Incidence
Increased incidence in those <2 years of age, with the peak incidence between 6–12 months of age

RISK FACTORS
- Exposure to environmental tobacco smoke is an independent risk factor.
- Risk is increased with exposure to large numbers of children (e.g., child care). Additive factors include number of hours spent in child care, younger age at child care entry, and type of child care setting (center vs. family child care).

GENERAL PREVENTION
- Breastfeeding decreases the risk of acute otitis media.
- Preventing exposure to environmental tobacco smoke can decrease the risk of otitis media.
- Decreasing exposure to multiple respiratory pathogens by delaying entrance to group child care or choosing settings with fewer numbers of children may be helpful.
- Vaccines: In addition to preventing invasive disease, conjugated pneumococcal vaccine significantly reduces the risk of AOM.

PATHOPHYSIOLOGY
- Dysfunction of the eustachian tube is the most important factor:
  - The eustachian tube in younger children is shorter, more compliant, and more horizontal than in older children and adults.
  - Children with craniofacial anomalies have an increased risk of eustachian tube dysfunction and subsequent otitis media.
- Viral upper respiratory tract infection often precedes or coincides with AOM. Viral infections may lead to development of AOM by several mechanisms:
  - Inducing inflammation in the nasopharynx and eustachian tube
  - Enhancing nasopharyngeal bacterial colonization
- Impairing host immune system and increasing susceptibility to secondary bacterial infection

ETIOLOGY
- *Streptococcus pneumoniae*: Up to 40%
- Nontypeable *Haemophilus influenzae*: 25–30%
- *Moraxella catarrhalis*: 10–20%
- Other organisms include group A streptococcus, *Staphylococcus aureus*, and gram-negative organisms, such as *Pseudomonas* species. Respiratory viruses are often noted as part of AOM, but are the sole pathogen in <10% of cases.

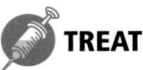 DIAGNOSIS

HISTORY
- History of current episode with presence of ear pain, fever, and associated symptoms
- Past medical history, including underlying disorders (e.g., cleft palate, Down syndrome), immune deficiency, and previous history of otitis media
- Recent treatment with antibiotics
- Exposure to large numbers of children (school, child care, large family)
- Ear pain
- Fever
- Irritability

PHYSICAL EXAM
- Look for other causes of fever and irritability in children: Upper respiratory tract infections, pharyngitis, lymphadenitis, meningitis, urinary tract infection (UTI), and bone and joint infections.
- Physical exam of the ear is best done with pneumatic otoscopy:
  - The patient should be adequately restrained if uncooperative.
  - Cerumen in the canal should be removed if view of the tympanic membrane is inadequate.
  - The tympanic membrane is visualized at rest, and with gentle positive and negative pressure via pneumatic otoscopy.
- The presence of a middle ear effusion is determined by the characteristics of the tympanic membrane:
  - Contour: Normal, retracted, full, or bulging; associated bulla(e)
  - Color: Gray, pink, yellow, white, or red; hemorrhagic
  - Translucency: Translucent or opaque
  - Mobility: Normal, decreased, or absent
- The presence of a middle ear effusion is suggested by abnormal color, opacification, decreased mobility, air–fluid levels, or visible air bubbles within fluid.
- A diagnosis of AOM is suggested if a middle ear effusion is present along with ear pain, fever, erythema, fullness, or bulging of tympanic membrane.
- The concomitant presence of conjunctivitis (otitis media–conjunctivitis syndrome) suggests the presence of *H. influenzae* or a virus as a causative organism.

DIAGNOSTIC TESTS & INTERPRETATION
Diagnostic Procedures/Other
- Tympanometry:
  - Easily performed by office personnel
  - Provides information on middle ear pressure and tympanic membrane compliance
  - Sensitive in detecting middle ear effusion, but poor positive predictive value
- Tympanocentesis:
  - For episodes of AOM that are resistant to antibiotic therapy, tympanocentesis and culture and sensitivity of the middle ear fluid may help guide antibiotic therapy.
- Tympanocentesis or myringotomy may also be required as part of the treatment of suppurative complications.

DIFFERENTIAL DIAGNOSIS
- OME: Tympanic membrane may appear dull with a diffuse light reflex, fluid bubbles may be visible, and mobility may be decreased.
- Otitis externa
- Auricular lesions like a furuncle or laceration
- Other causes of fever, including viral upper respiratory tract infections, pharyngitis, pneumonia, meningitis, UTIs, and bone and joint infections
- Pharyngitis and dental pain may be mistaken for otalgia.

TREATMENT

MEDICATION (DRUGS)
Note: Because as many as 80% of patients who have physical findings consistent with the diagnosis of AOM may recover without treatment, some experts recommend treating pain and fever 48–72 hours before starting antibiotics, especially in older patients. For patients <2 years of age, antibiotic treatment results in faster resolution than placebo and is recommended as initial therapy.

First Line
- Amoxicillin (80–90 mg/kg/d b.i.d.) is the drug of choice for most episodes of AOM. The higher doses are recommended to cover resistant *S. pneumoniae*.
- Recommended duration of therapy is 10 days, but a 5–7-day course, as well as lower dosing of amoxicillin (25–50 mg/kg/d divided b.i.d. or t.i.d.) may be considered for uncomplicated and isolated cases of AOM in children >2 years.
- Azithromycin may be used in patients who are allergic to penicillin (type I hypersensitivity). For patients who do not have type I reactions, a cephalosporin may be used. Clindamycin 30–40 mg/d divided into 3 doses is an alternative for the penicillin-allergic patient.

Second Line
- Failure of antibiotic therapy may be related to bacterial resistance or a viral etiology. The choice of a 2nd-line antibiotic depends on suspected mechanism of resistance. *H. influenzae* and *M. catarrhalis* produce β-lactamase. *S. pneumoniae* alters penicillin-binding proteins. Failure caused by a resistant pathogen is more likely due to *S. pneumoniae* than *H. influenzae* or *M. catarrhalis*.
- Amoxicillin–clavulanate (80–90 mg/kg/d of the amoxicillin component b.i.d.) is recommended for most treatment failures.
- Cefdinir, cefuroxime axetil, and IM ceftriaxone are also effective against resistant strains of bacteria.
- Amoxicillin–clavulanate or a second-generation cephalosporin may be used if *H. influenzae* (i.e., otitis media–conjunctivitis syndrome) or *M. catarrhalis* is suspected.
- The macrolides and trimethoprim–sulfa do not provide reliable coverage for resistant *S. pneumoniae*.

- Clindamycin 30–40 mg/d t.i.d. is effective against resistant pneumococci and is an alternative for penicillin-allergic patients.
- IM ceftriaxone:
  – Not recommended for routine treatment of AOM.
  – May be considered when PO therapy is impossible or when appropriate 1st- and 2nd-line therapies for *S. pneumoniae* have failed.
  – When used for treatment of resistant organisms, ceftriaxone 50 mg/kg IM should be given every 1–3 days for 3 doses.

ADDITIONAL TREATMENT
General Measures
- Antibiotics (see "Medication")
- Adjunctive therapy:
  – Fever relief may be provided with acetaminophen or other antipyretic.
  – Pain may be treated with acetaminophen, ibuprofen, or topical anesthetic drops.

ISSUES FOR REFERRAL
- Consider otolaryngology referral:
  – Persistent otitis media not responding to antibiotic therapy; tympanocentesis with culture of middle ear fluid may be helpful.
  – Recurrent acute otitis media with >4 episodes during a respiratory season, especially if earlier in the season
  – Persistent and/or recurrent otitis with abnormal hearing and/or speech

ONGOING CARE

FOLLOW-UP RECOMMENDATIONS
- Expect symptomatic improvement within 48–72 hours of treatment. May need to switch antibiotic therapy and/or re-evaluate for complications.
- Tympanic membrane may appear abnormal for some time after treatment. In infants or young children, initial follow-up exam should be scheduled 3–4 weeks after completion of antibiotic therapy. If effusion is present, follow monthly. For persistent effusions of >3 months' duration, a hearing evaluation is recommended.

PROGNOSIS
- Symptoms of acute infection (fever and otalgia) are relieved within 48–72 hours in most patients.
- Treatment failures are more likely with increased severity of disease and younger age.
- Development of another infection within 30 days usually represents a recurrence caused by a different organism, rather than a relapse.
- Recurrences are frequent and more common in younger children and if initial episode is severe.
- 30–70% of treated children will have an effusion at 2 weeks.
- Middle ear effusion may persist for weeks to months.

COMPLICATIONS
- Suppurative complications of AOM are much less common with current antibiotic therapy. The recent increase in resistant organisms could lead to a resurgence of suppurative complications.
- Hearing loss:
  – Acute conductive hearing loss is common and usually resolves as the effusion resolves.
  – Fluid of longstanding duration may lead to permanent conductive hearing loss.
  – Sensory-neural hearing loss may result from spread of infection into the labyrinth.
- Tympanic membrane perforation
- Chronic suppurative otitis media
- Tympanosclerosis
- Cholesteatoma
- Acute mastoiditis
- Petrositis
- Labyrinthitis
- Facial nerve paralysis
- Bacterial meningitis
- Epidural abscess
- Subdural empyema
- Brain abscess
- Lateral sinus thrombosis

ADDITIONAL READING

- AAP Subcommittee on Management of Acute Otitis Media. Clinical practice guideline. Diagnosis and management of acute otitis media. *Pediatrics*. 2004;113:1451–1465.
- Coker TR, Chan LS, Newberry SJ, et al. Diagnosis, microbial epidemiology, and antibiotic treatment of acute otitis media in children. *JAMA*. 2010: 2161–2169.
- Gould JM, Matz PS. Otitis media. *Pediatr Rev*. 2010;31:102–116.
- Hoberman A, Paradise JL, Rockette HE, et al. Treatment of acute otitis media in children under 2 years of age. *N Engl J Med*. 2011;364:105–115.
- Spiro DM, Tay KY, Arnold DH, et al. Wait-and-see prescription for the treatment of acute otitis media. *JAMA*. 2006;296:1235–1241.
- Takata GS, Chan LS, Morphew T, et al. Evidence assessment of the accuracy of methods of diagnosing middle ear effusion in children with otitis media with effusion. *Pediatrics*. 2003;112(pt 1): 1379–1387.

CODES

ICD9
- 381.00 Acute nonsuppurative otitis media, unspecified
- 381.4 Nonsuppurative otitis media, not specified as acute or chronic
- 382.9 Unspecified otitis media

ICD10
- H66.90 Otitis media, unspecified, unspecified ear
- H66.91 Otitis media, unspecified. right ear
- H66.92 Otitis media, unspecified, left ear

FAQ
- Q: When should children with acute otitis media be treated?
- A: The presence of a middle ear effusion may occur commonly with an upper respiratory tract infection. The presence of AOM, as described above, usually warrants treatment with antibiotics, especially in children <2 years, those who are prone to infection, and those with AOM during the winter season. Because a number of cases of acute otitis media resolve spontaneously in older children, treatment with antibiotics may be deferred for 48–72 hours while treating pain.
- Q: What is the antibiotic of choice for initial therapy of acute otitis media?
- A: Amoxicillin, 80–90 mg/kg/d, is recommended as initial therapy for most children. *S. pneumoniae* is currently the most important pathogen causing acute otitis media, being more common and more virulent than other bacteria isolated from middle ear fluid. Increased resistance of *S. pneumoniae* to lower doses of amoxicillin necessitate use of higher doses. Initial therapy with amoxicillin–clavulanate at 80–90 mg/kg of amoxicillin may be considered as initial therapy for patients recently treated with amoxicillin (i.e., within the past month) and for patients with more severe disease, including those with fever >39°C and/or those with severe otalgia.
- Q: What can be done to prevent the development of AOM in an individual child?
- A: A number of factors appear to put children at risk for AOM, including genetic, immune, and environmental factors and exposure to viral upper respiratory tract infections. Breastfeeding during the 1st year of life decreases the risk of AOM and is recommended. Eliminating exposure to environmental tobacco smoke may also be helpful. Development of upper respiratory tract infections at an early age is probably the most important factor in the development of otitis media. Limiting the exposure to large numbers of children by delayed entry to child care or by choosing a setting with smaller numbers of children should decrease a child's risk of otitis media. Pneumococcal vaccine has reduced the incidence of AOM. Administering influenza vaccine may also be helpful.

PALLOR
David T. Teachey

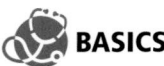 **BASICS**

DEFINITION
- Pallor is defined as paleness of the skin and may be a reflection of anemia or poor peripheral perfusion.
- The normal range for hemoglobin is age dependent.
- Anemia can be defined functionally as the inability of hemoglobin to meet cellular oxygen demand.
- Parents often fail to notice pallor of gradual onset.
  – Grandparents or others who see child less often may be the first to suspect pallor.

RISK FACTORS
- Age between 6 months and 3 years, or adolescent females:
  – Peak age ranges for iron deficiency
- Gender:
  – Some red cell–enzyme X-linked defects, such as glucose-6-phosphate dehydrogenase (G6PD) and phosphoglycerate kinase deficiencies are sex linked.
- Race:
  – Black: Hemoglobins S and C, - and -thalassemia trait, G6PD deficiency
  – Southeast Asian: Hemoglobin E and -thalassemia
  – Mediterranean descent: -thalassemia and G6PD deficiency

Genetics
Familial history:
- Some of the congenital hemolytic anemias are autosomal dominant.

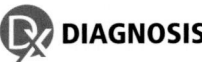 **DIAGNOSIS**

- Determine first that the child appears pale, not simply fair skinned. Second, decide if there is a medical emergency associated with circulatory failure. If not, the goal is to investigate the etiology and intervene appropriately.
- Phase 1: Assess for signs of shock.
  – If present, initiate emergency procedures as required to stabilize the patient, such as airway, breathing, and circulation.
- Phase 2: If patient is stable, perform history, physical examination, and CBC with reticulocyte count to establish time of onset of pallor, associated symptoms, and level of anemia.
- Phase 3: Follow specific diagnostic workup based on findings in phase 2.

SIGNS AND SYMPTOMS
- Pallor
- Other signs and symptoms dependent on etiology

HISTORY
- Acute versus chronic onset:
  – Helps with differential diagnosis.
- Associated symptoms: Weight loss, fever, night sweats, cough, and/or bone pain:
  – Suggest an underlying systemic illness, such as leukemia, infection, or rheumatologic disorder
- Jaundice, scleral icterus, dark urine:
  – Suggest hemolysis
- Age <6 months:
  – May represent a congenital anemia or isoimmunization
- Premature infant:
  – Increased risk of both iron and vitamin E deficiency.
  – Exaggerated hyperbilirubinemia can be the presenting symptom of isoimmune hemolytic or other congenital hemolytic anemia.
- Pica:
  – Often associated with plumbism and iron deficiency
- Medications:
  – Can cause bone marrow suppression and/or hemolysis
- Milk intake:
  – Cow's milk <12 months of age and high milk intake are associated with iron deficiency.
- Recent trauma and/or surgery:
  – Blood loss can result in iron deficiency.
- Recent infection:
  – Can be associated with hemolysis or bone marrow suppression
  – Most common form of mild anemia in childhood
- Family history:
  – Familial history of splenectomy and/or early cholecystectomy can be a clue for a previously undiagnosed hemolytic anemia.

PHYSICAL EXAM
- Rapid respiratory rate, decreased BP, weak pulses, slow capillary refill
  – Indications of uncompensated anemia and/or shock
- Frontal bossing and prominence of the malar and maxillary bones:
  – Extramedullary erythropoiesis
- Enlarged spleen:
  – Hemolytic anemias, malignancy, infection
- Glossitis:
  – Vitamin B$_{12}$ deficiency
- Scleral icterus or jaundice:
  – May indicate hemolysis
- Systolic flow murmur:
  – Anemia

- Bruits:
  – May indicate vascular malformations
- Petechiae and bruising:
  – May indicate an associated thrombocytopenia, coagulopathy, or vasculitis
- Dysmorphic features:
  – Diamond-Blackfan and Fanconi anemia are associated with other congenital defects, including thumb abnormalities, short stature, and congenital heart disease.

DIAGNOSTIC TESTS & INTERPRETATION
Lab
- CBC with red cell indices:
  – Establishes the diagnosis of anemia, distinguishes by size: Normocytic, macrocytic, microcytic
- Reticulocyte count:
  – Distinguishes between decreased production and increased destruction of red cells
- Coombs test and antibody screen:
  – Identifies immune-mediated red cell destruction
  – Can have false positives and negatives
- Peripheral blood smear:
  – Specific morphologic findings can be diagnostic.
- Iron studies: Iron-binding capacity, serum iron, ferritin, transferrin
  – Iron-deficiency anemia or anemia of chronic disease
- Hemoglobin electrophoresis with quantification:
  – Hemoglobinopathy
- Lead studies: Serum lead, free erythrocyte protoporphyrin:
  – Plumbism
- Stool guaiac:
  – Occult blood loss
- Osmotic fragility:
  – Red cell membrane defects (spherocytosis)
  – Any spherocytic anemia may be positive
- Quantitative red cell–enzyme assays:
  – Inherited RBC enzyme deficiencies
- Serum folate, RBC folate, and serum vitamin B$_{12}$ levels:
  – Deficiency

Diagnostic Procedures/Surgery
Bone marrow aspiration and biopsy:
- Malignancy or bone marrow failure syndrome

DIFFERENTIAL DIAGNOSIS
- Congenital:
  – Hemoglobinopathies: Sickle cell syndromes, thalassemia syndromes, other unstable hemoglobins
  – Erythrocyte membrane defects: Hereditary spherocytosis, elliptocytosis, stomatocytosis, pyropoikilocytosis, infantile pyknocytosis
  – Erythrocyte enzyme defects: G6PD deficiency, pyruvate kinase deficiency
  – Diamond–Blackfan anemia: Congenital pure red cell aplasia (rare)
  – Fanconi anemia: Constellation of varied cytopenias, multiple congenital anomalies, abnormal bone marrow chromosomal fragility

- Infectious:
  - Septic shock
  - Can get mild anemia after mild infections in childhood (anemia of inflammation)
  - Infection-related bone marrow suppression: Parvovirus B19 infection
  - Infection-related hemolytic anemias: Epstein-Barr virus, influenza, Coxsackievirus, varicella, cytomegalovirus, *Escherichia coli*, *Pneumococcus* species, *Streptococcus* species, *Salmonella typhi*, *Mycoplasma* species
- Nutritional/toxic/drugs:
  - Iron-deficiency anemia: Common cause of anemia in children, especially those <3 years of age and in female adolescents
  - Plumbism: Anemia usually due to coexisting iron deficiency. Very high lead levels associated with altered heme synthesis
  - Vitamin B$_{12}$ and/or folate deficiency: Results in a megaloblastic anemia
  - Medication-induced bone marrow suppression: Chemotherapy; antibiotics, especially trimethoprim–sulfamethoxazole
  - Drug-related hemolytic anemia: Antibiotics, antiepileptics, azathioprine, isoniazid, nonsteroidal anti-inflammatory drugs
- Trauma:
  - Acute blood loss
- Tumor:
  - Leukemia with bone marrow infiltration
  - Metastatic tumors with bone marrow infiltration
- Genetic/metabolic:
  - Metabolic derangements: Severe electrolyte disturbance, pH disturbance, inborn errors
  - Schwachmann–Diamond syndrome: Marrow hypoplasia with associated pancreatic insufficiency and associated failure to thrive
- Other:
  - Transient erythroblastopenia of childhood: Acquired pure RBC aplasia
  - Aplastic anemia: Bone marrow failure syndrome with at least 2 of the 3 blood cell lines eventually affected
  - Systemic diseases: Anemia of chronic disease, chronic renal disease, uremia
  - Hypothyroidism
  - Sideroblastic anemia: Defective iron utilization within the developing erythrocytes
  - Autoimmune and isoimmune hemolytic anemias
  - Microangiopathic hemolytic anemias: Thrombotic thrombocytopenic purpura (TTP), hemolytic uremic syndrome (HUS), disseminated intravascular coagulation (DIC)
  - Mechanical destruction: Vascular malformation, abnormal or prosthetic cardiac valves

 TREATMENT

ADDITIONAL TREATMENT
Initial Stabilization
- Severe anemia of unclear etiology with hemodynamic instability:
  - Transfuse with packed RBCs cautiously.
  - In an autoimmune hemolytic process, the child is at risk for a transfusion reaction and there may be delay in obtaining crossmatched blood
  - Obtain blood for diagnostic studies before transfusion if possible.
- Circulatory failure without anemia:
  - Requires intensive monitoring and access to critical care in an emergency department or intensive care unit
  - Fluid resuscitation and/or inotropic pressor support as needed
- Acute blood loss:
  - Treat circulatory failure as described.
  - Transfuse with packed RBCs, platelets, and fresh frozen plasma as needed.
- Malignancies:
  - Emergency care should be directed toward treatment of circulatory failure and possible associated infection, and then to rapid diagnosis and treatment of the malignancy.
  - Consultation with an oncologist should be sought as soon as possible.

General Measures
- Treat underlying cause.
- Consider packed RBC transfusion if in extremis or severe anemia and low likelihood of recovery in near future.
- Consider emergent plasmapheresis if microangiopathic hemolytic anemia.
- Consider immunosuppresive medications (corticosteroids, intravenous immunoglobulin (IVIgG) if autoimmune hemolytic anemia.
- Iron-deficiency anemia:
  - Elemental iron

MEDICATION (DRUGS)
Elemental iron:
- 4–6 mg/kg divided b.i.d.–t.i.d.
- Absorbed best with acidic drinks, including orange juice; dairy products decrease absorption.
- Reticulocyte should improve 72 hours after starting iron therapy; the hemoglobin may take a week to rise.
- Iron should be continued for at least 3 months to replenish iron stores.

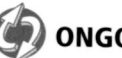 **ONGOING CARE**

ISSUES FOR REFERRAL
- Severe or unexplained anemia
- Anemias other than dietary iron deficiency or thalassemia trait
- Recurrent iron deficiency
  - May suggest ongoing bleeding or iron malabsorption.
- All bone marrow failure or infiltrative processes

ADDITIONAL READING

- Baker RD, Greer FR. Diagnosis and prevention of iron deficiency and iron-deficiency anemia in infants and young children (0-3 years of age). *Pediatrics.* 2010;126:1040–1050.
- Glader BE. Hemolytic anemia in children. *Clin Lab Med.* 1999;19:87–111.
- Graham EA. The changing face of anemia in infancy. *Pediatr Rev.* 1995;15:175–183.
- Monzon CM, Beaver D, Dillon TD. Evaluation of erythrocyte disorders with mean corpuscular volume (MCV) and red cell distribution width (RDW). *Clin Pediatr.* 1987;26:632–638.
- Segal G, Hirsh M, Feig S. Managing anemia in pediatric office practice, 1. *Pediatr Rev.* 2002;23; 75–84.
- Sills RH. Indications for bone marrow examination. *Pediatr Rev.* 1995;16:226–228.

 CODES

ICD9
782.61 Pallor

ICD10
R23.1 Pallor

PANCREATIC PSEUDOCYST

Raman Sreedharan
Devendra I. Mehta

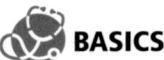 **BASICS**

DESCRIPTION

- Localized intrapancreatic or peripancreatic fluid collection that is rich in pancreatic enzymes but devoid of significant solid debris, enclosed by a wall of nonepithelialized granulation tissue
- Arises as a complication of acute or chronic pancreatitis

PATHOPHYSIOLOGY

- Pancreatic pseudocysts develop shortly after an attack of acute pancreatitis or insidiously in chronic pancreatitis.
- Disruption in the pancreatic ductular system results in the extravasation of pancreatic enzymes evoking an inflammatory response.
- The inflammatory reaction leads to a fluid collection that is rich in pancreatic enzymes and is termed *acute pancreatic fluid collection* (PFC).
- If the duration of the fluid collection is >4 weeks, becomes localized (intrapancreatic or extrapancreatic), and develops a fibrin capsule, it is called as a *pseudopancreatic cyst*.
- The pseudocyst does not have a true epithelial lining.
- If there is communication between the pseudocyst and the pancreatic duct, the enzyme level in the fluid remain elevated, and if there is no communication, the enzyme level falls with time.

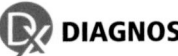 **DIAGNOSIS**

HISTORY

Acute or chronic pancreatitis: Suspect pancreatic pseudocyst in patients recovering from acute pancreatitis or in the patient with chronic pancreatitis who has recurrent/persistent abdominal pain, a palpable abdominal mass, or persistently elevated pancreatic enzymes in blood.

PHYSICAL EXAM

- Abdominal pain
- Abdominal mass
- Abdominal tenderness
- Nausea and vomiting
- Weight loss
- Jaundice
- Abdominal distention:
  - Mass/Ascites
- In many situations, no clinical signs are seen.
- Clinical signs may be secondary to complications:
  - Jaundice in hepatobiliary obstruction
  - Lower limb edema in compression of inferior vena cava
  - Ascites in peritonitis
  - Pleural effusion

DIAGNOSTIC TESTS & INTERPRETATION
Lab
Pancreatic enzyme levels:

- Persistently elevated enzymes in blood could be a clue, but is not an absolute indicator.
- The fluid drained from a pancreatic pseudocyst has high levels of amylase.

Imaging

- CT scan:
  - Reveals pseudopancreatic cyst and gauges size and relationship to adjacent organs
- Ultrasonography:
  - Visualizes pancreatic pseudocysts
  - Follow-up of cyst size
- Endoscopic ultrasonography:
  - Common modality in adult patients and increasingly used in pediatrics
- Endoscopic retrograde cholangiopancreatography (ERCP):
  - Used in some cases to delineate the pancreatic ductular system before drainage to distinguish ductal stenosis, stones, and other obstructions

DIFFERENTIAL DIAGNOSIS

- Congenital/Genetic:
  - Congenital cysts
  - Polycystic disease
  - Von Hippel-Lindau disease
  - Cystic fibrosis
- Infections:
  - Pancreatic abscess
  - Echinococcal (hydatid) cyst
  - Taenia solium cyst
- Tumor:
  - Serous cystadenoma
  - Mucinous cystadenoma
  - Cystic islet cell tumors
  - Teratoma
  - Pancreatoblastoma
  - Cystadenocarcinoma
  - Franz tumor
  - Angiomatous cystic neoplasms
  - Lymphangiomas
  - Hemangioendothelioma
- Miscellaneous:
  - Splenic cyst
  - Adrenal cyst
  - Enterogenous cyst
  - Duplication cysts
  - Endometriosis

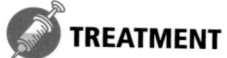
TREATMENT

ADDITIONAL TREATMENT
General Measures
- Medical management:
  - Most cases resolve with supportive care. If eating precipitates pain, short-term nasojejunal feedings or parenteral nutrition is warranted.
  - Follow-up with ultrasound or CT scan to make sure there are no complications.
  - >60% have complete resolution by the end of 1 year.
  - Usually no medications are used for managing pseudocysts. Somatostatin analogue (octreotide) has been reported to be used to decrease fluid collection along with drainage.
  - Antibiotics are used in situations of infected pseudocyst.
- Drainage:
  - Indications: Infection, rupture with cardiopulmonary compromise, biliary and gastric outlet obstruction, persistent symptoms, rapid enlargement, failure of large pseudocysts (>6 cm) to shrink after 6 weeks
  - Modalities:
    ○ Percutaneous drainage (aspiration or catheter drainage) is done in cases in which the pseudocyst has a less mature wall.
    ○ Percutaneous aspiration has a high recurrence rate of 63% and failure rate of 54%.
    ○ Continuous drainage has a recurrence rate of 8% and a failure rate of 19%.
    ○ Endoscopic procedures are becoming the 1st-line drainage modality, as they are less invasive than surgery.
    ○ Endoscopic procedures include transmural cystoenterostomies and transpapillary route procedures like stent placement for pseudocysts that communicate with the main pancreatic duct.
    ○ Endoscopic procedures in experienced hands report success rates of 82–89%, complication rates of 10–20%, and recurrence rates of 6–18%.

SURGERY/OTHER PROCEDURES
- Reserved for failed endoscopic procedures, complicated pseudocysts, and multiple pseudocysts
- Includes internal drainage (cystogastrostomy, cystoduodenostomy, and Roux-en-Y cystojejunostomy), resection, and external drainage
- Success rate is 85–90%.
- Recurrence rate is 0–17%.
- Mortality rate is between 3% and 5%.

ONGOING CARE

PROGNOSIS
Majority of pseudocysts resolve without intervention.

COMPLICATIONS
- Perforation/Rupture:
  - Cardiopulmonary compromise secondary to pleural effusion and ascites
  - Peritonitis and ascites, which can be fatal
- Hemorrhage:
  - Erosions of vessels lining the cyst cause intracystic bleeding and rapid increase in the cyst size.
  - Bleeding may occur directly into stomach, duodenum (clinically manifesting as GI bleeding), or peritoneal cavity.
- Obstruction:
  - Biliary obstruction: Jaundice
  - Portal obstruction: Portal hypertension
  - Gastric outlet obstruction
  - Inferior vena cava obstruction: Peripheral edema
  - Urinary obstruction
  - Colonic obstruction
- Infection is rare in children compared to adults:
  - High mortality rate for children and adults
  - Management usually requires surgical drainage.

ADDITIONAL READING

- Law NM, Freeman ML. Emergency complications of acute and chronic pancreatitis. *Gastroenterol Clin.* 2002;32:1169–1194.
- Reber HA. Surgery for acute and chronic pancreatitis. *Gastrointest Endosc.* 2002;56(Suppl):S246–S248.
- Vidyarthi G, Steinberg SE. Endoscopic management of pancreatic pseudocysts. *Surg Clin North Am.* 2001;81:405–410.
- Weckman L, Kylanpaa ML, Halttunen J. Endoscopic treatment of pancreatic pseudocysts. *Surg Endosc.* 2006;20(4):603–607.

CODES

ICD9
577.2 Cyst and pseudocyst of pancreas

ICD10
K86.3 Pseudocyst of pancreas

FAQ
- Q: How often does acute pancreatitis lead to pseudocyst formation?
- A: ~10% of cases of acute pancreatitis develop pseudocyst.
- Q: Can a pancreatic pseudocyst go unnoticed?
- A: Yes, as the natural history of the disease process is healing by itself.
- Q: What mode of therapy has the least recurrence rate?
- A: Surgical excision.

PANCREATITIS

Raman Sreedharan
Devendra I. Mehta

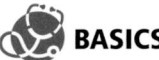

BASICS

DESCRIPTION
- Inflammation of the pancreas characterized by variable local and systemic inflammatory responses.
- Classified into acute and chronic:
  - Acute:
    - Characterized by abdominal pain, nausea, and vomiting with elevation of pancreatic enzymes
    - Usually self-limiting
    - Recurrent episodes of pancreatitis may occur, but the pancreatic function and morphology are restored between episodes.
    - Severe acute pancreatitis is rare in children and has a high mortality.
  - Chronic:
    - Characterized by recurrent or persistent abdominal pain with morphologic changes in the pancreas, leading to pancreatic exocrine or endocrine insufficiency in some patients

ETIOLOGY
- Idiopathic (20–25%)
- Trauma:
  - Bicycle handle injuries
  - Motor vehicle collisions
  - Child abuse
  - Postoperative:
    - Endoscopic retrograde cholangiopancreatography (ERCP)
    - Scoliosis surgery
- Infections:
  - Bacterial:
    - Typhoid
    - Mycoplasma
  - Viral: Measles, mumps, Epstein-Barr virus, Coxsackie B, rubella, influenza, echovirus, hepatitis A and B
  - Parasites (*Ascaris lumbricoides, Echinococcus granulosus, Cryptosporidium parvum, Plasmodium falciparum*)
- Biliary tract disease:
  - Gallstones
  - Sclerosing cholangitis
  - Congenital anomalies:
    - Pancreatic divisum
    - Annular pancreas
    - Anomalous choledochopancreatic–duodenal junction
    - Biliary tract malformations
    - Duplication cyst of the duodenum/gastropancreatic/common bile duct
  - Metabolic:
    - Hyperlipidemia
    - Hypercalcemia
    - Uremia
    - Inborn errors of metabolism
  - Systemic disease:
    - Shock/Hypoxemia
    - Hemolytic uremic syndrome
    - Crohn disease
    - Celiac disease
    - Malnutrition: Anorexia nervosa, bulimia, and refeeding syndrome
    - Diabetes mellitus
    - Mitochondropathy
    - Hemochromatosis
    - Vasculitis: Systemic lupus erythematosus (SLE), Henoch-Schönlein purpura, Kawasaki disease
  - Drugs: L-asparaginase, azathioprine/6-MP, mesalamine, sulfonamides, thiazides, furosemide, tetracyclines, valproic acid, corticosteroids, estrogens, procainamide, ethacrynic acid, and others
  - Toxins:
    - Alcohol, organophosphates, scorpion poison, snake poison
- Autoimmune pancreatitis: A relatively new entity mostly described in adults, but pediatric cases have been reported.

DIAGNOSIS

HISTORY
- Trauma:
  - Even trivial abdominal trauma should be a red flag.
  - Evaluate for evidence of child abuse.
  - Autoimmune pancreatitis can occur as a primary disorder or can be associated with other autoimmune diseases including Sjögren syndrome, primary sclerosing cholangitis, primary biliary sclerosis, sarcoidosis, rheumatoid arthritis, retroperitoneal fibrosis, and kidney diseases with autoimmune etiology.
- Family history:
  - Hereditary pancreatitis
  - Hypertriglyceridemia (I, IV, or V)
  - CFTR mutations/FH of CF
- Upper abdominal pain:
  - Usually epigastric with radiation to the back
  - May have some relief of pain on stooping forward
  - Aggravated by food intake
- Fever:
  - Low-grade fever
  - High-grade fever is usually due to infection.
- Nausea and vomiting common:
  - Vomiting may be bilious.

PHYSICAL EXAM
- General exam:
  - Growth parameters (weight and height), vital signs, capillary refill, pulse oximetry, pallor, jaundice, edema, and clubbing
  - Pallor could be due to chronic systemic disease or hemorrhage.
  - Clubbing could be an indicator of cystic fibrosis.
- GI:
  - Mouth: Presence of aphtous lesions; possibility of Crohn disease
    - Inspection: Abdominal distention or flank fullness (ascites or pseudopancreatic cyst); bluish discoloration of the flanks (Grey Turner sign) and periumbilical region (Cullen sign) in hemorrhagic pancreatitis.
    - Palpation: Guarding, tenderness, and rebound tenderness, especially in the epigastric region or upper abdomen; palpable mass could be a pancreatic pseudocyst; palpate for liver, gall bladder, spleen, and other masses.
  - Percussion: Dullness and fluid thrill in ascites
  - Auscultation: Bowel sounds decreased in ascites or absent in paralytic ileus
    - Rectal exam: Perianal region for skin tags, fistulas, abscesses, or healed scars, which could be indicative of inflammatory bowel disease; peri-rectal exam for mass, melena, or occult blood
- Respiratory system:
  - Pleural effusion and acute respiratory distress syndrome (ARDS)
  - Diffuse respiratory findings could be indicative of cystic fibrosis.
- CNS:
  - Stupor or coma

DIAGNOSTIC TESTS & INTERPRETATION
Lab
- CBC:
  - Hemoglobin may be decreased in hemorrhagic pancreatitis or intestinal hemorrhage.
- Basic metabolic panel:
  - Electrolyte imbalance due to fluid shift and renal complications
  - Calcium is decreased.
  - Glucose may be transiently elevated.
- Liver function tests:
  - Elevated transaminase levels suggest biliary cause.
  - Elevated bilirubin level
- Amylase level:
  - 3-fold elevation in the level increases the specificity for the diagnosis of pancreatitis.
  - Starts rising 2–12 hours after the insult and remains elevated for 3–5 days
  - Persistent elevation could be due to complication such as pseudocyst.
  - Degree of elevation does not have any correlation to the severity or the course of the illness.
  - Necrotizing and hemorrhagic pancreatitis may develop with normal amylase levels.
  - Other causes of elevated amylase levels include bowel obstruction, acute appendicitis, biliary obstruction, salivary duct obstruction, diabetic ketoacidosis, cystic fibrosis, pneumonia, salpingitis, ruptured ectopic pregnancy, ovarian cyst, cerebral trauma, burns, renal failure, and macroamylasemia.

- Lipase level:
  - Lipase levels are more specific than amylase for the diagnosis of pancreatitis.
  - Starts rising 4–8 hours after the insult and remains elevated for 8–14 days
  - 3-fold increase in the level is very sensitive and specific for pancreatitis.
  - Levels do not correlate with severity or with clinical outcome.
  - Other causes of elevated lipase levels include intestinal perforation, intestinal obstruction, appendicitis, mesentery infarction, cholecystitis, diabetic ketoacidosis, renal failure, and macrolipasemia.
- Serologic testing for autoimmune pancreatitis:
  - IgG4 levels are usually elevated but not specific.
  - Anti-PBP (plasminogen binding protein)

Imaging
- Abdominal x-rays:
  - Sentinel loop: Distended small intestinal loop near the pancreas
  - Colon cutoff sign: Absence of gas shadow in the colon distal to the transverse colon
  - Multiple fluid levels in paralytic ileus
  - Calcification or stones in pancreas or gallbladder
  - Diffuse haziness: Ascites
- Upper GI series
  - "Reverse 3 sign"/Frostberg sign: The curves of the "3" indicate swelling of the pancreas and the middLe apex of the "3" suggests the origin of the duct.
  - Anterior displacement of the stomach is seen in pseudopancreatic cyst or retroperitoneal swelling.
- Barium enema: Rarely indicated
- Chest x-ray:
  - Pleural effusion or ARDS
  - Diaphragmatic involvement
- US abdomen:
  - Pancreatic size, echogenicity, calcification, stones, abscess, and pseudocysts
  - Endoscopic US is more useful than the transabdominal US study but is difficult in children.
- CT scan:
  - In acute cases, as in trauma, to look at extent of injury to pancreas and other intra-abdominal structures
  - Can show complications such as abscess, hemorrhage, pseudocyst, etc.
  - Reveals pathology in the pancreaticobiliary system in most instances.
- Magnetic resonance cholangiopancreatography (MRCP):
  - More popular than CT for identifying pancreaticobiliary disorders.
  - Useful for delineation of the ductal structure of the pancreas and also to identify pathology in the hepatobiliary system
  - Serotonin stimulated MRCP (sMRCP) is becoming more popular in adults as it delineates the pancreatic ducts better.

- Endoscopic retrograde cholangiopancreatography (ERCP):
  - Indicated in persistent/chronic pancreatitis for delineation of pancreatic ducts and for therapeutic interventions.
  - Limitations include postprocedure complications and accessibility to gastroenterologist experienced with ERCP in children.

 TREATMENT

MEDICATION (DRUGS)
- Antibiotics:
  - Prophylaxis in severe cases when necrotizing pancreatitis is suspected
  - Few antimicrobials, such as imipenem–cilastatin, achieve adequate penetration.
- Pain management:
  - Narcotics
  - Meperidine is preferable to morphine because it has less effect on the sphincter of Oddi.
- H_2 blockade/PPI for acid suppression:
  - Prevents pancreatic stimulation in severe cases
- Autoimmune pancreatitis is treated with corticosteroids.

ADDITIONAL TREATMENT
General Measures
- NPO for pancreatic rest.
- In moderate to severe cases of pancreatitis and in cases with vomiting, nasogastric decompression by placement of nasogastric (NG) tube:
  - Pain management
- Acid suppression with H_2 blockers or PPI

SURGERY/OTHER PROCEDURES
- Peritoneal lavage rarely for salvage in necrotizing/hemorrhagic pancreatitis
- Management of pancreatic abscess and in some cases of pseudocysts

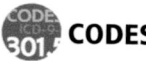 ONGOING CARE

DIET
- NPO initially
- Mild cases may be started on a low-fat diet after a few days.
- Nasojejunal feeds worth considering when oral feeding is not possible even after the 1st few days:
  - Alternative is total parenteral nutrition (TPN).

PROGNOSIS
Acute pancreatitis is usually a self-limiting disorder in children.

COMPLICATIONS
- Pancreatic edema
- Peripancreatic fat necrosis
- Pancreatic phlegmon
- Pancreatic abscess
- Pancreatic pseudocyst
- Hemorrhagic pancreatitis

- Necrotizing pancreatitis
- Pancreatic calculi
- Pancreatic fistula
- Pancreatic ductal strictures
- Pancreatic ductal dilatation
- Systemic complications
- Shock and multiorgan failure
- GI and hepatobiliary:
  - Paralytic ileus
  - Ascites, peritonitis
  - Stress ulcer
  - Intestinal hemorrhage
  - Portal vein thrombosis/splenic vein thrombosis/obstruction
  - Bile duct obstruction
- Pulmonary:
  - Atelectasis, pleural effusion, pneumonitis, ARDS
- Cardiovascular:
  - Hypotension/Circulatory collapse
  - Pericarditis/Pericardial effusion
  - EKG changes
- Sudden death

ADDITIONAL READING
- Chari ST, Takahashi N, Levy MJ, et al. A diagnostic approach to distinguish autoimmune pancreatitis from pancreatic cancer. *Clin Gastroenterol Hepatol*. 2009;7(10):1097.
- DeBanto JR, Goday PS, Pedroso MR, et al. Acute pancreatitis in children. *Am J Gastroenterol*. 2002;97:1726.
- Jackson WD. Pancreatitis: Etiology, diagnosis and management. *Curr Opin Pediatr*. 2001;13:447–451.
- Pietzak MM, Thomas DW. Pancreatitis in childhood. *Pediatr Rev*. 2000;21(12):406–412.
- Whitcomb DC. Clinical practice. Acute pancreatitis. *N Engl J Med*. 2006;354(20):2142–2150.

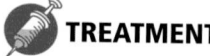 CODES

ICD9
- 577.0 Acute pancreatitis
- 577.1 Chronic pancreatitis

ICD10
- K85.9 Acute pancreatitis, unspecified
- K86.1 Other chronic pancreatitis

FAQ
- Q: What is hereditary pancreatitis?
- A: Hereditary pancreatitis presents as recurrent inflammation of the pancreas and runs in families over ≥2 generations. It is inherited as an autosomal dominant trait with variable penetrance.
- Q: Do normal findings on US or CT scan of the pancreas exclude a diagnosis of acute pancreatitis?
- A: No. Normal US and CT findings are common in mild cases.

PANHYPOPITUITARISM

Craig A. Alter
Jeffrey D. Roizen
Vaneeta Bamba (5th edition)

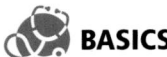

BASICS

DESCRIPTION
Deficiency of >1 pituitary hormone

EPIDEMIOLOGY
- Congenital forms affect both sexes equally and are diagnosed at a young age.
- The epidemiology of acquired or secondary forms depends on the underlying cause.

RISK FACTORS
Genetics
Most cases are not thought to be genetic; however, there are rare cases of autosomal recessive, autosomal dominant, and X-linked forms.

PATHOPHYSIOLOGY
- Pathology is based on specific deficiency.
- Growth hormone (GH): Hypoglycemia in newborns and poor growth in patients older than 6–12 months
- Adrenocorticotropic hormone: Hypercortisolism
- Thyroid-stimulating hormone (TSH): Hypothyroidism
- Luteinizing hormone (LH)/Follicle-stimulating hormone (FSH): Hypogonadism
- Antidiuretic hormone: Diabetes insipidus
- Prolactin: Hyperprolactinemia

ETIOLOGY
- Idiopathic (some may be due to hypophysitis)
- Congenital:
  - Absence of the pituitary (empty sella syndrome)
  - Genetic disorders due to mutations in genes or transcription factors (POUF1, HESX1, LHX3, LHX4, OTX2, SIX6, SOX2, SOX3, PTX2, PROP1, etc.)
  - Pituitary malformations (ectopic posterior pituitary, hypoplastic infundibular stalk, hypoplastic pituitary)
  - Familial panhypopituitarism
  - Rathke's cleft cyst
- Acquired:
  - Birth trauma or perinatal insult
  - Surgical resection of the gland or damage to the stalk
  - Traumatic brain injury
  - Hypophysitis
  - Child abuse or psychosocial deprivation
  - Iron deposition secondary to chronic transfusion therapy (e.g., β-thalassemia)
- Infection:
  - Viral encephalitis
  - Bacterial or fungal infection
  - Tuberculosis
- Vascular:
  - Pituitary infarction
  - Pituitary aneurysm
- Cranial irradiation
- Chemotherapy
- Tumors:
  - Craniopharyngioma
  - Germinoma
  - Glioma
  - Pinealoma
  - Primitive neuroectodermal tumor (medulloblastoma)
- Histiocytosis
- Sarcoidosis

COMMONLY ASSOCIATED CONDITIONS
- Midline defects such as cleft lip/palate, hypotelorism, single central maxillary incisor
- Septo-optic dysplasia (de Morsier syndrome)
- Holoprosencephaly

DIAGNOSIS

HISTORY
- Birth weight: Hypopituitary infants are usually normal or small for gestational age, in contrast to hyperinsulinemic infants, who are typically large for gestational age.
- Birth history:
  - Documented or symptoms of hypoglycemia, which include poor feeding, lethargy, irritability, or seizures
  - Hypoglycemia may be secondary to hyperinsulinism (HI), but HI babies are typically large for gestational age.
  - Hypopituitary babies are not large.
  - Midline defects are associated with hypopituitarism and not HI.
- Complications during pregnancy or delivery:
  - Birth trauma may be associated with pituitary injury.
  - Breech delivery or vacuum extraction has been associated.
- History of surgeries and previous diseases: Congenital hypopituitarism is often associated with midline facial defects, such as a single central incisor, bifid uvula, or cleft palate, which require repair.
- Growth pattern: Plot previous heights and look for growth pattern. GH deficiency usually manifests as poor linear growth by the end of the 1st year of life.
- Delayed puberty:
  - Children with delayed puberty show further growth failure in adolescence.
  - Sense of smell should be assessed to rule out Kallmann syndrome (isolated central hypogonadism and anosmia).
- Increased thirst and urination: Children with hypothalamic disorders may present with symptoms of diabetes insipidus.
- Special questions:
  - Complaints of headache and/or a visual defect: Headache can be a symptom of a brain tumor. Focal neurologic symptoms are highly suggestive of CNS pathology.

PHYSICAL EXAM
- Height and weight:
  - Patients with panhypopituitarism have normal size in the newborn period, whereas patients with hyperinsulinism are typically large for gestational age.
- Prolonged conjugated hyperbilirubinemia:
  - May be 1st sign of hypothyroidism with or without hypopituitarism. Some state newborn screens will not detect central hypothyroidism.
  - Hypopituitarism can lead to neonatal cholestasis.
- Micropenis in male newborns: Neonatal penis should be ≥ 2.5 cm in length; micropenis suggests gonadotropin and/or GH deficiency
  Physical exam tricks:
  - Penile and testicular size: Measure stretched phallic length (from pubic ramus to glans) with patient lying supine and phallus at 90 degrees to the body; use Prader beads to assess testicular volume.
  - Midline defects: Palpate for submucosal cleft palate, look for central incisor.
  - Visual field testing: Visual field defects suggest a brain tumor.

DIAGNOSTIC TESTS & INTERPRETATION
Lab
- Liver function tests: LFTs in newborns with congenital hypopituitarism are often elevated and accompanied by conjugated hyperbilirubinemia, as opposed to simple congenital hypothyroidism, in which unconjugated hyperbilirubinemia exists.
- Thyroid function tests including free thyroxine (FT_4): TSH may be normal, but free T_4 will be low.
- TSH stimulation test: Delayed, normal, or exaggerated TSH response is consistent with a hypothalamic lesion.
- Serum insulinlike growth factor-I (IGF-I) and insulinlike growth factor binding protein-3 (IGFBP-3): May be low, but normal growth factors do not exclude GH deficiency in children with brain tumors. IGF-1 may be low due to poor nutrition.
- Free T_4 by equilibrium dialysis: Must measure, not calculate, the free T_4 concentration in serum
- GH stimulation tests: Should be performed by a pediatric endocrinologist
- Cortrosyn stimulation test: More helpful in the diagnosis of primary adrenal insufficiency than secondary (adrenocorticotropic hormone) or tertiary (corticotropin-releasing hormone) deficiency
- Metyrapone or corticotropin-releasing hormone stimulation test:
  - Tests for adrenocorticotropic hormone or corticotropin-releasing hormone deficiency
  - Metyrapone not currently available in the U.S.
  - Must be performed by a pediatric endocrinologist
- Estradiol, testosterone, ultrasensitive LH, and FSH: Delayed puberty if no breast development by 13 years in girls, and no testicular enlargement by 14 years in boys
- Water deprivation test:
  - Definitive test for antidiuretic hormone deficiency (diabetes insipidus)
  - Should be performed by a pediatric endocrinologist
- Comments on testing: Measurement of water intake and urine output over 24 hours at home can help diagnosis of diabetes insipidus. Baseline serum tests (prolactin, 8AM cortisol, free-T4, IGF-1, IGF-BP3, serum and urine osmolality, testosterone for males in the first 6 months of life and again after the age of 11 years) can all be done in a nonfasting state:
  - Stimulation tests must be performed by a pediatric endocrinologist.

Imaging
- Bone age: Typically significantly delayed in GH deficiency or hypothyroidism
- MRI with contrast of brain with fine cuts through the hypothalamus and pituitary:
  – Look for tumors, but also size of pituitary, infundibulum and presence of normal "bright spot" in posterior pituitary.
  – Absence of the "bright spot" is highly associated with central diabetes insipidus of any etiology.
  – Ectopic pituitary consistent with GH deficiency and other anterior pituitary deficiencies

ALERT
- If adrenocorticotropic hormone deficient, stress dosing of glucocorticoids is necessary.
- A patient with diabetes insipidus who does not have an intact thirst mechanism and access to free water is at high risk for acute hypernatremia.

DIFFERENTIAL DIAGNOSIS
- Hyperinsulinism (HI) in newborns
- Isolated hormone deficiency, such as GH deficiency in newborns
- Constitutional growth delay

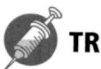 ## TREATMENT
MEDICATION (DRUGS)
- Recombinant human GH (rhGH) by SC injection daily: 0.15–0.3 mg/kg/wk
- Desmopressin acetate (DDAVP): Available in oral and intranasal formulations. Dose is variable.
- Estrogen/Testosterone: Started at puberty at low doses and slowly increased over 1–2 years to mimic endogenous secretion of sex steroids.
- Estrogen given as daily oral or topical forms to girls, whereas testosterone given as injection to boys every month
- Levo-thyroxine (Levo-T) PO: 25–200 levo-T$_4$ mcg daily, based on weight, age, and free T$_4$ levels
- TSH levels will not be useful in monitoring therapy, even after treatment is initiated.
- Hydrocortisone:
  – Replacement doses if needed: 8–15 mg/m^2/d PO, divided q8h (or t.i.d.)
  – In stress circumstances such as fever, severe illness, vomiting, or surgery, dose is increased to 50–100 mg/m^2/d PO
  – If dosed IV, provide a loading dose of 50–100 mg/m^2 IM or IV followed by 50–100 mg/m^2 divided q4h; oral stress doses should be divided q8h.
  – To calculate hydrocortisone dose, estimate body surface area (BSA) using a nomogram or the following formula: BSA (m^2) = square root of (height [cm] × weight [kg]/3,600)
- Duration: Long-term therapy: Monitored by a pediatric endocrinologist
  – rhGH: In children and adolescents: Until growth velocity drops to 2.5 cm/yr; once puberty is complete

– GH-deficient adults may benefit from lifelong rhGH because of the impact of GH on body composition, lipid profile, and cardiac function.
– Patient should again undergo GH provocative testing off rhGH therapy to determine if adult treatment is necessary.
– DDAVP: For life as needed to control symptoms of polyuria/polydipsia
– Acute hypernatremia may be managed with DDAVP, IV vasopressin, or fluids alone.
– Sex steroids: Around age 12; may be continued for lifetime
– Levo-thyroxine for life
– Hydrocortisone: Replacement dose based on individual's need
– Stress dose coverage for life
– Possible conflicts with other treatments: There is a theoretical risk that GH might stimulate tumor growth because of its mitogenic effect. Current data argue against GH as a tumor stimulant.

 ## ONGOING CARE
FOLLOW-UP RECOMMENDATIONS
- Initially, every 3 months by a pediatric endocrinologist
- When pituitary hormones are replaced, expect:
  – GH: Immediate resolution of hypoglycemia; and improved growth velocity within 3–6 months
  – T$_4$ levels should normalize within 4–6 weeks
  – Side effects of GH therapy: Headache, vision problems, seizures, changes in activity level, limp, knee or hip pain

PROGNOSIS
- For congenital forms, the prognosis is excellent with endocrine replacement.
- Diabetes insipidus in infants can be challenging to manage.
- For secondary forms, the overall prognosis depends on the primary disease.

COMPLICATIONS
- Hypoglycemia in the newborn period
- Short stature
- Adrenal crisis
- Dehydration/Hypernatremia

ALERT
- rhGH therapy is associated with idiopathic intracranial hypertension (pseudotumor cerebri), which usually improves whether or not medication is stopped.
- rhGH deficiency/therapy is associated with slipped capital femoral epiphysis (SCFE). Carefully evaluate any limp or knee or hip pain in patients on rhGH therapy. SCFE mandates orthopedic consultation.
- The diagnosis of panhypopituitarism must be considered in patients with hypoglycemic seizures.
- GH is a mitogenic factor, so there is a theoretical potential for increasing the incidence of leukemia. Clinical studies have not confirmed this hypothesis.
- The family and the patient must understand the importance of taking stress doses of steroid appropriately (e.g., with surgery, vomiting, or febrile illnesses).
- 20% of normal children will fail a single GH provocative test.

- A TSH level is generally not helpful when evaluating pituitary/hypothalamic causes of hypothyroidism. The unbound free T$_4$ level (by equilibrium dialysis) is the most useful test both to establish the diagnosis and to monitor L-thyroxine replacement therapy.

ADDITIONAL READING
- De Vries L, Lazar L, Phillip M. Craniopharyngioma: Presentation and endocrine sequelae in 36 children. *J Endocr Metab.* 2003;16:703–710.
- Jenkins PJ, Mukherjee A, Shalet SM. Does growth hormone cause cancer? *Clin Endocrinol (Oxf).* 2006;64(2):115–121.
- Maghnie M. Diabetes insipidus. *Horm Res.* 2003;59(Suppl 1):42–54.
- Parks JS, Brown MR, Hurley DL et al. Heritable disorders of pituitary development. *J Clin Endocrinol Metab.* 1999;84:4362–4370.
- Sklar CA, Constine LS. Chronic neuroendocrinological sequelae of radiation therapy. *Int J Radiat Oncol Biol Phys.* 1995;31:1113–1121.

 ### CODES
ICD9
253.2 Panhypopituitarism
ICD10
E23.0 Hypopituitarism

FAQ
- Q: When do I give stress doses of steroid, and for how long?
- A: Whenever the patient has fever, vomiting, serious illness, or surgery. Continue until 24 hours after stress resolves (e.g., the day after fever breaks or vomiting stops).
- Q: What are the chances of cretinism if hypopituitarism is congenital?
- A: Minimal, if medication is taken properly.

PARVOVIRUS B19 (ERYTHEMA INFECTIOSUM, FIFTH DISEASE)

Julia F. Shaklee
J. Nadine Gracia (5th edition)

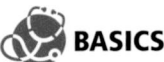 BASICS

DESCRIPTION
Parvovirus B19 (B19) is a common viral infection of school-aged children that is most commonly associated with an erythematous macular rash in an otherwise well-appearing patient. B19 is a single-stranded DNA virus, one of the smallest of the human viruses, 1st isolated from asymptomatic blood donors in 1975.

EPIDEMIOLOGY
- B19 infections are ubiquitous worldwide, occurring most often in school-aged children. Humans are the only hosts.
- Incubation period is 4–14 days.
- Modes of transmission:
  - Contact with respiratory secretions
  - Percutaneous exposure to blood or blood products (1,011 virions/mm of serum in patients with hereditary hemolytic anemias)
  - Vertical transmission from mother to fetus

Incidence
Attack rates: 15–60% of susceptibles (i.e., seronegative) will become infected upon exposure.

Prevalence
- Seroprevalence of B19 IgG antibodies:
  - >5 years old: 2–9%
  - 5–18 years old: 15–35%
  - Adults: 30–60%
  - Elderly: 90%

GENERAL PREVENTION
- B19 transmission can be decreased through routine infection-control practices, including hand hygiene and appropriate disposal of contaminated facial tissues.
- For hospitalized children with suspected aplastic crisis, immunocompromised patients with chronic infection and anemia, and patients with papulopurpuric gloves-and-socks syndrome secondary to B19, droplet precautions in addition to standard contact precautions are recommended.
- No additional measures are needed for normal hosts with rash.
- Due to the potential risks to the fetus from B19 infections, pregnant health care workers should pay attention to strict infection control procedures and avoid contact with immunocompromised hosts with B19 infection or those with aplastic crisis. Routine exclusion of pregnant women from the workplace where B19 infections is suspected is not recommended.

PATHOPHYSIOLOGY
- Parvovirus B19 inhibits erythropoiesis by lytically infecting RBC precursors in the bone marrow. It is associated with a number of clinical manifestations, ranging from benign to severe.
- There is no practical in vitro system for isolation or culture of the virus.

COMMONLY ASSOCIATED CONDITIONS
- Fifth disease, or erythema infectiosum, caused by B19 occurs in up to 35% of school-aged children.
- Transient aplastic crisis secondary to B19 may cause severe anemia in patients with hereditary hemolytic anemias or any condition that shortens the RBC lifespan, such as sickle cell disease or spherocytosis.
- Polyarthropathy syndrome, symmetric joint pain and swelling, especially of the hands, knees, and feet, is seen in adults more often than in children; among women with B19 infection, 80–100% develop polyarthritis.
- Hydrops fetalis may develop after maternal B19 infection with intrauterine involvement (typically within the first 20 weeks of pregnancy).
- Chronic anemia/pure red cell aplasia due to persistent B19 infection has been reported in immunocompromised patients.
- Papulopurpuric gloves-and-socks syndrome (PPGSS) consists of painful and pruritic papules, petechiae, and purpura localized to the hands and feet and is often associated with fever.
- Sporadic reports of extremity numbness and tingling, hemophagocytic syndrome, and Henoch-Schönlein purpura have been associated with B19 infection.

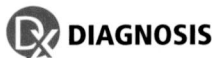 DIAGNOSIS

Diagnosis depends upon recognition of typical symptoms and the results of laboratory testing.

HISTORY
- Asymptomatic infection may occur in ~20% of children and adults.
- Erythema infectiosum (Fifth disease):
  - Most common form of parvovirus infection recognized
  - Characterized by an erythematous facial rash with a distinctive "slapped cheek" appearance, often accompanied by circumoral pallor.

- A symmetric, maculopapular, often lace-like rash occurs on the trunk, spreading outward to the rest of the body and extremities. The rash is often pruritic and may intensify with exposure to sunlight, heat, or exercise. It occasionally involves the palms and soles. Rarely, the rash can be papular, vesicular, or purpuric. It may last for ~7 days, but can persist >20 days.
- A brief, mild prodrome of systemic symptoms, including headache, sore throat, myalgias, and low-grade fevers, often precedes the appearance of rash by 7–10 days.
- The child is usually well-appearing and remains active and playful.
- Arthralgias and arthritis occur infrequently in children, but are seen in up to 80% of adults, especially women. Arthritis in children most commonly involves the knees.
- Aplastic crisis:
  - Prodromal symptoms in B19-infected children with sickle cell disease or other hereditary hemolytic anemias are nonspecific and consist of fever, malaise, and headache. Rash is usually absent.
  - Symptoms are usually self-limited, lasting 7–10 days.
  - Severe anemia, CHF, stroke, and acute splenic sequestration have also been associated.
- Chronic anemia/pure red cell aplasia:
  - In immunocompromised patients, B19 infection may persist for months, leading to chronic anemia with B19 viremia.
  - Low-grade fever and neutropenia may accompany anemia.

PHYSICAL EXAM
Fifth disease:
- An erythematous facial rash with a "slapped cheek" appearance, often associated with circumoral pallor
- Truncal, maculopapular, lacy-appearing rash spreading to the arms, buttocks, and thighs
  - Often pruritic and may become more intense with exercise or heat exposure
- Occasionally can be found on the palms and soles, and rarely can be papular, vesicular, or purpuric

DIAGNOSTIC TESTS & INTERPRETATION
Lab
- Antibodies:
  - Detection of parvovirus B19-specific IgM or IgG antibodies as determined by EIA or radioimmunoassay
  - The presence of B19-specific IgM antibodies is diagnostic in patients with symptoms of erythema infectiosum or aplastic crisis. IgM- and IgG-specific antibodies are detected in 90% of such patients by 3–7 days of illness.
  - B19-specific IgG antibodies persists for years, while specific IgM antibodies begin to decrease 30–60 days after onset of illness.
- Polymerase chain reaction (PCR) techniques:
  - Immunocompromised patients with chronic marrow suppression may be unable to produce B19-specific IgG or IgM antibodies. In such cases, B19 viral DNA can be detected using nucleic acid hybridization or PCR techniques. These techniques may also be used to detect virus in the fetus.
- Hematocrit and reticulocyte count in patients with aplastic crisis:
  - Laboratory studies reveal reticulocytopenia, usually with counts of <1%. During the illness, the patient's hematocrit may fall as low as 15%.

DIFFERENTIAL DIAGNOSIS
B19 infection should be considered in all patients with arthritis or viral exanthems with a consistent history and exam.

 ## TREATMENT

ADDITIONAL TREATMENT
General Measures
- There is no specific antiviral therapy for B19 infection.
- Most patients require supportive care only. However, transfusions may be required for treatment of severe anemia in patients with aplastic crisis.
- IV immunoglobulin (IVIG) therapy has been given with some success to a few patients with chronic marrow suppression secondary to B19 infection.

 ## ONGOING CARE

FOLLOW-UP RECOMMENDATIONS
Expected course of illness:
- The rash of erythema infectiosum in a child or adult may last up to 20 days. It may, at times, fade and/or intensify, depending on sunlight exposure, exercise, or body surface temperature changes (e.g., bathing).
- During aplastic crisis secondary to B19, the reticulocyte count usually remains low (often <1%) for ~8 days before spontaneous recovery.

PROGNOSIS
- The prognosis is quite good for all manifestations of B19 infections.
- Most patients recover spontaneously and require only supportive care.

COMPLICATIONS
- Parvovirus B19 during pregnancy:
  - 30–50% of pregnant women are susceptible to B19 infection.
  - Fetal loss, intrauterine growth retardation, or hydrops fetalis may result from maternal infection with B19 during pregnancy.
  - B19 has not been proven to cause congenital anomalies.
  - The greatest risk for B19 infection affecting the fetus exists in the first 20 weeks of gestation.
  - The risk of fetal death after exposure, if antibody status is unknown, is from 0.05–1%.
  - Fetal death occurs in 2–6% of cases.
  - There is no indication for elective abortion in cases of maternal infection.
  - The mainstay of treatment for an infected fetus is delivery, but intrauterine transfusions may be life-saving.
- Arthritis/Arthropathy:
  - Although most cases of polyarthritis resolve within 2 weeks, persistent symptoms for months to even years (rarely) have been reported.

ADDITIONAL READING

- de Jong EP, de Haan TR, et al. Parvovirus B19 infection in pregnancy. *J Clin Virol*. 2006;36:1–7.
- Kerr JR. Pathogenesis of human parvovirus B19 in rheumatic disease. *Ann Rheum Dis*. 2000;59:672–683.
- Lamont RF, Sobel JD, Vaisbuch E, et al. Parvovirus B19 infection in Pregnancy. *BJOG*. 2011;118:175–186.
- Nunoue T, Kusuhara K, Hara T. Human fetal infection with parvovirus B19: Maternal infection time in gestation, viral persistence, and fetal prognosis. *Pediatr Infect Dis J*. 2002;21:1133–1136.
- Smith-Whitley K, Zhao H, et al. Epidemiology of human parvovirus B19 in children with sickle cell disease. *Blood*. 2004;103:422–427.
- Young NS, Brown KE. Parvovirus B19. *N Engl J Med*. 2004;350:586–597.

 ## CODES

ICD9
057.0 Erythema infectiosum (fifth disease)

ICD10
B08.3 Erythema infectiosum [fifth disease]

FAQ
- Q: When may children with B19 infection return to school?
- A: Children are contagious only during the prodromal phase of illness, which is often unrecognized. Once the rash appears, they are no longer infectious and may return to school or day care.
- Q: What can be done to reduce risk of fetal infection?
- A: Because B19 infections during pregnancy may result in fetal death, and B19 infections often occur in community outbreaks, fetal risks following maternal exposure to persons with recognized B19 infection are a frequent concern. Risk to the fetus appears to be greatest if the infection occurs prior to the 20th week of gestation. Among pregnant women of unknown antibody status, the risk of fetal death after exposure to B19 is estimated to be <1.5%. Routine exclusion of pregnant women from the workplace when B19 infection is suspected is not recommended. However, pregnant teachers who are at risk for infection may consider a leave of absence during community outbreaks of B19.

PATENT DUCTUS ARTERIOSUS

Alexander Lowenthal
Ronn E. Tanel (5th edition)

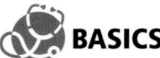 **BASICS**

DESCRIPTION

- Patent ductus arteriosus (PDA) is the persistence into postnatal life of the normal fetal vascular conduit between the central pulmonary and systemic arterial systems. Normally, the ductus arteriosus (DA) functionally closes within the 1st 1–3 days of life. Structural closure is usually completed by the 3rd week of life. If the DA remains patent beyond 3 months of life, it is considered abnormal and is unlikely to close spontaneously (spontaneous closure rate 0.6% per year).
- In the infant with a normal left aortic arch, the DA connects the main pulmonary artery (MPA) at the origin of the left pulmonary artery to the descending aorta, distal to the origin of the left subclavian artery.
- Many variations can occur, although they are less common. The main, proximal right, or proximal left pulmonary artery may be connected to virtually any location on the aortic arch or proximal portions of the brachiocephalic vessels.
- 5 distinct clinical conditions are associated with PDA:
  - Isolated cardiovascular lesion in premature infants
  - Isolated cardiovascular lesion in otherwise healthy term infants and children
  - Incidental finding associated with more significant structural cardiovascular defects
  - Compensatory structure in cases of neonatal pulmonary hypertension) without congenital heart disease (CHD)
  - Critical compensatory structure in some cyanotic or left-sided obstructed lesions

EPIDEMIOLOGY

- As an isolated defect, PDA is the 6th most common congenital cardiovascular lesion.
- Female : Male: 2:1

Incidence

- 1 per 2,000 (5% of all types of CHD)
- Increases with the degree of prematurity (50–80% in preterm infants <26 weeks' gestation)
- 60–70% of preterm infants of <28 weeks' gestation receive medical or surgical therapy for a PDA
- Varies significantly depending on management style (e.g., amount of maintenance fluid prescribed, surfactant administration), coexisting diseases (e.g., respiratory distress syndrome, hypoxemia, fluid overload, necrotizing enterocolitis, sepsis, hypocalcemia), and environmental factors (altitude).

PATHOPHYSIOLOGY

- Fetal blood flows from the MPA to the DA to the aorta, thus bypassing the pulmonary vascular bed and supplying systemic blood flow. With the 1st postnatal breaths, the pulmonary vascular resistance falls abruptly, the DA constricts, and pulmonary blood flow is directed into the lungs. With a PDA, excessive blood flow will continue from the aorta into the pulmonary artery, causing increased pulmonary blood flow and volume overloading of the left side of the heart.
- In premature infants and term infants with pulmonary hypertension, delayed closure represents an impaired developmental process, whereas in the healthy full-term infant, PDA probably reflects an anatomic abnormality of the ductal tissue.

ETIOLOGY

- Prematurity
- Rubella infection in the 1st trimester
- Genetic or familial factors
- High altitude
- Idiopathic

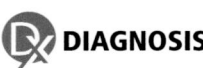 **DIAGNOSIS**

HISTORY

- Premature infants:
  - Variable: Ranging from asymptomatic to complete cardiovascular collapse
  - Increased ventilatory support, pulmonary hemorrhage, respiratory or metabolic acidosis from low cardiac output and excessive pulmonary blood flow
  - Tachypnea, feeding intolerance, apnea, bradycardia, necrotizing enterocolitis, and decreased urine output
- Infants and older children:
  - Small PDA: Usually asymptomatic, with incidental heart murmur found on routine exam
  - Moderate PDA: Possible CHF, poor feeding, and poor weight gain
  - Large PDA: Symptoms as above and recurrent respiratory infections

PHYSICAL EXAM

- Premature infants:
  - Tachypnea, rales, tachycardia (±S3 gallop)
  - Hyperdynamic precordium and bounding pulses with wide pulse pressure (due to diastolic "runoff" from the aorta to the pulmonary artery)
  - The typical PDA murmur in a premature infant is a pansystolic murmur audible at the left upper or midsternal border.

- With a large PDA and equalization of pressure between the MPA and the aorta, no murmur may be heard.
- Hepatomegaly may exist with heart failure (late sign).
- Infants and older children: Findings vary with size of shunt.
  - Small PDA:
    - ○ Pansystolic murmur may be heard at the 2nd left intercostal space. Murmur becomes continuous (i.e., extends into diastole) as the pulmonary vascular resistance decreases over the 1st months of life.
  - Moderate or large PDA:
    - ○ The murmur is louder, has a harsh quality, and acquires a machine-like quality often being heard posteriorly. In that case, a systolic thrill may be felt at the left upper sternal border.
    - ○ Tachycardia, bounding pulses with a wide pulse pressure, and a mid-diastolic low-frequency rumbling murmur may be audible at the apex with a large PDA.
    - ○ With severe left ventricular failure the classic PDA signs may disappear, but there will be findings consistent with CHF (tachycardia, S3 gallop at the apex, hepatomegaly, tachypnea, rales).
    - ○ In extreme cases, pulmonary hypertension may occur, with the murmur shortening, the diastolic component disappearing, and S2 becoming accentuated. At advanced stages of irreversible pulmonary vascular disease, cyanosis begins to appear, often more pronounced in the lower limbs, with reversal of shunting.

DIAGNOSTIC TESTS & INTERPRETATION

Imaging

- EKG:
  - Usually normal with a small PDA
  - Left atrial enlargement and left ventricular hypertrophy with moderate and large PDA
  - Biventricular hypertrophy in later stages
- Chest x-ray:
  - Usually normal with a small PDA, although prominence of main and peripheral pulmonary arteries may be seen
  - In moderate and large PDAs, these findings become more pronounced, along with an enlarged heart. Increased pulmonary vascular markings are proportionate to the left-to-right shunt. Pulmonary edema can be seen if CHF develops. In premature infants with respiratory distress syndrome, there is evidence of deteriorating lung disease with unclear cardiac borders.

- Echocardiogram:
  - Delineates the PDA and assesses the size of the left atrium and the left ventricle
  - Doppler techniques assess the ductal flow pattern and may be useful for estimating the pulmonary artery pressure
- Cardiac catheterization:
  - Most often not essential for diagnosis
  - Indicated for suspected concomitant pulmonary hypertension
  - Can be performed for treatment via transcatheter closure techniques

DIFFERENTIAL DIAGNOSIS
- Aortopulmonary window
- Systemic or pulmonary arteriovenous communications
- Ruptured sinus of Valsalva
- Coronary artery fistula
- Truncus arteriosus
- Innocent venous hum in older children
- Pulmonary atresia with collaterals
- Ventricular septal defect with aortic regurgitation
- Ventricular septal defect in infancy

 TREATMENT

ADDITIONAL TREATMENT
General Measures
- Premature infant:
  - Supportive treatment (careful use of oxygen, respiratory assistance, correction of metabolic acidosis)
  - Management of CHF with fluid restriction and diuretics
  - If PDA persists or patient is symptomatic, closure of PDA is indicated.
  - Medical closure: Indomethacin most often used; ibuprofen is as effective.
    - Contraindications to medical management include: Renal failure (creatinine >1.8 mg/dL), thrombocytopenia (platelets <100,000), associated conditions (necrotizing enterocolitis, intraventricular hemorrhage)
  - Surgical closure indicated if medical treatment fails or use of indomethacin is contraindicated.
- Infants and older children:
  - Medical management of CHF with digoxin and diuretics
  - PDA is no longer a stated indication for subacute bacterial endocarditis (SBE) prophylaxis, but clinical practice may vary.

- Spontaneous closure rate is low, and closure with indomethacin is not usually effective in this group of patients.
- Closure is indicated whenever a symptomatic or hemodynamically significant PDA exists.
- For asymptomatic audible PDA, closure can be performed electively and is primarily performed to reduce the risk of endocarditis. Recommendations for closure of an asymptomatic, incidentally found ("silent" ductus) are not standard.
- Most infants and children can have a PDA safely and effectively closed during cardiac catheterization, obviating the need for a surgical procedure.

SURGERY/OTHER PROCEDURES
Surgical closure of PDA can be achieved by 1 of 3 means:
- Open surgical ligation and division: Mostly in premature infants
- Video-assisted thoracoscopic ligation: Dependent on the institution
- Transcatheter occlusion with coils or other devices

 ONGOING CARE

PROGNOSIS
- Outcome in treated premature infants is generally good but depends mostly on the degree of prematurity and the presence of associated conditions.
- Outcome in term infants and older children is excellent if no complications have occurred.
- PDA among adults may be associated with significant mortality with or without surgery.
- After closure of PDA, no endocarditis prophylaxis is needed if complete obliteration of flow is achieved. Most cardiologists continue prophylaxis for 6 months after the procedure that closed the PDA.

COMPLICATIONS
- Pulmonary edema and CHF
- Pulmonary hemorrhage
- Pulmonary vascular obstructive disease
- Increased chronic lung disease
- Failure to thrive
- Recurrent respiratory infections
- Lobar emphysema or collapse
- Infective endarteritis
- Thromboembolism of cerebral arteries

- Aneurysm of the ductus
- Intracranial hemorrhage
- Necrotizing enterocolitis
- Renal dysfunction

ADDITIONAL READING

- Antonucci R, Bassareo P, Zaffanello M, et al. Patent ductus arteriosus in the preterm infant: New insights into pathogenesis and clinical management. *J Matern Fetal Neonatal Med*. 2010;23(Suppl 3): 34–37.
- Clyman RI, Chorne N. Patent ductus arteriosus: Evidence for and against treatment. *J Pediatr*. 2007;150(3):216–219.
- Evans N. Current controversies in the diagnosis and treatment of patent ductus arteriosus in preterm infants. *Adv Neonatal Care*. 2003;3:168–177.
- Hamrick SE, Hansmann G. Patent ductus arteriosus of the preterm infant. *Pediatrics*. 2010;125(5): 1020–1030.
- Knight DB. The treatment of patent ductus arteriosus in preterm infants. A review and overview of randomized trials. *Semin Neonatol*. 2001;6:63–73.
- Ohlsson A, Walia R, Shah SS. Ibuprofen for the treatment of patent ductus arteriosus in preterm and/or low birth weight infants. *Cochrane Database Syst Rev*. 2010(4):CD003481
- Schneider DJ, Moore JW. Patent ductus arteriosus. *Circulation*. 2006;114:1873–1882.
- Takami T, Yoda H, Kawakami T, et al. Usefulness of indomethacin for patent ductus arteriosus in full-term infants. *Pediatr Cardiol*. 2007;28(1): 46–50.
- Wyllie J. Treatment of patent ductus arteriosus. *Semin Neonatol*. 2003;8:425–432.

 CODES

ICD9
747.0 Patent ductus arteriosus

ICD10
Q25.0 Patent ductus arteriosus

PELVIC INFLAMMATORY DISEASE (PID)

Jonathan R. Pletcher

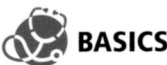 BASICS

DESCRIPTION

- PID is an ascending, polymicrobial infection of the female upper genital tract. It includes an array of inflammatory disorders, including endometritis, parametritis, salpingitis, oophoritis, tubo-ovarian abscess (TOA), peritonitis, and perihepatitis.
- Pelvic inflammatory disease (PID) is a clinical diagnosis.
- The CDC has established the minimal clinical criteria; if present and no other cause can be identified, empiric therapy for PID should be initiated in sexually active young women who have either:
  - Uterine tenderness, OR
  - Adnexal tenderness, OR
  - Cervical motion tenderness
- Additional criteria can be used to enhance the specificity of the diagnosis of PID in women with more severe clinical signs:
  - Oral temperature >38°C (101°F)
  - Abnormal cervical or vaginal mucopurulent discharge
  - Presence of WBCs on a wet mount of vaginal secretions
  - Elevated ESR or CRP
  - Laboratory-documented evidence of infection with *Neisseria gonorrhoeae* or *Chlamydia trachomatis*
- Definitive criteria:
  - Histopathologic evidence of endometritis on endometrial biopsy
  - Transvaginal sonography or MRI showing thickened fluid-filled tubes with or without free pelvic fluid or TOA
  - Laparoscopic abnormalities consistent with PID

EPIDEMIOLOGY

- Clinical diagnosis of PID is imprecise.
- Positive predictive value of clinical diagnosis ranges from 65–90% compared to laparoscopy.
- No single history item, physical exam finding, or laboratory test is either completely sensitive or specific for the diagnosis.

RISK FACTORS

- Adolescent women possess biologic factors that increase risk of PID:
  - Increased cervical ectopy
  - Decreased cervical immunity
- Risk also increases with:
  - Failure to use condoms
  - Prolonged menses or dysfunctional uterine bleeding (DUB)
  - Increasing number of lifetime partners
  - Having new partners in the last 3 months
  - History of STIs
- Lack of access to confidential health care

GENERAL PREVENTION

- Primary prevention involves early education and aggressive screening for STIs with onset of sexual activity or in high-risk populations.
- Abstinence should be advocated.
- For those individuals unable to commit to abstinence, consistent condom use should be advocated and facilitated.
- At a minimum, annual screening for STIs and treatment of sexual partners should be encouraged and facilitated. More frequent screening is indicated with new partners.

PATHOPHYSIOLOGY

- PID begins as an infection or inflammation of the cervix.
- Direct spread of bacteria to ascending structures, via migration, sperm transport, or refluxed menstrual blood
- Direct migration may be facilitated by menstrual flow, as there is loss of protective cervical mucus.
- Microbes invade epithelial cells, mucosa, and serosa, causing inflammation with subsequent scarring.

ETIOLOGY

- Although a polymicrobial infection, cervical infection, or vaginal bacterial overgrowth with the following organisms can lead to acute PID:
  - *N. gonorrhoeae* cervicitis
  - *C. trachomatis* cervicitis: Tends to be associated with less fever, pain, and systemic symptoms than PID due to gonococcus.
  - Organisms associated with bacterial vaginosis: Gram-negative rods, bacteroides, *Mobiluncus*, and *Peptostreptococcus* species.
  - CMV, *M. hominis*, *U. urealyticum*, and *M. genitalium* have all been associated with PID.

DIAGNOSIS

HISTORY

- Assessment begins with sensitive, confidential interview.
- Review of systems:
  - Presentation may be silent, with relatively few or mild symptoms.
- Complete medical, gynecologic, menstrual, sexual, GI, and urinary histories:
  - Associated symptoms may include dysmenorrhea, dyspareunia, vomiting, diarrhea, or constipation.
  - Supportive historic data include recent menstruation, use of IUD or douche, inconsistent condom use, and multiple or new sexual partners.
- Signs and symptoms: Classic presentation of PID includes:
  - Lower abdominal pain
  - Dyspareunia
  - Abnormal vaginal discharge
  - Dysuria
  - Irregular vaginal bleeding
  - Fever
  - Right upper quadrant abdominal pain

PHYSICAL EXAM

- Perform a thorough abdominal exam, noting tenderness, rebound or guarding, and signs of perihepatic involvement.
- Pelvic exam: Document the following:
  - Presence of external or vaginal lesions
  - Origin, quality, and quantity of discharge (e.g., "copious, mucopurulent cervical discharge," or "scant, thin vaginal discharge")
  - Signs of cervical inflammation (e.g., erythema, friability)
  - Cervical motion tenderness
  - Adnexal tenderness and/or fullness
  - Blot away discharge to better assess the source of new fluid accumulation

DIAGNOSTIC TESTS & INTERPRETATION

- Caution: Most bacteriologic studies are technique-dependent and require trained clinicians.
- All home pregnancy tests should be repeated.

Lab

- Urine β-human chorionic gonadotropin (β-hCG):
  - It is essential to know if the patient is pregnant, regardless of sexual history.
- CBC with differential
- ESR or CRP
- Wet prep of discharge for trichomonads, hyphae, clue cells, presence of WBCs (>10 WBC/high-power field is suggestive of infection)
- Gram stain of cervical discharge:
  - Testing for *N. gonorrhoeae* and *C. trachomatis*
  - Culture is technique-dependent, yielding 80% sensitivity with ideal collection technique.
- Antigen detection tests (e.g., direct fluorescent antibody [DFA], enzyme-linked immunosorbent assay [ELISA]) have lower sensitivities.
- Nucleic acid amplification tests (NAAT) require a single specimen for both organisms, offer a 24-hour turnaround time, and have >90% sensitivity.
- Syphilis serology in high-risk populations (e.g., rapid plasma reagin [RPR] testing) and HIV testing for all adolescents are recommended with appropriate counseling and follow-up.

Imaging
Pelvic US:

- Rule out TOA or other pelvic pathology.
- Pelvic US requires a full urinary bladder, unlike transvaginal US.

Diagnostic Procedures/Other
Laparoscopy: Not routinely used, but considered the gold standard for diagnosis

DIFFERENTIAL DIAGNOSIS

- Infection:
  - Cervicitis
  - Vulvovaginal candidiasis
  - Trichomoniasis
  - Bacterial vaginosis
  - Tubo-ovarian abscess (TOA)
  - Pyelonephritis or cystitis
  - Appendicitis

- Appendiceal abscess
- Tuberculosis
- Viral or bacterial enteritis
- Acute cholecystitis
- Mesenteric lymphadenitis
- Pelvic thrombophlebitis
- Gynecologic:
  - Dysmenorrhea
  - Pregnancy: Intrauterine or ectopic
  - Ovarian cyst or torsion
  - Chronic pelvic pain
  - Endometriosis
  - Teratoma or other mass
- Miscellaneous:
  - Foreign body or pelvic trauma
  - Functional pain

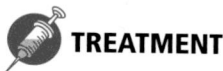 **TREATMENT**

MEDICATION (DRUGS)

- Inpatient management:
  - CDC regimen A:
    - Cefotetan 2 g IV q12h *OR* cefoxitin 2 g IV q6h
    - Plus, doxycycline 100 mg PO b.i.d. for 14 days
    - Regimen A should be continued for at least 24 hours after clinical improvement, and is followed by the completion of a 14-day course of doxycycline 100 mg PO b.i.d.
  - CDC regimen B:
    - Clindamycin 900 mg IV q8h
    - Plus, gentamicin loading dose 2 mg/kg IV or IM, followed by maintenance dose 1.5 mg/kg q8h
    - Regimen B should be continued for at least 24 hours after clinical improvement, and is followed by completion of a 14-day course of either doxycycline or clindamycin 450 mg PO b.i.d.
  - Alternative parenteral regimens include the following:
    - Ampicillin–sulbactam 3 g IV q6h
    - Plus, doxycycline 100 mg PO q12h
  - Regimen A versus regimen B: Choice based on availability and the drug allergy history of the patient. Data to support the use of alternative regimens are limited.
- Outpatient management:
  - Ceftriaxone 250 mg IM once *OR* cefoxitin 2 g IM with probenecid 1 g PO once or other parenteral 3rd-generation cephalosporins
  - Plus doxycycline 100 mg PO b.i.d. for 14 days
  - With or without metronidazole 500 mg PO b.i.d. for 14 days
- Because of the emergence of quinolone resistant *N. gonorrhoeae*, ofloxacin and levofloxacin are no longer recommended and should only be considered when the parenteral cephalosporins are not available.

ADDITIONAL TREATMENT
General Measures

- The goal of treatment is to eliminate infection and to reduce or prevent the likelihood of long-term adverse outcomes.
- A patient may be treated as an outpatient or inpatient based on a clinician's judgment as to the severity of the disease and the patient's ability to follow through with medical care.
- Hospitalization is recommended in the following cases:
  - Surgical emergency (e.g., appendicitis) cannot be ruled out.
  - Patient is pregnant.
  - Suspected TOA
  - Patient has failed or cannot comply with outpatient treatment (e.g., recurrent vomiting).
  - Patient is clinically ill or is at high risk for sequelae.
- When choosing outpatient treatment:
  - Repeat bimanual exam within 72 hours of initiating therapy.
  - Patient must be willing to take the medications and follow-up.
  - Patient should be given a full course of doxycycline (or other oral medications) and tolerate the 1st dose under supervision.
  - All patients with PID should receive intensive education about STI prevention and partner treatment.

 ONGOING CARE

FOLLOW-UP RECOMMENDATIONS

- For inpatients, substantial clinical improvement should occur within 3 days if the patient has been properly diagnosed and treated.
- Outpatients should have significant improvement after 72 hours of treatment.
- Test-of-cure exam and laboratory testing should be considered for all patients 6–8 weeks after diagnosis.

PROGNOSIS

- Excellent, if adequate treatment is obtained early and acute complications are absent
- One episode of PID increases the risk of future ectopic pregnancy 10-fold.
- Long-term sequelae are present in 25% of affected women, with a higher likelihood in adolescents owing to later presentation, delay in diagnosis, and inadequate treatment.

COMPLICATIONS

- Chronic pelvic pain or dyspareunia ($\leq$18%)
- Ectopic pregnancy
- Infertility:
  - 1 episode is associated with a 13–21% risk of infertility, 2 episodes with a 35% risk, and $\geq$3 episodes with a 55–75% risk.
- TOA
- Fitz-Hugh–Curtis syndrome (perihepatitis resulting from tracking of pus along the paracolic gutters)

ADDITIONAL READING

- Banikarim C, Chacko MR. Pelvic inflammatory disease in adolescents. *Adolesc Med*. 2004;15: 273–285.
- Centers for Disease Control and Prevention. Sexually transmitted diseases and treatment guidelines, 2010. *MMWR Morb Mortal Wkly Rep*. 2010; 59(RR-12):63–67. Available at http://www.cdc.gov/std/treatment/default.htm
- Erb T, Beigi RH. Update on infectious diseases in adolescent gynecology. *J Pediatr Adolesc Gynecol*. 2008;21(3):135–143.
- Hollier LM, Workowski K. Treatment of sexually transmitted diseases in women. *Obst Gynecol Clin North Am*. 2003;30:751–775.

 CODES

ICD9

- 614.4 Chronic or unspecified parametritis and pelvic cellulitis
- 614.9 Unspecified inflammatory disease of female pelvic organs and tissues
- 617.9 Endometriosis, site unspecified

ICD10

- N73.2 Unspecified parametritis and pelvic cellulitis
- N73.9 Female pelvic inflammatory disease, unspecified
- N80.9 Endometriosis, unspecified

FAQ

- Q: A patient states that she is not sexually active. Should I continue to consider PID?
- A: Yes. Because of the risk and severity of sequelae, PID should always be considered. Furthermore PID can occur in non–sexually active women. In fact, infections with *C. trachomatis* or *N. gonorrhoeae* are identified in <50% of PID cases.
- Q: A patient does not meet the criteria for PID; however, it is still the most likely diagnosis. Should I start therapy while other studies are pending?
- A: Yes. Appropriate therapy for PID may be initiated while further evaluation is in progress. Delay in therapy results in increased risk of adverse sequelae from PID.
- Q: An adolescent patient with PID has inquired about fertility. What should I tell her?
- A: Many clinicians would argue that an episode of PID could serve as a wake-up call to teenagers, inspiring them to abstain or comply with barrier contraception. However, a young woman who is told that she may have impaired fertility might try testing it through unprotected sex.
- Q: Does the absence of cervical motion tenderness exclude the diagnosis of PID?
- A: No. Cervical motion tenderness is only 1 of the 3 clinical signs that may be present in PID.

PENILE AND FORESKIN PROBLEMS

Caroline Mitchell
J. Christopher Austin (5th edition)

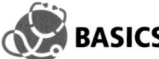 **BASICS**

DESCRIPTION
- Complaints relating to problems with retracting the foreskin, discharge from the foreskin, and circumcision. The most common diagnoses are listed below.
- Phimosis:
  - Physiologic attachment of the prepuce to the glans, which it protects and gradually separates from to allow retraction of the foreskin.
  - Ring of fibrotic scar tissue that prevents the foreskin from being retracted.
- Penile adhesions:
  - Attachments of the foreskin back to the glans after circumcision
- Meatal stenosis:
  - Narrowing of the urethral meatus
  - Significant narrowing will produce an upwardly deflected stream, which is tiny and strong. In severe cases, straining and prolonged voiding
- Epidermal inclusion cysts:
  - Small, enlarging white lesions growing subcutaneously along the scar from circumcision
- Balanitis:
  - Infection of the glans
  - May involve the prepuce (balanoposthitis)
  - Probably overdiagnosed owing to physiologic drainage of smegma or urea dermatitis from failure to retract foreskin during voiding in potty-trained boys
  - When infections do present, there can be significant cellulitis of the penis, edema, and fever.
  - Most common causative organisms are gram positive. Yeast is another causative organism.

RISK FACTORS
Genetics
Epidermal inclusion cysts may occur from congenital rests of skin cells buried during development, but these are rare and occur along the median raphe of the penis.

GENERAL PREVENTION
Some may be prevented with proper hygiene and education of the caretakers.

ETIOLOGY
- Phimosis:
  - Probably results from recurrent bouts of irritation of the foreskin from improper hygiene habits such as voiding through the foreskin.
- Penile adhesions:
  - Physiologic adhesions: The prepuce has adhered down to the glans after circumcision.
  - Surgical adhesions (skin bridges): Adherence between the scar of the circumcision and the glans due to healing of the crushed tissue where the foreskin was removed and the raw surface of the glans.
- Meatal stenosis:
  - Narrowing of the urethral meatus secondary to recurrent irritation of the meatus, likely from rubbing against moist diapers. Occurs almost exclusively in circumcised boys
- Epidermal inclusion cysts:
  - Caused by small islands of epithelium buried beneath the skin surface that progressively accumulate desquamated skin cells.

 DIAGNOSIS

HISTORY
- Problems associated with newborn circumcision
- Inquire as to when the changes occurred.
- Character of urinary stream
- Presence of fever
- Penile discharge in cases of balanitis
- Retraction of foreskin in uncircumcised males during voiding
- Ballooning of the foreskin with voiding
- In older boys, inquire about sexual activity.

PHYSICAL EXAM
- Circumcised males:
  - Size and position of meatus
  - Redundancy of inner preputial skin
  - Presence of adhesions to the glans and whether or not they involve the scar line between the shaft skin and the inner preputial skin
  - Lesions or erythema of glans or shaft
  - Watch patient void if meatal stenosis is suspected.
- Uncircumcised males:
  - Ability to retract foreskin with gentle retraction
  - Presence of phimotic ring
  - Lesions or erythema of prepuce

ALERT
Do not try to forcefully retract the foreskin. It can take 3–5 years before the foreskin can be retracted.

DIAGNOSTIC TESTS & INTERPRETATION
Lab
- In cases of balanitis with drainage, cultures may be taken.
- If urethral discharge is present, culture for gonorrhea and chlamydia in an adolescent male.

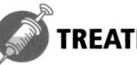 **TREATMENT**

MEDICATION (DRUGS)
Balanitis: If the child is afebrile, oral antibiotics such as a 1st-generation cephalosporin would be the 1st line of treatment. If the child develops fever or there is progression of cellulitis, then treatment with IV antibiotics (cefazolin or ampicillin–sulbactam).

ADDITIONAL TREATMENT
General Measures
- Phimosis:
  - Physiologic: No need for intervention
  - Good hygiene practices should be encouraged, such as pulling the foreskin back to expose the meatus when voiding and not voiding through the foreskin.

- Pamphlets or Web sites that explain the care of the penis for uncircumcised males are helpful to give to the parents.
- If there is a fibrotic ring of scar tissue preventing the retraction of the foreskin, a trial of betamethasone cream 0.05% applied to the foreskin b.i.d. for 4 weeks with daily gentle retraction may soften the scar tissue enough to resolve the phimosis. In cases where conservative measures fail, a circumcision is indicated.
- Penile adhesions:
  - Physiologic: Practices in the past have included separation using anesthetic (EMLA) cream. If there is redundancy of the foreskin or a prominent suprapubic fat pad that can tend to hide the penis in infants, adhesions often recur or require constant application of barrier creams or ointments to the penis and manual retraction of the redundant foreskin by the parents to prevent recurrence:
    ○ In many cases, no treatment is necessary, as the adhesions will break down over a period of years.
    ○ If there are extensive adhesions with significant redundancy of foreskin, consideration should be given to revision of the circumcision if the adhesions are to be treated.
  - Surgical (skin bridges):
    ○ These are due to scar tissue formation between the raw cut edge where the foreskin was removed and the raw surface of the glans.
    ○ As this represents true scarring and not 2 epithelial surfaces stuck together, the surfaces cannot be simply pulled apart like physiologic adhesions. They will not resolve with time, and if left in place, with growth, penile skin will be transferred to the glans, resulting in discoloration, especially in patients with darker skin tones.
    ○ These adhesions need sharp division either in the office with EMLA cream anesthesia or under general anesthesia if they are extensive.
- Meatal stenosis:
  - When the narrowing at the meatus is producing an upwardly deflected, narrow stream (which can make aiming into the toilet difficult) or is causing straining and prolonged voiding, treatment is indicated.
  - A meatotomy can be done in the office using EMLA anesthesia or as an outpatient surgical procedure.

- Epidermal inclusion cysts:
  - These subcutaneous islands of skin cells will progressively enlarge over time.
  - Complete excision is generally curative.
- Balanitis:
  - When the inflammation and irritation seem to be from chronic dampness and exposure to urine, treat with barrier creams or ointments.
  - Keeping the area clean and dry will help prevent future episodes.
  - If there are small whitish plaques (not smegma), associated with redness, yeast may be present and an antifungal cream such as 1% clotrimazole can be used to help speed the healing.
  - Antibiotics as necessary (see "Medication")
  - In cases where there is purulent drainage and cellulitis of the penis, which can often be rapidly spreading over 24 hours, treatment with antibiotics is recommended.
  - Genital infections of this nature should be taken quite seriously, and if treatment as an outpatient is attempted, close follow-up (return visit in 24–48 hours) is prudent.

 ## ONGOING CARE

PATIENT EDUCATION
- It is important that all parents of uncircumcised boys teach them proper hygiene habits during potty training.
- Do not forcibly retract the foreskin. Gently clean with warm water during baths and dry after. Retract the skin when voiding in potty-trained boys.

ADDITIONAL READING
- Blalock HJ, Vemulakonda V, Ritchey ML, et al. Outpatient management of phimosis following newborn circumcision. *J Urol*. 2003;169(6): 2332–2334.
- Orsola A, Caffaratti J, Garat JM. Conservative treatment of phimosis in children using a topical steroid. *Urology*. 2000;56:307–310.
- Van Howe RS. Incidence of meatal stenosis following neonatal circumcision in a primary care setting. *Clin Pediatr*. 2006;45(1):49–54.

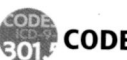 ## CODES

ICD9
- 605 Redundant prepuce and phimosis
- 607.1 Balanoposthitis
- 753.6 Atresia and stenosis of urethra and bladder neck

ICD10
- N47.1 Phimosis
- N47.5 Adhesions of prepuce and glans penis
- Q64.33 Congenital stricture of urinary meatus

FAQ

- Q: The foreskin is stuck down to my son's penis. Does that mean he needs another circumcision?
- A: Not necessarily. If there is minor redundancy and a small physiologic adhesion, then no treatment is needed.
- Q: My uncircumcised son had some thick white drainage from his foreskin. Is that from an infection?
- A: Probably not. The thick white material is probably shed skin cells, which have been slowly separating the foreskin from the glans.

P

PERICARDITIS
Meryl S. Cohen

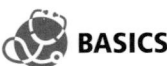 **BASICS**

DESCRIPTION
Inflammation of the pericardium, usually resulting in the accumulation of fluid in the pericardial space between the visceral (serosa tissue intimately related to the myocardium) and parietal (fibrosal layer composed of elastic fibers and collagen) pericardium. Pericarditis may be serous, fibrinous, purulent, hemorrhagic, or chylous.

EPIDEMIOLOGY
- Infectious pericarditis is more frequently seen in children <13 years, with predominance in children <2 years.
- Postpericardiotomy syndrome occurs in ~5–10% of children following uncomplicated cardiac surgery, particularly when the atrium has been entered.

PATHOPHYSIOLOGY
- Fine deposits of fibrin develop next to the great vessels, leading to altered function of the membranes of the pericardium, including changes in oncotic and hydrostatic pressure with subsequent accumulation of fluid in the pericardial space.
- Effusion is defined as excessive pericardial contents secondary to inflammation, hemorrhage, exudates, air, or pus.
- In postpericardiotomy syndrome, there appears to be a nonspecific hypersensitivity reaction to the direct surgical entrance into the pericardial space.

ETIOLOGY
- Infectious:
  – Viral: Coxsackievirus, echovirus, mumps, varicella, Epstein–Barr, adenovirus, influenza, human immunodeficiency virus
  – Bacterial: Streptococcus, pneumococcus, staphylococcus, meningococcus, mycoplasma, tularemia, *Haemophilus influenzae* type B, *Pseudomonas aeruginosa, Listeria monocytogenes, Pasteurella multocida, Escherichia coli*
  – Tuberculosis, atypical mycobacterium
  – Fungal: Candidiasis, histoplasmosis, actinomycosis
  – Parasitic: Toxoplasmosis, echinococcus, *Entamoeba histolytica*, rickettsia
- Rheumatologic/Inflammatory:
  – Acute rheumatic fever
  – Rheumatoid arthritis
  – Systemic lupus erythematosus
  – Systemic sclerosis
  – Sarcoidosis
  – Dermatomyositis
  – Kawasaki disease
  – Familial Mediterranean fever
  – Inflammatory bowel disease
- Metabolic/Endocrine:
  – Hypothyroidism
  – Uremia (chemical irritation)
  – Gout
  – Scurvy
- Neoplastic disease:
  – Lymphoma
  – Lymphosarcoma
  – Leukemia
  – Sarcoma
  – Metastatic disease to the pericardium
  – Radiation therapy induced
- Postoperative:
  – Postpericardiotomy syndrome (after cardiac surgery)
  – Chyolopericardium
- Other:
  – Trauma
  – Drug-induced (hydralazine, isoniazid, procainamide)
  – Aortic dissection
  – Postmyocardial infarction
  – Idiopathic

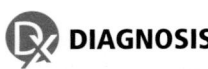 **DIAGNOSIS**

SIGNS AND SYMPTOMS
- Most common:
  – Precordial chest pain
  – Fever
  – Cough
  – Shoulder pain aggravated by changes in position
- Rapid accumulation of fluid:
  – Respiratory distress/dyspnea
  – Signs of hypotension
  – Change in mental status/loss of consciousness
- Pain: Often relieved if the child sits leaning forward
- Slow, chronic accumulation may be associated with no symptoms at all until tamponade develops.
- Other symptoms are dependent on the etiology of the pericarditis.

HISTORY
- Dependent on etiology
- Recent upper respiratory infection or gastroenteritis (viral pericarditis)
- Sepsis or other source of bacterial infection
- Symptoms of rheumatic disease
- Known thoracic neoplasm

PHYSICAL EXAM
- Pericardial friction rub is the pathognomonic finding (typically heard if only a small amount of fluid is in the pericardial space).
- Quiet precordium, tachycardia, hypotension and muffled heart sounds may be heard when there is a large amount of fluid and/or tamponade.
- Evidence of right-sided heart failure:
  – Peripheral edema, jugular venous distention, and hepatomegaly

- Pulmonary edema: Rare because the heart is underfilled, and left atrial pressure, although elevated, does not exceed right atrial pressure
- Pulsus paradoxus: An exaggerated decrease in systolic BP with inspiration
- Kussmaul sign: Paradoxical rise in jugular venous pressure during inspiration, often considered diagnostic of tamponade

DIAGNOSTIC TESTS & INTERPRETATION
EKG:
- Nonspecific, but generally demonstrates low-voltage QRS complexes secondary to dampening of the signal transmitted through the pericardial fluid
- One can also see diffuse ST segment elevation with or without T-wave inversion.
- These findings may be secondary to inflammation of the myocardium.
- Electrical alternans can be seen with large effusions.

Imaging
- Chest x-ray:
  – Often shows enlargement of the cardiac silhouette ("water bottle sign"), usually in association with normal pulmonary vascular markings. However, heart size may appear normal in acute pericarditis.
  – Calcification may be seen in constrictive pericarditis.
- CT
  – CT can also demonstrate calcification of the pericardium with excellent sensitivity
- Echocardiogram:
  – Most sensitive and specific test for pericardial thickening and fluid in the pericardial space
  – In the presence of a large effusion, the heart may appear to swing within the pericardial cavity.
  – In tamponade, diastolic collapse of the right atrium may be seen. Collapse of the left atrium and right ventricle occur in severe cases.
  – Tamponade can be diagnosed using Doppler inflow patterns of the tricuspid and mitral valves. In tamponade, mitral inflow E-wave velocity decreases by >30% during inspiration while the tricuspid inflow E-wave velocity increases by >50% during inspiration.

Diagnostic Procedures/Surgery
- Pericardiocentesis is performed when the etiology of the effusion is in question or tamponade has developed.
  – Fluid obtained should be sent to the lab for cell count, cytology, and culture (including bacteria, viruses, *Mycobacterium tuberculosis*, and fungi).
  – Complications include myocardial puncture, coronary artery/vein laceration, hemopericardium, and pneumothorax.
  – Echocardiogram or fluoroscopic guidance is useful for this procedure, but is not required if there is impending cardiovascular collapse.
- Pericardial window:
  – In cases of chronic pericardial effusion, removal of part or all of the pericardium may be performed (pericardial window).

DIFFERENTIAL DIAGNOSIS

- History, physical examination, and laboratory findings of acute pericarditis can be quite similar to those found in acute myocarditis. In addition, myocarditis can be associated with pericardial disease and vice versa. Echocardiogram is an excellent tool to help differentiate between these two entities.
- Acute myocarditis
- Restrictive cardiomyopathy
- Other causes of chest pain
- Myocardial infarction

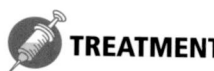 TREATMENT

ADDITIONAL TREATMENT
General Measures

- Treatment should be directed toward the etiology of the disease. However, no matter the cause, pericardiocentesis is required if there is an effusion that causes hemodynamic compromise. It may be life-saving in patients with bacterial pericarditis.
- Viral pericarditis usually resolves spontaneously in 3–4 weeks with bed rest and analgesics (NSAIDs).
- Bacterial pericarditis is potentially life threatening and requires immediate decompression of the pericardial space (often with open drainage and pericardial window creation), IV antibiotic therapy for at least 4 weeks, and supportive therapy (i.e., volume expansion, inotropes).
  - *Staphylococcus aureus* is the most common organism responsible for bacterial pericarditis.
- Rheumatologic causes of pericardial inflammation usually respond to corticosteroids and/or salicylates and rarely require pericardiocentesis.
- Uremic pericarditis usually responds to dialysis, but pericardiotomy (surgical removal of the pericardium) may be necessary in chronic situations.
- Neoplastic pericarditis is addressed by treating the primary disease and performing pericardiocentesis if indicated for diagnostic and/or hemodynamic reasons.
- Hemorrhagic pericarditis with effusion accumulation secondary to trauma should be drained because of the risk of subsequent development of constrictive pericarditis.
- Constrictive pericarditis is treated with complete stripping of the pericardium (pericardiectomy). Often, immediate clinical improvement is not seen because there has been myocardial damage. However, eventual full recovery is the norm.
- Postpericardiotomy syndrome occurs 1–4 weeks after cardiac surgery. Treat with anti-inflammatory drugs, bed rest, and occasionally steroids.
  - Pericardiocentesis is indicated if tamponade develops.

 ONGOING CARE

- Most forms of pericarditis resolve on their own, or with anti-inflammatory medication, over the course of several weeks.
  - Follow-up is necessary to ensure that effusions have resolved and to assess for recurrence (up to 15% relapse).
  - Patients with bacterial pericarditis require long-term antibiotic therapy and close follow-up to assess for the development of constrictive pericarditis.
- Signs to watch for include the following:
  - Postpericardiotomy syndrome: All cardiac surgical patients need an evaluation 2–4 weeks after surgery to assess for postpericardiotomy syndrome, with treatment and follow-up as necessary.
  - Signs of low cardiac output and right-sided heart failure indicate impending cardiac tamponade.
  - Constrictive pericarditis may present with a rapidly decreasing cardiac silhouette, calcifications on chest roentgenogram, and signs or symptoms of right-sided heart failure.

PROGNOSIS

- Most children recover fully from pericarditis, even if it is bacterial in etiology.
  - However, there is significant morbidity and mortality associated, especially in young infants, when the diagnosis is delayed and/or when *S. aureus* is the etiologic agent.
- Pericarditis can also recur in as many as 15% of patients.
- Prognosis varies with the cause of pericarditis, but generally is related directly to the primary disease.

COMPLICATIONS

- Cardiac tamponade:
  - Intrapericardial pressure increases at a rapid rate secondary to decreased compliance of the pericardial membranes, resulting in restriction of ventricular filling and eventual decrease in stroke volume and cardiac output.
  - The compliance of the pericardium is influenced by the disease process itself (i.e., the pericardium is thickened and stiff in bacterial and tuberculous pericarditis).
  - During cardiac tamponade, ventricular end-diastolic, atrial, and venous pressures are all equal.
  - In acute pericarditis, tamponade may occur with small amounts of fluid because of a rapid increase in the intrapericardial pressure. In contrast, large amounts of fluid may be tolerated if the accumulation is a chronic, slow process.
- Constrictive pericarditis:
  - Thick, fibrotic, and often calcified pericardium is seen, usually a late result of purulent or tuberculous pericarditis; it can occur months to years after the initial infection. It can also be seen in oncology patients with direct invasion of tumor into the pericardium or after significant radiation to the chest.

  - Poor compliance of the pericardium leads to diminished diastolic filling of the ventricle. Patients may complain of exercise intolerance and fatigue. Additionally, they may have signs of right heart failure.
  - This entity may be difficult to distinguish from restrictive cardiomyopathy.

ADDITIONAL READING

- Demmler GJ. Infectious pericarditis in children. *Pediatr Infect Dis J.* 2006;25(2):165–166.
- Towbin JA. Myocarditis and pericarditis in adolescents. *Adolesc Med.* 2001;12(1):47–67.

 CODES

ICD9
- 420.90 Acute pericarditis, unspecified
- 420.91 Acute idiopathic pericarditis
- 423.9 Unspecified disease of pericardium

ICD10
- I30.1 Infective pericarditis
- I30.9 Acute pericarditis, unspecified
- I31.9 Disease of pericardium, unspecified

FAQ

- Q: How does cardiac tamponade present?
- A: Patients with impending tamponade appear quite ill, with tachycardia, chest pain, and signs of right heart failure including jugular venous distention, hepatomegaly, ascites, and peripheral edema. They may also have signs of poor systemic perfusion secondary to low cardiac output. Chest x-ray may or may not show an enlarged cardiac silhouette, depending on how acutely the process occurs. It takes much less fluid to cause tamponade in an acute process than in a chronic process. Echocardiography is the standard diagnostic tool, and pericardiocentesis is the treatment.
- Q: What is pulsus paradoxus and how does one measure it?
- A: Pulsus paradoxus is an exaggerated response of the systolic BP to the normal respiratory cycle. Normally with inspiration, the systolic BP drops ~5 mm Hg secondary to the increased capacitance of the pulmonary veins from the increased systemic venous return. In tamponade, this response becomes more profound (>10 mm Hg), most likely secondary to diminished filling of the left heart. Pulsus paradoxus can also be seen in patients with severe respiratory distress associated with asthma and emphysema.
- To assess for pulsus paradoxus, measure the systolic BP first in expiration; then allow it to fall to the place where it is heard equally well in inspiration and expiration. A difference of >10 mm Hg is considered abnormal.

PERIODIC BREATHING

Richard M. Kravitz

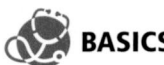 **BASICS**

DESCRIPTION
- A respiratory pattern consisting of regular oscillations in breathing amplitude.
- Typically, a respiratory pattern in which ≥3 apneas lasting ≥3 seconds occur, separated by <20 seconds of respiration.

ALERT
Don't confuse periodic breathing with obstructive and/or central apnea.

EPIDEMIOLOGY
- Usually absent in the 1st 48 hours of life
- More frequent during rapid eye movement (REM or active) sleep vs. non-REM (quiet) sleep
- Less common in prone vs. supine position
- In full-term infants:
  - Amount of periodic breathing usually <4% of sleep time
  - Amount gradually decreases through the 1st year of life
  - By 1 year of age, the mean amount of periodic breathing is <1% of total sleep time.
- In premature infants:
  - Amount of periodic breathing is higher than in full-term infants.
  - Amount correlates inversely with gestational age.

PATHOPHYSIOLOGY
- No common pathologic finding
- Abnormalities, when they exist, are related to the underlying disorder causing the periodic breathing.

ETIOLOGY
- Periodic breathing can be seen in healthy infants, children, and adults.
- Abnormalities in any component of the breathing control system may result in an increased amount of periodic breathing.
- Possible etiologies:
  - A delay in detecting changes in blood gas values by the chemoreceptors
  - Increased chemoreceptor gain

COMMONLY ASSOCIATED CONDITIONS
- Periodic breathing in infants is associated with the following:
  - Apnea of prematurity or infancy
  - Familial history of sudden infant death syndrome (SIDS)
  - Anemia of prematurity
  - Hypoxemia
  - Hypochloremic alkalosis
- Periodic breathing with adults is associated with:
  - Cardiac abnormalities (especially congestive heart failure [CHF])
  - Neurologic dysfunction (meningitis, encephalitis, brainstem dysfunction)
  - Exposure to high altitudes

DIAGNOSIS

HISTORY
- In most cases, parents notice periodicity in the child's respiratory pattern.
- An apparent life-threatening episode (ALTE) might precipitate an evaluation in which periodic breathing is documented.
- In otherwise healthy premature or term infants, there are no other symptoms.

PHYSICAL EXAM
In otherwise healthy premature or term infants, the physical exam is normal.

DIAGNOSTIC TESTS & INTERPRETATION
Imaging
Chest x-ray: Usually normal findings

Diagnostic Procedures/Other
- Polysomnography:
  - Assesses the extent of periodic breathing episodes
  - Determines if there is accompanying hypoxemia, hypercarbia, or bradycardia with the events
  - Distinguishes between periodic breathing and obstructive and/or central apnea
  - Useful for following response to treatment (i.e., normalization of polysomnography)
- pH probe done in combination with the polysomnogram (if gastroesophageal reflux is suspected): Record for a minimum of 6 hours
- 2-channel pneumogram:
  - Gives less information than polysomnography
  - Can document periodic breathing, but it may miss episodes of obstructive apnea
  - Monitors heart rate and respiratory effort (if oxygen saturation monitoring is desired, an additional channel is required)

DIFFERENTIAL DIAGNOSIS
- Other forms of apnea:
  - Central apnea
  - Mixed apnea
  - Obstructive apnea (or hypopnea)
- Other forms of periodic breathing:
  - Cheyne-Stokes respirations
  - Biot breathing
  - Kussmaul respirations
- Normal irregular respiration seen in infants

TREATMENT

MEDICATION (DRUGS)
- Stimulants
  - Caffeine:
    - Loading dose: 10 mg/kg
    - Maintenance dose: 2.5 mg/kg/d
    - Therapeutic level: 5–20 mg/L
  - Theophylline:
    - Loading dose: 4–5 mg/kg
    - Maintenance dose: 3–5 mg/kg/d divided t.i.d.
    - Therapeutic level: 6–10 mg/L

ADDITIONAL TREATMENT
General Measures
- Therapy should be directed at treating the underlying primary disease:
  - If periodic breathing is associated with apnea, hypoxemia, and/or other sleep disturbances, appropriate treatment should be instituted.
  - In cases secondary to CHF, appropriate cardiac interventions need to be instituted.
  - In cases associated with high altitude, treatment options include:
    - Acclimation (if tolerated)
    - Descent to lower altitude, then gradual ascent
    - Medication (acetazolamide most commonly used)
- Duration of therapy:
  - Depends on the underlying cause of the periodic breathing
  - Treatment does not change the natural course of periodic breathing in otherwise healthy infants.
  - Therapy should continue until the periodic breathing resolves or is no longer clinically significant.

Additional Therapies
- Supplemental oxygen: Useful if periodic breathing is secondary to hypoxemia
- Nasal continuous positive airway pressure (CPAP): Very effective in eliminating periodic breathing
- Home monitoring should be considered (although not absolutely indicated) in the following cases:
  - Significant amount of periodic breathing
  - Accompanying apnea
  - Associated hypoxia and/or bradycardia
  - History of a significant ALTE
  - Parental anxiety

 ONGOING CARE

FOLLOW-UP RECOMMENDATIONS
- Time to improvement depends on the underlying cause of the periodic breathing.
- Improvement is anticipated as the infant ages.
- When treatment is started, a decrease in the amount of periodic breathing should be seen almost immediately.

PROGNOSIS
- Excellent in otherwise healthy premature or term infants
- Governed by primary process in patients with an underlying cardiac or neurologic disorder

COMPLICATIONS
Relationship between periodic breathing and SIDS is controversial.

ADDITIONAL READING

- Carroll JL, Agarwal A. Development of ventilator control in infants. *Paediatr Respir Rev.* 2010;11:199–207.
- Horemuzova E, Katz-Salamon M, Milerad J. Breathing patterns, oxygen and carbon dioxide levels in sleeping healthy infants during the first nine months after birth. *Acta Paediatr.* 2000;89:1284–1289.
- Hunt CE, Corwin MJ, Lister G, et al. Longitudinal assessment of hemoglobin oxygen saturation in healthy infants during the first six months of age. *J Pediatr.* 1999;134:580–586.
- Poets CF. Apnea of prematurity: What can observational studies tell us about pathophysiology? *Sleep Med.* 2010;11:701–707.
- Schechter MS. Section on Pediatric Pulmonology, Subcommittee on Obstructive Sleep Apnea Syndrome. Technical report: Diagnosis and management of childhood obstructive sleep apnea syndrome. *Pediatrics.* 2002;109:e69.
- Sterni LM, Tunkel DE. Obstructive sleep apnea in children: An update. *Pediatr Clin North Am.* 2003;50:427–443.

CODES

ICD9
- 770.81 Primary apnea of newborn
- 786.04 Cheyne-Stokes respiration
- 786.9 Other symptoms involving respiratory system and chest

ICD10
- R06.3 Periodic breathing
- R09.02 Hypoxemia
- P28.4 Other apnea of newborn

FAQ

- Q: What is the risk of the patient dying of SIDS?
- A: The relationship between periodic breathing and SIDS is not clear, although most studies have not found a higher frequency of SIDS among patients with periodic breathing.

PERIORBITAL CELLULITIS

Scott M. Goldstein
Femida Kherani (5th edition)

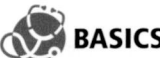 **BASICS**

DESCRIPTION
- Periorbital cellulitis is an acute infection of the superficial skin and subcutaneous tissues of the eyelids. It is also known as preseptal cellulitis because the inflammation is localized in the tissues anterior to the orbital septum. Thus, the eyeball and orbital structures are not involved.

EPIDEMIOLOGY
- Usually occurs in young children, commonly <5 years of age, but can occur at any age

RISK FACTORS
- Predisposing factors that may lead to infection include skin trauma, insect bites, and upper respiratory infections with paranasal sinusitis.

ETIOLOGY
- A variety of bacteria
  - Most common pathogens are *Staphylococcus aureus*, *Streptococcus pneumoniae*, and *Staphylococcus epidermis*.

COMMONLY ASSOCIATED CONDITIONS
- Periorbital cellulitis may be a secondary extension of another process such as sinusitis.

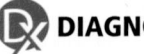 **DIAGNOSIS**

SIGNS AND SYMPTOMS
- The lids will be edematous, erythematous, warm to the touch, and typically tender on palpation.
  - The findings can start in one eyelid, but both the upper and lower eyelids are usually swollen.
  - May be signs of previous trauma, cutaneous injury, etc

HISTORY
- Onset, time course of symptom progression, and any predisposing factors
- Trauma or underlying respiratory infection
  - These types of questions have a low yield.
- The presence of pain supports cellulitis, whereas complaints of itching are more suggestive of an allergy.
- Quantify systemic symptoms such as fever and lethargy
  - These indicate a more severe, disseminated infection.

PHYSICAL EXAM
- Occasionally the eyelids are so swollen that it is difficult to examine the globe. To do so, place anesthetic eyedrops on the eye and fashion a paperclip into a lid retractor to lift the eyelid.
- The globe should be carefully examined. In preseptal cellulitis, the ocular exam is normal. The eye is usually white, although patients can have some conjunctival edema. Any change in vision or pupillary function, or limitations in eye motility suggest orbital involvement. Pediatric orbital cellulitis is an ophthalmologic emergency and requires prompt therapy.
- Many patients with preseptal cellulitis appear to have proptosis but actually do not. The presence of proptosis suggests deep orbital involvement.
- Evaluate for signs of fever, respiratory infection, and sepsis.

DIAGNOSTIC TESTS & INTERPRETATION
Lab
- Lab tests are usually not helpful or indicated.
- CBC is warranted only if bacteremia is suspected.
- Skin cultures and blood cultures have a low yield.
  - Blood cultures are obtained only when the child is febrile or appears septic.
  - Wound cultures can be obtained if there is an abscess.

Imaging
- CT scanning is a helpful modality to appreciate sinus and orbital disease. It is important to obtain imaging studies if orbital cellulitis is suspected, and especially in cases that do not respond to medical treatment.
  - CT scans will lag behind clinical findings once treatment is started. In fact, a repeat scan 24 to 48 hours after starting antibiotics will usually look worse than the preantibiotic scan. Thus, serial CT scanning should be done only if the child is not improving with treatment.

DIFFERENTIAL DIAGNOSIS
- Infectious
  - Early orbital cellulitis, dacryocystitis, stye, severe viral conjunctivitis
- Allergic
  - Periocular allergic reaction: insect bite, angioneurotic edema, contact dermatitis
- Other
  - Periocular trauma
  - Rhabdomyosarcoma
  - Idiopathic orbital inflammatory syndrome (IOIS)

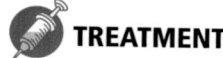

TREATMENT

ADDITIONAL TREATMENT
General Measures
* New antibiotics are constantly being introduced to replace older medications. Antibiotics that cover *gram-positive organisms and sinus pathogens*, such as second-generation cephalosporins or β-lactamase–resistant penicillins, should be started as soon as possible.
  – MRSA has become a leading cause of skin infections and must be considered when starting treatment
* Children <1 year of age should be hospitalized for IV therapy and very close observation.
* Children between the ages of 1 and 5 years should be watched closely.
  – Mild cases may be managed on an outpatient visit.
* Children >5 years of age can usually be treated with an oral regimen as long as they do not appear toxic or have orbital involvement.

MEDICATION (DRUGS)
* In nontoxic children, oral antibiotics (Clindamycin, Augmentin, cefaclor, Pediazole, Bactrim, etc.) are started on an outpatient basis; the child should be seen again within 24–48 hours.
* Children who do not improve or who deteriorate, and children who present with fever or septic symptoms, should be admitted for IV antibiotic (Clindamycin, Unasyn, ceftriaxone, etc.). These children should be watched closely.

SURGERY/OTHER PROCEDURES
* Surgical intervention is usually required when an abscess or a foreign body is present.

ONGOING CARE

* Patients usually take 24–48 hours to respond to therapy.
* Patients should be seen daily until a definite improvement is noted.

PROGNOSIS
* Excellent, with minimal incidence of long-term sequelae unless a complication is encountered

COMPLICATIONS
* Orbital extension (2.5–17%)
* Skin abscess (8%)
* Eyelid necrosis (1–2%)
* Sepsis
* Intracranial extension (2–3%)

Patient Monitoring
* Watch patients closely for signs of orbital extension, bacteremia, or other forms of disseminated infection.
* Neonates and infants can become septic very quickly, so they need to be closely monitored.

ADDITIONAL READING

* Donahue SP, Schwartz G. Preseptal and orbital cellulitis in childhood: A changing microbiologic spectrum. *Ophthalmology*. 1998;105:1902–1905.
* Foster JA, Katowitz JA. Pediatric orbital and periocular infections. In: Katowitz JA, ed. *Pediatric Oculoplastic Surgery*. Springer-Verlag; 2001.
* Georgakopoulos CD, Eliopoulou MI, Stasinos S, Exarchou A, Pharmakakis N, Varvarigou A. Periorbital and orbital cellulitis: A 10-year review of hospitalized children. *Eur J Ophthalmol*. 2010; 20(6):1066–1072.
* Lessner A, Stern GA. Preseptal and orbital cellulitis. *Infect Dis Clin North Amer*. 1992;6:933–952.
* Powell KR. Orbital and periorbital cellulitis. *Pediatr Rev*. 1995;16:163–167.
* Rutar T, Chambers HF, Crawford JB, Perdreau-Remington F, Zwick OM, Karr M, Diehn JJ, Cockerham KP. Ophthalmic manifestations of infections caused by the USA300 clone of community-associated methicillin-resistant Staphylococcus aureus. *Ophthalmology*. 2006;113: 1455–1462.
* Wald ER. Periorbital and orbital infections. *Pediatr Rev*. 2004;25(9):312–320.
* Vayalumkal JV, Jadavji T. Children hospitalized with skin and soft tissue infections: A guide to antibacterial selection and treatment. *Paediatr Drugs*. 2006;8:99–111.

CODES

ICD9
376.01 Periorbital sinusitis

ICD10
* H05.011 Cellulitis of right orbit
* H05.012 Cellulitis of left orbit
* H05.019 Cellulitis of unspecified orbit

PERIRECTAL ABSCESS

Calies Menard-Katcher
Judith Kelsen
Vera de Matos (5th edition)

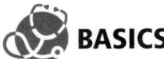 BASICS

DESCRIPTION
- Abscess in the perirectal area, most often arising from an anal gland.
- May be associated with fistula-in-ano.
- Classification of the abscess is based on the location in relation to the levator and sphincteric muscles of the pelvic floor.
- Classification by decreasing frequency: perianal, ischioanal, intersphincteric, and supralevator.

EPIDEMIOLOGY
- May occur at any age.
  - More common between the ages of 20–45 years.
  - In children, more common in infants.
- More common in boys.

PATHOPHYSIOLOGY AND ETIOLOGY
- Most often originate from occluded anal glands with subsequent bacterial overgrowth and abscess formation.
- Infection from within the anal glands penetrates through the internal sphincter and ends in the intersphincteric space.
- The most common *enteric* organism cultured is *Escherichia coli.*
- Chronic infection and inflammation may result in fistula-in-ano.
- May be a result of or associated with:
  - Nonspecific anal gland infection
  - Crohn disease
  - Immune deficiency (e.g., neutropenia, diabetes mellitus, AIDS)
  - Perforation by a foreign body
  - External trauma
  - Tuberculosis
  - Chronic granulomatous disease (CGD)
  - Tumor (e.g., carcinoma, rhabdomyosarcoma)

DIAGNOSIS

SIGNS AND SYMPTOMS
- Constant anal or perianal pain that often precedes local findings
- Localized swelling, erythema and fluctuance
- Painful defecation or ambulation
- Constitutional symptoms (e.g., fever or malaise)

PRESENTATION BY CLASSIFICATION
Perianal Abscess
- Result of distal vertical spread of the infection to the anal margin
- Presents as tender, fluctuant mass
- Most common type of perianal abscess

Ischiorectal Abscess
- Secondary to horizontal spread of infection across the external anal sphincter into the ischiorectal fossa
- Infection may track across the internal anal sphincter into the anal canal.
- Presents as diffuse, tender, indurated, fluctuant area
- Patients may have pain and fever prior to visible swelling.

Intersphincteric Abscess
- Limited to the intersphincteric space between the internal and external sphincters, therefore often does not cause perianal skin changes
- Associated with painful defecation
- Accounts for only 2–5 percent of all anorectal abscesses

Supralevator Abscess
- May arise from two different sources:
  - Proximal vertical spread from the gland through the intersphincteric space to the supralevator space
  - Pelvic inflammation or infection (e.g., Crohn disease)

- Presents with pelvic or anorectal pain, fever, and, at times, urinary retention
- Rectal exam usually reveals an indurated swelling above the anorectal ring.
- Imaging may be necessary to establish the diagnosis.

Horseshoe Abscess
- Secondary to abscessed anal gland located in the posterior midline of the anal canal
- Due to presence of anococcygeal ligament, the infection is forced laterally into the ischiorectal fossae and is therefore known as "horseshoe."
- May be unilateral or bilateral
- Presents with pain

DIAGNOSTIC TESTS & INTERPRETATION
Lab
- CBC
- Culture

Imaging
- CT scan
- MRI
- Rectal ultrasound

DIFFERENTIAL DIAGNOSIS
- Pilonidal infection
- Bartholin abscess
- Presacral epidermal inclusion cyst
- Hidradenitis suppurativa
- Rectal duplication cyst

 **TREATMENT**

ADDITIONAL TREATMENT
General Measures
- Abscess should be drained.
- Lack of fluctuation should not delay treatment.
- Antibiotics are reserved for situations in which infection does not appropriately respond to drainage or in the case of associated conditions such as adjacent cellulitis, immunocompromised patient, patient with abnormal cardiac valves, enteric organism on culture or in Crohn disease.
- Abscess should be cultured at time of drainage to direct therapy in the case antibiotics are needed.
- Sitz baths may be helpful with drainage.

SURGICAL TREATMENT
- Drainage may be performed either with conservative incision and drainage or with judicious probing for fistulae.
- It is a matter of debate as to whether a fistulotomy or fistulectomy should be performed at the time of drainage for an accompanying fistula.

 ONGOING CARE

- If abscess recurs, exploration for fistula-in-ano is recommended in an attempt to prevent recurrence.
- In the setting of recurrent abscess or fistula, consider other associated conditions (e.g., neutropenia, HIV, diabetes mellitus, Crohn disease, rectal duplication cyst).

PROGNOSIS
- Prognosis is good if there is early detection and drainage of abscesses.
- Patients typically recover well after surgical drainage without the need for antibiotics.

COMPLICATIONS
- Sepsis
- Fistula formation

SPECIAL CONSIDERATIONS
- Crohn disease should be considered in patients with perirectal abscess with or without fistula-in-ano.
- Signs and symptoms that increase suspicion for Crohn disease include: Weight loss or poor growth, chronic diarrhea or abdominal pain.
- Topical tacrolimus may be used in the treatment of perirectal abscess in the setting of Crohn disease.

ADDITIONAL READING

- Caliste X, Nazir S, Goode T, Street JH 3rd, Hockstein M, McArthur K, Trankiem CT, Sava JA. Sensitivity of computed tomography in detection of perirectal abscess. *Am Surg.* 2011;77(2):166–168.
- Chang HK, Ryu JG, Oh JT. Clinical characteristics and treatment of perianal abscess and fistula-in-ano in infants. *J Pediatr Surg.* 2010;45(9):1832–1836.
- Huang A, Abbasakoor F, Vaizey CJ. Gastrointestinal manifestations of chronic granulomatous disease. *Colorectal Dis.* 2006;8(8):637–644.
- Lejkowski M, Maheshwari A, Calhoun DA, et al. Persistent perianal abscess in early infancy as a presentation of autoimmune neutropenia. *J Perinatol.* 2003;23(5):428–430.
- Malik AI, Nelson RL, Tou S. Incision and drainage of perianal abscess with or without treatment of anal fistula. *Cochrane Database Syst Rev.* 2010;(7): CD006827.
- Marcus RH, Stine RJ, Cohen MA. Perirectal abscess. *Ann Emerg Med.* 1995;25(5):597–603.
- Niyogi A, Agarwal T, Broadhurst J, Abel RM. Management of perianal abscess and fistula-in-ano in children. *Eur J Pediatr Surg.* 2010;20(1):35–39.
- Rosen NG, Gibbs DL, Soffer SZ, et al. The nonoperative treatment of fistula-in-ano. *J Pediatr Surg.* 2000;35(35):938–939.
- Whiteford MH, Kilkenny J 3rd, Hyman N, et al. Practice parameters for the treatment of perianal abscess and fistula-in-ano (revised). *Dis Colon Rectum.* 2005;48(7):1337–1342.

 CODES

ICD9
- 565.1 Anal fistula
- 566 Abscess of anal and rectal regions

ICD10
- K60.3 Anal fistula
- K61.0 Anal abscess
- K61.1 Rectal abscess

FAQ

- Q: What are complications of this problem?
- A: Fistula formation is seen in ≤25% of patients with a predilection for males.
- Q: What are the most common organisms of the abscess?
- A: Staphylococcus species
- Q: What other disease may perirectal abscess be associated with?
- A: Crohn disease. If there has been exposure, tuberculosis should also be excluded.
- Q: What treatments can be done other than surgery?
- A: Sitz baths and warm compresses may be able to help with more superficial abscess.

PERITONITIS

Kathleen M. Loomes
Vera de Matos (5th edition)

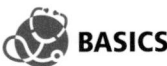 BASICS

DESCRIPTION
- Inflammation of the peritoneum in reaction to infection or chemical irritation by organic fluids (GI contents, bile, blood, or urine). Infectious peritonitis can be:
  - Primary or spontaneous bacterial peritonitis (SBP). Pathogens can reach the peritoneum by translocation from the intestinal lumen, from the bloodstream, from the lymphatics, from the vagina, from foreign bodies inserted in the peritoneal cavity, or from the pharyngeal or skin flora.
  - Secondary peritonitis occurs after bowel perforation, abscess formation, ischemic necrosis, or penetrating abdominal injury.
- Infectious organisms include aerobic gram-negative organisms (*Escherichia coli* [~50%] and *Klebsiella* species [~13%]) and aerobic gram-positive organisms (*Streptococcus* [~19%] and *Enterococcus* [5%] species).
- Anaerobes rarely cause SBP, and polymicrobial infections occur in relatively few patients (~8%).
- Urine cultures have been found to be positive for the same organism in ~44% of patients.
- Pneumonia and soft tissue infections have also been suggested as sources.

RISK FACTORS
- Liver cirrhosis (10–30% of adults hospitalized with cirrhosis have SBP), nephrotic syndrome (staphylococcal species, streptococci, enteric organisms, and fungi)
- Splenectomy (encapsulated organisms: Group A streptococci, *E. coli*, *Streptococcus pneumoniae*, *Bacteroides* sp.)
- Decreased serum complement levels
- Decreased ascitic protein and complement levels
- Presence of gastrointestinal hemorrhage

PATHOPHYSIOLOGY
- When bacteria or chemicals reach the peritoneal cavity, a local peritoneal and systemic response is initiated:
  - Hyperemia and exudation of fibrinogen, albumin, opsonins, and complement
  - Mesothelial cells secrete cytokines (interleukins [IL-6, IL-8], tumor necrosis factor-α [TNF-α]). IL-6 stimulates T- and B-cell differentiation, and IL-8 is a selective chemoattractant for polymorphonuclear (PMN) leucocytes.

- In SBP, pathogenic bacteria are cultured from peritoneal fluid without any apparent intra-abdominal surgical treatable source of infection. Recognized as a complication in patients with ascites as a result of cirrhosis of any etiology:
  - Generalized bacteremia and translocation of organisms from the gut (*E. coli, Klebsiella* sp.) into the portal veins or lymphatics or, less likely, directly into the ascitic fluid may account for the source of the infection.
  - Clearance of bacteria from the bloodstream may be impaired in patients with cirrhosis and ascites because of diminished phagocytic activity of the hepatic reticuloendothelial system secondary to cellular functional defects or shunting of blood away from the liver.
  - Complement, necessary for the opsonization of bacteria and ultimately clearance by phagocytes, is decreased in the ascitic fluid of patients with ascites.
- In secondary bacterial peritonitis, the underlying bacterial infection tends to be a complex polymicrobial infection with an average of 3 or 4 different isolates; the most common isolates are combinations of *E. coli* and *Bacteroides fragilis,* and the most common gram-positive organisms are nonenterococcal streptococci and enterococci.

ETIOLOGY
- Primary peritonitis: Liver cirrhosis (differential diagnosis in "Cirrhosis" chapter) or other conditions associated with ascites, such as:
  - Budd-Chiari syndrome
  - CHF
  - Nephrotic syndrome
  - Systemic lupus erythematosus
  - Rheumatoid arthritis
- The etiology of secondary peritonitis varies with age.
  - Neonate:
    - Necrotizing enterocolitis
    - Idiopathic gastrointestinal perforation
    - Perforation due to Hirschsprung disease
    - Spontaneous biliary perforation
    - Omphalitis
    - Perforation of a urachal cyst
  - Children and adolescents:
    - Secondary to appendicitis
    - Perforation of Meckel diverticulum
    - Gastric ulcer perforation
    - Pancreatitis
    - Traumatic perforation of the intestine
    - Intussusception
    - Neutropenic colitis (typhlitis)
    - Crohn disease with fistula and abscess formation
    - Toxic megacolon
    - Tuberculosis
    - Salpingitis

 DIAGNOSIS

HISTORY
- Dependent on stage, age, and etiology
- Fever, chills, vomiting
- Generalized abdominal pain with rebound tenderness
- Decreased bowel sounds
- In SBP, ~10% of cases are entirely asymptomatic.
- Other less common findings include:
  - Hypothermia
  - Hypotension
  - Diarrhea
  - Increased ascites despite diuretics
  - Worsening encephalopathy
  - Unexplained decrease in renal function

PHYSICAL EXAM
- Swollen rigid and painful abdomen
- Decreased bowel sounds
- Evidence of chronic liver disease
- Evidence of ascites

DIAGNOSTIC TESTS & INTERPRETATION
Diagnostic Procedures/Other
- Leucocytosis, increased C-reactive protein (CRP), leucopenia, and thrombocytopenia are also possible.
- Diagnosis may be confirmed with paracentesis. To improve culture yield, culture bottles should be inoculated immediately at the bedside in large-volume blood culture bottles.
- Elevated PMN count in ascitic fluid is important in the early diagnosis of SBP and is considered the most important laboratory indicator of SBP:
  - Diagnostic criteria for SBP include PMN leukocyte counts of >250/mm^3 in ascitic fluid. Culture is usually positive for a single organism.
  - Diagnostic criteria for secondary bacterial peritonitis include ascitic fluid culture positive for polymicrobial infection, total protein >1 g/dL, glucose <50 mg/dL, and lactate dehydrogenase (LDH) level >225 mU/mL.
  - Ultrasound, abdominal radiography, and CT scan may reveal fluid, thickening of bowel wall, abscesses, or pneumoperitoneum.

TREATMENT

MEDICATION (DRUGS)
- Empiric antibiotic coverage should be directed primarily toward enteric gram-negative aerobes and gram-positive cocci:
  - After the organism is identified, the antibiotic coverage may be optimized.
  - No particular antibiotic regimen has been shown to be superior in controlled clinical trials. Both single agents and combination regimens have been used.
- In SBP, cefotaxime has been shown to have higher resolution of infection and lower hospital mortality than the traditional ampicillin and an aminoglycoside as empiric coverage.

ADDITIONAL TREATMENT
General Measures
- Support the patient's cardiovascular and respiratory systems.
- Control the underlying infection with antibiotics or surgery (in secondary bacterial peritonitis).
- Decompression with nasogastric tube
- Patients at significant risk for SBP will benefit from selective intestinal decontamination as an effective preventive measure:
  - Antibiotics that have been studied for this use in adults include norfloxacin, ciprofloxacin, trimethoprim-sulfamethoxazole, and rifaximin.

SURGERY/OTHER PROCEDURES
In secondary bacterial peritonitis, surgery is the primary management tool with control of the source of the intra-abdominal infection:
- Control of the underlying source of the abdominal infection by repairing the affected bowel through laparotomy/laparoscopy should be considered.
- The degree of contamination may be decreased through intraoperative peritoneal lavage and débridement of loculations and abscesses.
- Adding antibiotics to lavage fluid has lost favor after the discovery that this procedure appears to impair neutrophil chemotaxis, inhibit neutrophil bactericidal activity, and increase the formation of adhesions.
- Catheters may be placed to drain a well-defined abscess cavity, form a controlled fistula, or provide access for continuous postoperative peritoneal lavage.

ONGOING CARE

PROGNOSIS
- SBP is associated with a high mortality. In reports from the 1970s, the mortality exceeded 90%. Currently with intensive treatment the in-hospital mortality in adults is still between 10% and 30%.
  - The combination of underlying disease and the infection causes acute decompensation in a marginally compensated host.
- Retrospective studies have indicated that SBP is a recurrent problem, with 60% of patients who survive the 1st episode going on to develop 1 or more recurrences.
- Severe secondary peritonitis is associated with a mortality rate of 30–55% in adults.

COMPLICATIONS
- Hypovolemia results from extravasation of fluid from the inflamed peritoneal membrane. Intravascular volume must be supported with crystalloids and blood products.
- Respiration may be impaired via mechanical mechanisms through diaphragmatic spasm and reflex abdominal rigidity and through increased permeability of the pulmonary vasculature in response to systemic inflammation.
- Long-term complications include adhesions.

ADDITIONAL READING
- de la Hunt MN. The acute abdomen in the newborn. *Semin Fetal Neonatal Med*. 2006;11(3):191–197.
- European Association for the Study of the Liver. EASL clinical practice guidelines on the management of ascites, spontaneous bacterial peritonitis and hepatorenal syndrome. *J Hepatol*. 2010;53(3):397–417.
- Hou W, Sanyal AJ. Ascites: Diagnosis and management. *Med Clin North Am*. 2009;93(4):801–817.
- Leonis MA, Balistreri WF. Evaluation and management of end-stage liver disease in children. *Gastroenterology*. 2008;134(6):1741–1751.

- Saab S, Hernandez JC, Chi AC, et al. Oral antibiotic prophylaxis reduces spontaneous bacterial peritonitis occurrence and improves short-term survival in cirrhosis: A meta-analysis. *Am J Gastroenterol*. 2009;104(4):993–1001.
- Sabri M, Saps M, Peters JM. Pathophysiology and management of pediatric ascites. *Curr Gastroenterol Rep*. 2003;5:240–246.
- Schaefer F. Management of peritonitis in children receiving chronic peritoneal dialysis. *Paediatr Drugs*. 2003;5:315–325.
- Thompson AE, Marshall JC, Opal SM. Intraabdominal infections in infants and children: descriptions and definitions. *Pediatr Crit Care Med*. 2005;6(3 Suppl):S30–S35.

CODES

ICD9
- 567.9 Unspecified peritonitis
- 567.21 Peritonitis (acute) generalized
- 567.23 Spontaneous bacterial peritonitis

ICD10
- K65.0 Generalized (acute) peritonitis
- K65.2 Spontaneous bacterial peritonitis
- K65.9 Peritonitis, unspecified

FAQ
- Q: Is peritonitis common in children with ascites?
- A: Despite the frequency of ascites from many different causes, peritonitis occurs rarely. In the setting of children with chronic liver disease and ascites, SBP may occur.
- Q: What are the most useful laboratory aids for this diagnosis?
- A: Paracentesis and analysis of the fluid for pH, glucose content, and number of inflammatory cells provides the most useful information regarding the diagnosis of peritonitis.

PERITONSILLAR ABSCESS
Nicholas Tsarouhas

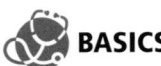 **BASICS**

DESCRIPTION
Infectious complication of tonsillitis or pharyngitis resulting in an accumulation of purulence in the tonsillar fossa. Also referred to as "quinsy"

EPIDEMIOLOGY
- Most common deep space infection of head and neck
- Seen most commonly in adolescents, but occasionally in younger children

RISK FACTORS
- Tonsillitis
- Pharyngitis

GENERAL PREVENTION
Abscess formation can often be prevented if appropriate antimicrobial therapy is initiated while the infection is still at the cellulitis stage.

PATHOPHYSIOLOGY
- Infectious tonsillopharyngitis progresses from cellulitis to abscess.
- The infection starts in the intratonsillar fossa, which is situated between the upper pole and the body of the tonsil, and eventually extends around the tonsil.
- The abscess is a suppuration outside the tonsillar capsule, in proximity to the upper pole of the tonsil, involving the soft palate.
- Purulence usually collects within 1 tonsillar fossa, but it may be bilateral.
- Tonsillar and peritonsillar edema may lead to compromise of the upper airway.

ETIOLOGY
- Most of these true abscesses are polymicrobial
- Group A β-hemolytic streptococci (GABHS)
- α-Hemolytic streptococci
- *Staphylococcus aureus*: Prevalence of methicillin-resistant *S. aureus* continues to increase.
- Anaerobic bacteria play an important role:
  - *Prevotella*
  - *Porphyromonas*
  - *Fusobacterium*
  - *Peptostreptococcus*
- Possible synergy between anaerobes and GABHS
- Gram negatives like *Haemophilus influenza*, and, more rarely, *Pseudomonas* species, may be isolated.

COMMONLY ASSOCIATED CONDITIONS
- Tonsillitis or pharyngitis usually precedes its development.
- Peritonsillar cellulitis is often associated with infectious mononucleosis.

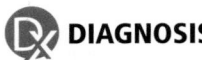 **DIAGNOSIS**

HISTORY
- Fever and sore throat:
  - Most common initial complaints
- Trouble swallowing, pain with opening the mouth (trismus), muffled ("hot potato") voice:
  - Classic presenting symptoms
- Unilateral neck or ear pain:
  - Other common presenting symptoms

PHYSICAL EXAM
- Unilateral peritonsillar fullness, or bulging of the posterior, superior, soft palate:
  - Diagnostic finding
- Uvular deviation:
  - Classic finding, though it may be absent in the more rare bilateral peritonsillar abscess
- Palpable fluctuance of palatal swelling:
  - Calls for urgent aspiration
- Erythematous, edematous pharynx, with enlarged and exudative tonsils:
  - Coexisting tonsillopharyngitis is common.
- Cervical adenopathy:
  - Common
- Drooling:
  - Often present
- Torticollis:
  - Sometimes seen

DIAGNOSTIC TESTS & INTERPRETATION
Lab
- WBC count:
  - Usually elevated with prominent left shift
- Rapid streptococcal throat antigen studies:
  - Helpful to diagnose GABHS infection
- Gram stain and culture of aspirate specimen:
  - Confirms causative microorganism

Imaging
- Radiographic studies are rarely necessary.
- CT scan or intraoral ultrasound:
  - Differentiation of peritonsillar cellulitis from peritonsillar abscess
  - CT scan most useful if patient cannot open mouth secondary to trismus
  - CT scan also important if deep neck extension is suspected

DIFFERENTIAL DIAGNOSIS
- Peritonsillar cellulitis:
  - Most common diagnostic consideration
  - Can be distinguished by its lack of peritonsillar space fullness, uvular deviation, dysphonia, and trismus
- Retropharyngeal abscess:
  - Minimal peritonsillar findings, along with a widened prevertebral space on lateral neck radiograph, are diagnostic of this airway-compromising disease, which usually occurs in preschool children.
- Epiglottitis:
  - This life-threatening airway emergency presents abruptly with fever, stridor, increased work of breathing, and drooling.
  - Usually occurs in toxic-appearing children 3–7 years old
  - Becoming a rare entity since the advent of the *Haemophilus influenzae* type B vaccine
- Other infectious causes of severe tonsillopharyngitis:
  - Epstein-Barr virus (infectious mononucleosis), coxsackievirus (herpangina), *Corynebacterium diphtheriae*, and *Neisseria gonorrhoeae*

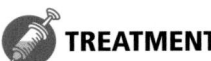 **TREATMENT**

MEDICATION (DRUGS)
First Line
- Clindamycin or ampicillin/sulbactam are the most commonly used 1st-line antibiotics owing to their efficacy versus GABHS, *Staphylococcus*, and anaerobes.
- As methicillin-resistant *S. aureus* isolates continue to increase, clindamycin becoming more popular as drug of choice
- Some initiate therapy with high-dose IV penicillin—in the presence of a positive strep antigen or culture study.

Second Line
- Nafcillin, oxacillin, and cefazolin are acceptable antibiotic alternatives.
- Steroids:
  - Some experts recommend steroids to decrease swelling, pain, and trismus.
  - Methylprednisolone, dexamethasone, and prednisone are all acceptable.

ADDITIONAL TREATMENT
General Measures
Treating a true abscess without incision and drainage is inadequate and can have airway-threatening implications:

- Abscesses should be urgently/emergently drained via either needle aspiration or surgical incision and drainage.
- Antibiotic therapy
- Steroid therapy debatable
- Surgical drainage
- Appropriate analgesia and adequate hydration should be ensured.

ISSUES FOR REFERRAL
Peritonsillar abscess: Otorhinolaryngology consultation for acute and chronic management

SURGERY/OTHER PROCEDURES
Surgical drainage with tonsillectomy: Consider in children not responding to parenteral antibiotics within 24–48 hours.

 ONGOING CARE

FOLLOW-UP RECOMMENDATIONS
- Patients may be discharged on oral antibiotics to complete a 10–14-day course when afebrile and peritonsillar swelling has subsided.
- Tonsillectomy should be considered after severe or recurrent peritonsillar abscesses.

PROGNOSIS
- Complete recovery with appropriate therapy.
- Recurrence of the abscess may occur.

COMPLICATIONS
- Upper airway obstruction is the most feared complication.
- Abscesses left untreated can rupture spontaneously into the pharynx, leading to aspiration and pneumonia.
- Other serious complications include parapharyngeal abscess, jugular vein thrombophlebitis, sepsis, cavernous sinus thrombosis, brain abscess, meningitis, and dissection into the internal carotid artery.
- Dehydration from decreased oral intake is the most common complication, however.
- Even after appropriate drainage, a small number of peritonsillar abscesses may reform.

ADDITIONAL READING

- Brook I. Microbiology and management of peritonsillar, retropharyngeal, and parapharyngeal abscesses. *J Oral Maxillofacial Surg.* 2004;62(12): 1545–1550.
- Brook I. The role of anaerobic bacteria in tonsillitis. *Int J Pediatr Otorhinolaryngol.* 2005;69(1):9–19.
- Brook I. Role of methicillin-resistant Staphylococcus aureus in head and neck infections. *J Laryngol Otol.* 2009;123:1301–1307.
- Hanna BC, McMullan R, Hall SJ. Corticosteroids and peritonsillar abscess formation in infectious mononucleosis. *J Laryngol Otol.* 2004;118(6): 459–461.
- Johnson RF, Stewart MG, Wright CC. An evidence-based review of the treatment of peritonsillar abscess. *Otolaryngol Head Neck Surg.* 2003;128:332–343.

- Marom T, Cinamon U, Itskoviz D, et al. Changing trends of peritonsillar abscess. *Am J Otol Head Neck Med Surg.* 2010;31:162–167.
- Megalamani SB, Suria G, Manickam U, et al. Changing trends in bacteriology of peritonsillar abscess. *J Laryngol Otol.* 2008;122:928–930.
- Naseri I, Jerris RC, Sobol SE. Nationwide trends in pediatric Staphylococcus aureus infections. *Arch Otolaryngol Head Neck Surg.* 2009;135(1):14–16.
- Rustom IK, Sandoe JAT, Makura ZGG. Paediatric neck abscesses: Microbiology and management. *J Laryngol Otol.* 2008;122:480–484.
- Watanabe T, Suzuki M. Bilateral peritonsillar abscesses: Our experience and clinical features. *Ann Otol Rhinol Laryngol.* 2010;119(10):662–666.

 CODES

ICD9
475 Peritonsillar abscess
ICD10
J36 Peritonsillar abscess

FAQ

- Q: Are radiographs necessary to make the diagnosis of peritonsillar abscess?
- A: No. The physical examination is diagnostic; a lateral neck radiograph is useful only if retropharyngeal abscess or epiglottitis is a diagnostic concern.
- Q: Is surgical consultation necessary in cases of peritonsillar abscess?
- A: Yes. Otorhinolaryngology consultation is indicated for both acute as well as chronic management.

PERSISTENT PULMONARY HYPERTENSION OF THE NEWBORN (PPHN)

Wendy J. Kowalski

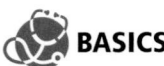 **BASICS**

DESCRIPTION
Clinical syndrome of severe respiratory failure and hypoxia in a neonate characterized by high systemic pulmonary arterial pressures, tricuspid regurgitation, and intracardiac shunting from right to left through persistent fetal pathways, including a patent foramen ovale and ductus arteriosus

EPIDEMIOLOGY
- Incidence of ~6.8 per 1,000 term live newborns
- Mostly occurs in full-term newborns owing to the presence of the muscular layer of arterioles, the risk of uteroplacental insufficiency, and the potential for the passage of meconium in utero, but it can complicate the course of an older premature baby with chronic lung disease
- Meconium aspiration is the number one cause of PPHN.
- PPHN complicates the course of about 10% of newborns with respiratory failure.

RISK FACTORS
Genetics
- Sporadic in occurrence
- Alveolar capillary dysplasia has been documented in 1 set of siblings; however, it too is primarily sporadic.
- Surfactant B deficiency has also been implicated but it is a rare, lethal, autosomal recessive disorder.

PATHOPHYSIOLOGY
- At a neonate's 1st breath after delivery, the pulmonary vascular resistance normally decreases to redirect ~50% of the cardiac output to the pulmonary circulation. This fails to occur in PPHN, hence the previous name of this condition, "persistent fetal circulation."
- Increased pulmonary vascular resistance increases right ventricular afterload, causing a backflow of blood to the right heart (and subsequent tricuspid regurgitation) and increased right heart pressures, which can lead to right ventricular failure.
- Increased pulmonary arterial pressures also cause intracardiac shunting across any patent foramen ovale, ductus arteriosus, or atrioseptal or ventriculoseptal defect that may be present. Blood shunts from right to left because of the supranormal systemic pulmonary arterial pressures. This causes more deoxygenated blood to go to the left heart and then to the body, which manifests as lower oxygen saturation in the lower extremities (postductally), cyanosis, and hypoxia.
- Deoxygenated blood in the left heart can lead to ischemic damage to the heart and right or left ventricular failure.
- If there is no shunting of blood, or the blood cannot get from the right to left heart because of a lack of persistent fetal pathways, a neonate may develop poor systemic perfusion, severe acidosis, shock, right ventricular failure, and even death.
- Any hypoxia, acidosis, or stress that occurs after birth further increases pulmonary vascular resistance.
- Usually, the pulmonary vasculature begins to relax within 3–5 days of life, and the process reverses. Sometimes, the pulmonary vascular resistance remains elevated as a result of an underlying disease process or anatomic abnormality.

ETIOLOGY
- Idiopathic: The pulmonary vasculature is remodeled due to chronic in utero stress or hypoxia, maternal use of NSAIDs near term, or maternal use of SSRIs in the 2nd trimester.
- Abnormally constricted pulmonary vasculature secondary to underlying disease: Infection, pneumonia, or meconium aspiration
- Secondary to an anatomic abnormality that has caused hypoplastic vasculature: Congenital diaphragmatic hernia, oligohydramnios and pulmonary hypoplasia, or alveolar capillary dysplasia

COMMONLY ASSOCIATED CONDITIONS
Related to the underlying disease or as a complication of treatment:
- Pneumothorax or air leak syndrome
- Chronic lung damage
- Long-term developmental delays
- Cerebral palsy
- Seizure disorder
- Sensorineural hearing loss

DIAGNOSIS

HISTORY
- Pregnancy history:
  - Congenital diaphragmatic hernia, congenital pulmonary airway malformation (CPAM), and congenital heart disease can all be diagnosed with a prenatal ultrasound.
  - History of oligohydramnios, which may be associated with pulmonary hypoplasia in the neonate
- Problems during labor and delivery:
  - Events that can cause fetal distress and/or hypoxia: Maternal chorioamnionitis, group B streptococcal infection, difficult delivery, or meconium aspiration
- Initial clinical course:
  - Infants with PPHN usually present with mild respiratory distress that worsens in the 1st minutes to hours of life, progressing to respiratory failure, labile oxygenation, hypoxia, and poor perfusion.
- Infants with cardiac disease, CPAM, or congenital diaphragmatic hernia are usually cyanotic and in significant distress from birth.

PHYSICAL EXAM
- The following physical exam findings suggest a diagnosis of PPHN:
  - Significant respiratory distress with nasal flaring, grunting, and retractions
  - Clear breath sounds (if idiopathic disease)
  - Pale, gray color with poor perfusion
  - Tricuspid regurgitation murmur heard at the left lower sternal border
- The following physical exam findings suggest diagnoses other than idiopathic PPHN:
  - Any murmur other than tricuspid regurgitation would suggest congenital heart disease.
  - Barrel chest shape suggests a pneumothorax or meconium aspiration.
  - Scaphoid abdomen suggests congenital diaphragmatic hernia.

DIAGNOSTIC TESTS & INTERPRETATION
Lab
- CBC with differential: Leukocytosis, leukopenia, bandemia, or neutropenia suggests bacterial infection.
- Blood culture: Should be performed in all cases of PPHN to rule out infection
- Frequent arterial blood gases:
  - Help to determine degree of hypoxia, hypercapnia, acidosis, and illness
  - Help manage ventilator support
  - Determine need for ECMO by calculating the oxygenation index (OI)
- OI:
  - $OI = (\text{mean airway pressure} \times FiO_2/PaO_2) \times 100$
  - Used to express severity of respiratory distress and to determine if neonate is a candidate for ECMO
  - Should be calculated with every blood gas. 3 OIs >40 suggest the need for ECMO.
- Hyperoxia test: While exposed to FiO_2 of 100% oxygen, a PaO_2 >250 mm Hg almost completely rules out cyanotic heart disease.

Imaging
- Chest radiograph:
  - In idiopathic disease, usually shows clear lungs
  - Will help to rule out pneumothorax, hyperinflation, meconium aspiration, and atelectasis
  - Assessing cardiac silhouette and pulmonary vascular markings may help rule out some congenital heart disease.
- Echocardiogram, important:
  - To diagnose PPHN and to rule out congenital heart disease
  - To follow cardiac output and function

DIFFERENTIAL DIAGNOSIS
- Congenital:
  - Cyanotic congenital heart disease
  - Total anomalous pulmonary venous return
  - Congenital diaphragmatic hernia
  - CPAM
  - Alveolar capillary dysplasia
- Infectious:
  - Pneumonia
  - Sepsis
- Pulmonary:
  - Surfactant deficiency (respiratory distress syndrome)
  - Meconium aspiration syndrome
  - Blood or amniotic fluid aspiration
  - Pneumothorax or air leak syndrome
  - Idiopathic pulmonary hypertension

TREATMENT

ADDITIONAL TREATMENT
General Measures
- All infants should be transferred to a Level III neonatal intensive care unit where high-frequency ventilation and inhaled nitrous oxide are available. If the neonate meets or nearly meets criteria for starting ECMO (OI >40 on 3 different blood gases), then ECMO should be available at the receiving institution.
- Support respiratory status:
  - Conventional ventilation or high-frequency ventilation to improve oxygenation and ventilation while minimizing lung damage
  - No set guidelines for ventilator management
  - Most institutions feel that high-frequency ventilation minimizes lung damage when high mean airway pressures (>15 cm H_2O) are needed.
  - Frequent monitoring to keep PaO_2 between 80 and 100 mm Hg, PCO_2 >35–45 mmHg, and OI below ECMO criteria (oxygen index >40 times 3)
  - Avoid hyperventilation, which has been associated with poor neurodevelopmental outcome.
- Lower the pulmonary vascular resistance and thus promote pulmonary blood flow:
  - Give 100% oxygen.
  - Keep blood gas pH alkalotic (pH >7.40) while keeping $PaCO_2$ >35–45 mm Hg by ventilator manipulation or bicarbonate infusion.
  - Keep systemic BP high (mean BP >45–50) with volume, transfusions, or medications.
  - Treat acidosis with fluid, blood, or bicarbonate infusion.
- Improve oxygen saturation and thus oxygen delivery to the tissues:
  - Initially 100% oxygen should be used to keep the PaO_2 >80–100 mmHg and the oxygen saturation around 99–100%. The oxygen can be weaned very slowly (2% per hour if saturation remains >98%).
  - Inhaled nitric oxide (iNO), a pulmonary vasodilator, should be used if the infant is on 100% (FiO_2) oxygen and the PaO_2 goal is not achieved. It is better to start iNO sooner rather than later:
    - Has been shown to decrease the need for ECMO in term neonates with hypoxic respiratory failure secondary to PPHN, except for those babies with congenital diaphragmatic hernia
    - Should be used only as a bridge to ECMO in babies with congenital diaphragmatic hernia
    - Wean slowly! If oxygen and iNO are weaned too quickly, the infant can become critically ill because PPHN is a very labile condition.
- Reduce oxygen demand:
  - Sedatives and paralytics may be given to prevent fluctuations in oxygenation during care. Minimize the use of paralytics because they have been shown to increase mortality.
  - Minimize stimulation.

- Treat any underlying lung disease with the following, if applicable:
  - Antibiotics
  - Surfactant
  - Chest tube placement
  - Surgery

ALERT
- Can be difficult to differentiate cyanotic congenital heart disease from PPHN. Infants who fail to improve should be re-evaluated for an underlying disease process.
- PPHN is a very labile condition. Neonates can change from being stable to being very sick and emergently needing ECMO.
- ECMO, though life saving and with a good survival rate, is not without problems. Side effects include:
  - Repeated exposure to blood products
  - Risk of intra-abdominal or intracardiac bleed
  - Potential for long-term neurologic sequelae
  - Long-term risk of having only 1 patent carotid artery

 ONGOING CARE

PROGNOSIS
- PPHN usually resolves either spontaneously or as the underlying parenchymal lung disease improves.
- Survival rate is good even for neonates who receive ECMO. Survival rate and incidence of long-term sequelae depend on underlying disease and severity of illness.
- Survival rate for all causes of PPHN in patients not requiring ECMO is >90%. ~10–20% have sensorineural hearing loss or an abnormal neurologic exam at follow-up.
- For those requiring ECMO, survival rate is 80% for idiopathic disease, 90% for meconium aspiration syndrome, 80% for disease secondary to sepsis, and only 50–60% for patients with congenital diaphragmatic hernia. Roughly 20% of these survivors have sensorineural hearing loss or abnormal neurologic examinations at follow-up.
- Even with advances in technology and the availability of ECMO, the prognosis is poor for those babies with severe underlying lung pathology, such as congenital diaphragmatic hernia.

COMPLICATIONS
- Myocardial dysfunction
- Congestive heart failure (CHF)
- Hypoxic ischemic insult

ADDITIONAL READING
- Cool CD, Deutsch G. Pulmonary arterial hypertension from a pediatric perspective. *Pediatr Dev Pathol*. 2008;11(3):169–177.
- Finner NN, Barrington KJ. Nitric oxide for respiratory failure in infants born at or near term. *Cochrane Database Syst Rev*. 2001;(2):CD000399.
- Lipkin PH, Davidson D, Spivak L, et al. Neurodevelopmental and medical outcomes of persistent pulmonary hypertension in term newborns treated with nitric oxide. *J Pediatr*. 2002;140:306–310.
- Sadiq HF, Mantych G, Benawra RS, et al. Inhaled nitric oxide in the treatment of moderate persistent pulmonary hypertension of the newborn: A randomized controlled trial. *J Perinatol*. 2003;23: 98–103.
- Vargas-Origel A, Gomez-Rodriguez G, Aldana-Valenzuela C, et al. The use of sildenafil in persistent pulmonary hypertension of the newborn. *Am J Perinatol*. 2010;27(3):225–230.

 CODES

ICD9
747.83 Persistent fetal circulation

ICD10
P29.3 Persistent fetal circulation

FAQ
- Q: Does iNO improve outcome in newborns with severe PPHN?
- A: Yes. iNO, used at a dose of 20 ppm, has been shown to decrease the need for ECMO and the incidence of death in term infants with PPHN without congenital diaphragmatic hernia. Follow-up studies have shown no difference in long-term disabilities between those babies treated and not treated with iNO. Long-term outcome is mainly determined by the underlying disease and the severity of illness.
- Q: Are there any other potential therapies for treating PPHN?
- A: Yes. Inhaled tolazoline, sildenafil (Viagra), other smooth muscle relaxants (dipyridamole, zaprinast, and E4021), iloprost, bosentan, and phosphodiesterase inhibitors have been studied and have been shown to be effective in enhancing the vasodilatory effects of iNO. Sildenafil is being used in select cases, particularly in older neonates, in centers without iNO or ECMO, or as an adjuvant to iNO, and it has shown the most promise for routine clinical use.

PERTHES DISEASE

Ali Al-Omari
Wudbhav Sankar
John P. Dormans (5th edition)

BASICS

DESCRIPTION
Self-limited osteonecrosis of the proximal femoral epiphysis of unknown etiology that can produce permanent deformity of the femoral head

EPIDEMIOLOGY
- Seen most commonly between ages 4–12 years
- Boys affected more than girls (5:1)
- 10–15% bilateral
- Most have delayed bone age

PATHOPHYSIOLOGY
- Disruption of blood supply to the femoral head
- Stages:
  – Synovitis
  – Necrosis: Sclerosis and density of the femoral head
  – Fragmentation: Fragmentation of necrotic bone with early revascularization
  – Reossification: Revascularization, resorption, and repair via creeping substitution
  – Healing: Remodeling

ETIOLOGY
- Unknown
- Factors that may contribute:
  – Trauma
  – Susceptible child (delayed bone age, low birth weight)
  – Hereditary factors
  – Coagulopathy
  – Hyperactivity
  – Smoke exposure

DIAGNOSIS

HISTORY
- Age at onset of symptoms/signs:
  – Older age at onset implies worse prognosis.
- Limping:
  – The most frequent complaint; especially after strenuous activities
  – Weeks to months duration
- Hip, thigh, or knee pain:
  – Hip pathology may cause referred pain at thigh or knee.
- There may be waxing and waning of symptoms for several months.
- There may be a history of trauma.
- Distribution of pain may follow the sensory distribution of the obturator nerve:
  – Medial thigh and knee (i.e., referred pain from hip pathology)

PHYSICAL EXAM
- Limping
- Trendelenburg gait:
  – Leaning over affected leg during stance phase of gait cycle
- Positive Trendelenburg test: As patient stands with weight on the affected hip, the pelvis on the opposite normal side drops owing to weakness of the hip abductor muscles.
- Limitation of range of motion:
  – Especially internal rotation and abduction
- Irritability and tenderness of hip joint area:
  – Usually early; related to synovitis from early repair
- Atrophy of thigh muscles:
  – Late finding
- Slight shortening of affected limb owing to collapse (real) or contracture (apparent)

DIAGNOSTIC TESTS & INTERPRETATION
Lab
Generally, labs are not helpful, but may be necessary to rule out other conditions, such as infection and juvenile rheumatoid arthritis (JRA).

Imaging
- The 1st plain radiographic sign of Perthes is smaller size of the femoral head epiphysis and a widened articular cartilage space compared with the other side; the 2nd sign is the subchondral fracture:
  – Incipient (or initial) stage (1st)
  – Aseptic or avascular stage (2nd)
  – Fragmentation stage (3rd)
  – Residual or remodeling stage (4th)
- Bone scan maybe helpful in the early stage of the disease when the diagnosis is questionable.

DIFFERENTIAL DIAGNOSIS
- Toxic synovitis
- Chondrolysis (idiopathic and secondary)
- Infection (Brodie abscess: Subacute osteomyelitis of proximal femoral epiphysis)
- Tuberculosis of the hip
- Juvenile rheumatoid arthritis
- Tumors (chondroblastoma of proximal femoral epiphysis)
- Bone dysplasias:
  – Multiple epiphyseal dysplasia
  – Trichorhinophalangeal syndrome
  – Spondyloepiphyseal dysplasia
- Hypothyroidism, juvenile cretinism
- Sickle cell disease, hemophilia
- Gaucher disease
- Hemophilia
- Traumatic aseptic necrosis

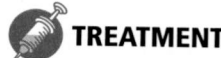

TREATMENT

MEDICATION (DRUGS)
NSAIDs for pain and inflammation

ADDITIONAL TREATMENT
General Measures
- Surgical treatment needed generally for those with more severe involvement (1/2 of head involved or late onset)
- 2 basic treatment principles:
  - Maintenance and/or restoration of range of motion
  - Containment of the femoral head epiphysis in the acetabulum
- General treatment modalities:
  - Bed rest early during collapse
  - Weight relief early during collapse (usually crutches)
  - Physical therapy to maintain range of motion
  - Traction (less popular now)
  - Bracing
  - Surgery to reposition acetabular or proximal femur

ISSUES FOR REFERRAL
Patients with Perthes disease preferably should be seen and followed by a pediatric orthopedic surgeon.

SURGERY/OTHER PROCEDURES
Younger patients with Perthes do not generally need surgery. Older patients with more significant collapse can benefit from surgical intervention. Early recognition and referral are key.

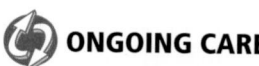

ONGOING CARE

FOLLOW-UP RECOMMENDATIONS
- Therapy generally continues until patient enters the reossification phase.
- The magnitude and duration of symptoms depend on the age of the patient at onset of the disease and the degree of involvement of the disease process. Most patients show improvement in symptoms by 6 months after the onset of disease.

Patient Monitoring
Signs to watch for:
- Stiffness: Loss of range of motion
- Limping
- Pain
- Subluxation of the hip joint

PROGNOSIS
- Overall, good prognosis for most patients
- Based on the following factors:
  - Age of the patient at onset of the disease (earlier onset gives better prognosis); if onset >8 years of age, poorer prognosis than if onset at younger age
  - Extent of femoral head involvement; if more than 1/2 of epiphysis involved, poorer prognosis
  - Subluxation of femoral head, poorer prognosis
  - Spherical congruency between the femoral head and acetabulum has good prognosis, and vice versa.
  - Growth disturbance of the physis, poorer prognosis

COMPLICATIONS
- Mild limb length discrepancy
- Restriction of hip range of motion
- Pain, limping
- Osteoarthritis (late)

ADDITIONAL READING
- Frick SL. Evaluation of the child who has hip pain. *Orthop Clin North Am.* 2006;37(2):133–140.
- Herring JA, Kim HT, Browne R. Legg-Calve-Perthes disease. Part II: Prospective multicenter study of the effect of treatment on outcome. *J Bone Joint Surg Am.* 2004;86-A(10):2121–2134.
- Herring JA, Sucato DJ. Legg-Calve-Perthes disease. In: *Tachdjian's Pediatric Orthopaedics*, 4th ed. New York: Saunders; 2007:771–838.
- Hubbard AM, Dormans JP. Evaluation of developmental dysplasia, Perthes disease, and neuromuscular dysplasia of the hip in children before and after surgery: An imaging update. *AJR Am J Roentgenol.* 164(5):1067–1073.
- Weinstein SL. Legg-Calve-Perthes syndrome. In: *Lovell and Winter's Pediatric Orthopaedics*, 6th ed. Philadelphia: Lippincott Williams & Wilkins; 2005: 1039–1084.

CODES

ICD9
732.1 Juvenile osteochondrosis of hip and pelvis

ICD10
- M91.10 Juvenile osteochondrosis of head of femur [Legg-Calve-Perthes], unspecified leg
- M91.11 Juvenile osteochondrosis of head of femur [Legg-Calve-Perthes], right leg
- M91.12 Juvenile osteochondrosis of head of femur [Legg-Calve-Perthes], left leg

FAQ

- Q: How long do you observe a patient with hip pain before ordering a radiograph?
- A: It depends on the presence or absence of abnormalities on the physical exam. If any of the signs mentioned are seen in conjunction with significant hip pain, a radiograph is indicated. A radiograph should be done early to establish the diagnosis and rule out other abnormalities.
- Q: Why do patients with hip pathology have knee pain?
- A: This is because the nerves that innervate the hip joint also have cutaneous sensory distributions. Both the obturator and femoral nerves innervate the hip joint, and both have cutaneous sensory distribution in the region of the thigh and knee joint.

P

PERTUSSIS

Laura K. Brennan
Louis M. Bell (5th edition)

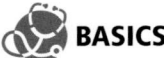 **BASICS**

DESCRIPTION
Pertussis is a classic "whooping cough" syndrome of prolonged paroxysmal coughing spells with a characteristic inspiratory whoop, caused by *Bordetella pertussis* infection.

EPIDEMIOLOGY
- Pertussis is one of the most highly communicable diseases with attack rates close to 80–90% in susceptible individuals.
- Humans are the only hosts of *B. pertussis*.
- Route of spread is primarily via large aerosolized respiratory droplets generated by coughing or sneezing.
- Pertussis occurs with seasonal peaks and 3–5-year cycles of increased incidence of disease.

Incidence
- Despite improved childhood vaccination rates in the US, pertussis infection rates have steadily risen since the early 1980s.
  - This may be in part because immunity to pertussis wanes ~5–10 years after completion of childhood vaccination, leading to a large susceptible adult population, who then are the major source of pertussis infection in children.
  - There also has been an increase in the detection and reporting of cases.
- Pertussis has been a disease of young children, with the highest incidence in infants <6 months of age, but rates in adolescents have been steadily increasing and now approach rates in infants.
- Disease in adolescents and adults often goes unrecognized:
  - In a recent Canadian study, the prevalence of pertussis in 422 adolescents and adults with prolonged cough illness was 20%.

GENERAL PREVENTION
- Infection control:
  - Isolation of hospitalized patient: Respiratory (droplet precautions) isolation for 5 days after starting appropriate antimicrobial therapy or until at least 3 weeks after the onset of the paroxysmal stage, if antibiotics were not given, is recommended.
  - Care of exposed people: Exposed individuals (all household contacts, other close contacts, other children in child care) should receive chemoprophylaxis to limit secondary transmission, regardless of immunization status. Immunization should be given to all unimmunized and underimmunized children <7 years of age, and to adolescents and adults who have not yet received the Tdap booster vaccination.

- Immunizations:
  - All pertussis vaccines available in the US are acellular vaccines in combination with diphtheria and tetanus toxoids, as this is the preferred vaccination product over previous whole-cell pertussis products.
  - Universal immunization of all children <7 years of age with DTaP vaccine is recommended as per CDC and AAP guidelines.
  - It is now also recommended that under-vaccinated children ages 7–10, all adolescents ages 11–18, adults ages 19–64, as well as certain adults ages 65 and older should receive a single dose of Tdap vaccine as this is paramount to control the rate of infection in infants and young children.

PATHOPHYSIOLOGY
- Replicates only in association with ciliated epithelium, causing congestion and inflammation of the bronchi; peribronchial lymphoid hyperplasia followed by a necrotizing process occurs and results in a bronchopneumonia; atelectasis can also occur owing to bronchiolar obstruction from accumulated secretions.
- The long incubation period (7–21 days) reflects the time necessary for *B. pertussis* to increase in numbers needed for progressive spread of infection in the respiratory tract and to produce enough toxin for eliciting damage and dysfunction of the respiratory epithelium.

ETIOLOGY
Infection with *B. pertussis*, a small, nonmotile, fastidious, gram-negative rod.

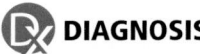 **DIAGNOSIS**

HISTORY
- The most likely source of pertussis in young infants is from the adolescent or adult with mild symptoms of pertussis. Therefore, a thorough history, including presence of cough in adult family members, must be taken and a high index of suspicion for pertussis must be maintained when evaluating infants and children for cough.
- 3 clinical stages:
  - Catarrhal stage (1–2 weeks) with symptoms of an upper respiratory infection
  - Paroxysmal stage (≥2–4 weeks) characterized by paroxysmal cough with increased severity and frequency producing the characteristic whoop during the sudden forceful inspiratory phase; posttussive vomiting is also observed during this stage.
  - The convalescent stage begins and lasts 1–2 weeks, but cough can persist for several months. In the adolescent or adult, long-standing cough of 2–3 weeks is the hallmark symptom. Most patients report a paroxysmal or staccato quality to the cough.
- Apnea is a common manifestation in infants <6 months. The characteristic whoop is typically absent.

PHYSICAL EXAM
- Rhinorrhea, lacrimation, conjunctival hyperemia, and fever can be seen in the early stage of disease.
- Cyanosis can be observed during the paroxysmal stage.
- Lung auscultatory examination is usually normal unless significant atelectasis or pneumonia has occurred.

DIAGNOSTIC TESTS & INTERPRETATION
Lab
- CBC:
  - Leukocytosis with predominant lymphocytosis (77%) is commonly observed at the end of the catarrhal stage and throughout the paroxysmal stage of illness, although this phenomenon is more common in infants and children than adolescents.
- Culture of *B. pertussis*:
  - Achieved using calcium alginate or Dacron swabs of the nasopharynx and plated onto selective media such as Regan–Lowe or Bordet–Gengou and incubated for 10 days
  - Most frequently successful during the catarrhal or early paroxysmal stages and is rarely found beyond the third week of illness.
  - Specificity 100%; overall sensitivity is 60–70% but can be lower in previously vaccinated individuals, if antibiotics have already been given, or if beyond the third week of illness.
- Polymerase chain reaction (PCR):
  - Available in most centers and have been shown to have a higher sensitivity than culture in the detection of *B. pertussis* from nasopharyngeal specimens, although specificity can vary
  - PCR techniques vary by institution; there is no FDA-licensed PCR test available, and there are no standardized protocols or reagents.
- Direct immunofluorescent assays (DFA) of nasopharyngeal specimens:
  - Can provide a rapid and specific diagnosis, but is generally less sensitive than culture and is limited by the experience of the laboratory personnel for interpretation
- Serology:
  - Has excellent sensitivity and specificity when the acute serum is collected early in the course of illness (≤2 weeks after cough onset) and compared with the convalescent serum specimen (collected ≥4 weeks after cough onset)

Imaging
Chest radiograph: May reveal perihilar infiltrates or a shaggy right-sided heart border, although these findings are neither sensitive nor specific.

DIFFERENTIAL DIAGNOSIS
- *Bordetella parapertussis* and adenoviruses
- Bronchiolitis
- Bacterial pneumonia
- Cystic fibrosis
- Tuberculosis
- Foreign-body aspiration
- Reactive airway disease

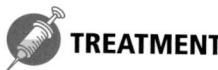 TREATMENT

MEDICATION (DRUGS)
First Line
Azithromycin (10 mg/kg as a single dose on day 1, then 5 mg/kg/d as a single dose on days 2–5) is recommended for ages ≥6 months.
- For infants <6 months of age, dosage is 10 mg/kg/d as a single dose for 5 days.
- For adolescents and adults, dosage is 500 mg as a single dose on day 1, followed by 250 mg as a single dose on days 2–5.

Second Line
- Erythromycin (50 mg/kg/d) in 4 doses for 14 days is recommended:
  – Alternative dose: 40 mg/kg erythromycin estolate b.i.d. for 14 days has shown equal efficacy.
  – *Note:* An association between oral erythromycin use and hypertrophic pyloric stenosis has been reported in infants <4 weeks, such that azithromycin is the drug of choice for treatment or prophylaxis of pertussis in that age group.
- Clarithromycin (15 mg/kg/d divided b.i.d for 7 days) has similar effectiveness to erythromycin, and can be used in children ≥1 month of age.
- Trimethoprim/Sulfamethoxazole is another alternative to erythromycin in children ≥2 months of age, although its efficacy is unproven.

ADDITIONAL TREATMENT
General Measures
- Patients with more severe disease manifestations (apnea, cyanosis, feeding difficulties) or other complications require hospitalization for supportive care:
  – Infants <6 months may develop apnea from fatigue secondary to excessive coughing. They need close observation, preferably in the hospital.
- If antibiotic treatment is initiated during the catarrhal stage, it can prevent disease from progressing. Antibiotics have not been shown to shorten the course of illness if begun during the paroxysmal stage, although they will eliminate the organism from the nasopharynx within 3–4 days, thus shortening the potential for contagion.

IN-PATIENT CONSIDERATIONS
Admission Criteria
- Young infant (<6 months of age) with concern for apnea or fatigue with coughing
- Patients with severe disease manifestations or complications

Discharge Criteria
- No evidence of cardiorespiratory instability
- Able to self-recover from coughing spells

 ONGOING CARE

FOLLOW-UP RECOMMENDATIONS
The paroxysmal stage can last up to 4 weeks, and the convalescent stage up to several months.

PROGNOSIS
Directly related to patient age:
- Highest mortality is observed in infants <6 months of age, with a 0.5–1% risk of death.
- In the older child, prognosis is good.

COMPLICATIONS
- The complications of pertussis are more likely to occur in infants <6 months of age and therefore tend to have a more serious, protracted course:
  – Pneumonia, which occurs in 22% of these infants, is responsible for >90% of deaths in young children with pertussis and is usually from secondary bacterial disease rather than *B. pertussis*.
  – Superinfections owing to viruses (adenovirus, respiratory syncytial virus, cytomegalovirus), bacteria (*Streptococcus pneumoniae*, *Staphylococcus aureus*), and gram-negative iatrogenic infections can complicate pneumonias.
  – Other pulmonary complications include atelectasis, pneumothorax, pneumomediastinum, and subcutaneous emphysema.
  – Seizures (2%) and encephalopathy (0.5%) have also been observed in infants with pertussis.
- Complications of pertussis in adolescents and adults include cough syncope, incontinence, rib fractures, and pneumonia.

ADDITIONAL READING
- Centers for Disease Control and Prevention. Updated Recommendations for Use of Tetanus Toxoid, Reduced Diphtheria Toxoid and Acellular Pertussis (Tdap) Vaccine from the Advisory Committee on Immunization Practices, 2010. *MMWR.* 2011;60(1):13–15.
- Cherry JD, Olin P. The science and fiction of pertussis vaccines. *Pediatrics.* 1999;104:1381–1384.
- Hoppe JE. Neonatal pertussis. *Pediatr Infect Dis J.* 2000;19:244–247.

 CODES

ICD9
- 033.0 Whooping cough due to *Bordetella pertussis*
- 033.9 Whooping cough, unspecified organism
- 484.3 Pneumonia in whooping cough

ICD10
- A37.00 Whooping cough due to Bordetella pertussis without pneumonia
- A37.01 Whooping cough due to Bordetella pertussis with pneumonia
- A37.90 Whooping cough, unspecified species without pneumonia

FAQ
- Q: Why is the transmission of pertussis difficult to control in the young infant?
- A: Unfortunately, many physicians do not consider pertussis in adolescents or adults because the symptoms can be nonspecific and often are not severe. They also assume that childhood immunization will protect adults against pertussis. Therefore, delays in antimicrobial treatment are common in adults owing to the lack of index of suspicion of pertussis by their providers. Finally, there was not a universal recommendation for adolescents and adults to receive pertussis boosters until 2005, even though the immunity protection by pertussis vaccination is limited. It is largely adolescents and adults with pertussis who then spread the disease to young infants and children.
- Q: When should adults get the Tdap vaccine?
- A: All adults ages 19–64 should receive a single dose of Tdap vaccine regardless of the interval since the last diphtheria or tetanus containing vaccine. Additionally, adults ages 65 years and older, especially those who have or anticipate having close contact with an infant aged <12 months, may receive a single dose of Tdap.

PHARYNGITIS
Mark L. Bagarazzi

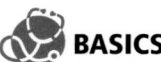

BASICS

DESCRIPTION
Pharyngitis (i.e., sore throat) is inflammation of the mucous membranes and underlying structures of the pharynx and tonsils, usually secondary to viral or bacterial infection.

GENERAL PREVENTION
- Long-term penicillin prophylaxis for patients with a history of rheumatic fever. Droplet precautions for hospitalized children with streptococcal pharyngitis until 24 hours after initiation of therapy
- Isolation of hospitalized patient with respiratory viruses and pharyngitis
- Control measures:
  - Children with group A streptococcal (GAS) pharyngitis can return to school or day care 24 hours after starting antimicrobial therapy.
  - Cultures of asymptomatic contacts of patients with streptococcal pharyngitis are not indicated except in outbreak situations in school or day care (where treatment of patients with positive rapid streptococcal antigen detection test [RADT] or culture is indicated) or in contacts with a history of nonsuppurative complications.

EPIDEMIOLOGY
- Streptococcal pharyngitis:
  - Most common in children 5–15 years of age, causing 15–20% of pharyngitis cases in this age group
  - Peak incidence in winter, early spring
- Viral disease is more common in younger children during winter months.

ETIOLOGY
- Viral:
  - Adenovirus types 1 through 7, 7a, 9, 14, 15, and 16
  - Epstein–Barr virus (EBV)
  - Influenza A, B: Usually associated with more severe systemic complaints
  - Parainfluenza 1, 2, and 3.
  - Enteroviruses: Coxsackievirus A and B and echoviruses
  - Measles and rubella and coronavirus, cytomegalovirus
  - Herpes simplex virus (HSV)
  - Rhinovirus and respiratory syncytial virus (RSV): not usually associated with pharyngeal inflammation
  - Human immunodeficiency virus (HIV)
- Bacterial:
  - *Streptococcus pyogenes* (group A β-hemolytic streptococcus)
  - Group C or G streptococci
  - *Fusobacterium necrophorum* (Lemierre syndrome)
  - *Corynebacterium diphtheriae* (diphtheria)
  - *Corynebacterium hemolyticum*
  - *Neisseria gonorrhoeae* and *Neisseria meningitidis*
  - *Mycoplasma pneumoniae*
  - *Mycoplasma hominis*
  - *Chlamydia pneumoniae, Chlamydia psittaci*
  - *Yersinia enterocolitica*
  - *Treponema pallidum* (syphilis)
  - Oral anaerobes (Vincent angina)
- Fungi: Candida species (oral thrush)

DIAGNOSIS

ALERT
- Caution: Diagnostic pitfalls:
  - Swabbing the throat from anywhere other than the tonsils and posterior pharyngeal wall
  - Use of clinical grounds alone, even experienced clinicians may overestimate the diagnosis of GAS pharyngitis by up to 80%.
  - About 20% of children with GAS pharyngitis who have mild symptoms may go unrecognized if cultures are not performed.
  - Failure to request identification of other organisms in the appropriate clinical setting. (e.g., *N. gonorrhoeae* or *A. hemolyticum, F. necrophorum*)
  - Reliance on monospot test in young children (<5 years) because of a high incidence of false-negatives (Consider EBV serology instead.)
  - Positive throat culture or RADT in patients with viral pharyngitis may represent streptococcal carrier state. Diagnostic tests for GAS should be used in patients suspected of having streptococcal disease on clinical and epidemiologic grounds, not on all patients who complain of a sore throat. In a meta-analysis, 9–14% of well children were found to be GAS carriers.

SIGNS AND SYMPTOMS
- Sore throat
- Fever
- Headache
- Nausea, vomiting, abdominal pain
- Rhinorrhea
- Cough
- Hoarseness
- Conjunctivitis
- Ulcerative pharyngeal lesions

HISTORY
- Sudden onset of fever, sore throat, with headache, nausea, and vomiting is frequent in streptococcal pharyngitis, which is usually exudative but cough or rhinorrhea is present in about 10% of cases
- Pharyngitis associated with rhinorrhea, cough, hoarseness, conjunctivitis, diarrhea, non-scarlatiniform exanthems, and ulcerative pharyngeal lesions: More likely to have a viral cause but GAS pharyngitis cannot be ruled out on this basis.
- Significant systemic complaints such as fever and malaise: Characteristic of EBV or HIV (acute retroviral syndrome)
- Appearance of papular eruption after administration of ampicillin or amoxicillin: Consider EBV.

PHYSICAL EXAM
- Tonsillar enlargement and moderate to severe pharyngeal erythema, which may be associated with petechiae, exudate, or ulceration.
- Follicular, exudative pharyngotonsillitis that may occur in association with conjunctivitis: Common with adenovirus infections (e.g., pharyngoconjunctival fever)
- Ulcerative lesions or characteristic enanthem consisting of 2–14 ulcers and vesicles (1– 2 mm) in the posterior pharynx: Common with enteroviral infections (e.g., Coxsackievirus A, B, echovirus)
- Ulcerative lesions on anterior oropharynx (gingivostomatitis): Characteristic of HSV infection, which can also cause an exudative pharyngitis in adolescents that may be difficult to differentiate from streptococcal or EBV pharyngitis
- Scarlatiniform rash: Strongly suggests diagnosis of GAS, but also reported with *A. hemolyticum.*
- Varying degrees of cervical adenopathy: Tender anterior lymphadenopathy more likely associated with streptococcal disease
- Splenomegaly and/or generalized adenopathy: Suggests EBV
- Presence of >6 palatal petechiae: Strongly associated with streptococcal pharyngitis

DIAGNOSTIC TESTS & INTERPRETATION
Because of the importance of its complications, streptococcal disease should be confirmed or excluded by laboratory testing, except in presentations suggestive of viral or other etiology of pharyngitis (e.g., a toddler with conjunctivitis and rhinorrhea, presence of gingivostomatitis, findings consistent with infectious mononucleosis, and so forth).

Lab
- RADT:
  - As effective as initial tests with >95% specificity and 50–80% sensitivity.
  - Cultures should be performed when rapid test is negative.
  - *Hint*: Culture throat using two swabs initially, keeping one for culture if the rapid test is negative.
  - Positive rapid tests do not require culture confirmation.
  - The best technique is to swab both tonsillar pillars and the retropharynx.
- Throat culture: Gold standard with best sensitivity (>90%) for group A β-hemolytic streptococci
- Monospot (heterophile antibody) test or EBV serology:
  - For infectious mononucleosis: Rate of heterophile antibody response appears to increase from infancy up to 4 years, after which the rate of response approaches values similar to that reported in young adult patients.
- Complete blood count (CBC) with differential:
  - May be helpful in diagnosing EBV if atypical lymphocytes are present

DIFFERENTIAL DIAGNOSIS
- Infectious:
  - Herpangina (enterovirus)
  - Hand-foot-and-mouth disease (enterovirus–coxsackievirus)
  - Peritonsillar abscess or cellulitis
  - Retropharyngeal abscess or cellulitis
  - Lemierre syndrome
  - Laryngitis
  - Epiglottitis
  - Kawasaki disease
  - Tularemia
- Ingestions:
  - Caustic or irritant ingestions
  - Inhaled irritant

- Tumors:
  - Leukemia
  - Lymphoma
  - Rhabdomyosarcoma
- Trauma:
  - Vocal abuse from shouting
- Inflammatory:
  - Allergy
- Miscellaneous:
  - PFAPA syndrome (periodic fever, aphthous ulcers, pharyngitis, and cervical adenitis)
  - Psychogenic pain (globus hystericus)
  - Vitamin deficiency (A, B complex, C)
  - Dehydration

 TREATMENT

MEDICATION (DRUGS)
First Line
- Oral penicillin V is the drug of choice for GAS pharyngitis except in penicillin-allergic individuals. Resistant strains have not been documented in vitro.
  - Children: 400,000 units (250 mg) b.i.d. or t.i.d. for 10 days
  - Adolescents/adults: 800,000 units (500 mg) b.i.d. for 10 days or 400,000 units (250 mg) t.i.d. or q.i.d. for 10 days
- Intramuscular (IM) benzathine penicillin G: Ensures compliance, useful in outbreaks
  - Children (<60 lb [27.2 kg]): 600,000 units IM (single dose)
  - Children (>60 lb [27.2 kg]) and adults: 1,200,000 units IM (single dose)
  - Procaine penicillin combinations are less painful.
  - Treatment failures with penicillin have risen steadily leading some experts to recommend other agents as first-line (e.g., cephalosporins). Failures occur even with benzathine penicillin (up to 37%) therefore compliance is not the cause. Potential causes include presence of β-lactamase-producing normal oropharyngeal flora that may be protecting GAS by inactivating penicillin.

Second Line
- Amoxicillin, clindamycin, and first-generation oral cephalosporins (≤10% of penicillin-allergic persons are also allergic to cephalosporins) are reasonable alternatives to penicillin in GAS pharyngitis:
  - Amoxicillin suspension is reported to be more palatable than penicillin VK.
  - Amoxicillin may be given in once daily 50 mg/kg (max 1 g) dose
- Clarithromycin and azithromycin have also been shown to eradicate streptococci; however, because of the broad spectra of these antibiotics and the increasing incidence of antibiotic-resistant bacteria, penicillin is still recommended by most experts except in cases of penicillin hypersensitivity, when patient nonadherence to a 10-day penicillin regimen is suspected, or for patients who fail therapy with a β-lactam:
  - Azithromycin, total dose of 60 mg/kg, given either as 12 mg/kg once daily for 5 days or 20 mg/kg once daily for 3 days
  - Clarithromycin, 15 mg/kg/d, given q12h for 10 days or 500 mg extended-release tablets given once a day for 5 days (studied in adolescents ≥12)
  - Oral erythromycin is indicated in penicillin-allergic individuals: Erythromycin ethyl succinate, 40–50 mg/kg/d in 2–4 divided doses. Resistance is rare in the US (<5% of isolates).

- Cefdinir, 14 mg/kg/day divided b.i.d. for 5 or 10 days or per day for 10 days (good palatability) and cefpodoxime proxetil, 10 mg/kg divided b.i.d. are approved for use in a more convenient 5-day dosing schedule.
- Clindamycin, 20 mg/kg per day divided in 3 doses (max 1.8 g/day) for 10 days
- Tetracyclines and sulfonamides should not be used owing to resistance of group A streptococci.

SURGERY/OTHER PROCEDURES
- Tonsillectomy for recurrent pharyngitis is still controversial, with only modest reductions in the number of subsequent episodes weighed against the morbidity of the procedure.

 ONGOING CARE

COMPLICATIONS
- Streptococcal pharyngitis:
  - Suppurative complications include peritonsillar abscess, cervical lymphadenitis, and mastoiditis.
  - Most significant nonsuppurative complication is acute rheumatic fever.
  - Post-streptococcal glomerulonephritis
- Lemierre syndrome:
  - Postanginal sepsis or necrobacillosis originates as pharyngitis or tonsillitis, then progresses to sepsis and suppurative thrombophlebitis of the internal jugular vein. Septic thromboemboli seed various organs, especially the liver, lungs, and joints.
  - Treatment requires anaerobic coverage, macrolides should be avoided.
- Pediatric autoimmune neuropsychiatric disorder associated with streptococcal infection (PANDAS) is a recently recognized nonsuppurative complication that now appears to be more common than rheumatic fever or glomerulonephritis.
  - Identified at National Institute of Mental Health (NIMH) while studying Sydenham chorea in setting of rheumatic fever.
  - NIMH Diagnostic Criteria for PANDAS
    ○ Presence of obsessive compulsive disorder (OCD) and/or tic disorder
    ○ Pediatric onset, usually between 3 and 12 years of age
    ○ Abrupt symptom onset and/or episodic course of symptom severity
    ○ Temporal association between symptom exacerbation and GAS infection
    ○ Presence of neurologic abnormalities during periods of symptom exacerbation
  - Treatment within 9 days of symptom onset appears to be necessary to halt progression of autoimmune antibody response.

ADDITIONAL READING
- Casey JR, Pichichero M. Meta-analysis of cephalosporin vs. penicillin treatment of group A streptococcal tonsillopharyngitis in children. *Pediatrics.* 2004;113:866–882.
- Feder HM. Periodic fever, aphthous stomatitis, pharyngitis, adenitis: A clinical review of a new syndrome. *Curr Opin Pediatr.* 2000;12:253–256.
- Gerber MA, Baltimore RS, Eaton CB, et al. Prevention of rheumatic fever and treatment of acute streptococcal pharyngitis: A scientific statement from the American Heart Association. *Circulation.* 2009;119:1541–1551.

 CODES

ICD9
- 034.0 Streptococcal sore throat
- 074.0 Herpangina
- 462 Acute pharyngitis

ICD10
- J02.0 Streptococcal pharyngitis
- J02.8 Acute pharyngitis due to other specified organisms
- J02.9 Acute pharyngitis, unspecified

FAQ
- Q: How many days after onset of GAS pharyngitis will therapy be effective in preventing acute rheumatic fever?
- A: Therapy started as late as 9 days after illness onset has been shown to be effective in preventing acute rheumatic fever.
- Q: Is there any benefit to starting therapy while waiting for culture results?
- A: Immediate therapy probably shortens the symptomatic period, but waiting for a positive test result avoids overuse of antibiotics.
- Q: Does an asymptomatic patient with a positive test for GAS from the pharynx (e.g., chronic carriers) require therapy?
- A: Usually not. Between 8% and 20% of children in school or day care will have asymptomatic carriage of GAS and generally do not require therapy. Exceptions are those with a history of acute rheumatic fever, outbreak situations, or to achieve eradication in families with recurrent episodes of GAS pharyngitis.
- Q: Is there any evidence of GAS resistance to penicillin and other β-lactam antibiotics?
- A: No, GAS has never been found to be resistant to penicillin, but some studies suggest tolerance to penicillin where penicillin is bacteriostatic rather than bactericidal. However, 2–8% of GAS strains will be resistant to macrolides.
- Q: Is tonsillectomy indicated for recurrent GAS pharyngitis?
- A: Rare patients in whom multiple symptomatic episodes of laboratory-confirmed GAS pharyngitis occur despite appropriate therapy may be considered for tonsillectomy.
- Q: Is continuous antimicrobial prophylaxis for recurrent GAS pharyngitis recommended?
- A: No, there is insufficient evidence to show that it is effective, except for preventing recurrences of acute rheumatic fever.
- Q: What is the association of pharyngitis and recurrent fever?
- A: There is an increasingly recognized syndrome of periodic fever, aphthous stomatitis, pharyngitis, and cervical adenitis, also known as PFAPA. The fever is usually high, recurs at fixed intervals of 2–8 weeks, and resolves spontaneously within 4 days. It does not appear to be familial, begins before the age of 5 years, the patient is well between episodes, and there are no known sequelae or etiology. Tonsillectomy was found to be effective treatment in a small randomized trial.

PHOTOSENSITIVITY

Leslie Castelo-Soccio
Albert Yan (5th edition)

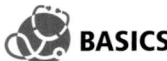 BASICS

DESCRIPTION
Adverse or abnormal reaction of the skin to sunlight

EPIDEMIOLOGY
- Variable for each disorder
- Photosensitivities with onset in childhood include albinism, hydroa aestivale, hydroa vacciniforme, the porphyrias (e.g., erythropoietic, erythropoietic protoporphyria, hepatoerythropoietic), and genetic disorders (e.g., xeroderma pigmentosa, Hartnup disease, poikiloderma congenitale, Bloom syndrome, and Cockayne syndrome).
- Photosensitivities that occur frequently in adults but can occur in childhood are vitiligo, chemically induced photosensitivities, polymorphous light eruption, and connective tissue disease.

RISK FACTORS
- Family history
- Disease
- Exposure to toxins

Genetics
- Genetic disorders include the porphyrias and others as previously listed:
  - The various porphyrias have variable inheritance patterns, whereas most of the other genetic disorders are inherited in an autosomal-recessive pattern.
  - There is a positive familial history in many cases of polymorphous light eruption.

PATHOPHYSIOLOGY
Findings are diverse for the different disorders and rarely diagnostic.

ETIOLOGY
- Combination of sunlight with some abnormality in the skin such as loss of pigment, a chemical agent, a metabolic product, another skin disorder, a genetic disease, or an unknown factor produces a cutaneous abnormality.
- Specific wavelengths of the radiant energy emitted by the sun and reaching the earth are usually responsible for each photosensitivity disorder, most commonly ultraviolet B (UVB, 290–320 nm), ultraviolet A (UVA, 320–400 nm), and visible light (400–800 nm).

DIAGNOSIS

HISTORY
- Age of onset of rash
- Occurrence:
  - Season: Spring and summer
  - Relation to sun exposure: Time frame, effect of sun through glass
- Oral medications:
  - May be related to oral contraceptives, tetracyclines (doxycycline in particular), sulfa drugs, iodines/bromides, or phenytoin
- New topical agents (e.g., perfumes, lemons, limes, sunscreens, etc.):
  - Photosensitivity may occur on neck or places where agents were placed on skin.
- Rash:
  - Accentuation of the rash on the nose, cheeks, and forehead with sparing of the eyelids and the submental portion of the chin
  - There is often a sharp cutoff in the nuchal area at the collar line.

PHYSICAL EXAM
- Distribution:
  - Distribution of lesions is the main sign of photosensitivity reactions.
  - Lesions are prominent on sun-exposed skin such as the face, pinnae of the ears, the V of the neck, the nuchal area, and the dorsa of the hands.
  - Often, sparing of the philtrum, the area below the chin, the eyelids, and other covered areas is seen.
  - In phytophotodermatitis, linear or bizarre shapes can occur, including, as an example, hand prints if a caregiver has been squeezing limes and then picks up a child and the child is then exposed to sunlight.
- Lesion characteristics:
  - Vary with the particular disease and can include papules, vesicles, and plaques (polymorphous light eruption), sunburn (chemical reaction to a systemic agent), linear areas of hyperpigmentation (chemical reaction to a topical agent), skin cancers (xeroderma pigmentosum), vesicles (porphyria)
  - In some cases, scarring can also be seen related to severe burns (porphyria).

DIAGNOSTIC TESTS & INTERPRETATION
- Phototesting:
  - Using an artificial source of light, can confirm the presence of certain photosensitivities. Procedures are of 2 types:
    - The 1st is exposure of skin to increasing doses of UVA and UVB to determine the erythema response (present at lower exposures than usual) and possibly reproduce lesions in certain diseases.
    - The 2nd is photopatch testing in which photoallergic chemicals are applied under patches in duplicate, and 1 set is subsequently exposed to UVA. Patients who have photoallergic contact dermatitis develop a reaction under only the exposed patch of the agent causing the problem.

Lab
Initial lab tests
- Genetic tests (optional): Find labs that perform genetic tests at www.genetests.org and enter disease name:
  - Cell culture: Evaluates DNA repair for xeroderma pigmentosum or shows chromosomal breaks in Bloom disease
  - Measurement of specific amino acid and indole excretion patterns in Hartnup disease
  - Measurements of antinuclear antibodies are helpful in connective tissue diseases.
- Biochemical tests:
  - Helpful for the diagnosis of the porphyrias, with elevated levels of various porphyrins specific to each type in the urine, blood, or stool
- Screening for connective tissue diseases should be done where appropriate.

DIFFERENTIAL DIAGNOSIS
- Photosensitivity resulting from pigment loss:
  - Albinism
  - Vitiligo
- Idiopathic photosensitivity:
  - Polymorphous light eruption
  - Solar urticaria
- Chemically induced reactions:
  - Topical agents: Perfumes, plant-associated phytophotodermatitis (e.g., lemons, limes, celery, parsnips, carrots, dill, parsley, figs, meadow grass, giant hogweed, mangos, wheat, clover, cocklebur, buttercups, shepherds purse, and pigweed), blankophores (e.g., optical brighteners in detergents), sunscreens, topical retinoids (e.g., tretinoin, adapalene, tazarotene)

- Systemic agents: Tetracyclines, sulfonamides, nalidixic acid, griseofulvin, phenothiazines, oral hypoglycemic agents, amiodarone, quinine, isoniazid, and thiazide diuretics
- Metabolic disorders:
  - Porphyrias: Disorders of hemoglobin synthesis producing various porphyrins that are photosensitizers
- Genetic disorders: See "Genetics"
- Cutaneous diseases aggravated by sunlight:
  - Connective tissue diseases

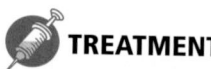 TREATMENT

ADDITIONAL TREATMENT
General Measures
- Protection against sun exposure:
  - Avoiding the sun, particularly between 10 a.m. and 3 p.m., and wearing protective clothing is important.
  - Sunscreens are helpful for those sensitive to UVB.
  - Sunscreens should be waterproof and reapplied q2h.
  - The higher the sun protection factor (SPF; ratio of minimal erythema dose of sunscreened skin to minimal erythema dose of unprotected skin), the better.
  - Sunscreens are less effective for blocking UVA and therefore less effective in helping patients with sensitivities to longer wavelengths.
  - Sunscreens that contain both UVA- and UVB-blocking capabilities offer better protection than most. These include sunscreens containing avobenzone, titanium dioxide, and zinc oxide. Avobenzone has a relatively short lifespan but is now available in a chemically stabilized form known by the trade names: Helioplex and Active Photobarrier Complex. Mexoryl is another long-acting broad-spectrum sunscreen that has especially good UVA protection.
  - Opaque formulations such as zinc oxide and titanium dioxide block UV and visible light, but may be less cosmetically appealing; however, new formulations made from microfine particles of titanium dioxide or zinc oxide make it more appealing,
  - Patients with severe photosensitivities may have to avoid any significant light exposure.
  - Most patients require chronic protection against sun exposure. However, the problem is generally more acute in spring and summer months.

- Removal of the offending agent is necessary in chemically induced photosensitivities:
  - Any severe and acute eruptions may require a short course of oral prednisone.
- Antimalarial agents have been used for polymorphous light eruption, lupus erythematosus, solar urticaria, and porphyria cutanea tarda and require the experience of a specialist.

ISSUES FOR REFERRAL
If possible, it is important to accurately document the specific wavelength of light and the degree of photosensitivity to accurately advise the patient. This requires phototesting by a specialist.

 ONGOING CARE

FOLLOW-UP RECOMMENDATIONS
Patient Monitoring
Skin exams for skin cancers routinely with frequency dependent on type of photosensitivity; for example, more monitoring for genetic causes like xeroderma pigmentosa

PATIENT EDUCATION
Education regarding significance of using sunscreen

PROGNOSIS
With the exception of chemically induced photosensitivities, most of the conditions are chronic.

ADDITIONAL READING

- Kuhn A, Ruland V, Bonsmann G. Photosensitivity, phototesting and photoprotection in cutaneous lupus erythematosus. *Lupus*. 2010;19:1036–1046.
- Morison WL. Clinical practice: Photosensitivity. *N Engl J Med*. 2004;350:1111–1117.
- Oh DH, Spivak G. Hereditary photodermatoses. *Adv Exp Med Biol*. 2010;685:95–105.
- Roelandts R. The diagnosis of photosensitivity. *Arch Dermatol*. 2000;136:1152–1157.
- Segal AR, Doherty KM, Leggott J, et al. Cutaneous reactions to drugs in children. *Pediatrics*. 2007; 120(4):e1082–1096.
- ten Berge O, Sigurdsson V, Brijinzeel-Koomen CA, et al. Photosensitivity testing in children. *J Am Acad Derm*. 2010;63:1019–1025.

 CODES

ICD9
- 270.2 Other disturbances of aromatic amino-acid metabolism
- 692.72 Acute dermatitis due to solar radiation
- 692.82 Dermatitis due to other radiation

ICD10
- L56.8 Other specified acute skin changes due to ultraviolet radiation
- L59.8 Other specified disorders of the skin and subcutaneous tissue related to radiation
- E70.30 Albinism, unspecified

FAQ

- Q: What is the best sunscreen to use?
- A: It depends on your particular problem. If you are sensitive to UVB, use a sunscreen with the highest SPF. If you are sensitive to UVA, sunscreens containing avobenzone, titanium dioxide, or zinc oxide are best.
- Q: I have heard that sunscreens with an SPF >15 are not necessary. Is this true?
- A: This is definitely not true for patients with photosensitivities, who have abnormal responses to light and require excessive protection. Even for the healthy person, it is often not true. An SPF of 15 suggests that someone may receive 15 times more sun exposure with the sunscreen applied than without and not become sunburned. Some physicians have suggested that this is more than anyone should need. However, this number is calculated by testing in a controlled laboratory. Normal outdoor conditions, such as wind, reflection from water and sand, perspiration, and water exposure can significantly decrease the effectiveness of the sunscreen.
- Q: What is "sun allergy"?
- A: This is a lay term for polymorphous light eruption, one of the most common photosensitivities, presenting with papules, vesicles, and plaques 1–2 days after sun exposure. It usually recurs every spring, and most patients learn to avoid sun exposure. However, ironically, it can improve with slow, gradual sun exposure.
- Q: Can I become allergic to sunscreens?
- A: Certain active agents in sunscreens can produce an allergic response in rare individuals. If the rash recurs with each use, switch to another sunscreen with different ingredients. If the problem continues, consult a specialist for evaluation.

PINWORMS

Terry Kind
Hope Rhodes

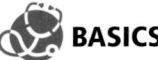 **BASICS**

DESCRIPTION
- Infection by a small, white nematode (roundworm), typically *Enterobius vermicularis*
- Pinworms may also be caused by *Enterobius gregorii* in Europe, Africa, and Asia.

EPIDEMIOLOGY
- Considered the most common helminthic infection of humans (the only known natural host) and the most common worm infection in US
- Occurs in school-aged children (5–10 years) and preschool children predominantly
- Does occur in adults, usually in those caring for infected children. Some individuals may be predisposed to having either heavy or light worm burdens.
- Independent of socioeconomic status

Incidence
- US infection rates: 5–15%
- Occurs worldwide, but is more prevalent in temperate climates

GENERAL PREVENTION
- Decontaminate the environment by washing underclothes, bedclothes, bed sheets, and towels.
- Maintain good hand hygiene, including handwashing and proper toileting.
- Keep fingernails short and avoid nail biting.
- Treat family members and close contacts.

PATHOPHYSIOLOGY
- *E. vermicularis* eggs are ingested and hatch in the human's stomach and duodenum. Then the larvae migrate to the ileum and cecum. Adult worms copulate in the cecum.
- The pregnant female pinworm migrates from the cecum to the anus ~5 weeks later and deposits eggs on the perianal skin (at which point the female pinworm usually dies). Thousands of eggs are laid, which may result in hundreds of worms.

- Pruritus is caused by the perianal deposition of eggs and a mucosal mastocytosis response. Other GI symptoms, such as anorexia or abdominal pain, may occur because of the mucosal inflammatory response.
- Granulomas may form if dead worms and eggs invoke an inflammatory response in ectopic locations such as the peritoneal cavity, vulva, cervix, uterus, and fallopian tubes.

ETIOLOGY
- Ingestion of organism via fecal–oral transmission
- Can be spread directly, hand to mouth, or via fomites, such as toys, bedding, clothing, toilet seats, and baths

DIAGNOSIS

HISTORY
- Prior pinworms or sibling with pinworms:
  - Eggs can survive for several days in the environment, and the incubation period can be 1–2 months.
  - Spread can occur between family members.
- Daytime itching:
  - Pinworm infections usually cause perianal itching during the night or just before waking in the morning.
  - Daytime perianal or perivulvar itching or irritation is likely due to other causes.
- Fevers, diarrhea, or vomiting:
  - Pinworms are highly unlikely to cause systemic symptoms (except in rare cases where they migrate aberrantly).
- Visible worms at night:
  - Pinworms may be seen 2–3 hours after the child has gone to sleep. Female worms are 8–13 mm, and males are 2–5 mm.
  - They may be visible as small, white worms in the perianal area at night.

PHYSICAL EXAM
- Exam may be normal, and the child may be well appearing.
- May have self-inflicted, perianal excoriation
- Pinworms may be visible perianally.
- Infection is characterized by perianal pruritus that occurs at night or just before waking.
- Difficulty sleeping, decreased appetite, and/or abdominal pain may occur.

DIAGNOSTIC TESTS & INTERPRETATION
Lab
- Stool or urine samples for ova or parasites:
  - Generally not helpful or recommended
  - Very few ova present in stool (even more rare in urine)
- Blood count for eosinophilia:
  - Generally not helpful or recommended
  - Eosinophilia is not observed because usually there is no tissue invasion.

Diagnostic Procedures/Other
- Transparent tape, Scotch tape test:
  - In the morning, prior to the child awakening and before defecation or washing, the adhesive side of transparent tape is applied to the perianal area.
  - After removal, the tape is applied to a glass slide and examined under light microscopy for pinworm ova. Several samples may be necessary to see the pinworms.

DIFFERENTIAL DIAGNOSIS
- Infection:
  - Other parasites (e.g., *Strongyloides stercoralis*)
  - Nonparasitic vulvovaginitis (due to bacterial, fungal, or viral causes)

- Dermatologic:
  - Contact or irritative diaper dermatitis
  - Hidradenitis suppurativa
  - Irritative vulvovaginitis secondary to soaps, bubble baths, or lotions
  - Anal fissures (usually cause pain rather than itching)
- Miscellaneous:
  - Behavioral: Self-touching (normal)
  - Sleep disorders not owing to nocturnal pruritus
  - Hemorrhoids

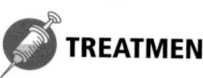 TREATMENT

MEDICATION (DRUGS)
Single-drug and -dose therapy with one of the following agents:

- Mebendazole, 100 mg (available as a chewable tablet) PO once, may repeat in 2 weeks if symptoms still present
- Pyrantel pamoate, 11 mg/kg (maximum 1 g) PO once, may repeat in 2 weeks
- Albendazole, 400 mg PO once, may repeat in 2 weeks
- Experience is limited in children <2 years of age. Consider risks and benefits before use.
- Caution in treating pregnant individuals with antihelminthic medications because mebendazole, pyrantel pamoate, and albendazole are all category C and are not recommended in pregnancy

ADDITIONAL TREATMENT
General Measures
- Reinfection is common especially if not all close contacts are treated.
- Treat all symptomatic contacts, and consider treating close household contacts, especially if repeated infections have occurred.
- Reinfection can occur if eggs remain on bed linen or clothing.
- Infection may be asymptomatic and transmitted to others.
- Autoreinfection can occur if eggs remain under the nails.

 ONGOING CARE

FOLLOW-UP RECOMMENDATIONS
Patient Monitoring
Watch for signs of reinfection.

PATIENT EDUCATION
National Library of Medicine's health information site: http://www.nlm.nih.gov/medlineplus/pinworms.html

PROGNOSIS
- Reinfection is common.
- With appropriate treatment, symptoms resolve within a few days.
- Any chronic symptoms are likely due to recurrence rather than chronic infection, because the life cycle of the adult worm is short, with eggs being laid by the adult worm within 5 weeks.

COMPLICATIONS
- Urethritis
- Vulvovaginitis
- Granuloma formation
- Pelvic inflammatory disease
- Bacterial superinfection of perianal excoriations
- Appendicitis (uncommon)

ADDITIONAL READING

- Arca MJ, Gates RL, Groner JI, et al. Clinical manifestations of appendiceal pinworms in children: An institutional experience and a review of the literature. *Pediatr Surg Int*. 2004;20(5):372–375.
- Elston DM. What's eating you? Enterobius vermicularis (pinworms, threadworms). *Cutis*. 2003;71:268–270.
- Grencis RK, Cooper ES. Enterobius, trichuris, capillaria and hookworm including Ancylostoma caninum. *Gastroenterol Clin North Am*. 1996;25:579–597.
- Stermer E, Sukhotnic I, Shaoul R. Pruritus ani: An approach to an itching condition. *J Ped Gastroenterol Nutr*. 2009;48:513–516.

 CODES

ICD9
127.4 Enterobiasis

ICD10
B80 Enterobiasis

FAQ
- Q: Could the child have acquired pinworms from a pet dog or cat?
- A: No. Household pets are not involved in the life cycles of pinworms.
- Q: When can an infected child return to day care?
- A: After receiving the 1st treatment dose, the child can return to school or day care. It is prudent to bathe the child and to trim and scrub his or her nails prior to school re-entry.
- Q: Is it necessary to re-evaluate and retest a child once treated?
- A: No. However, reinfection is common.
- Q: Can pinworm eggs survive on bedding, toilet seats, or clothing?
- A: Yes. Eggs can remain infectious in an indoor environment for up to 3 weeks.
- Q: Does pinworm infection cause nocturnal bruxism?
- A: There is no proof of any causal relationship.
- Q: How do the antihelminthic medications work?
- A: They inhibit microtubule function and cause glycogen deletion in the adult worms.

P

PLAGUE

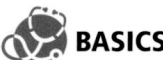

Genevieve L. Buser
Bruce Tempest (5th edition)
Jonathan Iralu (5th edition)

BASICS

DESCRIPTION
Plague is an enzootic disease transmitted by fleas from wild rodents and caused by *Yersinia pestis*. Humans and their pets can enter this cycle, resulting in human plague. Human plague has 3 forms: Bubonic, septicemic, and pneumonic.

EPIDEMIOLOGY
- >50% of contemporary cases of plague occur in persons <20 years of age, probably due to behavioral and environmental reasons.
- Worldwide: Enzootic in Africa, Asia, and Americas; 75% of cases are bubonic plague.
- *Y. pestis* is enzootic in the Western U.S., west of 100th meridian (ND to TX).
- In U.S., ~85% cases occur in AZ, NM, CA, CO.
- In U.S., most cases occur in spring/summer.
- 17 cases of plague occurred in the U.S. in 2006 including 5 septicemic, 8 bubonic, and 4 unknown. 2 developed plague pneumonia.
- 20% of U.S. cases with identified mode of transmission are acquired through direct contact with *Y. pestis*-infected animals, not via flea bite.
- No cases of person-to-person transmission of pneumonic plague have been reported in the U.S. since 1925.
- World-wide case fatality rate is 6.7% (WHO, 2010); U.S., 10.9% (estimate, 1987–2009).
- Untreated bubonic plague: >50% fatal.
- Untreated pneumonic plague: Nearly 100% fatal.

GENERAL PREVENTION
- Reduce rodent shelter and food sources in the immediate vicinity of the home by storing grain and animal food in rodent-proof containers.
- Flea disinfestation of cats and dogs, especially in endemic areas
- Hospital isolation precautions:
  – Patients with bubonic or septicemic plague and no evidence of pneumonia: standard precautions; add droplet precautions for 1st 24 hours of therapy, until chest radiograph persistently clear.
  – Patients with pneumonic plague: standard and droplet precautions. Continue droplet precautions until patient has completed 48 hours of appropriate antimicrobial therapy.
- Postexposure management:
  – All persons with exposure to known or suspected plague source in last 6 days:
    ○ Daily surveillance for fever or symptoms of disease for 7–10 days
    ○ Offer prophylaxis.
    ○ Initiate treatment if becomes ill.

  – Persons with close (<2 m) contact with a patient with pneumonic plague: Prophylaxis is strongly recommended, but isolation not necessary.
- Chemoprophylaxis ≥8 years:
  – Doxycycline (PO), *OR*
  – Ciprofloxacin (PO) at treatment doses for 7 days from last exposure (see "Medications" for dosing)
- Chemoprophylaxis <8 years:
  – Doxycycline or ciprofloxacin (PO) (weigh risks of adverse affects and disease exposure), *OR*
  – Trimethoprim–sulfamethoxazole (PO): TMP 20 mg/kg/d divided q6h, *OR*
  – Streptomycin (IM/IV): 30 mg/kg/d divided q8h, for 7 days from last exposure
- Notify State Public Health authorities of cases of suspected and proven *Y. pestis* infection.
- Vaccination is no longer available and is not considered useful to prevent plague from an enzootic source.

PATHOPHYSIOLOGY
- Skin portal of entry:
  – *Y. pestis* is transmitted from fleas to humans via the regurgitation of the organism into the bite during the flea's blood meal (*Y. pestis* blocks foregut, causing regurgitation).
  – Rodents, ground squirrels, cats, prairie dogs, marmots, rabbits, and occasionally dogs harbor infected fleas and are reservoirs of infection (enzootic).
  – Direct skin inoculation of organisms from infected animal tissue or blood occurs through breaks in the skin (e.g., cat scratch, skinning quarry).
  – Lymphatic spread of infection to the regional lymph nodes creates a localized inflammatory response (bubo, bubonic).
  – Subsequent hematogenous spread of the organism to other organs results in high levels of circulating bacterial endotoxin (septicemic plague).
  – By hematogenous spread to lungs, both bubonic and septicemic plague can cause secondary pneumonic plague.
- Respiratory portal of entry:
  – Primary pneumonic plague: Acquired via inhalation of respiratory tract droplets from a human or animal (e.g., cat) with pneumonic plague.
- Incubation period:
  – 2–6 days for bubonic or septicemic plague
  – 1–6 days for pneumonic plague

ETIOLOGY
Plague is caused by *Y. pestis,* a pleomorphic, bipolar staining, gram-negative coccobacilli from the Enterobacteriaceae family.

DIAGNOSIS

HISTORY
- A thorough travel history (especially to enzootic areas) is imperative to raise the index of suspicion for diagnosing plague.
- Environmental history should include epizootic deaths (die-offs) of rodents, ground squirrels, or prairie dogs in the patient's locale.
- In enzootic areas, a sick household cat or dog is an additional risk factor.
- Signs and symptoms:
  – Bubonic plague:
    ○ Initial symptom: Pain in the groin or axillae prior to lymph node swelling
    ○ Lymphadenitis (usually inguinal >axillary >cervical)
    ○ Fever, chills, prostration
  – Septicemic plague:
    ○ Tachycardia and hypotension
    ○ Abdominal symptoms
    ○ Hemorrhage
    ○ Fever, chills, prostration
  – Bubonic or septicemic plague may progress to secondary pneumonic plague.
  – Pneumonic plague:
    ○ Cough, dyspnea
    ○ Systemic manifestations
    ○ Fever, chills, shock
    ○ Rapidly progressive and often fatal

PHYSICAL EXAM
- Tachycardic, hypotensive, tachypneic, and toxic-appearing
- Flea-bite lymphadenitis classically affects inguinal nodes; cat-associated plague affects mostly axillary or cervical nodes secondary to handling infected cat.
- GI: Abdominal pain, nausea, and diarrhea are common, secondary to inflammatory mediators.
- Neurologic: Weakness, delirium, and coma, owing to the effects of the endotoxin of *Y. pestis*.
- Heme: Disseminated intravascular coagulation
- Renal: Glomerular parenchymal damage
- Rare: Meningitis, endophthalmitis, endocarditis and pleuritis.

DIAGNOSTIC TESTS & INTERPRETATION
Lab
- Total WBC count:
  – Usually 10,000–20,000, but may be as high as 100,000, with immature neutrophils
- Perform Gram, Wayson, Giemsa, or fluorescent antibody staining on specimen (blood, bubo, CSF, sputum) to look for gram-negative, bipolar staining organisms.

- *Y. pestis* culture (notify receiving lab):
  - Suspect bubonic plague: Needle aspiration of the bubo for stain and culture. Puncture center of bubo with a sterile syringe and inject 1 mL of nonbacteriostatic, sterile saline. Withdraw aspirate vigorously until blood-tinged liquid appears in syringe.
  - Suspect pneumonic plague: Sputum for stain and culture.
  - Blood cultures are usually positive, even with bubonic plague, and should always be done prior to therapy.
    - Slow-grower; may be misidentified as *Y. pseudotuberculosis* or *Acinetobacter* sp.
- Serology:
  - Single positive acute serology OR
  - At least a 4-fold increase in antibody titers by passive hemagglutination test between acute and convalescent sera taken 4–12 weeks apart
- Comprehensive testing and notification to State Public Health Lab and CDC

Diagnostic Procedures/Other
Pitfalls:

- Patients who present with a nonspecific febrile illness, tachycardia, tachypnea, rather than lymphadenitis, are at higher risk for delayed diagnosis and serious sequelae (e.g., septicemic plague, death).
- Failure to consider septicemic plague in the appropriate epidemiologic setting, and withholding appropriate antibiotics or using an empiric β-lactam regimen.
- Failure to treat suspected bubonic plague with antibiotics while awaiting culture results when needle aspiration of the bubo shows no organisms on direct stain.

DIFFERENTIAL DIAGNOSIS
- Diagnosis of plague follows a high index of suspicion and a thorough review of the patient's lifestyle, travel history, and recent activities. The appearance of septicemia and endotoxin-mediated shock includes a large differential diagnosis that includes sepsis owing to other bacteria or viruses, as well as distributive shock resulting from toxic ingestion or anaphylaxis.
- Infection:
  - Streptococcal and staphylococcal infections (especially between the toes) can result in tender inguinal lymph nodes, fever, shock.
  - Cat-scratch fever (*Bartonella henselae*) can present with a history of cat scratch or bite, regional lymphadenitis and fever.
  - Hantavirus in humans has a clinical presentation similar to septicemic and pneumonic plague, and occurs in many of the plague enzootic areas.
  - Rickettsial diseases: *Rickettsia, Orientia, Coxiella, Ehrlichia, Anaplasma* (e.g., Rocky Mountain spotted fever (*Rickettsia*) *rickettsii* and relapsing tick fever due to *Borrelia* sp. may mimic septicemic or pneumonic plague.
  - Recent reports of plague-like illnesses have been associated with infections by other organisms, such as *Pseudomonas pseudomallei* (melioidosis) and *Francisella tularensis* (tularemia).

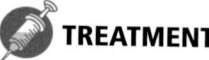 TREATMENT

MEDICATION (DRUGS)
- Use IV/IM forms for acute disease.
- Streptomycin is the drug of choice (IV/IM): Peds: 30 mg/kg/d divided q8–12h. Adult: 15 mg/kg q12h to max 1 gram q12h.
- Gentamicin, equally effective as streptomycin in recent study (IV): Peds: 2.5 mg/kg q8h. Adult: 5 mg/kg q24h.
- Meningitis or severe disease: Consider adding chloramphenicol (IV): 12.5–25 mg/kg q6h (max 4 grams). Monitor for toxicity.
- Alternatives:
  - Doxycycline: Peds <8 years (IV/PO): 2.2 mg/kg q12h. Peds ≥8 years (IV/PO): 2 mg/kg q12h up to adult dose. Adult: 200 mg IV × 1, then 100 mg IV/PO q12h. Some experts recommend adding it to gentamicin for severe disease.
  - Ciprofloxacin: Peds (IV/PO): 20–30 mg/kg/d divided q12h. Adults: 400 mg IV q12h; 500 mg PO q12h.
  - Tetracycline: Peds ≥8 years (PO): 25–50 mg/kg/d divided q6h (max 3 g). Adults (PO): 250–500 mg q6–12h.
- Continue antibiotic therapy for 7–10 days or until several days after lysis of fever.
- Severely ill patients may require a substantially longer course of therapy.
- TMP-SMZ should not be used for 1st-line treatment of bubonic plague or as monotherapy to treat septicemic or pneumonic plague, as some studies have shown higher failure rates and delayed treatment responses.
- Prolonged fever may suggest a pyogenic focus of *Y. pestis* infection (e.g., abscess).
- Foci (e.g., abscess) are infectious until sufficient appropriate antimicrobial therapy is given.

ADDITIONAL TREATMENT
General Measures
For septic patients in shock, initial attention should be given to airway management and fluid resuscitation, then antibiotics.

 ONGOING CARE

FOLLOW-UP RECOMMENDATIONS
Resolution of symptoms should begin in the first 3 days after initiation of therapy; however, the rate of clinical improvement depends on the initial severity of illness.

Patient Monitoring
None; most recover without sequelae

COMPLICATIONS
- Hematologic (disseminated intravascular coagulation)
- Renal (glomerular and parenchymal damage)

ADDITIONAL READING
- Boulanger LL, Ettestad P, Fogarty JD, et al. Gentamicin and tetracyclines for the treatment of human plague: Review of 75 cases in New Mexico. 1985–1999. *Clin Infect Dis.* 2004;38:663–669.
- Butler T. Plague into the 21st Century. *Clin Infect Dis.* 2009;49:736–742.
- CDC Plague Home Page. Available at www.cdc.gov.
- Centers for Disease Control and Prevention. Human plague—four states, 2006. *MMWR Dispatch.* 2006;55:1–3.
- Gage KL, Dennis DT, Orloski KA, et al. Cases of cat-associated human plague in the western US, 1977–1998. *Clin Infect Dis.* 2000;30:893–900.

 CODES

ICD9
- 020.0 Bubonic plague
- 020.2 Septicemic plague
- 020.9 Plague, unspecified

ICD10
- A20.0 Bubonic plague
- A20.7 Septicemic plague
- A20.9 Plague, unspecified

FAQ
- Q: Can one determine the risks of being exposed to plague during international travel?
- A: Yes. The CDC provides a service that contains updated information for international travel exposures at www.cdc.gov/travel.
- Q: Does persistent fever during treatment for plague warrant altering the antibiotic regimen?
- A: No. Fever can persist for up to 2 weeks despite appropriate 1st-line antibiotic therapy for *Y. pestis*. However, recommend an evaluation for a focus of infection requiring drainage.

PLEURAL EFFUSION

Richard M. Kravitz

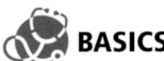 **BASICS**

DESCRIPTION
Accumulation of fluid in the pleural cavity

EPIDEMIOLOGY
- Depends on underlying cause
- Pneumonia (most common cause):
  - *Staphylococcus aureus* (increasing incidence of methicillin-resistant species)
  - *Streptococcus pneumoniae* (increasing incidence of penicillin-resistant species)
  - *Haemophilus influenzae* (decreasing incidence since introduction of *H. influenzae* type B [HiB] vaccine)
  - No identified organisms (all cultures sterile)
- Congenital heart disease
- Malignancy

PATHOPHYSIOLOGY
- Depends on the underlying disease
- 2 types of pleural effusion:
  - Transudate: Mechanical forces of hydrostatic and oncotic pressures are altered, favoring liquid filtration.
  - Exudate: Damage to the pleural surface occurs that alters its ability to filter pleural fluid; lymphatic drainage is diminished.
- Stages associated with parapneumonic effusions (infectious exudates):
  - Exudative stage:
    - Free-flowing fluid
    - Pleural fluid glucose, protein, lactate dehydrogenase (LDH) level, and pH are normal.
  - Fibrinolytic stage:
    - Loculations are forming.
    - Increase in fibrin, polymorphonuclear leukocytes, and bacterial invasion of pleural cavity are occurring.
    - Pleural fluid glucose and pH falls while protein and LDH levels increase.
  - Organizing stage (empyema):
    - Fibroblasts grow.
    - Pleural peal forms.
    - Pleural fluid parameters worsen.

ETIOLOGY
- Normally 1–15 mL of fluid in the pleural space
- Alterations in the flow and/or absorption of this fluid lead to its accumulation.
- Mechanisms that influence this flow of fluid:
  - Increased capillary hydrostatic pressure (i.e., congestive heart failure [CHF], overhydration)
  - Decreased pleural space hydrostatic pressure (i.e., after thoracentesis, atelectasis)
  - Decreased plasma oncotic pressure (i.e., hypoalbuminemia, nephrosis)
  - Increased capillary permeability (i.e., infection, toxins, connective tissue diseases, malignancy)
  - Impaired lymphatic drainage from the pleural space (i.e., disruption of the thoracic duct)
  - Passage of fluid from the peritoneal cavity through the diaphragm to the pleural space (i.e., hepatic cirrhosis with ascites)

DIAGNOSIS

HISTORY
- Underlying disease determines most systemic symptoms.
- Patient may be asymptomatic until the amount of fluid is large enough to cause cardiorespiratory compromise/distress.
- Dyspnea and cough are associated with large effusions.
- Fever (if infectious etiology)
- Pleuritic pain (pneumonia may cause irritation of the parietal pleura, causing pleural pain; as the effusion increases and separates the pleural membrane, the pain may disappear)

PHYSICAL EXAM
- Decreased thoracic wall excursion on the ipsilateral side
- Fullness of intercostal spaces on the ipsilateral side
- Trachea and cardiac apex displaced toward the contralateral side (may produce a mediastinal shift that can reduce venous return and compromise the cardiac output)
- Dull or flat percussion on the ipsilateral side (suggesting the presence of consolidation of pleural effusion)
- Decreased tactile and vocal fremitus
- Decreased whispering pectoriloquy
- Pleural rub during early phase (may resolve as fluid accumulates in the pleural space)
- Decreased breath sounds

DIAGNOSTIC TESTS & INTERPRETATION
- Cytologic exam of pleural fluid:
  - Fresh and heparinized specimen should be refrigerated at 4°C (39.2°F) until it can be processed.
  - Fixatives should not be added.
- Pleural fluid parameters to be routinely measured include:
  - pH
  - LDH
  - Protein
  - Glucose:
    - Note: Glucose of <40 mg/dL suggests a parapneumonic, tuberculosis, malignant, or rheumatic etiology to the effusion.

Lab
Initial lab tests
- Serology values to follow the degree of inflammation and the response to therapy:
  - Erythrocyte sedimentation rate (ESR)
  - C-reactive protein (CRP)

Imaging
- Chest radiograph:
  - Anteroposterior projection can show >400 mL of pleural fluid.
  - Lateral projection can show <200 mL of pleural fluid.
  - Lateral decubitus film to evaluate for free-flowing pleural fluid can show as little as 50 mL of pleural fluid.
- Ultrasound:
  - Reveals small (3–5 mL) loculated collections of pleural fluid
  - Useful as a guide for thoracentesis
  - Aids in distinguishing between pleural thickening and pleural effusion
- CT scan:
  - Clearly reveals effusions/empyemas, abscess, or pulmonary consolidations
  - Useful for defining the extent of loculated effusions

Diagnostic Procedures/Other
- Thoracentesis:
  - Indicated whenever cause is unclear or effusion causes symptoms (e.g., prolonged fever or respiratory distress)
- Pleural biopsy:
  - If thoracentesis is nondiagnostic
  - Most useful for diseases that cause extensive involvement of the pleura (i.e., tuberculosis, malignancies)
  - Confirms neoplastic involvement in 40–70% of cases

DIFFERENTIAL DIAGNOSIS
- Transudate:
  - Cardiovascular:
    - CHF
    - Constrictive pericarditis
  - Nephrotic syndrome with hypoalbuminemia
  - Cirrhosis
  - Atelectasis
- Exudate:
  - Infection:
    - Bacterial effusions (*S. aureus* is most common organism)
    - Tuberculous effusion
    - Viral effusions (adenovirus, influenza)
    - Fungal effusions: Most not associated with effusions; *Nocardia* and *Actinomyces* are most commonly seen.
    - Parasitic effusions
  - Neoplasm: Seen mostly in leukemia and lymphoma; uncommon in children

- Connective tissue disease:
  - ○ Rheumatoid arthritis
  - ○ Systemic lupus erythematosus
  - ○ Wegener granulomatosis
- Pulmonary embolus
- Intra-abdominal disease:
  - ○ Subdiaphragmatic abscess
  - ○ Pancreatitis
- Sarcoidosis
- Esophageal rupture
- Hemothorax
- Chylothorax
- Drugs
- Chemical injury
- Post-irradiation effusion

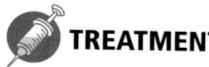 TREATMENT

MEDICATION (DRUGS)

Antibiotics:

- Used when effusion is caused by a bacterial infection
- Specific antibiotics dictated by organism identified
- If effusion is sterile, broad-spectrum antibiotics are indicated to cover for the usually seen organisms.
- Clinical improvement usually begins within 48–72 hours of therapy.
- Continue IV antibiotics until afebrile.
- Complete remainder of therapy on oral antibiotics.
- Duration of antibiotic therapy depends on the infectious organism and the degree of illness:
  - Total duration is controversial.
  - Usually, at least 2–4 weeks of total IV and PO

ADDITIONAL TREATMENT
General Measures

- Supportive measures:
  - Maintain adequate:
    - ○ Oxygenation
    - ○ Fluid status
    - ○ Nutritional balance
  - Antipyretic agents when febrile
  - Pain control
- Treat the underlying disease:
  - Antibiotics for infections
  - Cardiac medications for congestive heart failure
  - Chemotherapeutic agents for malignancies
  - Anti-inflammatory agents (i.e., steroids) for connective tissue diseases
  - Medium-chain triglycerides and low-fat diet for chylothorax
- Effective drainage of pleural fluid:
  - Thoracentesis
  - Chest tube drainage
  - Surgical drainage
- Duration of chest tube drainage:
  - Discontinue when patient is asymptomatic (afebrile, no distress) and drainage <50 mL/h
  - Thick, loculated empyema requires prolonged drainage (and possibly a video-assisted thoracic surgery [VATS] procedure if effusion not improving).

COMPLEMENTARY & ALTERNATIVE THERAPIES

- Thoracentesis:
  - For diagnosis purposes:
    - ○ To distinguish between a transudate and an exudate
    - ○ For culture material (if infection is suspected)
    - ○ For cytology (if malignancy is suspected)
  - For relief of dyspnea or cardiorespiratory distress

- Chest tube thoracostomy:
  - Reduce reaccumulation of fluid.
  - Drain parapneumonic effusion (before loculations develop which will prevent fluid drainage).
- Intrapleural fibrinolytics:
  - Adjunct to aid in drainage of complicated (i.e., multiloculated empyema) pleural effusions
- Streptokinase and urokinase are agents of choice.

SURGERY/OTHER PROCEDURES

- VATS:
  - Alternative to more invasive procedures (e.g., open thoracotomy/decortication)
  - Débridement through pleural visualization and lysis of adhesions/loculations
  - Useful when:
    - ○ Initial drainage is delayed
    - ○ Loculations prevent adequate drainage by chest tube alone
    - ○ Patient is failing more conservative therapy
- Pleurectomy:
  - Chylothorax
  - Malignant effusions
- Pleurodesis:
  - For recurrent effusions
  - Chemical agents frequently used include talc, tetracycline, doxycycline, and quinacrine.
  - Surgical methods include:
    - ○ Mechanical abrasion
    - ○ Pleurectomy via VATS
    - ○ Open thoracotomy route
  - In cases of malignant effusion:
    - ○ Sclerosing procedures are usually ineffective.
    - ○ Chest tube drainage can create a pneumothorax because the lung is incarcerated by the tumor.

 ONGOING CARE

FOLLOW-UP RECOMMENDATIONS

- Clinical improvement usually within 1–2 weeks
- With empyemas, the patient may have fever spikes for up to 2–3 weeks after improvement is noted.

DIET

When the effusion is a chylothorax:

- Medium-chain triglycerides
- Nutritional replacement
- At least 4–5 weeks on this regimen

PROGNOSIS

Dependent on underlying disease process:

- Properly treated infectious cause: Excellent prognosis
- Malignancy: Poor prognosis

COMPLICATIONS

- Hypoxia
- Respiratory distress
- Persistent fevers
- Decreased cardiac function
- Malnutrition (seen in chylothorax)
- Shock (secondary to blood loss in cases of hemothorax)
- Trapped lung

ADDITIONAL READING

- Beers SL, Abramo TJ. Pleural effusions. *Pediatr Emerg Care*. 2007;23(5):330–334.
- Buckingham SC, King MD, Miller ML. Incidence and etiologies of complicated parapneumonic effusions in children. *Pediatr Infect Dis*. 2003;22:499–504.
- Calder A, Owens CM. Imaging of parapneumonic pleural effusions and empyema in children. *Pediatr Radiol*. 2009;39:527–537.
- Doski JJ, Lou D, Hicks BA et al. Management of parapneumonic collections in infants and children. *J Pediatr Surg*. 2000;35:265–268; discussion 269–270.
- Heffner JE. Discriminating between transudates and exudates. *Clin Chest Med*. 2006;27:241–252.
- Krenke K, Peradzynska J, Lange J. Local treatment of empyema in children: A systematic review of randomized controlled trials. *Acta Paediatrica*. 2010;99(10):1449–1453.
- Merino JM, Carpinterol I, Alvarez T et al. Tuberculous pleural effusion in children. *Chest*. 1999;115:26–30.
- Proesma M, Boeck KD. Clinical Practice: Treatment of childhood empyema. *Eur J Pediatr*. 2009;168:639–645.
- Rocha G. Pleural effusions in the neonate. *Curr Opin Pulm Med*. 2007;13(4):305–311.

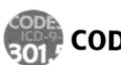 CODES

ICD9

- 511.81 Malignant pleural effusion
- 511.89 Other specified forms of effusion, except tuberculous
- 511.9 Unspecified pleural effusion

ICD10

- J11.1 Influenza due to unidentified influenza virus with other respiratory manifestations
- J90 Pleural effusion, not elsewhere classified
- J94.0 Chylous effusion

FAQ

- Q: When will the chest radiograph findings become normal?
- A: They may take up to 6 months (or longer) to return to normal appearance.
- Q: When will the pulmonary function tests normalize?
- A: Depending on extent of effusion, they may take up to 6–12 months.

PNEUMOYSTIC JIROVECI (PREVIOUSLY KNOWN AS PNEUMOCYSTIC CARINII PNEUMONIS)

Danna Tauber

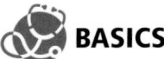 BASICS

DESCRIPTION
Opportunistic lung infection caused by *Pneumocystis jiroveci* (PJ). This organism is currently considered a primitive fungus based on DNA sequence analysis. It has two developmental forms (the cysts contain sporozoites that become trophozoites when excised).

- The acronym PCP is still in use and refers to *Pneumocystis* pneumonia. PCP occurs almost exclusively in the immunocompromised host. Children with congenital or acquired immune deficiency syndrome (AIDS) and recipients of suppressive therapy in the treatment of malignancies or after organ transplantation are at high risk.
- PCP is an AIDS-defining illness. It is the most common opportunistic life-threatening lung infection in infants with perinatally acquired HIV disease.
- PJ causes a diffuse pneumonitis characterized by fever, dyspnea at rest, tachypnea, hypoxemia, nonproductive cough, and bilateral diffuse infiltrates in the roentgenogram. It is a severe condition frequently leading to respiratory failure necessitating intubation and mechanical ventilation.
- Chemoprophylaxis against this microorganism has proven successful. Therefore, early identification of the HIV-infected mother becomes essential.
- Despite advances in therapy, the infection continues to be associated with significant morbidity and mortality.

EPIDEMIOLOGY
- Ubiquitous in mammals worldwide, particularly rodents
- Growth on respiratory tract surfaces
- Mode of transmission is unknown:
  - Airborne person-to-person transmission is possible, but case contacts are rarely identified.
  - Environmentally acquired
- Asymptomatic infection appears early in life; >70% of healthy individuals have antibodies by age 4 years.
- Primary infection is likely to be the mechanism in infants. Reactivation of latent disease with immunosuppression was proposed as an explanation for disease later in childhood; however, animal models of PCP do not support this proposition.
- PCP in the HIV patient can occur at any time, but usually presents during the 1st year of life. The highest incidence is between 3 and 6 months of age.
- In leukemic patients, the incidence of PCP has been directly related to the degree of immunodeficiency resulting from chemotherapy.
- Epidemics of PCP were reported in premature and malnourished infants and children in resource-limited countries and during times of famine.

PATHOPHYSIOLOGY
- In the immunodeficient child, the pathologic changes occur predominantly in the alveoli. Cysts and trophozoites are seen adhering to the alveolar lining cells or in the cytoplasm of macrophages.
- As infection progresses, the alveolar spaces are filled with a pink, foamy exudate containing fibrin, abundant desquamative cells, and a large number of organisms. Alveolar septal thickening with mononuclear cell infiltration is also seen.

℞ DIAGNOSIS

HISTORY
- Malnourishment:
  - Subacute onset with nonspecific manifestations:
    ○ Poor feeding, weight loss, and restlessness
    ○ Chronic diarrhea
    ○ Usually without fever
    ○ After 1–2 weeks, the patient develops progressive tachypnea, respiratory distress, and cough.
- Sporadic or immunocompromised host:
  - This form has a more abrupt onset, sometimes even fulminant:
    ○ Fever (>38.5°C)
    ○ Nonproductive cough
    ○ Dyspnea at rest
- These subtypes are characterized by general clinical guidelines. Symptoms may be superimposed and can be seen in infants, children, and adolescents.

PHYSICAL EXAM
- Fever and significant tachypnea are characteristic.
- Hypoxemia: Early in the course of disease and disproportionate to the auscultatory findings
- Rapidly progressive respiratory distress with cyanosis: Respiratory failure early in course
- Absence of crackles is a common initial finding.
- Chest auscultation can reveal decreased breath sounds, crackles, and rhonchi.
- Coryza and wheezing have infrequently been reported.

DIAGNOSTIC TESTS & INTERPRETATION
Diagnostic Procedures/Other
- Arterial blood gas:
  - pH is usually increased
  - Reduced PaO_2 in room air (<70 mm Hg)
  - Alveolar–arterial oxygen gradient (>35 mm Hg)
- Chest radiograph:
  - Most common radiologic presentation is diffuse bilateral alveolar infiltrates:
    ○ Initially a perihilar distribution that spreads to the periphery
    ○ Apices are the least affected.
    ○ Interstitial infiltrates and air bronchograms can be seen.
    ○ Rapid progression to whole lung consolidation
  - Presence of hilar or mediastinal adenopathy may indicate another process such as *Mycobacterium tuberculosis*, *Mycobacterium avium-intracellulare*, fungal infections, cytomegalovirus, or lymphoma.

- Other tests:
  - Lactate dehydrogenase (LDH) can be elevated in patients with AIDS and PCP, but this finding is nonspecific.
  - WBC count is usually normal.

Pathological Findings
- Definitive diagnosis can be obtained by demonstration of PJ in pulmonary specimens:
  - Induced sputum
  - Bronchoalveolar lavage (90% sensitivity), usually through flexible bronchoscopy
  - Open lung or transbronchial biopsy
- Staining (significance):
  - Cysts stain with methenamine-silver, toluidine blue-O stains, calcofluor white, and fluorescein monoclonal antibody.
  - Sporozoites and trophozoites are identified with Giemsa stain, modified Wright-Giemsa stain, and fluorescein-conjugated monoclonal antibody stain.
  - Polymerase chain reaction assays for detecting PJ are experimental. PCR is more sensitive but less specific than microscopic methods but is not US FDA approved for diagnosis.

DIFFERENTIAL DIAGNOSIS
- Viral infections:
  - Common viral respiratory pathogens
  - Cytomegalovirus
  - Epstein-Barr virus
- Bacterial infections:
  - *M. tuberculosis*
  - *M. avium-intracellulare*
- Other:
  - Lymphocytic interstitial pneumonitis

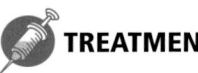 TREATMENT

MEDICATION (DRUGS)
First Line
- Minimum duration of therapy is 2 weeks; 3 weeks of therapy recommended in patients with AIDS.
- Antibiotics:
  - Trimethoprim-sulfamethoxazole (TMP-SMX) is the drug of choice:
    ○ TMP (15–20 mg/kg/d) and SMX (75–100 mg/kg/d) IV/PO divided q6h
    ○ Oral therapy is reserved for patients with mild illness who do not have malabsorption or diarrhea.

Second Line
- Minimum duration of therapy is 2 weeks; 3 weeks of therapy recommended in patients with AIDS.
- Pentamidine isethionate:
  - 3–4 mg/kg/d IV (or IM) given in a single daily dose
  - Used in patients who cannot tolerate TMP-SMX or are unresponsive after 5–7 days of therapy
  - If clinical improvement seen after 7–10 days of IV pentamidine, consider oral regimen to complete the 21-day course.

- Atovaquone:
  - 1–3 months and >24 months: 30 mg/kg/d PO divided into 2 doses
  - 4–24 months: 45 mg/kg/d PO divided into 2 doses
  - Maximum dose: 750 mg b.i.d.
- Dapsone plus trimethoprim
  - Dapsone: 2 mg/kg PO daily to a maximum of 100 mg daily
  - Trimethoprim: 15 mg/kg/d PO divided into 3 doses
- Primaquine plus clindamycin:
  - Primaquine: 0.3 mg/kg PO daily to a maximum of 30 mg PO daily
  - Clindamycin: 40 mg/kg/d PO divided into 4 doses to a maximum or 600 mg q6h.

ADDITIONAL TREATMENT
General Measures
- Supply oxygen as necessary to keep PaO_2 >70 mm Hg.
- Mechanical ventilation must be considered if PaO_2 is <60 mm Hg on FiO_2 of 0.5.
- Corticosteroids:
  - May be beneficial in HIV patients with moderate to severe PCP
  - Not systematically evaluated in children
  - Consider when PaO_2 is <70 mm Hg or the alveolar–arterial gradient is >35 mm Hg.
  - In patients >13 years of age, suggested dose is prednisone 40 mg PO b.i.d. for days 1–5, 40 mg PO once daily for days 6–10, and 20 mg PO once daily for days 11–21 with tapering. Doses of methylprednisolone or prednisone at 1 mg/kg given b.i.d.–q.i.d. for 5–7 days with a taper over the next 5 days have been suggested.

Additional Therapies
During high-risk periods, PCP can be effectively prevented in the immunodeficient host by chemoprophylaxis in the following groups:

- HIV exposed: 4–6 weeks to 4 months
- HIV infected or indeterminate: 4–12 months
- HIV infected: 1–5 years if $CD4^+$ T-lymphocyte count is <500 cells/μL or <15%
- HIV infected: ≥6 years if $CD4^+$ T-lymphocyte count is <200 cells/μL or <15%
- Severely symptomatic HIV patients or those with rapidly declining CD4 counts
- HIV patients who have had previous PCP illness
- Children who have received hematopoietic stem cell transplants (HSCTs)
- All HSCT recipients with hematologic malignancies (e.g., leukemia, lymphoma)
- All HSCT recipients receiving intense conditioning regimens or graft manipulation
- Prophylaxis is initiated at engraftment and administered for 6 months; longer than 6 months in children receiving immunosuppressive therapy or with chronic graft versus host disease

COMPLEMENTARY & ALTERNATIVE THERAPIES
Drug regimen for prophylaxis:

- TMP-SMX is the drug of choice.
  - 150 mg/m² body surface area per day of TMP or 750 mg/m² body surface area per day of SMX PO divided into 2 doses on 3 consecutive days per week
  - TMP-SMX can also be given 7 days a week when prevention against other bacterial infections is sought.
- For patients who cannot tolerate TMP-SMX:
  - Dapsone (>1 month of age): 2 mg/kg (maximum 100 mg) PO daily or 4 mg/kg (maximum 200 mg) PO weekly
  - Aerosolized pentamidine (>5 years of age): 300 mg via Respirgard II nebulizer inhaled monthly
  - Atovaquone (1–3 months and >24 months): 30 mg/kg PO daily (4β24 months): 45 mg/kg PO daily

ONGOING CARE
FOLLOW-UP RECOMMENDATIONS
- After 5–7 days of treatment
- If no improvement, TMP-SMX should be replaced with pentamidine.
- Standard precautions are required. Isolation from other immunodeficient patients is recommended.

PROGNOSIS
- 5–40% mortality in treated patients
- Near 100% mortality if patient is untreated
- ~35% of patients will have recurrence unless lifetime prophylaxis is instituted.

COMPLICATIONS
- High rate of respiratory failure necessitating intubation and mechanical ventilation (~60%)
- HIV-infected patients have a higher rate (40%) of adverse reactions to TMP-SMX than the general population. Rash is most common with fever, neutropenia, anemia, renal dysfunction, nausea, vomiting, and diarrhea occurring as well.
- Prophylactic medication protects the patient as long as the drug is administered. However, this does not eradicate PJ.

ADDITIONAL READING

- CDC. Guidelines for the prevention and treatment of opportunistic infections among HIV-exposed and HIV-infected children. *MMWR Recomm Rep.* 2009; 58(RR-11):1–166.
- Gigliotti F, Wright TW. In: Long SS, ed. *Principles and practice of pediatric infectious disease*, 3rd ed. Philadelphia: Elsevier; 2008:1203–1206.

- King SM. Evaluation and treatment of the human immunodeficiency virus-1–exposed infant. American Academy of Pediatrics Committee on Pediatric AIDS; American Academy of Pediatrics Infectious Diseases and Immunization Committee. *Pediatrics.* 2004; 114(2):497–505.
- Morris A, Wei K, Afshar K, et al. Epidemiology and clinical significance of Pneumocystis colonization. *J Infect Dis.* 2008;197(1):10–17.

CODES

ICD9
136.3 Pneumocystosis

ICD10
B59 Pneumocystosis

FAQ

- Q: Which are the most common side effects of pentamidine?
- A: They include hypoglycemia, impaired renal or liver function, anemia, thrombocytopenia, neutropenia, hypotension, and skin rashes. These side effects can be expected in 50% of patients.
- Q: How frequently is prophylaxis failure seen?
- A: Adequate TMP-SMX treatment has only a 3% failure rate.
- Q: How are adverse reactions to TMP-SMX during PCP therapy managed?
- A: Continuation of treatment, if the reactions are not severe, is recommended.

PNEUMONIA—BACTERIAL
Erica S. Pan
Michael D. Cabana

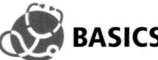 **BASICS**

DESCRIPTION
Pneumonia is an acute infection of the pulmonary parenchyma, which is associated with consolidation of alveolar spaces.

EPIDEMIOLOGY
Incidence
Highest incidence in children <5 years of age (annual incidence 3–4%)

RISK FACTORS
- Immune deficiency:
  - Immunocompromised status
  - Sickle cell anemia
- Increased aspiration risk:
  - Altered mental status
  - Tracheoesophageal fistula
  - Cerebral palsy
  - Seizure disorder
- Compromised lung function/anatomy:
  - Cystic fibrosis
  - Congenital pulmonary malformations
  - Bronchopulmonary dysplasia
  - Asthma

ETIOLOGY
- Etiology of bacterial pneumonia differs by age:
  - Neonates: Group B streptococcus, *Enterococcus*, *Listeria monocytogenes*, *Escherichia coli*, *Ureaplasma urealyticum*
  - 1–3 months: *Staphylococcus aureus*, *Haemophilus influenzae*, *Streptococcus pneumoniae*, *Bordetella pertussis*, *Chlamydia trachomatis*, *U. urealyticum*
  - 4 months to 4 years: *S. pneumoniae*, *S. aureus*, *H. influenzae*
  - >5 years of age: *S. pneumoniae*, *Mycoplasma pneumoniae*, *Mycoplasma tuberculosis*
- Etiology can also differ based on risk factors:
  - Aspiration as etiology increases the risk for oral flora including anaerobes such as *Bacteroides* and *Peptostreptococcus*.
  - Ventilator-dependent patients are at increased risk for *Pseudomonas* or *Klebsiella* infections, and infection with other gram-negative rods.
  - Cystic fibrosis increases the risk for *Pseudomonas* and other more unusual organisms.

DIAGNOSIS

HISTORY
- Fever and/or chills
- Rapid breathing is a sensitive but nonspecific finding in bacterial pneumonia.
- Difficulty breathing or shortness of breath is common and can lead to difficulty feeding in infants.
- Cough is often seen in bacterial pneumonia. *B. pertussis* pneumonia often presents after a catarrhal phase with a paroxysmal cough and posttussive vomiting.
- Pleuritic chest pain
- Abdominal pain and/or vomiting: Lower-lobe pneumonia can present with abdominal pain.
- Irritability, lethargy, and/or malaise
- Poor feeding or apnea in young infants

- Birth history, including maternal infections (e.g., *C. trachomatis* can be transmitted to an infant through a mother's genital tract at delivery)
- Immunization status: In a fully immunized child, *H. influenzae* type B, *B. pertussis*, and *S. pneumoniae* infections are less common.
- Recent history of upper respiratory tract infection (URI) or RSV can predispose to bacterial pneumonia.
- History of repeated bacterial infections suggests immunodeficiency or cystic fibrosis, which are risk factors for bacterial pneumonia.
- Exposure to contacts with pertussis, tuberculosis, or history of recent travel
- Travelers, health care workers, and persons working in prisons or institutional settings are at greater risk for tuberculosis.

PHYSICAL EXAM
- Ill appearance:
  - General examination can range from mildly ill appearing to toxic in appearance.
  - Infants may have a paucity of exam findings disproportionate to their appearance and tachypnea.
  - Patients may be dehydrated or in shock.
- Fever:
  - Most children with bacterial pneumonia have fever.
  - Patients with atypical bacterial pneumonia and pertussis are sometimes afebrile.
- Tachypnea or increased work of breathing: Nasal flaring, grunting, and/or retracting
- Decreased oxygen saturation; therefore, oxygen saturation should be obtained by pulse oximetry in children with tachypnea or other signs of distress.
- Localized rales, rhonchi, decreased breath sounds, or wheezing:
  - These are all significant clinical findings of pneumonia. Crackles suggest the diagnosis of pneumonia.
  - With increasing consolidation, dullness to percussion and decreased breath sounds may be noted.
  - In patients who are actively wheezing, it may be difficult to distinguish rales from other auscultated sounds.

DIAGNOSTIC TESTS & INTERPRETATION
- Not indicated for patients with uncomplicated pneumonia
- In toxic-appearing infants, blood, urine, and CSF cultures (i.e., a sepsis workup) should be considered.

Lab
- Blood culture:
  - Not usually indicated in healthy children with uncomplicated pneumonia
  - Rarely leads to identification of pathogen causing pneumonia
  - Should be obtained in toxic-appearing patients and infants <1 month old
  - Bacteremia has been noted in up to 30% of patients with pneumococcal pneumonia.
- Elevated peripheral WBC or range 15,000–40,000/mm^3 is associated with bacterial pneumonia or even higher WBC in pertussis, but should not be relied upon to distinguish etiology of pneumonia.

- Cold agglutinin test:
  - A positive test suggests *M. pneumoniae*. This test is usually not indicated because empiric treatment of this pathogen is typically safe and effective.
- Purified protein derivative (PPD) test or an interferon-gamma release assay (e.g., quantiFERON): Should be obtained in all patients in whom *M. tuberculosis* is suspected.

Imaging
- Chest radiograph (CXR), upright:
  - A CXR is not required for diagnosis if clinical symptoms and examination findings are consistent with pneumonia.
  - A CXR is typically obtained if pneumonia is suspected but clinical findings are unclear, if the patient has evidence of respiratory distress and if a complication (e.g., a pleural effusion) is suspected, or if the patient is not responding to treatment.
  - Characteristic CXR patterns include "alveolar or lobar infiltrate" with air bronchograms. "Round" infiltrates may be seen with *S. pneumococcus*. "Diffuse" interstitial infiltrates and hyperinflation may be seen with atypical pneumonia such as *M. pneumoniae* or chlamydial pneumonias.
  - More commonly, CXR cannot be reliably used to distinguish between viral and bacterial disease.
  - An infiltrate may not be seen (negative CXR) if the disease is diagnosed early or if the patient is dehydrated.
- CXR, lateral decubitus: More sensitive than an upright radiograph in detecting pleural effusions or foreign body aspiration
- CT scan: Not recommended as 1st-line imaging for suspected pneumonia. CT is mainly used as adjunct imaging for patients who are worsening (not improving) despite treatment, or have complications.

Diagnostic Procedures/Other
If diagnosis is unclear, consider the following:
- Flexible fiberoptic bronchoscopy with bronchoalveolar lavage or lung biopsy
- Thoracentesis if pleural fluid is present
- For empyema, drainage by aspiration or chest tube may be required.

DIFFERENTIAL DIAGNOSIS
- Infectious:
  - Sepsis
  - Viral pneumonia:
    - In infants: cytomegalovirus (CMV), metapneumovirus, herpes simplex virus (HSV)
    - From 1–3 months: CMV, respiratory syncytial virus (RSV), metapneumovirus
    - From 4 months to 4 years: RSV, adenovirus, influenza, metapneumovirus
  - Bronchiolitis
  - URI
  - Croup (laryngotracheobronchitis)
  - Fungal infection (if immunodeficiency or exposure history)
  - Parasitic infection (if immunodeficiency or exposure history)
- Pulmonary:
  - Asthma
  - Atelectasis
  - Pneumonitis (i.e., chemical)
  - Pneumothorax
  - Pulmonary edema
  - Pulmonary hemorrhage
  - Pulmonary embolism

- Congenital:
  - Pulmonary sequestration
  - Congenital pulmonary airway malformation
- Genetic: Cystic fibrosis
- Tumors:
  - Lymphoma
  - Primary lung tumor
  - Metastatic tumor
- Cardiac: CHF
- GI: Gastroesophageal reflux disease
- Miscellaneous:
  - Foreign body aspiration
  - Sarcoidosis

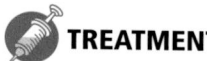 TREATMENT

ADDITIONAL TREATMENT
General Measures
Outpatient: Empiric Treatment
- Unlike adults, there is no validated tool to identify those patients at low risk who can be treated as outpatients. In general, neonates should be managed as inpatients.
- 2–4 months; if afebrile:
  - Azithromycin 10 mg/kg/d × 1 day then 5 mg/kg/d × 4 days
  - If febrile, hypoxic, or dehydrated, then admit (see "FAQ")
- 5 months to 5 years:
  - Amoxicillin 80–100 mg/kg/d divided q8–12h
  - Consider for additional coverage of *H. influenzae*, non–type B:
    - Amoxicillin/clavulanate 25–45 mg/kg/d divided b.i.d. or t.i.d.
    - Cefuroxime 30 mg/kg/d divided b.i.d., cefprozil 30 mg/kg/d divided b.i.d., cefdinir 14 mg/kg/d divided daily or b.i.d., or cefpodoxime 10 mg/kg/d divided b.i.d.
    - May consider use of ceftriaxone 50 mg/kg IM to initiate therapy
    - For penicillin-allergic patients, may use macrolide or cephalosporin
  - Age >5 years (unless organism other than atypical pathogen suspected; atypical pathogens are much more common in this age group):
    - Azithromycin 10 mg/kg/d × 1 day (max dose 500 mg) then 5 mg/kg/d (max dose 250 mg) × 4 days
    - May consider doxycycline 4 mg/kg/d divided by 2 doses in patients 9 years of age or older. Not to exceed 200 mg/d
    - May consider fluoroquinolones in patients ≥16 years of age if no other appropriate oral option is available
  - If specific pathogen is known or suspected, use appropriate antibiotic therapy.
  - For patients with more severe disease, may consider combining β-lactam antibiotic and macrolide

Inpatient Management
- Oxygen as needed to keep oxygen saturations >94–95%
- Intubation and positive pressure ventilation, if clinically indicated

- Empiric antibiotic treatment:
  - <1 month: Ampicillin 200 mg/kg/d divided q6–8h
  - Age 1–3 months: Erythromycin: 10 mg/kg IV q6h or azithromycin 2.5 mg/kg IV q12h
  - For infants <6 weeks, consider azithromycin instead of erythromycin owing to the associated increased risk of pyloric stenosis. If febrile, add cefotaxime 200 mg/kg/d divided q8h.
  - Age 4 months to 5 years (if atypical pathogens are not suspected): Ceftriaxone 50–75 mg/kg/d q12–24h or cefotaxime 200 mg/kg/d divided q8h
  - Age ≥5 years: Add macrolide to above therapy. For seriously ill patients, add vancomycin 60 mg/kg/d divided q6h. For antistaphylococcal coverage, add vancomycin 15 mg/kg/dose q6–8h or clindamycin 25–40 mg/kg/d divided q6–8h. If atypical pneumonia also suspected, may add macrolide. May also consider macrolides or clindamycin IV as alternative for cephalosporin-allergic patients.

 ONGOING CARE

FOLLOW-UP RECOMMENDATIONS
Patient Monitoring
- If treated as outpatient, consider telephone follow-up within 1–3 days.
- If worsening or not responding to treatment, consider repeated or additional diagnostic studies. For example, persistent fever may be due to loculated pleural fluid or an empyema.
- CXR may be abnormal for up to 10 weeks after successful treatment. Consider follow-up CXR only if indicated for severe disease or complications (e.g., effusion, empyema).
- For children with recurrent bacterial pneumonia, consider an underlying anatomic or immunologic disorder (e.g., abnormal antibody production, cystic fibrosis, tracheoesophageal fistula, pulmonary sequestration).

PROGNOSIS
Otherwise healthy children with uncomplicated pneumonia typically have rapid improvement with treatment (3–5 days).

COMPLICATIONS
- Pleural effusion
- Empyema
- Lung abscess
- Pneumatoceles
- Pneumothorax
- Bacteremia/sepsis

ADDITIONAL READING

- Bradley JS. Management of community-acquired pediatric pneumonia in an era of increasing antibiotic resistance and conjugate vaccines. *Pediatr Infect Dis J*. 2002;21:592–598.
- Gaston B. Pneumonia. *Pediatr Rev*. 2002;23: 132–140.
- Kabra SK, Lodha R, Pandey RM. Antibiotics for community acquired pneumonia in children. *Cochrane Database Syst Rev*. 2006;(3):CD004874.

- Lee GE, Lorch SA, Shffler-Collins S, et al. National hospitalization trends for pediatric pneumonia and associated complications. *Pediatrics*. 2010; 126:204–213.
- McIntosh K. Community-acquired pneumonia in children. *N Engl J Med*. 2002;346:427–437.
- Ranganathan SC, Sonnappa S. Pneumonia and other respiratory infections. *Pediatr Clin North Am*. 2009;56:135–156.

 CODES

ICD9
- 482.2 Pneumonia due to Hemophilus influenzae [H. influenzae]
- 482.9 Bacterial pneumonia, unspecified
- 482.30 Pneumonia due to Streptococcus, unspecified

ICD10
- J14 Pneumonia due to Hemophilus influenzae
- J15.3 Pneumonia due to streptococcus, group B
- J15.9 Unspecified bacterial pneumonia

FAQ

- Q: What are the indications for admission and inpatient treatment of pneumonia in children?
- A: Failure of outpatient therapy; hypoxemia; inability to maintain hydration orally or dehydration; respiratory distress; apnea; toxic appearance; presence of complications such as effusion or empyema and risk factors that predispose to complications, such as age <2 months; or immunocompromised status
- Q: What is the most common causative organism of pulmonary abscess, and what is the appropriate treatment?
- A: *S. aureus* is the most common causative organism. Treatment includes IV vancomycin, IV or PO clindamycin, or PO linezolid. If MSSA is confirmed cefuroxime may be used.
- Q: What is the case fatality rate for pneumonia in hospitalized children?
- A: Based on data from 1995–1997, case fatality rates for children differ by age and are as high as 4% for children <2 years of age and 2% for children aged 2–17 years.
- Q: Which children are most likely to have systemic complications from community-acquired pneumonia? Local complications?
- A: An analysis of inpatient data from pediatric hospitals from 1997–2006 suggests that children <1 year of age are more likely to have systemic complications (e.g., sepsis, acute respiratory failure), while patients aged 1–5 years are more likely to have local complications (e.g., empyema, abscess).
- Q: What are risk factors for invasive pneumococcal disease?
- A: Conditions associated with invasive pneumococcal disease include congenital immune deficiency (e.g., B- or T-lymphocyte deficiencies) diseases associated with immunosuppressive therapy or radiation therapy (including malignancies), and solid organ transplantation and chronic cardiac disease.

PNEUMOTHORAX
Richard M. Kravitz

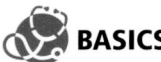 **BASICS**

EPIDEMIOLOGY
Depends on the underlying lung disease

Incidence
- Spontaneous pneumothorax:
  - Incidence: 7.4–18/100,000
  - Male >Female (6:1)
  - Peak incidence: 10–30 years
- Cystic fibrosis (CF):
  - Overall CF population: 3.5–8%
  - CF patients >18 years: 16–20%
  - Risk factors:
    o More severe disease
    o Decreased pulmonary function (i.e., forced expiratory volume in 1 second [FEV_1] <30–50%)
    o Colonization with *Pseudomonas aeruginosa*, *Burkholderia cepacia*, or *Aspergillus*

RISK FACTORS
- Asthma
- CF
- Pneumonia
- Collagen vascular diseases

PATHOPHYSIOLOGY
- Air can enter the pleural space via the following:
  - Chest wall (i.e., penetrating trauma)
  - Intrapulmonary (i.e., ruptured alveoli)
- Usually, collapse of the lung on the affected side seals the leak.
- If a ball valve mechanism ensues, however, air can accumulate in the thoracic cavity, causing the development of a tension pneumothorax (a medical emergency).

ETIOLOGY
- Spontaneous (secondary to rupture of apical blebs)
- Mechanical trauma:
  - Penetrating injury (i.e., knife or bullet wound)
  - Blunt trauma
- Barotrauma:
  - Mechanical ventilation
  - Cough (if severe enough)
- Iatrogenic:
  - Central venous catheter placement
  - Bronchoscopy (especially with biopsy)
- Infection: Most common organisms:
  - *Staphylococcus aureus*
  - *Streptococcus pneumoniae*
  - *Mycobacterium tuberculosis*
  - *Bordetella pertussis*
  - *Pneumocystis jiroveci*
- Airway occlusion:
  - Mucus plugging (asthma)
  - Foreign body
  - Meconium aspiration
- Bleb formation (i.e., idiopathic, secondary to CF)
- Malignancy

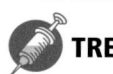 **DIAGNOSIS**

HISTORY
- May be asymptomatic (pneumothorax discovered on chest film obtained for other reasons)
- Cough
- Shortness of breath
- Dyspnea
- Pleuritic chest pain that is usually sudden in onset and localized to apices (referred pain to shoulders)
- Respiratory distress
- Underlying medical problems which increase risk for pneumothorax
- Activity prior to developing symptoms that might have caused the pneumothorax:
  - Heavy lifting
  - Increased coughing

PHYSICAL EXAM
- May be normal
- Decreased breath sounds on the affected side
- Decreased vocal fremitus
- Hyperresonance to percussion on the affected side
- Tachypnea
- Tachycardia
- Shortness of breath
- Respiratory distress
- Shifting of the cardiac point of maximal impulse away from the affected side
- Shifting of the trachea away from the affected side
- Subcutaneous emphysema
- Cyanosis
- Scratch sign (heard through the stethoscope): A loud scratching sound is heard when a finger is gently stroked over the area of the pneumothorax.

DIAGNOSTIC TESTS & INTERPRETATION
- EKG:
  - Diminished amplitude of the QRS voltage
  - Rightward shift of the QRS axis (if left-sided pneumothorax)

Lab
- Arterial blood gas:
  - pO_2 can frequently be decreased.
  - pCO_2:
    o Elevated with respiratory compromise
    o Decreased from hyperventilation
- Pulse oximetry:
  - Useful for assessing oxygenation

Imaging
- Chest radiograph:
  - Radiolucency of the affected lung
  - Lack of lung markings in the periphery of the affected lung
  - Collapsed lung on the affected side
  - Possible pneumomediastinum with subcutaneous emphysema
- Chest CT:
  - Useful for finding small pneumothoraces
  - Can help distinguish a pneumothorax from a bleb or cyst
  - Helpful for locating small apical blebs associated with spontaneous pneumothoraces

Diagnostic Procedures/Other
- Pitfalls:
  - Not considering the diagnosis in otherwise healthy patients
  - Confusing the symptoms with those of an underlying lung disease
  - Inserting a needle into a cyst or bleb (can cause a tension pneumothorax with rapid respiratory compromise)

DIFFERENTIAL DIAGNOSIS
- Pulmonary:
  - Congenital lung malformations:
    o Cysts (i.e., bronchogenic cysts)
    o Cystic adenomatoid malformation
    o Congenital lobar emphysema
  - Acquired emphysema
  - Hyperinflation of the lung
  - Postinfectious pneumatocele
  - Bullae formation
- Miscellaneous:
  - Diaphragmatic hernia
  - Infections (i.e., pulmonary abscess)
  - Muscle strain
  - Pleurisy
  - Rib fracture

TREATMENT

ADDITIONAL TREATMENT
General Measures
- Stabilization of the patient
- Evacuation of the pleural air:
  - Should be done urgently if tension pneumothorax is suspected
  - In small asymptomatic pneumothoraces, observation of the patient is indicated.
- Treat the underlying condition predisposing for the pneumothorax:
  - Antibiotics for any underlying infection
  - Bronchodilators and anti-inflammatory agents for asthma attacks
- Oxygen:
  - Used to keep $SaO_2 \geq 95\%$
  - Breathing 100% oxygen:
    o Can speed the intrapleural air's reabsorption into the bloodstream hastening lung reexpansion
    o Useful for treating smaller pneumothoraces, especially in neonates

SURGERY/OTHER PROCEDURES

- Needle thoracentesis: Useful for evacuation of the pleural air in simple, uncomplicated spontaneous pneumothorax
- Chest tube drainage:
  - Used for evacuation of the pleural air in recurrent, persistent, or complicated pneumothoraces, and cases with significant underlying lung disease
  - Chest tube should be left in (usually 2–4 days) until:
    - Most air is reabsorbed
    - No reaccumulation of air is seen on sealing of the chest tube
- Surgical removal of pulmonary blebs:
  - Blebs have a high rate of rupturing with resultant pneumothorax.
  - In patients with established pneumothoraces, the blebs should be removed or oversewn to prevent reoccurrence of the pneumothorax (blebs have a high rate of reoccurrence if not repaired).
  - Thoracotomy versus video-assisted thoracoscopic surgery (VATS)
- Pleurodesis:
  - Used to attach the lung to the intrathoracic chest wall to prevent reoccurrence of a pneumothorax
  - Useful in cases of recurrent pneumothorax or if the pneumothorax is unresponsive to chest tube drainage (i.e., CF, malignancy)
  - Mechanism of action: The surface of the lung becomes inflamed and adheres to the chest wall via the formation of scar tissue.
  - 2 commonly used methods:
  - Surgical pleurodesis:
    - Mechanical abrasion of part of the lung or pleurectomy
    - Advantages: Very effective; low reoccurrence rate; site specific (limits affected area)
    - Disadvantages: Requires surgery and general anesthesia; contraindicated if patient is unstable
  - Chemical pleurodesis:
    - Chemicals are used to cause inflammation.
    - Chemicals commonly used: Talc, tetracycline, minocycline, doxycycline, quinacrine
    - Advantages: Requires no surgery or general anesthesia
    - Disadvantages: Less effective than surgery; generalized inflammation (rather than site-specific; makes future thoracic surgery more difficult; painful)

 ONGOING CARE

FOLLOW-UP RECOMMENDATIONS
Symptomatic relief within seconds of the air being evacuated

Patient Monitoring
Sign to watch for: Inability to remove the chest tube without reaccumulation of air (suggestive of a bronchopulmonary fistula; requires surgical exploration if no improvement in 7–10 days)

PROGNOSIS
- Depends on the underlying cause of the pneumothorax
- If simple, spontaneous pneumothorax, recovery is excellent
- CF: Development of pneumothorax associated with increased morbidity and mortality (median survival after 1st pneumothorax is 4 years)

COMPLICATIONS
- Pain
- Hypoxia
- Respiratory distress
- Tension pneumothorax:
  - Hypoxia
  - Hypercarbia with acidosis
  - Respiratory failure
- Pneumomediastinum with subcutaneous emphysema
- Bronchopulmonary fistula

ADDITIONAL READING

- Baumann MH. Management of spontaneous pneumothorax. *Clin Chest Med*. 2006;27:369–381.
- Briassoulis GC, Venkataraman ST, Vasilopoulos AG, et al. Air leaks from the respiratory tract in mechanically ventilated children with severe respiratory disease. *Pediatr Pulmonol*. 2000;29:127–134.
- Flume PA, Strange C, Ye X, et al. Pneumothorax in cystic fibrosis. *Chest*. 2005;128:720–728.
- Johnson NN, Toledo A, Endom EE. Pneumothorax, pneumomediastinum, and pulmonary embolism. *Pediatr Clin N Am*. 2010;57:1357–1383.
- Noppen M. Management of primary spontaneous pneumothorax. *Curr Opin Pulm Med*. 2002;9:272–275.

- Sahn SA, Heffner JE. Primary care: Spontaneous pneumothorax. *N Engl J Med*. 2000;342:868–874.
- Ullman EA, Donley LP, Brady WJ. Pulmonary trauma emergency department evaluation and management. *Emerg Med Clin North Am*. 2003;21:291–313.

CODES

ICD9
- 512.81 Primary spontaneous pneumothorax
- 512.82 Secondary spontaneous pneumothorax
- 512.89 Other pneumothorax

ICD10
- J93.0 Spontaneous tension pneumothorax
- J93.1 Other spontaneous pneumothorax
- J93.9 Pneumothorax, unspecified

FAQ

- Q: Can a pneumothorax reoccur?
- A: Reoccurrence depends on the underlying cause of the pneumothorax. Spontaneous pneumothorax reoccurrence rates:
  - Observation alone: 20–50%
  - If thoracentesis performed: 25–50%
  - If chest tube drainage performed: 32–38%
  - Overall reoccurrence rate: 16–52%
- Chemical pleurodesis reoccurrence rates:
  - Tetracycline: 25%
  - Talc: 8–10%
- Surgical pleurodesis reoccurrence rates:
  - VATS: 13%
  - Thoracotomy: 3%
  - Thoracotomy with pleurectomy: 0–4%
- CF reoccurrence rates:
  - If no drainage attempted: 68%
  - Thoracentesis alone: 90%
  - Chest tube drainage alone: 72%
  - Chemical pleurodesis:
    - Tetracycline: 42–86%
    - Quinacrine:12.5%
    - Talc: 8%
  - Surgical pleurodesis: Thoracotomy with pleurectomy: 0–4%

POLYARTERITIS NODOSA

David D. Sherry

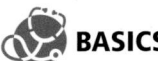 **BASICS**

DESCRIPTION
An inflammatory process of small- and medium-sized muscular arteries resulting in dysfunction of affected organs

EPIDEMIOLOGY
Incidence
Extremely rare in childhood
Prevalence
Prevalence equal in boys and girls

PATHOPHYSIOLOGY
Necrotizing arteritis of small- and medium-sized arteries resulting in segmental fibrinoid necrosis

ETIOLOGY
- Idiopathic
- Postinfectious (streptococcal, hepatitis B)

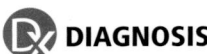 **DIAGNOSIS**

HISTORY
- Persistent constitutional symptoms
- Bilateral calf pain
- Abdominal pain
- Weight loss
- Unexplained fever
- Headache
- Arthralgia/Myalgia
- Rashes
- Seizures
- Weakness

PHYSICAL EXAM
- Check skin for livedo reticularis, splinter hemorrhages, erythema nodosum, and necrotic digits.
- Assess BP and pulses.
- Neurologic exam for findings consistent with neuropathy (mononeuritis multiplex)
- Ophthalmologic exam for cotton wool spots
- Check testes for tenderness or swelling.
- Check muscles for tenderness, especially calves.

DIAGNOSTIC TESTS & INTERPRETATION
Lab
Initial lab tests
- ESR:
  - Usually extremely elevated; leukocytosis and thrombocytosis are seen.
- Urine analysis:
  - Proteinuria and hematuria can be present.
- Creatinine and BUN levels:
  - May be elevated
- ANA and rheumatoid factor (RF):
  - Usually negative
- Muscle enzymes (creatine kinase, lactate dehydrogenase, aspartate aminotransferase, and aldolase levels):
  - Muscle involvement is common, especially in those with calf pain.
- Antineutrophil cytoplasmic antibody (ANCA):
  - Detectable in some; usually perinuclear (p) type, rarely cytoplasmic (c) type:
    - pANCA usually associated with anti-MPO, which is associated with microscopic angiitis
    - cANCA usually associated with anti-PR3, which is associated with Wegener vasculitis
  - Note: The detection of ANCA, previously thought to be highly specific for vasculitis, now appears to be less so. Hence, it remains important to confirm the diagnosis of polyarteritis nodosa with biopsy or angiography.
- Hepatitis B serologies:
  - Hepatitis B has been associated in some series of patients with polyarteritis nodosa.
- Streptococcal titers:
  - Polyarteritis nodosa may develop after streptococcal infections.

Imaging
- MRI of tender muscles:
  - Short TI inversion recovery (STIR) images may show edema, so a directed biopsy can be done to avoid false-negative muscle biopsy.
- MRA, CT angiography or angiography:
  - Can demonstrate vessel wall stenoses and aneurysm

Diagnostic Procedures/Other
Biopsy of affected tissue/organ: Usually skin, kidney, nerve, testicle

DIFFERENTIAL DIAGNOSIS
- Infection:
  - Bacterial endocarditis
  - Brucellosis
  - Influenza B (calf pain)
- Tumors:
  - Left atrial myxoma
  - Burkitt lymphoma
- Metabolic:
  - Homocystinuria
- Congenital
- Immunologic:
  - Systemic necrotizing vasculitis
  - Systemic lupus erythematosus

– Kawasaki disease
– Systemic juvenile rheumatoid arthritis
– Wegener granulomatosis
– Takayasu arteritis
– Cryoglobulinemia
– Antiphospholipid antibody syndrome
– Thrombotic thrombocytopenic purpura
• Psychologic:
– Münchausen syndrome
• Miscellaneous:
– Degos disease (malignant atrophic papulosis)

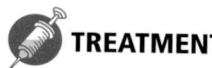 **TREATMENT**

MEDICATION (DRUGS)
• Corticosteroids are mainstay:
– Usually start at dose of 1–2 mg/kg/d and adjust based on response
– May initially give methylprednisolone 30 mg/kg up to 1 g/d IV for 3 days.
• Immunosuppressives such as methotrexate, azathioprine, and cyclophosphamide may be necessary.
• Hypertension should be managed aggressively.

ADDITIONAL TREATMENT
General Measures
• Medication
• Diet
• Caution:
– Do not initiate therapy before efforts to establish the diagnosis.

 ONGOING CARE

FOLLOW-UP RECOMMENDATIONS
• Initiation of steroid therapy may bring response in 1–2 weeks; however, management of specific organs affected during acute stage is essential.
• May require long-term therapy

Patient Monitoring
• Watch for the following:
– Rising creatinine and BUN levels
– Abdominal pain
– Uncontrolled hypertension
• Home testing:
– May wish to have patients monitor BP periodically if renal involvement suspected

DIET
• If renal system involved, diet low in sodium and potassium
• Possible conflicts with medications

PROGNOSIS
• May be extremely poor over the long term
• Risk is high for renal failure, hypertension, stroke, myocardial infarction, bowel infarction, and death.
• Owing to low incidence/prevalence, precise data are not available.
• Cutaneous polyarteritis nodosa is relatively benign.

COMPLICATIONS
• Hypertension
• Renal failure
• Digital necrosis
• Intestinal infarction
• Stroke

ADDITIONAL READING
• Cuttica RJ. Vasculitis in children: A diagnostic challenge. *Curr Probl Pediatr.* 1997;27:309–318.
• Hughes LB, Bridges SL Jr. Polyarteritis nodosa and microscopic polyangiitis: Etiologic and diagnostic considerations. *Curr Rheumatol Rep.* 2002;4:75–82.

• Khubchandani RP, Viswanathan V. Pediatric vasculitides: A generalists approach. [Review] *Indian J Pediatr.* 2010;77(10):1165–1171.
• Morgan AJ, Schwartz RA. Cutaneous polyarteritis nodosa: A comprehensive review. *Int J Dermatol.* 2010;49(7):750–756.
• Ozen S. The spectrum of vasculitis in children. *Best Pract Res Clin Rheumatol.* 2002;16:411–425.
• Ting TV, Hashkes PJ. Update on childhood vasculitides. *Curr Opin Rheumatol.* 2004;16(5):560–565.
• Yalcindag A, Sundel R. Vasculitis in childhood. *Curr Opin Rheumatol.* 2001;13:422–427.

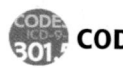 **CODES**

ICD9
446.0 Polyarteritis nodosa
ICD10
M30.0 Polyarteritis nodosa

FAQ
• Q: What is the difference between polyarteritis nodosa and systemic necrotizing vasculitis?
• A: Polyarteritis nodosa has a strict definition. Many children who clearly have vasculitis of the small- and medium-sized arteries do not fit precisely into the description of polyarteritis nodosa. In most ways, the search for organ involvement and therapy is the same.
• Q: Who should manage the patient with polyarteritis nodosa?
• A: Usually one discipline provides comprehensive management plan (either the pediatrician or rheumatologist). Subspecialist(s) of the affected organ systems provide management guidelines for specific organ issues.

POLYCYSTIC KIDNEY DISEASE

Christopher J. LaRosa
Andres J. Greco (5th edition)

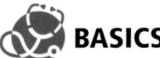 **BASICS**

DESCRIPTION
- Polycystic kidney disease (PKD) is a heritable disorder with diffuse cystic involvement of both kidneys without other dysplastic elements. The term PKD is generally used to describe 2 genetically distinct syndromes:
  - Autosomal dominant polycystic kidney disease (ADPKD):
    - Saccular, epithelial-lined, fluid-filled cysts of various sizes are derived from all segments of the nephron.
    - Cysts progressively enlarge and become disconnected from the tubule of origin.
    - Usually not clinically apparent until the 3rd or 4th decade of life
    - ~2–5% of patients have early-onset disease.
  - Autosomal recessive polycystic kidney disease (ARPKD):
    - Fusiform dilations arise from the collecting ducts and maintain contact with the nephron of origin.
    - Associated hepatic abnormalities are obligatory such as biliary dysgenesis and periportal fibrosis (congenital hepatic fibrosis), with portal hypertension.
    - Affects both the kidneys and the liver in approximately inverse proportions

EPIDEMIOLOGY
- ADPKD:
  - 1 of the most common human genetic disorders; the most common renal inherited disease
  - A major cause of end-stage renal disease (ESRD) in adults
  - Frequency 1 in 400–1,000
- ARPKD:
  - Incidence of 1 in 20,000–40,000 live births
  - Exact incidence unknown owing to perinatal deaths in severe cases

RISK FACTORS
Genetics
- ARPKD:
  - Mutations in the polycystic kidney hepatic disease 1 gene (PKHD1, chromosome 6)
- ADPKD:
  - Type I ADPKD accounts for 85–90% of cases of ADPKD and is caused by mutations in the PKD1 gene (chromosome 16).
  - Large genomic deletions may encompass PKD1 and TSC2 genes, resulting in early-onset ADPKD with tuberous sclerosis.
  - Type II ADPKD is caused by mutations in the PKD2 gene (chromosome 4) and accounts for 10–15% of the cases.

- Other:
  - Presymptomatic genetic screening for ADPKD is not recommended.
  - Normotensive women with ADPKD usually have uncomplicated pregnancies.
  - Higher risk for maternal/fetal complications if there is preexisting hypertension

PATHOPHYSIOLOGY
- ADPKD is produced by decreased functional polycystins:
  - Polycystin-1 is a membrane mechanoreceptor-like protein that forms multiprotein complexes at focal adhesions, cell–cell junctions, and cilia. It is involved in cell polarity, proliferation, cell–matrix interactions, and secretion.
  - Polycystin-2 is a divalent cation channel involved in calcium signaling and intracellular calcium homeostasis, and is likely critical for cytoskeletal organization, cell adhesion, migration, and proliferation.
- ARPKD is produced by loss of functional fibrocystin/polyductin:
  - Fibrocystin/polyductin is an integral membrane receptor with extracellular protein-interaction sites that transduce intracellular signals to the nucleus.
  - Proteins affected in cystic kidney disease localize to cilia on epithelial cells. Cilia are critical for cell architecture, proliferation, apoptosis, and polarity.

ETIOLOGY
- ADPKD is generally an adult-onset, systemic disorder with cystic and noncystic manifestations. Cysts occur in the kidneys and other epithelial organs (e.g., seminal vesicles, pancreas, and liver):
  - Polycystic liver disease is the most common extrarenal manifestation.
  - Intracranial aneurysms occur in ~8%.
  - Mitral valve prolapse is the most common valvular abnormality (demonstrated in up to 25% of affected individuals).
  - Colonic diverticula in 80% with ESRD
- ARPKD is a renal and hepatic developmental disorder. The hallmark of ARPKD liver diseases is congenital hepatic fibrosis and dilation of intrahepatic bile ducts (Caroli disease).
  - Severely affected infants may have the oligohydramnios sequence at birth, and associated pulmonary hypoplasia and respiratory complications convey a high mortality risk.

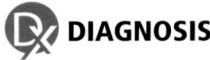 **DIAGNOSIS**

HISTORY
- ADPKD:
  - Detailed family history is essential.
  - Most common presenting complaint in adults is pain.
  - Hypertension, gross hematuria, nephrolithiasis, and UTIs are common.
- ARPKD:
  - Oligohydramnios sequence
  - Postnatal respiratory insufficiency
  - Renal insufficiency
  - Hypertension (may be severe)
  - Hepatobiliary manifestations (cholestasis, cholangitis, liver failure, portal hypertension, hypersplenism) evolve in older patients.
- Signs and symptoms:
  - ADPKD:
    - Older children are often asymptomatic, but may present with hypertension, abdominal pain, abdominal mass, gross hematuria after trauma, proteinuria, UTI/cyst infection, renal calculi, or decreased renal function.
  - ARPKD:
    - Presentation variable
    - Severely affected infants have "Potter" oligohydramnios sequence
    - Pulmonary hypoplasia/respiratory insufficiency a major cause of neonatal mortality
    - Renal insufficiency with neonatal survival
    - Hepatobiliary complications later in course (portal hypertension, hematemesis, hepatosplenomegaly hypersplenism with pallor, petechiae)

PHYSICAL EXAM
- Clinical spectrum variable, particularly in ARPKD
- Hypertension
- Abdominal pain; tenderness at flank or costovertebral angle
- Flank mass or palpable kidneys
- Hepatosplenomegaly, varices, jaundice/icterus, abdominal ascites in ARPKD

DIAGNOSTIC TESTS & INTERPRETATION
Lab
- Metabolic panel, to include BUN, creatinine, electrolytes
- Calcium, phosphorus
- Liver function tests
- CBC
- Urinalysis
- Note: Hyponatremia is often present in the neonatal period in ARPKD.

Imaging

- Ultrasonography is the preferred screening method. Should include liver and Doppler to evaluate for portal hypertension in ARPKD
- ARPKD:
  - Kidneys enlarged with increased echogenicity and loss of corticomedullary differentiation
  - The liver may be normal in infants and young children. Over time it becomes enlarged and hyperechoic. Dilated intrahepatic biliary ducts may be seen.
  - Prenatal ultrasound after 24–30 weeks' gestation may show hyperechoic enlarged kidneys, oligohydramnios, and absence of bladder filling.
- Ultrasound diagnostic criteria for ADPKD:
  - <40 years should have at least 2 cysts in 1 of the kidneys and 1 cyst in the other kidney or 3 cysts in a single kidney.
  - ≥40 and ≤59 years should have at least 2 cysts in each kidney.
  - >60 years should have at least 4 cysts in each kidney.
- CT scan with contrast has limited use in young children owing to exposure to ionizing radiation. It is mostly used in adults with ADPKD since it can distinguish between solid and liquid renal masses.
- MRI with gadolinium: Heavy-weighted T2 MRI is the most sensitive method currently available. Can be used in both conditions. Particularly useful to evaluate liver involvement in ARPKD

DIFFERENTIAL DIAGNOSIS

- Multicystic dysplastic kidney (MCDK)
- Glomerular cystic kidney disease (GCKD)
- Acquired cystic disease may occur in patients with ESRD.
- Genetic syndromes with cystic renal dysplasia: Meckel syndrome, Jeune syndrome, Ivemark syndrome, Zellweger syndrome, Bardet-Biedl syndrome, tuberous sclerosis, and others

TREATMENT

MEDICATION (DRUGS)

- Hypertension is common in PKD. Patients respond well to diuretics, ACE inhibitors, or calcium channel blockers. ACE inhibitors or angiotensin-receptor blockers are 1st line.
- In patients with PKD and nephrolithiasis, thiazide diuretics may be used for hypercalciuria, and potassium citrate supplements if hypocitraturia is found.
- Pyelonephritis in patients with PKD may lead to infected cysts. The treatment should include antibiotics that penetrate into the cysts (quinolones, trimethoprim) if cephalosporins and aminoglycosides fail to eradicate the infection.

ADDITIONAL TREATMENT

General Measures

- No currently approved targeted treatments to cure or slow progression
- Medical management is supportive.
- Pain is the most common symptom in ADPKD and can be difficult to treat.

Additional Therapies

Activity: Patients with PKD should not participate in high-contact athletics in which the abdomen may be traumatized repeatedly. Strenuous static exercise should be avoided in hypertensive patients.

 ONGOING CARE

FOLLOW-UP RECOMMENDATIONS

A pediatric nephrologist should be involved in the care of children with PKD.

DIET

In both conditions, dietary changes depend on the degree of renal failure. Sodium restriction is indicated in cases of hypertension and/or edema. Caffeine should be avoided in cases of ADPKD.

PATIENT EDUCATION

- Emotional support and education of patients with PKD and their families can be obtained through the Polycystic Kidney Foundation (www.PKDcure.org) and the PKD Alliance (www.arpkdchf.org).
- As in any genetic condition, genetic counseling is indicated in these disorders

PROGNOSIS

- ADPKD:
  - The probability of being alive and not having ESRD is about 77% at age 50, 57% at age 58, and 52% at age 73 years. Median onset of ESRD 53 years (PKD1) versus 69 years (PKD2).
  - Cystic expansion occurs at a consistent rate per individual, although it is heterogeneous in the population.
  - Larger kidneys associated with more rapid disease progression
  - PKD1 mutation is more severe because more cysts develop earlier, not because they grow faster.
- ADPKD:
  - Neonatal onset is fatal in up to 50% of infants because of pulmonary hypoplasia with associated respiratory failure.
  - Patients who survive the neonatal period have a 50–80% chance of surviving at least to age 15 years.

ADDITIONAL READING

- Avner ED, Sweeney Jr WE. Renal cystic disease: New insights for the clinician. *Pediatr Clin North Am*. 2006;53:889–909.
- Kaplan BS, Kaplan P, Rosenberg HK, et al. Polycystic kidney disease in childhood. *J Pediatr*. 1989;115:867.
- Sutters M. The pathogenesis of autosomal dominant polycystic kidney disease. *Nephron Exp Nephrol*. 2006;103:e149–e155.
- Wilson PD. Mechanism of disease: Polycystic kidney disease. *N Engl J Med*. 2004;350:151–164.

 CODES

ICD9

- 753.10 Cystic kidney disease, unspecified
- 753.19 Other specified cystic kidney disease

ICD10

- Q61.9 Cystic kidney disease, unspecified
- Q61.19 Other polycystic kidney, infantile type

FAQ

- Q: What can be done to slow the progression of renal insufficiency in ADPKD?
- A: Well-controlled BP and rapid treatment of UTIs may decrease the progression of renal failure.
- Q: Should asymptomatic older siblings of an infant with ARPKD be evaluated?
- A: Yes. An older child may have congenital hepatic fibrosis with minimal renal involvement.
- Q: Should one screen ADPKD-affected family members for the presence of cerebral vessel aneurysms if other family members have berry aneurysms?
- A: Although routine screening is not recommended, intrafamilial clustering of aneurysms has been reported and it may be advisable to screen children with MRI or cranial CT in a family with aneurysms.

POLYCYSTIC OVARY SYNDROME

Ernest M. Graham

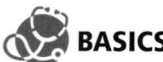 **BASICS**

DESCRIPTION
Polycystic ovary syndrome (PCOS) is an endocrinologic disorder characterized by chronic anovulation, excessive androgen production, and noncyclic gonadotropin secretion.

EPIDEMIOLOGY
PCOS is relatively common:
- Usually begins soon after menarche

Genetics
At least 1 group of patients with this condition inherits the disorder, possibly by means of an X-linked dominant transmission.

PATHOPHYSIOLOGY
- The ovaries of most women with PCOS are enlarged as much as 5 cm in diameter, and the ovarian capsule is smooth, white, and thickened:
  - Beneath the capsule are numerous small follicular cysts.
  - For years, it was erroneously believed that the thick sclerotic capsule acted as a mechanical barrier to ovulation.
- Instead of the characteristic picture of fluctuating hormone levels in the normal menstrual cycle, a steady state of gonadotropin and sex steroids is produced in association with persistent anovulation.
- There is increased pulse amplitude of gonadotropin-releasing hormone (GnRH) and tonically elevated levels of luteinizing hormone (LH).
- The polycystic ovary is a sign of these underlying endocrinologic abnormalities, not a disease intrinsic to the ovary.

ETIOLOGY
- The characteristic polycystic ovary emerges when a state of anovulation persists for any length of time.
- Although the ovaries of these women produce excessive amounts of androgens, there is no inherent endocrinologic abnormality in the ovaries.
- The tonically elevated LH levels cause the ovarian stromal tissue to produce more androgens, which in turn produce premature follicular atresia.
- Because there are many causes of anovulation, there are many causes of polycystic ovaries.
- It has been suggested that heredity, central catecholamine abnormalities, psychological stress, insulin resistance, and obesity may be involved.

 DIAGNOSIS

SIGNS AND SYMPTOMS
- Hirsutism
- Amenorrhea or oligomenorrhea
- Obesity

HISTORY
- Complete menstrual history
- Amenorrhea or irregular vaginal bleeding
- Infertility

PHYSICAL EXAM
- Hirsutism
- Most patients with this syndrome are obese:
  - Obesity probably enhances the syndrome because of the decrease in sex hormone–binding globulin, but is probably not important in its pathogenesis, because the syndrome occurs in some thin women and because many obese women do not have PCOS.

DIAGNOSTIC TESTS & INTERPRETATION
Lab
- Hormone levels:
  - Because follicle-stimulating hormone (FSH) levels are normal or low, an LH/FSH ratio >3 (provided the LH level is not <8 mIU/mL) may be used to suggest the diagnosis in women with clinical features of PCOS.
- Androgen levels:
  - Elevated
  - Serum testosterone levels are usually between 70 and 120 ng/dL
  - Androstenedione levels are usually between 3 and 5 ng/mL.

DIFFERENTIAL DIAGNOSIS
- Congenital adrenal hyperplasia
- Cushing syndrome
- Adrenal androgen-producing tumors
- Ovarian androgen-producing tumors
- Extragonadal sources of androgens

 TREATMENT

ADDITIONAL TREATMENT
General Measures
The best treatment for PCOS is oral contraceptives, unless pregnancy is desired, because these agents inhibit LH, decrease circulating testosterone levels, and increase levels of sex hormone–binding globulin, which binds and inactivates more of the testosterone in the circulation.

MEDICATION (DRUGS)
- Use oral contraceptives that contain <50 mcg estrogen and a progestin other than norgestrel, which is the most androgenic progestin in current use.
- Patients who desire fertility should be treated with ovulation-inducing agents, starting with clomiphene citrate and proceeding to human menopausal gonadotropin or GnRH agonists if unresponsive.
- If adrenal androgens (dehydroepiandrosterones [DHEAs]) are elevated, dexamethasone (0.25–0.5 mg at bedtime) should be given with the oral contraceptive to reduce adrenal androgen levels to normal.
- Patients with amenorrhea or irregular bleeding should be treated with monthly progestins, such as oral medroxyprogesterone acetate 10 mg daily for the 1st 10 days of the month, to prevent the effects of unopposed estrogens.
- Spironolactone 50–100 mg b.i.d. causes regression of the hirsutism in women with PCOS by decreasing androgenic action in the target organs.

SURGERY/OTHER PROCEDURES
Ovarian wedge resection was advocated in the past for treatment of androgen excess, but the decrease in circulating androgens occurred for only a short time, and this therapy should no longer be used.

 ONGOING CARE

In the patient who has long-standing anovulation, an endometrial biopsy, with extensive sampling, should be done because of the link between unopposed estrogen and endometrial cancer.

COMPLICATIONS
- The elevated levels of androgens that are produced are associated with hirsutism.
- The lack of a normal menstrual cycle leads to irregular bleeding, amenorrhea, and infertility.

- Because of the increased levels of unopposed estrogens, there is a 3-fold increased risk of endometrial cancer and a 3-fold greater risk of breast cancer appearing in the postmenopausal years.
- PCOS in early adulthood is associated with an increased long-term risk of diabetes and dysipidemia, independent of body mass index. ref 6

ADDITIONAL READING
- Olden NH, Carlson JL. The pathophysiology of amenorrhea in the adolescent. *Ann N Y Acad Sci*. 2008;1135:163–178.
- Blank SK, Helm KD, McCartney CR, et al. Polycystic ovary syndrome in adolescence. *Ann N Y Acad Sci*. 2008;1135:76–84.
- O'Brien RF, Emans SJ. Polycystic ovary syndrome in adolescents. *J Pediatr Adolesc Gynecol*. 2008; 21(3):119–128.
- Zidenberg N, Wright S. Care of the overweight adolescent including polycystic ovarian syndrome. *Clin Obstet Gynecol*. 2008;51(2):249–256.
- Wang ET, Calderon-Margalit R, Cedars MI, et al. Polycystic ovary syndrome and risk for long-term diabetes and dyslipidemia. *Obstet Gynecol*. 2011;117:6–13.

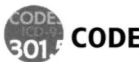 CODES

ICD9
- 256.4 Polycystic ovary syndrome
- 626.0 Absence of menstruation
- 704.1 Hirsutism

ICD10
- E28.2 Polycystic ovarian syndrome
- L68.0 Hirsutism
- N91.2 Amenorrhea, unspecified

FAQ
- Q: Can I still get pregnant if I have this syndrome?
- A: Yes. Although the best treatment for this syndrome is oral contraceptives, those patients who desire to become pregnant can be treated with ovulation-inducing agents.
- Q: I've noticed increased facial hair recently. Is there anything I can do about this?
- A: Yes. In most cases, the oral contraceptives will decrease circulating androgen levels sufficiently so that this will regress, but if increased body hair (hirsutism) persists, another drug, called spironolactone, which blocks the action of androgens, can be added to more effectively treat this.

POLYCYTHEMIA

David F. Friedman

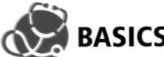 **BASICS**

DESCRIPTION
Polycythemia is an elevated hemoglobin and hematocrit level caused by an absolute increase in red cell mass. Polycythemia can be divided into subcategories, as follows:

- Primary polycythemia: Primary defect of bone marrow erythropoiesis, resulting in overproduction of red cells
- Secondary polycythemia: Stimulation of red cell production by increased levels of erythropoietin (EPO), which may be appropriately secreted in response to tissue hypoxia or may be inappropriately secreted because of renal disease or from a tumor
- Apparent or relative polycythemia: Increased hematocrit without true increase in red cell mass
- "Erythrocytosis" is another term describing increased red cell mass, which some authors prefer because it avoids confusion with the diagnosis of polycythemia vera (PCV).

EPIDEMIOLOGY
- Secondary causes of polycythemia are unusual:
  - Uncorrected cyanotic congenital heart disease
  - Chronic hypoxia due to lung disease
- Genetic causes of polycythemia are rare:
  - High oxygen-affinity hemoglobins
  - 2,3-Bisphosphoglycerate (2,3-BPG) dismutase deficiency
  - EPO receptor mutations
  - VHL, HIF2, PHD2, JAK2 mutations
  - PCV: <50 reported childhood cases (0.1% of cases of PCV are in children)

RISK FACTORS
Genetics
- High oxygen-affinity hemoglobins: Autosomal dominant
- PFCP:
  - Usually autosomal dominant
  - Finnish clusters described
- *VHL* gene mutation: Defect of oxygen sensing:
  - Autosomal recessive
  - Chuvash polycythemia
- 2,3-BPG mutase deficiency: Autosomal recessive

GENERAL PREVENTION
- There are no preventive measures for primary conditions such as PCV, hemoglobinopathies, or primary familial and congenital polycythemia (PFCP).
- Treatment of the underlying condition, such as correction of a cyanotic heart lesion or removal from high altitude, will prevent the development of secondary polycythemia.

PATHOPHYSIOLOGY
- Primary polycythemias:
  - PCV: Myeloproliferative disease with abnormal multipotent progenitor cells with abnormally high sensitivity to EPO; EPO levels are normal.
  - Mutation V617F in JAK2 gene found in most PCV but may not be initiating event
  - PFCP: Red cell precursors highly sensitive to EPO; usually autosomal dominant; some families have truncation mutations in the EPO receptor (EPOR), leading to a loss of down-regulation of EPO signaling.
- Secondary polycythemias: Relative tissue hypoxia resulting from reduced oxygen delivery:
  - Chronic lung disease and inadequate oxygenation
  - Cyanotic heart disease: Desaturation of arterial blood due to admixture of oxygen-poor venous blood from right-to-left shunt
  - Circulatory: Right-to-left shunting outside the heart
  - Hemoglobinopathy: Abnormal oxygen transport to tissues because of a mutant hemoglobin with higher than normal oxygen affinity and decreased oxygen delivery
  - At the partial pressure of oxygen of the tissues, high oxygen-affinity hemoglobins release less oxygen than normal, resulting in hypoxia.
  - Tissue hypoxia leads to supernormal secretion of EPO by the kidney and increased production of red cells from the marrow.
  - 2,3-BPG deficiency: Increased oxygen affinity of hemoglobin because of reduced level of red cell 2,3-BPG
  - Genetic defect of the hypoxia-sensing mechanism causes familial polycythemia: VHL—von Hippel-Lindau gene, HIF2—Hypoxia inducible factor, PHD2—prolyl hydroxylase domain
  - Inappropriate EPO secretion associated with kidney disease (not end stage, where EPO is usually deficient)
  - Malignant tumor that secretes EPO

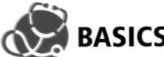 **DIAGNOSIS**

HISTORY
- Diagnosis of congenital heart disease, uncorrected or partially corrected
- History of cyanosis
- Delivery history
- Baby held below placenta
- Delayed clamping of cord
- Twins of disparate size
- Transfusion history
- Cigarette smoking
- Prolonged time spent at high altitude
- Family history of cyanosis, high hematocrit, need for phlebotomy
- Cobalt poisoning: Homemade beer and magnets may contain cobalt.

PHYSICAL EXAM
Signs and symptoms:
- Central and acral cyanosis
- Signs of dehydration:
  - Dry mucous membranes
  - No tears
  - Poor skin turgor
- Heart murmur
- Clubbing
- Plethora:
  - Conjunctival
  - Mucous membranes
  - Nail beds
- Splenomegaly:
  - Present in 75% of patients with PCV
- Headache, paresthesias, dizziness, syncope
- Transient blindness
- Decreased exercise tolerance, respiratory distress, dyspnea on exertion, oxygen requirement
- Pruritus
- Lethargy

ALERT
- Fingerstick CBC: Squeezing the finger to collect a specimen may give a falsely elevated hematocrit.
- Arterial blood gas: Cannot interpret low pO_2 if specimen is mixture of venous and arterial blood
- Relative polycythemia: Red cell mass normal
- Decreased plasma volume with normal red cell mass: Seen in adult cigarette smokers
- Dehydration: Elevated hematocrit due to hemoconcentration
- Hemoglobin electrophoresis does not identify all high-affinity hemoglobins:
  - Many co-migrate with normal hemoglobins.
  - Hemoglobin electrophoresis cannot be interpreted if the patient has been transfused within the past 3 months.
- Whole-blood P50: Fresh specimen required; normal samples different from red cell lysates, purified hemoglobin

DIAGNOSTIC TESTS & INTERPRETATION
Lab
- Initial:
  - CBC
  - Serum EPO: To distinguish primary from secondary polycythemia, but much overlap in EPO levels
  - Pulse oximetry: To determine percent saturation of hemoglobin
  - Arterial blood gas with co-oximetry: pO_2 low in lung disease or right-to-left shunt
- To investigate high oxygen-affinity hemoglobin:
  - Hemoglobin electrophoresis
  - Whole-blood P50 and red cell 2,3-BPG level
  - Met-hemoglobin level: Apparent cyanosis
- To investigate PCV:
  - Total red cell mass measurement by chromium 51–tagged red cells: Top normal range (adults) is <36 mL/kg in men, <32 mL/kg in women, or <25% above the predicted normal range normalized by body surface area; gold standard test for true polycythemia

– Bone marrow aspirate with chromosomes: Morphologic evidence of myelodysplastic syndrome; abnormal clone by karyotype or X-chromosome inactivation studies
– Serum B_{12}, unsaturated B_{12}-binding capacity (UB12BC): Markedly elevated in PCV
– Erythroid progenitor culture studies for burst-forming units–erythroid (BFU-E) that grow independent of EPO
– Genetic testing for V617F JAK2 mutation
• Other testing:
– Total blood viscosity: Rarely measured
– Iron studies: Serum iron (Fe), total iron-binding capacity (TIBC), ferritin
• BUN level, creatinine level, and urinalysis: Underlying renal disease

Imaging
• Echocardiography: To evaluate shunting
• Chest radiograph: To evaluate chronic lung disease, lung malignancies
• Abdominal ultrasound: To evaluate renal disease, spleen size, abdominal tumors
• Sleep study: To look for nighttime airway obstruction and desaturation

DIFFERENTIAL DIAGNOSIS
• Primary polycythemia:
– PCV
– Myeloproliferative disease
– Thrombocytosis or leukocytosis
– PFCP
• Secondary polycythemia:
– Cyanotic congenital heart disease
– Eisenmenger syndrome
– Pulmonary hypertension from long-standing uncorrected congenital heart disease with left-to-right shunting (acyanotic) leads to elevated right-sided pressures and reversal of shunt to flow right to left, leading to cyanosis.
– Extreme high altitude
– Compensation for low O_2 pressure includes an increase in red cell mass.
– Alveolar hypoventilation: Neuromuscular
– Muscular dystrophy
– Poliomyelitis
– Pickwickian syndrome
– Central hypoventilation
– End-stage lung disease
– Abnormal hemoglobins with high O_2 affinity
– 2,3-BPG mutase deficiency
– Inappropriate EPO secretion may occur in renal disease, including posttransplantation erythrocytosis after renal allografting; iatrogenic; excessive red cell transfusion, possible in trauma, resuscitations, neonatal blood exchange
– Excessive exogenous dosing of EPO (blood doping by competitive athletes)
– Neonatal polycythemia
– Twin-to-twin or placental transfusion
– Cobalt poisoning
• Relative polycythemia:
– May be seen in smokers
– Dehydration or diuretic use

 TREATMENT

MEDICATION (DRUGS)
• Hydroxyurea, alkylating agents, ^{32}P (in adults) to suppress red cell production in PCV
• Interferon: For PCV

ADDITIONAL TREATMENT
General Measures
• Observation only: Many patients require no therapy.
• Therapeutic phlebotomy:
– Removal of red cells every 3–4 weeks to maintain hematocrit below threshold for symptoms; usually <50–55%
– Patients with Eisenmenger syndrome and symptoms of hyperviscosity may not tolerate intravascular volume reduction if a large volume is removed at 1 time.
– Patients on a chronic phlebotomy program may require iron supplementation.
– Neonates with polycythemia may require therapeutic phlebotomy removing a series of small volumes of blood and replacing with plasma or albumin to reduce hematocrit while maintaining volume.
• Supplemental oxygen: Helpful for secondary polycythemia from underlying lung disease; may not help in right-to-left shunt

ISSUES FOR REFERRAL
• Persistent high hematocrit that is not clearly related to dehydration or neonatal causes
• Unexplained cyanosis

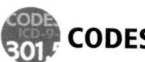 **ONGOING CARE**

FOLLOW-UP RECOMMENDATIONS
Patient Monitoring
Watch for the following:
• Insufficient phlebotomy
• Headache, dizziness, syncope
• Decreased exercise tolerance between phlebotomies
• Progression of myelodysplastic disease
• Thrombocytopenia
• Bleeding or thrombosis
• Stroke
• Severe headache
• Jaundice, ascites

PROGNOSIS
Depends on underlying condition:
• High oxygen-affinity hemoglobinopathies: Very good for normal life
• PCV: Guarded, as may progress to myelodysplastic syndrome
• Eisenmenger syndrome: Poor owing to progressive pulmonary hypertension and cor pulmonale

COMPLICATIONS
• Hyperviscosity:
– Blood viscosity increases dramatically when hematocrit is >65%.
– Decreased exercise tolerance, dyspnea, and mental status changes from slowed microcirculation in the CNS
• Thrombosis:
– Budd-Chiari syndrome from hepatic vein thrombosis, deep vein thrombosis, pulmonary embolus
– Seen especially in PCV
• Stroke: From hyperviscosity

ADDITIONAL READING
• Hodges VM, Rainey S, Lappin TR, et al. Pathophysiology of anemia and erythrocytosis. *Crit Rev Oncol Hematol.* 2007;64(2):139–158.
• Lee FS, Percy MJ. The HIF pathway and erythrocytosis. *Ann Rev Pathol.* 2011;6:165–192.
• Messinezy M, Pearson TC. The classification and diagnostic criteria of the erythrocytoses (polycythemias). *Clin Lab Haematol.* 1999;21: 309–316.
• Ozek E, Soll R, Schimmel MS. Partial exchange transfusion to prevent neurodevelopmental disability in infants with polycythemia. *Cochrane Database Syst Rev.* 2010;(1):CD005089.
• Prchal JT. Polycythemia vera and other primary polycythemias. *Curr Opin Hematol.* 2005;12: 112–116.

CODES

ICD9
289.0 Polycythemia, secondary

ICD10
D75.1 Secondary polycythemia

FAQ
• Q: Can a child with uncorrected cyanotic congenital heart disease be supported indefinitely with phlebotomy?
• A: No. Phlebotomy relieves the symptoms of hyperviscosity, but does not stop the progression of pulmonary hypertension.
• Q: When should a child with polycythemia be referred to a pediatric hematologist?
• A: If the high hematocrit is persistent and not clearly related to dehydration or neonatal causes (e.g., placental transfusion), the child should be referred to a pediatric hematologist. Unexplained cyanosis is also a reason for referral. In the case of congenital heart disease, the pediatric cardiologist may be comfortable managing polycythemia without consultation with a hematologist.

POLYPS, INTESTINAL

Steven Liu
Petar Mamula

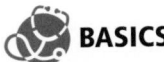 **BASICS**

DESCRIPTION
- Intestinal polyps are abnormal tissue growths protruding from the intestinal mucosa into the lumen. They are commonly solitary lesions, but may also be multiple in number and associated with various polyposis syndromes.
- Classification by gross appearance:
  - Pedunculated: Mushroom-like and attached to mucosa with a narrow stalk
  - Sessile: Elevated, flat lesions broadly attached to mucosa
- Types of polyps
  - Single, juvenile polyp
  - Juvenile polyposis syndrome (>3–5 juvenile polyps):
    - ○ Juvenile polyposis of infancy
    - ○ Juvenile polyposis coli (colonic involvement only)
    - ○ Generalized juvenile polyposis
  - Peutz-Jeghers syndrome
  - Familial adenomatous polyposis (FAP)
  - Other polyposis syndromes

EPIDEMIOLOGY
- Juvenile polyps are the most common childhood polyps:
  - Account for >90% of polyps seen in children
  - 1–2% of asymptomatic children are estimated to have juvenile polyps
  - Typically present between 2–5 years of age
  - Twice as common in boys than girls
  - >5 juvenile polyps should raise a suspicion for juvenile polyposis coli.
- Average age at onset of adenomatous polyps in FAP is 16 years.

Prevalence
- Juvenile polyposis syndrome: 1 in 100,000 to 1 in 160,000
- Peutz-Jeghers syndrome: 1 in 25,000 to 1 in 300,000
- FAP: 1 in 5,000 to 1 in 17,000

RISK FACTORS
Family history of polyposis syndrome

Genetics
Different genes and inheritance patterns with various polyposis syndromes:
- Juvenile polyposis syndrome:
  - Autosomal dominant with variable penetrance
  - Mutations in SMAD4 and BMPR1A genes, involved in transforming growth factor- (TGF-) signal transduction
- FAP:
  - Autosomal dominant
  - Mutation in adenomatous polyposis coli (APC) tumor suppressor gene

- Peutz-Jeghers syndrome:
  - Autosomal dominant
  - Mutations in STK11/LKB1 tumor suppressor gene are associated
- Cowden syndrome and Bannayan Riley Ruvalcaba syndrome (BRRS)
  - Autosomal dominant
  - Associated with mutations in PTEN gene

PATHOPHYSIOLOGY
Mutations in tumor suppressor genes likely lead to dysregulation of cell proliferation and apoptosis in polyposis syndromes.

COMMONLY ASSOCIATED CONDITIONS
- Juvenile polyposis syndrome, Cowden syndrome, and BRRS all have juvenile polyps as part of their manifestations.
- Peutz-Jeghers syndrome is characterized by multiple GI pedunculated hamartomatous polyps.
- FAP and Turcot syndrome are characterized by multiple adenomatous polyps.

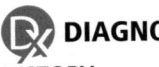 **DIAGNOSIS**

HISTORY
- Family history of polyps or polyposis syndromes is essential to obtain.
- Presence and amount of blood in stool
- Signs and symptoms:
  - Frequently asymptomatic
  - Painless rectal bleeding is typical presentation
  - Iron deficiency anemia
  - Prolapsing rectal lesion
  - Abdominal pain or obstruction from intussusception
  - Diarrhea

PHYSICAL EXAM
- Digital rectal exam may identify rectal polyp.
- Pigmentation of skin and mucous membranes consistent with Peutz-Jeghers syndrome
- Mucocutaneous lesions such as facial trichilemmoma, oral fibromas, and acral keratosis seen in Cowden syndrome
- Mental retardation, macrocephaly, lipomatosis, hemangiomas, and genital pigmentation seen in BRRS

DIAGNOSTIC TESTS & INTERPRETATION
Lab
- Stool test for occult blood may be positive.
- CBC can assess degree of anemia and also for baseline hemoglobin before polypectomy.
- PT/PTT should be considered before polypectomy due to risk of bleeding.
- Genetic testing can be considered if a polyposis syndrome is suspected.

Imaging
Radiologic studies are not the most effective methods of identifying polyps, but can be used:
- Barium enema may identify colonic polyps.
- Upper GI with small bowel study may locate presence of small bowel polyps.
- Use of CT and MR colonography has been studied mainly in adults.

Diagnostic Procedures/Other
- Full colonoscopy with polypectomy is the preferred test to perform.
- Flexible sigmoidoscopy may miss polyps in proximal colon:
  - 32% of juvenile polyps are located proximal to splenic flexure.
  - 12% of patients with juvenile polyps only had polyps located proximal to splenic flexure.
- Capsule endoscopy may be useful to identify small bowel polyps.

Pathological Findings
- Polyp pathology cannot be determined by gross visualization, hence polyps must be removed for histologic exam.
- Juvenile polyps:
  - Hamartomatous, but occasionally capable of adenomatous changes
  - Potential of malignancy in a solitary juvenile polyp is extremely low, but is increased in juvenile polyposis syndrome.
- Peutz-Jeghers syndrome:
  - Hamartomatous
  - Microscopically have hyperplasia of the smooth muscle layer, extending in an arborizing, tree-like manner
  - Relatively low potential of GI malignancy, but increased potential in other organs such as breast, pancreas, ovary, testicle, and uterus
- FAP:
  - Adenomatous polyps
  - Lifetime risk for colorectal cancer is 100%
  - Increased association with hepatoblastoma and desmoids tumors

DIFFERENTIAL DIAGNOSIS
- Because juvenile polyps often present with rectal bleeding, the differential diagnosis for lower GI bleeding should be considered:
  - Anal fissure
  - Meckel's diverticulum
  - Infectious enterocolitis
  - Inflammatory bowel disease
  - Intussusception
  - Vascular malformation
  - Hemorrhoids
  - Hemolytic uremic syndrome
  - Henoch-Schönlein purpura
  - Rectal trauma
  - Neoplasm

TREATMENT

MEDICATION (DRUGS)
Administration of some NSAIDs may slow progression of adenomatous polyps.

ADDITIONAL TREATMENT
General Measures
Full colonoscopy with polypectomy is an essential diagnostic and therapeutic tool. Removal of GI polyps can help to control symptoms and reduce the risk of malignancy.

ISSUES FOR REFERRAL
Patients suspected of having a polyp or polyposis syndrome should be referred to a gastroenterologist for evaluation. Patients with polyposis syndromes should be referred to a tertiary care center for genetic counseling.

SURGERY/OTHER PROCEDURES
- When adenomatous polyps are identified in FAP, prophylactic colectomy should be considered.
- Colectomy should also be considered in other polyposis syndromes with innumerable polyps or polyps showing premalignant changes.
- The main surgical options include a subtotal colectomy with ileorectal anastomosis (IRA) or a proctocolectomy with ileal pouch–anal anastomosis (IPAA).

ONGOING CARE

FOLLOW-UP RECOMMENDATIONS
- For solitary juvenile polyps, follow-up with stool guaiac check and CBC 6 months after polypectomy. Repeat colonoscopy is indicated with any abnormalities.
- For polyposis syndromes, screening recommendations differ depending on the syndrome:
  - Typically involve surveillance colonoscopies every 1–3 years depending on findings.
  - Asymptomatic children with an APC mutation for FAP should have annual colonoscopies starting at 10–12 years of age.
  - Published guidelines for follow-up of patients with various polyposis syndromes are available.
- Disposition:
  - Most uncomplicated polypectomies can be performed on an outpatient basis.

ADDITIONAL READING

- Barnard J. Screening and surveillance recommendations for pediatric gastrointestinal polyposis syndromes. *J Pediatr Gastroenterol Nutr.* 2009;(Suppl 48):S75–78.
- Chow E, Macrae F. Review of juvenile polyposis syndrome. *J Gastroenterol Hepatol.* 2005;20: 1634–1640.
- Erdman SH, Barnard JA. Gastrointestinal polyps and polyposis syndromes in children. *Curr Opin Pediatr.* 2002;14:576–582.
- Giardiello FM, Trimbath JD. Peutz-Jeghers syndrome and management recommendations. *Clin Gastroenterol Hepatol.* 2006;4(4):408–415.
- Gupta SK, Fitzgerald JF, Croffie JM, et al. Experience with juvenile polyps in North American children: The need for pancolonoscopy. *Am J Gastroenterol.* 2001;96:1695–1697.
- Merg A, Howe JR. Genetic conditions associated with intestinal juvenile polyps. *Am J Med Genet C Semin Med Genet.* 2004;129C(1):44–55.

CODES

ICD9
- 211.3 Benign neoplasm of colon
- 759.6 Other hamartoses, not elsewhere classified

ICD10
- D12.6 Benign neoplasm of colon, unspecified
- D13.9 Benign neoplasm of ill-defined sites within the digestive system
- Q85.8 Other phakomatoses, not elsewhere classified

FAQ

- Q: What is the potential of developing cancer from a polyp?
- A: Risk of neoplasia is dependent on the type of polyp:
  - Patients with solitary juvenile polyps have essentially no increased risk of colorectal carcinoma.
  - Patients with juvenile polyposis syndrome have been reported to have up to a 65% chance of developing GI cancer, with the risk of malignancy commencing from age 20.
  - Patients with Peutz-Jeghers syndrome have been reported to have almost a 50% chance of developing cancer in the intestinal tract or other organ systems.
  - Patients with FAP have a 100% lifetime risk of developing colorectal cancer.
- Q: Is a flexible sigmoidoscopy sufficient for the detection of polyps?
- A: ~37% of patients with juvenile polyps have polyps proximal to the splenic flexure, and 12% of patients have only proximal colon polyps. A flexible sigmoidoscopy would not identify these polyps, making it necessary to perform a full colonoscopy.
- Q: What is your management recommendation for a patient with painless rectal bleeding that stops on its own?
- A: It is widely believed that pedunculated polyps can auto-amputate after outgrowing their blood supply, although there is no objective evidence supporting this. If there is no family history of a polyposis syndrome, the patient can be followed with stool guaiac checks and a CBC in 6 months. If there is a family history, then referral to a gastroenterologist for full colonoscopy is indicated.
- Q: How many polyps can patients have?
- A: Patients with juvenile polyposis syndrome often have 50–200 polyps distributed throughout the colon. Patients with FAP may have a few to over a thousand polyps in the colon.

PORENCEPHALY CORTICAL DYSPLASIA/NEURONAL MIGRATION DISORDERS—MALFORMATIONS OF CORTICAL DEVELOPMENT

Irfan Jafree
Peter M. Bingham (5th edition)

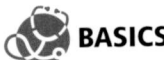 **BASICS**

DESCRIPTION

- Developmental brain malformations are associated with epilepsy and mental retardation.
- Associated features may include autism, learning difficulties, hypotonia, spasticity, movement disorders or orthopedic abnormalities.
- Blindness, hearing abnormalities and feeding difficulties may be present.
- Key histologic feature: Structural organization of the cerebral cortex is abnormal.
- Diffuse (lissencephaly, polymicrogyria, hemimegalencephaly) or focal regions of the brain as in focal cortical dysplasia (CD), tuberous sclerosis complex, neurofibromatosis, porencephaly
- General rule: The more extensive the malformation, the greater the degree of neurologic impairment.
  – Malformations of cortical development affecting wide regions of cortex: Etiologic agent likely <20 weeks' gestation.
    ○ Lissencephaly (smooth brain): Loss of cerebral cortical convolutions (sulci) and cortical laminations. May occur in combination with agyria–pachygyria.
    ○ Agyria–pachygyria: More heterogeneous pathologic classification in which there are broad regions of cortex without gyri (similar to lissencephaly), but focal areas of thickened cortical gyri also may be present.
    ○ Hemimegalencephaly: Rare condition in which 1 cerebral hemisphere is enlarged and may exhibit agyric–pachygyric features. Normal-sized hemisphere may also contain subtle, focal abnormalities.
  – Malformations of cortical development affecting focal regions of cortex: Etiologic agent likely >20 weeks' gestation
    ○ Dysplastic cortical architecture: Focal regions of disorganized cortical architecture and abnormally shaped neurons
    ○ Heterotopia: Clusters of neurons found within the white matter (where neurons are not typically found) May be nodular and confined to small region in cortex or adjacent to the ependyma (nodular forms) May extend across portions of a hemisphere (laminar heterotopia).
    ○ Schizencephaly: Nonloculated cavities or clefts (unilateral or bilateral) in the brain that communicate with the system and/or subarachnoid space.
  – Recent classification scheme for malformations of cortical development:
  – Disorders of cell proliferation: Tuberous sclerosis complex.
    ○ Focal CD
    ○ Hemimegalencephaly
    ○ Microcephaly syndromes
    ○ Dysembryoblastic neuroepithelial tumors
    ○ Ganglioglioma
    ○ Gangliocytoma.
  – Neural migration disorders (NMDs):
    ○ Lissencephaly type I (classical):
    ○ Miller–Dieker syndrome
    ○ X-linked lissencephaly

  – Lissencephaly type II (cobblestone):
    ○ Walker–Warburg syndrome
  – Muscle–eye–brain disease: Fukuyama congenital muscular dystrophy
  – Subcortical band heterotopia (double cortex syndrome)
  – Periventricular nodular heterotopia.
  – Disorders of brain organization:
    ○ Polymicrogyria
    ○ Schizencephaly
  – Taylor type I dysplasia: Microdysgenesis
  – Malformations, not otherwise classified:
    ○ Mitochondrial disorders
    ○ Peroxisomal disorders (e.g., Zellweger syndrome)

EPIDEMIOLOGY

- Incidence varies according to syndrome.
- Some children die at birth or in early childhood, owing to seizures, respiratory failure.
- Epilepsy may be associated with malformations of cortical development. Malformations of cortical development may underlie infantile spasms (especially tuberous sclerosis complex and lissencephaly).
- Estimated that 20–40% of specimens resected during epilepsy surgery contain malformations of cortical development

PATHOPHYSIOLOGY

- Most characteristic feature: Disruption of normal cerebral cortical architecture
- Lissencephaly:
  – Few cerebral convolutions (sulci and gyri) in the entire brain
  – Layering of cortex abnormal
  – Neurons often abnormally shaped, oriented incorrectly within cortex
- Heterotopias:
  – Clusters of neurons located inappropriately in the subcortical white matter
  – Large bilateral subcortical heterotopia found in patients with double cortex syndrome
  – Clusters of heterotopic neurons line the ventricles in periventricular nodular heterotopia.
- Disruption of the synaptic connections between various brain regions likely accounts for epilepsy and other neurologic problems such as mental retardation or autism associated with cortical malformations.

ETIOLOGY

CD/NMDs result from a variety of in utero causes, including infectious, toxic–metabolic, and ischemic insults. Several cortical malformations result from single gene mutations.

- Genetic:
  – Lissencephaly may occur as a sporadic syndrome, but has been associated with mutations in select genes.
  – Miller–Dieker lissencephaly syndrome: Chromosome 17p13.3
  – Lissencephaly with cerebellar hypoplasia: Chromosome 7q22
  – X-linked lissencephaly: Chromosome Xq22

  – Periventricular nodular heterotopia: Chromosome Xq28
  – Subcortical band heterotopia: Chromosome Xq22
  – Tuberous sclerosis complex: Chromosome 9q34, chromosome 16p13
  – Neurofibromatosis (NF) 1 Autosomal dominant, Chromosome 17q11.2 (Von Recklinghausen disease), Neurofibromin protein abnormal.
  – NF2 chromosome 22q12.2 Merlin gene, Autosomal dominant, associated with MEN syndromes.
  – Fukuyama congenital muscular dystrophy: Chromosome 9q31
  – Other lissencephaly-associated syndromes, including the Norman–Roberts, Neu–Laxova, and Walker–Warburg syndromes, are believed to have an autosomal recessive pattern of inheritance.
  – The HARD syndrome (hydrocephalus, agyria, retinal dysplasia and encephalocele) is autosomal recessive.
  – Cortical abnormalities also occur in trisomy 13, 18, and 21, chromosome 22q deletion syndrome.
- Infectious:
  – Polymicrogyria, pachygyria–agyria, and heterotopias may occur in the setting of toxoplasmosis, other agents, rubella, cytomegalovirus, and herpes virus (TORCH) infections of the CNS during early development. May also occur as a consequence of intrauterine hypoxic–ischemic injury.
- Ischemic/hemorrhagic:
  – Polymicrogyria and heterotopia may occur in the setting of in utero hypoxic–ischemic injury or hemorrhage.
  – Schizencephaly may reflect intrauterine infarction and is characterized by a large cleft in one or both hemispheres.
  – Porencephaly—porencephalic cysts—which may result from intrauterine hypoxic–ischemic injury, are intraparenchymal cavities that communicate with the ventricular system.
- Toxins:
  – Ethanol
  – Ionizing radiation
  – Carbon monoxide
  – Isotretinoin
  – Methyl mercury
  – Antiepileptic drugs (phenytoin/fosphenytoin, depakote)
- Metabolic:
  – CD/NMDs may be associated with Zellweger syndrome, neonatal adrenoleukodystrophy, Menkes disease, GM_2 gangliosidoses, and/or pyruvate dehydrogenase deficiency.
- Miscellaneous:
  – Cortical malformations may occur in syndromes featuring other anomalies: chromosome 22q11 deletion, Smith–Lemli–Opitz, Potter, and Meckel syndromes.

DIAGNOSIS

HISTORY

- Family history of genetic or chromosomal syndromes, family members with mental retardation, neurologic dysfunction or seizures, and infant deaths associated with profound neurologic impairment
- Parental consanguinity; maternal alcohol and drug use
- Subtle manifestations of neurocutaneous syndromes may be identified in family members with skin lesions or, in more overt cases, as individuals with CNS or other cancers, as in tuberous sclerosis or neurofibromatosis.
- Infants: Sudden head or truncal movements (infantile spasms)

PHYSICAL EXAM

- Some children with malformations of cortical developments have no overt signs of dysfunction, whereas others have global neurologic impairment.
- Developmental delay, seizures (especially infantile spasms), and focal neurologic signs may be observed.
- Plot head circumference: Microcephaly or macrocephaly is common.
- Some children will have dysmorphic facies characterized by hypotelorism, malformed skull, and midline deformities.
- Miller–Dieker lissencephaly syndrome: Thin upper lip and microcephaly
- Cutaneous manifestations such as hypomelanotic lesions (ash leaf spots), facial angiofibromas, a shagreen patch, or other regions of hyperpigmentation/hypopigmentation may identify patient with neurocutaneous disorders such as tuberous sclerosis. Neurofibromas, axillary and inguinal frecking, Café au lait spots, plexiform neurofibromas in neurofibromatosis.
- Funduscopic examination may reveal retinal hamartomas in tuberous sclerosis and Lisch nodules in NF1.
- A linear sebaceous nevus on the forehead is associated with hemimegalencephaly.
- Hypomelanosis of Ito: Associated with malformations of cortical development
  - Physical examination tricks:
    - ○ Wood lamp of skin: To identify subtle depigmented areas
    - ○ Tooth enamel pits: Tuberous sclerosis

DIAGNOSTIC TESTS & INTERPRETATION

- Routine blood tests and cerebrospinal fluid usually normal
- Lysosomal enzymopathies characteristic of disorders such as gangliosidoses may be identifiable via blood tests.
- Chromosomal karyotyping/fluorescence in situ hybridization (FISH) analysis: Miller–Dieker, chromosome 22q deletion, trisomies, for diagnosis and genetic counseling
- Screening for select gene mutations is available through several research labs and will become commercially available (http://www.genetests.org).

- EEG adjunct in diagnosing seizures. Characteristic findings may be sharp waves, spikes, hypsarrhythmia (in infantile spasms), and slow spike-wave discharges (Lennox–Gastaut syndrome). In children with developmental delay, formal neuropsychiatric assessment may be useful.

Imaging

- Brain MRI is essential to classify cortical malformations. Brain CT may be useful but has lower resolution.
- Research/quaternary epilepsy centers: Functional brain imaging, positron-emission tomography, to assess regional metabolic changes associated with epilepsy

DIFFERENTIAL DIAGNOSIS

- In patients presenting with even subtle neurologic symptoms or signs, consider a structural CNS abnormality.
- Some developmental anomalies may be difficult to distinguish from brain tumors.
- Epilepsy in pediatric patients may be a manifestation of a neurocutaneous disorder such as tuberous sclerosis.
- Tumors, vascular malformations, and in utero ischemic insults also should be considered.

TREATMENT

MEDICATION (DRUGS)

- Neurologic consultation is recommended to help manage children with cortical malformations and epilepsy.
- Virtually all children with malformations of cortical development and seizures will require anticonvulsant drugs for adequate seizure control. Regimens must be tailored to account for drug interactions, potential side effects, and long-term efficacy in seizure control.
- See chapter "Infantile Spasms."

SURGERY/OTHER PROCEDURES

- A significant proportion of children with cortical malformations and seizures will not respond to medications and will require epilepsy surgery to remove the seizure focus within the malformation of cortical development.
- In some cases, surgery is a small focal resection; in rare cases, removal of an entire hemisphere is indicated.
- Some cases are not amenable to epilepsy surgery; other treatment modalities include the vagal nerve stimulator or the ketogenic diet.

ONGOING CARE

- When to expect improvement:
  - Adequate seizure control may be difficult in these patients.
  - Cognitive, behavioral, and motor deficits may benefit somewhat from education, behavioral interventions, and physical therapy.
  - In children with a cortical malformation and refractory seizures, resective epilepsy surgery can provide a safe and successful alternative when anticonvulsant medications do not help.

- Signs to watch for:
  - Persistent change in mental status, which could indicate status epilepticus.
  - Development of new neurologic symptoms in patients with tuberous sclerosis could indicate tumor progression or hydrocephalus.

PROGNOSIS

Most patients with CD/NMDs will continue to suffer from seizures and cognitive impairment as well as from other neurologic and behavioral abnormalities.

ADDITIONAL READING

- Barkovich AJ, Kuzniecky RI. Gray matter heterotopia. *Neurology.* 2000;55:1603–1608.
- Barkovich AJ, Kuzniecky RI, Jackson GD, et al. A developmental and genetic classification for malformations of cortical development. *Neurology.* 2005;65:1873–1887.
- Bendavid C, et al. Holoprosencephaly: An update on cytogenetic abnormalities. *Am J Med Genet C Semin Med Genet.* 2010;154C(1):86–92.
- Crino PB, Chou K. Epilepsy and cortical dysplasias. *Curr Treat Options Neurol.* 2000;2:543–552.
- Di Rocco C. Hemimegalencephaly. In: Choux M, Di Rocco C, Hockey AD, Walker ML, eds. *Pediatric Neurosurgery.* New York: Churchill Livingstone; 1999:736–738.
- Eller KM, Kuller JA. Fetal porencephaly: A review of etiology, diagnosis and prognosis. *Obstet Gynecol Surv.* 1995;50:684–687.
- Rocco CD, et al. Hemimegancephaly: Clinical implications and surgical treatment. *Childs Nerv Syst.* 2006;22:852–866.
- Self L, Shevell MI. A registry-based assessment of cerebral palsy and cerebral malformations. *J Child Neurology.* 2010;25(11):1313–1318.

CODES

ICD9

- 742.2 Congenital reduction deformities of brain
- 742.4 Other specified congenital anomalies of brain
- 742.8 Other specified congenital anomalies of nervous system

ICD10

- Q04.6 Congenital cerebral cysts
- Q04.8 Other specified congenital malformations of brain
- Q07.8 Other specified congenital malformations of nervous system

PORTAL HYPERTENSION
Rose C. Graham

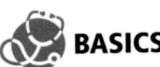 **BASICS**

DESCRIPTION
- Definition: Elevation of portal blood pressure greater than 5–10 mm Hg
- Portal hypertension may be pre-, intra-, or posthepatic in origin.
- A major cause of morbidity and mortality in children with chronic liver disease

PATHOPHYSIOLOGY
- An increase in portal resistance and increased portal blood flow are the main pathogenic factors initiating the process of portal hypertension:
  - Other factors including hyperdynamic circulation, expanded intravascular volume, systemic arteriolar vasodilatation, decreased splanchnic arteriolar tone, and humoral factors (i.e., nitric oxide) contribute to increased portal blood flow and pressure.
- Decompression of the high venous pressure through portosystemic collaterals leads to all the major sequelae of portal hypertension:
  - Splenomegaly
  - Varices (esophageal, gastric)
  - Hemorrhoids
  - Caput medusa (periumbilical varices)
  - Ascites
  - Hepatic encephalopathy

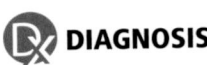 **DIAGNOSIS**

HISTORY
- History of umbilical catheterization
- History of hepatitis, abdominal trauma, clotting disorder, contraceptive pills, underlying medical problem such as cystic fibrosis, tyrosinemia, Wilson disease
- Ingestion of excessive amounts of vitamin A
- Hematemesis or melena: Upper GI tract bleed from varices may be the 1st sign of long-standing silent liver disease or previously undiagnosed portal vein thrombosis.

PHYSICAL EXAM
- Splenomegaly
- Hepatomegaly may or may not be present.
- Ascites (distension, fluid wave)
- Hemorrhoids
- Prominent vascular pattern on the abdomen (caput medusa)
- Digital clubbing
- Telangiectasia
- Palmar erythema
- Growth failure

DIAGNOSTIC TESTS & INTERPRETATION
Lab
- CBC and smear: Detect hypersplenism, GI tract blood loss, and chronic liver disease
- PT/INR and PTT: Detect coagulation defects
- Hepatic function panel includes liver enzymes (alanine aminotransferase [ALT], aspartate aminotransferase [AST]), albumin (measure of hepatic function), alkaline phosphatase, and γ-glutamyl transferase (GGT; may be elevated with cholestasis and bile duct injury)
- Additional laboratory testing to determine the cause of underlying liver disease, depending on clinical scenario (see chapter on "Cirrhosis" for more details)

Imaging
- Doppler ultrasound:
  - Liver size and echogenicity
  - Biliary anatomy
  - Spleen size
  - Renal cysts
  - Presence of ascites
  - Vessel diameter
  - Direction of blood flow
  - Presence of esophageal varices
- Esophagogastroduodenoscopy (EGD): Definitively identifies the presence of esophageal varices and determines if variceal rupture is the cause of GI tract bleeding

Diagnostic Procedures/Other
- Liver biopsy: Identify the underlying cause of the portal hypertension
- Hepatic venous wedge pressure gradient correlates and selective angiography are not used in pediatrics because of a lack of well-documented pediatric measurements and lack of a favorable risk–benefit ratio.

DIFFERENTIAL DIAGNOSIS
- Prehepatic causes:
  - Portal vein thrombosis with cavernous transformation (increased risk with umbilical vein catheterization, sepsis, dehydration, hypercoagulable state)
  - Splenic vein thrombosis
- Intrahepatic causes:
  - Hepatocellular disorders: Viral hepatitis, α_1-antitrypsin deficiency, chronic hepatitis, autoimmune hepatitis, Wilson disease, glycogen storage disease, tyrosinemia, schistosomiasis, peliosis hepatitis, vitamin A toxicity
  - Biliary tract disorders: Extrahepatic biliary atresia, ductal plate malformation/congenital hepatic fibrosis, intrahepatic cholestasis syndromes, primary sclerosing cholangitis, choledochal cyst, cystic fibrosis
- Posthepatic causes:
  - Budd-Chiari syndrome: Occlusion of suprahepatic inferior vena cava or hepatic veins by congenital web, tumor, or thrombus
  - Congestive heart failure
  - Veno-occlusive disease of hepatic venule

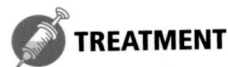 **TREATMENT**

MEDICATION (DRUGS)
- β-Blockade: Nonselective β-blockers, such as propranolol, have been shown to be effective in preventing both initial and recurrent variceal bleeds in adults. Data are limited on use of β-blockers in children with portal hypertension to prevent primary or secondary variceal bleeding. Use in children for this indication is empiric and mainly based on adult data:
  - Mechanisms include lowering portal blood flow and thus portal pressure by both β_2-blockade, which increases splanchnic tone, and β_1-blockade, which decreases cardiac output.
  - Propranolol, specifically, may also decrease collateral circulation.
  - β-Blocker effect on decreasing cardiac output may blunt an adaptive cardiovascular response (elevated heart rate) in the event of a hemorrhage; these medications should not be used in patients with asthma or diabetes.
  - Owing to lack of sufficient data, routine use of β-blockers in children for primary or secondary prevention of variceal bleeding cannot be recommended.
- Diuretic therapy (spironolactone +/– chlorothiazide) when ascites is present

ADDITIONAL TREATMENT
General Measures
Chronic management of varices:
- Surveillance endoscopy and primary prophylaxis in pediatric patients with portal hypertension who have not had a 1st variceal bleed are controversial and not yet recommended.
- Long-term management of patients with portal hypertension who have had a variceal bleed depends on the underlying cause of the portal hypertension and may include endoscopic sclerotherapy or ligation, portosystemic shunts, and liver transplantation.

Additional Therapies
- Endoscopic sclerotherapy: Reduces rebleeding episodes and long-term mortality when initiated after the 1st bleeding episode; it is unclear whether it will prevent occurrence of a 1st bleed.
- Endoscopic band ligation therapy may be as effective as and carry fewer complications compared with sclerotherapy. Endoscopic band ligation is limited in smaller patients by esophageal size.

SURGERY/OTHER PROCEDURES

- Portosystemic shunts:
  - May be helpful in the setting of prehepatic causes of portal hypertension to reduce portal pressure. Specifically, the Rex shunt (mesenteric-left portal bypass) has been used very successfully in the setting of cavernous transformation of the portal vein.
  - Does not improve long-term survival in patients with intrahepatic disease
  - Complications may include thrombosis and worsening of hepatic encephalopathy.
  - TIPS (transjugular intrahepatic portosystemic shunt) procedure may be an effective bridge to liver transplantation in pediatric patients with progressive liver disease and recurrent variceal bleeds.
  - Data in pediatric patients are limited.
- Liver transplantation:
  - The current approach at most institutions is liver transplantation for those patients with life-threatening bleeds not amenable to β-blockade or endoscopic therapies.

IN-PATIENT CONSIDERATIONS

Initial Stabilization

- Acute management of variceal bleed:
  - Vital signs: Remember that hemodynamic instability can be masked by β-blockers.
  - Fluid resuscitation: Two large-bore IV catheters or intraosseous needles, give crystalloid initially, then RBC transfusion with goal hemoglobin of 10 g/dL
  - Nasogastric tube placement: Lavage with room temperature saline or sterile water until clear; leave tube in place for evaluation and removal of continued or recurrent bleeding
  - Correction of coagulopathy: Parenteral vitamin K, fresh frozen plasma, platelet transfusion if platelets $<50,000/\mu L$
  - IV antibiotics: Acute variceal hemorrhage increases the risk of spontaneous bacterial peritonitis in the setting of ascites.
  - IV proton pump inhibitor or histamine receptor antagonist to decrease risk of bleeding from ulcers or erosions
  - Pharmacotherapy to control active bleeding:
    ○ Octreotide (somatostatin analog) decreases splanchnic blood flow via its inhibition of intestinal vasoactive peptide secretion. In turn, portal blood pressure is decreased. Somatostatin can be used but has a shorter half-life compared with octreotide.
    ○ Vasopressin decreases splanchnic blood flow via its vasoconstriction effects, but its use is limited owing to systemic vasoconstriction and a poor side effect profile. Nitroglycerin, a venodilator, has been used in conjunction to decrease the side effects. This combination is not preferred.
  - Lactulose to prevent hepatic encephalopathy in patients with cirrhosis
  - Endoscopy (after stabilization) to determine source of hemorrhage (variceal rupture or other, such as gastric ulcer) and perform therapeutic procedures such as sclerotherapy or band ligation for varices or electrocautery or clip placement for ulcer.

- Direct tamponade: Sengstaken-Blakemore tube for severe uncontrollable hemorrhage, but high rate of complications
- Surgical intervention: Portosystemic shunt, esophageal devascularization and/or transection, TIPS (transjugular intrahepatic portosystemic shunt)

ALERT

- The site of bleeding needs to be identified and managed appropriately: Not all GI bleeding in a patient with portal hypertension is an upper GI tract source (i.e., hemorrhoids); nasogastric lavage will help to determine if the problem is from the upper tract.
- Be careful not to overestimate the hemoglobin because equilibration may not have taken place at the time of presentation with an acute bleed.

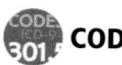 ONGOING CARE

FOLLOW-UP RECOMMENDATIONS

- Patients are followed closely for hepatic decompensation.
- Growth failure, recurrent life-threatening bleeds not controllable with prophylactic intervention, refractory ascites, and poor quality of life are indications for liver transplantation.

DIET

Sodium restriction when ascites is present

PROGNOSIS

- The disease course and prognosis depend on the underlying cause.
- Acute variceal bleeding is associated with a 6-week mortality of up to 30% in adults. The mortality rate in children is much lower.
- Variceal bleeding associated with prehepatic causes of portal hypertension such as portal vein thrombosis typically becomes less problematic as the child ages; these patients will most likely not require a shunt and may be easily managed with endoscopic therapy.
- Patients with congenital hepatic fibrosis also do very well, because the underlying disease is not progressive and bleeding may be easily managed with endoscopic therapy.
- Progressive liver disease has a worse prognosis and often requires liver transplantation.

COMPLICATIONS

- Hemorrhage from varices may present as hematemesis, hematochezia, or melena.
- Hypersplenism
- Malabsorption due to congestion of the intestinal mucosa
- Abnormal sodium retention
- Ascites: Presence of ascites increases risk of spontaneous bacterial peritonitis.

- Hepatorenal syndrome
- Hepatopulmonary syndrome (intrapulmonary right-to-left shunting) leads to hypoxemia, shortness of breath, exercise intolerance, and digital clubbing.
- Pulmonary hypertension can be a life-threatening complication of portal hypertension.

ADDITIONAL READING

- El-hamid NA, Taylor RM, Marinello D, et al. Aetiology and management of extrahepatic portal vein obstruction in children: King's College Hospital experience. *J Pediatr Gastroenterol Nutr.* 2008; 47:630–634.
- Mileti E, Rosenthal P. Management of portal hypertension in children. *Curr Gastroenterol Rep.* 2011;13:10–16.
- Molleston JP. Variceal bleeding in children. *J Pediatr Gastroenterol Nutr.* 2003;37:538–545.
- Ryckman FC, Alonso MH. Causes and management of portal hypertension in the pediatric population. *Clin Liver Dis.* 2001;5:789–818.
- Shashidhar H, Langhans N, Grand RJ. Propranolol in prevention of portal hypertensive hemorrhage in children: A pilot study. *J Pediatr Gastroenterol Nutr.* 1999;29:12–17.

CODES

ICD9
572.3 Portal hypertension

ICD10
K76.6 Portal hypertension

FAQ

- Q: What is my child's long-term prognosis?
- A: The disease course and prognosis depend on the underlying cause. Variceal bleeding associated with prehepatic causes of portal hypertension such as portal vein thrombosis typically becomes less problematic as the child ages and may be managed with endoscopic therapy.
- Q: Are there any medications I should avoid?
- A: Avoid aspirin and NSAID-containing products such as ibuprofen.

POSTERIOR URETHRAL VALVE

Shamir Tuchman

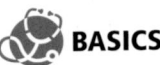 **BASICS**

DESCRIPTION
Valvular obstruction of the posterior urethra that results in variable dysfunction of all segments of the urinary tract, including the bladder, ureters, and renal parenchyma.

EPIDEMIOLOGY
- Most common congenital cause of obstructive uropathy resulting in renal failure in childhood
- Incidence: 1/5,000–8,000 male births
- Most boys with posterior urethral valve (PUV) present in the 1st year of life.
- By adolescence, ~30% of neonatally diagnosed patients will have renal insufficiency.
- There are rare reports of obstructive valves in the female urethra; however, they differ embryologically from those seen in males.

RISK FACTORS
Genetics
- Genetic basis remains unclear.
- Most cases are sporadic, although rare cases in siblings have been reported.

PATHOPHYSIOLOGY
- The embryogenesis is unclear.
- May arise from abnormal integration of the wolffian ducts into the urethra or from persistence of the urogenital membrane.
- The valve is a fold of fibrous connective tissue, extending between the verumontanum and the anterior urethral roof, which usually forms a diaphragm with a slit-like orifice.
- Children with PUV commonly have renal parenchymal dysplasia.
- With flow of urine from the bladder in patients with PUV, the valves balloon into the urethra, causing obstruction. As a result of the increased work of voiding, the bladder hypertrophies, with trabeculation and diverticulum formation. The bladder develops poor compliance, decreased capacity, increased pressure, and spastic hyperreflexia.
- Increased bladder volume and pressure causes incompetence of the ureterovesical junctions, with increased pressure transmitted into the upper urinary tract.
- The segment of the urethra proximal to the obstruction dilates and elongates.

COMMONLY ASSOCIATED CONDITIONS
- Hydroureteronephrosis, vesicoureteral reflux, perirenal urinoma, or urinary ascites may occur.
- Renal parenchymal damage may result.

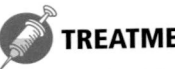 **DIAGNOSIS**

HISTORY
- Poor urinary stream
- Unexplained fevers
- Tachypnea from acidosis
- The clinical presentation depends on age of presentation and severity of obstruction:
  - Many severe cases are diagnosed postnatally as the result of evaluation of hydroureteronephrosis detected antenatally on maternal US.
  - Severely affected infants may present with respiratory distress and other sequelae of oligohydramnios, azotemia, sepsis, dehydration, acidosis, and electrolyte disorders.
  - Patients may present with delayed voiding after delivery, a palpable bladder, UTI, abnormal urinary stream, or failure to thrive because of renal failure.
  - Toddlers may present with UTI or voiding symptoms, such as dysuria and a weak urinary stream.
  - Older boys may present with daytime incontinence, nocturnal enuresis, or urinary frequency because of bladder hypertrophy coupled with polyuria secondary to a renal concentrating defect.
  - A strong urinary stream does not exclude the diagnosis of PUV because an adequate flow may be generated by the hypertrophied bladder.

PHYSICAL EXAM
Palpably enlarged bladder and kidneys are the most common physical finding.

DIAGNOSTIC TESTS & INTERPRETATION
Lab
Electrolytes: Infants with severe PUV may have UTIs and/or azotemia and fluid and electrolyte abnormalities such as dehydration, acidosis, hyperkalemia, and hyponatremia (type IV RTA).

Imaging
- Voiding cystourethrogram (VCUG):
  - Most important study for diagnosis
  - Will reveal a sharply defined lucency in the posterior urethra and bladder hypertrophy.
  - Bladder trabeculation, diverticuli, and vesicoureteral reflux may also be demonstrated.
- Abdominal US may demonstrate hydroureteronephrosis, evidence of renal dysplasia, dilatation of the posterior urethra with an enlarged, thickened bladder (keyhole sign), and urinary ascites.
- Hydronephrosis is present in 90% of infants with PUV.

Diagnostic Procedures/Other
- Urethroscopy
- Definitive diagnosis requires urethroscopic exam:
  - Caution: When a catheter is passed into the bladder, the valves flatten and are nonobstructive. This may give the misleading impression that there is no obstruction.

DIFFERENTIAL DIAGNOSIS
- Nonobstructive urinary tract dilatation may occur secondary to the following:
  - Vesicoureteral reflux
  - Prune belly syndrome
  - Detrusor sphincter dyssynergia
  - Polyuria
  - UTI
  - Ureteral stenosis
- Other entities that may mimic PUVs include the following:
  - Urethral strictures
  - Primary vesical neck contractures
  - Anterior urethral valves

TREATMENT

ADDITIONAL TREATMENT
General Measures
- Supportive:
  - Initial management in the neonate consists of inserting a fine urethral catheter into the bladder and treating any fluid and electrolyte disturbances and/or UTI.
  - A large postobstructive diuresis may occur, requiring ongoing management of fluids and electrolytes.

SURGERY/OTHER PROCEDURES
- Valve ablation (destruction of the obstructive valve leaflet) is the definitive treatment of the primary lesion. The most common approach is to incise the valves transurethrally through an endoscope.
- In utero drainage of the fetal bladder has yet to show improvement in long-term renal outcome compared to valve ablation after delivery.
- In utero drainage has been used in selected cases in an attempt to ameliorate pulmonary hypoplasia in the setting of oligohydramnios.
- Unless the patient has renal insufficiency that does not improve after fluid resuscitation and catheter drainage, the next step is endoscopic ablation of the valves.

- If the infant's urethra is too small for the endoscope, cutaneous vesicostomy may be necessary.
- If rapid recovery does not occur following placement of the catheter or after valve ablation, vesicostomy or supravesical urinary diversion (such as ureterostomy or nephrostomy) may be required.
- Supravesical diversion may be associated with poorer long-term bladder function.
- The optimal anatomic level of urinary diversion remains controversial.
- Following valve ablation, the posterior urethra will appear less dilated on VCUG. However, improvement in hydroureteronephrosis and vesicoureteral reflux occurs more slowly, over years.

ONGOING CARE

FOLLOW-UP RECOMMENDATIONS
- Growth problems, renal insufficiency, and end-stage renal disease can occur at any time during childhood, puberty, or beyond.
- Patients who require extensive urinary diversion, such as vesicostomy, pyelostomy, or ureterostomy, will require long-term reconstruction, including possible bladder reconstruction.
- Delayed obstruction may occur owing to urethral stricture.
- Patients with persistent incontinence require urodynamic evaluation to determine the cause and to dictate individualized therapy.

Patient Monitoring
Careful follow-up through childhood and puberty: Visits should include imaging for renal function and upper tract dilatation and drainage, urodynamic studies of bladder function, assessment of growth, blood pressure, urinary protein, and serum creatinine.

PROGNOSIS
- The prognosis for infants with severe PUV has improved owing to earlier recognition and improved management of pulmonary hypoplasia and fluid and metabolic derangements.
- Pulmonary hypoplasia and renal dysplasia account for most causes of death in infants with PUV.
- Oligohydramnios is a predictor of poor long-term renal function. The earlier and more severe the oligohydramnios occurs during pregnancy, the more guarded the prognosis for long-term renal function.
- Measures of renal function at the time of presentation may not correlate with ultimate outcome. Rather, the rate of improvement following relief of obstruction is more indicative of prognosis. An early nadir creatinine level <1.0 mg/dL does not preclude renal failure, as the child attains greater body mass.

- However, in patients diagnosed and treated in infancy, a creatinine level of <0.8 mg/dL at 1 year of age often portends a better long-term renal prognosis.
- During the course of many years, many children who seem to do well initially will suffer progressive renal failure and require renal transplantation.
- Patients with an abnormal serum creatinine at 2 years of age often develop end-stage renal disease by adolescence or young adulthood.
- Children who develop proteinuria have bilateral renal dysplasia, and/or bladder dysfunction are more likely to eventually develop renal insufficiency and hypertension.

COMPLICATIONS
- Severe cases may suffer the effects of intrauterine oligohydramnios, including Potter syndrome and pulmonary hypoplasia.
- The renal parenchymal damage results in the sequelae of progressive renal failure, such as anemia, acidosis, fluid and electrolyte abnormalities, and failure to thrive.
- UTIs and vesicoureteral reflux are common complications.
- Urinary incontinence may result from uninhibited bladder contractions, bladder noncompliance, and polyuria.

ADDITIONAL READING

- Chertin B, Cozzi D, Puri P. Long-term results of primary avulsion of posterior urethral valves using a Fogarty balloon catheter. *J Urol*. 2002;168(pt 2):1841–1843; discussion, 1843.
- Eckoldt F, Heling KS, Woderich R, et al. Posterior urethral valves: Prenatal diagnostic signs and outcome. *Urol Int*. 2004;73:296–301.
- Hodges SJ, Patel B, McLorie G, Atala A. Posterior urethral valves. *Sci World J*. 2009;9:1119–1126.
- Holmes N, Harrison MR, Baskin LS. Fetal surgery for posterior urethral valves: Long-term postnatal outcomes. *Pediatrics*. 2001;1:108.
- Krishnan A, De Souza A, Konijeti R, et al. The anatomy and embryology of posterior urethral valves. *J Urol*. 2006;175:1214–1220.
- Radhakrishnan J. Obstructive uropathy in the newborn. *Clin Perinatol*. 1990;17:215–239.

- Roth KS, Carter WH Jr, Chan JC. Obstructive nephropathy in children: Long-term progression after relief of posterior urethral valve. *Pediatrics*. 2001;107:1004–1010.
- Yiee J, Wilcox D. Management of fetal hydronephrosis. *Pediatr Nephrol*. 2008;23(3):347–353.

CODES

ICD9
- 753.6 Atresia and stenosis of urethra and bladder neck
- 753.8 Other specified anomalies of bladder and urethra

ICD10
- Q64.2 Congenital posterior urethral valves
- Q64.39 Other atresia and stenosis of urethra and bladder neck

FAQ

- Q: What can be done for children with long-term bladder dysfunction and incontinence?
- A: Voiding dysfunction may occur as the result of myogenic failure, detrusor hyperreflexia, and bladder hypertonia. Patients may require a combination of clean intermittent catheterization, pharmacologic therapy, and bladder augmentation. ~20% of patients with PUVs have secondary bladder pathology that is not reversible by primary therapy of the valve.
- Q: Are patients with PUVs good candidates for renal transplantation?
- A: Patients with valves have a 5-year graft survival rate of only 50%, compared with 75% for patients with other diagnoses. The main adverse factor is poor bladder function. Better results may follow more aggressive correction of the bladder anomalies. Transplantation has been successful in patients with bladder augmentation and in patients using clean intermittent catheterization.
- Q: Do patients with PUVs have impaired sexual and reproductive function?
- A: In a small study, patients had good sexual function and some were fertile. 95% had normal erections and were able to achieve penetration. 34% and 50% had normal and slow ejaculation, respectively. ~50% had normal semen.

PREMATURE ADRENARCHE

Andrew C. Calabria
Andrea Kelly
J. Nina Ham (5th edition)

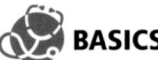 **BASICS**

DESCRIPTION
- Appearance of small amounts of pubic hair before age 8 years in girls and age 9 years in boys
- Recent data suggest that the onset of normal sexual development in girls is younger than previously recognized, but lowering of the traditionally accepted limits is subject to debate.
- With premature adrenarche, axillary hair, acne, and apocrine sweat gland secretion are not always present.
- No other signs of sexual development are exhibited. Presence of breast development suggests precocious puberty and not premature adrenarche.
- Occurs independently of hypothalamic–pituitary–gonadal axis.

Genetics
A familial pattern suggesting either recessive or dominant inheritance has been described.

PATHOPHYSIOLOGY
- Levels of dehydroepiandrosterone (DHEA) and dehydroepiandrosterone-sulfate (DHEAS) from the adrenal glands increase earlier than typically seen in normal puberty.
- Zona reticularis of the adrenals normally begins to increase androgen secretion at age 7–8 years.

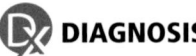 **DIAGNOSIS**

HISTORY
- Careful attention to presence of any other signs of sexual precocity as well as rate of progression
- Family history of pubertal development, infertility, irregular menses, hirsutism, polycystic ovarian syndrome, and premature male-pattern balding
- Birth weight that is small for gestational age (SGA) may predispose children to development of premature adrenarche.
- Obesity has been associated with an increased incidence of premature adrenarche.
- Girls with premature adrenarche are at increased risk for the development of polycystic ovarian syndrome.

PHYSICAL EXAM
- Linear growth velocity may be increased.
- The presence of pigmented, curly hairs in the pubic area is consistent with the androgen effect.
- In girls, clitoromegaly suggests congenital adrenal hyperplasia or androgen-secreting tumors.
- The finding of acanthosis nigricans suggests that insulin resistance and the risk of developing ovarian hyperandrogenism (polycystic ovarian syndrome) are present.

ALERT
Be careful to differentiate between true pubic hair (curly and short) and dark lanugo hair (straight, long, fine).

DIAGNOSTIC TESTS & INTERPRETATION
Lab
- Adrenal steroids: DHEA and DHEAS are often elevated for chronologic age but normal for pubertal stage (usually Tanner 2 or 3). However, testosterone and 17-OH progesterone (17-OHP) should be in prepubertal range.
- Gonadotropin-releasing hormone stimulation test: Not routinely recommended but would have a normal prepubertal response
- Children with systemic signs of virilization (such as a significantly advanced bone age) or elevated adrenal steroids (17-OHP or DHEA) should have adrenocorticotropic hormone (ACTH) stimulation testing to exclude congenital adrenal hyperplasia and other hyperandrogenic syndromes.

Imaging
- Bone age may be advanced by 1–2 years, but correlates with height age.
- Abdominal ultrasound, CT scan, or MRI should be considered if signs of significant virilization are present or if rapid progression has occurred; look for intracranial or intra-abdominal masses, especially if androgens are markedly elevated.

DIFFERENTIAL DIAGNOSIS
- Congenital: Nonclassic (late onset) congenital adrenal hyperplasia
- Tumors: Androgen-secreting tumors can arise in the gonads or adrenal glands.
- Miscellaneous:
  - Central precocious puberty
  - Familial male precocious puberty (testotoxicosis)
  - Exogenous male hormone exposure

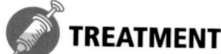

TREATMENT

ADDITIONAL TREATMENT
General Measures
- No treatment
- Reassure parents and children that this is a benign process.
- Reassess every 6 months to look for signs of virilization and pubertal progression.

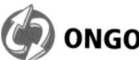

ONGOING CARE

- Regression does not occur.
- Watch for other signs of puberty, such as breast development, testicular enlargement (≥ 4 mL) or growth acceleration, that suggest onset of true precocious puberty.
- Increasing virilization suggests nonclassic congenital adrenal hyperplasia or early polycystic ovarian syndrome.
- Acanthosis nigricans or signs of insulin resistance have been reported in girls with a history of premature adrenarche.
- Monitor for glucose intolerance or early type 2 diabetes. Can check fasting glucose and insulin levels or oral glucose tolerance test if suspicion is high (e.g., obesity, acanthosis nigricans, polyuria, polydipsia).

PROGNOSIS
- Undergo puberty appropriately with normal fertility.
- Development of ovarian or adrenal hyperandrogenism during adolescence (also known as "polycystic ovarian syndrome") is more common in some girls with premature adrenarche. Insulin resistance, a common finding in ovarian hyperandrogenism, has been reported in some children and adolescents with a history of premature adrenarche.
- Final adult height is normal.

COMPLICATIONS
- Can be the first sign of true precocious puberty (i.e., development of breast tissue and advancement of bone age) and thus warrants careful observation.
- Boys with premature adrenarche and precocious puberty are more likely than girls to have an underlying CNS disorder.

ADDITIONAL READING

- Auchus RJ, Fainey WE. Adrenarche–physiology, biochemistry and human disease. *Clin Endocrinol*. 2004;60:288–296.
- Herman-Giddens ME, Slora EJ, Wasserman RC, et al. Secondary sexual characteristics and menses in young girls seen in office practice: A study from the pediatric research office in settings network. *Pediatrics*. 1997;99:505–512.
- Ibanez L, Jimenes R, de Zegher F. Early puberty-menarche after precocious pubarche: Relation to prenatal growth. *Pediatrics*. 2006;117: 117–121.
- Kaplowitz P. Clinical characteristics of 104 children referred for evaluation of precocious puberty. *J Clin Endocrinol Metab*. 2004;89:3644–3650.
- Kaplowitz P, Oberfield SE. Drug and Therapeutics and Executive Committees of the Lawson Wilkins Pediatric Endocrine Society. Reexamination of age limit for defining when puberty is precocious in girls in the United States: Implication for evaluation and treatment. *Pediatrics*. 1999;104:936–941.
- Kousta, K. Premature adrenarche leads to polycystic ovarian syndrome? Long-term consequences. *Ann NY Acad Sci*. 2006;1092:148–157.
- Midyett LK, Moore WV, Jacobson JD. Are pubertal changes in girls before age 8 benign? *Pediatrics*. 2003;111:47–51.
- Nebesio TD, Eugster EA. Pubic hair of infancy: Endocrinopathy or enigma? *Pediatrics*. 2006; 117:951–954.
- Neville KA, Walker JL. Precocious pubarche is associated with SGA, prematurity, weight gain, and obesity. *Arch Dis Child*. 2005;90:258–261.

 # CODES

ICD9
259.1 Precocious sexual development and puberty, not elsewhere classified

ICD10
E27.0 Other adrenocortical overactivity

FAQ

- Q: Is there a dietary cause of excess adrenal hormones?
- A: No.
- Q: Does premature adrenarche mean puberty will be early?
- A: The onset of puberty in these children is within the normal range and should follow the familial pattern.
- Q: Can anything be done to reverse the changes?
- A: This is a benign process that does not have long-term sequelae. Antiandrogen drugs are available but are not recommended.

PREMATURE THELARCHE

Andrew C. Calabria
Andrea Kelly
Olga T. Hardy (5th edition)

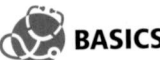 **BASICS**

DESCRIPTION
- Breast development <8 years of age in girls with no other signs of pubertal development
- A recent study suggested that African American girls are developing pubertal characteristics as early as age 6 and Caucasian girls as early as age 7. However, physicians should be cautious about using these as normal limits and should evaluate children on an individual basis because signs of puberty at these younger ages may not be normal.

EPIDEMIOLOGY
60–85% of cases noted between 6 months and 2 years of age

PATHOPHYSIOLOGY
- Transient increases in follicle-stimulating hormone levels causing follicular ovarian development
- Low levels of estrogen secretion by normal follicular cysts
- Increased sensitivity of breast tissue to low levels of estrogen

ETIOLOGY
Intermittent estrogen secretion by ovarian cysts or environmental sources of estrogen

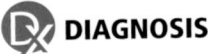 **DIAGNOSIS**

HISTORY
- Careful assessment of onset and progression of breast tissue
- Family history of early puberty
- Exposure to estrogens
- Be sure to ask about ingestion of foods with high estrogen levels.

PHYSICAL EXAM
- Areolar enlargement is usually not present.
- Galactorrhea is not present.
- Palpate carefully to distinguish fat from true breast tissue.
- Look carefully for other signs of puberty:
  – Menstrual blood
  – Dull, gray-pink, or rugose vaginal mucosa (vs. prepubertal appearance: Shiny, bright red, and smooth)
  – Pubic or axillary hair
- Inspect skin for birthmarks suggestive of McCune–Albright syndrome (café au lait spots in a coast of Maine pattern).
- Evaluate for signs of hypothyroidism: Goiter, short stature

DIAGNOSTIC TESTS & INTERPRETATION
Lab
- No test is specific.
- Serum follicle-stimulating hormone, inhibin B, and estradiol may be slightly higher than age-matched controls, but are not consistently elevated.
- In isolated premature thelarche, serum ultrasensitive luteinizing hormone is prepubertal.

Imaging
- Bone age is not significantly or is very mildly advanced (<1 year ahead of chronologic age). Useful in guiding the need for more intensive evaluation of true precocious puberty
- Pelvic ultrasonography may demonstrate presence and regression of small ovarian cysts (1–15 mm) and a prepubertal uterus.

DIFFERENTIAL DIAGNOSIS
- Environmental:
  – Exposure to exogenous estrogens in the form of creams or birth control pills
  – Intake of food with high estrogen levels (e.g., chicken liver)
- Tumors: Benign lipomas
- Congenital: Neonatal breast hyperplasia is benign breast enlargement in newborn boys or girls that is apparent shortly after birth and is caused by gestational hormones. This form of breast development usually regresses.
- Other:
  – Severe acquired hypothyroidism: High levels of thyroid-stimulating hormone may cross-stimulate gonadal follicle–stimulating hormone and/or luteinizing hormone receptors.
  – McCune–Albright syndrome: Triad of precocious puberty, café au lait spots, and polyostotic fibrous dysplasia due to gain of function mutations of G proteins
  – Thelarche variant or "exaggerated thelarche": lies on a spectrum between isolated premature thelarche and precocious puberty; occurs in up to 30% of premature thelarche cases, associated with moderate growth and bone age acceleration and increased uterine size, owing to unsustained estrogen secretion.
  – True precocious puberty

ALERT
- Must distinguish fat from breast tissue in obese girls
- Removal of a breast bud will result in failure of that breast to develop during adolescence

TREATMENT

ADDITIONAL TREATMENT
General Measures
- Observation
- Reassurance that this is a benign process

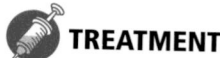 ONGOING CARE

- Regression often occurs by 2 years but may occur up to 6 years after onset.
- Evidence of pubertal progression should prompt additional evaluation by an endocrinologist:
  – Rapid increase in size of breast tissue
  – Vaginal bleeding
  – Growth spurt
  – Development of pubic and axillary hair

PROGNOSIS
- No known effects on growth or fertility
- Onset after age 2 years may be associated with increased risk of progression to precocious puberty.

COMPLICATIONS
May be the first sign of true precocious puberty

PATIENT EDUCATION

- No data to suggest that premature thelarche increases the risk of breast cancer
- Many newborn male and female infants have breast buds as a result of exposure to maternal estrogen in utero. This neonatal gynecomastia usually resolves quickly.

- Asymmetric breast development is quite common in the early stages of normal pubertal development. Malignant tumors of the breast during childhood are extremely rare. As mentioned earlier, any removal of breast tissue prior to or during puberty must be avoided if possible.

ADDITIONAL READING

- Crofton PM, Evans NEM, Wardhaugh B, et al. Evidence for increased ovarian follicular activity in girls with premature thelarche. *Clin Endocrinol*. 2005;62:205–209.
- Haber HP, Willmann HA, Ranke MB. Pelvic ultrasonography: Early differentiation between isolated premature thelarche and central precocious puberty. *Eur J Pediatr*. 1997;154:182–186.
- Herman-Giddens ME, Slora EJ, Wasserman RC, et al. Secondary sexual characteristics and menses in young girls seen in office practice: A study from the Pediatric Research Office in Settings Network. *Pediatrics*. 1997;99:505–512.
- Kaplowitz P, Oberfield SE, Drug and Therapeutics and Executive Committees of the Lawson Wilkins Pediatric Endocrine Society. Reexamination of age limit for defining when puberty is precocious in girls in the United States: Implication for evaluation and treatment. *Pediatrics*. 1999;104:936–941.
- Klein K, Mericq V, Brown-Dawson JM, et al. Estrogen levels in girls with premature thelarche compared with normal prepubertal girls as determined by an ultrasensitive recombinant cell bioassay. *J Pediatr*. 1999;134:190–192.

- Lebrethon MC, Bourguignon JP. Management of central isosexual precocity: Diagnosis, treatment, outcome. *Curr Opin Pediatr*. 2000;12:394–399.
- Midyett LK, Moore WV, Jacobson JD. Are pubertal changes in girls before age 8 benign? *Pediatrics*. 2003;111:47–51.
- Pasquino AM, Pucarelli I, Passeri F, et al. Progression of premature thelarche to central precocious puberty. *J Pediatr*. 1995;126:11–14. [Comment in *J Pediatr*. 1995;127:336–337.]
- Salardi S, Cacciari E, Mainetti B, et al. Outcome of premature thelarche: Relation to puberty and final height. *Arch Dis Child*. 1998;79:173–174.
- Stanhope R. Premature thelarche: Clinical follow-up and indication for treatment. *J Pediatr Endocrinol Metab*. 2000;13(suppl 1):827–830.
- Styne DM. New aspects in the diagnosis and treatment of pubertal disorders. *Pediatr Clin North Am*. 1997;44:505–529.
- Traggiai C, Stanhope R. Disorders of pubertal development. *Best Pract Res Clin Obstet Gynaecol*. 2003;17:41–56.

 CODES

ICD9
259.1 Precocious sexual development and puberty, not elsewhere classified

ICD10
E30.8 Other disorders of puberty

FAQ

- Q: Does premature thelarche predispose the child to abnormalities in pubertal development?
- A: If onset occurs after age 2 years, the girl may be more likely to enter puberty earlier. However, most girls with premature thelarche will have normal pubertal development and fertility.

PREMENSTRUAL SYNDROME (PMS)

Ann B. Bruner

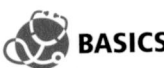 **BASICS**

DESCRIPTION

- Premenstrual syndrome (PMS), also called luteal phase disorder, is a disorder characterized by psychologic and physical symptoms that occur cyclically and consistently during the second half (luteal phase) of the menstrual cycle, negatively impact a woman's usual activities of daily living, and remit after the onset of menstruation.
- PMS is diagnosed through prospective symptom charting with symptoms present beginning at approximately day 13 of the cycle and resolving within 4 days of menses for 2 consecutive cycles.
  - At least 1 of the following symptoms must occur within 5 days of menses onset: Breast tenderness, bloating/weight gain, headache, swelling of hands/feet, aches/pains, mood symptoms (depression, anger, irritability, anxiety, social withdrawal), poor concentration, sleep disturbance, or change in appetite.
- Premenstrual dysphoric disorder (PMDD) is the extreme variant of PMS; defined in *DSM-IV-TR* as severe psychologic symptoms causing significant dysfunctions, which are not an exacerbation of symptoms of a chronic condition and are confirmed through prospective daily ratings of 3 consecutive cycles.
- Criteria for PMDD: At least 5 symptoms among the following must be present during most of the luteal phase, with at least 1 of the symptoms being among the first 4:
  - Depressed mood: Feeling sad, hopeless, or self-deprecating
  - Anxiety or tension: Feeling tense, anxious, or "on edge"
  - Affective lability: Fluctuating emotions interspersed with frequent tearfulness
  - Irritability or anger: Increased interpersonal conflicts
  - Decreased interest in usual activities, which may be associated with withdrawal from social relationships
  - Difficulty concentrating
  - Feeling fatigued, lethargic, or lacking in energy
  - Marked changes in appetite, which may be associated with binge eating or craving certain foods
  - Hypersomnia or insomnia
  - A subjective feeling of being overwhelmed or out of control
  - Physical symptoms such as breast tenderness/swelling, headaches, bloating or weight gain, arthralgias, or myalgias

EPIDEMIOLOGY

Prevalence

- 40–75% of women experience some PMS symptoms at some time.
- 15–30% of women report recurrent symptoms suggestive of PMS.
- 2–5% of women have symptoms that interfere with their usual activities (PMDD).
- 14–88% of adolescent girls have moderate to severe PMS; one study demonstrated a 5.8% prevalence of PMDD in young women ages 14–24.

RISK FACTORS

Genetics

Genetic factors may play a role in the development of PMS/PMDD: Twin studies show a 93% concordance rate in monozygotic twins, with only a 44% rate in dizygotic twins.

Age

More severe symptoms of PMDD may be seen in younger women.

Culture

PMS/PMDD appear to be more prevalent in Western cultures, possibly due to differences in socialization and symptom expectations.

Stress

PMS and PMDD may be associated with high levels of day-to-day stress and/or a history of stressful events, including sexual abuse.

PATHOPHYSIOLOGY

- Occurrence of symptoms is related to ovarian function/ovulation:
  - PMS does not occur before menarche, during pregnancy, or after menopause.
  - PMS can occur after hysterectomy, but not after bilateral oophorectomy.
- Research suggests altered cyclic interactions between sex hormones and neurotransmitters (in particular, relationships between sex hormones, prostaglandins, and serotonin): γ-aminobutyric acid (GABA) and opioid neurotransmitter systems have also been studied, along with trace elements, vitamins, and minerals.
- Women with PMS do not have abnormal serum concentrations of estrogen or progesterone or hormonal imbalance; research suggests that women with PMS have abnormal responses to normal variations in sex hormones.

ETIOLOGY

Etiology unknown, but presumed to be multifactorial

℞ DIAGNOSIS

SIGNS AND SYMPTOMS

Many women report that their PMS symptoms are not taken seriously.

HISTORY

- Complete medical history, including use of medications or illicit substances, cigarettes, dietary evaluation
- Gynecologic history: Age at onset of pubertal development, menstrual pattern, sexual activity, contraceptive use, dysmenorrhea
- Psychiatric history: Mental health disorders, medications
- Family history: Mental health and substance use/abuse
- Psychosocial history: Living situation, school/vocational activities and goals, hobbies, peers

- Complete review of systems including both physical symptoms (fatigue, breast tenderness/swelling, bloating, edema, weight gain, headache, arthralgias, myalgias, pelvic discomfort, changes in bowel habit, reduced coordination) and emotional/psychologic symptoms (depression, mood lability, irritability, tension, anxiety, tearfulness, restlessness, reduced concentration, fatigue, altered libido, altered appetite/eating habits, altered sleep)
- Chronologic review to determine if symptoms are recurrent with most menstrual cycles, isolated to luteal phase of cycle, and remit with onset of menses

PHYSICAL EXAM

There are no specific physical findings of PMS.

- Enlarged thyroid gland: May suggest hypothyroidism and need to evaluate for thyroid disease
- Virilization (hirsutism, clitoromegaly): May suggest hyperandrogenism and need to evaluate for adrenal disease, including Cushing syndrome, or other hormonal disorders such as polycystic ovarian syndrome
- Pallor: May suggest anemia
- Orthostatic hypotension: May suggest neurally mediated hypotension

DIAGNOSTIC TESTS & INTERPRETATION

PAF (Premenstrual Assessment Form), PRISM (Prospective Record of Severity of Menstruation), or COPE (Calendar of Premenstrual Experiences): Prospective symptom calendars can help establish diagnosis and provide information about symptom patterns (recurrence and relation to menses). Differences in symptom severity between the follicular and luteal phases (before and after ovulation) may be most diagnostic.

Lab

- CBC: Rule out anemia.
- Thyroid-stimulating hormone (TSH) assay: Rule out thyroid disease.

DIFFERENTIAL DIAGNOSIS

- Psychiatric:
  - Mood disorder, including major depression, dysthymia, bipolar disorder, postpartum depression, anxiety disorder
  - Substance abuse
  - Physical, sexual, or emotional abuse
  - Somatization disorder
  - Eating disorder
- Endocrinologic:
  - Thyroid disease
  - Cushing disease
  - Diabetes mellitus

- Gynecologic:
  – Dysmenorrhea (primary or secondary)
  – Pregnancy
  – Endometriosis
  – Hormonal contraceptive use
  – Perimenopause
- Immunologic/hematologic:
  – Anemia
  – Fibromyalgia
  – Systemic lupus erythematosus (SLE)
  – Chronic fatigue syndrome
- Neurologic:
  – Migraine headache
  – Neurally mediated hypotension

 # TREATMENT

ADDITIONAL TREATMENT
General Measures
- Treatment goals include reducing both symptom frequency and severity and the impact of symptoms on patients' activities.
- Patient education, counseling, and reassurance may be all that is needed for women with milder symptoms.
- Many pharmacologic and nonpharmacologic modalities have not been formally evaluated.

Diet
- Research supports reducing caffeine and alcohol intake and suggests that reductions in salt and refined sugars may also be beneficial.
- Meta-analyses of research to date have shown that some supplements are beneficial in reducing symptom frequency and severity, including calcium carbonate (1,200 mg/d), pyridoxine/vitamin B$_6$ (50 mg/d), and possibly magnesium (400 mg/d).
- Many herbal therapies are in use, including evening primrose oil, chaste berry, black cohosh, ginkgo, and St. John's wort. However, there is no strong evidence to support their use in PMS.

Activity
- Increasing physical activity, ensuring adequate and regular sleep, and maintaining a healthy diet are important first steps.
- Mind/body therapies are frequently used including individual psychotherapy, relaxation techniques, guided imagery, yoga, massage, biofeedback, and group therapy; to date, there is no strong evidence to support their use in PMS.

MEDICATION (DRUGS)
First Line
Many menstrually associated symptoms can be managed with nonsteroidal anti-inflammatory drugs (NSAIDs):
- NSAIDs (e.g., naproxen sodium 275–550 mg b.i.d.) relieve the majority of physical symptoms–premenstrual/menstrual cramping, headaches, and myalgias/arthralgias.
- Side effects include gastrointestinal upset and renal dysfunction.

Second Line
SSRIs are first line for PMDD and severe PMS, especially those with predominantly psychologic symptoms. SSRIs have been shown to improve mood, decrease irritability, ameliorate physical symptoms such as bloating and breast tenderness, and improve psychosocial function. Continuous and intermittent (during luteal phase) dosing can be used, and symptom amelioration can occur during the first cycle of treatment. Intermittent use includes administration during the last 14 days of the menstrual cycle or treatment begun at expected date of symptom onset:

- Fluoxetine (20–60 mg/d), sertraline (50–150 mg/d), paroxetine (10–30 mg/d), and citalopram (5–20 mg/d) are some of the most commonly used SSRIs for PMS/PMDD; side effects include gastrointestinal upset, insomnia, tremor/agitation, fatigue, dry mouth, and sexual dysfunction. SSRIs recently received a US FDA black box warning concerning an increased risk of suicidality among depressed children and adolescents; the warning was for the treatment of depression, not PMS/PMDD.
- Hormonal contraceptives (i.e., low-dose oral contraceptive pills, contraceptive patch) suppress ovulation, which may ameliorate hormonally mediated symptoms such as breast swelling/tenderness and bloating, but may exacerbate mood symptoms.
- Spironolactone (50 mg b.i.d.) is effective for breast tenderness and bloating; potassium levels must be monitored, and spironolactone is contraindicated in patients with abnormal renal function.

 # ONGOING CARE

- Frequent follow-up and the use of a prospective menstrual/symptom calendar are important.
- After the diagnosis of PMS is established, and after recommending appropriate lifestyle changes (and possibly NSAIDs), the patient should be re-evaluated after 3 months. If there has not been substantial improvement, secondary pharmacologic therapies (SSRIs) may need to be considered. When SSRIs are prescribed as first-line therapy for patients with more severe PMS or PMDD, response to SSRIs and any adverse reactions should be assessed at follow-up and dosage adjusted as needed.

ISSUES FOR REFERRAL
A gynecologist/reproductive endocrinologist can assist in the management of severe PMS/PMDD: Other pharmacologic agents that are used include gonadotropin-releasing hormone (GnRH) analogues, danazol, estrogen implants, and androgens.

COMPLICATIONS
Psychologic morbidity includes difficulty with interpersonal relationships (family and friends) and school absence/failure.

ADDITIONAL READING

- Claman F, Miller T. Premenstrual syndrome and premenstrual dysphoric disorder in adolescence. *J Pediatr Health Care*. 2006;29:1–12.
- Cronje WH, Studd JWW. Premenstrual syndrome and premenstrual dysphoric disorder. *Prim Care*. 2002;29:1–12.
- Dickerson LM, Mazyck PJ, Hunter MH. Premenstrual syndrome. *Am Fam Phys*. 2003;67:1743–1752.
- Girman A, Lee R, Kligler B. An integrative approach to premenstrual syndrome. *Clin J Women Health*. 2002;2:116–127.
- Halbreich U, Bornstein J, Pearlstein T, et al. The prevalence, impairment, impact, and burden of premenstrual dysphoric disorder (PMS/PMDD). *Psychoneuroendocrinology*. 2003;28(suppl 3):1–23.
- Halbreich U. The etiology, biology, and evolving pathology of premenstrual syndromes. *Psychoneuroendocrinology*. 2003;28(suppl 3): 55–99.
- Steiner M, Pearlstein T, Cohen L, et al. Expert guidelines for the treatment of severe PMS, PMDD, and comorbidities: The role of SSRIs. *J Womens Health (Larchmt)*. 2006;1:57–69.
- Vigod SN, Ross LE, Steiner M. Understanding and treating premenstrual dysphoric disorder: An update for the women's health practitioner. *Obstet Gynecol Clin N Am*. 2009;36:907–924.

CODES

ICD9
625.4 Premenstrual tension syndromes

ICD10
N94.3 Premenstrual tension syndrome

FAQ

- Q: Can adolescent girls have PMS and PMDD?
- A: The incidence of PMS and PMDD in adolescents is not well established. Although ≤50% of cycles are anovulatory during the first 1–2 years after menarche, younger patients experience many PMS symptoms, and menstrual problems are some of the most common reasons for school absence. Most experts believe that PMS/PMDD will not develop until a regular ovulatory pattern is established, ~2–3 years after menarche.
- Q: Is family history important?
- A: Genetic factors may play a role in the development of PMS/PMDD; twin studies show a 93% concordance rate in monozygotic twins, with only a 44% rate in dizygotic twins.
- Q: Are there any common comorbidities?
- A: The symptoms of PMS/PMDD are also seen with depression, anxiety, and other mood disorders. Psychiatric symptomatology can fluctuate, and symptoms may change in relation to the menstrual cycle. Careful and thorough history taking and prospective symptom diaries can help differentiate PMS/PMDD from another mental health disorder.

PRIMARY ADRENAL INSUFFICIENCY

J. Nina Ham
Lorraine E. Levitt Katz

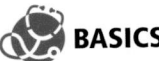 **BASICS**

DESCRIPTION
Deficiency in the secretion of cortisol by the adrenal glands

EPIDEMIOLOGY
- Age:
  - Addison disease is uncommon in children and usually presents between the ages of 20 and 50 years. In the pediatric population, it is most often seen in late childhood and adolescence.
  - Adrenoleukodystrophy typically presents late in the 1st decade of life with neurologic symptoms. Signs and symptoms of adrenal insufficiency may present at any age.
  - Adrenocorticotropic hormone (ACTH) unresponsiveness presents in late infancy or the toddler period.
  - Adrenal hypoplasia congenita presents in infancy or early childhood.
  - Adrenal insufficiency associated with congenital adrenal hyperplasia (CAH) presents in the newborn period.
- Sex:
  - Addison disease is more common in girls.
  - Adrenoleukodystrophy, an X-linked disorder, predominantly affects boys.
  - ACTH unresponsiveness and CAH affect both sexes equally.
  - Adrenal hypoplasia congenita, an X-linked disorder, predominantly affects boys.

RISK FACTORS
Genetics
- Addison disease:
  - Autoimmune adrenal insufficiency may be isolated or part of autoimmune polyglandular syndrome (APS) type 1 or 2. Mutations in the *AIRE1* gene have been identified as the cause of APS type 1. An association exists between idiopathic Addison disease and human leukocyte antigen (HLA)-B8 and DR3.
- Adrenoleukodystrophy:
  - X-linked recessive disorder of very-long-chain fatty acid metabolism due to ABCD1 gene mutation
  - An autosomal recessive form of the disease exists, with presentation during infancy.
- ACTH unresponsiveness: Autosomal recessive ACTH receptor defect
- Adrenal hypoplasia congenita: X-linked mutation in *DAX1* gene
- CAH: Autosomal recessive inheritance associated with a gene defect in 1 of multiple adrenal steroidogenic enzymes

PATHOPHYSIOLOGY
- Addison disease:
  - Primary hypoadrenalism due to bilateral destruction of the adrenal cortices; this can be due to autoimmune destruction (isolated or associated with APS), tuberculosis, hemorrhage, fungal infection, neoplastic infiltration, or AIDS.
- Adrenoleukodystrophy:
  - Inherited disorders of impaired peroxisomal degradation of very-long-chain fatty acids, resulting in adrenal insufficiency and progressive neurologic deterioration
- ACTH unresponsiveness:
  - Inherited defect in the ACTH receptor, resulting in isolated glucocorticoid deficiency with hypoglycemia in infancy and hyperpigmentation
- Adrenal hypoplasia congenita: A defect in adrenal organogenesis
- CAH: A group of enzymatic disorders of steroid metabolism, of which 21-hydroxylase deficiency is the most common
- Waterhouse-Friderichsen syndrome: Bilateral adrenal gland hemorrhage classically associated with fulminant meningococcemia, but also reported with *Staphylococcus aureus* and *Streptococcus pneumoniae*

COMMONLY ASSOCIATED CONDITIONS
- Deficiencies of other hormones, including aldosterone and adrenal sex steroids
- Adrenal hypoplasia congenita (*DAX1* mutation) is associated with hypogonadotropic hypogonadism.
- APSs are associated with other autoimmune disorders:
  - APS type 1: Mucocutaneous candidiasis, hypoparathyroidism
  - APS type 2: Autoimmune thyroid disease, type 1 diabetes
- Both types can also present in conjunction with multiple other autoimmune disorders (e.g., pernicious anemia, vitiligo, autoimmune hepatitis)

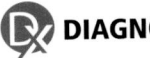 **DIAGNOSIS**

HISTORY
The symptoms of primary adrenal insufficiency are nonspecific and similar to those found in many disease processes. The electrolyte picture of adrenal insufficiency can be seen in renal disorders, obstructive uropathy, and isolated aldosterone deficiency:
- Weakness and fatigue
- Anorexia, weight loss
- Headache
- Nausea, vomiting, diarrhea, abdominal pain
- Orthostatic symptoms
- Muscle or joint pains
- Emotional lability
- Salt craving
- Hyperpigmentation
- Decreased axillary or pubic hair in females due to lack of adrenal androgens
- Amenorrhea in females

PHYSICAL EXAM
- Hyperpigmentation, especially on lip borders, buccal mucosa, nipples, and over skin creases
- Weight loss
- Hypotension
- Evaluate for other signs of autoimmune disease (e.g., thyromegaly, vitiligo).
- Pubertal staging
- Signs of virilization in females

DIAGNOSTIC TESTS & INTERPRETATION
Diagnostic Procedures/Other
- Specific:
  - Cosyntropin (Cortrosyn) stimulation test: Administer cosyntropin (synthetic ACTH) 250 mcg IV and measure cortisol at 30 and 60 minutes. A normal response is a final cortisol >18 mcg/dL. An insufficient cortisol response is diagnostic of adrenal insufficiency:
    - A baseline ACTH >200 pg/mL with inadequate cortisol is seen in primary adrenal insufficiency.
    - Serum adrenal antibodies may be positive in autoimmune Addison disease.
    - Very-long-chain fatty acids are elevated in adrenoleukodystrophy.
    - Low gonadotropin and sex steroid levels suggesting hypogonadotropic hypogonadism may be seen with adrenal hypoplasia congenita.
    - Adrenal steroid precursors will be elevated in CAH.

- Nonspecific:
  - Electrolytes:
    - Hyponatremia: Result of the mineralocorticoid defect and glucocorticoid deficiency; combination sodium loss from kidneys, and the inability to excrete a water load
    - Hyperkalemia and acidosis: Chronic mineralocorticoid deficiency with the inability to excrete potassium and acid
    - Hypercalcemia: Most likely a result of increased calcium absorption due to the lack of glucocorticoid effect on the gut
    - Hypoglycemia: Glucocorticoids have permissive effects on gluconeogenesis.
    - Renin levels are elevated when a mineralocorticoid deficiency is present.

DIFFERENTIAL DIAGNOSIS
- Autoimmune adrenal cortical destruction
- Infectious adrenal cortical destruction:
  - Tuberculous
  - Fungal
  - HIV
- Adrenal hemorrhage
- Neoplastic adrenal infiltration
- Adrenoleukodystrophy
- ACTH unresponsiveness
- Adrenal hypoplasia congenita
- CAH
- Withdrawal of chronic exogenous steroids

 TREATMENT

MEDICATION (DRUGS)
- Acute adrenal crisis:
  - Hydrocortisone (HC): Stress dosage of hydrocortisone: 100 mg/m^2 followed by 100 mg/m^2/24 hours of hydrocortisone divided q4-6h. Taper steroids rapidly to a physiologic replacement dosage when acute illness has resolved.
  - Mineralocorticoid replacement: Florinef 0.1 mg daily when able to take PO
- Chronic adrenal insufficiency:
  - Hydrocortisone 10–12 mg/m^2/d PO divided as t.i.d. Triple the dose for stress of fever, illness, or vomiting. For major stress (surgery, significant illness), give hydrocortisone 50–100 mg/m^2 IV/IM followed by 50–100 mg/m^2/24 hours IV divided q4–6h. IM hydrocortisone is recommended for emergency home use.
  - Florinef 0.1 mg PO daily

ADDITIONAL TREATMENT
General Measures
Chronic adrenal insufficiency:
- Daily maintenance HC replacement
- Increased HC dose for stress of fever, illness, vomiting
- Fludrocortisone acetate (Florinef): Mineralocorticoid agent
- Patient education on stress dosing in the event of illness

IN-PATIENT CONSIDERATIONS
Initial Stabilization
- Acute adrenal crisis:
  - An intercurrent illness or surgical procedure may provoke an episode of hypotension, tachycardia, and shock. Electrolytes reveal decreased serum sodium, elevated potassium, metabolic acidosis, and a decreased or normal glucose. Serum should be drawn and saved to aid in diagnosis, but emergent treatment should not be delayed for a diagnostic ACTH stimulation test.
- Treatment:
  - 5% dextrose in normal saline solution (D5NS) for volume repletion and treatment of salt wasting and hypoglycemia
  - HC or other glucocorticoid
  - Mineralocorticoid replacement

IV Fluids
D5NS for volume repletion and treatment of salt wasting

 ONGOING CARE

FOLLOW-UP RECOMMENDATIONS
An acute adrenal crisis usually improves rapidly with the administration of fluids and glucocorticoids. Once the acute phase of illness has resolved, steroids can be resumed at physiologic replacement doses.

Patient Monitoring
- Clinical status
- Reduction in hyperpigmentation
- Electrolytes, ACTH, and renin levels
- Screen for polyautoimmune disorders.
- Growth
- Very-long-chain fatty acid levels and neurologic function in adrenoleukodystrophy
- Pubertal development

PATIENT EDUCATION
- Stress dosing
- Importance of seeking medical attention for significant illness, persistent vomiting, or the inability to take fluids by mouth
- MedicAlert bracelet

PROGNOSIS
- Long-term prognosis of isolated adrenal insufficiency is good, provided adequate hydrocortisone is administered, particularly in times of illness.
- Adrenoleukodystrophy carries a poor prognosis.

COMPLICATIONS
- If not diagnosed and/or treated properly, a significant physical stress such as surgery or illness may result in a life-threatening adrenal crisis.
- Adrenoleukodystrophy results in severe neurologic impairment and death.
- Unrecognized ACTH unresponsiveness is associated with recurrent hypoglycemia, seizures, mental retardation, and death.
- Pubertal delay or hypogonadotropic hypogonadism is seen with adrenal hypoplasia congenita due to DAX1 mutations.
- CAH can cause virilization/ambiguous genitalia in female infants with the disease and can cause salt-wasting crises in infants of both sexes.

ADDITIONAL READING

- Achermann JC, Meeks JJ, Jameson JL. Phenotypic spectrum of mutations in DAX-1 and SF-1. Mol Cell Endocrinol. 2001;62(2):202–206.
- Adem PV, Montgomery CD, Husain AN, et al. Staphylococcus aureus sepsis and the Waterhouse-Friderichsen syndrome in children. N Engl J Med. 2005;353:1245–1251.
- Dorin RI, Qualls CR, Crapo LM. Diagnosis of adrenal insufficiency. Ann Intern Med. 2003;139:194–204.
- Husebye ES, Perheentupa J, Rautemaa R, et al. Clinical manifestations and management of patients with autoimmune polyendocrine syndrome type 1. J Intern Med. 2009;265:514–529.
- Perheentupa J. APS-I/APECED: The clinical disease and therapy. Endocrinol Metab Clin North Am. 2002;31(2):295–320.
- Selva KA, LaFranchi SH, Boston B. A novel presentation of familial glucocorticoid deficiency (FGD) and current literature review. J Pediatr Endocrinol Metab. 2004;17(1):85–92.
- Shulman DI, Palmert MR, Kepm SF. Adrenal insufficiency: Still a cause of morbidity and death in childhood. Pediatrics. 2007;119:e484–e494.
- Speiser PW, White PC. Congenital adrenal hyperplasia. N Engl J Med. 2003;349:776–788.
- Vaidya B, Pearce S, Kendall-Taylor P. Recent advances in the molecular genetics of congenital and acquired primary adrenocortical failure. Clin Endocrinol. 2000;53:403–418.

 CODES

ICD9
- 255.41 Glucocorticoid deficiency
- 277.86 Peroxisomal disorders
- 759.1 Anomalies of adrenal gland

ICD10
- E27.1 Primary adrenocortical insufficiency
- E71.529 X-linked adrenoleukodystrophy, unspecified type
- Q89.1 Congenital malformations of adrenal gland

FAQ
- Q: What are the indications for stress dosing and how rapidly can the stress hydrocortisone dose be tapered?
- A: Patients will require stress dosing of hydrocortisone for surgical procedures, fever (>37.7°C [100°F]), vomiting, diarrhea, and particularly vigorous exercise. The stress dose is typically given for 24 hours, after which the usual dose is resumed. Should it be necessary to administer the stress dosage for a more prolonged period, the dosage can usually be tapered rapidly to physiologic dosage, once the patient's clinical condition has improved.

PRION DISEASES (TRANSMISSIBLE SPONGIFORM ENCEPHALOPATHIES)

Jason Y. Kim

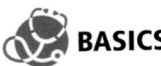 **BASICS**

DESCRIPTION

- Transmissible spongiform encephalopathies (TSEs) or prion diseases are a family of progressive neurodegenerative diseases of humans and animals that cause irreversible cumulative brain damage and are uniformly fatal.
- Prions are the infectious agents that cause TSE. The term *prion* was coined to denote "a small proteinaceous infectious particle resistant to inactivation by most procedures that modify nucleic acids."
- Prion proteins (PRP) are normal cellular glycoproteins (PRP^C) encoded by the *PRNP* gene, and are found on neurons and white blood cells.
- The infectious particles that cause TSEs are protease-resistant conformers of PRP^C (PRP^{RES} or PRP^{SC} for protease-resistant or scrapie-causing PRPs, respectively).
- Human TSEs include Creutzfeldt–Jakob disease (CJD), the more recently identified variant CJD (vCJD), kuru, Gerstmann–Sträussler–Scheinker syndrome, and fatal familial insomnia syndrome.
- Six TSEs in animals have been described: Bovine spongiform encephalopathy (BSE), also known as mad cow disease), scrapie in sheep and goats, feline spongiform encephalopathy, transmissible mink encephalopathy, exotic ungulate encephalopathy, and chronic wasting disease of cervids.

EPIDEMIOLOGY

- CJD:
  - CJD is the most prevalent form of TSE in humans and occurs as either a sporadic or a familial disease.
  - ~85% of cases are sporadic because there is no family history and no known source of transmission. Sporadic CJD occurs throughout the world at a rate 1/1,000,000 people.
  - Familial CJD (fCJD) cases are associated with a gene mutation in PRNP and account for ~10–15% of cases. fCJD shows an autosomal dominant inheritance, with >50 mutations in PRNP identified.
  - ~1% of CJD cases are iatrogenic, resulting from accidental transmission of the causative agent via contaminated surgical equipment, as a result of cornea or dura mater transplants, or administration of human-derived pituitary growth hormones.
  - No evidence confirms person-to-person transmission among family members via direct contact, droplet, or airborne spread.
  - Disease is characterized by progressive dementia, myoclonus, visual or cerebellar disturbance, pyramidal/extrapyramidal dysfunction, and/or akinetic mutism
  - Classic sporadic CJD most often occurs between the ages of 50–70 and affects both sexes equally; whites have about a 2-fold higher rate than blacks.
  - Death usually occurs within 1 year of onset of symptoms.

- Variant CJD (vCJD):
  - New form of CJD, 1st reported in 1994; has unique clinical features
  - In contrast to CJD, affects younger patients including adolescents (average age, 29 years) and has a longer duration of illness with median of 14 months as opposed to 4.5 months with CJD
  - Strong epidemiologic evidence links vCJD to BSE:
    - BSE is a TSE that affects cattle; it was 1st reported in the U.K. The most likely route of exposure is through bovine-based foods derived from BSE-infected cattle.
    - The highest incidence of vCJD is seen in the U.K., the country with the largest potential exposure to BSE.
    - 3 cases of vCJD have been confirmed in the U.S. (although each were likely to have been contracted outside the U.S.).
  - Clinical features, found early in the illness, include:
    - Prominent psychiatric symptoms (e.g., depression, schizophrenia-like psychosis) and ataxia
    - Other neurologic signs (e.g., paresthesia/dysesthesia, chorea, dystonia, myoclonus, and akinetic mutism) develop as the disease progresses.
  - Recently, clinical criteria for the diagnosis of vCJD were validated in the U.K. by autopsy/biopsy proven cases compared to non-cases

- Fatal familial insomnia (FFI):
  - An autosomal-dominant disorder, caused by mutation at codon 178 of PRNP, also identified in fCJD. If there are homozygous alleles at codon 129 encoding methionine in conjunction with the codon 178 mutation, FFI ensues. If codon 129 encodes valine in conjunction with the codon 178 mutation, then fCJD develops.
  - Clinical features include insomnia, dysautonomia, ataxia, myoclonus, and late dementia.
  - Pathology reveals minimal vacuolization and no plaques.

- Gerstmann–Straussler–Scheinker syndrome:
  - A disorder with autosomal-dominant inheritance
  - Clinical features include ataxia and dementia.
  - Pathology reveals amyloid plaques.

PATHOPHYSIOLOGY

- TSE arises when exogenous or endogenous PRP^{RES} cause PRP^C to misfold into the abnormal protease-resistant form associated with TSE.
- Progressive accumulation of PRP^{RES} in the CNS disrupts function, leading to vacuolization and cell death. There is no host-adaptive immune response beyond microglial cell activation involved in the pathologic process.
- Neuropathologic findings include neuronal loss, atrophy, vacuolization or spongiform change, reactive astroglosis, and cell death.
- PRP^{RES} also accumulate in the reticular endothelial system, mucosa-associated lymphoid tissues, and areas of chronic inflammation throughout the body.

ETIOLOGY

- Prions are infectious proteins lacking nucleic acids that are believed to cause TSE.
- Infection arises when normal protease-sensitive host proteins, involved in neuronal function, undergo spontaneous misfolding to yield the abnormal protease-resistant form associated with infectivity.
- Newly formed host PRP^{RES} recruit neighboring cellular PRP^C and convert it to the infectious conformer. The exact molecular and cellular mechanisms surrounding propagation of PRP^{RES} remains unknown.
- Although the presence of PRP^C is necessary for the migration of PRP^{RES} to the RES, the mechanism for migration to the CNS remains unknown.
- Prions reproduce by recruiting neighboring normal cellular PRP and stimulating its conversion to the infectious form.
- Whether PRP^{RES} reproduce without any genetic material, thus bypassing the central dogma, is still hotly debated.
- Not all scientists believe the prion hypothesis, and some have argued that the causative agent is virus-like and possesses nucleic acids although none has ever been isolated from TSE pathologic specimens.

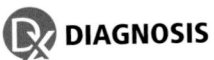 **DIAGNOSIS**

HISTORY

- Evidence of a familial form of TSE
- Potential iatrogenic exposures such as administration of human-derived pituitary growth hormones, implantation of dura mater or corneal grafts from humans, epilepsy surgery, or other CNS surgery involving stereotactic electrodes
- Duration of symptoms >6 months
- Afebrile illness
- In vCJD, progressive neuropsychiatric symptoms including:
  - Depression, anxiety, apathy, withdrawal, or delusions
  - Painful sensory symptoms including pain and/or dysesthesia
  - Ataxia
  - Myoclonus, chorea, or dystonia
  - Dementia

PHYSICAL EXAM

- Afebrile
- Abnormal mental status exam with defects in memory, personality, and other higher cortical functions, or psychosis
- Neurologic signs include unsteady gait and the presence of involuntary movements.
- Late findings include mutism and complete immobility.

DIAGNOSTIC TESTS & INTERPRETATION

Lab
- Most laboratory tests are of little value in the diagnosis of TSE. Exam of CSF fluid may reveal a mild elevation of protein, but otherwise the cerebrospinal fluid is normal.
- EEG:
  – In CJD, generalized slowing is seen early in the disease with progression to periodic burst of biphasic or triphasic sharp-wave complexes.
- In vCJD, the EEG does not show the waveforms characteristic of sporadic CJD. Although EEG abnormalities are seen in most patients, these findings are not specific.

Imaging
MRI:
- In patents with vCJD, abnormally high T2 signal in the bilateral pulvinar regions of the thalamus may be seen.
- In CJD, hyperintense signals in the basal ganglia are often seen.
- In later stages of CJD and vCJD, imaging studies such as MRI or CT scan reveal generalized atrophy with large ventricles.

Diagnostic Procedures/Other
- Diagnosis of TSE in humans can be confirmed only following pathologic exam of the brain.
- Microscopic exam of patients with all types of human TSEs reveals spongiform change accompanied by neuronal loss and gliosis.
- Amyloid plaques or immunohistochemical demonstration of abnormal PRP in the brain may also be seen.
- "Florid" plaques (amyloid plaques encircled by holes or vacuoles resulting in a daisy-like appearance) are consistently present in patients with vCJD.
- Tonsil biopsy revealing accumulation of PRP^{RES} may be helpful in confirming suspected cases of vCJD.

DIFFERENTIAL DIAGNOSIS
- Neurodegenerative disorders—mostly seen in older adults with the exception of Alpers disease:
  – Alzheimer disease
  – Parkinson disease
  – Frontotemporal dementia
  – Pick disease
  – Alpers disease (progressive cerebral hemiatrophy)
  – Amyotrophic lateral sclerosis
  – Huntington disease
  – Spinocerebellar ataxia
- Psychiatric disorders—especially when considering vCJD as a diagnosis:
  – Depression
  – Schizophrenia
  – Drug-induced psychosis
- Encephalitis, infectious
- Sydenham chorea
- Subacute sclerosing panencephalitis
- Progressive multifocal leukoencephalopathy
- Toxic encephalopathy
- Inborn errors of metabolism
- Hashimoto thyroiditis
- CNS vasculitis
- CNS tumors

TREATMENT

ADDITIONAL TREATMENT
General Measures
- No treatment is effective in slowing or stopping the progression of disease. Appropriate supportive care should be provided. Prognosis for patients with human TSEs is uniformly poor.
- Several compounds and methods have undergone testing in cell-free, tissue, and animal models of TSE. Some decrease the rate of PRP^{RES} accumulation and allow animals to reach their expected lifespan. None reverses the damage seen in the CNS after plaques have formed.
- Infection control:
  – Standard universal precautions are indicated for infection control.
  – Strict isolation is not necessary.
  – Caution should be used in obtaining cerebrospinal fluid and handling tissues obtained at autopsy.
  – Equipment contaminated by high-risk tissue should be soaked in ≥ 1 N sodium hydroxide solution for at least 1 hour and then autoclaved at 134°C for at least 1 hour.

ADDITIONAL READING

- Aguzzi A, Heikenwalder M. Pathogenesis of prion diseases: Current status and future outlook. *Nat Rev Microbiol*. 2006;4:765–775.
- Glatzel M, Soeck K, Seeger H, et al. Human prion disease: Molecular and clinical aspects. *Arch Neurol*. 2005;62:545–552.
- Hewitt PE, Llewelyn CA, MacKenzie J, et al. Creutzfeldt-Jakob disease and blood transfusion: Results of the UK Transfusion Medicine Epidemiological Review study. *Vox Sanguinis*. 2006;129:2241–2265.
- Holman RC, Belay ED, Christensen KY, et al. Human prion diseases in the United States. *PLoS One*. 2010;5:e8521.
- Johnson RT. Prion diseases. *Lancet Neurol*. 2005;4: 635–642.
- Kretzschmar HA. Diagnosis of prion diseases. *Clin Lab Med*. 2003;23:109–128.
- Prusiner SB. Shattuck Lecture—neurodegenerative diseases and prions. *N Engl J Med*. 2001;344: 1516–1526.
- Whitley RJ, MacDonald N, Asher DM. Technical report: Transmissible spongiform encephalopathies: A review for pediatricians. *Pediatrics*. 2000;106: 1160–1165.

CODES

ICD9
- 046.0 Kuru
- 046.19 Other and unspecified Creutzfeldt-Jakob disease
- 046.71 Gerstmann-Sträussler-Scheinker syndrome

ICD10
- A81.00 Creutzfeldt-Jakob disease, unspecified
- A81.09 Other Creutzfeldt-Jakob disease
- A81.81 Kuru

FAQ
- Q: Is transmission of TSEs from human blood possible?
- A: There have been 3 verified cases of vCJD attributed to transfusion of blood products in the U.K. There have been no cases of transfusion related vCJD in the U.S.
- Q: Is our food supply safe?
- A: No cases of BSE have been recognized in North America. The incidence in the U.K. has been low and is not increasing rapidly. Measures have been taken by the World Health Organization and the U.S. FDA to reduce the risk of TSE, including a ban on the use of ruminant tissues in animal feed and surveillance systems to detect TSE in animals and to prevent any part or product of an animal with suspected TSE to enter the human or animal food chain. The FDA has banned biologic agents of bovine origin produced in countries at risk of BSE. There have been 3 cases of vCJD in U.S. citizens, but each case was likely contracted outside the U.S. (U.K. and Saudi Arabia).

PROBIOTICS

Andi L. Shane
Michael D. Cabana

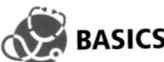 **BASICS**

DESCRIPTION
- Probiotics are defined by the World Health Organization as "live micro-organisms, which when administered in adequate amounts, confer a health benefit to the host."
- Just because a product contains "live cultures" does not make it a probiotic product. There has to be sufficient numbers of colonies, as well as a proven health benefit.
- Specific probiotic strains are generally regarded as safe. The Center for Food Safety and Nutrition (CFSAN) provides guidelines for the manufacture of probiotic products are not directly regulated as biologic drug products by the FDA, clinicians must carefully evaluate the agent selected.
- Probiotic strains are similar to the bacteria commonly found in fermented food products, such as yogurt, sour cream, sauerkraut, and buttermilk.
- Several formulations of probiotic products are available both in single-strain and multistrain preparations:
  - Probiotic organisms may be consumed as fermented dairy products or as supplements in the form of a capsule, tablet, liquid, or powder formulation.
  - Supplements theoretically provide a more consistent dose of colony-forming units (CFUs) of probiotic organisms than probiotics consumed in food products.
- Commonly used probiotic supplements contain single organisms, including the following strains:
  - *Bifidobacterium bifidum* strain YIT 4002
  - *Lactobacillus rhamnosus* ATCC 53103
  - *Lactobacillus delbrueckii* subsp. *bulgaricus*
  - *Streptococcus salivarius* subsp. *thermophilus*
  - *Escherichia coli* Nissle 1917
- Yeast, including *Saccharomyces boulardii*, is an alternative to bacterial probiotic formulations.
- Multistrain probiotics incorporate a combination of organisms in varying quantities.

PATHOPHYSIOLOGY
- Probiotics are hypothesized to exert their primary effects on the gut by re-establishing the intestinal microbiota balance, competing for receptor sites in the intestinal lumen and competing with pathogens for nutrients.
- The proposed immunomodulatory functions of probiotics include enhancing host immune defenses via strengthening tight junctions between intestinal enterocytes, increasing immunoglobulin A production, stimulating cytokine production, and producing substances (e.g., arginine, glutamine, and short-chain fatty acids) thought to secondarily act as protective nutrients.

 DIAGNOSIS

- The selection of a single-strain versus a multistrain probiotic product, or a bacterial probiotic versus a yeast probiotic, should be based on the underlying indication and whether the probiotic is administered for treatment or prophylaxis.
- The following probiotics have been shown to be efficacious for the treatment and/or prevention of the following conditions:

Probiotic	Indication
L. rhamnosus GG	Infectious diarrhea, especially of viral etiology
S. boulardii	Antibiotic-associated diarrhea
Combination therapy with lactobacilli, bifidobacteria, streptococci, *S. boulardii*	*Clostridium difficile*–associated diarrhea
Lactobacillus reuteri DSM 17938	Colic

- Efficacy with a probiotic strain or species does NOT imply that other strains will be equally efficacious. Host factors, dosing, and indication must be considered in formulating recommendations.

 TREATMENT

ADDITIONAL TREATMENT
General Measures
- The unit of dosing for oral probiotic supplements is the colony forming unit (CFU).
- Currently, there are no established dosing guidelines based on pharmacokinetic data for children.
- Studies, to date, in adults have used oral doses of 1–10 billion CFUs per dose, with administration frequency ranging from 3 times daily to weekly.
- Practitioners have used 1/2 of the adult dose for children of average weight and 1/4 of the adult dose for infants.

- There are no known reports of "toxicity" associated with probiotics in adults or children.
- The optimal dosing regimen with respect to timing of antimicrobials and probiotic supplements is not known. Currently available data suggest that temporal separation of probiotic and antimicrobial is not essential for efficacy. Furthermore, coadministration may improve compliance. For the treatment of antibiotic-associated diarrhea, there is no need to administer a probiotic at a different time from the administration of the antibiotic.

 ONGOING CARE

FOLLOW-UP RECOMMENDATIONS
- The use of probiotics for the treatment and prevention of disease and maintenance of health is a developing field. Specific probiotics may be beneficial for certain indications and hosts, but not for all.
- The American Academy of Pediatrics (AAP) has issued a clinical report summarizing the evidence for use of probiotics and supports their use on a case-by-case basis in children who may benefit from supplementation.
- Probiotics have been shown to be efficacious in randomized, double-blind, placebo-controlled studies for the following indications:
  - Decreasing the duration of infectious diarrheal episodes in hospitalized children, childcare attendees, and children with enteric viral infections in resource-poor areas
  - Reducing antibiotic-associated diarrhea in children receiving oral and intravenous antibiotics
  - Treating and preventing pouchitis, inflammation of a surgically created distal small bowel reservoir, and irritable bowel syndrome in children and adults
  - Treating atopic dermatitis (eczema)
- Probiotic applications currently being evaluated include:
  - Prevention of necrotizing enterocolitis
  - Maintenance of remission in persons with ulcerative colitis
  - Treatment and prevention of atopic disease including rhinitis and asthma
  - Improving tolerance of *Helicobacter pylori* eradication therapy
  - Prevention of genitourinary infections, such as urinary tract infections and candidiasis
  - Prevention of dental caries

- Future investigations to evaluate the efficacy and safety of probiotics in large-scale, multicenter trials; to monitor the potency and composition of probiotic formulations; to develop *in vitro* and *in vivo* systems to understand the molecular mechanisms of action; and to understand the balance among infection, immunity, and probiotics are in progress.
- The selection of a probiotic for pediatric use requires an understanding of the indication, the optimal formulation (single strain vs. multistrain), delivery system, and the host.

Patient Monitoring

- Currently available probiotic formulations are viable microorganisms and therefore have the potential to cause invasive infections in hosts who may have compromised mucosal epithelia.
- A recent review (2008) suggests that probiotics should be used with caution in children with major risk factors or multiple minor risk factors:
  - Major risk factors include immune compromise or prematurity.
  - Minor risk factors include the presence of a central venous catheter, impaired intestinal epithelial barrier, administration of a probiotic by jejunostomy, concomitant administration of a broad-spectrum antibiotic to which the probiotic organism is resistant, use of probiotic strains with high mucosal adhesion or known pathogenicity, and the presence of cardiac valvular disease (*Lactobacillus* strains only).
- An extremely low incidence of bacteremia has been observed with widespread use of probiotics in Finnish adults.
- To date, there have not been any adverse effects attributable to probiotic consumption in pregnant women consuming a probiotic supplement to prevent atopic dermatitis in their infants.
- HIV-infected adults taking a probiotic supplement to prevent diarrhea and improve tolerance of antiretroviral agents have not experienced adverse effects attributable to the probiotic supplement.

ADDITIONAL READING

- Alvarez-Olmos MI, Oberhelman RA. Probiotic agents and infectious diseases. *Clin Infect Dis*. 2001;32: 1567–1576.
- Boyle RJ, Robins-Browne RM, Tang ML. Probiotic use in clinical practice: What are the risks? *Am J Clin Nutr*. 2006;83:1256–1264.
- Land MH, Rouster-Steven K, Woods DR, et al. Lactobacillus sepsis associated with probiotic therapy. *Pediatrics*. 2005;115:178–181. Available at: www.cdc.gov/mmwr/pdf/RR/RR5216.pdf.
- Lin HC, Su BH, Chen AC, et al. Oral probiotics reduce the incidence and severity of necrotizing enterocolitis in very low birth weight infants. *Pediatrics*. 2005;115:1–4.
- *Report of a joint expert consultation on evaluation of health and nutritional properties of probiotics in food including powdered milk with live lactic acid bacteria*. FAO and WHO Joint and Expert Committee Report, 2001. Y6398/E. Available at: http://www.who.int/foodsafety/publications/fs_management/en/probiotics.pdf.
- Savino F, Pelle E, Palumeri E, et al. Lactobacillus reuteri (American Type Culture Collection Strain 55730) versus simethicone in the treatment of infantile colic: A prospective randomized study. *Pediatrics*. 2007;119:e124–e130.
- Thomas DW, Greer FR, Committee on Nutrition: Section on Gastroenterology, Hepatology, and Nutrition of the American Academy of Pediatrics. Clinical report: Probiotics and prebiotics in pediatrics. *Pediatrics*. 2010;126:1217–1231.
- Vanderhoof JA. Probiotics in allergy management. *J Pediatr Gastroenterol Nutr*. 2008;47(Suppl 2): S38–S40.

FAQ

- Q: Can children receive an adequate amount of probiotics by consuming yogurt?
- A: Although probiotic organisms are found in some foods such as yogurt, the dosage of active organisms provided via routine consumption may be inadequate for a therapeutic benefit. Food processing may result in variable viability and CFUs of probiotic organisms in food products. The availability of CFUs in commercially prepared probiotic formulations is theoretically more precise. Probiotic supplements may offer a higher dose of organisms in a more concentrated form. The volume of yogurt that one would need to ingest to match the CFUs of a nonfood probiotic supplement usually exceeds what an adult or child could consume in a single serving.
- Q: What is the difference between probiotic and prebiotic supplements?
- A: Probiotic supplements contain live microorganisms, while prebiotic supplements are substances that promote the growth of probiotic organisms. The most common prebiotic supplements are fructo-oligosaccharides and galacto-oligosaccharides, which are present in human milk.
- Q: What other factors should a clinician consider when recommending use of a probiotic supplement?
- A: The rate of adherence will affect the clinical effectiveness of probiotic supplementation. The addition of a probiotic supplement may complicate a treatment or maintenance regimen. "Per protocol" analyses of studies evaluating probiotic supplementation demonstrate statistical significance, while an "intention to treat analysis" may not. These results have implications regarding the importance of patient adherence for effectiveness.
- Q: What is the standard dose for a probiotic supplement?
- A: There are no uniform dosing recommendations for probiotics. The optimal dose depends on the indication, the host, and the species and strain of the probiotic being utilized.

PROLONGED QT INTERVAL SYNDROME

Ronn E. Tanel

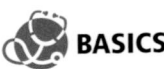 **BASICS**

DESCRIPTION
Prolonged QT interval syndrome, also known as *congenital long QT syndrome* (LQTS), is characterized by prolongation of the QT interval on the surface ECG, syncope, and sudden death as a result of malignant ventricular arrhythmias. The electrical instability is due to an abnormality of ventricular repolarization associated with a cardiac ion channelopathy.

EPIDEMIOLOGY
Incidence
Extrapolation from sudden death data suggests that the frequency may be ~1 in 2,500.

Prevalence
Exact prevalence of LQTS is not known, but it may be a relatively common cause of syncope and sudden unexplained death in children and young adults.

RISK FACTORS
Genetics
- Autosomal dominant (Romano-Ward syndrome)
- Autosomal recessive, sometimes associated with congenital nerve deafness (Jervell and Lange-Nielsen syndrome)
- Genetic linkage analysis studies have demonstrated that >400 genetic mutations among 12 cardiac channel genes account for nearly 3/4 of LQTS.
- Genotype-phenotype-based research studies have identified gene-specific electrocardiographic profiles, gene-specific arrhythmia triggers, gene-directed treatment strategies, and gene-specific risk stratification.

GENERAL PREVENTION
- Preventive measures focus on screening for the electrocardiographic abnormality, especially in individuals who appear to be at risk of having the diagnosis.
- Patients who have been diagnosed are advised to avoid exposure to stimulants, medications that are known to prolong the QT interval or provoke ventricular arrhythmias and situations that may aggravate the cardiac rhythm or induce torsades de pointes.

PATHOPHYSIOLOGY
2 hypotheses have been proposed to explain the pathogenesis of congenital long QT syndrome:
- An abnormality or imbalance in sympathetic innervation to the heart, which helps explain the findings of sinus bradycardia, abnormal repolarization, adrenergic dependence of arrhythmias, and response to adrenergic antagonist medications associated with the syndrome.
- Intrinsic cardiac ion (potassium and sodium) channel gene defects appear to be the mechanism responsible for cardiac repolarization abnormalities. Because some identified gene mutations that result in congenital long QT syndrome occur at loci that also encode a cardiac ion channel protein, ion channels have been proposed as the intrinsic abnormality that is responsible for abnormal repolarization.

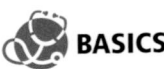 **DIAGNOSIS**

HISTORY
- Notable findings include:
  - Palpitations
  - Presyncope
  - Syncope
- These symptoms may be related to provocative stimuli, especially emotional or physical stress. Any use of medications known to prolong the QTc interval should be noted.
- Most importantly, a thorough family history for arrhythmia, syncope, epilepsy, or sudden unexplained death should be obtained.

PHYSICAL EXAM
Findings are usually normal, but bradycardia may be present.

DIAGNOSTIC TESTS & INTERPRETATION
Lab
- The Bazett formula: QTc = QT/(square root of RR interval). Generally, a QTc >480 msec is considered abnormal, although some clinicians allow a slightly longer QTc for infants <6 months of age.
- Some clinicians believe that the QTc should not be corrected at heart rates <60 beats per minute (bpm). The measurement should be taken in lead II without significant sinus arrhythmia.
- Children frequently have a prominent U wave. It should generally be included in the measurement of the QTc if it exceeds 1/2 the amplitude of the T wave.

- A single measured prolonged QTc interval does not confirm the diagnosis of long QT syndrome.
- Since 2004, genetic testing has been available as a commercial diagnostic test. Unfortunately, only 2/3–3/4 of all genetic causes of LQTS have been identified, so false-negative genetic testing is possible.
- Clinical scoring systems may help stratify patients into high, moderate, and low probability of having the diagnosis, based on symptoms, family history, and ECG findings.

Imaging
ECG:
- Atrioventricular block can be seen on the ECG in infants with relatively rapid heart rates and P waves that occur during the prolonged repolarization period (QT interval) of ventricular refractoriness.
- The echocardiogram should demonstrate normal cardiac structure and function.

Diagnostic Procedures/Other
- Other tests that may help confirm the diagnosis include 24-hour ambulatory Holter monitoring:
  - This recording may disclose asymptomatic ventricular ectopy or arrhythmias, T-wave alternans, or variability in the QTc interval during different periods of the day.
- Exercise stress testing may also be helpful in identifying ventricular arrhythmias or prolongation of the QTc interval, particularly during the early recovery phase.

DIFFERENTIAL DIAGNOSIS
- Congenital LQTS is most commonly misdiagnosed as vasovagal syncope or a seizure disorder. All patients who have a syncopal event or who are diagnosed with epilepsy should have a baseline screening ECG. Sudden infant death syndrome (SIDS) may be related to congenital long QT syndrome. Some studies have demonstrated that mutations of ion channel proteins that cause LQTS have been found in SIDS victims. QT interval prolongation may be subtle, such that ~10% of affected patients may have a normal result on routine ECG and ~40% may have borderline prolongation of the QT interval.
- Acquired forms of LQTS should be differentiated from the congenital and inherited form. Acquired LQTS may be due to the following:
  - Electrolyte abnormalities: Hypokalemia, hypocalcemia, hypomagnesemia, and metabolic acidosis
  - Toxins: Organophosphates
  - CNS trauma
  - Malnutrition: Anorexia

- Primary myocardial disease: Myocarditis, ischemia, cardiomyopathy
- Medication:
  - Cardiac medications: Quinidine, procainamide, disopyramide, sotalol, and amiodarone
  - Antibiotics/Antifungals: Erythromycin, trimethoprim–sulfamethoxazole, pentamidine, ketoconazole, and fluconazole
  - Psychotropic medications: Tricyclic antidepressants, phenothiazines, and haloperidol
  - Antihistamines: Terfenadine, astemizole, diphenhydramine
  - GI: Cisapride

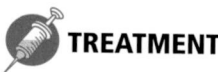

TREATMENT

MEDICATION (DRUGS)
- The primary therapy is β-blockade, most commonly with propranolol, atenolol, or nadolol.
- Class Ib antiarrhythmic medications (e.g., mexiletine) are also used in patients with congenital LQTS, especially in those with documented ventricular arrhythmia.
- Medications do not generally help treat patients with acquired LQTS.

ADDITIONAL TREATMENT
General Measures
Patients are usually treated based on symptoms and the clinical severity of the disease.

Additional Therapies
Automatic implantable cardioverter-defibrillators (ICDs) are usually reserved for older children and adolescents who have significant symptoms, documented ventricular arrhythmias, or other significant risk factors for sudden death.

SURGERY/OTHER PROCEDURES
- Occasionally, implantation of a permanent pacemaker is indicated based on the theory that the tachyarrhythmias (e.g., torsades de pointes) are dependent on bradycardia and/or pauses. Pacemaker implantation may be necessary to support the low heart rate that is a result of β-blocker therapy. Newborns and infants with a very prolonged QT interval, atrioventricular block, and low ventricular rates are historically treated with a pacemaker.
- An ICD may be recommended for patients thought to be at higher risk of developing ventricular arrhythmias.
- Left stellate ganglionectomy is controversially performed to eliminate the hyperactive left sympathetic ganglion output that has been proposed as a mechanism of ventricular arrhythmias.

IN-PATIENT CONSIDERATIONS
Initial Stabilization
Most clinicians treat diagnosed asymptomatic children with medications because of a high incidence of sudden death that occurs as the 1st symptom.

ONGOING CARE

FOLLOW-UP RECOMMENDATIONS
Patient Monitoring
- Follow-up outpatient appointments should review new or recurrent symptoms, including palpitations, near syncope or syncope, and the efficacy and adverse effects of medical therapy.
- ECG may demonstrate a normal or prolonged QTc.
- Follow-up 24-hour ambulatory Holter monitor recordings and exercise stress tests may help assess the adequacy of β-blocker therapy and identify ventricular arrhythmias.
- All family members of the patient should have an ECG, as a minimum screening measure.

PROGNOSIS
- Children have a higher incidence of sudden death than adults, which may reflect an inherent bias because adult patients have already survived childhood. The risk of cardiac events is higher in boys before puberty and in women during adulthood.
- Pediatric patients with greatest risk for sudden death are those with QTc >600 msec. Gender, environmental factors, genotype, and therapy are other factors that influence the clinical course.
- A particular clinical phenotype may be caused by different genetic substrates, while a single gene can cause very different phenotypes, even within the same family, by acting through different pathways.
- β-blocker therapy has been shown to reduce the incidence of sudden death.
- Current research may lead to the development of therapy specific to the precise ion channel defect.

COMPLICATIONS
- Complications, especially in untreated patients, include:
  - Ventricular tachyarrhythmias, specifically torsades de pointes
  - Syncope
  - Sudden death
- In patients with the congenital and inherited form of the condition, asymptomatic family members may be affected.

ADDITIONAL READING
- Ackerman MJ. Genotype-phenotype relationships in congenital long QT syndrome. *J Electrocard.* 2005;38:64–68.
- Hedley PL, Jorgensen P, Schlamowitz S et al. The genetic basis of long QT and short QT syndromes. *Hum Mutat.* 2009;30:1486–1511.
- Morita H, Wu J, Zipes DP. The QT syndromes: Long and short. *Lancet.* 2008;372:750–763.
- Priori SG, Napolitano C, Vicentini A. Inherited arrhythmia syndromes: Applying the molecular biology and genetic to the clinical management. *J Interv Card Electrophysiol.* 2003;9:93–101.
- Priori SG, Schwartz PJ, Napolitano C et al. Risk stratification in the long QT syndrome. *N Engl J Med.* 2003;348:1866–1874.
- Roden DM. Long-QT syndrome. *N Engl J Med.* 2008;358:169–176.

CODES

ICD9
426.82 Long QT syndrome

ICD10
I45.81 Long QT syndrome

FAQ
- Q: Should activity be restricted in patients with congenital LQTS?
- A: Because sudden rises in serum catecholamine levels may precipitate symptoms, it is appropriate to restrict competitive and vigorous athletics. Symptomatic patients may require greater restrictions. Documentation of appropriate β-blockade by a lower maximal heart rate at peak exercise on follow-up exercise stress test may be helpful.
- Q: If someone is identified as having LQTS, should family members be evaluated?
- A: Yes, with a high degree of suspicion. Most cases of congenital LQTS are inherited in an autosomal-dominant pattern, so that each child of an affected parent has a 50% chance of having the gene. This does not predict severity of symptoms, but parents, all siblings, and children of patients should be examined with an ECG. Holter monitor and exercise stress test. These studies may help reveal an abnormal QTc interval in suspected family members.

PROTEIN-ENERGY MALNUTRITION (KWASHIORKOR)

Robert D. Karch
Teena Sebastian

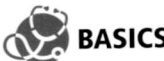 **BASICS**

DESCRIPTION

- The term "protein-energy malnutrition" (PEM) describes a general state of undernutrition and deficiency of multiple nutrients and energy.
- There are three clinical presentations of severe PEM: Kwashiorkor, marasmus, and marasmic kwashiorkor.
- Kwashiorkor results from protein deficiency and is characterized by hypoproteinemia, pitting edema, varying degrees of wasting and/or stunting, dermatosis, and fatty infiltration of the liver.
- Marasmus results from both energy and protein deficiency and is characterized by wasting, fatigue, and apathy.
- Marasmic kwashiorkor is caused by acute or chronic protein deficiency and chronic energy deficit and is characterized by edema, wasting, stunting, and mild hepatomegaly.
- The distinction between kwashiorkor and marasmus is frequently blurred and many children present with features of both.
- Severe PEM covers a broad clinical spectrum ranging from frank kwashiorkor to severe marasmus when the body's protein and energy requirements are not adequately met:
  - Primary:
    - Inadequate dietary intake
  - Secondary:
    - Result of other disease processes that limit food ingestion or reduce nutrient absorption, or those that increase nutrient requirements or losses
- Cicely Williams introduced the name "kwashiorkor" in 1935 in a classic description of her observations of the Ga tribe on the Gold Coast of Africa (currently Ghana).
- Kwashiorkor in the US:
  - In developed nations, symptoms of kwashiorkor have been described in chronic malabsorptive conditions such as cystic fibrosis.
  - In the US, few cases of kwashiorkor unrelated to chronic illness have been described.
  - Common reasons for the consumption of a protein-deficient milk alternative, sugar water or fruit juice, are nutritional ignorance, perceived milk or formula intolerance, or food fads.
  - Consumption of a low-protein health food milk alternative, such as rice milk, secondary to a history of chronic eczema and perceived milk intolerance, has occurred in the United States.
  - Symptoms like "flaky paint dermatitis," edema, and lab abnormalities suggestive of kwashiorkor have been seen in such cases.

EPIDEMIOLOGY

- Malnutrition underlies 55% of childhood mortality worldwide.
- Kwashiorkor may occur at any age, but is seen most frequently in children 1–3 years of age.
- Kwashiorkor is seldom seen in the 1st year of life. It is usually seen in the 2nd year or beyond, when the toddler is fully weaned or only partially breastfed and may have a low intake of dietary protein.

PATHOPHYSIOLOGY

- Temperature regulation is impaired, leading to hypothermia in a cold environment and hyperthermia in a hot environment.
- Increase in total-body sodium and decrease in total-body potassium
- Hypophosphatemia is associated with malnutrition and results in high mortality.
- Protein synthesis is reduced, particularly albumin, transferrin, and apolipoprotein B. Hypertriglyceridemia leads to fatty infiltration of the liver.
- Gluconeogenesis is reduced, which increases risk of hypoglycemia during infection.
- Reduced cardiac output leads to low blood pressure, compromised tissue perfusion, and a reduction in renal blood flow and glomerular filtration rate.
- Diminished inspiratory and expiratory pressures and vital capacity
- Reduction of gastric and pancreatic secretions
- Reduced intestinal motility
- Intestinal mucosa atrophy resulting in malabsorption of carbohydrates, fats, fat- and water-soluble vitamins
- Low circulating insulin levels
- Growth hormone secretion is increased while somatomedin activity is reduced.
  - Glucagon, epinephrine, and cortisol levels are increased.
  - Serum T_3 and T_4 levels are reduced.
- Immune system:
  - All aspects of immune function are diminished in malnutrition, thereby increasing susceptibility to infection.
  - Delayed wound healing may be seen owing to nutritional deficiencies.

ETIOLOGY

- There are two principal theories regarding the etiology of kwashiorkor: The classical theory of protein deficiency and the newer theory of free radical damage.
- Both theories emphasize different aspects of the environment: In the classical theory, nutrients, and in the free radical theory, oxidative stresses.
- The classical theory of protein deficiency was supported by Williams' original description of kwashiorkor developing in children who were weaned onto starchy gruels after being deposed from the breast and being cured by milk:
  - The free radical theory of kwashiorkor proposes that kwashiorkor results from an imbalance between the production of toxic free radicals and their safe disposal.
  - Golden and colleagues argue that inadequate diet leads to a state of impaired antioxidant defense.

- The free radical theory attempts to explain the entire spectrum of clinical findings in kwashiorkor by implicating a wide range of nutritional deficiencies, as well as environmental oxidative stressors (noxae):
  - Important noxae include infections and exogenous toxins such as aflatoxin and its metabolites.
  - Aflatoxin, from the fungus *Aspergillus flavus*, has been found in greater concentrations in the serum and urine of children with kwashiorkor than in controls.
  - There is a hierarchy of causes of PEM operating at different levels and interacting with one another; from food scarcity, infection, malabsorption, and neglect, to poverty and social disadvantage, to drought, war, or civil disturbance.
- The multiplicity of causes of PEM necessitates a multidisciplinary approach to its treatment and prevention.

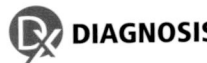 **DIAGNOSIS**

HISTORY

- Dietary history:
  - Diet before current illness episode
  - Adequacy of protein and total calories
  - Food and fluids taken in past few days
  - Assess whether parents and children adhere to special diets or whether health food milk alternatives, such as rice milk, are given.
- Determine duration and frequency of emesis or diarrhea.
- Loose stools with evidence of malabsorption are common. Stools may be watery and/or tinged with blood.
- Any death of siblings
- Cultural beliefs and practices regarding infant and childhood feeding
- Growth records: Decreased growth velocity commensurate with poor protein intake

PHYSICAL EXAM

- Weight and length/height:
  - Growth failure always occurs to some extent.
  - Wasting is also typical, although it may be masked by the presence of edema.
- Affected child is usually apathetic and irritable.
- Child is usually unsmiling and prefers to remain in one position.
- Hypothermia or hyperthermia
- There is some degree of edema in all cases of kwashiorkor:
  - Peripheral edema usually begins in the feet and ascends up the legs.
  - Pitting of the skin above the ankle is diagnostic.
  - The hands and face may become edematous.
  - Facial edema gives the characteristic "moon facies."

- Hair lacks luster and color may change to brown or reddish-brown.
- Hair is easily pluckable.
- Bands of discolored hair, representing periods of malnutrition, are termed the "flag sign."
- Dermatosis often develops in areas of friction or pressure.
- Hypo- or hyperpigmented patches may appear, which subsequently desquamate in scales or sheets, exposing atrophic ulcers resembling burns.
• Additional clinical signs of PEM:
  - Signs of B-vitamin deficiency, such as perioral lesions
  - Signs of vitamin A deficiency, such as xerosis and/or xerophthalmia
  - Pale, cold, and cyanotic extremities: Decreased vascular volume secondary to decreased protein concentration
  - Abdomen is frequently protuberant secondary to poor peristalsis, leading to distended stomach and intestinal loops.
  - Respiratory: Looks for signs of pneumonia or heart failure.
  - Enlargement of liver and jaundice may also be seen.

DIAGNOSTIC TESTS & INTERPRETATION
Lab
• Serum protein
• Prealbumin and serum transferrin may be useful in determining severity of kwashiorkor.
• Retinal binding protein may be reduced.
• Hemoglobin and hematocrit are usually low.
• Ratio of nonessential to essential amino acids in plasma is elevated in kwashiorkor and usually normal in marasmus.
• Increased serum elevation of free fatty acids
• Low serum and urine carnitine levels
• Stool exam to rule out infectious cause of chronic diarrhea
• Chest radiograph and PPD to rule out TB

DIFFERENTIAL DIAGNOSIS
• Nephrotic syndrome
• Hookworm anemia:
  - May cause edema alone. Commonly seen in association with kwashiorkor. It is not associated with the kwashiorkor-related dermatologic findings.
• Chronic dysentery
• Protein-losing enteropathy (PLE)
• Pellagra: Dermatosis of pellagra and kwashiorkor are similar. However, the dermatosis of pellagra is often seen in sun-exposed areas, not in areas such as the groin, as commonly seen in kwashiorkor. Kwashiorkor dermatosis is often described as "flaky paint" dermatosis.

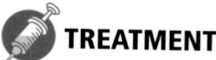 TREATMENT
WHO Guidelines
• Prevent and treat:
  - Hypoglycemia
  - Hypothermia
  - Dehydration
  - Electrolyte imbalances
  - Infection
  - Micronutrient deficiencies
• Provide special feeds for:
  - Initial stabilization
  - Providing catch-up growth
  - Providing loving care and stimulation
• Where guidelines have been fully implemented, mortality has been reduced by at least half.
• Management of the child with severe protein-energy malnutrition is divided into 3 phases: Initial treatment, rehabilitation, and follow-up.

ADDITIONAL TREATMENT
General Measures
• Whenever possible, a dehydrated child with malnutrition should be rehydrated orally or by nasogastric tube.
• IV infusion should be avoided except for when it is essential (e.g., severe dehydration and shock).
• Hypoglycemia is an important cause of death in the 1st 2 days of treatment.
• Suspected hypoglycemia should be treated with oral rehydration salts solution (ORS) or 10% glucose by mouth or nasogastric tube.
• Severely malnourished children have high levels of sodium and are deficient in potassium. Standard WHO ORS does not meet the special electrolyte requirements of the severely malnourished child.
• ReSoMal is a modified ORS that contains less sodium and more potassium than the standard WHO ORS and is the recommended ORS for severely malnourished children.
• Breastfeeding should not be interrupted during rehydration.

 ONGOING CARE
PROGNOSIS
• Treatment corrects the acute signs of the disease, but catch-up growth in height may never be achieved.
• Mortality rate in kwashiorkor can be as high as 40%, but adequate treatment can reduce it to <10%.
• Some of the factors that indicate poor prognosis:
  - Age <6 months
  - Infections
  - Dehydration and electrolyte abnormalities
  - Persistent tachycardia, signs of heart failure
  - Total serum protein <3 g/100 mL
  - Elevated serum bilirubin
  - Severe anemia with hypoxia
  - Hypoglycemia and/or hypothermia

• Several longitudinal studies have demonstrated associations between early childhood stunting and later cognitive function and academic attainment. Behrman et al. demonstrated that stunting at 72 months was related to cognition between 25 and 42 years of age.

ADDITIONAL READING
• Carvalho NF, Kenney RD, Carrington PH, et al. Severe nutritional deficiencies in toddlers resulting from health food milk alternatives. *Pediatrics.* 2001;107:E46.
• Golden MHN. Free radicals in the pathogenesis of kwashiorkor. *Proc Nutr Soc.* 1987;46:53–68.
• Grover Z, Ee LC. Protein energy malnutrition. *Pediatr Clin North Am.* 2009;56(5):1055–1068.
• Liu T, Howard RM, Mancini AJ, et al. Kwashiorkor in the United States: Fad diets, perceived and true milk allergy, and nutritional ignorance. *Arch Dermatol.* 2001;137:630–636.

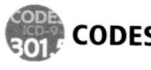 CODES
ICD9
• 260 Kwashiorkor
• 261 Nutritional marasmus
• 269.8 Other nutritional deficiency
ICD10
• E40 Kwashiorkor
• E41 Nutritional marasmus
• E61.8 Deficiency of other specified nutrient elements

FAQ
• Q: What are the signs and symptoms of kwashiorkor and how do these change over the course of the clinical spectrum of severe protein-energy malnutrition, from kwashiorkor to marasmus?
• A: Signs and symptoms of kwashiorkor:
  - Growth failure, wasting
  - Edema that is peripheral in onset and ascending
  - Hair changes including color change, "flag sign," and easy pluckability; "flaky paint" dermatosis of skin
  - In addition to above signs and symptoms child may also develop vitamin A and B deficiency, decreased peripheral circulation, and decreased peristalsis with distended bowel loops. Hepatomegaly/splenomegaly may also be observed. The child is at higher risk for developing other conditions such as pneumonia or congestive heart failure.
• Q: What are some common causes of severe undernutrition in the US that may present as kwashiorkor?
• A:
  - Chronic malabsorptive conditions such as cystic fibrosis
  - Consumption of protein-deficient milk substitutes such as rice milk, fruit juices, etc.

PROTEINURIA

Matthew G. Sampson
Andres J. Greco (5th edition)

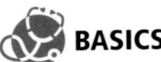 **BASICS**

DEFINITION

- Protein may be found in the urine of healthy children. The term proteinuria is used to indicate urinary protein excretion beyond the upper limit of normal (100 mg/m^2/d or 4 mg/m^2/hr in children and 150 mg/d in adults).
- Proteinuria >40 mg/m^2/hr is considered as nephrotic range.
- Classification:
  - Transient proteinuria: Often associated with high fever, cold stress, dehydration, and exercise. It is not associated with underlying renal disease and by definition is absent on subsequent urine examinations.
  - Orthostatic or postural proteinuria: Elevated protein excretion when the subject is upright and ambulating, but normal during recumbent position. It most commonly occurs in school-aged children and adolescents and rarely exceeds 1 g/m^2/d.
  - Persistent or fixed proteinuria: Urinary dipstick ≥1+ in the first morning urine specimen on multiple occasions for a period >3 months. Requires prompt referral to nephrology.
  - Glomerular proteinuria: The amount of proteinuria may range from <1 to >30 mg/d. It is usually found in the context of edema and hypoalbuminemia. If there is a mixed nephritic/nephrotic picture, there may be associated, hypertension, abnormal glomerular filtration rate, and hematuria. The major urinary component is albumin.
  - Tubular proteinuria: Rarely >1 g/d and is not associated with edema. It may be associated with other defects of proximal tubular function (e.g., glucosuria, phosphaturia, aminoaciduria) and tubular interstitial processes. The major marker is beta-2-microglobulin.

PATHOPHYSIOLOGY

- ~50% of the normally excreted protein consists of Tamm-Horsfall protein, a glycoprotein secreted by the ascending loop of Henle.
- Proteinuria may be the result of an increased permeability of the glomeruli to the passage of serum proteins (glomerular proteinuria) or decreased reabsorption of low molecular weight proteins by the renal tubules (tubular proteinuria).

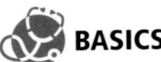 **DIAGNOSIS**

DIFFERENTIAL DIAGNOSIS

- **Idiopathic nephrotic syndrome**
  - Minimal change nephritic syndrome
  - Mesangial proliferation
  - Focal and segmental glomerulosclerosis
  - Membranous nephropathy
- **Nephrotic syndrome due to genetic causes**
  - Finnish-type congenital nephrotic syndrome
  - Familial focal and segmental glomerulosclerosis
  - Diffuse mesangial sclerosis
  - Denys-Drash syndrome (nephropathy, Wilms tumor, and genital abnormalities)
- **Chronic kidney disease**
- **Acquired glomerular disease**
  - Idiopathic glomerulonephritis (membranoproliferative glomerulonephritis)
  - Lupus-associated nephritis
  - IgA nephropathy
  - Systemic vasculitides
  - Subacute bacterial endocarditis
  - Diabetes mellitus
  - Hypertension
  - Hemolytic uremic syndrome
  - Hyperfiltration secondary to nephron loss (with or without sclerosis)
- **Genetic disorders**
  - Nail-patella syndrome
  - Alport syndrome
  - Fabry disease
  - Glycogen storage disease
  - Cystic fibrosis
  - Hurler syndrome (mucopolysaccharide type-1)
  - α-1-antitrypsin
  - Mitochondrial disorders (usually tubular proteinuria)
  - Gaucher disease
  - Dent disease (X-linked nephrolithiasis)
  - Cystinosis
  - Wilson disease
- **Oncologic/hematologic**
  - Sickle cell disease
  - Renal vein thrombosis
  - Leukemia
  - Lymphoma

- **Infectious**
  - Poststreptococcal glomerulonephritis
  - HIV-associated nephropathy
  - Hepatitis B and C virus infection
  - Malaria
  - Syphilis (can present as congenital nephrotic syndrome)
  - Pyelonephritis
- **Drugs/toxins**
  - Bee sting
  - Food allergens
  - Antibiotic-induced interstitial nephritis
  - Penicillamine
  - Gold salts
  - NSAIDs
  - Heavy metals (e.g., mercury, lead)
- **Miscellaneous**
  - Tubular interstitial nephritis
  - Acute tubular necrosis
  - Reflux nephropathy
  - Hypothyroidism
- **Congestive heart failure**

HISTORY

- **Question:** Changes in the aspect of the urine?
- *Significance:* Foamy or colored (red, tea-colored)
- **Question:** Recent illness?
- *Significance:* Pharyngitis and upper respiratory infections
- **Question:** Frequent episodes of fever?
- *Significance:* Lymphoma, malignancies
- **Question:** Medications or herbal/folk remedies?
- **Question:** Illicit drugs use and risk factors for STD in adolescent and adults?
- *Significance:* HIV, syphilis
- **Question:** Urinary tract infection in the past?
- *Significance:* Reflux nephropathy
- **Question:** Family history of renal, rheumatologic diseases or hearing loss?
- **Question:** Fatigue, general malaise, reduced appetite?
- **Question:** Weight changes?
- **Question:** Facial swelling (in the mornings) and lower limb swelling (in the afternoon)?
- **Question:** Symptoms related to rheumatologic conditions (skin rash, joint pain, joint stiffness)?
- **Question:** Cough, shortness of breath?

PHYSICAL EXAM
- General:
  - Hypertension
  - Growth and development
- HEENT:
  - Periorbital edema
  - Malar rash
- Chest:
  - Pericardial or pleural effusions
- Abdomen:
  - Ascites
  - Hepatosplenomegaly
  - Abdominal masses/organomegaly
- Genitalia:
  - Scrotal edema
  - Ambiguous genitalia (Denys-Drash syndrome)
- Skin:
  - Purpuric or petechial rash (leukemia, lymphomas)
  - Pallor (malignancies, chronic renal failure, HUS)
  - Angiokeratomas (Fabry disease)
- Extremities:
  - Pitting edema
  - Arthralgias/arthritis
- Dystrophic nails

DIAGNOSTIC TESTS & INTERPRETATION
- **Test:** Dipstick testing
- *Significance*:
  - Always to be performed in a first morning urine sample
  - A negative or trace result in a concentrated urine specimen (specific gravity >1.020) is normal.
- **Test:** 24-hour collection of urine for protein

- *Significance*:
  - It is indicated for quantification of proteinuria and to confirm the diagnosis.
  - Normal range: <100 mg/m^2/d or <4 mg/m^2/hr
- **Test:** Spot ratio for protein/creatinine
- *Significance*:
  - Always to be performed in a first morning urine sample
  - Normal values are <0.2 in children >2 years of age and <0.5 in children 6–24 months old.
  - It is the simplest method to quantitate proteinuria

ALERT
- Most patients with proteinuria will have orthostatic proteinuria that is identified with an early morning test for protein and a second test several hours later.
- It is important to check the urine sediment for red cell casts; this indicates a glomerular involvement and requires additional studies for nephritis and chronic renal disease.

ADDITIONAL READING
- Gipson DS, Massengill SF, Yao L, et al. Management of childhood onset nephrotic syndrome. *Pediatrics*. 2009;124(2):747–757.
- Hogg RJ, Portman RJ, Milliner D, et al. Evaluation and management of proteinuria and nephrotic syndrome in children: Recommendations from a pediatric nephrology panel established at the National Kidney Foundation Conference on proteinuria, albuminuria, risk, assessment, detection, and elimination (PARADE). *Pediatrics*. 2000;105:1242–1249.
- Quigley R. Evaluation of hematuria and proteinuria: How should a pediatrician proceed? *Curr Opin Pediatr*. 2008;20(2):140–144.

 CODES

ICD9
- 593.6 Postural proteinuria
- 791.0 Proteinuria

ICD10
- R80.1 Persistent proteinuria, unspecified
- R80.2 Orthostatic proteinuria, unspecified
- R80.9 Proteinuria, unspecified

FAQ
- Q: When to refer to nephrology?
- A: Patients with one of the following: Fixed proteinuria, associated hypertension, associated hematuria, clinical evidence of nephritic syndrome and patient with family history of renal diseases with proteinuria.
- Q: When are imaging studies indicated?
- A: Patients with abnormal renal function, hematuria, or nephrolithiasis. The best initial study is renal and bladder ultrasound.

PRUNE BELLY SYNDROME

Shamir Tuchman

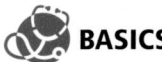 **BASICS**

DESCRIPTION
- Rare congenital disorder characterized by the triad of:
  - Deficiency of abdominal musculature
  - Bilateral cryptorchidism
  - Dilated, anomalous development of the bladder and upper urinary tract
- It presents with a broad-spectrum of severity, from mild hydroureter with an enlarged bladder and normal renal function to severe renal dysplasia and pulmonary hypoplasia.
- Also known as Eagle-Barrett syndrome

EPIDEMIOLOGY
- Incidence: 1/35,000–50,000 live births
- Most patients are detected during the neonatal period or prenatally during maternal ultrasound.
- Prune belly syndrome is much more common in males (>95%).

RISK FACTORS
Genetics
- The genetic basis of prune belly syndrome remains unclear.
- Most patients have normal karyotypes.
- Most cases are sporadic, although rare cases in sibs have been reported.

PATHOPHYSIOLOGY
The bladder in prune belly syndrome is large, irregularly shaped, and thick walled. Many patients have poor urinary flow and high residual volumes:
- Ureters are usually markedly dilated, tortuous, and elongated. Peristalsis is ineffective, and the distal ureters are most severely affected.
- Renal involvement is variable; the most severe dysplasia occurs in patients with extensive dilation of the urinary tract. Dysplastic changes are usually symmetric.
- Usually, the bladder neck is wide and the prostatic urethra is dilated and triangular.

ETIOLOGY
The cause of the prune belly syndrome remains unclear. 2 theories have been proposed:
- The triad of congenital defects may result from a primary mesodermal defect in development with congenital deficiency of smooth muscle in the bladder, ureter, and renal pelvis.
- Outflow obstruction of the bladder in utero may result in dilation of the bladder and upper urinary tract with subsequent renal injury. The expanded bladder may block the route of the descending testicles and may cause abdominal distention and abdominal wall muscle atrophy.

COMMONLY ASSOCIATED CONDITIONS
Many patients have associated anomalies:
- GI anomalies: Affect up to 30% of patients (e.g., imperforate anus and increased risk of volvulus)
- Musculoskeletal anomalies (e.g., talipes equinovarus, congenital hip dislocation, pectus excavatum, scoliosis).
- Respiratory (e.g., chronic respiratory tract infections due in part to impaired coughing, reactive airway disease, respiratory difficulty after general anesthesia)
- Genital anomalies in females (e.g., genital sinus, urethral atresia, vesicovaginal fistula, vaginal atresia, and bicornuate uterus). Ovaries in affected female patients are typically normal.
- Cardiac anomalies: Effect up to 10% of patients (e.g., patent ductus arteriosus [PDA], atrial septal defect [ASD], ventricular septal defect [VSD], tetralogy of Fallot [TOF])

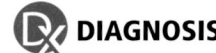 **DIAGNOSIS**

HISTORY
In patients with mild involvement of the abdominal wall that is not detected in the neonatal period, evaluation of UTIs may reveal the dilated urinary tract.

PHYSICAL EXAM
- Dilated urinary tract
- Abdominal wall is characterized by multiple wrinkles and redundant skin.
- A large, distended bladder creates a suprapubic mass.
- Ureters and kidneys are readily palpable.
- Intestinal loops and peristalsis may be observed.
- Testes are undescended.
- Myopathy results in difficulty in sitting up from a supine position.
- Abnormal gait secondary to congenital hip dislocation and abdominal muscular hypoplasia.
- Chronic constipation from abdominal muscular hypoplasia.

DIAGNOSTIC TESTS & INTERPRETATION
Lab
- Serum levels of creatinine and BUN may be elevated.
- Renal failure may result in anemia and elevated levels of potassium, phosphorus, hydrogen ion, and uric acid, and decreased concentrations of sodium, calcium, and bicarbonate.

Imaging
- Ultrasound will demonstrate dilatation and redundancy of the upper urinary tract.
- When considering a voiding cystourethrogram, assess possible risk of introducing infection into dilated, poorly draining urinary tract.
- Renal function and drainage of the dilated tract can be assessed by radioisotope renal scan or an excretory urogram.

Diagnostic Procedures/Other
Initial evaluation should include assessment of renal function.

DIFFERENTIAL DIAGNOSIS
- Distinctly abnormal findings of physical exam of the affected infant results in an early, accurate diagnosis in most cases.
- Pseudo–prune belly syndrome (e.g., prune belly syndrome uropathy, normal abdominal wall exam, and incomplete or absent cryptorchidism)

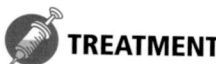# TREATMENT

SURGERY/OTHER PROCEDURES
- Some clinicians advocate minimal surgical intervention, based on lack of functional obstruction and that the dilated system has a low pressure owing to the deficient smooth musculature. If renal function deteriorates, urinary tract dilation progresses, or the patient develops a UTI despite antibiotic prophylaxis, cutaneous vesicostomy is recommended to facilitate drainage.
- Other physicians advocate extensive surgical remodeling. Possible procedures include, as indicated:
  - Internal urethrotomy, reduction cystoplasty
  - Excision of the redundant ureter with reimplantation of the remaining segment
  - Cutaneous ureterostomy
  - Pyelostomy
- Reconstruction of the abdominal wall has yielded good cosmetic results but only questionable improvements in physical function.
- Bilateral orchiopexy is indicated.

IN-PATIENT CONSIDERATIONS
Initial Stabilization
- Basic principles of supportive care and management of renal failure apply.
- Antibiotics in the neonatal period and antibiotic prophylactic of indefinite duration are indicated to prevent infection.

ONGOING CARE

FOLLOW-UP RECOMMENDATIONS
Regardless of how patients are managed, affected patients require long-term follow-up, with meticulous attention to renal function, pulmonary function, and urine bacteriology.

PROGNOSIS
- Patients with the most severe renal dysplasia and pulmonary hypoplasia (e.g., sequelae of severe, early oligohydramnios) succumb as neonates.
- Associated with a mortality rate of up to 20% in the neonatal period.
- ~25% of patients with prune belly syndrome who survive the neonatal period will progress to end-stage renal disease (ESRD).
- Those with a milder form do not require urinary tract surgery; renal function is usually stable and prognosis excellent.
- For patients with moderate involvement, the degree of renal dysplasia and insufficiency determines outcome. In addition, upper urinary tract stasis, poor bladder emptying, vesicoureteral reflux, and bacteriuria are factors that may combine to worsen the long-term prognosis.

COMPLICATIONS
- Pulmonary hypoplasia
- Frequent UTIs secondary to upper urinary stasis, vesicoureteral reflux, and bacteriuria
- Sequelae of progressive renal insufficiency

ADDITIONAL READING
- Dénes FT, Arap MA, Giron AM, et al. Comprehensive surgical treatment of prune belly syndrome: 17 years' experience with 32 patients. *Urology.* 2004;64(4):789–793.
- Jennings RW. Prune belly syndrome. *Semin Pediatr Surg.* 2000;9:115–20.
- Noh PH, Cooper CS, Winkler AC, et al. Prognostic factors for long-term renal function in boys with the prune-belly syndrome. *J Urol.* 1999;162:1399–1401.

- Strand WR. Initial management of complex pediatric disorders: Prunebelly syndrome, posterior urethral valves. *Urol Clin North Am.* 2004;31(3):399–415, vii.
- Sutherland RS, Mevorach RA, Kogan BA. The prune-belly syndrome: Current insights. *Pediatr Nephrol.* 1995;9:770–778.
- Wisanuyotin S, Dell KM, Vogt BA, et al. Complications of peritoneal dialysis in children with Eagle-Barrett syndrome. *Pediatr Nephrol.* 2003;18:159–163.
- Woodard JR, Zucker I. Lessons learned in 3 decades of managing the prune-belly syndrome. *Urol Clin North Am.* 1990;17:407.
- Woods AG, Brandon DH. Prune belly syndrome. A focused physical assessment. *Adv Neonatal Care.* 2007;7(3):132–143.

CODES

ICD9
756.71 Prune belly syndrome

ICD10
Q79.4 Prune belly syndrome

FAQ
- Q: Are patients with prune belly syndrome candidates for renal transplantation?
- A: Yes. However, special pretransplantation consideration should be given to patients with a dilated urinary tract to optimize function.
- Q: How does the urinary tract function in older children?
- A: A tendency for bladder tone and ureteral peristalsis to improve with age has been noted.
- Q: Are such patients infertile?
- A: Normal sexual activity has been described. However, there are no reports of fertility, and the patients usually have azoospermia.
- Q: What is the usual cause of morbidity in the newborn period?
- A: Respiratory failure.

PRURITUS

Mark L. Bagarazzi

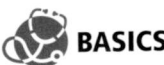 **BASICS**

DEFINITION
Itching—an unpleasant cutaneous sensation that provokes the desire to rub or scratch the skin to obtain relief

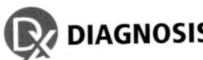 **DIAGNOSIS**

DIFFERENTIAL DIAGNOSIS
- **Congenital/anatomic**
  - Cholestasis secondary to biliary obstruction (e.g., Alagille syndrome)
- **Infectious**
  - Pinworms (*Enterobius vermicularis*):
    - ○ Pruritus that is worse at night is seen with scabies or pinworm.
  - Swimmer's itch (due to fresh water mammalian or avian schistosomes):
    - ○ If the child was recently swimming in fresh water, consider swimmer's itch, caused by fresh water mammalian or avian schistosomes.
  - Seabather eruption (affects swimmers and divers in marine waters off Florida, in the Gulf of Mexico, and the Caribbean, attributed to various organisms but more recently to the larvae of the thimble jellyfish), *Linuche unguiculata*
  - Herpes virus: Primary varicella infection or herpes zoster; herpes simplex
  - *Borrelia burgdorferi*: Erythema chronicum migrans lesion associated with Lyme disease
  - *Streptococcus pyogenes*: Sandpaper rash of scarlet fever
  - Tinea corporis
  - *Toxocariasis canis*
- **Toxic**
  - Contact dermatitis (see Table 1):

Table 1. Potential contact irritants

Medications (see below)	Plants (e.g., rhus dermatitis—poison ivy/oak, cacti)
Allergens	Foods
Cosmetics	Capsaicin in hot peppers*
Chemicals (e.g., soaps and detergents)	Animals
Dyes (for hair, etc.)	Clothing (e.g., wool)
Jewelry (nickel)	Shoes
Fiberglass	Diapers
Excrement	

*Acts as an irritant on first contact but may actually decrease pruritus if applied repeatedly over weeks

- **Environmental**
  - Papular urticaria: Bites of fleas, mosquitoes
  - Pediculosis (lice)
  - Mites: Scabies (*Sarcoptes scabiei*), chiggers (*Trombicula alfreddugesi*)
  - Subcutaneous foreign body
  - Phytophotodermatitis occurs when skin is exposed to sunlight after contact with an offending plant.
- **Drugs**
  - Systemic use of medications (e.g., aminophylline, aspirin, barbiturates, chloroquine, erythromycin, gold, griseofulvin, iodine contrast dyes, isoniazid, opiates, phenothiazines, vitamin A)
- **Allergic, inflammatory**
  - Atopic dermatitis (eczema)
  - Psoriasis (pruritus is often persistent)
  - Seborrheic dermatitis
- **Miscellaneous**
  - Burns
  - Nonspecific urticaria
  - Pityriasis rosea
  - Asteatotic eczema ("winter itch")
  - Xerosis (dry skin) due to excess bathing with or without strong detergents or low humidity; idiopathic

APPROACH TO THE PATIENT
Determine severity and if pruritus is isolated or due to an underlying systemic illness, primarily by assessing the presence or absence of associated signs and symptoms, especially rash.

- **Phase 1:** Assess severity of illness. Pruritus rarely constitutes a medical emergency except in cases of anaphylaxis or erythema multiforme major (i.e., Stevens–Johnson syndrome).
- **Phase 2:** A thorough review of potential precipitating events and the duration of symptoms will help determine if the itch is isolated or if there are any associated signs or symptoms. Pruritus is most frequently associated with rash. Pruritus with or without rash may be a manifestation of systemic illness. Underlying states may range from hepatic or renal diseases to pregnancy or psychiatric disease. As always, differential diagnosis should consider common causes first, then entertain less common and even rare causes.
- **Phase 3:** A thorough history and physical exam should narrow the differential diagnosis considerably, enabling the clinician to determine the underlying cause of the complaint in most cases. Laboratory tests may be indicated in cases where the diagnosis remains unclear.

HISTORY
- **Question:** New or recurrent problem?
- *Significance:* If it is new, one should ask if there is anything new in the child's life that may be associated with the onset of pruritus (with or without rash). This is often the most revealing question as one may find that the child recently came in contact with a new item, which is known to be a contact irritant.
- **Question:** How severe is the pruritus? On a scale of 1–10? Compared with a mosquito bite? Is it severe enough to interfere with the daily routine of the child (e.g., wakes the child from sleep)?
- *Significance:* Answers will provide some measure of the true severity of the problem. Waking from sleep may suggest a more severe form resulting from systemic disease.
- **Question:** Introduction of anything new or different, especially anything that comes in contact with the child's skin?
- *Significance:*
  - Frequency of baths and types of products used to bathe the child
  - Different soaps or detergents contain additives that may be allergenic. Changes in soaps may be important. Some soaps cause excessive dryness or contain heavy fragrances. Children who are bathed frequently with anything more than water may develop dry and irritated (pruritic) skin.
- **Question:** Hiking or camping in a wooded area?
- *Significance:* May be a clue to common skin irritation (rhus dermatitis) from contact with certain plants
- **Question:** Any underlying illness(es) or associated symptoms?
- *Significance:* Pruritus associated with night sweats and fever may point to hematopoietic malignancy. Many illnesses are associated with pruritus.
- **Question:** Complaints about itching from anyone who has frequent contact with the child?
- *Significance:* May identify a common source of a contact irritant. For example, one will often see multiple family members affected by scabies or lice.
- **Question:** Is the pruritus accompanied by rash or other signs and symptoms?
- *Significance:* This general question is meant to elicit additional signs and symptoms of any systemic disease. For instance, arthritis and arthralgias are seen in systemic lupus erythematosus and juvenile rheumatoid arthritis, and jaundice in the cholestatic disorders.
- **Question:** Itching has happened before?
- *Significance:* Atopic dermatitis will present as chronic or recurrent pruritic skin lesions.

P

PHYSICAL EXAM
* **Finding:** If rash is present, appearance of rash?
* *Significance*:
  – Lesions appear in crops with varicella zoster, scabies, and insect bites.
  – Lesions are in groups of 3 or 4 with a central punctum in scabies.
  – Papular lesions result from insect bites, chiggers, pediculosis, contact dermatitis, pityriasis rosea, urticaria (wheal), and atopic dermatitis.
  – Lichenification (i.e., plaque and scale formation) occurs with psoriasis, xerosis, tinea, and atopic dermatitis.
  – Serpiginous lesions occur with cutaneous larva migrans and myiasis (or maggots).
  – Vesicular lesions occur in varicella (generalized), scabies, poison ivy (linear), and atopic dermatitis.
  – Dry skin (xerosis) occurs in atopic dermatitis.
  – Christmas tree pattern occurs in pityriasis rosea.
* **Finding:** Location of the itch and/or rash?
* *Significance*:
  – Generalized distribution: Consider varicella
  – Anus: Consider pinworms
  – Back: Consider pityriasis rosea
  – Axillae and/or genital/diaper area: Consider seborrheic dermatitis and scabies
  – Dorsal foot: Consider shoe dermatitis from rubber or tanning agents
  – Exposed surfaces: Consider schistosomal dermatitis and poison ivy
  – Finger, earlobe, wrist, or necklace distribution: Consider irritant contact dermatitis (e.g., nickel)
  – Nipples: Consider scabies (burrows)
  – Interdigital areas and ulnar borders: Consider tinea pedis, scabies (burrows)
  – Palms and/or soles: Consider biliary cirrhosis
  – Plantar foot: Consider cutaneous larva migrans
  – Scalp: Consider pediculosis (nits found cemented to hair shaft) and tinea capitis
* **Finding:** Abnormal affect or mood?
* *Significance*: If after an exhaustive search there appears to be no physiologic basis for the itch, one must consider whether the complaint is a conversion disorder or due to neurotic excoriation, especially in cases of abnormal affect or mood.
* **Finding:** Enlargement of liver, spleen, or lymph nodes?
* *Significance*: Pruritus may be the initial manifestation of lymphoma.

DIAGNOSTIC TESTS & INTERPRETATION
* **Test:** Complete blood count with differential
* *Significance*: Presence of eosinophilia suggests atopy or parasitic infections.
* **Test:** Wood lamp examination, potassium hydroxide preparation
* *Significance*: Screen for tinea infections
* **Test:** Serum for hepatic and renal function
* *Significance*: Screen for underlying disease
* **Test:** Urinalysis for β-human chorionic gonadotropin
* *Significance*: Investigate presence of cholestasis associated with pregnancy

 ## TREATMENT

ADDITIONAL TREATMENT
General Measures
Antihistamines are the mainstay of symptomatic treatment of pruritus.

* Systemic and topical corticosteroids and topical pramoxine and doxepin have been shown to be effective in placebo-controlled trials.
* Some anecdotal references to other agents that are effective for pruritus include ursodeoxycholic acid in liver disease, opiate antagonists (e.g., naloxone and naltrexone), propofol at subhypnotic doses, cholestyramine, rifampin, gabapentin in burn-related pruritus, and serotonin antagonists (e.g., ondansetron).
* Tacrolimus and pimecrolimus have been used as second-line therapy for the short-term and noncontinuous chronic treatment of mild-to-moderate atopic dermatitis in non-immunocompromised children 2 years of age and older, who have failed to respond adequately to other topical prescription treatments, or when those treatments are not advisable. These drugs carry a "black box" warning about a possible risk of cancer and a Medication Guide. The Medication Guide is to be distributed with each prescription to help ensure that patients using these prescription medicines are aware of this concern.
* Exploratory studies of virtual reality immersion (VRI), an advanced computer-generated technique, show reduction of pruritus intensity before and during VRI.

Initial Stabilization
Pruritus due to anaphylaxis will require initial management of circulation, breathing and airway (CABs) followed by sympathomimetics (e.g., epinephrine), antihistamines (e.g., diphenhydramine), corticosteroids, and possibly fluid resuscitation.

ISSUES FOR REFERRAL
* Identification of an underlying disorder or state
* Some severe cases of atopic dermatitis or psoriasis may require dermatologic referral.
* Identification of pubic pediculosis may require investigation for child sexual abuse.

ADDITIONAL READING
* Charlesworth EN, Beltrani VS. Pruritic dermatoses: Overview of etiology and therapy. *Am J Med*. 2002;113(Suppl 9A):25S–33S.
* Greaves MW. Pathogenesis and treatment of pruritus. *Curr Allergy Asthma Rep*. 2010;10: 236–242.
* Millikan LE. Pruritus: Unapproved treatments or indications. *Clin Dermatol*. 2000;18:149–152.
* Paus R, Schmelz M, Biro T, et al. Frontiers in pruritus research: Scratching the brain for more effective itch therapy. *J Clin Invest*. 2006;116:1174–1186.
* Wahlgren CF. Itch and atopic dermatitis: An overview. *J Dermatol*. 1999;26:770–779.

CODES

ICD9
698.9 Unspecified pruritic disorder
ICD10
L29.9 Pruritus, unspecified

FAQ
* Q: Does the time course of a pruritic rash give any clue in identifying the offending agent?
* A: Yes, certain plants cause an immediate welt on the skin, but the urticaria is short-lived (immediate contact dermatitis). Skin that is traumatized mechanically (e.g., cactus spine) or chemically (e.g., capsaicin as found in hot peppers) produces more persistent skin reactions. Poison ivy or rhus dermatitis is a type of allergic contact dermatitis that only occurs in those previously sensitized. It is due to a cellular immune response and may persist for several weeks.
* Q: Are some antihistamines better than others for pruritus?
* A: Possibly; evidence is conflicting, but several studies have shown that older systemic antihistamines that cause greater somnolence are actually more effective at alleviating pruritus than newer, longer-acting antihistamines (e.g., astemizole, loratadine, terfenadine, cetirizine).
* Q: Do topical antihistamines alleviate pruritus?
* A: Not usually, except for widespread pruritus seen with insect bites and urticaria. Use of topical antihistamines for pruritus or rash that is widespread should be discouraged, because toxicity may result from systemic absorption.
* Q: Does scratching make the pruritus better or worse?
* A: Worse; scratching leads to the release of the mediators of inflammation including histamine which, in turn, leads to more pruritus, thus creating a vicious cycle.
* Q: Are there any useful adjuncts to reduce pruritus?
* A: Yes, keeping skin moist with moisturizers and avoiding dry environments. Avoid overwashing, especially with hot water and/or alkaline soaps.

PSITTACOSIS

Nicholas Tsarouhas

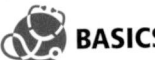 **BASICS**

DESCRIPTION
- An acute febrile disease characterized by pneumonitis and other systemic symptoms. The name is derived from the Greek for parrot, *psittakos*.
- Also known as *ornithosis*.

EPIDEMIOLOGY
- Birds (e.g., pigeons, parrots, parakeets, turkeys, chickens, ducks) are the major reservoir.
- Infecting agent present in bird nasal secretions, urine, feces, feathers, viscera, and carcasses.
- Inhalation of aerosols of feces, urine, and secretions of infected birds is the most common route of infection.
- Bird bites and mouth-to-beak contact also spread infection.
- Birds may be healthy or sick.
- Most reported cases (70%) are the result of exposure to pet caged birds (especially parrots, parakeets).
- Most common mammalian source of infection is sheep.
- Occupational hazard of workers in poultry plants, pet shops, zoos, farms
- Rarely transmitted person-to-person

Incidence
- Only 100–200 total cases reported in U.S. each year
- Very rare disease in young children

RISK FACTORS
Close human contact with birds, and in some cases, sheep

GENERAL PREVENTION
- Epidemiologic investigation is indicated in all suspected cases.
- Birds suspected to be infected should be killed, transported, and analyzed by qualified experts.
- Potentially contaminated living areas where bird was kept should be disinfected and aired.
- *Chlamydophila psittaci* is susceptible to most household disinfectants (rubbing alcohol, Lysol, bleach).

PATHOPHYSIOLOGY
- Inhalation of aerosolized organisms into the respiratory tract
- Incubation period 5–21 days
- Spreads via bloodstream to lungs, liver, and spleen
- Lymphocytic inflammatory alveolar response

ETIOLOGY
- Infection produced by *C. psittaci*, an obligate intracellular parasitic bacterium
- Antigenically and genetically different from *Chlamydia* species

COMMONLY ASSOCIATED CONDITIONS
Pneumonitis (with a severe headache) is a common presentation.

 DIAGNOSIS

HISTORY
- Mandatory to question parents about exposure of the patient to any type of bird—wild or domestic
- Signs and symptoms:
  - Abrupt onset of symptoms
  - Fever, headache, cough, weakness, chills, muscle aches, and joint pain
  - Nonproductive cough
  - Vomiting, confusion, and photophobia are less common findings.

PHYSICAL EXAM
- Ill-appearance, tachypnea, rales, and splenomegaly are common.
- A relative bradycardia is found in some cases.
- Rash, meningismus, pharyngeal injection, cervical adenopathy, hepatomegaly, and mental status changes are less common findings.

DIAGNOSTIC TESTS & INTERPRETATION
Lab
- Routine laboratory studies are rarely helpful.
- Complement fixation titers (see "FAQ")
- Microimmunofluorescence studies and polymerase chain reaction assays are more specific than complement fixation studies.
- Isolation of the organism is diagnostic.
- Complement fixation titers do not, however, distinguish between chlamydial infections (*C. trachomatis*), and the various chlamydophilal infections (*C. psittaci*, *C. pneumoniae*, and *C. pecorum*).

Imaging
- Chest x-rays are abnormal in 90% of hospitalized cases.
- Chest x-rays often demonstrate diffuse interstitial infiltrates, but may also have unilateral lower lobe consolidation.

DIFFERENTIAL DIAGNOSIS
- Psittacosis should be considered in all fevers of unknown origin or atypical pneumonitis.
- *Mycoplasma* and *Chlamydophila pneumoniae*, *Legionella* spp., *Coxiella burnetii* (i.e., Q fever), tuberculosis, viral and fungal pneumonitis, as well as pneumococcal pneumonia

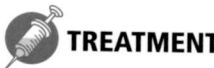 TREATMENT

MEDICATION (DRUGS)
First Line
- Tetracycline (40 mg/kg/d) or doxycycline (100 mg b.i.d.) in children >8 years of age
- Erythromycin (40 mg/kg/d) in children <8 years of age.
- Antibiotics should be continued for at least 10–14 days after defervescence.

Second Line
Azithromycin, clarithromycin, and chloramphenicol are additional options.

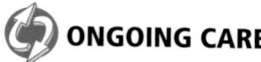 ONGOING CARE

PROGNOSIS
- Although complete recovery is the rule (even without antibiotic use), fatality rates as high as 15–20% have been reported.
- Resolution of fever and most other systemic symptoms can be expected within 48 hours of antibiotic therapy.
- Untreated patients may have severe pulmonary symptoms for 1–3 weeks.

COMPLICATIONS
- Hepatitis
- Anemia
- Thrombophlebitis
- Pulmonary embolus
- Adult respiratory distress syndrome
- Arthritis
- Keratoconjunctivitis
- Endocarditis
- Myocarditis
- Pericarditis
- Encephalitis: Agitation, delirium, confusion, stupor

ADDITIONAL READING

- American Academy of Pediatrics. Chlamydophila (formerly Chlamydia) psittaci. In Pickering LK, ed., *2009 Red Book: Report of the Committee on Infectious Diseases*, 28th ed. Elk Grove Village, IL: American Academy of Pediatrics, 2009:251–252.
- Cunha BA. The atypical pneumonia: Current clinical concepts focusing on legionnaires' disease. *Curr Opin Pulm Med*. 2008;14:183–194.
- Cunha BA. The atypical pneumonias: Clinical diagnosis and importance. *Clin Microbiol Infect*. 2006;12(Suppl 3):12–24.
- Gregory DW, Schaffner W. Psittacosis. *Semin Respir Infect*. 1997;12:7–11.
- Petrovay F, Balla E. Two fatal cases of psittacosis caused by Chlamydophila psittaci. *J Med Microbiol*. 2008;57:1296–1298.
- Scully RE. Weekly clinicopathological exercises: Psittacosis causing acute respiratory distress syndrome. *N Engl J Med*. 1998;338:1527–1535.
- Telfer BL, Moberley SA, Hort KP, et al. Probable psittacosis outbreak linked to wild birds. *Emerg Infect Dis*. 2005;11(3):391–397.

 CODES

ICD9
- 073.0 Ornithosis with pneumonia
- 073.8 Ornithosis with unspecified complication
- 073.9 Ornithosis, unspecified

ICD10
- A70 Chlamydia psittaci infections
- J17 Pneumonia in diseases classified elsewhere

FAQ
- Q: In children with pneumonia who have a pet bird, how is the diagnosis confirmed?
- A: An IgM titer of 1:16 or greater by microimmunofluorescence (MIF) assay, a 4-fold rise in IgG antibody titers by complement fixation or MIF assay (acute and convalescent specimens; 2–3 weeks apart); a single IgG titer of 1:32 or higher, or a positive culture.
- Q: Does the source bird usually exhibit signs of disease?
- A: No. The bird is often asymptomatic; it may, however, show some signs of illness (e.g., anorexia, ruffled feathers, depression, or watery green droppings).

P

PSORIASIS

Leslie Castelo-Soccio
Albert Yan (5th edition)

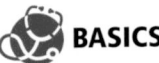

BASICS

DESCRIPTION
Skin disease characterized by a chronic relapsing nature and, most commonly, clinical features of scaly, erythematous papules, and plaques with thick white scale, usually involving elbows, knees, and scalp (i.e., psoriasis vulgaris). Other variants include guttate, erythrodermic, and pustular psoriasis (see "Physical Exam" for details).

EPIDEMIOLOGY
- No gender predilection
- Onset of psoriasis is bimodal, commonly presenting in the 3rd decade with a smaller 2nd peak of onset in the 6th decade; however, it can present at any age, with a mean age of onset in children of 8.1 years.
- Earlier onset is associated with more severe disease.

Prevalence
Psoriasis is universal in occurrence, but the prevalence varies in different populations. The average prevalence in the U.S. is estimated at 1–3%

RISK FACTORS
Genetics
- Although psoriasis has a strong genetic influence, mode of transmission is not defined. It is likely multifactorial with more than one gene involved and is modified by environmental influence.
- 1/3 of patients with psoriasis report a relative with the disease.
- In family studies, 8.1% of children develop psoriasis when 1 parent is affected.
- When both parents have psoriasis, the affected percentage increases to 41%.
- In twin studies, 65% of monozygotic twins are concordant for the disease, whereas only 30% of dizygotic twins are concordant.

PATHOPHYSIOLOGY
- Plaque-type psoriasis is characterized by a thickened parakeratotic epidermis with an absent granular layer above dermal papillae containing dilated tortuous capillaries.
- Collections of polymorphonuclear leukocytes extend from the dermal papillae into the epidermidis stratum corneum (i.e., Munro microabscesses).
- A mixed perivascular infiltrate is confined to the papillary dermis.

ETIOLOGY
The pathogenesis is unknown. Well-defined trigger factors include:
- Trauma to normal skin, producing psoriasis in the area (i.e., isomorphic response, sometimes called the Koebner phenomenon)
- Infections (e.g., upper respiratory infections, *Streptococcus pyogenes*, human immunodeficiency virus)
- Stress
- Winter in colder climates in northern hemisphere
- Some drugs (i.e., systemic corticosteroids, lithium, ®-adrenergic blockers, NSAIDs, and antimalarials)

COMMONLY ASSOCIATED CONDITIONS
Leukocytosis and hypocalcemia are associated with pustular psoriasis.

DIAGNOSIS

HISTORY
- 1st appearance of eruption
- Area involved
- Recent illness, particularly sore throat
- Recent medications, particularly systemic steroids
- Any appearance of lesions with trauma to skin
- Joint pain
- Previous treatments and response
- Improvement with sun exposure
- Family history of psoriasis
- Signs and symptoms:
  - Thick, flaky scales on skin
  - In psoriasis vulgaris, sharply demarcated erythematous plaques with white scale are located most commonly on the elbows, knees, scalp, lumbar area, and umbilicus, but they can cover any surface and large areas of the body. Intertriginous regions are often involved, but scale is absent.
  - Guttate psoriasis is a form that more often presents in children and young adults as small papules (0.5–1.5 cm), with limited scale over the trunk and proximal extremities, and is frequently associated with streptococcal infection.
  - Erythema with variable scale involving the majority of the body accompanied by chills is characteristic of erythrodermic psoriasis.
  - Generalized pustular psoriasis is the most serious variant, with sterile pustules as large as 23 mm arising on erythematous skin over large areas of the body. Usually, such appearance is accompanied by high fever.

- A chronic and localized variant of pustular disease, however, involves only the palms and soles.
  - Note: Classic plaque psoriasis is easily diagnosed, but variants and less virulent cases require careful exam for physical clues.
- Nails are frequently involved, with pinpoint pits, hyperkeratosis, and oil spots.
- Areas where disease is hidden are the retroauricular portion of the scalp and the perianal region.
- Swollen or deformed joints suggest associated psoriatic arthritis.

PHYSICAL EXAM
- A complete cutaneous exam is necessary.
- Removal of scale on plaques produces bleeding points, a feature known as the Auspitz sign.
- The Koebner phenomenon may produce linear or geometric lesions corresponding to areas of trauma.

DIAGNOSTIC TESTS & INTERPRETATION
Lab
- Common finding: Elevated uric acid level. *S. pyogenes* infection is frequent in guttate disease, and throat culture is appropriate.
- Other laboratory values are generally within normal ranges. However, in more severe variants, anemia, elevated ESR, and decreased albumin levels may be found.

DIFFERENTIAL DIAGNOSIS
- Classic plaque psoriasis is easily diagnosed. Variants of psoriasis, including guttate, erythrodermic, and pustular disease, are more difficult to recognize.
- The differential diagnosis varies with the type of psoriasis and includes:
  - Nummular eczema
  - Cutaneous T-cell lymphoma
  - Tinea corporis
  - Pityriasis rosea
  - Pityriasis lichenoides et varioliformis acuta
  - Secondary syphilis
  - Atopic dermatitis
  - Drug eruption
  - Candidiasis
  - Seborrheic dermatitis

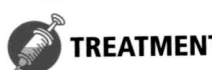

TREATMENT

ADDITIONAL TREATMENT
General Measures
- Phototherapy:
  - UVB:
    - Administered between 3–7 times weekly in a booth with bulbs that emit the appropriate wavelength of UV radiation
    - Effective for guttate and plaque psoriasis
    - Average treatment time: 3 months, with gradual increases in time of exposure. Sunscreen should be used on the face.
    - Narrow-band UVB represents a form of monochromatic UVB, using 311 nm wavelengths; appears to be a somewhat more effective form of delivering UVB phototherapy

– PUVA (psoralen and UVB):
  ○ PUVA and oral medications (e.g., methotrexate, acitretin) should be reserved for severe cases and carefully monitored by a dermatologist.

ALERT
- Possible conflicts with other drugs: Photosensitizing medication (e.g., tetracyclines, sulfa derivatives, phenothiazines, among others) should be avoided with phototherapy.
- Topical:
  – Topical corticosteroids
    ○ Mid- to high-potency topical corticosteroid ointments are applied b.i.d.
    ○ Mid-potency preparations (e.g., 0.025% fluocinolone ointment, 0.1% triamcinolone acetonide) are preferred in children.
    ○ Low-potency corticosteroids (e.g., 1.0% and 2.5% hydrocortisone) are used on the face and intertriginous regions to prevent atrophy.
    ○ Agents can also be found in shampoos (e.g., Derma-Smoothe FS and Capex).
  – Anthralin:
    ○ Anthralin, applied to plaques for a 30-minute application, should be carefully washed off.
    ○ Lower concentrations used initially (e.g., 0.1%, 0.25%) are increased gradually as tolerated (e.g., 0.5%, 1.0%).
    ○ Irritation and staining are common, so that the face and intertriginous regions cannot be treated with this approach.
  – Calcipotriene:
    ○ Calcipotriene ointment is a vitamin D_3 derivative often used to treat disease in adults.
    ○ It is applied b.i.d., avoiding the face and intertriginous regions.
    ○ Maximum weekly dosage in adults is 100 g.
    ○ Rare cases of hypercalcemia have been reported.
    ○ Although effective in children, safety guidelines have not been established.
  – Tazarotene gel:
    ○ A topical retinoid (i.e., 0.05% and 0.1%)
    ○ Can be mildly to moderately irritating when used as monotherapy
    ○ Often combined with topical steroids as adjunctive therapy applied once daily or b.i.d.
  – Coal tar:
    ○ A weak therapeutic agent as monotherapy
    ○ More effective when combined with UVB phototherapy
    ○ Used in various shampoo preparations, as well as in solution that can be added to the bath.
  – Systemic agents:
    ○ May be considered when the psoriasis is especially severe, or when joint symptoms are prominent. In these instances, consultation with a rheumatologist may be advisable.
    ○ Methotrexate
    ○ Isotretinoin or acitretin
    ○ Cyclosporine
    ○ Biologic agents, such as etanercept
    ○ Systemic corticosteroid should be avoided since withdrawal from steroid may be accompanied by a pustular psoriasis flare.

ISSUES FOR REFERRAL
- Pustules, a significant increase in degree or extent of erythema, or fever suggest progression of the disease to more serious variants and may require hospitalization and systemic therapy.
- Erythrodermic psoriasis may require hospitalization to address issues of impaired skin integrity, such as fluid–electrolyte imbalances, hypothermia, and sepsis.
- New evidence suggests that adult patients with psoriasis have an increased prevalence of cardiovascular disease and an increased risk for myocardial infarction. Patients should be monitored for increased cardiovascular risk factors and have blood pressure, glucose, weight and lipids under good control to decrease risk.

IN-PATIENT CONSIDERATIONS
Initial Stabilization
- Therapy is delivered by topical medications, phototherapy, or systemic medications.
- Localized disease is treated with topical therapy and more diffuse disease with phototherapy.
- Systemic medications are reserved for resistant cases.
- Except in the most severe cases, therapy for children should be limited to topical medication and UVB phototherapy.
- General skin care should include gentle washing, soaking to remove scale, and application of emollients, preferably ointments and creams.

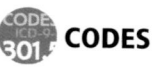 ONGOING CARE

FOLLOW-UP RECOMMENDATIONS
- Topical therapy is administered chronically, with breaks to minimize side effects.
- Remissions occur in summer with sun exposure, and medications may often be discontinued.
- The average treatment course with UVB therapy is 3 months; if the patient's skin clears, treatment may be followed by an average remission period of 5 months.

PROGNOSIS
- Once psoriasis appears, it generally persists throughout life.
- Spontaneous remissions of variable length and frequency occur but are unpredictable.
- Response depends on potency of medication and frequency of treatment.
- Improvement with topical medication is obvious at 2 weeks, and usually peaks at 2 months.
- 1 month of UVB therapy may produce a decrease in disease.
- If therapy is too aggressive, disease may worsen, due to irritation.
- Scrubbing by the patient to remove scales also irritates the disease.
- Psychologic aspects of the disease, particularly in children, should be addressed.

ADDITIONAL READING

- Al Robaee AA. Molecular genetics of psoriasis (Principles, technology, gene location, genetics polymorphisms and gene expression). *In J Health Sci.* 2010;4:103–127.
- Capella GL, Finzi AF. Psoriasis and other papulosquamous diseases in infants and children. *Clin Dermatol.* 2000;18:701–709.
- de Jong EM. The course of psoriasis. *Clin Dermatol.* 1997;15:687–692.
- Farber EM. Early intervention can reduce risks for problems later. *Postgrad Med.* 1998;103:89–92, 95–96, 99–100 passim.
- Gelfand JM, Mehta NN, Langan SM. Psoriasis and cardiovascular risk: Strength in numbers, part II. *J Invest Dermatol.* 2011;13:1007–1010.
- Kim NN, Lio PA, Morgan GA, et al. Double trouble: Therapeutic challenges in patients with both juvenile dermatomyositis and psoriasis. *Arch Dermatol.* 2011 March; epub ahead of print.
- Lapolla W, Yentzer BA, Bagel J, et al. A review of phototherapy protocols for psoriasis treatment. *J Am Acad Dermatol.* 2011;64:936–949.
- Leman J, Burden D. Psoriasis in children: A guide to its diagnosis and management. *Paediatr Drugs.* 2001;3:673–680.
- Silverberg NB. Update on pediatric psoriasis, part 1: Clinical features and demographics. *Cutis.* 2010;86: 118–124.
- Silverberg NB. Update on pediatric psoriasis, part 2: Therapeutic management. *Cutis.* 2010;86:172–176.

CODES

ICD9
696.1 Other psoriasis

ICD10
- L40.0 Psoriasis vulgaris
- L40.4 Guttate psoriasis
- L40.9 Psoriasis, unspecified

FAQ

- Q: Will my disease get worse?
- A: It is impossible to predict the course of any patient's disease, because it is influenced by both heredity and everyday factors in the environment. Although there is no cure, with treatment the disease can be kept under control. Remissions do occur and may be for prolonged periods of time.
- Q: When my disease is in remission, what can I do to prevent it from returning?
- A: Avoiding trauma and keeping skin moist are important. In the summer, controlled sun exposure is helpful. You may have to continue other treatments at less frequent intervals. Any cases of sore throat should be cultured and treated if streptococcal disease is present. However, frequently, it is impossible to prevent recurrence of the disease.
- Q: Will my other children get psoriasis?
- A: If neither parent has psoriasis, the chances are <10% that another child will develop the disease; if 1 parent is affected, the chances increase to 15%; if both parents are affected, the chances are 50%. Therefore, unless both parents are affected, it is more likely that other children will not get psoriasis.
- Q: Does stress make psoriasis worse?
- A: Some studies have suggested that flare-ups of psoriasis are associated with increased stress. It is difficult to evaluate whether stress is the cause or the result of the disease. Do all you can to reasonably relieve stress, but do not focus on this as the cause of your psoriasis.

PUBERTAL DELAY

Daniel H. Reirden
Kenneth R. Ginsburg (5th edition)

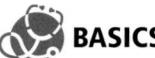 ## BASICS

DESCRIPTION
- Pubertal delay is the absence of secondary sexual characteristics by an age >2–2.5 standard deviations (*SD*) of the population mean. In the US, this is considered to be ~13 years of age for girls and 14 years of age for boys.
- Pubertal delay may also occur if progression through puberty stalls or takes longer than 2.5 *SD* from the mean time of the population.
- ~2.5% of healthy teens will meet criteria for pubertal delay.
- Most cases of pubertal delay can be ascribed to constitutional delay of growth and maturity (CDGM); however, missing the presentation of an underlying disease should be avoided.
- CDGM:
  - Likely an extreme normal variant of pubertal development
  - Children usually grow at or near the 5th%ile for most of childhood, enter puberty late, and usually reach normal adult height.
  - More common in boys than in girls
  - Strong familial component

GENERAL PREVENTION
- Begin conversations about pubertal development with both patients and parents in late childhood. Realistic expectations regarding timing can avoid undue stress and unnecessary testing.
- Examination of growth charts at routine visits can alert providers to potential problems or changes in growth.
- Children with chronic health conditions should receive counseling regarding the effect their illness may have on their puberty. For example, children with cystic fibrosis generally have delayed puberty.

EPIDEMIOLOGY
- By definition, delayed puberty will occur in 2.5% of the population.
- CDGM explains 90–95% of pubertal delay.
- >60% of patients with constitutional delay of puberty have a positive family history.

Genetics
- Pubertal timing is highly influenced by genetic factors. This is evidenced by high correlation within ethnic groups, families, and monozygotic twins.
- 50–80% of variation in timing can be explained by genetics
- Pubertal delay as a result of an underlying medical condition is influenced by the pathophysiology of each disorder.

ETIOLOGY
Deficiency of gonadal sex steroids, estrogen in girls or testosterone in boys, is the underlying cause of delayed puberty. Several pathways to the common etiology exist:
- Hypogonadotrophic hypogonadism: Delayed puberty as a result of a deficiency in secretion of gonadotropin-releasing hormone (GnRH):
  - Functional: Delay or transient decrease in GnRH secretion. Describes CDGM, hypothyroidism, chronic illness
  - Permanent: Irreversible deficiency of GnRH, such as in Kallman syndrome or panhypopituitarism
- Hypergonadotrophic hypogonadism: Generally failure of the gonad, as seen in Turner syndrome, Klinefelter syndrome, and anorchia

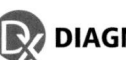 ## DIAGNOSIS

HISTORY
- A thorough history of past medical conditions, past growth patterns, and family history is essential.
- A complete review of systems to uncover an underlying chronic disorder, such as inflammatory bowel disease, is necessary.
- Request and examine a long-term growth chart:
  - CDGM will generally exhibit a consistent low percentile of growth throughout childhood.
  - Gonadotropin or gonadal causes will generally present with normal growth in childhood, but no increase in growth during the expected pubertal spurt.

- Obtain history of progression of secondary sex characteristics:
  - Adolescents with complete gonadal or gonadotropin deficiencies will not enter puberty unless initiated by exogenous or adrenal hormones, whereas those with constitutional delay will progress at a normal rate after initiation of puberty.
  - Adolescents with partial deficiencies may reach pubarche at a normal time, but will fail to progress.
- Medication history may be useful (e.g., use of glucocorticoids or cytotoxins).
- Assess nutrition and socioeconomic history: Rule out chronic malnutrition or eating disorder.

PHYSICAL EXAM
A thorough physical exam is essential. Pay particular attention to the following elements:
- Thyroid examination
- Neurologic and fundoscopic examinations to check for intracranial pathology
- Genital examination and sexual maturity rating (Tanner staging):
  - External examination for all patients
  - Breast exam for girls
  - Pubic hair
  - Penis/testicle exam for boys
  - Internal gynecologic examination for girls with amenorrhea may be indicated.
- The first sign of puberty in boys is when testicular size is >2.5 cm. Find which one of your finger segments is ~2.5 cm, and use it as a gross measure.
- As a means of screening size, using a finger is more subtle than using an orchidometer. However, when a clinician needs to follow pubertal progression closely, an orchidometer is necessary to establish testicular size accurately.

DIAGNOSTIC TESTS & INTERPRETATION
Lab
- Initial workup: routine screening tests for chronic or systemic disease:
  - CBC
  - Urinalysis
  - ESR
  - Electrolytes, renal function
  - Thyroid-stimulating hormone
  - Gonadotropin levels, follicle-stimulating hormone (FSH), and luteinizing hormone (LH)
    - Low levels suggest pre-puberty or hypothalamic-pituitary failure
    - High levels suggest gonadal failure or absence
    - If hypergonadotropic, obtain karyotype:
      - XX is suggestive of ovarian failure.
      - XO or abnormal X could be indicative of Turner syndrome or gonadal dysgenesis.
- If all of the aforementioned studies are normal, and there is no evidence to support constitutional delay, re-evaluation for cryptic chronic illness, substance abuse, eating disorder, or ongoing psychosocial stress should occur until puberty progresses or the underlying cause of delay becomes clear.

Imaging
- Bone age: Generally, an essential step in primary workup:
  - Plain film of the epiphyseal growth centers in the hand. Epiphyses change in response to growth hormone, thyroxine, and steroids of adrenal or gonadal origin.
  - Comparison to chronologic age can help to differentiate CDGM from organic disorders. A bone age that is >2 years delayed from chronologic age is consistent with CDGM but not specific, and can be found with any hypogonadotropic cause of delayed puberty.
- Pelvic ultrasound: Can be useful in locating intra-abdominal testicular structures or in determination of the presence or absence of Müllerian structures. Indicated when testes cannot be detected in patients with a male phenotype or when Müllerian structures cannot be confirmed on physical examination in patients with a female phenotype.
- CT or MRI of the head: Useful in assessing pituitary or hypothalamic structures, mass lesions, pathologic calcifications, or increased intracranial pressure if a central cause of delayed puberty is suspected

DIFFERENTIAL DIAGNOSIS
- Increased serum gonadotropins (LH/FSH):
  - Chromosomal abnormalities
  - Turner syndrome (gonadal dysgenesis)
  - Klinefelter syndrome
  - Bilateral gonadal failure
  - Cytotoxic therapy
  - Castration
  - Irradiation
  - Primary testicular failure
  - Vanishing testes syndrome
  - Trauma

- Normal or low serum gonadotropins:
  - CDGM
  - Hypothalamic dysfunction
  - Chronic illness
  - Strenuous exercise
  - Malnutrition
  - Eating disorders
  - CNS tumors
  - Hypopituitarism
  - Panhypopituitarism
  - Kallman syndrome
  - Hypothyroidism
  - Hyperprolactinemia
  - Pituitary adenoma
  - Drug associated

ALERT
- No test can make a definitive diagnosis of constitutional delay.
- Consultation with a specialist or experienced laboratory personnel is recommended before obtaining pituitary stimulation tests, as they may require special conditions.

 TREATMENT

ADDITIONAL TREATMENT
General Measures
Most patients with pubertal delay do not require drugs, but all need psychological and social support.

MEDICATION (DRUGS)
- In cases of presumed constitutional delay, hormones can be used to affect hypothalamic maturation, thereby initiating endogenous puberty.
- Referral to an endocrinologist or adolescent specialist is usually recommended before the initiation of hormonal therapy to aid in diagnosis and management.

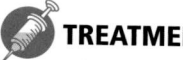 ONGOING CARE

In cases of permanent hypogonadism, because of gonadal absence, failure, or gonadotropin deficiency, long-term hormonal therapy is necessary.

ADDITIONAL READING
- Joffe A, Blythe, MJ. Abnormalities of growth and development. *Adolesc Med State Art Rev.* 2009;20: 434–441.
- Nathan BM, Palmert MR. Regulation and disorders of pubertal timing. *Endocrinol Metab Clin N Am.* 2005;34:617–641.

- Pinyerd B, Zipf WB. Puberty: Timing is everything. *J Pediatr Nurs.* 2005;20:75–82.
- Reiter EO, Lee PA. Delayed puberty. *Adolesc Med State Art Rev.* 2002;13:101–118, vii.
- Rosen DS, Foster C. Delayed puberty. *Pediatr Rev.* 2001;22:309–315.

 CODES

ICD9
- 253.4 Other anterior pituitary disorders
- 256.39 Other ovarian failure
- 259.0 Delay in sexual development and puberty, not elsewhere classified

ICD10
- E23.0 Hypopituitarism
- E28.39 Other primary ovarian failure
- E30.0 Delayed puberty

FAQ
- Q: As ~5% of pubertal delay is constitutional or physiologic, when can I avoid an expensive workup and just observe the patient?
- A: Unfortunately, only the spontaneous onset of puberty confirms the diagnosis of constitutional delay. Anxiety from delayed puberty may preclude waiting. To make a presumptive diagnosis of constitutional delay, pathology must be ruled out:
  - Physical examination, including genital anatomy and smell sense, must be normal.
  - There should be no signs or symptoms consistent with chronic disease.
  - History, including nutritional history and review of systems, must be negative.
  - Screening blood work must be negative.
  - Growth must progress ≥3.7 cm/yr.
  - Bone age must be delayed ≤4.0 years compared with chronologic age.
- Q: When should patients with pubertal delay be seen by an endocrinologist or adolescent specialist?
- A: Often, the initial workup of pubertal delay can be completed by the primary care provider. For complex stimulation tests, or if help is needed in interpreting test results, referral to an experienced specialist is warranted. If a specific chronic disease is suspected as the underlying cause, then referral should be made to the appropriate subspecialist.
- Q: Do racial differences affect pubertal onset and development?
- A: Several recent studies indicate that the mean ages for onset of breast development and menarche are younger for African American females than for Caucasian females. These differences are rarely, if ever, clinically relevant.

PULMONARY EMBOLISM
Akinyemi O. Ajayi

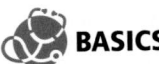 **BASICS**

DESCRIPTION
- Occlusion of a pulmonary vessel by a thrombus
- Pitfalls:
  - Failure to make the diagnosis is the most common mistake.
  - Pulmonary embolism must be suspected in critically ill children who have a central venous catheter in place and subsequently develop sudden respiratory failure. Because the symptoms of severe lung disease and pulmonary embolism are similar, the diagnosis might be missed if the index of suspicion is low.

EPIDEMIOLOGY
- Pulmonary embolism is seen more frequently in adults and tends to occur in postsurgical situations, especially when patients have been bedridden.
- ~10% of adults who present with an acute pulmonary embolus die within 1 hour of onset.
- Death occurs with 85% obstruction of the pulmonary artery.
- Risk factors vary according to age groups and gender.

Incidence
- Pulmonary embolism is rarely recognized in children; the incidence in children is 3.7%.
- Increasing incidence is secondary to increased central catheter use.
- Mortality rate can be as high as 30% if diagnosis is delayed.

RISK FACTORS
- In children:
  - Presence of a central venous catheter
  - Lack of mobility
  - Congenital heart disease
  - Ventriculoatrial shunt
  - Trauma
  - Solid tumors or leukemia
  - After surgical procedures (especially reparative intervention for scoliosis repair)
  - Hypercoagulable condition
- In adults: Most commonly due to the presence of a deep vein thrombosis, usually in the legs or pelvis.

PATHOPHYSIOLOGY
- Thromboemboli may develop anywhere in the systemic venous system.
- Pulmonary embolism is characterized by the triad of hypoxemia, pulmonary hypertension, and right ventricular failure.
- Diminished pulmonary perfusion causes a ventilation/perfusion (VQ) mismatch, resulting in hypoxemia.
- Hyperventilation occurs secondary to stimulation of proprioceptors in the lung.

- Hypercapnia is seen with severe occlusion of the pulmonary artery (often not seen with smaller emboli).
- Pulmonary infarction is uncommon owing to the presence of collateral pulmonary and bronchial arteries along with the airways providing additional sources of oxygen to the tissues.

ETIOLOGY
Blood clots appear as a result of deep vein thrombosis or other disease states.

 DIAGNOSIS

SIGNS AND SYMPTOMS
- Pulmonary embolism should be suspected in children who present with:
  - Pleuritic chest pain
  - Shortness of breath
  - Hemoptysis
  - Cough
  - Acute respiratory distress
  - Apprehension or anxiety
  - Syncope
  - Cardiovascular shock
- Symptoms may be nonspecific and indicative of other disorders.

HISTORY
Ask about chest symptoms: The clinician must have a high index of suspicion and recognize risk factors to establish the correct diagnosis.

PHYSICAL EXAM
- Findings on physical examination are nonspecific.
- General:
  - Fever
  - Diaphoresis
  - Nervousness or apprehension (altered mental status is uncommon)
- Cardiovascular:
  - Increased intensity of the pulmonic component of S2
  - Tachycardia
  - Gallop rhythm
  - New murmur
- Pulmonary:
  - Tachypnea
  - Rales
  - Cyanosis (present with 65% obstruction of the pulmonary artery)
  - Pleuritic chest pain
  - Dyspnea
  - Cough
  - Hemoptysis
  - Wheezing (uncommon)
- Extremities:
  - Deep venous thrombosis is frequently found in the adult population.
  - Phlebitis
  - Edema

DIAGNOSTIC TESTS & INTERPRETATION
Lab
- In general, blood tests are nonspecific and of no significant value in making the diagnosis of a pulmonary embolus.
- Arterial blood gases:
  - Decreased PaO_2 and $PaCO_2$
  - Increased alveolar-arterial (A-a) gradient

Imaging
- EKG:
  - Useful in ruling out other conditions
  - May show sinus tachycardia or nonspecific ST-T wave changes
- Echocardiogram:
  - Useful for identifying:
    - Abnormalities of cardiac anatomy
    - Thrombi on catheter tips
  - If emboli are seen on echocardiogram, mortality rate is 40–50%. Additionally, if signs of right ventricular dysfunction are noted (e.g., right ventricular dilatation, abnormal right ventricular wall motion, or increased tricuspid regurgitation jet velocity), risk of poor outcome is greater.
- Spiral CT:
  - New diagnostic modality
  - Greater sensitivity than ventilation/perfusion scan in the diagnosis of pulmonary embolism, due to the ability to image abnormal pulmonary pathology.
- Chest x-ray:
  - May be abnormal in 70% of patients with pulmonary embolus
  - Most frequent findings:
    - Parenchymal infiltrates
    - Atelectasis
    - Pleural effusions: Seen in 33% of cases, mostly unilateral
    - Hampton hump (pyramidal shape pointing toward the hilum)
- Ventilation/Perfusion scan
  - Results of a ventilation/perfusion scan performed to rule out a pulmonary embolus are reported in 1 of 5 categories, ranging from high probability to normal.
  - An abnormal ventilation/perfusion scan with normal ventilation and decreased perfusion in the appropriate clinical setting is 90% specific for a pulmonary embolus.
  - A normal result on ventilation/perfusion scan does not completely rule out pulmonary embolus, although if the patient is at low risk, a pulmonary embolus is highly unlikely.

- Pulmonary angiography:
  - Most sensitive and specific test
  - Not done as frequently in children as in adults because of complications of the procedure
  - With the introduction of newer, improved catheters and safer contrast solutions, this test can now safely be performed in the pediatric population.
  - Indicated for cases:
    ○ Intermediate-probability ventilation/perfusion scans
    ○ High-probability scans in patients who are: Poor candidates for anticoagulation, hemodynamically unstable, or require an embolectomy

Diagnostic Procedures/Surgery
- Pulmonary function testing:
  - Results are nonspecific.
- Evaluation of the lower extremities:
  - Diagnosing deep vein thrombosis via:
    ○ Impedance plethysmography
    ○ Doppler technology
    ○ Venography

DIFFERENTIAL DIAGNOSIS
- Cardiac:
  - Cardiac tamponade
  - Constrictive pericarditis
  - Restrictive cardiomyopathy
- Pulmonary:
  - Chronic cough
  - Status asthmaticus
  - Pneumonia with empyema
  - Pneumothorax

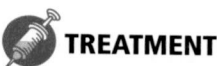 TREATMENT

ADDITIONAL TREATMENT
Initial Stabilization
- Stabilize patient before anticoagulation or thrombolytic therapy is begun:
  - Improve oxygenation.
  - Correct acidosis
  - Stabilize BP
  - Analgesia for severe pleuritic chest pain. Avoid prescribing opiates in cases of cardiovascular collapse.
- Goal of therapy is anticoagulation and/or thrombolysis.
- In patients with an intermediate or high suspicion, begin anticoagulation before investigations.

MEDICATION (DRUGS)
- Anticoagulation therapy to prevent further thrombus formation
  - Heparin:
    ○ Bolus dose: 100–200 U/kg
    ○ Maintenance dose: 10–25 U/kg/hr
    ○ Keep PTT at 55–60 seconds
    ○ Should be given for 7–10 days

- Coumadin:
  ○ Coumadin should be started 24–48 hours after heparin therapy is begun.
  ○ Maintenance dose: 2.5–10 mg/d
  ○ Keep PT twice normal and maintain the International Normalized Ratio between 2.0 and 3.0.
  ○ Should be continued for 36 months
- Thrombolytic therapy:
  - Agents available:
    ○ Streptokinase: No difference in outcome has been found using streptokinase over urokinase.
    ○ Urokinase
    ○ TPA (tissue plasminogen activator): Same efficacy as streptokinase and lower incidence of allergic reactions
  - Indications:
    ○ Hemodynamically unstable
    ○ Large embolus
- Low-molecular-weight heparin has been used as prophylaxis or as treatment for preexisting conditions in both adults and children.
  - A synthetic, nonthrombocytopenic heparin pentasaccharide with pure antifactor Xa activity is currently being tested.
- Ticlopidine and clopidogrel have been used successfully to prevent thrombotic strokes and arterial thrombotic syndromes.
- Contraindications to anticoagulation therapy:
  - Active internal bleeding
  - Recent cerebrovascular accident
  - Major surgery
  - Recent gastrointestinal bleed

SURGERY/OTHER PROCEDURES
- Embolectomy:
  - Indicated when hemodynamic instability persists; reserved for patients who have failed thrombolytic therapy or in whom medical treatment is contraindicated.
  - Late results are excellent if the patient has not suffered from a perioperative cardiac arrest, which is associated with early mortality.
- Percutaneous caval filtration:
  - Indicated if commencement or continuation of anticoagulation is strongly contraindicated, or if full anticoagulation has failed to prevent recurrent emboli.
  - This should be considered in patients undergoing venous thrombolysis, because up to 20% may develop embolization during treatment.

 ONGOING CARE

Patients receiving Coumadin therapy should have the usual follow-up for those receiving an anticoagulant.

PROGNOSIS
- If treated promptly, prognosis is good
- If treatment is delayed, especially if the patient is hemodynamically unstable, prognosis is poor.

ADDITIONAL READING
- Biss TT, Brandao LR. Clinical features and outcome of pulmonary embolism in children. *Br J Haem.* 2008;142(5):808–818.
- Fedullo PF, Tapson VF. Clinical practice. The evaluation of suspected pulmonary embolism. *N Engl J Med.* 2003;349:1247–1256.
- Goldhaber SZ, Elliott CG. Acute pulmonary embolism: Part I: Epidemiology, pathophysiology, and diagnosis. *Circulation.* 2003;108:2726–2729.
- Kruip MJ, Leclercq MG, van der Heul C, et al. Diagnostic strategies for excluding pulmonary embolism in clinical outcome studies. A systematic review. *Ann Intern Med.* 2003;138:941–951.
- Meister B, Kropshofer G, Klein-Franke A, et al. Comparison of low-molecular-weight heparin and antithrombin versus antithrombin alone for the prevention of symptomatic venous thromboembolism in children with acute lymphoblastic leukemia. *Pediatr Blood Cancer.* 2008;50(2):298–303.
- Patocka C, Nemeth J. Pulmonary embolism in pediatrics. *J Emerg Med.* 2012;42(1):105–116.
- Snow V. Management of venous thrombo-embolism in primary care: A clinical practice guideline from the American Academy of Family Physicians and the American College of Physicians. *Ann Fam Med.* 2007;5:74–80.
- Zierler BK. Ultrasonography and diagnosis of venous thromboembolism. *Circulation.* 2004;109(suppl 1): I9–I14.

 CODES

ICD9
415.19 Other pulmonary embolism and infarction

ICD10
I26.99 Other pulmonary embolism without acute cor pulmonale

FAQ
- Q: Is it safe for children on Coumadin to play contact sports?
- A: The general recommendation is that no contact sports should be allowed while children are on Coumadin therapy, because of the increased risk of bleeding.

PULMONARY HYPERTENSION
Richard M. Kravitz

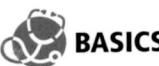 **BASICS**

DESCRIPTION
Increased pulmonary vascular resistance

EPIDEMIOLOGY
Incidence
Incidence in children is unknown.

PATHOPHYSIOLOGY
- Structural alterations in pulmonary vessel architecture (remodeling)
- Smooth muscle hypertrophy
- Extension of blood vessel's smooth muscle into smaller vessels
- Inflammation

ETIOLOGY
- Hypoxemia-induced pulmonary hypertension
- Chronic lung disease:
  - Cystic fibrosis
  - Bronchopulmonary dysplasia
  - Interstitial lung disease
  - Diaphragmatic hernia with secondary pulmonary hypoplasia
- Upper airway obstruction:
  - Tonsillar and/or adenoid hypertrophy
  - Obesity
- Hypoventilation:
  - Neurologically mediated process
  - Secondary to muscular weakness
- High pulmonary blood flow secondary to left-to-right shunting (seen in congenital heart disease):
  - Patent ductus arteriosus
  - Atrial septal defect
  - Ventricular septal defect
- Left-sided cardiac disorders that increase pulmonary venous pressure:
  - Left ventricular failure
  - Mitral valve stenosis
  - Obstructed anomalous pulmonary veins
- Occlusion of pulmonary vessels:
  - Sickle cell disease
  - Veno-occlusive disease
  - Thromboembolism
- Pulmonary vasculitis:
  - Systemic lupus erythematosus
  - Rheumatoid arthritis
  - Scleroderma
- Persistent pulmonary hypertension of the newborn
- Idiopathic cases (primary pulmonary hypertension)

DIAGNOSIS

HISTORY
- Dyspnea (usually earliest complaint reported)
- Fatigue:
  - Seen early in course of illness with exercise or exertion (but not at rest)
  - Seen at rest in the later stages of the illness or in severe cases
- Exercise intolerance
- Feeding intolerance
- Failure to thrive
- Excessive sleeping
- Diaphoresis
- Chest pain
- Syncope
- Palpitations (late finding)
- Signs and symptoms pitfalls:
  - Signs and symptoms of pulmonary hypertension are not specific and can easily be missed.
  - Consider obstructive sleep apnea as a possible cause of pulmonary hypertension (ask about snoring if suspecting pulmonary hypertension in the absence of overt cardiac or pulmonary disease).

PHYSICAL EXAM
- Typically governed by the signs and findings related to underlying lung or heart disease
- Tachypnea
- Arrhythmias
- Narrowed splitting of S2 heart sound
- Increased P2 heart sound
- Presence of S3 and/or S4 heart sounds
- Murmur of pulmonary or tricuspid insufficiency; tricuspid insufficiency more common
- Jugular venous distention
- Peripheral edema
- Hepatomegaly

DIAGNOSTIC TESTS & INTERPRETATION
Lab
Arterial blood gases:
- Measurement of pO_2 assesses degree of hypoxia.
- Evaluation of pCO_2 determines presence or absence of hypoventilation.

Imaging
Chest x-ray:
- Will vary according to the underlying disorder and extent of pulmonary hypertension
- Degree of pulmonary hypertension correlates poorly with chest x-ray findings.
- In primary pulmonary hypertension:
  - Cardiomegaly
  - Enlarged pulmonary artery
  - Peripheral lung appears underperfused ("pruning" of pulmonary vessels)

Diagnostic Procedures/Other
- EKG:
  - Can be normal if cor pulmonale has not yet developed
  - If cor pulmonale present, EKG can demonstrate:
    - Right QRS axis deviation
    - Right ventricular hypertrophy
    - Right atrial hypertrophy
- Echocardiogram with Doppler flow:
  - Increased pulmonary artery pressure
  - Right ventricular hypertrophy
  - Paradoxical movement of the intraventricular septum
  - Pulmonic and tricuspid valve regurgitation
  - Right-to-left shunting via an open foramen ovale
- Cardiac catheterization:
  - Most accurate measurement of pulmonary artery pressure is accomplished by right heart catheterization.
  - Criteria for pulmonary hypertension in children:
    - Mean pulmonary arterial pressure >25 mm Hg (at rest)
    - Mean pulmonary arterial pressure >30 mm Hg (with exercise)
    - Pulmonary vascular resistance >3 U/m^2
    - Systolic pulmonary artery pressure >1/2 systolic systemic pressure
  - Pressures should be measured before and after various vasodilators to assess potential reversibility of pulmonary hypertension.
  - Caution: In patients with severe disease, catheterization is associated with increased risk of complications.

DIFFERENTIAL DIAGNOSIS
- Pulmonary:
  - Asthma
  - Cystic fibrosis
  - Chronic obstructive pulmonary disease
  - Emphysema
  - Pulmonary arteriovenous malformations
- Miscellaneous:
  - Congestive heart failure (CHF)
  - Noncardiogenic pulmonary edema
  - Fatigue
  - Syncope

TREATMENT

MEDICATION (DRUGS)
- Oxygen:
  - Acts as a vasodilator
  - Keep $SaO_2 \geq 95\%$
  - Supplemental O_2 may prove useful even with normal resting SaO_2 (supplemental O_2 will cover for desaturations associated with exertion, exercise, or illness).
  - Caution: Supplemental oxygen can sometimes cause hypercapnia by blunting the hypoxia-driven respiratory drive.
- Anticoagulation therapy (i.e., Coumadin):
  - Prevents clot formation in the narrowed pulmonary vessels
  - Helpful even in the absence of thromboembolic disease
- Vasodilators:
  - Methods of action:
    - Decreases pulmonary arterial pressures
    - Improves right-sided cardiac function
  - Available agents:
    - Oxygen
    - Calcium-channel blocker (i.e., nifedipine)
    - Nitric oxide (continuous inhalation)
    - Prostacyclin (continuous IV infusion) (i.e., epoprostenol)
    - Endothelin receptor antagonist, PO (i.e., bosentan)
    - Phosphodiesterase inhibitor PO (i.e., sildenafil)
  - Caution: Vasodilators should be used under close supervision because of their effect on systemic BP (systemic hypotension can be a significant problem).

ADDITIONAL TREATMENT
General Measures
- Provide for patient stabilization.
- Treat the primary disease process.
- Treat underlying hypoxia (supplemental O_2).
- Treat underlying hypoventilation:
  - Useful for correcting hypoxia and hypercarbia secondary to hypoventilation
  - Available methods:
    - Noninvasive positive pressure ventilation (bi-level ventilation)
    - Mechanical ventilation (tracheostomy with mechanical ventilation)

SURGERY/OTHER PROCEDURES
- Tonsillectomy and/or adenoidectomy if obstructive sleep apnea is the underlying etiology
- Atrial septostomy may be considered when inadequate right-to-left shunting is present with syncopal episodes and/or right-sided heart failure
- Transplantation (lung or heart-lung transplantation): Reserved for patients with refractory, severe pulmonary hypertension

ONGOING CARE

PROGNOSIS
- Depends on underlying disease, but generally poor
- In cases of primary pulmonary hypertension, improvement of pulmonary hypertension with administration of vasodilators during initial catheterization is associated with a better survival rate than if no response occurs.
- 10–40% mortality in treated patients
- Near 100% mortality if patient is untreated
- Treatment can be lifelong unless the primary cause of the pulmonary hypertension can be corrected.
- In acute pulmonary hypertension, response to most treatment modalities is almost immediate.
- Oxygen has been shown to reverse hypoxia-related remodeling of the airways after 1 month of therapy.

COMPLICATIONS
- Chronic hypoxia
- Exercise intolerance
- Right-sided heart failure (cor pulmonale)
- Death

ADDITIONAL READING

- Chatterjee K, De Marco T, Alpert JS. Pulmonary hypertension: Hemodynamic diagnosis and management. *Arch Intern Med.* 2002;162: 1925–1933.
- Hawkins A, Tulloh R. Treatment of pediatric pulmonary hypertension. *Vasc Health Risk Manag.* 2009;5:509–524.
- Klings ES, Farber HW. Current management of primary pulmonary hypertension. *Drugs.* 2001;61: 1945–1956.
- Mourani PM, Sontag MK, Younoszai A, et al. Clinical utility of echocardiography for the diagnosis and management of pulmonary vascular disease in young children with chronic lung disease. *Pediatrics.* 2008;121:317–325.
- Ravishankar C, Tabbutt S, Wernovsky G. Critical care in cardiovascular medicine. *Curr Opin Pediatr.* 2003;15:443–453.
- Rosenzweig EB, WidLitz AC, Barst RJ. Pulmonary arterial hypertension in children. *Pediatr Pulmonol.* 2004;38:2–22.
- Simonneau G, Galie N, Rubin LJ, et al. Clinical classification of pulmonary hypertension. *Am J Coll Cardiol.* 2004;43:5S–12S.
- WidLitz A, Barst RJ. Pulmonary arterial hypertension in children. *Eur Respir J.* 2003;21:155–176.
- Yeh TF. Persistent pulmonary hypertension in preterm infants with respiratory distress syndrome. *Pediatr Pulmonol.* 2001;23(Suppl):103–106.

CODES

ICD9
- 416.0 Primary pulmonary hypertension
- 416.8 Other chronic pulmonary heart diseases
- 747.83 Persistent fetal circulation

ICD10
- I27.0 Primary pulmonary hypertension
- I27.2 Other secondary pulmonary hypertension
- P29.3 Persistent fetal circulation

FAQ

- Q: How many hours per day should supplemental oxygen be used?
- A: Studies have shown decreased mortality in patients using oxygen 24 hours per day compared with patients using supplemental oxygen for only part of the day.
- Q: Should the dosage of oxygen be adjusted during the day according to the patient's activity?
- A: Increasing supplemental oxygen should be considered for activities that require increased oxygen consumption (i.e., exercise, eating, sleeping).
- Q: Can an echocardiogram replace the need for a cardiac catheterization?
- A: No. Although an abnormal echo can confirm the presence of pulmonary hypertension, it does not inform one of its severity or the (acute) response to therapy. Furthermore, a normal study does not rule out pulmonary hypertension (especially mild cases).

PURPURA FULMINANS

David F. Friedman

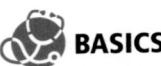 **BASICS**

DESCRIPTION
- Congenital, acquired, or idiopathic condition of rapidly progressive microvascular hemorrhage into the skin
- Associated with an underlying acquired or congenital disorder of coagulation
- May lead to skin necrosis as well as acral amputations

EPIDEMIOLOGY
Incidence
- Neonatal purpura fulminans related to homozygous protein C deficiency: 1 in 2–4 million births
- Clinical protein C deficiency: 1 in 20,000 individuals
- Homozygous protein S deficiency is more rare.

Prevalence
Purpura can be seen in bacterial sepsis with meningococcus and other pathogens, as well as other causes of disseminated intravascular coagulation.

RISK FACTORS
Genetics
- Deficiencies of protein C and protein S are autosomally inherited with variable penetrance.
- Over 150 different genetic mutations of protein C have been described, leading to both qualitative and quantitative defects of the proteins.
- Heterozygous protein C and S deficiency states usually cause a hypercoagulable condition, with increased risk of venous or arterial thrombosis throughout life.
- Homozygous protein C or S deficiency states lead to severe deficiency (<1% of normal factor activity) and neonatal purpura fulminans and are often fatal.
- Factor V Leiden:
  - Known risk factor for thrombosis
  - May predispose to infection-associated purpura fulminans
  - May also predispose to purpura fulminans in patients who are heterozygotes for protein C or S deficiency
- Other genetic predispositions to thrombosis, such as prothrombin mutations, may also contribute to risk for purpura fulminans.

PATHOPHYSIOLOGY
Common features of purpura fulminans:
- Inflammation: Endothelial injury from bacterial endotoxin or other trigger may initiate secretion of inflammatory cytokines or activation of coagulation and complement proteins.
- Purpura: Extravasation of formed elements of the blood from injured capillaries into the skin
- Dermal vascular thrombosis: Formation of microthrombosis in blood vessels of the skin, leading to hemorrhage in the skin (purpura), necrosis of skin, and gangrene

ETIOLOGY
- Infection-associated purpura fulminans:
  - Overwhelming sepsis, usually bacterial; *Neisseria meningitidis* most common
  - May be a complication of varicella infection
  - Disseminated intravascular coagulation: State of sustained activation of coagulation cascade and fibrinolytic mechanisms, leading to consumption of platelets, fibrinogen, and often formation of microthrombosis
- Inherited defect of coagulation presenting as neonatal purpura fulminans:
  - Deficiency of protein C: Loss of important inhibitory regulation of coagulation and uncontrolled clotting
  - Protein C slows ("brakes") the coagulation cascade at two steps: By degrading activated coagulation factor Va in the common part of the coagulation pathway and by degrading factor VIIIa in the intrinsic pathway
  - Also plays a role in inflammatory cascade
  - Protein S is a cofactor for protein C.
- Idiopathic:
  - Postinfectious complication: Formation of antibodies to protein S causing protein S deficiency has been described as a postinfectious autoimmune phenomenon.
  - Complication of warfarin (Coumadin) therapy
  - Other unknown mechanisms

 DIAGNOSIS

HISTORY
- Current bacterial sepsis: Fever, weakness, dizziness, nausea, vomiting, onset of petechial rash:
  - Family history suggestive of hypercoagulable state
  - Blood clots or thromboses at an early age, such as stroke, deep vein thrombosis, pulmonary embolism
  - Family members taking warfarin (Coumadin) or low-molecular-weight heparin or other anticoagulation
- Previous affected child with purpura fulminans or hypercoagulable state
- Prior exposure to heparin, therapeutically or via IV Hep-Lock
- Medications, including anticoagulation

PHYSICAL EXAM
- Signs of sepsis:
  - Fever
  - Hypotension
  - Tachycardia
  - Poor perfusion
  - Cool extremities
  - Decreased pulses
  - Shock
- Nonblanching purpura
- Acral purpura and necrosis: Check fingers, nose, toes, and penis for black areas.
- An erythematous border may surround purpuric areas.
- Bullae may form over purpuric skin.
- Oozing at sites of venipuncture

- Pain, ischemia, and edema of extremities or internal organ dysfunction may result from deep vein thrombosis or arterial thrombosis, depending on location and severity.
- Physical exam trick: Depress the purpuric area with a glass slide to determine whether it blanches.

DIAGNOSTIC TESTS & INTERPRETATION
Lab
Screening:
- CBC:
  - Platelet count may be low.
  - Hemoglobin may be low.
- Prothrombin time and INR: Prolonged as in disseminated intravascular coagulation
- Partial thromboplastin time: Prolonged as in disseminated intravascular coagulation
- Fibrinogen: Decreased with consumption and fibrinolysis
- D-Dimer: Increased fibrinolysis as in disseminated intravascular coagulation
- Etiologic:
  - Protein C activity in patient and parents
  - Protein S antigen (total and free) in patient and parents
- Test for antiphospholipid antibodies: Usually lupus anticoagulant or anticardiolipin antibody
- Factor V Leiden mutation assay
- False positives:
  - Protein C and S levels may decrease because of consumption during a thrombotic episode that is not related to an underlying deficiency. Low measurements often need to be repeated at baseline after recovery. Protein C and S levels may be below adult normal ranges for the first 3–6 months of life in healthy infants.

Imaging
To document presence and extent of suspected large-vessel thrombosis: The most useful imaging strategy depends on location and clinical situation:
- Ultrasound with Doppler flow study
- CT scan
- MRI: Better for visualization of vessels
- Angiography: Most invasive, requires vascular injury for access
- Imaging is potentially useful to:
  - Distinguish thrombosis from other pathology
  - Judge age of thrombus (based on collateralization)
  - Assess clot size prior to anticoagulant or thrombolytic therapy
  - Distinguish baseline old clot from new thrombosis

DIFFERENTIAL DIAGNOSIS
- Infection:
  - *N. meningitidis*, most common infectious cause of purpura fulminans
  - Streptococci
  - *Haemophilus* species
  - Staphylococci
  - Gram-negative bacteremia: *Escherichia coli*, *Klebsiella*, *Proteus*, *Enterobacter*
  - Rickettsia: Rocky Mountain spotted fever
  - Varicella

- Environmental:
  - Warfarin-induced skin necrosis: 1 in 500–1,000 individuals starting warfarin therapy develops necrosis in subcutaneous fat.
  - Thought to be caused by relative depletion of anticoagulant protein C (a vitamin K–dependent factor) during the initial phase of warfarin effect
- Tumor: Myeloid leukemia
- Congenital: Inherited deficiencies of protein C and protein S:
  - Only severe, homozygous (<1% activity) deficiencies of proteins C and S are associated with purpura fulminans.
  - Milder, heterozygous deficiencies of protein C and protein S as well as deficiency of antithrombin III, dysfibrinogenemias, the carrier state for factor V Leiden, and other prothrombotic defects all give rise to hypercoagulable states, but usually not neonatal purpura fulminans.
  - Patients with 1 or more risk factors for thrombosis may be more likely to develop purpura fulminans with an environmental stimulus.
  - Immune: Heparin-induced thrombocytopenia: Antibody to heparin–platelet complex causes platelet activation, thrombocytopenia, and microthrombosis, including dermal vessels.
- Antiphospholipid antibody syndrome: Predisposition to thrombosis can include skin necrosis.
- Miscellaneous:
  - Thrombotic thrombocytopenic purpura
  - Paroxysmal nocturnal hemoglobinuria
  - Henoch-Schönlein purpura

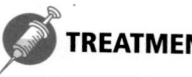 TREATMENT

MEDICATION (DRUGS)
Contraindications, precautions, and significant possible interactions:
- Many drugs can affect warfarin metabolism.
- Chronic protein C concentrate infusion therapy for neonates may run into access problems.

First Line
- Anti-infective agents depending on underlying cause
- Fresh frozen plasma q12h to replace proteins C and S in acute disseminated intravascular coagulation of purpura fulminans
- Periodic fresh frozen plasma infusions for chronic replacement
- Prothrombin complex concentrates also have thrombogenic potential.
- Protein C concentrates are available and probably of benefit in meningococcemia.
- Protein C has half-life of 6–10 hours in circulation.
- Protein C replacement by periodic infusion of protein C concentrate
- Oral warfarin therapy indefinitely usually recommended for documented severe protein C or S deficiency with thrombosis
- Low-molecular-weight heparin given subcutaneously is also a commonly used option for long-term anticoagulation therapy.

 ONGOING CARE

FOLLOW-UP RECOMMENDATIONS
Patient Monitoring
- When to expect improvement: Related to underlying cause of purpura fulminans
- Signs to watch for:
  - Spread of purpura
  - Hypotension
  - Gangrene
- Pitfalls:
  - Individuals with protein C and protein S deficiency may have increased risk of warfarin-induced skin necrosis when starting warfarin. Patients should be heparinized for several days prior to the start of oral anticoagulation.
  - Management of an infant on oral anticoagulation is difficult because of the practical problem of obtaining reliable measurements of PT, the increased risk associated with deep venipunctures for blood samples, and difficulty in establishing a stable warfarin dose. Low-molecular-weight heparin by injection is usually the preferred anticoagulant therapy in infants.

DIET
Patients on warfarin therapy may need to avoid foods with high vitamin K content, especially if there is variation in the dose of warfarin required to maintain adequate anticoagulation.

PROGNOSIS
- Related to underlying cause of purpura fulminans
- Overall, poor for homozygous deficiencies of proteins C and S

COMPLICATIONS
- Skin necrosis and gangrene
- Scarring
- Acral amputations, from tips of digits to whole limbs
- Thrombosis in internal organs
- Death

ADDITIONAL READING

- Canavese F, Krajbich, JI, LaFleur BJ. Orthopaedic sequelae of childhood meningococcemia: Management considerations and outcomes. *J Bone Joint Surg Am*. 2010;92:2196–2203.
- de Kleijn ED, de Groot R, Hack CE, et al. Activation of protein C following infusion of protein C concentrates in children with severe meningococcal sepsis and purpura fulminans: A randomized, double-blinded, placebo-controlled dose-finding study. *Crit Care Med*. 2003;31:1839–1847.
- Goldenberg NA, Manco-Johnson MJ. Protein C deficiency. *Haemophilia*. 2008;14:1214–1221.
- Leclerc F, Leteurtre S, Cremer R, et al. Do new strategies in meningococcemia produce better outcomes? *Crit Care Med*. 2000;28:S60.

- Patha N, Faust SN, Levin M. Pathophysiology of meningococcal meningitis and septicaemia. *Arch Dis Child*. 2003;88:601–607.
- Veldman A, Fischer D, Wong FY, et al. Human protein C concentrate in the treatment of purpura fulminans: A retrospective analysis of safety and outcome in 94 pediatric patients. *Crit Care*. 2010;14:R156.
- Vincent JL, Nade S, Kutsogiannis DJ, et al. Drotrecogin alfa (activated) in patients with severe sepsis presenting with purpura fulminans, meningitis, or meningococcal disease: A retrospective analysis of patients enrolled in recent clinical trials. *Crit Care*. 2005;9:R331–R343.

 CODES

ICD9
286.6 Defibrination syndrome

ICD10
D65 Disseminated intravascular coagulation [defibrination syndrome]

FAQ

- Q: What is the risk of a 2nd affected child with protein C or S deficiency?
- A: If the diagnosis is confirmed by family studies that show both parents to be carriers of the deficiency and the affected child to be homozygous, there is a 25% chance that each subsequent infant would have purpura fulminans and a 50% chance that each child would be a carrier. However, other hypercoagulable states have been described that may be risk factors for purpura fulminans.
- Q: Should a child with purpura fulminans be followed by a specialist?
- A: Generally yes, with a pediatric hematologist, to assist in acute management of purpura, establishment of diagnosis, and management of long-term anticoagulation.

PYELONEPHRITIS

Shamir Tuchman
Kevin E. C. Meyers

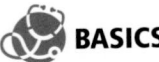 **BASICS**

DESCRIPTION
Acute pyelonephritis (upper urinary tract infection [UTI]) is defined clinically by fever, a positive urine culture, and urinary symptoms (e.g., dysuria, frequency/urgency, and/or flank pain) and histologically by acute renal parenchymal (interstitial) inflammation secondary to bacterial invasion.

EPIDEMIOLOGY
- UTIs are more likely to involve the upper renal tracts in children <3 years of age.
- UTIs are more common in females, except in uncircumcised males <3 months of age.

Incidence
Cumulative incidence of UTIs (1st 6 years of life):
- 6.6% for girls
- 1.8% for boys

Prevalence
- 5–7% of febrile infants <8 weeks of age
- 1% of all school-aged children
- 1–3% of girls between 1–5 years
- 0.03% in school-aged boys

RISK FACTORS
- Previous history of UTI
- Sibling with a history of a UTI
- Female sex
- Indwelling urinary catheter
- Structural abnormalities of the kidneys and lower urinary tract
- Vesicoureteral reflux (VUR): Present in ~30–40% of children with febrile UTIs.
- The majority (>95%) of VUR associated with febrile UTIs is low-moderate grade (grade I–III). Although, there is a stronger statistical association of febrile UTI with high grade (grade >IV) VUR.

PATHOPHYSIOLOGY
Specific factors related to development of pyelonephritis:
- Host related:
  - Anatomic abnormalities (e.g., obstruction, fistula)
  - Functional abnormalities (e.g., dysfunctional voiding, vesicoureteral reflux)
- Pathogen related:
  - Adherence factors (P and type 1-fimbriae, adhesins)
  - Virulence factors (e.g., lipopolysaccharide, capsular antigen)
- Adhesion of bacteria to uroepithelium induces cytokine release and a subsequent inflammatory response.
- Patchy infiltration of the medullary parenchyma by polymorphonuclear leukocytes and lymphocytes leads to degradation of extracellular matrix, tubular disruption, and interstitial edema.
- Parenchymal scarring may result as a consequence of the infection.

ETIOLOGY
- Enterobacteriaceae: *Escherichia coli* most frequent cause (90% of initial infections and in up to 66% of recurrent infections); *Proteus, Klebsiella, Enterobacter* spp. are also implicated.
- Gram-positive organisms cause 10–15% of cases: *Staphylococcus aureus*, *S. epidermidis*, *S. saprophyticus*, *Enterococci* spp.
- Other organisms: *Pseudomonas, Haemophilus influenzae, Streptococcus* group B

COMMONLY ASSOCIATED CONDITIONS
- Struvite kidney stones: Associated with urease-producing bacteria (e.g., *Proteus* sp.)
- Anatomic or physiologic abnormality of the collecting system: Found in up to 50% of infants with pyelonephritis

 DIAGNOSIS

HISTORY
- A fever of 38.5°C may be the only presenting complaint.
- In the neonate, inquire of caregivers about vomiting, lethargy, poor feeding, irritability, fever, hypothermia, and jaundice.
- Older children are more likely to present with flank pain, dysuria, frequency, urgency, and incontinence.
- Important factors that predispose to the development of UTI that should be specifically inquired about:
  - Constipation
  - Incorrect toilet training
  - Perineal skin irritation
  - Antibiotic exposure
  - Uncircumcised males
  - Previous UTIs
  - Investigations already performed
  - A family history of UTIs or reflux nephropathy
  - A history of structural abnormalities of the kidneys and/or lower urinary tract
  - Symptoms suggestive of dysfunctional voiding, such as that the bladder always feels full, infrequent use of the toilet, double-voiding, and urgency incontinence
  - Previous surgery or trauma to the lower back
- Lower-motor milestones
- Signs and symptoms:
  - Fever
  - Chills
  - Flank pain
  - Urination problems: Dysuria, frequency, urgency

PHYSICAL EXAM
- Findings may be nonspecific.
- Fever, irritability, rigors, lethargy
- Flank tenderness:
  - May be related to an underlying renal tract abnormality, such as flank mass due to obstruction with hydronephrosis or cystic kidney disease, spina bifida apparent or occult (as evidenced by a dimple), pilonidal sinus, or hemangioma
- Gentle posterior punch test will reveal tenderness at the costovertebral angle.
- Bimanual palpation of kidneys to assess tenderness and size
- Careful neuromuscular exam of lower limbs and back to evaluate for the presence of a neurogenic bladder
- Assess rectal tone.

DIAGNOSTIC TESTS & INTERPRETATION
Lab
- Collect urine using sterile methods (e.g., midstream in toilet-trained children, catheter or suprapubic for infants).
- Urine dipstick for measurement of leukocyte esterase and nitrites as a rapid screen for infection.
- WBC casts on urine microscopy are diagnostic.
- As a screening test, an unspun clean-catch urine specimen with bacteria on stained microscopic exam correlates (80–90%) with culture results exceeding 100,000 colonies/mL.
- Urine for culture and sensitivity: A positive culture result is defined by the growth of a single pathogenic organism of clean-catch 100,000 colonies/mL, catheter 1,000 colonies/mL, and by *any* growth in a suprapubic specimen.
- CBC with an elevated WBC count
- ESR and C-reactive protein (CRP) levels are often increased.

Imaging
- Renal ultrasound to rule out obstruction and assess renal size and parenchyma
- Voiding cystourethrogram (VCUG) to rule out anatomic anomalies including obstruction (e.g., posterior urethral valves) and vesicoureteric reflux
- ^{99m}Tc-dimercaptosuccinic acid (DMSA) test can be done to confirm the presence of acute pyelonephritis and to look for renal scarring. This is a sensitive and specific test that some clinicians believe to be the imaging study of choice for diagnosing acute pyelonephritis and renal scarring.

Diagnostic Procedures/Other
- Imaging evaluation of the urinary tract after a UTI should be individualized based on the child's clinical presentation and clinical judgment.
- All children <36 months of age should have an ultrasound and VCUG.
- A VCUG should be done in all males with a confirmed 1st pyelonephritis and a VCUG or nuclear cystogram in all females ≤7 years of age.

- After the urine is sterile, a VCUG can be performed; there is no need to wait 4 weeks.
- Administer antibiotic prophylaxis before the VCUG.

ALERT
- False-positive test results:
  - May be due to nonsterile collection techniques (bagged urine specimen) or allowing urine to stand unrefrigerated.
- False-negative test results:
  - The rapid test for nitrites requires urine to stay in the bladder for several hours and is therefore not useful in infants who do not store urine in the bladder.
  - Precollection antibiotic exposure

DIFFERENTIAL DIAGNOSIS
- Cystitis
- Sterile pyuria:
  - Vulvovaginitis
  - Balanitis
  - Systemic viral illness
  - Post-vaccination
  - Pregnancy
  - Appendicitis
  - Cystic renal disease
  - Tuberculosis
- Lower-lobe pneumonia
- Acute appendicitis

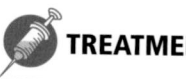 ## TREATMENT

MEDICATION (DRUGS)
- Give IV antibiotics (especially in children who appear toxic, are dehydrated, or vomiting) until afebrile for at least 24 hours, then change to an oral formulation.
- In total, 7–14 days of antibiotic therapy are required.
- Patients with 1st-time urinary infections should receive low-dose antibiotic prophylaxis until their workup is completed.
- Children with frequent symptomatic recurrences of UTI and those with high-grade vesicoureteric reflux require long-term antibiotic prophylaxis.
- Antibiotics such as co-trimoxazole (Bactrim), amoxicillin–clavulanate (Augmentin), and the 2nd-generation cephalosporins
- Familiarity with local antibiotic patterns of resistance is particularly important in treating hospital-acquired infections.
- Antipyretics (e.g., acetaminophen)

ALERT
- Removing struvite calculi during active infection may precipitate bacteremia/urosepsis.
- High index of suspicion is required for pyelonephritis associated with cystic renal disease as urine cultures may be negative when the infection is intracystic.

IN-PATIENT CONSIDERATIONS
IV Fluids
- May be necessary when children are hospitalized with fever and vomiting, to maintain hydration and urine output.
- Underlying anatomic or functional urinary collecting system abnormality should be evaluated/treated by a urologist.

 ## ONGOING CARE

FOLLOW-UP RECOMMENDATIONS
Patient Monitoring
Requirements for testing: Educate caregivers in the use and interpretation of the dipstick, and about the symptoms and signs of UTI.

PROGNOSIS
- Fever usually resolves in 3–5 days.
- Ongoing fever or persistent flank pain requires further evaluation to exclude a drug-resistant organism, kidney stone, kidney abscess or another unrecognized urinary tract obstruction.
- Diagnosis and treatment of any underlying voiding dysfunction and constipation are required for successful management of UTIs in children.
- Outcome of acute pyelonephritis is usually good but may result in parenchymal scarring.
- Pyelonephritis associated with struvite renal stones requires removal of the infectious stones after antibiotic treatment is completed.
- Risk factors for renal damage include obstruction, reflux with dilation, young age, delay in treatment, number of episodes of pyelonephritis, and bacterial virulence factors.

COMPLICATIONS
- Acute:
  - Reduced concentrating ability, hyperkalemic renal tubular acidosis
  - Bacteremia: Highest risk in young infants (23% of children <2 months)
  - Perinephric abscess formation
- Chronic:
  - Focal renal scarring, hypertension, proteinuria, azotemia, xanthogranulomatous pyelonephritis

ADDITIONAL READING
- Agarwal S. Vesicoureteral reflux and urinary tract infections. *Curr Opin Urol*. 2000;10:587–92.
- Bloomfield P, Hodson EM, Craig JC. Antibiotics for acute pyelonephritis in children. *Cochrane Database Syst Rev*. 2003;(3):CD003772.
- Committee on Quality Improvement: Sub-committee on Urinary Tract Infection. Practice parameter: The diagnosis, treatment, and evaluation of the initial urinary tract infection in febrile infants. *Pediatrics*. 1999;103(4):843–852.
- Greenbaum LA, Mesrobian HO. Vesicoureteral reflux. *Pediatr Clin North Am*. 2006;53:413–427.

- Hewitt IK, Zucchetta P, Rigon L, et al. Early treatment of acute pyelonephritis in children fails to reduce renal scarring: Data from the Italian Renal Infection Study Trials. *Pediatrics*. 2008;122(3):486–490.
- Hoberman A, Charron M, Hickey RW, et al. Imaging studies after a first febrile urinary tract infection in young children. *N Engl J Med*. 2003;348(3):195–202.
- Keren R, Carpenter M, Greenfield S, et al. Is antibiotic prophylaxis in children with vesicoureteral reflux effective in preventing pyelonephritis and renal scars? A randomized, controlled trial. *Pediatrics*. 2008;122(6):1409–1410.
- Martinell J, Hansson S, Claesson I, et al. Detection of urographic scars in girls with pyelonephritis followed for 13–38 years. *Pediatr Nephrol*. 2000;14:1006–1010.
- Raszka WV, Khan O. Pyelonephritis. *Ped Rev*. 2005;26:364–369.
- Weir M, Brien J. Adolescent urinary tract infections. *Adolesc Med State Art Rev*. 2000;11:293–313.

 ## CODES

ICD9
- 590.10 Acute pyelonephritis without lesion of renal medullary necrosis
- 590.80 Pyelonephritis, unspecified

ICD10
- N10 Acute tubulo-interstitial nephritis
- N12 Tubulo-interstitial nephritis, not specified as acute or chronic

FAQ
- Q: Should a DMSA scan be used to help diagnose acute pyelonephritis?
- A: Routine use of the DMSA scan to diagnose acute pyelonephritis is controversial because disagreement exists about the therapeutic implications of a positive test result, and such routine testing is expensive. Children with hypertension and previous UTIs require a DMSA scan to look for renal cortical scarring.
- Q: Does renal parenchymal scarring occur *without* reflux?
- A: Yes. The causal relationships among reflux, acute pyelonephritis, and renal parenchymal scarring are complex.

PYLORIC STENOSIS

Joy L. Collins

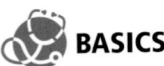 **BASICS**

DESCRIPTION
Hypertrophy of the muscular layers of the pylorus with elongation and thickening, leading to obstruction of the gastric outlet

EPIDEMIOLOGY
- Exceedingly rare in newborns, as well as in patients >6 months of age
- More common in Caucasians

Incidence
~1 in 950 live births

PATHOPHYSIOLOGY
- Diffuse hypertrophy and hyperplasia of the pylorus lead to narrowing of the gastric antrum.
- The antrum becomes thickened, elongated, and firm.
- Hypergastrinemia associated with hyperactivity, elevations of prostaglandins, and deficiency of nitric oxide as a smooth muscle neurotransmitter have been suggested as etiologic factors.

ETIOLOGY
- Unknown
- No specific pattern of inheritance established
- Multifactorial inheritance likely
- Neonatal hypergastrinemia and gastric hyperacidity are involved.
- An association between infantile hypertrophic pyloric stenosis and the administration of oral erythromycin given for postexposure prophylaxis for pertussis has been described.

COMMONLY ASSOCIATED CONDITIONS
Increased occurrence of esophageal atresia and malrotation was noted in 5% of infants with pyloric stenosis.

DIAGNOSIS

HISTORY
- The infant is typically a "hungry vomiter," refeeding immediately, only to vomit yet again.
- Signs and symptoms:
  - Nonbilious vomiting, classically projectile in an otherwise well and hungry child between 2–8 weeks of age
  - Possible weight loss
  - Varying degrees of dehydration and lethargy

PHYSICAL EXAM
- Visible peristalsis may be appreciated just after the infant feeds, which is seen as a waveform proceeding from the left upper quadrant toward the pylorus in the right upper quadrant.
- A palpable, hard, mobile, and nontender mass in the epigastrium to the right of the midline, referred to as an "olive"
- Best confirmed by palpation after the stomach has been emptied and with the infant quiet and comfortable

DIAGNOSTIC TESTS & INTERPRETATION
Lab
- Hypochloremia and alkalosis
- Hyponatremia
- Hypokalemia
- 1–2% of infants have indirect hyperbilirubinemia associated with jaundice.

Imaging
- Ultrasound:
  - Ultrasonography identifies the hypertrophic pyloric musculature as a broad ring with low echo density and an inner layer of high echo density corresponding to the mucosa.
  - To confirm the diagnosis, muscle thickness should be >4 mm or pyloric length >15 mm.
- GI studies:
  - An upper GI study can differentiate antral webs, pylorospasm, and other obstructive lesions.
  - Vigorous gastric peristalsis with little or no gastric emptying is seen in association with pyloric stenosis.
  - An elongated, narrow pyloric anal canal can be seen as a single or sometimes a double tract of barium, commonly known as the "string sign."
  - A pyloric bulge into the distal antrum, producing an umbrella appearance, also may be seen.

DIFFERENTIAL DIAGNOSIS
- Gastroesophageal reflux
- Gastroenteritis
- Pyloric atresia
- Antral or duodenal web

TREATMENT

SURGERY/OTHER PROCEDURES
- Pyloromyotomy (Ramstedt procedure): Longitudinal incision of the antropyloric muscle
- Laparoscopic pyloromyotomy is a minimally invasive version of pyloromyotomy and is favored by many surgeons over an open approach.
- Pyloric stenosis is a medical emergency, but not a surgical emergency.

IN-PATIENT CONSIDERATIONS
Initial Stabilization
- Early identification of electrolyte abnormalities and correction with appropriate IV fluids
- Correction of metabolic abnormalities by replacing (i.e., maintaining levels of) sodium, chloride, and potassium
- Postoperative vomiting is well recognized and is most likely caused by persistent local edema.
- Most patients can resume feedings 6–8 hours after surgery.

ONGOING CARE

FOLLOW-UP RECOMMENDATIONS
Vomiting may persist for several days after surgery.

ALERT
- Do not fail to appreciate that chloride loss is the most significant electrolyte disorder when replacing fluids and electrolytes.
- Do not fail to appreciate that this disorder occurs in girls as well as boys.

PROGNOSIS
Morbidity and mortality rates are low; surgery is curative.

COMPLICATIONS
- Dehydration
- Electrolyte abnormalities, primarily hypochloremic metabolic alkalosis that results from loss of hydrochloric acid caused by persistent vomiting
- Postoperative complications:
  – Incomplete pyloromyotomy
  – Mucosal injury; may lead to leak and sepsis if not immediately recognized and repaired

ADDITIONAL READING

- Adibe OO, Nichol PF, Flake AW, et al. Comparison of outcomes after laparoscopic and open pyloromyotomy at a high-volume pediatric teaching hospital. *J Pediatr Surg.* 2006;41(10):1676–1678.
- Aspelund G, Langer JC. Current management of hypertrophic pyloric stenosis. *Semin Pediatr Surg.* 2007;16(1):27–33.
- Hernanz-Schulman M. Pyloric stenosis—role of imaging. *Pediatr Radiol.* 2009;39(Suppl 2): S134–S139.
- Letton RW Jr. Pyloric stenosis. *Pediatr Ann.* 2001;30: 745–750.
- Sola J, Neville H. Laparoscopic vs. open pyloromyotomy: A systematic review and meta-analysis. *J Pediatr Surg.* 2009;44:1631–1637.

CODES

ICD9
- 537.0 Acquired hypertrophic pyloric stenosis
- 750.5 Congenital hypertrophic pyloric stenosis

ICD10
- K31.1 Adult hypertrophic pyloric stenosis
- Q40.0 Congenital hypertrophic pyloric stenosis

FAQ
- Q: Can ultrasound help make the diagnosis?
- A: Yes. Many clinicians order this test 1st, to avoid possible aspiration of contrast material.
- Q: Why is so much chloride lost?
- A: The chloride loss occurs with the loss of gastric acid, which contains hydrochloric acid.
- Q: What plan should I follow when replacing electrolytes?
- A: Correct the deficiency of fluids with twice maintenance fluid volumes. Correct chloride loss with normal saline, and correct potassium loss with potassium chloride.

P

RABIES
Edmund A. Milder
Louis M. Bell (5th edition)
Suzanne Dawid (5th edition)

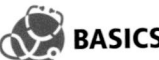 **BASICS**

DESCRIPTION
Viral infection of CNS transmitted from animals to humans

EPIDEMIOLOGY
- Although the current annual incidence of reported human rabies in the U.S. is ~1–2 cases per year, incidence rates elsewhere in the world are much higher.
- In addition, thousands of infected animals are identified each year in the U.S.
- Endemic regions of the U.S. include the mid-Atlantic, southeast, south central, and north central areas, and the state of California.
- Common vectors: 7 species of animals account for 98% of all reported animal rabies cases in the U.S.: Skunk (38–43%), raccoons (28–31%), bats (14%), cats (4%), foxes (4%), cattle (4%), dogs (3%), and all other (2%).

Prevalence
- From 2000–2007, there were 20 cases of rabies acquired in the U.S. 17 of these were associated with bat rabies strains.
- Despite widespread infection of raccoons, there has been only 1 documented human death.

RISK FACTORS
- Travel to areas where canine rabies is endemic
- Exposure to a wild animal, typically through a bite. In the U.S., bats, raccoons, skunks, foxes, and coyotes are the principal reservoir.
- Exposure to an unimmunized domestic animal, especially through a bite.
- Transmission from transplanted corneas and organs has occurred.
- Working with animals (e.g., veterinarians), or working in a laboratory with the virus.

GENERAL PREVENTION
- Immunoprophylaxis: Preexposure vaccines are offered to those at high risk (e.g., veterinarians, animal handlers).
- Because wild animals account for 90% of new rabies cases in the U.S. today, avoiding unnecessary contact is helpful.
- Attempts are being made in several areas of the U.S. to vaccinate wild animals orally by using vaccine-baited food.
- Pets should be vaccinated.

PATHOPHYSIOLOGY
- Except for rare cases, the rabies virus enters the body through a bite that breaks the skin and introduces infected saliva:
  - From there, the virus gains access to muscle, where it is sequestered.
  - The virus then enters the peripheral nerves, where it moves centripetally to the CNS at a rate of ~3 mm/h.
  - Once in the CNS, infection spreads rapidly to involve nearly all neurons.
  - This state, if untreated, leads to cardiopulmonary arrest and death shortly thereafter, as a result of still poorly understood mechanisms.
- The incubation period is typically 4 weeks but can be days to years, with the longest documented incubation being 6 years.

ETIOLOGY
Rabies virus is a rhabdovirus containing single-stranded RNA.

 DIAGNOSIS

HISTORY
- Behavior of animal: Although signs of rabies in animals vary greatly, atypical behavior for the animal is the norm (e.g., passive animals become aggressive, nocturnal animals roam in daylight).
  - Foaming at the mouth and lack of coordination may be present.
- A few humans with rabies have no identifiable preceding animal exposure.
- Type of animal inflicting the bite (domestic vs. wild)
- Location of the animal and availability for observation
- History of previous rabies vaccination of the animal and patient
- Signs and symptoms:
  - Prodrome: 2–10 days with vague and insidious symptoms (e.g., sore throat, malaise, anxiety, depression, fever, nausea). A fairly specific prodromal symptom is itching, pain, or tingling at the site of the bite.
  - Acute neurologic phase: Furious (80%) vs. paralytic (20%) rabies:
    - Furious rabies: Agitation, hyperactivity, bizarre behavior, nuchal rigidity, sore throat, and hoarseness. The pathognomonic sign is hydrophobia and, at times, aerophobia.
    - Paralytic rabies: Initial finding is flaccid paralysis in the limb that was bitten; subsequently spreads to other limbs. Cranial nerve involvement can give complete lack of facial affect.
    - Coma: Onset follows acute neurologic phase; may persist up to 2 weeks and is followed by death almost universally.

PHYSICAL EXAM
- Although neurologic findings can vary, cranial nerve paralysis (e.g., palate, vocal cords) is common. Therefore, hoarseness and stridor can be seen.
- Meningismus is also fairly common, along with involuntary movements. Beyond this, findings depend on type of presentation (furious vs. paralytic).

DIAGNOSTIC TESTS & INTERPRETATION
Lab
- There are no known methods for identification of rabies virus infection before onset of clinical signs. However, after signs appear, laboratory diagnosis is now possible as early as day 5 of illness by several techniques:
  - Enzyme-linked antibodies stain of brain tissue from captured animal
  - Fluorescent antibody stain of corneal epithelial cell smears or a section of skin from the neck at the hairline of patient
  - Serologic diagnosis is possible if the patient survives beyond the acute period. A rise in virus-neutralizing antibody will be seen.
  - Viral isolation in suckling mice or tissue culture from saliva, CSF, urine sedimentation, and brain is, at times, possible between days 4–24.
- Postmortem diagnosis is made by the presence of pathognomonic cytoplasmic inclusions (i.e., Negri bodies) in brain tissue (sensitivity, 80%).

DIFFERENTIAL DIAGNOSIS
- Other causes of encephalitis (e.g., herpes simplex virus, enterovirus) can mimic rabies.
- Paralytic rabies can present much like Guillain-Barré syndrome or poliomyelitis.
- Pseudorabies is conversion-related (hysteria) in someone who believes she or he has rabies but does not. In such patients, however, normal blood gases and lack of variation in bizarre behavior are diagnostic for no finding of rabies.

TREATMENT

MEDICATION (DRUGS)
- Immunization: Both passive and active immunization should be initiated concurrently
- Passive:
  - Human rabies immune globulin derived from the plasma of volunteers hyperimmunized with rabies vaccine should be given to anyone bitten by any species of wild animal known to be at high risk for rabies infection (e.g., skunk, raccoon, fox, coyote, bat) and any domestic dog or cat not in good health and in the custody of someone able to observe the animal for a 10-day period. Local health departments can advise about the risk of specific animal exposures.
  - The present recommendation for human rabies immune globulin vaccination is 20 IU/kg instilled locally into the tissue at the site of the bite.
    - Remaining vaccine can be given IM.
    - In cases of multiple wounds, to ensure that all wounds receive an injection of human rabies immune globulin, dilution in saline (2–3-fold) is acceptable.
    - Using more than the recommended dosage is contraindicated because it may interfere with the immune response to the active vaccine.
- Active:
  - 2 forms of rabies vaccine are commercially available. These include human diploid cell rabies vaccine (HDCV) and purified chicken embryo cell vaccine (PCEC). These should be administered by the same criteria given above for passive immunization. In addition, preexposure vaccination is recommended for those at high risk for exposure (e.g., veterinarians, animal handlers, trappers).
- Dosage: 1 mL IM in the deltoid region on days 0, 3, 7, 14, and 28 postexposure. The anterolateral thigh can be used in infants or young children. Discontinue the vaccine series if fluorescent antibody testing of the animal is conducted and result is negative.

IN-PATIENT CONSIDERATIONS
Initial Stabilization
Local wound care:
- The 1st step in preventing infection is washing out the virus mechanically or inactivating it before it has a chance to attach to and enter a neuron.
- The wound should be flushed with copious amounts of soap and water or saline solution.
- For puncture wounds, insertion of a catheter (i.e., angiocatheter) and irrigation with fluid by means of an attached syringe should be performed. If irrigation is too painful, infiltration of the area with local anesthetic can help.

ONGOING CARE

PROGNOSIS
- After the patient is infected with the rabies virus, prognosis is poor. There is no medical therapy available once the nervous system is infected
- Without postexposure rabies immunization, the disease is uniformly fatal.
- 1 patient survived following intensive care and induced coma (see www.mcw.edu/rabies). 2 other patients survived the acute illness using this regimen, but died of complications during rehabilitation.

ADDITIONAL READING
- Gomez-Alonso J. Rabies: A possible explanation for the vampire legend. *Neurology*. 1998;51:856–859.
- Jackson AC. Rabies. *Neurol Clin*. 2008;26(3): 717–726.
- NASPHV Compendium Committee. Compendium of animal rabies control. *MMWR Morb Mortal Wkly Rep*. 1987;35:815.
- Nicholson KG. Modern vaccines. *Lancet*. 1990;335: 1201.
- Plotkin SA. Rabies. *Clin Infect Dis*. 2000;30:4–12.
- Rabinowitz PM, Gordon Z, Odofin L. Pet-related infections. *Am Fam Phys*. 2007;76(9):1314–1322.
- US Centers for Disease Control and Prevention. First human death associated with raccoon rabies: Virginia 2003. *MMWR Morb Mortal Wkly Rep*. 2003;52:1102–1103.

CODES

ICD9
071 Rabies

ICD10
A82.9 Rabies, unspecified

FAQ
- Q: Does a wild squirrel or rabbit bite necessitate rabies prophylaxis?
- A: In general, rodents (e.g., squirrels, rats, mice, hamsters, gerbils), lagomorphs (e.g., rabbits and hares), and opossums are not known to serve as natural rabies reservoirs. They should not be considered rabid unless they exhibit unusual behavior.
- Q: Is there any evidence of human-to-human spread?
- A: No. However, health care workers or others exposed to a patient with known or suspected rabies should receive vaccination if they have suffered a bite wound or if mucosal surfaces or open wounds have been exposed to the patient's body fluids.
- Q: Are there any countries that require routine rabies vaccination?
- A: Yes, Nepal.
- Q: What if a severe allergic reaction occurs during postexposure rabies prophylaxis?
- A: The reaction should be treated at the time, as you would any systemic anaphylactic reaction. Subsequently, the rabies vaccine adsorbed (RVA), produced in rhesus diploid cells, can be given on the same schedule as human diploid cell rabies vaccine.
- Q: If a bat is found in the house, should the family members receive immunoprophylaxis?
- A: If a bat is found in the room of a sleeping person, previously unattended child, or mentally disabled person, prophylaxis should be considered. The injury inflicted by a bat bite or scratch may not be noticed in the above situations.

R

RECTAL PROLAPSE

Joel Friedlander
Andrew F. Zigman

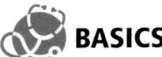 **BASICS**

DESCRIPTION

3 types exist:
- Complete: Full thickness of rectum prolapses through anus (2 layers of rectum with an intervening peritoneal sac, which may contain small bowel).
- Incomplete/Mucosal: Prolapse limited to only 2 layers of mucosa
- Concealed: Internal intussusception of upper rectum into lower, which does not, however, emerge through anus

EPIDEMIOLOGY
- Most cases occur in children <4 years of age around time of toilet training, equal incidence in boys and girls.
- Common in developing countries, perhaps because of poor nutrition and parasitic infection; uncommon in the Western world
- It usually presents between 6 months–3 years of age in patients with cystic fibrosis (CF). Incidence is 20%. Presentation in such children >5 years of age is rare. Highest incidence is in the 1st year of life.
- In older children and adults, strong (6-fold) female predilection

RISK FACTORS
Genetics
No known inheritance pattern aside from the association with CF, which is an autosomally recessive inherited disease

ETIOLOGY
Exact etiology uncertain, but the following are usually related findings and predisposing conditions:
- Excessive straining with bowel movements from constipation and toilet training (hips and knees flexed)
- Diarrhea; may be more of a cause in tropic and subtropical countries
- Malnutrition; can cause loss of the ischiorectal fat pad
- Complete prolapse is rarer in children, but when it occurs it may be related to poor fixation of rectum to sacrum and to weak pelvic and anal musculature.
- Complication of past surgery, such as imperforate anus repair
- Infections: Hookworms and other parasitic infections
- CF
- Ulcerative colitis
- Hirschsprung disease
- Ehlers–Danlos syndrome
- Meningomyelocele
- Pertussis
- Rectal polyp
- Pneumonia
- Anorexia
- Rectal neoplasm

 DIAGNOSIS

HISTORY
- Usually 1st noted by a parent after child has defecated; may be associated with minimal, painless rectal bleeding
- Often reduces spontaneously; if not, usually easily reduced manually by parent
- Rectal prolapse may cause some discomfort during bowel movements.
- Trauma to the recurrently prolapsed mucosa may lead to ulceration and mucus discharge.
- Ask whether this patient has CF or symptoms of the above conditions.
- Signs and symptoms:
  – Protrusion of rectal layers through anus, usually found during defecation or attempted defecation
  – Although the history of rectal prolapse may be evident, it is often difficult to elicit on examination, and by the time the patient is seen after a prolapse at home, it may already be spontaneously reduced. Thus, the assumption of the diagnosis may have to rest primarily on the parental history.
  – Although usually benign, rectal prolapse is distressing to both the parents and the child.

PHYSICAL EXAM
- Usually, prolapse is not seen on examination while the patient is at rest, unless it is irreducible (dark or bright red mass protruding from child's anus without discomfort).
- May see poor anal tone and/or large anal orifice, especially within hours after the prolapse
- In complete rectal prolapse, concentric mucosal rings can be seen, whereas incomplete (mucosal) prolapse reveals radial folds. If clinician sees >5 cm of rectum emerging, it is most likely a complete prolapse. Asking the patient to strain may allow the mucosa to prolapse. However, this is obviously not helpful in a very young patient.
- A polyp is differentiated in that it is plum-colored and does not involve the entire anal circumference.
- In an intussusception, it is possible to insert the finger around the prolapsing apex of the intussusception, between it and the lining of the anal canal.

DIAGNOSTIC TESTS & INTERPRETATION
Lab
- Sweat test: All children with rectal prolapse should have a sweat test to rule out CF. This is a simple, noninvasive, inexpensive test with good specificity and sensitivity when performed by an experienced clinician in a qualified facility.
- Stool cultures for bacterial and parasitic infestations, if diarrhea could be causative
- Other tests for the above conditions as clinically indicated

Imaging
Evacuation proctography: A barium enema is given, and movement of barium is observed under fluoroscopy during defecation. This may reveal an internal prolapse not easily recognizable on physical examination. This is not commonly used in children, because full cooperation is essential.

DIFFERENTIAL DIAGNOSIS
- Tumors
- Prolapsing rectal tumor: Very rare
- Trauma
- Sexual abuse (e.g., result of anal penetration)
- Metabolic
- CF: From 10–50% of patients diagnosed with CF >4 years of age have experienced rectal prolapse (either at the time of the diagnosis or as a past event), but few individuals with rectal prolapse have CF.
- Anatomic abnormality (such as absence of Houston valves in infants)
- Solitary rectal ulcer syndrome: An uncommon benign condition usually affecting older children (teenagers). Rectal bleeding on defecation is common. Some studies report an association between this entity and rectal prolapse.
- Prolapsing polyp
- Large hemorrhoids
- Colonic intussusception
- Constipation
- Ehlers–Danlos syndrome
- Hirschsprung disease
- History of imperforate anus
- Pertussis/Pneumonia
- Ulcerative colitis
- History of meningomyelocele

TREATMENT

MEDICATION (DRUGS)
- Stool softeners (i.e., polyethylene glycol) to relieve constipation or medication with the associated condition
- In a patient with CF, addition of pancreatic enzyme supplementation, if not already a part of the regimen, has been shown to improve rectal prolapse dramatically.

ADDITIONAL TREATMENT
General Measures
- Rectal prolapse has a tendency to resolve spontaneously over time (90%; unlikely if 1st episode is in patient >4 years of age)
- Patients who present with a prolapsed rectum should undergo manual reduction in a prone position:
  – Parents should be provided with gloves and lubricant and taught how to reduce the prolapse.
  – The prolapsed bowel may be grasped with lubricated gloved fingers and pushed back in with gentle steady pressure.

– If the bowel has become edematous, firm steady pressure for several minutes may be necessary to reduce the swelling and allow for reduction.
– Digital rectal examination should always follow this procedure to verify complete reduction.
– If the prolapse immediately recurs, it may be reduced again and the buttocks taped together for several hours.

- The prolapse will resolve more successfully and quickly if the patient is treated for constipation:
  – This should include both dietary manipulations (e.g., increased fiber, hydration) and improved defecation methods.
  – It also will usually require the use of supplemental aids such as laxatives (polyethylene glycol).
- A small child should try to defecate with his hips at 90 degrees, his buttocks at toilet seat level, not hunched over, and on an appropriately sized toilet. If a child-sized toilet is unable to accomplish this, then an adult commode can be tried.
- In the rare case of stool infection with diarrhea as the underlying etiology, the appropriate therapy for that infection should be instituted.

SURGERY/OTHER PROCEDURES

Numerous (>130) approaches have been attempted and advocated with varying degrees of enthusiasm, suggesting that none is perfect. These include:

- Perianal sutures: Poor results and high complication rate
- Delorme procedure: Rectal mucosa is excised, and underlying rectal muscle is plicated with sutures.
- Laparoscopic suture rectopexy: Rectal wall is exposed and then sutured to the fascia of the sacral promontory; 5% full thickness recurrence rate.
- Abdominal rectopexy: Rectum is mobilized and attached to the sacrum by prosthetic material. Although the procedure provides good results, it has a high complication rate of constipation (>50%).
- Anterior resection rectopexy: Resection of the sigmoid loop and upper rectum; good results, but again, high complication rate.
- Perineal resection: Perineal rectosigmoidectomy with a coloanal anastomosis; good results
- Circumferential injection procedures (90–100% success rate): Injection of phenol, oil, hypertonic saline, dextrose 50% solution (500 g/L), or ethyl alcohol to promote adhesion and stabilization of the rectum
- Lockhart–Mummery operation (near 100% success): Mesh pack is placed temporarily in the retrorectal space (8–10 days) to promote adhesions that stabilize rectum.

IN-PATIENT CONSIDERATIONS
Initial Stabilization
Palliative:

- Reassurance of patient and/or family and caregivers
- Although surgery seems to be a quicker and more definite solution, in most cases it is more prudent to allow time and medical management to solve the problem. Surgical procedures are not without risk and may lead to further complications (>130 procedures exist, more effective in patients <4 years of age).

 ONGOING CARE

FOLLOW-UP RECOMMENDATIONS
Patient Monitoring
Ask caregiver to watch whether the child is beginning to strain to defecate.

DIET
- Increase consumption of liquids.
- Add larger amounts of fiber to diet (5 g + age in years)

PROGNOSIS
- With proper medical management, excellent prognosis; surgery is not usually required.
- Treatment of constipation should continue indefinitely, or until the child has demonstrated regular bowel habits on a high-fiber diet on his or her own without evidence of prolapse for at least several months.
- Over a period of months to years on a good dietary and behavioral regimen

COMPLICATIONS
- In some older patients who may also have an overactive external sphincter, the need to generate high rectal pressures to defecate, together with the rectal prolapse, may cause venous congestion; it may lead to the solitary rectal ulcer syndrome.
- Repetitive trauma to mucosa can produce proctitis.
- Surgical complications of repair
- Frequent recurrence

ADDITIONAL READING

- Antao B, Bradley V, Roberts JP, et al. Management of rectal prolapse in children. *Dis Colon Rectum*. 2005;48(8):1620–1625.
- Laituri CA, Garey CL, Fraser JD, et al. 15-year experience in the treatment of rectal prolapse in children. *J Pediatr Surg*. 2010;45(8):1607–1609.
- Potter DD, Bruny JL, Allshouse MJ, et al. Laparoscopic suture rectopexy for full-thickness anorectal prolapse in children: An effective outpatient procedure. *J Pediatr Surg*. 2010;45(10): 2103–2107.
- Sajid MS, Siddiqui MR, Baig MK. Open vs laparoscopic repair of full-thickness rectal prolapse: A re-meta-analysis. *Colorectal Dis*. 2010;12(6): 515–525.
- Siafakas C, Vottler TP, Andersen JM. Rectal prolapse in pediatrics. *Clin Pediatr (Phila)*. 1999;38(2):63–72.
- Steele SR, Goetz LH, Minami S, et al. Management of recurrent rectal prolapse: Surgical approach influences outcome. *Dis Colon Rectum*. 2006; 49(4):440–445.

CODES

ICD9
569.1 Rectal prolapse

ICD10
K62.3 Rectal prolapse

FAQ

- Q: What should I do if my child has a rectal prolapse but I cannot reduce it?
- A: You should wrap the prolapse in moist towels and bring your child to the emergency department. Physicians there will try to reduce it. Rarely, if a prolapse is irreducible and left for a period of time, it can cause bowel ischemia and may require surgery.
- Q: My child has rectal prolapse and now he is supposed to have a sweat test to determine whether he has CF. Is this very likely?
- A: No. Although it is important to rule out this disease, most patients with rectal prolapse do not have CF. However, many children with CF suffer from rectal prolapse.
- Q: My child, who has rectal prolapse, is in daycare. How will I know if he is having the prolapse?
- A: You should inform someone in the school (a teacher or guardian) of his condition, and he or she should check the child for prolapse after a bowel movement. Although, if present, it usually resolves spontaneously, the teacher should inform you so you can do a manual reduction, if necessary.

REFRACTIVE ERROR

Monte D. Mills

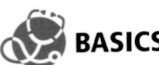 **BASICS**

DESCRIPTION

To allow vision, light coming into the eye must focus on the retina. Refractive errors are aberrations in the optic components of the eyes that cause the eye to lose focus. Uncorrected refractive error blurs vision in 1 or both eyes, and may also cause strabismus and amblyopia in children (see "Amblyopia" and "Strabismus").

GENERAL PREVENTION

- Early detection and correction of refractive errors is important to prevent amblyopia and strabismus. Recognition visual acuity testing using charts should start by age 4 years.
- Children with significant refractive errors are not necessarily symptomatic. All children should be screened for visual acuity in each eye.
- Glasses may not reverse amblyopia, even if the refractive error is appropriately corrected. Patients with suspected amblyopia (i.e., anisometropia, unilateral poor vision, and strabismus) should be rechecked often even if wearing glasses.

EPIDEMIOLOGY

Because of the age-related growth of the optic components of the eye, prevalence of refractive errors varies during childhood. At birth, usual median refractive error is low hyperopia, approximately +2.00 diopters. In adults, the median is emmetropia. The incidence of refractive error requiring correction increases with age.

Prevalence

- In school-aged children in the US, 7–25% have refractive error significant enough to affect visual acuity. ~25% of the adult population of the US have myopia, and ~5% have hyperopia.
- Some ethnic groups have increased prevalence of myopia, including people of Native American, Chinese, and Japanese descent.

RISK FACTORS

Genetics

- Both genetic and environmental factors are important in refractive status. ~60% of myopia can be predicted by parental degree of refraction, although inheritance seems to be polygenic in most cases.
- Some genetic syndromes associated with refractive errors include:
  - Myopia:
    ○ Stickler syndrome
    ○ Albinism
    ○ Marfan syndrome
    ○ Down syndrome
    ○ Ehlers–Danlos syndrome
  - Hyperopia:
    ○ Senior–Loken syndrome
    ○ WAGR (Wilms tumor, *a*niridia, *g*enitourinary malformations, and mental *r*etardation) syndrome
  - Astigmatism:
    ○ Down syndrome
    ○ Crouzon syndrome
    ○ Albinism

- Environmental:
  - Environmental factors associated with refractive error in childhood include premature birth, eye surgery, and eye trauma.

PATHOPHYSIOLOGY

- The most important optic components of the eye are the cornea and the lens, which refract light coming into the pupil to focus an image on the retina. The cornea and lens determine the focal length of the eye, which must match the actual eye length (distance from cornea to retina). A sharply focused image on the retina is necessary for recognition of small objects and normal visual acuity; refractive errors cause blurring.
- Refractive errors can be classified in three groups based on the optic effects:
  - Myopia, also called "near-sightedness," is correctable with concave lenses with negative diopteric power. Myopic eyes may be in focus for closer targets, but blurred for more distant.
  - Hyperopia, correctable with convex lenses with positive diopteric power.
    ○ Although hyperopia is sometimes called "far-sightedness," this is a misnomer in children.
    ○ Small hyperopic refractive errors are easily overcome by focusing the eye, or accommodation, and many hyperopic children have no difficulty seeing near or distant targets.
    ○ Larger amounts of hyperopia may blur both near and distant targets, or cause eye strain or esotropia because of the focusing effort required for focusing (see "Strabismus").
  - Astigmatism, correctable with toric lenses, is caused by aspheric aberration. Uncorrected astigmatism creates images that are not focused for near or distant targets.
    ○ Astigmatism may occur simultaneously with myopia and hyperopia.
- Other terms related to refractive error include:
  - Emmetropia, or neutral refraction (no refractive error)
  - Anisometropia, or unequal refractive error between the 2 eyes
  - Accommodation, the ability to refocus eyes for near targets, and to overcome hyperopia
- In children <8 years of age, because of visual development and plasticity, uncorrected refractive errors may have a significant effect on life-long vision. Amblyopia, which may cause permanent uncorrectable vision loss, and strabismus are among the risks of untreated refractive errors in young children (see "Strabismus" and "Amblyopia").

PATHOPHYSIOLOGY

- The refractive components of the eye (e.g., cornea, lens, eye length) normally develop simultaneously during early childhood to allow focused images. Factors determining the relative growth and development of these ocular features are not completely understood, and abnormal growth of any component may result in refractive error.
- High myopia (>5 diopters in children) is associated with pathological thinning of the retina and sclera, and is associated with an increased risk of retinal detachment later in life.

COMMONLY ASSOCIATED CONDITIONS

Refractive errors are frequently associated with other ocular conditions. These include:

- Myopia:
  - Childhood glaucoma
  - Retinitis pigmentosa
  - Coloboma
  - Microphthalmia
  - Retinopathy of prematurity
  - Congenital cataract
  - Achromatopsia
  - Retinal detachment
  - Retinal hole
- Hyperopia:
  - Esotropia
  - Leber congenital amaurosis
  - Surgically treated cataracts (aphakia)
- Astigmatism:
  - Congenital ptosis
  - Coloboma
  - Forceps birth injury
  - Glaucoma
  - Retinopathy of prematurity

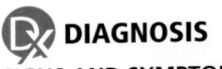 **DIAGNOSIS**

SIGNS AND SYMPTOMS

- Loss of vision
- Blurred vision
- Headache
- Squinting

HISTORY

- Age of onset of vision loss
- Associated ocular abnormalities, trauma, injury, or surgery
- History of strabismus, amblyopia
- History of prematurity, genetic disorders, collagen disorders (e.g., Ehlers–Danlos, Marfan syndromes)
- History of headaches, squinting, or subjective vision problems
- Family history of glasses or refractive error, amblyopia, strabismus

PHYSICAL EXAM

- Visual acuity is the most effective diagnostic tool for detecting refractive errors.
- Vision must be tested with each eye separately, using a patch, opaque card, or plastic occluder.
- Testing charts are available with letters as well as pictures and for children who cannot yet read figures (Es). In children who are too young to test with charts, the Bruchner simultaneous red reflex examination can detect high refractive errors and anisometropia, which appear as an asymmetric or distorted red pupillary reflex using the direct ophthalmoscope.
- Strabismus is frequently a secondary sign of refractive error in children and can be detected by cover test, Hirschberg corneal light reflex test, or Bruchner test. Photoscreening, which uses the principle of red reflex testing, is also effective in detecting high or asymmetric refractive errors.

DIFFERENTIAL DIAGNOSIS

- Any cause of monocular or binocular vision loss can simulate refractive error. Because refraction is not easily measured without eye drops and special equipment, possibility of refractive error must be considered in all children with reduced visual acuity and should also be considered in children with strabismus and normal vision. Cycloplegic refraction (measuring refraction after the use of eye drops to relax accommodation), and, in younger children, a trial of correction with glasses, is necessary to eliminate the possibility of residual amblyopia or other cause of poor vision.

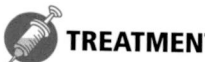 TREATMENT

ADDITIONAL TREATMENT
General Measures

- Refractive errors are treated by corrective lenses. In young children, this is usually glasses, although contact lenses are frequently used in teenagers.
- Unlike adults, children with neglected refractive error are at great risk for significant long-term complications, including amblyopia and strabismus. Hyperopia and anisometropic hyperopia pose the greatest risk for amblyopia. Therefore, smaller amounts of hyperopia and anisometropia are generally corrected with glasses. Glasses are prescribed to improve vision and treat or prevent amblyopia in children for:
  - Myopia, −3.00 diopters or more in infants and young children, −1.00 diopter or more in school-age children
  - Hyperopia, +4.00 diopters or more in infants, +3.00 diopters or more in school-age children, or +1.50 diopters or more anisometropia (difference between eyes)
  - Any hyperopia in accomodative esotropia. Bifocals may also be prescribed to treat residual esotropia for near targets (high AC/A ratio).
  - Astigmatism of >3.00 diopters in infants and young children, or >1.50 diopters in school-age children
- In general, children accept full correction of all refractive error, although undercorrection of hyperopia by 0.50–1.00 diopter may enhance the acceptance of new glasses. Occasionally, if hyperopic correction is not well accepted, a brief period of cycloplegia with topical atropine can reinforce use of the glasses.
- In suspected amblyopia, vision should be retested to measure visual improvement after glasses have been worn for several weeks. Children wearing glasses must be remeasured regularly, usually at least annually, until they have reached visual maturity and the risk of amblyopia has passed (i.e., 8–10 years of age).
- Hyperopic patients may develop accommodative esotropia when their glasses are off, after wearing the glasses for some time. Full correction of hyperopia and continuous correction are key approaches to this unusual complication.

 ONGOING CARE

Refractive errors change over time due to growth of the eye and its optic components. In general, younger children will need rerefraction and new glasses more frequently. All children wearing glasses should have acuity tested and be rerefracted at least annually.

PROGNOSIS

With treatment, generally glasses in younger children but including contact lenses in older children and teenagers, refractive errors rarely lead to significant functional limitations for daily activities and school. Amblyopia and strabismus must also be treated, if present. Special frames for sports and athletic activities should be considered for children if standard glasses are interfering with those activities.

COMPLICATIONS

In children, the most significant complications of uncorrected refractive errors are strabismus and amblyopia.

- Accommodative esotropia: Uncorrected hyperopia in young children can be overcome by focusing, or accommodation.
  - This involuntary focusing of the eyes is controlled reflexively and integrated with convergence (i.e., crossing the eyes inward).
  - Usually, accommodation is used to focus on near targets, and convergence keeps both eyes pointed at the near target.
  - If excessive hyperopia is present, or an abnormal ratio of accommodative convergence to accommodation exists (AC:A ratio), the eyes may cross with accommodation, producing accommodative esotropia (see "Strabismus").
- Amblyopia: Poor visual development results from a poorly focused image. Anisometropia (unequal refractive error), which blurs vision in 1 eye and is the most frequent cause of unilateral amblyopia, causes ~35% of amblypia. Less frequently, bilateral high refractive errors may cause bilateral amblyopia (see "Amblyopia").

ADDITIONAL READING

- American Academy of Ophthalmology. *Preferred Practice Pattern: Pediatric Eye Examination*. San Francisco: American Academy of Ophthalmology; 2002.
- American Academy of Ophthalmology. *Preferred Practice Pattern: Refractive Errors*. San Francisco: American Academy of Ophthalmology; 2002.
- Kuo A, Sinatra RB, Donahue SP. Distribution of refractive error in healthy infants. *J Am Assoc Pediatr Ophthalmol Strabismus*. 2003;7:174–177.
- Mills MD. The eye in childhood. *Am Fam Phys*. 1999;60:907–918.
- Paysse EA, Williams GC, Coats DK, et al. Detection of red reflex asymmetry by pediatric residents using the Bruchner reflex versus the MTI photoscreener. *Pediatrics*. 2001;108.
- Thorn F. Development of refraction and strabismus. *Curr Opin Ophthalmol*. 2000;11:301–305.

 CODES

ICD9
- 367.1 Myopia
- 367.31 Anisometropia
- 367.9 Unspecified disorder of refraction and accommodation

ICD10
- H52.7 Unspecified disorder of refraction
- H52.10 Myopia, unspecified eye
- H52.11 Myopia, right eye

FAQ

- Q: Will my child always need glasses?
- A: Not necessarily. Many children who wear glasses are able to see well without correction as adults. Contact lenses and refractive surgery are also possible in older children or adults, if correction remains necessary.
- Q: Will wearing glasses weaken my child's eyes?
- A: No, wearing correction for refractive errors will not weaken the eyes or vision, and is important to prevent amblyopia and permanent vision loss. Occasionally, children with hyperopia will develop accommodative esotropia when the glasses are removed, after wearing correction for some time. This is rarely a problem as long as the glasses are worn continuously.
- Q: Is my child too young for glasses?
- A: Glasses can be worn in children as young as a few months old, with appropriate frames. Usually, children get used to glasses quickly and accept correction easily.
- Q: My child can see well, why does he need glasses?
- A: Some children with hyperopia can see charts well, but the accommodation (i.e., focusing) necessary to overcome the refractive error may cause eye strain, fatigue, and esotropia. Others may need glasses for unilateral refractive error and seem to see well with both eyes open. In these children, wearing correction may treat or prevent problems even though they may seem to see well without correction.
- Q: Everyone in my family has needed glasses for myopia in childhood. Is there anything we can do for my child that will prevent the development of myopia?
- A: Unfortunately, few environmental factors have been clearly identified to affect the development of myopia. Reading, particularly at an early age; excessively close visual targets (holding books or toys too close to the face); and light exposure during nighttime have been suggested as factors in myopia development. Avoiding long periods of reading, avoiding intensive near work, using a reasonable reading distance (i.e., 16–18 inches), and avoiding use of night lights may reduce some environmental stimuli.

RENAL ARTERY STENOSIS

Danielle Soranno
Michelle Denburg
Thomas L. Kennedy (5th edition)

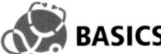 **BASICS**

DESCRIPTION
Narrowing of 1 or both renal arteries and/or their more distal branches, resulting in decreased perfusion, increased renin release, increased vascular resistance, and systemic hypertension.

EPIDEMIOLOGY
- Hypertension in infants and young children is often secondary to some identifiable cause. Of those with secondary hypertension, most have intrinsic renal disease (e.g., renal scarring, dysplasia, chronic nephritis).
- Most older children and adolescents with hypertension (i.e., readings consistently exceeding 95th percentile for age and height) have primary or idiopathic hypertension.
- Up to 5% of adults with hypertension have RAS.
- Renal artery stenosis accounts for ~10% of secondary hypertension in children. Its importance clinically is not its frequency, but its potential curability.

RISK FACTORS
Include any condition associated with thromboembolic events (such as a complication of an umbilical artery catheter in newborns), renal trauma including renal artery surgery (e.g., transplantation), or extrinsic compression of the renal artery (e.g., Wilms tumor, neuroblastoma, or pheochromocytoma).

GENERAL PREVENTION
Reduce risk factors, such as thromboembolic events, which can lead to renal artery narrowing.

PATHOPHYSIOLOGY
Arterial narrowing leads to diminished perfusion of the affected kidney, leading to signals in the juxtaglomerular apparatus, which lead to renin release and results in increased vascular resistance and BP.

ETIOLOGY
- Majority are caused by fibromuscular dysplasia. The cause is unknown and is usually an isolated finding.
- Arterial narrowing by atheroma is common in adults, but rare in children.

COMMONLY ASSOCIATED CONDITIONS
- Renal artery stenosis may occur in many other conditions, including congenital anomalies (e.g., renal artery hypoplasia), neurocutaneous disorders (neurofibromatosis [type 1], tuberous sclerosis), vasculitis (Wegener, polyarteritis nodosa, Kawasaki disease, Takayasu arteritis, moyamoya disease), syndromes (Williams, Marfan, Alagille), and infections (e.g., congenital rubella and fungal infection [immunocompromised hosts]).
- The nephrotic syndrome may accompany renal artery stenosis and is probably secondary to it.
- Renal artery stenosis has been associated with multicystic dysplasia in the contralateral kidney.

 DIAGNOSIS

Prehospital
Obtain multiple BP readings with an appropriate-size cuff in an upper extremity. Avoid using automated devices (oscillometers). Consider renal artery stenosis in a child with very high BP readings (i.e., at or above the 99th percentile).

HISTORY
- Ask about prior BP determinations, family history of hypertension, previous renal disease, symptoms of hypertension, and preexisting conditions associated with renal artery stenosis.
- Signs and symptoms:
  - Symptoms of hypertension in infants are not specific and include irritability, poor feeding, and vomiting.
  - In children, symptoms include headache, nausea/vomiting, visual disturbance, dizziness, and seizure.
  - Many affected children remain asymptomatic and 1/3 of children with RAS are diagnosed incidentally.

PHYSICAL EXAM
- Obtain multiple accurate BP readings using an appropriate-size cuff in the right upper extremity and compare to the BP nomogram for age, sex, and length/height percentile.
- BP must be repeated until patient is completely relaxed with baseline heart rate.
- Most accurate readings obtained with either a mercury column or an aneroid sphygmomanometer.
- The inflatable bladder of the cuff should almost completely encircle the arm.
- Determine the BP in all extremities. A gradient from the upper to lower extremities should prompt evaluation for aortic coarctation or midaortic syndrome.
- Examine the skin for lesions suggestive of vasculitis or neurocutaneous disorder (e.g., café-au-lait macules).
- Assess the child's facies and habitus for features of associated syndromes.
- View the optic fundi for hypertensive vascular changes.
- Auscultate the lower back and abdomen for the presence of a bruit (suggesting turbulent flow).
- In infancy, signs of heart failure may be present.

DIAGNOSTIC TESTS & INTERPRETATION
ECG and echocardiogram to assess for left ventricular hypertrophy and function

Lab
- BUN and creatinine to evaluate for renal insufficiency
- Electrolytes to assess possible hyperaldosteronism with hypokalemia and metabolic alkalosis. Hyponatremia may sometimes occur.
- ESR or CRP to screen for vasculitis

Imaging
- The definitive diagnostic test remains the selective renal arteriogram. If the diagnosis is made, angioplasty may be part of the same procedure. Angiography should not be delayed in any child in whom the diagnosis is strongly suspected.
- Renal ultrasound with Doppler to identify a smaller kidney and/or increased resistance to flow is simple and not invasive, but it is neither sensitive nor specific. Length discrepancy of >1 cm in children can increase suspicion for RAS.
- Contrast-enhanced CT or MR angiography also is not completely diagnostic and is not therapeutic.
- Nuclear renal scans using DMSA or MAG-3 enhanced with captopril (and more recently angiotensin-receptor blockers) also are not diagnostic for all children.
- Diagnostic accuracy of various imaging studies:

Technique	Sensitivity (%)	Specificity (%)
Ultrasound	73–85	71–92
DMSA with ACE	52–93	63–92
CTA	64–94	62–97
MRA	64–93	72–97

Diagnostic Procedures/Other
- Avoid excessive investigation in children whose BP is minimally or episodically elevated and therefore in whom the diagnosis of renal artery stenosis is less likely.
- Selective renal vein renin determinations suggest unilateral stenosis if the affected side is 1.5 times the contralateral (normal) side. However, the procedure is invasive and requires catheterization of the femoral vein.
- Random renin determinations have little value and may be misleading. If obtained, renin levels should be interpreted in the context of the urine sodium concentration.

Pathological Findings
- Fibromuscular dysplasia is a segmental sclerotic process involving smooth muscle hyperplasia of the media layer of the artery. It is unilateral in 75%.
- Stenosis is usually distal in the renal artery, sometimes involving intrarenal branches.
- The stenotic area(s) of the artery may be associated with distal aneurysms.
- In neurofibromatosis arterial narrowing is at the vessel's ostium and usually involves the intimal layer.

DIFFERENTIAL DIAGNOSIS
- Renal artery stenosis should be suspected and investigated in children with severe, progressive, and/or difficult-to-manage hypertension.
- The differential diagnosis consists of other causes of significant hypertension, including increased intracranial pressure, coarctation of the aorta, midaortic syndrome, rapidly progressive glomerulonephritis, vasculitis, and pheochromocytoma.

TREATMENT

Treat children immediately who are symptomatic (e.g., severe headaches, seizures, blurred vision, facial palsy).

MEDICATION (DRUGS)

- Hypertension accompanying renal artery stenosis is often difficult to control and may worsen over time. Multiple medications given in high doses are common until the diagnosis is made and angioplasty can be done.
- Because renal artery stenosis results in increased renin levels, renin-angiotensin blockade with ACE inhibitor therapy (e.g., enalapril, lisinopril) and/or angiotensin receptor blockers (ARBs, e.g., losartan) is often effective. In children where bilateral renal artery stenosis is known or suspected, ACE inhibitor and ARB therapy must be avoided to prevent acute renal failure. 50% of children will have bilateral disease. Renal function should be checked before and after initiation of ACE inhibition or ARB therapy.
- If BP is easy to control on monotherapy, may consider medical management alone rather than angioplasty
- β-Blockers, calcium channel blockers, diuretics, and direct vasodilators (e.g., minoxidil, hydralazine) are all possibly effective.

ADDITIONAL TREATMENT
General Measures
- If renal artery stenosis is suspected, begin the diagnostic evaluation and pharmacotherapy together.
- If BP is very high, use bed rest until BP is better controlled.

ISSUES FOR REFERRAL
- Nephrology
- Cardiology follow-up for echo changes, if indicated
- Ophthalmologic follow-up for resolution of vascular changes, if indicated

SURGERY/OTHER PROCEDURES
- Actual surgery on the stenotic renal artery has been replaced by angioplasty, which has been successfully carried out in very young infants. Stents are occasionally used.
- Surgery must sometimes be performed, especially in children with neurofibromatosis where the stenosis is frequently at the renal artery's ostium.

IN-PATIENT CONSIDERATIONS
Initial Stabilization
- If symptomatic, use potent, rapidly acting medications such as labetalol or nicardipine.
- Be prepared to have difficulty adequately controlling the BP using a single medication.

Admission Criteria
- Children who present with a BP at or above the 99th percentile
- Children who appear to have symptomatic hypertension
- Children with progressive renal insufficiency

Nursing
- Obtain BP levels frequently and carefully.
- Notify MD if high or low limits exceeded.
- Monitor intake of salt, I&O, and weight.

Discharge Criteria
BP in the 90th–95th percentile

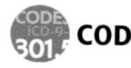 **ONGOING CARE**

FOLLOW-UP RECOMMENDATIONS
- The child's BP must be followed closely, both before and after the angioplasty. Response to angioplasty may be immediate, but may require continued antihypertensive therapy at some level for weeks to months.
- Medical therapy should be monitored closely. Until correction, the need for progressively higher doses and/or additional medications is common.
- Disposition:
  – Close follow-up by the primary care provider, mainly for monitoring BP, and a specialist comfortable with the evaluation and treatment of childhood hypertension.
  – Patient and/or family must be familiar with medication, exercise program, and diet.

Patient Monitoring
- Long-term follow-up of the BP is most important. If on no medications, the BP should be checked monthly, preferably somewhere the child is comfortable and the correct cuff is employed. Begin to space visits after 6 months.
- Checking renal growth on serial renal ultrasounds is important (e.g., at 6 months postangioplasty and then yearly). If the child is fully grown, check ultrasound at 6 months.
- Check renal function annually.

DIET
Limit salt intake.

PROGNOSIS
Long-term outcome of percutaneous angioplasty is excellent; most children require no long-term antihypertensive medications.

COMPLICATIONS
- Restenosis of the renal artery, either ipsilateral or contralateral, is uncommon but possible.
- When renal artery stenosis causes severe hypertension, it may cause encephalopathy, severe headache, seizures, or stroke.
- If untreated, chronic hypertension may cause end-organ damage, including heart and kidney.
- Angiography may lead to contrast-induced renal failure. The procedure may also cause injury to the kidney and/or renal artery.
- Rare cases of subarachnoid hemorrhage secondary to coexisting intracranial aneurysm may occur.

ADDITIONAL READING

- Airoldi F, Palatresi S, Marana I, et al. Angioplasty of atherosclerotic and fibromuscular renal artery stenosis: Time course and predicting factors of the effects on renal function. *Am J Hypertension*. 2000;13:1210–1217.
- Konig K, Gellerman J, Querfeld U, et al. Treatment of severe renal artery stenosis by percutaneous transluminal renal angioplasty and stent implantation: Review of the pediatric experience: Apropos of two cases. *Pediatr Nephrol*. 2006; 21(5):663–671.
- Rountas C, Vlychou M, Vassiou K, et al. Imaging modalities for renal artery stenosis in suspected renovascular hypertension: Prospective intraindividual comparison of color Doppler US, CT angiography, GD-enhanced MR angiography, and digital substraction angiography. *Ren Fail*. 2007;29(3):295–302.
- Sethna CB, Kaplan BS, Cahill AM, et al. Idiopathic mid-aortic syndrome in children. *Pediatr Nephrol*. 2008;23(7):1135–1142.
- Shahdadpuri J, Frank R, Gauthier BG, et al. Yield of renal arteriography in the evaluation of pediatric hypertension. *Pediatr Nephrol*. 2000;14:816–819.
- Spyridopoulos T, Kaziani K, Balanika AP, et al. Ultrasound as a first line screening tool for the detection of renal artery stenosis: A comprehensive review. *Med Ultrason*. 2010;12:228–232.
- Tullus K. Renal artery stenosis: Is angiography still the gold standard in 2011? *Pediatr Nephrol*. 2011;26:833–837.
- Vade A, Agrawal R, Lim-Dunham J, et al. Utility of computer tomographic renal angiogram in the management of childhood hypertension. *Pediatr Nephrol*. 2002;17:741–744.

CODES

ICD9
- 440.1 Atherosclerosis of renal artery
- 747.62 Renal vessel anomaly

ICD10
- I70.1 Atherosclerosis of renal artery
- Q27.1 Congenital renal artery stenosis

R

RENAL TUBULAR ACIDOSIS

Christopher P. Bonafide
Christopher J. LaRosa
Andres J. Greco (5th edition)

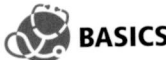

BASICS

DESCRIPTION

- Renal tubular acidosis (RTA) syndromes are renal transport defects characterized by normal anion gap metabolic acidosis, hyperchloremia, and normal renal function.
- Acidification of the blood occurs when there is an inability to excrete the daily endogenous metabolic acid load (distal RTA), a failure to reabsorb filtered bicarbonate (proximal RTA), or aldosterone deficiency/resistance (hyperkalemic RTA).
- Distal RTA (type I):
  - Caused by impaired acidification of the urine in the distal tubule of the kidney
  - Main defect is either a failure of the apical H^+-ATP pump, back-leak of secreted hydrogen ions, or insufficient negative charge in the distal tubule.
  - Characterized by an inability to lower urinary pH maximally (<5.5), even in severe systemic acidemia
- Proximal RTA (type II):
  - Caused by impaired bicarbonate reabsorption in the proximal tubule of the kidney
  - Main defect is a more acidic serum threshold for proximal tubular bicarbonate reabsorption ($\sim$15 mEq/L vs. the normal threshold of $\sim$22 mEq/L).
  - Distinguished from distal RTA in that urinary acidification mechanisms are intact in severe systemic acidemia (these patients can decrease urine pH <5.5, although the setpoint for appropriate acidification is altered).
  - May occur as an isolated defect or as part of the Fanconi syndrome (generalized proximal tubular dysfunction resulting in glycosuria with a normal plasma glucose, phosphaturia, hypophosphatemia, aminoaciduria, and tubular proteinuria)
- Hyperkalemic RTA (type IV):
  - Caused by impaired action of aldosterone on hydrogen and potassium excretion.
  - Main defect is either aldosterone deficiency or resistance, which may occur in the context of renal parenchymal damage.
  - Characterized by hyperkalemia and mild acidosis (serum bicarbonate >17 mEq/L).

EPIDEMIOLOGY

- Primary RTA is very rare.
- The most common forms of RTA in children are proximal and distal.

Genetics

- Distal RTA can be observed sporadically or as an autosomal dominant (chromosome 17q21–22) or recessive transmission with deafness (chromosome 2p13) or without deafness (chromosome 7q33–34). The genes affected encode the chloride-bicarbonate exchanger or the hydrogen-ATPase pump.
- Isolated proximal RTA can occur secondary to mutations in the gene encoding the sodium bicarbonate cotransporter.
- Proximal RTA with Fanconi syndrome occurs in several genetic conditions: cystinosis, Lowe syndrome, Wilson disease, Dent disease, tyrosinemia, hereditary fructose intolerance, galactosemia, and mitochondrial myopathies.
- Hereditary hyperkalemic RTA is most frequently observed in children with congenital adrenal hyperplasia, aldosterone synthase deficiency, and pseudohypoaldosteronism type 1 or type 2 (Gordon syndrome).

COMMONLY ASSOCIATED CONDITIONS

- Distal RTA may also be caused by autoimmune conditions, obstructive uropathy, interstitial renal disease, and medications including lithium, cisplatin, and amphotericin B.
- Osteopenia, rickets, growth failure, nephrocalcinosis, and nephrolithiasis may develop in patients with distal RTA.
- Isolated proximal RTA may also be caused by medications including sulfonamides.
- Proximal RTA with Fanconi syndrome may also be caused by interstitial renal disease, heavy metal exposure, and medications including aminoglycosides, cisplatin, and ifosamide.
- Proximal RTA can occur with vitamin D deficiency and hyperparathyroidism.
- Rickets can occur due to the phosphate wasting in Fanconi syndrome.
- Proximal and distal RTA may occur in the setting of renal transplantation.
- Hyperkalemic RTA may also be caused by HIV infection, obstructive uropathy, interstitial renal disease, diabetes mellitus, and medications including heparin, NSAIDS, ACE inhibitors, calcineurin inhibitors, and sulfonamides.

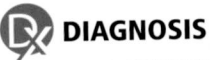

DIAGNOSIS

SIGNS AND SYMPTOMS

- Children with RTA often present with growth failure, polyuria, constipation, and anorexia. Other associated signs and symptoms may include:
- Dehydration
- Vomiting
- Bone pain or deformities
- Renal colic
- Severe metabolic acidosis and electrolyte imbalance resulting from mild gastroenteritis
- Photophobia (in cystinosis)
- Hypertension (in RTA type IV secondary to renal parenchymal disease or Gordon syndrome)

HISTORY

- Weight loss or poor weight gain
- Urine concentration deficits (polyuria, polydipsia, enuresis)
- Constipation
- Anorexia
- History of hospitalization for dehydration or metabolic acidosis with mild gastroenteritis
- Medications as noted earlier
- Family history of RTA
- Deafness (autosomal recessive distal RTA)
- Developmental delay (autosomal recessive proximal RTA)

PHYSICAL EXAM

- General: Failure to thrive
- Head and neck: Frontal bossing, abnormal eye examination (cystine deposition, glaucoma, cataracts, Kaiser–Fleischer rings)
- Chest: Rachitic rosary (rickets)
- Abdomen: Hepatomegaly, enlarged kidneys
- Extremities: Bowing of legs, widening of epiphysis of wrists

DIAGNOSTIC TESTS & INTERPRETATION

The hallmark of RTA is a hyperchloremic metabolic acidosis with normal anion gap and normal renal function.

Lab
- Serum electrolytes:
  – Helps to identify the presence of metabolic acidosis, hypokalemia, or hyperkalemia.
  – Permits calculation of serum anion gap (SAG).
    ○ SAG = $Na^+ - [Cl^- + HCO_3^-]$
    ○ Normal anion gap = 8–16 mEq/L
  – When assessing for RTA, this test should be run STAT to decrease the chance of a falsely low bicarbonate result from cell lysis.
- Serum creatinine: Helps to exclude renal failure.
- Urinalysis: Evaluates for features of Fanconi syndrome (glycosuria) or renal disease (proteinuria).
- Urine electrolytes and pH:
  – If urine pH is <5.5, then type I RTA can be ruled out.
  – Permits calculation of urine anion gap (UAG)
    ○ UAG = [urine Na^+] + [urine K^+] − [urine Cl^-].
  – Negative urine anion gap is seen in GI losses and proximal RTA.
  – Positive urine anion gap is seen in distal and hyperkalemic RTA.
- Urine spot for calcium/creatinine ratio: Patients with RTA can have hypercalciuria.
- Tubular reabsorption of phosphate (TRP): TRP <60% can be seen in Fanconi syndrome and other causes of proximal RTA.
- 24-hour urine for citrate, calcium, potassium, and oxalate: Hypercalciuria and hypocitraturia are risk factors for nephrocalcinosis and/or nephrolithiasis.

Imaging
- Long bone films/rickets survey: Evaluates for rachitic changes, osteopenia, bone age.
- Renal ultrasound: Evaluates for renal dysplasia, obstructive uropathy, nephrocalcinosis, nephrolithiasis, or hydronephrosis.

DIFFERENTIAL DIAGNOSIS
- GI fluid losses: Diarrhea, ileal conduits, fistulas draining the small bowel, biliary tract, or pancreas
- Use of acetazolamide and other carbonic anhydrase inhibitors
- Parenteral nutrition

 ## TREATMENT

- Alkali administration is the primary therapy for children with RTA, with the dose titrated to maintain normal bicarbonate levels.
- Sodium/potassium citrate is preferable for children with distal or proximal RTA, because hypokalemia may also be present.
- Sodium citrate or sodium bicarbonate is used in children with hyperkalemic RTA who require potassium restriction.
- Patients with distal RTA usually require 1–4 mEq/kg alkali therapy per day in 3–4 divided doses.
- Patients with proximal RTA require considerably more alkali therapy (5–20 mEq/kg/d in 4–6 divided doses).
- The dosage of alkali in children with hyperkalemic RTA ranges 1–5 mEq/kg/d, which is usually sufficient to correct the potassium level.
- Sodium polystyrene sulfonate (kayexalate) may be needed for patients with hyperkalemic RTA whose potassium level does not normalize with alkali therapy.
- Mineralicorticoids should be given to treat underlying hypoaldosteronism in hyperkalemic RTA.
- All patients with secondary causes of RTA should be treated for the underlying disease.
- All patients with RTA due to medications should have them withdrawn if the risks of RTA outweigh the benefits of the medication.

 ## ONGOING CARE

- Patients with RTA should be closely monitored with frequent potassium and bicarbonate levels until a steady state is reached.
- Normal growth may be attained after the metabolic acidosis is corrected.
- Untreated distal RTA can lead to renal failure by causing progressive nephrocalcinosis. Adequate alkali therapy is usually enough to avoid this complication.
- Patients with hypercalciuria should be monitored with spot urine calcium/creatinine ratio. Alkali therapy should be adjusted to maintain a ratio <0.2 mg/mg.
- Renal ultrasound follow-up is recommended in patients with nephrocalcinosis.

Patient Monitoring
- Avoid hemolyzed specimens that may artificially increase the serum potassium and reduce the plasma bicarbonate levels.
- Administer alkali over several divided doses.
- Closely monitor patients during episodes of gastroenteritis to avoid dehydration and severe metabolic acidosis.

ADDITIONAL READING

- Alper SL. Familial renal tubular acidosis. *J Nephrol.* 2010;23(suppl)16:S57–76.
- Chan J, Scheinman JI, Roth K. Consultation with the specialist: Renal tubular acidosis. *Pediatr Rev.* 2001;22:277–287.
- Rodriguez-Soriano J. Renal tubular acidosis: The clinical entity. *J Am Soc Nephrol.* 2002;13: 2160–2170.

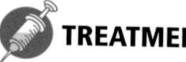 ## CODES

ICD9
588.89 Other specified disorders resulting from impaired renal function Other specified disorders resulting from impaired renal function

ICD10
N25.89 Other disorders resulting from impaired renal tubular function

R

RENAL VENOUS THROMBOSIS

Christine B. Sethna

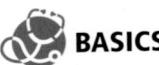 **BASICS**

DESCRIPTION
- Renal venous thrombosis is a thrombotic process that begins in the intrarenal venous radicals that usually progresses forward toward the main renal vein and may extend to the inferior vena cava.
- Rarely, the thrombosis may progress in the opposite direction.
- Usually presents clinically as a triad of macroscopic hematuria, palpable abdominal mass and thrombocytopenia in a newborn.

EPIDEMIOLOGY
- Renal venous thrombosis is predominantly a disease of the newborn.
- Slight male predilection
- More frequently unilateral than bilateral
- Left-sided predominance

Incidence
- Poorly defined
- 2.2 per 100,000 live births in a German registry study

Prevalence
Accounts for 20% of neonatal thromboembolism

RISK FACTORS
- Hyperosmolar state after angiocardiography
- Coagulopathy
- Sepsis
- Acute blood loss/shock
- Dehydration/Diarrhea
- Maternal diabetes
- Sickle cell disease
- Maternal lupus anticoagulant
- Central venous lines
- Prematurity
- In utero fetal distress

Genetics
Inherited prothrombotic risk factors are found in 50% of patients with neonatal RVT.

GENERAL PREVENTION
- The infant of a mother with diabetes should be observed for evidence of renal venous thrombosis.
- Patients with nephrotic syndrome are at increased risk of thrombosis in general when treated with diuretics.
- If cyanotic congenital heart disease is present, contrast agents should be used judiciously.
- Parents and caregivers should be educated about the importance of adequate intake and good hydration in the newborn and infant.
- There should be an increased index of suspicion among medical staff when examining an infant with diarrhea or a hyperosmolar state.

PATHOPHYSIOLOGY
- Renal venous thrombosis in newborns and infants is commonly associated with asphyxia, dehydration due to diarrhea, shock, sepsis, hypertonicity, coagulation abnormalities, and hemoconcentration.
- Additional predisposing factors in the newborn include congenital renal anomalies and maternal diabetes.
- In older children, associated with the nephrotic syndrome, cyanotic heart disease, and hyperosmolar states such as with the use of angiographic contrast agents
- In many children, no underlying cause is apparent.
- The slow double circulation of the kidney is especially vulnerable to thrombosis.
- Thrombus formation may be initiated by vascular endothelial cell injury in conjunction with diminished vascular flow.
- Renal venous thrombosis usually starts in the small venous radicals, with progression through the arcuate and interlobular veins toward the main renal vein.
- Renal venous thrombosis causes renal congestion and occasionally infarction.

 DIAGNOSIS

HISTORY
- Most patients are newborns.
- Renal venous thrombosis is usually heralded by the sudden onset of hematuria, unilateral or bilateral flank masses, and thrombocytopenia; however, only a fraction will have this "triad" on presentation
- Signs and symptoms:
  - Pallor
  - Tachypnea
  - Abdominal distention
  - Shock
  - Flank pain
  - Fever
  - Oliguria
  - Anuria
  - Hematuria

PHYSICAL EXAM
- 60% of affected patients have a palpably enlarged kidney.
- If lower limbs become edematous, cyanotic, and hypothermic during thrombosis, the inferior vena cava is involved.
- Hypertension at presentation is uncommon/rare, but it may develop later on.

DIAGNOSTIC TESTS & INTERPRETATION

Lab
- Urine:
  - Proteinuria is common.
  - Most patients have macroscopic hematuria.
- CBC:
  - 90% have progressive thrombocytopenia, and most also have microangiopathic hemolytic anemia.
- Fibrin split products:
  - Fibrin split products may be elevated, with low plasma fibrinogen levels.
- Electrolytes and BUN:
  - Azotemia and other biochemical evidence of acute kidney injury may be present.
  - Variations in plasma electrolytes depend on the presence of diarrhea or renal injury.
- Workup for procoaguable states, such as Factor V Leiden and maternal lupus anticoagulant, should be done.

Imaging
- Ultrasonography: Most useful study; will differentiate renal enlargement and extrarenal masses; will also identify obstruction, cystic changes, and many congenital anomalies; will show renal enlargement, increased echogenicity, calcification and loss of corticomedullary differentiation.
- Doppler ultrasound: Useful to detect resistance of absence of flow in renal veins.
- Radioisotopic reperfusion and excretion studies may also be helpful.

DIFFERENTIAL DIAGNOSIS
- Exclude other causes of renal enlargement (e.g., hydronephrosis, cystic renal disease, renal tumors, abscess, hematoma).
- Hemolytic-uremic syndrome should also be considered because renal venous thrombosis may also result in fragmented erythrocytes and thrombocytopenia.

 TREATMENT

MEDICATION (DRUGS)
- Recommendations from the American College of Chest Physicians Evidence-Based Clinical Practice Guidelines (8th edition) for Antithrombotic Therapy in Neonates and Children include:
  - For unilateral renal vein thrombosis in the absence of renal impairment or extension into the IVC, supportive care with monitoring of the RVT for extension or anticoagulation with unfractionated heparin (UFH)/low-molecular-weight heparin (LMWH), or LMWH in therapeutic doses for 3 months is suggested.
  - For unilateral RVT that extends into the IVC, anticoagulation with UFH/LMWH or LMWH for 3 months is suggested.
  - For bilateral RVT, anticoagulation with UFH and initial thrombolytic therapy with tPA, followed by anticoagulation with UFH/LMWH is suggested.

ADDITIONAL TREATMENT
General Measures
- Correction of underlying pathophysiologic abnormalities should be attempted.
- Management includes supportive therapy, anticoagulant therapy or thrombolysis. Renal outcomes are similar between supportive therapy and anticoagulant therapy.

ISSUES FOR REFERRAL
Patients with renal venous thrombosis should be followed regularly by a nephrologist.

SURGERY/OTHER PROCEDURES
- A surgical approach in the acute phase is rarely indicated. Surgery, complicated by disturbed fluid balance and acid–base status and altered coagulation, is risky.
- Because the thrombosis begins deep within the kidney and spreads to the larger veins, thrombectomy should be considered only in the event of bilateral involvement with involvement of inferior vena cava.
- Ultimately, if the kidney has negligible function and contributes to hypertension or recurrent infections, nephrectomy may be indicated.

IN-PATIENT CONSIDERATIONS
Initial Stabilization
Treatment is supportive and includes correction of fluid and electrolyte disturbances and treatment of infection.

Admission Criteria
- Neonates with renal venous thrombosis should be admitted to the NICU for close observation and management.
- Fibrinolytic therapy should be initiated in an ICU setting.

Discharge Criteria
Stabilization of renal function and blood pressure

 ## ONGOING CARE

FOLLOW-UP RECOMMENDATIONS
Patient Monitoring
- All patients should be observed closely for evidence of hypertension.
- Renal size should be monitored by US.

PROGNOSIS
- Patients must be followed closely for development of hypertension, atrophy, functional loss, and chronic kidney disease.
- Degree of irreversible renal damage depends on the degree of involvement and associated conditions.
- Rare deaths in these patients seem to be unrelated to the renal venous thrombosis and are usually the result of an underlying comorbid condition.
- Recovery of function may occur in affected kidneys. Varying degrees of renal impairment are seen in 30% of patients.
- Hypertension is seen in 20%.
- Most patients have residual renal structural abnormalities (e.g., atrophy, coarse renal scarring).
- Kidney size >6 cm at the time of presentation may correlate negatively with renal outcome.

COMPLICATIONS
- Bilateral renal venous thrombosis may lead to chronic kidney disease.
- Scarring may result in hypertension.

ADDITIONAL READING
- Goldenberg NA. Long-term outcomes of venous thrombosis in children. *Curr Opin Hematol*. 2005;12(5):370–376.
- Kuhle S, Massicotte P, Chan A, et al. A case series of 72 neonates with renal vein thrombosis. Data from the 1-800-NO-CLOTS Registry. *Thromb Haemost*. 2004;92:929–933.

- Lau KK, Stoffman JM, Williams S, et al. Neonatal renal vein thrombosis: Review of the English-language literature between 1992 and 2006. Canadian Pediatric Thrombosis and Hemostasis Network. *Pediatrics*. 2007;120(5):e1278–e1284.
- Messinger Y, Sheaffer JW, Mrozek J, et al. Renal outcome of neonatal renal venous thrombosis: Review of 28 patients and effectiveness of fibrinolytics and heparin in 10 patients. *Pediatrics*. 2006;118:1478–1484.
- Monagle P, Chalmers E, Chan A, et al. Antithrombotic therapy in neonates and children: American College of Chest Physicians Evidence-Based Clinical Practice Guidelines (8th Edition). *Chest*. 2008;133:887S–968S.
- Winward PJ, Bharucha T, DeBruyn R, et al. Perinatal renal venous thrombosis: Presenting renal length predicts outcome. *Arch Dis Child Fetal Neonatal Ed*. 2006;91(4):F273–F278.

 ## CODES

ICD9
453.3 Other venous embolism and thrombosis of renal vein

ICD10
I82.3 Embolism and thrombosis of renal vein

FAQ
- Q: Can renal venous thrombosis occur in the absence of gross hematuria?
- A: Most patients do have hematuria that may be gross. However, hematuria is often microscopic or absent.
- Q: Do patients with renal venous thrombosis usually have hypertension during the acute phase?
- A: Hypertension is uncommon at presentation.

RESPIRATORY SYNCYTIAL VIRUS (RSV)

Kathleen Wholey Zsolway
Alyssa Siegel

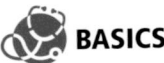 **BASICS**

DESCRIPTION
- A pleomorphic, enveloped RNA virus of the family Paramyxoviridae. There are 2 major groups, A and B, which differ in the largest surface glycoprotein, the G protein. The fusion protein, F protein, is ~95% homologous between the 2 subgroups.
- It is the most common cause of bronchiolitis, a viral lower respiratory tract disease of infants and young children.

EPIDEMIOLOGY
- Incubation period is 2–4 days.
- Virus is detected in secretions 4 days prior to clinical symptoms and 7 days following the resolution of symptoms (viral shedding is demonstrated for as long as 20 days).
- Most effective mode of transmission is via person-to-person spread—by droplet or hand-to-nose contact.
- Nosocomial spread occurs from infected hospital personnel to patients.
- There is a worldwide distribution. Temperate climates experience an annual mid-winter epidemic, whereas epidemics are less predictable in the tropics.
- In the U.S., epidemics may begin in November (or as late as May) and last as long as 12 weeks in urban areas.
- One antigenic strain predominates during any given epidemic.

Incidence
Peak incidence is the 1st 2 years of life.

Prevalence
- 50% of children are infected by their 1st birthday, with a similar attack rate for the uninfected child during the 2nd year of life.
- 40–70% of preschool children and 20% of school-aged children are reinfected with exposure.

RISK FACTORS
Those at greatest risk for severe infection include:
- Children <1 year of age, especially those between the ages of 6 weeks–6 months
- Children with compromised cardiorespiratory status (e.g., bronchopulmonary dysplasia, congenital heart disease)
- Those born prematurely
- Those with immune deficits
- Those with neuromuscular disease
- Those with malignancy

GENERAL PREVENTION
- Nosocomial and household spread can be minimized by strict hand washing and avoidance of contact with infected individuals.
- Routine use of gowns and gloves has been shown to decrease RSV nosocomial spread.
- Patients with RSV infection should be isolated in private or RSV-cohorted rooms.
- Nursing care should be cohorted so that nurses are not caring for both RSV-infected and noninfected patients.
- 2 products are available for the prevention of RSV infection: RSV immune globulin IV (RSV-IGIV), made from RSV antibody-positive donor serum, and palivizumab, a humanized monoclonal antibody produced by recombinant DNA technology:
  - Both products are approved for the prevention of RSV disease in select children <2 years of age with bronchopulmonary dysplasia or with a history of prematurity (birth at <35 weeks' gestation).
  - Specific recommendations are available from the American Academy of Pediatrics (AAP) Committee on Infectious Diseases and Committee on Fetus and Newborn for the use of palivizumab and RSV-IGIV, and these criteria should guide the use of these products.
  - RSV-IGIV is given 1 month prior to and monthly throughout RSV season, whereas palivizumab is given IM monthly throughout RSV season.

PATHOPHYSIOLOGY
- The F protein is responsible for fusing infected cells to adjacent cells, generating a syncytium.
- Infection is initiated in the upper respiratory tract with inoculation of the nose or eyes, and may spread to the lower respiratory tract.
- Obstruction of smaller airways occurs secondary to edema, necrotic tissue, and inflammatory cells.
- Virus-induced epithelial damage may expose certain receptors to environmental irritants. Receptor–irritant complexes may contribute to the signs and symptoms of reactive airway disease.

DIAGNOSIS

HISTORY
- Initial symptoms are nasal discharge, cough, and fever.
- Cough typically progresses over 1–2 days, with tachypnea developing.
- Duration of symptoms will help in the assessment of the typical clinical progression of illness and the anticipated time course for the child.
- Other significant points within the history:
  - Lethargy, apnea, and possible cyanotic episodes
  - Dehydration is secondary to decreased oral intake, as well as to increased insensible losses. Assess oral intake and urine output to rule out dehydration.
  - Increasing respiratory distress
  - Child stopped breathing/had apnea

PHYSICAL EXAM
- Nasal discharge
- Acute otitis media or otitis media with effusion
- Pharyngeal injection
- Conjunctivitis
- Respiratory distress with nasal flaring and retractions, grunting, rales, rhonchi, and expiratory wheezing noted on auscultation
- Risk for hypoxemia increases as the respiratory rate approaches and surpasses 60 breaths per minute.
- Chest may become barrel-shaped as respiratory distress increases.
- Hyperinflation of the lungs will push liver and spleen into palpable positions within the abdomen.

DIAGNOSTIC TESTS & INTERPRETATION
Lab
- A definitive diagnosis of RSV can be made by viral isolation, but RSV takes up to 5 days to grow on viral culture medium. Sensitivity may vary among laboratories.
- Rapid diagnostic antigen assays are used for RSV detection, usually with a sensitivity of 80–90%:
  - Immunochromatographic assay
  - Enzyme immunoassay
  - Immunofluorescent assay
- Polymerase chain reaction (PCR) may be superior to rapid antigen testing for low viral loads, but it is not widely available.
- Nasopharyngeal aspirate/washings are specimens of choice for testing.
- Pulse oximetry to rule out hypoxemia

ALERT
- RSV is labile at room temperature. Samples should be placed in viral transport medium at the bedside and transported to the laboratory for immediate inoculation to cell culture.
- Instillation and aspiration of 5 mL of isotonic saline is the preferred method of viral collection, as opposed to nasal swabs.

Imaging
- Chest x-rays are obtained for clinical concerns of pneumonia.
- Significance: Reveals hyperinflation, increased bronchial markings, and areas of atelectasis/infiltrate.
- Note: The pulmonary densities, referred to as "RSV pneumonia," are frequently areas of atelectasis but may represent bacterial infection, especially in the seriously ill patient.

DIFFERENTIAL DIAGNOSIS
- Infection:
  - Influenza virus
  - Parainfluenza virus type 3
  - Adenovirus
  - Human metapneumovirus
  - Human bocavirus
  - *Chlamydia*
- Environmental: Foreign body in airway
- Tumors: Mass compressing upper airway
- Congenital: Tracheomalacia

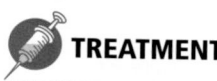# TREATMENT

MEDICATION (DRUGS)
- Ribavirin: An antiviral agent; has in vitro antiviral activity against RSV, but ribavirin aerosol treatment for RSV infections is controversial. Ribavirin should not be used routinely in the treatment of children with bronchiolitis.
- Corticosteroids have not been proven to be efficacious in bronchiolitis and should not be used routinely.
- β-adrenergic agents: There is some evidence of effectiveness in some patients with RSV bronchiolitis. A trial of a bronchodilator is frequently recommended, but continues to be controversial.
- Mist use is considered controversial because it may irritate the airways.
- Antibiotics are rarely indicated because bacterial disease (lung or blood) is uncommon in hospitalized infants with RSV bronchiolitis.
- Heliox, an inhaled mixture of helium and oxygen, is under investigation for use in cases of severe respiratory distress in the pediatric intensive care unit setting.

ADDITIONAL TREATMENT
General Measures
- Supportive care: Hydration therapy and supplemental oxygen as needed to maintain oxygen saturation >94%
- Cardiorespiratory monitoring and pulse oximetry are necessary for infants at risk for apnea and hypoxemia. Duration of hospitalization monitoring depends on the clinical course.
- Mechanical ventilation as clinically indicated

IN-PATIENT CONSIDERATIONS
Initial Stabilization
Life-threatening apnea may require emergency support with mechanical ventilation.

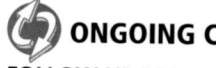# ONGOING CARE

FOLLOW-UP RECOMMENDATIONS
- Bronchiolitis peaks in severity over 48–72 hours; therefore, reassess the patient if seen early in the disease course.
- Symptoms usually last 7 days but may last up to 2–3 weeks, with evidence of reactive airway disease persisting for months to years.
- Periodic breathing may occur 48–72 hours post-extubation, but recurrent apneic episodes are rare, and home monitoring is usually not indicated.

- Fever commonly resolves over 48 hours.
- Respiratory symptoms commonly improve between days 2–5 of illness.
- Evidence of airway hyperactivity may continue for months to years in patients who have had bronchiolitis.

Patient Monitoring
Signs to watch for:
- Increased respiratory rate and increased work of breathing (i.e., use of accessory muscles)
- Lethargy, altered mental status
- Prolonged high fever

PROGNOSIS
- The majority of patients have a mild to moderate disease course with symptomatic support.
- Some infected children proceed to more serious illness, necessitating hospitalization. An average hospital stay for previously healthy children is 5–7 days; full recovery is 2 weeks.
- Infants with underlying cardiac or pulmonary disease are at increased risk for more severe and longer duration of disease; mortality is as high as 30%.
- Reinfections occur throughout life.
- An association between RSV infection and long-term asthma symptoms has been speculated, but remains unclear.

COMPLICATIONS
- Apneic episodes in very young and premature patients
- Pneumonia, rarely bacterial
- Pneumonitis
- Croup
- Respiratory failure
- Hypoxemia
- Hypercarbia
- Asthma
- Acute otitis media
- Dehydration

ADDITIONAL READING
- AAP Committee on Diagnosis and Management of Bronchiolitis. Diagnosis and management of bronchiolitis. *Pediatrics*. 2006;118:1774–1793.
- AAP. Respiratory syncytial virus. In: Pickering LK, ed. *Red Book: 2009: Report of the Committee on Infectious Diseases*, 27th ed. Elk Grove Village, IL: American Academy of Pediatrics, 2009:560–569.
- Liet JM, Ducruet T, Gupta V et al. Heliox inhalation therapy for bronchiolitis in infants. *Cochrane Database of Syst Rev*. 2010;4:CD006915.
- McBride JT. Dexamethasone and bronchiolitis: A new look at an old therapy? *J Pediatr*. 2002;140:8–9.
- Nokes JD, Cane PA. New strategies for control of respiratory syncytial virus infection. *Curr Opin Infect Dis*. 2008;21(6):639–643.
- Van den Hoogen BG, Osterhaus DM, Fouchier RA. Clinical impact and diagnosis of human metapneumovirus infection. *Pediatr Infect Dis J*. 2004;23(Suppl.1):S25–S32.

CODES

ICD9
- 079.6 Respiratory syncytial virus (RSV)
- 490 Bronchitis, not specified as acute or chronic

ICD10
- B97.4 Respiratory syncytial virus as the cause of diseases classified elsewhere
- J20.5 Acute bronchitis due to respiratory syncytial virus

FAQ
- Q: How did my child get this illness?
- A: RSV bronchiolitis is caused by respiratory syncytial virus, which is passed from one person to another by contact with nasal secretions and through airborne transmission of droplets.
- Q: For how long is my child contagious?
- A: Viral shedding occurs for 24 hours prior to the onset of clinical symptoms and for up to 21 days from the onset of symptoms.
- Q: Will my child develop asthma because of the wheezing that is occurring now?
- A: Evidence of airway hyperactivity following RSV bronchiolitis may continue for months or even years in some children. It is impossible to predict future episodes of reactive airway disease, but the child should be monitored clinically over time.
- Q: If a patient has severe chronic lung disease with a supplemental oxygen requirement and is <2 years of age at the onset of the RSV season, should RSV-IGIV or palivizumab be recommended for this patient?
- A: The risks and benefits of each therapy must be evaluated on a patient-by-patient basis. RSV-IGIV provides additional protection against other respiratory viral illnesses and may be considered for some selected high-risk infants. However, palivizumab is preferred for most high-risk children secondary to its ease of administration, safety, and effectiveness.

RETINOBLASTOMA

Kelly C. Goldsmith

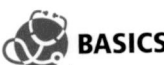 **BASICS**

DESCRIPTION
- The most common primary intraocular tumor of childhood
- Malignant tumor of the embryonic neural retina

EPIDEMIOLOGY
- 1:16,000–25,000 live births
- The most common primary intraocular tumor of childhood (ocular leukemia most common overall)
- Represents 3% of all pediatric malignancies
- No sex, race, geographic, or socioeconomic predilection
- 90% diagnosed <4 years of age
- Median age at diagnosis for unilateral disease is 24 months and 12 months for bilateral disease (see "Genetics")

RISK FACTORS
Genetics
Tumor development depends on loss of function of both copies of the *RB1* gene (located on chromosome 13) in a retinoblast. Hereditary and nonhereditary (sporadic) forms exist.
- Hereditary retinoblastoma (RB):
  - 45% of all RB
  - 1 *RB1* gene is dysfunctional in all cells (germline mutation); mutation in remaining *RB1* gene in any retinal cell will lead to development of a tumor.
  - 90% probability of second mutation occurring in at least 1 (but usually more) retinal cells leading to tumor development (high penetrance)
  - Therefore, multiple tumors are common (Usually bilateral and/or multifocal, but may be unilateral).
  - Mean age at diagnosis: 12 months
  - Only 8% have positive familial history; remainders are new germline mutations.
  - ~40–45% of offspring will develop RB the most common being osteosarcoma (autosomal-dominant transmission, 90% penetrance).
  - *RB1* gene mutation in all cells predisposes to second (non-RB) malignancies as well.
- Nonhereditary RB:
  - 55% of all RB
  - No germline *RB1* mutation; 2 acquired (somatic) *RB1* mutations must occur in a single retinal cell (a rare event).
  - Always unilateral
  - Rarely diagnosed before 6 months (mean, 24 months)
  - No increased risk of RB in offspring
  - No increased risk of second malignancy

PATHOPHYSIOLOGY
- Originates in retinal cell precursor (retinoblast)
- Histology: Small round blue cells with large hyperchromatic nuclei and scant cytoplasm
- Growth of tumor may be endophytic (from inner surface of retina to vitreous) or exophytic (from outer layer of retina into subretinal space); may cause retinal detachment.
- Spread is via optic nerve (common) with potential to invade CNS, direct extension beyond the eye, and lymphatic or hematogenous spread (uncommon).
- Tumor cells may break off from primary mass and grow independently within the eye (called "vitreous seeding"); single tumor with seeding may be confused with multifocal disease.

 DIAGNOSIS

HISTORY
- Familial history of RB or any eye tumors: Hereditary RB; siblings may require eye exam
- Leukocoria (white pupil, "cat's eye reflex"): Often noted in photographs of children with advanced intraocular RB (60%)
- Strabismus, either eso- or exotropic (20%): Esotropia is more common in the general population, so exotropia is more suspicious.
- Eye complaints: RB is rarely painful (unless secondary glaucoma or inflammation is present); vision problems are rare complaints because tumor is usually unilateral
- Inflammation, heterochromia, and glaucoma: Rare presentations (<10%)
- Neurologic signs, orbital/periorbital masses, bone pain, anorexia, signs of cytopenias: May represent metastatic disease
- Associated conditions: 13q deletion syndrome has RB, dysmorphism, mental retardation, and genitourinary (GU) or other anomalies.

PHYSICAL EXAM
- Only 3% discovered with routine funduscopic examination.
- Leukocoria or strabismus more common as presenting sign.
- Proptosis and orbital/periorbital masses: Late sequelae of mass effect
- Check for red reflex in darkened room: Screen for RB in office.
- Evaluate for anisocoria.
- Cover test to assess for strabismus (20%)
- Test vision of each eye independently to identify unilateral RB.

DIAGNOSTIC TESTS & INTERPRETATION
Lab
- Ophthalmologic examination: Confirmation of diagnosis based on ophthalmologic examination by a specialist in pediatric ocular tumors via direct and indirect ophthalmoscopy (and examination under anesthesia [EUA]) and by imaging modalities (MRI or CT). Parents and siblings should also undergo ophthalmologic screening in many cases.
- Biopsy: Biopsy confirmation is rarely necessary (risk for tumor seeding).
- CBC: Assess for bone marrow involvement.
- CSF cytology: Evaluate for leptomeningeal spread (only necessary if tumor has spread beyond the globe).
- Chromosome analysis: Should be performed, but even in hereditary cases, only 5% have mutations detectable by this means.

Imaging
CT or MRI: Evaluate primary tumor (80% have calcification) and optic nerve extension, leptomeningeal spread, pineal blastoma (in 4% of hereditary RB, patients will have bilateral RB and pineal tumor noted on MRI = "trilateral RB").

Diagnostic Procedures/Surgery
- Biopsy rarely done due to risk for visual damage and spreading tumor cells
- Diagnosis based on dilated ophthalomologic evaluation (often under anesthesia)
- Intraocular and extraocular staging systems exist: The International Classification of Retinoblastoma (ICRB) was introduced in 2003 that more simply stages the extent of disease. Reese–Ellsworth is still in wide use.
- Most RB in the US is intraocular without metastatic disease.
- Patients with tumor extension outside the globe should have a lumbar puncture to assess for tumor cells in CSF and bone marrow evaluation for complete staging.

Pathological Findings
- Biopsy rarely done due to risk of visual damage and spreading of tumor cells

DIFFERENTIAL DIAGNOSIS
- Coats disease: Acquired anomaly, males, retinal telangiectasias
- Persistent hyperplastic primary vitreous (PHPV)
- Inflammatory conditions: Hypopyon, uveitis, iritis, endophthalmitis
- Toxoplasmosis, *Toxocara canis*, other ocular infections
- Retinopathy of prematurity (ROP)

TREATMENT

ADDITIONAL TREATMENT
General Measures
- Primary goals:
  - Eradicate tumor
  - Prevent metastasis
- Secondary goals:
  - Salvage the eye and retain useful vision.
  - Cosmetic considerations
- Treatment must be individualized, depending on bilateral or unilateral disease, potential for salvageable vision, and evidence of local extension or metastatic disease. Referral to a center with oncologic and ophthalmologic specialists is essential.
- Minimal (nonbulky) intraocular disease:
  - Plaque radiotherapy (radioactive seeds sewn to episcleral surface above RB lesion): This provides local radiation to tumor in selected solitary RBs, up to 16 mm in diameter with or without vitreous seeds
  - Photocoagulation (laser directed at tumor blood vessels): For selected small RBs, usually <3 mm
  - Transpupillary thermotherapy (TTT; laser aimed directly at tumor with lower temp vs. photocoagulation): Treatment of peripapillary tumors for which photocoagulation cannot be used
  - Cryotherapy (topical freeze technique): For selected RBs <3–4 mm in diameter without vitreous seeding, which are located anteriorly in the eye
  - Locally delivered chemotherapy: Subtenon/subconjunctival chemotherapy (usually carboplatin) delivered by direct intraocular injection
- Bulky intraocular disease:
  - Current trend is toward eye salvage therapy: Initial systemic chemotherapy for tumor reduction followed by local definitive therapy (as for nonbulky disease)
  - Tumor resection without enucleation is not possible because of risk of tumor spillage; enucleation of involved eye (with long segment of optic nerve removal to ensure tumor-free margins) may be required for large tumors refractory to chemoreduction or when vision is not salvageable.
  - External beam radiation therapy (EBRT): RB is extremely radiosensitive; however, increases risk of second malignancy (especially in hereditary RB). Other effects: Dry eye, cataract, retinopathy, and cosmetic deformity from bone maldevelopment. EBRT is still an important modality but is avoided whenever effective alternative therapies are available.
  - Experimental treatments are available in referral centers
- Metastatic disease:
  - Multiagent chemotherapy with or without autologous bone marrow transplantation; poor results to date
  - Effective treatment requires multidisciplinary collaboration between ophthalmologists, oncologists, and radiation oncologists.

 ONGOING CARE

- Frequent ophthalmologic examinations (including EUA) are mandatory to evaluate response to therapy and to screen for disease progression, particularly in hereditary RB.
- Therapy must include genetic counseling regarding the risk of second malignancies (with or without adjuvant XRT), risk to siblings, as well as the risk to future children of affected patients with hereditary RB.
- Primary care physicians must be aware of the risks of second malignancies (see "Prognosis") and maintain an appropriately high index of suspicion for their development.
- Primary care physicians should be aware of the genetics of RB and screen siblings appropriately.
- Pitfalls:
  - Missed or delayed diagnosis: Ophthalmologic examination by a specialist in pediatric ocular tumors required to establish diagnosis and follow regression or recurrence in treated eyes, follow for development of new tumors in hereditary cases
  - Failure to recognize the possibility that a child with RB has a genetic predisposition, especially in the frequent setting where there is no familial history of RB
  - Failure to refer for appropriate genetic counseling

PROGNOSIS
- Mortality from RB is 3–5% for the US, Japan, and Europe
- Mortality is more concerning for developing countries due to late detection (20–70% in Asia, Africa, and Latin America/Caribbean nations).
- Survival depends on extent (stage) of disease.
- Metastatic disease is uncommon in the US but can occur up to 5 years after diagnosis and has a poor outcome (same for hereditary and nonhereditary).
- Prognosis for vision depends on size and location of tumor(s).
- Second malignancy is most common cause of death in hereditary RB:
  - These include osteosarcoma (most frequent), pineal blastoma, melanoma, fibrosarcoma, and others.
  - Rates of second malignancy in hereditary RB are 10% at 10 years and as high as 40% at 30 years in patients who received EBRT (70% of second tumors occur in the field of radiation, 30% elsewhere).

COMPLICATIONS
- Metastatic spread: Local spread within orbit, through the optic nerve to brain, or to distant sites (uncommon)
- Loss of eye: Surgical enucleation in advanced cases
- Blindness: In advanced, bilateral disease; bilateral enucleation rarely required
- Cosmetic deformity: From enucleation, ocular prosthesis lacks normal eye movements; potential orbital bone hypoplasia secondary to EBRT
- Second malignancy: Patients with hereditary RB have a predisposition to cancer; this risk is greatly increased by exposure to radiotherapy.

ADDITIONAL READING
- Abramson DH, Schefler AC. Update on retinoblastoma. Retina. 2004;24(6):828–848.
- Kivela T. The epidemiological challenge of the most frequent eye cancer: Retinoblastoma, an issue of birth and death. Br J Ophthalmol. 2009;93:1129–1131.
- MacPherson D, Dyer MA. Retinoblastoma: From the two-hit hypothesis to targeted chemotherapy. Cancer Res. 2007;67(16):7547–7550.
- Nahum MP, Gdal-On M, Kuten A, et al. Longterm follow-up of children with retinoblastoma. Pediatr Hematol Oncol. 2001;18(3):173–179.
- Rao A, Rothman J, Nichols KE. Genetic testing and tumor surveillance for children with cancer predisposition syndromes. Curr Opin Pediatr. 2008;20(1):1–7.
- Shields CL, Shields JA. Retinoblastoma management: Advances in enucleation, intravenous chemoreduction, and intra-arterial chemotherapy. Curr Opin Optho. 2010;21:203–212.

CODES

ICD9
190.5 Malignant neoplasm of retina

ICD10
- C69.20 Malignant neoplasm of unspecified retina
- C69.21 Malignant neoplasm of right retina
- C69.22 Malignant neoplasm of left retina

FAQ
- Q: What is the risk that a child with RB will become blind?
- A: Vision is salvageable in 100% of eyes with low-stage involvement, and in 81% overall. In <10% of patients are both eyes affected severely enough to threaten vision (bilateral disease only occurs in hereditary RB).
- Q: What is the chance that a child with RB in 1 eye will get it in the other?
- A: Bilateral disease is seen with hereditary RB. A child with unilateral disease has a 15% chance of having hereditary RB, which would put the contralateral eye at risk; this risk is much higher if the child has multifocal involvement or is <1 year of age.
- Q: What happens to the eye socket after an enucleation?
- A: Prostheses can be made to fit the socket of the enucleated eye to give excellent cosmetic results.
- Q: Is there a test to identify hereditary cases?
- A: Routine chromosome analysis does not reveal a defect related to the RB gene in the majority (95%) of hereditary cases. Specialized molecular tests may be used in research labs, but because there are many possible mutations, this is costly and time-consuming. In general, hereditary cases are determined clinically because of young presentation, family history, and/or bilateral or multifocal unilateral disease.

RETROPHARYNGEAL ABSCESS

Richard M. Rutstein

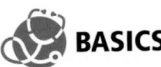 **BASICS**

DESCRIPTION
A relatively rare but potentially life-threatening infection occurring in the potential space bounded by the layers of cervical fascia posterior to the esophagus and anterior to the deep cervical fascia.

EPIDEMIOLOGY
Children <6 years of age are most at risk, with 50% of the cases occurring in those <48 months of age.

Incidence
Most large children's hospital centers report 1–5 cases per year.

PATHOPHYSIOLOGY
- Most infections result from pharyngitis or supraglottitis and occur because of suppuration of the retropharyngeal lymph nodes, which lie in 2 paramedial chains and drain various nasopharyngeal structures.
- Other sources of infection in this space include penetrating trauma (e.g., foreign object aspiration, dental procedures, attempts at intubation).
- Extension of infection into this space can arise from vertebral body osteomyelitis or petrositis.

ETIOLOGY
- Infectious: Cultures frequently reveal multiple organisms.
- The predominant organisms isolated include:
  - *Streptococcus* (group A and others)
  - *Staphylococcus aureus*
  - Various anaerobic species (e.g., *Bacteroides, Peptostreptococcus, Fusobacterium*)
  - One pediatric study cultured *Haemophilus influenzae* type b in 20% of cases; however, the study took place before the routine use of *H. influenzae* type b conjugate vaccines.
- Many of the isolates are β-lactamase producers.

 DIAGNOSIS

HISTORY
- Symptoms may be present from hours to days before correct diagnosis. Many patients will have been taking oral antibiotics for presumed pharyngitis/sinusitis.
- Ask about neck trauma, especially penetrating injuries, recent surgery (especially dental), and history consistent with aspiration of a foreign object.
- Physicians must maintain a high index of suspicion. The presentation of a retropharyngeal abscess can be subtle, with the most frequent initial diagnostic impression usually epiglottitis or severe pharyngitis.

- Signs and symptoms:
  - Most frequent symptoms include sore throat, decreased oral intake, muffled voice, drooling, stiff or painful neck, fever, dysphagia, and stridor.
  - Fever
  - Stridor (seen in up to 50% of children in 1 study, but only 5% in a more recent series)
  - Drooling
  - A tender cervical neck region/mass and restricted range of motion
  - Classic diagnostic finding of a bulging posterior pharyngeal wall; may be absent or difficult to appreciate in an ill, apprehensive child

PHYSICAL EXAM
- Muffled voice
- Drooling
- Stiff or painful neck
- Fever
- Dysphagia
- Stridor

DIAGNOSTIC TESTS & INTERPRETATION
Lab
CBC may reveal an elevated total leukocyte level, with a significant left shift.

Imaging
- Lateral neck x-ray: Widening of retropharyngeal space and at times an air–fluid level. Negative plain neck film does not rule out retropharyngeal abscess.
- CT scan or MRI of the neck: Most definitive modality; can usually differentiate abscess from local cellulitis/adenitis
- Both plain films and CT scan have false positives and false negatives.

DIFFERENTIAL DIAGNOSIS
- Pharyngitis
- Peritonsillar or lateral wall abscess
- Epiglottitis/Supraglottitis

 TREATMENT

ADDITIONAL TREATMENT
General Measures
- Start broad-spectrum parental antibiotics, active against *Streptococcus pneumoniae*, *S. aureus*, and oral anaerobic organisms. If patient does not improve, broaden coverage to include drugs active against β-lactamase-producing organisms and anaerobic organisms. Clindamycin or ampicillin–sulbactam are good initial choices.
- Immediate consultation with otolaryngology surgical team:
  - Be prepared to schedule incision/aspiration of abscess for severe cases associated with airway compromise with team experienced in airway management of small children.
  - CT-guided aspiration of the abscess has aided the surgical approach at many sites.
  - Recent data suggest that up to 50% of patients can be successfully managed without surgical intervention.
  - Patients with a well-defined abscess on admission CT are most likely to require surgical intervention.
  - Patients treated with antibiotics alone must be followed closely for signs of worsening clinical status.

ISSUES FOR REFERRAL
After diagnosis is confirmed, urgent consultation with experienced surgical staff is mandatory.

IN-PATIENT CONSIDERATIONS
Initial Stabilization
Emergency therapy requires maintaining patent airway; be wary of sudden spontaneous drainage of the abscess, with catastrophic aspiration.

 ONGOING CARE

PROGNOSIS
Excellent with appropriate antibiotics, expectant care, and surgery, if needed, at optimal time.

COMPLICATIONS
- Spontaneous rupture with aspiration of infected material, with subsequent asphyxia or overwhelming pulmonary infection
- Hemorrhage from extension into local arteries, and/or venous thrombosis from involvement of major neck vessels
- Extension of the infection inferiorly can occur, leading to a subdiaphragmatic or psoas abscess.

ADDITIONAL READING
- Daya H, Lo S, Papsin BC, et al. Retropharyngeal and parapharyngeal infections in children: The Toronto experience. *Int J Pediatr Otolaryngol*. 2005;69: 81–86.
- Elsherif AM, Park AH, Alder SC, et al. Indicators of a more complicated clinical course for pediatric patients with retropharyngeal abscess. *Int J Pediatr Otolaryngol*. 2010;74:198–201.

- Grisaru-Soen G, Komisar O, Aizenstein O, et al. Retropharyngeal and parapharyngeal abscess in children: Epidemiology, clinical features and treatment. *Int J Pediatr Otolaryngol*. 2010;74: 1016–1020.
- Loftis L. Acute infectious upper airway obstructions in children. *Semin Pediatr Infect Dis*. 2006;17(1): 5–10.
- Rafei K, Lichenstein R. Airway infectious disease emergencies. *Pediatr Clin North Am*. 2006;53(2): 215–242.
- Wang LF, Kuo WR, Tsai SM, et al. Characterizations of life-threatening deep cervical space infections: A review of one hundred ninety-six cases. *Am J Otolaryngol*. 2003;24:111–117.

 CODES

ICD9
478.24 Retropharyngeal abscess

ICD10
J39.0 Retropharyngeal and parapharyngeal abscess

R

REYE SYNDROME

Seth L. Ness
Andrew Mulberg (5th edition)

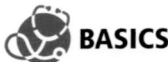 BASICS

DESCRIPTION
- Acute encephalopathy and fatty degeneration of the liver
- The CDC description is of an illness that meets all the following criteria:
  - Acute, noninflammatory encephalopathy that is documented clinically by (a) an alteration in consciousness and, if available, (b) a record of the CSF containing ≤8 leukocytes/mm³ or a histologic specimen demonstrating cerebral edema without perivascular or meningeal inflammation
  - Hepatopathy documented by either (a) a liver biopsy or an autopsy considered to be diagnostic of Reye syndrome or (b) a 3-fold or greater increase in the levels of the serum glutamic-oxaloacetic transaminase (SGOT), serum glutamic-pyruvic transaminase (SGPT), or serum ammonia
  - No more reasonable explanation for the cerebral and hepatic abnormalities

EPIDEMIOLOGY
- Peak incidence age 6 years
- Most children range from 4–12 years of age.
- Association with ingestion of aspirin-containing medicines by children with varicella or influenza B
- In 1982, the U.S. Surgeon General issued an advisory on the use of salicylates and Reye syndrome.

Incidence
- Peak incidence of 555 cases in children in the U.S. in 1980
- From 1994–1997, there were no more than 2 cases of Reye syndrome annually.

PATHOPHYSIOLOGY
- Mitochondrial injury of unknown etiology in a viral-infected host results in dysfunction of oxidative phosphorylation and fatty acid oxidation.
- Mitochondrial toxins, usually salicylates, exacerbate the condition when ingested after mitochondrial injury.
- Postmortem:
  - Liver: Grossly yellowish-white, due to increased triglyceride levels; foamy cytoplasm with increased microvesicular fat, decreased glycogen
  - Brain: Marked edema with increased intracellular fluid and loss of neurons
  - Abnormal-looking mitochondria can be detected in many tissues.

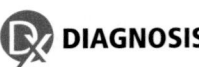 DIAGNOSIS

HISTORY
- Prodromal illness: Upper respiratory infection (73%)—influenza B, influenza A, and varicella
- Abrupt-onset vomiting within 47 days of initial illness
- Natural history: Neurologic deterioration in which delirium may progress to seizures, coma, or death

PHYSICAL EXAM
- Slight liver enlargement without jaundice
- Absence of focal neurologic signs
- Neurologic exam varies with stage of disease:
  - Stage 0: Alert, wakeful
  - Stage 1: Difficult to arouse, lethargic, sleepy
  - Stage 2: Delirious, combative, with purposeful or semipurposeful motor responses
  - Stage 3: Unarousable, with predominantly flexor motor responses, decorticate
  - Stage 4: Unarousable, with predominantly extensor motor responses, decerebrate
  - Stage 5: Unarousable, with flaccid paralysis, areflexia, and pupils unresponsive
  - Stage 6: Treated with curare or equivalent drug, and therefore unclassifiable

DIAGNOSTIC TESTS & INTERPRETATION
Lab
- Ammonia test: Result may be normal at the onset of vomiting. Serum level >45 g/dL suggests higher mortality.
- CSF: Normal except for elevated intracranial pressure

Imaging
EEG: Characteristic of metabolic encephalopathy with generalized slow-wave abnormalities

Diagnostic Procedures/Other
- Liver and muscle function testing: Elevated levels of transaminases, creatinine kinase, lactate dehydrogenase, and ammonia; increased PT
- Metabolic workup: Abnormalities of organic and amino acids may be present if symptoms are caused by a metabolic disorder.

DIFFERENTIAL DIAGNOSIS
- It is important to distinguish between so-called classic Reye syndrome, associated with aspirin (acetylsalicylic acid) therapy, and Reye-like syndromes, often due to metabolic disorders and other causes, as mentioned subsequently.
- Metabolic diseases: In a report by Hou et al., Reye-like syndrome was secondary to hereditary organic acidemias (n = 13), urea cycle defects (n = 4), mitochondrial disorders (n = 3), fulminant hepatitis (n = 2), tyrosinemia (n = 1), and valproate-associated hepatotoxicity (n = 1). In the U.K., 12% of Reye syndrome cases between 1981–1996 were subsequently reclassified as metabolic disorders.
- CNS infections (e.g., meningitis, encephalitis)
- Toxins
- Drug ingestion (e.g., salicylates, valproate)

ALERT
Failure to recognize early and control or prevent cerebral edema is the immediate cause of death.

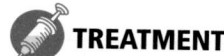 **TREATMENT**

ADDITIONAL TREATMENT
General Measures
Vitamin K, fresh-frozen plasma, and platelets as needed for treatment of secondary coagulopathy

IN-PATIENT CONSIDERATIONS
Initial Stabilization
- Should be tailored based on severity of presentation
- IV glucose to counteract effects of glycogen depletion
- Fluid restriction in patients with cerebral edema (1,500 mL/m²/d), along with mannitol to increase serum osmolality and induce cerebral dehydration

 ONGOING CARE

FOLLOW-UP RECOMMENDATIONS
Cerebral function at presentation is the best predictor of outcome.

PROGNOSIS
- Most patients suffer only mild illness without progression.
- Patients with milder disease (stages 0, 1, 2) tend to recover completely.
- Patients with stage 3 disease are equally likely to recover completely or die.
- Patients with stage 4–5 disease usually do not survive.

COMPLICATIONS
- Elevated intracranial pressure secondary to cerebral edema
- Cardiovascular collapse
- Overall mortality of 31%

ADDITIONAL READING
- Belay ED, Bresee JS, Holman RC et al. Reye's syndrome in the United States from 1981 through 1997. *N Engl J Med*. 1999;340:1377–1382.
- Chow EI, Cherry JD, Harrison R et al. Related articles, reassessing Reye syndrome. *Arch Pediatr Adolesc Med*. 2003;157(12):1241–1242.
- Duerksen DR, Jewell LD, Mason AL et al. Co-existence of hepatitis A and adult Reye's syndrome. *Gut*. 1997;41:121–124.
- Glasgow JF, Middleton B. Reye syndrome—insights on causation and prognosis. *Arch Dis Child*. 2001;85:351–353.
- Green Cl, Blitzer MG, Shapiro E. Inborn errors of metabolism and Reye's syndrome: Differential diagnosis. *J Peidatr*. 1988;113–156.
- Schrör K. Aspirin and Reye syndrome: A review of the evidence. *Paediatr Drugs*. 2007;9(3):195–204.
- van Bever HP, Quek SC, Lim T. Related articles, aspirin, Reye syndrome, Kawasaki disease, and allergies: A reconsideration of the links. *Arch Dis Child*. 2004;89(12):1178.

 CODES

ICD9
331.81 Reye's syndrome
ICD10
G93.7 Reye's syndrome

FAQ
- Q: Is Reye syndrome fatal?
- A: ~30% of children will die, usually due to cerebral edema. Mortality rates are best predicted by neurologic state at the onset of presentation.
- Q: How can the neurologic findings of Reye syndrome be differentiated from those of meningitis?
- A: Aside from elevated intracranial pressure, the lumbar taps of patients with Reye syndrome are at best unremarkable. Elevated leukocyte count is not seen in these cases.

R

RHABDOMYOLYSIS

Divya Moodalbail
Thomas L. Kennedy (5th edition)

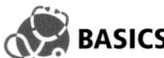 **BASICS**

DESCRIPTION
Skeletal muscle injury results from trauma, infection, or from inadequate delivery, production, or consumption of energy or oxygen relative to demands. Release of intracellular contents may cause severe electrolyte disturbances including life-threatening hyperkalemia, hyperphosphatemia, and hypocalcemia. The resulting myoglobinuria can cause obstruction of renal tubules and pigment-induced acute renal failure.

EPIDEMIOLOGY
- Rhabdomyolysis is more common in adults, where it is seen most frequently in patients in comas resulting from heroin or cocaine abuse and long periods of remaining motionless.
- Rhabdomyolysis is uncommon in childhood and unusual in the 1st decade.
- It may be seen in heat exhaustion.
- Rhabdomyolysis may be a common clinical problem in a catastrophic disaster (e.g., an earthquake).

RISK FACTORS
Genetics
Many unusual causes of rhabdomyolysis, including muscle enzyme deficiencies, muscular dystrophy, and disorders of mitochondrial metabolism, are heritable disorders.

ETIOLOGY
- The most common causes include physical causes such as muscle trauma from crush or compression injury (crush syndrome), burns, or electric shock. Others include viral illnesses (e.g., influenza, Epstein–Barr virus infection), heat stroke, severe exertion, status epilepticus, and vasculitis with myositis.
- A common cause in adolescents is exercise which is novel, intense, or prolonged, often the result of competition or punitive measures, especially in the presence of extremely hot, humid weather conditions (so-called "March Myoglobinuria").
- Less common causes in childhood include penetrating trauma (e.g., gun shot); congenital metabolic myopathies; acute dystonic reactions; malignant hyperthermia syndrome; other infections; exposure to some medications, toxins, or illicit drugs; and severe electrolyte disturbances.
- Myopathies involving muscle enzyme or energy substrate deficiencies include carnitine palmitoyltransferase deficiency type II (CPT II deficiency), type V glycogenosis, mitochondrial deficiency disorders, and phosphofructokinase deficiency. Usual triggers for rhabdomyolysis in such conditions are fasting, exertion, or viral illness.

- Rhabdomyolysis is more likely to occur after exertion in association with the dystrophinopathies, which include all forms of muscular dystrophy.
- Infections, in addition to the viral illnesses listed above, include Coxsackievirus, HIV, *Plasmodium*, *Legionella* sp., mycoplasma, SARS, and toxic shock syndrome.
- Causative medications include the lipid-lowering "statin" inhalation anesthetics, propofol, cyclosporine, amphotericin B, itraconazole, and isotretinoin. An overdose of epinephrine and high-dose IV norepinephrine are also on the list.
- Hyperthermia: Malignant hyperthermia, is a rare inherited condition that results in hyperthermia, muscle breakdown, and subsequent rhabdomyolysis, on receiving halogenated hydrocarbon-containing anesthetics or muscle relaxants such as succinylcholine. Neuroleptic malignant syndrome is a rare neurological disorder characterized by hyperthermia, rhabdomyolysis, and autonomic changes in patients receiving neuroleptic or antipsychotic medications
- Toxins and illicit drugs include snake, spider, and vespid venoms, fish toxins, some mushrooms, hydrocarbons, ethanol, methanol, cocaine, heroin, amphetamines, phencyclidine (PCP), and ecstasy. Rhabdomyolysis has also been reported, possibly due to copper toxicity, in Wilson disease.
- Electrolyte disturbances include hypokalemia, severe hypophosphatemia, hypernatremia, hyponatremia, hypocalcemia, and hyperosmolar states such as diabetic ketoacidosis. Hypokalemia can cause rapid muscle ischemia leading to rhabdomyolysis, as potassium is essential for causing vasodilation of the microvasculature supplying the muscles to maintain adequate perfusion.
- It is important to remember that the muscle injury caused by severe hypokalemia (e.g., Bartter syndrome) may rapidly lead to life-threatening hyperkalemia.
- The insult may lead to muscle cell destruction or failure of membrane function with release of intracellular contents including proteins and electrolytes and uptake of large amounts of extracellular water leading to severe hypovolemia and decreased renal perfusion.
- The list of causes here is not exhaustive. Any child with sudden onset of muscle pain, tenderness, or weakness should be suspected of having rhabdomyolysis, and any child with dark urine suspected of myoglobinuria.

COMMONLY ASSOCIATED CONDITIONS
In addition to the previously mentioned causes, rhabdomyolysis has also been reportedly associated with diverse conditions, including asthma, hemolytic-uremic syndrome, and diabetes mellitus. It may also occur in Kawasaki disease and adrenal insufficiency, associations which are rare, but must not be missed.

 DIAGNOSIS

- Muscle pain or weakness; rarely focal or diffuse muscle swelling can be seen
- Brownish urine

HISTORY
- Increased exertion, viral illness, muscle injury, and electric shock are conditions associated with muscle breakdown and rhabdomyolysis.
- Rhabdomyolysis is associated with muscular dystrophy and reaction to drugs (e.g., anesthetic agents).
- Any prior history of illness or insult associated with rhabdomyolysis may follow certain illnesses (e.g., influenza) and insults (e.g., crush injury), and thus a history positive for these should be sought.
- Muscle pain or weakness may result from rhabdomyolysis and help suggest diagnosis if present.
- Brownish discoloration of the urine

PHYSICAL EXAM
- Palpate muscle for tenderness and, less commonly, swelling or fullness
- Test for motor strength
- Elicit reflexes to exclude neuropathy
- Examine skin and mucous membranes for signs of vasculitis
- The child with evidence of rhabdomyolysis must be examined looking for signs of child abuse.
- Examine for signs of a concomitant precipitating illness

Lab
- Serum creatine phosphokinase will be elevated to over 100 times normal in rhabdomyolysis.
- CK levels peak within the first 24 hours of insult and trend down over the next few days. If the CK levels continue to rise, it should raise suspicion for ongoing muscle damage or development of compartment syndrome.
- Serum electrolytes, calcium, and phosphorus to reveal hypo/hyperkalemia, hyperphosphatemia, and/or hypocalcemia. There may be metabolic acidosis with a wide anion gap in those conditions associated with lactate production.
- BUN and creatinine: Creatinine level may be elevated out of proportion to that of BUN, secondary to conversion of liberated muscle creatine to creatinine.
- CBC and smear because many of the metabolic disorders causing rhabdomyolysis cause a hemolytic anemia as well.

- Patients with rhabdomyolysis are at increased risk for disseminated intravascular coagulation (DIC) secondary to thromboplastin released from the injured myocytes. It is essential to obtain PT/INR, PTT, platelets, and fibrinogen levels.
- Abnormal plasma acylcarnitine profile and free carnitine level in CPT II deficiency
- Serum uric acid may be elevated secondary to increased purine metabolism.
- LDH, AST, aldolase, and other muscle enzyme levels will be elevated secondary to muscle injury.
- Urinalysis: Urine may appear brown and test positive for blood on dipstick without erythrocytes on microscopy. In this instance the diagnostic possibilities are hemoglobinuria or myoglobinuria. Granular pigmented casts are common.
- Definitive tests for myoglobinuria:
  - Ammonium sulfate solubility testing is a reasonable screening test to help differentiate myoglobin from hemoglobin.
- Other tests:
  - EKG may reveal changes associated with acute hyperkalemia, such as peak T waves, prolongation of PR, absent P wave with prolonged QRS interval or even ventricular tachycardia/fibrillation in severe untreated hyperkalemia

Imaging
Use of radiocontrast in imaging studies as part of diagnostic evaluation can worsen acute renal failure. Use only if absolutely necessary and be certain the child is well hydrated and voiding briskly.

Diagnostic Procedures/Other
Muscle biopsy: Necessary to diagnose metabolic myopathies. A biopsy will demonstrate immunohistochemical features of a myopathy. Immunoblotting is helpful in evaluating the dystrophinopathies.

DIFFERENTIAL DIAGNOSIS
- Any condition associated with muscle pain, tenderness, and/or weakness. Many causes of rhabdomyolysis may be associated with these signs and symptoms but demonstrate no elevation in creatine phosphokinase levels.
- Many viral illnesses
- Lyme disease
- Suppurative myositis
- Guillain–Barré syndrome
- Collagen vascular diseases

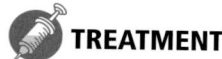 TREATMENT

INITIAL STABILIZATION
Treatment is supportive. If an underlying cause is identified, it should be corrected or removed.

General Measures
- Fluid resuscitation is very essential in the management of rhabdomyolysis. Vigorous hydration with crystalloid IV fluids followed by adequate maintenance fluids (e.g., 2–3 times maintenance) should be sufficient to provide brisk urine flow (e.g., >4 mL/kg/h). Myoglobinuric nephrotoxicity is the one of the very few clinical situations in which acute renal failure can be averted by maintaining good urine flow. Alkalinization of the urine is probably beneficial. Furosemide and/or mannitol may be helpful to maintain urine output.

MEDICATION (DRUGS)
- With myoglobinuria, bicarbonate therapy should be given IV to maintain the urine pH >7.0.
- If urine output declines despite adequate hydration, furosemide (1–4 mg/kg/dose IV) should be given to attempt to prevent oliguric renal failure—furosemide will also maximize potassium elimination by the kidney.
- If severe hyperkalemia occurs, measures should be taken to prevent cardiac dysrhythmias with IV calcium gluconate, sodium bicarbonate, insulin, and glucose. Kayexalate can be given by mouth or per rectum, in order to eliminate potassium through the GI tract.
- With hypocalcemia, give calcium only if symptoms are present.
- Indications for dialysis:
  - Oliguric acute renal failure
  - Severe hyperkalemia refractory to medical management
  - Severe metabolic acidosis
  - Respiratory distress secondary to pulmonary edema

 ONGOING CARE

Close monitoring of labs with serial measurements of CK levels, creatinine, and electrolytes is essential. Also the patient should be watched closely for signs of ongoing muscle injury, compartment syndrome, DIC, or oliguria.

PROGNOSIS
- Depends on extent of pre-existing irreversible renal disease, prompt recognition and institution of appropriate therapy, and the diuretic response to fluid replacement. In general, however, outlook for recovery is good.
- Prompt cessation of rhabdomyolysis may be expected when the inciting cause is corrected or resolves.
- Although most children recover promptly, severe muscle injury may cause prolonged muscle weakness and warrant follow-up by physical and occupational therapy.
- With resolution of myoglobinuria, return to normal renal function is the rule.

COMPLICATIONS
- Electrolyte release from muscle can lead to hyperkalemia, hyperphosphatemia, and secondary hypocalcemia.
- Acute renal failure may occur due to myoglobinuria and does in ~20–40% of patients. Dialysis is required in ~50% of those with acute renal failure. Myoglobin may exert direct renal cytotoxicity, tubular obstruction with myoglobin casts, as well as decreased renal blood flow and glomerular filtration rate as a result of hypovolemia.
- Compartment syndrome may result from muscle swelling.
- Furosemide may interfere with alkalinization of the urine.
- Use of bicarbonate may precipitate symptomatic hypocalcemia.
- Calcium therapy for severe hyperkalemia is necessary, but its use with hyperphosphatemia increases risk of vascular calcification.
- Risk factors for acute renal failure include pre-existing renal disease, delay in recognition and treatment, concurrent use of potentially nephrotoxic agents (e.g., NSAIDs), volume depletion, and either hypotension or hypertension.
- Failure to discontinue IV fluids if oligoanuric renal failure develops could produce iatrogenic fluid overload.

ADDITIONAL READING
- Celik A, Ergun O, Ozok G. Pediatric electrical injuries: A review of 38 consecutive patients. *J Pediatr Surg*. 2004;39(8):1233–1237.
- DiGiacomo JC, Frankel H, Haskell RM, et al. Unsuspected child abuse revealed by delayed presentation of periportal tracking and myoglobinuria. *J Trauma*. 2000;49:348–350.
- Hollander AS, Olney RC, Blackett PR, et al. Fatal malignant hyperthermia-like syndrome with rhabdomyolysis complicating the presentation of diabetes mellitus in adolescent males. *Pediatrics*. 2003;111(6 Pt 1):1447–1452.
- Malinoski DJ, Slater MS, Mullins RJ. Crush injury and rhabdomyolysis. *Crit Care Clin*. 2004;20:171–192.

 CODES

ICD9
728.88 Rhabdomyolysis (idiopathic)

ICD10
M62.82 Rhabdomyolysis

RHABDOMYOSARCOMA

Edward F. Attiyeh

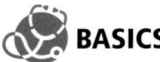 **BASICS**

DESCRIPTION
Malignant tumor of immature mesenchymal cells committed to skeletal muscle lineage

EPIDEMIOLOGY
- 3rd most common extracranial solid tumor of childhood, after neuroblastoma and Wilms tumor
- ~1.2 times more common in boys than girls

Incidence
- ~350 new cases are diagnosed each year in the US.
- Most cases (~60–70%) are diagnosed in children <6 years of age.

RISK FACTORS
Genetics
- Most cases occur sporadically.
- Several predisposing conditions:
  - Li-Fraumeni syndrome:
    - Family cancer syndrome associated with germline mutations of the p53 gene (17p13)
    - The syndrome was 1st described after examining the family records of children with rhabdomyosarcoma.
    - Autosomal dominant inheritance
    - Also predisposes to other soft tissue sarcomas, leukemia, brain tumors, adrenocortical carcinoma, and early-onset breast carcinoma
  - Beckwith-Wiedemann syndrome:
    - Fetal overgrowth syndrome characterized by an abnormality at chromosome 11p15
    - Primarily have an increased incidence of Wilms tumor and hepatoblastoma
  - Neurofibromatosis type I:
    - Autosomal dominant genetic disorder characterized by mutation of the NF1 gene (17q11)
    - Also associated with other soft tissue sarcomas (e.g., malignant nerve sheath tumors, neurofibrosarcomas), leukemia, Wilms tumor, and brain tumors
  - Previous radiation exposure, especially in patients with Li-Fraumeni, neurofibromatosis type I, or hereditary retinoblastoma (RB1 germline mutation)
  - Congenital anomalies of the genitourinary system and CNS are more frequent than expected in children with rhabdomyosarcoma.

PATHOPHYSIOLOGY
- 1 of the "small round blue cell" tumors of childhood
- 2 major subtypes:
  - Embryonal (70% of cases):
    - Spindle-shaped cells, less densely cellular with stroma-rich appearance
    - Associated with a chromosomal abnormality at chromosome band 11p15
  - Alveolar (20% of cases):
    - Small round cells with dense appearance lined up along spaces resembling pulmonary alveoli
    - Associated with translocation between chromosomes 2 and 13 (PAX3-FKHR), or less commonly 1 and 13 (PAX7-FKHR)
- Undifferentiated and pleomorphic types make up the remaining cases.

COMMONLY ASSOCIATED CONDITIONS
- Fetal alcohol syndrome
- CNS and genitourinary anomalies
- Tobacco smoking in fathers
- Marijuana and cocaine use in mothers and fathers in the year before child's birth

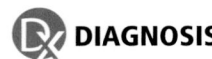 **DIAGNOSIS**

HISTORY
- A painless firm swelling or mass is the most common presentation.
- Other symptoms depend on site of origin:
  - Head/neck: Nasal congestion or discharge, epistaxis, snoring, sinusitis, dysphagia, otorrhea, chronic otitis media, cranial nerve palsies, proptosis, headache, vomiting, or systemic hypertension (with intracranial growth of tumor)
  - Trunk: Usually few symptoms until tumor widespread
  - Genitourinary/pelvic: Urinary frequency or retention, hematuria, constipation, vaginal discharge or bleeding
  - Extremity: Painful or painless lumps or erythema

PHYSICAL EXAM
- Condition can occur in any location, even in sites in which skeletal muscle is not normally found.
- Distribution of primary tumor sites include:
  - Head and neck (38%): Parameningeal (e.g., middle ear, nasal cavity, paranasal sinuses, nasopharynx, infratemporal fossa, pterygopalatine fossa, parapharyngeal area), orbit (e.g., orbit, eyelid), nonparameningeal (e.g., scalp, parotid, oral cavity, larynx, oropharynx, cheek, hypopharynx, thyroid, parathyroid, neck)
  - Genitourinary tract (21%): Bladder, prostate, uterus, vagina, vulva, and paratesticular region
  - Extremity (18%)
  - Trunk (7%)
  - Retroperitoneum (7%)
- Special attention should be given during physical exam to lymphatic structures and surrounding tissues, because this may identify local invasion and/or lymphatogenous spread.

DIAGNOSTIC TESTS & INTERPRETATION
Lab
- CBC
- Electrolytes, liver function tests, and renal function tests in anticipation of starting chemotherapy

Imaging
- To evaluate primary site and confirm diagnosis: CT scan or, preferably, MRI scan
- To evaluate for evidence of distant metastases (present in 20% of patients at diagnosis):
  - Chest radiograph and CT scan
  - ^{99}Tc-diphosphonate bone scan
  - PET scan

Diagnostic Procedures/Other
- Biopsy:
  - Should be performed by an experienced surgeon:
    - Avoid contamination of surrounding tissues.
    - Ensure adequate tissue sampling to make the diagnosis.
  - In addition to routine morphologic and immunohistochemical stain assessments, analysis of tumor genetics by traditional cytogenetics, fluorescence in situ hybridization, or reverse transcriptase-polymerase chain reaction (RT-PCR) is helpful in making the diagnosis and may provide information regarding prognosis.
  - Because of the importance of these studies, consultation with a pediatric oncologist before the biopsy is essential.
- Bilateral bone marrow aspirates and biopsies
- Lumbar puncture for cerebrospinal fluid cytology (parameningeal tumors only; to determine whether CNS is involved)

DIFFERENTIAL DIAGNOSIS
- Malignant:
  - Ewing sarcoma
  - Neuroblastoma
  - Non-Hodgkin lymphoma
  - Leukemic chloroma
  - Germ cell tumor
  - Rare soft tissue sarcomas
- Nonmalignant:
  - Trauma
  - Benign tumors: Lipoma, rhabdomyoma, neurofibroma
  - Langerhans cell histiocytosis
  - Abscess

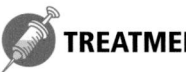 **TREATMENT**

MEDICATION (DRUGS)
- Chemotherapy: Common pharmacotherapeutic agents used include vincristine, dactinomycin, cyclophosphamide, doxorubicin, etoposide, and ifosfamide. Other agents (e.g., topotecan, irinotecan) are being investigated.
- Most patients require placement of an indwelling central venous catheter for the duration of their therapy.

ADDITIONAL TREATMENT

General Measures

- Therapy is multimodal with chemotherapy, radiation therapy, and surgery. Typically structured as:
  - Neoadjuvant chemotherapy
  - Local control (surgery, radiation therapy)
  - Adjuvant chemotherapy
- Most children are treated at pediatric oncology centers using large cooperative group protocols
- Treatment is characterized by significant side effects, including increased susceptibility to infection, severe mucositis, and poor nutritional status.
- Experimental therapies such as immunotherapy (vaccination with fusion-gene peptide products) are being investigated in clinical trials for patients with high-risk or relapsed disease.

Additional Therapies

Radiotherapy

- Radiation therapy can be used to aid in local control and for control of metastatic disease.

ISSUES FOR REFERRAL

Consultation with a pediatric oncologist is essential before any attempt is made at a diagnostic biopsy.

SURGERY/OTHER PROCEDURES

Trend is toward less radical surgical interventions.

 ## ONGOING CARE

PROGNOSIS

- Overall ~70% of patients can be cured.
- Tumor stage and clinical group are used to predict survival and guide therapy:
  - Staging is based on the anatomic site of the tumor and the extent of spread:
    - Favorable sites include orbit, nonparameningeal head and neck, nonbladder/prostate genitourinary
    - Unfavorable sites include extremities, parameningeal, bladder/prostate
  - Clinical grouping is based on extent of surgical resection. Generally:
    - Stage I: Completely resected
    - Stage II: Gross total resection with microscopic residual disease
    - Stage III: Biopsy only, gross residual disease
    - Stage IV: Distant metastases
- Tumors with alveolar histology (typically extremity lesions) tend to metastasize early.
- The presence of the *PAX3-FKHR* or *PAX7-FKHR* gene rearrangement (seen in tumors with alveolar histology) is an adverse prognostic factor, associated with older patients and more advanced disease stage.
- Recurrence can occur many years after completion of therapy but is rare after 3 years.

COMPLICATIONS

- Rhabdomyosarcoma can compromise the function of surrounding organs.

- Metastatic spread may occur to lymph nodes, lung, bone, bone marrow, liver, or brain.
- Acute effects of therapy:
  - Frequent hospital admissions for chemotherapy or complications of therapy
  - Bone marrow suppression:
    - Transfusions are usually necessary.
    - Neutropenia: Increased risk of bacterial and fungal infections; granulocyte colony-stimulating factor is usually administered daily after chemotherapy to shorten duration of neutropenia.
  - Complications from the GI side effects of chemotherapy or radiotherapy:
    - Nausea and vomiting: Relieved with ondansetron and other antiemetic agents
    - Malnutrition secondary to reduced appetite and mucosal ulcerations
- Late effects of therapy:
  - Cardiomyopathy:
    - Anthracyclines (doxorubicin) weaken cardiac muscle, leading to reduced left ventricular function many years after therapy.
    - ~5% of patients receiving cumulative doses of doxorubicin exceeding 500 mg/m^2 develop CHF.
    - Radiation to the heart can reduce the cumulative dose threshold to 300 mg/m^2.
  - Kidney and bladder damage:
    - Urinalysis should be performed to detect hemorrhagic cystitis or tubular damage.
    - BP should be monitored in patients who received irradiation to the kidneys; vascular damage and hypertension may develop many years after therapy.
  - Infertility and delayed puberty:
    - Reduced or absent gonadal function is related to high doses of alkylating agents (e.g., cyclophosphamide, ifosfamide): Boys are at high risk of azoospermia; girls may be fertile but are at risk for premature menopause.
    - Low-dose estrogen therapy with oral contraceptive medications may be necessary for amenorrheic women.
  - 2nd malignant neoplasms:
    - Sarcomas may occur within the radiation field.
    - Myelodysplastic syndromes and acute myeloid leukemia may occur secondary to radiation or chemotherapy.
  - Bowel obstruction and enteritis (abdominopelvic tumors):
    - Adhesions as a consequence of surgery or radiation
    - A history of failure to gain weight or symptoms of malabsorption suggest a need for additional evaluation.
  - Growth abnormalities/functional defects at the primary site:
    - Radiation doses >20 Gy will cause growth retardation in prepubertal children.
    - Scoliosis can occur if the vertebrae are involved in the radiation field.
    - Cataracts can occur after irradiation involving the head.
  - Learning difficulties: Radiotherapy directed to the CNS in children <3 years old with head/neck primary cancers may produce significant cognitive deficits.

ADDITIONAL READING

- Herzog CE, Stewart JMM, Blakely ML. Pediatric soft tissue sarcomas. *Surg Oncol Clin North Am.* 2003;12:419–447.
- McCarville MB, Spunt SL, Pappo AS. Rhabdomyo-sarcoma in pediatric patients: The good, the bad, and the unusual. *Am J Roentgenol.* 2001;176:1563–1569.
- McDowell HP. Update on childhood rhabdomyo-sarcoma. *Arch Dis Child.* 2003;88: 354–357.
- Parham DM, Ellison DA. Rhabdomyosarcomas in adults and children: An update. *Arch Pathol Lab Med.* 2006;130(10):1454–1465.
- Paulino AC, Okcu MF Rhabdomyosarcoma. *Curr Probl Cancer.* 2008;32(1):7–34.
- Ruymann FB, Grovas AC. Progress in the diagnosis and treatment of rhabdomyosarcoma and related soft tissue sarcomas. *Cancer Invest.* 2000;3: 223–224.

 ## CODES

ICD9

- 171.9 Malignant neoplasm of connective and other soft tissue, site unspecified
- 188.9 Malignant neoplasm of bladder, part unspecified

ICD10

- C49.9 Malignant neoplasm of connective and soft tissue, unspecified
- C67.9 Malignant neoplasm of bladder, unspecified

FAQ

- Q: Can a child with rhabdomyosarcoma attend school?
- A: Because chemotherapy for rhabdomyosarcoma is intensive, many children are unable to continue with school during this time but benefit from educational instruction at home.
- Q: Is the treatment associated with infertility?
- A: The present chemotherapy regimens include high cumulative doses of alkylating agents placing boys, in particular, at high risk for infertility. Sperm banking is recommended for adolescent boys before starting chemotherapy.

RHEUMATIC FEVER
David Hehir

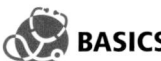

BASICS

DESCRIPTION
A postinfectious inflammatory disease caused by rheumatogenic strains of group A β-hemolytic *Streptococcus* (GABHS). Clinically diagnosed using the Jones criteria, acute rheumatic fever (ARF) results in a wide range of disease, from mild joint involvement to chronic carditis. The most significant health care and socioeconomic impact is caused by its most severe form, rheumatic heart disease (RHD).

EPIDEMIOLOGY
• Occurs following pharyngitis with rheumatogenic GABHS strains
• GABHS strains that cause skin infections are classically thought to be associated with glomerulonephritis; however, there is some evidence that ARF can be associated with skin infections in tropical and underdeveloped areas of the world.
• Initial episode seen primarily in patients 5–15 years of age
• No racial or ethnic predilections

Incidence
• Historically, untreated GABHS infection results in ARF in 0.1–0.3% of cases, with attack rates as high as 3% in endemic areas.
• Recent incidence data reveal 0.5/100,000 school-aged children in industrialized countries are affected. Incidence is as high as 500/100,000 in tropical and underdeveloped countries.
• Decrease in incidence due to increased use of antibiotics, improved environmental factors such as overcrowding, and changing virulence patterns of GABHS strains.

Prevalence
12 million people are affected by ARF worldwide, with 400,000 cases of RHD. This accounts for 25–40% of all cardiac disease worldwide.

RISK FACTORS
Genetics
No specific genetic risk factor identified, although numerous studies have demonstrated an association of ARF with specific human leukocyte antigen (HLA) alleles

PATHOPHYSIOLOGY
• GABHS triggers a complex inflammatory host response affecting the heart, joints, brain, blood vessels, and subcutaneous tissue.
• Classic example of molecular mimicry, in which the host produces antibodies to certain GABHS M proteins, which are similar in structure to host proteins such as myosin, resulting in autoimmune tissue damage.
• Aschoff nodules are proliferative lesions noted in the myocardium that may persist for months to years after initiation of disease.

ETIOLOGY
Immune-mediated inflammatory reaction to specific rheumatogenic strains of GABHS.

DIAGNOSIS

HISTORY
• A clinical diagnosis based on the modified Jones criteria (updated 1992): Evidence of recent GABHS infection with the presence of either 2 major or 1 major and 2 minor criteria:
• Major criteria (% affected):
  – Polyarthritis (70%): Migratory arthritis of major joints; more common in adults
  – Carditis (50%): 85% of those with carditis have mitral regurgitation, and 54% have aortic valve involvement. Symptoms range from asymptomatic murmur to fulminant heart failure; carditis is more common and more severe in children
  – Sydenham chorea (15%): Abnormal behavior and/or involuntary, purposeless movements
  – Erythema marginatum (10%): Evanescent, pink rash with serpiginous borders
  – Subcutaneous nodules (2–10%): Painless nodules over extensor surfaces of large joints, the occiput, and/or vertebral processes
• Minor criteria:
  – Fever
  – Arthralgia (mild pain without objective findings): Can only be considered without finding of arthritis
  – Elevated acute-phase reactants: ESR, C-reactive protein
  – Prolongation of the PR interval on electrocardiogram
• Exceptions to the Jones criteria include:
  – Sydenham chorea alone
  – Subclinical carditis (echocardiogram evidence of RHD) in the absence of other criteria should be treated as ARF.
  – Jones criteria cannot be applied to recurrence; World Health Organization (WHO) recommends treating recurrence in a patient with RHD and presence of any major or minor criterion.

PHYSICAL EXAM
• Cardiac:
  – Murmur of valvulitis: Holosystolic mitral regurgitant murmur, Carey-Coombs apical middiastolic murmur, or a basal diastolic murmur of aortic insufficiency (major criterion)
  – Pericardial friction rub: Pericardial effusion
• Musculoskeletal:
  – Pain, limited motion, erythema, warmth of 2 or more large joints: Arthritis (major criterion)
• Neurologic: Choreiform movements (must be differentiated from tics, athetosis, and hyperkinesis): Sydenham chorea (major criterion)
• Dermatologic:
  – Evanescent, pink rash with pale centers and serpiginous borders on the trunk and proximal extremities: Erythema marginatum (major criterion)
  – Firm, painless nodules over the extensor surface of large joints, occiput, and/or spinous processes: Subcutaneous nodules (major criterion)

DIAGNOSTIC TESTS & INTERPRETATION
Lab
• Specific tests: No specific diagnostic test is available.
• Nonspecific tests:
  – Throat culture: Neither sensitive nor specific. False negative in up to 2/3 of affected patients, or false positive in patients who are colonized
  – Elevated or rising streptococcal antibody titers, antistreptolysin O, anti-DNase B, antihyaluronidase
  – ESR and C-reactive protein elevation

Imaging
• ECG: Prolonged PR interval (minor criterion), junctional rhythm, transient arrhythmias, ST-T wave changes
• Chest radiograph: Cardiomegaly may indicate carditis or pericardial effusion. Pulmonary edema may reflect left heart failure due to valvulitis.
• Echocardiogram: Assess valve involvement, ventricular dilatation, function, and pericardial effusion.

DIFFERENTIAL DIAGNOSIS
• Carditis:
  – Viral
  – Bacterial
  – Rickettsial
  – Parasitic
  – Mycoplasma myocarditis
  – Kawasaki disease
• Arthritis:
  – Poststreptococcal reactive arthritis (PSRA)
  – Serum sickness
  – Septic arthritis (i.e., gonococcal)
  – Lyme disease
• Collagen vascular disease:
  – Juvenile rheumatoid arthritis (small joints, not migratory, and not relieved promptly with aspirin)
  – Systemic lupus erythematosus
  – Bacterial endocarditis
• Chorea:
  – Congenital choreoathetosis
  – Brain tumors
  – Huntington chorea
  – Wilson disease
  – Pediatric autoimmune neuropsychiatric disorders associated with streptococcus (PANDAS)
• Hematologic disorders with joint involvement:
  – Sickle cell anemia
  – Leukemia
• Congenital heart defects: Previously undiagnosed valvular heart disease
• Mitral valve prolapse with regurgitation

TREATMENT

MEDICATION (DRUGS)
First Line
- Anti-inflammatory
  - Aspirin 60–100 mg/kg/d; may be reduced when fever and acute-phase reactants have normalized for 6–8 weeks
- Antibiotics in ARF:
  - Penicillin Vpotassium (Pen VK):
    - Children: 250 mg 2–3 times/day for 10 days
    - Adolescents, adults: 500 mg 2–3 times/day for 10 days
- Secondary prophylaxis:
  - Benzathine penicillin G IM (600,000 U for weight <27 kg or 1,200,000 U for weight >27 kg) every 3–4 weeks

Second Line
- Anti-inflammatory:
  - Prednisone 2 mg/kg/d for 2 weeks, then taper
- Antibiotics in ARF:
  - Erythromycin, amoxicillin, 1st-generation cephalosporin
- Secondary prophylaxis:
  - Penicillin V 250 mg b.i.d.
  - Erythromycin, sulfadiazine

ADDITIONAL TREATMENT
General Measures
- Primary prevention: Appropriate and early treatment of GABHS pharyngitis
- Interventions to address poverty, crowding, and housing challenges
- Treatment of ARF:
  - Antibiotics: Full course of penicillin or equivalent to eradicate active infection; does not alter course of carditis
  - Anti-inflammatory: High-dose aspirin is standard; steroids may help for severe carditis but remain controversial.
  - Cardiac support: Aggressive support of cardiac function and use of systemic afterload reduction for severe disease
  - Surgical valvuloplasty or valve replacement may be necessary in severe cases.
  - Bed rest: Controversial; still recommended for severe cases
- Secondary prevention:
  - Ideally administered as benzathine penicillin G as a monthly IM injection, but oral daily penicillin or erythromycin is acceptable in areas of low prevalence.
  - Duration based on clinical presentation and degree of cardiac involvement:
    - ARF without cardiac involvement: 5 years or until age 18, whichever is longer
    - ARF with mild or resolved carditis: 10 years or until age 25, whichever is longer
    - ARF with severe carditis or cardiac surgery: Lifelong

- Treatment of chorea:
  - Usually supportive
  - Phenobarbital and haloperidol are most commonly used; chlorpromazine, diazepam, or valproic acid also used

ISSUES FOR REFERRAL
Patients with new murmurs or clinical evidence of heart failure should be referred to a cardiologist.

IN-PATIENT CONSIDERATIONS
Initial Stabilization
Full treatment of streptococcal pharyngitis infection and cardiac support if heart failure present. Treatment phases include primary prevention, management of ARF, and secondary prevention of recurrence.

ONGOING CARE

FOLLOW-UP RECOMMENDATIONS
- Patients without carditis:
  - Close follow-up is needed for 2–3 weeks to assess patient's condition for development of acute carditis.
  - Long-term pediatric follow-up is needed to diagnose patients with indolent carditis.
  - Long-term follow-up is needed to evaluate patients who develop chorea.
  - Prophylaxis should be stressed even in patients without carditis.
- Patients with carditis:
  - Cardiology follow-up is needed to assess development or evolution of RHD.
  - Symptoms of worsening heart failure suggest progression of valvular or myocardial disease, recurrent ARF, or endocarditis.
  - Secondary prophylaxis and bacterial endocarditis prophylaxis should be stressed.

PROGNOSIS
- ARF recurrence rate as high as 36% without prophylaxis
- Chorea may last weeks to months and has a similarly high recurrence rate.
- Carditis may resolve spontaneously (70–80%) or progress. Severity of the initial carditis is a major determinant of progression.

COMPLICATIONS
Long-term complications related to evolution of RHD:
- Mitral stenosis
- Mitral regurgitation
- Aortic stenosis
- Aortic regurgitation
- Chronic heart failure

ADDITIONAL READING
- Carapetis JR, McDonald M, Wilson NJ. Acute rheumatic fever. *Lancet*. 2005;366:155–168.
- Cilliers AM, Manyemba J, Saloojee H. Cochrane review: Anti-inflammatory treatment for carditis in acute rheumatic fever. *The Cochrane Library*. 2006;4:1–37.
- Kerdemelidis M, Lennon DR, Arroll B, et al. The primary prevention of rheumatic fever. *J Paediatr Child Health*. 2010;46:534–548.
- Stollerman GH. Rheumatic fever in the 21st century. *Clin Infect Dis*. 2001;33:806–814.

CODES

ICD9
- 390 Rheumatic fever without mention of heart involvement
- 398.90 Rheumatic heart disease, unspecified
- 729.89 Other musculoskeletal symptoms referable to limbs

ICD10
- I00 Rheumatic fever without heart involvement
- I09.9 Rheumatic heart disease, unspecified

FAQ

- Q: Does a negative throat culture rule out ARF?
- A: No. Throat cultures may be negative in 2/3 of patients.
- Q: Is there a vaccine available to prevent ARF?
- A: Not at present. However, research efforts to develop a recombinant multivalent vaccine have been promising. Note that >90 antigenic strains of group A *Streptococcus* have been identified; any vaccines developed ought to focus on those with the greatest virulence.
- Q: What genetic factors predispose to ARF?
- A: Several studies done worldwide have reported a high incidence of certain HLA-DR antigens in patients with rheumatic fever. The specific antigen/allele involved varies with the ethnic group studied.
- Q: Can ECG evidence of carditis alone be used to diagnose rheumatic fever?
- A: This is currently under debate. An ECG finding of carditis without a murmur cannot be used to fulfill the Jones criteria. However, many experts would agree to treat subclinical carditis as ARF, especially in areas of high prevalence.
- Q: Can intravenous γ-globulin be used as a treatment for ARF?
- A: One study revealed that intravenous γ-globulin did not alter the natural history of ARF, with no detectable difference in the cardiac outcome, laboratory findings, or ECG parameters when compared to placebo.

RHINITIS, ALLERGIC

Esther K. Chung
Karen P. Zimmer

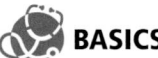 **BASICS**

DESCRIPTION
- Inflammation of the nasal and sinus mucosae, associated with sneezing, swelling, increased mucus production, and nasal obstruction; may be classified as seasonal, perennial, or a combination
- Seasonal: Periodic symptoms, involving the same season for at least 2 consecutive years; most often due to pollens (e.g., trees, grass, weeds) and outdoor spores
- Perennial: Occurring at least 9 months of the year; may be more difficult to detect because of overlap with other infections; may be due to multiple seasonal allergies or continual exposure to allergens (such as dust mites, cockroaches, molds, and animal dander)
- Perennial, with seasonal exacerbations

EPIDEMIOLOGY
Prevalence
Most common allergic disease, affecting ~40 million Americans; affects 40% of children and 15–30% of adolescents

RISK FACTORS
Genetics
- Increased incidence in families with atopic disease
- If 1 parent has allergies, each child has a 30% chance of having an allergy; if both parents have allergies, each child has a 70% chance of having an allergy.

GENERAL PREVENTION
- Minimize exposure to dust mites: Consider removing carpets, upholstered furniture, and curtains; washing bedding in hot water frequently, at least every 1–2 weeks; use pillow and mattress covers.
- Minimize exposure to animal dander:
- Minimize exposure to all animals; consider using solutions containing tannic acid, which will denature animal allergens; shampoo pets frequently if pets cannot be removed from the household; use air-vent filters.
- Minimize exposure to pollens: Keep windows closed, use air conditioning, and avoid leaf raking or lawn mowing.
- Minimize exposure to molds: Keep houseplants out of the bedroom; avoid spending time in the basement, keep humidity at 35–50%.

ETIOLOGY
- Indoor allergens: House dust mite, cockroaches, animal dander, cigarette smoke, hair spray, paint, molds
- Pollens: Tree pollens in early spring, grass in late spring and early summer, ragweed in late summer and autumn
- Multiple environmental factors
- Changes in air temperature

COMMONLY ASSOCIATED CONDITIONS
- Asthma
- Allergic conjunctivitis
- Atopic dermatitis (eczema)
- Urticaria
- Otitis media with effusion
- Sleep, taste, and/or smell disturbance
- Nasal polyps

- Mouth breathing
- Snoring
- Adenoidal hypertrophy and sleep apnea
- Decreased appetite
- Delayed speech

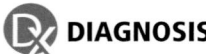 **DIAGNOSIS**

HISTORY
- Typical symptoms: Patient often reports stuffy nose, sneezing, itching, runny nose, noisy breathing, snoring, cough, halitosis, and repeated throat clearing. Sensation of plugged ears and wheezing may occur.
- Red and itchy eyes
- Symptom occurrence: Seasonal, perennial, or episodic
- Exacerbating factors, including pollen, animals, cigarette smoke, dust, molds
- Family history of atopic disease, such as asthma or atopic dermatitis
- Any related illnesses: Asthma, urticaria, eczema, ear infections, and delayed speech are commonly associated conditions.

PHYSICAL EXAM
- Allergic shiners:
  - Dark discoloration beneath the eyes due to obstruction of lymphatic and venous drainage, chronic nasal obstruction, and suborbital edema
- Dennie–Morgan lines:
  - Creases in the lower eyelid radiating outward from the inner canthus; caused by spasm in the muscles of Müller around the eye due to chronic congestion and stasis of blood
- Allergic salute:
  - A gesture characterized by rubbing the nose with the palm of the hand upward to decrease itching and temporarily open the nasal passages
- Allergic crease:
  - Transverse crease near the tip of the nose, secondary to rubbing
- Nasal mucosa may appear pale and/or edematous; mucoid or watery material may be seen in the nasal cavity; check for nasal polyps, septal deviation.

DIAGNOSTIC TESTS & INTERPRETATION
- Audiometry and tympanometry when indicated
- Sweat test if cystic fibrosis is suspected or if nasal polyps are present

Lab
- Nasal cytology
- Specimen of nasal discharge to check for the presence of eosinophils. Have the patient blow his or her nose into a piece of nonporous paper or collect discharge with a cotton swab and transfer the discharge to a glass slide. >10% eosinophils are considered positive for nasal eosinophilia. Note: Use of intranasal steroids may reduce the number of eosinophils found in nasal discharge.
- Radioallergosorbent tests (RAST):
  - In vitro test to measure allergen-specific IgE; expensive; useful in patients who have diffuse atopic dermatitis. The ImmunoCAP system (Pharmacia Diagnostics) is the preferred method for specific IgE testing; uses a single blood sample to identify levels of specific IgE to a number of common respiratory allergens (available as a

profile specific to the region of the country where the patient resides), food antigens (food allergy profile), or both (childhood allergy profile).
- Total IgE: Elevated in allergic rhinitis; not routinely indicated, but may come as part of specific IgE testing; >100 kU/L is considered elevated.
- CBC: May show eosinophilia; not routinely indicated
- Skin testing:
  - Prick test: Percutaneous, qualitative test in which antigen concentrate is placed on the skin of the volar surface of the arm or upper back, and a needle is inserted; the skin reaction is graded subjectively from 0–4.
  - Intradermal test: Qualitative test in which antigen is introduced intradermally (0.02 mL with a 26–30-gauge needle); more sensitive than the prick test and often used if prick test is negative or equivocal; the degree of swelling and erythema is graded from 0–4.
  - Caution: Skin tests may be difficult to interpret in patients with diffuse eczema and dermatographism.

Diagnostic Procedures/Other
Rhinoscopy to assess the nasal turbinates and to look for nasal polyps

DIFFERENTIAL DIAGNOSIS
- Infection:
  - Viral upper respiratory tract infection
  - Bacterial sinusitis
- Environmental:
  - Foreign body
  - Temperature
  - Odors
- Tumors:
  - Nasal polyps
  - Dermoid cyst
  - Nasal glioma
- Congenital:
  - Cystic fibrosis
  - Choanal atresia
  - Immotile cilia syndrome
  - Septal deviation
  - Primary atrophic rhinitis
- Immunologic:
  - Sarcoidosis
  - Wegener granulomatosis
  - Systemic lupus erythematosus
  - Sjögren syndrome
- Allergic:
  - Nonallergic perennial rhinitis
  - Idiopathic (vasomotor) rhinitis
  - Drug-induced rhinitis
  - Food-induced rhinitis
- Miscellaneous:
  - Rhinitis medicamentosa
  - Rhinitis associated with pregnancy/other hormonal rhinitis
  - Hypothyroidism
  - Idiopathic neonatal rhinitis

TREATMENT

MEDICATION (DRUGS)

- Caution: Cardiac arrhythmias have been seen with patients taking terfenadine and astemizole.
- Improve mucociliary flow:
  – Steam inhalation
  – Normal saline drops
  – Bicarbonate spray
  – N-acetylcysteine (orally or inhaled)
  – Oral guaifenesin
- Antihistamines: Competitively blocking histamine (H_1) receptors; suppress itching, ocular symptoms, sneezing, and rhinorrhea; not very effective against nasal congestion:
- Intranasal 2nd-generation antihistamine:
  – Azelastine: Age ≥5 years; 137 mcg; 1 spray per nostril b.i.d. The efficacy of this dose has not yet been established in the pediatric population but rather extrapolated from adult data.
- 2nd-generation antihistamines: Tend not to cross the blood–brain barrier and therefore do not have CNS side effects such as drowsiness
  – Loratadine (Claritin, Schering): FDA-approved for children as young as 2 years. Dose: Ages 2–5 years, 5 mg/d PO; ages 6 years or older, 10 mg/d PO
  – Desloratadine (Clarinex, Schering): FDA-approved for children ≥6 months. Dose: 6–12 months, 1 mg/d PO; 12 months–5 years, 1.25 mg/d PO; 6–12 years, 2.5 mg/d PO; >12 years, 5 mg/d PO.
  – Cetirizine HCl (Zyrtec, Pfizer): FDA-approved for children as young as 6 months of age. Dose: Age 6 months–5 years, 2.5 mg = 1/2 tsp/d (1 mg/mL banana–grape flavored syrup) PO with maximum dose of 5 mg/d (must be divided into 2.5 mg b.i.d. for children <2 years of age). Age ≥6 years, 5–10 mg/d
  – Levocetirizine (Xyal): FDA-approved for children as young as 6 years. Dose: 6–11 years, 2.5 mg/d (half tab) PO; ≥12 years, 5 mg/d PO.
  – Fexofenadine (Allegra, Aventis): Age 6–11 years, 30-mg tab b.i.d.; age ≥12 years, 60 mg/d b.i.d. or 180 mg/d PO.
- 1st-generation antihistamine side effects include drowsiness, performance impairment, and paradoxical excitement; anticholinergic (e.g., dry mouth, tachycardia, urinary retention, and constipation): Diphenhydramine (Benadryl) 5 mg/kg/d PO divided q.i.d.
- Intranasal steroids: Blunt early-phase reactions and block late-phase reactions; may not be fully effective until several days to 2 weeks after initiation of therapy. Must be used regularly and best when administered lying down with the head back:
  – Beclomethasone (Vancenase, Beconase): For use in children ≥6 years of age
  – Flunisolide (Aerobid): For use in children ≥6 years of age
  – Fluticasone propionate (Flonase 0.05%): For use in children ≥4 years of age
  – Budesonide (Rhinocort): For use in children ≥6 years of age
  – Triamcinolone acetonide (Nasacort): For use in children ≥6 years of age
  – Mometasone furoate monohydrate (Nasonex): For use in children ≥2 years of age
- Intranasal antihistamines: Azelastine hydrochloride (Astelin; approved for children ≥5 years; dose: 1–2 sprays per day) or olopatadine (Patanase; approved for children ≥6 years; dose: 2 sprays per day) are FDA-approved for use in seasonal allergic rhinitis

- Topical cromolyn (Nasalcrom): Mast-cell stabilizer; minimal side effects; does not provide immediate relief (may take 2–4 weeks to see clinical effect): For use in children ≥2 years of age
- Oral decongestants: 1- and 2-Adrenergic agonists (i.e., ephedrine, pseudoephedrine, and phenylephrine) act to cause vasoconstriction, decreased blood supply to the nasal mucosa, and decreased mucosal edema. Cardiovascular and CNS side effects include tremors, agitation, hypertension, insomnia, and headaches.
- Topical decongestants: Sympathomimetics such as short-acting phenylephrine (Neo-Synephrine) and long-acting oxymetazoline (Afrin) may be useful for a few days to open nasal passages to allow for delivery of topical steroids; side effects include drying of the mucosa and burning. Use for more than a few (3–5) days may result in rebound vasodilatation and congestion (rhinitis medicamentosa).
- Combined oral decongestants and antihistamines: Numerous preparations on the market
- Leukotriene receptor antagonist (montelukast/Singulair): For use in children ≥6 months. Dose for 12 mos to 5 years, 1 granule packet daily; age 2–5 years, 4 mg chewable tab daily; 6–14 years, 5 mg chewable tab daily; age ≥15 years, 10 mg chewable tab daily.
- Immunotherapy: Also referred to as hyposensitization or desensitization. Consists of a series of injections with specific allergens, with increasing concentrations of allergens, once or twice weekly. Recommended for patients who have not responded to pharmacologic therapy:
  – Extremely effective and long lasting. After several months to years of treatment, total serum IgE levels decrease, and the intensity of the early-phase response is reduced.
  – Side effects include urticaria, bronchospasm, hypotension, and anaphylaxis.

ADDITIONAL TREATMENT
General Measures
Avoidance therapy: Identify and eliminate known/suspected allergens.

SURGERY/OTHER PROCEDURES
- Removal of allergic polyps
- Inferior turbinate surgery to reduce the size of the turbinate and relieve obstruction
- Endoscopic sinus surgery to relieve obstruction

 ONGOING CARE

FOLLOW-UP RECOMMENDATIONS
Patient Monitoring
Watch for fever, prolonged or severe headache, dizziness, pain, or purulent discharge; should suggest a diagnosis other than allergic rhinitis alone.

PROGNOSIS
Generally good: Complete recovery occurs in 5–10% of patients.

COMPLICATIONS
- Chronic sinusitis
- Recurrent otitis media
- Hoarseness
- Loss of smell
- Loss of hearing
- High-arched palate and dental malocclusion from chronic mouth breathing

ADDITIONAL READING

- Kaari J. The role of intranasal corticosteroids in the management of pediatric allergic rhinitis. *Clin Pediatr*. 2006;45:697–704.
- Mahr TA, Ketan S. Update on allergic rhinitis. *Pediatr Rev*. 2005;26:284–288.
- Phan H, Moeller ML, Nahata MC. Treatment of allergic rhinitis in infants and children: Efficacy and safety of second-generation antihistamines and the leukotriene receptor antagonist montelukast. *Drugs*. 2009;69(18):2541–2576.
- Prenner BM, Schenkel E. Allergic rhinitis: Treatment based on patient profiles. *Am J Med*. 2006;119:230–237.
- Wallace DV, Dykewicz MS, Berstein DI, et al. The diagnosis and management of rhinitis: An updated practice parameter. *J Allergy Clin Immunol*. 2008;122(2 Suppl):S1–84.

CODES

ICD9
- 477.0 Allergic rhinitis due to pollen
- 477.2 Allergic rhinitis due to animal (cat) (dog) hair and dander
- 477.9 Allergic rhinitis, cause unspecified

ICD10
- J30.1 Allergic rhinitis due to pollen
- J30.2 Other seasonal allergic rhinitis
- J30.9 Allergic rhinitis, unspecified

FAQ

- Q: How does one minimize exposure to dust mites?
- A: Keep household temperature low; maintain humidity at ~40–50%; wash linens weekly at hot temperatures; use a microfilter when vacuuming; place mattress and box spring in tightly woven casing; use air conditioning; use high-efficiency particulate air filter units.
- Q: How often are nasal polyps associated with cystic fibrosis?
- A: In up to 40% of children, nasal polyps are associated with cystic fibrosis. <0.5% of children with asthma and rhinitis have nasal polyps.
- Q: When used on a daily basis, are intranasal steroids safe?
- A: Yes. It is generally accepted that inhaled steroids are safe. Growth suppression has been reported in children using certain intranasal steroids; however, this effect does not appear to be an effect of all intranasal steroids. Importantly, one should use the lowest effective dose of intranasal steroids when treating allergic rhinitis.

RICKETS

Maria Mascarenhas
Sara Karjoo
Alisha J. Rovner (5th edition)

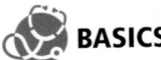

BASICS

DESCRIPTION
- Failure or delay in the mineralization of growing bone and cartilage, caused primarily by a deficiency of vitamin D, calcium, or phosphorus
- See for classification of rickets and vitamin D metabolite levels

EPIDEMIOLOGY
Children at risk for rickets:
- Low-birth-weight and/or premature infants
- Breast-fed infants who do not receive supplemental vitamin D
- Darker skinned infant
- Mother who is deficient in vitamin D during pregnancy
- Higher latitudes, and seasons
- Use of sunscreens and UVR blocking agents
- Chronic renal insufficiency
- Inadequate dietary vitamin D intake (see table)
- Illnesses with malabsorption
  - Cholestatic liver disease
  - Celiac disease
  - Cystic fibrosis

GENERAL PREVENTION
Start vitamin D supplements in breastfed infants, if intake low or patient at risk (see table for at-risk conditions).

PATHOPHYSIOLOGY
Overproduction and deficient calcification of osteoid tissue, with associated osseous deformities; alterations in growth patterns. In addition, there is abnormal organization of cartilaginous growth plates and impairment of cartilage mineralization.

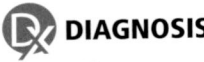

DIAGNOSIS

HISTORY
- Symptoms of hepatic, renal, or GI disease
- Prolonged breastfeeding without vitamin D supplementation:
  - Little or no sunlight exposure (or being covered up when exposed to sunlight)
  - Born to mother who is vitamin D-deficient
- Calcium intake
- Strict vegetarian diet
- Factors influencing calcium absorption:
  - Low vitamin D intake
  - Steatorrhea
  - Antacids
  - Anticonvulsants
- Diet high in foods containing oxalic acid
- Dietary history of Vitamin D–fortified milk in children >1 year of age
- Amount of exposure to sunlight
- Prolonged use of cholestyramine
- Factors influencing calcium excretion: Diuretics, polyuria, or glycosuria suggests renal tubular dysfunction.
- Bone pain
- Delayed standing or walking
- Anorexia
- Seizures

- Pathologic fractures
- Tetany
- Familial history of rickets
- Signs and symptoms:
  - Anomalies of osteoid tissue
  - Skeletal and dental deformities
  - Growth disturbances and delayed gross motor development
  - Hypocalcemia
  - Tetany
  - Seizures
  - Irritability
  - Listlessness
  - Generalized muscular weakness
  - Bone pain
  - Increased risk of infections

PHYSICAL EXAM
- Failure to thrive
- Long-bone deformities (i.e., varus or valgus deformity)
- Fractures following minimal trauma
- Skull abnormalities (i.e., delay in closure of anterior fontanelle, craniotabes, and frontal bossing)
- Chest deformities (i.e., enlargement of costochondral junctions leading to rachitic rosary)
- Muscular hypotonia
- Waddling gait

DIAGNOSTIC TESTS & INTERPRETATION
Lab
- Circulating vitamin D metabolites (25-hydroxyvitamin D, 1,25-dihydroxyvitamin D)
- Circulating levels of parathyroid hormone
- Serum calcium, phosphorous, magnesium, alkaline phosphatase, and total CO_2
- Urinary calcium, phosphorous, magnesium, pH, creatinine, and amino acids, to rule out Fanconi syndrome and proximal renal tubular acidosis

Imaging
- Order 1 view because rickets is symmetrical.
- Knee or wrist films (the earliest sign at the wrist is a loss of clear demarcation between the growth plate and the metaphysis, with loss of the provisional zone of calcification).
- Radiographic findings: Irregular cortices and bony margins, widened metaphyses, widened growth plates, osteopenia

DIFFERENTIAL DIAGNOSIS
- Blount disease
- Fanconi syndrome
- Metastatic bone disease
- Neurofibromatosis type 1
- Proximal renal tubular acidosis

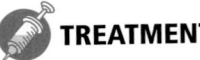

TREATMENT

ADDITIONAL TREATMENT
General Measures
- Studies suggest difference in potency between vitamin D_3 and D_2
- Once intake of vitamin D surpass 4,000 IU/d and 2,000 mg/d calcium, the risk for harm also increases.
- See table "Causes and Management of Rickets."

ISSUES FOR REFERRAL
- To look for other causes of rickets other than low vitamin D intake; these include:
  - No radiographic evidence of healing by 3 months
  - Radiologic evidence of rickets at <6 months of age and between 3–10 years of age
  - Findings of normal alkaline phosphate, 25(OH)-D, very high or low 1,25(OH)-D, high BUN, creatinine.

IN-PATIENT CONSIDERATIONS
Admission Criteria
- Tetany
- Severe hypocalcemia
- Seizures

Discharge Criteria
- Stable laboratory values
- Mental status and neurology exam improvement

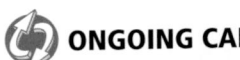

ONGOING CARE

FOLLOW-UP RECOMMENDATIONS
Patient Monitoring
- Monitor serum calcium, alkaline phosphatase, and phosphorus levels every 2–4 weeks; reimage bones radiographically monthly until stabilized.
- 1 early radiographic sign of healing is the appearance of the provisional zone of calcification at the boundary between the physis and metaphysis.

PROGNOSIS
- Generally good with vitamin D treatment
- Skeletal changes improve over time with adequate treatment.

COMPLICATIONS
- Fractures
- Seizures
- Failure to thrive, poor motor development
- Frequent infections

ADDITIONAL READING

- Gartner LM, Greer FR; Section on Breastfeeding and Committee on Nutrition. Prevention of rickets and vitamin D deficiency: New guidelines for vitamin D intake. *Pediatrics.* 2003;111:908–910.
- Jewell JA, McElwain LL, Blake AS. Nutritional rickets. *Arch Pediatr Adolesc Med.* 2006;160:983–985.
- Misra M, Pacaud D, Petryk A et al. Vitamin D deficiency in children and its management: Review of current knowledge and recommendations. Drug and Therapeutics Committee of the Lawson Wilkins Pediatric Endocrine Society. *Pediatrics.* 2008; 122(2):398–417.
- Ross C, Abrams S, Aloia J et al. Dietary reference intakes for calcium and vitamin D. *Institute of Medicine Report Brief.* November 2010.
- Weisberg P, Scanlon K, Li R et al. Nutritional rickets among children in the United States: Review of cases reported between 1986 and 2003. *Am J Clin Nutr.* 2004;80(6 Suppl):1697S–1705S.

Dietary reference intake for calcium and vitamin D

Age	Estimated average requirement (mg/day)	Recommended dietary allowance (mg/day)	Upper level intake (mg/day)	Estimated average requirement (IU/day)	Recommended dietary allowance (IU/day)	Upper level intake (IU/day)
0–6months	200	200	1,000	400	400	1,000
6–12 months	260	260	1,500	400	400	1,500
1–3 years	500	700	2,500	400	600	2,500
4–8 years	800	1,000	2,500	400	600	3,000
9–13 years	1,100	1,300	3,000	400	600	4,000
14–18 years	1,100	1,300	3,000	400	600	4,000
19–30 years	800	1,000	2,500	400	600	4,000
31–50 years	800	1,000	2,500	400	600	4,000
51–70 years males	800	1,000	2,000	400	600	4,000
51–70 years females	1,000	1,200	2,000	400	600	4,000
>70 years	1,000	1,200	2,000	400	800	4,000
14–18 pregnant & lactating	1,100	1,300	3,000	400	600	4,000
19–50 pregnant & lactating	800	1,000	2,500	400	600	4,000

*Adapted from the 2010 institute of medicine report brief on dietary reference intakes for calcium and vitamin D

Causes and management of rickets

Causes	Management
Calcium deficiency	–
Low intake	<6 months of age 400 mg/day 6–12 months of age 600 mg/day 1–10 years of age 800 mg/day
Extreme prematurity (birth weight <1,500 g)	Adjust intake to 200 mg/kg/day
Steatorrhea	25-OH-D3 (5–7 mcg/kg/d) if serum levels are low and supplement dietary calcium between 25–100 mg/kg/day
Anticonvulsant (Phenobarbital or phenytoin)	Calcium <6 months of age 400 mg/day 6–12 months of age 600 mg/day 1–10 years of age 800 mg/day vitamin D 200 IU/day of ergocalciferol
Renal tubular acidosis	Base supplement: 3–10 mM/kg/d as NaHCO$_3$ or citrate
Vitamin D deficiency	
Insufficient UV light exposure	200 IU/day of vitamin D of ergocalciferol
Breastfeed infants who are not supplemented with vitamin D	200 IU/day of vitamin D of ergocalciferol
Liver disease	4,000–8,000 IU/day ergocalciferol
Renal disorders	4,000–40,000 IU/day of Calcitriol
Nutritional rickets and osteomalacia	1,000–5,000 IU/day of ergocalciferol
Vitamin D-dependent rickets	3,000–5,000 IU/day of Calcitriol
Vitamin D-resistant rickets	40,000–80,000 IU/day of ergocalciferol with phosphate supplements, daily dosage is increased at 3–4 month intervals in 10,000–20,000 IU increments
Phosphorus deficiency	
Diet (limited to premature infants)	Adjust formula or parenteral source to give 10 mg/kg/d
Antacid excess	Alternative gastric acid control
Excessive phosphaturia from tubular dysfunction	Supplemental P and calcitriol if low

Classification of rickets and vitamin D metabolite levels

	Calcium	Phosphorus	Alkaline phosphate	25-(OH)-D
Deficient synthesis and supply like: No sunlight Poor diet Immaturity	N or ↓	↓	↑	↓
Malabsorption	N or ↓	↓	↑	↓
Liver disease	N or ↓	↓	↑	↓
Chronic renal failure	N or ↓	↑	↑	N
Vitamin D-dependent rickets (recessively inherited)	↓	↓	↑	N
Vitamin D-resistant rickets (sex-linked dominant)	N	↓	↑	N
Renal tubular disorders (defect of phosphate reabsorption)	N	↓	↑	N

N, normal; ↓, decreased; ↑, increased.

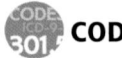

CODES

ICD9
- 268.0 Rickets, active
- 269.3 Mineral deficiency, not elsewhere classified
- 275.3 Disorders of phosphorus metabolism

ICD10
- E55.0 Rickets, active
- E55.9 Vitamin D deficiency, unspecified
- E58 Dietary calcium deficiency

FAQ

- Q: What is the best way to diagnose rickets?
- A: Laboratory investigation and x-rays are the best ways to make the diagnosis. The most common biochemical findings of children with vitamin D–deficient rickets are hypocalcemia, hypophosphatemia, low 25-(OH)-D concentrations, and elevated levels of parathyroid hormone and alkaline phosphatase. The classic radiographic findings occur at the growth plate of long bones and are best seen at the distal end of the radius and ulna or at the tibia and femoral growth plates around the knee. Widening of the physis, with fraying, cupping, and splaying of the metaphyses and underdevelopment of the epiphysis are common findings.
- Q: What are the recommendations for vitamin D supplementation in infants and children?
- A: To prevent rickets and vitamin D deficiency in healthy infants and children, and acknowledging that adequate sunlight exposure is difficult to determine, the American Academy of Pediatrics recommends a supplement of 200 IU/d for the following:
  - All breastfed infants unless they are weaned to at least 500 mL/d of vitamin D–fortified formula or milk
  - All non–breastfed infants who are ingesting <500 mL/d of vitamin D–fortified formula or milk
  - Vitamin D needs to be started by the 1st 2 months of life because vitamin D stores last 8 weeks post birth.
  - Children and adolescents who do not get regular sunlight exposure, do not consume at least 500 mL/d of vitamin D–fortified milk, or do not take a daily multivitamin supplement containing at least 200 IU of vitamin D
- Q: What are the distinguishing features of vitamin D–deficient and calcium-deficient rickets?
- A: The biochemical features (e.g., hypocalcemia, high alkaline phosphatase, and high parathyroid hormone) and radiographic features (i.e., growth-plate changes) are similar. The distinguishing feature is the difference in vitamin D status. In vitamin D–deficient rickets, 25-(OH)-D levels are low. Typically, in calcium-deficient rickets, 25-(OH)-D levels are normal (>10 ng/mL) and 1,25-(OH)2-D levels are high.

RICKETTSIAL DISEASE

Abby M. Green
Suzanne Dawid (5th edition)

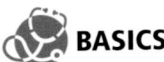 **BASICS**

DESCRIPTION
- Disorders caused by the Rickettsiae family of organisms including those which cause Rocky Mountain spotted fever and other similar tick-borne illnesses, the typhus group, the organism responsible for Q fever, and the organisms that cause ehrlichiosis.
- All organisms are obligate intracellular gram-negative bacteria and therefore are difficult to grow in culture.
- The diseases caused by each group of organisms are similar, encompassing a syndrome including fever, rash, headache, and capillary leak and, with the exception of Q fever, all are transmitted via an insect vector.

GENERAL PREVENTION
- Fleas, ticks, and mites should be controlled in endemic areas with the appropriate insecticides.
- Clothing to cover the entire body should be worn in tick-infested areas. In the case of a recognized bite, ticks should be removed from human skin properly with care not to expel the contents of the tick's stomach into the site of the bite.
- In areas where louse-borne typhus is epidemic, periodic delousing and dusting of insecticide into clothes are recommended.
- Paradoxic effect of rodenticides: Fleas, mites will seek alternate hosts (i.e., humans) when mice or rats are not present. Therefore, rodenticides should not be the only prevention measure taken in endemic areas.
- Except for *Orientia tsutsugamushi* (scrub typhus) and *Ehrlichia*, all rickettsial diseases produce long-term immunity to the etiologic organisms within the same group.

PATHOPHYSIOLOGY
- Spotted fever, typhus, and ehrlichiosis groups cause vasculitis as a result of organisms invading the endothelial cells of small blood vessels or white blood cells. This manifests as rash in cutaneous tissues, and systemic illness due to capillary leak throughout other organs.
- Q fever, caused by *Coxiella burnetii*, causes pneumonitis initially due to proliferation of inhaled organisms in lungs, followed by bloodstream infection and distant organ involvement including hepatitis, endocarditis, and neurologic disease.

ETIOLOGY
- Spotted fever group rickettsia and the agents of ehrlichiosis (*Ehrlichia* and *Anaplasma*) are transmitted to humans by ticks.
- Rickettsialpox and scrub typhus are transmitted by mites associated with mice.
- Epidemic typhus is a louse-borne illness, and endemic typhus, also known as murine typhus, is transmitted by fleas.
- Q fever is acquired via inhalation of the organisms from body fluid or tissue of infected mammals.
- The rickettsial diseases that occur in the U.S. are Rocky Mountain spotted fever, murine typhus, rickettsialpox, epidemic typhus, Q fever, and ehrlichiosis.

 DIAGNOSIS

HISTORY
- In general, rickettsial disease should be considered as a diagnosis in a patient with fever, headache, and rash. Progression of rash can be particularly helpful in considering the diagnosis.
- Signs and symptoms:
  - Spotted fever group:
    - Illness often begins with fever, myalgia, and headache
    - Rash occurs 3–5 days following onset of symptoms and is typically described as centripetal, beginning on hands and feet and moving towards the trunk. Rash is variable and may not always follow this pattern.
    - Other symptoms include headache, neurologic changes, hypotension, hyponatremia, and consumptive coagulopathy
    - Fulminant RMSF may cause cardiovascular collapse.
  - Rickettsialpox:
    - Similar to spotted fever group though less severe and with fewer systemic symptoms; rash often includes an inoculation eschar
  - Q fever:
    - Pneumonia is most common; also may cause endocarditis, hepatitis, or osteomyelitis.
    - Rash is not a hallmark of this disease.
    - Also may be a self-limited febrile illness.
  - Typhus group:
    - Epidemic typhus is transmitted by the human body louse and causes fever, headache, and rash that can progress to pulmonary symptoms, neurologic disease, and death.
    - Endemic typhus is transmitted by fleas associated with rodents and causes symptoms similar to epidemic typhus, although with a less prevalent rash.
    - Scrub typhus is also similar but causes marked neurologic symptoms including mental status changes.

- Ehrlichiosis:
  - Spectrum of illnesses including human monocytotropic ehrlichiosis and human granulocytotropic anaplasmosis that cause fever, headache, and myalgias similar to the spotted fever group.
  - Rash is less common in ehrlichiosis and occurs in <50% of patients. Vasculitis is also not present in ehrlichiosis.

PHYSICAL EXAM
- All rickettsial diseases cause fever and the majority cause rash. Differentiating clinical findings of each group are described subsequently in this section, and the rashes associated with each illness are given in a table in Section VI.
- These 3 findings suggest illness caused by the spotted fever group:
  - Hypotension, cardiovascular instability
  - Hepatosplenomegaly
  - Tache noire (French for black spot): The earliest finding in the spotted fever group, this lesion originates at the site of the infecting bite and may form eschar with regional lymphadenopathy related to the eschar. The lesion is usually found on the head in children and on the legs in adults; present in 30–90% of cases
- These 3 findings suggest illness caused by the typhus group:
  - Impaired level of consciousness
  - Pulmonary and renal involvement
  - Brill-Zinsser disease is actually a recrudescence of a previous infection with epidemic (louse-borne) typhus caused by *R. prowazekii*; can occur years after the initial infection and is usually less severe than the initial episode of louse-borne typhus.
- These 4 findings suggest illness caused by *C. burnetii*, the organism responsible for Q fever:
  - Pulmonary symptoms: Mild pneumonitis/cough; radiographically confirmed pneumonia in moderately ill patients; rapidly progressive pneumonia
  - Endocarditis
  - Hepatitis of varying severity
  - Nervous system findings range from headache to meningitis and encephalitis.
- These 5 findings suggest ehrlichiosis:
  - Acute febrile illness characterized by headache and myalgia
  - Rash in ~50%, spares palms, soles, and face
  - Cytopenia, particularly leukopenia

DIAGNOSTIC TESTS & INTERPRETATION
Lab
- Serologic testing is the standard for laboratory diagnosis of rickettsial disease because the organisms are obligate intracellular bacteria and do not grow in culture.
- Serologic tests are available for all rickettsial organisms. There is some cross-reactivity among similar organisms.
- Serologic testing is often negative at the start of illness and requires a convalescent (paired) sample done 2–3 weeks later for comparison. If the convalescent titer is 4-fold or greater than the acute, it is considered positive.
- Polymerase chain reaction (PCR) tests are rarely done in clinical labs and have significant inaccuracy given the similarities in genomes of these organisms.
- The Weil-Felix agglutination test has poor sensitivity and specificity and is not used in the U.S.
- Nonspecific general lab tests may help to make the diagnosis; for example, patients with RMSF often have hyponatremia and thrombocytopenia and may have features of disseminated intravascular coagulation (DIC). Patients with ehrlichiosis often have leukopenia.

DIFFERENTIAL DIAGNOSIS
- Before rash appears, constitutional symptoms associated with the spotted fevers result in a broad differential diagnosis. After rash appears, the diagnoses are more limited.
- Infectious: Measles, meningococcemia, secondary syphilis, Coxsackievirus (e.g., hand-foot-and-mouth disease), infectious mononucleosis, enteroviral infection.
- Environmental (poisons): Drug hypersensitivity reaction (i.e., toxicodermatosis)
- Tumors: Leukemia with thrombocytopenia
- Immunologic: Idiopathic thrombocytopenia purpura
- Miscellaneous: Leukocytoclastic angiitis, erythema multiforme/Stevens-Johnson syndrome

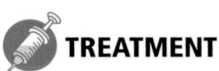 TREATMENT

MEDICATION (DRUGS)
- The 1st-line antibiotic treatment for all rickettsial diseases is doxycycline. Recommended dosage depends on the specific rickettsial infection being treated.
- Therapy is most effective if instituted within the 1st week of illness.
- Antibiotics should be given for 7 days. If the patient is still febrile at that point, antibiotics should be continued until several days after defervescence.

- Studies have shown that there is little risk of tooth staining in children <8 years old who receive <3 courses of doxycycline. In the case of rickettsial disease, the benefit of giving doxycycline far outweighs the risk of side effects.
- Macrolides, trimethoprim–sulfamethoxazole, and the fluoroquinolones have been used with variable success against rickettsial infections but should not be given as 1st-line therapy.

IN-PATIENT CONSIDERATIONS
Initial Stabilization
- Fluid resuscitation, respiratory support as indicated
- Antimicrobial therapy should be instituted as soon as the diagnosis is suspected and should not be delayed while awaiting serologic confirmation.
- Patients may require blood product transfusion in the case of consumptive coagulopathy or severe thrombocytopenia.

 ONGOING CARE

PROGNOSIS
Improvement in the patient's clinical status usually takes place within 1–2 weeks after therapy starts, depending on the severity of illness. This improvement may also be delayed if treatment is begun after the 1st week of illness.

COMPLICATIONS
- Venous thrombosis
- Disseminated intravascular coagulopathy
- Cardiac injury including endocarditis
- Severe disease is more common in patients with G6PD deficiency, cardiac insufficiency, or immunodeficiency.

ADDITIONAL READING

- American Academy of Pediatrics. *2009 Red Book: Report of the Committee on Infectious Diseases*, 28th ed. Elk Grove Village, IL: American Academy of Pediatrics, 2009.
- Brunette GW, Ed. Rickettsial (spotted and typhus fevers) and related infectious (anaplasmosis and ehrlichiosis). *CDC Health Information for International Travel 2010*. Spain: Elsevier, 2009.
- Dumler JS, Dey C, Meier F. Human monocytic ehrlichiosis: A potentially severe disease in children. *Arch Pediatr Adolesc Med*. 2000;154:847–849.
- Mandell GL. Rickettsioses, Ehrlichioses, and Anaplasmosis. In Mandell GL, Bennet JE, Dolin R, eds., *Principles and practice of infectious diseases*, 7th edition. Philadelphia: Churchill Livingstone/Elsevier, 2010.
- Purvis JJ, Edward MS. Doxycycline use for rickettsial disease in pediatric patients. *Pediatr Infect Dis J*. 2000;19:871–874.

 CODES

ICD9
- 083.0 Q fever
- 083.8 Other specified rickettsioses
- 083.9 Rickettsiosis, unspecified

ICD10
- A77.0 Spotted fever due to Rickettsia rickettsii
- A79.89 Other specified rickettsioses
- A79.9 Rickettsiosis, unspecified

FAQ

- Q: Should my child receive antibiotics if he is bitten by a tick in an area endemic to rickettsial disease?
- A: There is no role for prophylaxis against rickettsial diseases for patients who have suffered tick bites.
- Q: Are there differences between typhoid and typhus?
- A: Typhoid, or typhoid fever, is a separate entity from typhus. Typhoid is an enteric infection caused by *Salmonella typhi* and is unrelated to the rickettsial diseases.
- Q: If I contract a rickettsial illness, can I get that illness or a similar illness again?
- A: With the exception of scrub typhus and diseases involving *Ehrlichia*, infection with a rickettsial organism confers immunity to other rickettsia within the same group.

ROCKY MOUNTAIN SPOTTED FEVER

Carolyn A. Paris
Jennifer R. Reid
George A. Woodward

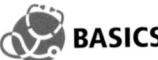 **BASICS**

DESCRIPTION
- Life-threatening systemic illness (i.e., small vessel vasculitis) caused by infection with *Rickettsia rickettsii*, an obligate intracellular gram-negative bacterium, transmitted by *Ixodidae* tick
- Member of spotted fever subgroup of rickettsial diseases
- Seasonal endemic disease, but may occur in other areas and throughout the year
- Classic symptoms of fever, headache, rash following tick exposure are often not present

EPIDEMIOLOGY
- Most common rickettsial disease in the U.S.
- Seasonal: April–September accounts for 90% of cases
- Geographic:
  - Restricted to countries of western hemisphere
  - Cases reported from all states except Alaska, Hawaii, and Maine; occurs most often in southern Atlantic and south central regions. 1994–2003 >50% of cases in North Carolina, South Carolina, Tennessee, Oklahoma, Arkansas
  - Less often seen in Rocky Mountain states
  - Also occurs in Western Canada, Mexico, Central and South America
- Single isolated cases most common in U.S.; reported in clusters infrequently in U.S. (4.4% familial), more typical in certain endemic areas (e.g., Brazil)
- Up to 2/3 of patients <15 years

Incidence
- Annual Incidence: 7 million cases per million people (2002–2007)
- More common and specific pediatric population
- 250–1,200 cases reported per year; likely many unreported cases
- More often reported in American Indians, whites, males and children; incidence highest in 5–9 year olds
- Fatal outcome reported in 20% of untreated, and 5% of treated, cases
- Geographic variations in case fatality occur, likely due to different levels of pathogenicity, host factors and delayed recognition in less endemic regions
- 15% reported deaths in children <10 years

Prevalence
4–22% of children show significant antibody titers in endemic areas, likely representative of subclinical disease

RISK FACTORS
R. rickettsii-infected tick exposure or rural environment or occupation increasing forest exposure in endemic region

GENERAL PREVENTION
- Avoid tick-infested areas; limit skin exposure with long, light-colored clothing, tucked-in socks or boots, inspect frequently
- Use tick repellants or impregnated clothing.
- Remove ticks promptly
  - Do not crush; may increase transmission
  - Avoid direct contact; remove with tweezers or gloved fingers close to skin
  - Apply steady upward traction until tick's grip is released
  - Clean wound
  - Matches, petroleum jelly, nail polish, and rubbing alcohol are not effective for removal
- Vaccine not available in U.S.; may not prevent disease but does prevent deaths

PATHOPHYSIOLOGY
- Transmission usually occurs from tick bite (reservoir):
  - Usually >4 hours of attachment needed to transmit disease (often 24 hours)
  - Can be by transfusion or aerosol route
- Incubation period 2–14 days, average 7 days
- *R. rickettsia* spreads through the lymphatic system, causing a small-vessel vasculitis that affects all organs, especially skin and adrenals. Increased vascular permeability and focal areas of endothelial proliferation cause hyponatremia, hypoalbuminemia, edema, and hypotension
- Immunity is conferred following disease

ETIOLOGY
Wood tick (*Dermacentor andersoni*) in Rocky Mountain states and southwest Canada; dog tick (*Dermacentor variabilis*) in east central region and areas of Pacific coast; Lone Star tick (*Amblyomma americanum*) in Southwest; *Rhipicephalus sanguineus* in Southwest and Mexico; *Amblyomma cajennense* in Central and South America

COMMONLY ASSOCIATED CONDITIONS
- Patients with glucose-6-phosphate dehydrogenase (G6PD) deficiency account for a disproportionate number of deaths
- Serious biological weapon threat due to virulence causing severe disease, difficulty establishing diagnosis, low levels of immunity, agent available in nature, high infectivity, and feasibility of propagation, stabilization, and dispersal; thus development of a cross-protective vaccine against all *Rickettsia* is desirable for biodefense, as well as for travel medicine

DIAGNOSIS

HISTORY
- History: Classic triad of fever, headache, and rash seen in ~50% of cases
- Abdominal pain common mainly in children
- Symptoms usually appear 2–8 days after tick bite
- Gradual fever onset to >40°C (104°F), often unresponsive to antipyretics or antibiotics

- Headache: Intense, retrobulbar or frontal, persistent and difficult to treat; young children may not describe
- Cough, dyspnea
- Nausea, vomiting, abdominal pain, diarrhea
- Tick bite is reported by only 50–60% of cases

PHYSICAL EXAM
- Fever and rash present in 85% of patients
- Skin:
  - Rash: Usually appears by illness day 2–3, may be >6th day; 10–15% never develop rash so absence should not delay therapy
  - Usually small, irregular, erythematous blanching macules, become maculopapular then petechial and confluently hemorrhagic
  - Usually on wrists and ankles first, spreads within hours to trunk, neck, and face; may involve palms, soles, and scrotum:
    - May appear first on trunk or diffusely; can progress to necrosis of ears, nose, scrotum, fingers, or toes
    - Difficult to detect in people with dark skin
- CNS: Meningismus, restlessness, irritability, apprehension, confusion, delirium, lethargy, stupor, coma, ataxia, opisthotonos, aphasia, papilledema, seizures, cortical blindness, central deafness, spastic paralysis, cranial nerve palsy
- Cardiac: CHF, myocarditis, arrhythmias, hypovolemic vascular collapse
- Pulmonary: Pneumonitis, dyspnea, pulmonary edema, hypoxemia, pleural effusions, alveolar infiltrates
- GI: Diarrhea, hepatomegaly, splenomegaly, anorexia, jaundice, mild pancreatitis
- Ocular: Conjunctivitis, venous engorgement, papilledema, cotton wool spots, retinal hemorrhages, retinal artery occlusion, uveitis
- Other: Edema, myalgias (especially calf or thigh), parotitis, orchitis, pharyngitis

DIAGNOSTIC TESTS & INTERPRETATION
Presumptive diagnosis based on signs, symptoms, exposure history, and epidemiologic considerations rather than laboratory aids

Lab
- Nonspecific:
  - CBC: Anemia (30%), thrombocytopenia (from consumptive coagulopathy); normal or low leukocytes days 4–5, subsequent leukocytosis associated with secondary bacterial disease; bandemia common
  - Electrolytes: Hyponatremia
  - Elevated BUN, creatinine, liver function tests, bilirubin, creatine kinase
  - Screen for disseminated intravascular coagulation (DIC), prolonged prothrombin time, decreased fibrinogen (consumption),
  - Arterial blood gases: Acidosis
  - Hypoalbuminemia
  - CSF: Usually clear (leukocyte count <10), may see pleocytosis in 1/3 and increased protein in 1/2 of patients

- Specific serologic tests:
  – Indirect immunofluorescence assay (IFA):
    o Best and most widely available method
    o 2 serum samples obtained weeks apart showing 4-fold increase in IgG and IgM anti-R. rickettsii antibody titers
    o Positive 6–10 days after onset of disease, sensitivity increases to 94% with convalescence serum sample from days 14 to 21 days; specificity 100%
  – PCR, immunohistochemical staining, and culture are best done on biopsy specimen (of rash site or at autopsy) due to low circulating organism levels
  – Routine hospital blood cultures will not detect; available only at specialty labs
  – Weil–Felix test: Oldest specific test, but nonspecific and insensitive so no longer recommended
  – No early specific laboratory tests; serologic data reliable by days 10–12 of illness; negative results do not exclude diagnosis
  – All test results normalize with early intervention

Imaging
Chest radiograph, ECG, and electrocardiogram recommended

DIFFERENTIAL DIAGNOSIS
Measles, meningococcemia, ehrlichiosis, typhoid fever, leptospirosis, rubella, scarlet fever, disseminated gonococcal disease, infectious mononucleosis, secondary syphilis, rheumatic fever, enteroviral infection, immune thrombocytic purpura, thrombotic thrombocytopenic purpura, immune complex vasculitis, drug hypersensitivity reaction, murine typhus, rickettsialpox, and recrudescent typhus

ALERT
Do not exclude diagnosis even if there is no history or evidence of tick bite and/or results of serologic tests are negative.

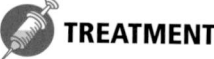 TREATMENT

MEDICATION (DRUGS)
Treatment should be initiated based on clinical and epidemiological information as laboratory confirmation may not be available during acute illness. All agents are rickettsiostatic (hinder replication), not rickettsicidal, so host can eradicate disease. Treat until there is evidence of clinical improvement and at least 3 days without fever, standard duration is 5–10 days of therapy

First Line
- Doxycycline (usual tetracycline antibiotic):
  – Adults: 100 mg q12h PO/IV
  – Children under 45 kg (100 lbs): 4 mg/kg/d divided b.i.d.
  – Also treats ehrlichiosis (similar presentation)
  – Side effects: Less likely to stain teeth than tetracycline; contraindicated for pregnancy

- Chloramphenicol (advised with pregnancy):
  – Adult: 50–100 mg/kg/d divided q6h (max 4 g/d)
  – Child >1 month: 50–100 mg/kg/d IV divided q6h
  – Side effects: Peripheral neuropathy, aplastic anemia, "gray baby syndrome" with high dosage, possible association with leukemia, hemolytic anemia with G6PD
  – Not as effective as tetracyclines, or against ehrlichiosis

Second Line
- Quinolones (ciprofloxacin, pefloxacin), macrolide (clarithromycin) with in vitro effect, no clinical evidence of efficacy
- Corticosteroids:
  – May be helpful in severe cases, although no controlled studies published
  – Not advised for mild or moderately ill patients

ADDITIONAL TREATMENT
General Measures
- Treat empirically if clinical suspicion
- Platelets as indicated for thrombocytopenia
- Vitamin K (IM) for prolonged clotting time
- Manage hyponatremia with fluid restriction; avoid sodium supplements
- Albumin if indicated
- Report to state health department

IN-PATIENT CONSIDERATIONS
Initial Stabilization
Volume, electrolyte support as indicated

 ONGOING CARE

FOLLOW-UP RECOMMENDATIONS
Expect improvement in 24–36 hours and defervescence in 2–3 days with treatment, especially if initiated <5 days after onset of symptoms

PROGNOSIS
- Related to early recognition of disease and initiation of appropriate therapy
- Case fatality 2–4% if treated <6 days from onset of symptoms
- Case fatality 15–22.9% if treated >6 days from onset of symptoms:
  – Higher mortality if <4 years, G6PD deficiency, CNS involvement, renal failure, jaundice, cardiovascular collapse, hepatomegaly, thrombocytopenia, DIC, GI symptoms, inappropriate antibiotics, late rash, absence of headache, or male gender
  – Death usually between 8th–15th days (fulminant cases with death in 5–6 days)

COMPLICATIONS
- Uncommon with early appropriate treatment
- Neurologic sequelae:
  – Behavioral disturbances, learning disabilities (more common), emotional lability, hyperactivity, memory loss, seizures
- Dermatologic sequelae:
  – Gangrene of extremities, end organs, skin necrosis
  – Skin rash usually heals without sequelae
- Hematologic sequelae: DIC

- GI sequelae:
  – Hepatic dysfunction
  – Hypoalbuminemia from hepatic dysfunction, protein loss from damaged vessels
- Cardiac sequelae: Can have persistent cardiac findings, CHF, cardiovascular collapse
- Metabolic sequelae: Hyponatremia from water shift to intracellular spaces, sodium loss in urine
- Renal sequelae: Acute tubular necrosis

ADDITIONAL READING
- Buckingham SC, Marshal GS, Schutze GE et al. Clinical and laboratory features, hospital course, and outcomes of Rocky Mountain spotted fever in children. *J Pediatr.* 2007;150:180–184.
- Centers for Disease Control and Prevention. Rocky Mountain spotted fever. Available at: Http://www.cdc.gov/ncidod/dvrd/rmsf/index.htm
- Chen LF, Sexton DJ. What's new in Rocky Mountain spotted fever? *Infect Dis Clin N Amer.* 2008;22:415–432.
- Dantas-Torres F. Rocky Mountain spotted fever. *Lancet Infect Dis.* 2007;7:724–732.
- Openshaw JJ, Swerdlow DL, Krebs JW, et al. Rocky Mountain spotted fever in the United States, 2000–2007: Interpreting contemporary increases in incidence. *Am J Trop Med Hyg.* 2010;83(1):174–182.
- Walker DH. The realities of biodefense vaccines against Rickettsia. *Vaccine.* 2009;27:D52–D55.

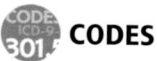 CODES

ICD9
082.0 Spotted fevers

ICD10
A77.0 Spotted fever due to Rickettsia rickettsii

FAQ
- Q: In which patients should Rocky Mountain spotted fever be considered in the differential diagnosis?
- A: Anyone with a fever during the spring and summer who has been in an endemic area, regardless of presence of rash or history of tick bite. Nonspecific symptoms (e.g., GI, respiratory, rashes) may lead to misdiagnosis and thus delay therapy.
- Q: Should a child with a tick bite receive antibiotic prophylaxis when a tick is discovered?
- A: There is no evidence that prophylaxis is necessary or efficacious in preventing disease. To contract disease, one must be bitten by a tick that carries the disease (low risk), the tick must transmit the Rickettsia (low risk, usually requires >6 hours of attachment), and the *Rickettsia* must be pathogenic if inoculated (low risk).

R

ROSEOLA

Ross Newman
Jason Newland
Louis M. Bell (5th edition)

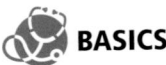 **BASICS**

DESCRIPTION
Roseola infantum is a common illness in preschool-aged children characterized by fever lasting 3–7 days followed by rapid defervescence and the appearance of a blanching maculopapular rash (usually on the 4th day of illness) lasting only 1–2 days.
- Incubation period is 5–15 days.
- No gender predilection

EPIDEMIOLOGY
- Roseola affects children from 3 months to 4 years. The peak age is 7–13 months.
- 90% of cases occur in the 1st 2 years of life.
- Roseola can occur throughout the year; outbreaks have occurred in all seasons of the year.

GENERAL PREVENTION
- The virus associated with roseola infantum is usually transmitted via respiratory secretions or the fecal–oral spread.
- Outbreaks in hospitals have been reported, and standard infection control precautions are recommended.

PATHOPHYSIOLOGY
- Unknown
- The typical pattern of rash that appears as the fever disappears may represent virus neutralization in the skin.

ETIOLOGY
- Roseola-like illnesses have been associated with a number of different viruses including enterovirus (coxsackievirus A and B, echoviruses), adenoviruses (types 1, 2, 3), parainfluenza virus, and measles vaccine virus.
- A major cause of roseola is human herpesvirus 6 and 7 (HHV-6 and HHV-7).
- HHV-6 was 1st associated with roseola infantum in 1988.
- HHV-6 and HHV-7 account for 20–40% of unexplained febrile illness in emergency department visits by febrile infants 6 months to 2 years of age.
- Almost all children will acquire a primary infection and be seropositive for HHV6 by the age of 4 years.
- ~30% of children infected with HHV6 will present with the classic manifestations of roseola.

DIAGNOSIS

HISTORY
- Affected children do not look sick.
- Rash
- Fever, typically >39.5°C
- Mild cough
- Acute rhinitis
- Lymphadenopathy
- Eyelid edema
- Bulging fontanelle can occur occasionally

DIAGNOSTIC TESTS & INTERPRETATION
Lab
- Not helpful in diagnosis. PCR tests are available for detecting HHV-6 and HHV-7.
- CBC: Occasionally, leukopenia with lymphocytosis is noted. Thrombocytopenia is likely secondary to viral bone marrow suppression.

DIFFERENTIAL DIAGNOSIS
- Roseola has a distinctive presentation, but does resemble other viral exanthems.
- Antibiotic-associated rash in a child taking oral antibiotics when rash develops after defervescence
- Rubella and enteroviral infections
- Viral exanthems in preschool-aged children are sometimes called roseola even when fever is concomitant with rash.

ONGOING CARE

PROGNOSIS

Most children with roseola infantum recover without sequelae.

COMPLICATIONS

- Seizures are the most common complication of roseola; between 10–15% of children have a generalized tonic–clonic seizure associated with fever.
- Aseptic meningitis with <200 cells, primarily mononuclear cells, have been reported.
- Encephalitis
- Thrombocytopenic purpura

ADDITIONAL READING

- Jackson MA, Sommeraver JF. Human herpes virus 6 and 7. *Pediatr Infect Dis J*. 2002;21:565–566.
- Leach CT. Human herpes virus 6 and 7 infections in children: Agents of roseola and other syndromes. *Curr Opin Pediatr*. 2000;12(3):269–274.

- Leach CT, Sumaya CV, Brown NA. Human herpes virus-6: Clinical implication of a recently discovered, ubiquitous agent. *J Pediatr*. 1991;121:173–181.
- Stoeckle MY. The spectrum of human herpes virus 6 infection: From roseola infantum to adult disease. *Annu Rev Med*. 2000;51:423–430.
- Vianna RA, de Oliveira SA, Camacho LA, et al. Role of human herpes virus 6 infection in young Brazilian children with rash illnesses. *Pediatr Infect Dis J*. 2008;6(27):533–537.

CODES

ICD9

- 058.10 Roseola infantum, unspecified
- 058.11 Roseola infantum due to human herpesvirus 6
- 058.12 Roseola infantum due to human herpesvirus 7

ICD10

- B08.20 Exanthema subitum [sixth disease], unspecified
- B08.21 Exanthema subitum [sixth disease] due to human herpesvirus 6
- B08.22 Exanthema subitum [sixth disease] due to human herpesvirus 7

FAQ

- Q: When can a child with roseola return to daycare?
- A: As soon as fever subsides; there is no infectious risk of spread afterward. The child may return to daycare even with the rash visible.
- Q: Will there be long-term sequelae in the child who has a seizure associated with roseola?
- A: In general, these seizures are typical febrile seizures that hold only a slightly higher risk than the general population for long-term neurologic sequelae (e.g., epilepsy).

R

ROTAVIRUS

Sheila M. Nolan
Suzanne Dawid (5th edition)

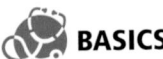

BASICS

DESCRIPTION
Infection with rotavirus causes high fever, profuse nonbloody diarrhea, and vomiting lasting 3–8 days. It is the most common cause of severe gastroenteritis in children in both the developed and developing worlds. All children have serologic evidence of infection by 5 years of age.

EPIDEMIOLOGY
- Rotavirus is the most common cause of severe gastroenteritis throughout the world.
- Rotavirus has a predictable seasonality depending on location:
  – In North America, peaks occur in the early winter in the west, moving northward and eastward.
  – In the northeastern U.S. and Canada, the highest incidence of disease occurs in late winter and early spring.
  – In tropical regions, disease occurs throughout the year.
- Majority of severe disease occurs in children 6–24 months old.
- All children have serologic evidence of disease by the age of 5 years.
- Incubation period is 12 hours to 4 days.
- Exposure to as few as 200 viral particles can result in disease. The virus can persist on surfaces for prolonged periods of time.
- Virus can be shed asymptomatically, but shedding may precede disease by 2 days and typically persists for 10 days.

Incidence
- Infection accounts for 20–50% of pediatric hospitalizations for gastroenteritis.
- Causes >500,000 deaths per year in developing countries
- In the U.S., in the pre-vaccine era, rotavirus infection caused at least 50,000 hospitalizations per year and 20–40 deaths per year.

GENERAL PREVENTION
- Reduction of person-to-person transmission by proper hygiene, especially in child care settings.
- 2 vaccines are currently available in the U.S.:
- A live, oral human/bovine reassortant pentavalent vaccine (RotaTeq) was licensed for use in infants in 2006. Vaccination is indicated at 2, 4, and 6 months of age
- A live, attenuated human rotavirus vaccine (Rotarix) was licensed in the U.S. in 2008:
  – Numerous studies have demonstrated significant reductions in rotavirus gastroenteritis (both inpatient and outpatient) in areas where these vaccines have been introduced.
  – A recent study from Mexico demonstrated a 35% reduction in diarrhea-related deaths in children <5 years of age for the 2008 and 2009 rotavirus seasons after the introduction of rotavirus vaccine in 2006.
  – Small studies on hospitalized patients have suggested that the prophylactic use of probiotics may decrease the incidence of nosocomially acquired rotavirus infection.

PATHOPHYSIOLOGY
The cause of diarrhea is unknown but is believed to be a result of multiple disruptions in the normal mechanisms of water reabsorption in the gut:
- Peptides encoded in the viral genome disrupt the transport of glucose and salt, resulting in increased water within the gut.
- Decreased levels of intestinal disaccharidases, including lactase, result in malabsorption of sugars.
- Viral replication within enterocytes results in atrophy and ischemia of small intestinal villi.
- Infection with rotavirus results in activation of the enteric nervous system, resulting in abnormal stimulation of water secretion into the GI tract.

DIAGNOSIS

HISTORY
- Presents with high fever and vomiting, with as many as 20 watery stools a day
- Diarrhea may test heme positive, but is not grossly bloody.
- Up to 10% of children present with vomiting and/or fever without diarrhea.
- 50% of parents of infected infants are also infected; however, only 1/3 of these are symptomatic.

PHYSICAL EXAM
Consistent with dehydration

DIAGNOSTIC TESTS & INTERPRETATION
Lab
- Rotavirus ELISA for the presence of viral protein in the stool is highly sensitive and specific.
- PCR is also used in some clinical laboratories.
- Stool tends to be negative for leukocytes; however, this testing is rarely useful.
- Testing for malabsorption via stool assays for reducing substances or by D-xylose absorption assays is often positive.
- 67% of hospitalized children have mild elevations in their transaminases.

DIFFERENTIAL DIAGNOSIS
- Viral infections:
  – Adenovirus
  – Astrovirus
  – Caliciviruses (Norovirus and Sapovirus)
- Bacterial infections:
  – *Salmonella*
  – *Shigella*
  – *Campylobacter*
  – *Escherichia coli*
  – *Yersinia*
  – *Vibrio*
  – *Plesiomonas*
  – *Aeromonas*
  – *Clostridium difficile*
- Parasitic infections:
  – *Giardia*
  – *Cyclospora*
  – *Isospora*
  – *Cryptosporidium*

 ## TREATMENT

IN-PATIENT CONSIDERATIONS
Initial Stabilization
- Supportive care with either oral or IV rehydration, depending on disease severity
- Limited studies have suggested that the addition of lactobacillus early in infection may decrease the duration of symptoms.

 ## ONGOING CARE

COMPLICATIONS
- Disease is typically self-resolving; however, 20% of 1st-time infections are moderate to severe and require medical attention. Severe dehydration may occur, resulting in acidosis and electrolyte disruptions.
- Diarrhea may be more severe and protracted in immunocompromised hosts.

ADDITIONAL READING

- Bernstein DI. Rotavirus overview. *Pediatr Infect Dis J*. 2009;28(3 Suppl):S50–S53.
- Cortese MM, Parashar UD. Prevention of rotavirus gastroenteritis among infants and children: Recommendations of the Advisory Committee on Immunization Practices (ACIP). Centers for Disease Control and Prevention (CDC). *MMWR Recomm Rep*. 2009;58(RR-2):1–25.5.
- Cortese MM, Tate JE, Simonsen L, et al. Reduction in gastroenteritis in United States children and correlation with early rotavirus vaccine uptake from national medical claims databases. *Pediatr Infect Dis J*. 2010;29:489–494.
- Richardson V, Hernandez-Pichardo J, Quintanar-Solares M, et al. Effect of rotavirus vaccine on death from childhood diarrhea in Mexico. *N Engl J Med*. 2010;362:299–305.
- Rosenfeldt V, Michaelsen KF, Jakobsen M, et al. Effect of probiotic Lactobacillus strains in young children hospitalized with acute diarrhea. *Pediatr Infect Dis J*. 2002;21:411–416.

- Szajewska H, Kotowska M, Mrukowicz JZ, et al. Efficacy of Lactobacillus GG in prevention of nosocomial diarrhea in infants. *J Pediatr*. 2001;138:361–365.
- Wang FT, Mast TC, Glass RJ, et al. Effectiveness of the pentavalent rotavirus vaccine in preventing gastroenteritis in the United States. *Pediatrics*. 2010;125:e208–e213.

 ## CODES

ICD9
- 008.61 Enteritis due to rotavirus
- 008.69 Enteritis due to other viral enteritis
- 079.0 Adenovirus infection in conditions classified elsewhere and of unspecified site

ICD10
- A08.0 Rotaviral enteritis
- A08.2 Adenoviral enteritis
- A08.32 Astrovirus enteritis

FAQ

- Q: When should children with rotavirus infection resume feeding?
- A: Feeding early in the course of disease promotes intestinal healing and should be instituted within 24 hours of illness. Infants should be given breast milk or diluted or regular-strength formula. Children should be given lactose-free carbohydrate-rich foods. Juices and sodas should be avoided because of their high sugar content.
- Q: Are antiemetics or antidiarrheal agents useful in the treatment of children with rotavirus infection?
- A: No. There have been no studies demonstrating efficacy of these medications in children.
- Q: Is natural infection protective against subsequent infections?
- A: Somewhat. The 1st episode of rotavirus infection tends to be the most severe; however, reinfection may occur, although it is often asymptomatic.

R

SALICYLATE POISONING (ASPIRIN)

Kevin C. Osterhoudt

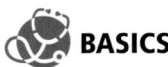 **BASICS**

DESCRIPTION
- May occur with acute or chronic overdosage of:
  - Acetylsalicylic acid (aspirin)
  - Methyl salicylate (oil of wintergreen)
  - Bismuth subsalicylate (Pepto Bismol)
  - Salicylic acid (a keratolytic)
- The potentially toxic acute oral dose of acetylsalicylic acid is >150 mg/kg.

EPIDEMIOLOGY
- Analgesics are the most common drugs implicated in human exposures reported to US poison control centers.
- Salicylate preparations constitute ~9% of all analgesic poisoning exposures reported to poison control centers.

PATHOPHYSIOLOGY
- Ingested drug is absorbed in stomach and proximal intestine.
- With therapeutic aspirin dosing, serum levels peak in 1–2 hours (standard preparations) or 4–6 hours (enteric coated).
- After oral overdose, absorption may be prolonged and erratic.
- Acetylsalicylate ingestion may produce gastritis and may trigger centrally mediated vomiting.
- After overdose, the elimination half-life of salicylate becomes prolonged.
- As blood pH falls, the proportion of nonionized salicylate rises, and more salicylate shifts into tissues, including brain.
- Toxic salicylate exposures uncouple mitochondrial oxidative phosphorylation and increase oxygen consumption.
- Direct stimulation of the medullary respiratory center leads to hyperventilation and respiratory alkalosis.
- Multiple metabolic derangements produce a wide anion gap metabolic acidosis.
- Dehydration and electrolyte shifts are common.
- Low cerebral glucose concentrations may exist despite normal serum glucose concentrations.
- Pulmonary and/or cerebral edema may occur.

COMMONLY ASSOCIATED CONDITIONS
- Aspirin is often marketed in combination with other pharmaceuticals, which may complicate drug overdose situations.
- Adolescents frequently overdose on more than 1 drug preparation.
- Therapeutic use of acetylsalicylic acid among children with influenza has been associated with the occurrence of Reye syndrome.

DIAGNOSIS

HISTORY
- Aspirin poisoning mimics many illnesses, and chronic overdosage often results in delayed diagnosis.
- Enteric coating may lead to significantly delayed drug absorption.
- Timing of ingestion allows for proper consideration of the risks versus benefits of gastrointestinal decontamination.
- Tinnitus frequently associated with serum salicylate levels >25 mg/dL

PHYSICAL EXAM
- Hyperpnea indicates primary central hyperventilation and/or compensation for metabolic acidosis.
- Hyperpyrexia: Presence of "fever" may confuse salicylism with infection.
- Hypoxia: Pulmonary edema complicates therapy of aspirin overdose.
- Hypotension indicates severe dehydration, likely complicated by metabolic acidosis and salicylate-mediated myocardial inefficiency.
- Encephalopathy: CNS depression or seizures represent grave toxicity.

DIAGNOSTIC TESTS & INTERPRETATION
Lab
- Serum electrolytes: A wide anion gap metabolic acidosis is common, and hypoglycemia or hyperglycemia may occur.
- Arterial blood gas: May show mixed respiratory alkalosis/metabolic acidosis
- Salicylate level: Serum salicylate levels >60–100 mg/dL (acute) or 30–40 mg/dL (chronic) portend serious toxicity.
- Urine pH: Allows monitoring of adequacy of urinary alkalinization
- Acetaminophen level: Acetaminophen may be a coingestant.
- Ferric chloride test: A few drops of 10% ferric chloride will turn brown or purple in 1 mL of urine that contains salicylate.

ALERT
- Respiratory acidosis suggests central nervous system depression and is an ominous sign.
- Salicylate levels after chronic or acute-on-chronic overdose correlate poorly to clinical condition.
- Serial salicylate levels may be necessary to rule out ongoing drug absorption.

DIFFERENTIAL DIAGNOSIS
- Gastroenteritis
- Pneumonia
- Metabolic disease
- Ketoacidosis
- Sepsis
- Meningitis/encephalitis

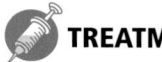 **TREATMENT**

ADDITIONAL TREATMENT
General Measures
- Fluids/alkalinization:
  - Intravascular volume should be repleted with intermittent boluses of 10–20 mL/kg of isotonic crystalloid.
  - Altered mentation may imply CNS hypoglycemia and should be treated with dextrose.
  - Acidemia should be treated with sodium bicarbonate to limit salicylate distribution to the brain. Serum pH of 7.5 is reasonable goal.
  - With significant poisoning, an IV infusion of 5% dextrose with 100–150 mEq/L of sodium bicarbonate and 20–40 mEq/L of potassium chloride should be initiated at 1.5–2 times maintenance requirements. Titrate fluid volume to produce urine output of 2–3 mL/kg/h. Titrate alkalinization to produce urine pH between 7.5 and 8, which greatly increases the urinary elimination of salicylate via "ion-trapping" effect.
- Hemodialysis indications:
  - Acute serum salicylate level >100 mg/dL
  - Chronic serum salicylate level >60 mg/dL
  - Severe acidosis or severe electrolyte disturbance
  - Renal failure
  - Persistent neurologic dysfunction
  - Progressive clinical deterioration

ALERT
- Hypokalemia may interfere with the ability to achieve urinary alkalinization.
- Sedating a salicylate-poisoned patient may lead to respiratory depression and clinical deterioration.
- Endotracheal intubation is dangerous and, if performed, must be accompanied by sodium bicarbonate intravenous bolus and hyperventilation to prevent worsening acidemia and salicylate distribution to the brain.
- Hemodialysis equipment must be carefully primed to prevent worsening hypovolemia and cardiovascular collapse.
- If hemodialysis is performed, adjust dialysate to maintain alkalemia.
- Pulmonary edema and/or cerebral edema may complicate fluid management.

IN-PATIENT CONSIDERATIONS
Initial Stabilization
GI decontamination:
- Activated charcoal 1 g/kg (maximum 75 g) may be administered if aspirin is judged to be present in the stomach or proximal intestine.
- Many authorities suggest a 2nd charcoal dose 2–4 hours after the 1st, or if salicylate levels continue to rise.
- Whole-bowel irrigation may reduce drug absorption after large overdoses.

 ONGOING CARE

FOLLOW-UP RECOMMENDATIONS
- Drug administration education should be offered to victims of chronic overdose.
- Mental health services should be provided to victims of intentional overdose.

PROGNOSIS
- Chronic therapeutic misuse often leads to delayed diagnosis and has the most serious prognosis.
- Single acute ingestion of >300 mg/kg acetylsalicylic acid should be considered life threatening.

COMPLICATIONS
- Nausea and vomiting
- Dehydration
- Metabolic acidosis
- Electrolyte abnormalities
- Disorientation, coma, seizures
- Noncardiogenic pulmonary edema
- Renal failure
- Cerebral edema and death

ADDITIONAL READING
- Chyka PA, Erdman AR, Christainson G, et al. Salicylate poisoning: An evidence-based consensus guideline for out-of-hospital management. *Clin Toxicol*. 2007;45:95–131.

- Curry S. Salicylates. In: Brent J, Wallace KL, Burkhart KK, et al., eds. *Critical care toxicology: Diagnosis and management of the critically poisoned patient*. Philadelphia: Elsevier Mosby; 2005:621–630.
- O'Malley GF. Emergency department management of the salicylate-poisoned patient. *Emerg Med Clin North Am*. 2007;25:333–346.
- Stolbach AI, Hoffman RS, Nelson LS. Mechanical ventilation was associated with acidemia in a case series of salicylate-poisoned patients. *Acad Emerg Med*. 2008;15:866–869.

 CODES

ICD9
965.1 Poisoning by salicylates

ICD10
- T39.014A Poisoning by aspirin, undetermined, initial encounter
- T39.014D Poisoning by aspirin, undetermined, subsequent encounter
- T39.014S Poisoning by aspirin, undetermined, sequela

FAQ
- Q: What amount of the candy-scented oil of wintergreen is toxic to a toddler?
- A: Oil of wintergreen may contain as much as 98% methyl salicylate. 1 mL of methyl salicylate is the equivalent of 1,400 mg of aspirin. Therefore, 1 teaspoon of oil of wintergreen represents a very serious "aspirin" overdose.
- Q: Is there a prognostic nomogram for aspirin poisoning similar to that used for acetaminophen overdose?
- A: The Done nomogram is applicable only to ingestion of non–enteric-coated aspirin by children with normal mentation and normal blood pH, and the validity of its prognostication is suspect. Its use is not widely recommended.

S

SALMONELLA INFECTIONS

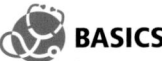

Edmund A. Milder
Suzanne Dawid (5th edition)

BASICS

DESCRIPTION
Salmonella has a wide range of clinical manifestations from asymptomatic infection to a life-threatening febrile illness.

EPIDEMIOLOGY
- Reservoirs:
  - *Salmonella* species other than *S. typhi*: Animals and animal products (mammals, birds, reptiles, and insects); contaminated food and water; infected humans (fecal shedding may persist for several months)
  - Humans are the only natural reservoir for *S. typhi*: Most commonly transmitted via fecally contaminated food and water; may be transmitted congenitally; chronic carriers may shed *S. typhi* in stool for years.
- Incubation period:
  - *Salmonella* gastroenteritis; symptoms typically begin within 24 hours (12–48 hours).
  - Incubation period of *S. typhi* is 1–3 weeks.
- Age distribution: Children <5 years are most commonly infected with nontyphoidal *Salmonella*; *S. typhi* is most common in 5–25-year-olds.

GENERAL PREVENTION
Personal hygiene (especially hand hygiene) and sanitation measures are the primary means by which to prevent *Salmonella* infections.

- Carriers of *Salmonella* pose a public health risk:
  - Hospitalized patients: Contact precautions for length of illness
  - Outpatients: Should be restricted from preparing food for others, and diapered patients should not attend daycare settings until cleared by public health.
- 3 vaccines against *S. typhi* are licensed for use in persons living in high-risk environments, including those residing with a chronic carrier or living in an endemic area:
  - The Ty21a vaccine is a live attenuated strain that is given orally in 4 doses on alternating days. It is approved only for children >6 years.
  - Typhoid vaccine is a parenteral heat-phenol-inactivated vaccine.
  - The Vi capsular polysaccharide vaccine is a parenteral vaccine that is licensed for children >2 years.
- All vaccines require booster dosing.

ETIOLOGY
3 species are responsible for most human salmonellosis: *S. enteritidis* (>2,000 serotypes exist), *S. choleraesuis*, and *S. typhi*.

COMMONLY ASSOCIATED CONDITIONS
- Acute asymptomatic infection:
  - No clinical signs or symptoms become apparent.
  - Probably most common *Salmonella* syndrome
  - Patients can be identified only by recovery of organisms in stool.

- Acute gastroenteritis:
  - Salmonellosis is the most common type of infectious food poisoning in the US.
  - Symptoms begin 12–48 hours after *Salmonella* ingestion.
  - Predominant manifestations are nausea, vomiting, cramps (often severe), abdominal pain, and diarrhea (rarely, gross blood may be found).
  - Other common features are malaise, myalgia, headache, and fever.
  - Symptoms usually resolve spontaneously in 2–7 days.
- Bacteremia:
  - *Salmonella* organisms may produce acute or intermittent bacteremia.
  - Symptoms: Fever/chills, diaphoresis, myalgia, anorexia
  - Bacteremia may occur before clinical gastroenteritis, and, in infants, may present as a persistent bacteremic state with failure to thrive.
  - Up to 1/20 patients with *Salmonella* gastroenteritis may develop bacteremia (perhaps as high as 1/4 in infants).
  - ~10% of patients with bacteremia will develop focal infections (e.g., osteomyelitis, meningitis).
- Enteric fever (typhoid fever, paratyphoid fever):
  - Caused by *S. typhi* and several other *Salmonella* serotypes
  - Incubation period is 1–3 weeks.
  - Insidious onset of symptoms over 2–7 days: Fever as high as 41°C, malaise, anorexia, abdominal pain, constipation, or diarrhea
  - Additional symptoms and signs: Lethargy, myalgia, headache, cough, rigors, delirium, lymphadenopathy, organomegaly, rose spots
  - Progression of illness: When untreated, illness with high fevers may last weeks; severe morbidity or death may result from especially virulent *Salmonella* strains.
- Asymptomatic chronic carriage: ~1% of patients infected with *Salmonella* gastroenteritis or enteric fever will continue to shed *Salmonella* in the stool for >1 year.

DIAGNOSIS

HISTORY
- Exposure:
  - History of eating raw or undercooked meat or eggs
  - Exposure to pet lizard, turtle, or snake. Less common outbreaks have been tied to exposure to infected pet rodents (hamsters, mice, and rats).
- Common historical features of *Salmonella* gastroenteritis:
  - Nausea and vomiting begin 12–48 hours after ingestion.
  - Diarrhea and abdominal pain with tenesmus follow; pain is typically periumbilical and in the right lower quadrant.
  - Diarrhea lasts 2–7 days.
  - Fever seldom exceeds 39°C; occurs in 50% of affected patients.

- Common historical features of enteric fever:
  - Symptoms begin 3–60 days after exposure.
  - Commonly acquired during foreign travel
  - Diarrhea uncommon early in course
  - Fever ensues, which gradually increases in magnitude.
  - Malaise, anorexia, myalgia, headache, abdominal pain, and vomiting may occur.

PHYSICAL EXAM
- *Salmonella* GI disease may display certain features:
  - Dehydration may be evident.
  - Abdominal pain may closely mimic appendicitis and/or cholecystitis.
  - Stools may be bloody, watery, or contain mucus.
- Important signs of enteric fever:
  - Enlarged liver and spleen
  - Relative bradycardia for height of fever
  - Rose spots: 2–4 mm in diameter; blanching pink papules; most commonly found on anterior thorax; 5–20 are generally apparent at a time; fade 3–4 days after appearance; characteristic of enteric fever, but not specific

DIAGNOSTIC TESTS & INTERPRETATION
Lab
- There are several nonspecific laboratory aids to diagnosis:
  - Stool examination: May have hemoccult-positive stools; stool may be positive for fecal leukocytes in enterocolitis.
  - CBC with differential: Normal in simple gastroenteritis; neutropenia, thrombocytopenia, and mild anemia are common in enteric fever.
  - Serum chemistries: Metabolic acidosis and electrolyte abnormalities may occur with severe enteritis; a mild hepatitis is frequently found in enteric fever.
  - Stool and blood culture and identification of *Salmonella* organisms: The gold standard method for laboratory confirmation of infection
  - Bone marrow aspirate culture is positive in ~90% of patients with enteric fever, blood culture in 60%, and stool culture is often negative.
  - Urine culture: May be a source of *Salmonella* organisms in the young or elderly population and in those with enteric fever
  - Biopsy: Needle aspiration of purulent material may yield positive cultures; punch biopsy and culture of rose spots may confirm diagnosis of *S. typhi*.
  - False positives: Leukocytes in the stool are suggestive of colitis, but are more typical of *Campylobacter*, *Shigella*, or milk allergy.
- Pitfall: Enteric fever may precede enteritis symptoms and fecal shedding of bacteria.

DIFFERENTIAL DIAGNOSIS
- The following illnesses may mimic *Salmonella* gastroenteritis and/or enterocolitis:
  - Shigellosis: Severe abdominal pains often are present; associated with high fevers; ulcers of the GI lining are common; stools are often grossly bloody, with sheets of fecal leukocytes.
  - Staphylococcal food poisoning
  - Other bacterial infections of the GI tract

- Viral enteritis: Rotavirus, Norwalk virus, norovirus, and other viruses
- Parasitic infections
- Toxic ingestion
- Noninfectious systemic illnesses marked by inflammatory colitis
- Enteric fever from *Salmonella* infection may be confused with:
  - Other causes of invasive bacterial disease
  - Other causes of fever in a return traveler (e.g., malaria)
  - Other causes of prolonged fever (e.g., viral, *Bartonella*)
  - Spirochetal infection

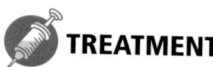 TREATMENT

MEDICATION (DRUGS)
Various antibiotics may be used to treat *Salmonella* infection:

- *Salmonella* gastroenteritis at high risk of invasive disease: Increasing resistance to amoxicillin, ampicillin, and trimethoprim/sulfamethoxazole; parenteral third-generation cephalosporins or fluoroquinolones are preferred empirically.
- Invasive *Salmonella* disease: IV ampicillin for 2 weeks has been first-line therapy; chloramphenicol, a third-generation cephalosporin, or a quinolone may be used for resistant organisms; cefotaxime for treatment of meningitis; meningitis or osteomyelitis may require 4–6 weeks of parenteral antibiotic therapy.
- Some authorities treat chronic carriers of *S. typhi* who shed for >1 year with high-dose parenteral ampicillin; high-dose oral amoxicillin (with or without probenecid) or ciprofloxacin; consider cholecystectomy for refractory cases.

IN-PATIENT CONSIDERATIONS
Initial Stabilization
- Acute asymptomatic infection: Should not be treated with antibiotics. Antibiotics do not have an impact on duration of diarrhea and may lengthen duration of carrier state and contagious shedding.
- Acute gastroenteritis (see "FAQ"):
  - Supportive care: Maintain intravascular volume, correct electrolyte abnormalities
  - Do not administer antidiarrheal agents; they prolong GI transit time.
  - Consider antibiotics in individuals at high risk of subsequent systemic invasive illness: Children <3 months, immunocompromised hosts, patients with hemoglobinopathies or chronic GI tract disease
- Bacteremia, enteric fever, and/or chronic carrier state:
  - Supportive care
  - Antibiotics are indicated; initial therapy usually to be administered intravenously.
  - Surgical drainage of local suppuration is indicated as in most other infections.
  - Corticosteroids (3 mg/kg load, 1 mg/kg q6h) may be beneficial to critically ill patients with enteric fever exhibiting neurologic complications.
  - Antipyretics are controversial in enteric fever syndromes because they may cause precipitous declines in temperature and shock.

 ONGOING CARE

FOLLOW-UP RECOMMENDATIONS
- Acute GI illness:
  - Symptoms usually resolve spontaneously within 7 days.
  - Supportive care to prevent or treat dehydration may be required.
  - Young children and those with underlying disease processes may be at higher risk of complications.
- Enteric fever:
  - Untreated, this illness will have a prolonged course over weeks.
  - Life-threatening complications are most common during the 2nd or 3rd week of illness, often after a period of apparent clinical improvement.
  - Even with appropriate treatment, up to 20% of patients may suffer relapse which require retreatment with antibiotics.
- Chronic carriage:
  - 1% of patients with *Salmonella* infection will shed bacteria in the stool for >1 year.
  - Chronic carriers should be identified because they pose a public health risk.

ALERT
- More people with *Salmonella* infestation are asymptomatic than are symptomatic.
- Antibiotic resistance is a growing problem.
- Even with appropriate therapy, patients may shed bacteria on a persistent basis or may suffer relapse.

PROGNOSIS
- Most normal hosts with *Salmonella* gastroenteritis will recover spontaneously.
- Some individuals will develop a chronic carrier state, persistently shedding bacteria in the stool.
- The relapse rate of enteric fever may approach 20% of patients, even when adequately treated.

COMPLICATIONS
- Dehydration and/or electrolyte imbalance is the most common complication arising from acute gastroenteritis.
- Invasive *Salmonella* may lead to complications of bacteremia:
  - Sepsis: Most common in neonates and immunosuppressed individuals
  - Meningitis: Vast majority of cases occur in 1st month of life.
  - Osteomyelitis: Most common in patients with sickle cell anemia
  - Other local infections: Pneumonia, pericarditis
- Complications of enteric fever include intestinal or splenic rupture (at areas of lymphoid hypertrophy), hepatitis, pancreatitis, parotitis, orchitis, arthritis, and myocarditis.
- A postinfectious form of hemolytic uremic syndrome may occur following *Salmonella* infection.

ADDITIONAL READING
- Fierer J, Swancutt M. Non-typhoid salmonela: A review. *Curr Clin Top Infect Dis.* 2000;20:134–157.
- Nataro JP. Treatment of bacterial enteritis. *Pediatr Infect Dis J.* 1998;17:420–421.
- Sirinavin S, Garner P. Antibiotics for treating salmonella gut infections. *Cochrane Database Syst Rev.* 2000;CD001167.
- Stephens I, Levine MM. Management of typhoid fever in children. *Pediatr Infect Dis J.* 2002;21: 157–158.
- Swanson SJ, Snider C, Braden CR, et al. Multidrug-resistant Salmonella enterica serotype Typhimurium associated with pet rodents. *N Engl J Med.* 2007;356:21–28.

 CODES

ICD9
- 003.0 Salmonella gastroenteritis
- 003.9 Salmonella infection, unspecified
- 558.9 Other and unspecified noninfectious gastroenteritis and colitis

ICD10
- A02.0 Salmonella enteritis
- A02.9 Salmonella infection, unspecified
- K52.9 Noninfective gastroenteritis and colitis, unspecified

FAQ
- Q: Should all infants with *Salmonella* gastroenteritis be treated with antibiotics?
- A: Clinicians caring for children <1 year with proven, or suspected, *Salmonella* infection face many treatment dilemmas. Any toxic-appearing infant and any infant with proven *Salmonella* bacteremia should be admitted to the hospital for parenteral antibiotics. High-risk infants (<3 months of age) with positive stool cultures should be treated with antibiotics after blood cultures are obtained. Well-appearing infants >3 months of age with *Salmonella* enterocolitis and fever should be observed off antibiotics after surveillance blood cultures are obtained.

S

SARCOIDOSIS

Peter Weiser
Randy Q. Cron
Frank Pessler (5th edition)

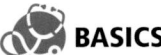 BASICS

DESCRIPTION
A multisystem chronic granulomatous disease that has 2 distinct variations often differentiated by age of onset

EPIDEMIOLOGY
More common in the southeastern part of the US. Disease occurs before age 4 years as arthritis, uveitis, and dermatitis, and in adolescence as Löfgren syndrome with erythema nodosum, polyarthritis, and hilar adenopathy. Adult-type disease with marked pulmonary involvement may also occur in older adolescents. CNS involvement (rare): Seizures, cranial neuropathy, hypothalamic dysfunction.

RISK FACTORS
Genetics
- Blacks are more commonly affected than whites; specific genetic tendencies not identified.
- Early childhood cases of arthritis, uveitis, and dermatitis may result from mutation of the CARD15/NOD2 gene—either spontaneous or hereditary—familial form, the latter also known as Blau syndrome (AD). Some of the mutation-negative patients have systemic/visceral involvement.

PATHOPHYSIOLOGY
T-cell-mediated disease resulting in noncaseating epithelioid giant cell granulomas in affected organs

ETIOLOGY
Unknown (possibly infectious); resembles pulmonary borreliosis; possible association with substantial dust inhalation (e.g., collapse of World Trade Center towers in New York).

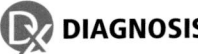 DIAGNOSIS

HISTORY
Prolonged malaise, fever, weight loss, rash, painful arthritis, swollen lymph nodes, chronic cough, and hematuria (can be microscopic) may be initial complaints.

PHYSICAL EXAM
- Peripheral lymphadenopathy is most common manifestation.
- Conjunctival injection
- Bilateral parotid gland enlargement and hepatosplenomegaly may be present.
- The arthritis, usually in the ankles, is extremely tender and boggy.
- Rash is diffuse, erythematous, and macular or plaque-like. Can also be erythema nodosum.

DIAGNOSTIC TESTS & INTERPRETATION
Lab
- CBC:
  - Mild anemia, leukopenia, lymphopenia
- ESR elevated
- ACE level elevation:
  - Produced in most granulomatous diseases, but is useful in cases in which index of suspicion is high
- Lysozyme level elevation:
  - May be more sensitive than ACE level for detecting sarcoidosis
- Serum calcium and creatinine levels:
  - Important in baseline evaluation
- Urine test for blood:
  - Seen in patients with hypercalciuria
- Synovial effusion are typically mildly inflammatory.
- Biopsy of affected organ, such as peripheral lymph node, parotid gland, skin, conjunctivae, or minor salivary gland or synovium (demonstrating noncaseating granuloma), is helpful.

Imaging
- Chest radiography:
  - May demonstrate hilar adenopathy
- Gallium scan:
  - Demonstrates uptake diffusely in lungs (extremely sensitive test)
- False-positives:
  - ACE level: May be elevated in patients with miliary tuberculosis and biliary cirrhosis. Not a perfect screening test; however, can follow levels in response to treatment.
  - Lysozyme level: Also elevated in lymphoma. May be useful to follow disease activity in proven cases, if ACE levels cannot be used.

ALERT
Uveitis may be occult; ophthalmology evaluation is important.

DIFFERENTIAL DIAGNOSIS
- Infection:
  - Tuberculosis, bacterial sepsis, mumps, HIV, gonorrhea, Lyme disease, pulmonary mycoses
- Tumors:
  - Leukemia, neuroblastoma, lymphoma
- Immunologic: Sjogren disease
  - Oligoarticular juvenile idiopathic arthritis (for early-onset type), systemic juvenile idiopathic arthritis, systemic lupus erythematosus, dermatomyositis, Behcet disease, Crohn disease
  - Immunodeficiency: CVID
- Skin
  - Granuloma annulare; erythema nodosum due to streptococcus/hepatitis B

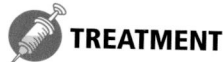

TREATMENT

Medical therapy during times of disease activity causing clinical symptoms

MEDICATION (DRUGS)

- Corticosteroids may provide rapid improvement; NSAIDs/analgesics have roles.

In cases of chronic disease:

- Immunosuppressive medications such as methotrexate can be used in addition to corticosteroids
- The tumor necrosis factor-α inhibitors, specifically antibodies, infliximab, and adalimumab, show promising preliminary results.
- In cases of hypercalciuria/hypercalcemia, consider hydration and furosemide.
- Cyclophosphamide for neurosarcoid

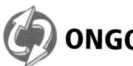

ONGOING CARE

FOLLOW-UP RECOMMENDATIONS
Patient Monitoring

- Referral to rheumatologist indicated, also regular ophthalmologic assessment:
- Signs to watch for:
  - Climbing creatinine, shortness of breath, or persistent uveal tract inflammation, neurologic deficit
- Pitfalls:
  - Overtreating asymptomatic lymphadenopathy and not detecting hypercalciuria

PROGNOSIS

Variable in early onset. Severe organ involvement, joint and eye damage can occur—needs close follow-up. Löfgren syndrome can resolve after a couple of years. More than 40% of older children with adult-type disease have persistent pulmonary changes, but only a few will have pulmonary symptoms.

COMPLICATIONS

- In children, usually related to uveitis or from hypercalciuria resulting in renal injury. Lung, CNS, and ocular involvement can bring long-term defects.
- In older adolescents, pulmonary problems, such as restrictive lung disease, as well as severe growth delay, may occur.

ADDITIONAL READING

- Baumann RJ, Robertson WC Jr. Neurosarcoid presents differently in children than in adults. *Pediatrics.* 2003;112:e480–e486.
- Iannuzzi MC, Rybicki BA, Teirstein AS. Sarcoidosis. *N Engl J Med.* 2007;357:2153–2165.
- Lindsley CB, Petty RE. Overview and report on international registry of sarcoid arthritis in childhood. *Curr Rheumatol Rep.* 2000;2:343–348.
- Rose CD, Wouters CH, Meiorin S, et al. Pediatric granulomatous arthritis: An international registry. *Arthritis Rheum.* 2006;54:3337–3344.
- Shetty AK, Gedalia A. Childhood sarcoidosis: A rare but fascinating disorder. *Pediatr Rheumatol Online J.* 2008;6:16.

CODES

ICD9
- 135 Sarcoidosis
- 517.8 Lung involvement in other diseases classified elsewhere
- 695.2 Erythema nodosum

ICD10
- D86.0 Sarcoidosis of lung
- D86.9 Sarcoidosis, unspecified
- L52 Erythema nodosum

FAQ

- Q: Why is the outcome better in childhood sarcoid compared with adults with sarcoid?
- A: These may be 2 distinct granulomatous diseases. The 2 have clearly different patterns of organ involvement.

S

SCABIES

Kathleen Wholey Zsolway
Alyssa Siegel

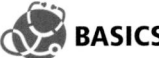 **BASICS**

DESCRIPTION
- Results from infestation of stratum corneum by the human mite, *Sarcoptes scabiei* (subspecies Hominis, phylum Arthropoda, class Arachnida, and order Acarina)
- Animal scabies, or sarcoptic mange, occurs from contact with an infested canine and produces only a transient rash in humans.
- Crusted scabies, formerly known as Norwegian scabies, is a highly contagious variant of human scabies that occurs in institutional settings, developmentally disabled and immunocompromised patients, including those using long-term topical steroids and with HIV. It requires isolation measures and diligent use of medications for elimination.
- Post-scabetic syndrome consists of persistent pruritus caused by hypersensitivity to mite antigen and may persist for several days after live mite has been eliminated.

EPIDEMIOLOGY
- Affects all age groups, but particularly children
- Epidemics are reported to occur in 15-year cycles.
- Sole reservoir of *S. scabiei* is the human.
- Close, personal contact with an infested human (with or without clinical symptoms) is required for transmission.
- Mites can live isolated from the human body for 2–3 days; extent of fomite transmission is unclear.

Incidence
~300 million cases of scabies in the world annually

GENERAL PREVENTION
- Bedding, clothing, and items of close contact should be washed and dried in hot temperatures at time of treatment.
- All family members and close contacts, symptomatic and asymptomatic, should be treated concurrently to eliminate mite and prevent immediate reinfestation. Contacts may be infested without symptoms.

PATHOPHYSIOLOGY
- Female mite burrows into stratum corneum, rarely penetrating epidermis, for 15–30 days, traveling 2–4 mm/day and laying 1–3 eggs/day.
- Egg laying is completed in 4–5 weeks when female dies within a burrow.
  - Eggs, hatching within a burrow, will undergo several molts and emerge on skin surface as nymphs.
  - After a 2–3-week maturation period, mating will occur; male will die, and gravid female will restart cycle with burrowing.
- Following first exposure, signs and symptoms will develop 10–30 days after scabies infestation; perhaps time lag necessary for body to develop humoral or cellular hypersensitivity to mite and/or its byproducts or time necessary for adequate mass of mites to develop.
- Previously infested patients are immunologically sensitized, leading to development of symptoms 1–4 days after re-exposure.

ETIOLOGY
Etiologic agent is gravid female mite, *S. scabiei*, 0.2–0.4 mm in size.

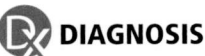 **DIAGNOSIS**

HISTORY
- Pruritus: Intensity worse at night when mite activity increases secondary to increase in body temperature
- Evolution of rash:
  - Characteristically changes over time both in appearance and distribution
  - May consist of burrows, papules, and vesicular lesions
  - Recurrent clusters of vesicles and pustules can occur over time.
  - In older children, rash may involve webs of fingers, axillae, arms, wrists, waistline, and genitalia. In young children, may include palms, soles, head, neck, and face.
- Symptoms in other family members or close contacts: Close contact required for transmission

PHYSICAL EXAM
- Distribution of rash usually from neck down in infants; in children, neck and face may also be involved.
- Lesions typically more numerous on hands, especially web spaces, as well as thenar and hypothenar eminences in older children and adults
- Palms, proximal half of foot, and heel are sites of numerous lesions in infants.
- Lesions also seen on wrists, in axillae, around waistline, on gluteal cleft, and surrounding nipples and genitalia
- A burrow, the characteristic lesion of scabies, is present in 90–95% of all symptomatic patients, and forms a "lazy S" shape with a broad base and a punctate brown-black dot at leading edge of mite's path. If burrows are not easily identified, washable felt-tip marker can be rubbed across web space, and after superficial ink is removed with alcohol or water, ink will have penetrated through stratum corneum outlining burrow.
- Secondary lesions are more numerous and obvious than burrows and may consist of crusted papules, small vesicles, pustules, excoriated broad areas of dermatitis, and areas of secondary infection from impetigo and folliculitis.

DIAGNOSTIC TESTS & INTERPRETATION
Lab
- Skin scrapings may be obtained to secure definitive diagnosis.
  - The burrows most commonly found on hands and feet should be moistened with alcohol or mineral oil.
  - Scrape a no. 15, round-bellied blade attached to a scalpel handle briskly across burrows
  - Place scraped material on a slide with a drop of potassium hydroxide or mineral oil with a cover slip
  - Under a scanning microscope, presence of gravid female, eggs, larvae, and/or feces is diagnostic.
- New diagnostic methods include detection of *S. scabiei* DNA from cutaneous scales by PCR or ELISA.

DIFFERENTIAL DIAGNOSIS
- Infection:
  - Impetigo
  - Papular viral exanthem
- Environmental: Contact dermatitis
- Immunologic:
  - Atopic dermatitis
  - Papular urticaria
- Miscellaneous:
  - Drug eruption
  - Psoriasis
  - Infantile acropustulosis

 TREATMENT

MEDICATION (DRUGS)
- 5% permethrin cream (Elimite 5%):
  - Drug of choice due to effectiveness and safety profile
  - Used for infants >2 months and children
  - Apply to entire body surface and leave on for 8–14 hours, then wash off. One application is usually effective, though some recommend a second application 1 week later.
- 1% lindane cream:
  - All members of the affected household should be treated at the same time.
  - Should remain on body for 8–12 hours
  - Effective for older children and nonpregnant women. No longer recommended for use in children due to potential absorption and toxicity.
- 10% crotamiton cream:
  - Not approved for use in children
  - Can be applied for 2 consecutive days followed by cleansing bath 48 hours after last application
  - Treatment failures have been reported.
- 6% sulfur in a petrolatum base:
  - May be used in older children and adults
  - Apply for 3 consecutive days

- Mild-to-moderate topical steroids (e.g., 1% hydrocortisone, 0.025–0.1% triamcinolone) may be beneficial in post-scabetic syndrome.
- Oral agents such as ivermectin:
  - Not approved for treatment of scabies by the U.S. Food and Drug Administration, but has been used in adult patients for resistant cases, particularly in crusted scabies and in institutional-setting outbreaks.
  - Has been used in solution of propylene glycol as topical agent in some trials

 ONGOING CARE

FOLLOW-UP RECOMMENDATIONS
Patient Monitoring
- Pruritus may take up to 4 weeks to resolve after effective treatment. Use of mild-to-moderate topical steroid may improve this symptom.
- Continued appearance of new burrows may indicate ineffective treatment (most commonly misapplication) and warrants repeat evaluation by healthcare professional.

PROGNOSIS
Excellent outcome with topical therapy; resistant cases, necessitating referral to a dermatologist and consideration for oral therapy, have been increasing worldwide.

COMPLICATIONS
- Secondary infections, including impetigo and folliculitis
- Id eruption or auto-sensitization
- Pruritus

ADDITIONAL READING
- Angeles RM. A closer look at Sarcoptes scabiei. *Arch Pathol Lab Med*. 2005;129:810.
- Chosidow O. Scabies and pediculosis. *Lancet*. 2000;355:819–826.
- Chouela E, Abeldano A, Pellerano G, et al. Diagnosis and treatment of scabies: A practical guide. *Am J Clin Dermatol*. 2002;3:9–18.

- Elston DM. Controversies concerning the treatment of lice and scabies. *J Am Acad Dermatol*. 2002;46:794–796.
- Hicks M, Elston D. Scabies. *Dermatol Ther*. 2009;22:279–292.
- Huynh TH, Norman RA. Scabies and pediculosis. *Dermatol Clin*. 2004;22:7–11.
- Strong M, Johnstone PW. Interventions for treating scabies. *Cochrane Database Syst Rev*. 2007;3:CD000320.

 CODES

ICD9
133.0 Scabies

ICD10
B86 Scabies

FAQ
- Q: How did my child get scabies?
- A: From close contact with an infected person
- Q: How long will my child continue to itch?
- A: Pruritus may continue for weeks; the use of topical hydrocortisone may be helpful.
- Q: Do I need to wash my child's bedding in a special detergent?
- A: Simply wash all bedding in hot, soapy water after your child has been treated.

S

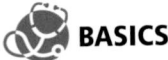 **SCARLET FEVER**

Mark L. Bagarazzi

BASICS

DESCRIPTION
- A clinical syndrome consisting of fever, pharyngitis, cervical lymphadenitis, and the characteristic "sandpaper rash," which results from infection with a strain of *Streptococcus pyogenes* (group A β-hemolytic streptococcus) that elaborates streptococcal pyrogenic toxin
- Toxins include A, B, and C. Toxin A is associated with more virulent disease.
- Similar syndrome may also be seen after infection with certain toxin-producing (enterotoxin G, I) strains of *Staphylococcus aureus*; known as staphylococcal scarlet fever.

GENERAL PREVENTION
- Prompt treatment leads to fewer secondary cases of streptococcal disease.
- Chemoprophylaxis with penicillin is recommended by some experts in children with repeated documented episodes occurring at short intervals.
- Control measures, including hygiene advice and exclusion of pupils for 24 hours while initiating penicillin treatment, were ineffective in a school outbreak.

EPIDEMIOLOGY
- No sex predilection
- Occurs uncommonly before the age of 3 years or after the age of 15 years, possibly related to the requirement for prior sensitization and toxin-specific immunity
- All forms of streptococcal pharyngitis (i.e., with or without pyrogenic toxin) are more common in temperate and cold climates and winter and spring months, with some areas reporting an increased incidence in the fall.
- Incubation period is usually 24–48 hours.

Incidence
Peak incidence during the first few school years

Prevalence
By age 10, 80% of children have developed toxin-specific antibodies.

PATHOPHYSIOLOGY
- Susceptible individuals thought to lack toxin-specific immunity. Supported by results of Dick test, in which a small amount of toxin introduced intradermally produces local erythema in susceptible individuals but no reaction in those with toxin-specific immunity.
- Rash and other toxic manifestations of scarlet fever have been attributed to the development of hypersensitivity to the toxin, which therefore would require prior exposure to the toxin.
- Toxin production depends on lysogeny of the infecting streptococcus by a temperate bacteriophage.

- Pharyngitis is characterized by mucosal erythema and frequently by small crypt abscesses with punctate exudate in enlarged tonsils.
- Edematous papillae protrude from coated mucosa to produce a strawberry tongue.
- Histologic examination of affected skin shows dilated blood and lymphatic vessels and engorged capillaries, most prominently around hair follicles.
- Acute, edematous polymorphonuclear inflammatory reaction is seen microscopically within affected tissues.
- Epidermal inflammatory reaction is usually followed by hyperkeratosis, which accounts for scaling during defervescence.

DIAGNOSIS

HISTORY
- Sudden onset of fever up to 40.5°C, sore throat, headache, nausea, vomiting, and toxicity are classic symptoms for group A streptococcal disease.
- Texture of rash (e.g., feels like sandpaper) is more important than appearance.
- Characteristic rash typically occurs 12–48 hours after onset of fever.
- Patient may complain of abdominal pain or muscle aches before onset of rash, as well as aching in extremities or back.
- There may be close contacts with streptococcal infection.

PHYSICAL EXAM
- Fine maculopapular (sandpaper texture) rash on erythematous background: usually begins on the trunk and spreads to involve almost the entire body within hours to days. Although the rash seen with scarlet fever is generally fine and sandpaperlike, larger papules and petechiae may be seen.
- Deep, red, nonblanching lesions in the antecubital and popliteal areas: "Pastia lines" develop in the skin folds of joints.
- Circumoral pallor: Classic finding
- Rash blanches with pressure and ultimately desquamates: Desquamation occurs within 7–21 days from onset of illness.
- Characteristic toxin-induced scarlet fever exanthem: may rarely be seen without pharyngitis in the setting of pyoderma or an infected wound (known as surgical scarlet fever).
- Systemic toxicity: May indicate incorrect diagnosis
- Dorsum of tongue: Has white coat early in illness with edematous red papillae. White covering desquamates and reveals swollen, red, and mottled strawberry tongue.
- Other findings:
  – Pharynx and tonsils are beefy red and may contain exudate.
  – Hemorrhagic spots on interior pillar of tonsils and soft palate
  – Large, tender anterior cervical nodes

DIAGNOSTIC TESTS & INTERPRETATION
Lab
- Rapid streptococcal antigen tests: effective as screening tests; 50–80% sensitivity and >95% specificity. Positive rapid tests do not require culture confirmation.
- Throat culture: The gold standard with best sensitivity (>90%) for group A β-hemolytic streptococci. A culture should be performed when rapid test is negative.
- White blood cell count: usually elevated, although may be elevated in viral pharyngitis as well. Low count would be rare with streptococcal infection.
- Eosinophilia (up to 30%): Common in the recovery phase
- Dick test: of historic interest; no longer used clinically
- Pitfalls:
  – A positive throat culture may be evidence only of carriage in some cases of acute pharyngitis that are actually viral (e.g., Epstein–Barr virus).
  – Milder disease is becoming more common and is easier to miss. Rash may involve only the bridge of the nose, face, shoulders, and upper chest. Circumoral pallor and severe exudative pharyngitis are being seen less frequently.

DIFFERENTIAL DIAGNOSIS
- Nonscarlatinal streptococcal pharyngitis/tonsillitis
- Viral exanthems (measles, rubella, erythema infectiosum)
- Drug eruptions
- Staphylococcal scalded skin syndrome
- Toxic epidermal necrolysis
- Toxic shock syndrome (streptococcal or staphylococcal)
- Kawasaki disease
- Uncommon entities:
  – Infection with *Corynebacterium hemolyticum*
  – Mercury poisoning (acrodynia)
  – Atropine intoxication
  – Boric acid poisoning
  – Rifampin overdose

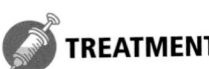 **TREATMENT**

ADDITIONAL TREATMENT
Initial Stabilization
- Identical to therapy for streptococcal pharyngitis
- Therapy started as late as 9 days after illness onset should be effective in preventing acute rheumatic fever.
- May withhold treatment until throat culture result is available
- Immediate therapy probably shortens symptomatic period.

MEDICATION (DRUGS)

- Oral penicillin VK:
  - Drug of choice except in penicillin-allergic individuals
  - Resistant strains have not been documented in the US.
  - Dose: 25,000 to 50,000 units/kg (1,600 units = 1 mg) divided into 3–4 doses for 10 days
  - 400,000 units (250 mg) b.i.d. for children <27 kg (or 60 lbs) and 800,000 units (500 mg) twice daily for children ≥27 kg (60 lbs) for 10 days has also been shown to have comparable efficacy and is endorsed by the American Academy of Pediatrics.
- Intramuscular benzathine penicillin G:
  - Equally effective as oral penicillin
  - Dose: 600,000 units for children <27 kg (<60 lbs); 1,200,000 units in larger children and adults
  - Ensures compliance
  - Bringing to room temperature reduces discomfort.
  - Benzathine/procaine penicillin combinations are less painful.
- Clarithromycin and azithromycin have also been shown to eradicate streptococci; however, because of the broad spectra of these antibiotics and the increasing incidence of antibiotic-resistant bacteria, penicillin is still recommended by most experts, except in cases of penicillin hypersensitivity, when patient nonadherence to a 10-day penicillin regimen is suspected, or for patients who fail therapy with a β-lactam:
  - Azithromycin, total dose of 60 mg/kg, given either as 12 mg/kg once daily for 5 days or 20 mg/kg once daily for 3 days
  - Clarithromycin, 15 mg/kg/d, given b.i.d. for 10 days, or 500 mg extended-release tablets given once a day for 5 days (studied in adolescents ≥12 years)
  - There are reports of acute rheumatic fever after the 3-day course of azithromycin.
- Oral erythromycin is indicated in penicillin-allergic individuals. Erythromycin ethyl succinate (40 to 50 mg/kg/d in 2–4 divided doses). Resistance is rare in the US (<5% of isolates).
- Amoxicillin, clindamycin, and first-generation oral cephalosporins (up to 15% of penicillin-allergic persons are also allergic to cephalosporins) are reasonable alternatives to penicillin.
- Recent trials comparing 10-day course of penicillin with shorter duration of therapy with newer oral cephalosporins have shown similar bacteriologic and clinical cure rates, but efficacy in prevention of nonsuppurative sequelae is unknown.
- Cefdinir and cefpodoxime proxetil are approved for use in a more convenient 5-day dosing schedule.
- Tetracyclines and sulfonamides should not be used because of resistance of group A streptococci.
- Positive posttreatment cultures in asymptomatic patients: Retreatment is not recommended.

 ## ONGOING CARE

- Fever and symptoms usually resolve within 24–48 hours of antibiotic treatment.
- Nonsuppurative complications occur after unrecognized disease and when treatment is delayed for >9 days. Acute rheumatic fever occurs an average of 18 days after untreated infection. Acute postinfectious glomerulonephritis occurs an average of 10 days after untreated infection. The risk of glomerulonephritis is not reduced by treatment with antibiotics.

PROGNOSIS

- Overall prognosis is excellent.
- Few patients suffer suppurative complications.
- Risk of developing acute rheumatic fever in untreated streptococcal infections is about 3% under epidemic conditions (0.3% in endemic situations).
- Risk of developing acute postinfectious glomerulonephritis depends on nephritogenicity of infecting strain. Attack rate is 10–15% with nephritogenic strains.

COMPLICATIONS

- Acute otitis media
- Sinusitis
- Suppurative cervical lymphadenitis
- Pneumonia with or without effusion/empyema
- Peritonsillar cellulitis/abscess
- Retropharyngeal abscess
- Meningitis
- Brain abscess
- Thrombosis of intracranial venous sinuses
- Osteomyelitis
- Hepatitis
- Arthritis
- Acute rheumatic fever
- Acute postinfectious glomerulonephritis
- Erythema nodosum, possibly

ADDITIONAL READING

- Altemeier WA. A pediatrician's view. A brief history of group A beta hemolytic strep. *Pediatr Ann*. 1998;27:264–267.
- Duncan SR, Scott S, Duncan CJ. Modeling the dynamics of scarlet fever epidemics in the 19th century. *Eur J Epidemiol*. 2000;16:619–626.
- Lamden K. An outbreak of scarlet fever in a primary school. *Arch Dis Child*. 2011;96:394–397.

- Richardson M, Elliman D, Maguire H, et al. Evidence base of incubation periods, periods of infectiousness and exclusion policies for the control of communicable diseases in schools and preschools. *Pediatr Infect Dis J*. 2001;20:380–391.
- Shiseki M, Miwa K, Nemoto Y, et al. Comparison of pathogenic factors expressed by group A streptococci isolated from patients with streptococcal toxic shock syndrome and scarlet fever. *Microb Pathog*. 1999;27:243–252.

 ## CODES

ICD9
- 034.0 Streptococcal sore throat
- 034.1 Scarlet fever

ICD10
- A38.9 Scarlet fever, uncomplicated
- J02.0 Streptococcal pharyngitis

S

FAQ

- Q: Should household contacts have throat cultures performed?
- A: Obtain cultures only from symptomatic household contacts. Cultures should not routinely be obtained in asymptomatic contacts.
- Q: Should posttreatment throat cultures be performed?
- A: Only in symptomatic individuals and patients at risk for acute rheumatic fever and acute postinfectious glomerulonephritis
- Q: Can scarlet fever recur?
- A: Yes, there have been documented reports of recurrent scarlet fever.
- Q: Have there been documented child care outbreaks of scarlet fever?
- A: Yes, outbreaks have been traced back to a single strain.
- Q: How soon can children return to school or child care?
- A: When they are afebrile, and after at least 24 hours of antibiotic therapy.
- Q: Is there any known association between scarlet fever or other group A streptococcal infections and neuropsychiatric disorders?
- A: Retrospective epidemiologic studies have shown that subjects with newly diagnosed obsessive compulsive disorder, attention deficit hyperactivity disorder, major depressive disorder, Tourette syndrome and other tic disorders were more likely to have had a diagnosis of streptococcal infection in the previous year.

SCLERODERMA

Peter Weiser
Randy Q. Cron

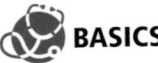 **BASICS**

DESCRIPTION
Scleroderma means "hard skin." It can be systemic or localized.
- Systemic sclerosis (SSc) or progressive systemic sclerosis (PSS):
  - CREST: A variant form of systemic sclerosis, almost nonexistent in children
- Localized:
  - Morphea
  - Linear
  - En Coup de Sabre
  - Parry-Romberg syndrome

EPIDEMIOLOGY
- Systemic:
  - Age of onset: 30–50 years; very rare in children
  - Sex ratio: <7 years, Male = Female; >7 years, Female > Male (3:1); 15–44 years, Female > Male (15:1)
- CREST:
  - Earlier age of onset than systemic sclerosis
  - Female > Male

Incidence
- Systemic: 0.27 per million annually
- CREST: Affects ~1/2 of patients with systemic disease
- Localized: Approximately 10× more common than systemic sclerosis

PATHOPHYSIOLOGY
- Systemic involvement:
  - Vasculopathy: Based on high association with Raynaud phenomenon; vascular injury leading to fibrotic changes as a part of overcorrection
  - Serum factors: Endothelin
  - Immune dysfunction: Autoimmunity directed against connective-tissue antigen such as laminin or type IV collagen, PDGF receptor stimulating fibrosis
- Localized form:
  - Alteration of normal glycosylation and hydroxylation of collagen
  - May represent distinct early and late processes:
    - Early: Increased hydrophilic glycosaminoglycan; increased T cells, macrophages, and plasma cells; mast-cell hyperplasia
    - Late: Increased collagen content; collagen is embryonic with narrow fibrils and immature cross-banding; atrophy of rete pegs

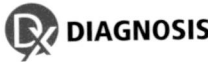 **DIAGNOSIS**

HISTORY
- Thickening of skin
- Tightness of joints
- Discoloration of skin
- Often insidious onset
- Morning stiffness
- Heartburn, dysphagia, reflux, cough with swallowing

Signs and symptoms:
- Systemic sclerosis:
  - Diagnostic criteria (1 major criterion or 2 minor criteria required)
  - Major: Sclerodermatous changes (tightness, thickening, induration) proximal to metacarpophalangeal or metatarsophalangeal joints
  - Minor: Sclerodactyly-sclerodermatous changes limited to digits (unable to pinch skin over the digit), digital pitting, bibasilar pulmonary fibrosis not due to primary lung disease
  - CREST:
    - Calcinosis
    - Raynaud phenomenon
    - Esophageal dysmotility
    - Sclerodactyly
    - Telangiectases
  - Same characteristics as systemic scleroderma, but calcinosis is more severe
  - Distal symptoms are more severe.
  - Associated with anti-centromere antibody
- Localized:
  - Fibrosis limited to skin, SC tissue, and muscle; comes with loss of subcutaneous tissue pulp of the fingers
  - Systemic features:
    - Rare: Visceral involvement later in disease
    - Occasional: Evolution into another connective tissue disease such as mixed connective tissue disease or systemic lupus erythematosus (SLE)
    - Very rare: Raynaud phenomenon
  - Forms:
    - Morphea: ≥1 oval or round indurations that become hard and whitish early on, have active inflammatory border with violaceous color. Forms: Plaque or guttate; limited number of lesions; generalized: extensive; nodular: SC
  - Linear: ≥1 linear areas affecting subcutaneous tissue, muscle, and bone; can cross joint lines
  - En Coup de Sabre: Involves face or scalp; may be associated with seizures
  - Parry-Romberg syndrome: Form of linear scleroderma; congenital dysplasia of subcutaneous tissue; neurologic changes such as TIAs in the corresponding brain matter under the lesion without its direct extension into the scull

PHYSICAL EXAM
- Findings:
  - Skin:
    - Stage 1: Edema. Tense, non-pitting, perhaps warm or tender, but often asymptomatic
    - Stage 2: Sclerosis. Waxy, hard texture; bound to SC structures, back of digits, face (loss of forehead wrinkles, reduced mouth orifice)
    - Stage 3: Atrophy. Shiny appearance, hypopigmented or hyperpigmented, calcium deposits in SC tissue. Telangiectases: Macular dilatations that fill slowly, unlike spider telangiectasias
    - Ulcerations on finger tips with prolonged healing

- Pitfalls:
  - Failure to appreciate limited mouth opening
  - 2 conditions:
    - Primary phenomenon or Raynaud disease
    - Secondary Raynaud phenomenon
  - Primary Raynaud phenomenon is not associated with underlying disease:
    - Milder form
    - 75% are women.
  - Secondary Raynaud phenomenon is associated with underlying disease such as lupus, Sjögren syndrome, mixed connective tissue disease, dermatomyositis, and polymyositis; more serious:
    - Triple phase: Blanching of digits with sharp border to normal colored skin, cyanosis erythema, tingling/numb sensation of the digits
    - Present in ~90% of patients with systemic sclerosis
    - Usually fingers; also toes, nose, ears, and tongue; often spares thumb
  - Pathophysiology: Arterial vasoconstriction, venous stasis to cyanosis, reflex vasodilatation to erythema
  - Calcinosis, especially over extensor joint surfaces in systemic form only
  - Musculoskeletal:
    - "Creaking" of thickened tendons
    - Contractures, especially proximal interphalangeal joints and elbows
    - No intra-articular inflammation
    - Muscle inflammation in ~30% of cases
  - GI:
    - Mucosal telangiectasias of mouth
    - Decreased incisor distance/mouth opening secondary to skin tightness of the lips
    - Sicca syndrome with parotitis
    - Loosening of teeth secondary to periodontal membrane disease
    - Esophageal disease: Esophagitis, occasional ulceration or stricture
    - Large-bowel disease less common
  - Cardiac:
    - Primary cause of morbidity
    - Possibly due to Raynaud phenomenon of coronary arteries and pulmonary artery hypertension
  - Pulmonary:
    - Interstitial fibrosis with gradual obliteration of vascular bed and resulting cor pulmonale
    - Parenchymal disease is almost universal; frequently asymmetric; may have hacking cough, dyspnea on exertion, pleural rub
    - Combined pulmonary vascular and pulmonary parenchymal disease
    - Primary pulmonary vascular disease with right ventricular failure
  - Renal: Due to decreased renal plasma flow, proteinuria, hypertension
  - CNS: Cranial nerve involvement, especially sensory branch of trigeminal nerve
  - Sicca syndrome:
    - Xerostomia (dry mouth)
    - Keratoconjunctivitis sicca (dry eyes)

DIAGNOSTIC TESTS & INTERPRETATION
Lab
There are no specific diagnostic tests.

- Nonspecific tests:
  - Systemic form:
    - ANA: Often positive
    - Hemoglobin: 25% have anemia due to chronic disease or vitamin B12 and folate deficiencies resulting from chronic malabsorption in sclerodermatous gut.
    - Eosinophilia: Present in 50%
    - Sclero-70 (Scl-70 or topoisomerase 1) antibodies: Present in 26% of adults; more common with diffuse disease than with peripheral vascular disease
    - Anti-centromere antibody: Present in 22%, almost exclusively with CREST
    - Muscle biopsy
  - Localized forms:
    - Eosinophilia: Present in 25–50% during active disease
    - ANA: Positive in 37–67%

Imaging
- Chest radiograph:
  - Bibasilar pulmonary fibrosis
  - Rib notching
  - Calcifications (in CREST)
- High-resolution chest CT:
  - Ground-glass attenuation
  - Honeycombing
- Bone radiograph:
  - Acro-osteolysis: Resorption of tufts of distal phalanges, especially with severe Raynaud phenomenon
  - Periarticular or subcutaneous calcification (15–25% patients)
  - Bony erosions

Diagnostic Procedures/Other
- For sicca syndrome:
  - Schirmer test for dry eyes
  - Lip biopsy
  - Rose bengal staining of cornea
- ECG:
  - First-degree block
  - Right and left bundle-branch block
  - Premature atrial contractions (PACs) and premature ventricular contractions (PVCs): Nonspecific T-wave changes, ventricular hypertrophy
- Pulmonary function tests:
  - Restrictive lung disease: Present in 34% of patients with systemic sclerosis
  - Earliest changes are decreased FVC and small airway disease.
  - Decreased diffusing capacity of the lung for carbon monoxide (DLCO): Present in 18% of patients with systemic sclerosis at the time of diagnosis

Pathological Findings
- Periungual nailfold changes: Capillary dropout and dilated loops; occasional redundant cuticular growth and digital pitting
- Histologic:
  - Skin: Loss of subcutaneous fat, increased amount of fibroblasts
  - Muscle: Increased collagen and fat; negative immunofluorescence
  - Esophagus: Atrophic muscle replaced by fibrous tissue more commonly affects smooth muscle of lower 2/3 of esophagus.

- Esophageal manometry and pH probe: Decreased or absent peristalsis of distal esophagus—distal dilatation, hiatus hernia, stricture
- Dilatation of second and third part of duodenum and proximal jejunum

DIFFERENTIAL DIAGNOSIS
- Graft vs. host disease
- Phenylketonuria
- Borrelia infection: Acrodermatitis chronica atrophicans
- Porphyria cutanea tarda
- Scleredema
- Stiff skin syndrome (mucin deposition in the dermis, hardening of the subcutaneous tissue with normal looking epidermis)
- Eosinophilic fasciitis

 ## TREATMENT
MEDICATION (DRUGS)
Disease modification: Many agents have been tried; however, there are few controlled trials and no proven treatment exists. Medications include:

- Localized:
  - Imiquimod, calcitriol ointment, PUVA therapy; methotrexate
- Systemic:
  - Colchicine: Inhibits fibroproliferative process
  - Immunosuppressives:
    - Steroids, chlorambucil, methotrexate, cyclosporine, cyclophosphamide, rituximab
- Pitfall: Avoid excessive use of immunosuppressive therapy late in disease when inflammatory component has resolved.

ADDITIONAL TREATMENT
General Measures
- Supportive care: Avoid trauma and excessive cold—keep extremities warm AND dry
- Management of Raynaud phenomenon:
  - Avoid beta-blockers, caffeine, and stimulating ADHD medications

Additional Therapies
- Physical therapy
  - Helps retard development of contractures and muscle atrophy
  - Pitfall:
    - Insufficient physical therapy resulting in permanent joint contractures

 ## ONGOING CARE
FOLLOW-UP RECOMMENDATIONS
Patient Monitoring
- Localized forms:
  - Physical exam for joint mobility, muscle bulk, and growth
  - Difficult to follow slow disease progression, thus photography of lesions every 3–6 months is recommended
- Systemic forms:
  - Physical exam for digital ulcerations, joint mobility, muscle bulk, and growth
  - Yearly pulmonary function tests
  - Yearly barium swallow
  - ECHO

PROGNOSIS
- Natural course includes several phases:
  - Initial: Inflammation
  - Late: Sclerosis
  - Occasional regression over 3–5 years
- Ultimate prognosis depends on severity of skin tightness, joint contracture, and visceral involvement.
- Mortality:
  - Males > Females
  - Nonwhites > Whites
- Most common cause of death in pediatric patients is secondary to cardiac, renal, and pulmonary complications.

COMPLICATIONS
- Localized:
  - Skin thickening
  - Joint contractures
  - Leg length discrepancies
  - CNS bleed in Parry-Romberg

ADDITIONAL READING

- Fitch PG, Rettig P, Burnham JM, et al. Treatment of pediatric localized scleroderma with methotrexate. *J Rheumatol.* 2006;33:609–614.
- Foeldvari I. Update on pediatric systemic sclerosis: Similarities and differences from adult disease. *Curr Opin Rheumatol.* 2008;20:608–612.
- Foeldvari I. Methotrexate in juvenile localized scleroderma. *Arthritis Rheum.* 2011;63:1779–1781.
- Herrick AL, Ennis H, Bhushan M, et al. Incidence of childhood linear scleroderma and systemic sclerosis in the UK and Ireland. *Arthritis Care Res.* 2010;62: 213–218.
- Marini G, Foeldvari I, Russo R, et al. Systemic sclerosis in childhood: Clinical and immunological features of 153 patients in an international database. *Arthritis Rheum.* 2006;54:3971–3978.
- Zulian F. New developments in localized scleroderma. *Curr Opin Rheumatol.* 2008;20:601–607.

 ## CODES

ICD9
- 447.6 Arteritis, unspecified
- 710.0 Systemic lupus erythematosus
- 710.1 Systemic sclerosis

ICD10
- M34.89 Other systemic sclerosis
- M34.9 Systemic sclerosis, unspecified
- L94.0 Localized scleroderma [morphea]

FAQ

- Q: Is a biopsy necessary?
- A: Biopsy is often useful to confirm diagnosis and assess degree of inflammation.
- Q: Is the sclero-70 antibody useful?
- A: Not for diagnosis; it is positive only in a subset of individuals with the systemic form and, therefore, useful for predicting more severe disease.

S

SCOLIOSIS (IDIOPATHIC)

Ali Al-omari
John P. Dormans

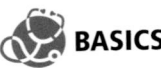 **BASICS**

DESCRIPTION

- Scoliosis: Lateral curvature of spine exceeding 10 degrees (with rotation of spine); curves <10 are termed spinal asymmetry; considered idiopathic only after other causes have been excluded
- Kyphosis: Anteriorly concave curvature of vertebral column

EPIDEMIOLOGY

- Female-to-male ratios:
  – 1.4:1 for curves 11–20 degrees
  – 5.4:1 for curves >20 degrees

Prevalence

- Generally considered 1.5–3% for curves ≥10 degrees
- 0.3–0.5% for curves >20 degrees

RISK FACTORS

Genetics

Positive familial history for idiopathic scoliosis in 30% (not predictive of severity)

ETIOLOGY

By definition, unknown; listed are some theories, none proven in isolation:

- Genetic:
  – Positive familial history for scoliosis in 30% (not predictive of severity)
- Connective tissue disorder:
  – Associated with several connective tissue disorders
  – Alterations in connective tissue of the spine, paraspinous muscles, and platelets
  – May be related to osteopenia (decreased mineral bone density) of vertebral bodies
- Neurologic (equilibrium system):
  – Abnormalities noted in vestibular, ocular, proprioceptive, and vibratory functions
- Hormonal:
  – Lower levels of melatonin secreted from pineal body in those with adolescent idiopathic scoliosis
  – Growth-stimulating hormone: More of an influential factor than etiologic factor studies
  – Vertebral growth abnormalities
  – Asymmetric growth rates between the right and left sides of the spine

COMMONLY ASSOCIATED CONDITIONS

Connective tissue disorders

DIAGNOSIS

HISTORY

- Onset: Consider when first noted, by whom, rate of worsening, previous treatment, patient recent growth, the physical change of puberty, associated signs or symptoms, familial history, etc.
- Patients with idiopathic scoliosis usually should not have pain, although they might have a discomfort or mild pain.
- Back pain in scoliotic patients must be investigated thoroughly and taken seriously.
- If night pain, consider tumor such as osteoid osteoma.
- Other signs or symptoms: Review of systems (especially neurologic)

PHYSICAL EXAM

- General inspection to look for skin changes such as café au lait spots, pigmentation, or other signs of neurofibromatosis; also dysraphic signs (e.g., hairy patches, midline hemangioma, skin dimpling)
- Assess for skeletal maturity, hyperelasticity, contracture, congenital anomalies
- Assess for deformity; asymmetry of spine, shoulders, and trunk, including decompensation; abnormalities of thoracic kyphosis or cervical or lumbar lordosis
- Adam forward-bending test used to look for rib or paraspinous elevations
- Assess for leg length discrepancy, congenital anomalies, and neurologic abnormalities (including abnormal abdominal reflex)
- Special finding:
  – Crankshaft phenomenon:
    ○ Progression of curve size and rotation following posterior spinal fusion in a young child, result of continued anterior spinal growth
    ○ Patient is Risser 0, open triradiate cartilages, <10 years old, and prior to occurrence of peak height velocity (time of maximum spinal growth)
    ○ Consider anterior fusion in addition to posterior fusion
- Physical exam tricks:
  – Measure rib rotation with scoliometer test
  – Abnormal abdominal reflex may suggest intraspinal pathology, including syrinx
- Perform Adams forward test after the pelvis is leveled by inserting appropriately sized block underneath the short leg in patients with scoliosis and leg length discrepancy

---

DIAGNOSTIC TESTS & INTERPRETATION

Pulmonary function testing is useful preoperatively for more severe curves

Lab

Usually not helpful unless to rule out associated metabolic conditions

Imaging

- Plain standing posterior–anterior and lateral scoliosis films on long 3-foot radiograph cassette
- One must look for soft tissue and congenital bony abnormalities (Wedge vertebrae, bars, hemivertebrae)
- Curve is measured using Cobb method.
- The status of the triradiate cartilage and Risser classification of iliac apophysis ossification are indicators of maturity.
- The triradiate cartilage usually closes before the iliac apophysis appears (Risser 0).
- Risser sign is defined by the amount of calcification present in the iliac apophysis and measures the progressive ossification from anterolaterally to posteromedially.
  – A Risser grade of 1 signifies up to 25% ossification of the iliac apophysis, proceeding to grade 4, which signifies 100% ossification.
  – A Risser grade of 5 means the iliac apophysis has fused to the iliac crest after 100% ossification.
- MRI not routinely necessary for adult idiopathic scoliosis without back pain
- 7% prevalence of intraspinal abnormalities found in left thoracic curves, so MRI maybe indicated
- Curve patterns classified according to King or Lenke classifications
- Renal ultrasound or IVP used for evaluation of patient with congenital scoliosis (look for associated renal abnormalities)

DIFFERENTIAL DIAGNOSIS

- Adolescent idiopathic scoliosis (11–17 years)
- Juvenile idiopathic scoliosis (4–10 years)
- Infantile idiopathic scoliosis (0–3 years)
- Congenital scoliosis—due to bony abnormalities of the spine that are present at birth (failure of formation or segmentations of vertebrae)
- Scoliosis associated with neurofibromatosis

- Scoliosis associated with tumors (e.g., osteoid osteoma)
- Neuromuscular scoliosis (e.g., cerebral palsy, spina bifida, muscle disorders)
- Postural scoliosis (e.g., from leg length discrepancy):
  - No rib hump or rotation
  - Does not have fixed deformities
  - Disappears with forward bending
  - Long curve
  - No progression

 TREATMENT

ADDITIONAL TREATMENT
General Measures
- Treatment:
  - Concepts for treatment are based on severity of deformity and on likelihood of progression.
- Observation:
  - Curves <25 degrees:
    ○ Immature patients (Risser 0, 1, 2) should be re-evaluated in 4–6 months.
    ○ Skeletally mature patients (Risser 4 or 5) usually do not require ongoing follow-up unless special circumstances exist.
  - Curves 25–45 degrees in skeletally mature patients:
    ○ Risser 4 or 5 patients usually re-evaluated in 6 months to 1 year
    ○ Mature patients usually re-evaluated yearly

Additional Therapies
- Brace treatment:
  - Curves 25–45 degrees (Risser 0, 1) and 30–45 degrees (Risser 2 or 3):
    ○ Brace on initial evaluation
  - Curves ≥25 degrees (in Risser 0–3 patient) that have demonstrated >10 degrees progression during period of observation
    ○ Continue brace treatment until maturity (2 years postmenarchal and Risser 4 in females, Risser 5 in males)
- Brace types:
  - Thoracolumbosacral orthosis: Success reported when used >16–18 hours daily; significantly improved outcome when compared with natural history
  - Milwaukee: Seldom needed except for higher thoracic or cervical curves
  - Nighttime bending brace

SURGERY/OTHER PROCEDURES
- Recommended when curves exceed 45–50 degrees:
  - Exception: Balanced thoracic and lumbar curves <55 degrees may be observed for progression.
- Thoracic curves and double major curves:
  - Posterior segmental fixation instrumentation remains current state of the art.
  - Anterior spinal instrumentation for selected curves
  - The role of thoracoscopic technique being defined
- Isolated thoracolumbar and lumbar curves:
  - Anterior spinal fusion using solid rod segmental constructs

 ONGOING CARE

FOLLOW-UP RECOMMENDATIONS
Patient Monitoring
- Watch for back pain associated with idiopathic scoliosis (may indicate other diagnosis):
  - Present in 23% at time of initial evaluation (additional 9% during follow-up)
  - Of those with back pain, only 9% found to have identifiable cause such as spondylolysis, Scheuermann, syrinx, disc herniation, tumor, tether cord

PROGNOSIS
- Overall, good for most patients
- Risk of curve progression related to patient's maturity (Risser sign, menarchal status) and to size of curve
- Curves <20–25 degrees have low risk of progression, even if patient is immature.
- Curves 25–45 degrees have higher risk of progression, particularly in the immature patients.
- Curves >45–50 degrees have much higher risk of progression, regardless of maturity.

COMPLICATIONS
Natural history:
- Reduced pulmonary function for patients with thoracic curves >60 degrees
- Progression of lumbar curves >50 degrees in adult life with degenerative disc disease and pain in some
- Cosmetic and emotional issues

ADDITIONAL READING
- Kim YJ, Noonan KJ. What's new in pediatric orthopaedics. *J Bone Joint Surg Am.* 2009;91(3):743–751.
- Lowe TG, Edgar M, Margulies JY, et al. Etiology of idiopathic scoliosis: Current trends in research. *J Bone Joint Surg.* 2000;82:1157–1168.
- Shelton YA. Scoliosis and kyphosis in adolescents: Diagnosis and management. *Adolesc Med State Art Rev.* 2007;18(1):121–139.

 CODES

ICD9
- 737.30 Scoliosis idiopathic
- 737.32 Scoliosis infantile progressive
- 754.2 Congenital musculoskeletal deformities of spine

ICD10
- M41.20 Other idiopathic scoliosis, site unspecified
- M41.119 Juvenile idiopathic scoliosis, site unspecified
- M41.129 Adolescent idiopathic scoliosis, site unspecified

FAQ
- Q: How long do you observe a patient with spinal asymmetry before ordering a radiograph?
- A: It depends on the presence or absence of abnormalities on the physical exam. If any of the signs mentioned here are seen or significant back pain is present, a radiograph or referral is indicated. The scoliometer is also a useful tool in screening patients.
- Q: If a child presents with scoliosis and back pain that occurs especially at night and is relieved with aspirin, what diagnosis is suggested?
- A: Scoliosis is associated with osteoid osteoma.

S

SEBORRHEIC DERMATITIS

Kara N. Shah

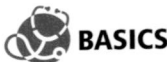 **BASICS**

DESCRIPTION
- An erythematous, scaly, greasy dermatitis that favors the sebaceous areas of the body, including the scalp, face, postauricular, central chest, and intertriginous areas
- The distribution pattern and clinical course varies with age. Infants commonly manifest predominantly self-limiting scalp involvement ("cradle cap"), while adults and adolescents more commonly demonstrate chronic involvement of the face, ears, and scalp.

GENERAL PREVENTION
Frequent washing with a medicated shampoo containing sulfur, selenium sulfide, salicylic acid, tar, corticosteroid, an antifungal agent, or zinc pyrithione or application of a medicated lotion, foam, gel or cream containing either one of the aforementioned compounds can reduce disease flares. There are no other preventive measures and modulation of dietary intake is of no benefit.

EPIDEMIOLOGY
- There are 2 populations in whom seborrheic dermatitis develops: Infants, in which seborrheic dermatitis usually develops after the first 3–4 weeks of life, peaks at age 3 months, and usually resolves by 1 year of age; and adolescents and adults, in whom it usually persists, although the disease may be seen in children of all ages.
- In adults, seborrheic dermatitis is more common in males.
- The development of seborrheic dermatitis during infancy does not predict the development of adolescent and/or adult disease.

Incidence
Although it is one of the more common skin diseases seen in infants as well as in adolescents and adults, the incidence of seborrheic dermatitis is unknown.

Prevalence
- Affects 2–5% of the adult population.
- Affects ~6% of children 2 to 10 years of age.
- Affects ~ 18% of infants <2 years of age.

RISK FACTORS
Genetics
Controversy exists as to whether there is a genetic predisposition. There is evidence that it is more common in families, but not spouses, of affected patients.

PATHOPHYSIOLOGY
- Although not an infection per se, there is increasing acceptance that the lipophilic yeast *Malassezia*, a commensal skin organism, is a contributing factor. Increased sebaceous gland activity likely favors the growth of *Malassezia*. The use of topical antifungal agents such as ketoconazole significantly decreases the number of *Malassezia* yeast in seborrheic dermatitis patients with subsequent clinical improvement.

- The local host immune response to *Malassezia* toxins or enzymes also plays a probable role in the development of seborrheic dermatitis. Seborrheic dermatitis is one of the most common cutaneous manifestations of AIDS in adults, where it can be particularly severe and recalcitrant to standard therapy.
- Androgen-mediated stimulation of sebaceous gland activity is likely important, given that seborrheic dermatitis presents in infancy and puberty.
- The histopathologic findings are nonspecific and include parakeratosis, acanthosis, spongiosis, elongation of the rete ridges, and a mild lymphocytic dermal inflammatory infiltrate.

ETIOLOGY
- A multifactorial disease influenced by both genetic and environmental factors
- It is not clear whether the infantile and adolescent/adult forms share a common etiology or whether they are distinct disorders.

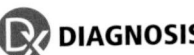 **DIAGNOSIS**

HISTORY
- Infants usually present after 3–4 weeks of life, with a peak prevalence at age 3 months and resolution usually by 1 year of age. It is generally asymptomatic. There may be a coexistent atopic dermatitis.
- Adolescents and adults usually present with a chronic, recurrent, often pruritic rash that begins sometime after puberty. Many patients have tried multiple treatments, including shampoos and medicated creams and/or lotions, with initial improvement but prompt recurrence after discontinuation.

PHYSICAL EXAM
- The characteristic lesions are erythematous scaling patches often with an orange/yellow hue and greasy in appearance. In persons with darker skin complexion, affected areas may appear as hypopigmented, scaling patches resembling tinea versicolor.
- In infants, seborrheic dermatitis most commonly involves the scalp ("cradle cap") but can also involve the face, neck, umbilicus, diaper area, and intertriginous areas. Cradle cap may appear as thick, greasy adherent scaling of the scalp. Rarely, infants may present with diffuse involvement of the head, neck, body and extremities.
- Adolescents and adults may present with a pruritic, scaling scalp dermatitis or with involvement of the face (favoring the perinasal areas, beard area, and eyebrows), postauricular area and external ear canals, and presternal area. Blepharitis with erythema and scaling of the eyelid margins may also occur.

DIAGNOSTIC TESTS & INTERPRETATION
Lab
- There are no specific tests for seborrhea.
- Microscopic examination with a potassium hydroxide wet mount preparation or a fungal culture of skin scrapings will differentiate seborrheic dermatitis from a dermatophyte infection.

Diagnostic Procedures/Surgery
Skin biopsy may be helpful if the presentation is unusual or in cases not responding to conventional therapy; however, findings are not necessarily diagnostic for seborrheic dermatitis.

DIFFERENTIAL DIAGNOSIS
- Infection:
  - Fungal infections with dermatophytes are commonly confused with seborrheic dermatitis. Tinea facei, tinea corporis, and tinea barbae usually cause localized scaly circinate inflammatory patches, although infection of hair follicles can result from misdiagnosis and treatment with topical steroids and often presents as an inflammatory plaque.
    - Tinea capitis presents most commonly with diffuse or patchy fine white adherent scaling on the scalp with broken hairs and/or patchy or diffuse hair loss. Cervical adenopathy is often present. Tinea capitis is primarily a disease of infants and prepubertal children.
    - Tinea versicolor presents with multiple small round to oval hypopigmented or hyperpigmented macules favoring the upper chest and back and typically sparing the face. Tinea versicolor is generally seen in adolescents and adults.
  - Dermatophyte infections can be differentiated by microscopic examination of hairs or skin scarapings using a potassium hydroxide wet mount preparation and by fungal culture.
- Malignancy:
  - Langerhans cell histiocytosis is an uncommon infiltrative disorder of monocytes, macrophages, and dendritic cells that may present with a scaly erythematous eruption on the scalp, behind the ears, or in the intertriginous regions. It is differentiated from seborrheic dermatitis by the presence of small reddish-brown crusted papules or vesicles, purpuric lesions, hepatosplenomegaly, and adenopathy. It is currently not clear whether Langerhans cell histiocytosis is a reactive or a neoplastic disease.

- Immunologic:
  - Atopic dermatitis usually begins in infancy and is characterized by a chronic, recurrent pruritic dermatitis that is usually seen in the context of a personal or family history of atopy.
    ○ Atopic dermatitis in infants favors the face (but typically spares the perinasal and periocular areas) and extensor aspects of the extremities and spares the diaper area.
    ○ In children and adults, atopic dermatitis favors the flexural aspects of the extremities but may also involve the face, scalp, and trunk.
    ○ Some infants and adolescents manifest features of both atopic dermatitis and seborrheic dermatitis.
  - Psoriasis vulgaris in children and adults is characterized by symmetric, well-demarcated erythematous plaques with a thick white micaceous scale
    ○ Lesions favor the extensor aspects of the extremities.
    ○ Scalp involvement is common and present with erythematous scaly plaques in the scalp.
    ○ Other features of psoriasis include characteristic nail changes such as nail pitting and onycholysis.
    ○ In infants, psoriasis may involve the diaper area and other intertriginous areas or may present with diffuse involvement of the trunk, face, and extremities.
    ○ It is generally accepted that there is often an overlap in the clinical manifestations of psoriasis and seborrheic dermatitis, which is often referred to as "sebopsoriasis."
  - Leiner disease results in a severe generalized erythematous, exfoliative dermatitis accompanied by severe diarrhea, recurrent infections, and failure to thrive. It may result from a number of nutritional and immunologic disorders, such as acrodermatitis enteropathica, severe combined immunodeficiency syndrome, and complement deficiencies.

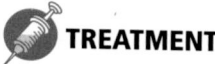 **TREATMENT**

ADDITIONAL TREATMENT
General Measures
- In infants, mild scalp seborrhea can be treated with intermittent use of a mild shampoo.
  - A sulfur or salicylic acid shampoo (i.e., Sebulex) may be used for several days as needed.
  - Scales can be loosened with application of mineral oil or baby oil followed by gentle brushing or combing of the scalp to loosen scales.
- Persistent scalp seborrhea and seborrheic dermatitis involving the face, diaper area, and body will usually respond to treatment with a short course of a low-potency topical corticosteroid lotion or cream or to a topical antifungal such as ketoconazole cream.
- Adolescents with mild scalp seborrhea often respond to intermittent use of a shampoo with zinc pyrithione (e.g., Head & Shoulders), selenium sulfide (e.g., Selsun), a topical corticosteroid (e.g. Capex) or tar (e.g., Neutrogena T-Gel).
  - Those with more erythema, scaling, and/or and severe pruritus may consider treatment with a medium-potency topical corticosteroid solution or foam.

- Dense, diffuse scalp involvement may be treated overnight for several days as needed with a topical corticosteroid such as Derma-Smoothe/FS lotion, Luxiq foam or fluocinonide 0.05% solution.
  - Ketoconazole or clobetasol shampoo is an alternative therapy.
- Seborrheic dermatitis of the face and body may be treated with a low-potency topical corticosteroid lotion, foam, gel or cream, a topical antifungal cream such as ketoconazole; with a topical sulfur/sulfacetamide wash, lotion, or cream (e.g. Clenia; or with one of the topical calcineurin inhibitors, tacrolimus ointment and pimecrolimus cream, which have anti-inflammatory properties and have also been shown to have potent antifungal activity against *Malassezia in vitro*.
- If the seborrheic dermatitis is particularly widespread, severe, or is refractory to topical treatment, oral ketoconazole has been shown to be effective.
- Blepharitis should be treated with warm water compresses, cleansing with a gentle shampoo, and if necessary, application of sodium sulfacetamide ophthalmic ointment or cautious application of a topical calcineurin inhibitor such as Elidel 1% cream or Protopic 0.1% ointment to the eyelid margins.
  - Topical steroids may be effective, but the side effects of its use around the eye (such as glaucoma) make this a poor choice for chronic therapy.

 ONGOING CARE

- In infants, seborrheic dermatitis self-resolves by the age of 1 year, but often requires intermittent therapy until resolution occurs.
- Although some improvement should be seen with treatment by 10–14 days, long-term intermittent therapy may be required, especially in adolescents in whom seborrheic dermatitis is often chronic.
- Seborrhea may rarely be complicated by secondary bacterial or candidal infections, which present with erythema, tenderness, and ulceration.
- Patients who are intermittently using topical corticosteroids should be monitored for the development of adverse effects, including local cutaneous atrophy, dyspigmentation, and striae.
- Seborrhea may be caused or complicated by associated underlying disorders, including immunodeficiency diseases such as AIDS, which should be considered in cases that are resistant to treatment.

PROGNOSIS
- The infantile form will self-resolve by the end of the first year of life.
- The adolescent form may persist into adulthood.

ADDITIONAL READING
- Cohen S. Should we treat infantile seborrheic dermatitis with topical antifungals or topical steroids? *Arch Dis Child*. 2004;89:288–289.
- Gupta AK, Bluhm R, Cooper EA, et al. Seborrheic dermatitis. *Dermatol Clin*. 2003;21:401–412.
- Gupta AK, Madzia SE, Batra R. Etiology and management of seborrheic dermatitis. *Dermatology*. 2004;208:89–93.
- Poindexter GB, Burkhart CN, Morrell DS. Therapies for pediatric seborrheic dermatitis. *Pediatr Ann*. 2009;38:333–338.
- Williams JV, Eichenfield LF, Burke BL, et al. Prevalence of scalp scaling in prepubertal children. *Pediatrics*. 2005;115:e1–e6.

 CODES

ICD9
- 690.10 Seborrheic dermatitis, unspecified
- 690.11 Seborrhea capitis
- 690.12 Seborrheic infantile dermatitis

ICD10
- L21.0 Seborrhea capitis
- L21.1 Seborrheic infantile dermatitis
- L21.9 Seborrheic dermatitis, unspecified

FAQ
- Q: Does therapy speed resolution of the disorder?
- A: Treatment does not appear to influence the underlying cause of this disorder, which appears to be caused by hormonally-mediated sebaceous gland activity, skin colonization with the lipophilic yeast *Malassezia* and the resultant local inflammatory response.
- Q: Shouldn't the use of topical corticosteroids worsen the dermatitis if it is caused by a fungal infection?
- A: Topical corticosteroids are commonly used to treat seborrheic dermatitis. These agents seem to work because of their anti-inflammatory effect. Although in the past high-potency steroids were used for this indication, adverse effects are associated with their prolonged use. Currently, low-potency corticosteroids or non-steroidal therapies are preferred.
- Q: Does seborrheic dermatitis cause permanent hair loss?
- A: Patients can be reassured that it does not cause permanent hair loss.

SEIZURES-FEBRILE

Juliann Paolicchi
Eric Masch (5th edition)
Amy R. Brooks-Kayal (5th edition)

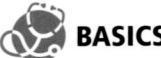 **BASICS**

DESCRIPTION
- Simple febrile seizures (FS): Single, brief (<15 minutes), generalized seizures during fever (rise or fall) in developmentally and neurologically normal children usually between 6 months and 5 years of age without intracranial infection
- Complex febrile seizures: Febrile seizures that either last >15 minutes, have focal features or postictal focal weakness, or recur within 24 hours
- Febrile status epilepticus: continuous or intermittent seizures without neurologic recovery for a period of 30 minutes or longer. (See status epilepticus.)
- Febrile seizure syndrome: Generalized epilepsy with febrile seizures plus (GEFS+): Febrile seizures with generalized tonic–clonic seizures, complex partial seizures, and absence seizures. Strong family history of similar seizures.

EPIDEMIOLOGY
Strongly age dependent: 90% between 6 months and 3 years with the peak period between 12 and 18 months. 4% occur before 6 months, and 6% after age 3.

Incidence
Typically, 2–4% of children <5 years of age; however, in certain populations, the incidence can be as high as 15%.

Genetics
- Inheritance: Multifactorial in most cases. To date, at least 5 different genetic loci have been identified.
- Febrile seizure syndrome: Multiple genes identified including *SCN1A*, *SCN2A*, *SCN1B*, and GABA(A) gamma 2 subunit genes

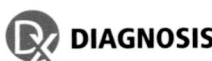 **DIAGNOSIS**

HISTORY
- Previous history of FS, afebrile seizures, neurologic or developmental abnormality

Presence of neurologic and developmental abnormality increases risk of subsequent epilepsy. Occurrence of previous afebrile seizures suggests a seizure precipitated by fever, as opposed to febrile seizure.

- Diagnosis of FS after age 6 years is unusual.
- Precipitating factors: Degree and duration of fever; symptoms and duration of intercurrent illness, recent history of head trauma, possibility of ingestion of toxic substance
  - Degree of fever is variable, and 25% of FS occurs between 38 and 39C.
  - FS is most common at the onset of fever and may be the first sign of illness.
  - Low fever, ingestion, head trauma, or prolonged illness before seizure suggest cause other than fever alone.
- Past medical history: Gestation, birth, general health, growth and development, and current medications.
- Family history: Both febrile and afebrile seizures can be hereditary. A family history of febrile seizures is typically present.
- Neurologic findings: Recent onset of headaches, vomiting not in the setting of GI illness, lethargy, weakness, sensory deficits, or changes in vision, behavior, balance, or gait suggests underlying brain pathology or infection and the need for neuroimaging and/or lumbar puncture.

PHYSICAL EXAM
- Vital signs:
  - Degree of fever
  - Tachycardia or hypotension (suggests sepsis)
  - Tachypnea (suggests respiratory infection)
  - Head circumference
- Signs of head trauma or possible abuse: Retinal hemorrhages and evidence of intracranial hypertension such as bulging fontanelle should be noted on head, eyes, ears, nose, and throat (HEENT) exam
- Possible meningitis: Kernig and Brudzinski signs, nuchal rigidity,
  - NOTE: These signs are less reliable in children <12 months of age, especially if <6 months of age.
- Careful neurologic examination: Specific attention should be directed to mental status and any focal abnormalities of motor strength, tone, sensation, or gait if relevant.

DIAGNOSTIC TESTS & INTERPRETATION
EEG:
- Not indicated after simple febrile seizure, and not indicated acutely
- Should be considered in children who are neurologically abnormal, experience recurrent complex febrile seizures or in whom the history is suggests a cause other than fever alone.
- EEG abnormalities have not been shown to have a correlation with either recurrence of FS or the development of epilepsy.

Lab
- Routine testing:
  - Not indicated for simple FS
  - May be indicated for the cause of the fever: i.e., tox screen if ingestion identified in history, electrolytes and glucose in the setting of fever, vomiting, and diarrhea.
- Lumbar puncture: Should be performed in any child in whom CNS infection is suspected, especially children <12 months of age because clinical signs of meningitis are less reliable. Any older child who appears toxic and has meningeal or other clinical signs suggesting CNS infection should undergo a lumbar puncture.
- AAP recommendations for LP in FS include:
  - Meningeal signs
  - Infants 6–12 months in whom the immunization status for *Haemophilus influenzae* type B or *Streptococcus pneumoniae* is deficient or unknown
  - Children on antibiotic therapy

ALERT
- Infants presenting with FS may have serious bacterial infections (bacteremia, meningitis, or sepsis) underlying fever without meningeal signs.
- Prolonged FS with focal features can be associated with HSV encephalitis. Both conditions are indications for lumbar puncture.

Imaging
Acute imaging (CT or MRI) recommended in children with febrile status epilepticus, have a large head circumference, or a persistent neurologic deficit including unresponsiveness, focal features on neurologic examination, and signs of increased intracranial pressure.

Non-emergent head MRI:

- Reserved for children with:
  - Complex (focal or prolonged) febrile seizures
  - Focal neurologic deficits, even transitory, after seizure
  - Focal abnormality on EEG other than postictal slowing.

DIFFERENTIAL DIAGNOSIS

- History, physical exam, and as indicated earlier, lumbar puncture and acute neuroimaging are usually sufficient to exclude non-epileptic causes of seizures:
  - Chills due to fever in an ill child
  - CNS infection
  - Anoxia/stroke/hemorrhage
  - Trauma
  - Intoxication
  - Metabolic encephalopathy
  - Neurodegenerative disorder
  - Brain lesion or tumor
  - Epileptic conditions
    - Previous history of afebrile seizures
    - Certain neurogenetic conditions present with seizures in the setting of high fevers, i.e., Angelman and Dravet syndrome
    - Neurocutaneous syndromes (tuberous sclerosis, Sturge–Weber, neurofibromatosis)
    - Previous brain injury (history of stroke, CNS infection, hemorrhage, birth asphyxia, cerebral palsy)

 TREATMENT

ADDITIONAL TREATMENT
General Measures
- Treatment of single FS not indicated
- Antiepileptic medication is typically reserved for children in whom diagnosis of epilepsy is established with neurologic evaluation.
  - Anti-epileptic medication does not prevent the subsequent development of epilepsy.
- Abortive therapy is recommended in children with complex FS, and recurrent simple FS.
- Treatment with antipyretics does not significantly affect the recurrence rate of FS.
- The AAP does not recommend continuous or intercurrent treatment with anti-epileptic medication for recurrent simple FS, but does recognize that recurrence "can increase anxiety in some parents and their children and as such appropriate educational and emotional support should be provided."

MEDICATION (DRUGS)
- Primary therapy is abortive. Rectal diazepam, 0.3–0.5 mg/kg, can be administered at time of febrile seizure if it persists for >5 minutes.
  - Focality and a prolonged FS, >10 minutes; more likely to have recurrence; Therapy with abortive medication should be considered with the first incidence of FS.

- Oral administration or diazepam, 0.3 mg/kg q8h, during febrile illnesses reduces risk of recurrent febrile seizures; however, causes sedation, and is typically useful only for children with a history of recurrent FS within an illness.
- Antiepileptic medications that have been studied to be effective in recurrent FS include phenobarbital, valproate, and primidone but had limiting side effects in 40% of patients in a recent analysis.
- Phenytoin and carbamazepine are ineffective as prophylaxis.
- There is limited data to support the use levetiracetam for FS.

 ONGOING CARE

PROGNOSIS
- Recurrent FS occur in 30% of children with FS, and 50% of children with recurrence have a third FS.
- The four predictors of occurrence are age at onset, FS in a first degree relative, low precipitating fever, and short duration between fever onset and seizure. The risk factors are cumulative: 70% with 4 factors, 20% with none.
- Age of presentation is the strongest predictor of recurrence: 50–60% of infants <12 months have recurrence.
- 90% of recurrences occur within 2 years, 75% within 1 year, and 50% within 6 months
- Overall, the risk of children with FS developing epilepsy is 2%, compared with 1% in the general population.
- Risk factors for the development of epilepsy include: focal, prolonged, and recurrent seizures. The risk factors were cumulative: 25% higher in children with 3 factors compared with none.
- No evidence that occasional febrile seizures or even febrile status epilepticus causes subsequent neurologic or cognitive deficits.

OTHER
NIH Febrile Seizures Fact Sheet: http://www.ninds.nih.gov/disorders/febrile_seizures/detail_febrile_seizures.htm

ADDITIONAL READING

- Baumann RJ, Duffner PK. Treatment of children with simple febrile seizures: The AAP practice parameter. American Academy of Pediatrics. *Pediatr Neurol*. 2000;23:11–17.
- Norgaard M, Ehrenstein V, Mahon BE, et al. Febrile seizures and cognitive function in young adult life: A prevalence study in Danish conscripts. *J Pediatr*. 2009;155:404.
- Patient Information Web site: http://www.epilepsy.com
- Strengell T, Uhari M, Tarkka R, et al. Antipyretic agents for preventing recurrences of febrile seizures: Randomized controlled trial. *Arch Pediatr Med*. 2009;163:799.
- Subcommittee on Febrile Seizures. Neurodiagnostic evaluation of the child with a simple febrile seizure. *Pediatrics*. 2011;127:389.

 CODES

ICD9
- 780.31 Febrile convulsions (simple), unspecified
- 780.32 Complex febrile convulsions

ICD10
- R56.00 Simple febrile convulsions
- R56.01 Complex febrile convulsions

FAQ

- Q: What should be done if the child has another febrile seizure?
- A: Emergency measures include placement of the child recumbent or supine with head turned to avoid aspiration. Place nothing in the mouth. Abortive therapy should be initiated at 5 minutes of seizure activity. If not available, EMT services should be activated. For children who have had prolonged or recurrent series of seizures, instructions to administer rectal diazepam are recommended.
- Q: What restrictions should be placed on general activity of a child with recurrent febrile seizures?
- A: No specific activity restrictions are recommended. Children at risk for recurrent seizures are recommended not to swim or bathe unattended, sleep in a top bunk bed, climb to high places, and wear a helmet when biking or using any wheeled toy.

S

SEIZURES, PARTIAL AND GENERALIZED

Juliann M. Paolicchi
Eric Masch (5th edition)
Amy R. Brooks-Kayal (5th edition)

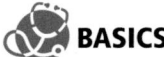 **BASICS**

DESCRIPTION
Seizures arise from abnormal, excessive, electrical neuronal discharges in the cerebral cortex that lead to alterations of consciousness, behavior, motor activity, sensation, or autonomic function. Epilepsy is defined as 2 or more seizures without acute provocation.

Seizures are classified as partial (begin in local area of cerebral cortex) and primary generalized (begin simultaneously in both hemispheres).

- Partial seizures types:
  - Simple partial (consciousness not impaired)
  - Complex partial (consciousness impaired)
  - Partial seizures evolving to generalized tonic–clonic convulsions
- Primary generalized seizure types:
  - Absence, atypical absence, myoclonic, tonic, atonic, tonic–clonic

EPIDEMIOLOGY
Incidence
1% of children will have 1 seizure by age 14 years. The highest incidence is in infancy. In childhood, 30% of 1st seizures occur before age 4 years and nearly 80% occur before age 20 years.

Prevalence
4–9 per 1,000 children in developed countries have epilepsy.

RISK FACTORS
- Developmental disability present in 35% of children who develop epilepsy
- Active neurologic disease/illness (CNS infection, trauma, hemorrhage/stroke)
- History of previous seizure
- Recent withdrawal of anticonvulsant medication
- History of remote neurologic insult (stroke, intracranial hemorrhage, cerebral palsy, head trauma, meningitis)
- Family history of seizures
- Brain tumor
- Neurodegenerative disorder

Genetics
- Idiopathic seizures: A multifactorial pattern
- Epilepsy syndromes with defined genetic loci: Generalized epilepsy with febrile seizures, autosomal dominant nocturnal frontal lobe epilepsy, benign familial neonatal convulsions, severe myoclonic epilepsy of infancy
- Other epilepsy syndromes (benign rolandic, childhood, juvenile absence, juvenile myoclonic epilepsy) are heterogeneous or show autosomal dominant pattern with variable penetrance.

DIAGNOSIS

HISTORY
- Age, family history of seizures/epilepsy, developmental status
- Health at seizure onset: Febrile, ill, exposed to illness, complaints of not feeling well, sleep deprived.
- Precipitating events other than illness: Trauma, toxins, ingestion, previous head injury

- Current medications and change in antiepileptic medication
- Other neurologic signs: Confusion, encephalopathy, weakness, sensory deficits, and change in vision, behavior, balance, or gait
- Detailed history of symptoms during seizure
  - Aura: Subjective sensations
  - Behavior: Preceding and during seizure
  - Loss of consciousness
  - Vocal: Cry, gasp, speech
  - Motor: Head or eye turning or deviation; jerking, posturing, stiffening, automatisms. Important to determine if generalized or focal
  - Respiration: Cyanosis, change in breathing pattern
  - Autonomic: Papillary dilatation, drooling, incontinence, pallor, vomiting
- Symptoms after seizure: Amnesia, confusion, sleepiness, lethargy, transient focal weakness (Todd's paresis)

PHYSICAL EXAM
- Vital signs: ABCs need to be checked immediately, and recurrently, if child continues to seize or be unresponsive.
- Fever, tachycardia/bradycardia, or hypertension
- Signs of head trauma and child abuse: Retinal hemorrhages, evidence of intracranial hypertension, presence of fractures, bruising
- Head circumference/abnormal head growth: Microcephaly
- Signs of systemic infection: Meningismus (CNS infection), unresponsiveness
- Skin examination: Café au lait or ash leaf spots; facial hemangioma, suggesting neurocutaneous disorders
- Neurologic examination: Pupillary asymmetries, altered mental status, fixed eye deviations, and focal motor weakness (Todd's paralysis) suggest focal onset of seizures and possible underlying structural lesion.
- Seizures: If there is a question of continuing seizures, proceed with recommendations for "Status Epilepticus."

ALERT
- Attention to adequate airway and breathing and need for oxygenation or ventilatory support is the primary focus at presentation. A serum glucose level should be assessed as soon as possible.
- If the child continues to seize or has recurrent seizures, administration of an abortive benzodiazepine should be administered either rectally or IV.

DIAGNOSTIC TESTS & INTERPRETATION
Lab
- Glucose
- Oximetry or arterial blood gas indicated if child is actively seizing
- The standard laboratory evaluation of electrolytes, blood urea nitrogen. CBC, liver enzymes, calcium, and magnesium did not show unsuspected abnormalities or contribute to the diagnosis or management in 2 Class 1, and 2 Class 2 studies.
- Antiepileptic drug (AED) levels if indicated. Few of the newer AEDs have relevant serum levels.

- Testing should be based on clinical history (i.e., vomiting, diarrhea, dehydration, or continued unresponsiveness) and toxicology screening in any child in whom there is a question of drug exposure from substance abuse.

Imaging
- Neuroimaging: Based on evidence-based reviews that showed low yields of emergent CT or MRI in children presenting with seizures without focal signs or deficits, current recommendations are:
  - MRI is the preferred modality overall.
  - Emergent neuroimaging, either CT or MRI, should be performed in any child with a postictal focal deficit (Todd's paresis) or who remains unresponsive postictally.
  - Nonurgent MRI recommended for children with: cognitive or motor impairment of unknown etiology, abnormalities on neurologic examination, focal seizures, children <1 year of age, or abnormal EEG findings other than benign partial epilepsy or a primary generalized epilepsy.

Diagnostic Procedures/Other
- EEG:
  - Indicated urgently if the patient fails to awaken within hours after convulsions cease (children with neurologic deficits may have longer recovery), or if there is concern that child may be continuing to seize.
  - Nonurgent EEGs indicated for 1st afebrile seizure or complicated febrile seizure.
- Lumbar puncture: Meningeal signs, infants <6 months of age, or alteration of consciousness; if intracranial hypertension, mass lesion, or hydrocephalus suspected, defer lumbar puncture until after neuroimaging.

DIFFERENTIAL DIAGNOSIS
- Nonepileptic events:
  - Syncope
  - Breath-holding spells
  - Hyperventilation
  - Psychogenic seizures
  - Movements related to gastroesophageal reflux (Sandifer syndrome)
  - Sleep disorders: Benign sleep myoclonus, night terrors, somnambulism, narcolepsy–cataplexy
  - Migraine/headache syndromes, especially complicated migraine
  - Nonepileptic movements: Startle disease, shuddering spells, paroxysmal dyskinesias, tics, drug-induced dystonia
  - Behavioral: Stereotypies, self-stimulatory behaviors, inattention/ADHD
- Definite seizure or epilepsy (e.g., generalized tonic–clonic, complex partial, absence, myoclonic, tonic, atonic):
  - Idiopathic (presumed genetic)
  - Remote symptomatic (previous history of stroke, intracranial hemorrhage, birth asphyxia, head trauma, meningitis)
  - Acute symptomatic: CNS infection, anoxia, trauma, stroke/hemorrhage, intoxication, metabolic encephalopathy, anticonvulsant withdrawal
  - Neurodegenerative disorder
  - Brain tumor
  - Malformations of cortical development (lissencephaly, agenesis of corpus callosum, holoprosencephaly)

– Neurocutaneous syndromes (tuberous sclerosis, Sturge-Weber syndrome, neurofibromatosis)
– Febrile seizure: Seizure associated with fever in children <6 years of age with no history of afebrile seizures. Children younger than 6 months should undergo lumbar puncture (see "Seizures, Febrile" chapter).

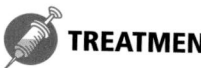

TREATMENT

MEDICATION (DRUGS)
- The choice of AED for long-term management of epilepsy depends on the specific seizure type. Monotherapy always preferred
- Many formulations, such as liquid, sprinkle capsules, and extended-release forms are available, and should be individualized to the patient. For teenagers, extended-release forms are recommended for compliance.
- Partial-onset seizures (with or without secondary generalization):
  – Oxcarbazepine: 20–40 mg/kg/d
  – Levetiracetam: Initial dosing of 10–20 mg/kg/d and increase to 60 mg/kg/d
  – Additional options:
    ○ Lamotrigine: 5–15 mg/kg/d in patients not taking valproate, 1–5 mg/kg/d in patients on valproate
    ○ Topiramate: 4–10 mg/kg/d; build up dose slowly to minimize cognitive side effects.
    ○ Valproate: 10–15 mg/kg/d, increased to 20–60 mg/kg/d for blood levels of 50–100 mg/d
    ○ Zonisamide: Initial dosing 1–2 mg/kg/d and increase to maximum dose of 10 mg/kg/d in nightly or b.i.d. dosing
- Acute treatment of seizures:
  – Fosphenytoin: 20 mEq of phenytoin per kg IM/IV and phenobarbital 10–20 mg/kg IV used less for chronic maintenance therapy (cognitive, behavioral, cosmetic effects)
- Primary generalized epilepsies (including absence, myoclonic, tonic, or clonic seizures): Ethosuximide, 15–40 mg/kg/d in 2 divided doses = initial AED for absence seizures. Titration is based on efficacy (seizure freedom) and EEG normalization.
- Alternatives for generalized seizures: Valproate, lamotrigine, topiramate, levetiracetam, rufinamide, and zonisamide. Adverse effects of valproate include thrombocytopenia, pancreatitis, hyperammonemia, and fatal hepatotoxicity. CBC and liver function tests should be routinely monitored. Children <5 years and on polytherapy (more than 1 AED) have an increased risk of hepatotoxicity from valproate, and children <10 years have an increased risk of serious rash from lamotrigine.
- Prolonged seizures (>5 minutes) or acute repetitive seizures: Rectal diazepam (0.3–0.5 mg/kg per dose) can be administered by parents/caregivers. Effective at stopping the seizure with minimal risk of respiratory depression.
- Patients refractory to AED treatment: Other options—ketogenic diet, vagus nerve stimulator, surgical resection

ALERT
- Hyponatremic seizures: Serum sodium <120 mEq/dL in infants with gastroenteritis. Slow sodium correction indicated
- Apnea and hypoventilation from excessive administration of benzodiazepines, phenobarbital for seizures. Monitor ventilation and oxygenation; avoid large doses.

ADDITIONAL TREATMENT

General Measures
- Chronic AED therapy is not indicated after acute symptomatic seizures (transient metabolic disturbances [e.g., hyponatremia, intoxication]) or after a single unprovoked seizure in a child with normal neurologic examination and EEG.
- Chronic AED therapy may be considered after 1st seizure symptomatic of an acute, structural brain lesion (i.e., brain tumor).

ALERT
A 2-fold risk of increased suicidality has been associated with AED use, with an FDA black box warning on product labeling. Monitoring for suicidal ideation and mood changes is warranted in all patients taking AEDs.

ONGOING CARE

PROGNOSIS
- In a child who is neurologically normal with an unprovoked seizure, the risk of recurrence is 24% in 1 year and 45% in 14 years.
- If there is evidence of prior neurologic insult, the risk of recurrence is 37% in 1 year.
- If the patient has 2 seizures separated by >24 hours, risk is 70% in 1 year.
- The EEG is the most significant predictor of recurrence: 15% risk in 1 year in a child with a normal EEG and 41% with an abnormal EEG.
- The risk is increased (up to 80%) in children with abnormal examinations, focally abnormal EEGs, onset of seizure in sleep, positive familial history of seizures, partial seizures, or postictal (Todd's) paralysis.

COMPLICATIONS
- Brain damage:
  – From brief seizures: No convincing evidence
  – From prolonged seizures (>30 minutes): Brain injury may occur secondary to hypoxia (respiratory compromise).
  – Untreated or poorly controlled epilepsy: Increased risk of intractable epilepsy syndromes, sudden unexplained death (SUDEP)
- Injuries: Rarely, serious injury occurs with brief seizures from loss of consciousness and resultant falls (see "Safety" below).
- Daily precautions: Few restrictions are needed with the exceptions of driving (see state laws), operating heavy machinery, or dangerous sports, such as scuba diving, parachuting, or rock climbing.
- Supervised bathing and swimming, showering safer than bathing, helmets with all wheeled toys (bikes, scooters, skateboards); avoid top bunk beds or locked bedrooms, and heights.
- Chronic epilepsy is associated with inattention, depression, and deficits in memory and academic performance.
- Patient monitoring: Dependent on treatment and as mentioned above

ADDITIONAL READING

- Arthur TM, deGrauw TJ, Johnson CS, et al. Seizure recurrence risk following a first seizure in neurologically normal children. *Epilepsia*. 2008; 49:1950–1954.
- Epilepsy Foundation. *Answer place: Parent information on the Internet*. Available at: http://www.epilepsyfoundation.org/answerplace.
- Glauser TA, Cnaan A, Shinnar S, et al. Ethosuximide, valproic acid, and lamotrigine in childhood absence epilepsy. *N Engl J Med*. 2010;362:790.
- Hamiwka LD, Wirrell ED. Comorbidities in pediatric epilepsy: Beyond "just" treating the seizures. *J Child Neurol*. 2009;24(6):734–742.
- Hirtz D, Ashwal S, Berg A, et al. Practice parameter: Evaluating a first nonfebrile seizures in children. *Neurology*. 2000;55:616–623.
- Sogawa Y, Masur D, O'Dell C, et al. Cognitive outcomes in children who present with a first unprovoked seizures. *Epilepsia*. 2010;51(12): 2432–2439.

S

CODES

ICD9
- 345.90 Epilepsy, unspecified, without mention of intractable epilepsy
- 780.39 Other convulsions

ICD10
- G40.101 Localization-related (focal) (partial) symptomatic epilepsy and epileptic syndromes with simple partial seizures, not intractable, with status epilepticus
- G40.109 Localization-related (focal) (partial) symptomatic epilepsy and epileptic syndromes with simple partial seizures, not intractable, without status epilepticus
- G40.901 Epilepsy, unspecified, not intractable, with status epilepticus

FAQ

- Q: How do I know my child has epilepsy?
- A: The term "epilepsy" is applied to children with 2 or more seizures without an acute cause.
- Q: Will my child always have epilepsy?
- A: The likelihood of outgrowing epilepsy depends on the syndrome. In many cases, anticonvulsants can be discontinued if the child has been seizure free for 2 years.
- Q: Why take an antiepileptic medication?
- A: The purpose of antiepileptic medication is to decrease further seizures. They do not, however, affect the long-term course of epilepsy.
- Q: Why did my child's seizures change?
- A: Generalized tonic–clonic seizures may arise in childhood absence epilepsy; children may develop different epilepsy syndromes. Medications may make seizures milder, or can become less effective.

SEPARATION ANXIETY DISORDER

Ushama Patel

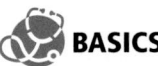 **BASICS**

DESCRIPTION
- Separation anxiety is characterized by developmentally inappropriate and excessive anxiety about being apart from the individuals to whom a child is most attached.
- Frequently, the individual worries excessively that harm may come either to a parent or an attachment figure or himself or herself, which would result in their separation.

EPIDEMIOLOGY
The prevalence is 3.5%. It is slightly higher in females than males.

ETIOLOGY
- Temperament is that of behavioral inhibition which is a child's tendency to approach unfamiliar situations with distress, restraint, and avoidance
- Insecure attachment between mother and child
- Increased parental anxiety
- Parenting style of being excessively controlling and overprotective
- Exposure to negative life events

COMMONLY ASSOCIATED CONDITIONS
- Depression (62%)
- Simple phobia (46%)
- Social phobia (34%)
- Generalized anxiety disorder (29%)
- Obsessive compulsive disorder (10%)
- Alcohol abuse in adolescence

 DIAGNOSIS

- Separation anxiety is a normative part of development, typically beginning around 6 or 7 months of age, peaking around 18 months and decreasing after 30 months.
- DSM IV criteria are:
  - Developmentally inappropriate and excessive anxiety concerning separation from home or from those to whom the individual is attached, as evidenced by 3 (or more) of the following:
    - Recurrent excessive distress when separation from home or major attachment figures occurs or is anticipated
    - Persistent and excessive worry about losing, or about possible harm befalling, major attachment figures
    - Persistent and excessive worry that an untoward event will lead to separation from a major attachment figure (e.g., getting lost or being kidnapped)
    - Persistent reluctance or refusal to go to school or elsewhere because of fear of separation
    - Persistently and excessively fearful or reluctant to be alone or without major attachment figures at home or without significant adults in other settings
    - Persistent reluctance or refusal to go to sleep without being near a major attachment figure or to sleep away from home
    - Repeated nightmares involving the theme of separation
    - Repeated complaints of physical symptoms (such as headaches, stomachaches, nausea, or vomiting) when separation from major attachment figures occurs or is anticipated
  - Duration of disturbance is at least 4 weeks.
  - Onset is before age 18 years.
  - Disturbance causes clinically significant distress or impairment in social, academic, or other important areas (occupational).

HISTORY
- Overwhelming fear of losing or becoming separated from a parent
- Child fears that separation could be due to death, kidnapping, or serious accident.
- Nightmares about separation
- Avoidance behaviors such as procrastination during the morning routine before school or refusing to leave the side of a parent
- Somatic complaints such as stomachaches and headaches
- Interferes with normative development in a number of ways such as difficulty attending school, participating in extracurricular activities, and attending sleepovers

PHYSICAL EXAM
There are no pertinent findings on physical exam.

DIAGNOSTIC TESTS & INTERPRETATION
Lab
- There are no pertinent findings on lab work.
- Scales:
  - CGI (Clinical Global Impressions) improvement scale
  - Pediatric anxiety scale

DIFFERENTIAL DIAGNOSIS
- Generalized anxiety disorder where anxiety is generalized
- Social anxiety where anxiety is during social situations
- Specific phobia where anxiety is due to a specific object
- Panic disorder where anxiety is focused on the fear of having a panic attack

TREATMENT

MEDICATION (DRUGS)
- Selective serotonin reuptake inhibitors (SSRIs; first-line): Initiate half the starting dose for children with anxiety disorders
- Side effects include GI upset, headaches, dizziness, and agitation.
- There is a black-box warning by the FDA indicating that all antidepressants may increase suicidal thinking and behavior in children and adolescents.
- Fluoxetine (Prozac) (10–60 mg)
- Sertraline (Zoloft) (25–200 mg)
- Paroxetine (Paxil) (10–40 mg)
- Benzodiazepines—side effects include sedation, dizziness, and weakness.
- Lorazepam
- Clonazepam
- Alprazolam

ADDITIONAL TREATMENT
General Measures
- Psychosocial
  - Psychosocial treatment of choice is cognitive behavioral therapy.
- Pharmacological
  - First-line choice of pharmacological treatment is SSRI.
  - Second line of choice is a tricyclic antidepressant (trials show less compliance due to side effects).
  - Benzodiazepines can be considered on a short-term basis alone or in combination with SSRI or TCA while waiting for SSRI or TCA to reach a therapeutic level.

Additional Therapies
- Psychosocial treatment:
  - Cognitive behavioral therapy
  - Individual psychotherapy
  - Group therapy
  - Behavior modification
  - Psychoeducation
  - Family therapy

 ONGOING CARE

FOLLOW-UP RECOMMENDATIONS
Patient Monitoring
- Monitoring of response to psychosocial treatment should be performed routinely every 2–3 months.
- If medication is initiated, close monitoring on a weekly basis is recommended for the first 4 weeks followed by monthly monitoring.
- Cognitive behavioral therapy is performed on a weekly or twice weekly regimen.
- Monitoring of any emerging comorbidities is suggested.

PROGNOSIS
- Generally favorable course and outcome
- Separation anxiety disorder may be a precursor to panic disorder in adulthood.

ADDITIONAL READING
- Albano AM, Chorpita BF, Barlow DH. Childhood anxiety disorders. In: Mash EJ, Barkley RA, eds. *Child psychopathology*. New York: Guilford, 1996:196–241.
- Allen AJ, Leonard H, Swedo SE. Current knowledge of medications for the treatment of childhood anxiety disorders. *J Am Acad Child Adolesc Psychiatry*. 1995;34:976–986.
- American Psychiatric Association. *Diagnostic and statistical manual of mental disorders*, 4th ed. Washington, DC: American Psychiatric Association, 1994.

CODES

ICD9
309.21 Separation anxiety disorder

ICD10
F93.0 Separation anxiety disorder of childhood

S

SEPSIS

Virginia M. Pierce
Christine S. Cho (5th edition)

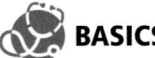 **BASICS**

DESCRIPTION
The terms SIRS (systemic inflammatory response syndrome), infection, sepsis, severe sepsis, and septic shock are defined as:

- SIRS: nonspecific inflammatory response to bodily injury, defined as at least 2 of the following 4 criteria (one of which must be abnormal temperature or leukocyte count):
  - Temperature >38.5 or <36°C
  - Tachycardia (mean HR >2 SDs above normal)
  - Tachypnea (mean RR >2 SDs above normal)
  - Leukocytosis, leukopenia, or >10% bands
- Infection: suspected or proven infection or clinical syndrome associated with high probability of infection
- Sepsis: SIRS in the presence of infection
- Severe sepsis: sepsis accompanied by evidence of altered end-organ perfusion (cardiovascular dysfunction OR acute respiratory distress syndrome [ARDS] OR 2 or more other organ dysfunctions)
- Septic shock: sepsis with cardiovascular dysfunction (hypotension, need for vasoactive drug to maintain normal BP, or any combination of unexplained metabolic acidosis, increased arterial lactate, oliguria, prolonged capillary refill, and core-to-peripheral temperature gap)

EPIDEMIOLOGY
Incidence
The incidence of severe sepsis varies with age, with significantly higher rates in infants (5.2 per 1,000 infants <1 year of age) than in older children (0.5 per 1,000 children age 1–4 years, about 0.2 per 1,000 children age 5–14 years, and 0.4 per 1,000 age 15–19 years).

Prevalence
Sepsis is among the most common (10–25%) medical diagnoses on admission to PICUs.

RISK FACTORS
- Although sepsis may occur in previously healthy children, it is a particular concern for children with chronic underlying conditions that render them immunosuppressed or vulnerable to invasive infections.
- Hyposplenism, either surgical or functional (e.g., sickle cell anemia)
- Neutropenia (<1,000 neutrophils/mm³ of blood, and especially <500/mm³)
- Primary or acquired syndromes of immunodeficiency (e.g., AIDS, severe combined immunodeficiency)
- Malignancy
- Organ transplant recipients
- Chronic use of high doses of steroids
- Indwelling central venous catheters
- Extensive burns
- Multiple trauma injuries
- Prematurity
- Unimmunized children

GENERAL PREVENTION
- Routine vaccination for *Haemophilus influenzae* type b (Hib), *Streptococcus pneumoniae*, and *Neisseria meningitidis*, particularly in high-risk patients (e.g., asplenia)
- Antibiotic prophylaxis for household or daycare exposure to Hib or *N. meningitidis*
- Prompt evaluation for fever in immunosuppressed patients
- Aseptic technique for insertion and care of vascular catheters, minimizing duration of use

ETIOLOGY
- Sepsis is caused by microbial invasion of the bloodstream or by the release of microbial products/toxins into the bloodstream. The responsible pathogens vary with age, host immune status, and location of the child (community or hospital setting).
- The most common causes in the first 4 weeks of life are group B streptococcus and Gram-negative enterics (e.g., *Escherichia coli*). Other important pathogens include *Listeria monocytogenes*, *Enterococcus* spp., herpes simplex virus, and enterovirus.
- In neonates with a history of hospitalization, instrumentation, or mechanical ventilation, consider *Staphylococcus aureus*, coagulase-negative staphylococci, Gram-negative bacilli, and *Candida* spp.
- In otherwise healthy older infants and children, leading sepsis pathogens include *S. pneumoniae*, *N. meningitidis*, and *S. aureus*. Group A streptococci, *Salmonella* spp., and rickettsiae are other causes.
- Patients with underlying immune defects are also susceptible to a broad range of additional organisms.

DIAGNOSIS

Have a high suspicion for sepsis; presenting signs of fever and tachycardia are nonspecific. Hypotension is not a sensitive sign of septic shock.

HISTORY
- Identify children with "Risk Factors"
- Duration of illness before presentation:
  - Abrupt onset of symptoms more typical of invasive bacterial infection
- Change in behavior may be initial sign of systemic infection

PHYSICAL EXAM
All patients with suspected sepsis should have a full set of vital signs (e.g., temperature, pulse, respiratory rate, BP, pulse oximetry).
- Temperature:
  - Fever is the hallmark of an infection; infants may demonstrate hypothermia.
- Stertor, stridor:
  - Assess for signs of airway obstruction
- Auscultation of the chest:
  - Assess adequacy of breathing (tachypnea, rales)
- Tachycardia, hypotension, poor skin perfusion, delayed capillary refill, presence of mottling, weak or bounding peripheral pulses:
  - Evidence of inadequate circulatory function
- Altered mental status (somnolence, confusion, disorientation, agitation, irritability):
  - Evidence of severe systemic disease, possible poor cerebral perfusion
- Presence of petechiae and purpura:
  - May be associated with meningococcemia or disseminated intravascular coagulation (DIC)
- Thorough physical exam:
  - Look for focus of infection

DIAGNOSTIC TESTS & INTERPRETATION
Lab
Patients with suspected sepsis should have:
- Blood culture:
  - Prior to starting antibiotics when possible
  - Culture yield is related to sample volume.
- CBC with differential:
  - Elevated WBC count with increased band count suggestive of invasive infection
  - Depressed WBC count may also be seen.
- Electrolytes, glucose, ionized calcium:
  - Metabolic acidosis, hypoglycemia, hypocalcemia
- BUN, creatinine, liver function tests:
  - Evaluate for end-organ injury
- Arterial blood gas (ABG) and lactate:
  - Monitor acid–base status
- PT, PTT, fibrinogen, fibrin degradation products, platelets, peripheral smear:
  - Screen for DIC
- Urinalysis and urine culture:
  - Potential source of infection
- Lumbar puncture (when hemodynamically stable):
  - Required for diagnosis of meningitis
- Gram stain and culture of petechiae, abscess contents, purulent wound drainage, indwelling devices, sputum, tracheal aspirate (especially within a few hours after intubation), other body fluids suspected to be infected:
  - May yield causative organism

DIFFERENTIAL DIAGNOSIS
- Congenital heart disease (e.g., ductal-dependent disease, or defects resulting in congestive heart failure)
- Myocarditis, pericarditis, cardiomyopathy
- Cardiac dysrhythmia
- Myocardial infarction
- Pulmonary embolus
- Congenital adrenal hyperplasia
- Thyrotoxicosis, hypothyroidism
- Inborn error of metabolism
- Hypoglycemia
- Diabetic ketoacidosis

- Severe anemia
- Methemoglobinemia
- Neoplasm
- Hemophagocytic lymphohistiocytosis
- Macrophage activation syndrome
- Dehydration
- Pyloric stenosis
- Necrotizing enterocolitis
- Volvulus
- Intussusception
- Pancreatitis
- Infant botulism
- Toxic ingestion/poisoning
- Trauma (accidental or nonaccidental)

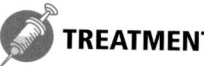 **TREATMENT**

Rapid recognition of sepsis is critical. Early reversal of shock is associated with reduced mortality.

ADDITIONAL TREATMENT
General Measures
- Ensure a patent airway (consider endotracheal intubation)
- Provide supplemental oxygen
- Assist ventilation (e.g., bag-valve-mask device) as needed
- Obtain large-bore peripheral intravenous access (consider central venous line or intraosseous line)
- Volume resuscitation: Bolus 20 mL/kg of normal saline, repeat as needed; consider blood after initial 60–80 mL/kg of crystalloid
  - Early, aggressive fluid resuscitation is imperative. Inadequate early fluid resuscitation is associated with increased mortality.
- Inotropic agents: If hemodynamic instability persists despite fluid resuscitation, start dopamine (begin at 5 μg/kg/min, titrate up to 20 μg/kg/min as needed). If the child has fluid refractory/dopamine-resistant shock, then start epinephrine (0.05–0.3 μg/kg/min) for cold shock or norepinephrine for warm shock to restore normal BP and perfusion.
- Consider stress-dose hydrocortisone for catecholamine-resistant hypotension and in patients at risk for adrenal insufficiency.
- Correct hypoglycemia (0.5–1 g/kg of dextrose) and hypocalcemia.
- Broad-spectrum intravenous antibiotics that cover the likely causative pathogens should be initiated promptly. Once the causative pathogen is identified, antibiotic therapy can be targeted appropriately. Empiric choice should include consideration of patient age, immune status, need for penetration into certain tissues (e.g., CNS), and whether the infection was community- or nosocomially-acquired.
  - Neonates ≤4 weeks: ampicillin and gentamicin (no meningitis); ampicillin and cefotaxime (with meningitis). Add acyclovir to either regimen if herpes simplex virus infection suspected. Switch ampicillin to vancomycin if CSF Gram stain or culture reveals Gram-positive cocci.
  - Infants and children ≥4 weeks: cefotaxime or ceftriaxone (no meningitis); vancomycin and cefotaxime or ceftriaxone (with meningitis)

- Patients with immunosuppression and/or central venous catheters: vancomycin plus aminoglycoside plus advanced generation cephalosporin (e.g., cefepime)
- Patients with an intra-abdominal focus of infection: carbapenem; ticarcillin-clavulanate or piperacillin-tazobactam; ceftriaxone, cefotaxime, or cefepime plus metronidazole; ampicillin plus gentamicin plus metronidazole or clindamycin
- Drainage or eradication of focus of infection
- Pitfalls:
  - Recognize the patient with "Risk Factors"
  - Initial priorities in management are ensuring adequate airway, breathing, and circulation.
  - Provide adequate initial volume resuscitation; early reversal of shock is associated with improved outcome.
  - Evaluate for a focus of infection amenable to source control and eradicate it if is possible (e.g., drainage of infected fluid collection, debridement of infected tissue, removal of implanted devices/foreign bodies).
  - Consider meningitis when appropriate.
  - Continuous monitoring and reassessment of the patient are essential.

IN-PATIENT CONSIDERATIONS
Admission Criteria
- Patients with sepsis should be admitted for close monitoring.
- Patients with severe sepsis or septic shock should be admitted to an ICU.

 ONGOING CARE

FOLLOW-UP RECOMMENDATIONS
Patient Monitoring
- Admit all patients with suspected sepsis to the hospital; consider ICU admission.
- Continuous BP monitoring for the development of refractory shock
- Serial vital signs and physical exams to monitor response to therapy
- Monitoring for complications of sepsis and the development of multiple organ dysfunction syndrome (MODS):
  - Chest radiograph and serial ABGs for evidence of acute lung injury/ARDS
  - Urine output, BUN, creatinine for acute renal failure
  - Serial coagulation studies (PT/PTT) and platelets for development of DIC
  - Serial blood glucose levels for hypo- or hyperglycemia
  - Serial liver function tests for evidence of hepatic dysfunction
  - Serial neurologic examinations for evidence of CNS dysfunction

PROGNOSIS
- Case fatality rates have improved from nearly 50% to ~10%. With implementation of clinical practice guidelines focused on early reversal of shock, several recent studies have demonstrated reduction of in-hospital mortality rates to ~4–8% for patients with severe sepsis.
- Mortality is higher in children with chronic illnesses than in previously healthy children.
- Development of ARDS or MODS is associated with increased mortality.

COMPLICATIONS
- Sepsis is one of the leading causes of pediatric mortality, accounting for 7% of deaths in children.
- The most common complications are those resulting primarily from either acute hypoperfusion of vital organs or from organ injury incurred by the uncontrolled systemic inflammatory response:
  - Acute lung injury
  - Acute renal failure
  - DIC
  - Hypoglycemia
  - ARDS
  - Refractory shock
  - MODS

 ADDITIONAL READING

- Bateman SL, Seed PC. Procession to pediatric bacteremia and sepsis: Covert operations and failures in diplomacy. *Pediatrics*. 2010;126: 137–150.
- Brierley J, Carcillo JA, Choong K, et al. Clinical practice parameters for hemodynamic support of pediatric and neonatal septic shock: 2007 update from the American College of Critical Care Medicine. *Crit Care Med*. 2009;37:666–688.
- Butt W. Septic shock. *Pediatr Clin North Am*. 2001;48:601–625, viii.
- Buttery JP. Blood cultures in newborns and children: Optimising an everyday test. *Arch Dis Child Fetal Neonatal Ed*. 2002;87:F25–F28.
- Carcillo JA. Pediatric septic shock and multiple organ failure. *Crit Care Clin*. 2003;19:413–440.
- Odetola FO, Gebremariam A, Freed GL. Patient and hospital correlates of clinical outcomes and resource utilization in severe pediatric sepsis. *Pediatrics*. 2007;119:487–494.
- Rivers E, Nguyen B, Havstad S, et al. Early goal-directed therapy in the treatment of severe sepsis and septic shock. *N Engl J Med*. 2001; 345:1368–1377.

 CODES

ICD9
- 785.52 Septic shock
- 995.90 Systemic inflammatory response syndrome, unspecified
- 995.91 Sepsis

ICD10
- A41.9 Sepsis, unspecified organism
- R65.10 SIRS of non-infectious origin w/o acute organ dysfunction
- R65.21 Severe sepsis with septic shock

SEPTIC ARTHRITIS

Sujit S. Iyer
Rakesh D. Mistry

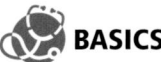 **BASICS**

DESCRIPTION
Microbiologic infection and inflammation of the usually sterile joint space

EPIDEMIOLOGY
- Toddler and school age (2–6 years) most commonly affected
- Predominant sex: Male > Female, 2:1
- Lower extremities (knee and ankle) and large joints (shoulder, hip, elbow) commonly affected

PATHOPHYSIOLOGY
- Entry of bacteria into joint space:
  - Hematogenous spread
  - Direct inoculation (penetrating trauma)
  - Extension from bone infection (mainly in children <1 year old when vessels cross from metaphysis to epiphysis)
- Influx of inflammatory cells within the joint capsule
- Rapid destruction of cartilaginous structures within the joint by bacterial and lysosomal enzymes:
  - If untreated, may progress to necrosis of the intra-articular epiphysis

ETIOLOGY
- Bacteria:
  - *Staphylococcus aureus* most common etiology outside of perinatal period (methicillin-sensitive and methicillin-resistant)
  - Streptococci
  - *Kingella kingae*
  - *Haemophilus influenzae*
  - *Salmonella*
  - *N. gonorrhoeae*
  - *Neisseria meningitidis*
  - *Borrelia burgdorferi* (Lyme)
- Aseptic arthritis:
  - Rubella
  - Parvovirus
  - Hepatitis B or C
  - Mumps
  - Herpesviruses (Epstein–Barr virus, cytomegalovirus, herpes simplex virus, varicella zoster virus)
  - Epstein–Barr virus
  - Varicella
  - *Candida albicans* (neonatal)

COMMONLY ASSOCIATED CONDITIONS
- Neonatal septic arthritis may be associated with *S. aureus*, group B streptococcus, *Escherichia coli*, and *Candida*.
- Sickle cell disease is associated with *Salmonella* infection, although *S. aureus* is still the most common.
- Immunocompromised patients: *Mycoplasma*, *Ureaplasma*, *Klebsiella*, or *Aspergillus* infection

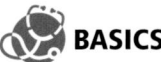 **DIAGNOSIS**

HISTORY
- Fever, rigors
- Affected joint pain, or refusal to walk or move joint in preverbal children
- History of recent trauma does not rule out septic arthritis.
- Pain of bacterial arthritis worsens over 1–3 days and does not wax and wane.
- Septic arthritis is rarely polyarticular.
- Lyme arthritis is typically more subacute, without constitutional symptoms.

PHYSICAL EXAM
- Fever occurs within the first few days of illness in 75% of patients but less commonly in infants. Only 50% of children with gonococcal arthritis have fever.
- Children with septic arthritis usually appear ill.
- The joint appears warm and swollen.
- Infants may demonstrate "pseudoparalysis."
- Hip involvement causes the leg to be held flexed, abducted, and externally rotated.
- The child with septic arthritis usually has pain through any range of motion. In contrast, most traumatic injuries allow some painless range of motion of that joint.
- Lyme infection is characterized by a painless joint that is warm, swollen, and tender.
- There is usually a more delayed presentation with minimal external findings when the hip or shoulder joints are infected.
- Consider hip involvement when the patient complains of knee or thigh pain.
- In the frightened or uncooperative child, it is possible to have the parent perform an examination for tenderness and range of motion while the physician observes from a distance.

DIAGNOSTIC TESTS & INTERPRETATION
Lab
- Synovial fluid analysis in septic arthritis:
  - The WBC count is often >100,000/mm^3, but may be as low as 50,000/mm^3 in early infections.
  - The glucose level in the synovial fluid is <50% that of the serum.
  - Culture of the joint reveals an organism in 70–80% of cases (except for gonorrhea).
  - Inoculation of joint fluid into blood culture bottle facilitates recovery of *K. kingae*.
    - Emerging technology of real-time PCR for *K. kingae* toxin from joint fluid may show higher yield of identification than routine Gram stain or culture alone.
  - A Gram stain of synovial fluid reveals pathogens in 50% of cases.

- Other supportive tests:
  - ESR is elevated (>30 mm/h) in 95% of cases. Retain suspicion if >20 mm/h.
  - The C-reactive protein (CRP) is increased. In one study, a CRP <1.0 mg/dL had a negative predictive value of 87% in a population in which the prevalence of septic arthritis in tested patients was 29%.
  - Blood cultures are positive in 30–40% of cases.
  - A high peripheral WBC count is neither sensitive nor specific for septic arthritis.
- An immunofluorescent antibody assay for *B. burgdorferi*, when available, may be helpful in the rapid differentiation between bacterial arthritis and Lyme disease. Modest inflammation (25–50,000 WBC) is usually evident in the synovial fluid.

Imaging
- Radiography is rarely helpful in diagnosis; may show widening of joint space and/or displacement of the normal fat pads in the knee or elbow; and is less often positive in the shoulder or hip.
- Ultrasound of the affected joint usually delineates the amount of fluid within the joint capsule. Increased blood flow on color Doppler may suggest infection. However, this test cannot differentiate between an infectious and a purely inflammatory disease.
- A technetium-99 bone scan reveals increased uptake in the perimeter of the joint during the "blood pool" phase of the study.
- False-positives:
  - Bone scan cannot easily differentiate septic arthritis from epiphyseal osteomyelitis.
  - Evaluation of synovial fluid from patients with rheumatologic disease may mimic that of infectious arthritis; however, the clinical picture should allow differentiation of these entities.

DIFFERENTIAL DIAGNOSIS
- Osteomyelitis with contiguous spread
- Cellulitis causing decreased range of motion of joint secondary to inflammation
- Tuberculous arthritis
- Psoas abscess or retroperitoneal abscess with associated hip pain
- Prepatellar bursitis (knee)
- Tumors:
  - Osteogenic sarcoma (long-bone pain spreading to joint space)
  - Leukemia/lymphoma
- Trauma:
  - Occult fracture in proximity to growth plate
  - Ligamentous injury (sprain)
  - Foreign-body synovitis
  - Traumatic knee effusion/hemarthrosis
- Immunologic:
  - Toxic synovitis
  - Postinfectious
  - Acute rheumatic fever
  - Reactive arthritis
  - *Campylobacter*, *Shigella*, *Yersinia*, *Chlamydia* infection
  - Reiter syndrome (after GI or chlamydial infection), arthritis, uveitis, urethritis
  - Collagen vascular
  - Systemic lupus erythematosus
  - Juvenile rheumatoid arthritis

- Henoch–Schönlein purpura
- Behçet syndrome (iridocyclitis, genital and oral ulcerations)
- Inflammatory bowel disease (Crohn disease, ulcerative colitis)
- Serum sickness
- Erythema multiforme/Stevens–Johnson syndrome
- Miscellaneous:
  – Knee
  – Apophysitis (e.g., Osgood–Schlatter disease)
  – Patellofemoral pain syndrome (chondromalacia patella)
  – Osteochondritis dissecans
  – Hip
  – Slipped capital femoral epiphysis
- An algorithm using 4 or more of the following factors has been used to successfully differentiate septic arthritis and transient synovitis of the hip:
  – Fever
  – ESR >20 mm/h
  – CRP >1.0 mg/dL
  – WBC >11,000 cells/mL
  – Joint space fluid apparent on plain radiograph
  – The absence of all of these parameters is strongly associated with the absence of septic arthritis.
- Pitfalls:
  – Clinical examination in conjunction with the history of acute onset should raise the suspicion of septic arthritis, even in the face of "negative" laboratory screening tests. The most accurate determinations can be inferred from analysis of the synovial fluid.
  – Realize that some children, especially neonates and young infants, will not manifest signs of systemic disease early in the course of the illness.
  – Observe failure or success of therapy, especially when the extremity is immobilized.

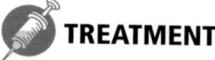 TREATMENT

MEDICATION (DRUGS)
- Choice of antibiotics depends on age of child as outlined.
- Antistaphylococcal penicillin and first-generation cephalosporins are usual first-line antibiotics.
- The incidence of methicillin-resistant *S. aureus* (MRSA) septic arthritis is increasing in many communities. Therefore, in areas where prevalence of MRSA is high (>15%), vancomycin or clindamycin should be considered as first-line treatment until susceptibilities are identified. Addition of ceftriaxone in sickle cell patients. Duration of therapy (intravenous and by mouth) for various organisms:
  – Treat for at least 2 weeks after resolution of fever and joint effusion
  – At least ≥28 days: *S. aureus*, Gram-negative organisms, group B streptococcus, and for infections of the shoulder and hip
  – At least ≥4 days: *H. influenzae*, *N. meningitidis*, streptococci
  – At least ≥7 days: *N. gonorrhoeae*
- Intra-articular injection of antibiotics is not recommended.
- Unproven therapies:
  – Steroid therapy in the first 4 days has been shown in small studies to reduce residual dysfunction; however, this has yet to be proven effective in larger studies.

IN-PATIENT CONSIDERATIONS
Initial Stabilization
- Drainage of infection: Should occur as soon as possible if bacterial cause is suspected
- Indications for open surgical drainage/irrigation:
  – Hip involvement
  – Shoulder involvement (controversial)
  – Thick, purulent, or fibrinous exudate unable to pass through 18-gauge needle
  – All other joints not undergoing open drainage should undergo needle aspiration.
- Antibiotic administration immediately after joint aspiration is performed.
- Immobilization of extremity
- Pain management

 ONGOING CARE

FOLLOW-UP RECOMMENDATIONS
Patient Monitoring
- Involve orthopedic surgery and physical therapy services in follow-up
- Once the patient is receiving oral therapy, serum bactericidal titers (SBTs) must be monitored on a weekly basis if possible. Oral antibiotic titers should be kept at 8 times the SBT.
- When to expect improvement: With appropriate antibacterial therapy, one should see improvement of symptoms with 2 days of initial administration.
- Signs to watch for:
  – Continued pain, fever, or lack of improvement of range of motion after 3–4 days of appropriate antibiotic treatment
  – Rising ESR or CRP in the face of antibiotic treatment
  – Severe cases of septic arthritis may require serial drainage and debridement.

PROGNOSIS
- Depends on duration of illness prior to institution of appropriate therapy
- Incidence of residual joint dysfunction increased if antibiotic therapy not instituted within first 4 days of illness

COMPLICATIONS
- Permanent limitation of range of motion due to tissue destruction and scarring
- Growth disturbance if the epiphysis is involved

ADDITIONAL READING
- Caird MS, Flynn JM, Leung YL, et al. Factors distinguishing septic arthritis from transient synovitis of the hip in children: A prospective study. *J Bone Joint Surg Am.* 2006;88:1251–1257.
- Ceroni D, Cherkaoui A, Ferey S, et al. *Kingella kingae* osteoarticular infections in young children: Clinical features and contribution of a new specific real-time PCR assay to the diagnosis. *J Pediatr Orthop.* 2010;30(3):301–314.
- Harel L, Prais D, Bar-On E, et al. Dexamethasone therapy for septic arthritis in children: Results of a randomized double-blind placebo-controlled study. *J Pediatr Orthop.* 2011;31(2):211–215.

- Jung ST, Rowe SM, Moon ES, et al. Significance of laboratory and radiologic findings for differentiating between septic arthritis and transient synovitis of the hip. *J Pediatr Orthop.* 2003;23:368–372.
- Kocher MS, Mandiga R, Murphy JM, et al. A clinical practice guideline for treatment of septic arthritis in children. *J Bone Joint Surg.* 2003;85-A:994–999.
- Martinez-Aguilar, Avalos-Mishaan A, Hulten K, et al. Community-acquired, methicillin-resistant and methicillin-susceptible *Staphylococcus aureus* musculoskeletal infections in children. *Pediatr Infect Dis J.* 2004;23:701–706.
- Shaw BA, Kasser JR. Acute septic arthritis in infancy and childhood. *Clin Orthop.* 1990;257:212–215.
- Sultan J, Hughes PJ. Septic arthritis or transient synovitis of the hip in children: The value of clinical prediction algorithms. *J Bone Joint Surg Br.* 2010;92(9):1289–1293.
- Taekema HC, Landham PR, Maconochie I. Towards evidence based medicine for paediatricians. Distinguishing between transient synovitis and septic arthritis in the limping child: How useful are clinical prediction tools? *Arch Dis Child.* 2009;94(2):167–168.
- Tory HO, Zurakowski D, Sundel RP. Outcomes of children treated for Lyme arthritis: Results of a large pediatric cohort. *J Rheumatol.* 2011;37(5):1049–1055.
- Willis AA, Widmann RF, Flynn JM, et al. Lyme arthritis presenting as acute septic arthritis in children. *J Pediatr Orthop.* 2003;23:114–118.

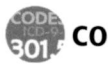 CODES

ICD9
- 711.00 Pyogenic arthritis, site unspecified
- 711.05 Pyogenic arthritis, pelvic region and thigh
- 711.06 Pyogenic arthritis, lower leg

ICD10
- M00.861 Arthritis due to other bacteria, right knee
- M00.869 Arthritis due to other bacteria, unspecified knee
- M00.9 Pyogenic arthritis, unspecified

FAQ
- Q: How can one differentiate toxic synovitis from septic arthritis on the initial visit?
- A: Although this is sometimes a difficult diagnosis to make with certainty, patients with toxic synovitis usually exhibit certain characteristics that patients with septic arthritis do not:
  – Almost always involves the hip joint
  – History of previous viral infection
  – Some painless range of motion of the involved joint is possible.
  – The ESR is <20 mm/h.
  – Fever is low grade.

SERUM SICKNESS
Denise A. Salerno

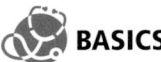

BASICS

DESCRIPTION
- Serum sickness:
  - Type III hypersensitivity reaction that occurs 7–21 days after injection of foreign protein or serum (usually in the form of antiserums)
  - Immune complexes deposit in the skin, joints, and other organs.
  - Clinical syndrome consists of skin rash, itching, fever, malaise, proteinuria, vasculitis, and joint pain.
- Serum sickness-like reactions:
  - Characterized by fever, rash, lymphadenopathy, and arthralgia
  - Occur 1–3 weeks after drug exposure
  - Immune complexes, vasculitis, and hypocomplementemia are absent.
  - This type of reaction, most commonly associated with medications, is commonly referred to as serum sickness also.
  - More common than true serum sickness because equine serum antitoxins have been replaced with human antitoxin sera
- Clinically, these entities present and are treated the same.

EPIDEMIOLOGY
- Limited information is available regarding the incidence of adverse drug reactions in children; generally believed to occur less frequently in children than in adults.
- >90% of serum sickness cases are drug-induced.
- <5% of serum sickness cases are fatal.

RISK FACTORS
Genetics
People with a genetic predisposition to produce IgE are more susceptible.

GENERAL PREVENTION
- No known way to prevent first occurrence
- Take careful history of previous allergic reactions
- Skin testing prior to antiserum administration will prevent anaphylaxis but not serum sickness.
- When the need for antiserum arises, consider prophylactic antihistamines.

PATHOPHYSIOLOGY
- Serum sickness—type III immune complex, antigen–antibody complement reaction:
  - Antibodies form 6–10 days after the introduction of foreign material.
  - Antibodies interact with antigens, forming immune complexes that diffuse across the vascular walls.
  - They become fixated in tissue and activate the complement cascade.
  - C3a and C5a are produced, resulting in increased vascular permeability and activated inflammatory cells.
  - Polymorphonuclear cells and monocytes cause diffuse vasculitis.
- Serum sickness-like reaction
  - Abnormal inflammatory reaction in response to defective metabolism of drug byproducts

ETIOLOGY
- Common causative agents:
  - Horse antithymocyte globulins
  - Human diploid-cell rabies vaccine
  - Streptokinase
  - Hymenoptera venom
  - Penicillins
  - Cephalosporins (especially cefaclor)
  - Sulfonamides
  - Hydralazine
  - Thiouracils
  - Metronidazole
  - Naproxen
  - Dextrans
- Case-reported agents:
  - Minocycline
  - Amoxicillin
  - Infliximab
  - Bupropion

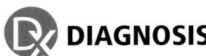

DIAGNOSIS

HISTORY
- Suspect in any patient who has been taking any new drug during the past 2 months, and who has an unexplained vasculitic rash.
- Presentation and evolution of rash: Typically, the rash first appears on the sides of the fingers, hands, and feet before becoming widespread.
- Associated pruritus is often present.
- Fever is present in 10–20% of cases, and is usually mild.
- Arthritis or arthralgia is present >50% of the time; usually involves the metacarpophalangeal and knee joints.
- Associated abdominal pain: Some cases may have visceral involvement.
- History of hematuria: There can be modest renal involvement, usually presenting as proteinuria and microscopic hematuria.
- Patient reports any neurologic symptoms: Peripheral neuropathy, brachial plexus involvement, and Guillain–Barré syndrome have been reported associations.
- Previous history of a similar rash: Was it associated with any medications in the past? The rash and symptoms of serum sickness will occur sooner on repeat exposure. Try to differentiate from simple drug rash; timing of rash after exposure is important in differentiating the two.
- Has patient had any drug or antitoxin exposure in the past month, especially to penicillins, cephalosporins, sulfonamides, hydralazine, thiouracils, streptokinase, metronidazole, naproxen, or dextrans?

PHYSICAL EXAM
- Erythematous purpuric rash starts at the sides of the feet, toes, hands, and fingers and then becomes more widespread.
- Erythema multiforme, maculopapular, purpuric, or urticarial type rash
- Mild-to-severe fever
- Generalized lymphadenopathy; may be localized to lymph nodes that drain the injection site
- Splenomegaly, occasionally
- Edema of the face and neck
- Joint pain

DIAGNOSTIC TESTS & INTERPRETATION
Lab
- Not extremely helpful in establishing diagnosis because no abnormality is universally present. Diagnosis usually apparent by classic findings and history of foreign protein or drug exposure:
  - Urinalysis: May show proteinuria and/or hematuria
  - Complement levels variably reduced before returning to normal
  - Leukocytosis or leukopenia with or without eosinophilia
  - Erythrocyte sedimentation rate may be slightly elevated.
  - Direct immunofluorescent staining of rash biopsy (not routinely recommended as part of workup) shows deposits of IgM and C3 complement in capillary walls.

DIFFERENTIAL DIAGNOSIS
- Erythema multiforme
- Mononucleosis
- Systemic lupus erythematosus
- Rocky Mountain spotted fever
- Henoch–Schönlein purpura
- Hypersensitivity syndrome reaction
- Drug-induced pseudoporphyria
- Acute generalized exanthematous pustulosis
- Wegener granulomatosis
- Pitfalls:
  - A history of fever, rash, and arthralgias is commonly seen with many childhood illnesses. One must always consider differential diagnoses.
  - Symptoms may be so minimal that patient does not seek medical attention.
  - Often misdiagnosed as simple drug allergy

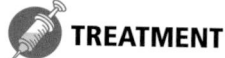

TREATMENT

ADDITIONAL TREATMENT

General Measures

- Stop suspected medication/antigen immediately and avoid its future use
- Topical steroids to relieve itching
- Antihistamines to inhibit the action of vasoactive mediators
- Antipyretics for fever
- NSAIDs to relieve joint pain
- Oral corticosteroids for severe cases:
  - Recommended to administer and taper over 10–14-day period
  - Shorter course may result in relapse, and recurrent symptoms are more difficult to alleviate.
- Admit if symptoms are severe or diagnosis is unclear
- Future avoidance of triggering agent if identified

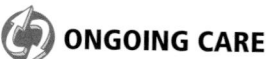

ONGOING CARE

FOLLOW-UP RECOMMENDATIONS

When to expect improvement:

- Usually self-limited illness that resolves in a few days to weeks
- If symptoms persist for >1 month, reconsider the diagnosis.

PATIENT EDUCATION

- An initial episode of serum sickness cannot be prevented. Future episodes can be prevented by avoiding the causative medication (and class of medications) if it has been identified.

PROGNOSIS

Excellent. Most cases are mild and transient with no long-term sequelae.

COMPLICATIONS

- Shock
- Digital necrosis
- Guillain–Barré syndrome (rare)
- Generalized vasculitis (rare)
- Peripheral neuropathy (rare)
- Glomerulonephritis (rare)
- Acute flaccid paralysis (case report)
- Increased risk of anaphylaxis with repeat exposure to precipitating substance
- Fatality (rare, usually due to continued administration of antigen)

ADDITIONAL READING

- Bettge AM, Gross G. A serum sickness-like reaction to a commonly used acne drug. *JAAPA*. 2008;21(3):33–34.
- Guidry MM, Drennan RH, Weise JW, et al. Serum sepsis, not sickness. *Am J Med Sci*. 2011;341(2):88–91.
- McCollum R, Elbe DH, Ritchie AA. Bupropion indirect serum sickness-like reaction. *Ann Pharmacother*. 2000;34:471–473.
- Mener D, Negrini C, Blatt A. Itching like mad. *Am J Med*. 2009;122(8):732–734.
- Roujeau J, Stern RS. Severe adverse cutaneous reactions to drugs. *N Engl J Med*. 1994;331:1272–1285.
- Swanson JK, English JC III. Serum sickness-like reaction to Pamabrom. *J Drugs Dermatol*. 2006;5:284–286.

CODES

ICD9

- 999.51 Other serum reaction due to administration of blood and blood products
- 999.52 Other serum reaction due to vaccination

ICD10

- T80.61XA Oth serum reaction due to admin blood/products, init
- T80.62XA Other serum reaction due to vaccination, initial encounter

FAQ

- Q: My child broke out all over her body with an itchy rash and hives a few days after taking cefaclor, was this serum sickness?
- A: It is more likely that she is allergic to cefaclor. The difference is that drug allergies are type I IgE-mediated hypersensitivity reactions that occur very soon after drug exposure in a previously sensitized individual. Serum sickness is a type III antibody–antigen immune complex and complement amplified hypersensitivity reaction that occurs 1–3 weeks after an initial exposure.
- Q: If my child has had serum sickness, is she at risk for getting it again?
- A: Yes, if she receives the same medication or related medications again. The symptoms will occur more quickly, usually in 2–4 days, and may be more severe.
- Q: Can the vaccines that my doctor recommends for my child give my child serum sickness?
- A: It is possible but pretty rare. There have been a few reports of serum sickness-like reactions occurring after receiving vaccines submitted to the Vaccine Adverse Event Reporting System (VAERS).
- Q: Is there any way to prevent my child from getting serum sickness?
- A: Unfortunately, there is no way to predict if your child will have a serum sickness-like reaction to a particular medication. It is extremely important to be aware of your child's exact allergies to medications and to inform all healthcare providers caring for your child.
- Q: My oldest child had serum sickness after taking cefaclor. Is it true that all my children should now avoid taking cefaclor?
- A: No, there is no known genetic predisposition to serum sickness. Your other children do not need to avoid the medication that caused serum sickness.
- Q: How is the Arthus reaction different from serum sickness?
- A: The Arthus reaction is also a type III hypersensitivity reaction but causes only a local reaction. It is a local vasculitis caused by formation of antigen–antibody complexes in local vessel walls, which then activate the inflammation process. The reaction occurs within hours after an individual is injected intradermally with an antigen against which he or she has been actively immunized.
- Q: My child was diagnosed with serum sickness 1 year ago. He still gets episodes of rash, fever, and joint pain every now and then. How can this be cured?
- A: Serum sickness is a self-limited disease, and as long as the offending agent is stopped your child will completely recover. If there are continuing symptoms and your child is no longer taking the offending agent, then other causes for these symptoms need to be considered.

S

SEVERE ACUTE RESPIRATORY SYNDROME (SARS)

Nicholas Tsarouhas

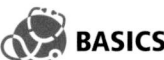 **BASICS**

DESCRIPTION

Clinical criteria for severe acute respiratory syndrome (SARS) must be interpreted in the context of the prevailing epidemiologic laboratory criteria as published by the World Health Organization (WHO) and the Centers for Disease Control and Prevention (CDC).

- WHO clinical criteria (5/01/03):
  - Suspect SARS case:
    - A person presenting after November 1, 2002, with high fever (>38°C), and
    - Cough or difficulty breathing, and
    - Close contact with SARS patient or travel criteria to SARS area (see "History")
  - Probable SARS case:
    - A suspect case with radiographic pneumonia or respiratory distress syndrome, or
    - A suspect case with confirmatory laboratory studies (see "Lab"), or
    - A suspect case with autopsy findings
- CDC clinical criteria (12/12/03):
  - Early illness:
    - 2 or more constitutional symptoms—fever, chills, rigors, myalgia, headache, diarrhea, sore throat, or rhinorrhea
  - Mild-to-moderate illness:
    - Temperature >100.4°F (>38°C)
    - 1 or more lower respiratory findings—cough, shortness of breath, or difficulty breathing
  - Severe illness:
    - Clinical criteria of mild-to-moderate illness, and
    - 1 or more of the following—radiographic evidence, acute respiratory distress syndrome, or autopsy findings
- SARS time line:
  - November 2002: A series of severe idiopathic respiratory illnesses begin occurring in Southeast Asian countries (China, Hong Kong, Vietnam, and Singapore).
  - February 11, 2003: The Chinese Ministry of Health notifies the WHO that 305 cases of acute respiratory syndrome of unknown etiology have occurred in Guangdong province in southern China from November 16, 2002 to February 9, 2003.
  - Late February: SARS outbreak in Toronto
  - March 12: WHO issues global SARS alert as number of reported cases steadily increases.
  - March 14: CDC activates emergency operations center with first confirmed death of SARS patient.
  - March 15: WHO issues travel advisories and warnings.
  - March 17: 167 cases and 4 deaths reported in 7 countries
  - March 24: CDC implicates a coronavirus as the causative SARS agent.
  - April 10: The New England Journal of Medicine e-publishes "A Novel Coronavirus Associated with SARS."
  - April 13: Vancouver team sequences the coronavirus.

- April 16: WHO confirms coronavirus as the cause of SARS as a Netherlands team infects monkeys with the virus. The monkeys go on to develop SARS, and then have the coronavirus recovered from them.
- April 18: Worldwide cases rapidly multiplying—3,461 cases, 170 deaths, 27 countries
- May 17: Deaths dramatically rise—7,761 cases, 623 deaths, 31 countries
- June 9: Reported cases slow—8,421 cases, 784 deaths, 32 countries
- July 5: WHO declares the SARS epidemic over.
- Since July 2003: <12 confirmed new cases, including a "second SARS mini-outbreak" in March 2004, started by a young postgraduate student who was working at an institute of virology in Beijing.
- Overall statistics to date:
  - Worldwide: >9,000 cases, nearly 1,000 deaths, 29 countries affected
  - US: 134 suspected cases, 19 probable cases, 8 confirmed cases, no deaths, 17 states
- Transmission:
  - Direct or indirect contact of mucous membranes with infectious respiratory droplets or fomites
  - Period of infectivity: Most likely during period with active symptoms (fever, cough)
  - Incubation period: 2–10 days; mean 6 days
  - All cases can be traced to contact with individuals from Asian countries or community, spread from an individual whose illness could be traced to Asia.
  - There have been no suspected SARS cases among casual contacts of the US cases.
  - Many healthcare workers were infected after providing care to SARS patients.
  - No evidence that SARS is transmitted from asymptomatic individuals
  - However, healthcare workers who developed SARS may have been a source of transmission within healthcare facilities during early phases of illness, when symptoms were mild and not recognized as SARS.
  - There is no evidence that SARS can be spread after recovery from the disease.
  - Pediatric population:
    - Children pose a lower risk of transmission than do adults; only 1 reported case of transmission of SARS from pediatric patient.
    - Vertical transmission of SARS-CoV from infected mothers to their newborns has not been observed.
    - None of the newborns had clinical, laboratory, or radiological evidence suggestive of SARS-CoV infection.

GENERAL PREVENTION

- Vaccine:
  - Human clinical trials in China continue to show promise for vaccine development.
  - Safety concerns exist, however, for vaccine production workers.
- Hospital infection control precautions:
  - Hospitalized patients meeting SARS case definition should be placed in a negative-pressure, single examination room.
  - Protective equipment appropriate for standard, contact, and airborne precautions (e.g., hand hygiene, gown, gloves, and N95 respirator) in addition to eye protection are recommended for healthcare workers to prevent transmission of SARS in healthcare settings.
- Pediatric patients with potential SARS exposure:
  - Children who have been exposed to an ill individual who is suspected of having SARS, or children who have traveled to an area where SARS is occurring, should be evaluated based on the following:
    - If well, parents should self-monitor the child's condition for fever or respiratory tract illness. Attendance at child care or school is not restricted.
    - If the child is not well, parents should contact their physician and the child should be isolated at home.
    - If the child is not well and is experiencing breathing difficulty, he or she should be hospitalized. Healthcare workers should be informed before the admission, so SARS precautions can be initiated.
  - Children who have been exposed to individuals who are not ill but have traveled to areas where SARS is occurring do not require isolation.

PATHOPHYSIOLOGY

The virus attaches itself to human receptor cells and initiates a nonspecific acute lung injury response leading to diffuse, severe alveolar damage.

ETIOLOGY

- A previously unrecognized coronavirus (a single-strand RNA virus)
- Coronaviruses are a common cause of mild-to-moderate upper respiratory infections in humans and have occasionally been linked to pneumonia.
- Many believe that the virus originated in an animal species in China, then mutated in such a way that it was able to attach itself to human receptor cells.

DIAGNOSIS

HISTORY
- Recent travel:
  - Travel (including transit in an airport) within 10 days of onset of symptoms to an area with recently documented or suspected transmission of SARS is an important epidemiologic criterion for the diagnosis of a SARS case.
  - At the height of the SARS epidemic, these areas included China, Hong Kong, Singapore, Taiwan, Toronto, and Hanoi.
- Recent contact with a SARS patient:
  - Close contact within 10 days of onset of symptoms with a person known or suspected to have SARS infection is another important epidemiologic criterion.
- The clinical presentation of SARS in children >12 years of age is similar to that of adults.
- Constitutional symptoms, such as fever, chills, rigors, headache, malaise, myalgias, and diarrhea, are common in older patients.
- One meta-analysis (Stockman et al.) of 6 pediatric case series of 135 SARS cases noted the following symptom prevalence: Fever (98%), cough (60%), and nausea or vomiting (41%).
- Respiratory symptoms:
  - At the onset of illness, most cases have mild respiratory symptoms.
  - After 3–7 days, the onset of a dry, nonproductive cough begins, often with dyspnea that may be accompanied by, or progress to, hypoxemia.

PHYSICAL EXAM
- Fever: The illness generally begins with fever.
- Tachypnea, increased work of breathing, or rales
- Adult patients generally present with evidence of respiratory distress.
- Importantly, however, although some children present with cough or difficulty breathing, many have remarkably normal examinations. Thus, the case definitions above may not be sufficiently sensitive for young children.

DIAGNOSTIC TESTS & INTERPRETATION
Lab
- Detection of SARS coronavirus: Confirmatory laboratory criteria for the diagnosis of SARS:
  - Antibody by ELISA or indirect fluorescent-antibody assay (IFA)
  - RNA by reverse transcriptase polymerase chain reaction (RT-PCR) assays
  - Viral culture
- SARS virus may be detected in blood, nasopharyngeal aspirates, throat, and stool samples.
- CBC: Hematologic abnormalities are common in children with SARS.
  - Leukopenia (lymphopenia or neutropenia)
  - Thrombocytopenia
- Liver enzymes: Some patients have elevated transaminases.
- Raised serum lactate dehydrogenase is also commonly seen.

Imaging
- The characteristic feature of pulmonary SARS-CoV infection is patchy airspace consolidation predominantly located at the periphery of the lungs and in the lower lobes.
- Many patients, however, have normal chest radiographs.
- Pitfalls: Not searching for alternative diagnoses, even during an epidemic of SARS; other microbiologic studies should still be performed to confirm or rule out other infectious diseases.
  - Not performing convalescent antibody testing in equivocal cases; undetectable antibody >28 days after onset of illness excludes the diagnosis.

DIFFERENTIAL DIAGNOSIS
- Bacterial infections:
  - *Pneumococcus*
  - *Staphylococcus*
  - *Legionella*
  - *Mycoplasma*
  - *Chlamydophila pneumoniae*
- Viral infections:
  - Respiratory syncytial virus
  - Influenza A and B

 TREATMENT

IN-PATIENT CONSIDERATIONS
Initial Stabilization
- There is no proven effective treatment.
- CDC currently recommends that patients with SARS receive the same treatment and supportive care that would be used for any patient with serious community-acquired atypical pneumonia of unknown cause.
- Steroids, interferon, ribavirin, oseltamivir, and other antivirals have been used without consistent success.

ONGOING CARE

PROGNOSIS
- Patients 12 years of age and younger:
  - Milder disease
  - Fewer ICU admits
  - Decreased need for supplemental oxygen
  - Less likely to receive methylprednisolone
- No pediatric deaths were reported.
- Overall fatality rate: 11%
  - Highest: 27% (Taiwan)
  - Lowest: 0 (US)

COMPLICATIONS
- Overall, in 10–20% of cases, the respiratory illness was severe enough to require mechanical ventilation.
- In children, only 5% required admission to an ICU, and <1% required mechanical ventilation.

ADDITIONAL READING

- Bitnun A, Allen U, Heurter H, et al. Children hospitalized with SARS-related illness in Toronto. *Pediatrics*. 2003;112:e261–e268.
- Bitnun A, Read S, Tellier R, et al. Severe acute respiratory syndrome—associated coronavirus infection in Toronto children: A second look. *Pediatrics*. 2009;123(1):97–101.
- Booth CM, Matukas LM, Tomlinson GA, et al. Clinical features and short-term outcomes of 144 patients with SARS in the greater Toronto area. *JAMA*. 2003;289:2801–2809.
- Hon KLE, Leung CW, Cheng PKS, et al. Clinical presentations and outcome of SARS in children. *Lancet*. 2003;361:1701–1703.
- Li AM, Ng PC. Severe acute respiratory syndrome (SARS) in neonates and children. *Arch Dis Child*. 2005;90(6):F461–F465.
- Peiris SM, Phil D, Yuen KY, et al. The severe acute respiratory syndrome. *N Engl J Med*. 2003;349:2431–2441.
- Stockman L, Massoudi MS, Helfand R, et al. Severe acute respiratory syndrome in children. *Pediatr Infect Dis J*. 2007;26(1):68–74.
- Zhong N, Zeng G. What we have learned from SARS epidemics in China. *BMJ*. 2006;333(7564):389–391.

CODES

ICD9
- 079.82 SARS-associated coronavirus
- 480.3 Pneumonia due to SARS-associated coronavirus

ICD10
- B97.21 SARS-associated coronavirus causing diseases classd elswhr
- J12.81 Pneumonia due to SARS-associated coronavirus

FAQ
- Q: Is the clinical presentation and course different in children?
- A: Fortunately, younger children tend to have a shorter and milder course, consisting mainly of low-grade fever, cough, and rhinorrhea. Adolescents, conversely, follow a more severe course, similar to that of adults.
- Q: What constitutes close contact with a SARS patient?
- A: Close contact includes having cared for or lived with a person known to have SARS, or having a high likelihood of direct contact with respiratory secretions and/or body fluids of a patient known to have SARS.

S

SEVERE COMBINED IMMUNODEFICIENCY

Michael Keller
Timothy Andrews (5th edition)

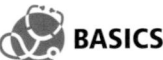

BASICS

DESCRIPTION
Severe combined immunodeficiency (SCID) is characterized by onset of severe, life-threatening infections in infancy owing to defects in development or survival of T lymphocytes. It is the most profound form of primary immunodeficiency, and the diagnosis is a medical emergency.

EPIDEMIOLOGY
- Most patients present within the first year of life.
- The most common four molecular defects are:
  - X-linked SCID (IL2-Rα): 45% of cases.
  - Adenosine deaminase (ADA) deficiency: roughly 16% of cases
  - Interleukin-7 receptor deficiency: 10%.
  - Janus-associated kinase 3 (JAK3): 7%.

Incidence
- Estimated at: 1 in 50,000–100,000 live births (though may be underestimated due to associated early mortality).
- SCID due to Artemis defects (Anthabascan SCID) occurs in 1 in 2,500 live births in the Navajo population due to a founder mutation.

Genetics
- X-linked and autosomal recessive inheritance
- Digeorge syndrome is autosomal dominant, but only a very rare subset of these patients has complete athymia and SCID.
- See table in Section VI

ETIOLOGY
- Results from defects in signaling pathways required for development or survival of T lymphocytes. These include:
  - DNA repair mutations preventing VDJ recombination (RAG1/2, Lig4, Artemis)
  - Defects in IL2/7 signaling pathway (X-linked SCID, IL-7Ra, JAK3)
  - Athymia (Digeorge syndrome)
  - Accumulation of metabolites toxic to lymphocytes (ADA, PNP deficiency)

DIAGNOSIS

HISTORY
- Patients present with both severe illnesses due to common infections (chronic rotavirus, adenovirus, influenza, oral candidiasis), and opportunistic infections (pneumocystis, CMV).
- Chronic diarrhea and failure to thrive are common.
- There may be a family history of early, unexplained deaths, or consanguinity.

PHYSICAL EXAM
- Evaluation should focus on the presence of infection.
- Often an emaciated-appearing infant
- Absent or hypoplastic lymphoid tissue (lack of thymic shadow on CXR, lack of tonsils or lymph nodes).
- Dermatologic evaluation may reveal atypical rashes (morbilliform or eczema-like).

DIAGNOSTIC TESTS & INTERPRETATION
- CBC with differential to assess for degree of lymphopenia; the lower limit normal absolute lymphocyte count in the neonatal period is $>2,800/\text{mm}^3$. Of note, many infants with SCID will still have a normal ALC.
- Lymphocyte enumeration:
  - T lymphocytes (CD3+) are markedly decreased or absent.
  - B lymphocytes (CD20+) and NK cells (natural killer, CD16/56+) vary on the basis of the type of SCID (see table in section VI).
- Mitogen and antigen stimulation tests (T/B-cell functional assays) are markedly decreased or absent.
- Immunoglobulin levels are usually low or absent, although patients can have normal IgG levels in the first few months of life owing to transplacentally derived maternal IgG.

- TRECs: T-cell recombination excision circles are a reflector of lymphocyte recombination and thymic output. They are used in prenatal screening (presently in WI, MA, and NY), and are uniformly absent in SCID. They are run off of a standard Guthrie blood spot card. Of note, they are known to be decreased in premature infants, but not to the degree seen in SCID (<30 copies/reaction).
- Appropriate cultures to identify pathogens

DIFFERENTIAL DIAGNOSIS
- Reticular dysgenesis
- Bone marrow or thymic infiltrative processes (hematologic or other malignancies).
- HIV infection
- Iatrogenic immunodeficiency

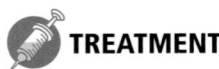

TREATMENT

ADDITIONAL TREATMENT
General Measures
- Bone marrow transplant is the definitive treatment in most cases. Because of the underlying lack of T-cell function, preconditioning (chemotherapy) is not strictly required, though reduced-intensity conditioning is often given to attempt to ensure complete engraftment.
- Aggressive and early specific antibiotic/antifungal/antiviral therapy for infections
- *Pneumocystis carinii* prophylaxis
- If required, patients should receive only irradiated, leukocyte reduced blood products. There is a risk of graft versus host disease owing to viable donor leukocytes that may survive in nonirradiated products.
- IV immunoglobulin replacement: This may be required even after bone marrow transplant because of variable B-lymphocyte reconstitution.
- Enzyme replacement therapy has been used in adenosine deaminase-deficient patients.
- Gene therapy has been successful in clinical trials for X-linked and ADA forms, though development of vector-associated leukemia remains a major concern.

ONGOING CARE

- Close monitoring of clinical status should be done before bone marrow transplant. This may be every 2–4 weeks, depending on the patient's status.
- The posttransplant course is variable:
  - Overall success rate for matched bone marrow transplant in severe combined immunodeficiency is >70%, and is highly dependent on the age and health of the patient at transplantation, and the type and degree of matching of the graft. Success in early transplants (<2 months old) has been reported to be as high as 95%.
  - Patients should still be followed closely for signs of infection, graft failure, and graft versus host disease.

COMPLICATIONS

- Untreated, nearly all patients will succumb to infection prior to 2 years of age.
- Graft versus host disease may result from maternal T cells that cross into fetal circulation or from transfusion of nonirradiated blood products.
- Omenn syndrome is an autoimmune phenomenon caused by clonal, autoreactive T-cells, and resembles graft-versus-host disease. It occurs most commonly in patients with RAG1/2 mutations.
- Clinical disease can be caused by live vaccines in previous undiagnosed severe combined immunodeficiency patients (including BCG or rotavirus).
- Increased risk of hematologic malignancy (30×)
- Radiation sensitivity is present in forms of SCID caused by DNA repair defects (Artemis, Ligase-4, DNA-PKcs, Cernunnos).

ADDITIONAL READING

- Buckley RH. Molecular defects in human severe combined immunodeficiency and approaches to immune reconstitution. *Annu Rev Immunol.* 2004;22:625–655.
- Dvorak CD, Cowan MJ. Radiosensitive Severe combined immunodeficiency. *Immuno All Clin N Am.* 2009;30: 125–142.
- Gaspar HB, Gilmour KC, Jones AM. Severe combined immunodeficiency—molecular pathogenesis and diagnosis. *Arch Dis Child.* 2001;84:169–173.
- Puck JM. Neonatal screening for severe combined immune deficiency. *Curr Opin Allergy Clin Immunol.* 2007;7(6):522–527.
- Winkelstein JA, Blease RM, et al., eds. Immune Deficiency Foundation. *Patient and Family Handbook for the Primary Immune Deficiency Diseases.* 3rd ed. Towson, MD: Immune Deficiency Foundation; 1999–2000.

CODES

ICD9
279.2 Combined immunity deficiency

ICD10
- D81.0 Severe combined immunodeficiency with reticular dysgenesis
- D81.1 Severe combined immunodeficiency w low T- and B-cell numbers
- D81.9 Combined immunodeficiency, unspecified

FAQ

- Q: How should children with severe combined immunodeficiency be managed before bone marrow transplant?
- A: Children suspected to have severe combined immunodeficiency should be isolated from potential sources of infection. They should not attend public places, and should be kept away from any relatives who are ill. Prophylactic antibiotics to prevent opportunistic infections such as *pneumocystis* are usually given, and replacement of immunoglobulin is also commonly provided prior to transplant.
- Q: Should patients with severe combined immunodeficiency receive live viral vaccines?
- A: Live viral vaccines are contraindicated in severe combined immunodeficiency. Patients suspected of severe combined immunodeficiency should not receive live viral vaccines until their immunodeficiency is defined. If the patient is receiving IV immunoglobulin therapy, vaccinations are not required. In addition, siblings of patients with severe combined immunodeficiency who live in the same household should generally not receive live viral vaccines because of the risk of viral shedding in the siblings.
- Q: What is the chance of another child being affected with severe combined immunodeficiency?
- A: The risk of another child being born with severe combined immunodeficiency in a family with a previously affected child will depend on the type of SCID, and would depend on whether a mutation is de novo or transmitted. A mother who carried the gene for X-linked SCID would have a 50% chance of an affected male or carrier female; autosomal recessive causes would carry a 25% chance of an affected child. Genetic counseling should be offered to female carriers of X-linked severe combined immunodeficiency.
- Q: Can SCID be diagnosed prenatally?
- A: Prenatal testing is available. Amniocentesis can be performed, and fetal cells can be tested for known genetic cause of severe combined immunodeficiency.
- Q: Can SCID be screened for via newborn testing?
- A: Newborn testing is done in several states (WI, NY, MA) via analysis of TRECs from Guthrie blood spot cards (see Tests above). TRECs can also be sent electively in other states.

S

SEXUAL ABUSE

Sarah M. Frioux
Cindy W. Christian

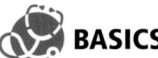 **BASICS**

DESCRIPTION
Sexual abuse is the involvement of children in sexual activities that they cannot understand, for which they are not developmentally prepared, to which they cannot give informed consent, and/or that violate societal norms.
- Associated problems:
  - Physical abuse
  - Domestic violence
  - Neglect
  - Emotional abuse
- Pitfalls:
  - Failing to consider sexual abuse in the differential diagnosis of nonspecific behavioral and physical complaints

EPIDEMIOLOGY
- Children of all ages may be victimized, with a peak age of vulnerability between 7 and 13 years.
- Girls are victimized more than boys, although abuse of boys is thought to be underreported. Boys represent ~20% of cases reported to child protection agencies.
- Race and socioeconomic status are not believed to play a role in the epidemiology of sexual abuse.

Incidence
~150,000 substantiated cases are identified each year in the US. This is likely to be a significant underestimation of the actual numbers.

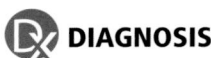 **DIAGNOSIS**

HISTORY
- The physician interview should be detailed enough to know whether a report to child protection or law enforcement is needed, especially if it is the first professional interview of the child:
  - Prior to the examination, however, the child may have been interviewed by the police, social service workers, or a forensic interviewer.
- The interview should be conducted with the child separate from family members; diagnosis often depends on the history obtained from the child.
- Ask open-ended, nonleading questions.
- Use developmentally appropriate language.
- Special questions:
  - Identity of alleged perpetrator/relationship to child
  - Time of last possible contact
  - Method of disclosure
  - Specific types of sexual contact included in the abuse
  - Previous official reports of the abuse
  - Review of systems including genital pain, bleeding, dysuria, constipation, painful bowel movements, and behavioral changes

PHYSICAL EXAM
- Most sexually abused children have normal genital examinations:
  - The abuse may not have caused injury to tissues.
  - Mucosal injuries heal quickly and may be resolved by the time the child is examined.
- Prepubertal children require detailed external genital inspection only:
  - Genital examination can be done with child in supine frog-leg position.
  - Use of the techniques of labial separation and labial traction will allow complete examination of the vulvar structures.
- Adolescent girls usually do not require a full pelvic examination:
  - Prepubertal girls should not have speculum examination unless anesthesia is used.
- Few physical findings are diagnostic of abuse:
  - These include the presence of semen or sperm, acute genital/anal injuries without an adequate accidental explanation, syphilis, and *Neisseria gonorrhoeae* (excluding perinatal infection).
  - Look for acute genital injuries and marked disruptions in hymenal tissue.
- Many genital findings are unlikely to be related to abuse. These include small labial adhesions, *Candida albicans* dermatitis, erythema of the vestibule, and small mounds or projections on an otherwise normal hymen.

DIAGNOSTIC TESTS & INTERPRETATION
Lab
- Universal STI screening is not necessary:
  - If child has disclosed high-risk contact or child/parent desires, consider testing for *N. gonorrhoeae, Chlamydia trachomatis, Trichomonas vaginalis*, syphilis, hepatitis B virus infection, and HIV.
- Testing for *N. gonorrhoeae* and *C. trachomatis* may be performed with vaginal/urethral culture or nucleic acid amplification techniques (NAATs):
  - Cultures have historically been the gold standard method for diagnosing STIs in prepubertal children. Recently, NAAT has proven to be sensitive and specific for *N. gonorrhoeae* and *C. trachomatis* infection in this age group.
  - Be familiar with your laboratory's methods of identification and confirmation. Some labs no longer process cultures for these pathogens.
- The unestrogenized hymen is very sensitive; therefore, great care should be taken when inserting a swab through the hymenal opening. Allow 10–15 seconds for swabs to absorb secretions:
  - Cultures for *N. gonorrhoeae* from rectum, vagina (prepubertal), cervix (adolescent), penile urethra, and/or throat; misidentification of *N. gonorrhoeae* can be a problem if confirmatory tests (e.g., sugar fermentation, latex agglutination) are not properly done.

- Chlamydia cultures from rectum, vagina (prepubertal), cervix (adolescent), and/or penile urethra; obtain cells for chlamydia culture by gently scraping the vaginal wall with a swab (in young children).
- NAAT has higher sensitivity than culture. Repeat NAAT should be performed prior to treatment to confirm infection in young children.
- Rapid plasma reagin (RPR), hepatitis B serology, HIV, if indicated
- Forensic evidence collection (for an acute assault)

Diagnostic Procedures/Other
- The labial traction technique (gently grasping the posterior portion of the labia majora and pulling laterally, down, and toward the examiner) allows for the best visualization of the hymenal edges.
- When available, the use of colposcopy is generally recommended for purposes of magnification and photodocumentation of the examination.

DIFFERENTIAL DIAGNOSIS
- Infection with genital discharge:
  - *N. gonorrhoeae*
  - *C. trachomatis*
  - *T. vaginalis*
  - Group A streptococcus
  - *Haemophilus influenzae*
  - *Staphylococcus aureus*
  - *Corynebacterium diphtheriae*
  - *Mycoplasma hominis*
  - *Gardnerella vaginalis*
  - *Shigella flexneri* (discharge may be bloody)
- Infection with genital bleeding:
  - UTI
  - Vulvovaginitis
- Infection with genital inflammation/pruritus:
  - STIs
  - Pinworms
  - Scabies
  - *C. albicans* (in pubertal girls)
  - Group A streptococcal vulvovaginitis or perianal cellulitis
- Trauma:
  - Accidental trauma, including straddle and impaling injuries
  - Mechanical friction from tight clothing or obesity
  - Accidental tourniquet of genitals by hair
- Congenital:
  - Variations in hymenal configuration (septated, cribriform, microperforate, imperforate hymens)
  - Urethral caruncles; vestibular bands
  - Ectopic ureterocele; hemangiomas
  - Syndromes associated with anogenital anomalies
- Psychosocial:
  - Normal behaviors (masturbation, playing doctor)
  - Exposure to sexual activity (e.g., in which the child witnesses sexual acts)
  - False allegations of sexual abuse

- Dermatologic:
  - Contact dermatitis
  - Seborrhea
  - Diaper dermatitis
  - Lichen sclerosis et atrophica
  - Balanitis xerotica
  - Nevi
- Miscellaneous:
  - Nonspecific vulvovaginitis
  - Rectovaginal fistula
  - Labial adhesion (agglutination)
  - Urethral prolapse
  - Phimosis, paraphimosis
  - Foreign body

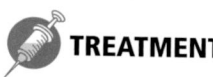 **TREATMENT**

MEDICATION (DRUGS)
- Prophylactic antibiotics are effective against common STIs, such as gonorrhea, chlamydia, and trichomonas:
  - Generally not used for prepubertal children, because these infections are uncommon and rarely result in more serious outcomes like pelvic inflammatory disease
  - Prophylaxis against STIs may be considered for acute sexual assaults, stranger assaults, or children with severe genital injuries.
- Identified STIs should be treated with the appropriate regimen according to published guidelines from the Centers for Disease Control and Prevention (CDC).
- Consider pregnancy prevention (e.g., emergency hormonal contraceptive) for adolescents, after ensuring the patient is not pregnant
- Tetanus booster for patients with acute, serious genital or other injuries
- Hepatitis B vaccination for unimmunized patients
- Hepatitis B immune globulin for patients with recent sexual contact with known positive perpetrator
- Sitz baths for comfort

ADDITIONAL TREATMENT
General Measures
- Report suspected abuse to the local child welfare agency.
- Report suspected sexual abuse to law enforcement.
- Consult a social worker.
- Inform the parents of the report.

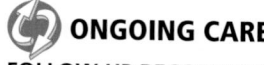 **ONGOING CARE**

FOLLOW-UP RECOMMENDATIONS
Patient Monitoring
- Cases will be investigated by child welfare and/or the police.
- Need for foster care placement and/or ongoing supervision is decided by child welfare investigators.
- Most children are referred for short- or long-term counseling.
- Persistent physical/genital complaints may indicate ongoing abuse, an STI, or psychological problems.
- Patient victimizing younger child: Young perpetrators are often victims of previous abuse.

PROGNOSIS
- Varies greatly depending on specifics of abuse sustained, available support systems
- More extensive injuries (e.g., deep lacerations, tears) may take weeks to months to heal.
- The emotional impact of sexual abuse may take years to resolve.

COMPLICATIONS
- STIs, such as gonorrhea, genital warts, *C. trachomatis*, syphilis, HIV, and herpes simplex virus, are identified in only a small percentage of sexually abused children.
- Emotional problems such as posttraumatic stress disorder (PTSD), feelings of helplessness, impaired trust, low self-esteem, depression, adolescent substance abuse, and suicide attempts are seen in some victims of sexual abuse.
- Aggressive, hypersexual, withdrawn behavioral problems may be consequences of having been abused.

ADDITIONAL READING

- Berenson AB, Chacko MR, Wiemann CM, et al. A case-control study of anatomic changes resulting from sexual abuse. *Am J Obstet Gynecol.* 2000; 182:820–834.
- Black CM, Driebe EM, Howard LA, et al. Multicenter study of nucleic acid amplification tests for detection of Chlamydia trachomatis and Neisseria gonorrhoeae in children being evaluated for sexual abuse. *Pediatr Infect Dis J.* 2009;28(7):608–613.
- Centers for Disease Control and Prevention. Sexually transmitted diseases treatment guidelines. *MMWR Morb Mortal Wkly Rep.* 2010;59(R-12):1–110.
- Kellogg N, American Academy of Pediatrics Committee on Child Abuse and Neglect. The evaluation of sexual abuse in children. *Pediatrics.* 2005;116:506–512.
- Kellogg ND, American Academy of Pediatrics. Committee on Child Abuse and Neglect. The evaluation of sexual behaviors in children. *Pediatrics.* 2009;124:992–998.
- Legano L, McHugh MT, Palusci VJ. Child abuse and neglect. *Curr Probl Pediatr Adolesc Health Care.* 2009;39(2):31.e1–26.

 CODES

ICD9
995.53 Child sexual abuse

ICD10
- T74.22XA Child sexual abuse, confirmed, initial encounter
- T74.22XD Child sexual abuse, confirmed, subsequent encounter
- T74.22XS Child sexual abuse, confirmed, sequela

FAQ
- Q: What does "intact hymen" mean?
- A: "Intact hymen" is not a medical term and should be avoided in describing the medical examination of the genitals. The hymen should be inspected for signs of trauma. There is a wide variation of normal hymenal appearances, and caution should be used in interpreting findings.
- Q: Can there be penetration without physical findings?
- A: Yes. Although full penetration of an erect penis into the prepubertal vaginal canal (through the hymen) will likely leave injury, the healing properties of the vulvar tissues are great, so that past injuries are sometimes difficult or impossible to identify. Furthermore, penetration may be partial (as in vulvar coitus) and may not leave any injuries to the tissue. Physical injuries may not be identified despite a history of penetration.
- Q: Are STIs always transmitted sexually?
- A: No. All STIs may be transmitted vertically (from mother to infant). The incubation periods of different infections vary, so they are expressed at different ages accordingly. Casual transmission of STIs is postulated for some organisms, but not for others. Gonorrhea and syphilis are considered diagnostic of sexual abuse outside of congenital infection. Chlamydia, herpes simplex virus 2, and trichomonas are probably due to sexual abuse and should be reported for evaluation. Condyloma acuminata is probably related to sexual abuse in school-aged and older children but may be transmitted to younger children innocently during toileting or diaper changes. Nevertheless, children presenting with condyloma should be referred for evaluation. Herpes simplex virus type 1 and bacterial vaginosis are nonspecific infections that are not usually related to sexual abuse. Candida is unlikely to be related to sexual abuse.
- Q: How often do sexually abused children have physical evidence of the abuse?
- A: In most cases, there are no specific physical indicators of abuse.

S

SEXUAL AMBIGUITY

J. Nina Ham
Lorraine E. Levitt Katz

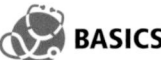 **BASICS**

DESCRIPTION
Genitalia can be defined as ambiguous when it is not possible to categorize the gender of the child based on outward appearances.
- "Disorders of sexual development" (DSD) is the preferred terminology to replace terms such as "intersex," "hermaphroditism," or "pseudohermaphroditism," which are perceived as pejorative by patients:
  - Preferred terms include 46XX DSD; 46XY DSD; ovotesticular DSD; 46XX testicular DSD; and 46XY complete gonadal dysgenesis.
  - These represent general categorizations, however, and when available, specific diagnoses are preferable.
- Pitfalls: Girls with congenital adrenal hyperplasia (CAH) may appear quite virilized at birth and be mistaken for boys. Nevertheless, they have good female reproductive potential with adequate control of their disease and should be assigned a female sex.

EPIDEMIOLOGY
- CAH is the most common cause of sexual ambiguity, with a worldwide incidence of 1/10,000–20,000.
- Disorders causing sexual ambiguity occur congenitally, and the time of presentation is the newborn period. Children with 5α-reductase deficiency demonstrate virilization with puberty.

RISK FACTORS
Genetics
- CAH is caused by defects in the genes encoding adrenal steroidogenic enzymes. It follows an autosomal recessive inheritance pattern:
  - The most common form is 21-hydroxylase deficiency (due to mutations in the gene CYP21A).
  - Sexual ambiguity can also be seen in defects in 17-hydroxylase (CYP17), 3β-hydroxysteroid dehydrogenase (HSD3B2), 17-ketosteroid reductase (HSD17B3), and 11β-hydroxylase (CYP11B1).
  - Congenital lipoid adrenal hyperplasia has been associated with defects in steroidogenic acute regulatory protein (StAR) and, less commonly, cholesterol desmolase.
- Gonadal dysgenesis is associated with chromosomal aberrations.
- Syndromes of gonadal dysgenesis can also arise from mutations in the Wilms tumor suppressor gene (WT-1), steroidogenic factor 1 (SF-1), sex-determining region Y (SRY), and the SRY homeobox gene SOX9.
- 5α-Reductase deficiency is an autosomal recessive disorder that manifests only in genetic males.
- Androgen resistance syndromes are due to defects in the androgen receptor gene, located on the X chromosome. Thus, inheritance follows an X-linked recessive pattern.

GENERAL PREVENTION
- Avoid the use of androgenic steroids during pregnancy.
- Prenatal diagnosis of CAH and maternal steroid treatment to prevent virilization of female fetuses is possible, but is still best considered on a research basis.

PATHOPHYSIOLOGY
- 46XX DSD:
  - Masculinization of the female fetus is usually caused by androgens produced by the fetus or transferred across the placenta from the mother. The most common cause is CAH in which the fetal adrenal glands overproduce androgens in an attempt to correct cortisol deficiency.
- 46XY DSD:
  - Incomplete masculinization of the male fetus can be caused by enzyme disorders of testosterone synthesis (e.g., CAH and 5α-reductase deficiency), unresponsiveness to testosterone action (androgen insensitivity syndromes), or defects in testicular development (complete or partial gonadal dysgenesis).
- Ovotesticular DSD:
  - Includes patients with both ovarian and testicular elements. These patients can be 46XX/46XY (chimeric) or 45X/46XY (mixed gonadal dysgenesis).
  - Phenotypically, individuals may exhibit a range from female external genitalia to ambiguous to normal male.
- Gonadal dysgenesis:
  - Partial dysgenesis of the gonads following differentiation into testes will result in a spectrum of abnormalities ranging from phenotypically female external genitalia with the absence of müllerian structures to micropenis or cryptorchidism.
  - Mixed gonadal dysgenesis: Individuals with the mosaic genotypes XO/XY and XX/XY have gonads containing both ovarian and testicular elements and external genitalia ranging from normal female to ambiguous to normal male.

DIAGNOSIS

Ambiguous genitalia in the neonate should be treated as an emergency, and the diagnostic evaluation undertaken as soon as possible.

HISTORY
Obtain a careful pregnancy and family history addressing:
- Drug ingestion
- Exposure to teratogens
- Infections during the pregnancy
- Androgenic changes in the mother
- Family history suggestive of CAH

PHYSICAL EXAM
Notable features:
- Palpable gonads: Imply the presence of Y-chromosome material
- Fusion of the labia
- Existence of a vagina
- Position of the urethra
- Length and diameter of the penis or clitoris
- Development of the scrotum
- Other dysmorphic features
- Hypertension is seen with 17α-hydroxylase and 11-hydroxylase deficiencies.
- Features of the classic disorders of adrenal steroidogenesis

DIAGNOSTIC TESTS & INTERPRETATION
Lab
- Specific tests:
  - Karyotype
  - Steroid levels: 17-hydroxyprogesterone, 17-hydroxypregnenolone, dehydroepiandrosterone (DHEA), testosterone, dihydrotestosterone (DHT), 11-deoxycortisol, androstenedione
  - In the case of suspected CAH, ACTH-stimulated values may aid in diagnosis.
- Nonspecific tests: Electrolytes: Hyponatremia, hyperkalemia, and metabolic acidosis are associated with several adrenal enzyme deficiencies.

Imaging
- Pelvic ultrasound
- Urethrogram

DIFFERENTIAL DIAGNOSIS
- Gonadal dysgenesis:
  - Partial dysgenesis of the gonads
  - Mixed gonadal dysgenesis
  - Ovotesticular DSD
- 46XX DSD:
  - CAH: Inherited adrenal enzymatic defects, including 21-hydroxylase, 11-hydroxylase, and HSD3B2 deficiencies can cause virilization of females.
  - Maternal androgen exposure
  - Exogenous androgens or endogenous production (e.g., maternal virilizing tumor)
  - Multiple congenital anomalies
  - Ambiguous genitalia can be a part of a spectrum of congenital anomalies, especially those of the urologic system and rectum.
  - Idiopathic
- 46XY DSD:
  - CAH: Deficiencies in HSD3B2, 17α-hydroxylase, StAR protein, and cholesterol desmolase result in insufficient androgen synthesis potentially causing undervirilization of boys:
    - 5α-Reductase deficiency prevents the conversion of testosterone to DHT, which is necessary for the development of the male external genitalia.
    - Syndromes of androgen resistance are due to abnormalities in androgen receptor or postreceptor defects. Patients with incomplete forms of androgen resistance may present with sexual ambiguity.
- Multiple congenital anomalies
- Idiopathic

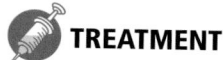

TREATMENT

ADDITIONAL TREATMENT
General Measures
- Treatment of CAH:
  - Acute salt-wasting adrenal crisis
  - Volume resuscitation with 5% dextrose in normal saline (D5NS)
  - Chronic management of CAH consists of cortisol replacement 12–25 mg/m^2 per 24 hours divided as q8h and fludrocortisone 0.05–0.3 mg/d.
- Counseling of families

SURGERY/OTHER PROCEDURES
Surgery may be necessary so that the sexual phenotype and gonads are consistent with the gender assignment. Dysgenetic testes and ovotestes should be removed.

IN-PATIENT CONSIDERATIONS
Initial Stabilization
- Gender assignment: The results of the diagnostic evaluation should be available within 48–72 hours. Parents should be counseled that the diagnostic information as well as surgical factors, prediction of hormone function, and potential for fertility will be taken together as a whole. Gender assignment should be made through a multidisciplinary team approach with consultations from endocrinology, urology, genetics, psychiatry/psychology, and social work.
- Treatment of CAH:
  - Acute salt-wasting adrenal crisis
  - Volume resuscitation with D5NS
  - Stress hydrocortisone 25–50 mg IV immediately after the serum studies are drawn. This should be followed by 100 mg/m^2 per 24 hours of hydrocortisone intravenous divided q4h.
  - Hydrocortisone is gradually tapered over the next few days.
  - Fludrocortisone 0.05–0.3 mg/d when able to take PO

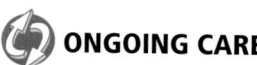

ONGOING CARE

FOLLOW-UP RECOMMENDATIONS
Patient Monitoring
- Hormone replacement therapy at puberty may be necessary.
- Long-term follow-up may involve monitoring hormone levels, linear growth, and sexual development.

PROGNOSIS
The cosmetic outcome from surgery is usually good. The potential for gender-appropriate sexual function is usually good with therapy. The potential for reproductive function depends on the diagnosis. Long-term studies of psychological adjustment are under way.

COMPLICATIONS
- 21-Hydroxylase-, HSD3B2-, and StAR protein–deficient forms of CAH are associated with mineralocorticoid deficiency and consequent life-threatening salt-losing adrenal crises presenting in the 1st 2 weeks of life.
- CAH is also associated with cortisol deficiency, requiring emergent and chronic cortisol replacement.
- Dysgenetic testes and ovotestes have an increased risk of malignant degeneration and should be removed.
- An incorrect or hastily made sexual assignment can cause family members additional emotional stress.

ADDITIONAL READING

- Hyun G, Kolon TF. A practical approach to intersex in the newborn period. *Urol Clin North Am.* 2004;31:435–443.
- Kohler B, Lumbroso S, Leger J, et al. Androgen insensitivity syndrome: Somatic mosaicism of the androgen receptor and consequences for sex assignment and genetic counseling. *J Clin Endocrinol Metab.* 2005;90:106–111.
- Lee PA, Houk CP, Ahmed SF, et al. Consensus statement on management of intersex disorders. *Pediatrics.* 2006;118:e488–e500.
- MacLaughlin DT, Donahoe PK. Sex determination and differentiation. *N Engl J Med.* 2004;350:367–378.
- Nabhan ZM, Lee PA. Disorders of sex development. *Curr Opin Obstet Gynec.* 2007;19:440–445.
- New MI. Inborn errors of adrenal steroidogenesis. *Mol Cell Endocrinol.* 2003;211:75–83.
- New MI, Carlson A, Obeid J, et al. Prenatal diagnosis for congenital adrenal hyperplasia in 532 pregnancies. *J Clin Endocrinol Metab.* 2001;86:5651–5657.
- Ogilvy-Stuart AL, Brain CE. Early assessment of ambiguous genitalia. *Arch Dis Child.* 2004;89:401–407.

- Speiser PW, Azziz R, Baskin LS, et al. Congenital adrenal hyperplasia due to steroid 21-hydroxylase deficiency: An Endocrine Society Clinical Practice Guideline. *J Clin Endocrinol Metab.* 2010;95:4133–4160.
- Speiser PW, White PC. Congenital adrenal hyperplasia. *N Engl J Med.* 2003;349:776–788.
- Yong EL, Lim J, Qi W, et al. Molecular basis of androgen receptor diseases. *Ann Med.* 2000;32:15–22.

CODES

ICD9
- 255.2 Adrenogenital disorders
- 259.8 Other specified endocrine disorders
- 752.7 Indeterminate sex and pseudohermaphroditism

ICD10
- E25.0 Congenital adrenogenital disorders associated with enzyme deficiency
- Q56.0 Hermaphroditism, not elsewhere classified
- Q56.4 Indeterminate sex, unspecified

FAQ

- Q: Should a child's sex assignment be consistent with the karyotype?
- A: In the past, surgery was performed when the team decision focused on sexual function potential. Recently, there is a trend to raise the child consistent with the karyotype. This is a major decision that should involve the family and the treatment team.
- Q: What clues can the physical exam give to the timing of in utero events causing sexual ambiguity?
- A: In the virilized female, labioscrotal fusion results from androgen exposure prior to 12 weeks' gestation. Thereafter, androgen exposure can cause only clitoromegaly.

S

SEXUAL PRECOCITY

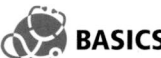

Andrew C. Calabria
Andrea Kelly
Rachana Shah (5th edition)

BASICS

DESCRIPTION
- Sexual precocity has traditionally been defined as physical signs of sexual development before age 8 years in girls and age 9 in boys.
- Recently, new guidelines were proposed for lowering the age considered to be normal for sexual development in girls:
  - Signs of puberty as young as age 7 in white girls and age 6 in black girls may be normal.
  - These new guidelines have not been universally adopted.
- The entire clinical picture, including rate of progression and the presence of neurologic symptoms, must be taken into account.

EPIDEMIOLOGY
- Precocious puberty is 5–6 times more common in girls.
- 80–90% of affected girls have idiopathic central precocious puberty.
- Precocious puberty in boys is more likely to be associated with underlying pathology.
- ~50% of affected boys have idiopathic central precocious puberty.
- Increased incidence seen in internationally adopted children and in children born premature or small for gestational age

Incidence
Precocious puberty occurs in 1 in 5,000 children

Genetics
- Familial male precocious puberty (testitoxicosis): Sex-limited, autosomal dominant inheritance of activating mutation in the luteinizing hormone (LH) receptor
- McCune–Albright syndrome: Sporadic, postzygotic, somatic mutation in the stimulatory subunit of G-protein receptor; precocious puberty more common in girls

PATHOPHYSIOLOGY
- Central precocious puberty can be associated with CNS disorders
- Peripheral precocious puberty arises from peripheral sex hormone sources, including gonadal and adrenal disorders, abdominal or pelvic tumors, or exogenous sex steroids.
- Peripheral precocious puberty can progress to central precocious puberty due to maturation of the hypothalamic–pituitary axis by sex steroids.

ETIOLOGY
Central precocious puberty (gonadotropin-releasing hormone [GnRH]–dependent):
- Associated with gonadotropin (LH and/or follicle-stimulating hormone [FSH]) levels that are elevated beyond the normal prepubertal range. Results from activation of hypothalamic–pituitary–gonadal axis.
- Peripheral precocious puberty (GnRH-independent): Gonadotropin-independent elevation of sex steroids arising (i) directly from gonads and/or adrenals, (ii) through stimulation of gonads by GnRH-independent mechanism, or (iii) from an exogenous source

DIAGNOSIS

SIGNS AND SYMPTOMS
- Careful chronology of physical changes, growth spurt, onset of menses
- Presence of neurologic, visual, or behavioral changes to suggest a CNS lesion

HISTORY
Family history of early puberty or hyperandrogenic disorders (e.g., congenital adrenal hyperplasia)
- Presence of exogenous sex steroids in the home

PHYSICAL EXAM
- Plot accurate height (using wall-mounted stadiometer), weight, and growth velocity. Growth acceleration within the past year may be strong evidence for puberty.
- Carefully stage breasts, color of vaginal mucosa, and pubic hair in girls.
- Carefully stage testicular volume (with Prader gonadometer), penile size, and pubic hair in boys.
- Carefully evaluate for abdominal masses.
- Examine skin for acne and café au lait spots.
- Perform comprehensive neurologic evaluation to assess for possible CNS pathology.

DIAGNOSTIC TESTS & INTERPRETATION
Lab
- Sex steroids: Estradiol, total testosterone
- Adrenal steroids: 17-OH progesterone, dehydroepiandrosterone sulfate (DHEA-S), androstenedione
- Gonadotropins: FSH, LH (ultrasensitive or immunochemiluminometric [ICMA]-LH most accurate; also listed as "pediatric")

- Prolactin: May be elevated with CNS tumors
- Thyroid-stimulating hormone (TSH) and free thyroxine (T_4)
- Human chorionic gonadotropin (hCG) levels
- Provocative tests should be done when the aforementioned tests are abnormal or equivocal:
  - GnRH test for central precocious puberty; prepubertal GnRH response is predominantly FSH, whereas pubertal response is predominantly LH
  - Adrenocorticotropic hormone (ACTH) stimulation test for adrenal abnormalities. Exogenous corticosteroid therapy will interfere with ACTH test, but does not interfere with GnRH test of pituitary–gonadal axis.

Imaging
- Bone age: If advanced, further studies are warranted, guided by history and physical examination. If not advanced, or if the patient has only mild breast or pubic hair development (but not both), premature thelarche or premature adrenarche, respectively, is the most likely diagnosis.
- MRI of head: As indicated by history, physical examination, and laboratory tests; almost always done in boys because they are much less likely than are girls to have idiopathic sexual precocity
- Ultrasound of gonads/adrenals: As indicated by examination and studies. Look for tumors in both sexes; in girls, ultrasound can also evaluate development of ovaries and uterus.

ALERT
- Obese children often have advanced bone age.
- Palpation of breast tissue (buds) can be difficult due to adiposity.

DIFFERENTIAL DIAGNOSIS
- Causes of central precocious puberty:
  - Often idiopathic (girls more often than boys)
  - Any cause of peripheral precocious puberty
  - Tumors:
    - CNS tumors
    - Hypothalamic hamartoma: Most common CNS mass to cause precocious puberty; benign (nonprogressive), congenital malformation of neurons that secrete GnRH
    - Hypothalamic–chiasmatic glioma: Often associated with neurofibromatosis
    - Astrocytoma
    - Ependymoma

- Post-CNS trauma or damage:
  - Surgery
  - Radiation: May occur after 18-Gy exposure
  - Hydrocephalus and other CNS malformations
  - Infection: Brain abscess, meningitis, encephalitis, granuloma. Lesions may result in stimulation or lack of inhibition of the GnRH-secreting area of the hypothalamus, resulting in early activation of the pituitary
- Mimickers of central precocious puberty:
  - Human chorionic gonadotropin-secreting tumors (pineal gland or liver): Ectopic hCG activates LH receptors in testes
  - Severe acquired hypothyroidism: High levels of TSH may cross-stimulate gonadal FSH and/or LH receptors
- Causes of peripheral precocious puberty:
  - Tumors:
    - Gonadal tumors
    - Adrenal tumors
  - Environmental: Exogenous estrogens (creams and oral forms) and/or exogenous androgens (anabolic steroids or testosterone formulations)
  - Congenital adrenal hyperplasia: Poorly controlled CAH can activate the hypothalamic–pituitary–gonadal axis in either gender
  - Severe acquired hypothyroidism: High levels of TSH may cross-stimulate gonadal FSH and/or LH receptors.
  - McCune–Albright syndrome: Triad of precocious puberty, café au lait spots, and polyostotic fibrous dysplasia
  - Familial male precocious puberty (familial testitoxicosis)
  - Refeeding after severe malnutrition during early development (such as adopted children who had kwashiorkor)
- Incomplete pubertal development:
  - Premature thelarche
  - Premature adrenarche

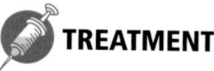

TREATMENT

MEDICATION (DRUGS)
- Central precocious puberty: GnRH agonists are the treatment of choice. Adjunctive therapy with growth hormone may improve final adult height.
- Calcium supplementation may preserve bone mass accretion during GnRH agonist therapy.
- Peripheral precocious puberty: Aromatase inhibitors and antiandrogens (spironolactone or ketoconazole). Glucocorticoids for congenital adrenal hyperplasia

 ONGOING CARE

- When to expect improvement:
  - Depends on cause. For example, sexual changes of McCune–Albright syndrome are due to autonomously functioning ovarian cysts, which regress variably over time.
  - Treatment of central precocious puberty with a GnRH agonist usually results in cessation of menses within 2 months, slowing or nonprogression of pubertal changes over 4–6 months, and decreased acceleration of bone age within 12 months.
- Typically, GnRH agonists such as leuprolide (Lupron) are administered in a depot form every 28 days. Some children require shortening of the interval, often prompted by reports of moodiness, development of acne, or breakthrough menses. A new longer-acting formulation of leuprolide is now available for every 3 month injection. An 12-month duration implantable formulation (histrelin) is also available.
- The length of treatment is highly individualized but typically continues until the age of normal pubertal onset.

PROGNOSIS
- With treatment, improvement in predicted height may be achieved, but most children do not reach target height predicted by midparental height measurements.
- Earlier treatment results in improved final height.
- Treatment may decrease psychosocial distress.
- Effect of GnRH agonists on fertility has not been fully elucidated.

COMPLICATIONS
- Short stature
- Psychosocial stresses of early puberty

ADDITIONAL READING

- Antoniazzi F, Bertoldo F, Lauriola S, et al. Prevention of bone demineralization by calcium supplementation in precocious puberty during gonadotropin-releasing hormone agonist treatment. *J Clin Endocrinol Metab.* 1999;84:1992–1996.
- Carel JC, Eugster EA, Rogol A, et al. Consensus statement on the use of gonadotropin-releasing hormone analogs in children. *Pediatrics.* 2009; 123(4):e752–e762.
- Carel JC, Léger J. Clinical practice. Precocious puberty. *N Engl J Med.* 2008;358(22): 2366–2377.
- Herman-Giddens ME, Slora EJ, Wasserman RC, et al. Secondary sexual characteristics and menses in young girls seen in office practice: A study from the Pediatric Research Office in Settings Network. *Pediatrics.* 1997;99:505–512.
- Ibanez L, Zegher F. Puberty after prenatal growth restraint. *Horm Res.* 2006;65(suppl 3):112–115.

- Kaplowitz P, Oberfield SE, Drug and Therapeutics and Executive Committees of the Lawson Wilkins Pediatric Endocrine Society. Reexamination of the age limit for defining when puberty is precocious in girls in the United States: Implications for evaluation and treatment. *Pediatrics.* 1999;104:936–941.
- Kaplowitz PB. Treatment of central precocious puberty. *Curr Opin Endocrinol Diabetes Obes.* 2009;16(1):31–36.
- Nathan BM, Palmert MR. Regulation and disorders of pubertal timing. *Endocrinol Metab Clin North Am.* 2005;34:617–641.
- Oostidjk W, Rikken B, Schreuder S, et al. Final height in central precocious puberty after long term treatment with a slow release. GnRH agonist. *Arch Dis Child.* 1996;75:292–297.
- Styne DM. New aspects in diagnosis and treatment of pubertal disorders. *Pediatr Clin North Am.* 1997;44:505–529.
- Teilmann G, Pederson CB, Skakkebaek NE, et al. Increased risk of precocious puberty in internationally adopted children in Denmark. *Pediatrics.* 2006;1818:391–398.

 CODES

ICD9
259.1 Precocious sexual development and puberty, not elsewhere classified

ICD10
E30.1 Precocious puberty

FAQ
- Q: If my child is treated with GnRH agonists, will he/she go through puberty when we stop the medication?
- A: Yes, children on GnRH agonist treatment do proceed through normal puberty when the medication is stopped. Effects on fertility have not been fully studied long-term.
- Q: If my child already has some pubertal changes, can they be reversed?
- A: If GnRH agonists are used, menses will cease, and breast tissue and pubic hair will often regress.

SHORT-BOWEL SYNDROME

Maria R. Mascarenhas
Judith Kelsen

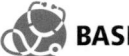 **BASICS**

DESCRIPTION
Malnutrition, malabsorption, and/or fluid and electrolyte loss after extensive small-bowel resection

PATHOPHYSIOLOGY
- Markedly decreased mucosal surface area due to resection
- Loss of trophic hormones
- Loss of peptide hormones that regulate motility
- Abnormal transit
- Malabsorption of protein, fat, carbohydrate, vitamins, electrolytes, and trace elements, depending on site of resected intestine (see "Follow-Up"). The patient can lose as much as half of the intestine if the duodenum, distal ileum, and ileocecal valve (ICV) are present. If the ICV is gone, patients may not be able to tolerate even a 25% loss of intestine without the help of total parenteral nutrition (TPN).
- Normal bowel length: 150–200 cm (26 weeks gestation); 200–300 cm (at birth in full-term infant); 600–800 cm (adult)
- Infants have no intestinal reserve and do not tolerate small-bowel resection as well as do adults. However, long-term prognosis may be better because of hypertrophy and hyperplasia of the intestine.
- Gastric acid hypersecretion occurs soon after intestinal resection, but is transient.
- Bowel adaptation can occur over time. Increased surface area due to bowel dilatation, villus hypertrophy, and bowel lengthening can occur. Stimulation of luminal contents is needed for bowel growth and factors such as glutamine, short-chain fatty acids, tropic hormones, and growth factors may be important for bowel growth.

ETIOLOGY
- Infants: Intestinal resection for necrotizing enterocolitis
- Congenital anomalies include intestinal atresias, gastroschisis, omphalocele, apple peel syndrome, and meconium ileus.
- Malrotation may result in volvulus with bowel resection secondary to ischemic injury.
- Older children: Neoplasms and radiation enteritis
- Intestinal resection secondary to Crohn disease, trauma, pseudo-obstruction syndrome

 **DIAGNOSIS**

HISTORY
- Stooling pattern: Number, size, nature (watery, bulky, foul smelling), presence of blood and mucus
- Weight loss or gain: Gaining length/height
- Abdominal distention and flatulence
- Intense perianal rashes related to stool acidity and malabsorption of carbohydrates
- Abdominal pain and characteristics
- Vomiting and characteristics
- Diet history: Appetite, oral intake, tube feeds, parenteral nutrition (PN)
- Medication history
- Surgical history

PHYSICAL EXAM
- Weight, length, and head circumference measurements (if applicable); try to get previous growth chart if available
- Look for signs of vitamin deficiencies in examination of mouth, lips, skin, hair loss, and healing difficulties
- Abdominal examination: Surgical scars, ostomies, distention, hepatosplenomegaly, bowel sounds
- Rectal examination: Consistency of stool, heme positivity, perianal rash

DIAGNOSTIC TESTS & INTERPRETATION
Lab
- Blood tests:
  - CBC: Check for anemia and mean corpuscular volume
  - Electrolytes: Check for losses and adequacy of replacement
  - Minerals: Calcium, phosphorus, magnesium, iron; check for losses and adequacy of replacement therapy
  - Albumin and prealbumin: Check for protein stores and nutritional status
  - Prothrombin time/partial thromboplastin time and protein induced by vitamin K absence (PIVKA): Assess vitamin K status
    - A new test known as the PIVKA-II assay is a more sensitive measure of vitamin K status; however, it is more useful in adolescents.
  - Liver function tests: Alanine transaminase (ALT), γ-glutamyl transpeptidase (GGT), bilirubin if on PN to check for TPN-associated liver disease
  - Vitamin levels: Vitamin A, 25-hydroxy vitamin D, vitamin E, folic acid, B12; check for adequacy
  - Zinc level: Check status and adequacy of supplementation
  - Carnitine: Check status if on long-term PN and presence of liver disease
  - Breath tests: Lactose and lactulose breath test to check for lactase deficiency and bacterial overgrowth, respectively

- Stool tests:
  - Stool for pH and reducing substances: Check for carbohydrate malabsorption
  - Stool smear for fat (Sudan stain—qualitative): Check for excessive fat loss
  - Stool for blood: Check for mucosal damage
  - Stool elastase: Measure of pancreatic insufficiency
- Tests of absorption:
  - Xylose absorption test and lactose breath test to check for carbohydrate malabsorption
  - 72-hour quantitative fecal fat collection along with concomitant diet record
  - Carotene levels to check for fat absorption
  - 24-hour stool collection for α-1-antitrypsin clearance to check for protein absorption

Imaging
Upper GI series with small-bowel follow-through and barium enema to evaluate length, caliber, and location of remaining bowel

Diagnostic Procedures/Other
Endoscopy:
- Upper endoscopy: Look for presence of inflammation that may be contributing to malabsorption; get cultures for bacterial overgrowth
- Lower endoscopy: Look for presence of colitis, especially eosinophilic colitis, as well as caliber of anastomotic site if in colon

DIFFERENTIAL DIAGNOSIS
- Infants: Necrotizing enterocolitis, volvulus, atresia (jejunal and ileal), gastroschisis, meconium peritonitis, congenital short-bowel syndrome
- Older children: Mid-gut volvulus (due to malrotation), Crohn disease, adhesions causing intestinal obstruction, strictures, trauma, aganglionosis of the intestine

 **TREATMENT**

MEDICATION (DRUGS)
- Supplementation of vitamin (E, D, K, B12, folic acid) deficiency, calcium, magnesium, iron, and zinc
- H_2-receptor antagonists and proton pump inhibitors decrease gastric acid hypersecretion and reduce gastric secretory volume.
- Antidiarrheal drugs: Codeine, diphenoxylate, and anticholinergic drugs (e.g., loperamide) to decrease motility (caution in patients with slow transit or bacterial overgrowth)
- Ion-exchange resins: Cholestyramine binds intraluminal dihydroxy bile acids to prevent bile acid-induced diarrhea.
- Octreotide/somatostatin: Decreases gastric, pancreatic, and intestinal secretions; slows GI motility and splanchnic blood flow
- Bacterial overgrowth: Commonly used oral antibiotics are metronidazole, trimethoprim–sulfamethoxazole, vancomycin, and gentamicin.

- Prokinetic agents: Reglan to treat delayed gastric emptying
- Miscellaneous: Sucralfate to treat bile reflux, probiotics to treat bacterial overgrowth, ursodiol for cholestasis, Polycitra for electrolyte losses, dietary fiber to enhance absorption-caution in infancy
- Duration of treatment: Depends on amount and site of bowel resected and degree of intestinal adaptation that occurs. The more the resection, the longer is the therapy. Successful enteral feeds decrease the duration of PN. Macronutrient losses decrease with intestinal adaptation. Micronutrient supplementation may be lifelong (e.g., vitamin B12).

SURGERY/OTHER PROCEDURES
- Surgery is useful in patients who develop strictures and partial obstruction or in those who have very short intestine length.
- Intestinal interpositions (isoperistaltic or antiperistaltic) can be used to delay gastric emptying, slow intestinal transit, and increase absorption, intestinal valves, and reversed intestinal segments.
- Intestinal lengthening and tapering procedures, including the Bianchi and step enteroplasty procedures, increase absorptive surface area.
- In patients with extremely short intestines and PN dependency, small-bowel transplantation or small-bowel/liver transplantation is considered.

ONGOING CARE

FOLLOW-UP RECOMMENDATIONS
Patient Monitoring
- When to expect improvement: Depends on site and extent of bowel resection
- Signs to watch for:
  - Vomiting, diarrhea, weight loss, severe fluid and electrolyte abnormalities, sepsis, bowel dilatation, intestinal obstruction
- Major cause of death: Sepsis and cholestatic liver disease

DIET
- Fluid and electrolyte therapy: Extremely important in the acute phase immediately after bowel resection. In the chronic phase, it is important to keep up with ongoing losses, especially when enteral feeds are started.
- Oral diet: In those patients who are able to avoid PN or tube feeds, a low-lactose diet may be well tolerated. Low-oxalate diets are helpful in preventing oxalate stones. In general, a high-calorie diet regardless of carbohydrate and fat composition should be the mainstay of treatment.
- Enteral feeds: More successful in the patient with less extensive resection, intact ICV, and colon in continuity. In extensive loss, feeds initiated after electrolytes are stabilized.
  - Feeds started very slowly, often started with elemental diet to facilitate absorption, and for concern for allergic injury.
  - Enteral feeds stimulate intestinal adaptation. Before 1 year of age formula should have low osmolality: Higher fat content than carbohydrate.
  - After >1 year of age there is no advantage of elemental formulas over intact formulas with respect to tolerance, unless small-bowel damage is present.

- Enteral feeds are important for development of developmental milestones, with suck and swallow.
- PN: Important in the acute phase postoperatively, when nutrition must be maintained in the face of paralytic ileus; indispensable in the chronic phase when full enteral feeds cannot be instituted and nutrition needs to be maintained.
  - Balanced solutions of protein, glucose, and fat should be administered.
  - Prophylactic measures to prevent PN-induced liver damage should be instituted (e.g., prevention of overfeeding, early introduction of enteral feeds, cycling of PN when patient is stable). If cholestasis is present, it is necessary to modify amount of trace elements in PN.
  - Need permanent central access to deliver concentrated PN solutions
- Intravenous fish-based oil emulsion (composed of omega-3 polyunsaturated fatty acids) has been studied as a preventive measure against PN-associated liver disease with promising results.

PROGNOSIS
- Depends on site and amount of bowel resected
- The greater the amount of bowel resected, the worse is the prognosis.
- Loss of ICV portends a worse prognosis.
- Loss of jejunum and ileum creates a poorer clinical condition than loss of colon.
- The longer it takes to tolerate full enteral feeds in a patient, the worse is the prognosis. Most progress is made in the 1st year after bowel resection.
- Development of severe TPN liver disease: Poor prognosis

COMPLICATIONS
- Fluid and electrolyte loss, resulting in diarrhea, dehydration, and metabolic acidosis
- Calcium and magnesium deficiency, resulting in bone disease and osteoporosis
- Carbohydrate malabsorption
- Fat malabsorption
- Vitamin A deficiency: Increased susceptibility to infections
- Vitamin D deficiency: Bone disease (e.g., rickets)
- Vitamin E deficiency: Peripheral neuropathy, hemolysis
- Vitamin K deficiency: Prolonged clotting time, bruising
- Vitamin B12: Macrocytic anemia and thrombosis
- Folic acid: Macrocytic anemia
- Gallstones: Due to disturbed enterohepatic circulation of bile salts and lithogenic bile formation
- Renal stones: Due to fat malabsorption and increased oxalate absorption
- Failure to thrive
- TPN-dependent liver disease: Cholestasis, end-stage cirrhosis and portal hypertension
- Zinc deficiency: Poor growth, infections
- Carnitine deficiency: Contributes to development of steatosis
- Sepsis
- Small-bowel bacterial overgrowth and D-lactic acidosis due to stasis, causing encephalopathy, ataxia, and other neurologic symptoms

ADDITIONAL READING

- Duro D, Kamin D, Duggan C. Overview of pediatric short bowel syndrome. J Pediatr Gastroenterol Nutr. 2008;47(Suppl 1):S33–S36.
- Fallon EM, Le HD, Puder M. Prevention of parenteral nutrition-associated liver disease: Role of omega-3 fish oil. Curr Opin Organ Transplant. 2010;15(3): 334–340.
- Goulet O. Irreversible intestinal failure. J Pediatr Gastroenterol Nutr. 2004;38:250–269.
- Goulet O, Ruemmele J. Causes and management of intestinal failure in children. Gastroenterology. 2006;130:S16–S28.
- Hwang S, Shulman R. Recent advances in neonatal gastroenterology, update on the management and treatment of short gut. Clin Perinatol. 2002;29: 181–194.
- Olieman JF, Penning C, Ijsselstijn H, et al. Enteral nutrition in children with short bowel syndrome: Current evidence and recommendations for the clinician. J Am Diet Assoc. 2010;110(3):420–426.
- Rudolph JA, Squires R. Current concepts in the management of pediatric intestinal failure. Curr Opin Organ Transplant. 2010;15(3):324–329.
- Sigalet DL. Short bowel syndrome in infants and children: An overview. Semin Pediatr Surg. 2001;10(2):49–55.
- Vanderhoof JA, Young RJ. Enteral and parenteral nutrition in the care of patients with short-bowel syndrome. Best Pract Res Clin Gastroenterol. 2003;17(6):997–1015.

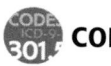 CODES

ICD9
579.3 Other and unspecified postsurgical nonabsorption

ICD10
K91.2 Postsurgical malabsorption, not elsewhere classified

FAQ

- Q: What are the favorable prognostic factors in short-bowel syndrome?
- A: Poor prognosis is related to the greater length of the bowel resected, loss of the ICV, loss of jejunum and ileum, longer time to tolerate full enteral feeds, and development of severe TPN–liver disease. Neonates have greater chances of bowel adaptation than do adults.
- Q: Are elemental formulas better than intact formulas in the management of patients with short-bowel syndrome in patients >1 year of age?
- A: Recent studies have shown similar rates of absorption, stomal output, and electrolyte losses between elemental and intact formulas. The disadvantages of elemental formulas include high osmolality and cost.

SHORT STATURE

Jeffrey D. Roizen
Vaneeta Bamba
Mitchell Schwartz (5th edition)

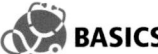 **BASICS**

DEFINITION
- Growth failure, which ultimately leads to short stature, occurs when height crosses percentiles downwards over the normal growth curves. Evidence of growth failure necessitates diagnostic evaluation even if short stature is not yet present.
- Failure to thrive refers to infants and children who fail to gain weight along their growth percentile curves. They may or may not be short and are underweight for height.
- Idiopathic short stature is defined as height below the 3rd percentile.

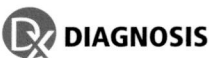 **DIAGNOSIS**

DIFFERENTIAL DIAGNOSIS
Extremes of normal growth:
- **Familial short stature**
  - Normal exam, no systemic illness
  - Short parent(s)
  - Normal height velocity (HV)
  - Normal age of onset of puberty
  - Normal bone age
  - Short stature throughout childhood
  - Final adult height close to the midparental height and around the 3rd or 5th percentile
- **Constitutional short stature/delay of growth**
  - Normal exam, no systemic illness
  - Height percentile below the target range defined by parental heights
  - Delayed bone age
  - Reduced HV (especially in late childhood—below 25th percentile)
  - Associated with delay of puberty, positive family history, usually boys
  - Final adult height in the normal range and commensurate with target height
- **Idiopathic short stature**
  - Categorizes otherwise normal patients who cannot be diagnosed with a variant of normal growth or any of the causes of short stature. May not always turn out to be a true normal variant.
  - This is a diagnosis of exclusion and groups patients whose calculated predicted height is >2 standard deviations (SD) below the midparental height, whose height is below the 3rd percentile, with or without delay of skeletal maturation, and without identifiable diagnosis after appropriate evaluation.

Primary short stature: Usually the consequence of an abnormality of the skeletal system. Bone age often not delayed or only delayed mildly.
- **Skeletal defect:** Can be primary or secondary to a metabolic abnormality. This may lead to disproportionate short stature and/or significant dysmorphism. Occasionally, the skeletal abnormalities are subtle and do not lead to disproportionate short stature.

- **Skeletal dysplasia**
  - Achondroplasia, hypochondroplasia
  - Osteochondrodysplasia
  - Genetic transmission (may be new mutation)
  - Defects in growth of tubular bones and/or axial skeleton
  - Typical radiologic findings on skeletal survey radiograph
- **Short stature due to congenital error of metabolism**
  - Diffuse skeletal involvement
  - Mostly autosomal-recessive inheritance
  - Dysmorphic features
  - Typical biochemical abnormalities
  - More common type (mucopolysaccharidosis)
- **Chromosomal abnormalities**
  - Autosomes or sex chromosomes
  - Usually associated with other somatic abnormalities or mental retardation
  - Clinical findings may be subtle (mosaicism).
  - More common forms: Trisomy 21, trisomy 18, trisomy 13, Turner syndrome
- **Intrauterine growth restriction (IUGR) and small for gestational age (SGA)**
  - Often with poor postnatal growth
  - Etiology may be due to maternal, fetal, or placental problems.
  - IUGR is seen in congenital infection, fetal exposure to toxin, placental abnormalities, maternal disease, Russell–Silver syndrome, and other congenital anomalies.
  - Risk for SGA is increased with maternal cigarette smoking and cocaine use, maternal medical history of chronic hypertension, renal disease, antiphospholipid syndrome, and malaria
  - Patients with SGA have lab values consistent with mild growth hormone (GH) resistance (elevated GH concentrations but low IGF and IGFBP3 concentrations) in the neonatal period.
- **Primordial dwarfism:** Due to intrinsic fetal defect leading to both prenatal and postnatal growth failure (may be associated with specific genetic anomaly)

Secondary short stature:
- **Malnutrition**
  - Especially <2 years of age (most common in first 6 months of life)
  - Caloric (malnutrition and/or protein) malnutrition
  - Vitamin and mineral deficiencies (vitamin D, iron, zinc deficiency)
- **Chronic illness**
  - Many chronic diseases initially present with poor growth.
  - Cardiovascular: Ventricular septal defect, patent ductus arteriosus, tetralogy of Fallot, transposition of the great vessels, aortic stenosis, pulmonic stenosis, aortic coarctation, atrioventricular (AV) canal
  - Pulmonary: Asthma, cystic fibrosis, bronchopulmonary dysplasia
  - GI/liver: Inflammatory bowel disease, celiac disease, malabsorption, short-bowel syndrome, chronic gastroenteritis, cystic fibrosis
  - Renal: Nephrotic syndrome, chronic glomerulonephritis, renal tubular acidosis, chronic renal failure, nephrogenic diabetes insipidus, uropathy, congenital anomalies

  - Metabolic: Poorly controlled diabetes mellitus, storage disorders, chronic infections (HIV), and immune deficiencies
  - Hematopoietic: Anemia, leukemia, sickle cell disease
- **Medications**
  - Corticosteroids
  - Sex steroids
  - Methylphenidate, dextroamphetamine
- Psychosocial growth retardation
- GH deficiency or resistance, hypothyroidism, Cushing syndrome, adrenal disorder, rickets
- Among secondary short stature, endocrine causes are least frequent.

HISTORY
- **Question:** Child short for their midparental height?
- *Significance:* Gender-adjusted midparental height is calculated to estimate the target height.
  - Calculate mean parental height (MPH)
  - For boys, add 6.5 cm (2.5 inches) to MPH
  - For girls, subtract 6.5 cm (2.5 inches) from the MPH. The 2 SD range for this calculation is 10 cm.
  - If the child's height percentile is dramatically decreased relative to this range, an evaluation may be warranted.
- **Question:** Height velocity?
- *Significance*: HV for an interval of at least 6 months should be annualized and plotted on a HV curve. This is an important measure of a patient's growth and is separate from height at any point in time, which may only reflect prior events. Normal HV is at least 4 cm/year from age 4 to puberty.
- **Question:** Weight-to-height ratio?
- *Significance*:
  - Increased in hypothyroidism, Cushing syndrome, pseudohypoparathyroidism, and GH deficiency
  - Normal or decreased in emotional deprivation, anorexia, and chronic diseases such as chronic renal failure, renal tubular acidosis, inflammatory bowel disease, malabsorption, malnutrition, lung and heart disease
- **Question:** Complications during pregnancy, labor, and delivery?
- *Significance*: Clues from the pregnancy may provide information about possible maternal disorders, intrauterine drug exposure, or placental abnormalities that lead to IUGR and/or SGA. Birth trauma can be associated with hypopituitarism.
- **Question:** Family history?
- *Significance*:
  - Heights of grandparents, siblings, and other relatives?
  - Any family members with short stature? What was the timing of puberty in parents and siblings? Any history of endocrine disorders or chronic illnesses affecting a major organ system?
    - If short stature runs in the family, this may lend evidence to familial or genetic short stature, isolated GH deficiency, or skeletal dysplasia.
    - Delayed pubertal maturation in parents may lend support to a diagnosis of constitutional growth delay.
    - Disorders such as diabetes mellitus, diabetes insipidus, thyroiditis, hypophosphatemic rickets, arthritis, and inflammatory bowel disease can lead to short stature

- **Question:** Social situation?
- *Significance:* Emotional stressors affect growth and development, either directly (abnormal GH production) or indirectly (inadequate nutrition).
- **Question:** Current and past dietary history (evidence of underuse of calories ingested)?
- *Significance:* Estimate approximate total daily caloric intake. Low caloric intake or inefficient use of calories may point to nutritional disorders such as malabsorption, rickets, anorexia, or other calorie restriction.
- **Question:** Chronic illness or any hospitalization, surgery, or head trauma?
- *Significance:* Growth failure may be the only sign of a chronic disorder such as rheumatoid arthritis, celiac disease, and inflammatory bowel disease. Previous hospitalizations or surgery may be a sign of underlying pathology. Chronic inflammation or treatment with exogenous steroids can also lead to growth failure, as in asthma. Head trauma may be cause for pituitary insufficiency.
- The history should be completed by obtaining a detailed review of systems, specifically inquiring about the occurrence of headache, vomiting, visual disturbance, anorexia, diarrhea or constipation, polyuria and polydipsia, medications, activity pattern, sleep hygiene, and general development.
- While boys are more frequently referred for short stature, girls may be more likely to have a pathologic reason for short stature.

PHYSICAL EXAM
- **Finding:** Abnormal upper to lower segment ratio?
- *Significance:* Primary short stature (short stature due to an intrinsic defect in the skeletal system)
- **Finding:** Low weight to height ratio?
- *Significance:* Points toward malnutrition
- **Finding:** Edema?
- *Significance:* Chronic renal failure, malnutrition
- **Finding:** Frontal bossing, flat nasal bridge, and truncal fat deposition?
- *Significance:* GH deficiency
- **Finding:** General dysmorphism?
- *Significance:* Underlying genetic disorder such as Russell–Silver syndrome or 22q11 deletion syndrome
- **Finding:** Abdominal distention and gluteal wasting?
- *Significance:* Malabsorption and celiac disease
- **Finding:** Webbed neck, increased carrying angle, shield chest?
- *Significance:* Turner syndrome
- **Finding:** Abnormal trunk-to-limb ratio?
- *Significance:* Achondroplasia or a mutation in the SHOX gene
- **Finding:** Smooth tongue?
- *Significance:* Iron deficiency
- **Finding:** Round face, ear lobe abnormality, and mental retardation?
- *Significance:* Pseudohypoparathyroidism
- **Finding:** Temporal thinning of the hair, sparse hair, dry hair?
- *Significance:* Hypothyroidism, GH deficiency, hypopituitarism

- **Finding:** Midline abnormalities?
- *Significance:* Hypopituitarism
- **Finding:** Delayed pubertal maturation?
- *Significance:* Turner syndrome, constitutional delay, hypopituitarism, hypothyroidism, inflammatory bowel disease, chronic renal disease
- **Finding:** Leg bowing, rachitic rosary, widening of wrists?
- *Significance:* Rickets, malabsorption

DIAGNOSTIC TESTS & INTERPRETATION
- **Test:** Celiac panel
- *Significance:* May reveal asymptomatic celiac disease
- **Test:** CBC with differential
- *Significance:* Anemia, infection, lymphoma, or leukemia
- **Test:** C-reactive protein and erythrocyte sedimentation rate
- *Significance:* Infection, inflammation
- **Test:** Electrolyte panel, glucose
- *Significance:* Renal disorders, diabetes mellitus, and diabetes insipidus
- **Test:** Metabolic panel
- *Significance:* Malnutrition, liver disease, bone disorder, pseudohypoparathyroidism
- **Test:** Urinalysis
- *Significance:* Urinary tract infection, diabetes, renal disorder, metabolic problem
- **Test:** Thyroxine and thyroid-stimulating hormone
- *Significance:* Hypothyroidism, hypopituitarism
- **Test:** X-ray study of the left hand and wrist
- *Significance:* Bone age determination
- **Test:** Karyotype or genome wide array
- *Significance:* Turner syndrome in short girls, SHOX deletion, other chromosomal disorders
- **Test:** IGF-I and IGFBP-3 concentrations
- *Significance:* These are a proxy for GH secretion. Unlike GH secretion which is pulsatile and diurnal, IGF-1 and IGFBP3 show little fluctuation, although they vary with age and Tanner stage. While classically IGF-I and IGFBP-3 are low in GH deficiency, they can also be low in hypothyroidism, chronic illness, or states of poor nutrition. Normal IGF-I and IGFBP-3 concentrations make GH deficiency less likely.

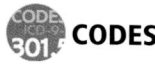 **TREATMENT**

ADDITIONAL TREATMENT
General Measures
Overall goal: Determine if the patient has short stature and/or growth failure. Identify significant changes in weight and head circumference.

- Determine if patient's profile fits normal variant of growth or if profile fits with pathologic short stature.
- Screening evaluation, referral to pediatric endocrinologist, or observation
- For endocrine disease, replacement of the absent hormone (thyroid hormone for hypothyroidism, rhGH for GH deficiency, hydrocortisone for adrenal insufficiency) or removal of the excess hormone (removal of the ACTH-secreting or glucocorticoid-secreting tumor or gradual decrease in exposure to glucocorticoid therapy) will enable normalization of growth rate.

ISSUES FOR REFERRAL
- It is critical to obtain accurate measurements of height, weight, and head circumference to adequately evaluate the abnormally growing child.
- Slow growth velocity, plateau in growth, delayed bone age, abnormal thyroid tests, poorly controlled diabetes, physical findings consistent with GH deficiency, hypothyroidism, or rickets
- Protein-losing enteropathy, malabsorption, hepatic disorder
- Chronic lung disease, abnormal sweat chloride test
- Congenital heart disease, occult cardiac disease
- Elevated creatinine, low serum bicarbonate, abnormal urinalysis
- Growth failure is usually a relatively slow or subacute process and therefore does not require emergency workup.

ADDITIONAL READING
- Deodati A, Cianfarani S. Impact of growth hormone therapy on adult height of children with idiopathic short stature: Systematic review. *BMJ.* 2011; 342:c7157.
- Grimberg A, Kutikov JK, Cucchiara AJ. Sex differences in patients referred for evaluation of poor growth. *J Pediatr.* 2011;146(2):212–216.
- Grote FK, Oostdijk W, de Muinck Keizer-Schrama SM, et al. The diagnostic work up of growth failure in secondary health care: An evaluation of consensus guidelines. *BMC Pediatr.* 2008;8(1):21.
- Grote FK, van Dommelen P, Oostdijk W, et al. Developing evidence-based guidelines for referral for short stature. *Arch Dis Child.* 2008;93(3): 212–217.
- Lee JM, Davis MM, Clark SJ, et al. Threshold of evaluation for short stature in a pediatric endocrine clinic: Differences between boys versus girls? *J Pediatr Endocrinol Metab.* 2007;20(1):21–26.
- Lee PA, Kendig JW, Kerrigan JR. Persistent short stature, other potential outcomes, and the effect of growth hormone treatment in children who are born small for gestational age. *Pediatrics.* 2003; 112(1 pt 1):150–162.
- Oostdijk W, Grote FK, de Muinck Keizer-Schrama SM, et al. Diagnostic approach in children with short stature. *Horm Res.* 2009;72(4):206–217.

CODES

ICD9
783.43 Short stature

ICD10
- E34.3 Short stature due to endocrine disorder
- R62.52 Short stature (child)

SICKLE CELL DISEASE

Kim Smith-Whitley

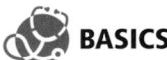 **BASICS**

DESCRIPTION

Sickle cell disease (SCD), a group of inherited hemoglobin disorders in which sickle hemoglobin (HbS) predominates, is characterized by hemolysis, vascular occlusion, and an increased risk of bacterial infection with encapsulated organisms.

EPIDEMIOLOGY

- The frequencies of SCD genotypes from highest to lowest are SCD-SS (60%), SCD-SC (25–30%), SCD-$S\beta^+$ thalassemia, SCD-$S\beta^0$ thalassemia, and other relatively infrequent variants.
- Although population data indicate that patients with SCD-SS and SCD-$S\beta^0$ thalassemia experience more complications than patients with other variants, disease severity varies widely among all individuals with SCD regardless of disease genotypes.

Prevalence

- 1 in 375 African American newborns has SCD.
- 1 in 12 African Americans has sickle cell trait.

RISK FACTORS

Genetics

- SCD has an autosomal recessive inheritance.
- Common genotypes include SCD-SS, SCD-SC, SCD-$S\beta^+$ thalassemia, and SCD-$S\beta^0$ thalassemia.

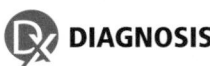 **DIAGNOSIS**

HISTORY

- SCD genotype
- Baseline hemoglobin and reticulocyte count
- Baseline pulse oximetry values (SpO_2)
- Interval history of SCD complications
- Onset of pain, location of pain
- Prior blood transfusions and complications
- Current medications, including analgesics and hydroxyurea

PHYSICAL EXAM

- Fever
- Pallor (may be accentuated at time of splenic sequestration or transient aplastic episode)
- Scleral icterus
- Signs of respiratory distress (due to acute chest syndrome)
- Flow murmur may be present.
- Splenomegaly
- Warmth, tenderness, decreased range of motion at site of pain
- Abnormal neurologic findings suggestive of CNS infarction or hemorrhage

DIAGNOSTIC TESTS & INTERPRETATION

Lab

- Diagnostic:
  - Hemoglobin electrophoresis: Definitive test along with DNA analysis
  - Screening test: "Sickledex" or "shake" tests are not recommended to establish a diagnosis or carrier status; do not use for screening in children <12 months of age or those who have been transfused recently, because of false-negative results.
- Monitoring:
  - CBC: Hemoglobin values vary depending on age and SCD genotype; peripheral blood smear—sickled forms, targets, nucleated RBCs, and increased polychromasia are common (sickle forms may be absent in transfused patients, patients with high hemoglobin F levels, or patients with phenotypes other than SCD-SS).
  - Reticulocyte count: Increased
  - Quantitative hemoglobin electrophoresis
  - Chemistry panel: Elevated lactate dehydrogenase (LDH), unconjugated bilirubin, aspartate aminotransferase (AST) (evidence of hemolysis)
  - Transcranial Doppler (TCD) ultrasonography annually to determine stroke risk in children with SCD-SS or $S\beta^0$ thalassemia aged 2–16 years
  - Ophthalmologic examinations to screen for retinopathy
  - Neurocognitive testing to detect neurocognitive deficits should be considered.

 TREATMENT

General Measures

- Infection prophylaxis with penicillin starting by 2 months of age
- Pneumococcal vaccines (13-valent as per American Academy of Pediatrics [AAP] recommendations and 23-valent at 2 and 5 years of age)
- Meningococcal vaccines (MedImmune and Menactra) as per AAP recommendations
- Routine immunizations, including hepatitis B series and yearly influenza vaccine.
- Consider folic acid supplementation.
- Teach parents to monitor for fever, splenomegaly, pain (including dactylitis), and increased pallor.
- Encourage good oral hydration and supply family with medications to treat uncomplicated painful episodes at home.

COMPLEMENTARY & ALTERNATIVE THERAPIES

- Transfusion therapy can prevent the development of SCD complications and decrease associated morbidity or recurrence of complications when used appropriately:
  - When children with SCD-SS receive erythrocyte transfusions, avoid posttransfusion hemoglobin levels >12 g/dL.
  - Erythrocyte antigen matching for ABO as well as C, D, E, and Kell is recommended.
  - Monitor children carefully for erythrocyte antibodies and/or delayed transfusion reactions.

Measures for Specific Complications

- Fever (rule out sepsis):
  - History, physical exam, CBC, reticulocyte count, blood culture (urine culture, CSF culture, throat culture as indicated by exam)
  - Parenteral antibiotics to provide 24–48-hour coverage until blood cultures are negative
  - Close monitoring for other SCD complications
- Pain (vaso-occlusive episode):
  - Hydration: Avoid excessive hydration and encourage incentive spirometer use for acute chest syndrome prevention.
  - Analgesics:
    ○ Patients and their families can often tell physicians what therapies have been helpful in the past.
    ○ In general, for mild pain, start with mild nonnarcotic medications (acetaminophen, ibuprofen) and mild oral opioids (codeine, oxycodone).
    ○ Consider stronger agents such as oral ketorolac, hydromorphone, and morphine for initial management of moderate pain.
    ○ For severe pain, use parenteral medications such as morphine, hydromorphone, and ketorolac.
  - Comfort measures (massage, heating pad, warm soaks)
  - Frequent reassessment for pain control and side effects of medications is mandatory.
- Acute chest syndrome:
  - Initial findings: Chest tenderness, cough, hypoxia, fever, infiltrate on chest radiography, leukocytosis, exacerbation of anemia
  - Parenteral antibiotics
  - Pain management
  - Supplemental oxygen for hypoxia
  - Incentive spirometry or chest physiotherapy
  - RBC cell transfusion for moderate to severe illness

- Splenic sequestration:
  - History, physical examination, CBC, reticulocyte count, blood culture as indicated, type, and screen
  - Initial findings: Increased spleen size, acute pallor, shock (if episode severe), anemia, thrombocytopenia, elevated reticulocyte count
  - Sequestration episode may have a more insidious onset or be chronic in nature.
  - Fever management (if indicated)
  - Close, frequent observation of hemoglobin level, reticulocyte count, spleen size, and cardiovascular status
  - Fluid bolus and maintenance hydration
  - RBC transfusion: Avoid transfusing to hemoglobin values >10 g/dL, as hemoglobin may increase as the episode resolves and RBCs are released from the spleen.
  - Repeated sequestration episodes may be an indication for splenectomy.
- Transient aplastic episode:
  - History, physical exam, CBC, reticulocyte count (blood culture as indicated), type and screen, human parvovirus B19 serology
  - Initial findings: Pallor, tachycardia, absent or low reticulocytes unless recovery phase
  - Fever management (if indicated)
  - Close observation of hemoglobin level, reticulocyte count, and cardiovascular status
  - Respiratory isolation (95% of cases are due to infection with human parvovirus B19)
  - RBC transfusion for evidence of cardiovascular compromise
- Stroke (acute care):
  - History, physical exam, CBC, reticulocyte count, blood culture as indicated, type, and screen
  - Initial findings: Syncope, weakness, numbness, limpness, hemiparesis, seizure, headache, slurred speech, aphasia, somnolence, coma
  - Imaging: Head CT, brain MRI and MRA; consider arteriogram if aneurysm suspected
  - IV fluid bolus and maintenance hydration
  - Supplemental oxygen
  - RBC transfusion (given as simple or exchange transfusion)
  - Supportive (e.g., anticonvulsives)
- Stroke (primary and secondary stroke prevention), chronic care: Monthly RBC transfusions to keep HbS level <30%

ONGOING CARE

PROGNOSIS

Population estimates of life expectancy from 1978–1988 data range from 42–48 years for SCD-SS and from 60–68 years for SCD-SC. However, many believe that early SCD diagnosis (newborn screening), penicillin prophylaxis, comprehensive medical care, hydroxyurea therapy, and broader indications for chronic RBC transfusions (using chelation therapy or RBC exchange to treat transfusional iron overload) may increase life expectancy.

COMPLICATIONS

- Acute:
  - Painful episodes
  - Dactylitis: Painful swelling of hands and feet
  - Bacterial infection:
    - *Streptococcus pneumoniae* in young patients
    - Gram-negative organisms in older children and adults
    - *Salmonella* infections are problematic for patients of all ages.
  - Acute chest syndrome: A pneumonia-like illness defined as a new infiltrate on chest radiography
  - Neurologic: Including stroke (infarctive and hemorrhagic) and transient ischemic attack
  - Acute splenic sequestration: Acute enlargement of the spleen, with a decreased hemoglobin and increased reticulocyte count
  - Aplastic episode: Transient decrease in RBC production characterized by a decrease in hemoglobin and reticulocyte count; human parvovirus B19 is most common cause.
  - Cholecystitis: Risk is greatest after age 10 years.
  - Priapism: A prolonged penile erection, which can be seen in males of all ages
  - Hematuria
- Chronic:
  - Delayed linear growth and puberty
  - Cholelithiasis
  - Retinopathy: Particularly in children with SCD-SC
  - Neurologic: Sequelae of stroke, "silent" cerebral infarction, cerebral vasculopathy, and/or abnormal cerebral blood flow velocity
  - Hypersplenism: Particularly in young children or patients with SCD-SC or SCD-Sβ^{0+} thalassemia
  - Avascular necrosis: Particularly of the hips
  - Pulmonary hypertension
  - Renal: Proteinuria, microalbuminuria, nephrotic syndrome, acute glomerulonephritis
  - Pulmonary function abnormalities
  - Primary nocturnal enuresis
  - Leg ulcers

ADDITIONAL READING

- Adams RJ. Lessons from the stroke prevention trial in sickle cell anemia (STOP) study. *J Child Neurol.* 2000;15:344–349.
- Driscoll MC. Sickle cell disease. *Pediatr Rev.* 2007; 28(7):259–268.
- National Institutes of Health, National Heart, Lung and Blood Institute. *The management of sickle cell disease,* 4th ed. NIH Publication No. 02-2117. National Institutes of Health, National Heart, Lung and Blood Institute; 2002.
- Wang CJ, et al. Quality-of-care indicators for children with sickle cell disease. *Pediatrics.* 2011;1–10.

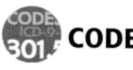

CODES

ICD9
- 282.5 Sickle-cell trait
- 282.60 Sickle-cell disease, unspecified

ICD10
D57.1 Sickle-cell disease without crisis

FAQ

- Q: How long will my baby with SCD live?
- A: No one can predict how long a child with SCD will live. When studies were done on a large number of individuals with SCD almost 2 decades ago, these individuals were living, on average, into their 40s if they had the SS type of SCD and into their 60s if they had the SC type of SCD.
- Q: Is there any "cure" for SCD?
- A: Bone marrow transplantation (BMT) is the only known cure for SCD in children.
- Q: What is hydroxyurea therapy?
- A: Hydroxyurea is a medication that has been shown to reduce the number of painful episodes and acute chest syndrome events in adults with SCD. Hydroxyurea therapy in children >5 years of age has a similar safety profile to that of adults.

SINUSITIS

Esther K. Chung
Karen P. Zimmer

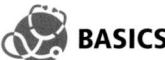 **BASICS**

DESCRIPTION
- Sinusitis is inflammation of the mucous membranes lining the paranasal sinuses, but most commonly is used to describe bacterial rhinosinusitis, which is a clinical diagnosis made by the presence of upper respiratory tract symptoms that have not improved in 10 days or have worsened after 5–7 days. Diagnosis of sinusitis should be considered based on persistence and/or severity of symptoms.
- Classification based on duration of symptoms:
  - Acute: Persistent nasal and sinus symptoms for 10–30 days
  - Subacute: Clinical symptoms for 4–12 weeks
  - Chronic: Symptoms lasting at least 12 weeks
  - Recurrent: Acute sinusitis with complete resolution of 10 days between episodes; 3 episodes in 6 months or 4 episodes in 1 year
- Classification by severity of illness:
  - Persistent symptoms: With >10–14 days but <30 days; nasal discharge and/or daytime cough
  - Severe: Temperature of >39°C (102.2°F) with concurrent purulent nasal discharge for 3 days and/or, facial pain, headache, and/or periorbital edema

GENERAL PREVENTION
- Avoid allergen exposure and treat allergies if present.
- Practice daily nasal hygiene through the use of normal saline drops/spray.
- Improve mucociliary clearance by increasing ambient humidity with a humidifier.

PATHOPHYSIOLOGY
- Normal sinus function depends on patency of paranasal sinus ostia, function of the ciliary apparatus, and secretion quality.
- A buildup of secretions is due to ostial obstruction, reduction in ciliary function, and overproduction of secretions.

ETIOLOGY
- Viral pathogens (e.g., rhinovirus, parainfluenza virus) have been recovered in respiratory isolates, but their significance is unknown.
- Most illnesses of short duration (<7 days) are thought to be from viral infections and should not be treated with antibiotics.
- Bacterial pathogens: Increasing prevalence of penicillin resistance:
  - *Streptococcus pneumoniae* (30–40%)
  - *Haemophilus influenzae*, nontypeable (~20–28%)
  - *Moraxella catarrhalis* (~20–28% in children)
  - Group A Streptococci
  - Group C Streptococci
  - Peptostreptococci
  - Other Moraxella species
  - *Streptococcus viridans*
  - *Eikenella corrodens*
  - *Staphylococcus aureus*
  - *Pseudomonas aeruginosa* (in patients with cystic fibrosis)
  - Anaerobic organisms
  - Fungal pathogen: Aspergillus

 DIAGNOSIS

HISTORY
- Some or all of the following may be present:
  - Nasal discharge: consistency, color. In older patients, nasal discharge may not be the primary complaint, but concurrent rhinitis is a common feature.
  - Postnasal drainage, nasal congestion
  - Fever
  - Recent history of a upper respiratory tract infection (URI)
  - Sore throat from mouth breathing due to nasal obstruction
  - Cough present during the day; may be worse at night
  - Malodorous breath
  - Hyposmia/anosmia
  - Maxillary dental pain
  - Ear pressure or fullness
  - Headache and facial pain are uncommon in young children with sinusitis, but may be seen in older children and adolescents
  - Fatigue
  - Irritability
  - Snoring
  - Hyponasal speech

PHYSICAL EXAM
- Fever may be present.
- Nasal-sounding voice may be present.
- Malodorous breath may be noted.
- Purulent drainage in the nose and/or oropharynx may be appreciated.
- Nasal mucosa may be erythematous, pale, and/or boggy.
- Frontal, maxillary, and ethmoid areas may be tender to palpation/percussion.
- Headache and/or facial pain may change with position, increasing in intensity as the patient leans forward.
- Transillumination is not a reliable aid in diagnosis.
- Proptosis, eye swelling, and impaired extraocular movements suggest orbital infection.

DIAGNOSTIC TESTS & INTERPRETATION
Lab
- For chronic or recurrent sinusitis, consider:
  - Sweat chloride test to rule out cystic fibrosis
  - Immunoglobulin levels, IgG subclass levels, complement levels, and testing for HIV
  - Mucosal biopsy to assess ciliary function

Imaging
- Imaging is not recommended in uncomplicated cases of sinusitis in children ≤6 years of age; and it is controversial in children >6 years of age.
- Sinus radiographs:
  - Caldwell view (anteroposterior) for identifying frontal sinusitis
  - Waters view (occipitomental) for identifying maxillary sinusitis
  - Plain radiographs do not adequately identify ethmoid sinusitis.
  - Findings suggestive of sinusitis include complete sinus opacification, mucosal thickening ≥4 mm, and air–fluid levels.
- CT scans of the paranasal sinuses: Useful in complicated, recurrent and chronic sinusitis; poor response to medical therapy; and/or history of polyposis
- CT scan of the head with contrast: Indicated when sinusitis is accompanied by signs of increased intracranial pressure, meningeal irritation, proptosis, toxic appearance, limited extraocular movements, or focal neurologic deficits, or in patients being considered for sinus-related surgery
- MRI of the sinuses: Reserve for complicated cases; will show mucosal thickening and fluid; imaging modality of choice for fungal sinusitis
- Pitfalls:
  - Sinus radiographs may be abnormal in asymptomatic children or those with mild URIs
  - Studies have shown a relatively high incidence of sinus abnormalities on CT scan in asymptomatic children, especially in infants <12 months of age. The significance of opacified sinuses in asymptomatic children is not well understood.
  - Up to 1/3 of patients with symptoms of chronic sinusitis may have normal CT scans.

DIFFERENTIAL DIAGNOSIS
- Infection: Viral URI with or without mucopurulent rhinitis
- Environmental: Allergic rhinitis
- Drug-induced: Rhinitis medicamentosa
- Tumors:
  - Nasal polyps
  - Hypertrophied adenoids
  - Neoplasms
- Trauma: Foreign body (e.g., bead, cotton, tissue)
- Congenital:
  - Septal deviation
  - Unilateral choanal atresia
  - Immotile cilia
- Other: Vasomotor rhinitis

TREATMENT

ADDITIONAL TREATMENT
General Measures
- If orbital or CNS infection is suspected by history and examination, antibiotics should be started immediately, and emergency CT studies should be performed.
- Pitfalls:
  - Diagnosis of sinusitis is being made with increasing frequency and may result in overtreatment, given that up to 45% will have spontaneous resolution.
  - With widespread antibiotic use, there are increasing numbers of resistant organisms.

MEDICATION (DRUGS)
- Antibiotics:
  - Appropriate drug choice is dependent on local resistance patterns.
  - High-risk children include: Age <2 years, antibiotic use within 3 months, and child care attendance

- First-line treatment (no major risk factors): Amoxicillin 45–90 mg/kg/d divided b.i.d. 10–21 days or 7 days symptom-free
- First-line treatment (high-risk children): Amoxicillin/clavulanic acid (80–90 mg/kg/d of amoxicillin component with 6.4 mg/kg/d of clauvulanate divided b.i.d. × 10–21 days or 7 days symptom-free
- Second-line treatment: Second–generation or higher cephalosporins (i.e., cefuroxime axetil 30 mg/kg/d divided b.i.d.), macrolides (i.e., clarithromycin 15 mg/kg/d divided b.i.d., azithromycin 10 mg/kg/d on day 1 then 5 mg/kg/d for 4 days)
- Course of therapy is controversial, but treatment to 7 days beyond symptom resolution is generally accepted.
- Complicated sinusitis (CNS or orbital involvement): IV antibiotics and hospitalization; ceftriaxone (100 mg/kg/d divided b.i.d.) or ampicillin–sulbactam (200 mg/kg/d divided q.i.d.); vancomycin (60 mg/kg/d divided q.i.d.) is added to cefotaxime if source of infection is known or highly likely to be caused by penicillin-resistant *Streptococcus pneumoniae*
- Chronic sinusitis: Use a broad-spectrum antibiotic for 4 weeks; amoxicillin/clavulanate (80–90 mg/kg/d of amoxicillin component with 6.4 mg/kg/d of clavulanate divided b.i.d.); macrolides (clarithromycin, azithromycin); or cefuroxime axetil (250–500 mg divided b.i.d.)
- Other pharmaceuticals:
  - Decongestants: These decrease nasal airway resistance and increase ostia patency in some studies, but the overall effect on acute sinusitis is unknown.
    - Topical decongestants should be used only for short-term therapy (5–7 days), because rebound mucosal congestion may occur.
    - Systemic decongestants (e.g., pseudoephedrine) have side effects that include tachycardia, hypertension, jitteriness, and insomnia.
  - Mucolytics, such as guaifenesin, may improve mucous clearance.
  - Topical nasal steroids: May reduce and prevent mucosal swelling, that can lead to ostial occlusion; particularly useful for patients with allergic rhinitis.
- Other:
  - Humidifier: Improves mucociliary clearance
  - Normal saline: Squirt into each nostril daily or b.i.d.; removes sensitizing agents, increases humidity, and enhances mucociliary transport; vasoconstricts, and improves drainage and ventilation.

SURGERY/OTHER PROCEDURES

- Maxillary sinus aspiration: If unresponsive to multiple antibiotics, severe facial pain, and orbital or intracranial complications; should be performed by a trained ear, nose, and throat (ENT) specialist.
- Surgery: Performed as a last resort after medical therapy attempted and in patients with orbital or CNS complications

 ## ONGOING CARE

PROGNOSIS

- Spontaneous resolution in up to 50% of patients
- Usually improves within 72 hours of initiation of antibiotics
- Excellent for those who are otherwise healthy

COMPLICATIONS

- Periorbital cellulitis
- Orbital cellulitis
- Orbital abscess
- Meningitis
- Intracranial abscess
- Optic neuritis
- Cavernous or sagittal sinus thrombosis
- Epidural, subdural, and brain abscesses
- Osteomyelitis of the maxilla
- Osteomyelitis of the frontal bone (Pott puffy tumor)

PATIENT MONITORING

- Immediate referral is indicated if there are CNS symptoms, periorbital edema, visual changes, facial swelling, extraocular muscle involvement, or proptosis
- Radiographic soft tissue changes may last for up to 8 weeks; therefore, reimaging is of limited value.
- Referral to an otolaryngologist when the sinusitis is chronic and not responsive to medical therapy; recurrent; complicated; or when there is polyposis

ADDITIONAL READING

- American Academy of Pediatrics Subcommittee on Management of Sinusitis and Committee on Quality Improvement. 2001; Clinical practice guideline: Management of sinusitis. *Pediatrics*. 2001;108:798–808.
- Dyskewicz M. Rhinitis and sinusitis. *J Allergy Clin Immunol*. 2003;111:S520–S529.
- Ioannidis JPA, Lau JL. American Academy of Pediatrics: Technical report: Evidence for the diagnosis and treatment of acute uncomplicated sinusitis in children: A systematic overview. *Pediatrics*. 2001;108(3):e57.
- Leung AKC, Kellner JD. Acute sinusitis in children: Diagnosis and management. *J Pediatr Health Care*. 2004;18:72–76.
- Principi N, Esposito S. New insights into pediatric rhinosinusitis. *Pediatr Allergy Immunol*. 2007; 18(Suppl 18):7–9.
- Slavin RG, Spector SL, Berstein IL, et al.; American Academy of Allergy Asthma and Immunology; American College of Allergy, Asthma, and Immunology; Joint Council of Allergy, Asthma, and Immunology. The diagnosis and management of sinusitis: A practice parameter update. *J Allergy Clin Immunol*. 2005;116:S13–S47.
- Zacharisen M, Casper R. Pediatric sinusitis. *Immunol Allergy Clin North Am*. 2005;25:313–332.

 ## CODES

ICD9

- 461.9 Acute sinusitis, unspecified
- 473.9 Unspecified sinusitis (chronic)

ICD10

- J01.90 Acute sinusitis, unspecified
- J01.91 Acute recurrent sinusitis, unspecified
- J32.9 Chronic sinusitis, unspecified

FAQ

- Q: Are all of the sinuses present at birth?
- A: No, the maxillary and ethmoid sinuses form during the third and fourth gestational month, and are present at birth. They continue to enlarge until the preteen years. The sphenoid sinuses are pneumatized by 5 years; isolated sphenoid sinusitis is rare. The frontal sinuses are present at age 7–8 years and are not completely developed until late adolescence.
- Q: Does the nasal discharge seen with sinusitis have to be purulent and thick?
- A: No. Although the nasal discharge is often described as purulent and thick, it may also be clear or mucoid, or thick or thin. Multiple studies have shown that a change in color or consistency is not a specific sign of a bacterial infection.
- Q: Are radiographic studies useful in the diagnosis of sinusitis?
- A: There is evidence to suggest that plain radiographs (x-rays) have limited value in the diagnosis of sinusitis, and are not recommended in cases of uncomplicated sinusitis. Mucosal thickening may be seen with viral upper respiratory tract infections and allergic rhinitis. Studies have shown that x-rays do not correlate well with CT scans in the diagnosis of chronic sinusitis.
- Q: Can one make the diagnosis of sinusitis based on CT scan results alone?
- A: No. Up to 50% of patients who had CT scans performed for other reasons had soft tissue changes in their sinuses. Mucosal thickening and opacification on CT imaging have been seen in large numbers of asymptomatic patients. These findings seem to occur more frequently in infants <12 months of age. Given the poor specificity of CT imaging of the paranasal sinuses, results must be used in the context of the patient's clinical presentation.

S

SLEEP APNEA–OBSTRUCTIVE SLEEP APNEA SYNDROME

Akinyemi O. Ajayi

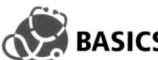 **BASICS**

DESCRIPTION

- Sleep-disordered breathing encompasses a range of breathing disorders occurring during sleep. These conditions include primary snoring (PS), respiratory events related to arousals (RERA), and obstructive sleep apnea syndrome (OSAS).
- Obstructive apnea is defined as the cessation of air flow at the nose and mouth despite respiratory effort, associated with some gas-exchange abnormality and/or loss of regular sleep patterns.
- Distinct from central apnea (cessation of air flow that is not accompanied by respiratory effort), which indicates brain immaturity or dysfunction
- Many children with OSAS exhibit partial airway obstruction. This is known as obstructive hypoventilation or hypopnea and is more commonly seen in children than is complete obstruction.
- OSAS may be subdivided into mild, moderate, and severe forms according to degree of severity.
- Upper airway resistance syndrome is a respiratory disorder characterized by partial airway obstruction and arousals leading to sleep fragmentation, and is not associated with gas-exchange abnormalities.
- In infants, OSAS is uncommon; however, it may exist with craniofacial anomalies, neurologic disorders associated with low muscle tone, laryngomalacia or tracheomalacia, and gastroesophageal reflux.
- Impaired arousal mechanisms also contribute to abnormalities seen in OSAS.
- In older children, OSAS may be associated with obesity. This form may resemble the adult type of OSAS.
- PS or habitual snoring implies snoring that does not lead to abnormalities in gas exchange or sleep fragmentation.
- Central apnea up to 20 seconds may be a normal finding in premature or newborn infants during the first months of life.
- Periodic breathing: 3 or more episodes of central apnea lasting at least 3 seconds each, separated by <20 seconds. Periodic breathing may be found in the newborn; however, it should not exceed >4% of sleep time (from a sleep study) and is not associated with bradycardia or hypoxemia.

ALERT

- Normal-size tonsils do not exclude OSAS.
- Tonsillar size does not predict the presence of OSAS.
- Treatment of gastroesophageal reflux in infants with obstructive apnea may be helpful even in the absence of obvious symptoms of reflux.

Genetics

- Several genetic disorders with associated craniofacial anomalies, hypotonia, and obesity may lead to OSAS. These include:
  – Pierre Robin syndrome
  – Treacher Collins syndrome
  – Down syndrome
  – Mucopolysaccharide disorders
  – Arnold–Chiari malformations
  – Prader–Willi syndrome
  – Hereditary neuromuscular disorders

COMMONLY ASSOCIATED CONDITIONS

- Adenotonsillar hypertrophy
- Craniofacial anomalies including midfacial hypoplasia and mandibular hypoplasia.
- Laryngomalacia
- Neurologic and neuromuscular disorders that cause hypotonia may underlie poor ventilation during sleep.
- Gastroesophageal reflux
- Obesity
- Metabolic disorders
- Allergic rhinitis, nasal septum deviation, nasal polyps
- Sedatives, seizure medications, and anesthesia

DIAGNOSIS

HISTORY

- Nocturnal symptoms include difficulty breathing when asleep, snoring, apnea, and restless sleep with frequent arousals.
- Daytime symptoms: Excessive sleepiness, frequent upper respiratory/ear infections, conductive hearing loss, mouth breathing, poor appetite, and a hyponasal voice
- Other concerns: ADHD, gastroesophageal reflux, poor school performance, and headaches (especially in the morning and upon awakening)
  – OSAS rarely produces these symptoms acutely, but tends to occur over weeks to months.
  – Parents may notice that symptoms worsen with upper respiratory infections.
- The possibility of sleep-disordered breathing or a primary sleep disorder should be considered in children evaluated for attention deficit hyperactivity disorder.

PHYSICAL EXAM

- Assessment of the child's growth. In severe cases of OSAS, failure to thrive has been reported.
- Obesity remains a risk factor, especially in older children.
- Assessment of tonsillar size
- Presence of mouth breathing, hyponasal speech, adenoidal facies, midfacial hypoplasia, retrognathia, micrognathia, or other craniofacial anomalies may be present at times and may suggest the diagnosis.
- Nasal obstruction due to polyps, nasal septum deviation, turbinate hypertrophy, or congestion

- Tongue size
- Mobility and elevation of the soft palate; hard palate integrity
- In extreme cases, cardiac involvement may lead to cor pulmonale and heart failure. Examination may suggest signs of pulmonary hypertension or congestive heart failure, such as an increased second heart sound.
- A neurologic examination to evaluate general muscle strength, tone, and developmental status, especially in infants and children who do not improve after adenotonsillectomy

DIAGNOSTIC TESTS & INTERPRETATION
Lab

- Polysomnography:
  – The gold standard for the diagnosis of OSAS is nocturnal polysomnography, to differentiate the type of sleep apnea and to assess severity.
  – Polysomnography is an 8–10-hour-long multichannel study performed in a controlled setting that can assess respiratory and/or sleep abnormalities.
  – Indices such as oxygenation, ventilation, apnea index (AI), apnea hypopnea index (AHI), arousal index, arousal awakening index, and periodic limb movements index are determined along with sleep parameters such as sleep efficiency and sleep stages.
  – Monitoring includes EEG, electro-oculogram, electromyogram, arterial oxygen saturation, end tidal CO_2 tension, air flow, respiratory effort, and EKG.
  – Normative respiratory and sleep variables for children have recently been published and include an apnea-hypopnea index of <1 being normal.
  – Scoring for pediatric polysomnography differs from that of adults. This includes using 2 respiratory cycles to define both obstructive apnea and central apnea or 2 respiratory cycles associated with a 30% decline in airflow and a >4% decline in oxygen level to define hypopnea. Lower AHI values are considered significant in children, compared with adults.
- Other studies:
  – Validated questionnaires are helpful to screen for OSAS in the office.
  – Routine blood work is generally noncontributory; in severe forms, polycythemia, hypercarbia, and elevated bicarbonate may be noted.
  – Evaluation for gastroesophageal reflux may include pH monitoring during sleep, barium swallow, or radionuclide studies (milk scan).
  – Home testing is not approved for use in children with suspected obstructive sleep apnea syndrome

Imaging

- Lateral neck x-ray is easy to perform to assess adenoid and tonsillar size, as well as patency of the nasopharyngeal airway.
- Nocturnal audio- and videotaping, as well as abbreviated nap polysomnography, are useful studies if the results are positive, but generally have a poor negative predictive value.
- Upper airway endoscopy as well as bronchoscopy may be performed to evaluate anatomic or dynamic causes for airway obstruction (pharyngeal hypotonia, pharyngeal stenosis, laryngotracheomalacia, vocal cord polyps, papilloma).

- Head or neck CT or MRI should be considered for complex craniofacial anomalies. If central apnea is noted, then MRI studies should also evaluate the brain stem to evaluate for an Arnold–Chiari malformation.
- In severe cases of OSAS, a cardiac evaluation, including ECG, chest x-ray, and Doppler ECG, may be indicated.

DIFFERENTIAL DIAGNOSIS

- PS or habitual snoring: By definition is not associated with sleep-disordered breathing, but may progress to OSAS. Between 20% and 50% of children with habitual snoring may have OSAS.
- Upper airway resistance syndrome: This condition is associated with sleep fragmentation and daytime sleepiness.
- Obesity–hypoventilation syndrome: A variant of OSAS
- Central apnea and periodic breathing
- Congenital central hypoventilation syndrome
- Other causes of excessive daytime sleepiness include:
  - Disorganized home environment, emotional stress
  - Substance abuse/drug intoxication: Psychotropic medications, antihistamines, anticonvulsants, narcotics
  - Narcolepsy: Onset typically around adolescence, but cataplexy may occur later and delay the diagnosis.
    - Classic tetrad of symptoms of narcolepsy includes excessive daytime somnolence, cataplexy, hypnagogic hallucinations, and sleep paralysis.
    - In addition, fragmented night time sleep may be seen.
  - Epilepsy: Absence spells of unresponsiveness, electroencephalogram changes
- Causes of obstructive apnea include any cause of lymphoidal hypertrophy in the upper airway (allergies viral/bacterial tonsillitis, neoplasm, epiglottitis, retropharyngeal abscess); chronic phenytoin exposure; and excessive storage material in upper airway submucosa.
- Causes of abnormal laxity of upper airway soft tissues: Down syndrome, acute polyneuropathy (Guillain–Barré syndrome), chronic neuromuscular disease, Prader–Willi syndrome, myasthenia gravis
- Causes of abnormal control/coordination of upper airway musculature: Almost any cause of diffuse CNS dysfunction, including cerebral palsy, and acquired lesions of the CNS such as stroke and head trauma
- Causes of central apnea: Beyond infancy, most commonly due to drugs that suppress ventilatory drive; in premature infants may be due to nonspecific immaturity of neural ventilatory control mechanism, sepsis, and, rarely, seizures, brainstem compression, brain tumors, Arnold–Chiari type 2 (although increasingly seen with type 1)
- Reflux may potentiate central apnea and should be investigated (see "Gastroesophageal Reflux" topic).
- Androgen steroids may cause central apnea in adults.

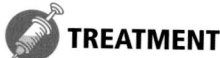 TREATMENT

INITIAL STABILIZATION

- Severe cases may require urgent intervention.
- Severe cases of upper airway obstruction are usually diagnosed during polysomnography or during procedures involving sedation or anesthesia.
  - Ensure adequate ventilation and oxygenation, with quick assessment of the cause.
  - Temporary relief of the obstruction should be undertaken by an experienced team.
  - Transfer to an intensive care unit where the airway can be monitored carefully.
  - Following relief of airway obstruction, pulmonary and airway edema, as well as copious secretion production, may develop.
  - Modalities of care should include placement of a nasopharyngeal airway, noninvasive ventilation with continuous positive airway pressure/bilevel positive airway pressure (CPAP/BiPAP), or placement of an endotracheal tube for mechanical ventilation.
- Risk factors for postoperative complications in children with OSAS include age <3 years, severe OSAS, pulmonary hypertension, obesity, prematurity, failure to thrive, craniofacial or neuromuscular disorders, and/or upper respiratory tract infection.

General Measures

- In most cases, adenotonsillectomy is first-line therapy. However, some patients continue to have significant postoperative OSAS that requires further evaluation.
- Noninvasive ventilatory support with CPAP or BiPAP may be helpful.
- In complicated cases, when craniofacial malformations are involved, surgical procedures such as tongue reduction, uvulopalatopharyngoplasty, or mandibular or maxillary advancement may be indicated.
- When there is evidence of gastroesophageal reflux, treatment with acid-suppression agents and chalasia precautions are indicated.
- Weight loss may be useful in obese children.
- Laser surgery and dental appliances may be useful in adults with mild OSAS, but there is no experience with these approaches in children.
- In extreme cases, a tracheostomy may be indicated, especially when significant craniofacial abnormalities exist.

 ONGOING CARE

COMPLICATIONS

Complications are due to chronic hypoxemia, hypercarbia, acidosis, as well as impaired sleep and include:

- Pulmonary hypertension, later cor pulmonale (rare)
- Systemic hypertension has been reported in adults and a few pediatric cases.
- Congestive heart failure; arrhythmias are common in adults with underlying coronary artery disease.
- Neurodevelopmental complications: Daytime somnolence, poor school performance, hyperactivity, and social withdrawal
- Poor growth and failure to thrive
- Postanesthesia respiratory failure and death have been reported in children with OSAS.

PATIENT MONITORING

- Clinical improvement is expected soon after adenotonsillectomy. In children <1 year of age with severe forms of OSAS, underlying craniofacial anomalies, or neurologic disorders, repeat overnight polysomnography is indicated 6–8 weeks after surgery.
- Regrowth of adenoid tissue may occur months to years after adenoidectomy. Therefore, if clinical symptoms, such as snoring, difficulty breathing while asleep, or a decline in school performance recur, a re-evaluation is indicated.

ADDITIONAL READING

- American Academy of Sleep Medicine. *International Classification of Sleep Disorders*, 2nd ed. Westchester, IL: American Academy of Sleep Medicine; 2005:56–60.
- American Sleep Apnea Association. Available at http://www.sleepapnea.org.
- D'Andrea LA. Diagnostic studies in the assessment of pediatric sleep-disordered breathing: Techniques and indications. *Pediatr Clin North Am*. 2004; 51(1):169–186.
- Pandit C, Fitzgerald DA. Respiratory problems in children with Down syndrome. *J Paed Child Health*. 2011 Apr 29.
- Rosen CL. Obstructive sleep apnea syndrome in children: Controversies in diagnosis and treatment. *Pediatr Clin North Am*. 2004;51(1):153–167, vii.
- Witmans M, Young R. Update on Pediatric sleep disordered breathing. *Pediatr Clin North Am*. 2011;58(3):571–589.

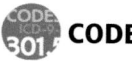 CODES

ICD9

- 327.20 Organic sleep apnea, unspecified
- 327.23 Obstructive sleep apnea (adult)(pediatric)

ICD10

- G47.30 Sleep apnea, unspecified
- G47.33 Obstructive sleep apnea (adult) (pediatric)

FAQ

- Q: Can my child still have OSAS after adenotonsillectomy?
- A: Yes, at times the adenoid tissue can grow back again. In addition, some cases of OSAS are related to a small upper airway that is restricted by anatomic or neurologic conditions. In these cases, adenotonsillectomy will not always resolve OSAS.
- Q: Does OSAS cause neurologic problems?
- A: Several studies suggest neurocognitive deficits in children with OSAS. The most common findings include reduced school performance and ADHD.

SLIPPED CAPITAL FEMORAL EPIPHYSIS

David D. Sherry

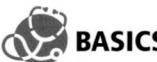 **BASICS**

DESCRIPTION
- Slipped capital femoral epiphysis (SCFE) is displacement of the epiphysis of the head of the femur.
- Pitfall: Hip pain may be absent; there may be no pain, or only thigh or knee pain due to referred pain

EPIDEMIOLOGY
- Males > Females (3:2)
- Left hip twice as often as right, 25% bilateral
- Associated with obesity, increased height, genital underdevelopment, pituitary tumors, growth hormone therapy

Incidence
- 1–5 per 100,000
- Age of onset: Boys, 14–16 years; girls, 11–13 years (essentially, premenarche)

RISK FACTORS
Genetics
5% of children affected have a parent with SCFE

PATHOPHYSIOLOGY
- Unclear: Abnormal stress on normal physeal plate vs. a process that weakens the plate
- The femoral head slips posteriorly and inferiorly, exposing the anterior and superior aspects of the metaphysis of the femoral neck.
- Associations: Obesity, endocrine dysfunction, primary hypothyroidism, pituitary dysfunction, hypogonadism, cryptorchidism, chemotherapy, pelvic radiotherapy, renal rickets

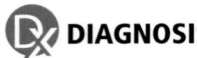 **DIAGNOSIS**

HISTORY
- Pain in hip or knee
- Occasional history of trauma; however, usually not sufficient to explain the findings
- 3 patterns
  - Chronic: Most common, onset of symptoms >3 weeks, lack of full internal rotation of hip
  - Acute: Sudden onset with inability to walk or severe pain and difficulty walking
  - Acute-on-chronic: Sudden exacerbation of symptoms that have been present for a while

PHYSICAL EXAM
- Limp if unilateral, or waddling gait if bilateral
- Tenderness and occasional palpable thickening over hip
- Thigh atrophy
- Lack of full internal rotation of hip and decreased motion in all planes secondary to mechanical limitation due to the slip
- Procedure: When the hip is flexed, the thigh is forced into external rotation.

DIAGNOSTIC TESTS & INTERPRETATION
Imaging
- Anteroposterior and lateral view (frog leg or Lowenstein)
- Measure degree of displacement
  - Minimal: Alteration in plane of epiphysis relative to femoral neck; significant if angle <82 degrees
  - Mild: Displacement <1 cm
  - Moderate: Displacement >1 cm, <2/3 diameter of femoral neck

- Epiphyseal plate widened and irregular
- Decreased height of physis
- "Blanch sign": Dense area in femoral neck
- A "Klein line" drawn along the superior femoral neck on the anteroposterior view should transect the epiphysis but not on the slipped side.
- Hormonal evaluation if suspected

Pathological Findings
Histologic findings include widening of the epiphyseal plate, large clefts, and necrotic debris in the cartilage and synovitis

DIFFERENTIAL DIAGNOSIS
- Septic arthritis of the hip
- Ischemic necrosis
- Tuberculosis of the hip; however, pain is associated with movement in all directions, and there should be other evidence of disease.
- Renal rickets
- Achondroplasia
- Shwachman syndrome: Metaphyseal chondrodysplasia with pancreatic insufficiency

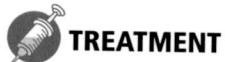 TREATMENT

ADDITIONAL TREATMENT
General Measures
- Designed to prevent complications and further slipping; urgent orthopedic consultation mandatory
- Conservative: Bed rest with traction; probably does not reduce slipping; temporizing until surgery can be scheduled
- Manipulative reduction: Risk of damage to epiphyseal vessels or breakdown of callus; probably only to be considered if within 24 hours of acute slip
- Epiphyseal fixation: Risk of damage to articular surface or growth plate
- Intertrochanteric osteotomy
- Salvage: Hip fusion

 ONGOING CARE

FOLLOW-UP RECOMMENDATIONS
Patient Monitoring
Chondrolysis and avascular necrosis are uncommon side effects of slipped capital femoral epiphysis.

COMPLICATIONS
- Ischemic necrosis of epiphysis: Usually due to manipulative reduction of the slippage; more common in males; x-rays reveal increased density, irregularity, and ultimately collapse of epiphysis.
- Chondrolysis (acute cartilage necrosis): 1–40%, more common in females and blacks; etiology unclear; x-rays reveal narrowed joint space, sclerosis of acetabular rim, and osteoporosis of femoral head.

ADDITIONAL READING
- Hotchkiss BL, Engels JA, Forness M. Hip disorders in the adolescent. *Adolesc Med State Art Rev*. 2007;18(1):165–81, x–xi.
- Lehmann CL, Arons RR, Loder RT, et al. The epidemiology of slipped capital femoral epiphysis: An update. *J Pediatr Orthop*. 2006;26(3):286–290.

- Loder RT. Controversies in slipped capital femoral epiphysis. *Orthop Clin North Am*. 2006;37(2): 211–221, vii.
- Peck D. Slipped capital femoral epiphysis: Diagnosis and management. *Am Fam Physician*. 2010; 82(3):258–262.
- Tosounidis T, Stengel D, Kontakis G, et al. Prognostic significance of stability in slipped upper femoral epiphysis: A systematic review and meta-analysis. *J Pediatr*. 2010;157(4):674–680, 680.e1.

 CODES

ICD9
732.2 Nontraumatic slipped upper femoral epiphysis

ICD10
- M93.001 Unsp slipped upper femoral epiphysis, right hip
- M93.002 Unsp slipped upper femoral epiphysis, left hip
- M93.003 Unsp slipped upper femoral epiphysis, unsp hip

S

SMALLPOX (VARIOLA VIRUS)

Hamid Bassiri
Joanne N. Wood (5th edition)

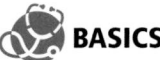

BASICS

DESCRIPTION
- Smallpox is a life-threatening, acute eruptive, contagious disease caused by the variola virus.
- The disease is characterized by a febrile prodrome followed by the development of a rash.
- Rash evolves in a characteristic fashion: macules → papules → vesicles → pustules. Scabs form and fall off leaving scars called pockmarks.
- There are 2 clinical forms of smallpox:
  - Smallpox minor is a less common and less severe form of the disease.
  - There are 5 types of smallpox major, the more common and serious form of the disease.
    ○ Ordinary smallpox
    ○ Modified smallpox
    ○ Flat smallpox
    ○ Hemorrhagic smallpox
    ○ Variola sine eruptione

EPIDEMIOLOGY
- The last documented case of endemic smallpox was in Somalia in 1977. The last case in the US was in the late 1940s.
- Smallpox was declared eradicated by the World Health Organization in 1979.
- Historically in unvaccinated individuals ordinary smallpox accounted for 90% of cases and hemorrhagic accounted for 7% of cases. Flat and modified smallpox accounted for the remainder of cases.
- Modified smallpox was rare in unvaccinated individuals but accounted for 25% of cases of disease in vaccinated individuals.

GENERAL PREVENTION
- Prior to 1972, all children in the US were vaccinated.
- Vaccines were produced from the vaccinia virus, an orthopoxvirus that is closely related to the variola virus.
- Historically, the vaccine was prepared from virus grown on the skin of animals and in some cases the vaccine was contaminated with animal proteins, bacteria, and adventitial viruses.
- Newer smallpox vaccines are developed from vaccinia clones grown in tissue culture and therefore are free of contamination from bacteria and other viruses.
- Laboratories in the US and Russia have stockpiles of smallpox virus. There is concern that scientists in the Soviet Union may have illegally transported samples of this virus to other nations.
- Due to concern regarding the possible use of smallpox as a bioterrorism weapon, the US has increased the production of smallpox vaccine.
- The only currently FDA-licensed smallpox vaccine, ACAM2000, is used for active immunization of persons determined to be at highest risk for infection. ACAM2000, which replaced Dryvax in the US, is currently provided for Strategic National Stockpile use.
- The Advisory Committee on Immunization Practices recommends smallpox vaccination for:
  - Public-health response teams responsible for investigating suspected smallpox cases
  - Hospital-based healthcare teams responsible for assessing and caring for suspected smallpox cases

- Vaccine efficacy:
  - 95% efficacious in preventing disease if given prior to exposure
  - May prevent smallpox or decrease severity if given 1–3 days after exposure
  - May decrease severity of disease if given 4–7 days after exposure
- Length of immunity after vaccination is estimated to be 3–10 years. Vaccine may decrease the severity of disease for 10–20 years.
- Vaccine administration:
  - A skin abrasion is created using a bifurcated needle dipped in the vaccine.
  - The vaccine site should be loosely covered to prevent the spread of virus to others.
  - After 3–4 days a red pruritic papule appears at the vaccination site. A vesicle and then a pustule forms. After a few weeks a scab forms that falls off leaving a scar.
- Contraindications to vaccine:
  - Atopic dermatitis or exfoliative skin disorder
  - Immunosuppression
  - Pregnancy or breastfeeding
  - Close contact of someone who is pregnant, immunosuppressed, or has skin disease
  - Allergy to vaccine component
  - Moderate or severe acute illness
  - Inflammatory eye disease
  - Heart disease (myocardial infarction, stroke, cardiomyopathy, heart failure, or angina)
  - 3 or more risk factors for heart disease
  - Age <1 year
  - These contraindications may be re-evaluated if smallpox is reintroduced into the population.
- Common adverse reactions to vaccination:
  - Fever, swelling, lymphadenitis, and headache are seen in 2–16% of adults receiving the vaccine for the first time.
  - A mild rash occurs in ~8% of cases.
- Less common vaccine reactions:
  - Vaccinia keratitis and vision loss
  - Accidental inoculation with blister formation
  - Moderate-to-severe generalized rash
  - Eczema vaccinatum
  - Encephalitis
  - Congenital vaccinia and generalized vaccinia
  - Myopericarditis
  - Progressive vaccinia/vaccinia gangrenosum
  - Bacterial superinfection

PATHOPHYSIOLOGY
- The virus infects the upper respiratory tract and replicates. Rarely, primary infections via skin, conjunctiva, or placenta can occur.
- The virus then enters the bloodstream causing primary viremia and is taken up by macrophages.
  - Patient is asymptomatic during this time.
- Next the virus enters the reticuloendothelial system where it continues to replicate.
- Secondary viremia occurs as the virus enters the bloodstream and the organs.
  - Virus enters the epidermis causing necrosis and swelling.
  - Virus infects the bone marrow, kidneys, liver, lymph nodes, spleen, and other organs.
  - The virus causes coagulopathy and multiorgan system failure.

- Exact mechanisms of viral toxicity are not understood but may involve both direct viral cytopathic effects and inflammatory mediators.

ETIOLOGY
- The variola virus, a member of the poxvirus family and the orthopox genus, causes smallpox.
- Variola is a double-stranded DNA virus. It is usually transmitted during face-to-face contact via respiratory aerosol or direct contact with the virus via skin lesions.
- Transmission of the virus via air in enclosed settings or via infected fomites is uncommon.
- Humans are the only vectors.

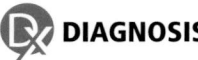

DIAGNOSIS

- Ordinary smallpox:
  - Incubation period of 7–17 days, followed by febrile prodrome lasting 1–4 days.
    ○ The prodrome is characterized by high fever, headache, back pain, chills, abdominal pain, and emesis.
  - Eruptive phase begins with lesions of the mouth, tongue, and oropharynx.
  - Then the rash develops:
    ○ Often starts on face and spreads to rest of body within 24–48 hours.
    ○ On day 1 the rash is macular.
    ○ On day 2 the rash becomes papular.
    ○ On days 4–5 the rash is vesicular.
    ○ By day 7 the rash has become pustular.
    ○ By 2–3 weeks the scabs have formed.
    ○ Scabs fall off and leave scars.
- Modified smallpox:
  - Milder than ordinary smallpox
  - Accelerated course
  - Lesions are not as deep.
- Flat smallpox:
  - Characterized by a soft, flat, semiconfluent or confluent rash that does not progress to pustules
  - Can result in significant skin loss
- Hemorrhagic smallpox:
  - Shorter incubation time
  - Skin becomes dusky.
  - Bleeding occurs in the skin and mucous membranes.
  - Can be difficult to diagnose unless exposure to variola virus is known
- Variola sine eruptione:
  - May be asymptomatic or cause a febrile influenza-like illness
  - Noncontagious
  - Seen in infants with protective maternal antibodies and in vaccinated individuals
- If there has not been a release or circulation of smallpox, the CDC Protocol for evaluating patients for smallpox can be used to guide the assessment of a suspicious rash illness.
- CDC protocol for evaluating patients for smallpox:
  - If a patient has an acute, generalized rash on the body, with vesicles or pustules:
    ○ Use the major and minor criteria to assess the likelihood of smallpox

- Major criteria:
  - Febrile prodrome: 1–4 days prior to rash onset including a temperature $\geq 101°F$ and 1 or more of the following: prostration, headache, backache, chills, vomiting, or severe abdominal pain
  - Classic smallpox lesions are deep-seated, firm/hard, round, well-circumscribed vesicles or pustules that can become umbilicated or confluent as they evolve on any one part of the body (e.g., the face or arm); all the lesions are in the same stage of development
- Minor criteria:
  - Centrifugal distribution: greatest concentration of lesions on face and extremities
  - First lesions appear on the oral mucosa, palate, face, or forearms.
  - Patient appears toxic or moribund.
  - Slow evolution: lesions evolve from macules to papules to pustules over days (each stage lasts 1–2 days).
  - Lesions on the palms and soles
- High risk of smallpox:
  - Febrile prodrome and classic smallpox lesions in same stage of development
- Moderate risk of smallpox:
  - Febrile prodrome and 1 other major smallpox criterion, or
  - Febrile prodrome and ≥ 4 minor smallpox criteria
- Low risk of smallpox:
  - No febrile prodrome, or
  - Febrile prodrome and <4 minor smallpox criteria
- Online tool for evaluation risk of smallpox is available at: http://www.bt.cdc.gov/agent/smallpox/diagnosis/riskalgorithm/

DIAGNOSTIC TESTS & INTERPRETATION
Diagnostic Procedures/Other
- Use the CDC smallpox evaluation protocol to guide testing
  - If high risk of smallpox:
    - Consult infectious disease and/or dermatology
    - Public-health agency will advise on management and collection of samples.
    - Variola testing will be performed at an approved laboratory prior to other testing.
  - If moderate risk of smallpox:
    - Consult infectious disease and/or dermatology
    - Perform testing for varicella and other disorders including herpes simplex virus as indicated
    - If no diagnosis made after testing and consultation ensure adequacy of specimen and have consultants re-evaluate
    - If still cannot rule out smallpox, then classify case as high-risk case
  - If low risk of smallpox, and history and physical exam are highly suggestive of varicella then varicella testing is optional.
  - If low risk of smallpox and diagnosis is uncertain then testing should be done for varicella and other disorders as indicated.
- Variola testing:
  - Should not be performed in low- and moderate-risk cases because of risk of false positives
  - Should only be performed in high containment facilities designated by national authorities
  - Lesion specimens (fluid, cells, and scabs) are preferred for testing but blood, tonsillar swabs, and biopsy specimens may be used.
  - Serologic studies and electron microscopy cannot distinguish between the variola virus and other orthopoxviruses.

- PCR assays can distinguish variola virus from other orthopoxviruses.
- Variola virus can be cultured.
- Historically variola was identified by the characteristic pocks it produced when grown on chorioallantoic membranes of chick embryos.

DIFFERENTIAL DIAGNOSIS
- Multiple rash illnesses, including the following, can be confused with smallpox:
  - Varicella and Herpes zoster
  - Herpes simplex virus
  - Measles
  - Rubella
  - Monkeypox and Tanapox
  - Viral exanthema including Enterovirus
  - Disseminated Molluscum contagiosum
  - Impetigo, insect bites, or scabies
  - Post-smallpox vaccine rash (Vaccinia)
  - Secondary syphilis
  - Acne and contact dermatitis
  - Drug reactions including erythema multiforme
  - Meningococcemia can be confused with the hemorrhagic form of smallpox.

ALERT
- Varicella can be confused with smallpox.
- Lesions in varicella are in different stages, superficial, concentrated on the trunk and face, and often spare palms and soles.
- Lesions of smallpox are all at the same stage, deep, concentrated on face and limbs, and often involve palms and soles.

 TREATMENT

MEDICATION (DRUGS)
- Patients suspected of having smallpox should be vaccinated against smallpox, especially if they are in the early stages of the disease.
- No treatment has been proven to be effective.
- The efficacy of antivirals developed since the eradication of smallpox is unknown. Although cidofovir has been suggested for therapy of smallpox infections, there is currently not enough data to support its use.
- Several new medications are under investigation (e.g., ST-246, CI-1033) for therapy, but have not yet been approved for use.
- The use of vaccinia immune globulin (VIG) can be considered for complications from vaccinia immunization but not for therapy of smallpox infection.

ADDITIONAL TREATMENT
General Measures
- Suspected cases of smallpox require notification of state and local authorities, who should then notify the CDC.
- Use CDC smallpox evaluation protocol to guide reporting and infection control measures.
  - For all patients with acute, generalized vesicular or pustular rash:
    - Institute airborne and contact precautions
    - Alert infection control at time of admission
  - If high risk: Report to state and local public-health agency immediately

- Individuals recently exposed (within 3–4 days) to someone with contagious smallpox (e.g., someone with oral or skin lesions) should receive postexposure vaccination, as this offers the potential to limit disease but also provides significant protection from death.
- Individuals with smallpox may be contagious during the febrile prodrome and are most contagious during the early rash phase. They remain contagious until all the scabs have fallen off.

 ONGOING CARE

PROGNOSIS
- The mortality rate for variola minor was <1%.
- Historically the overall mortality rate for variola major was 30% but was close to 100% for the flat and hemorrhagic forms of the disease.
- The highest mortality rates occurred among young children, pregnant women, elderly individuals, and those with immunodeficiencies.
- Long-term sequelae include pockmarks, vision loss, and limb deformities.

COMPLICATIONS
- Secondary bacterial infections: Skin, lung, joint, bone, sepsis, etc.
- Corneal ulcers and keratitis
- Arthritis
- Encephalitis

ADDITIONAL READING

- Besser JM, Crouch NA, Sullivan M. Laboratory diagnosis to differentiate smallpox, vaccinia, and other vesicular/pustular illnesses. *J Lab Clin Med*. 2003;142:246–251.
- Breman JG, Henderson DA. Diagnosis and management of smallpox. *N Engl J Med*. 2002;346:1300–1308.
- Fulginiti Vam Papier A, Lane M, Neff JM, et al. Smallpox vaccination: A review, part I. *Clin Infect Dis*. 2003;37:241–250.
- Fulginiti Vam Papier A, Lane M, Neff JM, et al. Smallpox vaccination: A review, part II. *Clin Infect Dis*. 2003;37:251–271.
- McFadden G. Killing a killer: What next for smallpox? *PLoS Pathog*. 2010;6:e1000727.
- Moore ZS, Seward JF, Lane JM. Smallpox. *Lancet*. 2006;367:425–435.

 CODES

ICD9
- 050.0 Variola major
- 050.2 Modified smallpox
- 050.9 Smallpox, unspecified

ICD10
B03 Smallpox

SNAKE AND INSECT BITES

Payal S. Kadia
Jill C. Posner

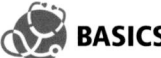 **BASICS**

DESCRIPTION

- Injury to the human skin and/or subcutaneous tissues caused by bite, envenomation, or sting, causing usually local, but in some cases systemic, effects
- Snake bites:
  - Crotalinae (pit vipers: Cotton mouths, copperheads, and rattlesnakes)
  - Elapidae (coral snakes)
- Spider bites:
  - Black widow (*Latrodectus mactans*)
  - Brown recluse (*Loxosceles reclusa*)
- Insect stings: Hymenoptera: Fire ants (*Solenopsis*), yellow jackets, wasps, bees

EPIDEMIOLOGY

- Only 15% of all snake bites are from poisonous snakes, and only ~2/3 of those involve true envenomation. Crotaline snakes are the most common cause of venomous snake bites in the US. Coral snake bites constitute <1% of all snake bites.
- The black widow spider is found in most areas of North America but especially in southern New England. The brown recluse spider is found mainly in southern and midwestern states.
- 1–4% of the US population is at risk for anaphylaxis from Hymenoptera stings.

Incidence

- Annually, ~8,000 people sustain a poisonous snake bite in the US, 99% of which are from crotaline snakes, and 12–15 fatalities occur.
- The incidences of black widow and brown recluse spider bites are unknown.
- 50–150 people die each year from sting anaphylaxis.

PATHOPHYSIOLOGY

- Snake bites:
  - Although there are ~120 snake species in the US, only 15% envenomate substances are capable of causing fatal reactions.
  - Snake venom consists of numerous enzymes and polypeptides that are neurotoxic, cytotoxic, and hemotoxic.
  - Pit viper venom produces significant local inflammation and injury to the vascular endothelium, and may lead to coagulopathy, thrombocytopenia, and shock.
  - The venom of the coral snake is primarily neurotoxic and may produce neuromuscular paralysis and respiratory depression.
- Spider bites:
  - Most of the 20,000 species of predominantly venomous spiders in the US lack fangs capable of penetrating human skin or toxin strong enough to produce more than a mild reaction. However, the black widow and brown recluse spiders can cause significant harm.
  - The black widow venom, α-latrotoxin, is a neurotoxin that stimulates myoneural junctions and nerve terminals by increasing synaptic release of acetylcholine and by initiating a massive influx of calcium, causing severe skeletal muscle pain and cramping and autonomic disturbances such as hypertension and sweating. Pediatric patients are more severely inflicted given the ratio of mg of venom to kg of body weight.
  - The brown recluse venom, mainly sphingomyelinase D, acts on RBC membranes, platelets, endothelial cells, and other cells, resulting in tissue infarction and necrosis. Systemic symptoms are more likely to occur in children, presumably because of a smaller ratio of body weight to venom volume. Hemolysis, hemoglobinuria, disseminated intravascular coagulation, shock, seizures, and death rarely may occur.
- Insect stings:
  - The fire ant bites with its jaws and then swings its head around to inflict multiple stings. The venom has a direct toxic effect on mast cell membranes, causing an immediate wheal-and-flare reaction at the bite site.
  - The venoms of the bee, hornet, yellow jacket, and wasp contain antigens that trigger an IgE antibody response, resulting in allergic reactions that vary in severity from mild local effects to profound anaphylactic reactions.

DIAGNOSIS

HISTORY

ALERT

- If the snake is brought in for identification, use caution! The head of a dead snake can deliver a venomous bite for up to 1 hour after death/decapitation.

- Snake bites:
  - Poisonous snakes have triangular-shaped heads, a pit (heat sensor in front of each eye), fangs, slitlike pupils, and a single row of subcaudal plates, and may have a rattle:
    - The corals have oval heads, yet are still poisonous.
  - Nonpoisonous snakes have oval heads, no pits, rows of small teeth, round pupils, a double row of subcaudal plates, and no rattles.
  - In the Elapidae family, the coral snake can be differentiated from the benign king snake by the pattern of the colored bands: "Red on yellow, kill a fellow; red on black, venom lack."
- Spider bites: Identification of spider (rare): The black widow is about the size of a quarter, glossy black, gray, or brown, with a red, orange, or yellow hourglass-shaped marking on the ventral surface. A single bite can deliver a lethal dose of venom. The brown recluse is small (1–1.5 cm), gray or reddish/brown, with a brown violin-shaped mark on the dorsum of the cephalothorax.
- Insect bites:
  - Type of insect
  - Previous history of insect bite allergy

PHYSICAL EXAM

- Crotalinae (pit viper) bites:
  - Intense local pain and burning occur in the 1st few minutes, followed by edema and perioral numbness that may extend to the scalp and periphery. Paresthesias may be accompanied by a metallic taste in the mouth.
  - Local ecchymosis and vesicles appear within the 1st few hours, and by 24 hours hemorrhagic blebs are present. Lymphadenitis may result.
  - Without treatment, necrosis extending throughout the bitten extremity generally ensues. Compartment syndrome is uncommon.
  - Nausea, vomiting, weakness, chills, and sweating can also occur with systemic absorption of venom.
  - Neuromuscular involvement (e.g., diplopia, dysphagia, lethargy) can develop within several hours.
  - Signs of hypovolemic shock, hemorrhagic diathesis, and neuromuscular dysfunction may occur in life-threatening envenomations.
- Elapidae (coral snake) bites:
  - Mild, often unimpressive local signs and symptoms (pain, swelling), but significant neurologic effects that include extremity paresthesias, weakness, fasciculations, and bulbar dysfunction that can progress to flaccid paralysis and respiratory failure.
  - Inspect bite wound for fang punctures.
  - Carefully assess neurovascular integrity, and consider compartment pressures if severe edema.
- Black widow spider bites:
  - No local symptoms associated with bite
  - Within 8 hours after bite, regional or generalized pain and muscle cramping, fasciculations; abdominal rigidity without tenderness is a hallmark sign.
  - Children often have nausea and vomiting.
  - Respiratory difficulty may occur.
  - Hypertension, tachycardia, and cholinergic effects (diaphoresis, salivation, lacrimation, and bronchorrhea)
  - Death may occur from respiratory or cardiovascular collapse.
  - Syndrome can last 3–6 days.
- Brown recluse spider bites:
  - Spectrum from minor local reaction to severe necrosis
  - Local reaction: Pain, erythema, swelling, and pruritus, classic "bull's eye" lesion
  - Ischemia and skin necrosis: A bright red papule appears within a few hours of the bite and can evolve within 48–72 hours into a hemorrhagic vesicle surrounded by purple discoloration (necrosis) or blanching (vasospasm), "the bull's eye." Shortly after, a firm, purple necrotic lesion appears, and within 7–14 days black eschar is visible. Ulcer healing can take weeks to months, leaving a deep scar.
- Insect bites:
  - Small local reactions: Painful, pruritic, urticarial lesion at the sting site
  - Large local reaction: Swelling and erythema, may become several centimeters in diameter
  - Anaphylaxis is rare with fire ants but occurs more frequently with bee stings

DIAGNOSTIC TESTS & INTERPRETATION
Lab
- Snake bites: CBC, platelet count, PT/PTT, fibrinogen, fibrin split products, serum electrolytes, creatine kinase, creatinine, urinalysis
- Spider bites: CBC, PT/PTT, fibrinogen, serum electrolytes, creatinine, creatine kinase, urinalysis
- Insect bites: No tests done routinely

DIFFERENTIAL DIAGNOSIS
- Black widow spider bites: Acute abdomen, renal colic, opioid withdrawal, tetanus
- Poisonous snake bites: Nonpoisonous snake bite (leaves scratches, not punctures), rodent bites, thorn wounds
- Brown recluse spider bite: Other spider bites, insect bites and stings (including Lyme), cellulitis, poison ivy/oak, Stevens-Johnson syndrome, toxic epidermal necrolysis, erythema nodosum, chronic herpes simplex, purpura fulminans, diabetic ulcer, gonococcal hemorrhagic lesion, pyoderma.

 TREATMENT

- Crotalinae (pit vipers) bites:
  - Remove constrictive items (jewelry or clothing) and immobilize extremity at or below level of heart. Cryotherapy, arterial tourniquets, excision, and incision are not recommended. Oral suctioning is never recommended!
  - Rapid transport to medical facility
  - Address airway, breathing, and circulation.
  - The use of a constrictive band is controversial. Main indication is for cases of prolonged transport time to a medical facility or rapid progression of systemic symptoms. A flat band is placed 5–10 cm proximal to the bite, with enough pressure to impede lymphatic and superficial venous flow but not arterial flow. 1–2 fingers should fit easily between the band and the patient's extremity.
- Elapidae (coral snakes): Constriction bands, suction, and drainage do not prevent coral snake venom absorption.

ADDITIONAL TREATMENT
General Measures
- Crotalinae (pit vipers) bites:
  - Wound care: Irrigation and dressing
  - Determine if envenomation has occurred via serial examinations (q30min) and laboratory studies (q4h).
  - Antivenom: Administration of antivenom should be made in consultation with a toxicologist and/or herpetologist. General indications include progressive local swelling, pain or ecchymosis, and any systemic signs or symptoms.
  - 2 Crotalinae antivenom products used to be available: Antivenin (Crotalidae) Polyvalent (ACP) (Wyeth Laboratories) and Crotalidae Polyvalent Immune Fab (Ovine) (Altana, Inc.), approved by the FDA in October 2000. However, administration of ACP antivenom was commonly associated with serum sickness and anaphylaxis and it is now no longer manufactured.

- Some hospitals (in endemic areas) and many zoos stock antivenoms. In addition, the regional poison control center may have access to the Antivenom Index and will be able to help locate the nearest supply.
- Data suggest that the use of Fab preparations is safe and effective and is associated with fewer immediate and delayed hypersensitivity reactions than ACP, though they do occur and must be monitored.
- Early administration of Fab within 6 hours is advised. Initial dose is 4–6 vials of Fab diluted in 250 mL normal saline infused over 1 hour.
- Supportive care: Volume replacement, packed red blood cells, platelets, fresh-frozen plasma, cryoprecipitate as indicated for hypovolemia and bleeding diathesis. Observe closely for respiratory and renal failure.
- Frequent assessment of tissue perfusion; fasciotomy only for elevated compartment pressures
- Empiric antibiotics are controversial but may be indicated in cases of extensive tissue involvement
- Analgesia and tetanus prophylaxis
- Elapidae (coral snakes):
  - Crotalinae antivenom is ineffective in treating Elapidae envenomation. Antivenom that was formerly manufactured by Wyeth Laboratories is no longer in production, but an alternative formulation from Mexico (Coralmyn) is being tested.
  - Any degree of flaccid paralysis is an indication for antivenom therapy.
  - Local wound care, supportive care, analgesia, and tetanus vaccination as above
- Black widow spider bites:
  - To alleviate muscle pain and cramping, parenteral opioids and benzodiazepines can be administered.
  - 10% calcium gluconate had been used anecdotally, but is no longer recommended.
  - Latrodectus-specific antivenom is available for more severe envenomations given via IV infusion. Specific indications include young age, pregnancy, life-threatening hypertension and tachycardia, or severe symptoms refractory to other treatment measures. Administration of an equine serum preparation has been associated with hypersensitivity reactions and occasionally death. 1 vial is generally all that is needed.
- Brown recluse spider bites:
  - Most bites can be treated on an outpatient basis with local wound care with Burrow solution or hydrogen peroxide and symptomatic treatment for pain and pruritus.
  - No specific antivenom is available in the US.
  - Patients with systemic symptoms, serious infection, or extensive necrosis warrant hospitalization, IV fluids, and aggressive supportive care.
  - Surgical excision advocated in the past, but is no longer indicated
  - Neither dapsone nor hyperbaric oxygen therapy has proved to be effective; dapsone in children is associated with methemoglobinemia.

- Insect bites or stings:
  - Rarely require more than ice, and antihistamine for pruritus
  - If stinger remains in skin, remove by pinching with forceps or scraping. Emphasis should be on quick removal to decrease exposure to venom. Do not squeeze venom gland.
  - Life-threatening anaphylaxis should be treated with subcutaneous epinephrine (0.01 mL/kg 1:1,000, max 0.3 mL), methylprednisolone (2 mg/kg), and/or diphenhydramine (1.25 mg/kg).
- Bacterial superinfection is rare, but if present can usually be treated with oral and/or topical antibiotics.

 ONGOING CARE

PROGNOSIS
- Snake bites: Because the majority of snake bites are from nonvenomous snakes, and ~1/3 of bites from venomous snakes do not involve envenomation, the majority of bites cause only local injury. However, once serious injury is established, prognosis becomes unclear.
- Spider bites: Children have severe reactions and rare fatalities.
- Insect bites: Most bites and stings cause minimal local effects, although some cause serious systemic reactions and, rarely, death.

ADDITIONAL READING
- Dart RC, McNally J. Efficacy, safety, and use of snake antivenoms in the United States. *Ann Emerg Med.* 2001;37:181–188.
- Goto CS, Feng SY. Crotalidae polyvalent immune Fab for the treatment of pediatric crotaline envenomation. *Pediatr Emerg Care.* 2009;25: 273–282.
- Offerman SR, Bush SP, Moynihan JA, et al. Crotaline Fab antivenom for the treatment of children with rattlesnake envenomation. *Pediatrics.* 2002; 110:968–971.
- Peterson ME. Brown spider envenomation. *Clin Tech Small Anim Pract.* 2006;21:191–193.
- Schmidt JM. Antivenom therapy for snakebites in children: Is there evidence? *Curr Opin Pediatr.* 2005;17(2):234–238.

 CODES

ICD9
- 919.4 Insect bite, nonvenomous, of other, multiple, and unspecified sites, without mention of infection
- 989.5 Toxic effect of venom

ICD10
T63.001A Toxic effect of unsp snake venom, accidental, init

SOCIAL ANXIETY DISORDER
C. Pace Duckett

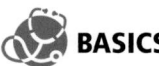 **BASICS**

DESCRIPTION
- Social anxiety disorder, also known as social phobia, is a psychiatric condition with developmental underpinnings. The disorder is characterized by marked and persistent fear of social situations in which the person is exposed to unfamiliar people or possible scrutiny by others.
- Diagnostic types:
  - Generalized: Individuals experience anxiety and fear across most social situations.
  - Non-generalized: Individuals experience anxiety and fear towards specific situations (such as public speaking).
- DSM-IV criteria:
  - A marked and persistent fear of one or more social or performance situations in which the person is exposed to unfamiliar people or to possible scrutiny by others.
  - The feared situation provokes anxiety and may precipitate a panic attack.
  - The feared social situation or performance is avoided.
  - Symptoms have persisted for >6 months.
  - The anxiety, avoidance, or distress leads to significant impairment in social or academic functioning.
  - There must be evidence of the capacity for age-appropriate social relationships with familiar people and the anxiety must occur in peer situations, not just in interactions with adults.

EPIDEMIOLOGY
Incidence
Approximately 5% of youths suffer from social anxiety disorder. The prevalence is somewhat higher in girls than in boys. It is the third most common psychiatric disorder in the US.

RISK FACTORS
- Shyness
- Avoidant temperament
- Behavioral inhibition
- Familial heritability pattern
- Moderate genetic component based on twin studies

COMMONLY ASSOCIATED CONDITIONS
- Anxiety disorders (36%)
  - Generalized anxiety disorder (10%)
  - Specific phobia (10%)
  - Selective mutism (8%)
  - Obsessive compulsive disorder (6%)
  - Panic disorder (2%)
- ADHD (10%)
- Depression (2%)

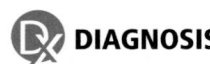 **DIAGNOSIS**

HISTORY
- The diagnostic evaluation should entail gathering of data through separate interviews with the child/adolescent and the parents.
- Current symptoms should be elicited with attention to severity, duration, and level of functional impairment.
- Core symptoms of marked anxiety in social situations, fear of negative scrutiny by others, and avoidance of these situations should be present.
- Distress can be manifested by physical symptoms such as blushing, palpitations, trembling, or GI upset.
- Younger children may exhibit periods of selective mutism in social situations, while having the ability to talk freely while at home.
- Older children may appear oppositional and exhibit school refusal.
- Symptoms may be exacerbated by environmental transitions such as a new school or the family moving.

PHYSICAL EXAM
There are no pertinent findings on physical exam.

DIAGNOSTIC TESTS & INTERPRETATION
Lab
There are no pertinent findings on physical exam.

Diagnostic Procedures/Other
- Diagnostic scales:
  - Social Anxiety Scale for Adolescent (SAS-A)—self-administered for adolescents aged 13–17
  - Multi-Dimensional Anxiety Scale for Children (MASC)—broad anxiety scale self-administered for ages 8–19
  - Liebowitz Social Anxiety Scale for Adolescents (LSAS-A)—clinician-administered scale for ages 13–17

DIFFERENTIAL DIAGNOSIS
- Anxiety disorders
- Depression
- Autistic spectrum disorders

 TREATMENT

MEDICATION (DRUGS)
- SSRIs (first-line): Initiate half the starting dose for children with anxiety disorders
  - Side effects include GI upset, headaches, dizziness, and agitation.
  - There is a black-box warning by the FDA indicating that all antidepressants may increase suicidal thinking and behavior in children and adolescents.
  - Close monitoring is recommended following initiation.
    - Fluoxetine (Prozac) (10–60 mg)
    - Sertraline (Zoloft) (25–200 mg)
    - Paroxetine (Paxil) (10–40 mg)
    - Citalopram (Celexa) (10–60 mg)
    - Escitalopram (Lexapro) (10–20 mg)
    - Fluvoxamine (Luvox) (25–200 mg)

- SNRIs (second-line):
  - Side effects include somnolence, insomnia, dizziness, anxiety, headache, sweating, and tremor.
  - There is a black-box warning by the FDA indicating that all antidepressants may increase suicidal thinking and behavior in children and adolescents.
  - Venlafaxine extended release (Effexor XR) (25–225 mg)
- Benzodiazepines (second-line):
  - Side effects include sedation, dizziness, and weakness.
  - Lorazepam (Ativan)
  - Clonazepam (Klonopin)
  - Alprazolam (Xanax)
  - Alprazolam XR (Xanax XR)

ADDITIONAL TREATMENT
General Measures
- There are 2 types of treatment for social anxiety disorder—psychosocial treatment and pharmacotherapy.
  - The psychosocial treatment with the strongest evidence is cognitive behavioral therapy (CBT).
  - The SSRIs are the first-line agents for medication management.
  - Combination treatment with SSRIs and CBT is superior to either treatment alone.
- Psychosocial treatments: There is an emphasis on relaxation techniques such as breathing exercises and progressive muscle relaxation.
  - Exposure to a hierarchy of avoided situations with concomitant cognitive reframing is core to CBT.
  - Psychoeducation with the family is imperative for decreasing parental accommodation of avoidant patterns.

Additional Therapies
- CBT
- Individual psychotherapy
- Group therapy
- Psychoeducation

 ## ONGOING CARE
FOLLOW-UP RECOMMENDATIONS
Patient Monitoring
- Monitoring of response to psychosocial treatment should be performed routinely every 2–3 months.
- If medication is initiated, close monitoring on a weekly basis is recommended for the first 4 weeks followed by monthly monitoring.
- CBT is performed on a weekly or twice weekly regimen.
- Monitoring of any emerging comorbidities is suggested.

PROGNOSIS
- Social anxiety disorder is generally considered a chronic condition that does not remit without intervention.
- Serious comorbidities may develop in adulthood, such as depression and alcohol dependence.

ADDITIONAL READING

- Beidel DC, Ferrell C, Alfano CA, et al. The treatment of childhood social anxiety disorder. *Psychiatr Clin North Am.* 2001;24(4):831–846.
- Khalid-Khan S, Santibanez MP, McMicken C, et al. Social anxiety disorder in children and adolescents: Epidemiology, diagnosis, and treatment. *Paediatr Drugs.* 2007;9(4):227–237.
- Walkup JT, Albano AM, Piacentini J, et al. Cognitive behavior therapy, sertraline, or a combination in childhood anxiety. *N Engl J Med.* 2008;359(18):1–14.

 ## CODES
ICD9
300.23 Social phobia

ICD10
- F40.10 Social phobia, unspecified
- F40.11 Social phobia, generalized

CLINICAL PEARLS
- Pitfalls:
  - Incomplete assessment of the comorbid psychiatric illnesses
  - Parental accommodation of the child's avoidant patterns

S

SORE THROAT

Cynthia R. Jacobstein

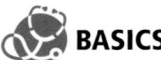 **BASICS**

DEFINITION

Sore throat or pain with swallowing is a common presenting complaint in the pediatric population. The majority of cases have an infectious etiology, with viral causes being the most common.

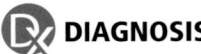 **DIAGNOSIS**

DIFFERENTIAL DIAGNOSIS

- **Infectious**
  - Pharyngitis/tonsillitis
  - Viral: Adenovirus/influenza/parainfluenza, Epstein–Barr virus (EBV), cytomegalovirus (CMV), human immunodeficiency virus
  - Bacterial: Group A β-hemolytic Streptococcus (*Streptococcus pyogenes*), groups C and G Streptococci, diphtheria, *Neisseria gonorrhoeae*, anaerobic bacteria, tularemia, *Arcanobacterium haemolyticum*
  - Stomatitis: Herpes simplex virus, coxsackievirus
  - Other infectious etiologies include peritonsillar cellulitis/abscess, retropharyngeal abscess, epiglottitis/supraglottitis, Lemierre syndrome
- **Environmental**
  - Irritative pharyngitis: Exposure to smoke or dry air
- **Trauma**
  - Foreign body: Either retained or causing laceration to posterior pharynx
  - Burns: Hot liquids/foods
  - Voice overuse
- **Tumor**
  - Rare in pediatric population
- **Allergic/inflammatory**
  - Allergens causing chronic postnasal drip that leads to irritant pharyngitis
- **Miscellaneous**
  - Kawasaki disease
  - PFAPA: Periodic fever, aphthous stomatitis, pharyngitis, adenitis
  - Psychogenic pain
  - Referred pain

APPROACH TO THE PATIENT

The majority of cases of sore throat have an infectious cause, with most (~70–80%) of these having a viral etiology. Once the life-threatening and/or noninfectious causes have been excluded, the goal is to determine if the pharyngitis is caused by group A β-hemolytic Streptococci (GABS), which should be treated with antibiotics, or one of the many other infectious etiologies.

- **Phase 1:** Use history and physical exam to separate infectious from noninfectious causes. If etiology seems infectious, consider testing for group A Streptococcal infection.
  - The clinical appearance of GABS pharyngitis may be indistinguishable from pharyngitis of viral etiologies. The therapy for these illnesses is different:
    - Antibiotics for group A Streptococcus vs. symptomatic care for viral pharyngitis. The practitioner should perform diagnostic testing (i.e., rapid Strep antigen and/or culture) when GABS pharyngitis is considered.
    - In general, it is not recommended to treat pending the culture results; rather, wait until the GABS pharyngitis is confirmed with a positive antigen or culture before starting antibiotics.

HISTORY

- **Question:** Sore throat in association with fever, headache, and/or abdominal pain?
- *Significance*: Common association of symptoms present in group A Streptococcal pharyngitis
- **Question:** Sore throat in association with fever, upper respiratory infection symptoms (cough, rhinorrhea, conjunctivitis)?
- *Significance*: More suggestive of viral pharyngitis
- **Question:** Presence of drooling, voice changes?
- *Significance*: Possibility of more severe infectious etiology, including retropharyngeal or peritonsillar abscess, epiglottitis
- **Question:** Foreign body exposure?
- *Significance*: Retained foreign body (e.g., fishbone) or laceration/irritation from foreign body
- **Question:** Irritant exposure (e.g., dry air from heating or cooling system)?
- *Significance*: Pharyngeal mucosal drying
- **Question:** Immunization status and travel history?
- *Significance*: Possibility of diphtheria in the non- or incompletely immunized patient, especially if recent travel to countries of the former Soviet Union
- **Question:** Sexual activity (including oral sex and possibility of abuse)?
- *Significance*: Gonococcal pharyngitis

PHYSICAL EXAM

- **Finding:** Pharyngeal erythema with or without exudate?
- *Significance*: Suggestive of infectious etiology, though does not reliably differentiate viral from bacterial causes
- **Finding:** Tender cervical adenopathy?
- *Significance*: Suggestive of infectious etiology; anterior cervical nodes described in classic GABS infection; posterior cervical nodes +/− hepatosplenomegaly suggest possibility of EBV.
- **Finding:** Concomitant pharyngitis and conjunctivitis?
- *Significance*: Suggestive of adenovirus infection
- **Finding:** Stridor/drooling?
- *Significance*: Raises concern for etiologies that may cause airway obstruction
- **Finding:** Asymmetric enlargement of tonsillar pillar with deviation of uvula away from enlarged side +/− trismus?
- *Significance*: Peritonsillar abscess
- **Finding:** Mild erythema with cobblestoning of posterior pharyngeal mucosa?
- *Significance*: Suggests allergic or irritant etiology
- **Finding:** Vesicular or ulcerative lesions in oropharynx?
- *Significance*: Suggestive of viral etiologies including herpes simplex (lesions commonly in anterior oropharynx) or coxsackievirus (lesions commonly in posterior oropharynx).
- **Finding:** Diffuse fine blanching erythematous papular rash?
- *Significance*: Suggestive of scarlet fever, which is caused by GABS

DIAGNOSTIC TESTS & INTERPRETATION

- **Test:** Throat swab for Strep antigen test with subsequent culture if antigen test is negative
- *Significance*: Useful for definitive diagnosis of group A Streptococcal infection. A negative antigen test should be followed by throat culture to improve sensitivity. The sensitivity of current rapid antigen tests ranges from 80% to 90%. The sensitivity of a correctly obtained throat culture swab ranges from 90% to 95%.

- **Test:** CBC and Mono spot if indicated
- *Significance*: Atypical lymphocytosis/presence of heterophil antibodies suggestive of EBV infection. EBV titers (if indicated) should be sent in those <4 years of age because of low sensitivity (~50%) of Mono spot in this age group.

Imaging
- Lateral neck x-ray:
  - Enlarged epiglottis suggests epiglottitis; widened prevertebral soft-tissue space suggestive of retropharyngeal abscess
- CT scan of neck:
  - For diagnosis of retropharyngeal abscess in setting of suggestive lateral neck x-ray

TREATMENT

ADDITIONAL TREATMENT
General Measures
- The treatment of viral pharyngitis is largely supportive care, including fluids and pain control.
- Penicillin is the drug of choice for treatment of GABS pharyngitis. PO and IM regimens are available. A once-daily amoxicillin regimen has been endorsed as an alternative treatment option. Macrolide antibiotics (e.g., azithromycin), clindamycin, or some first-generation cephalosporins (provided no allergy in the form of immediate-type hypersensitivity to β-lactam antibiotics) may be used for those with penicillin allergy.

ISSUES FOR REFERRAL
- Fluctuant peritonsillar abscess: Drainage may be done by otolaryngologist
- Presence of foreign body: May need removal by otolaryngologist, or x-ray to look for air in retropharyngeal soft tissue

IN-PATIENT CONSIDERATIONS
Initial Stabilization
- Factors that make sore throat an emergency include:
  - Airway compromise: Epiglottitis, retropharyngeal abscess, peritonsillar abscess, significant tonsillar hypertrophy, diphtheria
- The patient may present with toxic appearance, fever, drooling, voice change, and sitting in the sniffing position (to optimize airway). Make NPO, supplemental oxygen; consider airway adjuncts (e.g., nasal pharyngeal airway), IV access to facilitate airway management (if patient able to tolerate). Consider anesthesia consult for endotracheal intubation in most controlled setting.

Admission Criteria
- Signs/symptoms of airway compromise: General toxicity, stridor, drooling. Patient may need emergency airway protection/stabilization
- Significant dehydration secondary to poor oral intake

ADDITIONAL READING

- Attia MW, Bennett JE. Pediatric pharyngitis. *Pediatr Case Rev*. 2003;3(4):203–210.
- Baltimore RS. Re-evaluation of antibiotic treatment of streptococcal pharyngitis. *Curr Opin Pediatr*. 2010;22:77–82.
- Bisno AL. Acute pharyngitis. *N Engl J Med*. 2001; 344(3):205–211.
- Gerber MA. Diagnosis and treatment of pharyngitis in children. *Pediatr Clin N Am*. 2005;52:729–747.

- Shulman ST. Acute streptococcal pharyngitis in pediatric medicine: Current issues in diagnosis and management. *Pediatr Drugs*. 2003;5(Suppl 1): 13–23.
- Wessels MR. Streptococcal pharyngitis. *N Engl J Med*. 2011;364(7):648–655.
- Young BJ, Steele RW. A teenager with sore throat and neck pain. *Clin Pediatr*. 2010;49(11): 1088–1089.

 CODES

ICD9
- 034.0 Streptococcal sore throat
- 462 Acute pharyngitis
- 784.1 Throat pain

ICD10
- J02.0 Streptococcal pharyngitis
- J02.9 Acute pharyngitis, unspecified
- R07.0 Pain in throat

FAQ

- Q: What is the incidence of group A Streptococcal disease as the cause of pharyngitis?
- A: Group A Streptococcus is the most common bacterial etiology of infectious pharyngitis. The incidence of this disease is ~15–30% of all cases of infectious pharyngitis.
- Q: When must antibiotic therapy begin in group A Streptococcal pharyngitis in order to prevent rheumatic fever?
- A: Antibiotics should be started within 9 days from the onset of symptoms in order to prevent this nonsuppurative complication of group A Streptococcal pharyngitis.

S

SPEECH DELAY
Maureen McMahon

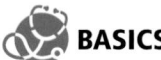 **BASICS**

DEFINITION
- Speech delay is delay in the acquisition of spoken language.
- Language is a system of symbols through which humans communicate thoughts, feelings, and ideas. It has 3 components—receptive, expressive, and visual language.
  - Receptive language is the ability to process and understand language.
  - Expressive language is the ability to communicate through speech, written, or formal sign language.
- Speech delay can be primary, as in specific language impairment (SLI) or developmental language disorder (DLD); or secondary to another condition, such as a syndrome or neurologic disorder. SLI is impaired speech/language in an otherwise normally developing child who lacks signs or stigmata of other conditions.
- Constitutional language delay, a retrospective diagnosis, is language delay associated with eventual achievement of normal speech and language milestones by school age. There are no subsequent difficulties with learning to read or write.
- Expressive language disorders include the following:
  - Verbal dyspraxia: Little speech produced with great effort, very dysfluent, single words most commonly
  - Speech programming deficit disorder: Poorly organized difficult-to-understand speech
- Mixed receptive and expressive disorders:
  - Verbal auditory agnosia: Impaired ability to decode speech, resulting in a severe expressive impairment. Can often learn language visually.
  - Phonologic/syntactic deficit disorder: Most common type of DLD. Comprehension exceeds spoken ability. Speech is dysfluent, grammatically incorrect with short utterances.
  - Most frequent causes of speech delay:
    o Hearing loss
    o Specific language impairment
    o Autism spectrum disorder
    o Intellectual disability (formerly mental retardation)

EPIDEMIOLOGY
- Up to 15% of 2-year olds have speech and language delays.
- 5% of school-aged children have speech and language delays.
- 3:1 male-to-female ratio in DLD

RISK FACTORS
- Family history of speech/language delay or disorder
- Male gender
- Low maternal education
- Maternal depression
- Prematurity
- Birth weight <1,000 g

DIAGNOSIS

DIFFERENTIAL DIAGNOSIS
- **Hearing loss**
  - Isolated genetic hearing loss
  - Hearing loss secondary to in utero CMV infection: Full syndrome at birth or asymptomatic infection with delayed onset of progressive hearing loss
  - Acquired hearing loss: Following head trauma, tumor-associated, following bacterial meningitis, as the result of frequent acute otitis media or chronic otitis media with effusion
- **Intellectual disability**
- **Autism spectrum disorder**
- **Specific language impairment**
- **Constitutional language delay**
- **Environmental**
  - Lack of stimulation and/or poor linguistic environment
  - Child abuse or neglect
  - Lead poisoning
- **Congenital**
  - Cerebral palsy
  - Hydrocephalus
  - Down syndrome
  - Fragile X syndrome
  - 22q11 Microdeletion syndrome
  - Fetal alcohol syndrome
  - Turner syndrome
  - Klinefelter syndrome
  - Prader–Willi syndrome
  - Angelman syndrome
  - Muscular dystrophy
  - Tuberous sclerosis
  - Neurofibromatosis
  - Williams syndrome
  - Branchio-oto-renal (BOR) syndrome
  - Craniofacial anomalies such as Treacher Collins, Goldenhar syndromes
- **Nutritional**
  - Malnutrition
  - Iron deficiency
- **Infectious**
  - HIV encephalopathy
  - Other in utero viral infection
  - Congenital toxoplasmosis
  - Congenital syphilis

ALERT
- Avoid late referral of congenital hearing loss: Amplification and therapy by 6 months of age can result in near normal rate of speech/language acquisition.
- Constitutional language delay is a retrospective diagnosis. Do not assume that a delayed toddler is a "late bloomer" and avoid missing a language disorder.
- Avoid overlooking fine or gross motor delays.
- Avoid missing a genetic or neurologic diagnosis.

HISTORY
Does the family note a concern about speech delay or hearing impairment?
- **Question:** Perinatal history?
- *Significance*: Prenatal care, maternal illness, NICU admission, hyperbilirubinemia requiring exchange transfusion, treatment with ototoxic drugs such as gentamicin, newborn hearing screen results
- **Question:** Full developmental history?
- *Significance*: To determine if global delay or isolated speech and language delay
- **Question:** Parental concern about delayed expressive language?
- *Significance*: Often the presentation of autism
- **Question:** History of feeding, swallowing difficulties, or poor acceptance of textured foods?
- *Significance*: Signs of oromotor dysfunction and may indicate a neurologic problem
- **Question:** Family history of speech delay, hearing loss, neurologic disorder, or syndrome?
- *Significance*: May direct further evaluation
- **Question:** Any regression or loss of language milestones?
- *Significance*: Should prompt a neurologic and metabolic workup
- **Question:** What is the social interaction of the child?
- *Significance*: Lack of interest in playing is a red flag for autism.
- **Question:** Any concern regarding child abuse or neglect, or psychosocial deprivation?
- *Significance*: May have occurred as the result of a parental, genetic, or developmental disorder, drug or alcohol abuse, poverty, child malnutrition, or environmental toxins like lead
- **Question:** History of frequent acute otitis media or otitis media with effusion and conductive hearing loss?
- *Significance*: May precede speech delay
- **Question:** Visual impairments?
- *Significance*: May impact speech development since interpretation of facial expressions and gestures is a component of infant receptive language development
- **Question:** History of traumatic brain injury?
- *Significance*: Speech delay may occur with a seizure disorder.

PHYSICAL EXAM
Complete examination looking for signs that may be associated with speech delay.
- **Finding:** Microcephaly?
- *Significance*: Associated with intellectual disability, in utero CMV infection, or dysmorphic features
- **Finding:** Macrocephaly?
- *Significance*: Associated with hydrocephalus, various syndromes
- **Finding:** Dysmorphic features?
- *Significance*: Suggestive of a syndrome
- **Finding:** Excess drooling and open-mouth posture?
- *Significance*: Signs of poor oral motor control of muscles used for speech production

- **Finding:** Craniofacial abnormalities?
- *Significance*: Articulation difficulty may be due to velopalatal insufficiency (VPI) seen with unrepaired cleft lip or palate.
- **Finding:** Scarred tympanic membranes or middle ear fluid?
- *Significance*: May be clue to acquired intermittent or chronic conductive hearing loss
- **Finding:** Macroorchidism?
- *Significance*: Fragile X syndrome
- **Finding:** Neurologic exam—hypertonia or hypotonia, abnormal reflexes, other focal findings?
- *Significance*: Suggestive of neurologic impairment
- **Finding:** Café-au-lait spots, hypopigmented macules, Shagreen patch, axillary or inguinal freckling?
- *Significance*: Skin findings suggestive of a neurocutaneous syndrome

DIAGNOSTIC TESTS & INTERPRETATION

- The American Academy of Pediatrics recommends a specific development screening tool be administered at the 9, 18, and 24 or 30-month well-child care visits, and an autism-specific tool be administered at the 18 and 24-month visits.
- Office development screening tools:
  - Denver Developmental Assessment II
- Early Language Milestone Scale (ELMS)
- Clinical Linguistic and Auditory Milestone Scale (CLAMS)
- Hearing evaluation:
  - 41 states have mandated Universal Newborn Hearing Screening Programs.
  - Automated Auditory Brainstem Response (AABR) and Transient Evoked Otoacoustic Emissions (OAEs) are the methods used for screening hearing.
  - Hearing should be tested in all speech-delayed children, even if the newborn hearing screen was normal.
  - <6 months of age: The definitive test is Brainstem Auditory Evoked Response (BAER).
  - >6 months of age in a neurologically normal child: The definitive test is behavioral audiometry, such as visual reinforcement audiometry (VRA), performed by a trained audiologist.
- Selected speech/language milestones:
  - 2 months: Cooing, response to voice
  - 6 months: Babbling
  - 4–9 months: Turns to sound, responds to name
  - 9 months: Dada/mama nonspecific, begins to understand "no"
  - 9–12 months: Jargon
  - 12 months: Dada, mama specific, 1 additional word, jargon is complex, points to gesture, follows 1-step command
  - 18 months: 10 words, knows body parts
  - 2 years: 50 words, 2-word phrases, 50% intelligible by strangers, pronouns, can point to specific objects in a picture, may know 1 color, follows 2-step commands
  - 3 years: 300–500 words, tells stories, 75% intelligible by strangers
  - 4 years: Grammatically correct sentences, 100% intelligible by strangers
- Routine cranial imaging or screening tests for metabolic diseases are not recommended.
- **Test:** Full speech and language evaluation
- *Significance*: To delineate the disorder and determine therapy

- **Test:** Individuals with Disabilities Education Act (IDEA) mandates Early Intervention services from birth to 3 years.
- *Significance*: Children can get a full developmental evaluation and appropriate therapy if sufficient delays are demonstrated.
- **Test:** EEG
- *Significance*: Indicated if there is concern for seizures
- **Test:** Genetics evaluation
- *Significance*: Should be obtained for congenital hearing loss or if there is concern for a syndrome or genetic diagnosis
- **Test:** Prolonged sleep EEG
- *Significance*: Indicated with loss of language milestones (consider the diagnosis of Landau–Kleffner syndrome)

TREATMENT

ADDITIONAL TREATMENT
General Measures
- Congenital hearing loss is managed by a team consisting of an otolaryngologist, audiologist, and speech/language therapist who individualize management. Options are amplification, cochlear implant for the severely impaired, or use of sign language.
- Speech and language therapy can be provided through physician referral or parent-generated referral to early intervention programs.
- Sign language can be used as a bridge to promote communication while the child learns verbal skills. It will not preclude or delay the development of speech.
- Augmentative communication devices such as picture boards or programmed computers with voice synthesizers can be used by children with physical impairments such as cerebral palsy.

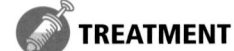 ONGOING CARE

- Children with DLD usually speak adequately by school age. Some percentage will go on to have difficulty reading and writing
- Children with constitutional language delay will achieve normal milestones by the time they start school.

ADDITIONAL READING

- Agin M. The "late talker"—when silence isn't golden. *Contemp Pediatr*. 2004;21(11):22–32.
- Campbell T, Dollaghan C, Rockette H, et al. Risk factors for speech delay of unknown origin in three-year old children. *Child Dev*. 2003;74: 346–357.
- Coplan J. Normal speech and language development: An overview. *Pediatr Rev*. 1995;16:91–100.
- Coplan J. Language delays. In: Parker S, Zuckerman B, Augustyn M, eds. *Developmental and behavioral pediatrics*, 2nd ed. Philadelphia: Lippincott Williams & Wilkins, 2005:222–226.

- Feldman H. Evaluation and management of language and speech disorders in preschool children. *Pediatr Rev*. 2005;26:131–140.
- Rapin I. Practitioner review: Developmental language disorders—a clinical update. *J Child Psychol*. 1996;37:643–655.
- Sokol J, Hyde M. Hearing screening. *Pediatr Rev*. 2002;23:155–161.
- U.S. Preventive Services Task Force. Screening for speech and language delay in preschool children: Recommendation statement. *Pediatrics*. 2006; 117(2):497–501.

CODES

ICD9
- 315.34 Speech and language developmental delay due to hearing loss
- 315.39 Other developmental speech or language disorder

ICD10
- F80.4 Speech and language development delay due to hearing loss
- F80.9 Developmental disorder of speech and language, unspecified

FAQ

- Q: Do second- and third-born children speak later than first-born children?
- A: No, the norms for expected speech/language development are the same regardless of birth order. Second- and third-born children should have the same degree of motivation to speak as their first-born sibling.
- Q: When should I refer a child for speech/language evaluation?
- A: If the parents or physician have any concern for speech delay, then referral for evaluation is wise. Some speech-delayed children will eventually normalize and meet all milestones. It is difficult to distinguish who is constitutionally delayed from those who have another disorder. There are several indications for a prompt referral. No pointing or babbling by 1 year, no single words by 16 months, no 2-word spontaneous phrases by 2 years, no sentences by 3 years, poor intelligibility for age, or any regression in language skills.
- Q: Do children raised in bilingual households have expressive language delay?
- A: No, living in a bilingual household is not a cause of expressive language delay. However, toddlers who are learning 2 languages may interchange words in both languages. Total vocabulary and phrase length are typically normal in these children by 2–3 years of age.

S

SPEECH PROBLEMS

Judith A. Turow

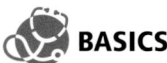 **BASICS**

DEFINITION

- Language: A system of symbols with a systematic relationship that is used to communicate new ideas
- Speech: The expression of language in a verbal fashion
- Phonemes are the units of sound in speech.
- Phonology is the order in which speech sounds form words.
- Articulation: The process by which words are expressed through muscular movements controlled by complex neuromuscular changes with the production of vocal and articulate sounds
- Children can have central, structural, or functional reasons for speech disorders. The most common speech problems include:
  - Disorders of articulation: Articulation disorders can be organic or functional and occur when children misarticulate words by:
    - Using substitutions of 1 sound for another, commonly "W" for "R"
    - Omitting sounds commonly at the beginning of a word "kip" for "skip"
    - Distorting or adding sounds as "puhlay" for "play"
    - Apraxia is a motor disorder of speech involving central programming for the production of phonemes and the sequencing of voluntary muscle movements for the production of words. Also called "apraxic dysarthria"
    - Dysarthria is a disorder of speech sound production with demonstrable dysfunction or structural abnormality of the tongue, lips, teeth, or palate.
    - Phonologic disorders are functional problems with multiple phoneme errors.
  - Disorders of voice are noted to be disorders of pitch, loudness, quality, and resonance.
    - Dysphonia: A disorder of the voice
    - Rhinolalia: Altered speech due to some abnormality of nasal structures
    - Hoarseness is the most common problem, and results from problems with the vocal folds or their nerve supply. The most common condition in childhood is vocal nodules, which can be removed, but need to be followed by a period of voice rest.
    - Hypernasal speech is the result of a short, cleft or paralyzed palate as a result of an incompetent palatopharyngeal sphincter. It may also occur with a profoundly deaf child because nasal sounds provide the maximal feedback.
    - Hyponasal speech is often acutely due to nasal congestion as seen with viral upper respiratory tract infections or in association with adenoidal hypertrophy when chronic.

- Disorders of fluency include pauses, hesitations, repetitions, interjections, or prolongations.
  - Aphasia is a loss or impairment of ability to produce and/or comprehend language owing to brain damage. It is usually due to damage of the language centers of the brain (Broca aphasia is due to damage in the frontal lobe, and Wernicke aphasia is due to damage of the temporal lobe).
  - Dysrhythmia: A disorder of coordination between respiration and articulatory function (see "Stuttering" chapter)
- Secondary speech disorders are speech disorders not associated with dysfunction or structure but due to other diseases or adverse environmental factors, including mental retardation, hearing defects, psychiatric disorders, and extreme social deprivation, isolation, or institutionalization.
- Mixed speech disorder: A mixture of 2 or more of the categories above (e.g., a cleft lip with abnormal hearing and mental retardation)
- Developmental language impairment and specific language impairment (see "Speech Delay" chapter)

EPIDEMIOLOGY

Communication disorders are the most common developmental problems in preschool-aged children:

- Nearly 20% of 2-year-olds are thought to have delayed onset of speech.
- By age 5, 19% of children are considered to have speech and language disorders—6.4% from speech impairment, 4.6% from speech and language impairment, and 8% from language impairment.
- 50% of mentally retarded children fail to acquire any symbolic communication skills.
- The majority of language disorders, up to 85%, are seen in boys.

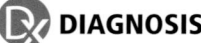 **DIAGNOSIS**

HISTORY

- Is there a history of prolonged feeding time, tongue thrusts, choking on foods, and/or nasal reflux during feeding? Dysarthria is often preceded by dysphasia.
- Persistent nasal reflux during feeding is always a pathologic sign and may be indicative of velopharyngeal insufficiency due to an anatomic or neurologic abnormality.
- Frequent pneumonia, recurrent upper respiratory tract infections, or nasal congestion? Is there evidence for palatal insufficiency?
- Recurrent ear infections, or recent infections implying chronic or acute middle ear fluid?
- Any disorders of the mouth, palate, or tongue? Is there a structural reason for dysarthria?
- Prematurity, intrauterine growth retardation, or meningitis? Are there factors that predispose the child to deafness or mental retardation?
- Family history of speech problems?
- Family history of deafness?
- History of lower motor neuron damage or trauma to the pharynx?

- History of hearing loss?
- Voice overuse?
- Odd/stereotypic behavior, unusual social interactions, or limited play skills? Is there evidence for autism spectrum disorder, pervasive developmental disorder?
- Discrepancy among the areas of skill sets, or regression of skills? Is there any evidence of autistic regression or Landau-Kleffner syndrome (epileptic aphasia)?

PHYSICAL EXAM

Finding:

- Iris heterotropia, white forelock (piebaldism), or dystopia canthorum: Seen in Waardenburg syndrome and with associated deafness
- Microcephaly: May be associated with brain damage from underlying in utero infection, toxin exposure, or genetic disorder
- Enlarged tonsils: Potential reason for abnormal resonance, such as hyponasal speech
- Any impaired sucking or swallowing, bifid or notched uvula, drooling, abnormal gag reflex, tongue thrusts, evidence of tracheotomy scar, potential reason for functional or structural dysarthria, potential reason for damage to vocal cords?
- Upper motor neuron signs, such as involuntary grimacing, drooling, abnormalities of the gag reflex, impairment of sucking and swallowing: May be seen with cerebral palsy, Möbius syndrome

DIAGNOSTIC TESTS & INTERPRETATION
Diagnostic Procedures/Other

- Formal testing to examine overall cognitive level, language related to the cognitive level, and other atypical features (including stereotypies, poor socialization skills, sensory aversions)
- Speech and language pathologist
- Psychoeducational testing
- Hearing evaluations
- Screening audiometry: High false-negative rate and inappropriate for the younger child
- Formal audiologic testing including tympanometry and audiometry and possible brainstem evoked response testing for hearing loss
- Speech evaluation
- Videofluoroscopic speech study
- Nasometer: Microchip-based instrument to measure sound coming from the oral and nasal cavities; test to aid in the evaluation of resonance
- Language evaluation:
  - The Early Language Milestone (ELM) Scale (revised ELM 2 now available): Covers language development from birth through age 36 months and intelligibility of speech from ages 24–48 months
  - The Clinical Linguistic and Auditory Milestone Scale (CLAMS): Tests language development from birth through 36 months, confirming normal language in the 14–36-month age range, although less useful for confirming receptive language delay in 14–36-month-old children, or expressive language delay in children <25 months
- Metabolic and cytogenetic testing for disorders including Fragile X syndrome

- Apex SNHL (sensorineural hearing loss) microarray for molecular diagnosis of genetic deletions in nonsyndromic SNHL
- Central nervous system (CNS) imaging is rarely helpful, except with autistic regression or Landau-Kleffner syndrome (epileptic aphasia)

DIFFERENTIAL DIAGNOSIS
- Infectious:
  - Prenatal: Toxoplasmosis, rubella, cytomegalovirus, or herpes virus (TORCH) infections
  - Postnatal infections, particularly bacterial meningitis caused by:
    o *Neisseria meningitidis*
    o *Haemophilus influenzae*
    o *Streptococcus pneumoniae*
  - Recurrent throat infections
  - Recurrent ear infections
- Environmental: Isolation and/or social deprivation
- Structural:
  - Cleft lip or palate
  - Notched uvula
- Genetic:
  - Waardenburg, branchio-oto-renal, or Stickler syndromes; neurofibromatosis type 2
  - Autosomal recessive (AR) inheritance
    o Refsum disease, Usher syndrome, Pendred syndrome, Biotinidase deficiency
  - X-linked recessive
    o Alport syndrome
    o Mohr-Tranebjaerg syndrome
- Developmental:
  - Mental retardation
  - Autism spectrum disorder
  - Apraxia
- Neuromuscular:
  - Cerebral palsy
  - Broca or Wernicke aphasia
  - Möbius syndrome
  - Landau-Kleffner syndrome
- Nutritional: Malnutrition
- Acquired hearing loss
  - Noise exposure
  - Aminoglycoside-acquired hearing loss
  - Hyperbilirubinemia, severe
  - Trauma to the head and neck
  - Cholesteatoma
- Acquired voice loss/dysfunction:
  - Trauma to the head and neck
  - Tracheotomy
  - Adenoid enlargement
  - Chronic/recurrent nose and/or throat infections
  - Nasal allergies
  - Voice abuse

 TREATMENT

ADDITIONAL TREATMENT
General Measures
- Home-based programs through early intervention for preschool children up to age 5.
- Special education enrollment for school-aged children
- Audiologic assessment for all children with speech disorders is a must and should include hearing testing. Referral to an otolaryngologist to evaluate the function and structure of anomalies of the head and neck
- Referral to a speech therapist: Children who have oral–motor deficits (especially speech apraxia) and require intensive speech and language therapy

- Signing and/or picture card system may be helpful with severe speech and language problems to teach child how to communicate:
  - Use of signing by nonverbal children has been shown to be an effective bridge to spoken language. Picture exchange is another method of communicating.
- Referral to psychologist/child developmentalist
- Referral to an occupational therapist trained in sensory integration techniques: Can assist in management of children who show aversive behaviors
- American Sign Language teacher

 ONGOING CARE

FOLLOW-UP RECOMMENDATIONS
- The prognosis for most children with expressive language problems is excellent. Most will have normal language skills by the time they enter primary school.
- However, if there are persistent speech and/or language problems by 5 years of age, there is a 70–80% chance of continued communication difficulty and reading disorders.
- Pearls:
  - "Rule of 4s": Divide the child's age in years by 4; the quotient is approximately equal to the percentage of the child's speech that should be intelligible to strangers:
    o A 1-year-old should be intelligible to strangers 1/4 of the time
    o A 2-year-old, 1/2 of the time
    o A 3-year-old, 3/4 of the time
    o A 4-year-old, essentially 100% of the time
    o The average 1-year-old should be speaking at least 1 word (other than mama, dada, or family names), following at least a 1-step command not accompanied by physical gestures, and pointing with 1 finger to desired objects.
    o A 2-year-old will be speaking 2-word phrases and following 2-step commands.
    o Between ages 2 and 3, the average child uses "telegraphic speech" (e.g., "go home now").
    o The average 3-year-old should be fluent in the present tense and have a speaking vocabulary of 500–1,000 words.
    o The average 5-year-old follows 3-step commands, names 5 colors, has a vocabulary of >2,000 words, and makes up rhymes.

ADDITIONAL READING
- Coplan J. Evaluation of the child with delayed speech or language. *Pediatr Ann*. 1985;14:203–208.
- Coplan J. Normal speech and language development: An overview. *Pediatr Rev*. 1995;16: 91–100.
- Feldman HM. Evaluation and management of language and speech disorders in preschool children. *Pediatr Rev*. 2005;26:131–142.

- Sharp HM, Hillenbrand K. Speech and language development and disorders in children. *Pediatr Clin North Am*. 2008;55:1150–1173.
- Simms M, Schum R. Preschool children who have atypical patterns of development. *Pediatr Rev*. 2000;21:147–158.
- Smith RJH, Van Camp G. Deafness and hereditary hearing loss overview. Available at: http://www.geneclinics.org/profiles/deafness-overview/details.html.

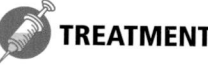 **CODES**

ICD9
- 315.31 Expressive language disorder
- 315.32 Mixed receptive-expressive language disorder
- 315.39 Other developmental speech or language disorder

ICD10
- F80.0 Phonological disorder
- F80.9 Developmental disorder of speech and language, unspecified
- R47.9 Unspecified speech disturbances

FAQ
- Q: Does ankyloglossia make a difference in the emergence of language?
- A: The tongue has to move freely for speech with such sounds as /t/, /d/, /n/, and /l/, but misarticulation caused by ankyloglossia is quite rare.
- Q: Does "signing" delay speech?
- A: In fact, signing may promote speech development and progression owing to the increased ability of the child to communicate.
- Q: Is gender or birth order a risk factor for delayed speech?
- A: Studies show male children lag 1–2 months behind in vocabulary and grammar when compared to females. Studies on birth order are inconclusive.
- Q: Does bilingualism make a difference in speech progression?
- A: Toddlers from bilingual homes may show some delays early on. Speech progression is enhanced if the two languages are spoken in separate contexts (e.g., the 1st language is spoken at home all the time and the 2nd language is spoken out of home all the time, rather than a mixture of both languages in the same environment), but this is not always practical for families.

S

SPINAL MUSCULAR ATROPHY

Jennifer A. Markowitz
Peter B. Kang (5th edition)

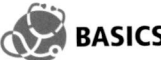 BASICS

DESCRIPTION
- Spinal muscular atrophy (SMA) is a progressive disorder of motor neurons in the spinal cord and brainstem.
- Major symptom is proximal weakness.
- 3 forms are described based on clinical features:
  - Type I, also known as Werdnig-Hoffman disease, typically presents by 6 months; these children never sit.
  - Type II typically presents between 6 and 18 months; these children sit independently but never walk.
  - Type III, also known as Kugelberg-Welander disease, may be diagnosed later; these children stand and walk at some point.
- There appears to be a spectrum of severity within and between each type.

EPIDEMIOLOGY
The most common genetic cause of infant mortality

Incidence
Incidence estimated at 1 in 6,000–10,000 live births; carrier frequency 1 in 40–50, though some variation between populations seems to exist

RISK FACTORS
Genetics
- Genetic testing is recommended in all cases, even when the diagnosis appears clear.
- Genetic counseling is critical for all families with children affected by SMA, as the chance of recurrence is 25%.
- SMN2 copy number varies among the general population and is loosely correlated with SMA type (type I likely to have fewer copies); however, all copies of SMN2 are not equal (some make more SMN protein than others) and an individual patient's SMN2 copy number should not be used for prognostic purposes.
- Universal newborn screening is strongly recommended by some but is not yet in place.

ETIOLOGY
- All 3 types of proximal SMA follow an autosomal recessive inheritance and are caused by mutations in the survival motor neuron (SMN) gene on 5q11.2 to 13.3.
- 2 copies of SMN on each chromosome. SMN1 (SMNt), the telomeric copy, produces stable SMN protein. SMN2 (SMNc), the centromeric copy, is an inverted duplication of SMN1 with a single nucleotide change in an exonic splice enhancer, which produces mostly an unstable, truncated protein product and a smaller percentage of stable, full-length SMN protein. Individuals with SMA harbor homozygous deletions of exon 7 in the SMN1 gene, which renders it nonfunctional. The presence of SMN2 essentially "rescues" individuals with SMN1 deletions, since complete absence of SMN protein appears to be embryonically lethal. The level of SMN protein roughly correlates with the severity of disease.

- The SMN protein plays a role in RNA processing; it is unclear why motor neurons (anterior horn cells) are selectively vulnerable to this defect, although a role in axonal mRNA trafficking and splicing is being explored.

COMMONLY ASSOCIATED CONDITIONS
Other anterior horn cell diseases:
- SMARD (SMA with respiratory distress) or diaphragmatic SMA, due to mutations in the IGHMBP2 gene on chromosome 11q
- Distal SMAs, a group of disorders with distal weakness, genetically heterogeneous
- Other variants are associated with arthrogryposis, pontocerebellar hypoplasia, congenital fractures, and congenital heart disease. Few such cases have been shown to have SMN mutations.
- Fazio-Londe disease: Rare degeneration of anterior horn cells in the brainstem, childhood onset
- Kennedy disease, or X-linked spinal and bulbar muscular atrophy: Anterior horn cell disease with adult onset; affected men have gynecomastia, bulbar weakness, and reduced fertility.

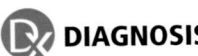 DIAGNOSIS

HISTORY
- Hypotonia and weakness are the primary features. Infants with SMA I will be floppy and less active and have delayed motor milestones, with preserved language/social interaction (a bright, alert demeanor is often remarked upon).
- Some babies with type I present with feeding problems and failure to thrive.
- History of reduced vigor of prenatal movements

PHYSICAL EXAM
- Weakness and absent or reduced reflexes suggest a neuromuscular rather than central etiology for hypotonia. A proximal pattern of weakness is consistent with SMA, myopathies, and muscular dystrophies; a distal pattern usually suggests polyneuropathies.
- Weakness is almost universally symmetric, but occasional cases of asymmetric weakness have been reported in SMA III.
- Extraocular movements remain intact in SMA.
- Facial strength diminishes in children with type I over time, and jaw contractures may be present in type II.
- Dysmorphic features, or involvement of other organs, may point to alternative diagnoses. Occasionally, SMA presents with contractures (spectrum of arthrogryposis multiplex congenita).
- Tongue fasciculations strongly suggest SMA, but their absence does not exclude the diagnosis.
- Tremor of a specific type, polyminimyoclonus, is often present in type II.

DIAGNOSTIC TESTS & INTERPRETATION
Lab
- Initial screening tests: Serum creatinine kinase may be mildly elevated.
- Genetic testing:
  - Genetic testing of DNA extracted from blood (SMN deletions): Now the gold standard in diagnosis, may be done prenatally, >95% sensitive
  - Genetic testing for Prader-Willi syndrome (fluorescence in situ hybridization and methylation) may be indicated if there is no SMN gene deletion and electromyography (EMG) is normal in an infant who appears to have SMA.
- Other testing:
  - EMG may be helpful if the clinical presentation is atypical for SMA or if genetic testing is negative. EMG shows high-amplitude, long-duration motor units with a reduced recruitment pattern.
  - With the advent of molecular testing, muscle biopsy is rarely performed. Use when genetic testing is unrevealing. The characteristic findings are fiber-type grouping with generalized atrophy of muscle fibers.
  - If the entire evaluation is negative, MRI of the spine may be indicated to evaluate for an anomaly or mass lesion.

DIFFERENTIAL DIAGNOSIS
- Other genetic neuromuscular disorders include congenital muscular dystrophy, congenital myopathy, glycogen storage disorders (Pompe disease), myotonic dystrophy, mitochondrial disease, congenital myasthenia gravis, and Prader-Willi syndrome.
- More acute course may suggest infant botulism or Guillain-Barré syndrome, although the latter is rare in this age group.
- Systemic disorders: Sepsis, meningitis, acute bowel syndromes
- SMA II differential: Congenital muscular dystrophy, congenital myopathy, and congenital myasthenia gravis
- SMA III differential includes Duchenne, Becker, and the limb girdle muscular dystrophies.
- Spinal cord mass lesions may rarely resemble SMA.

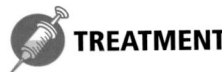 TREATMENT

ALERT
An apparently minor respiratory infection may carry a higher risk of respiratory failure in SMA I and later stages of SMA II and III. Depending on family/patient wishes regarding respiratory support, consider admitting such a patient to the hospital for observation. Infants with SMA may be exquisitely sensitive to postural shifts—watch for hypoventilation, for example, with forward truncal flexion associated with some seating arrangements.

ADDITIONAL TREATMENT
General Measures

- A multidisciplinary approach to care is recommended, with early and proactive involvement of orthopedics, nutrition, pulmonary, and physical and occupational therapy, as well as social work and psychological support for families and patients.
- Physical therapy is appropriate for all 3 types; though it may not affect the course in SMA I, it can lessen discomfort and make care easier by improving range of motion and preventing contractures
- A wheelchair provides mobility in SMA II. Children as young as age 2 may be considered for a motorized wheelchair, depending on developmental level. Adults with SMA III may require the use of a wheelchair later in their course.
- Bracing of ankles, wrists, and back can help reduce contractures and slow progression of scoliosis.
- Spinal fusion surgery may preserve respiratory function.
- Low threshold for empiric antibiotics for respiratory infection is appropriate.
- Chest physiotherapy and early implementation of cough assist device can help prevent pneumonia and atelectasis.
- Be wary of symptoms of hypoventilation (disturbed sleep, daytime fatigue, moodiness, morning headaches), which may occur prior to other symptoms of respiratory insufficiency.
- Low threshold to order a sleep study if hypoventilation is suspected
- In acute respiratory illness, supplemental oxygen is appropriate, as long as the patient is also evaluated and treated for hypercarbia.
- Noninvasive positive-pressure ventilation (BiPAP and other regimens) may improve quality of life and life expectancy in patients with decreased respiratory function. More aggressive respiratory management is becoming more common and accepted among families and physicians, but the extent of interventions varies widely. Start discussions about family/patient preferences early, as respiratory decompensation can occur very quickly.
- Avoid catabolic state with proactive nutritional support, including tube feeding.
- However, note that type II patients may have increased adiposity, and overweight is also a risk.
- Monitor for osteopenia, which is almost universal in types I and II, and ensure adequate calcium and vitamin D intake.
- Social and psychological support for caregivers and patients

 ONGOING CARE

PATIENT EDUCATION
- Families of SMA: http://www.fsma.org
- Fight SMA: http://www.fightsma.org
- Muscular Dystrophy Association: http://www.mdausa.org
- Spinal Muscular Atrophy Foundation: http://www.smafoundation.org

PROGNOSIS
- Survival in all 3 forms has been increasing with improved supportive care and, in type I, ventilatory support.
- Most children with SMA type I die by 2 years without major pulmonary interventions. With ventilatory support, patients may survive several years longer; survival as long as 2 decades has been observed with tracheostomy and full mechanical ventilation.
- Children with SMA type II typically survive into late adolescence or early adulthood; this life expectancy is increasing with more aggressive pulmonary management.
- Individuals with SMA type III survive well into adulthood, and often have a normal life expectancy. In 1 study of patients with SMA type III with onset <3 years, 50% could not walk 20 years later; for those with onset >3 years, 30% could not walk 20 years later.
- Intelligence is generally preserved.
- Death typically ensues from respiratory complications. Discuss the level of respiratory interventions, including resuscitation, early in SMA I and in the advanced stages of SMA II and III.

COMPLICATIONS
- Recurrent pneumonias, hypoventilation
- Swallowing difficulties may require tube feeding.
- Scoliosis may require surgery.

ADDITIONAL READING

- Chung BH, Wong VC, Ip P. Spinal muscular atrophy: Survival pattern and functional status. *Pediatrics*. 2004;114(5):e548–e553.
- Hardart MKM, Truog RD. Spinal muscular atrophy—type I. *Arch Dis Child*. 2003;88:848–850.
- Hirtz D, Iannaccone S, Heemskerk J, et al. Challenges and opportunities in clinical trials for spinal muscular atrophy. *Neurology*. 2005;65:1352–1357.
- Iannaccone ST, Burghes A. Spinal muscular atrophies. *Adv Neurol*. 2002;88:83–98.
- Kolb SJ, Kissel JT. Spinal muscular atrophy: A timely review. *Arch Neurol*. 2011;74:E1–E6.
- Lunn MR, Wang CH. Spinal muscular atrophy. *Lancet*. 2008;371(9630):2120–2133.
- Messina S, Pane M, De Rose P, et al. Feeding problems and malnutrition in spinal muscular atrophy type II. *Neuromusc Disord*. 2008;18:389–393.
- Ogino S, Leonard DG, Rennert H, et al. Genetic risk assessment in carrier testing for spinal muscular atrophy. *Am J Med Genet*. 2002;110:301–307.
- Petit F, Cuisset JM, Rouaix-Emery N, et al. Insights into genotype-phenotype correlations in spinal muscular atrophy: A retrospective study of 103 patients. *Muscle Nerve*. 2011;43:26–30.
- Prasad AN, Prasad C. The floppy infant: Contribution of genetic and metabolic disorders. *Brain Dev*. 2003;25(7):457–476.
- Prior TW, Snyder PJ, Rink BD, et al. Newborn and carrier screening for spinal muscular atrophy. *Am J Med Genet Part A*. 2010;152A:1608–1616.
- Wang CH, Finkel RS, Bertini ES, et al. Participants of the International Conference on SMA Standard of Care. Consensus statement for standard of care in spinal muscular atrophy. *J Child Neurol*. 2007;22(8):1027–1049.
- Zerres K, Rudnik-Schoneborn S. Natural history in proximal spinal muscular atrophy. Clinical analysis of 445 patients and suggestions for a modification of existing classifications. *Arch Neurol*. 1995;52(5):518–523.

S

 CODES

ICD9
- 335.0 Werdnig-Hoffmann disease
- 335.10 Spinal muscular atrophy, unspecified
- 335.19 Other spinal muscular atrophy

ICD10
- G12.0 Infantile spinal muscular atrophy, type I [Werdnig-Hoffman]
- G12.1 Other inherited spinal muscular atrophy
- G12.9 Spinal muscular atrophy, unspecified

FAQ

- Q: Can routine vaccinations be given to children with SMA?
- A: Yes. In addition to routine vaccinations, yearly influenza and RSV vaccinations are recommended.
- Q: How much respiratory support should a child with SMA receive?
- A: Standards of care are evolving rapidly, and a consensus remains elusive. However, noninvasive respiratory interventions are becoming more widely accepted. Noninvasive respiratory options should be offered to all patients with SMA I and those in the later stages of SMA II. Tracheostomy is more controversial.
- Q: Are more effective therapies for SMA being developed?
- A: There are ongoing studies in animal models and on humans, involving both pharmacologic and gene-based therapies. Families of SMA, the Muscular Dystrophy Association, and other groups are sources of information on such research.

SPLENOMEGALY
Matthew J. Ryan

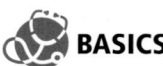 **BASICS**

DEFINITION
- A palpable spleen is found in most premature infants and in 30% of term infants. A spleen tip is still palpable in 10% of infants at 1 year of age and in 1% of children at 10 years of age.
- Normal spleens are not greater then 6 cm at 3 months, 7 cm at 12 months, 9.5 cm at 6 years, 11.5 cm at 12 years, and not greater then 13 cm for adolescents.
- The clinical significance of splenomegaly found on radiologic study, but not palpable on physical exam, is unclear in the absence of other laboratory or clinical data.
- Normal spleens are soft at the midclavicular line, nontender, and often palpable only on deep inspiration.
- Dullness on percussion beyond the 11th intercostal space suggests splenomegaly.
- A spleen edge palpated >2 cm below the costal margin is always an abnormal finding.
- Splenic tenderness is abnormal.

PATHOPHYSIOLOGY
- The spleen is a hematopoietic organ with 2 main parts:
  - White pulp is the lymphoid tissue.
  - Red pulp is the red cell mass.
- Splenic sinusoids are lined with macrophages that destroy abnormal red cells.
- The spleen also serves as a reservoir for platelets. A normal-sized spleen can hold 1/3 of the circulating platelets; an enlarged spleen can hold up to 90% of the circulating platelet mass.

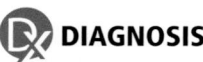 **DIAGNOSIS**

DIFFERENTIAL DIAGNOSIS
- **Infectious**
  - Bacterial:
    - Bacteremia
    - Pneumonia
    - Sepsis
    - Subacute bacterial endocarditis
    - Salmonellosis
    - Tuberculosis
    - Brucellosis
    - Staphylococcal shunt infections
    - Tularemia
    - Syphilis
    - Leptospirosis

  - Viral:
    - Epstein–Barr virus (mononucleosis)
    - Cytomegalovirus
    - HIV
    - Rubella
    - Herpes
    - Hepatitis A, B, C
  - Rickettsial/protozoan:
    - Rocky Mountain spotted fever
    - Malaria
    - Toxoplasmosis
    - Trypanosomiasis
    - Babesiosis
    - Schistosomiasis
    - Visceral larval migrans
    - Kala azar
  - Fungal:
    - Histoplasmosis
    - Coccidioidomycosis
- **Hematologic disorders**
  - Hereditary spherocytosis
  - Sickle cell disease in early childhood or during splenic sequestration crisis
  - Hemoglobin C disease
  - Thalassemia major
  - Autoimmune hemolytic anemia
  - Glucose-6-phosphate dehydrogenase deficiency
  - Isoimmunization disorders
  - Infantile pyknocytosis
  - Iron-deficiency anemia (rare)
  - Thrombocytopenic purpura
- **Vascular disorders**
  - Cavernous transformation of the portal vein
  - Budd–Chiari syndrome
  - Splenic vein thrombosis
  - Congenital portal vein stenosis or atresia
  - Splenic hematoma
  - Splenic hemangioma
- **Liver disease/cirrhosis** (examples include, but are not limited to)
  - Biliary atresia
  - Wilson disease
  - Cystic fibrosis
  - α-1-Antitrypsin deficiency
  - Hereditary hemochromatosis
  - Congenital hepatic fibrosis
  - Autoimmune hepatitis
  - Primary sclerosing cholangitis

- **Metabolic diseases (storage)**
  - Gangliosidoses
  - Mucolipidoses
  - Metachromatic leukodystrophy
  - Wolman disease
  - Gaucher disease
  - Niemann–Pick disease
  - Amyloidosis
- **Neoplastic diseases**
  - Leukemia
  - Lymphoma
  - Lymphosarcoma
  - Neuroblastoma
  - Histiocytosis X
  - Familial hemophagocytic lymphohistiocytosis
- **Miscellaneous**
  - Serum sickness
  - Connective-tissue disorders
  - Juvenile rheumatoid arthritis
  - Systemic lupus erythematosus
  - Sarcoidosis
  - Splenic hamartoma
  - Splenic cysts: Congenital and post-traumatic
  - Trauma: Subcapsular hematoma
- **Nonsplenic upper left quadrant abdominal masses**
  - Large kidney
  - Retroperitoneal tumor
  - Adrenal neoplasm
  - Ovarian cyst
  - Pancreatic cyst
  - Mesenteric cyst
  - Rib anomaly

ALERT
- Life-threatening causes: Sepsis, severe hemolytic anemia, trauma, splenic sequestration
- A large-bore IV access route should be rapidly placed when a life-threatening cause is suspected.

APPROACH TO THE PATIENT
General goal is to determine the etiology of the large spleen.
- **Phase 1:** Establish the presence of enlarged spleen, not a palpable spleen that is pushed down by inflated lungs
- **Phase 2:** Rule out common causes such as a viral infection, bacterial infection, or anemia
- **Phase 3:** Rule out malignancy or storage disease or other rare causes of large spleen

HISTORY

- **Question:** History of acute illness?
- *Significance:* Suggests infection
- **Question:** History of GI bleeding with splenomegaly?
- *Significance:* Suggests portal hypertension
- **Question:** Familial history of hematologic or immune disease?
- *Significance:* Suggests genetic etiology
- **Question:** An enlarged liver, developmental delay, or neurologic findings?
- *Significance:* May suggest a storage disease or metabolic disorder

PHYSICAL EXAM

Begin the abdominal examination in the lower left quadrant, because an enlarged spleen may be missed in the upper quadrant exam. Stand to the right of the patient; use the right hand to palpate and the left hand to support the patient's left lower rib cage. Flexing the legs at the knees may help to relax the abdominal musculature.

- **Finding:** Auscultate?
- *Significance:* For rub or bruit
- **Finding:** Look for signs of storage disease?
- *Significance:* Retinal exam, coarse facies
- **Finding:** Complete evaluation of lymph nodes?
- *Significance:* Enlargement suggests infection or neoplasia.
- **Finding:** Palpate for ascites or hepatomegaly?
- *Significance:* Suggests underlying hepatic disease
- **Finding:** Prominent abdominal veins or hemorrhoids?
- *Significance:* Suggest increased portal venous pressure
- **Finding:** Pain/tenderness?
- *Significance:* Suggests capsular distention secondary to perisplenitis or trauma; also raises the question of splenic infarct.
- **Finding:** Asthmatic patients may have palpable spleen?
- *Significance:* Secondary to overinflation of lungs and depressed diaphragm

DIAGNOSTIC TESTS & INTERPRETATION

Discriminating laboratory tests: If no hemolytic disease, with signs of infection

- Blood culture
- Thick smear of blood for malaria
- Viral testing
- **Test:** CBC with manual differential and smear
- *Significance:* For sickle cell disease, hemolytic anemia, leukemia
- **Test:** Decreased WBC count and platelets
- *Significance:* Often seen with splenic sequestration or portal hypertension
- **Test:** Reticulocyte count
- *Significance:* For hemolytic anemia
- **Test:** Hepatic function panel (liver enzymes, albumin, bilirubin) and PT/INR, PTT
- *Significance:* For cirrhosis, hepatic obstruction
- **Test:** Serum LDH
- *Significance:* For hemolysis or tumor screen

Imaging

- If no hemolytic disease, no sign of infection, no sign of congestion:
  - Ultrasound with Doppler
  - Liver spleen scan
  - Biopsy of lymph node, liver, or other tissue, depending on findings
- If no hemolytic disease, no sign of infection, but signs of congestion:
  - Ultrasound with Doppler
  - MRI; consider MRA/MRV
  - CT scan

 TREATMENT

ADDITIONAL TREATMENT

General Measures

Depends on underlying etiology

ISSUES FOR REFERRAL

- Disproportionate size of spleen
- Increasing size over serial examinations
- Unexplained lymphadenopathy
- Liver dysfunction
- Ascites
- Signs of storage or metabolic disease
- Howell–Jolly bodies on peripheral smear, suggesting splenic dysfunction

ADDITIONAL READING

- Donnelly LF, Foss JN, Frush DP, et al. Heterogeneous splenic enhancement patterns on spiral CT images in children: Minimizing misinterpretation. *Radiology.* 1999;210:493–497.
- Imrie J, Wraith JE. Isolated splenomegaly as the presenting feature of Niemann-Pick disease type C. *Arch Dis Child.* 2001;84:427–429.
- McCormick PA, Murphy KM. Splenomegaly, hypersplenism and coagulation abnormalities in liver disease. *Best Pract Res Clin Gastroenterol.* 2000;14:1009–1031.
- Pozo AL, Godfrey EM, Bowles KM. Splenomegaly: Investigation, diagnosis and Management. *Blood Rev.* 2009;23:105–111.
- Rosenberg HK, Markowitz RI, Kolberg H, et al. Normal splenic size in infants and children: Sonographic measurements. *Am J Roentgenol.* 1991;19:1465.

S

 CODES

ICD9

- 289.51 Chronic congestive splenomegaly
- 789.2 Splenomegaly

ICD10

- R16.1 Splenomegaly, not elsewhere classified
- D73.2 Chronic congestive splenomegaly

FAQ

- Q: How long will the enlarged spleen secondary to a viral infection be present?
- A: The enlarged spleen may persist for several months.
- Q: Should a child with an enlarged spleen refrain from sports?
- A: Contact sports should be avoided for a child with an enlarged spleen. An enlarged spleen is engorged with blood, and a splenic rupture would be a catastrophic event. Children with persistent splenomegaly should be considered for a spleen guard.

STAPHYLOCOCCAL SCALDED SKIN SYNDROME (SSSS)

Mark L. Bagarazzi

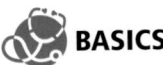 **BASICS**

DESCRIPTION

- A spectrum of generalized exfoliative skin eruptions, that resemble scalding injuries but are caused by an epidermolytic toxin produced by certain strains of *Staphylococcus aureus*
- Known as Ritter disease or pemphigus neonatorum in neonates
- Spectrum of disease includes:
  - Bullous impetigo: Characterized by discrete, flaccid bullae containing clear or cloudy yellow fluid localized to the site of staphylococcal infection
  - Staphylococcal scarlet fever: A mild generalized scarlatiniform eruption with exfoliation, but without the strawberry tongue and palatal enanthem of streptococcal scarlet fever. Evidence based on toxin production now suggests that staphylococcal scarlet fever often represents an abortive form of toxic shock syndrome.
  - Classic staphylococcal scalded skin syndrome (SSSS): Characterized by abrupt onset of fever, irritability, and diffuse, blanchable erythema in association with marked skin tenderness in which toxin circulates throughout the body, causing blisters at and distant to the site of infection
- Pitfalls
  - Differentiation from streptococcal disease with need for penicillinase-resistant antibiotic therapy (e.g., nafcillin)
  - A methicillin-resistant strain of *S. aureus* has been reported to cause SSSS.
  - Adhesive occlusive dressings used to apply topical local anesthetic prior to venipuncture have been shown to cause injury and discomfort in areas previously free of blistering in patients with SSSS.
  - Diagnosis should be made clinically and should not be delayed several days while waiting for the results of cultures or other diagnostic tests, that are largely confirmatory.

GENERAL PREVENTION

- Eradication of staphylococci to prevent recurrences after first attack
- Preventing skin from becoming overly moist or macerated
- Scrupulous care in performance of even minimally invasive health promotion measures such as vitamin K prophylaxis and metabolic screening can reduce neonatal cases.
- Isolation of hospitalized patient
  - Suspected or documented cases should be placed in contact isolation.

EPIDEMIOLOGY

- The vast majority of cases occur in neonates or even in the intrauterine environment (as in Ritter disease) and children <5 years of age.
- Antibodies to exfoliative (epidermolytic) toxin A (ETA) (see below) have been found in 88% of cord blood samples and are absent in acute sera of patients with SSSS.
- Most cases are caused by type 71 (75% of cases) or type 70, with occasional cases due to types 3A, 3B, 3C, and 55.
- Large screening experiments reveal toxin-producing strains in 5–6% of individuals.
- Occurs rarely in adults, due to increased circulating antibodies and adult kidney excretion of the toxin
- Occurs most frequently in adults in association with immunosuppression or renal impairment

Incidence

No differences in incidence based on gender or socioeconomic status

PATHOPHYSIOLOGY

- The soluble exotoxins referred to as exfoliative (epidermolytic) toxin A or B (ETA or ETB), produced by certain strains of *S. aureus* and usually belonging to phage group II in the United States, are responsible for SSSS.
  - The exotoxins are glutamate-specific trypsin-like serine proteases. The active site of the exfoliative toxins appears to be conformationally blocked in its native state. The target for the toxins has been identified as desmoglein-1, a desmosomal glycoprotein that plays an important role in maintaining cell-to-cell adhesion in the superficial epidermis. It is speculated that binding of the exfoliative toxin's active site to desmoglein-1 results in a conformational change than opens the active site of the toxin to cleave the extracellular domain of desmoglein-1, resulting in disruption of intercellular adhesion and formation of superficial blisters.
- Generalized desquamation with early intra-epidermal bullae demonstrating a cleavage plane just beneath the granular cell layer
- Nikolsky sign develops within 12 hours to 3 days, accompanied by flaccid thin-walled bullae. Bullae rupture spontaneously within hours, separating the superficial epidermis into large sheets revealing moist red surfaces resembling burns. 1–3 days later, the denuded areas dry and the entire body surface undergoes a secondary flaky desquamation. The entire skin heals within 10–14 days.

 DIAGNOSIS

- Pitfall: Confusion with toxic epidermal necrolysis (TEN) may lead to possible use of corticosteroids or simple discontinuation of antibiotics, resulting in enhanced infection from prolonged toxin production.

HISTORY

- Nonspecific virus-like prodrome with irritability is the typical presentation of SSSS.
- Rash typically begins perorally, then extends to the trunk and extremities and finally desquamates.
- Recent, seemingly trivial, localized extracutaneous infection
  - Infections involving the nasopharynx, middle ear, conjunctivae, pharynx, tonsils, umbilicus, or urinary tract are frequently recalled.
- Recent medication use: A history of recent drug use suggests TEN.

PHYSICAL EXAM

- Erythroderma: Usually extremely painful
- Fever: Usually abrupt onset after prodrome
- Large flaccid bullae that leave behind denuded skin resembling a burn after rupturing; bullae often appear in areas of trauma, or in areas that are rubbed or touched, including intertriginous zones.
- Distribution of lesions: Usually involve perineal, periumbilical, and intertriginous areas of the neonate; in older children, the extremities are usually involved.
- Crusting seen in a radial pattern (sunburst) around the mouth, nose, and eyes; occurs without mucous membrane involvement
- Sandpaper texture of rash and increased erythema or petechiae in skin creases; Pastia lines are seen in the scarlatiniform variant.
- Nikolsky sign: Gentle friction applied obliquely to apparently healthy skin will cause wrinkling, then sloughing.

DIAGNOSTIC TESTS & INTERPRETATION
Lab

- Skin biopsy: Used to differentiate SSSS from TEN; the cornified skin layer is recovered in SSSS, whereas the entire necrotic epidermis should be recognized in TEN.
- Excision of some exfoliated skin for frozen or permanent histologic section; easier to obtain than a biopsy; often useful in arriving at the diagnosis

DIFFERENTIAL DIAGNOSIS
- Toxic epidermal necrolysis (TEN)
- Kawasaki disease
- Erythema multiforme bullosum
- Erythema multiforme major (Stevens-Johnson syndrome)
- Streptococcal or staphylococcal toxic shock syndrome (TSS)
- Bullous varicella
- Burns, including inflicted burns in suspected child abuse
- Primary bullous disorders (e.g., bullous mastocytosis)
- Chronic bullous disease of childhood
- Pemphigus vulgaris or foliaceus
- Epidermolysis bullosa

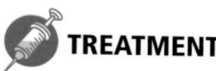 TREATMENT

General Measures
- Apply principles of good burn care in severe cases, including:
  - Cases affecting large areas of skin should be managed in a critical care setting.
  - Fluid and electrolyte management should include daily maintenance requirements as well as replacement of "third-space" fluid loss based on the percentage of affected body surface area (BSA). Fluid should be replaced as an isotonic solution calculated at 3 mL/kg of affected BSA. Most experts recommend replacement of one half of losses over the first 8 hours and the other half over the next 16 hours.
  - Children should be allowed to rest unclothed on sterilized linens, and handling of the child should be kept to a minimum. Wound care should focus on maintenance of developing eschars. This is usually followed by débridement, and affected areas are eventually dressed with silver sulfadiazine or a similar agent.
  - FDA-approved absorbable, synthetic wound dressing with properties of natural epithelium appear to reduce pain, accelerate epithelialization and reduce nursing time in SSSS.

MEDICATION (DRUGS)
- Antistaphylococcal agents: Parenteral antibiotic therapy (e.g., nafcillin, oxacillin, cephalosporins, clindamycin) should be used for extensive skin involvement or serious systemic disease. Oral therapy (e.g., dicloxacillin, cloxacillin, amoxicillin/clavulanate, cephalexin, clindamycin) is generally sufficient for bullous impetigo. Duration of therapy is typically 7–10 days. Topical preparations are of no benefit.
- Corticosteroids have been shown to be detrimental both in experimental animal models as well as clinical trials.

 ONGOING CARE

PROGNOSIS
- Exfoliated areas eventually dry with a flaky desquamation within 3–5 days of initiating appropriate antibiotic therapy.
- Usually, complete recovery within 10–14 days without scarring
- Prognosis is more guarded in infants and those with underlying illness.
- Mortality reported as 1–10% in neonates and 3% in children but as high as 60% in adults with underlying disease

COMPLICATIONS
- Occasional shedding of hair and nails
- Fungal or bacterial superinfection following desquamation
- Serious fluid and electrolyte disturbances in cases involving large surface areas, which may lead to poor temperature control, hypovolemia, sepsis syndrome, and death. Neonates are particularly susceptible.

PATIENT MONITORING
Patients may be followed via telephone as long as lesions are healing well and parents do not report significant complications.

ADDITIONAL READING
- Anbu AT, Williams S. Miliaria crystallina complicating Staphylococcal scalded skin syndrome. *Arch Dis Child*. 2004;89:94.
- D Eichenfield, LA. Images in clinical medicine. Staphylococcal scalded skin syndrome. *N Engl J Med*. 2000;342:1178.
- Kress DW. Pediatric dermatology emergencies. *Curr Opin Pediatr*. 2011 Jun 8.
- Patel NN, Patel DN. Staphylococcal scalded skin syndrome. *Am J Med*. 2010;123(6):505–507.
- Stanley JR, Amagai M. Pemphigus, bullous impetigo, and the Staphylococcal Scalded-Skin Syndrome. *N Engl J Med*. 2006;355:1800–1810.

 CODES

ICD9
- 695.81 Ritter's disease

ICD10
- L00 Staphylococcal scalded skin syndrome

FAQ
- Q: Can SSSS recur?
- A: Yes
- Q: Is SSSS contagious?
- A: Yes, the staphylococci are spread primarily from person to person (familial clusters have been reported), even from mother to fetus, most efficiently by someone with lesions, but asymptomatic carriers may also spread infection. Spread of organisms does not necessarily lead to signs of toxin production in those acquiring infection.
- Q: How can one distinguish TEN from SSSS?
- A: TEN is frequently confused with SSSS and may be differentiated by skin biopsy showing cleavage plane at the dermal–epidermal junction. TEN or Lyell disease is more common in adults and is usually secondary to drug hypersensitivity (e.g., sulfonamides, barbiturates, pyrazolone derivatives).
- Q: Can staphylococcus be isolated from the bullae?
- A: SSSS bullae are sterile, although organisms may be found in a distant focus, such as the nares or conjunctivae. In bullous impetigo, however, staphylococci may be isolated from the bullae.

S

STATUS EPILEPTICUS

Juliann Paolicchi
Eric Marsh (5th edition)
Amy R. Brooks-Kayal (5th edition)
Keith Nagle (5th edition)

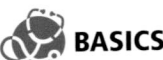 **BASICS**

DESCRIPTION
- Status epilepticus (SE) is defined as >30 minutes of continuous seizure activity or sequential seizures in 30 minutes without full recovery of consciousness. In practice, convulsive seizures >5 minutes in duration are treated as presumptive SE, since it is uncommon for convulsive seizures to continue >5 minutes and more likely to continue into SE.
- SE presents in several forms:
  - Generalized SE: Continuous or repeated generalized convulsion(s) with persistent loss of consciousness and neurologic function
  - Nonconvulsive SE or absence SE: Persistent encephalopathy, often with variable subtle motor signs such as myoclonus or nystagmus
  - Repeated partial seizures with an alteration of consciousness (focal status epilepticus) or preserved consciousness (epilepsia partialis continua)
  - SE is also classified by etiology:
    ○ Acute symptomatic (26%)
    ○ Remote symptomatic (33%) prior history of CNS disease
    ○ Progressive encephalopathy (underlying, progressive CNS disorder)
    ○ Febrile (22%)
    ○ Cryptogenic (15%)

ALERT
- The most common etiology for SE in children with epilepsy is low antiepileptic medication (AED) levels. Check levels on any patient on AED treatment.
- Neuromuscular blockers used in intubation may obscure ongoing seizures. EEG monitoring is mandatory for all patients who have had pharmacologic paralysis for airway control during SE.
- Continued encephalopathy after convulsions have ended may indicate continued electrographic seizures (non-convulsive SE)
- Nonepileptic SE (psychogenic) is often mistaken for SE. EEG establishes the diagnosis.
- Rhabdomyolysis may complicate SE. Hydration should be maintained, and creatine kinase levels can be followed.

GENERAL PREVENTION
- Need for long-term antiepileptic drug (AED) therapy after SE depends on the etiology, patient's age, and circumstances in which SE occurred.
  - Chronic AED therapy is indicated when SE is caused by structural brain lesions or in patients with known epilepsy.
  - Chronic AED therapy is generally not needed in children who have SE from transient metabolic disturbances (e.g., hyponatremia, intoxication, fever), or in idiopathic SE as a first seizure.

- Educate family members regarding first aid for seizures. Discuss potential risks of seizure recurrence even if the child is taking an AED. Review risks of climbing, swimming, bathing, and not having head protection for wheeled toys (bikes, skateboards, scooters).
- Provide caregivers with rectal diazepam with instructions for its use for seizure >5 minutes in duration.
- Neurology consultation is recommended.

EPIDEMIOLOGY
Incidence
- Incidence in the pediatric population is 17–23/100,000. In children <1 year old, incidence is 135–156/100,000.

RISK FACTORS
- History of epilepsy most common (10–20% of children with epilepsy have had SE) with AED withdrawal the most common cause
- Other: Brain tumor, neurodegenerative disorder, history of remote neurologic insult (stroke, intracranial hemorrhage, birth asphyxia, head trauma, meningitis) or condition (cerebral palsy)

Genetics
Some inherited conditions increase risk of SE, including neurocutaneous syndromes (tuberous sclerosis, Sturge–Weber) and familial epilepsy syndromes, especially GEFS+. There is evidence for a genetic predisposition to SE.

PATHOPHYSIOLOGY
SE can be due to acute and chronic factors.
- Most common inciting acute factors are fever, metabolic derangements (e.g., electrolyte imbalances, renal failure), intoxications, trauma, neoplasm, anoxia and stroke/hemorrhage, discontinuation of seizure medications.
- Chronic causes include pre-existing epilepsy, neurodegenerative disorders, brain tumors, and neurocutaneous syndromes (tuberous sclerosis, Sturge–Weber), familial epilepsy syndromes (GEFS+).

DIAGNOSIS

HISTORY
- Ask about prior seizures, treatment with AEDs, and other neurological abnormality.
- Ask specifically about precipitating factors: Fever, preceding illness, head trauma, change in antiepileptic medication, and family history of seizures.

PHYSICAL EXAM
- Vital signs: Fever, respiratory rate/O_2 sats (adequacy of air exchange and abnormal breathing patterns), heart rate, BP (hypertension suggests intracranial hypertension)
- Signs of head trauma: Retinal hemorrhages, excess bruising, bone fractures, evidence of intracranial hypertension such as bulging fontanelle

- Meningismus signals CNS infection, intracranial hemorrhage or spine trauma. May be absent in young infants with meningitis
- Signs of systemic infection: Fever (also potentiates seizure activity), petechiae, mucosal lesions, lymphadenopathy
- Skin examination: Check for neurocutaneous disorders.
- During convulsions: Observe for focal features or asymmetry.
- Postictal exam: Transient neurologic abnormalities (e.g., pupillary asymmetries, eye deviation, and focal motor weakness [Todd paresis]) may not correlate with the underlying structural lesion. After seizure has stopped, a neurological examination should be performed, with attention to mental status, focal weakness, tone, or sensation.

DIAGNOSTIC TESTS & INTERPRETATION
Lab
- Initial:
  - STAT glucose, electrolytes, calcium, magnesium, and arterial blood gas
  - AED levels if indicated
  - CBC, liver function tests
  - Toxicology screen, urinalysis
  - TESTS:
  - LP: Indicated to evaluate CNS infection. Contraindications include intracranial hypertension known or suspected from exam or CT scan; cerebral mass lesion; obstructive hydrocephalus. Lumbar puncture may be deferred if suspicion of CNS infection is low, i.e., patient is afebrile, and an alternate etiology is present.
  - Neuroimaging, CT or MRI: Indicated for SE, especially with partial-onset seizures (including aura), focally abnormal EEG, focal neurological signs, or history of head trauma. MRI is the preferred neuroimaging test, but CT may be more appropriate for urgent imaging or if the patient is medically unstable.
  - EEG: Recommended to determine focal versus generalized abnormalities and continued electrographic seizures. Urgent EEG recommended in patients with persistent SE or encephalopathy, and in those with concern for nonconvulsive SE and nonepileptic SE.

DIFFERENTIAL DIAGNOSIS
- Nonepileptic SE (psychogenic or pseudo SE). Clinically suspected with eye closure; asynchronous, thrashing limb movements; purposeful resistance to passive movement; and normal concurrent EEG. Induction of a seizure by suggestion further supports this diagnosis.
- Movement disorders (including dystonia, chorea, and very frequent tics) can be mistaken for persistent seizure activity.
- Postanoxic myoclonus: Status after prolonged cardiopulmonary arrest. These movements are usually nonrhythmic and segmental but can appear rhythmic at times. EEG is recommended for diagnosis.

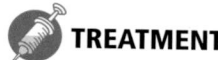

TREATMENT

INITIAL STABILIZATION

- ABCs (stabilization of airway, supporting respiration, maintaining BP, and gaining intravascular access)
- BP, EKG, and respiratory function should be monitored.
- Airway control may be maintained by head positioning, and oral airway placement and oxygen supplementation provided via nasal cannula, mask, or bag–valve–mask ventilation. If the need for respiratory assistance persists, endotracheal intubation may be required.
- For hypoglycemia: 2–4 mL/kg of D25 (25% dextrose)
- Rectal acetaminophen and a cooling blanket for fever

General Measures

- AED administration should be initiated whenever seizure activity persists for >5 minutes
- Benzodiazepines are initial management of patients with active convulsions.

Lorazepam IV (0.05–0.1 mg/kg/dose at 2 mg/min maximum, up to a total dose of 0.3–0.5 mg/kg) more effective and with less respiratory depression than diazepam (0.1–0.2 mg/kg/dose at 5 mg/min, up to a total dose of 1.0 mg/kg, not to exceed a total dose of 10 mg).

Midazolam (0.1–0.3 mg/kg IV followed by infusion if needed of 1 mcg/kg/min)

Respiratory depression and hypotension are common side effects of benzodiazepine administration.

- SE persists: Administer an IV loading dose fosphenytoin (20 mg/kg "phenytoin equivalents" at a rate of 3 mg/kg/min, max rate 150 mg/min, max daily dose, 1500 mgPE). Additional 5-mg/kg doses may be given if needed to stop convulsions (to maximum total dose of 30 mgPE/kg)
- Alternative treatment choices:
- IV phenobarbital at a loading dose of 20 mg/kg (maximum rate, 50 mg/min). Additional 5–10-mg/kg increments (to total maximum dose of 30–40 mg/kg) may be given as necessary to stop convulsions. Respiratory depression and hypotension are potential serious side effects.
- IV valproate at a loading dose of 20–40 mg/kg (over 5–10 minutes) May be followed by infusion if needed of 5 mg/kg/hr or repeated doses up to 60 mg/kg/dat divided 2–4 times a day. Monitoring to keep total valproate levels between 50 and 100 mg/L is recommended. Thrombocytopenia, pancreatitis, hepatitis, and skin rashes are potential side effects. IV valproate should be changed to a PO formulation before 14 days.

- If IV access is difficult to obtain, diazepam (0.5 mg/kg to a maximum of 20 mg), IM fosphenytoin, or buccal midazolam can be administered.
- Refractory SE exists if the above medications fail and the patient continues to have convulsions or is in nonconvulsive SE.
- Alternative agents for this situation include the use of IV AEDS, i.e., valproate, levetiracetam, and/or the induction of pharmacologic coma with midazolam, pentobarbital, phenobarbital, or propofol or inhalational anesthetics (isoflurane) administered in an intensive care unit with neurologic consultation. EEG monitoring is required, with the goal of inducing a suppression-burst pattern for the first 24 hours.

ONGOING CARE

PROGNOSIS

The morbidity and mortality of SE reflect etiology and are lower in children than in adults. Recent mortality estimates in children range from 2–5% with risk of new neurological sequelae estimated at 15%, and subsequent epilepsy at 30%. Refractory status epilepticus, however, has a morbidity estimated at 32%, and a mortality of 17%.

ADDITIONAL READING

- Abend NS, Dlugos DJ. Treatment of refractory status epilepticus: Literature review and a proposed protocol. *Pediatr Neurol.* 2008;38(6):377–390.
- Appleton R, Macleod S, Martland T. Drug management for acute tonic-clonic convulsions including convulsive status epilepticus in children. *Cochrane Database Syst Rev.* 2008;(3):CD001905.
- Chin RD, Neville BG, Peckham C, et al. Treatment of community-onset, childhood convulsive status epilepticus: A prospective, population-based study. *Lancet Neurol.* 2008;7:696.
- Raspall-Chaure M, Chin RF, Neville BG, et al. The epidemiology of convulsive status epilepticus in children: A critical review. *Epilepsia.* 2007;48:1652.
- Riviello JJ, Ashwal S, Hirtz D, et al. Practice parameter: Diagnostic assessment of the child with status epilepticus (an evidence-based review). *Neurology.* 2006;67:1542–1550.

- Singh RK, Stephens S, Berl MM, et al. Prospective study of new-onset seizures presenting as status epilepticus in childhood. *Neurology.* 2010;74:636.
- Sofou K, Kristjansdottir R, Papachatzakis NE, et al. Management of prolonged seizures and status epilepticus in childhood: A systematic review. *J Child Neurol.* 2009;24:918–926.

CODES

ICD9
345.3 Grand mal status

ICD10
G40.901 Epilepsy, unsp, not intractable, with status epilepticus

FAQ

- Q: Does SE cause brain injury?
- A: Research suggests that neuronal loss may occur at 30 minutes of SE. This illness represents a neurologic emergency. Other determinants of outcome are hypoxic brain injury due to hypoventilation during a seizure and brain injury because of an identifiable underlying cause of SE, such as encephalitis. Outcome in children with idiopathic SE without hypoxia is usually very good. Outcome of SE due to other brain injury (e.g., hypoxia, encephalitis, trauma) depends on the severity of the inciting process.
- Q: How safe is administration of rectal diazepam for children with cluster seizures?
- A: Studies suggest that when dosing guidelines are followed, this agent is safe and effective in terminating clusters of seizures, obviating a trip to the emergency room.
- Q: How likely is SE likely to recur?
- A: It is estimated at 17% in the first year, and predominantly in children with other neurologic conditions.

S

STEVENS-JOHNSON SYNDROME AND TOXIC EPIDERMAL NECROLYSIS

Alexis Weymann
James R. Treat
Paul S. Matz (5th edition)

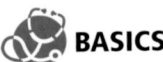 **BASICS**

DESCRIPTION

Stevens–Johnson syndrome (SJS) and toxic epidermal necrolysis (TEN) are severe, potentially fatal mucocutaneous drug reactions, characterized by epidermal necrosis involving skin and at least 2 mucous membranes. The cutaneous necrosis leads to widespread epidermal detachment and loss of skin barrier function. Given the potential risk for infection and fluid and electrolyte imbalances with widespread denudation, SJS and TEN are considered medical emergencies.

EPIDEMIOLOGY
Incidence
- Overall annual risk of 0.5–1.9 per million in the general population
- The precise incidence in children is unknown.
- Patients with HIV have a 1,000-fold increased risk.

RISK FACTORS
- Exposure to inciting medications
- Infection with *Mycoplasma pneumoniae*, HIV
- Genetic background
- Coexistence of cancer
- Concomitant radiotherapy

Genetics
- Recently, strong associations have been made between HLA alleles and SJS/TEN.
- HLA-B*1502 (most commonly found in Han Chinese and Thai populations) has been linked to significantly increased risk of carbamazepine- and phenytoin-related SJS/TEN.
- HLA-B*5801 has been associated with allopurinol-related SJS/TEN in Han, Thai, and Japanese populations.

GENERAL PREVENTION
- The FDA recommends checking for HLA-B*1502 in Asian populations where this HLA subtype is highly prevalent before prescribing carbamazepine.
- Once SJS/TEN has occurred, the inciting medication and any cross-reacting medications should be avoided.

PATHOPHYSIOLOGY
- Widespread keratinocyte and mucosal cell death occurs secondary to CD8+ T-cell mediated apoptosis via Fas and Fas Ligand pathways and/or direct granulysin secretion. Fas receptors are located on keratinocytes and when activated with Fas Ligand, induce apoptosis and therefore necrosis of epidermal cells. Granulysin is released from cytotoxic T cells and induces apoptosis by creating holes in target cell membranes.
- The exact mechanism by which the implicated drug or infection triggers activation of cytotoxic T cells and the upregulation of the Fas/FasL pathway is unknown.
- Soluble Fas Ligand is increased in patients with SJS/TEN.

- IVIG theoretically acts to block the Fas–FasL ligand connection, thereby interrupting keratinocyte death and epidermal necrosis. Trials that show a benefit of IVIG use, demonstrate improvement of disease severity but not complete abolition of symptoms; this may be due to IVIG being started too late in the disease progression or because there may be an alternative pathway to keratinocyte destruction as well.

ETIOLOGY
- Over 100 medications have been implicated in causing SJS/TEN. High-risk drugs include: Aromatic amine anticonvulsants such as carbamazepine, phenobarbital and phenytoin, lamotrigine, beta-lactam antibiotics, sulfa medications (including trimethoprim-sulfamethoxazole and sulfasalazine), minocycline, cephalosporins, quinolones, NSAIDs in the oxicam class, allopurinol, and nevirapine.
- A greater risk of developing SJS/TEN is seen in the first 8 weeks of treatment with these medications with the highest risk being 1–3 weeks after exposure.
- *M. pneumoniae* is a well-established non-drug cause of SJS/TEN and is more commonly implicated in children and adolescents.
- There is scant evidence that vaccines, neoplastic syndromes, and autoimmune disease such as systemic lupus erythematosus (SLE) may play a role in etiology.
- <5% of cases have no known cause.
- Herpes simplex virus-associated erythema multiforme (EM) was historically categorized on the spectrum with SJS and TEN, but new classification schemes place EM as a separate entity.

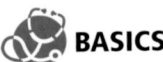 **DIAGNOSIS**

HISTORY
- Prodromal period of 1–7 days of low-grade fever, sore throat or upper respiratory infection or dysphagia, and general malaise; patient may also complain of pain or stinging in the eyes.
- Subsequent development of targetoid red papules and plaques with dusky, blistered or eroded center as well as mucosal (lip, intraoral, conjunctival, urethral, anal) pain with blistering and erosions
- Recent initiation of high-risk agent (see above list) or upper respiratory symptoms such as chronic cough indicative of mycoplasma infection

PHYSICAL EXAM
- Acute phase: Early skin lesions are flat, erythematous targetoid lesions with a dusky center that usually start on the face, pre-sternal area of chest, and palms and soles. >90% of patients also have ocular and/or genital mucosa involvement consisting of erythema and erosions as well as hemorrhaging, crusting, and blisters. The skin and mucosal lesions are very tender. Intraoral lesions may precede the cutaneous rash.

- Ocular involvement at the onset of disease is common. Early ocular disease ranges from acute conjunctivitis, eyelid edema, and ocular discharge to pseudomembrane formation and corneal erosion.
- Secondary phase: As the lesions progress over hours to days, they necrose, blister, and slough off, causing large areas of epidermal detachment. Lesions are characterized by a positive Nikolsky sign (epidermal detachment upon mechanical stress).
- Extensive mucosal involvement may also include the esophagus, distal regions of the GI tract, and the respiratory epithelium.
- Occasionally mycoplasma-induced SJS can only involve the mucosal surfaces with little or no cutaneous involvement.

DIAGNOSTIC TESTS & INTERPRETATION
Lab
Initial lab tests
- CBC with differential, metabolic panel, hepatic function test, coagulation studies, urinalysis, mycoplasma serology or PCR if indicated
- Anemia and lymphocytopenia are common and indicate a poor prognosis.

Imaging
- Chest x-ray and abdominal x-ray may be indicated depending on the extent of mucosal and systemic involvement.

Clinical Diagnosis
- The diagnosis of SJS and TEN is largely clinical, based on history and physical exam.
- By definition, <10% affected body surface area (BSA) is SJS; 10–30% affected BSA is SJS/TEN overlap; >30% affected BSA is TEN.

Diagnostic Procedures
- Skin biopsy with cryosection should be performed to confirm the clinical diagnosis if in doubt.
- Histological examination with direct immunofluorescence (DIF) should be performed to rule out other autoimmune blistering diseases such as paraneoplastic pemphigus if in doubt.

Pathological and Diagnostic Findings
- Skin biopsy shows full-thickness epidermal necrosis and few inflammatory cells; the skin biopsy in TEN may additionally show skin lysis at the subepidermal level.
- DIF shows no immunoglobulin or complement deposition in the epidermis or in the epidermal-dermal zone.

DIFFERENTIAL DIAGNOSIS

- Staphylococcal-scalded skin syndrome (SSSS)
- Linear IgA dermatosis
- Pemphigus—paraneoplastic pemphigus, pemphigus vulgaris, and bullous pemphigus
- Acute generalized exanthematous pustulosis
- Disseminated fixed bullous drug eruption
- Drug-induced hypersensitivity syndrome
- Drug reaction with eosinophilia and systemic symptoms (DRESS)

 TREATMENT

MEDICATION (DRUGS)

First Line

- Stop all potentially offending medications.
- Early admission to burns unit or pediatric intensive care unit (PICU) for initial stabilization and management of fluid, electrolytes, and nutritional requirements, airway stability, and eye care
- Early ophthalmology and dermatology consultations
- Meticulous wound care with bland emollients; avoid silver sulfadiazine as it may cause SJS due to its sulfa moiety. Topical antibiotics should be used in areas of superinfection. The prophylactic use of topical antibiotics is somewhat controversial. Most agree that they should be applied to areas with a higher risk of superinfection, such as the perioral, periocular, and intertriginous areas.

Medications/Therapeutics

- 0.5–1 gram/kg per dose given for 2–4 days for total of 2–3 grams/kg total
- There have been variable results from a limited number of quality studies looking at the effects of IVIG. Most studies, however, have demonstrated a beneficial effect especially if started early in the course, and so early administration of high-dose IVIG is recommended.
- Adverse effects of IVIG include acute renal failure, DIC, osmotic nephrosis, anaphylaxis, serum sickness, aseptic meningitis, PE, and DVT, among others.
- Steroids (prednisolone, dexamethasone, methylprednisolone) were the mainstay of therapy in the 1990s but now are less commonly used because of the increased risk of sepsis, infection, and other complications when used especially in TEN when there is widespread epidermal loss. Pulse steroid use is being investigated.
- Thalidomide, cyclosporine, TNF antagonists, plasmapheresis, and cyclophosphamide are other therapeutics that have been studied in the treatment of SJS/TEN but none have sufficient amounts of reliable data to support their use.
- Prophylactic systemic antibiotics are not recommended, as they place the patient at an increased risk of candidemia and resistant infections.

ADDITIONAL TREATMENT

- Pain control is key to patient comfort.
- Good oral care using agents such as "magic mouthwash" helps debride dead skin and provide oral anesthesia.

SURGERY/OTHER PROCEDURES

- +/– Surgical debridement: Studies have shown surgical debridement of wounds prior to wound care yielded no additional benefit.
- +/– Synechial and vaginal adhesion breakup

Discharge Criteria

- When afebrile, the loss of skin is clearly done and re-epithelialization has occurred; cleavage of synechiae in the eyes is no longer needed and the patient can eat and drink appropriately.

 ONGOING CARE

FOLLOW-UP RECOMMENDATIONS

- Follow up with a dermatologist and/or wound care specialist. Re-epithelialization often starts within days and may take up to 3 weeks to be completed.

Patient Monitoring

- SCORTEN is a well-validated, widely used scoring system in adults used for its predictive value, which is best at day 3. Variables include age, percentage BSA affected, BUN, serum glucose, HR, serum bicarbonate, associated malignancy.
- Monitor for skin, urinary tract, and pulmonary infections, synechiae in the eyes as well as vaginal and urethral adhesions.

PROGNOSIS

- Mortality is 1–5% in SJS; 25–35% in TEN.
- Largely depends on amount of BSA affected, time to cessation of offending medication, and time to initiation of supportive care
- More severe disease often seen in elderly patients
- Children have lower mortality and faster re-epithelialization.

COMPLICATIONS

- Mucosal complications occur in >70% of patients with acute phase mucosal involvement. Ocular complications occur in 50% of patients with TEN.
- Systemic—sepsis, multiorgan failure, major metabolic dysregulation
- Mucosal—respiratory failure, pneumonia, pulmonary embolus, UTI, GI hemorrhage, obstruction, and perforation
- Cutaneous—skin infections, scarring, hypo-/hyperpigmentation, nail dystrophies
- Ocular—synechiae, dry eyes, bacterial conjunctivitis, suppurative keratitis, endophthalmitis, impaired tear ducts, corneal ulcers, vision loss

ADDITIONAL READING

- Bastuji-Garin S, Razny B, Stern RS, et al. Clinical classification of cases of toxic epidermal necrolysis, Stevens–Johnson syndrome, and erythema multiforme. *Arch Dermatol*. 1993;129(1):92–96.
- Del Pozzo-Magana BR, Lazo-Langner A, Carleton B, et al. A systematic review of treatment of drug-induced Stevens–Johnson syndrome and toxic epidermal necrolysis in children. *J Popul Ther Clin Pharmacol*. 2011;18(1):e121–e133.
- Harr T, French L. Toxic epidermal necrolysis and Stevens–Johnson syndrome. *Orphanet J Rare Dis*. 2010;5:39.
- Momin S, Del Rosso J. Review of intravenous immunoglobulin in the treatment of Stevens–Johnson syndrome and toxic epidermal necrolysis. *J Clin Aesth Dermatol*. 2009;2(2):51–58.
- Phillips E, Mallal S. Pharmacogenetics of drug hypersensitivity. *Pharmacogenomics*. 2010; 11(7):973–987.
- Treat J. Stevens–Johnson syndrome and toxic epidermal necrolysis. *Pediatr Ann*. 2010;39(10): 667–674.

 CODES

ICD9

- 695.13 Stevens-Johnson syndrome
- 695.15 Toxic epidermal necrolysis

ICD10

- L51.1 Stevens-Johnson syndrome
- L51.2 Toxic epidermal necrolysis [Lyell]

CLINICAL PEARLS

- The progression of disease from flat, targetoid lesions to sheets of widespread epidermal necrosis and sloughing may be hours. As such, SJS and TEN are true medical emergencies.
- The systemic severity of SJS and TEN is often underestimated based on the severity of skin disease.
- Ocular involvement is often early and severe.
- The key to therapy is cessation of the offending medication and supportive care, and in many areas IVIG has become first line therapy.

S

STOMATITIS

Lee R. Atkinson-McEvoy

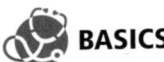 **BASICS**

DESCRIPTION
- Inflammation of the mucous membranes of the mouth
- Gingivostomatitis is when stomatitis is accompanied by inflammation of the gingiva.
- Recurrent aphthous stomatitis, known more commonly as canker sores, does not have an identified infectious agent.
- Herpangina is a disease caused by coxsackievirus group A and marked by stomatitis consisting of 1–2 mm oral vesicles and ulcers, and systemic symptoms, most notably fever.

EPIDEMIOLOGY
- Enteroviral infections occur commonly in summer and fall months.
- Recurrent aphthous stomatitis has a prevalence of 20–37% in children.
- Herpes simplex virus (HSV) type 1:
  - Up to 90% of the adult population has serologic evidence of previous infection.
- Age of child:
  - Herpangina and herpetic gingivostomatitis occur in infants, toddlers, and preschool-aged children.
  - Coxsackievirus (hand-foot-and-mouth disease) occurs most frequently in toddlers and young school-aged children.
  - Aphthous stomatitis occurs in older children and adults.

GENERAL PREVENTION
- Hand washing can prevent spread of viral infections.
- Due to the long life of enterovirus on surfaces, toys and other objects used by affected children should be sterilized before being used by other children.
- Contact isolation should be observed for children with viral stomatitis in the hospital setting.

PATHOPHYSIOLOGY
- Infection, inflammation, or trauma leads to interruption of the integrity of the mucosal epithelium.
- Ongoing inflammation leads to further denudation of the epithelium.
- Inflammatory cells and mediators can produce exudates and erythema of the ulceration.

ETIOLOGY
- Multiple etiologies, with viral infections (e.g., HSV type 1), and recurrent aphthous stomatitis being the most common in children
- Recurrent aphthous stomatitis is believed to be mediated by antibody-dependent cell-mediated cytotoxicity due to multifactorial insults, including trauma, stress, hormonal fluctuations, infections, vitamin or nutritional deficiencies, and allergens. There is also a familial tendency in 40% of cases.
- Herpangina is caused by coxsackievirus group A.
- Stomatitis:
  - Enterovirus, including coxsackievirus
  - HSV, particularly type 1

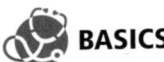 **DIAGNOSIS**

HISTORY
- Ask about associated symptoms:
  - Fever, malaise, diarrhea, and other constitutional symptoms occur with coxsackievirus infection, herpangina, and primary herpetic gingivostomatitis.
- Ask about chronic medical problems:
  - Immunodeficiency states (e.g., HIV and neutropenia), poor nutritional status, and inflammatory bowel disease are associated with development of mucosal ulceration.
- Ask about medications and possible exposures to medications:
  - Medications, particularly penicillins, sulfa-containing drugs, and antiepileptics, have been associated with Stevens–Johnson syndrome, which has oral mucositis as part of its constellation of symptoms.
- Signs and symptoms:
  - Inflammation
  - Pain in the mouth
  - Decreased intake
  - Drooling
  - Fever
  - Malaise
  - Diarrhea
  - Constitutional symptoms

PHYSICAL EXAM
- Recurrent aphthous stomatitis lesions are usually well demarcated, round to oval, and have a white-yellow fibrinous pseudomembranous cap with surrounding erythema.
- Enteroviral infections are associated with small shallow ulcerations with smooth borders on the posterior oral cavity structures such as the tonsils, soft palate, and pharynx. In addition, vesicular lesions may be present on the palms and soles.
- Hand-foot-and-mouth disease, due to coxsackievirus (a type of enterovirus), consists of lesions in the mouth as well as the palms and soles.
- Herpangina consists of oral vesicles and ulcers, typically around the fauces, near the tonsillar pillars.
- HSV infections cause shallow ulcers with irregular, erythematous borders that coalesce; these lesions are found on the lips, tongue, and gingiva.
- Gingivitis in association with stomatitis is usually present in drug-induced causes of stomatitis, as well as with HSV.
- Herpetic whitlow is the transmission of HSV with development of lesions on the extremities, notably the fingers, due to direct contact with lesions in the mouth.
- Varicella presents with grouped vesicles or erosions on the tongue, gingival and buccal mucosae, and the lips. The lesions are shallow ulcers with erythematous borders that usually do not coalesce. In addition, diffuse vesicles in varying stages of healing can be found on the skin, particularly the trunk and extremities. In severe cases, there may be lesions in the oral cavity, particularly on the soft palate.

- Smallpox may also present with small red spots on the tongue and in the oral mucosa following a prodromal period with fever. These spots then can become ulcerated. This is followed by the development of a diffuse erythematous rash that becomes papular over the entire body, including the palms and soles. The rash becomes pustular, then crusted.
- Stevens–Johnson syndrome presents with large irregular ulcers, which may occasionally be deep. There is occasionally a hemorrhagic component to these ulcers. Ulcers are also sometimes present on other mucosal surfaces. Target lesions, bullae, and urticarial lesions may also be present.
- Behçet syndrome and Reiter syndrome may have painless ulceration of the oral mucous membranes. Generally these oral lesions are accompanied by skin lesions and diffuse systemic symptoms.
- Oral lichen planus is a chronic inflammatory disease usually seen in adults, but can occur in children. It causes bilateral white striations, papules, or plaques on the buccal mucosae, tongue, and gingivae. Erythema, erosions, and blisters may or may not be present.
- Familial Mediterranean fever syndrome is an autosomal recessive disease that presents with painful febrile episodes. Associated with these episodes are recurrent oral aphthae.

DIAGNOSTIC TESTS & INTERPRETATION
Lab
- HSV can be diagnosed with direct fluorescent antibody staining, rapid enzyme immunoassay, or viral culture of the lesion.
- Enterovirus can be cultured from stool, nasopharyngeal, throat, CSF, and blood specimens.
- Polymerase chain reaction testing of CSF fluid can also diagnose an enteroviral infection.

Diagnostic Procedures/Other
Usually there is no need for laboratory testing for simple stomatitis. If there are other systemic signs of illness (e.g., diarrhea or arthritis), a more thorough workup for more severe illnesses such as Crohn disease, Reiter syndrome, or cyclic neutropenia should be done.

DIFFERENTIAL DIAGNOSIS
- Infection:
  - Enterovirus, including coxsackievirus
  - HSV
  - Varicella
  - Smallpox (variola)
  - Candidal infection
  - HIV-associated aphthous ulcers
- Hematologic:
  - Cyclic neutropenia
- Trauma
- Medications (e.g., chemotherapeutic agents)
- Miscellaneous:
  - Stevens–Johnson syndrome
  - Oral lichen planus
  - Reiter syndrome or disease (reactive arthritis, rash, conjunctivitis, urethritis, diarrhea, and stomatitis with painless erosive ulcers)
  - Behçet syndrome (associated with ulcerations of the oral and genital mucous membranes)
  - Crohn disease
  - PFAPA syndrome: Periodic fever, aphthous stomatitis, pharyngitis, and adenitis

TREATMENT

MEDICATION (DRUGS)

- Analgesics:
  - Acetaminophen or ibuprofen
  - Acetaminophen with codeine may be used in severe cases, when intake of fluids is greatly affected by pain. Codeine should be used cautiously, as it may cause constipation and CNS depression.
  - Viscous lidocaine 2% (but see "General Measures")
  - Silver nitrate in a single application for recurrent aphthous stomatitis has been shown to reduce the severity of pain without altering healing time.
  - Topical nonsteroidal anti-inflammatory agents or corticosteroids may be required for severe recurrent aphthous ulcers.
- Acyclovir may be given orally for HSV infections to decrease the length of infection, but in order to be effective it needs to be given within the first 48 hours of development of oral lesions. Acyclovir is usually more beneficial when used for household contacts who begin to exhibit symptoms, and when treatment can be initiated early. Topical acyclovir has not been shown to be effective.

ADDITIONAL TREATMENT
General Measures
Rinses:

- Salt-water rinses (normal saline or 1 tsp of table salt mixed with 16 oz of tepid water or 1 tsp of baking soda with 32 oz of water) q1–2h while ulcers are present may aid in reducing pain and shortening the duration of the ulceration.
- Magic mouthwash: Equal parts of diphenhydramine and Maalox™ or Kaopectate™. In severe cases, 2% viscous lidocaine can be added in an equal amount, but care must be taken to limit the application of lidocaine on ulcerated mucosa, as it may be absorbed and possibly result in arrhythmias. In addition, when applied to the posterior pharynx, lidocaine can decrease the gag reflex, increasing the risk of aspiration.
- Avoid certain foods that can trigger eruption of new lesions or prolong the course of the existing lesions. Acidic, hard, salty, or spicy foods should be avoided. In addition nuts, chocolate, citrus fruits, and carbonated beverages can worsen outbreaks.

 ONGOING CARE

FOLLOW-UP RECOMMENDATIONS
Patient Monitoring
Young children should be followed closely. If dehydration occurs due to poor oral intake, IV rehydration should be considered.

PROGNOSIS
- Most cases of stomatitis are mild and resolve within 1–2 weeks.
- HSV stomatitis is most severe during the initial infection; however, it tends to recur in response to stress or trauma, as the virus has a long latent period within the nerves of the face, particularly the trigeminal nerve.
- Recurrent aphthous stomatitis also recurs in response to stress or trauma.

COMPLICATIONS
- Infectious:
  - Cellulitis
  - Lymphadenitis
- Miscellaneous:
  - Dehydration, particularly in young children
  - Pain

ADDITIONAL READING

- Bruce AJ, Rogers RS. Acute oral ulcers. *Dermatol Clin*. 2003;21:1–15.
- Faden H. Management of primary herpetic gingivostomatitis in young children. *Pediatr Emerg Care*. 2006;22(4):268–269.
- Munoz-Corcuera M, Esparaza-Gomez G, Gonzalez-Moles MA, et al. Oral ulcers: Clinical aspects. A tool for dermatologists. Part I. Acute ulcers. *Clin Exp Dermatol*. 2009;34:289–294.
- Siegel MA. Strategies for management of commonly encountered oral mucosal disorders. *J Calif Dent Assoc*. 1999;27:210–227.
- Zunt SL. Recurrent aphthous stomatitis. *Dermatol Clin*. 2003;21:33–39.

CODES

ICD9
- 523.10 Chronic gingivitis, plaque induced
- 528.00 Stomatitis and mucositis, unspecified
- 528.2 Oral aphthae

ICD10
- B00.2 Herpesviral gingivostomatitis and pharyngotonsillitis
- K12.1 Other forms of stomatitis

FAQ

- Q: Is stomatitis contagious?
- A: Yes, this is a contagious infection. To avoid spreading the illness, careful hand washing should be done. In cases of suspected enteroviral infections, careful sterilization of toys and surfaces with which the affected child has contact should be done before use by unaffected children.
- Q: How can I get my child to take food and liquids if stomatitis is painful?
- A: The inability to stay hydrated is one of the complications of stomatitis. Children will not have their regular intake of solids due to mechanical effects of these on painful ulcers. Using regular analgesics, such as acetaminophen or ibuprofen, can help decrease pain. Topical administration of magic mouthwash (see "General Measures") before offering fluids may be helpful. Small amounts of nonacidic, cool liquids (and popsicles) frequently may be better tolerated than large amounts given all at once. If your child has decreased urine output or altered mental status, seek medical attention.
- Q: When should I take my child to seek medical care?
- A: Children with stomatitis are at high risk for dehydration if they have many lesions. If your child won't take even sips of liquids, has marked decreased urine output, or is lethargic and difficult to arouse, bring him in to be evaluated. If the lesions do not heal in 7–10 days, bring your child in to be evaluated.
- Q: When can my child return to school/day care?
- A: Young children with herpes or enteroviral stomatitis can infect others via oral secretions. In cases of young children who drool frequently or place toys in their mouths, there is a high risk for transmitting the illness. Children become less contagious when the lesions heal. In the case of varicella, children are contagious until all vesicles are crusted over.

S

STRABISMUS

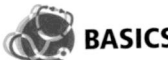

Monte D. Mills

BASICS

DESCRIPTION
- From the Greek *strabismos* (to squint), strabismus is abnormal misalignment of the eyes. The misalignment can be constant or intermittent, and the eyes can be misaligned in any direction.
- When the deviation between the eyes is constant in all gaze positions, the deviation is comitant.
  - Most childhood strabismus is comitant.
- Incomitant strabismus, with a variable angle depending on the direction of gaze, is seen with palsy of cranial nerve III, IV, or VI, and in some strabismus syndromes such as Duane and Brown syndromes and Graves ophthalmopathy.
- Patients with intermittent strabismus may benefit from treatment, even if the deviation is not present constantly.

EPIDEMIOLOGY
Most patients with idiopathic comitant strabismus are otherwise developmentally and neurologically normal.

Prevalence
Strabismus of all types has an overall prevalence of 4–5%.

RISK FACTORS
- Premature birth
- Cerebral palsy
- Seizure disorders
- Developmental delays
- Congenital or acquired loss of vision
- Other ocular abnormalities

Genetics
- ~30% of strabismus patients have affected family members.
- Inheritance appears to be multigenic.
- No specific genes have been associated with idiopathic childhood strabismus syndromes.
- Genetic causes have been identified for some rarer strabismus syndromes, including congenital fibrosis syndromes (chromosome 12p) and Kearn Sayer syndrome (mitochondrial deletion).

PATHOPHYSIOLOGY
- No specific pathologic abnormality of the motor nerves, extraocular muscles, or orbits is seen in most patients with idiopathic, comitant strabismus.
- Patients with paretic strabismus demonstrate atrophy of cranial nerves and extraocular muscles.
- Graves disease, myasthenia, and other neuromotor diseases that cause strabismus have specific pathologic features in the extraocular muscles.
- The pathophysiology of the most common forms of childhood strabismus is poorly understood. Infants with strabismus demonstrate subtle abnormalities in both motor function (asymmetric smooth pursuit movements) and binocular sensory function (suppression, anomalous retinal correspondence). No neuroanatomic abnormalities have been consistently demonstrated in infants with idiopathic strabismus.

- Accommodative esotropia, a common strabismus syndrome, is caused by abnormalities in the reflexive convergence that is necessary for looking at near objects.
  - If the ratio of accommodation (focusing for near) to convergence (rotating eyes inward to keep each eye on the target) is abnormally high, focusing on near targets leads to excessive convergence and esotropia.
- Less often, strabismus syndromes are caused by anatomic restriction to extraocular rotation (Graves disease, Brown syndrome), congenital or acquired paresis, or palsy of extraocular muscles (III, IV, or VI palsy, Duane syndrome, Moebius syndrome) or abnormalities of vision (sensory strabismus).

COMMONLY ASSOCIATED CONDITIONS
- Strabismus can be a sign of more significant ocular or neurologic abnormality. Retinoblastoma, retinal detachment, brain tumor, and other treatable conditions may initially present with ocular misalignment.
- Frequent coincident ophthalmic diagnoses are amblyopia (30–60%), nystagmus (8–10%), and refractive error (30–50%).

DIAGNOSIS

- Patients rarely "grow out of" strabismus.
- Infants as young as 3 months of age can have careful examinations of eye movement and alignment.
- Delayed diagnosis may worsen prognosis.

SIGNS AND SYMPTOMS
- The strabismus is identified by the relative direction of the eyes. Esotropia is an inward deviation or crossing; exotropia is an outward deviation; hypertropia and hypotropia are deviations up and down.
- Strabismus is frequently recognized by parents and primary care practitioners, but amblyopia may be asymptomatic.

HISTORY
- Age of onset of deviation
- Frequency, duration, and direction of deviation
- Subjective vision problems or complaints
- History of eye or head trauma, premature birth, seizure disorder, neurologic abnormality, or other motor problems
- Previous use of glasses, patching, or other therapy
- Family history of strabismus, amblyopia, refractive error, or childhood vision problems

PHYSICAL EXAM
- Patients capable of recognition are tested with charts (letters, pictures, Es), younger patients are tested by the ability to fixate and hold visual fixation on targets (toys, lights) in each eye. It is very important to test each eye separately, in order to detect possible amblyopia and other causes of monocular vision loss (see Amblyopia). Patients capable of reading charts should have complete ophthalmic examination if they cannot recognize at least the 20/40-size target with each eye, or if there is a difference of >1 chart line between eyes.

- Ocular alignment:
  - Hirschberg test: With patient looking at a flashlight, observe the location of the reflection of the light on the corneal surface. Normally, the reflection should be centered in the pupil and symmetric. In strabismus, the reflection will be displaced laterally (esotropia) or medially (exotropia) in 1 eye.
  - Bruchner test: With a direct ophthalmoscope using the largest light, and the patient looking directly at the light, the light is shone into the patient's eyes. Normally, the pupils should be orange or red and the pupils should symmetrically fill with light. Asymmetric brightness or color between the 2 eyes or shadows in the pupil of either eye is abnormal and may indicate strabismus or other eye problems.
  - Cover test (alternate cover test): With the patient holding his or her visual attention on a single target, the eyes are alternately occluded to force the patient to switch fixation between eyes. Normally, switching fixation should not cause the eyes to move. Movement of the eyes with alternate occlusion signifies strabismus and merits complete evaluation.
- Ocular rotations:
  - Comitant strabismus will demonstrate a consistent angle of deviation in all gaze directions. Incomitant strabismus, including cranial nerve palsies, thyroid ophthalmopathy, and Duane and Brown syndromes, will be greater in one direction and smaller or absent in others. Ductions (movements of each eye) may be restricted in certain directions with incomitant strabismus.
- Complete ophthalmic examination, including evaluation of vision, alignment, ocular anatomy, and cycloplegic refraction, is indicated whenever there is suggestion or suspicion of strabismus or abnormal vision based on history, screening tests, or examination.

DIAGNOSTIC TESTS & INTERPRETATION
The diagnosis of strabismus is based on clinical examination, and no laboratory or radiologic tests are routinely necessary.

Lab
Serologic testing for antiacetylcholine receptor antibodies is a specific test for myasthenia gravis, a very rare cause of strabismus.

Imaging
Depending on the clinical situation, imaging studies of the orbits and brain may be helpful in evaluating cranial nerve palsies, suspected traumatic strabismus, and strabismus associated with neurologic disease.

DIFFERENTIAL DIAGNOSIS
- The differential diagnosis of abnormal eye movement in childhood includes palsy of cranial nerve III, IV, or VI, orbital fracture or craniofacial anomaly, systemic or localized motor abnormalities such as myasthenia gravis, orbital fibrosis syndrome, infantile botulism, and idiopathic orbital pseudotumor.
- The most common reason for mistaken referral of infants for esotropia is "pseudoesotropia," caused by wide epicanthal folds giving the false appearance of esotropia.
  - This can be easily recognized by the normal corneal light reflex (Hirschberg test) and normal cover test.
- Sensory strabismus, due to reduced vision in 1 or both eyes, can be comitant or incomitant and can be caused by any ocular, optic nerve, or central cause of vision loss.
  - Sensory deviations are most frequently exotropic, but may be in any direction.
- Special strabismus syndromes include Duane syndrome (congenital aberrant innervation of cranial nerve III), Moebius syndrome (congenital absence of cranial nerve VI and VII), Brown syndrome (congenital or acquired monocular elevation defect due to abnormality of the trochlea-superior oblique tendon complex), myasthenia gravis, and thyroid ophthalmopathy (Graves disease).

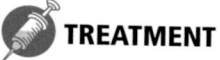 TREATMENT

ADDITIONAL TREATMENT
General Measures
- Prompt diagnosis and treatment are important for successful outcome from childhood strabismus.
- Depending on the diagnosis, treatment may include glasses, patching, orthoptic exercises, surgery, or a combination of these therapies.
- Glasses are useful, and may be curative, in certain forms of strabismus, especially accommodative esotropia.
  - With accommodative esotropia, glasses reduce or eliminate esotropia by reducing the need to focus the eyes to overcome hyperopia.
- Occlusive therapeutic patching is used to treat amblyopia.
  - In addition to the improved prognosis for long-term stability of surgical correction after amblyopia is treated, patching may sometimes improve alignment even without surgery. However, patching and other amblyopia treatments are usually only an adjunct to strabismus treatment.

- Eye excercises (orthoptic excercises) are useful in certain patients with convergence insufficiency, but are generally not effective in the common forms of childhood esotropia and exotropia.
  - Vision therapy (aside from orthoptic exercises noted earlier) is not effective for strabismus.

SURGERY/OTHER PROCEDURES
- Surgery is frequently necessary to realign the eyes to treat strabismus.
  - The ocular insertions of the extraocular muscles are shifted, either weakening or strengthening the muscle's effectiveness relative to the other muscles.
- In most patients, strabismus surgery can be performed in an ambulatory setting with minimal operative risk and postoperative morbidity.
- In large case series, ~20% of patients require >1 surgery for satisfactory alignment.

 ONGOING CARE

Visual acuity testing with each eye separately, and long-term follow-up until patients reach the age of visual maturity (~10 years) is important even after successful surgical correction.

ADDITIONAL READING
- Donahue SP. Clinical practice: Pediatric strabismus. *New Eng J Med*. 2007;356(10):1040–1047.

 CODES

ICD9
- 378.00 Esotropia, unspecified
- 378.9 Unspecified disorder of eye movements
- 378.10 Exotropia, unspecified

ICD10
- H50.00 Unspecified esotropia
- H50.9 Unspecified strabismus
- H50.10 Unspecified exotropia

FAQ
- Q: Does strabismus interfere with learning?
- A: No. Patients with normal vision and childhood strabismus should not necessarily have difficulty learning. Learning problems should not be blamed solely on strabismus.
- Q: Is "vision training therapy" an effective treatment for strabismus?
- A: Eye exercises are sometimes helpful in treating a limited number of patients with childhood strabismus. Orthoptic exercises have been effective in only certain specific conditions including convergence insufficiency, and are not effective in the majority of patients with more common types of esotropia and exotropia. There is very little practical or scientific evidence that vision training therapy as commonly practiced has value in patients with comitant childhood strabismus, except for treatment of amblyopia with patching or penalization (see "Amblyopia").
- Q: Does early surgical correction of strabismus improve the long-term outcome?
- A: Correction of esotropia prior to 2 years of age has been demonstrated to improve the chance of developing normal binocularity. However, not all patients develop binocularity even after early treatment. Many other factors influence the visual outcome in strabismus patients.
- Q: Is correction of strabismus in older children and adults just cosmetic?
- A: No. Older children and adults may have measurable visual improvement after treatment of strabismus, including expansion of visual fields and restoration of binocularity. In addition, the psychologic and social effects of disfiguring strabismus may justify corrective surgery even if no visual improvement is expected.
- Q: In patients with accommodative esotropia treated with glasses, will the glasses be necessary for the rest of the patient's life?
- A: Many patients wearing glasses for accommodative esotropia are able to stop wearing glasses later in childhood (age 12–14 years) without recurrence of esotropia.

STREP INFECTION: INVASIVE GROUP A β-HEMOLYTIC STREPTOCOCCUS

Avani Shah Mehta
Jill C. Posner

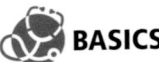 **BASICS**

DESCRIPTION

- Infection associated with isolation of group A β-hemolytic Streptococci (GABHS) from a normally sterile body site or from wound specimen in patient with necrotizing fasciitis (NF) or streptococcal toxic shock syndrome (STSS)
- Infection can result in a number of syndromes: Deep and systemic infections (e.g., bacteremia, endocarditis, meningitis, pneumonia, osteomyelitis, septic arthritis, surgical wound infection), NF, and STSS. Case definition for STSS includes the following:
- (I) Isolation of GABHS:
  - (A) From a normally sterile site (e.g., blood, CSF, tissue, peritoneal fluid)
  - (B) From a nonsterile site (e.g., throat, vagina, sputum)
- (II) Clinical signs of severity:
  - (A) Hypotension
  - (B) 2 or more of the following signs:
    - ○ Renal impairment
    - ○ Coagulopathy
    - ○ Hepatic involvement
    - ○ Adult respiratory distress syndrome
    - ○ A generalized erythematous macular rash that may desquamate
    - ○ Soft-tissue necrosis, including NF or myositis, or gangrene
- A definite case is an illness fulfilling criteria IA and II (A and B).
- A probable case is an illness fulfilling criteria IB and II (A and B) and no other identifiable cause.

EPIDEMIOLOGY

The rate of STSS and fatal cases of invasive GABHS appear to be lower in children as compared with adults.

Incidence

- During the mid-1980s and early 1990s, there was a notable increase in the incidence, morbidity, and mortality. However, these statistics have been stable since 1996.
- It is estimated that the annual incidence in the US is 3.5 cases per 100,000 persons, ~8,950–11,500 cases per year.
- In infants <1 year old, incidence is 5.3 cases per 100,000 persons.
- Increased incidence in winter/early spring

RISK FACTORS

- Prior to varicella vaccine, the most common antecedent in children was varicella.
- Several reports have suggested an association between the use of NSAIDs and invasive GABHS infection. There are no data to support a causal link.
- A recent case series (Jean 2010) reported an increased morbidity and mortality with coinfection of invasive GABHS and H1N1 influenza, even in previously healthy patients.
- Other high-risk groups include patients with diabetes mellitus, chronic cardiac or pulmonary disease, HIV infection or AIDS, and those with a history of IV drug use.

GENERAL PREVENTION

- Routine immunization against varicella
- Isolation of hospitalized patients: In addition to standard precautions, droplet precautions are recommended for children with pneumonia, and contact precautions should be used for children with extensive or draining cutaneous infections for at least 24 hours after the start of antimicrobial therapy.
- Multivalent GABHS vaccine (covering 26 serotypes) currently in phase 2 trial

PATHOPHYSIOLOGY

- The pathogenic mechanism has not been fully elucidated; however, an association with streptococcal pyrogenic exotoxin (SPE) has been suggested. These toxins, especially SPE A, B, and C, as well as mitogens and superantigens, stimulate large numbers of T cells to release a variety of cytokines, leading to capillary leak, hypotension, and organ damage.
- Portal of entry may be inapparent or unimpressive.
- Shock and multiorgan system failure may ensue.
- In NF, an area of cellulitis develops initially, followed by bullous skin changes and rapid progression of subcutaneous tissue necrosis involving fat and fascia. Skeletal muscle is rarely involved.

ETIOLOGY

Streptococcus pyogenes is the only species within this group of β-hemolytic Streptococci.

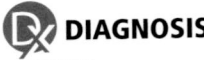 **DIAGNOSIS**

HISTORY

- Historic features vary depending on the GABHS syndrome.
- Consider GABHS infection in any child with varicella who has any of the following:
  - Return of fever after defervescence
  - A temperature of ≥39°C (102.7°F) beyond the 3rd day of illness
  - A fever persisting beyond the 4th day of illness
- In children without varicella, presentation can be nonspecific with fever, chills, myalgias, malaise, pain, and/or macular erythematous rash.
- Severe pain and hyperesthesia out of proportion to the clinical findings
- Portal of entry is unknown in 25–50% of cases.
- A preceding clinical pharyngitis is not common.
- Children <10 years old are less likely to present with cutaneous/soft-tissue infection, and are more likely to present with abscesses, osteomyelitis, epiglottitis, otitis media, meningitis, or primary bacteremia.
- Incubation period for STSS is unknown.

PHYSICAL EXAM

- Vital signs:
  - Elevated temperature
  - Tachycardia
  - Hypotension is a later sign.
- Toxic appearance is common but not the rule, especially early in the disease course.
- Skin exam varies:
  - In many instances, there are no cutaneous findings or, in cases of varicella, the lesions may not appear superinfected.
  - Alternatively, there may be an initial erythematous cellulitic area that rapidly progresses to a violaceous color with bullous formation.
  - A generalized macular erythematous rash is sometimes observed with STSS.
- Deep infections will have physical exam findings consistent with the specific focus (e.g., joint pain and limitation of mobility in septic arthritis, respiratory symptoms in GABHS pneumonia).

DIAGNOSTIC TESTS & INTERPRETATION

Lab

- CBC
- Electrolytes, BUN, creatinine (Cr), and glucose levels
- Liver function tests
- Screen for disseminated intravascular coagulation (DIC)
- Creatine kinase level: May be helpful in differentiating NF from cellulitis
- WBC count: Not elevated in all pediatric case series
- Blood culture: Positive for *S. pyogenes* in >50% of cases
- Culture of wound and tissue aspirates
- Throat culture: Positive in 50% of cases:
  - A rise in antibody titers to streptolysin O, deoxyribonuclease B, or other streptococcal extracellular products 4–6 weeks after infection may help confirm the diagnosis if culture results are negative. These antibodies may remain elevated for several months and indicate an infection in the recent past (not current).

Imaging

MRI: Defines the extent of involvement in NF

DIFFERENTIAL DIAGNOSIS

- Bacterial sepsis
- STSS
- Other soft-tissue infections:
  - Cellulitis
  - Erysipelas
  - Clostridial or mixed anaerobic and aerobic fasciitis/gangrene
- Diagnostic pitfalls include the following:
  - Not considering the diagnosis until hemodynamic instability is apparent
  - Do not exclude diagnosis even in the absence of rash, cellulitis, or superinfected varicella lesions. Rash is only 1 of 6 clinical signs of severity in the criteria for STSS.
  - Recognize that the involvement of subcutaneous structures in NF may be much more extensive than what might be suggested on physical exam.
  - Failing to search for a localized infection as a source of toxin in STTS

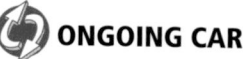

TREATMENT

MEDICATION (DRUGS)

- IV antibiotic therapy for both GABHS and *Staphylococcus aureus* should be instituted promptly.
- Oxacillin (150 mg/kg/d divided q6h) or nafcillin (200 mg/kg/d divided q4–6h; maximum, 12 g/d) *plus* clindamycin (25–40 mg/kg/d divided q6h or q8h). In penicillin-allergic patients, consider vancomycin (40 mg/kg/d divided q6h) *plus* clindamycin. Vancomycin should be used in place of β-lactamase-resistant penicillins in areas with high prevalence of community-acquired methicillin-resistant *S. aureus*.
- Following the identification of GABHS from blood, body fluid, or tissue specimens, the drugs of choice are high-dose penicillin G (200,000–400,000 U/kg/d in 4–6 divided doses) plus clindamycin (helps stop toxin production via protein synthesis inhibition).
- No penicillin G-resistant isolates of GABHS have been reported. There are strains resistant to clindamycin, so this drug should not be used alone until it is shown to be sensitive.
- Large numbers of GABHS organisms can overcome the efficacy of penicillin: The synergistic use of clindamycin should be considered in cases of NF and STSS.
- Inotropes should be administered as indicated.
- The use of IV immunoglobulin may be considered in patients with STSS who remain unresponsive to other treatment modalities and for patients with infection in an area that precludes drainage. Various regimens have been used: 150–400 mg/kg/d for 5 days; 1–2 g/kg as single dose.
- However, a recent multicenter, retrospective cohort study (Shah 2009) suggested that the use of IVIG for STSS was associated with higher costs but no improved outcomes in children.
- At this time, the optimal regimen is unknown.

ADDITIONAL TREATMENT

General Measures

- Volume resuscitation
- Replete electrolytes as indicated
- Blood products as indicated for anemia or thrombocytopenia
- Airway support for severe depression of level of consciousness or respiratory insufficiency

SURGERY/OTHER PROCEDURES

- Consider surgical consult early in management of NF.
- Fasciotomy to relieve compartment syndrome.
- Extensive debridement of necrotic tissue is often indicated.

ONGOING CARE

PROGNOSIS

- Fulminant course with rapid deterioration is characteristic of invasive GABHS infections.
- Improved prognosis with early recognition and aggressive management
- Case fatality rate in pediatric series is 13.7% (36.7% for STSS and 24% for NF)
- Emm/M strain types 1, 3, 12 have worse prognosis.
- Increasing age, occurrence in winter/early spring, or development of GI symptoms have worse prognosis.

COMPLICATIONS

- From deep and systemic infections:
  – Sepsis syndrome
  – Hematologic seeding and development of focal infection
  – Complications associated with specific site of involvement (e.g., meningitis—neurologic impairment; septic arthritis—joint destruction)
- From NF:
  – Severe tissue necrosis usually requires extensive surgical debridement and often results in amputation of involved extremities.
  – Compartment syndrome
  – Functional disabilities
  – Cosmetic sequelae
- From STSS:
  – Multiorgan system failure from systemic hypotension and direct effects of inflammatory mediators
  – Adult respiratory distress syndrome
  – DIC
  – Acute tubular necrosis resulting in renal failure
  – Hepatic failure
  – Cardiac insufficiency
  – Cerebral ischemia and edema
  – Metabolic derangements

ADDITIONAL READING

- American Academy of Pediatrics. *Group A streptococcal infections. Red Book: Report of the Committee on Infectious Diseases*, 28th ed. Washington, DC: American Academy of Pediatrics, 2009:616–628.
- Ibia EO, Imoisili M, Pikis A. Group A beta-hemolytic streptococcal osteomyelitis in children. *Pediatrics*. 2003;112(pt 1):e22–e26l.
- Jean C, Louie JK, Glaser CA, et al. Invasive group A streptococcal infection concurrent with 2009 H1N1 Influenza. *Clin Infect Dis*. 2010;50(10):e59–e62.
- Lamagni TL, Neal S, Keshishian C, et al. Predictors of death after severe Streptococcus pyogenes infection. *Emerg Infect Dis*. 2009;15:1304–1307.
- O'Loughlin RE, Roberson A, Cieslak PR, et al. The epidemiology of invasive group A streptococcal infection and potential vaccine implications: United States, 2000-2004. *Clin Infect Dis*. 2007;45:853–862.
- Shah SS, Hall M, Srivastava R, et al. Intravenous immunoglobulin in children with streptococcal toxic shock syndrome. *Clin Infect Dis*. 2009;49:1367–1376.

CODES

ICD9

- 040.82 Toxic shock syndrome
- 041.01 Streptococcus infection in conditions classified elsewhere and of unspecified site, streptococcus, group A
- 728.86 Necrotizing fasciitis

ICD10

- A48.3 Toxic shock syndrome
- A49.1 Streptococcal infection, unspecified site
- B95.0 Streptococcus, group A, causing diseases classd elswhr

FAQ

- Q: For whom should the diagnosis of invasive GABHS be entertained?
- A: Consider GABHS in any child with varicella who experiences recrudescence of fever, fever ≥39°C (102.2°F) beyond the 3rd day of illness, or any fever beyond the 4th day of illness. A high index of suspicion should be maintained in patients with septicemia, and in febrile patients with pain and hyperesthesia out of proportion to the clinical findings.
- Q: Should the use of NSAIDs be restricted in patients with varicella?
- A: There are several reports suggesting an association between the use of NSAIDs and the development of invasive group A streptococcal diseases, but there has been no study to establish a causal relationship. It has been demonstrated that NSAIDs inhibit immune-mediated defense mechanisms, enhance the production of cytokines, and suppress the pain and fever that might encourage a patient with invasive GABHS infection to seek medical attention sooner. No formal recommendations for restricting the use of NSAIDs are being made at this time.
- Q: Should close contacts of patients with invasive GABHS infections receive chemoprophylaxis?
- A: Chemoprophylaxis of household contacts of people with invasive GABHS remains controversial. Although the risk of developing disease for household contacts is elevated in comparison to the risk of sporadic disease development, the overall frequency of invasive GABHS disease remains small. Testing for GABHS colonization and chemoprophylaxis of household contacts of people with invasive GABHS is not routinely recommended. However, in high-risk populations (people >65 years or those suffering from HIV infection, chickenpox, or diabetes mellitus), targeted chemoprophylaxis may be considered. Chemoprophylaxis is not recommended in schools or child care facilities.

S

STROKE

Irfan Jaffree
Peter M. Bingham (5th edition)

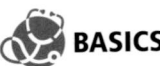 **BASICS**

DESCRIPTION
A neurologic deficit progressing over minutes to hours, due to insufficient perfusion of the brain or spinal cord. Also, otherwise "asymptomatic," remote strokes may present as epilepsy.

EPIDEMIOLOGY
Incidence
- Overall incidence is ~2.5 per 100,000, but certain groups are at higher risk (those with heart disease, sickle cell disease, hereditary thrombophilias).
- Neonatal stroke incidence 1 in 4,000 live births.

RISK FACTORS
Genetics
Various hereditary and metabolic disorders: Neurocutaneous diseases, Down syndrome, collagen disorders, congenital heart disease syndromes, coagulation disorders, hereditary cavernoma or telangiectasia, hyperhomocysteinemia, mitochondrial diseases (MELAS), and others

ETIOLOGY
- Underlying causes of stroke include hematologic, circulatory, and cardiac disorders.
- Hematologic:
  - Factor V mutation
  - Prothrombin gene mutation
  - Anticardiolipin/antiphospholipid syndrome
  - Sickle cell
  - Hemolytic uremic syndrome
  - Hyperhomocysteinemia
  - Dyslipidemia
  - Protein S or C
  - Antithrombin III deficiency
  - Asparaginase treatment
  - Hyperviscosity syndromes (including leukemia)
  - Thrombocythemia ± iron deficiency
  - Extreme dehydration
  - Mixed connective tissue disease
  - Systemic lupus erythematosus
  - Methyl-tetrahydrofolate reductase (MTHFR) mutation
- Vascular:
  - Carotid or vertebral dissection (MTHFR associated with vertebral dissections in children)
  - Arteriovenous malformation (AVM)
  - Carotid trauma
  - Moyamoya
  - Cavernous angioma ("occult cerebrovascular malformations")
  - Vasculitis (especially due to bacterial meningitis)
  - Brain tumor surgery
  - Rarely, aneurysm, Takayasu arteritis, chronic meningitides (tuberculosis, Lyme disease, lupus, or sarcoidosis)
  - Infective endocarditis
- Cardiac:
  - Rheumatic heart disease, cyanotic congenital heart disease, heart failure, cardiomyopathy
  - Possible association with mitral prolapse, atrial septal defects
  - Atrial myxoma, aortic dilatation (Marfan syndrome), pulmonary AVM
  - Single ventricle

DIAGNOSIS

HISTORY
- Inquire about substance use, prior trauma (including head, neck, seat belt injury for dissection and cardiac contusion), infection, excessive bleeding or spontaneous clotting, or history of heart disease.
- Prior surgical history of ASD or VSD repair, PFO closure, cardiac catheterization, or prosthetic heart valves
- Family history of premature thrombosis, hemoglobinopathy, or vascular malformations (e.g., cavernous hemangioma or hereditary hemorrhagic telangiectasia)
- Perinatal stroke frequently presents with neonatal seizures: May be associated with multiple gestation
- Complications of labor or fetal exposure to vasoactive compounds may be associated.
- Recent travel to/from areas of endemic infections.

PHYSICAL EXAM
- Note level of alertness and capacity for sustained attention; fluency, appropriateness, and construction of speech; comprehension; emotional state; and subjective or objective pain.
- Vital signs, color, and respiratory pattern may disclose existing or impending respiratory failure due to loss of protective airway reflexes.
- General examination should include peripheral pulses and perfusion; palpation and auscultation of the precordium and cervical area may reveal evidence of dysrhythmia or anatomic lesions.
- Note confrontation visual fields, funduscopy (especially for papilledema, retinal hemorrhage for shaken baby), eye movements, facial symmetry, pattern of movement of affected limbs, and extensor response of great toe to plantar stimulation (Babinski sign).
- In the absence of sensory complaints, detailed sensory exam is often fruitless. Conversely, isolated sensory complaints are rarely an indication of stroke.
- Examine for signs of neurocutaneous syndromes (neurofibroma, shagreen patch, ash lesions, axillary freckling, telangiectasia, nevi, facial angiomas).

DIAGNOSTIC TESTS & INTERPRETATION
Lab
- Blood chemistry, particularly glucose; mild hyperglycemia may reflect stress response.
- Toxin screen
- Carbon monoxide poisoning in winter months.
- CBC, PT, and PTT may prompt important therapeutic decisions.
- Consider lumbar puncture (if neuroradiologic findings show no risk of incipient herniation) to look for evidence of inflammatory/infectious basis (vasculitis, though CSF occasionally normal).

- ESR, CRP for endocarditis
- TSH and free T_4 (atrial fibrillation)
- More extensive testing in undiagnosed cases may include the following:
  - Tests for specific coagulopathies (see "Etiology and Differential Diagnosis")
  - Varicella serology (may be a common cause of stroke in children, postvaricella angiopathy)
  - Toxin screen (association with cocaine, amphetamines, OCP)
  - Amino acid screening (for homocysteine)
  - Hemoglobin electrophoresis (sickle hemoglobin)
  - Lipid profile (hypercholesterolemia)
  - RPR

Imaging
- Individuals with stable vital signs and suspected stroke should undergo a brain imaging study promptly:
  - Non–contrast-enhanced images to look for possible hemorrhage, may be followed by contrast-enhanced images to evaluate for possible focal encephalitis or underlying vascular lesions (MR/conventional angiography)
  - Many diagnostic questions can be resolved equally well by CT or MRI, although CT may be preferable in suspected subarachnoid hemorrhage; MRI—especially diffusion-weighted MRI—is much more sensitive in the 1st 24 hours after symptom onset and may identify venous or sinus thrombosis or smaller bilateral lesions pointing to systemic embolization.
  - Cervical spine imaging may help in posterior circulation infarcts to look for vertebral abnormalities.
- More extensive testing in undiagnosed cases may include the following:
  - ECG to assess for rhythm dysfunction
  - Echocardiography (atrial–septal defect, luminal lesion transthoracic/transesophageal)
  - Carotid Doppler (stenosis/dissection)
  - Specialized vascular neuroradiologic studies (MRA, CTA, conventional angiography)

ALERT
- AVMs may not be seen on angiography immediately after a primary intracerebral hemorrhage. Consider repeat angiography weeks or months later.
- CT scan may be normal in the 1st 24 hours after nonhemorrhagic stroke. A follow-up study may be necessary.
- Suspected transient ischemic attack (TIA) should prompt a vigorous diagnostic evaluation.

DIFFERENTIAL DIAGNOSIS

Several disorders may mimic the presentation of stroke:

- Migraine
- Demyelinating disease
- Focal encephalitis
- Postepileptic paralysis (Todd paresis)
- Conversion disorder
- Brachial plexus palsy, spinal cord lesion, intracranial neoplasm, abscess, subdural empyema, or mitochondrial disease may present as stroke.

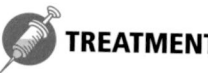 TREATMENT

MEDICATION (DRUGS)

- Investigational therapies include hypervolemic hemodilution, thrombolytic agents, calcium channel antagonists, and neuroprotective agents such as glutamate receptor antagonists.
- In most cases, there is no contraindication to pharmacotherapy appropriate to any identified underlying condition; the decision to use antiplatelet or thrombolytic therapy or anticoagulation is complex and depends on risk of hemorrhage, experience of the clinician, and potential side effects.

ADDITIONAL TREATMENT
General Measures

- Patients with radiologically documented or clinically suspected stroke who have stable airway, breathing, and circulation are most often hospitalized for observation and supportive therapy:
  - Those with a diminished or fluctuating level of alertness or with radiographically extensive area(s) of infarction are often monitored in an intensive care unit for changes in respiratory status or signs of increased intracranial pressure.
- Strokes involving the posterior fossa or cerebellum, or affecting a large area of the cerebrum, are of particular concern because of the risk of tentorial or subfalcine herniation: A neurosurgical consult should be obtained for these cases and for those with intracranial hemorrhage above or below the tentorium.
- Consultation with neurology, cardiology, hematology, other pediatric subspecialists

Additional Therapies

Rehabilitation and physical therapy may improve outcome: Institute as soon as the patient's condition permits.

IN-PATIENT CONSIDERATIONS
Initial Stabilization

- Stroke may present as new-onset seizures: Follow protocol for emergency treatment of seizures.
- Urgent neurosurgical evaluation indicated in cases of large cerebral hemispheric stroke, intracranial hemorrhage, or posterior fossa ischemic stroke
- Empiric antibiotics indicated in the setting of stroke and fever (abscess, septic emboli, empyema)

 ONGOING CARE

FOLLOW-UP RECOMMENDATIONS

The usual course in stroke of any cause is for gradual improvement after the acute onset of symptoms: Significant recovery of neurologic function may continue for months after the ictus, especially in infants and toddlers.

PATIENT EDUCATION

- Internet information for families: National Stroke Association: www.stroke.org
- Children's Hemiplegia and Stroke Association: www.chasa.org
- Pediatric Stroke Network: www.pediatricstrokenetwork.com

COMPLICATIONS

- Remote sequelae that may not be evident for months or years after stroke include epilepsy, hydrocephalus, learning difficulties, depression, short attention span, posture disturbances (especially cerebral palsy), sphincter disturbances, pressure sores, and susceptibility to infection if airway protective reflexes are impaired.
- Other complications include the following:
  - Seizures
  - Respiratory insufficiency
  - Intracranial hypertension
  - Motor, visual, cognitive deficits and neglect syndromes
  - Autonomic disturbances
  - Infection susceptibility

ADDITIONAL READING

- Dicuonzo F, Palma M, Fiume M. Cerebrovascular disorders in the prenatal period. *J Child Neurol*. 2008;23(11):1260–1266.
- Ganesan V, Chong WK, Cox TC, et al. Posterior circulation stroke in childhood: Risk factors and recurrence. *Neurology*. 2002;59:1552–1556.
- Gunther G, Junker R, Strater R, et al. Symptomatic ischemic stroke in full-term neonates: Role of acquired and genetic prothrombotic risk factors. *Stroke*. 2000;31:2437–2441.
- Jayawant S, Parr J. Outcome following subdural haemorrhages in infancy. *Arch Dis Child*. 2007;92:343–347.
- Mackay MT, Wizniter M, Benedict SL, et al. Arterial ischemic stroke risk factors: The International Pediatric Stroke Study. *Ann Neurol*. 2011;69:130–140.

 CODES

ICD9

- 436 Acute, but ill-defined, cerebrovascular disease
- 779.89 Other specified conditions originating in the perinatal period

ICD10

- I67.8 Other specified cerebrovascular diseases
- P96.89 Other specified conditions originating in the perinatal period

FAQ

- Q: Will my child have another stroke?
- A: The chance of recurrence depends on remediation of the underlying cause. Available evidence suggests that children with no identifiable underlying basis for stroke have a very low recurrence risk.
- Q: Are there any medications for acute stroke?
- A: Tissue plasminogen activator (TPA) appears to be useful in some cases of adult nonhemorrhagic stroke, but its usefulness in childhood stroke has not been studied. Depending on the presence or degree of secondary cerebral hemorrhage, many specialists favor the use of heparin or low-molecular-weight heparin in the setting of stroke due to venous sinus thrombosis.
- Q: What can be done to reduce the risk of future strokes?
- A: Risk factor modification like diet, exercise, BP control, and treating underlying cause of stroke if identified. Medication compliance.

S

STUTTERING

Gary A. Emmett

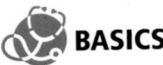 **BASICS**

DESCRIPTION

Stuttering is an involuntary disturbance in the normal fluency and timing of speech which is not appropriate for the age of the speaker. Various patterns are seen:

- Prolongation of sounds or syllables
- Repetition of sounds or syllables or even whole words
- Pauses in the middle of words
- Blocking—either silence or pauses filled with nonsense sounds in the middle of words, as if considering what to say next
- Avoidance—word substitutions that are used to skip known problem words; also called circumlocution
- Overemphasis of some syllables or words; also called tension
- Stuttering is significant when it interferes with the patient's life in academic, occupational, or social arenas. Many children with developmental delays have disfluencies of speech, but it is not considered stuttering unless the disfluencies are present more frequently than expected for the level of disability.

EPIDEMIOLOGY

- At least 1% of all studied populations affected
- Males stutter 3 times more often as females.
- Stuttering is found in every culture and language. The language spoken in the home does not increase or decrease the amount of stuttering.
- Stuttering begins between 2 and 7 years of age with 98% of cases presenting by age 10.
- Girls start stuttering several months earlier on average than boys; but they also speak, in general, earlier than boys do.

RISK FACTORS
Genetics
Stuttering does cluster in families:

- Monozygotic twins have a higher concordance for stuttering than dizygotic twins.
- The more closely related one is to a stutterer, the more likely one is to stutter.
- Identical twins have a concordance for stuttering of ≥30%.
- In specific families with a high propensity for stuttering, Kang et al. (and others) have shown single gene defects that correlate highly with dysfluency.

GENERAL PREVENTION
There is no known prevention strategy for stuttering.

PATHOPHYSIOLOGY

Stuttering appears to be associated with an excessive amount of dopamine, or closely related vasoactive compounds, in the brain:

- Patients with Parkinson disease often develop adult-onset stuttering.
- PET scans show increased vasoactive substances in the brains of those who stutter.
- Medications that increase brain dopamine (antidepressants) or are dopaminergic (major tranquilizers) can induce stuttering in non-stutterers; medications that lower dopamine (e.g., clomipramine) may stop stuttering.
- Many differences exist between the brains of stutterers and non-stutterers in glucose uptake, dopamine release, and metabolic activity of the basal ganglia, but no single physiologic process has been well defined as the cause of stuttering.

ETIOLOGY

- Specific etiology is not known, but many factors contribute. Stuttering may be more pronounced when a child is fatigued, excited, upset, rushed, or exposed to some other stressor.
- Environmental factors are thought to have a role. Children adopted by a parent who stutters are more likely to stutter than children adopted by a parent who does not stutter.

COMMONLY ASSOCIATED CONDITIONS

- Other language problems: Articulation disorders, phonologic disorders, learning disabilities, dyslexia, ADHD
- Students with developmental delay or intellectual impairment are found to stutter up to 25% of the time.

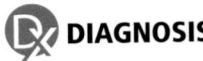 **DIAGNOSIS**

HISTORY

- Stuttering runs in families by both nature and nurture.
- Age of onset and length of persistence:
  - Onset is insidious, with the child often unaware of the problem.
  - If stuttering starts after the 10th birthday, suspect an intracranial mass or brain ischemia.
- Physiologic stuttering is rarely present during oral reading, singing, acting, and reciting in rhythm, or while talking to pets or inanimate objects.
- Medications, especially those that increase dopamine, may activate stuttering.
- Increased intracranial pressure from disease or trauma may lead to stuttering.

PHYSICAL EXAM

- There are no specific physical exam findings of stuttering. Observations of children improve the ability to make this diagnosis. Stuttering is 2 or more repetitions of a speech unit.
- Stutterers often improve in one-to-one situations with familiar people, so ask the parents to bring in a video recording of the child in a variety of situations: when talking in public, singing, and talking to a pet or infant.
- Observations that may be made in the office and correlate strongly with the diagnosis of stuttering include:
  - Multiple repetitions and/or prolongations
  - Rising pitch with difficult words
  - Grimacing or other physical tension, such as taking deep breaths or jerking the head back when speaking
  - Inappropriate emphasis of words not normally emphasized, extremely slow speech, or speech without intonation
- Although unwillingness to speak to the examiner is normal, unwillingness to speak to the parent is not.

DIAGNOSTIC TESTS & INTERPRETATION
Diagnostic Procedures/Other

- None currently available, but PET scan may be a useful modality in the future
- If stuttering begins after the age of 10, or if the patient has additional neurologic or developmental problems, a workup for brain abnormalities should be considered.

DIFFERENTIAL DIAGNOSIS

- Developmental:
  - Normal development: Disfluencies associated with rapid onset of full speech capabilities that will usually resolve very quickly
  - Transitory dysfluency is an ill-defined term but generally means stuttering in preschool-aged children that lasts <1 year.
  - Cluttering: Patients with extremely rapid speech will have disfluencies that resolve with slowing down of speech.
  - Pervasive developmental disorder (autism spectrum disorder): May also have echolalia, tonelessness, and poor eye contact
- Neurologic:
  - Tics/Tourette syndrome: Similar time of onset, initially somewhat similar symptoms. Stuttering is usually not associated with simultaneous physical movement.
  - Trauma, tumor, or major CNS disease, such as Parkinson disease, may cause late-onset stuttering.
- Medications:
  - Any medication that increases the presence of dopamine may worsen (or cause) stuttering. Examples are SSRI-type antidepressants or major tranquilizers.

TREATMENT

ADDITIONAL TREATMENT

General Measures

- Therapy must work on improving the child's fluency and increasing acceptance and tolerance of this problem by the patient and his or her family.
- In a multicultural learning atmosphere, sensitivity to the learning styles of each social group is paramount in achieving successful results.

Additional Therapies

- Speech therapy:
  - Stuttering in young children can be resolved with very short courses of therapy, often ≤3 months. Stuttering remains resolved in ≥95% of these early treatment cases. The younger the patient is at the time of referral to speech therapy, the shorter the course of therapy needed, and the more likely that the therapy will be successful.
  - Many experts in dysfluency believe that early intervention is more likely to be successful than waiting to start therapy if the stuttering has not spontaneously resolved by the 7th birthday.
  - Among the more successful new programs for young children who stutter is the Lidcombe Program of Early Stuttering Intervention, an intense behavioral therapy program in which the belief is that stuttering is physical in nature. The program teaches parents and caregivers how to praise the child for speaking fluently and how to correct them occasionally when they stutter. Parents are supported throughout the process by the clinician. The therapy ultimately enables the child to speak fluently and to monitor his or her own speech.
- Other therapies:
  - A successful new therapy for adolescents and adults is a hearing-aid type device (SpeechEasy, www.speecheasy.com) that feeds the individual's speech directly back into an earpiece.
  - Devices that make hearing monaural or provide a white noise background in the ear also improve stuttering.
  - Information for families is available through organizations such as The Stuttering Foundation, a nonprofit organization (www.stutteringhelp.org).

ALERT

- Because stuttering waxes and wanes with time, temporary improvement does not equal cure.
- Any behavioral therapy must be done under the guidance of a well-trained professional because inappropriate criticism may worsen stuttering.
- Waiting to see if stuttering goes away by age 7 is not the best strategy for young children, as was often taught in the past.
- The literature does not give a clear time frame for how long stuttering in preschool children should last before requiring evaluation and treatment, but a significant stutter that lasts for >1 year should be referred to a speech therapist.
- No medications are known to reduce stuttering safely. Acupuncture, hypnosis, and yoga have been used with some success, but not in controlled studies.

ONGOING CARE

FOLLOW-UP RECOMMENDATIONS

If stuttering is reported by the parents in a preschool-aged child, follow up in 1–2 months to see if it was only a transitory dysfluency that has resolved. If not, obtain a speech therapy consult for evaluation.

Patient Monitoring

- Periodic follow-up to ensure that speech therapy is in place and that progress is being made
- Reassessment to ensure that child is adapting to social situations and interacting with others

PATIENT EDUCATION

The following suggestions, though helpful to parents, should be recommended in conjunction with, but not in place of, speech therapy. Parents may be too critical of their own children.

- Take time out of each day to speak with the child one-on-one.
- Model slow speech
- Wait for the child to speak. Take turns speaking.
- Allow for transition time between activities and tasks.
- Keep a notebook of things that help make speech better and things that elicit stuttering.

PROGNOSIS

- Up to 80% of stuttering cases spontaneously regress by age 16.
- Severity of stuttering does not relate to persistence of stuttering.
- The longer stuttering exists, the more likely it will persist.

COMPLICATIONS

- Anxiety and depression, often far out of proportion to the degree of dysfluency
- Blocking and hesitation, giving an impression of delayed intellectual development
- Voluntary withdrawal from social interaction to avoid embarrassment

ADDITIONAL READING

- Battle DE. Communication disorders in multicultural populations, 3rd ed. Boston, MA: Butterworth-Heinemann, 2002.
- Craig A, Hancock K, Tran Y, et al. Epidemiology of stuttering in the community across the entire life span. *J Speech Lang Hear Res.* 2002;45:1097–1105.
- Gordon N. Stuttering: Incidence and causes. *Dev Med Child Neurol.* 2002;44:278–281.
- Jones M, Onslow M, Packman A, et al. Randomised controlled trial of the Lidcombe programme of early stuttering intervention. *BMJ.* 2005;331:659–661.
- Kang C, Riazuddin S, Mundorff J, et al. Mutations in the lysosomal enzyme: Targeting pathway and persistent stuttering. *N Engl J Med.* 2010; 362(8):677–685.
- Rosenfield DB, Viswanath NS. Neuroscience of stuttering. *Science.* 2002;295:973–974.
- The Stuttering Foundation. Videotape No. 70: Stuttering and the preschool child. Help for families. Memphis, TN: Stuttering Foundation of America, 2000. www.stutteringhelp.org.
- Ward D. The aetiology and treatment of developmental stammering in childhood. *Arch Dis Child.* 2008;93(1):68–71.

S

CODES

ICD9
315.35 Childhood onset fluency disorder

ICD10
F80.81 Childhood onset fluency disorder

FAQ

- Q: Are some children more prone to stuttering?
- A: Yes, "sensitive" children (many different definitions in many different studies) are more likely to stutter, as are the children of highly critical parents.
- Q: Should family and friends complete the sentences of children who stutter?
- A: No, children who cannot complete a thought should be gently asked to slow down and try again with no time limit set; or, others should simply wait until the child has completed his or her sentence. Children with a stuttering problem should also be praised when they do not stutter.

SUBDURAL HEMATOMA

Dennis J. Dlugos
Sabrina E. Smith

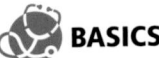 **BASICS**

DESCRIPTION
A subdural hematoma (SDH) is a collection of blood between the outer pial and inner dural meningeal layers. The bleeding is usually venous in origin, although either cortical arteries or bridging veins may be torn.

EPIDEMIOLOGY
- Heterogeneous causes; occur in all age groups
- Incidence in infants <1 year old estimated at 20–25/100,000

RISK FACTORS
- In infants and young children, SDHs are frequently the result of abusive head trauma.
- In older children, SDHs are often the result of motor vehicle collisions.
- Neonatal SDHs occur with spontaneous deliveries, but may be more frequent following deliveries with forceps or vacuum extraction. SDHs related to birth usually resolve.
- Risk factors for abusive head trauma include disability or prematurity of the child, unstable family situations, parents of young age, and low socioeconomic status.
- 1 study found that fathers were the most frequent perpetrators, followed by boyfriends, female babysitters, and mothers, in descending order of frequency.
- Accidental trauma

Genetics
There is no clear genetic predisposition, except when hereditary coagulopathy or metabolic disease is implicated.

GENERAL PREVENTION
- Parents should be counseled about appropriate methods to channel frustration and anger toward infants and children. Shaking an infant when the parent is angry is never appropriate.
- Bicycle helmets, car seats, and seat belts are all valuable in preventing head injuries in children.

PATHOPHYSIOLOGY
- SDHs may be acute or chronic:
  - Arterial SDHs grow quickly, whereas venous SDHs may accumulate slowly, remaining undetected for weeks or months.
  - Acute SDHs contain blood, whereas chronic SDHs contain proteinaceous exudate and blood-breakdown products.
  - Rebleeding may be the underlying cause of many chronic SDHs.
- Significant force is usually required for SDH unless there are predisposing circumstances; SDH is only rarely due to trivial or minor trauma. However, SDH can occur with relatively minor trauma in individuals with bleeding disorders, children on chronic dialysis, and those with enlarged extracerebral spaces or cortical atrophy.

- SDHs in abusive head trauma may be due to the striking of the infant's head against a surface (such as a mattress):
  - The sudden deceleration associated with the impact may tear bridging veins traveling in the subdural space.
- The term shaking-impact syndrome may be more accurate than shaken-baby syndrome.

ETIOLOGY
- See "Risk Factors."
- SDHs can also occur after ventricular shunting and extracorporeal membrane oxygenation (ECMO).

COMMONLY ASSOCIATED CONDITIONS
- Some metabolic disorders, such as glutaric aciduria type I and Menkes disease, can be associated with both acute and chronic SDHs.
- Victims of motor vehicle collisions with SDH may have other intracranial injuries, such as diffuse axonal injury.
- Traumatic SDHs are often associated with cerebral contusions. Other associated injuries include skull fractures, diffuse axonal injury, and penetrating injuries.
- Sequelae: Epilepsy, developmental delay, cerebral palsy

 DIAGNOSIS

A careful history and detailed physical exam are essential to explore possible causes of the SDH, assess the child's neurologic status, and look for evidence of other injuries. Prompt neuroimaging is critical.

HISTORY
- Newborns: SDHs due to birth trauma may present with lethargy, pallor, poor feeding, apnea, and seizures. However, many term newborns with small SDHs are asymptomatic.
- Infants and young children: SDHs may also present with a nonspecific history of lethargy, irritability, vomiting, poor feeding, apnea, and seizures.
- Older children: Present with a history of trauma and alteration of consciousness
- Caution:
  - Be suspicious if the stated history does not fit with the pattern or severity of the injury.
  - Physicians and other health care professionals with experience in child abuse should be consulted early if abuse is suspected.

PHYSICAL EXAM
- Newborns may present with decreased responsiveness, a bulging fontanelle, hypotonia, or hypertonia. Retinal hemorrhages are not specific at this age, because they are seen in up to 40% of newborns following a vaginal delivery.
- Infants and young children may also present with nonspecific physical signs, but focal neurologic signs may be present. Retinal hemorrhages are most often associated with abusive head trauma, but they have been reported after accidental trauma leading to SDH. Bilateral retinal hemorrhages with retinal folds or detachments are particularly associated with abusive head trauma.

- Other signs of child abuse include burns, lacerations, and bruises in various stages of healing, and belt marks, choke marks, and multiple fractures of different ages.
- Older children present with signs of external head trauma, decreased responsiveness, and focal neurologic signs.
- SDHs present with nonspecific signs, such as vomiting, irritability, lethargy, failure to thrive, anemia, and seizures.

DIAGNOSTIC TESTS & INTERPRETATION
Imaging
- CT scan is the imaging study of choice in acute head trauma with neurologic signs:
  - SDH appears as an extra-axial area of increased density, crescentic in shape, and often associated with cerebral contusion or mass effect.
  - CT also may show evidence of cerebral edema, with loss of gray matter/white matter differentiation and small ventricles.
  - Subacute SDHs may be difficult to distinguish from adjacent gray matter on CT scan.
  - Loss of gray/white matter differentiation may occur.
  - Chronic SDHs appear as areas of low density on CT scan, often bilateral.
- MRI is helpful to clarify subacute and chronic SDHs and to identify small SDHs missed by CT.
- Ultrasound is less helpful, because it may be difficult to distinguish the subdural space from the subarachnoid space.
- If child abuse is suspected, a skeletal survey or bone scan is useful to look for fractures of different ages.
- Incidental SDH may be found on neuroimaging studies in newborns; frequently no intervention is required other than close follow-up.

DIFFERENTIAL DIAGNOSIS
- SDHs are usually traumatic, but separating accidental from nonaccidental trauma may be difficult: Falls in infants may cause linear skull fractures, rarely SDHs. On noncontrast head CT, homogeneous hyperdense subdural hematoma is more common following accidental trauma, while mixed-density subdural hematoma is more common following nonaccidental trauma.
- Macrocephaly or other signs/symptoms since birth may help to date the origin of the SDH to the perinatal or neonatal period.
- Epidural hematomas, subarachnoid hemorrhages, and acute SDHs cannot be distinguished clinically:
  - The lucid interval sometimes seen with epidural hematomas in adults is not a reliable sign.
  - A head CT should differentiate.
- Chronic SDHs must be differentiated from benign enlargement of the subarachnoid spaces, a self-limited condition characterized by progressive macrocrania and extra-axial fluid collections with the density of spinal fluid:
  - MRI can differentiate benign enlargement of the subarachnoid spaces from SDH.
  - Rarely SDH can also occur in children with benign enlargement of the subarachnoid spaces.

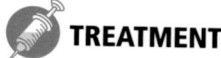 **TREATMENT**

MEDICATION (DRUGS)

Seizures:

* Phenytoin and levetiracetam are good choices if IV medication is needed, with phenobarbital as a reasonable alternative, especially in neonates.
* Prophylactic anticonvulsants given for a few weeks are effective in reducing early posttraumatic seizures but may not affect long-term risk of epilepsy.

ADDITIONAL TREATMENT

General Measures

* The treatment of choice for large, acute SDHs is surgical evacuation. Smaller SDHs may be managed conservatively, with careful monitoring for signs of neurologic deterioration.
* While awaiting surgery, attention to airway, breathing, and circulation (ABCs) is critical. Tracheal intubation should be performed if the child's Glasgow Coma Scale score is <8 or if airway protective reflexes are impaired.
* Measures to control intracranial pressure (ICP) include elevating the head of the bed 30° to promote venous drainage and osmotic therapy with mannitol:
  – ICP monitoring should be considered.
  – Mild hyperventilation (PcO_2 30–35 mm Hg) may be helpful but should not be instituted prophylactically.
  – The efficacy of these measures in improving long-term outcome following large SDHs has not been established. Mild hypothermia and hypertonic saline have been used in some cases of traumatic brain injury in adults, but these are not proven therapies in children.
* Seizures should be treated promptly.
* Treatment of chronic SDHs is more controversial:
  – If there are no signs of elevated ICP, conservative treatment is reasonable, and most collections will resolve.
  – Subdural taps are indicated if ICP rises.
  – If taps are not successful, a subdural peritoneal shunt may be placed.
* Treatment of SDHs that develop after ventricular shunting is particularly challenging.

ISSUES FOR REFERRAL

Social work services should be consulted in cases of known or suspected child abuse.

SURGERY/OTHER PROCEDURES

The treatment of choice for large, acute SDHs is surgical evacuation.

IN-PATIENT CONSIDERATIONS

Initial Stabilization

* Children with SDHs may be critically ill on presentation.
* The aggressiveness of acute therapy depends on the child's clinical condition.
* Neuroimaging studies and, if necessary, prompt neurosurgical consultation should be performed.

IV Fluids

Isotonic fluids should be given, because hypotonic fluids may worsen cerebral edema.

 ONGOING CARE

FOLLOW-UP RECOMMENDATIONS

Children with neurologic sequelae from head injury may benefit from admission to a rehabilitation hospital.

PROGNOSIS

* In general, long-term outcome is related to the condition of the child at time of presentation. Prolonged elevation of ICP, concomitant ischemic brain injury, or significant cerebral edema before treatment is worrisome and indicates a poor prognosis.
* Children typically have a better outcome from head injury than do adults, but children <7 years of age often do worse than older children, especially if the SDH is the result of abusive head trauma.

COMPLICATIONS

* SDHs may result in mass effect, focal neurologic signs, and coma.
* Increased ICP and seizures are other serious complications.
* Neurologic sequelae of SDHs are more severe than epidural hematomas because of associated cerebral contusions.
* Long-term problems include headache, seizures, hydrocephalus, cerebral palsy, difficulty concentrating, poor school performance, fixed neurologic deficits, and neurobehavioral problems.
* Epilepsy eventually develops in ~10–15% of patients after severe head injury: This risk generally does not warrant the use of prophylactic anticonvulsants.

ADDITIONAL READING

* Foerster BR, Petrou M, Lin D, et al. Neuroimaging evaluation of non-accidental head trauma with correlation to clinical outcomes: A review of 57 cases. *J Pediatr.* 2009;154(4):573–577.
* Matschke J, Voss J, Obi N, et al. Nonaccidental head injury is the most common cause of subdural bleeding in infants <1 year of age. *Pediatrics.* 2009;124(6):1587–1594.
* McNeely PD, Atkinson JD, Saigal G, et al. Subdural hematomas in infants with benign enlargement of the subarachnoid spaces are not pathognomonic for child abuse. *AJNR Am J Neuroradiol.* 2006; 27(8):1725–1728.
* Swift DM, McBride L. Chronic subdural hematoma in children. *Neurosurg Clin North Am.* 2000; 11:439–446.
* Tung GA, Kumar M, Richardson RC, et al. Comparison of accidental and nonaccidental traumatic head injury in children on noncontrast computed tomography. *Pediatrics.* 2006;118: 626–633.

 CODES

ICD9

* 432.1 Subdural hemorrhage
* 852.20 Subdural hemorrhage following injury without mention of open intracranial wound, unspecified state of consciousness

ICD10

* S06.5X0A Traumatic subdural hemorrhage without loss of consciousness, initial encounter
* S06.5X0D Traumatic subdural hemorrhage without loss of consciousness, subsequent encounter
* S06.5X0S Traumatic subdural hemorrhage without loss of consciousness, sequela

FAQ

* Q: When did the bleed occur?
* A: With chronic SDHs, the time and type of injury may be difficult to establish, because no trauma may be reported and the trauma may have occurred weeks or months before. Neuroimaging can give some indication of the injury's timing.
* Q: What limitations should be imposed after an acute SDH?
* A: Because SDH may recur with minor trauma, it is prudent to avoid any activities that have significant risk of fall or a blow to the head for weeks to months or until neuroradiologic resolution of the hematoma.
* Q: Why are anticonvulsants not used to prevent seizures following SDHs?
* A: Seizure medications may be given for a few weeks to prevent early seizures following an SDH. After a few weeks, the risks and side effects of the medications outweigh the risk of developing seizures. If seizures begin at a time remote to the injury, then seizure medications can be restarted.
* Q: My baby twisted out of my arms, fell head-first onto a tile floor, and suffered a head injury. Will I be reported for child abuse?
* A: Not if the injuries fit with the stated history. In this case, the most likely injury would be a linear skull fracture. If more serious intracranial injuries occur, they will probably not be associated with retinal hemorrhages or other injuries, such as older fractures in multiple stages of healing.

SUBSTANCE USE DISORDERS

Matthew L. Prowler

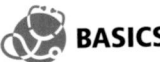

BASICS

DESCRIPTION
DSM-IV-TR criteria:
- Substance abuse—a maladaptive pattern of substance use leading to significant impairment or distress: Failure to fulfill role obligations at home and school (absences, suspensions, expulsions); physically hazardous situations (in car with driver impaired by substance use); legal/criminal problems; continued use despite social or interpersonal problems
- Substance dependence—differentiated from abuse by the presence of:
  - Tolerance—a need for markedly increased amounts of substance to achieve intoxication; diminished effect with continued use of same amount
  - Withdrawal symptoms develop, and use of same (or similar) substance is necessary to avoid withdrawal.
  - Efforts to cut back are unsuccessful; substance taken in larger amounts than intended; a great deal of time is spent in activities necessary to obtain substance; important social/recreational activities are given up or reduced.

EPIDEMIOLOGY
- Estimated rates for substance use vary by substance. Most recent epidemiologic data from the annual survey, "Monitoring the Future," a long-term study sponsored by the National Institute on Drug Abuse (NIDA):
  - Cigarettes: Approximately 40% of American youth have tried cigarettes by 12th grade, and about 1 in 5 those reporting lifetime prevalence >20% of 12th graders is a current smoker.
  - Alcohol: More than 20% of 12th graders surveyed admitted to having ≥5 drinks in a row on at least one occasion in the 2 weeks prior to the survey (considered "binge drinking").
  - Marijuana: More than 5% of 12 graders reported daily use of marijuana and more than 1/3 have used in the last 12 months.
  - Prescription drugs: The adolescent misuse of addictive prescription drugs has become a growing problem in the US in recent years. The proportion of 12th graders in 2010 who reported use of these prescription drugs (amphetamines, sedatives, tranquilizers, and narcotics other than heroin) without medical supervision in the prior year was 15%, those reporting lifetime prevalence >20%.

RISK FACTORS
- Social and familial environmental factors: Lack of parental supervision or discipline, minimal peer affiliation, lack of engagement in structured activities, low socioeconomic status
- Familial heritability pattern: Genetic heritability as high as 0.8 in twin studies

COMMONLY ASSOCIATED CONDITIONS
- ADHD
- Conduct disorder
- Mood disorders
- Post-trauma states

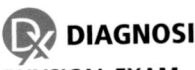

DIAGNOSIS

PHYSICAL EXAM
- Fatigue/malaise: Cannabis, sedative-hypnotic, opiate intoxication, stimulant withdrawal
- Increased heart/respiratory rate: Stimulants, cannabis
- Increased blood pressure: Stimulants, cannabis, PCP
- Decreased blood pressure/respiratory rate: Opiates
- Injected conjunctiva: Cannabis
- Nystagmus: PCP
- Pupillary constriction: Opiates
- Pupillary dilatation: Opiate withdrawal, cocaine, PCP

DIAGNOSTIC TESTS & INTERPRETATION
Lab
- Drug screens are available for urine and blood samples. Urine drug screens (UDS) are the most commonly used.
- When administered, care should be given to individual drug half-lives, as a negative screen may not indicate that a patient is not using drugs.
- Pay attention to lab cutoff concentrations for sensitivity of positive findings. For instance, some labs use 50 ng/mL and 500 ng/mL for cannabis and amphetamine, respectively, while other labs use 100 ng/mL and 1,000 ng/mL.
- For alcohol intoxication:
  - Blood levels >100 mg/dL: Impaired balance and drowsiness
  - >200 mg/dL: Marked muscular incoordination, vomiting, stupor
  - >300 mg/dL: Loss of consciousness, incontinence
  - >400 mg/dL: Can be fatal

Diagnostic Procedures/Other
- Screening tools: CRAFFT substance abuse screening test—a brief, validated tool (6 items) designed for screening in pediatric primary care settings. Multiple longer screening instruments exist for use in subspecialty offices (e.g., POSIT, PESQ, AADIS).
- Interview:
  - A thorough substance use history includes: Age of onset, duration, frequency, and route of ingestion for each drug used. It may be helpful to outline a brief timeline or drug chart.
  - Note if there are any temporally related events in patient's life that correspond to increased use.
  - Other questions that help ascertain severity: Ask about context of use; does the patient use alone or with peers; have there been negative consequences of use or clear functional impairment.
  - Explore the motivation to quit or change behavior.
  - Explore adolescent's attitudes and beliefs regarding substance use and perceived risks or benefits of continued use.

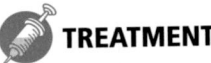

TREATMENT

ADDITIONAL TREATMENT
General Measures
- Inpatient rehabilitation: Acute stabilization in cases of substance abuse severely affecting functioning; high-risk behavior or severely symptomatic comorbid states are demonstrated.
- Partial hospitalization: Child remains in the home, but attends daily therapeutic program.
- After-school intensive outpatient programs: Usually 2–3 times/week, group therapy based.
- Outpatient therapy: Less acute, but may be intensive with several visits a week, consisting of psychotherapy and/or psychopharmacology.

Additional Therapies

- Psychotherapeutic treatments: The most efficacy has been shown for the following therapeutic approaches:
  - Cognitive behavioral therapy (CBT)
  - Family therapy
  - Motivational interviewing/enhancement
- Pharmacologic treatments:
  - Limited research has focused on medication management of substance use disorders in adolescents.
  - While off-label, there have been positive findings for nicotine replacement therapy (NRT) and bupropion for smoking cessation in adolescents.
  - There is early evidence that buprenorphine is a safe and effective treatment for opiate-dependent adolescents and young adults.
  - Treating comorbid conditions: There is evidence that treatment of comorbid ADHD and Bipolar Disorder leads to better outcomes of substance use.
- Support groups:
  - 12-Step model: Multi-step approach to recovery, group-support, utilizes higher power concept; usually adverse to psychopharmacologic treatments
    - Alcoholics Anonymous (AA)/Narcotics Anonymous (NA): Adult groups, but some fellowships may welcome younger members.
    - Teen Anon/Family Teens Support Group: Designed specifically for teens and families of teens with substance use disorders
    - Local community/Religious support group
    - There is evidence of higher rates of abstinence in adolescents engaged in support groups compared to those not participating in such groups.

 ## ONGOING CARE

Patient Monitoring/Prognosis

- Substance use disorders may be chronic conditions, and relapse is common.
- Long-term monitoring, including regular follow-up visits to assess for relapse and/or signs of continued substance use into adulthood.
- Engagement in treatment is a good prognostic factor.

ADDITIONAL READING

- American Psychiatric Association. *Diagnostic and statistical manual of mental disorders*, revised 4th ed. Washington, DC: Author, 2000.
- Bukstein OC, Deas D. Substance abuse and addictions. In: *Dulcan's textbook of child and adolescent psychiatry*. Arlington, VA: American Psychiatric Publishing, 2010:241–258.
- Hopfer C, Riggs P. Substance use disorders. In: *Lewis' child and adolescent psychiatry*. Philadelphia, PA: Lippincott Williams and Wilkins, 2007:615–623.
- Johnston LD, O'Malley PM, Bachman JG, et al. *Monitoring the future national results on adolescent drug use: Overview of key findings, 2010*. Ann Arbor, MI: Institute for Social Research, The University of Michigan, 2011.
- Kaminer Y, Marsch LA. Pharmacotherapy of adolescent substance use disorders. In: Kaminer Y, Winters KC, eds. *Clinical manual of adolescent substance abuse treatment*. Washington, DC: American Psychiatric Association, 2010.
- Knight JR, Sherritt L, Shrier LA. Validity of CRAFFT substance abuse screening test among adolescent clinic patients. *Arch Pediatr Adolesc Med*. 2002;156:607–614.

 ## CODES

ICD9

- 292.0 Drug withdrawal
- 304.90 Unspecified drug dependence, unspecified
- 305.90 Other, mixed, or unspecified drug abuse, unspecified

ICD10

- F19.10 Other psychoactive substance abuse, uncomplicated
- F19.20 Other psychoactive substance dependence, uncomplicated
- F19.230 Other psychoactive substance dependence withdrawal, uncomplicated

CLINICAL PEARLS

- As compared to adult users, adolescents may experiment with many drugs, rather than identify a single drug of choice.
- As opposed to regular daily use, adolescents may demonstrate great variability in the use of drugs—periods of abstinence, interrupted by rapid transitions to binge-like consumption.

S

SUDDEN INFANT DEATH SYNDROME (SIDS)

Norman Lewak

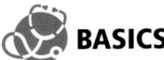 **BASICS**

DESCRIPTION

- Sudden infant death syndrome (SIDS) is the sudden death of an infant <1 year of age, which remains unexplained after a thorough case investigation, including performance of a complete autopsy, examination of the death scene, and review of the clinical history.
- SIDS always occurs during a sleep period.

EPIDEMIOLOGY

- Most common cause of death in postneonatal infancy
- Peak age of incidence: 2–4 months; uncommon after 6 months; rare before 2 weeks
- Incidence has been decreasing over the years:
  - 1970s: ~2.5 SIDS deaths per 1,000 live births
  - 1980s: ~1.4 per 1,000—reduced both by improved perinatal care and by identifying diseases that had appeared to be SIDS but were not (e.g., infant botulism)
  - 1992: "Back to Sleep" campaign started in the US with a subsequent reduction in the 1990s from 1.13 cases per 1,000 births in 1992 to 0.62 per 1,000 in 1999.
  - 2000s: Leveled off at 0.51 SIDS deaths per 1,000 live births
- Recurrence in families is rarely seen: There is no evidence for a genetic factor.

RISK FACTORS

Etiology unknown by definition; risk factors include:
- Male sex
- Poverty
- Poor prenatal care
- Low birth weight
- Prematurity
- Maternal smoking
- Maternal drug abuse
- Prone sleep position
- Exposure of infant to 2nd-hand smoke
- Exposure of infant to increased warmth
- Bed sharing with parent
- Soft bedding
- Nonuse of pacifier
- Although African American infants are at higher risk for SIDS, this is not thought to be related to genetic factors.

Genetics

- Genetic studies have been inconclusive in SIDS. However, most seem to agree that there are data to support a slight increased risk for SIDS siblings. The best explanation for this is that the populations studied, although all with a diagnosis of SIDS, were probably made up of varying subpopulations. It is likely that there is a large group of classic SIDS that is not genetic as well as much smaller populations made up of other entities.

- 2 of the previous subgroups already considered new diseases are medium-chain acylcoenzyme A dehydrogenase (MCAD) deficiency, a metabolic genetic entity, and infant botulism, a nongenetic environmental entity. There are probably other subgroups that will prove to have familial abnormalities, perhaps related to serotonin metabolism or the depth of sleep. There are probably also other environmental factors aside from the ones already noted as risk factors: Smoking, drugs, poverty, and prematurity. Whether new findings establish a new disease or simply establish the boundaries of a distinct subgroup will be argued, but if such divisions do arise, genetic counseling for the parents will be more accurate.

GENERAL PREVENTION

- Avoid maternal tobacco use and drug abuse during pregnancy.
- Avoid 2nd-hand smoke exposure to infant.
- Use supine (back) sleep position on a firm surface.
- Avoid overheating infant from excess room temperature, clothing, and/or bedding.
- Offer a pacifier to infant during sleep times. For those infants that are breastfeeding, introduce a pacifier after breastfeeding is well established.
- Encourage breastfeeding among expectant women and new mothers as it is associated with a reduced risk of SIDS.
- Apnea monitors or intercoms are not recommended for routine use, but may be indicated on a case-by-case basis for infants with a history of apnea or chronic disease associated with apnea. Apnea monitors have not been shown to be associated with a reduced risk of SIDS.

PATHOPHYSIOLOGY

- As a syndrome defined by only a limited number of similar epidemiologic and pathologic findings, it is not surprising that a number of recently described entities have been separated from the SIDS umbrella. These include infant botulism, MCAD deficiency, and long QT syndrome. Current thought supports a **"triple risk model" of SIDS**. This model envisions that SIDS occurs when a vulnerable infant during a vulnerable developmental period is stressed by an environmental challenge.
- Findings consistent with **biologic vulnerability** have been seen in SIDS. Tissue changes have been found in (research) postmortem exams of SIDS infants. Recently these changes have been related to a decrease of serotonin. Some investigators have postulated that these changes may be genetic; others point to the evidence that tobacco exposure to the fetus has been implicated in the brainstem changes. Also, many investigators have pointed out that prematurity, poverty, and poor nutrition during pregnancy, along with drug abuse, could probably join tobacco use in pregnancy as precursors of the brainstem pathology in the fetus.
- There is a **developmental vulnerable period** of brainstem control of respiration, which peaks at 2–4 months. During this transition period when control of respiration changes from an infantile to an adult pattern, it is postulated that a vulnerable infant is less likely to resume breathing during the usual apneas of infantile sleep—resulting in fatal obstructive apnea.

- Any theory on the pathophysiologic mechanism of the **environmental challenge** must explain how that theory relates to known risk factors. There are currently 2 major theories: Failure of arousal and carbon dioxide rebreathing:
  - Failure of arousal of a sleeping infant: It is postulated that deep sleep is the trigger for failure of the respiratory center during the vulnerable period. Even mildly increased warmth during sleep deepens the sleep; prone sleeping babies are warmer than supine ones; and soft bedding and/or sleeping in the parental bed increases the warmth. Also, not using a pacifier may cause deeper sleep.
  - Carbon dioxide rebreathing caused by prone sleeping in a soft bed or bed sharing could also affect the respiratory center
- Another commonality in SIDS is that there is obstructive apnea, long described as the "final common pathway" in all infants who carry the SIDS label:
  - Obstructive apnea is consistent with the intrathoracic petechiae found in SIDS infants.
  - This obstructive apnea can be related to an anomalous "dive reflex," postulated by some investigators to be the final event in SIDS. The "dive reflex" is seen in certain birds and amphibians as a protective mechanism when the animal dives into the water. Water in the airway causes laryngeal spasm (closure) to protect the lungs from the immersion. It is thought that infants are born with this residual phylogenetic tendency, which may be stimulated under certain conditions by saliva.

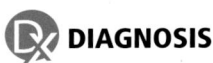 **DIAGNOSIS**

ALERT

- Being misled by the current concerns about missing child abuse. Physicians should be aware that in the infant whose death appears to be typical SIDS, the final diagnosis will be SIDS in ~80% of cases and only 3–6% will be attributable to child abuse.
- The physician should state clearly to the family that this death appears to be SIDS and give no suggestion that abuse is a consideration. In the families whose babies die of SIDS, even a hint of such suspicion can be devastating. If abuse is found later, nothing has been lost by initially treating that family as if their baby died of SIDS. This is also true in the ~15% in which another medical condition will be the final diagnosis.
- The Consumer Product Safety Commission, a federal agency, has added crib safety to its area of interest. They have joined with the American Academy of Pediatrics and Keeping Babies Safe to publicize a "Safe Sleep Initiative." Although their focus is generally on accidental morbidity and mortality from cribs (thus adding a new meaning to "crib death"), they have included supine (back) sleeping in their list of safe sleeping actions. Thus, preventing SIDS has been rightfully included in their initiative. However, this confluence of entities (which also includes "suffocation") adds unnecessary guilt to SIDS parents. Thus, once again physicians must be aware of the information that is disseminated to families in our society.

HISTORY

Previously healthy infant found dead during a time of sleep:

- Typical case: Between 1 and 6 months of age; no family history; no history of an apparent life-threatening event (ALTE); no history suggestive of child abuse; may have had an antecedent mild upper respiratory tract infection
- Atypical case (but still probably SIDS): Outside the typical age range; a family history of a sibling with SIDS; history of an ALTE; had a severe preexisting medical problem, but one that usually does not cause death

PHYSICAL EXAM

Normal-appearing infant without obvious reason for death:

- May have postmortem lividity and/or a pink, frothy discharge from the mouth or nose
- May have bruising from resuscitation attempts

DIAGNOSTIC TESTS & INTERPRETATION
Lab

These may be done as indicated:

- Toxicology screen
- Individual testing, such as test for infant botulism
- Skeletal survey: May reveal fresh rib fractures consistent with resuscitation attempts

Pathological Findings

A death scene review, review of the history, and a complete autopsy must be performed in all SIDS cases:

- External exam: Many have a pink, frothy discharge from the nose and mouth. May have bruising and/or fractured ribs from resuscitation attempts.
- Internal exam: Most have intrathoracic petechiae and some have mild pulmonary inflammatory changes (that are insufficient and not the cause of death)

DIFFERENTIAL DIAGNOSIS

Many proposed etiologies for "crib death" over the centuries have been proposed for sociopolitical purposes (i.e., society has difficulty accepting that healthy babies die for "no reason"):

- Various terms for proposed causes that are "mother blaming": overlying, suffocation, infanticide, and child abuse
- Proposed causes advanced to "absolve" the mother: Sepsis, pneumonia, heart disease, metabolic disease, an enlarged thymus (status thymolymphaticus)
- Of all unexpected infant deaths that appear clinically to be SIDS, ~15% will be caused by another medical condition:
  - Infections: Infant botulism, sepsis, myocarditis, overwhelming pneumonia
  - Metabolic disease: MCAD deficiency (a familial condition)
  - Cardiac arrhythmia: Long QT syndrome (a familial condition)

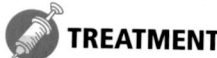 TREATMENT

ADDITIONAL TREATMENT
General Measures

- Resuscitation attempts by the 1st responders have proved to be futile by definition.
- Immediate physician management and follow-up
- Suggestions for a community SIDS plan (public health department; may be mandated by state law):
  - Autopsy in all infants who die suddenly and unexpectedly
  - Immediate results of initial autopsy findings given to family
  - Use of the term SIDS by coroner rather than the proxy terms of "undetermined," "unknown," or "sudden unexpected infant death" (SUID)
  - Continuing public health contact for the family
- Immediate physician management:
  - After taking the history and evaluating the physical findings, if it appears to be SIDS, the family should be told that "it looks like SIDS."
  - Explain to the family what happens in that community following such a death.
  - Provide immediate emotional support to the involved family members and others, including child care provider.
  - Ensure that the family has resources available during the immediate grief period.
  - Arrange physician follow-up within 2–3 days to discuss the initial autopsy results and the emotional status of the family.
- Ongoing management, follow family closely:
  - Inform family of the initial autopsy findings.
  - Inform family of the final autopsy report.
  - If the coroner uses a proxy term for SIDS, tell the family that some coroners are avoiding the term SIDS but that current pediatric practice warrants the SIDS terminology.
  - Refer family to a SIDS support group.
  - Continue contact with the family.
  - Refer family for emotional counseling as needed.
- Siblings (or any children who are close to the family) should not be forgotten. They should participate in all events around the death. They should be assured that this only happens to infants and that they (the sibling or other child) are in no way responsible. Be aware that siblings often get upset with this new infant who is "taking their place" and at such times "wish that the new infant would 'go away.'"

ADDITIONAL READING

- Beckwith JB. Defining the sudden infant death syndrome. *Arch Pediatr Adolesc Med.* 2003;157: 286–294.
- Blair PS, Fleming PJ. Recurrence risk of sudden infant death syndrome. *Arch Dis Child.* 2008; 93:267–270.

- Hauck FR, Omojokum DO, Siadaty MS, et al. Do pacifiers reduce the risk of sudden infant death syndrome? A meta-analysis. *Pediatrics.* 2005; 116:e716–e723.
- Lewak N. Prone sleeping is a risk for SIDS, not for suffocation. Available at: http://www.pediatricsdigest.mobi/content/128/5/1030/reply#pediatrics_el_51774.
- Malloy MH, MacDorman M. Changes in the classification of sudden unexpected infant deaths: United States, 1992–2001. *Pediatrics.* 2005; 115:1247–1253.
- Sahni R, Fifer WP, Myers MM. Identifying infants at risk for sudden infant death syndrome. *Curr Opin Pediatr.* 2007;19:145–149.
- SIDS and Other Sleep-Related Infant Deaths: Expansion of Recommendations for a Safe Infant Sleeping Environment 128(5):1030–1039. doi:10.1542/peds.2011–2284.

 CODES

ICD9
798.0 Sudden infant death syndrome

ICD10
R99 Ill-defined and unknown cause of mortality

FAQ

- Q: How does one tell the difference between SIDS and intentional suffocation?
- A: Victims of child abuse are usually identified by history or signs of previous abuse, such as old healed rib fractures on radiography, or signs of current abuse, such as bruises other than those related to resuscitation attempts. Although it is possible to suffocate an infant without leaving marks or other evidence, such an act would have to be premeditated. Because abusive parents act impulsively in fits of rage, this would not be consistent with a premeditated act of infanticide.
- Q: Does a 2nd SIDS death in a family indicate abuse?
- A: No. According to an American Academy of Pediatrics (AAP) report, 2nd SIDS deaths in a single family are SIDS in 87% of cases.
- Q: Do all families who experience a SIDS death require counseling?
- A: What they need above all else is an accurate diagnosis and explanation that their child's SIDS death was neither predictable nor preventable. All families also require support from other family members and friends. Being there to facilitate the (probably gradual) return of the normal activities of daily living is what others can do for them. This is the role for the SIDS support groups—not as counselors but as new friends who can understand what needs to be done. The SIDS support groups can be found through the state or local health department.
- Q: Is the flattened head from putting infants in a "back to sleep" position a reason for concern?
- A: The skull shape in almost all babies with a flattened occiput, positional plagiocephaly, almost always returns to a normal configuration by 1–2 years of age. Cosmetic surgery is possible but it is unclear if it is ever needed.

SUICIDE

Leonard J. Levine
Jonathan R. Pletcher

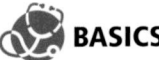 BASICS

DESCRIPTION
- Suicidal behavior is a voluntary self-harming act with the goal of ending one's own life.
- Attempted suicide occurs when the act does not succeed in its goal (also, failed or near-suicide).
- Suicidal ideation is any thought, with or without a specific plan, to end one's life.
- Suicidality can include suicidal ideation, preparatory acts, and/or attempts.

EPIDEMIOLOGY
- Suicide is the third leading cause of death for the 10–14, 15–20, and 20–24-year-old age groups.
- Adolescent mortality from suicide tripled between the 1950s and the 1990s.
- Females attempt suicide at a rate 2–4 times that of males. Females are most likely to attempt suicide through ingestion.
- Males 15–24 are 5 times as likely to die by suicide as females.
- Males are most likely to use more lethal methods, such as firearms and hanging, when attempting suicide.
- Completed suicide rates are highest in non-Hispanic white (13.5/100,000) and Native American (14.3/100,000) adolescents. Suicide rates for black males 10–19 years old doubled between the years 1980 and 1995.
- Gay, lesbian, bisexual, and questioning youth report higher rates of suicide thoughts and attempts than their heterosexual peers.

Incidence
- Annually in the US ~2,000 adolescents die from suicide and over a million suicide attempts come to medical attention; there as many as 11 times the number of attempts as completed suicides.
- Overall, suicide accounted for 6.9 deaths per 100,000 persons aged 15–19 years in 2007.
- In 2007, suicide accounted for 0.9 deaths per 100,000 persons aged 10–14 years, and 12.7 deaths per 100,000 persons aged 20–24 years.
- In 2009, 14% of youth surveyed in grades 9–12 reported seriously considering suicide at some point in the preceding year: >6% reported attempting suicide in the previous year.

RISK FACTORS
- Previous suicide attempt(s)
- Mood disorders
- Disruptive behavior
- Substance/alcohol abuse
- Family history of suicide
- Family history of mental illness or substance abuse
- History of sexual or physical abuse
- Family conflict or disruption
- Presence of firearms in the home

GENERAL PREVENTION
- Universal screening of all adolescents for suicidality and its primary root cause of depression should occur in primary and acute care settings. As many as 4 out of 5 adolescent suicide attempters were not identified by healthcare providers in the months leading up to the attempt.
- Brief, validated screening tools are available for medical settings.
- Warning signs, aside from obvious emotional distress, can include:
  - Chronic physical symptoms, with or without discrete physiologic etiology (e.g., chronic headache, abdominal pain)
  - Change in level of functioning in school, work, or home
  - Changes in mood or affect
  - Direct inquiry about suicidal ideation and plans
- If suicidal ideation is reported, components of risk assessment include the following:
  - Frequency and timing of suicidal thoughts
  - Active planning
  - Access to lethal means such as firearms
  - History of past suicide attempt(s)
  - History of mental health problems, including substance abuse, and treatment
  - Acute or anticipated psychosocial stressor
  - Family history of suicide
  - Family violence
  - Exploration of coping strategies and social support
- Referral or consultation with a psychiatrist or mental health professional is indicated with any question or risk for suicide attempt

PATHOPHYSIOLOGY
- Decreased central serotonergic activity may result in aggressive or impulsive behaviors, which may be aimed at oneself.
- An underlying psychiatric or personality disorder acutely worsened by a stressful life event may trigger a suicidal act.
- Feelings of isolation and lack of external support (particularly from caregivers) may result in hopelessness and despair.
- Suicide may be an impulsive act designed to punish loved ones or express frustration or rage. All suicidal behaviors must be carefully evaluated and taken seriously.

ETIOLOGY
Suicidal behavior in adolescents results from the interaction of longstanding individual and family conditions, social environment, and acute stressors:
- Psychiatric disorders:
  - Suicidal behavior is included in the diagnostic criteria for major depressive episode and borderline personality disorder (DSM-IVTR).
  - Additionally, psychotic disorders, conduct disturbance, adjustment disorder, and panic disorders have all been found to be associated with suicidal behavior.
- Intense emotional state, in particular shame or humiliation, can be "trigger events" for a suicidal act.
- Personality and social factors, such as antisocial behavior, aggressive or impulsive proclivities, and social isolation, can also contribute.

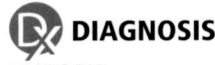 DIAGNOSIS

HISTORY
- The provider should sensitively ascertain if the patient has a weapon or access to lethal method of self-harm.
- A comprehensive history should always be obtained or reviewed by a trained mental health worker. Components of a comprehensive history include:
  - Method and timing (particularly if method is ingestion)
  - Lethality of attempt (e.g., number of pills, seriousness of physical injury)
  - Circumstances of attempt (e.g., remote site, public display)
  - History of prior attempts
  - Level of planning of attempt
  - Current affect and psychological status (e.g., feelings and/or level of depression, hopelessness, impulsivity, self-esteem)
  - Family consistency and dynamics
  - Pharmaceuticals available at home; what is missing
  - History of interpersonal conflict or personal loss
  - Family history of suicide
  - History of substance use
  - History of psychological disorder or disease state
  - History of abuse, neglect, or incest
  - Social supports and coping strategies
  - Feelings of regret or continued desire for self-harm
- The following historical information increases the risk for a future, potentially lethal suicide attempt:
  - History of potentially lethal attempt
  - Family history of suicide or attempted suicide
  - Unstable family structure
  - Poor social support system, lack of feeling connected

PHYSICAL EXAM
- Even without a history of ingestion, closely observe vital signs, skin, mucous membranes, and pupils for evidence of toxidrome.
- Examine the skin for signs of physical abuse or self-mutilation
- A complete neurologic examination is essential for the evaluation of intracranial processes, acute mental status changes, and ingestions.

DIAGNOSTIC TESTS & INTERPRETATION
Different laboratories offer different spectra and sensitivities in their toxicology screens.

Lab
- Serum and urine toxicology screens
- Urine pregnancy test to assess pregnancy as a potential precipitating factor and to recognize potential danger to the fetus
- Acetaminophen level, as it is highly hepatotoxic and is used frequently by teenagers
- EKG is indicated for many pharmacologic ingestions, including antidepressants and benzodiazepines.

Imaging
Abdominal plain film: If history of iron or vitamin ingestion, or severe trauma

DIFFERENTIAL DIAGNOSIS

- CNS trauma: Any insult to the cerebral cortex can result in disinhibitory behaviors.
- Psychiatric disorders, with particular attention to depression, personality disorder, and substance abuse
- Psychosocial trauma or maladjustment:
  – Emotional or physical abuse, with the suicide attempt being a way to gain attention, obtain help, or to serve as a means of escape
  – Feelings of isolation or abandonment, such as following the revelation of pregnancy or homosexuality

 TREATMENT

MEDICATION (DRUGS)

- For recent ingestions, GI decontamination with activated charcoal may be appropriate, as is the administration of pertinent antidotes (e.g., naloxone for opioids, N-acetylcysteine for acetaminophen).
- Although psychotherapy is an essential component to the care of the suicidal adolescent, pharmacotherapy with antidepressants can also play a role, especially given the high association with comorbid mood disorders.
  – Keep in mind when prescribing tricyclic antidepressants (TCAs) their high lethality potential. TCAs are typically not indicated in treating depression in children and adolescents.
  – Several SSRIs (fluoxetine, sertraline, and citalopram) have been shown to be effective in treating depressive disorders in adolescents. Use of SSRIs in patients with the potential for suicidal behavior requires close monitoring. In general, SSRIs may cause an increase from 1% to 2% in the risk of suicidality in depressed teens.

ADDITIONAL TREATMENT

General Measures

- Parents and professionals should avoid minimizing attempts as "not serious" or as "just seeking attention."
- Psychiatric disposition should be determined by, or in conjunction with, a mental health professional. Considerations for admission include the following:
  – Historical factors indicating high risk for repeated attempt
  – Ongoing suicidal ideation and/or planning
  – Family instability and lack of support
  – Altered mental status
  – Lack of alternative interventions (e.g., intensive psychiatric follow-up, day treatment program)
  – Medication initiation that has risk for increasing suicidal thoughts, e.g., SSRIs
- When discharge to a caregiver is being considered, the following minimal criteria should be in place at the time of discharge:
  – The patient reliably expresses regret and denies ongoing suicidal thoughts.
  – The patient is medically stable.
  – The patient's family is involved and reports understanding of the seriousness of the attempt.
  – The patient and parents agree to contact a health professional or go to the emergency department if suicidal intent recurs. The patient and family must have 24-hour access to mental health or physical health professionals.

– The patient must not have impaired mental status (e.g., severely depressed, psychoses, delirium, intoxication).
– Lethal methods of self-harm are not immediately available to the patient.
– Follow-up and treatment of underlying mental health disorders have been arranged. This ideally involves much more than providing a phone number to psychiatric services or asking the family to contact their insurer.
– Acute precipitants and crises have been addressed.
– Caregivers and patients are in agreement with the discharge plan.
– Barriers to obtaining follow-up treatment, in particular insurance and fear of stigma, have been addressed and will not preclude the next step toward ongoing treatment.

Additional Therapies

In addition to medication, important psychiatric interventions include acute, short-term, inpatient psychiatric hospitalization, partial hospitalization (with intensive treatment and support), and outpatient therapy.

IN-PATIENT CONSIDERATIONS

Initial Stabilization

- Circulation, airway, breathing (CABs)
- Monitoring of behavior and vital signs if history of ingestion. One-to-one monitoring is typically indicated until formal mental health evaluation is obtained.
- Decontamination of GI tract and circulation as indicated
- When available, a Poison Control Center may be helpful with evaluation and treatment of most drug ingestions.
- Ongoing safety is of primary concern: Provide immediate physical protection (remove all weapons) and enforce around-the-clock observation.

 ONGOING CARE

FOLLOW-UP RECOMMENDATIONS

Long-term psychotherapy (individual and family therapy) is often needed for adolescents who attempt suicide. Improvement may be slow and punctuated by frequent setbacks.

PROGNOSIS

- 20–50% of those attempting suicide will try again.
- Psychiatric hospitalization has not been shown to decrease risk of attempted suicide in patients with a history of mood disorder or substance abuse.
- Multiple reports show that a majority of adolescents who attempt suicide disengage with treatment after a few visits.

COMPLICATIONS

- Long-term organ damage or physical disability, depending on the method used
- Long-lasting emotional scars in families of victims, resulting from frustration, anger, and guilt
- Repeat suicide attempt or completion

ADDITIONAL READING

- Centers for Disease Control and Prevention, Youth Risk Behavior Survey. http://www.cdc.gov/HealthyYouth/yrbs/pdf/us_overview_yrbs.pdf [Accessed February 27, 2011].
- Horowitz LM, Ballard ED, Pao M. Suicide screening in schools, primary care and emergency departments. *Curr Opin Pediatr*. 2009;21:620–627.
- National Institute of Mental Health. http://www.nimh.nih.gov/health/publications/suicide-in-the-us-statistics-and-prevention/index.shtml#intro [Accessed February 29, 2011].
- Shain BN, American Academy of Pediatrics Committee on Adolescence and the American Academy of Child and Adolescent Psychiatry. Suicide and suicide attempts in adolescents. *Pediatrics*. 2007;120(3):669–676.
- Williams SB, O'Connor EA, Eder M, et al. Screening for child and adolescent depression in primary care settings: A systemic evidence review for the US Preventive Services Task Force. *Pediatrics*. 2009;123:e716–e735.

 CODES

ICD9

- 300.9 Unspecified nonpsychotic mental disorder
- V62.84 Suicidal ideation

ICD10

- R45.851 Suicidal ideations
- T14.91 Suicide attempt
- Z91.5 Personal history of self-harm

FAQ

- Q: Should I ever keep suicide attempts or plans confidential?
- A: No. The limits of confidentiality should be clearly outlined to patients and families at the first visit or early in the patient's adolescence. These limits include anything that will directly place the patient's life in danger, such as suicidal intent, ongoing or recent abuse, or homicidal intentions.
- Q: If I directly question my patients about suicide, won't that put the idea in their head?
- A: No. In the majority of cases, patients will be relieved by having a professional who wants to talk about suicide. There is only risk in asking if nothing is done with the answer. Appropriate referral to mental health services or counseling will save patients' lives.
- Q: Is a patient who is engaging in self-injurious behavior but denies suicidal ideation actually suicidal?
- A: Certainly any adolescent who is practicing self-mutilation to cope with emotional distress is at risk of developing additional unhealthy coping behaviors. Furthermore, they are likely suffering from a mood disorder that places them at risk for developing suicidality. There is no evidence to support management of self-injurious behavior as if the patient has a secret agenda.

SUPERIOR MESENTERIC ARTERY SYNDROME

Henry Lin
Tracie Wong
Vera de Matos (5th edition)

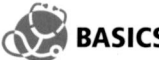 **BASICS**

DESCRIPTION
Superior mesenteric artery (SMA) syndrome is extrinsic obstruction of the distal duodenum by the superior mesenteric artery or its branches; it is also called Wilkie syndrome, cast syndrome, or aortomesenteric duodenal compression syndrome.

EPIDEMIOLOGY
Incidence
- Rare, incidence in general population between 0.013% and 0.3% (based on GI barium series)
- More common in adolescents and following corrective scoliosis surgery
  - Increased incidence rate following scoliosis surgery of 0.5–2.4%

ETIOLOGY
- The superior mesenteric artery arises from the aorta at the L1 vertebral body level and forms an acute downward aortomesenteric angle that is normally between 25–60°.
- The third portion of the duodenum lies within the aortomesenteric angle and narrowing of the angle (6–25°) can lead to duodenal compression by the SMA anteriorly and the vertebra posteriorly.
- Any factor that narrows the aortomesenteric angle can cause duodenal compression. Common conditions that predispose to narrowing of this angle are:
  - Illnesses associated with significant weight loss leading to loss of the mesenteric fat pad
    ○ Anorexia nervosa, malignancy, spinal cord injury, trauma or burns
  - Rapid linear growth in children
  - Increase in lordosis of the back, such as from immobilization by body cast, scoliosis surgery, or prolonged bed rest in a supine position
    ○ Weight percentile for height of <5% is a risk factor for development of SMA syndrome following scoliosis surgery.
  - Variations of the ligament of Treitz: A short ligament lifts the third or fourth part of the duodenum into the narrower segment in the aortomesenteric angle.

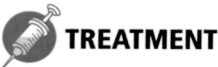 **DIAGNOSIS**

HISTORY
- Clinical presentation can be acute or chronic with gradual, progressive symptoms.
- Symptoms are generally consistent with proximal small bowel obstruction, including the following:
  - Nausea, vomiting (bilious and nonbilious), postprandial nausea and vomiting, epigastric abdominal pain, eructation, weight loss, early satiety, dehydration, bloating, failure to thrive

PHYSICAL EXAM
- Nonspecific findings of small bowel obstruction include the following:
  - Abdominal distension
  - Succussion splash
  - High-pitched bowel sounds
- No pathognomoic signs or symptoms, but a history of weight loss, immobilization, or back surgery followed by symptoms of early satiety, bloating, and vomiting after meals would suggest the diagnosis.

Imaging
- Imaging should show duodenal obstruction with dilated stomach and proximal duodenum, active peristalsis, and a narrow angle between the aorta and the SMA.
- Abdominal radiograph is usually the initial diagnostic imaging test.
  - Findings can be nonspecific, but may also reveal suggestive findings of obstruction including a distended stomach or a dilated proximal duodenum with a sharp cutoff of the third portion of the duodenum where the SMA crosses the duodenum
- Additional evaluation with upper gastrointestinal series.
  - Passage of contrast is typically delayed and often stops at the third portion of the duodenum. Contrast passes when the patient is moved to a prone position, where gravity will increase the aortomesenteric angle
  - Similar findings can be seen with CT

- Additional imaging may be required if the diagnosis remains unclear.
  - Superior mesenteric arteriography with simultaneous barium contrast radiography to show SMA superimposed on duodenum.
  - CT and MR angiography have now replaced superior mesenteric arteriography.
- Determination of the aortomesenteric angle in severe cases may help with decision for surgery.

DIFFERENTIAL DIAGNOSIS
- Causes of small bowel obstruction
  - Luminal obstruction: Foreign body
  - Intramural obstruction: Duplication cyst, web, tumor, bezoar, stricture
  - Extramural obstruction: Tumor, annular pancreas, bands, adhesions, volvulus, intussusception
- Duodenal dysmotility
  - Intrinsic neuronal disorder, muscular weakness (holovisceral myopathy, diabetes), fibrosis (scleroderma, lupus retroperitoneal fibrosis), collagen vascular diseases, chronic idiopathic intestinal pseudo-obstruction
- Anorexia nervosa/bulimia

TREATMENT

General Measures
- Correct fluid and electrolyte imbalances
- Decompress obstruction
  - Insert nasogastric tube to decompress stomach and proximal duodenum
- Feed to improve nutrition and weight gain
  - Feeding in a prone position may help, but may require a jejunal tube to bypass the obstruction
  - Decreasing viscosity of feedings has a theoretical advantage

- If a patient had recent spinal surgery:
  - Frequent repositioning of patients in body casts
  - Reversal of back surgery may be necessary in some patients
- Surgery is typically unnecessary and only indicated if supportive care is ineffective. Usually performed in patients with a prolonged history of weight loss or pronounced duodenal dilation
  - Surgery options include duodenojejunostomy, Roux-en-Y duodenojejunostomy, gastrojejunostomy, and anterior transposition of the third part of the duodenum.
- Definitive treatment is aimed at correcting the precipitating factor.

 ONGOING CARE

PROGNOSIS
- Delay in diagnosis of SMA syndrome can result in electrolyte disturbances, dehydration and malnutrition, and in severe cases, possible intestinal perforation or death.
- Most patients do not require surgery and improve with supportive care alone.

ADDITIONAL READING

- Agrawal GA, Johnson PT, Fishman EK. Multidetector row CT of superior mesenteric artery syndrome. *J Clin Gastroenterol*. 2007;41:62–65.
- Jain R. Superior mesenteric artery syndrome. *Curr Treat Options Gastroenterol*. 2007;10:24–27.
- Kadji M, Naouri A, Bernard P. Superior mesenteric artery syndrome: A case report. *Ann Chir*. 2006;131:389–392.
- Kim IY, Cho NC, Kim DS, et al. Laparoscopic duodenojejunostomy for management of superior mesenteric artery syndrome: Two case reports and a review of the literature. *Yonsei Med J*. 2003;44:526–529.
- Kurbegov A, Grabb B, Bealer J. Superior mesenteric artery syndrome in a 16 year-old with bilious emesis. *Curr Opin Pediatr*. 2010;22:664–667.
- Okugawa Y, Mikihiro I, Uchida K, et al. Superior mesenteric artery syndrome in an infant: case report and literature review. *J Pediatr Surg*. 2007;42:E5–E8.
- Schwartz A. Scoliosis, superior mesenteric artery syndrome, and adolescents. *Orthop Nurs*. 2007;26:19–24.
- Scovell S, Hamdan A. Superior mesenteric artery syndrome. In: Basow, DS, ed., *UpToDate*, Waltham, MA: UpToDate; 2011.
- Stamatakos M, Kontzoglou K, Stefanaki C, et al. Wilkie syndrome. What is this? *Chirurgia (Bucur)*. 2009;104:11–15.
- Welsch T, Büchler MW, Kienle P. Recalling superior mesenteric artery syndrome. *Dig Surg*. 2007;24:149–156.

 CODES

ICD9
557.1 Chronic vascular insufficiency of intestine

ICD10
K55.1 Chronic vascular disorders of intestine

FAQ

- Q: When the diagnosis of superior mesenteric artery syndrome is suspected, what are the next steps in management?
- A: The logical sequence is to confirm the diagnosis with an imaging study such as an upper GI contrast study and also to initiate supportive care of refeeding and mobilization.
- Q: The following treatment modalities are known to be useful in treatment of superior mesenteric artery syndrome: Do nothing, or feed with a jejunal tube, a liquid diet, prone feeding, or total parenteral nutrition. Which program works?
- A: All of the above have been used in superior mesenteric artery syndrome. Weight gain has also been accomplished with total parenteral nutrition.
- Q: Does radiographic testing or a feeding clinical trial help in confirming the diagnosis?
- A: Yes, it may be helpful to confirm the diagnosis and look at the aortomesenteric angle with a CT or MR angiography. In addition, a clinical trial of feeding and weight gain often becomes the criterion for confirmation of the diagnosis.

S

SUPRAVENTRICULAR TACHYCARDIA

Francesca Byrne
Jonathan R. Kaltman (5th edition)

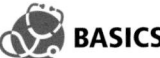

BASICS

DESCRIPTION
- Supraventricular tachycardia (SVT) is a tachycardia originating at or above the atrioventricular (AV) node. The heart rate in infants generally ranges from 220–320 beats per minute (bpm) and in older children from 150–250 bpm.
- Most infants and children with SVT have structurally normal hearts.
- Of patients who present in infancy, 40–70% will be asymptomatic by 1 year of age. However, ~1/3 of these patients may experience a reappearance of their tachycardia at an average age of 8 years. Most older children who present with SVT will have persistent recurrence of their tachycardia.

EPIDEMIOLOGY
- SVT is the most common arrhythmia in childhood.
- 50–60% of pediatric patients present in the 1st year of life.

RISK FACTORS
Genetics
- Wolff-Parkinson-White (WPW) syndrome has been noted in several families, and an autosomal dominant mode of inheritance has been demonstrated:
  - ~20% of cases of WPW have associated congenital heart disease, with Ebstein anomaly, L-looped transposition of the great arteries, and hypertrophic cardiomyopathy being the most common.
- ~50% of the cases of junctional ectopic tachycardia occur in a familial setting with an autosomal dominant mode of inheritance.

PATHOPHYSIOLOGY
There are 2 major mechanisms for SVT:
- Re-entry tachycardia: This is the most common mechanism for SVT. It involves a circuit rhythm within the atria (atrial flutter), within the AV node (AV nodal re-entry tachycardia), or using an accessory pathway (AV re-entrant tachycardia). Re-entrant tachycardias are characterized by sudden onset and termination, regular rate, and responsiveness to pacing maneuvers and direct current cardioversion.
- Automatic tachycardia: Automaticity refers to a cell's or group of cell's enhanced ability to spontaneously depolarize, which can overdrive suppress the sinus node. Examples are ectopic atrial tachycardia, multifocal atrial tachycardia, and junctional ectopic tachycardia. Automatic tachycardias are characterized by warm-up and cool-down phases, an irregular rate that is sensitive to the body's catecholamine state, and lack of responsiveness to pacing and cardioversion.

ETIOLOGY
SVT can frequently be precipitated by exercise, infection, fever, or drug exposure (e.g., cold medications).

COMMONLY ASSOCIATED CONDITIONS
- SVT is commonly observed in patients who have undergone surgery for congenital heart disease.
- SVT is frequently observed after the Mustard/Senning procedure, the Fontan operation, and repair of an atrial septal defect.

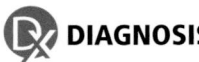

DIAGNOSIS

HISTORY
- Infants will manifest signs and symptoms of low cardiac output if the tachycardia has gone unnoticed for a prolonged period: Findings may include tachypnea, retractions, irritability, decreased feeding, excessive sweating, hypotension, poor perfusion, and decreased urine output. Most infants with tachycardia for >48 hours present with evidence of congestive heart failure.
- The toddler and older child may experience palpitations, shortness of breath, chest pain, and dizziness or syncope:
  - It is important to know what the child was doing at the time the arrhythmia started and whether the rhythm had an abrupt onset and termination.
  - Older children often report being able to terminate episodes of tachycardia by performing a vagal maneuver (e.g., Valsalva, gagging, or standing on their head).

PHYSICAL EXAM
The following need to be assessed in all patients presenting with SVT:
- Heart rate
- Respiratory rate
- BP
- Hydration status
- Peripheral perfusion
- Liver size
- Mental status
- Presence of gallop rhythm on auscultation

DIAGNOSTIC TESTS & INTERPRETATION
Imaging
A chest radiograph may reveal cardiomegaly if there is CHF or underlying structural heart disease.

Diagnostic Procedures/Other
- Diagnosis is made by recording an electrocardiogram during the arrhythmia. This can be accomplished with a 12-lead electrocardiogram, 24-hour Holter recording, or transtelephonic event monitor.
- Patients with WPW syndrome have diagnostic ventricular pre-excitation (short PR interval and a delta wave) on the surface electrocardiogram during sinus rhythm.
- An exercise stress test and/or electrophysiologic testing may be indicated in older patients with WPW syndrome to help determine the risk of rapid conduction through the accessory pathway.
- Nonpharmacologic maneuvers (ice, vagal) and pharmacologic maneuvers (e.g., IV adenosine, 50–300 mcg/kg/dose) may distinguish tachycardias that involve the AV node from other types of SVT.

DIFFERENTIAL DIAGNOSIS
- Narrow-complex SVT needs to be distinguished from sinus or junctional tachycardia and sick-sinus syndrome with tachyarrhythmia.
- Structural heart disease should be excluded in all cases of newly diagnosed SVT.
- Wide-complex tachycardia from either aberrantly conducted SVT or SVT with antegrade conduction down an accessory pathway can be seen in a small percentage of patients and may be difficult to distinguish from ventricular tachycardia. Generally, unless there are preexisting data that the patient has SVT, wide-complex tachycardia should always be interpreted as ventricular tachycardia until proven otherwise.
- Differentiating between types of SVT (re-entrant vs. automatic) can be accomplished by evaluating the regularity of the rate, modes of onset and termination, and the tachycardia's responsiveness to pacing and cardioversion.

TREATMENT

ADDITIONAL TREATMENT
General Measures
- Re-entrant SVT:
  - In a stable child, adenosine (IV rapid bolus, 0.1 mg/kg and may increase by 0.1 mg/kg to a maximum of 0.3 mg/kg) 50–300 mcg/kg) may be used to block the AV node and achieve pharmacologic cardioversion for re-entrant SVT that requires the AV node as part of the circuit. The half-life of the drug is <10 seconds. Because of the risk of atrial fibrillation, DC cardioversion should be available for back-up. Use adenosine with caution in patients with asthma as it can cause acute bronchospasm.

– Verapamil should be avoided for acute treatment of SVT in children <12 months of age because of its vasodilating and negative inotropic effect.
– Nonpharmacologic vagal maneuvers, including ice to the face without obstructing respiration, Valsalva, gag, and headstand, may be helpful. In younger children, Valsalva can be achieved by having the child blow into an obstructed straw or thumb. Pacing maneuvers via an esophageal catheter may also be used.
– Oral digoxin is an option in patients with hemodynamically stable SVT needing chronic therapy. Digoxin, however, is contraindicated in patients with WPW because it may potentiate faster conduction down the accessory pathway, making ventricular fibrillation more likely in some patients.
– β-Blockers (propranolol or nadolol) are the treatment of choice in individuals with WPW. Procainamide and amiodarone may be used in cases that are more resistant. β-Blockers are usually given to patients with exercise-induced SVT.
– Atrial flutter may be treated with digoxin, procainamide, sotalol, or amiodarone as a single agent or in combination.
– Catheter ablation using radiofrequency energy or cryoenergy is an alternative to long-term drug therapy and may be used for the following reasons:
  ○ SVT refractory to medical therapy
  ○ Side effects from the medical regimen
  ○ Patient choice
  ○ Life-threatening arrhythmias
  ○ Rapid conduction properties of an accessory pathway (e.g., WPW)
  ○ Concomitant congenital or acquired heart disease
• Automatic SVT: Automatic tachycardias may be responsive to antiarrhythmics such as procainamide, flecainide (should generally be avoided if the patient has structural heart disease), amiodarone, or β-blockers either alone or in different combinations. Ectopic atrial tachycardia and junctional ectopic tachycardia are also amenable to catheter ablation.

IN-PATIENT CONSIDERATIONS
Initial Stabilization
• Always assess the child's ABCs (airway, breathing, and circulation).
• Initial management of SVT depends on the child's hemodynamic condition.
• Presentation with cardiovascular collapse warrants treatment with synchronized DC cardioversion (0.5–2.0 J/kg).

 ## ONGOING CARE
FOLLOW-UP RECOMMENDATIONS
• As SVT may recur, neonates and infants generally should receive maintenance therapy for the 1st year of life and then be observed off medications if they are not having breakthrough episodes of SVT.
• Patients with recurrences in the 1st year of life or those requiring multiple medications may ultimately have their medications discontinued if they have a prolonged period of time without episodes.
• In children who present beyond infancy, spontaneous resolution of the tachycardia substrate is less likely, and treatment may need to be continued into adulthood. These patients may be considered for catheter ablation therapy.
• Over-the-counter sympathomimetic cold medications and caffeine should be avoided, as they may increase the likelihood of SVT

COMPLICATIONS
Complications from SVT can arise from 1 of 3 causes:
• Persistent tachycardia can lead to CHF and cardiovascular collapse. This is especially true of the infant whose symptoms go unrecognized for 24–48 hours.
• Some patients with WPW syndrome (<5%) can have rapid conduction through the accessory pathway. A rapid ventricular response to atrial flutter/fibrillation can potentially cause ventricular fibrillation and sudden death. Patients with WPW syndrome who receive digoxin and/or verapamil are at increased risk.
• Side effects of pharmacologic agents used to treat SVT include bradycardia, other arrhythmias due to proarrhythmic effects (digoxin, procainamide, amiodarone, flecainide), and noncardiac side effects (GI, liver, pulmonary, and thyroid dysfunction).

ADDITIONAL READING
• Drago F. Paediatric catheter cryoablation: Techniques, successes and failures. *Curr Opin Cardiol.* 2008;23(2):81–84.
• Fox DJ, Tischenko A, Krahn AD, et al. Supraventricular tachycardia: Diagnosis and management. *Mayo Clin Proc.* 2008;83(12):1400–1411.
• Friedman RA, Walsh EP, Silka MJ, et al. Radiofrequency catheter ablation in children with and without congenital heart disease. *Pacing Clin Electrophysiol.* 2002;25:1000–1017.
• Manole E, Saladino RA. Emergency department management of the pediatric patient with supraventricular tachycardia. *Pediatr Emerg Care.* 2007;23(3):176–185.
• Paul T, Bertram H, Bökenkamp R, et al. Supraventricular tachycardia in infants, children and adolescents: Diagnosis, and pharmacological and interventional therapy. *Paediatr Drugs.* 2000;2:171–181.

 ## CODES

ICD9
• 426.7 Anomalous atrioventricular excitation
• 427.89 Other specified cardiac dysrhythmias

ICD10
• I45.6 Pre-excitation syndrome
• I47.1 Supraventricular tachycardia

FAQ
• Q: How should infants on chronic therapy be monitored?
• A: Parents with infants on chronic therapy for SVT should be educated about counting the heart rate by palpation or auscultation at least 1 or 2 times daily. This method of surveillance is just as effective as apnea/bradycardia monitors. Because alarm monitors can increase parental anxiety with frequent false alarms, they are generally not recommended.
• Q: What is the concern with verapamil?
• A: Verapamil is an L-type calcium channel blocker that blocks conduction in the AV node and is very effective in treating SVT in adults. Because myocardial contractility in infants depends mostly on the trans-sarcolemmal L-type calcium channels, hypotension and cardiovascular collapse have been reported in children <1 year of age.
• Q: What are the indications, success rates, and risks of catheter ablation?
• A: Refractory arrhythmias, the need for multiple medications, undesirable side effects from the medications, life-threatening events (syncope, cardiac arrest), wide-complex tachycardia (cannot differentiate SVT from VT), and elective ablation are some of the indications. The success rate of radiofrequency catheter ablation varies from 80–97%, depending on the location of the bypass tract or ectopic focus. The incidence of major complications is <2%, with the most common being heart block requiring a pacemaker, cardiac perforation, brachial plexus injury, and embolization. The risk of complete heart block is greater in patients whose accessory pathway is located close to the AV node. In such patients, cryoablation is a safer ablation technique because of its potentially reversible electrical and thermal effects.

S

SYMPATHOMIMETIC POISONING

Robert J. Hoffman
Doug Finefrock
Yuki Yasaka (5th edition)

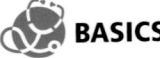 **BASICS**

DESCRIPTION

- Excess autonomic stimulation by adrenergic agents produces the clinical syndrome typically described as "sympathomimetic."
- Overdose from sympathomimetic agents occurs secondary to the use of prescription drugs, nonprescription drugs such as OTC cold medicine (e.g., pseudoephedrine), dietary supplements (e.g., ephedra, synephrine) and illicit drugs such as cocaine, amphetamine, and methamphetamine.
- The sequelae of sympathomimetic overdose are generally related to the neurological and cardiovascular systems.
- Severe problems may include agitation-induced hyperthermia, cardiac dysrhythmia, hypertension, myocardial ischemia and infarction; CVA; seizure; and cardiovascular collapse.

EPIDEMIOLOGY

- Cocaine, methamphetamine, and MDMA (ecstasy) are the 3 most common illicit stimulant drugs causing emergency visits in the US.
- Prescription stimulants such as methylphenidate and albuterol are often are frequent causes of intentional as well as unintentional poisoning.

RISK FACTORS

- Prescription sympathomimetics, such as methylphenidate, pose some risk factor for both the recipient of the prescription as well as siblings.
- Adolescents are at increased risk for using drugs of abuse.

PATHOPHYSIOLOGY

- Relevant pathophysiology is based on the adrenergic receptor type stimulated by the drug in question. The adrenergic receptors of relevance include $\alpha 1$, $\beta 1$, and $\beta 2$ receptors.
- Ephedrine and pseudoephedrine stimulate both α and β receptors:
  - Excessive cardiovascular stimulation results in symptoms qualitatively similar to those that occur with catecholamines.
  - Ephedrine and pseudoephedrine have weaker penetration of the CNS relative to drugs of abuse.
  - As a result, users may suffer from systemic complications of the relatively larger doses necessary to achieve the CNS "high" of other stimulants.
- Nonelective β-adrenergic agonists
- Isoproterenol, rarely used, is the prototypical nonselective β-agonist causing the following:
  - Tachycardia, hypotension, tachydysrhythmia, myocardial ischemia and flushing due to its cardiostimulatory and vasodilatory properties
  - Commonly CNS effects of anxiety, fear, and headache occur.

- Selective $\beta 2$ adrenergic agonists are commonly used, and these include albuterol, levalbuterol, salmeterol, terbutaline, and others.
- Common adverse effects include the following:
  - Tachycardia, palpitations, and tremor
  - Hypotension, often with widened pulse pressure
  - Nausea, vomiting, and sometimes diarrhea
  - Hyperglycemia and hypokalemia
  - Elevation of CPK as well as troponin, though myocardial infarction is never expected to occur in otherwise healthy children with selective $\beta 2$ agonist exposure.
  - Anxiety, fear, and headache also may occur.
- $\alpha 1$ selective agonists include phenylephrine and phenylpropanolamine, though the latter is no longer commercially produced in any meaningful quantity in the US.
  - Hypertension due to direct vasoconstrictive effects is the most common effect.
  - Reflex bradycardia may occur, particularly with phenylpropanolamine.
  - Headache due to elevated BP and even CVA may occur.

ETIOLOGY

Causative agents:

- Agents with combined α- and β-adrenergic activity: Epinephrine, norepinephrine, dopamine, ephedrine, and pseudoephedrine
- $\alpha 1$ adrenergic agonists: Phenylephrine, phenylpropanolamine
- β-adrenergic agonists: Nonselective β-agonist isoproterenol
- Selective $\beta 1$ agonists: Dobutamine
- Selective $\beta 2$ agonists: Albuterol, salmeterol, terbutaline, ritodrine
- OTC agents: Ephedrine-containing cold medicine, ephedra, Ma Huang
- Illicit drugs: Cocaine, amphetamine, methamphetamine, MDMA (ecstasy)
- Theophylline and caffeine may cause a clinical syndrome of sympathomimetic poisoning.

COMMONLY ASSOCIATED CONDITIONS

- Many sympathomimetic agents are capable of producing psychiatric symptoms, particularly psychosis.
- This psychosis is similar to or indistinguishable from schizophrenia.
- 2 rare results of MDMA use include serotonin syndrome and SIADH with symptomatic hyponatremia.

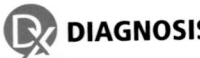 **DIAGNOSIS**

SIGNS AND SYMPTOMS

- The clinical effects of these agents' overdose vary based on their receptor selectivity.
- Most agents have some degree of combined α- and β-adrenergic activity (ephedrine, pseudoephedrine).
  - Hypertension, tachycardia, dysrhythmia, acute coronary syndromes, pulmonary edema and cerebrovascular injury, anxiety, a sense of impeding doom, apprehension, fear, and headache may occur.
  - At very high doses, agents cross the blood–brain barrier, which results in central nervous system symptoms, such as headache, seizures, and intracranial hemorrhage.

HISTORY

- History of exposure may be helpful, but is often unavailable or deliberately concealed, particularly use of illicit drugs such as cocaine, methamphetamine, and ecstasy.
- The use of OTC medicines, such as multisymptom cold preparations or dietary supplements may be obtained.
- High suspicion of sympathomimetic overdose especially in patients with the sympathomimetic toxidrome.
- The onset of symptoms usually occurs within 1 hour.
  - Typically, prescription and OTC sympathomimetic agents are inhaled or orally administered.
  - Inhalation or injection results in immediate symptoms.
  - Cocaine, amphetamine, and methamphetamine or the sympathomimetics most commonly used in this manner.
  - Sympathomimetic toxicity following ingestion typically peaks 1–4 hours and last 4–8 hours, but sustained-release preparations may alter this time course.

PHYSICAL EXAM

Sympathomimetic toxicity is a clinical diagnosis.

- Vital sign derangement is the most common and most reliable indicator of toxicity.
- Mental status changes are also common though less reliable as they do not occur with the same regularity and may be the result of toxicologic or psychiatric phenomenon.
- The patient's general appearance (e.g., agitation, diaphoretic, delirium, psychotic) is often suggestive of toxicity.
- HEENT: Headache, mydriasis, visual changes, epistaxis

- Chest: Chest pain due to dysrhythmia, myocardial ischemia, myocardial infarction, etc. may be a complaint.
- Tachycardia and hypertension are the most common vital sign abnormalities.
- Skin: Diaphoresis, flushing, the track marks associated with IV drug use.
- CNS: Focal neurologic findings may occur. Focal cranial nerve abnormalities are particularly concerning for the possibility of cerebrovascular accident. CNS stimulation or agitation is very common.

DIAGNOSTIC TESTS & INTERPRETATION
- Sympathomimetic overdose is a clinical diagnosis and assays are only adjunctive.
- Unless there are specific forensic indications, such as malicious poisoning or child abuse, drug of abuse screening is not recommended and is not useful.
- Serum acetaminophen level should be considered in patients with ingestion with intent of self harm.
- The measurement of electrolytes, BUN, creatinine, and blood sugar may be useful.
- Cardiac markers (e.g., CPK-MB, troponin) are appropriate to screen for cardiac injury.
- An EKG should be obtained to assess for ischemia as well as dysrhythmias

Imaging
A noncontrast head CT should be obtained in unresponsive patients or those with focal neurologic deficits.

DIFFERENTIAL DIAGNOSIS
- Hyperthyroidism/Thyroid storm
- Anticholinergic syndrome
- Pheochromocytoma
- Withdrawal syndromes
- Mania
- Subarachnoid hemorrhage
- Serotonin syndrome
- Neuroleptic malignant syndrome
- Other situations of increased endogenous catecholamine release

TREATMENT

INITIAL STABILIZATION
Managing ABCs should be addressed first, but sympathomimetic toxicity usually does not result in illness requiring any specific airway, breathing, or circulation issues.

General Measures
Maintaining vital signs within acceptable limits and controlling patient agitation are commonly required.
- Managing ABCs is paramount.
- If protocol permits, sedation of agitated patients with a benzodiazepine may be appropriate.
- Use of benzodiazepines is helpful to address both cardiovascular stimulation as well as psychomotor agitation.
- Use of specific cardiovascular medications may be needed.
- Use of antipsychotics, such as haloperidol or droperidol, is relatively contraindicated both because these medications may lower seizure threshold, impair heat dissipation, and increase risk of cardiac dysrhythmia.

SPECIAL THERAPY
- Severe hyperthermia should be treated with active cooling.

- Patients with core temperature of $\geq 107°$F should be placed in an ice bath and have core temperature monitored.

IV Fluids
- Unless there is a contraindication, at least maintenance IV fluid should be administered.
- This may serve to protect against rhabdomyolysis as well as potential dehydration that may occur with stimulant exposure.

MEDICATION (DRUGS)
Agitation, vasoconstrictive effects, chronotropic and inotropic effects, and psychomotor agitation are the most common issues requiring mediation therapy for sympathomimetic toxicity.

First Line
- Psychomotor agitation may be managed with benzodiazepines.
- The quantity of benzodiazepine required will directly depend on degree of adrenergic stimulation.
- In some cases, large doses may be required for sedation.
  - Lorazepam in doses of 0.1 mg/kg IV q15min titrated to effect is preferred due to predictable duration of action.
  - Diazepam 0.1 mg/kg IV q15min titrated to effect may also be used.
- Vasoconstrictive effects may be managed with a variety of medications.
  - Phentolamine 0.1 mg/kg/dose (up to 5 mg/dose) IV repeated q10min PRN
  - A dihydropyridine calcium channel blocker, such as nifedipine or amlodipine, may be used.
  - Sodium nitroprusside 0.3–10 mcg/kg/min IV, titrated to effect
- Chronotropic and inotropic effects may be managed with conduction-modulating calcium channel blockers such as diltiazem or verapamil.

Second Line
- A β-blocker may be used only if an α-adrenergic antagonist is concomitantly administered.
- Use of a β-blocker without α-adrenergic blockade may result in paradoxical increase in BP and death.
  - Labetalol has some α-adrenergic blockade and may be used alone as a second-line agent: 0.2–0.5 mg/kg/dose IV, maximal dose 20 mg, followed by infusion of 0.25–1 mg/kg/h
  - Esmolol: 500 mcg/kg/min IV bolus followed by infusion 50 mcg/kg/min titrated to effect up to 500 mcg/kg/min
- Severe cardiovascular symptoms resulting from β-agonists or methylxanthines such as theophylline or caffeine may be treated with a β-blocker.
  - This treatment may seem counter-intuitive in the management of hypotension.
  - Severe $\beta2$ agonist effects resulting in hypotension may be counteracted by using a β-blocker.
  - Such therapy should only be undertaken under the direction of a medical toxicologist, intensivist, or other clinician familiar with and experienced with use of such cardiovascular medications.

ONGOING CARE

DISPOSITION
Admission Criteria
Any patient with severely deranged vital signs, end-organ manifestations such as chest pain, severe headache, focal neurologic deficit, or agitation should be admitted.

Discharge Criteria
Any patient with vital signs within safe limits, normal mental status, and no evidence of end-organ damage or manifestations may be discharged from the emergency department or inpatient unit.

PROGNOSIS
If end-organ damage such as myocardial infarction or CVA are prevented, prognosis for full recovery to premorbid status is excellent.

COMPLICATIONS
The most common catastrophic complications are cardiovascular, including dysrhythmia, myocardial infarction, and CVA.

ADDITIONAL READING

- Carr BC. Efficacy, abuse, and toxicity of over-the-counter cough and cold medicines in the pediatric population. *Curr Opin Pediatr*. 2006;18(2):184–188.
- Haller CA, Meier KH, Olson KR. Seizures reported in association with use of dietary supplements. *Clin Toxicol (Phila)*. 2005;43(1):23–30.
- Haynes JF Jr. Medical management of adolescent drug overdoses. *Adolesc Med Clin*. 2006;17(2):353–379.
- Kuehn BM. Citing serious risks, FDA recommends no cold and cough medicines for infants. *JAMA*. 2008;299(8):887–888.
- Thirthalli J, Benegal V. Psychosis among substance users. *Curr Opin Psychiatry*. 2006;19(3):239–245.

CODES

ICD9
971.2 Amphetamine or related acting sympathomimetic abus

ICD10
- T44.901A Poisn by unsp drugs aff the autonm nervous sys, acc, init
- T44.902A Poisn by unsp drugs aff the autonm nrv sys, slf-hrm, init

S

SYNCOPE
Nancy Drucker

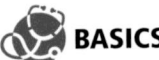 **BASICS**

DEFINITION
Loss of consciousness, typically lasting no longer than 1–2 minutes, due to a transient drop in cerebral perfusion pressure

GENERAL PREVENTION
- Avoiding circumstances predisposing to the most common form of syncope (vasovagal)
- Sitting or lying down when warning signs occur
- Maintaining adequate hydration, especially during illness/exertion

PATHOPHYSIOLOGY
Most common mechanism is vasovagal or neurocardiogenic, in which a variety of stimuli and conditions—pain, dehydrated state, emotional upset, carotid pressure—trigger increased vagal tone, leading to slowed heart rate and peripheral vasodilatation and decreased cerebral perfusion.

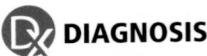 **DIAGNOSIS**

DIFFERENTIAL DIAGNOSIS
- **Cardiac**
  - Congenital heart defect, myocarditis, cardiomyopathy, coronary artery anomaly, heart block (congenital or acquired complete heart block, status post cardiac surgery), arrhythmia secondary to Long QT syndrome, Brugada syndrome, arrhythmogenic right ventricular dysplasia, catecholaminergic polymorphic ventricular tachycardia, Wolff–Parkinson–White. Syncope due to an arrhythmia may be familial, may occur as unprovoked syncope, or as exercise-induced syncope that may resemble an epileptic convulsion.
- **Neurologic**
  - Migraines (predisposed to orthostatic intolerance), arteriovenous malformation; pulmonary hypertension; intracranial hypertension due to hydrocephalus, mass, pseudotumor

- **Pulmonary**
  - Pulmonary hypertension
- **Other**
  - Medications/toxins
- Other causes of syncope by age group include the following:
  - Toddlers:
    - Pallid or cyanotic breath-holding spells; these occur in response to pain, fear, excitement, or frustration, begin with a deep inspiration or exhalation, although the precipitating "gasp" may not be apparent (anemia may be associated).
  - Older children:
    - Adrenal insufficiency
    - Dysautonomia, orthostatic hypotension
    - Dehydration
- Syncopal spells in children may be accompanied by a convulsion (nonepileptic) that usually lasts <1 minute (EEG shows normal findings).
- Alternative causes of loss of consciousness not due to syncope include:
  - Head trauma
  - Epilepsy ("temporal lobe syncope")
  - Psychogenic
  - Stroke
  - Hypoglycemia (rare except in certain metabolic disorders)

HISTORY
- **Question:** Detailed history of the spell (focus on signs/symptoms prior to the event)?
- *Significance*: Most important information used to distinguish syncope from seizure or head trauma
- **Question:** The child or observers may recall "presyncopal" signs?
- *Significance*: Often present in patients with benign syncope—such as warmth, diaphoresis, light-headedness, nausea, palpitations, auditory or visual changes—all lasting only a few seconds before loss of consciousness

- **Question:** Family history?
- *Significance*: Obtaining a careful history is essential. Family history of sudden unexpected death, seizures, syncope, cardiomyopathy, or arrhythmias especially at younger ages or requiring pacemaker/implantable defibrillator should trigger further testing and investigation.
- **Question:** Syncope during exercise or without warning?
- *Significance*: May indicate an underlying arrhythmia
- **Question:** Generalized tonic–clonic movements?
- *Significance*: May occur with syncope—presyncopal signs point to the nonepileptic nature of the event
- **Question:** Increasing duration of unconsciousness?
- *Significance*: Suggests increasing probability that the event is epileptic, rather than syncope
  - Caution: Syncope may be associated with a convulsion in an epileptic patient.
  - Epilepsy may rarely mimic a syncopal episode or recurrent presyncopal symptoms; "temporal lobe syncope" seems to occur principally in adults or adolescents.
- **Question:** Details of body position, eye movements, and respiratory pattern?
- *Significance*: May help determine etiology
- **Question:** Carbon monoxide poisoning?
- *Significance*: May cause syncope-like spells; ask about potential exposure

PHYSICAL EXAM
Key findings to document include the following:
- Vital signs with orthostatic pulse and BP changes
- Right and left arm BPs
- Funduscopy: Possible papilledema
- Cranial bruits
- Precordial thrill
- Heart sounds (gallop, click, rub, significant murmur)

DIAGNOSTIC TESTS & INTERPRETATION

Often only a thorough physical exam, detailed history, and family history are needed if findings are consistent with vasovagal syncope.

- **Test:** EKG* and cardiac consultation
- *Significance*: If the event is suspected to be symptomatic of a heart condition or there is a concerning history/family history, an EKG* and cardiac consultation may be indicated.
- **Test:** Treadmill electrocardiogram, Holter monitoring, echocardiogram, EEG, MRI (Chiari malformation)
- *Significance*: Children with unexplained syncope may undergo more extensive testing.
- **Test:** Glucose, CBC, blood gases, spinal tap
- *Significance*: Laboratory testing may be appropriate based on clinical suspicion of underlying causes.

ALERT

Pitfall: Recurrent syncope due to prolonged QT interval may be missed on routine EKG; prolongation of QT interval may only be noted on treadmill testing or cardiac monitoring.

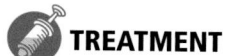 TREATMENT

ADDITIONAL TREATMENT
General Measures

- Clinical intervention is aimed primarily at training the patient in prevention/anticipation:
  - Avoiding circumstances predisposing to the most common form of syncope (vasovagal)
  - Sitting or lying down when warning signs occur
  - Maintaining adequate hydration, especially during illness/exertion
- Therapy is otherwise addressed to underlying causes, in the unusual circumstance that one is found.
- Syncope during exercise always warrants a cardiovascular evaluation, with EKG as initial step.

 ONGOING CARE

- Many children experience a developmental stage in which for unknown reasons they have frequent vasovagal episodes; they may retain a tendency to syncopal spells through adulthood.
- Persistent and frequent spells may prompt more extensive laboratory testing, as described above.

ADDITIONAL READING

- Batra AS, Hohn AR. Consultation with the specialist: Palpitations, syncope, and sudden cardiac death in children—who's at risk? *Pediatr Rev.* 2003;24:269–275.
- DiVasta AD, Alexander ME. Fainting freshmen and sinking sophomores: cardiovascular issues of the adolescent. *Curr Opin Pediatr.* 2004;16(4):350–356.
- Friedman MJ, Mull CC, Sharieff GQ, et al. Prolonged QT syndrome in children: An uncommon but potentially fatal entity. *J Emerg Med.* 2003;24:173–179.
- Kapoor WN. Syncope. *N Engl J Med.* 2000;343:1856–1862.
- McVicar K. Seizure-like states. *Pediatr Rev.* 2006;27(5):e42–e44.
- Sapin SO. Autonomic syncope in pediatrics: A practice-oriented approach to classification, pathophysiology, diagnosis, and management. *Clin Pediatr.* 2004;43:17–23.
- Strickberger SA, Benson DW, Biaggioni I, et al. AHA/ACCF scientific statement on the evaluation of syncope. *Circulation.* 2006;113:369–370.
- Strieper MJ. Distinguishing benign syncope from life-threatening cardiac causes of syncope. *Semin Pediatr Neurol.* 2005;12:32–38.

 CODES

ICD9
- 780.2 Syncope and collapse
- 992.1 Heat syncope

ICD10
- R55 Syncope and collapse
- T67.1XXA Heat syncope, initial encounter
- T67.1XXD Heat syncope, subsequent encounter

S

FAQ

- Q: Do breath-holding spells cause brain damage?
- A: Pallid breath-holding spells appear to be uniformly benign; in rare cases, older children with cyanotic breath-holding spells have had neurologic sequelae of recurrent hypoxemia.
- Q: What limitations in activity are appropriate for children with recurrent syncope who have normal heart structure and function?
- A: Precautions should be taken similar to those for children of similar age who have epilepsy—closely monitored water recreation and restrictions on climbing; however, most children with recurrent syncope do not experience spells in the midst of vigorous activity.

SYNOVITIS–TRANSIENT

David D. Sherry

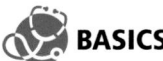 **BASICS**

DESCRIPTION
Transient inflammatory process resulting in arthralgia and arthritis (especially affecting the hip) and occasionally rash precipitated by an exposure to an infectious agent

EPIDEMIOLOGY
Any age at risk, common in ages 3–10 years, with males affected 1.5 times more commonly

RISK FACTORS
Genetics
No specific associations

PATHOPHYSIOLOGY
A type III hypersensitivity reaction mediated by immune complex deposition within the skin and joint spaces

ETIOLOGY
Usually viral (especially upper respiratory, but also enterovirus)

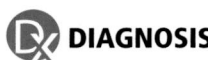 **DIAGNOSIS**

HISTORY
- Preceding viral syndromes
- Day care
- Relatively rapid onset of symptoms, with refusal to bear weight, in a nontoxic-appearing child
- Recent nonspecific upper respiratory or GI infection

PHYSICAL EXAM
- General examination usually benign, with occasional low-grade fever
- Child refuses to bear weight but may tolerate limited ranging of joint.
- Effusions in peripheral joints are rare and usually small and evanescent.
- Pitfalls:
  - Distinctions between transient synovitis and a septic joint may be impossible.
  - Extreme pain and guarding on passive ranging raises suspicion for septic joint.

DIAGNOSTIC TESTS & INTERPRETATION
Lab
- CBC:
  - Usually mild leukocytosis
- ESR:
  - Usually midrange elevation (35–50 mm/h)

Imaging
- Radiography:
  - Usually normal findings or demonstrates small effusion; no evidence of periosteal changes
- Ultrasound:
  - Affected hip joints may have demonstrable effusions.
- MRI:
  - Normal signal intensity may help differentiate transient synovitis from septic hip.

Diagnostic Procedures/Other
- Joint aspirate culture is usually not needed.
- Be wary of contaminated joint aspiration cultures
- Up to 50% of infected joints are negative on culture.

DIFFERENTIAL DIAGNOSIS
- Infection:
  - Lyme disease
  - Septic
  - Tuberculosis
  - Gonorrhea
- Environment
- Trauma (fracture or soft-tissue injury):
  - Slipped capital femoral epiphysis
  - Avascular necrosis
- Tumors:
  - Osteoid osteoma
- Immunologic:
  - Juvenile rheumatoid arthritis
  - Spondyloarthropathy
- Psychological:
  - Psychogenic limp
  - Imitative limp
- Miscellaneous:
  - Hypothyroidism

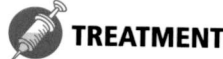 **TREATMENT**

MEDICATION (DRUGS)
- Usually responsive to NSAIDs such as ibuprofen (up to 10 mg/kg/dose q.i.d.)
- Very rarely, a short course of oral steroids is necessary.
  - Usually 1–3 weeks of a tapering course of NSAIDs are effective.

ADDITIONAL TREATMENT
General Measures
Pitfalls:

- Missing a septic hip or, alternatively, overinvestigating transient synovitis with invasive procedures
- Avoid initiation of therapy until septic joint is not in the differential.

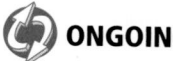 **ONGOING CARE**

FOLLOW-UP RECOMMENDATIONS
Usually significant improvement in 24–48 hours

Patient Monitoring
Ongoing synovitis despite therapeutic levels of NSAIDs or any bony changes indicates need to change diagnosis.

PROGNOSIS
Excellent, although on occasion patients will experience recurrence of symptoms with subsequent viral syndromes or if there is an underlying spondyloarthropathy.

COMPLICATIONS
Questionably associated with subsequent avascular necrosis of femoral head and coxa magna

ADDITIONAL READING

- Delbaccaro MA, Champoux AN, Bockers T, et al. Septic arthritis verus transient synovitis of the hip: The value of screening laboratory tests. *Ann Emerg Med*. 1992;21:1418–1422.
- Do TT. Transient synovitis as a cause of painful limps in children. *Curr Opin Pediatr*. 2000;12:48–51.
- Luhmann SJ, Jones A, Schootman M, et al. Differentiation between septic arthritis and transient synovitis of the hip in children with clinical prediction algorithms. *J Bone Joint Surg*. 2004;86-A:956–962.

- Taekema HC, Landham PR, Maconochie I. Towards evidence based medicine for paediatricians: Distinguishing between transient synovitis and septic arthritis in the limping child—how useful are clinical prediction tools? *Arch Dis Child*. 2009;94(2):167–168.
- Uziel Y, Butbul-Aviel Y, Barash J, et al. Recurrent transient synovitis of the hip in childhood: Long-term outcome among 39 patients. *J Rheumatol*. 2006;33:810–811.

 CODES

ICD9
727.09 Other synovitis and tenosynovitis

ICD10
- M67.30 Transient synovitis, unspecified site
- M67.351 Transient synovitis, right hip
- M67.359 Transient synovitis, unspecified hip

FAQ

- Q: Are there any chronic sequelae from transient synovitis?
- A: Not usually. This is generally a benign disease, but there is a questionable association with avascular necrosis of the femoral head.
- Q: Is there an association with chronic arthritis?
- A: No, there is no known increased risk for chronic arthritis in affected children unless this is the first manifestation of a spondyloarthropathy.

S

SYPHILIS
Esther K. Chung

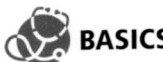 **BASICS**

DESCRIPTION
- Systemic infection caused by the spirochete, *Treponema pallidum*
- Can be congenital or acquired
- Consider sexual abuse when syphilis is diagnosed in young children.

EPIDEMIOLOGY
- Congenital syphilis is transmitted from an infected mother to her unborn or newborn baby.
- Acquired syphilis is sexually transmitted from an infected to an uninfected individual.
- Infection transmitted to the fetus at any stage of disease; during primary and secondary syphilis, rate of transmission is 60–100%.
- Nasal secretions are highly infectious in congenital syphilis, and open, moist skin lesions are infectious in congenital and acquired syphilis.

RISK FACTORS
- Lack of prenatal care
- Maternal use of illicit drugs
- Sexual abuse
- Infection with HIV

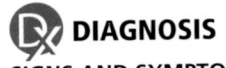 **DIAGNOSIS**

SIGNS AND SYMPTOMS
- Congenital syphilis:
  - Clinical manifestations range from asymptomatic to death or stillbirth.
  - Clinical signs include periostitis, osteochondritis, persistent rhinorrhea, or maculopapular rash.
- Acquired syphilis:
  - Primary stage: Painless, indurated ulcers (chancres), single or multiple, at the site of inoculation ~3 weeks after exposure (range 10–90 days); lesions usually resolve without treatment in 3–6 weeks.
  - Secondary stage: Generalized rash, which is often maculopapular and involves the palms and soles; condyloma lata, hypertrophic papular lesions; fever, malaise, lymphadenopathy; signs appear 3–6 weeks after initial chancre and may last 2–10 weeks
  - Relapse: Symptoms of secondary syphilis may recur 1 or more times before the latent period.
  - Latent period: Untreated, illness may enter a latent stage; patients are asymptomatic, not contagious; lasts 1–40 years or more; patients seroreactive but without other evidence of disease.
    ○ Early latent period: first 4 years of latent period
    ○ Late latent period: Subsequent years
  - Tertiary stage: Up to 1/3 of untreated secondary syphilis cases progress to tertiary or late disease; can occur many years after the primary infection; may see gummatous changes of the skin, bone, and/or viscera, or cardiovascular syphilis
  - Neurosyphilis: CNS involvement in 3–7% of untreated cases; can develop at any stage of disease; signs include changes in mood/behavior, hyperactive reflexes, impaired memory and/or judgment, and Argyll–Robertson pupils

HISTORY
- Newborn/infants:
  - Obtain a detailed prenatal history; inquire about all syphilis testing done on the mother; if mother has a history of syphilis, ensure documented treatment. The local department of health should have detailed records that include titers and treatment on all cases of syphilis.
  - Newborns should be evaluated for congenital syphilis if the mother is not adequately treated for syphilis—mother treated with nonpenicillin regimen, such as erythromycin; mother treated adequately but without a 4-fold decrease in antibody titers in early or high-titer syphilis; maternal syphilis treated <1 month (30 days) before delivery; maternal syphilis treated prior to pregnancy with insufficient follow-up to assess serologic response to treatment; maternal titer has increased 4-fold, if the infant's titer is 4-fold greater than the mother's titer, or if the infant is symptomatic.
- Older children/adolescents:
  - Ask about possible sexual abuse in children.
  - Ask about sexual activity in adolescents, including experience, number of lifetime partners, ages of partners, history of other STDs.
  - Ask about other risk behaviors.
  - Ask about risk factors for HIV exposure.

PHYSICAL EXAM
- Early congenital syphilis:
  - Low birth weight; irritability, bulging fontanel, if neurosyphilis is present
  - Alopecia (scalp and eyebrows)
  - Fissures in the lips, nares, anus; mucocutaneous lesions
  - Rhinitis ("snuffles") may occur at one to several weeks of age and may be blood-tinged and purulent
  - Lymphadenopathy
  - Pneumonia: Check for tachypnea and/or respiratory distress.
  - Myocarditis
  - Hepatosplenomegaly with or without jaundice
  - Pseudoparalysis of an extremity
  - Rash: bullous ("syphilitic pemphigus") and/or maculopapular ("blueberry muffin") lesions symmetrically distributed on palms, soles, and other parts of the body
  - Condyloma lata: Flat, wartlike, moist lesions around the anus/vagina, chancres
- Late congenital syphilis:
  - Bony deformities, such as short maxilla, high-arched palate, saddle nose, mulberry molars, Higoumenaki sign (enlargement of the sternoclavicular portion of the clavicle), protuberance of the mandible, saber shins, scaphoid scapulae
  - Rhagades, neurologic involvement

- Acquired syphilis:
  - Primary syphilis:
    ○ Chancre (painless ulcer), single, most commonly located on the genitalia, and/or
    ○ Painless inguinal adenopathy
  - Secondary syphilis: Flulike illness with fever, headache, sore throat, nasal discharge, generalized arthralgias and myalgias, malaise, generalized painless and mobile lymphadenopathy; hepatosplenomegaly; maculopapular rash involving the palms and soles that may involve mucous membranes; condyloma lata (moist, papular lesions); alopecia; signs of meningitis, hepatitis, nephropathy, ocular involvement

DIAGNOSTIC TESTS & INTERPRETATION
- Pitfalls:
  - Mothers of infants with congenital syphilis should also be tested for gonorrhea, chlamydia, HIV, and hepatitis B virus infection.
  - In newborns, cord blood testing may result in false-positive and false-negative results; therefore, serum from the infant is the preferred source of testing.
  - False-positive nontreponemal test (e.g., rapid plasma reagin [RPR]) results may be seen with lab error, autoimmune disease, tuberculosis, lymphoma, viral infections (including Epstein–Barr, hepatitis, varicella, HIV, and measles viruses), endocarditis, malaria, and IV drug abuse.
  - False-positive treponemal tests may be seen in other spirochetal diseases (i.e., Lyme disease, leptospirosis), and rarely in autoimmune disease (i.e., systemic lupus erythematosus) and viral infections.

Lab
- Nontreponemal tests:
  - VDRL (Venereal Disease Research Laboratory) or RPR test to measure nonspecific antibodies
  - Used for routine screening; quantitative serum titers generally correlate with disease activity; need to confirm positive results with a treponemal antibody test. 4-fold titer change (e.g., from 1:8–1:32) necessary to document clinically significant change. Titers for different nontreponemal tests are not equivalent; therefore, use same test (and preferably same lab) when following serial titers.
  - VDRL (not RPR) used on CSF to rule out neurosyphilis.
- Treponemal antibody tests:
  - FTA-ABS (fluorescent treponemal antibody-absorption), TPHA (*T. pallidum* hemagglutination), MHA-TP (microhemagglutination assay for *T. pallidum* antibodies), or EIA (enzyme immunoassay for antitreponemal IgG)
  - Treponemal tests remain positive for life once infected; not useful for measuring treatment effectiveness
- Dark-field microscopy

- CSF analysis:
  - Findings include mononuclear pleocytosis, moderately elevated protein, normal glucose
  - Should be performed in all patients with acquired syphilis of >1 year's duration.
  - Perform on infants when congenital syphilis suspected, if the physical examination is consistent with syphilis, if infant's titer is 4-fold greater than that of mother, if dark-field or fluorescent antibody test positive on body fluids, and on all children being treated with antibiotics for syphilis.
  - Remember that CSF protein levels in normal newborns are higher than in older children; some are as high as 150–200 mg/dL.

Imaging
Long-bone plain films: Rule out metaphyseal osteochondritis and/or diaphyseal periostitis.

DIFFERENTIAL DIAGNOSIS
- Congenital syphilis:
  - Herpes simplex virus (HSV)
  - Toxoplasmosis
  - Cytomegalovirus
  - Rubella
  - Neonatal hepatitis
  - Osteomyelitis
- Acquired syphilis:
  - Chancroid (Haemophilus ducreyi)
  - Granuloma inguinale
  - Calymmatobacterium granulomatis
  - Lymphogranuloma venereum (Chlamydia trachomatis)
  - Scabies
  - Mycotic infections
  - Genital herpes (HSV)
  - Venereal warts (human papillomavirus, HPV)
  - Viral exanthem (e.g., enteroviruses may cause a maculopapular rash involving the palms and soles)

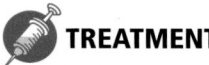 **TREATMENT**

MEDICATION (DRUGS)
- Infants <28 days of age:
  - Aqueous crystalline penicillin G (50,000 U/kg/dose) IV q12h for first 7 days of life, then q8h for a total of 10 days or procaine penicillin G (50,000 U/kg/dose) IM daily for 10 days
  - If >1 day of treatment is missed, restart 10-day course.
- Infants >28 days of age:
  - Aqueous crystalline penicillin G (50,000 U/kg/dose) IV q4–6h for 10 days
- Primary and secondary syphilis:
  - Benzathine penicillin G 50,000 U/kg IM (maximum, 2.4 million units), single dose
  - Doxycycline 100 mg PO b.i.d. or tetracycline 500 mg PO q.i.d. for 14 days for nonpregnant, penicillin-allergic patients
- Early latent syphilis (<1 year's duration):
  - Benzathine penicillin G 50,000 U/kg IM (maximum, 2.4 million units), single dose
  - Doxycycline 100 mg PO b.i.d. or tetracycline 500 mg PO q.i.d. for 14 days for nonpregnant, penicillin-allergic patients
- Late latent syphilis or disease of unknown duration:
  - Benzathine penicillin G 50,000 U/kg IM (maximum 2.4 million U) weekly for 3 consecutive weeks
  - Doxycycline 100 mg PO b.i.d. or tetracycline 500 mg PO q.i.d. for 4 weeks for nonpregnant, penicillin-allergic patients
- Alternative therapy can be found at www.cdc.gov/nchstp/dstd/penicillinG.htm.

 ONGOING CARE

DISPOSITION
Issues for Referral
All cases should be reported to the local department of (public) health.

PROGNOSIS
- The prognosis is better the earlier syphilis is detected and treated.
- Following appropriate therapy, the disease is usually totally arrested.
- With late findings of syphilis involving the nervous and/or cardiovascular systems, there may not be clinical improvement.
- Untreated infection in the neonate progresses to neurosyphilis within 1 year.
- Osteochondritis and periostitis in the newborn are usually self-limited and heal in the first 6 months of life.
- Hemolytic anemia seen in congenital syphilis may persist for weeks.

COMPLICATIONS
- Stillbirth or spontaneous abortion
- Perinatal death in 40% of pregnancies in mothers with untreated early syphilis
- Hydrops fetalis
- Prematurity
- Nephrosis
- Failure to thrive
- Disseminated intravascular coagulation
- Pseudoparalysis of Parrot: Paralysis of one of the limbs of an infant affected by congenital syphilis; usually unilateral
- Acute syphilitic leptomeningitis
- Cranial nerve palsies
- Interstitial keratitis—5–20 years after birth
- Cerebral infarction
- Seizure disorder, mental retardation
- Rhagades: Cluster of scars radiating around the mouth
- Mulberry molars: Maldevelopment of the cusps in the first molars
- Clutton joints: Painless arthritis of the knees and, rarely, other joints
- Hutchinson triad: Hutchinson teeth (notched upper central incisors), interstitial keratitis, eighth-nerve deafness
- Saber shins: Anterior bowing of the midportion of the tibia

PATIENT MONITORING
- Congenital syphilis:
  - Clinical follow-up and serial nontreponemal serologic testing every 2–3 months until titer decreases 4-fold or test is nonreactive
  - After adequate treatment, nontreponemal tests should be nonreactive after 6 months; infants with a history of abnormal CSF findings need serial CSF analyses every 6 months until CSF is normal.
  - Treated infants, follow-up at 1, 2, 4, 6, and 12 months of age; serologic tests should be performed at 2, 4, 6, and 12 months after therapy until they become nonreactive or the titer has decreased 4-fold.
  - If titers have not shown a decline by 6–12 months, require reevaluation and treatment.

- Primary and secondary syphilis:
  - Clinical follow-up and serial nontreponemal titers at 6 and 12 months after treatment (more often, if at high risk for reinfection or treatment failure): Nontreponemal titers should drop 4-fold within 6 months of treatment of primary or secondary syphilis, and within 12–24 months after treatment of latent or tertiary syphilis.

ADDITIONAL READING

- American Academy of Pediatrics. Syphilis. In: Pickering LK, ed. Red Book 2009: Report of the Committee on Infectious Diseases. 28th ed. Elk Grove Village, IL: AAP; 2009:638–651.
- Centers for Disease Control and Prevention. Congenital syphilis: United States, 2003–2008. MMWR Morb Mortal Wkly Rep. 2010;59:413–417.
- Centers for Disease Control and Prevention. Primary and secondary syphilis: United States, 2003–2004. MMWR Morb Mortal Wkly Rep. 2006;55:269–273.
- Chakraborty R, Luck S. Managing congenital syphilis again? The more things change. Curr Opin Infect Dis. 2007;20:247–252.
- Chakraborty R, Luck S. Syphilis is on the increase: The implications for child health. Arch Dis Child 2008;93:105–109.
- Ferran M, Martin-Ezquerra G, Vicente A, et al. Picture of the month. Acquired secondary syphilis. Arch Pediatr Adolesc Med. 2007;161(2):199–200.
- Hyman EL. Syphilis. Pediatr Rev. 2006;27:37–39.
- Tobian AA, Serwadda D, Quinn TC, et al. Male circumcision for the prevention of HSV-2 and HPV infections and syphilis. N Engl J Med. 2009;360: 1298–1309.

 CODES

ICD9
- 090.9 Congenital syphilis, unspecified
- 091.2 Other primary syphilis
- 097.9 Syphilis, unspecified

ICD10
- A50.9 Congenital syphilis, unspecified
- A51.2 Primary syphilis of other sites
- A53.9 Syphilis, unspecified

FAQ

- Q: Can an infant have congenital syphilis if the mother had a negative RPR during pregnancy?
- A: A mother with a negative RPR during pregnancy may have acquired syphilis late in pregnancy and transmitted it to her fetus. If the mother was not tested at delivery, then the diagnosis may have been missed.
- Q: What is the prozone phenomenon?
- A: When a nontreponemal test is falsely negative due to high concentrations of antibody to T. pallidum; diluting the serum will result in positive test results.

TAPEWORM

Jessica K. Hart
Samir S. Shah

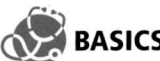 **BASICS**

DESCRIPTION

- Tapeworms cause 2 major types of zoonotic disease syndromes, depending on whether humans are the definitive or intermediate host. When humans serve as definitive hosts, adult tapeworms infect the GI tract and interfere with nutrition. These infections are often asymptomatic. When humans serve as intermediate hosts for the larval cestode, serious pathology results.
- Causative organisms include:
  - *Taenia saginata* (beef tapeworm)
  - *Taenia solium* (pork tapeworm)
  - *Diphyllobothrium latum* (fish tapeworm)
  - *Dipylidium caninum* (dog tapeworm)
  - *Echinococcus granulosus*

EPIDEMIOLOGY

- Beef tapeworm:
  - Widespread in cattle-breeding areas of the world, with a prevalence of >10% in areas of Africa, such as Ethiopia and Kenya, and the former Soviet Union.
- Pork tapeworm:
  - Cysticercosis has a high prevalence in developing areas of Central and South America.
  - In the US, immigrants account for >90% of cases.
- Fish tapeworm:
  - Infection is most prevalent in temperate climates of Europe, North America, and Asia. Persons who prepare raw fish are most at risk.
  - In the US, infected salmon have been implicated in most cases.
- Dog tapeworm:
  - Found in dogs and cats worldwide
- Echinococcosis:
  - Associated with the practice of feeding sheep viscera to dogs.
  - It is hyperendemic in sheep-raising areas of South America, Australia, areas of Africa, China, central Asia, and the western US.

GENERAL PREVENTION

- Adult tapeworms:
  - Proper cooking of meat and fish prevents transmission of beef, pork, and fish tapeworms.
- Pork tapeworm:
  - The refrigeration of pork infested with cysticerci at temperatures >0°C (32°F) does not affect parasite survival. However, storage of pork for 4 days at −5°C (21.2°F) or 1 day at −24°C (−11.2°F) kills most cysticerci.
- Fish tapeworm:
  - Brief cooking (at 56°C [132.8°F] or higher for 5 minutes) or freezing (−18°C [−0.4°F] for 24 hours) renders the fish safe for consumption.
- Dog tapeworm:
  - Periodic deworming of pets prevents infections.
- Echinococcosis:
  - Careful disposal of sheep viscera and mass chemotherapy of dogs can interrupt the life cycle of *E. granulosus* as the cestode moves between sheep and carnivore hosts.

PATHOPHYSIOLOGY

- Beef tapeworm:
  - Cattle (intermediate host) ingest the eggs of *T. saginata* in contaminated feeds. The eggs hatch, releasing embryos. The embryos penetrate intestinal mucosa, enter the bloodstream, and settle in various tissues, where they develop into larvae. Larvae in undercooked meat are consumed by humans and mature into adult tapeworms within the human (definitive host) GI tract. They grow up to 25 m long.
- Pork tapeworm: Humans are the only definitive host for the adult pork tapeworm, whereas both humans and pigs are intermediate hosts for its embryonic form, cysticercus.
  - Pigs (intermediate host) ingest *T. solium* eggs. In the intestine, the eggs release embryos that penetrate the mucosa, enter the bloodstream, and settle in various tissues to differentiate into cysticerci (infective larvae). Cysticerci are ingested by humans (definitive host) who consume undercooked pork.
  - Humans (intermediate host) ingest food contaminated with human feces containing *T. solium* eggs. The eggs hatch, liberating embryos (oncospheres). Penetration through the intestinal mucosa leads to blood-borne distribution to the brain, subcutaneous tissues, muscle, and eye, where they develop into cysticerci.
- Fish tapeworm:
  - When sewage containing *D. latum* eggs contaminates freshwater lakes and streams, larvae hatch into the water. These larvae are eaten by crustaceans and fish. Humans are infected when they consume these undercooked fish. The larvae mature into adult tapeworms in the intestines of humans.
- Dog tapeworm:
  - Larvae develop in fleas (intermediate host) after ingestion of the eggs; humans are infected through accidental ingestion of infected fleas.
- Echinococcosis (hydatid disease):
  - Humans ingest eggs of *E. granulosus* through contaminated dog feces. After ingestion, the eggs hatch and release embryos (oncospheres) in the small intestine. Penetration through the mucosa leads to blood-borne distribution to the liver, lungs, and other sites, where development of cysts begins. Within the cysts, new larvae (scolices) develop, accumulate fluid, and encroach on surrounding structures.

DIAGNOSIS

HISTORY

- Recent travel or immigration:
  - Tapeworm infections are more prevalent in other countries.
- GI tract:
  - Nausea, weight loss, diarrhea, abdominal tenderness or distention.
  - Fish and, rarely, dog tapeworm infections can be complicated by intestinal obstruction.
  - May observe proglottids that resemble rice or seeds in stool from dog tapeworm infections.

- Jaundice:
  - Hepatic cysts from echinococcosis may be palpable in the right upper quadrant.
  - Biliary tree extension can lead to obstructive jaundice and cholangitis.
- Respiratory tract:
  - Pulmonary hydatid cyst due to *E. granulosus* causes cough, dyspnea, and hemoptysis; rupture of a cyst can cause anaphylaxis.
- Hematologic:
  - Anemia from vitamin B12 deficiency occurs in 2% of fish tapeworm infections. Other signs of pernicious anemia include glossitis, peripheral neuropathy, decreased vibration sense, and ataxia.
- CNS:
  - New-onset seizures (partial or generalized) occur with neurocysticercosis and some species of *Echinococcus*.
  - Neurocysticercosis may present with alteration in mental status, signs of elevated intracranial pressure (headache, vomiting, visual changes), or meningitis
  - Neurocysticercosis and vitamin B12 deficiency due to fish tapeworm can mimic psychotic illness with delirium or hallucinations.
  - CNS symptoms in neurocysticercosis typically appear 5–7 years after initial infection (range: 6 months to 30 years).
- Note: For echinococcosis, a presymptomatic stage may last for years before the enlarging cysts cause symptoms. The variability of signs and symptoms depends on the target organ.

DIAGNOSTIC TESTS & INTERPRETATION
Lab

- Beef tapeworm:
  - Identification of scolex in stool.
  - Ziehl–Neelsen stain of stool or perianal adhesive tape preparations identifies eggs.
  - Collection of proglottids in saline with microscopic examination.
  - ELISA test detects *Taenia* antigens in stool.
- Pork tapeworm:
  - Enzyme immunotransfer blot (most sensitive) and serologic assays.
  - Stool samples for intestinal worms as for beef tapeworm.
- Fish tapeworm:
  - Stool samples for eggs and proglottids are diagnostic.
  - Mild eosinophilia (5–15%).
  - Low vitamin B12 levels (50%).
  - Megaloblastic anemia 2%.
- Dog tapeworm
  - Characteristic egg packets (loose membrane containing up to 20 eggs) may be identified in stool or perianal adhesive tape preparations.

- Echinococcosis:
  - IgE levels are elevated. Eosinophilia is present in <25% of infected persons.
  - Polymerase chain reaction (PCR) of stool
  - Mild elevation of hepatic enzymes may be present with hepatic hydatid cysts.
  - The Casoni skin test (injection of hydatid fluid into the dermis) yields an erythematous papule in <60 minutes in 50–80% of infected patients. There is a false-positive result in 30% of uninfected patients.
- Serologic testing is falsely negative in 10–50% of cases. False-negative results are more likely in patients with pulmonary hydatid cysts and in children. No serologic test excludes the diagnosis of hydatid cysts.

Imaging
- Pork tapeworm:
  - Contrast-enhanced CT or MRI of the brain may reveal cysticerci; ring-enhancing lesions with surrounding edema represent a dying parasite; calcification represents a resolved infection.
  - Imaging is usually diagnostic.
- Echinococcosis:
  - On x-ray, pulmonary cysts demonstrate a sharply demarcated, smooth-bordered cyst; there is a crescent-shaped air level after cyst rupture. Liver and spleen lesions may calcify over time.
  - Hydatid cysts: Internal septa or daughter cysts after cyst rupture are detected by CT, MRI, or ultrasound; present in ~50% of patients with unilocular liver cysts.

Diagnostic Procedures/Other
Echinococcosis: In seronegative persons, a presumptive diagnosis can be confirmed by demonstrating protoscolices or hydatid membranes in liquid obtained by ultrasound-guided percutaneous cyst aspiration. This procedure is controversial because anaphylaxis may occur with cyst rupture.

DIFFERENTIAL DIAGNOSIS
- Non-tapeworm gastroenteritis.
- Inflammatory bowel disease.
- Cholecystitis or biliary obstruction (i.e., gallstones, neoplasms, or liver disease).
- B12 deficiency from dietary deficiency, decreased ileal absorption, pancreatic insufficiency
- Idiopathic epilepsy.
- Echinococcal cysts must be differentiated from benign cysts, cavitary tuberculosis, abscesses, and neoplasms.

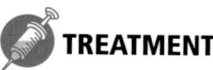 **TREATMENT**

MEDICATION (DRUGS)
- Beef tapeworm, pork tapeworm, fish tapeworm, dog tapeworm, and most other intestinal cestodes:
  - Praziquantel: 5–10 mg/kg as a single dose; no safety profile exists for children <4 years of age.
  - Niclosamide (second line for beef tapeworm): Children 11–34 kg, 1 g as a single dose; children >34 kg, 1.5 g as a single dose (not available in the US).
  - Supplement with vitamin B12 for fish tapeworm.

- Neurocysticercosis:
  - Treatment should be individualized based on number, location, and viability of cysticerci on MRI or CT scan. Although antiparasitic drugs are cysticercidal and hasten radiologic resolution, most symptoms result from the host inflammatory response and may be exacerbated by treatment.
  - Treatment may not be indicated for single degenerating cysts, calcifications, or encephalitis. Most experts recommend therapy for patients with nonenhancing or multiple cysticerci.
  - Albendazole: 15 mg/kg/d (maximum, 800 mg/d) in 2 divided doses for 8–30 days or praziquantel 50–100 mg/kg/d in 3 divided doses for 30 days.
  - Symptomatic therapy includes anticonvulsants for seizures and shunt placement for hydrocephalus.
  - Corticosteroids control host inflammation in the first 2–3 days of therapy for certain forms of neurocysticercosis. Data on optimal dose or duration are lacking but 1 mg/kg/day of prednisone or 0.5 mg/kg/day of dexamethasone is often used.
  - Antiparasitic therapy is contraindicated in patients with diffuse cerebral edema ("cysticercal encephalitis") because the inflammatory response that follows treatment may worsen cerebral edema. These patients should be treated with high-dose corticosteroids.
  - No definite recommendations exist regarding the use of corticosteroids alone.
- Echinococcosis:
  - Albendazole 15 mg/kg for 1–6 months.
  - May require 3 courses of therapy with drug-free intervals of 14 days between courses.
- Note: The benzimidazoles, including albendazole, are contraindicated in patients with blood dyscrasia, leukopenia, and liver disease. Prolonged courses require monitoring of liver function and hematopoiesis.

SURGERY/OTHER PROCEDURES
Echinococcosis: Surgical resection of intact hydatid cysts, especially if >10 cm or secondarily infected

 ONGOING CARE

FOLLOW-UP RECOMMENDATIONS
Patient Monitoring
- Beef tapeworm:
  - Stool should be checked for eggs and proglottids 1 month after therapy.
- Pork tapeworm:
  - Repeat CNS imaging studies at 2-month intervals (with continued therapy) until successful elimination of parenchymal brain cysticerci.
- Fish tapeworm:
  - Perform stool examination 6 weeks after therapy to test for cure.
- Dog tapeworm:
  - No follow-up stool examination required, but the appearance of proglottids >1 week after therapy indicates treatment failure.
- Echinococcosis:
  - Requires prolonged follow-up with ultrasound or other imaging procedures.

COMPLICATIONS
- Cysticercosis:
  - Cysticerci develop in the brain, muscle, eye, or other organs.
- Echinococcosis:
  - Cysts grow slowly, causing symptoms only when relatively large.
  - They frequently develop in the liver (50–70%) and lung (20–30%); 5–10% of cysts involve other organs, including the eye, brain, spleen, heart, bone, and kidneys.
  - Spontaneous rupture of cysts can cause anaphylaxis.
  - Bone involvement can cause pathologic fractures.
  - Renal involvement causes pain or hematuria.

ADDITIONAL READING

- Bruckner DA. Helminthic food-borne infections. *Clin Lab Med*. 1999;19:639–660.
- Garcia HH, Evans CA, Nash TE, et al. Current consensus guidelines for treatment of neurocysticercosis. *Clin Microbiol Rev*. 2002;15:747–756.
- Moon TD, Oberhelman RA. Antiparasitic therapy in children. *Pediatr Clin N Am*. 2005;52:917–948.
- Schantz PM. Tapeworms (cestodiasis). *Gastroenterol Clin*. 1996;25:637–653.
- Sinha S, Sharma BS. Neurocysticercosis: A review of current status and management. *J Clin Neuroscience*. 2009;16:867–876.

 CODES

ICD9
- 123.0 Taenia solium infection, intestinal form
- 123.2 Taenia saginata infection
- 123.9 Cestode infection, unspecified

ICD10
- B68.0 Taenia solium taeniasis
- B68.1 Taenia saginata taeniasis
- B71.9 Cestode infection, unspecified

FAQ

- Q: Can vegetarians develop neurocysticercosis?
- A: Yes, because neurocysticercosis results from ingestion of *T. solium* eggs in products contaminated with infected fecal matter. GI symptoms result from infected pork consumption.
- Q: Is treatment for neurocysticercosis always indicated?
- A: The findings are controversial. In many children, the lesion disappears spontaneously within 2–3 months. Guidelines for treatment depend on the number and location of lesions, as well as the viability of the parasites within the nervous system. A growing parasite deserves active management, either with antiparasitic drugs or surgical excision.

TEETHING

Julie A. Boom

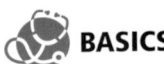

BASICS

DEFINITION
Teething is the normal developmental process of primary tooth eruption, often characterized by parental reports of fever, fussiness, increased drooling, increased finger sucking, alterations in bowel pattern, and/or decreased appetite.

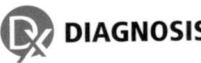

DIAGNOSIS

DIFFERENTIAL DIAGNOSIS
- **Congenital/anatomic**
  - Natal teeth, neonatal teeth
  - Gastroesophageal reflux resulting in esophagitis with decreased appetite
- **Infectious**
  - Primary herpes gingivostomatitis causing pain or drooling
  - Human herpesvirus 6 causing fever
  - Coxsackievirus oral infection causing fever or drooling
  - Epiglottitis causing severe drooling with fever
  - Viral illness causing fever >38.3°C (101°F), diarrhea, or upper respiratory symptoms
- **Toxic ingestion causing drooling**
- **Trauma**
  - "Lancing" of gums (i.e., incising the gum to expose the erupting tooth) causing pain
  - Hair tourniquet syndrome causing pain and irritability
  - Corneal abrasion causing pain
- **Miscellaneous:** Drooling, gum rubbing, and finger sucking may be normal developmental behaviors.

APPROACH TO THE PATIENT
The overall goal is to determine if the infant has any other signs or symptoms of another illness that would require additional investigation (e.g., fever 38.8°C [102°F], diarrhea, or irritability); avoid overdiagnosing teething, which might delay diagnosis of a more serious illness.
- **Phase 1:** Careful history and physical exam
- **Phase 2:** Workup of specific signs or symptoms that are not consistent with teething
- **Phase 3:** Provide relief of discomfort for the child who is teething

ALERT
Of note, fever >38.8°C (102°F), irritability, or diarrhea should not be attributed to teething, and other etiologies should be considered, such as acute otitis media, urinary tract infection (UTI), septicemia, meningitis, septic arthritis, or viral infection.

HISTORY
- **Question:** Age?
- *Significance:* The average age for the eruption of the first tooth is ~6 months.
  - 1% of infants acquire the first tooth before 4 months of age, and 1% after 12 months of age.
  - Rule of thumb: Age (months) − 6 = average number of teeth (up to 2 years of age)
  - Eruption usually begins with the lower central incisors.
- **Question:** Swelling or bluish discoloration of the gums?
- *Significance:*
  - Primary tooth eruption is frequently associated with swelling of the gums.
  - A bluish area of gum swelling may represent an eruption cyst secondary to a hematoma. This condition requires parental reassurance only.
- **Question:** Consolability?
- *Significance:*
  - Infants who are teething may be fussy but should be consolable.
  - An infant who is irritable and not consolable should be evaluated for serious systemic illness such as septicemia, meningitis, septic arthritis, or UTI.
- **Question:** Fever?
- *Significance:* Several studies suggest that mild temperature elevation may occur 1–3 days before tooth eruption.
- **Question:** Other symptoms?
- *Significance:*
  - One recent study found that the following symptoms may be seen 4 days before and 3 days after tooth eruption: Increased biting, drooling, gum rubbing, sucking, irritability, wakefulness, ear-rubbing, facial rash, decreased appetite for solid foods, and mild temperature elevation.
  - In this study, congestion, sleep disturbance, stool looseness, increased stool number, decreased interest in drinking, cough, nonfacial rashes, vomiting, and fever >38.8°C (102°F) were not associated with the teething period. Another recent study did not validate these findings.

- **Question:** Sleeping habits?
- *Significance:*
  - A teething child should be able to sleep with minimal disturbance.
  - Changes in sleeping habits, such as frequent nighttime awakening, should suggest common problems with sleep associations often seen in young children 6–12 months old.
- **Question:** Illness in the home?
- *Significance:* An acute illness should be investigated as the cause of the child's symptoms.

PHYSICAL EXAM
- **Finding:** Swelling with slight pallor over the gum where the tooth will erupt?
- *Significance:* Normal finding
- **Finding:** Bluish discoloration overlying the gum where a tooth is expected?
- *Significance:* This represents a hematoma, known as an "eruption cyst," which is a normal finding.
- **Finding:** Irritability?
- *Significance:* Irritability on physical exam suggests a more serious illness than teething. In addition to the infectious etiologies noted, the child should be evaluated for hair tourniquet syndrome and/or corneal abrasion.
- **Finding:** Oral ulcers?
- *Significance:* Viral enanthems, such as those seen with herpes simplex virus or coxsackievirus, should be considered.
- **Finding:** Presence of cervical lymphadenopathy?
- *Significance:* Oral, dental, or pharyngeal infections should be considered.
- **Finding:** Signs of dehydration, such as dry mucous membranes, absent tears, sunken fontanel, or tenting of the skin?
- *Significance:* Infectious etiologies that result in poor oral intake or diarrhea should be considered.
- **Finding:** Oral erythema and abrasions with excessive drooling?
- *Significance:* The possibility of caustic ingestion should be explored.

DIAGNOSTIC TESTS & INTERPRETATION
No laboratory tests are indicated in the otherwise healthy child with teething.

TREATMENT

ADDITIONAL TREATMENT
General Measures
- Application of cold/frozen objects locally onto the gums: Many find that cold objects work well, but care must be taken because direct contact with a frozen object may result in local irritation.
  - Liquid-filled teething rings should be chilled but not frozen. Extreme temperatures may alter the integrity of the plastic cover and result in bacterial contamination with organisms such as *Pseudomonas*.
- Objects for chewing: Choking hazards, such as raw carrots, must be avoided.
- Teething rings should not be attached to a tether around the child's neck, as they represent a strangulation hazard. Teething rings made prior to 1998 should be discarded as they might contain diisononyl phthalate, a softening agent now thought to be toxic.
- Acetaminophen (15 mg/kg PO q4h) or ibuprofen (10 mg/kg PO q6h) may be used for pain relief as needed, but should not be given around-the-clock so as not to mask fever.
- Home remedies or treatments given by parents:
  - Most over-the-counter preparations marketed for the relief of teething symptoms contain 7.5–10% benzocaine as the active ingredient. Excessive use of benzocaine preparations has been associated with methemoglobinemia.
  - Homeopathic remedies may contain a variety of ingredients including belladonna alkaloids, chamomile, and ground coffee. Depending on the size of the child and the amount of medication or herb ingested, toxicity is possible.
- Remedies that have been used in the past and are no longer recommended include: Alcoholic liquors, paregoric, 2% lidocaine solution (excess may result in seizures), honey, emetics, purgatives, lancing the gums, and rubbing the gums with a thimble until the tooth breaks through the gum.

ISSUES FOR REFERRAL
- Children who have delayed eruption of their first primary tooth beyond 12 months require additional investigation for the following: Anodontia, hypothyroidism, hypopituitarism, rickets, Gaucher disease, and multiple syndromes such as osteodystrophies, Apert syndrome, and Down syndrome. Most of these conditions require referral to a specialist for management.
- Children with premature eruption may have a familial cause; however, referral for evaluation of hyperpituitarism should be considered.
- Referral to a dentist should be considered for children with significant variation in eruption caused by dental infections, additional teeth in the path of eruption, insufficient space in the dental arch, and/or ectopic placement of teeth.
- Natal teeth that are stable and do not interfere with breastfeeding may remain. Loose natal teeth may need to be removed to prevent choking and aspiration. Natal teeth can interfere with breastfeeding and cause ulceration, which is another indication for removal.

PATIENT EDUCATION
- Information available at: www.ada.org/public/topics/tooth_eruption.asp
- Parent handout available at: http://contpeds.adv100.com/contpeds/data/articlestandard/contpeds/332004/112042/article.pdf

ADDITIONAL READING

- Anderson J. "Nothing but the tooth": Dispelling myths about teething. *Contemp Pediatr*. 2004;21:75–87.
- Ashley MP. It's only teething—a report of the myths and modern approaches to teething. *Br Dent J*. 2001;191:4–8.
- Macknin ML, Piedmonte M, Jacobs J, et al. Symptoms associated with infant teething: A prospective study. *Pediatrics*. 2000;105:747–752.
- Markman L. Teething: Facts and fiction. *Pediatr Rev*. 2009;30:e59–e64.
- Wake M, Hesketh K, Lucas J. Teething and tooth eruption in infants: A cohort study. *Pediatrics*. 2000;106:1374–1379.

 # CODES

ICD9
520.7 Teething syndrome

ICD10
K00.7 Teething syndrome

FAQ

- Q: What is the difference between natal teeth and neonatal teeth?
- A: Natal teeth are present at birth, whereas neonatal teeth erupt during the 1st month of life. The incidence of natal teeth is 1:2,000–6,000 live births and usually involves the lower central incisor. Natal teeth can be associated with various conditions including Pierre Robin sequence, cleft lip and/or palate, chondroectodermal dysplasia, and Hallermann–Streiff, Ellis–van Creveld, and Sotos syndrome. There is often a familial history of natal or neonatal teeth. 95% of natal teeth are normal primary incisors that may have formed superficially and erupted early. Only 5% of natal teeth are supernumerary (extra) teeth. Therefore, if a natal tooth is removed, a primary tooth will not erupt in its place in most cases. Because primary teeth act as space holders for the secondary teeth, early loss of a primary tooth may result in significant crowding of the secondary teeth.
- Q: Does primary tooth eruption in preterm infants occur at the same time as in full-term infants?
- A: In healthy preterm infants who had relatively uneventful neonatal courses, the first primary tooth erupts at the usual chronological age. Premature infants requiring prolonged oral intubation and/or who experience inadequate nutrition due to the severity of neonatal disease may have delays in tooth eruption. The initial eruption sequence remains the same (lower central incisors first).
- Q: Does obesity affect dental development?
- A: Obese children, ages 8–15, have been shown to have advanced dental development compared to their nonobese peers. This can have important implications for planning the timing of orthodontic treatment.

T

TENDONITIS

David D. Sherry

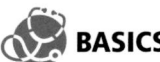 **BASICS**

DESCRIPTION
Inflammation of a tendon or along the tendon sheath

EPIDEMIOLOGY
- Increases with age and at time of puberty
- May be slightly more common in girls

RISK FACTORS
Genetics
Hypermobile individuals may be prone to tendonitis.

PATHOPHYSIOLOGY
Inflammation and microtearing may be present.

ETIOLOGY
Frequently associated with repetitive motion/overuse activities

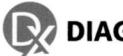 **DIAGNOSIS**

HISTORY
- Trauma or overuse:
  - Verify acute nature of injury
- Signs and symptoms:
  - Pain
  - Tenderness

PHYSICAL EXAM
- Evidence of hematoma:
  - Palpate around and about affected areas, detecting point tenderness especially at tendon insertions as well as over bony prominences
- Evidence of bursitis or arthritis:
  - Systemic conditions, such as spondyloarthropathy, can lead to inflammation of tendons, bursa, and joints, and bursitis can mimic the pain of tendonitis.
- Pop or snap felt at the time of the event:
  - Sometimes this is felt when tendons and ligaments are torn or avulsed.

- Caution: False-positives:
  - Patients may have torn ligaments, fractures, or arthritis, not just tendonitis on examination.
- Pitfalls:
  - Overdiagnosis in young children, in whom overuse is rare and other diagnoses should be considered
- Underdiagnosis in older children in whom repetitive activities are likely to occur

DIAGNOSTIC TESTS & INTERPRETATION
Lab
ESR: Occasionally helpful to rule out inflammatory conditions if history and/or physical exam are suggestive

Imaging
Plain radiograph: Affected area may be indicated to rule out a fracture, avulsion, or identify a bone spur.

DIFFERENTIAL DIAGNOSIS
- Infection:
  - Especially gonococcal disease, septic arthritis, or osteomyelitis
- Environmental:
  - Fracture
- Metabolic:
  - Homocystinuria

- Congenital:
  - Generalized hypermobility
  - Marfan syndrome
  - Ehlers–Danlos
- Immunologic:
  - Ankylosing spondylitis and the reactive spondyloarthropathies (inflammatory bowel disease, reactive arthritis)
  - Inflammatory arthritides
- Psychological:
  - Amplified musculoskeletal pain

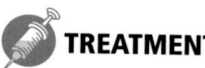 **TREATMENT**

MEDICATION (DRUGS)
- NSAIDs
- Rarely do soft-tissue steroid injections have a role in children

ADDITIONAL TREATMENT
General Measures
- Rest/reduced use of the affected tendon/muscle group is essential, occasionally requiring splinting.
- Duration of therapy:
  - 1–4 weeks

Additional Therapies
- Physical or occupational therapy
- Either self-directed or formal help with resumption of desired activity, through gentle range of motion exercises against low resistance and advanced as tolerated

 ONGOING CARE

FOLLOW-UP RECOMMENDATIONS
Improvement often takes 2–6 weeks.

Patient Monitoring
If the provocative activity is resumed too soon, the irritation will recur.

PROGNOSIS
Usually good for children; however, many will suffer recurrences if proper exercises before desired activity are not continued.

COMPLICATIONS
Ongoing pain and predisposition for recurrence

ADDITIONAL READING
- Almekinders LC, Temple JD. Etiology, diagnosis, and treatment of tendonitis: An analysis of the literature. *Med Sci Sports Exerc*. 1998;30:1183–1190.
- Marsh JS, Daigneault JP. Ankle injuries in the pediatric population. *Curr Opin Pediatr*. 2000;12:52–60.
- Pommering TL, Kluchurosky L. Overuse injuries in adolescents. *Adolesc Med State Art Rev*. 2007;18(1):95–120.

 CODES

ICD9
726.90 Tendonitis

ICD10
M77.9 Enthesopathy, unspecified

FAQ
- Q: Which activities can result in overuse syndromes and tendonitis?
- A: Virtually any repetitive activity in which children engage can cause tendonitis. For example, pain in the tendons of the thumb has occurred in children overusing video games.

T

TERATOMA

Jane E. Minturn

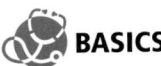 ## BASICS

DESCRIPTION
Embryonal neoplasm composed of tissue derived from all 3 germ layers (endoderm, mesoderm, and ectoderm):
- Gonadal or extragonadal location
- Mature or immature and may occur with or without associated malignant elements
- A subset of the broader class of germ cell tumors

GENERAL PREVENTION
There is no known prevention for the development of teratomas and other germ cell tumors.

EPIDEMIOLOGY
- Gonadal and extragonadal germ cell tumors account for ~3% of childhood malignancies (<15 years) and 15% of malignancies of ages 15–19 years.
- Incidence of germ cell tumors as a whole is ~2.5 cases per million in white children and 3 cases per million in black children <15 years of age.
- One suggestive epidemiologic association is with high maternal hormone levels during pregnancy.
- More controversial associations include younger gestational age; viral infections including herpes simplex virus, varicella-zoster virus, cytomegalovirus, mumps; other congenital anomalies; maternal urinary tract infection or tuberculosis; and paternal occupation in chemical industries.
- Sacrococcygeal teratoma: Accounts for 50% of all childhood teratomas and up to 78% of extragonadal germ cell tumors. Most prevalent in infants (1:40,000 live births); girls more frequently affected (4:1 female to male)
- Testicular and ovarian teratomas account for 5% and 25% of childhood teratomas, respectively.
- Vaginal tumors: Most prevalent in girls <3 years old
- Mediastinal tumors: Arise in anterior mediastinum, rarely heart or pericardium. Average age of the pediatric patient is 3 years, but also found in adolescents; most common extragonadal germ cell tumor in adults
- Intracranial teratoma: Midline, primarily pineal or suprasellar. Comprise 50% of congenital brain tumors (≤60 days of life)

Genetics
- Isochromosome 12p [i(12p)] is characteristic in adult mixed germ cell tumors. Pediatric tumors show no clear pattern of genetic aberration.
- No pattern of inheritance is known.

PATHOPHYSIOLOGY
- Absence of normal mitotic/meiotic arrest of primordial germ cells in gonads leading to gonadal tumor formation. Aberrant migration of primordial germ cells during embryonal development, causing germ cells to come to rest outside the gonads leading to extragonadal tumors.
- Mature teratoma: Contains well-differentiated, nonmitotic tissues from all 3 germ layers, such as squamous epithelium, neuronal tissue, muscle, teeth, cartilage, bone, GI, and respiratory epithelium.
- Immature teratoma: Contains various embryonic elements representative of all 3 germ layers, such as neuroepithelial tissues; divided histologically into 4 grades, 0–3, dependent on degree of immaturity and mitotic activity.
- Teratoma with malignant germ cell elements: Foci of malignant tissue that resemble other germ cell tumors such as embryonal carcinoma, yolk sac tumor (endodermal sinus tumor), and choriocarcinoma, in addition to mature or immature tissues. Prone to local recurrence and metastasis.

DIAGNOSIS

HISTORY
- External mass, constipation, urinary abnormalities, lower extremity weakness:
  - Sacrococcygeal mass may impinge on nerve structures.
  - Anterior sacrococcygeal mass may have no external component.
  - Fetal sacrococcygeal teratoma often initially picked up on prenatal ultrasonography.
- Cough, wheeze, dyspnea, superior vena cava syndrome suggest anterior mediastinal mass.

- Blood-tinged vaginal discharge: Vaginal teratoma
- Abdominal pain, nausea, vomiting, constipation, urinary tract symptoms: Ovarian tumors present late with a large mass. Symptoms mimicking acute abdomen may indicate ovarian torsion.
- Painless scrotal swelling or painful testicular torsion: Testicular mass may be teratoma.
- Cryptorchidism: Associated with germ cell tumors in boys

PHYSICAL EXAM
- Palpable mass either externally or internally, signs of spinal cord compression: Sacrococcygeal tumor
- Vaginoscopy reveals a polyploid lesion arising from the vaginal wall: Examination under anesthesia is usually necessary.
- Palpable abdominal mass, peritoneal symptoms: Ovarian mass may be large.
- Palpable mass in scrotum: Testicular origin
- Decreased breath sounds, consolidation, wheezing, superior vena cava syndrome: Mediastinal mass may be an emergency.

DIAGNOSTIC TESTS & INTERPRETATION
Lab
- Serum α-fetoprotein (AFP) and β-human chorionic gonadotropin (β-HCG): Pure teratomas are not associated with elevated tumor markers. Elevation of either of these markers indicates the presence of more malignant germ cell elements and requires review of the histologic material.
- CBC and chemistry profile, with electrolytes, BUN, creatinine, liver function tests, uric acid, and lactate dehydrogenase: Workup to rule out other malignancies or associated organ dysfunction

Imaging
- Plain radiograph: May reveal mature calcified tissues, such as bone or teeth, within tumor
- Chest radiograph: Shows mediastinal mass
- CT scan: Necessary to evaluate the primary site and regional disease
- Transscrotal ultrasound as initial imaging for testicular mass shows heterogeneous mass with calcifications

- Prenatal MRI for fetal sacrococcygeal teratoma diagnosed by ultrasound: Allows more accurate prenatal counseling and improved preoperative planning
- Chest CT and bone scan: If malignancy is suspected or proven, these are indicated for evaluation of metastasis.
- Ultrasound, if CT is not readily available:
  - May be helpful, but will rarely suffice as the sole imaging study of the primary site
  - May be first evidence of anterior sacrococcygeal mass or to differentiate testicular mass from hydrocele

DIFFERENTIAL DIAGNOSIS

- Sacrococcygeal: Pilonidal cyst, meningocele, lipomeningocele, hemangioma, abscess, bone tumor, epidermal cyst, chondroma, lymphoma, ependymoma, neuroblastoma, glioma
- Abdominal: Wilms tumor, neuroblastoma, lymphoma, rhabdomyosarcoma, hepatoblastoma, retained twin fetus
- Vaginal: Rhabdomyosarcoma (sarcoma botryoides), clear cell carcinoma
- Ovarian: Cyst, appendicitis, pregnancy, pelvic infection, hematocolpos, sarcoma, lymphoma, other ovarian tumors
- Testicular: Epididymitis, testicular torsion, infarct, orchitis, hernia, hydrocele, hematocele, rhabdomyosarcoma, lymphoma, leukemia, other testicular tumors
- Mediastinal: Hodgkin and non-Hodgkin lymphoma, leukemia, thymoma

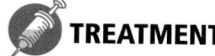 **TREATMENT**

SURGERY/OTHER PROCEDURES

- Every effort should be made to preserve fertility in gonadal teratomas. An experienced pediatric–gynecology oncologic surgeon is critical.
- Sacrococcygeal teratomas should undergo complete resection to include the coccyx for definitive therapy and patients followed closely postoperatively with tumor markers. Fetal surgery indicated when early signs of hydrops develops
- Mature teratoma: Full surgical excision, irrespective of site, is curative in prepubescent patients. One exception is in postpubescent testicular germ cell tumor (with high-risk of mature teratoma relapse in lymph nodes), where orchidectomy, post-adjuvant chemotherapy and +/− post-chemotherapy lymph node dissection are recommended.
- Immature teratoma:
  - Complete surgical resection is therapy of choice. Close observation and tumor marker evaluation for normalization
  - In cases of elevated AFP and incomplete surgical resection; chemotherapy should be offered given risk of microscopic foci of endodermal sinus tumor.
- Teratoma with malignant components:
  - Surgery plus chemotherapy with etoposide, cisplatin or carboplatin, and bleomycin
  - Patients with residual disease should have additional surgery and additional chemotherapy if total resection is not possible.
  - High-dose chemotherapy with autologous stem cell support and radiation are reserved for salvage therapy in recurrent disease.

 ONGOING CARE

- Serial physical exams and imaging studies of primary site
- Tumor markers (AFP or β-HCG) if elevated at diagnosis
- If chemotherapy or radiation therapy used, need to monitor for secondary malignancies, long term. Short term, need to monitor blood counts, chemistries, renal function, and audiology

ADDITIONAL READING

- Barksdale EM, Obokhare I. Teratomas in infants and children. *Curr Opin Pediatr.* 2009;21:344–349.
- Hedrick HL, Flake AW, Crombleholme TW, et al. Sacrococcygeal teratoma: Prenatal assessment, fetal intervention, and outcome. *J Pediar Surg.* 2004;39:430–438.
- Koulouris CR, Penson RT. Ovarian stromal and germ cell tumors. *Semin Oncol.* 2009;36:126–136.
- Lakhoo K. Neonatal teratomas. *Early Hum Devel.* 2010; 86:643–647.
- Mannuel HD Hussain A. Update on testicular germ cell tumors. *Curr Opin Oncol.* 2010;22:236–241.

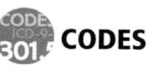 **CODES**

ICD9

- 183.0 Malignant neoplasm of ovary
- 220 Benign neoplasm of ovary
- 222.0 Benign neoplasm of testis

ICD10

- D27.9 Benign neoplasm of unspecified ovary
- D29.22 Benign neoplasm of left testis
- C56.9 Malignant neoplasm of unspecified ovary

FAQ

- Q: What is the chance of cure for immature/malignant teratomas?
- A: With current chemotherapy as outlined above, overall survival is 85–97% (dependent on disease stage).
- Q: Can a benign tumor recur? If so, can it then be malignant?
- A: Yes. If there is residual tissue left behind, the tumor can recur. If there were unrecognized areas of malignancy, the recurrence can be a malignant teratoma. The greatest risk for the latter is with the immature teratomas.

TETANUS

Hamid Bassiri
Joanne N. Wood (5th edition)

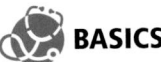 **BASICS**

DESCRIPTION
- Tetanus is a disease characterized by muscle rigidity and spasms due to a neurotoxin produced by *Clostridium tetani* in infected wounds.
- There are 4 clinical forms of tetanus: Generalized, localized, cephalic, and neonatal.

EPIDEMIOLOGY
- Tetanus remains a major problem in developing countries but is rare in the developed world because of widespread immunization.
- Rare cases have been reported in patients with protective levels of anti-tetanus antibodies.
- In the US 40 or fewer cases of tetanus are reported per year.
- Generalized tetanus is the most common form of disease. Neonatal tetanus is rare in the US but common in countries in which women are not immunized and nonsterile care of the umbilical cord is practiced.

RISK FACTORS
- Inadequate immunization
- Neonate born to unimmunized mother
- Elderly with declining immune status
- Injection drug use
- Chronic wounds
- Acute traumatic injury
- Nonsterile delivery conditions and practice of applying mud or feces to umbilical cord

GENERAL PREVENTION
- All wounds should be cleaned with soap and water and foreign bodies should be removed.
- Universal immunization with tetanus toxoid is vital.
  - Primary series: DTaP given at 2, 4, 6, 15–18 months and 4–6 years
  - Booster dose: Tdap at 11–12 years
  - Unimmunized pregnant women should complete primary series prior to delivery if possible or at least receive 2 doses of Td 4 weeks apart.
- Tetanus prophylaxis should be initiated at the time of injury, depending on the nature of the wound. For clean, minor wounds:
  - If the patient has had ≥3 prior doses of tetanus toxoid and it has been <10 years since the last dose, no tetanus prophylaxis is indicated. If it has been ≥10 years since the last dose, tetanus toxoid is indicated.
  - If the patient has had <3 prior doses of tetanus toxoids, tetanus toxoid is indicated.
- For all other wounds:
  - If the patient has had ≥3 prior doses of tetanus toxoid and it has been <5 years since the last dose, no tetanus prophylaxis is indicated. If it has been ≥5 years since the last dose, tetanus toxoid is indicated.
  - If the patient has had <3 doses of tetanus toxoid, tetanus toxoid and tetanus immune globulin (TIG) should be given at separate sites.

- Type and dose of IM tetanus toxoid for wound prophylaxis:
  - For a child <7 years old use DTaP. If pertussis vaccine is contraindicated use DT.
  - For a child 7–10 years old use Td.
  - For an adolescent 11–18 years old who has not received Tdap, give Tdap. For those who have received Tdap or for whom pertussis is contraindicated, administer Td.
- TIG dose is 250 U IM (regardless of age or weight).
- If TIG is unavailable, IV immunoglobulin (IVIG) or equine tetanus antitoxin (after testing for sensitivity) can be used.

PATHOPHYSIOLOGY
- *C. tetani* produces tetanospasmin, a powerful metalloprotease neurotoxin.
- Tetanospasmin can be absorbed directly into skeletal muscles adjacent to the injury.
- Tetanospasmin can travel to the CNS, via retrograde axonal transport through peripheral nerves, or via lymphocytes.
- Tetanospasmin affects the CNS, and the peripheral and autonomic nervous systems:
  - In the CNS, tetanospasmin prevents the release of gamma-aminobutyric acid (GABA) into the post-synaptic cleft, thereby removing the inhibitory control of alpha motor neurons, resulting in sustained excitatory discharges (motor spasms).
  - In the peripheral nervous system, tetanospasmin binds to gangliosides and blocks inhibitory impulses to motor neurons.
  - The mechanism by which tetanospasmin causes autonomic instability (cardiac arrhythmias, blood pressure lability, and respiratory failure) is not as well understood.
- Tetanospasmin does not directly affect cognitive processes.
- Infection with tetanus does not confer immunity, and thus all patients with tetanus need to be immunized with 3 doses of tetanus toxoid starting at diagnosis.

ETIOLOGY
- Tetanus is caused by *C. tetani*, a spore-forming, anaerobic, Gram-positive bacillus.
- *C. tetani* is found in soil, animal and human feces, house dust, salt and fresh water.
- Under anaerobic conditions inoculated spores become vegetative and produce tetanospasmin.
- Anaerobic conditions in wounds are promoted by large amounts of necrosis, foreign bodies, and other ongoing infections with suppuration.

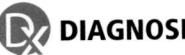 **DIAGNOSIS**

HISTORY
- Incubation period is usually 3–21 days but can vary.
  - Sites of inoculation farther from the CNS are associated with longer incubation periods.
- Generalized tetanus:
  - "Lockjaw" or trismus is initial symptom in 50–75% of cases.
  - Other early complaints include dysphagia, neck pain and stiffness, stiffness and pain in other muscle groups, urinary retention, restlessness, irritability, and headache.
  - More muscles groups involved as disease progresses.
  - Noise, light, touch, and other stimuli can trigger painful spasms.
- Local tetanus:
  - Painful muscle contractions and stiffness limited to the area near the wound.
  - Can persist for several weeks.
  - Can progress to generalized tetanus.
- Cephalic tetanus:
  - Caused by *C. tetani* infections of head and neck wounds.
  - May complicate chronic infections of the head and neck including chronic otitis media.
  - Affects cranial nerves, especially cranial nerve VII.
  - Can progress to generalized tetanus.
- Neonatal tetanus:
  - Occurs following vaginal delivery to unimmunized mothers.
  - Presents at around 1 week of life with irritability and poor feeding.
  - Rapidly progresses to generalized tetanic spasms.

PHYSICAL EXAM
- Vital sign abnormalities:
  - Severe and labile episodes of hypertension and tachycardia.
  - Hypotension may be a late feature.
  - Initially, patients are afebrile.
    - Fever may develop with sustained contractions or from superinfections.
- Trismus is often initial presenting sign.
- Persistent trismus causes *risus sardonicus*, wrinkling of the forehead and distortion of the eyebrows and the corners of the mouth
- As the disease progresses, other muscle groups develop tetanic contractions and spasms:
  - Can lead to a severe opisthotonic posture.
  - Can mimic seizures.
  - Can be extremely painful.
  - Can be associated with potentially fatal laryngospasm and tetany of the respiratory musculature.
  - The anxiety and pain associated with these spasms may precipitate additional spasms.
- Sweating can occur from autonomic instability.
- Normal mental status usually seen.
- Cephalic tetanus:
  - Cranial nerve palsies and muscle spasms including trismus can be seen.
  - Look for underlying wound or chronic infection of the face, scalp, neck, or ear.

DIAGNOSTIC TESTS & INTERPRETATION

Diagnostic Procedures/Other
- Laboratory tests often yield little information.
- Gram stain and anaerobic wound cultures yield *C. tetani* in <1/3 of cases.
- The WBC count is usually normal or mildly elevated.
- Presence of protective tetanus antibody titer does not exclude possibility of disease.
- CSF studies are unremarkable.
- EEG and electromyelogram findings are nonspecific.

DIFFERENTIAL DIAGNOSIS
- Infections:
  – Dental infections, retropharyngeal and peritonsillar abscesses, poliomyelitis, viral encephalitis, and meningoencephalitis may present with trismus and/or cranial nerve findings.
- Toxins and medications:
  – Dystonic reactions to phenothiazine medications may resemble tetanus. Diphenhydramine will effectively treat these reactions.
  – Strychnine poisoning may mimic generalized tetanus.
  – Malignant neuroleptic syndrome can cause increased muscular rigidity resembling titanic spasms.
- Metabolic:
  – Hypocalcemic tetany is usually not as severe as the contractions seen with tetanus.
- Stiff-man syndrome can result in fluctuating tonic muscle contractions resembling titanic spasms.
- Bell's palsy may resemble cephalic tetanus.

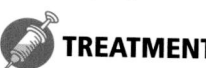 TREATMENT

MEDICATION (DRUGS)
First Line
- Neutralization of unbound neurotoxin:
  – Human TIG 3,000–6,000 U IM as a single dose. Part of the dose may be infiltrated around the wound.
  – Administer prior to antibiotics and wound manipulation.
- Tetanus toxoid should be administered IM at a site contralateral to where TIG is given.
- Antibiotics—used to decrease the number of vegetative *C. tetani* that produce tetanospasmin:
  – First line: Metronidazole 30 mg/kg/d PO or IV in 4–6 divided doses. Maximum 4 g/d.
  – Alternative: Penicillin G 100,000–200,000 U/kg/d IV in 4–6 divided doses.
  – Treat for 10–14 days.
  – Do not use cephalosporins as they are not effective.
- Sedation and muscle relaxation:
  – Diazepam 0.1–0.2 mg/kg IV q4–6h.
  – Phenothiazines, especially chlorpromazine, may be helpful.
  – Carefully titrate sedation to desired effect and monitor for respiratory depression.
- Nondepolarizing neuromuscular blockade and mechanical ventilation—use if spasms cannot be adequately controlled or if spasm of airway and respiratory musculature compromises ventilation:
  – Vecuronium 0.08–0.1 mg/kg IV followed by a continuous infusion or hourly dosing intervals.
  – Pancuronium or doxacurium can be used.
  – Avoid use of succinylcholine because of increased risk of hyperkalemia and arrhythmia.

- Management of autonomic dysfunction:
  – Beta-blockers (such as labetalol 0.4–1.0 mg/kg/hr) may be needed to control hypertension and arrhythmias.
  – Magnesium sulfate has been shown to significantly reduce cardiovascular instability and act as an adjunctive agent to control muscle spasms.

Second Line
If TIG is not available:
- IVIG 200–400 mg/kg may be used but is not FDA approved for this use.
- Equine tetanus antitoxin (TAT) can be given in doses of 1,500–3,000 U IM or IV (to achieve a serum concentration of 0.1 IU/mL), but only after a skin test for sensitization is negative or desensitization has been performed:
  – TAT is not available in the US.
  – Anaphylactic reactions can occur with varying severity in up to 20% of patients.

ADDITIONAL TREATMENT
General Measures
- Keep patient in a quiet, darkened room with minimum stimulus.
- Monitor cardiac and respiratory status closely.
- Be prepared to perform a tracheotomy to prevent fatal laryngospasm.
- Monitor for and treat urinary retention and constipation.
- Parenteral nutrition is usually required to maintain adequate nutrition and hydration.
- Monitor for and correct electrolyte abnormalities, especially hyperkalemia.

SURGERY/OTHER PROCEDURES
Aggressive surgical debridement and removal of foreign bodies from the infected wound is crucial.

IN-PATIENT CONSIDERATIONS
Initial Stabilization
- Prompt recognition of clinical signs of tetanus and initiation of emergency care are critical.
- All suspected cases of tetanus should be rapidly transferred to a tertiary care center capable of providing sophisticated ventilatory and cardiovascular support in an intensive care setting.
- In the emergency department, treatment with TIG should be initiated to neutralize unbound neurotoxin. However, supportive care including aggressive airway management, ventilatory support, and pharmacologic interventions (sedation, muscle relaxation) are also critical to ameliorate the effects of bound neurotoxin.

ONGOING CARE

PROGNOSIS
- Signs and symptoms usually progress for ~1 week. The patient's condition plateaus for ~1 week and then gradually improves over the next 2–6 weeks.
- Overall mortality rates have decreased with advances in the ability to provide respiratory support in an intensive care setting.
- Mortality rates vary from 1–18% for localized tetanus, 15–30% for cephalic tetanus, 45–55% for generalized tetanus to 50–100% for neonatal tetanus.

- Children and young adults have a better prognosis than older individuals.
- A more rapid onset and progression of disease from trismus to generalized spasms is associated with a more severe course.
- In the absence of complications, survivors usually recover fully without long-term sequelae.

COMPLICATIONS
- Most complications are related to the severe tetanic muscle contractions:
  – Rhabdomyolysis and hyperkalemia
  – Vertebral body and other fractures
  – Muscle hemorrhages
- Respiratory failure from spasms of the upper airway or diaphragm is the most common cause of death in acute phase.
- Arrhythmias and myocardial infarctions are most common cause of death later in disease.
- Cerebrovascular hemorrhages may be seen in rare cases, especially in neonatal tetanus.
- Pneumonia, including aspiration, can occur.

ADDITIONAL READING
- American Academy of Pediatrics. Tetanus. In: Pickering LK, Baker CJ, Kimberlin DW, et al., eds. *Red Book: 2009 Report of the Committee on Infectious Diseases*, 28th ed. Elk Grove Village, IL: American Academy of Pediatrics, 2009:655–660.
- Brook I. Tetanus in children. *Pediatr Emerg Care*. 2004;20:48–51.
- Howdieshell TR, Heffernan D, Dipiro JT. Surgical infection society guidelines for vaccination after traumatic injury. *Surg Infect*. 2006;3(3):275–303.
- Rhee P, Nunley MK, Demetriades D, et al. Tetanus and trauma: A review and recommendations. *J Trauma*. 2005;58:1082–1088.
- Thwaites CL, Farrar JJ. Preventing and treating tetanus. *BMJ*. 2003;326:117–118.

CODES

ICD9
- 037 Tetanus
- 771.3 Tetanus neonatorum

ICD10
- A33 Tetanus neonatorum
- A35 Other tetanus

FAQ
- Q: What are characteristics of a tetanus-prone wound?
- A: Punctures and avulsion wounds; crush injuries and burns; wounds from frostbite or missiles; wounds contaminated with saliva, soil, or feces; all wounds—even minor ones—may be inoculated with spores and lead to the development of tetanus.

TETRALOGY OF FALLOT

Christopher J. Petit

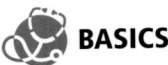 **BASICS**

HISTORY
Described by Fallot of Marseills in 1888, and classified by Mavde Abbott in 1936. Tetralogy of Fallot is the most common form of cyanotic congenital heart disease. It was first successfully palliated in 1944. Now, infants with tetralogy of Fallot commonly undergo complete repair.

DESCRIPTION
Anatomic hallmark is anterior malalignment of infundibular septum:
- A large and unrestrictive ventricular septal defect (VSD)
- Various degrees of right ventricular outflow tract obstruction (RVOTO)
- Overriding aorta
- Right ventricular hypertrophy (RVH): secondary to unrestrictive VSD

Prevalence
3.5–8% of all congenital heart disease

Genetics
- Tetralogy of Fallot (TOF) is associated with a chromosome 22q11 microdeletion in 5–16% of cases
- May be associated with other syndromes including Trisomy 21, Alagille syndrome, CHARGE syndrome, VACTERL syndrome, fetal alcohol syndrome, and those syndromes involving a variety of limb abnormalities. May also affect infants of diabetic mothers. TOF may also be associated with midline abdominal defects (e.g., omphalocele) as in the pentalogy of Cantrell.

PATHOPHYSIOLOGY
Severity of clinical signs and symptoms depends on the degree of RVOTO and resulting cyanosis due to right-to-left shunting. Most infants present with cyanosis due to right → left shunting, while rarely patients can present with overcirculation.

 DIAGNOSIS

SIGNS AND SYMPTOMS
Heart murmur in the newborn period:
- Various degrees of progressive cyanosis reflect severity of RVOT obstruction
- History of paroxysmal cyanosis, especially when crying or during and after physical exercise
- Rarely, a history of tachypnea and feeding intolerance (in "Pink Tetralogy") reflecting overcirculation

PHYSICAL EXAM
Various degrees of cyanosis may be present at birth or may appear later during infancy or childhood as a result of progression of the RVOT/pulmonary stenosis.
- Normal S1 and single loud S2 secondary to a more anteriorly located aorta
- Systolic ejection murmur at left upper sternal border secondary to RVOTO

DIAGNOSTIC TESTS & INTERPRETATION
Imaging
- Electrocardiography: Right axis deviation (+90–180°), RVH
- Chest radiograph: Right aortic arch (30%), decreased pulmonary vascular markings, boot-shaped heart (coeur en sabot) with concave main pulmonary artery (PA) segment
- Echocardiography: Anterior malalignment VSD, infundibular stenosis, overriding aorta, RVH. May also see: Other (muscular) VSDs, valvular pulmonary stenosis and/or branch PA stenosis, abnormal (right-sided) aortic arch anatomy, coronary artery anomalies, ASD.
- Cardiac catheterization: Generally not indicated unless concern is present regarding branch PA anatomy, coronary anatomy, or multiple additional VSDs that need to be defined before surgery
- MRI: Magnetic resonance imaging is commonly performed in older children/adults with repaired TOF to evaluate RV size and function and to determine severity of pulmonery value leakage.

DIFFERENTIAL DIAGNOSIS
- TOF should be considered in all cyanotic infants with a heart murmur, or in children with a history of hypercyanotic spells.
- Important subtypes of TOF include:
- TOF with pulmonary atresia: Pulmonary blood flow arises from the ductus arteriosus. These infants are prostaglandin-dependent and always require neonatal intervention.
- TOF with absent pulmonary valve. These patients are often acyanotic, but may have significant airway complications due to bronchial compression/hypoplasia due to enlarged main and branch pulmonary arteries.
- Differential diagnosis if cyanotic: Transposition of the great arteries (TGA), tricuspid atresia (TA), total anomalous pulmonary venous return (TAPVR), truncus arteriosus, double-outlet right ventricle (DORV)
- Differential diagnosis if not cyanotic: VSD, DORV, peripheral pulmonic stenosis (PPS), valvular pulmonic stenosis (PS)

TREATMENT

MEDICATION (DRUGS)
Hypercyanotic spells (aka "tet spells"): Profound cyanosis due to infundibular spasm and decreased pulmonary blood flow.
- Knee–chest position:
- Oxygen
- Morphine sulfate (0.1 mg/kg IV or IM)
- IV fluid bolus and/or NaHCO3
- Elevate the systemic blood pressure (fluids pressors, etc.)

- β-blocker (esmolol infusion for immediate therapy, propranolol for long-term prophylaxis)
- Phenylephrine (0.02 mg/kg IV)
- Presurgical management:
  - Polycythemia: Oral iron supplement for iron deficiency to avoid microcytosis
  - β-blocker for "tet spell" prophylaxis
  - Subacute bacterial endocarditis (SBE) prophylaxis

SURGERY/OTHER PROCEDURES

- Palliative surgery: Systemic-pulmonary shunt
- Corrective surgery: VSD patch closure and right ventricular outflow tract reconstruction (either an RV-to-PA conduit or a patched reconstruction of the MPA segment)

 ONGOING CARE

PROGNOSIS

Generally good if condition treated surgically in a timely manner:

- >90% of children with TOF are expected to survive to adulthood.
- Surgical mortality is low in most centers: 5-year survival >95%, 20-year survival ~94%
- Long-term quality of life in adulthood is comparable with that of the general population.
- Young patients with TOF have a greater risk of requiring additional help in school.
- Residual hemodynamic abnormalities are quite common
- Pulmonary insufficiency (PI) is common with transannular patch repair:
- Residual RVOTO may occur.
- Right ventricular dysfunction +/− ventricular arrhythmias in adulthood from right ventricular volume overload secondary to PI

- In the setting of severe RV dysfunction and dilatation due to severe PI, some patients require surgical revision of the right ventricular outflow tract in adolescence or adulthood
- Left PA stenosis
- Residual VSD occurs rarely
- Conduction abnormalities (e.g., complete heart block, right bundle branch block [RBBB])
- Supraventricular and ventricular arrhythmias

COMPLICATIONS

Preoperatively:

- Paroxysmal hypoxic spells (i.e., hypercyanotic spells, "tet spell")
- Bacterial endocarditis
- Cerebrovascular accident (CVA) secondary to cyanosis, polycythemia, and microcytic anemia
- Postoperatively: Right ventricular dysfunction and ventricular arrhythmia. Postoperative sudden death (ventricular arrhythmias and/or complete heart block). Exercise intolerance and dyspnea due to severe RV dilatation/dysfunction in the setting of PI

ADDITIONAL READING

- Cobanoglu A, Schultz JM. Total correction of tetralogy of Fallot in the first year of life: Late results. *Ann Thorac Surg.* 2005;74:133–138.
- Nollert G, Fischlein T, Bouterwek S, et al. Long-term survival in patients with repair of tetralogy of Fallot: 36-year follow-up of 490 survivors of the first year after surgical repair. *J Am Coll Cardiol.* 1997;30:1374–1383.
- Neill CA, Clark EB. Tetralogy of Fallot. The first 300 years. *Texas Hert Inst J.* 1994;21(4):272–279.
- Walker WT, Temple IK, Gnanapragasam JP, et al. Quality of life after repair of tetralogy of Fallot. *Cardiol Young.* 2002;12:549–553.

 CODES

ICD9
745.2 Tetralogy of fallot

ICD10
Q21.3 Tetralogy of Fallot

FAQ

- Q: What is the etiology of the "tet spell"?
- A: There is an increased impedance to flow through the RVOT and/or pulmonary vascular bed that leads to a dramatic decrease in pulmonary blood flow and an increased right→left shunt at the level of the VSD. Therefore, treatment should be aimed at increasing pulmonary blood flow either by decreasing pulmonary vascular resistance (e.g., O_2, morphine) or increasing systemic vascular resistance (e.g., knee–chest position, phenylephrine) or decreasing dynamic obstruction by decreasing heart rate and thus increasing RV preload (e.g., β-blockers).
- Q: When is an optimal time for surgical repair of TOF?
- A: At The Children's Hospital of Philadelphia, elective repair of "typical" TOF is performed in early infancy (3–6 months). Progressive hypoxemia or recurrent "tet spell" indicates a need for earlier surgical intervention. Patients with TOF with pulmonary atresia are treated in the newborn period or infancy, and patients with TOF with absent pulmonary valve are treated on a patient-by-patient basis dictated by the degree of airway disease.

T

THALASSEMIA

Peter de Blank
Janet Kwiatkowski (5th edition)

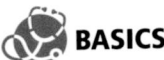 **BASICS**

DESCRIPTION

Thalassemia syndromes are hereditary microcytic anemias that result from mutations that quantitatively reduce globin synthesis.

- Normal hemoglobin is a tetramer of 2 α and 2 β chains:
  - α-Thalassemia: Reduced or absent α-globin production
  - β-Thalassemia: Reduced or absent β-globin production

GENERAL PREVENTION

Thalassemia can be prevented by identifying and counseling potential parents who can have children with thalassemia. Diagnosis can be made in early pregnancy by chorionic villus sampling.

EPIDEMIOLOGY

- α-Thalassemia: Predominantly in Chinese subcontinent, Malaysia, Indochina, and Africa, and in African Americans
- β-Thalassemia: Mediterranean countries, Africa, India, Pakistan, Middle East, and China

Genetics

- α-Thalassemia:
  - Normally, there are 4 α-globin genes, 2 on each chromosome 16.
  - Most mutations in α-thalassemia are large deletions.
  - Deletions may be in *trans* conformation (1 deletion on each chromosome, common in African Americans) or *cis* conformation (2 genes deleted on same chromosome, common in Asians).
  - Hemoglobin Constant Spring is an α-globin gene mutation caused by a point mutation that reduces or eliminates production of α-globin, leading to a more severe phenotype.
  - The 4 α-thalassemia syndromes reflect the inheritance of molecular defects affecting the output of 1, 2, 3, or 4 α genes.
- β-Thalassemia:
  - Normally, there are 2 β-globin genes, 1 on each chromosome 11.
  - Most mutations in β-thalassemia are point mutations.
  - Many mutations abolish the expression completely (β^0), whereas others variably decrease quantitative expression ($\beta+$).
  - Heterozygous state for β-globin mutation produces β-thalassemia trait.
  - Homozygous state produces β-thalassemia major or β-thalassemia intermedia.
  - NOTE: Rare dominant β-thalassemia mutations exist, causing ineffective erythropoesis with a single mutation (due to creation of unstable β-globin variants)

Genotype	Name	Degree of anemia
α thalassemia		
$\alpha\alpha/\alpha -$	Silent carrier	Asymptomatic
$\alpha -/\alpha -$ or $\alpha\ \alpha/- -$	α-thalassemia trait	Asymptomatic
$\alpha -/- -$	α-thalassemia intermedia, HbH disease	Moderate to severe
$- -/- -$	α-thalassemia major	Hydrops fetalis
β-thalassemia		
$\beta/\beta+$ or β/β^0	β thalassemia trait	Asymptomatic
β/β^0 or $\beta+/\beta+$	β thalassemia intermedia	Variable, intermittent or chronic transfusions
$\beta^0/\beta+$ or β^0/β^0	β thalassemia major	Severe, chronic transfusions

PATHOPHYSIOLOGY

- Decrease in either α- or β-globin synthesis leads to fewer completed $\alpha_2-\beta_2$ tetramers produced per RBC, which results in a decrease in intracellular hemoglobin and microcytosis.
- Unpaired globin chains precipitate resulting in apoptosis of red cell precursors (ineffective erythropoiesis) and damage to the RBC membrane leading to hemolysis.
- Ineffective erythropoiesis causes hepatosplenomegaly and osseous changes.
- The erythrocyte's life span is shortened by hemolysis and splenic trapping.
- Degree of anemia varies depending on the specific gene defect.
- Chronic transfusion therapy, and to a lesser degree, increased absorption of dietary iron in thalassemia major lead to iron accumulation.
- Increased absorption of dietary iron and intermittent transfusions in thalassemia intermedia lead to iron accumulation.
- Iron overload leads to cardiac arrhythmias and congestive heart failure (CHF) that can be fatal, liver inflammation and fibrosis, and endocrinopathies (e.g., diabetes mellitus, hypothyroidism, gonadal failure), osteoporosis.

 **DIAGNOSIS**

HISTORY

- Severe α-thalassemia (4 gene deletion) presents prenatally by ultrasound or at birth with hydrops fetalis and severe anemia.
- Severe β-thalassemia usually presents between 3 and 12 months old, as the production of the normal fetal hemoglobin decreases.
- α-Thalassemia syndromes will present with microcytosis in infancy. Hemoglobin H disease may present later, with mild to moderate anemia on screening or after worsening hemolysis related to intercurrent infection.
- Mediterranean, African, or Asian are common ethnic backgrounds in patients with thalassemia.
- Familial history of anemia, long-term transfusions, recurrent iron therapy for presumed iron-deficiency anemia, or splenectomy. Siblings and/or parents may be affected.

PHYSICAL EXAM

- Pallor indicates anemia.
- Heart murmur: Flow murmurs are often heard in significant anemia. Patients with severe anemia may present with CHF.
- Variable degrees of icterus: Hemolysis leads to increased bilirubin production.
- Abnormal facies (frontal bossing and maxillary hyperplasia): Facial bone expansion by hypertrophic marrow in poorly transfused patients with β-thalassemia
- Failure to thrive: Related to anemia and energy expended in ineffective erythropoiesis
- Variable degrees of hepatosplenomegaly (or CHF) due to extramedullary hematopoiesis

DIAGNOSTIC TESTS & INTERPRETATION

Lab

- CBC with RBC indices:
  - Mean cell volume, mean cell hemoglobin, and mean cell hemoglobin concentration are all decreased in both α- and β-thalassemia.
  - RBC volume distribution width is usually normal.
  - Mentzer index [MCV/(RBC count)] can distinguish thalassemia trait from iron-deficiency anemia:
    - <13 suggests thalassemia
    - >13 suggests iron deficiency anemia
  - Peripheral smear may reveal microcytosis, hypochromia, anisocytosis, poikilocytosis, target cells, nucleated RBCs, and/or polychromasia.
  - Hemoglobin 9–12 g/dL in α- or β-thalassemia trait
  - Hemoglobin usually 7–10 g/dL in HbH disease
  - Hemoglobin usually 7–10 g/dL in β-thalassemia intermedia
  - Hemoglobin <7 g/dL in thalassemia major (without transfusions)
- Reticulocyte count: Usually mildly elevated in HbH and β-thalassemia intermedia and major
- Indirect bilirubin: May be elevated in severe thalassemia where there is significant red cell destruction

- Hemoglobin electrophoresis:
  - α-Thalassemia trait (2 defective genes) will have 5–10% Hb Barts (a tetramer of 4 γ chains) at birth, which should be detected on the newborn's screen. This disappears in 1–2 months, after which time the electrophoresis will be normal in α-thalassemia trait.
  - β-Thalassemia trait: HbF 1–5%, HbA2 3.5–8%, remainder HbA. The elevated HbA2 will distinguish α- from β-thalassemia trait.
  - HbH disease (3 defective α genes): 5–30% HbH (β_4), remainder HbA
  - Hydrops fetalis (4 defective α genes): Mainly Hb Barts(γ_4)
  - β-Thalassemia major (2 defective β genes): HbF 20–100%, HbA2 2–7%. In most cases, little or no HbA is detected, unless recently transfused.
- Iron studies, serum ferritin: Useful to help distinguish thalassemia from iron deficiency

DIFFERENTIAL DIAGNOSIS
- Iron deficiency anemia can be distinguished with iron studies.
- Anemia of chronic inflammation (can be distinguished with soluble transferrin receptor assay)
- Lead poisoning

 TREATMENT

- Silent carriers (single α gene deletion) and α-and β-thalassemia trait:
  - Genetic counseling only
  - Distinguish from iron deficiency microcytosis to avoid excess iron supplementation.
- For HbH disease:
  - Folic acid daily
  - Transfusions whenever necessary (aplastic episode, infection)
  - Splenectomy if evidence of hypersplenism
  - Cholecystectomy if necessary
- For β-thalassemia intermedia:
  - Folic acid daily
  - No iron supplements
  - Transfusions whenever necessary (aplastic episode, infection, acute complication)
  - Splenectomy less commonly performed due to increased risk of thrombosis and pulmonary hypertension.
  - Cholecystectomy if necessary
  - HbF-inducing agents such as hydroxyurea may be beneficial.
  - Monitoring and treatment of iron overload
- β-Thalassemia major:
  - Stem cell transplantation (umbilical cord blood or bone marrow) using histocompatible sibling donor can cure the disease and is being used more frequently.
  - Regular transfusions of RBCs every 3–4 weeks to maintain Hb at 9–10 g/dL
  - Chelation therapy: It is important to balance the treatment of iron overload with the dangers of overchelation (toxicity to ears, eyes, bone).

- Chelation options include:
  - Deferoxamine (SC or IV infusion over 8–24 hours)
  - Deferasirox (once daily PO chelator). Side effect include GI discomfort, rash, renal failure +/− proteinuria, hepatic failure
  - Deferiprone (currently available in the US only through compassionate use protocol). Especially good for cardiac iron removal. Side effects include arthropathy, GI upset, agranulocytosis.
- Folic acid daily
- Penicillin prophylaxis (125–250 mg b.i.d.) for splenectomized patients
- *Pneumococcus, Meningococcus,* and *Haemophilus influenzae* vaccines before splenectomy and annual influenza A vaccination
- Cholecystectomy if indicated
- No iron supplements
- Genetic counseling for those with any thalassemia syndrome

> ### ALERT
> Thalassemia trait is often treated incorrectly as presumptive iron-deficiency anemia. Iron studies should be performed to confirm the diagnosis if there is no improvement in Hb level after a few weeks of iron therapy.

 ONGOING CARE

For patients with thalassemia major and intermedia:
- Serum ferritin, blood chemistries, and liver function tests should be monitored.
- Annual monitoring for cardiac complications (echocardiogram, EKG) and endocrine function is recommended.
- Liver iron quantitation by biopsy, MRI, or other techniques are necessary intermittently to quantitate the status of iron overload accurately.
- Newer cardiac T_2* MRI techniques to assess the degree of cardiac iron loading, which correlates with risk of cardiac complications.
- Annual audiologic and ophthalmologic screening is recommended for persons receiving chelation therapy (to monitor for chelator toxicity).
- DXA scan or bone peripheral quantitative computed tomography (PQCT) annually

PROGNOSIS
- Life expectancy for patients with β-thalassemia major has improved over the years because of regular transfusions and chelation therapy.
- Bone marrow transplant from a histocompatible sibling donor may be curative.

COMPLICATIONS
Most complications occur in patients with β-thalassemia intermedia or major and can be divided into 2 categories
- Complications related to anemia/ineffective erythropoiesis and hemolysis (seen mostly in thalassemia intermedia):
  - Skeletal abnormalities secondary to hyperplastic marrow
  - Osteopenia, osteoporosis, and fractures
  - Growth retardation

- Extramedullary hematopoiesis
- Leg ulcers
- CHF owing to severe anemia
- Thrombophilia, particularly in thalassemia intermedia after splenectomy
- Hypercoaguability: DVT, PE
- Gallstones from hemolysis
- Pulmonary hypertension
- Allo- or auto-immunization with RBC antibodies
- Complications of iron overload:
  - Cardiac abnormalities: Pericarditis, arrhythmias, CHF
  - Hepatic abnormalities: Cirrhosis and liver failure (onset usually after second decade)
  - Endocrine disturbances: Delayed puberty, growth retardation, diabetes mellitus, hypothyroidism, hypoparathyroidism
  - Infection: Particularly Yersinia species

ADDITIONAL READING

- Cohen AR, Galanello R, Pennell DJ, Cunningham MJ, Vinchinsky E. Thalassemia. *Hematology Am Soc Hematol Educ Program.* 2004:14–34.
- Cunningham MJ. Update on thalassemia: Clinical care and complications. *Pediatr Clin North Am.* 2010; 24:215–227.
- Gu X, Zeng Y. A review of the molecular diagnosis of thalassemia. *Hematology.* 2002;7:203–209.
- Lo L, Singer ST. Thalassemia: Current approach to an old disease. *Pediatr Clin North Am.* 2002;49: 1165–1191.
- Rund D, Rachmilewitz E. β-Thalassemia. *N Engl J Med.* 2005;353:1135–1146.

 CODES

ICD9
- 282.40 Thalassemia, unspecified
- 282.43 Alpha thalassemia
- 282.44 Beta thalassemia

ICD10
- D56.0 Alpha thalassemia
- D56.1 Beta thalassemia
- D56.9 Thalassemia, unspecified

FAQ
- Q: Is prenatal testing available?
- A: Yes.
- Q: In a transfused patient, when does iron overload become a problem and when is chelation started?
- A: Usually after the age of 3–4 years.
- Q: At what age should monitoring for cardiac iron overload begin in β-thalassemia major?
- A: 6–10 years of age.

THORACIC INSUFFICIENCY SYNDROME

Fiona M. Healy
Robert M. Campbell, Jr.
Oscar H. Mayer

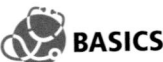 **BASICS**

DESCRIPTION
- Thoracic insufficiency syndrome (TIS) is the inability of the thorax to support normal respiration or lung growth.
- Patients are skeletally immature with varied anatomic deformities that often include:
  - Flail chest syndrome: Rib absence due to a congenital malformation or chest wall tumor resection, rib instability in cerebrocostomandibular syndrome, and others
  - Constrictive chest wall syndrome, including rib fusion and scoliosis: VACTERL association, chest wall scarring from radiation treatment, windswept deformity of the chest from progressive scoliosis, and others
  - Hypoplastic thorax syndrome including Jeune syndrome, Jarcho-Levin syndrome, Ellis–van Creveld syndrome, spondylothoracic dysplasia (STD), and others
  - Progressive congenital scoliosis (without rib anomaly) or neuromuscular scoliosis
- The recognizable anatomic abnormalities often occur before respiratory insufficiency, with patients compensating for low lung volumes and poor respiratory mechanics with an increased respiratory rate.
- Subsequently decreased activity and chronic respiratory insufficiency

PATHOPHYSIOLOGY
- The thorax is the respiratory pump, requiring an adequate diaphragm (abdominal) and chest wall movement. Limitation in resting volume (functional residual capacity [FRC] and/or the ability of the rib cage to expand during respiration can significantly alter respiratory function and cause TIS.
- The window of rapid lung growth and alveolar development is during the first 3 years of life, although alveolar development is felt to continue through 5 or 8 years of age, if not longer. Without concurrent thoracic growth, however, the lung cannot grow normally.
- Growth of the thoracic pump is also necessary so that the respiratory system can continue to meet a patient's metabolic demands. Thoracic spinal height (TSH) directly contributes to thoracic volume and lung volume. At birth, the TSH is 13 cm normally, then during the first 5 years of life, thoracic spinal growth is 1.4 cm/year, 0.6 cm/year from 5–10 years, and 1.2 cm/year from 10–18 years of age. A thoracic length of 22 cm at skeletal maturity, the normal TSH of a 10 year old, appears to be the minimum height necessary for normal respiration.

- Complex scoliosis spinal rotation with spinal lordosis into the convex hemithorax, the "windswept" deformity of the thorax, can further diminish transverse volume available for lung growth.
- Unilateral caudal rotation of the ribs in neuromuscular disease, the "collapsing parasol deformity," typically occurs on the convex side of the scoliosis and may also severely narrow the thorax, worsen thoracic mechanics, and further increase work of breathing.

ETIOLOGY
- The etiologies of TIS can be grouped into unilateral or bilateral volume depletion deformities (VDDs) of the thorax that reduce the volume available for the lungs in certain subsets of patients with rare syndromes. This causes primary TIS, or deformity of the chest from scoliosis.
- In addition, progressive congenital scoliosis without rib anomalies can result in TIS from a variant of type II VDD of the thorax.
- Type IIIB VDD of the thorax can also develop in neurogenic scoliosis, as in spinal muscular atrophy with marked intercostal muscle weakness.
- Spinal deformity, such as lumbar kyphosis in spina bifida, collapses the torso into the pelvis, raising abdominal pressure that blocks diaphragm excursion, causing secondary TIS.

COMMONLY ASSOCIATED CONDITIONS
- Congenital renal abnormalities can occur in 33% of congenital scoliosis.
- Cervical spine abnormalities, causing stenosis and proximal instability
- Spinal cord abnormalities, including spinal cord syrinx and tethered cord, which are especially prevalent in meningomyelocele
- Jeune syndrome:
  - Congenital renal abnormalities
  - Hepatic fibrosis
  - Cervical spinal stenosis in 60% of cases
- Ellis–van Creveld syndrome
- STD:33% have congenital diaphragmatic hernia
- Cerebrocostomandibular syndrome, Pierre Robin syndrome: Mmicrognathia
- Severe tracheal compression and severe narrowing can occur in advanced scoliosis or severe anteroposterior narrowing.

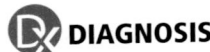 **DIAGNOSIS**

HISTORY
- Onset of clinical scoliosis
- Onset of respiratory symptoms:
  - Relative exertional intolerance
  - Ineffective cough
  - Pneumonia
  - Hospitalizations for respiratory symptoms
  - Need for supplemental oxygen or ventilator support (BiPAP or CPAP)
- Progression of the spinal or chest wall deformity
- Current symptoms:
  - Chronic respiratory insufficiency
  - Exertional limitation relative to age and gross motor capability
  - Recurrent respiratory illnesses
  - Balance problems
  - Back pain

PHYSICAL EXAM
- Comprehensive respiratory examination:
  - Assessment of work of breathing including accessory muscle use and thoracoabdominal asynchrony
  - Qualitative assessment of chest wall compliance and motion
- Visual assessment
- Thumb excursion test: The palms of each hand are loosely positioned posteriorly over each side of the chest with the thumbs aligned on either side of the spinal column, and relative excursion is assessed by the amount of lateral thumb movement.
- Assessment of rib hump by having the patient bend forward while standing upright
- Measure of liver size to evaluate for hepatomegaly and possible cor pulmonale

DIAGNOSTIC TESTS & INTERPRETATION
Lab
- Serum bicarbonate as an indirect assessment for chronic hypoventilation
- Arterial blood gas if there is a concern for acute respiratory failure
- Liver function testing to assess for coincident liver failure
- Brain-type natriuretic peptide to help assess for progressive heart strain or failure
- Genetic testing as indicated based on suspected underlying condition

Imaging

- Standing anteroposterior and lateral radiographs to establish severity of scoliosis in the sagittal and coronal planes; bending films to establish the flexibility of the curve
- Chest CT scan with 5-mm cuts noncontrast with optimal pediatric settings to minimize radiation, with spinal and chest wall reconstruction to assess in 3-dimensional orientation
- MRI of spine and spinal cord to look for spinal cord abnormality
- Additional radiologic testing may be employed in certain cases (e.g., ventilation-perfusion scan of the lungs to quantify right vs. left functional perfusion asymmetry)
- Echocardiogram to evaluate for cor pulmonale and pulmonary hypertension

Diagnostic Procedures/Other

- Pulmonary assessment:
  - Pulmonary function testing
  - Dynamic lung volumes and flows:
    - Forced vital capacity (FVC)
    - Timed expiratory volume (forced expiratory volume in 0.5 or 1 second) and the ratio to FVC
    - Forced expiratory flow between 25% and 75% of vital capacity (FEF 25–75%)
  - Static lung volume measurements:
    - Total lung capacity (TLC), FRC, residual volume (RV), and RV/TLC
  - Specialized measurements of respiratory system compliance (stiffness) and partitioned measurements of chest wall and lung compliance
  - Pulse oximetry and end-tidal carbon dioxide measurement
  - Overnight polysomnography to assess the degree of underlying respiratory insufficiency and need for supplemental oxygen or noninvasive ventilation
  - Exercise testing adapted for the capabilities of the patient (6-minute walk test) can be used to assess for exertional limitation.
- Genetic assessment:
  - If there is significant thoracospinal abnormality and certainly if there is other dysmorphology, a genetics assessment is very helpful to comprehensively assess for an underlying disorder.

 TREATMENT

ADDITIONAL TREATMENT

General Measures

- Bracing and halo-gravity traction can be used as a temporizing procedure and at best has been shown to control some forms of scoliosis or partially improve, but not correct, scoliosis.
- Physical and occupational therapy

SURGERY/OTHER PROCEDURES

- The goal of surgical treatment of TIS is to gain the biggest, most symmetrical, and most functional thorax by skeletal maturity through repeated expansions of the chest wall along with spinal growth and correction of spinal deformity without the growth inhibition effects of spinal fusion.
- Vertical expandable prosthetic titanium rib (VEPTR) expansion thoracoplasty techniques enable five types of acute thoracic reconstructions to handle each of the subtypes of TIS. The procedure can be performed as early as 6 months of age to exploit the growth potential of the developing lungs and provide additional thoracic volume and compensatory lung growth. After implantation to stabilize the initial thoracospinal reconstruction, it can then be expanded about every 6 months commensurate with patient growth until skeletal maturity.

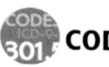 **ONGOING CARE**

FOLLOW-UP RECOMMENDATIONS

- After TIS surgery, patients are followed with radiographs at regular intervals.
- Pulmonary follow-up should include careful assessment for respiratory insufficiency.
- Longitudinal measure of lung function and growth to demonstrate an improvement in respiratory status or lung function, or at the very least a decrease in the rate of decline, in the most severely affected patients

PROGNOSIS

- Prognosis will vary depending on the underlying cause of TIS, severity of respiratory insufficiency, and the age of the patient at surgery.
- For older patients near skeletal maturity, the focus is chest wall reconstruction and spinal stabilization, hopefully with stabilization in pulmonary function. Significant improvement in vital capacity is doubtful because of late onset in treatment.
- The expectation in infancy would be for growth preservation and an increase in lung volume above the preoperative value as a percent of predicted. There does appear to be an inverse relationship between the age of the patient at the time of surgery and the level of positive impact of VEPTR insertion on lung function.

- Jeune syndrome is one of the more severe forms of TIS with 60–70% mortality in early infancy from respiratory failure. However, after VEPTR insertion, the outcomes are more favorable.
- Of those patients with TIS due to an STD, 47% die in infancy from respiratory complications and pulmonary hypertension. VEPTR treatment of STD is controversial.

COMPLICATIONS

- In the immediate postoperative period——wound infection, skin slough, and bleeding
- Migration of fixation over 3–5 years
- Device breakage is very uncommon.
- Neurologic complications are rare.

ADDITIONAL READING

- Campbell RM Jr, Smith MD. Thoracic insufficiency syndrome and exotic scoliosis. *J Bone Joint Surg Am.* 2007;89(Suppl 1):108–122.
- Cornier AS, Ramirez N, Arroyo S, et al. Phenotype characterization and natural history of spondylothoracic dysplasia syndrome: A series of 27 new cases. *Am J Med Genet A.* 2004;128(2):120–126.
- Mayer OH. Management of thoracic insufficiency syndrome. *Curr Opin Pediatr.* 2009;21(3):333.

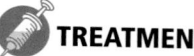 **CODES**

ICD9

- 518.82 Other pulmonary insufficiency, not elsewhere classified
- 786.09 Other respiratory abnormalities

ICD10

R06.89 Other abnormalities of breathing

T

THROMBOSIS
Char Witmer

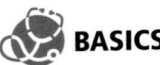 **BASICS**

DEFINITION
Pathologic arterial or venous intravascular occlusion secondary to abnormal thrombus formation.
The following are common thrombotic events:
- Deep venous thrombosis (DVT): Involves large systemic veins outside CNS
- Cerebral sinovenous thrombosis: Involves intracranial venous sinuses
- Ischemic stroke: CNS arterial occlusion with infarction of brain tissue
- Intracardiac thrombosis: Mural, valvular, or foreign body associated
- Femoral artery thrombosis: Can be associated with vessel catheterization
- Renal vein thrombosis: Commonly in the neonatal period; may be unilateral or bilateral
- Myocardial infarction: Kawasaki disease, antiphospholipid antibody syndrome or with severe familial hypercholesterolemia
- Budd–Chiari syndrome: Thrombosis of the hepatic vein
- Portal vein thrombosis

EPIDEMIOLOGY
- Incidence of venous thrombosis in children is estimated at 0.7 per 100,000 per year. It is likely that the actual incidence is higher.
- Age distribution is bimodal, peak rates in the neonatal and adolescent age groups
- Idiopathic thrombosis is rare in children.
- >90% of pediatric venous thrombosis is associated with additional risk factors.
- Central venous lines are the most common risk factor for venous thrombosis in children.

RISK FACTORS
- **Neonatal**
  - Prematurity
  - Maternal diabetes
  - Umbilical catheters or other central lines
  - Sepsis
  - Polycythemia
  - Perinatal asphyxia
- **Malignancy/bone marrow disorders**
  - Leukemia (hyperleukocytosis, acute promyelocytic leukemia)
  - Myeloproliferative disorders
  - Paroxysmal nocturnal hemoglobinuria
- **Medications**
  - L-Asparaginase
  - Oral contraceptives
  - Heparin-induced thrombocytopenia
  - Steroids
- **Anatomic**
  - Indwelling catheters
  - Congenital heart disease
  - Prosthetic heart valves
  - Intracardiac baffles
  - Tumor compression
  - Atresia of the inferior vena cava
  - Thoracic outlet obstruction (Paget–Schroetter syndrome)
  - May–Thurner syndrome (compression of the left iliac vein by the artery crossing over it)

- **Miscellaneous**
  - Infection
  - Trauma
  - Surgery
  - Obesity
  - Prolonged immobilization or paralysis
  - Dehydration
  - Antiphospholipid syndrome
- **Risk factors/conditions specific for arterial disease**
  - Kawasaki disease
  - Takayasu arteritis
  - Hyperlipidemia
  - Antiphospholipid syndrome

COMMONLY ASSOCIATED CONDITIONS
- Nephrotic syndrome
- Inflammatory disorders
- Liver disease
- Sickle cell disease
- Diabetes mellitus

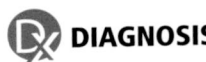 **DIAGNOSIS**

DIFFERENTIAL DIAGNOSIS
Primary prothrombotic states:
- **Inherited**
  - Factor V Leiden gene mutation
  - Prothrombin 20210A gene mutation
  - Protein C deficiency
  - Protein S deficiency
  - Antithrombin deficiency
  - Homocystinemia (mild to moderate) from minor defects in enzymes such as methylenetetrahydrofolate reductase or severe in homocystinuria
  - Elevated lipoprotein(a)
  - Plasminogen deficiency
  - Dysfibrinogenemia
  - Heparin cofactor II deficiency
- **Acquired:** Antiphospholipid antibody syndrome

ALERT
- Normal ranges for coagulation tests are age dependent: Diagnosing an inherited deficiency in any of the anticoagulant proteins can be difficult in the neonatal period. Repeat testing at 6–12 months of age is necessary.
- Consumption can occur during acute thrombosis; therefore, low levels of the anticoagulant proteins must be repeated.
- Warfarin will decrease the levels of protein C, protein S, and clotting factors II, VII, IX, and X.

APPROACH TO THE PATIENT
- **Phase 1:** Perform complete history and physical exam; establish diagnosis using the appropriate radiographic study
- **Phase 2:** Send initial laboratory studies (CBC, PT/aPTT, D-dimer, β-hCG testing in postmenarchal females and antithrombin) and begin anticoagulation therapy with unfractionated heparin or low-molecular-weight heparin. Patients with life- or limb-threatening thrombosis may require thrombolysis.
- **Phase 3:** Complete lab workup for hypercoagulable state; outpatient anticoagulation; follow thrombosis radiologically

HISTORY
Presence of risk factors previously listed
- **Question:** Current (or recent) central venous or arterial catheter?
- *Significance:* Most significant risk factor for thrombosis
- **Question:** Family history of thrombosis?
- *Significance:* May be an inherited thrombophilia
- **Question:** Personal history of thrombosis?
- *Significance:* Patients with history of thrombosis are at increased risk of recurrence.
- **Question:** Neonatal seizure?
- *Significance:* Common and often the only presenting sign for cerebral sinovenous thrombosis or arterial ischemic stroke
- **Question:** Chest pain or shortness of breath?
- *Significance:* Suggestive of pulmonary embolism

PHYSICAL EXAM
- **Finding:** Unilateral swelling/edema of a limb?
- *Significance:* Extremity DVT
- **Finding:** Bilateral lower extremity edema of a limb?
- *Significance:* Thrombosis of the inferior vena cava
- **Finding:** Plethoric, swollen head and neck?
- *Significance:* Superior vena cava syndrome
- **Finding:** Pale extremity with decreased perfusion/pulses?
- *Significance:* Arterial thrombosis
- **Finding:** Abdominal mass in neonate with hematuria?
- *Significance:* Renal vein thrombosis
- **Finding:** Tachypnea, shallow respirations?
- *Significance:* Pulmonary embolism
- **Finding:** Unexplained hepatosplenomegaly?
- *Significance:* Hepatic or portal vein thrombosis
- **Finding:** Superficial dilated cutaneous veins distal to the site of venous occlusion?
- *Significance:* Post-thrombotic syndrome
- **Finding:** Chronic discoloration (darkening) of the skin, ulcerations, pain, intermittent swelling?
- *Significance:* Post-thrombotic syndrome

DIAGNOSTIC TESTS & INTERPRETATION
- General evaluation of the hemostatic system:
  - PT, aPTT, fibrinogen
  - CBC with platelet count
  - D-dimer
  - β-hCG in postmenarchal female
- The following tests are used to investigate for a prothrombotic state:
  - Phase 1:
    ○ Factor V Leiden mutation analysis
    ○ Prothrombin 20210A mutation analysis
    ○ Lupus anticoagulant screen (dilute Russell viper venom time, aPTT)
    ○ Anticardiolipin antibodies (IgG, IgM)
    ○ Anti-β2-glycoprotein antibodies (IgG, IgM)
    ○ Protein C activity
    ○ Protein S activity
    ○ Antithrombin activity
    ○ Fasting homocysteine
    ○ Fasting lipoprotein(a)
    ○ Factor VIII activity

– Phase 2: For patients whose phase 1 studies are normal, but there is a strong family history of thrombosis:
  ○ Plasminogen
  ○ Thrombin time or dysfibrinogenemia screen
  ○ Activated protein C resistance clotting assay
  ○ Heparin cofactor II
  ○ Plasminogen activator inhibitor type 1
  ○ Factor IX and XI activity

Imaging

Radiologists should be consulted for choosing the best imaging study for diagnosis and follow-up.

- Contrast angiography: Gold standard, but invasive and sometimes technically difficult to perform in small children
- Ultrasound: Most commonly used imaging study because of noninvasiveness, absence of radiation, and ability to be performed at the bedside
- In the diagnosis of upper extremity-related DVT, often a combination of ultrasound and venography is necessary:
  – Compression ultrasound of the upper central veins may be impeded by the distal end of the clavicle.
  – Venography has poor sensitivity for diagnosing thrombosis of the internal jugular veins.
  – Recommended approach for diagnosis of an upper extremity thrombosis is to start with ultrasound and proceed to venography if the ultrasound is normal and there is a high clinical suspicion for thrombosis.
- Echocardiogram may be useful in evaluating atrial thrombi, which may result from central venous catheters.
- Pulmonary angiography, ventilation–perfusion scans, and spiral CT scans are the imaging studies used for the diagnosis of pulmonary embolism, although none of these have been studied in children.
- In patients with a pulmonary embolism, it is important to look for a source of thrombosis in the upper and lower extremities.
- Other diagnostic imaging options include CT or MRV:
  – Noninvasive
  – Sensitivity and specificity not known
  – May be helpful in evaluating proximal thrombosis
- For diagnosis of cerebral sinovenous thrombosis, the most sensitive imaging study is a brain MRI with venography.

TREATMENT

- Unfractionated heparin:
  – Given as a bolus followed by an infusion, adjusted to maintain the aPTT at 1.5–2.5 times baseline
  – Younger children require higher doses of heparin to achieve a therapeutic level secondary to physiologically decreased antithrombin levels.
- Low-molecular-weight heparin:
  – More predictable dose response
  – Given subcutaneously twice a day
  – Equivalent in efficacy to unfractionated heparin in the acute management of uncomplicated DVT
  – Renal clearance
- Thrombolytic therapy:
  – Recombinant tissue plasminogen activator
  – May be given systemically or locally
  – High risk of bleeding

- Warfarin:
  – Oral anticoagulant
  – Initially started when a patient is already receiving a form of heparin. The heparin is discontinued when the warfarin is in the therapeutic range.
  – Warfarin is adjusted to maintain an international normalized ratio (INR) of 2.0–3.0 for treatment of DVT
  – Used for outpatient management
- Aspirin:
  – Beneficial in stroke and other arterial events
  – Irreversibly inhibits platelet function

General Measures

- Therapy for acute thrombosis and long-term management is individualized.
- Consult a pediatric hematologist or someone with expertise in pediatric anticoagulant therapy.

ONGOING CARE

COMPLICATIONS

- Inferior vena cava filters are used to prevent pulmonary embolism. There are limited pediatric studies. They should only be considered in the setting of a lower extremity DVT with a contraindication to anticoagulation (i.e., recent extensive surgery or active bleeding) or if a patient experiences a pulmonary embolism while on therapeutic anticoagulation. Temporary filters should be placed and removed as soon as possible as they are a nidus for further thrombosis formation. The risk/benefit ratio needs to be considered individually.
- Vary depending on the location and severity of the thrombosis
- In DVT, pulmonary embolism is the most significant acute complication. Recurrent thrombosis and post-thrombotic syndrome are common chronic complications.
- In arterial thromboembolic disease, the ischemic injury to the involved organ determines the acute and long-term complications.

ALERT

- Central venous catheter-related thrombosis may be subtle despite extensive damage to the venous system. Recurrent line infection, line occlusion, and prominent venous collaterals on the chest suggest upper extremity DVT. The long-term consequences of this are not known.
- Warfarin can cause purpura fulminans if started in a non-heparinized patient.

ADDITIONAL READING

- Goldenber N, Bernard T. Venous thromboembolism in children. *Pediatr Clin N Am.* 2008;55:305–322.
- Kearon C. Natural history of venous thromboembolism. *Circulation.* 2003; 107(23 Suppl 1):I22–I30.
- Line BR. Pathophysiology and diagnosis of deep venous thrombosis. *Semin Nucl Med.* 2001;31: 90–101.
- Monagle P, Chalmers E, Chan A, et al. Antithrombotic therapy in neonates and children. Antithrombotic and thrombolytic therapy: ACCP Evidence-Based Clinical Practice Guidelines (8th edition). *Chest.* 2008;133:887s–968s.
- Raffini L. Thrombolysis for intravascular thrombosis in neonates and children. *Curr Opin Pediatr.* 2009;21(1):9–14.
- Witmer CM, Ichord R. Crossing the blood brain barrier: Clinical interactions between neurologists and hematologists in pediatrics. Advances in childhood arterial ischemic stroke and cerebral venous thrombosis. *Curr Opin Pediatr.* 2010; 22:20–27.

CODES

ICD9

- 325 Phlebitis and thrombophlebitis of intracranial venous sinuses
- 453.9 Other venous embolism and thrombosis of unspecified site
- 453.40 Acute venous embolism and thrombosis of unspecified deep vessels of lower extremity

ICD10

- I82.90 Acute embolism and thrombosis of unspecified vein
- I82.409 Acute embolism and thombos unsp deep vn unsp lower extremity
- G08 Intracranial and intraspinal phlebitis and thrombophlebitis

FAQ

- Q: If an inherited prothrombotic condition is identified, should family members be tested?
- A: Yes, if they have other risk factors for thrombosis such as malignancy, major surgery, oral contraceptives, or obesity.
- Q: When is it appropriate to use low-molecular-weight heparin rather than unfractionated heparin?
- A: There are several potential advantages to low-molecular-weight heparin. The pharmacokinetics is much more predictable, and frequent monitoring is not necessary. It is administered subcutaneously, not intravenously. The risk of bleeding may be slightly lower. Low-molecular-weight heparin cannot be completely reversed with protamine and it is renally cleared.
- Q: When is it appropriate to use thrombolytic therapy?
- A: Studies do not clearly demonstrate a role for thrombolytic therapy in deep venous thrombosis. However, if a thrombus is high risk (i.e., limb-threatening), thrombolytic therapy can be used. Intracranial bleeding, other active bleeding and surgery within 7 days are contraindications to thrombolytic therapy. For arterial thrombotic events, thrombolytic therapy is often the treatment of choice because of the rapid resolution of the clot and restoration of blood flow.
- Q: What precautions should be taken for invasive procedures and for athletics when a patient is on anticoagulant therapy?
- A: Lumbar punctures, arterial punctures, and surgical procedures should be avoided. If they are necessary, then the child should have the anticoagulant reversed or held before the procedure. The child should not participate in contact sports such as football, karate, and boxing.

T

TICK FEVER

Brian T. Fisher

BASICS

DESCRIPTION
- Both endemic relapsing fever and Colorado tick fever (CTF) will be discussed in this chapter.
- Relapsing fever in its endemic form is a vector-borne infection with characteristic recurrent fevers caused by several species of spirochetes of the genus *Borrelia*. In the US, the vector for endemic relapsing fever is ticks of the genus *Ornithodoros*. Epidemic relapsing fever is transmitted by the body louse and is no longer found in the US.
- CTF is a febrile, usually benign, systemic illness caused by a double-stranded RNA coltivirus in the family Reoviridae and transmitted by a tick bite. Although the primary reservoir for infection is the *Dermacentor andersoni* tick, the causative organism has been isolated from many other ticks. The virus is referred to as Colorado tick fever virus.

EPIDEMIOLOGY
- Endemic relapsing fever:
  - Reported in almost all western states up to and including Texas.
  - Sites of high exposure include limestone caves and forested areas.
  - Most cases present during June through September; ~450 cases were reported in the US between 1977 and 2000.
  - Infection in the United States most commonly occurs after exposure to *Ornithodoros hermsi* and *Ornithodoros turicata*. The former feeds on rodents in forests at elevations of 1,500–8,000 feet, while the latter prefer drier locations at lower elevations.
- CTF:
  - Human infections typically occur in areas where *D. andersoni* is found: Western US and southwestern Canada at elevations of 4,000–10,000 feet
  - Cases usually occur between April and July when adult ticks are most active. There are 200–400 reported cases in the US annually, but this may be an underestimation.
  - Infection is more common in males and the median age of those infected is 43 years but 25% of cases occur in those younger than 20 years.
- Transfusion-related and laboratory-associated infection are rare but have been reported.

GENERAL PREVENTION
- Both of these infections can be prevented by avoidance or protection from the tick vector.
- Light-colored, long-sleeved shirts and pants should be worn when tick-infested areas cannot be avoided.
- Permethrin should be applied to clothing and diethyltoluamide (DEET) applied to exposed skin to help repel ticks.
- Persons who enter endemic areas should inspect themselves and each other frequently for adherent ticks.
- Avoid rodent-infested homes in endemic areas. If necessary, rodent-nesting materials should be removed with protective gloves.
- Confirmed cases should be reported to health authorities so that control measures can be instituted.

PATHOPHYSIOLOGY
- Endemic relapsing fever:
  - When an Ornithodoros tick feeds on a natural host (e.g., squirrels, chipmunks, and rodents), Borrelia subsequently invade all tissues of the tick including the salivary glands. Once infected, ticks remain capable of transmitting disease for many years. Transovarial infection of tick offspring is possible but is thought to be rare.
  - Ticks in the larval stage are unlikely to be infectious.
  - Borrelia is transmitted to humans when the tick takes a blood meal and then detaches itself. Transmission is possible after only 30 seconds of feeding.
  - Ornithodoros ticks typically feed at night and for short periods. The exposed person is often unaware of the tick bite.
  - After transmission, spirochetemia develops resulting in systemic symptoms. Antibody production ultimately leads to agglutination and phagocytosis of the spirochetes with symptom resolution.
  - The spirochete is capable of various strategies (e.g., spontaneous antigenic variation and sequestration in certain organs) to evade the immune system. This results in recurrent spirochetemia with associated febrile episodes. Tick-borne disease may relapse 10–15 times before final resolution.
  - Between episodes of spirochetemia, organisms likely persist in the CNS, bone marrow, liver, and spleen.
  - Pathologic findings in humans include petechial hemorrhages on visceral surfaces, hepatosplenomegaly, and a histiocytic myocarditis.
- CTF:
  - Ticks are infected during their larval stage when they feed on viremic, intermediate hosts such as chipmunks, ground squirrels, and porcupines.
  - Once infected, ticks remain infected for life (as long as 3 years)
  - Human infection typically takes place when the adult *D. andersoni* wood tick attaches and ingests a blood meal from an incidental human host.
  - CTF virus is thought to infect hematopoietic cells, causing leukopenia and prolonged viremia for up to 3–4 months.

ETIOLOGY
- Endemic relapsing fever is caused by several species of spirochetes in the genus *Borrelia*. *B. hermsii* and *B. turicatae* are the 2 most common species found in the US. Epidemic relapsing fever is caused by *B. recurrentis*, which is transmitted by *Pediculus humanus* (human body louse).
- CTF is caused by CTF virus, a double-stranded RNA coltivirus in the family Reoviridae.

DIAGNOSIS

HISTORY
- Both endemic relapsing fever and CTF most commonly present with symptoms including high fever, headache, myalgias, and chills. A thorough history documenting recent travel and a description of the fever curve are necessary to help direct the clinician to either diagnosis.
- Endemic relapsing fever:
  - Fevers present after a mean incubation period of 5–7 days (range 4–>18 days). Symptoms resolve after 3–6 days but then recur within 7 days. Relapses may be less severe than the initial episode with prolonged asymptomatic intervals.
  - Patients commonly complain of headache, myalgia, nausea, vomiting, arthralgias, and abdominal pain. Less commonly, patients are symptomatic with confusion, dry cough, diarrhea, photophobia, rash, dysuria, or hepatosplenomegaly.
  - Patients rarely are aware of a recent tick bite.
- CTF:
  - CTF has a usual incubation period of 3–5 days (range 1–14 days):
    ○ In ~50% of patients, fever will present in a "saddleback" pattern. The fever persists for 2–3 days with resolution for 2–3 days. Fever then recurs and lasts for another 2–3 days. Some patients will have a 3rd febrile period.
    ○ Patients may complain of lethargy, photophobia, retro-orbital pain, and conjunctival injection.
    ○ Less commonly, patients will have gastrointestinal symptoms, pharyngitis, nuchal rigidity, and a rash.
    ○ Unlike endemic relapsing fever, 90% of patients presenting with CTF will have a previous history of tick exposure.

PHYSICAL EXAM

High fevers (39–41°C) are common to both endemic relapsing fever and CTF:

- Endemic relapsing fever:
  - In addition to the typical fever curve and symptoms described above, the clinical presentation is varied and the physician's exam should evaluate for, but not be limited to, the following:
    ○ Elevated pulse and BP are common.
    ○ Tender hepatosplenomegaly with jaundice
    ○ Nuchal rigidity suggesting meningitis
    ○ Gallop on cardiac auscultation suggesting underlying myocarditis
    ○ A macular rash starting on the trunk that becomes generalized and or petechial in nature
    ○ Neurologic deficits are less common but can include delirium, cranial nerve deficits (7th or 8th nerve palsy), and visual impairment from iridocyclitis.
- CTF:
  - Similar to that of endemic relapsing fever, the clinical presentation for CTF is varied but may include the following:
    ○ A small, red painless papule may be seen.
    ○ A maculopapular rash with petechial lesions has been reported in ~10% of cases.
    ○ Pharyngitis is reported in 20% of cases.
    ○ Hepatosplenomegaly has been found in some patients.
    ○ Nuchal rigidity and delirium are rare but, if present, suggest meningitis or encephalitis.

DIAGNOSTIC TESTS & INTERPRETATION

- Endemic relapsing fever:
  - The diagnosis can be readily made by identification of loosely coiled spirochetes on thin and thick smears of the peripheral blood. Blood samples taken at the time of fever have the highest yield.
  - Increased sensitivity can be obtained by examining Acridine orange–stained preparations of dehemoglobinized thick smears or buffy coat preparations.
  - The organism can only be cultured on special culture medium. Intraperitoneal inoculation of mice with the patient's blood can lead to spirochetemia in the mice.
  - Multiple serologic antibody studies exist, including direct and indirect immunofluorescence, ELISA, and immunoblot analysis:
    ○ A 4-fold rise in titers between acute and convalescent studies is considered confirmatory.
    ○ These studies may have false-positive reactions in patients with prior spirochete infections such as Lyme disease.
  - Polymerase chain reaction (PCR) analysis can be useful in identifying the causative organism but is not readily available.
  - Other nonspecific laboratory findings may include leukocytosis, anemia, thrombocytopenia, unconjugated hyperbilirubinemia, elevated hepatic transaminases, and proteinuria.
  - If myocarditis is present, an electrocardiogram can reveal abnormalities such as a prolonged corrected Q-T interval.
  - In cases complicated by meningitis, the CSF will typically have moderately elevated protein and a mononuclear pleocytosis.
- CTF:
  - PCR testing and viral cultures are available in certain laboratories. PCR testing is the most sensitive and timely approach for diagnosing acute infection.

- Various techniques (e.g., complement fixation, indirect immunofluorescence, EIA and Western blot) have been used to establish a serologic diagnosis:
  ○ Serologic testing for antibody presence is not diagnostic in the acute phase because antibodies are slow to rise. Presence of a 4-fold rise in neutralizing antibody titers at >2 weeks after onset can be confirmatory.
  ○ Associated laboratory findings include leukopenia and thrombocytopenia.
- In patients with meningitis or encephalitis, CSF studies may also reveal elevated protein and a lymphocytic pleocytosis.

DIFFERENTIAL DIAGNOSIS

- Endemic relapsing fever and CTF resemble each other clinically. Presence of biphasic or relapsing fever along with a history of travel to an area where appropriate vectors are found are helpful clues in diagnosing either disease. Leukopenia and a history of a tick bite may differentiate CTF from endemic relapsing fever.
- Relapsing fever and CTF may be misdiagnosed as influenza or enteroviral infections, especially with the 1st febrile episode.
- Other infectious illnesses that may present with recurrent fevers include but are not limited to yellow fever, dengue fever, lymphocytic choriomeningitis, brucellosis, malaria, leptospirosis, rat bite fever, and chronic meningococcemia. The patient travel history and animal exposure should help differentiate among some of these diagnoses.

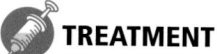 **TREATMENT**

MEDICATION (DRUGS)

- Endemic relapsing fever:
  - The treatment of choice is oral tetracycline/doxycycline for 7–10 days. Children <8 years of age and pregnant women should receive erythromycin or penicillin.
  - Newer macrolides may be effective but are not routinely recommended.
  - In >50% of cases, treatment results in a Jarisch-Herxheimer reaction (severe fevers, rigors, diaphoresis, and hypotension) related to rapid clearing of the spirochetemia. Close observation, IV fluids, and good supportive care are important in treating possible reactions.
  - Some experts support the use of an initial single dose of oral penicillin (7.5 mg/kg) or IV penicillin G (10,000 U/kg given over 30 minutes) in patients presenting with systemic symptoms. It is thought that this initial dose of penicillin leads to gradual clearance of spirochetes decreasing the risk of the Jarisch-Herxheimer reaction. These patients should then receive a 10-day course of tetracycline or erythromycin because penicillin has been associated with an increased rate of relapse.
  - Single-dose tetracycline or erythromycin has been successful for the treatment of louse-borne epidemic relapsing fever in Ethiopia.
- CTF:
  - There is no specific therapy for patients with CTF Treatment is primarily supportive.
  - Thrombocytopenia should be monitored closely because generalized bleeding rarely results in death of children.
- Ribavirin has been shown in animal studies to be helpful and thus could be considered in certain severe situations.

 ONGOING CARE

PROGNOSIS

- Endemic relapsing fever:
  - Generally responds rapidly to appropriate antibiotic therapy.
  - Mortality in patients treated appropriately is thought to be <1%.
  - Untreated louse-borne relapsing fever is associated with a much higher rate of fatality.
- CTF:
  - Usually a self-limiting illness without sequelae
  - Death is rare but has been reported in children with generalized bleeding likely secondary to thrombocytopenia.
  - Prolonged weakness may persist for ≥3 weeks and is more likely in those patients >30 years old.

COMPLICATIONS

- Endemic relapsing fever:
  - May be associated with splenic rupture, diffuse histiocytic interstitial myocarditis, hepatitis, pneumonia, ARDS, and iridocyclitis
  - CNS complications include meningitis, meningoencephalitis, and focal deficits such as cranial nerve palsy.
  - In utero infection may result in fetal loss or severe neonatal infection.
- CTF:
  - Complications are rare but most commonly occur in children.
  - May lead to aseptic meningitis, encephalitis, myocarditis, pneumonitis, hepatitis, hemorrhage, and epididymo-orchitis

ADDITIONAL READING

- Brackney MM, Marfin AA, Staples JE, et al. Epidemiology of Colorado tick fever in Montana, Utah, and Wyoming, 1995–2003. *Vector Borne Zoonotic Dis.* 2010;10:381–385.
- Dworkin MS, Schwan TG, Anderson DE Jr, et al. Tick-borne relapsing fever. *Infect Dis Clin N Am.* 2008;22:449–468.
- Larsson C, Andersson M, Bergstrom S. Current issues in relapsing fever. *Curr Opin Infect Dis.* 2009;22:443–449.
- Romero JR, Simonsen KA. Powassan encephalitis and Colorado tick fever. *Infect Dis Clin N Am.* 2008;22:545–559.
- Roscoe C, Epperly T. Tick-borne relapsing fever. *Am Fam Physician.* 2005;72:2039–2044.

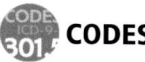 **CODES**

ICD9
- 066.1 Tick-borne fever
- 087.1 Relapsing fever, tick-borne

ICD10
- A68.1 Tick-borne relapsing fever
- A93.2 Colorado tick fever

TICS

Rebecca K. Lehman
Mohammad M. Qasaymeh (5th edition)
Jonathan W. Mink (5th edition)

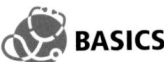

BASICS

DESCRIPTION

- A tic is a sudden, repetitive, stereotyped, involuntary movement (e.g., blinking, grimacing) or vocalization (e.g., throat clearing, grunting, barking). Tics can be further classified as simple (e.g., nose twitching, grunting) or complex (e.g., head shaking, trunk flexion, echolalia, neologism). Tics characteristically change in anatomic location, frequency, type, complexity, and severity over time, although each tic has a stable appearance from one occurrence to the next. Most individuals are able to suppress their tics for brief periods of time, and some endorse having premonitory sensory urges preceding tics. Tics typically abate during sleep but can persist in some cases.
- *DSM-IV-TR* classification of tic disorders:
  - Tourette syndrome (TS): Onset before age 18 years and at least 2 motor tics and 1 vocal tic present in some combination over the course of ≥ 1 year
  - Chronic motor or vocal tic disorder: Onset before 18 years and single or multiple motor or vocal tics, but not both, for ≥ 1 year
  - Transient tic disorder: Onset before 18 years and motor and/or vocal tics that have been present ≥ 4 weeks but ≤ 1 year
  - Tic disorder not otherwise specified (NOS): Motor and/or vocal tics that do not fit a specific tic disorder (e.g., lasting <4 weeks, onset >18 years)
- Pediatric autoimmune neuropsychiatric disorder associated with streptococcus (PANDAS):
  - A controversial entity first described in 1998. In theory, group A β-hemolytic streptococcal (GABHS) infection triggers antibodies that cross-react with the basal ganglia and cause obsessive-compulsive disorder (OCD) symptoms and/or tics in some individuals.
  - The National Institute of Mental Health (NIMH) defines PANDAS as follows:
    - Presence of OCD and/or a tic disorder
    - Prepubertal onset
    - Sudden, explosive onset of symptoms and a course of dramatic exacerbations and remissions
    - Temporal relationship between symptom onset and exacerbations and GABHS infections
    - Presence of neurologic abnormalities (hyperactivity, choreiform movements, tics) during exacerbations
  - These diagnostic criteria do not always prove helpful in distinguishing PANDAS from other "standard" tic disorders. The high incidence of GABHS infections and high prevalence of asymptomatic carriers make it difficult to prove a link between GABHS infection and tics.

EPIDEMIOLOGY

- Described in almost all ethnic groups
- Affects males > females
- Typical onset is between ages 5 and 7 years.

Prevalence

- The prevalence of chronic tics and TS in school-age children is 3–6% and 0.1–1%, respectively.
- Transient tics occur in 20–25% of children.

RISK FACTORS

Genetics

No single gene has been associated with tics or TS; however, the family history is often positive for tics. The prevalence of TS in 1st-degree relatives is 10 times that in the general population.

GENERAL PREVENTION

Tics cannot be prevented, but educating patients, families, and school personnel about tics can help to minimize their impact. Identification and aggressive management of comorbid conditions strongly influences patient outcomes.

PATHOPHYSIOLOGY

The pathophysiology of underlying tics and TS is not completely understood but is thought to involve abnormal dopamine neurotransmission within the basal ganglia. Evidence also implicates problems with serotonin, norepinephrine, and acetylcholine.

ETIOLOGY

Theory: Environmental or hormonal perturbations trigger tics in genetically susceptible individuals.

COMMONLY ASSOCIATED CONDITIONS

- ~50% of children with chronic motor tics or TS meet diagnostic criteria for attention deficit hyperactivity disorder (ADHD), and ~50% have OCD or obsessive-compulsive traits.
- Anxiety, learning disabilities (LD), oppositional defiant disorder, conduct disorder, and rage episodes are also associated with TS.

DIAGNOSIS

The diagnosis of tics is clinical. Physical examination, laboratory tests, and imaging studies typically are normal.

HISTORY

- Document a description of the patient's past and current tics, including age of onset, type, anatomic location(s), duration, number, frequency, complexity, severity, and exacerbating (stress/anxiety) or alleviating factor(s).
- Determine the degree to which the tics are causing interference and/or impairment.
- Assess for comorbid conditions, including ADHD, anxiety disorders (including OCD), LD, and disruptive behaviors.
- In prepubertal patients with severe, sudden-onset OCD symptoms and/or tics, inquire about recent GABHS infections.

PHYSICAL EXAM

Physical examination is usually normal. Tics may not be seen; thus, it may be necessary to depend on history. Having the child intentionally reproduce the sound(s) and/or movement(s) of concern and/or having the parents provide video can aid in differentiating tics from other movement disorders.

DIAGNOSTIC TESTS & INTERPRETATION

Lab

There is little evidence to support routine testing for GABHS in children suspected of having PANDAS. Throat cultures should be obtained in children with symptoms of pharyngitis.

Diagnostic Procedures/Other

Diagnosis depends largely on history. Diagnostic tests are unnecessary. Psychological testing may elucidate comorbid conditions (ADHD, OCD, LD).

DIFFERENTIAL DIAGNOSIS

- Usually, diagnosis is straightforward. Complex or dystonic tics can be more difficult to diagnose because they can resemble purposeful, normal movements or other abnormal movements. In general, tics can be distinguished from other movement disorders based on their stereotyped appearance, waxing and waning course, associated premonitory urges, and ability to be suppressed for brief periods of time.
- Hemifacial spasm (HFS) is a rare condition that results in frequent, involuntary muscle contractions involving one side of the face. Initially, the spasms are intermittent and are restricted to a few muscles; over time, they become continuous and spread to involve the entire hemiface. Early cases of HFS may be difficult to distinguish from motor tics. However, HFS is limited to one side of the face, and the spasms last longer than tics.
- Chorea is characterized by rapid, random, purposeless movements that often have a "dance-like" quality. Unlike tics, chorea is not stereotyped.
- Myoclonus is a sudden, brief, shock-like movement. "Sleep starts" that often occur in normal individuals as they drift off to sleep are a typical example. Myoclonus is not suppressible and is not associated with a premonitory sensation.
- Stereotypies are patterned, episodic, repetitive, purposeless, rhythmic movements. The movements are constant in pattern and location, without variation over time.
- Fasciculations are fine, random, spontaneous worm-like or twitching movements that occur in the setting of chronic denervation. They reflect spontaneous firing of single motor units and are easily distinguished from tics based on their clinical appearance and electrophysiologic signature.
- Myokymia refers to involuntary, spontaneous, localized twitching of a few muscle bundles. It results from hyperexcitability of peripheral nerve motor axons and is readily distinguished by its clinical and electrophysiologic appearance.

- Tremor is a regular oscillatory movement around a central point or plane, whereas tics are repetitive but irregular and nonoscillatory.
- Dystonia is characterized by repetitive, sustained muscle contractions that cause abnormal postures and movements, often with a twisting quality. A dystonic tic (i.e., tic that results in a sustained posture) can be difficult to distinguish from dystonia; however, the presence of a premonitory urge would suggest the former diagnosis.
- Periodic limb movement disorder (PLMD) is associated with repetitive, often stereotyped limb movements during non–rapid eye movement (non-REM) sleep. Since the movements only occur during sleep and are generally restricted to the lower limbs, they are easily distinguished from tics. PMLD can be associated with restless leg syndrome; however, the diagnosis is made by polysomnography.
- Partial seizures may be confused with tics. The automatisms accompanying partial seizures may look like tics, but they are not associated with premonitory sensations, nor are they under partial voluntary control. EEG is normal in children with tics but may be abnormal in those with seizures.

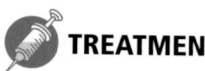 **TREATMENT**

Many tics do not interfere with children's lives and therefore do not require specific treatment. Educating the child and family about tics is often sufficient. Clinical decisions must take comorbid symptoms into account, and treatments must target the most impairing symptoms first. The waxing and waning nature of tics confounds treatment; it may take weeks to identify whether an intervention is helping.

MEDICATION (DRUGS)
- Mild/Occasional tics: Medication not needed
- Moderate or severe: α-2 agonist or dopamine antagonist may reduce severity/frequency.
- With OCD: Selective serotonin reuptake inhibitors can be helpful. Fluoxetine, fluvoxamine, and sertraline appear to be equally effective.
- With ADHD: Guanfacine (or clonidine) may help hyperactivity/impulsivity. Consider addition of a stimulant if symptoms are refractory or if inattention is the primary complaint.
- PANDAS: As above. There is insufficient evidence to support the use of long-term antibiotics and/or immunomodulation.

First Line
- Clonidine and guanfacine are considered 1st-line (off-label) medications. Avoid abrupt discontinuation, which can cause rebound hypertension.
- Clonidine: Start 0.05 mg at bedtime. Increase by 0.05 mg every week as needed and as tolerated to a maximum of 0.3–0.4 mg/day, divided 3 or 4 times/day. Sedation and orthostatic hypotension are common initial adverse effects. A transdermal clonidine patch is an alternative to oral preparations.
- Guanfacine: Start 0.5 mg at bedtime. Increase by 0.5 mg every week as needed and as tolerated to a maximum of 3–4 mg/day, divided twice a day. Guanfacine is less likely than clonidine to cause sedation and hypotension.

Second Line
- Atypical and typical antipsychotic medications are considered 2nd-line medications. Weight gain is common with all antipsychotic medications, but the atypical agents are generally preferred because they are better tolerated overall and are less likely to cause extrapyramidal side effects.
- Commonly used atypical agents include:
  – Risperidone: Start 0.01 mg/kg daily. Increase by 0.02 mg/kg/day every week as needed and as tolerated to a maximum of 0.06 mg/kg/day.
  – Ziprasidone or olanzapine: Reasonable alternatives
- Typical antipsychotics (haloperidol, pimozide) are potent medications for tics but are associated with troublesome side effects, such as sedation, weight gain, metabolic syndrome, and galactorrhea. More serious side effects include extrapyramidal reactions, neuroleptic malignant syndrome, and tardive dyskinesia. Pimozide is associated with QT prolongation, which can lead to ventricular arrhythmias. The use of typical antipsychotic should be limited to refractory and disabling tics.

ADDITIONAL TREATMENT
General Measures
There is no evidence that lifestyle changes or restriction of activities modify the course of tic disorders.
Additional Therapies
- A recent randomized controlled trial of children and adolescents with TS and chronic tic disorder demonstrated that a comprehensive behavioral intervention—consisting of awareness training, competing response training, relaxation training, and social support—resulted in greater improvement in tic severity than supportive therapy and education alone. The effect size of the intervention was on par with that of medication.
- Focal motor (or vocal) tics may be treated with injections of botulinum toxin into the affected muscles (especially useful for focal dystonic tics).

SURGERY/OTHER PROCEDURES
Recent experimental data have shown deep brain stimulation (DBS) as a potential treatment for adults with severe and refractory tics.

 ONGOING CARE

DIET
There is no evidence that dietary modifications alter the course of tic disorders.

PATIENT EDUCATION
The Tourette Syndrome Association (www.tsa-usa.org) is a valuable resource for information. There are many local chapters.

PROGNOSIS
Although common, tics cause impairment in a minority of children. Peak severity occurs in preadolescence. Most patients have partial or complete resolution of tics as adults. Long-term outcome depends on associated comorbidities.

COMPLICATIONS
Tics can be emotionally distressing and can result in social disability. Injuries—due to complex tics, compulsions, impulsivity, inattention, and other factors—may be more common in patients with TS that in the general population. Chronic repetitive, and forceful tics can cause musculoskeletal problems (e.g., cervical spine arthritis, disc herniation) or other neurologic problems (e.g., cervical myelopathy, stroke secondary to vertebral artery dissection).

ADDITIONAL READING
- Deckersbach T, Rauch S, Buhlmann U, et al. Habit reversal versus supportive psychotherapy in Tourette's disorder: A randomized controlled trial and predictors of treatment response. *Behav Res Ther*. 2006;44:1079–1090.
- Mink JW, Walkup J, Frey KA, et al. Patient selection and assessment recommendations for deep brain stimulation in Tourette syndrome. *Mov Disord*. 2006;21(11):1831–1838.
- Piacentini J, Woods DW, Scahill L, et al. Behavior therapy for children with Tourette disorder: A randomized controlled trial. *JAMA*. 2010;303(19):1929–1937.
- Snider LA, Seligman LD, Ketchen BR, et al. Tics and problem behaviors in schoolchildren: Prevalence, characterization, and associations. *Pediatrics*. 2002;110:331–336.
- Tourette Syndrome Study Group. Treatment of ADHD in children with tics: A randomized controlled trial. *Neurology*. 2002;58:527–536.
- Shprecher D, Kurlan R. The management of tics. *Mov Disord*. 2009;24(1):15–24.

 CODES

ICD9
- 307.20 Tic disorder, unspecified
- 307.21 Transient tic disorder
- 307.22 Chronic motor or vocal tic disorder

ICD10
- F95.2 Tourette's disorder
- F95.9 Tic disorder, unspecified
- G25.69 Other tics of organic origin

FAQ
- Q: Can a child with tics and ADHD be treated with stimulant medication?
- A: Although there have been concerns of stimulants making tics worse, there is no evidence that stimulants cause chronic tics. Furthermore, several recent studies have shown that treatment of ADHD with stimulants does not worsen tics and may lead to improvement.
- Q: Should mild tics be treated if they lead to teasing?
- A: The best approach is to educate the child, parents, and teacher about tics. The child can be armed with a response to questions, such as "Those are tics. They are just something I do, and I can't help it."

T

TOXIC ALCOHOLS

Thomas Nguyen
Robert J. Hoffman
Khalid Alansari (5th edition)

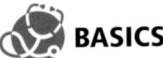

BASICS

DESCRIPTION
- Toxic alcohols discussed here include ethylene glycol, isopropyl alcohol, and methanol.
- Ethylene glycol is a sweet, odorless, colorless liquid commonly used as automobile antifreeze solution as well as for other uses.
- Isopropyl alcohol is used as rubbing alcohol as well as in liquid soaps, hand sanitizers, and for other uses.
- Methanol is used in windshield wiper fluid, Sterno, paint removers, and other products.

EPIDEMIOLOGY
- Exposure to toxic alcohols is common; mild morbidity occurs regularly.
- Severe morbidity or death occurs without treatment but is uncommon in treated patients.

RISK FACTORS
Toxicity via dermal absorption rarely occurs in infants or young children with permeable skin.

GENERAL PREVENTION
Poison proofing homes and giving parents poison prevention advice is the most effective way to prevent toxic alcohol exposures in children.

PATHOPHYSIOLOGY
All toxic alcohols have direct effects as intoxicants. More importantly, ethylene glycol and methanol are metabolized to toxic by-products that result in severe morbidity or mortality:
- Ethylene glycol is metabolized to oxalic acid and glycolic acid, ultimately forming calcium oxalate crystals, which may precipitate in the renal tubules and cause renal failure.
- Methanol is metabolized to formaldehyde and then formic acid, which may damage the retina and cause visual impairment or blindness.
- The metabolism of ethylene glycol and methanol to their toxic metabolites may be prevented by competitively inhibiting alcohol dehydrogenase with either fomepizole or ethanol.
- Therapy to inhibit alcohol dehydrogenase is used for ethylene glycol and methanol exposure.
- Isopropyl alcohol is metabolized to acetone and causes ketosis without acidosis.
- Inhalational absorption of isopropyl alcohol may rarely occur.

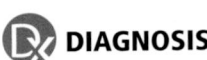

DIAGNOSIS

HISTORY
- Typically, a history of exposure is available.
- In absence of this history, an osmolar gap or anion gap with metabolic acidemia is suggestive of toxic alcohol exposure.
- Signs and symptoms:
  - Inebriation may occur after exposure.
  - Isopropyl alcohol may cause severe gastrointestinal irritation or hemorrhage.

PHYSICAL EXAM
- Tachycardia and hypotension are the most frequent vital sign abnormalities that occur.
- Hyperpnea or tachypnea often accompanies metabolic acidemia.
- Cardiovascular effects may include hypocalcemic QT prolongation and myocarditis.
- Neurologic abnormalities may include ataxia, CNS depression, coma, dysarthria, focal neurologic changes, hyporeflexia, hypotonia, nystagmus, or seizure.
- Gastrointestinal effects may include gastritis emesis, hematemesis, pain, or pancreatitis.
- Ophthalmologic findings may include blurred vision, diplopia, hazy vision, or nystagmus.
- Constricted visual fields, hyperemic optic disc with retinal edema, and transient or permanent blindness may result from methanol exposure.
- Hematuria, renal insufficiency, or renal failure may occur, particularly from ethylene glycol.
- Fluid and electrolyte abnormalities from ethylene glycol or methanol may include hypokalemia, hypocalcemia, hypomagnesemia, and elevated anion gap metabolic acidosis.
- Acetonemia and ketonemia may result from isopropyl alcohol ingestion.
- Hypoglycemia may be associated with toxic alcohol exposure as well as with ethanol therapy.
- Respiratory irritation from isopropyl alcohol inhalation or respiratory depression from any toxic alcohol ingestion may occur.

DIAGNOSTIC TESTS & INTERPRETATION
Diagnostic Procedures/Other
- Check serum electrolytes, BUN, creatinine, and glucose:
  - As metabolism occurs, an increased anion gap metabolic acidemia results with ethylene glycol or methanol toxicity.
  - Absence of this gap early after ingestion is expected and does not rule out ingestion.
  - Elevated anion gap metabolic acidemia supports the diagnosis of ethylene glycol or methanol exposure.
  - Acidemia is an indication for use of fomepizole or ethanol as well as potential indication for hemodialysis.
  - Fomepizole treatment should not be delayed waiting to determine if acidemia will develop.
  - Anion gap metabolic acidemia does not result from isopropyl alcohol poisoning.
- Blood gas analysis should be performed to assess for degree of metabolic acidemia in any patient with low serum bicarbonate:
  - Initial use of venous blood gas to screen for abnormality is acceptable.
  - Repeated blood gas analysis should occur every 1–2 hours if acidemia results.
- Serum level of ethylene glycol, isopropyl alcohol, or methanol should be obtained:
  - An ethylene glycol or methanol level >20 mg/dL is an indication for fomepizole or ethanol infusion.
  - An ethylene glycol or methanol level >50 mg/dL is an indication for hemodialysis.

- Serum ionized calcium is useful in managing ethylene glycol toxicity.
- Urinalysis with microscopic examination is recommended with ethylene glycol exposure:
  - Presence of oxalate crystals corroborates poisoning.
  - Absence of crystals does not exclude the possibility of ethylene glycol toxicity.
  - Fluorescence of urine is unreliable and is neither sensitive nor specific for exposure.
- Proteinuria and hematuria may be present with ethylene glycol or isopropyl alcohol exposure.
- Serum osmolality or osmolarity may be useful in predicting the level of ethylene glycol, isopropyl alcohol, or methanol if rapid laboratory quantification cannot be performed.
- Serum ethanol level should simultaneously be performed to determine quantity of ethanol contribution to osmolar gap.
- An elevated osmolar gap can be used to rule in, but not exclude, toxic alcohol exposure.
- An elevated osmolar gap indicates the presence of unmeasured solute such as ethanol, ethylene glycol, isopropyl alcohol, or methanol.
- Absence of an osmolar gap does not exclude the possibility of toxic alcohol exposure.
- Osmolar gap is calculated as follows: Osmolar gap = Measured serum osmolality − Calculated osmolarity.
- The measured osmolality is determined by the laboratory.
- The calculated osmolarity is determined as follows: $2 \times [\text{Na (mEq/L)}] + [\text{BUN (mg/dL)}/2.8] + [\text{glucose (mg/dL)}/18]$.
- Normal osmolar gap is <15 mEq/L.
- Any patient with increased osmolar gap should be presumed to have toxic alcohol exposure.
- Additional tests may include ECG to detect cardiac conduction disturbance (prolonged QTc) or serum acetaminophen and salicylate levels in patients with intentional ingestion or with presumed intent of self-harm.
- Tests necessary to rule out differential diagnoses should be obtained when appropriate.

DIFFERENTIAL DIAGNOSIS
Drugs and disorders that may alter laboratory values include acetone, diethylene glycol, ethanol, iron, isoniazid, lactic acidemia, mannitol, methanol, propylene glycol, renal failure, salicylates, toluene, and various forms of ketoacidosis.

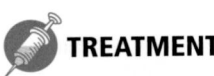

TREATMENT

MEDICATION (DRUGS)
- For ethylene glycol or methanol poisoning, either fomepizole or ethanol is used to competitively inhibit alcohol dehydrogenase, thus preventing the formation of toxic metabolites.
- Fomepizole is highly preferable to ethanol in children, as ethanol has many severe adverse side effects such as hypoglycemia, CNS depression, and hypothermia.

- Indications for fomepizole or ethanol include:
  - Serum level of ethylene glycol or methanol >20 mg/dL
  - Metabolic acidemia, urine oxalate crystals, pH <7.3 with any quantity of detectable ethylene glycol or methanol
- Use of fomepizole or ethanol will prolong the half-life of ethylene glycol and methanol:
  - Without therapy, the ethylene glycol half-life is 3–4 hours, while methanol is 14–20 hours.
  - With fomepizole or ethanol, the ethylene glycol half-life is 12 hours, while methanol is 30–50 hours.
- Some clinicians consider a necessary duration of therapy longer than several days to be an indication for hemodialysis. Successful use of prolonged therapy with fomepizole to avoid hemodialysis has been reported.
- Fomepizole is contraindicated in patients with documented allergic reaction to the drug.
- Ethanol should be used with extreme caution in Asians because aldehyde dehydrogenase deficiency may result in flushing, severe illness, and hypotension.
- The loading dose of fomepizole is 15 mg/kg IV.
- Maintenance dosing is 10 mg/kg q12h for 4 doses.
- Fomepizole induces its own metabolism, and after 4 maintenance doses the maintenance dose is increased to 15 mg/kg q12h thereafter.
- Each dose is diluted into 100 mL of normal saline or D5W and infused over 30 minutes to prevent burning at the infusion site.
- Each time after hemodialysis is performed, a loading dose must be readministered.
- Ethanol is administered as a 10% solution in D5W. This dilution requirement often results in a very large quantity of free water administration.
- The ethanol loading dose is 10 mL/kg of a 10% solution infused IV over 1 hour.
- A maintenance dose of 1.0–2.0 mL/kg of 10% ethanol is then given IV.
- Target blood ethanol level is 100–125 mg/dL.
- Patients receiving ethanol should have the ethanol level and serum glucose checked hourly.
- Oral ethanol may be used when IV is not available or if the patient is willing and capable of drinking. This is possibly feasible in adolescents.
- Adjunctive treatment with folate or Leucovorin for methanol, and thiamine and pyridoxine for ethylene glycol, may be given IV q6h:
  - This continues until methanol or ethylene glycol levels are undetectable.
  - Folate or tetrahydrofolate (Leucovorin) may hasten the elimination of formic acid resulting from methanol exposure.
  - Leucovorin 1–2 mg/kg may be administered IV q6h.
  - Pyridoxine and thiamine hasten elimination of ethylene glycol metabolites.
  - Pyridoxine may be given as 1–2 mg/kg up to 100 mg maximum IV q6h.
  - Thiamine may be given as 50 mg to children <20 kg or 100 mg to children >20 kg, administered IV over at least 5 minutes and repeated q6h.

ADDITIONAL TREATMENT
General Measures
Supportive care is the most important general principle. The illness is managed with intent of close monitoring and addressing issues as they arise:

- For ingestion <1 hour previously, an attempt to aspirate gastric contents with a nasogastric tube is reasonable.
- Treatment for ethylene glycol or methanol exposure should focus on acid-base correction and preventing organ damage.
- Hemodialysis should be considered for the following:
  - Any patient with severe metabolic acidemia from ethylene glycol or methanol
  - Any patient with evidence of end-organ damage, particularly if metabolic acidemia is present
  - Any patient with profound hypotension or life-threatening symptoms resulting from isopropyl alcohol toxicity

IN-PATIENT CONSIDERATIONS
Initial Stabilization
- Prompt evaluation of airway, breathing, circulation, serum glucose, and ECG (A,B,C,D,E) is critical.
- Consultation with a medical toxicologist or poison center is recommended.

Admission Criteria
- Any patient requiring therapy with fomepizole, ethanol, or hemodialysis
- Any patient with renal impairment, visual impairment, or other organ effect
- Any patient for whom consequential ingestion is suspected and ethylene glycol or methanol levels are unavailable

IV Fluids
- IV fluid to maintain adequate blood pressure may be necessary.
- Maintenance IV fluid may be required in patients who are unable to take PO.
- IV fluid may be necessary to aid in prevention of calcium oxalate crystals in the urine.
- IV fluid may be helpful to prevent renal injury if rhabdomyolysis occurs.

Nursing
- Protect inebriated patients from falls.
- For the duration of inebriation or therapy with ethanol, vigilance for detection of hypoglycemia should be maintained.

Discharge Criteria
- Inpatients who have received therapy with fomepizole, ethanol, or hemodialysis must be medically and metabolically stable for at least 12–24 hours prior to discharge.
- Patients with ethylene glycol or methanol exposure who have not developed symptoms or metabolic derangement may be discharged within 24 hours.

ONGOING CARE

FOLLOW-UP RECOMMENDATIONS
- Asymptomatic patients with undetectable ethylene glycol or methanol levels and no metabolic acidemia may be safely discharged.
- Most exposures for which ethylene glycol or methanol levels cannot be obtained should be followed for 12–24 hours to detect development of metabolic acidemia or other symptoms.

- From the hospital, patients with ethylene glycol or methanol level <20 mg/dL, no anion gap, no metabolic academia, and stable renal function and vision may be discharged.
- Patients with isopropyl alcohol exposure who develop no symptoms or have only mild symptoms may be discharged within 4–6 hours.

Patient Monitoring
Symptomatic exposure to ethylene glycol or methanol may warrant intensive care monitoring.

PROGNOSIS
- For ethylene glycol and methanol exposure, prognosis depends upon the degree of toxin metabolism as well as adequacy of care.
- Speed and adequacy of therapy with fomepizole or ethanol, as well as prompt hemodialysis when indicated, is critical.
- For isopropyl alcohol, prognosis depends upon severity of intoxication and adequacy of supportive care.

COMPLICATIONS
Blindness, coma, hepatic injury, hypertension or hypotension, myocarditis, temporary or permanent neurologic injury, pancreatitis, renal failure, respiratory depression, rhabdomyolysis, or seizure may occur as a result of toxic alcohol exposure.

ADDITIONAL READING
- Howland MA. Antidotes in depth: Ethanol. In: Goldfrank LR, Flomenbaum NE, Lewin NA, et al., eds. *Goldfrank's Toxicologic Emergencies*. 8th ed. Stamford, CT: Appleton & Lange; 2006.
- Howland MA. Antidotes in depth: Fomepizole. In: Goldfrank LR, Flomenbaum NE, Lewin NA, et al., eds. *Goldfrank's Toxicologic Emergencies*. 8th ed. Stamford, CT: Appleton & Lange; 2006.
- Patil N, Lai-Becker M, Ganetskty M. Toxic alcohols: Not always a clear cut diagnosis. *EM Practice*. 2010;12:11.
- Weiner S. Toxic alcohols. In: Goldfrank LR, Flomenbaum NE, Lewin NA, et al., eds. *Goldfrank's Toxicologic Emergencies*. 8th ed. Stamford, CT: Appleton & Lange; 2006.

CODES

ICD9
- 980.1 Toxic effect of methyl alcohol
- 980.2 Toxic effect of isopropyl alcohol
- 982.8 Toxic effect of other nonpetroleum-based solvents

ICD10
- T51.1X4A Toxic effect of methanol, undetermined, initial encounter
- T51.2X4A Toxic effect of 2-Propanol, undetermined, initial encounter
- T52.3X4A Toxic effect of glycols, undetermined, initial encounter

T

TOXIC SHOCK SYNDROME

Mark L. Bagarazzi

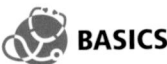 **BASICS**

DESCRIPTION

- Toxic shock syndrome (TSS) is an acute febrile illness characterized by myalgia, vomiting, diarrhea, pharyngitis, diffuse desquamating macular erythroderma, erythema of mucous membrane and conjunctiva, multiorgan system involvement by direct inflammatory damage or ischemia, disseminated intravascular coagulopathy (DIC), and hypotension.
- TSS is most commonly caused by group A β-hemolytic streptococci (GABS or *Streptococcus pyogenes*) or TSS toxin-1 (TSST-1)–producing strains of *Staphylococcus aureus* (including methicillin-resistant isolates). Cases have also been reported in association with group B, C, and G1 streptococci and *Streptococcus mitis*.

GENERAL PREVENTION

- Avoidance of tampon use after first episode of TSS
- Scrupulous wound care
- Limitation of intravaginal foreign body use (e.g., tampon, sponge) and strict adherence to manufacturer's directions

EPIDEMIOLOGY

- Early 1980s: >90% of cases (almost exclusively owing to *S. aureus*) occurred in menstruating women; associated with superabsorbent tampon use. The frequency of cases occurring in menstruating women dropped in the mid-1980s because of changes to less absorbent or tampons of different composition. In 1996, <50% of cases were associated with menstruation.
- Mean age: 22 years
- Incubation period for postoperative *S. aureus*–mediated TSS can be <12 hours.
- Preceding varicella infection dramatically increases the risk for acquiring invasive disease owing to group A β-hemolytic streptococci including TSS.
- Currently, about 60% of cases occur in girls and women.

Incidence

- Current incidence of menses-related disease: 1–5/100,000 women of menstrual age per year
- In US from 2000–2004, case-fatality rate in patients aged <10 years with streptococcal TSS was 7.7%. Streptococcal TSS incidence is highest among young children.

RISK FACTORS

- Use of superabsorbent tampon, diaphragm, or contraceptive sponge; local or invasive staphylococcal or streptococcal infection
  - Including but not limited to bacteremia, endocarditis, pyogenic arthritis, sinusitis, osteomyelitis, pneumonia, pharyngitis, pancreatitis, cholecystitis, abscess, cervical adenitis
- Superficial and surgical wounds; childbirth; abortion, varicella infections; immunosuppressive (including corticosteroids and nonsteroidal anti-inflammatory drugs) or immunomodulatory therapy.

DIAGNOSIS

SIGNS AND SYMPTOMS

- U.S. Centers for Disease Control and Prevention (CDC) criteria for diagnosis of staphylococcal TSS:
  - Fever 38.9°C (102.0°F) or higher
  - Diffuse macular erythroderma
  - Desquamation 1–2 weeks after onset, particularly affecting palms and soles
  - Hypotension below fifth percentile for children, orthostatic changes >15 mm Hg or orthostatic syncope, or dizziness
  - Involvement of three or more organ systems: gastrointestinal, muscular, mucous membrane, renal, hepatic, hematologic, or neurologic.

All 5 of the aforementioned criteria with blood culture(s) positive for *S. aureus* only and negative serology for Rocky Mountain spotted fever (RMSF), leptospirosis, and measles. 4 of 5 criteria termed probable. 4 criteria plus death before desquamation yields complete syndrome.

- U.S. Centers for Disease Control and Prevention criteria for diagnosis of streptococcal TSS:
  - Hypotension or shock
  - Any 2 of the following: Renal impairment, DIC, thrombocytopenia, hepatic impairment, adult respiratory distress syndrome, erythematous macular rash that may desquamate, or soft-tissue necrosis
  - Isolation of group A β-hemolytic streptococci from a normally sterile site constitutes a definite case. Isolation of group A β-hemolytic streptococci from a nonsterile site constitutes a probable case.
- Pitfalls:
  - Production of TSST-1 by isolate is only presumptive evidence unless case meets diagnostic criteria.
  - Failure to meet US Centers for Disease Control and Prevention's diagnostic criteria
  - Failure to identify soft-tissue or muscular site of local infection
  - Failure to identify or remove foreign body
  - Erythroderma may not be appreciated if patient is already hypotensive.
  - Diagnosis still must be considered in the absence of an identifiable focus.

HISTORY

- Recent use of tampons, contraceptive sponge, or diaphragm are all known risk factors.
  - May occur at any time during menses
- Any surgical procedures including catheters (e.g., intravenous, peritoneal dialysis)
  - Incubation period for postoperative TSS may be as short as 12 hours
- Nonsurgical wounds, burns, childbirth, abortion, or puerperal infections.
- Other active streptococcal or staphylococcal infections:
  - History frequently elicits probable recent infections.

- Abrupt onset of high fever, rapid-onset hypotension, rapidly accelerated renal failure, and multisystem organ failure are all historical findings associated with either staphylococcal or streptococcal TSS. Chills, malaise, headache, pharyngitis, fatigue, and dizziness or syncope are also seen frequently.
- Profuse watery diarrhea (often with fecal incontinence), vomiting, abdominal pain, generalized erythroderma, conjunctival injection, and severe myalgias are all historical findings seen commonly in staphylococcal TSS but less frequently in streptococcal TSS. The presence of a foreign body is also more common with staphylococcal TSS than with streptococcal TSS.
- Evidence of increasingly painful local soft tissue infection (e.g., abscess, cellulitis, myositis, or necrotizing fasciitis) are all historical findings seen commonly in streptococcal TSS but less frequently in staphylococcal TSS.
- Tampons with ingredients such as polyacrylate, polyester foam, cross-linked carboxymethylcellulose; or claims of superabsorbency are associated with TSS.

PHYSICAL EXAM

- Any sign of soft-tissue infection (e.g., cellulitis, necrotizing fasciitis, myositis, soft-tissue abscesses, sinusitis):
  - Often seen before onset of TSS
- Overall appearance:
  - Patients with TSS are always moderately to severely ill.
- Altered vital signs:
  - Fever, tachycardia, tachypnea, orthostasis, or frank hypotension. Tachycardia is the prelude to hypotension.
- Abnormal skin, mucous membranes, and soft tissues:
  - Erythroderma, peripheral cyanosis and edema, bulbar conjunctival hyperemia, subconjunctival hemorrhages, beefy red mucous membranes, and muscle tenderness are seen with TSS.
- Mental status changes:
  - Altered mental status, including somnolence, agitation, disorientation, and obtundation within 24–72 hours are seen with TSS.
- Intensity of erythroderma:
  - May be most intense surrounding the infected focus (e.g., perineum)
- Desquamation:
  - Begins on trunk and extremities 5–7 days after symptom onset. Full thickness desquamation of fingers, toes, palms, and soles begins 10–12 days after onset.
- Vesicle or bullae formation, or presence of violaceous hue:
  - Ominous findings associated with increased fluid loss and potentially hypotensive shock

DIAGNOSTIC TESTS & INTERPRETATION
Lab
- Antibodies to TSST-1 (available for informational purposes/research only from Toxin Technology, Inc., www.toxintechnology.com):
  - Test result will be positive several weeks after acute presentation.
- Antibodies to antistreptolysin O (ASO), antideoxyribonuclease B, or other streptococcal extracellular products:
  - May increase 4–6 weeks after infection in streptococcal-mediated disease
- Complete blood count:
  - Usually reveals thrombocytopenia early in the course of disease, thrombocytosis during the recovery phase, anemia early in disease, normal or slightly elevated leukocyte count with left shift, and absolute lymphopenia. Neutropenia is more ominous than lymphopenia.
- Blood cultures:
  - Positive in 60% of streptococcal TSS, rarely (<5%) positive in staphylococcal TSS
- Local cultures:
  - S. aureus may be isolated from vagina or cervix in menstrual TSS, or from other infectious focus in nonmenstrual cases. Isolation of group A streptococci from a sterile site is a definite case, whereas isolation from a nonsterile site constitutes a probable case.
- Pitfall:
  - S. aureus isolated from nares or vagina may represent a false-positive finding because 10–30% of those affected are healthy carriers.
- Coagulation studies:
  - May reveal prolonged prothrombin and partial thromboplastin times (PT/PTT) with or without evidence of DIC; low fibrinogen, elevated fibrin degradation products.
- Urinalysis:
  - May reveal sterile pyuria
- Lumbar puncture:
  - May reveal cerebrospinal fluid pleocytosis
- Creatine phosphokinase (CPK):
  - May be elevated, reflecting skeletal muscle involvement

DIFFERENTIAL DIAGNOSIS
- Septic shock owing to Neisseria meningitidis
- Streptococcal and staphylococcal scarlatiniform eruptions
- Leptospirosis
- RMSF without characteristic rash
- Fulminant viral infection (e.g., adenovirus)
- Kawasaki disease, although TSS may present simultaneously with Kawasaki disease. Coronary artery dilatation has been reported in cases presenting as TSS.
- Toxic epidermal necrolysis (TEN)
- Drug-induced hypersensitivity (e.g., vancomycin)

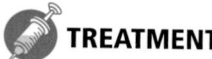 TREATMENT

SPECIAL THERAPY
- Remove all foreign bodies.
- Surgical débridement with myositis and necrotizing fasciitis; abscess drainage
- Antibiotics: Parenteral administration with antistreptococcal and staphylococcal therapy eradicates source of the toxin, but does not affect the course of the acute illness.

MEDICATION (DRUGS)
- Use both a bacterial cell wall inhibitor, such as semisynthetic antistaphylococcal penicillins (i.e., nafcillin, oxacillin, dicloxacillin, and cefuroxime or ampicillin/sulbactam) as well as a protein synthesis inhibitor (e.g., clindamycin, linezolid) to end production of toxins, enzymes, and cytokines.
- Continue therapy for 10–15 days or until causative bacteria is eradicated on follow-up cultures.
- Clindamycin or erythromycin if patient is allergic to penicillin
- Intravenous immunoglobulin (IVIG) remains controversial with no adequately powered prospective studies:
  - Placebo-controlled multicenter study did not show a significant benefit in 28-day survival in patients with definite streptococcal TSS.
  - Anecdotal reports of efficacy for streptococcal TSS
  - May be considered for infections refractory to aggressive therapy or in patients with infection in an area that cannot be drained.
  - Optimal regimen is not known, although single doses of 1–2 g/kg, as well as several days of 150–450 mg/kg/d have been studied.
- Corticosteroids: Have not been systematically studied

 ONGOING CARE

- Poor prognosis is often heralded by development of pulmonary edema, falling cardiac index, and rising pulmonary capillary wedge pressure.
- Temperature usually returns to normal within 2 days.
- Toxin-mediated cardiomyopathy should resolve if fatal arrhythmia does not occur during decompensated stage.
- Gastrointestinal, hepatic, and musculoskeletal changes resolve rapidly with rare permanent sequelae except for muscle weakness.
- Hair and nail loss may occur 4–16 weeks after illness onset; should resolve within 5–6 months.
- Encephalopathy is common, rarely causes seizures; both usually resolve within 4–5 days.

PROGNOSIS
- Recurrences are associated with inadequate treatment.
- Mortality 5–7% for staphylococcal disease. Myocardial and pulmonary failure are the most common causes of death.
- Mortality is higher in nonmenstrual TSS (men and women >45 years of age) owing to delayed recognition.
- Death usually occurs within the first few days; may occur as late as 2 weeks following onset.
- Permanent renal damage is extremely rare.

COMPLICATIONS
Multisystem organ failure secondary to distributive shock/hypotension including:
- Pulmonary edema
- DIC
- Acute renal failure (oliguric and nonoliguric)
- Hepatic failure
- Myocardial edema and decreased contractility with or without arrhythmias
- "Stunned" myocardium demonstrating severe ventricular contractile dysfunction
- Cerebral edema with toxic or ischemic encephalopathy
- Metabolic disturbances
- Telogen effluvium; temporary hair and nail loss
- Neuropsychologic disturbances including memory loss; abnormal electroencephalogram (EEG) rare

ADDITIONAL READING

- American Academy of Pediatrics. Staphylococcal and Group A Streptococcal Infections. In: Pickering LK, ed. Red Book: 2009 Report of the Committee on Infectious Diseases, 28th ed. Elk Grove Village, IL: American Academy of Pediatrics; 2009:601–628.
- Bisno AL, Stevens DC. Streptococcal infection of skin and soft-tissues. N Engl J Med. 1996;334:240–245.
- Darenberg J, Ihendyane N, Sjolin J, et al., and the Streptlg Study Group. Intravenous immunoglobulin G therapy in streptococcal toxic shock syndrome: A European randomized, double-blind, placebo-controlled trial. Clin Infect Dis. 2003;37:333–340.
- O'Loughlin RE, Roberson A, Cieslak PR, et al. The epidemiology of invasive group A streptococcal infection and potential vaccine implications: United States, 2000–2004. Clin Infect Dis. 2007;45: 853–862.
- Reich HL, Crawford GH, Pelle MT, et al. Group B streptococcal toxic shock-like syndrome. Arch Dermatol. 2004;140:163–166.

 CODES

ICD9
040.82 Toxic shock syndrome

ICD10
A48.3 Toxic shock syndrome

FAQ

- Q: Can toxic shock syndrome recur?
- A: Yes. Inadequate eradication of the nidus of infection, as in continuing sinusitis or a case that involves a foreign body, can lead to recurrent staphylococcal toxic shock syndrome. Moreover, some people with some immune system defects may develop recurrent toxic shock syndrome.
- Q: Can toxic shock syndrome be diagnosed in patients who have no risk factors?
- A: Yes, there have been reports meeting the case definition where none of the known associated factors was present.

TOXOPLASMOSIS

Richard M. Rutstein

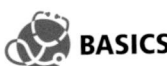 **BASICS**

DESCRIPTION

Toxoplasma gondii is an intracellular protozoan parasite with a complex life cycle; its definitive host is the cat. In addition to causing asymptomatic infection and clinical disease in humans, the organism is capable of causing asymptomatic and symptomatic infections in a wide range of other mammals and birds:

- Pitfalls:
  - Failure to consider diagnosis in an at-risk or symptomatic infant
  - Failure to consider the significant risk of late sequelae in an asymptomatic exposed/infected neonate and therefore failure to offer therapy to the asymptomatic infected neonate

EPIDEMIOLOGY

- The rate of acquired infection, usually asymptomatic, varies widely through the world and increases with age.
- At birth, 70–90% of children with congenital toxoplasmosis are asymptomatic. Late sequelae (e.g., chorioretinitis, mental retardation, seizures, sensorineural hearing loss) occur in 25–50% of untreated infants considered asymptomatic at birth.

Incidence

Worldwide, the incidence of congenital infection ranges from 1–7/1,000 live births; in the US, incidence is estimated at 0.1–1/1,000 live births. It is believed that 400–4,000 infants are born annually in the US with congenital toxoplasmosis.

Prevalence

Seroprevalence rates among pregnant women vary from 4–80% worldwide; in the US, a serologic survey found that 15% of women of child-bearing age were seropositive.

GENERAL PREVENTION

- Avoidance of undercooked meats
- Seronegative women need to exercise caution in caring for cats as well as eating undercooked meat.
- Maternal/Neonatal antibody screening is important in areas with a significant incidence of toxoplasmosis.

- Treatment of pregnant women with documented seroconversion to prevent congenital infection is generally offered, although its efficacy is not proven. If fetal infection is established, aggressive treatment during pregnancy with spiramycin, pyrimethamine, and sulfonamide may palliate the severity of the disease in the infant; however, recent evidence has not shown a protective effect of prenatal treatment against the development of neurologic or ocular sequelae.

PATHOPHYSIOLOGY

- Toxoplasmosis is acquired by the ingestion of oocysts or intact viable tissue cysts in inadequately cooked meat.
- After ingestion, the oocysts and cysts are disrupted by the digestive process, and viable infective organisms cross the GI lining. Hematologic spread leads to infection of multiple organs, most notably the heart, skeletal muscle, and the brain. There, slowly growing or dormant cysts remain for the patient's lifetime.
- Congenital toxoplasmosis generally occurs during a primary maternal infection. An exception may be when the pregnant woman is severely immunocompromised; congenital infection has occurred in children of HIV-infected women with latent toxoplasmosis infection.
- Primary infection in the 1st trimester is associated with a higher incidence of symptomatic congenital disease, although most congenital infections occur late in pregnancy and affected neonates have subclinical infection at birth. Overall, 30–40% of infants born to mothers with primary infection during pregnancy will be congenitally infected; 25% of those will have ocular or intracranial disease noted in infancy.

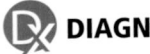 **DIAGNOSIS**

HISTORY

- For acquired infection: History of contact with cats; eating raw or undercooked meat (especially pork)
- For congenital infection: History of maternal exposure or positive titers (IgG and/or IgM)

PHYSICAL EXAM

- Acquired infection: Adenopathy, rash, fever, malaise, hepatosplenomegaly
- Congenital infection: Microcephaly or macrocephaly, hydrocephalus, chorioretinitis, hepatosplenomegaly, petechiae, sensorineural hearing loss, intracerebral calcifications

DIAGNOSTIC TESTS & INTERPRETATION

Lab

- Screen all pregnant women or their infants in high-incidence areas by use of toxoplasmosis-specific IgM or rise in IgG titer over time.
- PCR analysis of amniotic fluid may assist in diagnosis; in 1 study, the specificity and positive predictive values were 100% and sensitivity was 92%.
- Several states now mandate neonatal screening; filter paper test for IgM detects 75% of cases, many asymptomatic.
- For the at-risk neonate, diagnosis is made by demonstration of specific IgM, IgA, or IgE titers, or rise in IgG titers, and/or clinical symptoms in the infant of a mother with recent primary infection.
- Thrombocytopenia
- Elevated result on liver function tests

Imaging

Head CT or MRI demonstrating calcifications

Diagnostic Procedures/Other

Early and frequent audiologic and ophthalmic evaluations are a necessity. Many affected infants will have normal results of neonatal examinations.

DIFFERENTIAL DIAGNOSIS

- Primary infection: Acute disease symptoms of adenopathy, fever, rash: Primary Epstein-Barr virus, cytomegalovirus, HIV infection
- For the newborn with micro/macrocephaly, hepatosplenomegaly, eye disease; other congenital infections: Cytomegalovirus, syphilis, rubella

 ## TREATMENT

MEDICATION (DRUGS)

Pyrimethamine and sulfadiazine for the 1st year of life for all congenitally infected infants whether symptomatic or not, although the efficacy of treatment, for preventing or limiting sequelae, is controversial:

- Folic acid is given during the course of therapy to minimize hematologic side effects.

 ## ONGOING CARE

FOLLOW-UP RECOMMENDATIONS

- Continued attention to neurologic development and frequent audiologic and ophthalmic evaluations throughout the 1st few years of life
- For children with early symptomatic disease, careful attention to neurologic condition and early intervention services to optimize outcome

PROGNOSIS

- Most acquired infections are asymptomatic or associated with mild short-lived symptoms.
- Most congenital infections are asymptomatic, although late sequelae occur in >50% of untreated infants.
- Symptomatic newborns are at significant risk for sequelae, most frequently neurologic (e.g., hydrocephalus, retardation) or ophthalmologic (e.g., retinitis, blindness).
- Prenatal treatment appears to decrease risk to newborn; therapy of all infected infants, symptomatic or not, for 1 year, improves outcome.

COMPLICATIONS

- Congenital infection: Retardation, retinitis, hydrocephalus, seizures, microcephaly, sensorineural hearing loss
- Acquired infection (all rare): Adenopathy, mononucleosis-like syndrome, myocarditis, pneumonia, meningitis/encephalitis

ADDITIONAL READING

- Berrebi A, Assouline C, Bessieres M-H, et al. Long-term outcome of children with congenital toxoplasmosis. *Am J Obstet Gynecol.* 2010;203: 552.e1–e6.
- Freeman K, Tan HK, Prusa A, et al. Predictors of retinochoroiditis in children with congenital toxoplasmosis: European Prospective Cohort Study. *Pediatrics.* 2008;121:e1215–e1221.
- Gilbert R, Gras L; European Multicentre Study on Congenital Toxoplasmosis. Effect of timing and type of treatment on the risk of mother to child transmission of Toxoplasma gondii. *BJOG.* 2003;110:112–120.
- Hill D, Dubey JP. Toxoplasma gondii: Transmission, diagnosis and prevention. *Clin Microbiol Infect.* 2002;8:634–640.
- Jones JL, Lopez A, Wilson M, et al. Congenital toxoplasmosis: A review. *Obstet Gynecol Surv.* 2001;56:296–305.
- SYROCOT Study Group. Effectiveness of prenatal treatment for congenital toxoplasmosis: A meta-analysis of individual patients' data. *Lancet.* 2007;369:115–122.

 ## CODES

ICD9

- 130.7 Toxoplasmosis of other specified sites
- 130.9 Toxoplasmosis, unspecified
- 771.2 Other congenital infections specific to the perinatal period

ICD10

- B58.00 Toxoplasma oculopathy, unspecified
- B58.9 Toxoplasmosis, unspecified
- P37.1 Congenital toxoplasmosis

FAQ

- Q: What is the risk of congenital infection in a mother with stable toxoplasmosis?
- A: The risk of congenital infection in the child of a mother with long-standing toxoplasmosis infection is considered low; the exception is for mothers with a significant degree of immunosuppression or deficiency.
- Q: What is the risk of congenital infection in children of a mother with documented primary infection during pregnancy?
- A: ~30–40% of infants born to mothers with primary infection during pregnancy will be infected themselves. This rate may be lower if the mother receives therapy (spiramycin or pyrimethamine/sulfadiazine) prenatally. Of the infected infants, most (70–90%) are normal at birth; with treatment for 12 months, it appears most will have a favorable outcome.

T

TRACHEITIS

Charles A. Pohl

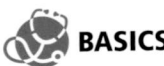

BASICS

DESCRIPTION
Infection of the trachea associated with airway inflammation and obstruction:
- Acute tracheitis: Sudden onset; higher morbidity and mortality
- Subacute tracheitis: Indolent presentation and course; more common among children with prolonged intubation, tracheostomy, and/or underlying respiratory or neurologic conditions

EPIDEMIOLOGY
- Viral prodrome common
- Increased incidence during viral respiratory season (fall and winter): Up to 75% coinfected with influenza A
- Gender predisposition unclear (2:1 male-to-female ratio has been reported)
- 3% mortality rate

GENERAL PREVENTION
- Routine childhood immunization with *Haemophilus influenzae* type B, influenza, and pneumococcal vaccines
- Avoid overaggressive suctioning of children with artificial airways.

PATHOPHYSIOLOGY
- Epithelial damage from a viral infection or mechanical trauma (e.g., endotracheal intubation, surgical procedure) occurs in the trachea at the level of the cricoid cartilage. As a result, the damaged tissue is more susceptible to bacterial superinfection.
- Mucosal damage characterized by marked subglottic edema, copious purulent secretions, and a pseudomembrane (mucosal lining, inflammatory products, and bacteria). These changes lead to marked airway obstruction.
- Toxic shock syndrome may be a consequence if the infection is associated with toxin-producing strains of *Staphylococcus aureus* or *Streptococcus pyogenes*.

ETIOLOGY
- Bacteria:
  – *S. aureus* (most common), group A *β*-hemolytic streptococcus, *Moraxella catarrhalis*, nontypeable *H. influenzae*, *Streptococcus pneumoniae*
  – *Pseudomonas aeruginosa* and other gram-negative enteric bacteria have been associated with nosocomial infections.
  – *Mycobacterium tuberculosis*, *Mycoplasma pneumoniae*, *Corynebacterium diphtheria*, *H. influenzae* type B, and respiratory anaerobic bacteria are uncommon pathogens.
- Viruses: Influenza, parainfluenza, respiratory syncytial, herpes simplex, and measles viruses have been found with bacterial pathogen(s).
- Fungi: Seen with underlying immunodeficiency disorders or chronic steroid use

DIAGNOSIS

HISTORY
- Hyperpyrexia; nonpainful, brassy cough; noisy respirations; lethargy; dyspnea; rapid progression of airway occlusion (hours to a few days)
- Hoarseness, dysphagia, neck pain, drooling, and croupy cough are less common.
- Presence of upper airway infection
- Lack of clinical improvement with racemic epinephrine should raise the suspicion for tracheitis.
- An indolent progression of symptoms, including increase of supplemental oxygen requirement and tracheal secretions (thicker and color changes), may be seen in subacute tracheitis.
- Affects any age (peak age 2–6 years)

PHYSICAL EXAM
- Toxic appearance; anxious, agitated, or lethargic; labored breathing with signs of severe respiratory distress (e.g., air hunger posture, retractions); pallor or cyanosis; severe stridor; concomitant signs of pneumonia
- Deviated uvula suggests a peritonsillar abscess.
- Asymmetric lung sounds are often found in patients with foreign bodies in the airway.
- Generalized lymphadenopathy and splenomegaly are clues for infectious mononucleosis.

DIAGNOSTIC TESTS & INTERPRETATION
Imaging
- Radiographs must be completed in controlled settings by personnel who are trained in airway management.
- Lateral and anteroposterior neck films: Findings include distention of the hypopharynx, subglottic narrowing, and irregularity of the tracheal wall owing to mucosal sloughing or the presence of a pseudomembrane.
- Chest radiograph: Obtain if pneumonia, which may be concurrent, is suspected.

Diagnostic Procedures/Other
- Laryngoscopy or bronchoscopy:
  – Direct visualization and suctioning of obstructed airway is both diagnostic and therapeutic.
  – Findings include a red, edematous, and/or eroded trachea and bronchi with purulent secretions and pseudomembrane.
  – Consider in an ill-appearing child with an unclear diagnosis or when the child's condition does not respond to current management.
- Tracheal bacterial culture (for aerobic and anaerobic bacteria): The gold standard for diagnosis
- Tracheal gram stain for pathogens and white blood cells (especially polymorphonuclear leukocytes): Helps differentiate bacterial infection from colonization

- Blood culture: Occasionally may be helpful in diagnosis (<50% positive)
- CBC: Little diagnostic value but may show leukocytosis with a left shift
- ESR and/or C-reactive protein: May be elevated

DIFFERENTIAL DIAGNOSIS
- Infectious:
  – Epiglottitis/Supraglottitis (presence of supraglottic inflammation)
  – Peritonsillar and parapharyngeal abscesses
  – Retropharyngeal abscess
  – Infectious mononucleosis (Epstein-Barr virus)
  – Diphtheria (rare)
- Environmental:
  – Aspiration or inhalation of a caustic substance, including alkali products (e.g., oven cleaner) or smoke
  – Foreign body aspiration
  – Generalized allergic reaction or anaphylaxis leading to angioedema
- Tumors (rare):
  – Papillomas secondary to human papillomavirus
  – Hamartoma and inflammatory pseudotumor
  – Laryngeal tumors
- Trauma:
  – Posttraumatic tracheal stenosis
  – Blunt trauma to neck
- Congenital:
  – Tracheal stenosis
  – Vascular ring and slings
  – Laryngotracheal web and clefts
  – Laryngotracheomalacia
  – Vocal cord paralysis
  – Arnold-Chiari malformation

ALERT
- Watch for sudden deterioration from tracheal inflammation and secretions. Continuous monitoring is necessary.
- Bacterial tracheitis must be considered in all children with sudden upper respiratory distress and hyperpyrexia.

TREATMENT

MEDICATION (DRUGS)

Select antibiotic therapy based on gram stain and culture results of tracheal secretions. Also consider known prior colonization and institutional pathogens in children with pre-existing artificial airway and hospital-acquired infections:

- Mild illness:
  - Empiric therapy with amoxicillin–clavulanic acid or a 2nd-generation cephalosporin for 10–14 days (50 mg/kg/24 hours depending on the antibiotic used)
  - Consider a semisynthetic penicillin such as dicloxacillin (40 mg/kg/24 hours) if *H. influenzae* type B vaccine completed and clindamycin (10–30 mg/kg/24 hours) if presence of a penicillin allergy
- Moderate to severe illness:
  - Empiric therapy with a 2nd- or 3rd-generation cephalosporin or with ampicillin-sulbactam
  - Consider vancomycin (40 mg/kg/24 hours) if a hospital-acquired infection is present or if pneumococcal resistance is suspected.
- Anaerobic, pseudomonas, and other gram-negative coverage should be considered in children not responding to initial therapy or having pre-existing artificial airways.
- In contrast to croup, nebulized racemic epinephrine and steroids do not provide significant relief.
- Duration: Based on clinical response; usually 10–14 days

ADDITIONAL TREATMENT
General Measures

- Support by stabilizing circulation, airway, breathing (CABs).
- Maintain airway.
- Initiate IV, O_2, and monitor.
- Rapid assessment of CABs is essential with emphasis on airway control.
- Supplemental oxygen is usually needed.
- Anticipate and prepare for emergent endotracheal intubation and tracheostomy.
- Endoscopy with suctioning and debridement is often necessary for diagnosis and therapy.
- Subsequent airway suctioning and monitoring prevents adverse outcomes.
- Increased ventilatory support is often required for children with pre-existing artificial airways.

 ONGOING CARE

FOLLOW-UP RECOMMENDATIONS

- Routine surveillance cultures in children with artificial airways are not recommended. They usually represent colonization in an asymptomatic patient.
- Signs to watch for:
  - Toxic appearance, excessive secretions, persistent fever, or worsening respiratory distress after introducing antibiotics suggest a resistant organism, an unusual pathogen, or a different diagnosis.
  - Recurrent respiratory distress, especially stridor, with subsequent respiratory tract infections suggests underlying tracheal stenosis.
  - Sudden deterioration on a ventilator may indicate endotracheal tube obstruction, pneumothorax, or mechanical problems.

DIET
NPO until the airway is stabilized and the patient is able to tolerate oral foods

PROGNOSIS
- Most children recover without any sequelae.
- Younger patients are more likely to require intubations and longer hospital stays.
- Children at risk for subacute tracheitis are more likely to have recurrent episodes.

COMPLICATIONS
- Atelectasis
- Pulmonary edema and pneumonia
- Septicemia
- Staphylococcal toxin syndromes (e.g., toxic shock syndrome)
- Prolonged mechanical ventilation with associated complications (including air leak, infection, pneumothorax, and tracheal stenosis)
- Subglottic stenosis
- Respiratory failure and arrest
- Death (<3.7%)

ADDITIONAL READING

- Hopkins A, Lahiri T, Salerno R, et al. Changing epidemiology of life-threatening upper airway infections: The reemergence of bacterial tracheitis. *Pediatrics*. 2006;118:1418–1421.
- Graf J, Stein F. Tracheitis in pediatric patients. *Semin Pediatr Infect Dis*. 2006;17(1):11–13.

- Salamone FN, Bobbit DB, Myer CM, et al. Bacterial tracheitis reexamined: Is there a less severe manifestation. *Otolaryngol Head Neck Surg*. 2004;131:871–876.
- Tebruegge M, Pantazidou A, Thorburn K, et al. Bacterial tracheitis: A multi-centre perspective. *Scand J Infect Dis*. 2009;41:548–557.
- Tebruegge M, Pantazidou A, Yau C. Bacterial tracheitis—tremendously rare, but truly important: A systemic review. *J Pediatr Infect Dis*. 2009; 4:199–209.
- Ward MA. Emergency department management of acute respiratory infections. *Semin Respir Infect*. 2002;17:65–71.

CODES

ICD9
464.10 Acute tracheitis without mention of obstruction

ICD10
- J04.10 Acute tracheitis without obstruction
- J04.11 Acute tracheitis with obstruction

FAQ

- Q: How can you differentiate a child with severe croup from one with tracheitis?
- A: Infectious croup and tracheitis can present with similar features of fever, toxic appearance, respiratory distress, and stridor. Direct endoscopic visualization and culture of the upper airway is the test of choice to distinguish these medical conditions. Croup is commonly associated with parainfluenza virus and a "steeple sign" of the upper trachea on an anteroposterior neck radiograph.
- Q: Is influenza A virus a common pathogen of tracheitis?
- A: This subject is controversial. Influenza A virus is frequently recovered from tracheal cultures in children who present with tracheitis. It remains unclear, though, whether this virus is a pathogen or predisposing factor in tracheitis.
- Q: Is the supraglottic area usually involved in tracheitis?
- A: No. Unlike with epiglottitis, the supraglottic region is usually spared in tracheitis. Lack of supraglottic involvement suggests bacterial tracheitis rather than epiglottitis.

T

TRACHEOESOPHAGEAL FISTULA AND ESOPHAGEAL ATRESIA

Wendy J. Kowalski

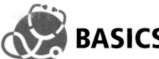 **BASICS**

DESCRIPTION
- Esophageal Atresia (EA) is a congenital malformation of the esophagus where the esophagus ends in a blind pouch. There is a complete disconnection between the proximal pouch and the distal esophagus.
- Tracheoesophageal fistula (TEF) is a congenital malformation in which there is an abnormal connection between the esophagus and the trachea.
- There are 5 basic types of TEFs with varying incidences:
  – Proximal esophageal atresia with a fistula between the distal esophagus and the trachea (86%).
  – Esophageal atresia without a fistula (7%). There is typically a long gap between the 2 esophageal ends.
  – H-type fistula: TEF between the esophagus and cervical trachea without any atresia (4%).
  – Esophageal atresia with a proximal TEF (2%).
  – Esophageal atresia with both a proximal and a distal fistula (<1%).

EPIDEMIOLOGY
- Incidence 1/3000 to 1/4500 live births with slight male predominance
- 30–40% are born prematurely due to the polyhydramnios
- Increased incidence among twins

RISK FACTORS
- TEF generally accepted to be a multifactorial disorder. No specific environmental factor has been identified.
- Environmental: Prenatal methimazole, exogenous sex hormones, diethylstilbestrol, maternal alcohol and smoking, working in horticulture, insulin-dependent diabetes mellitus in the first trimester, anthracycline, and vitamin A deficiency.
- Intrauterine anoxia or vascular compromise of the tracheobronchial tree.
- A baby who has other anomalies or gastrointestinal atresias should be evaluated closely for TEF or EA.
- 50–75% of patients with TEF have other associated anomalies (cardiac, genitourinary, musculoskeletal, and CNS). Of these with associated anomalies, 15–25% of these will be a part of the VATER, VACTERL, or CHARGE association).
  – **VACTERL: V**ertebral defects, **A**nal atresia, **C**ardiac defects, **TE**F, **R**adial or **R**enal anomalies, and **L**imb anomalies
  – **CHARGE: C**oloboma, **H**eart disease, **C**hoanal **A**tresia, **R**etarded growth, **G**enital hypoplasia, and **E**ar anomalies with deafness

Genetics
- The role of genetics is unclear especially when assessing the incidence in identical twins. Usually only 1 twin is affected.
- Recent isolation and identification of new genetic mutations that cause syndromic forms of inherited TEF include the following: SOX2, FOX, NMYC, FANCA, FANCB, and CHD7.
- Occurs as part of a known genetic syndrome in 6–10% of patients, including full trisomies, Opitz syndrome, Feingold syndrome, Fanconi anemia, and Pallister–Hall syndrome.

PATHOPHYSIOLOGY
The trachea and the esophagus develop from a common foregut during the 3rd and 4th weeks of embryogenesis. The foregut divides into a ventral and a dorsal tube. The underlying mechanism of separation is unknown. When this process of division is abnormal due to genetic factors, as part of a syndrome or because of compression by extrinsic structures, EA and/or TEF may result.

ETIOLOGY
There is no consensus on the exact etiology or underlying mechanism.

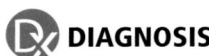 **DIAGNOSIS**

HISTORY
- Prenatal:
  – History of polyhydramnios
  – Absent stomach bubble or a proximal esophageal pouch may be seen on prenatal ultrasound though usually the anatomy looks normal. Absent stomach bubble has a 56% positive predictive value for EA.
- Postnatal:
  – Respiratory symptoms at or shortly after birth due to aspiration of gastric contents which can cause a pneumonitis or compression of trachea/lungs by dilated or air-filled distended pouch or fistula
- Excessive salivation that requires frequent suctioning
  – Choking, coughing, or emesis during feedings
  – Inability to pass a catheter through the esophagus and into the stomach

PHYSICAL EXAM
- Vital signs: Tachypnea, hypoxia, or fever may indicate aspiration.
- Head: Abnormal ocular findings (coloboma) or ear anomalies may suggest associated syndrome
- Lungs: Persistent cough; recurrent cough with feeds; retractions, crackles, and/or wheezes with pneumonitis or pneumonia
- Cardiac: Thorough exam for a murmur that may suggest associated cardiac disease
- Abdominal: Flat or scaphoid abdomen if there is no fistula to the stomach or abdominal distension if there is a fistula between the trachea and the distal esophagus and the baby has been crying or received positive pressure ventilation

- Genitourinary: Assess for associated anomalies of the genitalia or palpable, large kidneys.
- Perianal: Document patent anus.
- Musculoskeletal: Inspection of spine, palpation of radial bone, and thumb to rule-out their absence.

DIAGNOSTIC TESTS & INTERPRETATION
Lab
- Electrolytes/BUN/Creatinine: If poor feeding, on intravenous fluids, as part of a preoperative evaluation or if there is excess loss of fluid through oral secretions
- CBC with differential: If concern for aspiration or other infection or for preoperative evaluation
- Blood type and screen: For preoperative evaluation

Imaging
- Prenatal ultrasound: Findings that suggest EA or TEF are only present 40% of the time.
- Anteroposterior/lateral chest radiograph: First line to make the diagnosis after a nasogastric or orogastric feeding tube is passed.
  – Feeding tube curled up in esophageal pouch and absence of GI gas are highly suggestive of EA;
  – Feeding tube curled up in esophageal pouch with presence of GI gas suggests TEF;
  – Right upper lobe pneumonia or pneumonitis may also be seen due to aspiration of gastric contents
- Abdominal radiograph: Absence of air in the stomach and lower GI tract suggests EA without fistula
- Upper GI with contrast is contraindicated because of the risk of aspiration; however, it is useful for the diagnosis of H-type fistulas
- Bronchoscopy and/or endoscopy: Useful for suspected H-type fistulas
- Echocardiogram and Renal Ultrasound to evaluate for any associated anomalies and to determine the side of the aortic arch before surgery
- Radiographs of limbs if any abnormalities are noted on exam and of the vertebrae to look for any defects

DIFFERENTIAL DIAGNOSIS
- Gastroesophageal reflux
- Esophageal duplication
- Esophageal web/stricture
- Trauma to proximal esophagus
- Vascular ring/sling
- Pulmonary hypoplasia
- Tracheomalacia
- Central or neurologic cause of the feeding disorder and drooling

TREATMENT

ADDITIONAL TREATMENT
General Measures
Preoperative Management:

- Make the patient NPO and administer intravenous fluids
- Place a Replogle suction catheter into the upper esophageal pouch and elevate the head of the bed 30 degrees to minimize the secretions and risk for aspiration of gastric contents.
- Administer broad spectrum antibiotics.
- Avoid positive pressure ventilation if possible.
- Monitor closely for abdominal distention especially if there is a known distal TEF. The baby may need an emergent, venting gastrostomy to prevent gastric perforation, respiratory failure and death.
- Use comfort measures to reduce crying and subsequent gastric distention.
- Assess for associated anomalies as noted in the physical exam and imaging sections.

SURGERY/OTHER PROCEDURES
- Definitive treatment is surgical correction.
- The surgical options depend on the medical condition of the baby, the type of defect, and the distance between the esophageal segments.
- Primary end-to-end anastomosis and fistula ligation via thoracotomy is the desired method of correction; may not be feasible in long-gap atresias, in patients who are severely ill from associated problems, such as cardiac disease or in premature infants.
- If the distance between the 2 esophageal segments is too long, the stretching to make them meet will cause excessive tension on the anastomosis and is a risk for anastomotic leak or esophageal stricture.
- Delicate closure of the TEF is needed to prevent tracheal stenosis.
- An intra-operative chest tube is often placed to drain any potential leaks from the esophageal anastomosis.
- An intra-operative oral-gastric tube is often passed through the anastomosis and firmly secured to the baby's face.
- Gastrostomy is recommended when primary anastomosis is not immediately feasible and a gastrostomy tube is necessary for feeding or it may be placed emergently if there is a concern for gastric distention and perforation.
- Closure, even in severe cases, can occur within 8–12 weeks of life with esophageal elongation procedures as well as natural lengthening of esophagus as infant grows.
- If primary end-to-end anastomosis is not achievable, other suboptimal surgical options exist (e.g., gastric pull-up, creation of neoesophagus with colonic tissue, extrathoracic elongation), all of which are associated with a higher complication rate.

ONGOING CARE

FOLLOW-UP RECOMMENDATIONS
- Immediate (postoperative):
  - Aggressive pulmonary treatment to minimize risk of respiratory infection.
  - Low pressure ventilation and respiratory support.
  - Empiric postoperative antibiotics to reduce infection risk especially if a chest tube is in place.
  - Frequent oral suctioning.
  - Low intermittent suction on orogastric tube that was passed intraoperatively
  - Total parenteral nutrition
  - Perform a dye study about 7 days post-op to look for any anastomotic leaks that would drain into the chest tube or oral-gastric tube
  - If no anastomotic leaks are present, the chest tube can be removed and the infant can be fed either orally or through the orogastric tube
  - Feedings can be advanced rather quickly once the anastomoses are proven intact and patent
- Long term:
  - Management of nonsurgical and surgical complications—airway issues like tracheomalacia, wheezing, or stridor; feeding issues like reflux and esophageal dysmotility; weight gain; infections
  - Coordination of care if associated with other congenital anomalies
  - Genetic evaluation and counseling

PROGNOSIS
- Several prognostic classifications have been developed which take into account birth weight, and the presence of associated anomalies.
- Survival is nearly 100% for infants with birth weight >1500 g, no major cardiac disease, no other congenital anomalies and no respiratory complications who have EA with a distal TEF.
- In premature infants with associated anomalies, only a 50% survival is reported.
- In infants with severe associated anomalies, especially cardiac, survival has been reported at 30–50%.

COMPLICATIONS
- The course of a premature baby is typically more complicated and has the potential for more adverse outcomes.
  - Anastomotic leak: Early complication following surgical repair, in up to 15%; most resolve spontaneously but half of the cases will end up developing an esophageal stricture. Worst case scenario is mediastinal sepsis with the need for re-exploration and possible esophageal ligation.
  - Esophageal stricture: Seen in 5–40% of cases about 2–3 weeks post-op, especially after repair of long-gap atresias as tension on anastomosis increases stricture risk or after an anastomotic leak; often requires dilatation.
  - Esophageal dysmotility/dysphagia: Seen in >75% of patients (100% of those requiring colonic interposition).
  - Gastroesophageal reflux: Seen in 40–60% of patients with TEF and persists into adulthood; may contribute to strictures, poor growth, aspiration, and development of lung disease; treated with aggressive medical management.
  - Recurrent TEF: Uncommon complication following initial repair; increased risk following anastomotic leak; should be suspected when choking, coughing, and wheezing recur.

  - Tracheomalacia: Reported in up to 75% of patients, but only 10–20% manifest clinical symptoms (i.e., barking cough, stridor, difficulty breathing with feeds); usually improves as the tracheal rings harden
  - Injured recurrent laryngeal nerve: Especially with H-type fistula repair; presents with hoarse cry and recurrent aspiration
  - Long term: Poor growth, chronic respiratory infections, wheezing, chest wall deformities and scoliosis

ALERT
- Meticulous postoperative care is essential for successful recovery after tracheoesophageal reconstruction. The fresh suture lines need to be protected so that they can heal properly.
- Mechanical ventilation with low pressures.
- Extubation only when the likelihood of requiring re-intubation is low.
- Careful manipulation of the head and the neck. Avoid hyperextension and forceful turning of the head.
- Careful oral suctioning—do not go too deep into the esophagus or the trachea so as to avoid injury to the surgical sites.
- Pay close attention to the depth of insertion of the oral-gastric tube and be sure it is secure since it usually ends right at or passes through the anastomosis site.

ADDITIONAL READING

- Berrocal T, Madrid C, Novo S, et al. Congenital anomalies of the tracheobronchial tree, lung, and mediastinum: Embryology, radiology, and pathology. *Radiographics*. 2004;24(1):e17.
- deJong E, Felix J, deKlein A, et al. Etiology of Esophageal Atresia and Tracheoesophageal Fistula: "Mind the Gap." *Curr Gastroenterol Rep*. 2010;12:215–222.
- Konkin DE, O'Hali WA, Webber EM, et al. Outcomes in esophageal atresia and tracheoesophageal fistula. *J Pediatr Surg*. 2003;38(12):1726–1729.
- Seo J, Kimdo Y, Kim AR, et al. An 18-year experience of tracheoesophageal fistula and esophageal atresia. *Korean J Pediatric*. 2010;53(6):705–710.
- Stringel G, Lawrence C, McBride W. Esophageal atresia without anastomosis. *J. Pediatr Surg*. 2010;45(5):872–875.

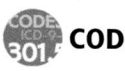 ## CODES

ICD9
750.3 Tracheoesophageal fistula, esophageal atresia and stenosis

ICD10
Q39.1 Atresia of esophagus with tracheo-esophageal fistula

TRACHEOMALACIA/LARYNGOMALACIA

Marleine Ishak
Sumit Bhargava
Ronn E. Tanel (5th edition)

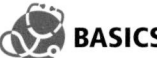 BASICS

DESCRIPTION
- Laryngomalacia:
  - Narrowing and collapse of the supraglottic structures of the larynx
  - Most common congenital anomaly of the larynx
  - Most common noninfectious cause of stridor in children
- Tracheomalacia:
  - Narrowing and collapse of the extrathoracic or intrathoracic trachea
  - Common cause of chronic wheezing in infants and children
  - Classified as primary or secondary:
    ○ Primary: Congenital; results from immature development of the tracheal structures; may occur with other congenital anomalies such as tracheoesophageal fistula, laryngomalacia, and facial anomalies
    ○ Secondary: Acquired in a normally developed trachea after some insult such as prolonged positive pressure ventilation, recurrent infection or aspiration, or external compression

ETIOLOGY
- Laryngomalacia:
  - Multiple factors likely involved
  - Inward collapse of aryepiglottic folds (cuneiform cartilages) during inspiration
  - Elongated, flaccid, omega-shaped epiglottis prolapses posteriorly into the pharynx during inspiration.
  - Immaturity of the laryngeal cartilage results in weakness and collapse during inspiration.
  - Immaturity of neuromuscular control results in hypotonia of pharyngeal muscles.
- Tracheomalacia:
  - Weakness of the tracheal wall secondary to softening of the anterior cartilaginous rings and to decreased tone of the posterior membranous wall
  - During exhalation, increased collapsing pressure across a compliant airway wall causes invagination of the posterior membrane.
  - With increasing age, the length, area, thickness, and amount of cartilage increases in the anterior rings as well as the size and contractility of the membranous wall.

Dx DIAGNOSIS

HISTORY
- Laryngomalacia:
  - Symptoms may be present at birth or delayed until 1–2 months of age.
  - Inspiratory stridor
  - May be asymptomatic during sleep or quiet breathing
  - Worsens with crying, agitation, feeding, upper respiratory infections, supine positioning
- Tracheomalacia:
  - Primary: Symptoms may be delayed until 2–3 months of age.
  - Secondary: Symptoms delayed until after causative insult occurs
  - Expiratory wheeze (or inspiratory stridor if extrathoracic trachea involved)
  - Harsh barking cough
  - May be asymptomatic during sleep or quiet breathing
  - Worsens with crying, agitation, feeding, and upper respiratory infections

PHYSICAL EXAM
- Laryngomalacia:
  - High-pitched or vibratory, low-pitched inspiratory stridor
  - Suprasternal retractions
  - Positional changes noted: Usually worsens with flexion of neck, supine position
  - Stridor transmitted throughout the chest on auscultation
- Tracheomalacia:
  - Homophonous expiratory wheeze (intrathoracic)
  - High-pitched inspiratory stridor (extrathoracic)
  - Intercostal retractions, worse during acute respiratory infections

DIAGNOSTIC TESTS & INTERPRETATION
Diagnostic Procedures/Other
- Flexible fiberoptic laryngo/bronchoscopy:
  - Performed during spontaneous breathing
  - Most efficient method to evaluate stridor or chronic wheezing
  - Visualize the degree and extent of laryngomalacia and/or tracheomalacia.
  - Evaluate for other airway lesions in the differential diagnosis.

- Barium swallow:
  - Best noninvasive test to evaluate stridor or chronic wheeze
  - Especially of value in evaluation of patients with concomitant swallowing abnormalities
  - May see external compression of esophagus from vascular malformation
- Chest radiograph:
  - Usually normal in both laryngomalacia and tracheomalacia
  - Important to rule out other causes of chronic cough or abnormalities that may cause external airway compression
- Airway fluoroscopy:
  - Lateral views are the most useful to visualize the defect.
  - May be normal; does not rule out diagnosis
  - Inspiratory collapsing larynx may be seen in laryngomalacia.
  - Expiratory narrowing or collapse of the trachea may be seen in tracheomalacia.
- MRI:
  - Evaluates for thoracic/vascular anomalies that may cause external compression of the airway
  - May provide more precise measurements of airway size
  - May be performed dynamically to show changes in airway caliber during respiratory cycle
- Pulmonary function tests:
  - Might show diminished expiratory flow, typical notching on the flow volume loop, a biphasic flow volume loop, or flow oscillations.

DIFFERENTIAL DIAGNOSIS
- Laryngomalacia: Differential diagnosis of chronic stridor:
  - Abnormalities of the vocal cords: Vocal cord paralysis
  - Laryngeal abnormalities: Laryngeal cleft, laryngeal web, subglottic hemangioma, papilloma
  - Subglottic stenosis (biphasic stridor)

- Tracheomalacia: Differential diagnosis of chronic homophonous wheeze:
  - Structural abnormalities: Vascular compression/ring, tracheal stenosis/web, cystic lesion, mass/tumor
  - External compression from mediastinal mass, vascular ring
  - Nonstructural abnormalities: Gastroesophageal reflux disease, retained foreign body, chronic bacterial bronchitis

ALERT
- Do not miss other causes for presenting symptoms (see Differential Diagnosis above).
- Investigate lower airway in more severe cases of laryngomalacia for other airway anomalies.
- Treat diseases that may exacerbate symptoms and delay spontaneous resolution.
- The use of bronchodilators may increase the tracheal wall collapsibility by decreasing muscular tone, thereby making the symptoms worse.
- Bronchoscopy should ideally be done under conscious sedation during spontaneous breathing to avoid altering vocal cord movement and airway dynamics.
- The use of rigid bronchoscopy may stent open the trachea, making tracheomalacia more difficult to identify.

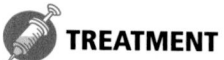

TREATMENT

ADDITIONAL TREATMENT
General Measures
- Laryngomalacia:
  - Usually resolves spontaneously by 15–18 months of age
  - Observation and reassurance
  - Treatment of exacerbating factors, such as upper respiratory infections, asthma, or gastroesophageal reflux disease
  - Tracheostomy may be needed in severe cases to bypass airway obstruction.
  - In rare situations, laryngeal surgery is necessary: Epiglottoplasty, resection of arytenoids
- Tracheomalacia:
  - Usually resolves spontaneously by 18–24 months of age
  - Observation and reassurance
  - Treatment of exacerbating factors, such as upper respiratory infections, asthma, or gastroesophageal reflux disease
  - Bronchoconstrictor therapy to increase tone of airway wall: Bethanechol chloride, ipratropium bromide
  - Continuous positive airway pressure may be needed in more severe cases.

- Tracheostomy may be needed in severe cases to bypass lesion or to provide continuous positive airway pressure.
- Humidification of secretions may help some patients, especially during respiratory infections.
- Aortopexy may be needed in severe cases to suspend the anterior trachea and widen the airway.

ONGOING CARE

FOLLOW-UP RECOMMENDATIONS
Monitor for recurrent respiratory symptoms, poor growth, and other exacerbating conditions (asthma, gastroesophageal reflux disease).

PROGNOSIS
- In cases of isolated laryngomalacia and/or tracheomalacia, prognosis is usually excellent.
- In patients with history of tracheoesophageal fistula, vascular ring, or other airway anomalies, tracheal dysfunction may persist after corrective surgery.

ADDITIONAL READING

- Carden KA, Boiselle PM, Waltz DA, et al. Tracheomalacia and tracheobronchomalacia in children and adults: An in-depth review. *Chest.* 2005;125:984–1005.
- Daniel SJ. The upper airway: Congenital malformations. *Paediatr Respir Rev.* 2006;7: S260–S263.
- Jaquiss RD. Management of pediatric tracheal stenosis and tracheomalacia. *Semin Thorac Cardiovasc Surg.* 2004;16:220–224.
- Masters IB, Chang AB. Tracheobronchomalacia in children. *Expert Rev Respir Med.* 2009;3(4); 425–439.
- Masters IB. Congenital airway lesions and lung disease. *Pediatr Clin North Am.* 2009;56(1): 227–242.
- Murgu SD, Colt HG. Tracheobronchomalacia and excessive dynamic airway collapse. *Respirology.* 2006;11:388–406.

 CODES

ICD9
- 519.19 Other diseases of trachea and bronchus
- 748.3 Other anomalies of larynx, trachea, and bronchus
- 748.3 Other anomalies of larynx, trachea, and bronchus

ICD10
- J38.7 Other diseases of larynx
- Q32.0 Congenital tracheomalacia
- Q31.8 Other congenital malformations of larynx

FAQ

- Q: When will the symptoms improve?
- A: As anatomic structures mature with age, laryngomalacia symptoms may improve by 6 months of age with usual resolution by 18 months of age. Tracheomalacia may last longer, but in both entities symptoms usually resolve completely by age 2 years.
- Q: Should all patients have an endoscopic evaluation?
- A: No. Diagnosis is usually made based on the appropriate history and physical examination. Infants with mild to moderate typical presentation need only careful monitoring for recurrence or worsening of symptoms and for poor growth. However, airway evaluation should be performed in all cases where a different pathology is considered or when symptoms worsen or persist past the expected age of resolution.
- Q: What should I do when symptoms worsen?
- A: Calm the patient; provide humidification of secretions and treatment of intercurrent infection. In cases where associated bronchospasm is suspected, a trial of steroids or bronchodilators may be considered.

T

TRANSFUSION REACTION

Cynthia F. Norris

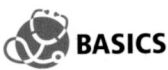 **BASICS**

DESCRIPTION
Any acute or subacute adverse reaction that develops as a consequence of the administration of blood components:
- Types include:
  - Acute reactions: Hemolytic, febrile, allergic, anaphylactic, hypervolemia, bacterial sepsis, transfusion-related acute lung injury (TRALI)
  - Delayed reactions: Delayed hemolytic, transfusion-associated graft-versus-host disease (TA-GVHD)
  - Late complications of transfusion: Infection, alloimmunization, iron overload

EPIDEMIOLOGY
Incidence
10% of blood product recipients develop some type of transfusion reaction.

GENERAL PREVENTION
- Acute hemolytic: Proper labeling of blood specimens and products and adherence to procedures for correct identification of product and recipient will eliminate most acute hemolytic transfusion reactions.
- Febrile: Pretransfusion antipyretic or administration of leukodepleted products; the latter is recommended for long-term transfused patients who have a high incidence of febrile transfusion reactions.
- Allergic: Pretransfusion antihistamine or administration of washed erythrocyte products (in patients with repeated or severe allergic reactions)
- Hypervolemia: Administer appropriate volumes (typically 10–15 mL/kg) at appropriate rate, usually over 3–4 hours unless hypovolemic or actively bleeding; patients with chronic anemia are euvolemic and should be transfused with smaller volumes over longer time periods.
- Bacterial sepsis: Sterile technique in blood collection, storage, and administration; inspection of product before transfusion; bacterial screening of platelet products before they are transfused
- Delayed hemolytic: Appropriately performed antibody screen and cross-match as pretransfusion testing; check blood bank records for previous antibodies
- Anaphylactic: If due to anti-IgA in an IgA-deficient recipient, provision of IgA deficient products may be possible.
- TRALI: Deferral of donors is implicated in proven TRALI cases.
- GVHD: Patients at risk must receive irradiated blood products.

PATHOPHYSIOLOGY
- Acute hemolytic:
  - Antigen–antibody interaction leads to complement activation on the surface of the transfused RBCs, resulting in acute intravascular hemolysis and vasomotor instability.
  - Usually, ABO blood group incompatibility
  - Most commonly due to medical error
- Febrile:
  - Prior exposure to blood products may result in the formation of antibodies to leukocytes or plasma protein antigens; on re-exposure, the antigen–antibody interaction releases pyrogens; cytokines released into the product can also cause fever in the recipient.
  - More frequent in patients with past transfusions or pregnancy
- Allergic:
  - Recipient allergic response to donor plasma proteins or other constituents of plasma
  - Sporadic and donor dependent
- Hypervolemia: Also called TACO (transfusion-associated circulatory overload)
  - Circulatory overload leading to heart failure
  - Administration of an excessive volume of a blood product or infusion at an excessive rate
- Bacterial sepsis:
  - Intravascular infusion of viable bacteria and endotoxins leads to fever, chills, and/or acute septic shock.
  - Contaminated blood product; most commonly a platelet product near the end of shelf life
- Delayed hemolytic:
  - Previously transfused patients who are sensitized to a minor blood group antigen develop an anamnestic response on re-exposure. Antibody is below detectable levels in antibody screen and cross-match; after transfusion, titers rise (usually within 3–10 days) and extravascular hemolysis occurs.
- Anaphylactic:
  - Overwhelming acute allergic reaction. Can be mediated by anti-IgA formed by a recipient who is IgA deficient and receives blood products containing IgA.

- TRALI:
  - Antibodies to white cell antigens in the donor or recipient cause leukocyte aggregates that deposit in the lung.
  - Multiparous female donors with HLA sensitization often are implicated.
- GVHD:
  - Patients with inherited or acquired T-cell immunodeficiency can develop TA-GVHD from transfused immunocompetent T cells; can also occur if the donor and recipient are related and share HLA types.

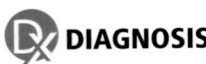 **DIAGNOSIS**

HISTORY
- Acute hemolytic: Fever, chills, abdominal or flank pain, pink or tea-colored urine, tachycardia, hypotension, oliguria
- Febrile: Fever, chills
- Allergic: Urticaria; sometimes bronchospasm; rarely anaphylaxis
- Hypervolemia: Hypertension, dyspnea, rales, cardiac arrhythmia
- Bacterial sepsis: Fever, chills, hypotension
- Delayed hemolytic: Fever, malaise, dark urine, jaundice; rarely shock, renal failure
- TRALI: Acute dyspnea, tachypnea, rales, decreased oxygenation

DIAGNOSTIC TESTS & INTERPRETATION
Lab
- Acute hemolytic:
  - Direct Coombs test: Positive
  - CBC: Anemia
  - Urinalysis: Hemoglobinuria
  - PT, PTT, fibrinogen, fibrin split products: Disseminated intravascular coagulation (DIC)
- Febrile:
  - Direct Coombs test: Negative or no change from pretransfusion
  - Immediate Gram stain of the product
  - Blood culture of the patient and product
  - All results should be negative; a diagnosis of exclusion.
- Allergic:
  - No specific testing
- Bacterial sepsis:
  - Immediate Gram stain and blood culture of the transfused product: Result positive for bacteria

- Delayed hemolytic:
  - CBC: Anemia
  - Bilirubin: Elevated
  - Indirect Coombs test (antibody screen): Positive
  - Direct Coombs test: Positive (mixed field) if done early
- TRALI:
  - Leukocyte antibody testing in the implicated donor(s)
- Anaphylaxis:
  - IgA level in recipient. If undetectable, test for anti-IgA antibody (of the IgE class).

Imaging
Hypervolemia (TACO) and TRALI:
- Chest radiograph: Increased pulmonary vascular markings or infiltrates

 # TREATMENT

ADDITIONAL TREATMENT
General Measures
- Acute hemolytic:
  - Stop transfusion immediately.
  - Hydration, pressors, and diuretics to maintain circulation and urine output
  - Treat disseminated coagulation with plasma.
- Febrile:
  - Stop transfusion.
  - Antipyretics (acetaminophen)
  - May resume transfusion if patient is stable and acute hemolytic transfusion reaction and bacterial sepsis are ruled out
- Allergic:
  - Stop transfusion.
  - Antihistamine (diphenhydramine)
  - Steroids or epinephrine in severe reactions
- Hypervolemia: Diuretics (furosemide)
- Bacterial sepsis:
  - Stop transfusion.
  - Fluids if hypotensive
  - Antibiotics to eradicate *Staphylococcus* and Gram negatives including *Yersinia* species
- Delayed hemolytic: Depends on degree of hemolysis; if profound, management as acute hemolytic reaction. If mild, no therapy may be needed.
- TRALI: Supportive care, usually resolves in 12–24 hours
- Anaphylaxis: Epinephrine STAT, IV fluids, pressors, respiratory support

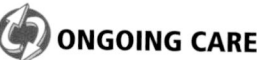 # ONGOING CARE

COMPLICATIONS
- Posttransfusion hepatitis: Caused by hepatitis B or C viruses, others
- AIDS: Caused by HIV
- Cytomegalovirus (CMV):
  - Symptomatic infection in patients with inherited or acquired immunodeficiency states, premature neonates
  - These individuals should receive CMV-safe products.
- Other transfusion transmissible infections: Epstein-Barr virus, syphilis, malaria, toxoplasmosis, human T-lymphotropic virus I (HTLV-I), Chagas disease, babesiosis, filariasis, West Nile virus, parvovirus B19
- Alloimmunization:
  - Formation of antibodies to erythrocyte, platelet, and HLA antigens can develop in some multiply transfused patients; may cause delays in pretransfusion testing, febrile transfusion reactions, delayed hemolytic transfusion reactions, and platelet transfusion refractoriness.
  - HLA alloimmunization may also affect eligibility and organ procurement for solid organ transplantation.
- Iron overload: Long-term transfusion recipients will accumulate iron as a by-product of erythrocyte breakdown; an iron-chelating drug (deferoxamine or deferasirox) will enhance its excretion.

ADDITIONAL READING
- AuBuchon JP, Kruskall MS. Transfusion safety: Realigning efforts with risks. *Transfusion*. 1997;37:1211–1216.
- Capon SM, Goldfinger D. Acute hemolytic transfusion reaction, a paradigm of the systemic inflammatory response: New insights into pathophysiology and treatment. *Transfusion*. 1995;35:513–520.
- Dodd RY, Notari EP, Stramer SL. Current prevalence and incidence of infectious disease markers and estimated window-period risk in the American Red Cross blood donor population. *Transfusion*. 2002;42:975–979.
- Manno CS. What's new in transfusion medicine? *Pediatr Clin North Am*. 2002;43:793–808.

- Quirolo KC. Transfusion medicine for the pediatrician. *Pediatr Clin North Am*. 2002;49: 1211–1238.
- Schreiber GB, Busch MP, Kleinman SH, et al. The risk of transfusion transmitted infection. *N Engl J Med*. 1996;96:1685–1690.
- Cherry T, Steciuk M, Reddy VVB, et al. Transfusion-related acute lung injury: Past, present and future. *Am J Clin Pathol*. 2008;129:287–297.

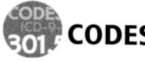 # CODES

ICD9
- 999.80 Transfusion reaction, unspecified
- 999.83 Hemolytic transfusion reaction, incompatibility unspecified
- 999.89 Other transfusion reaction

ICD10
- T80.89XA Other complications following infusion, transfusion and therapeutic injection, initial encounter
- T80.92XA Unspecified transfusion reaction, initial encounter
- T80.919A Hemolytic transfusion reaction, unspecified incompatibility, unspecified as acute or delayed, initial encounter

FAQ
- Q: What is the risk of acquiring certain viral infections?
- A: Hepatitis B: 1:350,000 transfused units; hepatitis C: 1:1,935,000 transfused units; HIV: 1:2,135,000 transfused units
- Q: What is the risk of developing bacterial sepsis?
- A: 1:50,000 red cell units; 1:5,000–10,000 platelet units
- Q: Is directed donor blood safer?
- A: No, there is no evidence that the infection risk is lower, and some studies suggest that the infection risk may be higher.
- Q: Is it safe to give a transfusion to a patient with fever?
- A: Yes. However, if the temperature rises during the transfusion or if symptoms such as chills or hypotension develop, the transfusion should be stopped and the patient evaluated for a transfusion reaction.

TRANSIENT ERYTHROBLASTOPENIA OF CHILDHOOD

Julie W. Stern

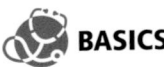 **BASICS**

DESCRIPTION
An acquired, self-limited suppression of red cell production in an otherwise healthy child

EPIDEMIOLOGY
- Mean age at diagnosis is 26 months; <10% are >3 years of age at diagnosis.
- Slight male predominance (male/female 5.1:3.1)
- No seasonal predominance

RISK FACTORS
Genetics
There is no simple genetic pattern; familial transient erythroblastopenia of childhood has been reported (rarely), suggesting a combination of environmental factors and genetic propensity.

GENERAL PREVENTION
There is no known way to prevent transient erythroblastopenia of childhood.

ETIOLOGY
- Unknown
- Possible viral causes include parvovirus B19 and human herpesvirus 6 (HHV-6), but this remains hypothetical.
- A serum inhibitor, such as an IgG directed at the committed erythroid stem cell progenitor, has also been proposed but not yet proven.

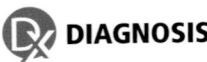 **DIAGNOSIS**

HISTORY
- Pallor: Typically slow in onset and therefore often missed by parents; often noted by an adult who sees the child less frequently
- Activity level:
  - Often preserved because of slow onset of anemia
  - An extremely anemic child may be irritable, sleepy, and/or lethargic.
- History of fever, easy bruisability, or frequent/severe infections (especially bacterial): Should alert the clinician to consider other diagnoses such as leukemia and bone marrow failure syndromes

PHYSICAL EXAM
- Child is generally well appearing and not chronically ill.
- Pallor
- Tachycardia secondary to anemia
- Usually no organomegaly, ecchymosis, petechiae, or jaundice

DIAGNOSTIC TESTS & INTERPRETATION
Diagnostic Procedures/Other
- CBC:
  - Low hemoglobin, normal mean corpuscular volume, normal RBC morphology
  - Total WBC count/morphology and platelet count should be normal; if not, consider leukemias.
  - Absolute neutrophil count may be decreased (rarely $<500/\mu L$), but morphology must be normal.
  - Red cell distribution width may be elevated during recovery.
- Reticulocyte count: Low to zero during anemic phase; should be high during recovery
- Chemistry/Blood bank: Bilirubin, lactate dehydrogenase, ferritin, iron levels, and direct and indirect Coombs testing should be normal to rule out iron-deficiency anemia and immune hemolysis.
- Parvovirus titers, parvovirus PCR testing
- Immunoglobulin (Ig) levels in some cases
- Hemoglobin electrophoresis with quantitative fetal hemoglobin: Should be normal in transient erythroblastopenia of childhood, fetal Hgb elevated in Diamond-Blackfan anemia
- Chest radiograph: To determine degree of cardiomegaly

- Bone marrow aspiration:
  - Not mandatory to make diagnosis
  - May be necessary to rule in transient erythroblastopenia of childhood and rule out other diagnoses such as Diamond-Blackfan and the leukemias
  - Presence or absence of early RBC precursors may help predict time to recovery.
  - Maturation of megakaryocytes and the myeloid cell line must be normal, especially if neutropenia is present.

DIFFERENTIAL DIAGNOSIS
- Environmental: Iron-deficiency anemia
- Metabolic: Hypothyroidism
- Congenital: Diamond-Blackfan anemia (this diagnosis usually made within 1st year of life)
- Neoplasm: Leukemia, myelodysplastic syndromes
- Miscellaneous: Renal disease, anemia of chronic disease, blood loss (usually GI)

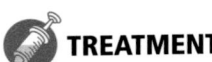 **TREATMENT**

MEDICATION (DRUGS)
- No role for prednisone, iron supplements, anabolic steroids, or other immunosuppressive agents
- Short-term folic acid may be indicated during reticulocytosis.

ADDITIONAL TREATMENT
General Measures
- Initial inpatient observation for complications of severe anemia; daily CBC at least initially to gauge rate of fall of hemoglobin/rise of reticulocyte count and to estimate time to recovery

- Packed RBC transfusion:
  - Only if there is evidence of cardiovascular compromise
  - If a transfusion is needed, transfuse slowly to prevent fluid overload. A good rule of thumb is to transfuse the same number of mL/kg as the patient's hemoglobin over 3–4 hours. Should a 2nd transfusion be needed, attempt to use a 2nd aliquot of the same unit to decrease donor exposure.
- Normal activity and diet for age, as tolerated
- Instruct family on signs and symptoms of severe anemia.

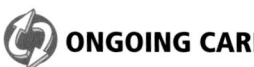 ## ONGOING CARE

FOLLOW-UP RECOMMENDATIONS
- Clinic visits weekly to monitor hemoglobin and reticulocytes. These visits may need to be more frequent in the beginning of the illness and less frequent as recovery becomes evident.
- Elevation of reticulocyte count is the 1st sign of recovery.

PROGNOSIS
- All children recover usually within 1–2 months from diagnosis (up to 8 months to recovery).
- Prognosis is excellent.
- Recurrence is rare.

COMPLICATIONS
- Cardiovascular compromise secondary to severe anemia is often less than expected given the level of anemia. High-output CHF is unusual.
- Neurologic symptoms including confusion and transient hemiparesis have been reported but are rare.

- A significant number of patients also have neutropenia (absolute neutrophil count $\leq 1,500/\mu L$) during either the acute or recovery phase of the illness.

ALERT
- Isolation is necessary because of possible teratogenicity of parvovirus 19 and contagion within the hospital.
- Transient erythroblastopenia of childhood must be an isolated normocytic, normochromic anemia. If the other cell lines are affected (except for mild neutropenia) or if the anemia is macrocytic, consider bone marrow failure syndromes.
- Iron therapy has no place in the treatment of transient erythroblastopenia of childhood. Be sure to check RBC indices and reticulocyte count prior to instituting iron therapy for anemia.

ADDITIONAL READING

- Bhambhani K, Inoue S, Sarnaik SA. Seasonal clustering of transient erythroblastopenia of childhood. *Am J Child Dis*. 1988;142:175–177.
- Shaw J, Meeder R. Transient erythroblastopenia of childhood in siblings: Case report and review of the literature. *J Pediatr Hematol Oncol*. 2007;29(9): 659–660.
- Skeppner G, Kreuger A, Elinder G. Transient erythroblastopenia of childhood: Prospective study of 10 patients with special reference to viral infections. *J Pediatr Hematol Oncol*. 2002;24: 294–298.

 ## CODES

ICD9
284.81 Red cell aplasia (acquired)(adult)(with thymoma)

ICD10
D60.1 Transient acquired pure red cell aplasia

FAQ

- Q: Can other children in a family get this illness?
- A: The cause(s) of this illness in otherwise normal children is unknown. It is very rare for other family members to be affected. It is appropriate to reassure parents with regard to this issue.
- Q: Are transfusions always necessary?
- A: No. Only in cases of heart failure is a transfusion necessary. Most often, children can be managed with watchful waiting.
- Q: How can transient erythroblastopenia of childhood be distinguished from Diamond-Blackfan syndrome?
- A: Children with Diamond-Blackfan syndrome are usually <1 year old and can have elevated hemoglobin F levels. If a bone marrow aspirate is obtained during the recovery phase of transient erythroblastopenia of childhood, the diagnosis will be clear. Often, however, only time will tell. Children with transient erythroblastopenia of childhood always recover; those with Diamond-Blackfan syndrome do not.
- Q: Is transient erythroblastopenia of childhood a precursor to leukemia?
- A: No. However, if recovery does not occur in a timely manner, or if neutropenia worsens, a bone marrow aspirate may be indicated if not previously completed.

T

TRANSIENT TACHYPNEA OF THE NEWBORN (TTN)

John I. Takayama

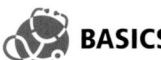 **BASICS**

DESCRIPTION

Early onset of tachypnea (respiratory rate >60 breaths/minute) in the newborn following uneventful, normal preterm or term, vaginal, or cesarean delivery; sometimes with retractions, expiratory grunting, or nasal flaring; rarely with cyanosis; relieved by minimal oxygen (FIO$_2$ <40%)

EPIDEMIOLOGY

Incidence

- 4–6 per 1,000 live births (common)
- Incidence is higher in males than females.

RISK FACTORS

Early gestational age and cesarean section delivery have been identified as major risk factors. Other factors include maternal diabetes, macrosomia, and parental history of asthma.

GENERAL PREVENTION

- When possible, infants should be delivered by vaginal birth because TTN is seen more in infants born by cesarean section.
- Elective cesarean section should be postponed until 39 weeks' gestation or later.

ETIOLOGY

- Slow or decreased absorption of fetal lung fluid, including fluid accumulation in the interstitial space, resulting in decreased pulmonary compliance, decreased tidal volume, and increased dead space. Disruption of sodium transport by lung epithelia has been postulated recently as reason for ineffective transepithelial alveolar fluid movement.
- Mild immaturity of the surfactant system may contribute to decreased pulmonary compliance and result in increased respiratory rate. In some infants with TTN, a decreased amount of phosphatidylglycerol has been found in their amniotic fluid.

DIAGNOSIS

HISTORY

- Usually presents as early onset of tachypnea (within 1st few hours of life)
- Maternal risk factors: TTN is twice as likely for infants of mothers with asthma compared with infants of mothers without asthma.
- Birth-related risk factors (mechanisms unknown):
  – Maternal sedation
  – Maternal fluid administration
  – Maternal exposure to sympathomimetics
  – Prolonged labor
  – Cesarean section
  – Preterm birth
  – Fetal asphyxia
- Presence of risk factors for other conditions (e.g., maternal fever) may make the diagnosis of TTN less likely and other diagnoses more likely (e.g., pneumonia or sepsis).

PHYSICAL EXAM

- Respiratory rate >60/minute
- Grunting, nasal flaring, intercostal retractions; at times, cyanosis
- Barrel-chest appearance
- Lungs clear on auscultation; sometimes rales or crackles but not rhonchi
- Absence of signs and symptoms more specific for infection and neurologic as well as cardiac conditions (e.g., fever, cyanosis without respiratory distress)

DIAGNOSTIC TESTS & INTERPRETATION

- Pulse oximetry: Oxygen saturation should be maintained at >96%.
- Arterial blood gas: Metabolic acidosis with base deficit suggests asphyxia; not usually ordered.
- CBC: Decreased or increased WBC count and increased immature forms (e.g., bands) suggest infection; not usually ordered.
- If febrile, blood culture: Positive results indicate infection.

Imaging

Chest radiograph: TTN is indicated by prominent central pulmonary vascular markings (central perihilar streaking), fluid lines in the interlobar fissures, hyperaeration, flat diaphragms, and, occasionally, pleural fluid.

DIFFERENTIAL DIAGNOSIS

- Respiratory:
  – Meconium aspiration
  – Respiratory distress syndrome
  – Pneumothorax
  – Pneumomediastinum
- Infection:
  – Pneumonia
  – Sepsis
- Neurologic:
  – Cerebral hypoventilation
  – Birth asphyxia
- Cardiac:
  – Congenital cyanotic heart disease
- Metabolic:
  – Conditions manifesting as metabolic acidosis
- Miscellaneous:
  – Congenital cystic adenomatoid malformation (CCAM)
  – Congenital diaphragmatic hernia

ALERT

Because TTN is a diagnosis of exclusion, it is important to consider and exclude other diagnoses by carefully relying on history, examination, and appropriate laboratory aids.

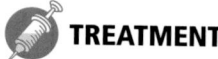
TREATMENT

ADDITIONAL TREATMENT
General Measures
- Emergency care: Usually not required
  - Initially, nothing by mouth until respiratory status is stabilized and diagnosis is clarified.
  - Oxygen: May help reduce respiratory distress if the patient is hypoxic
  - Antibiotics if pneumonia or sepsis suspected
  - Neither furosemide (diuretic) nor racemic epinephrine has been shown to improve TTN.
- Supportive care:
  - IV fluids if NPO
  - Monitoring of respiratory status using continuous pulse oximetry and respiratory and heart rate surveillance
- Duration of therapy:
  - Typically 2–5 days

ONGOING CARE

FOLLOW-UP RECOMMENDATIONS
- When to expect improvement:
  - Rapid respirations slow gradually.
  - 12–72 hours
- Signs to watch for:
  - Fever, lethargy, poor feeding, early jaundice
  - Persistent or increased need for oxygen

PATIENT EDUCATION
Infant can go home when the breathing rate is low enough so that he or she feeds well and when oxygen is no longer required.

PROGNOSIS
- Generally considered a self-limited condition with no recurrence and no residual pulmonary dysfunction. Some studies, however, have demonstrated associations with persistent pulmonary hypertension of the newborn.
- Infant may be at risk for breathing problems such as asthma. Recent evidence indicates a higher incidence of wheezing and asthma in children with TTN diagnosis.

COMPLICATIONS
- Hypoxia
- Rarely, respiratory failure requiring continuous positive airway pressure or mechanical ventilation

ADDITIONAL READING

- Birnkrant DJ, Picone C, Markowitz W, et al. Association of transient tachypnea of the newborn and childhood asthma. *Pediatr Pulm*. 2006;41: 978–984.
- Consortium on Safe Labor; Hibbard JU, Wilkins I, Sun L, et al. Respiratory morbidity in late preterm births. *JAMA*. 2010;304:419–425.
- Guglani LG, Lakshminrusimha S, Ryan R. Transient tachypnea of the newborn. *Pediatr Rev*. 2008;29: e59–e65.
- Jain L, Eaton DC. Physiology of fetal lung fluid clearance and the effect of labor. *Semin Perinatol*. 2006;30:34–43.
- Lewis V, Whitelaw A. Furosemide for transient tachypnea of the newborn. *Cochrane Database Syst Rev*. 2002;1:CD003064.
- Miller MJ, Fanaroff AA, Martin RJ. Respiratory disorders in preterm and term infants. In: Fanaroff AA, Martin RJ, eds. *Neonatal-Perinatal Medicine: Diseases of the Fetus and Infants*. 7th ed. St. Louis, MO: Mosby–Year Book; 2002:1030–1031.
- Tutdibi E, Gries K, Bucheler M, et al. Impact of labor on outcomes in transient tachypnea of the newborn: Population-based study. *Pediatrics*. 2010;125: e577–e583.
- Yurdakok M. Transient tachypnea of the newborn: What is new? *J Matern Fetal Neonatal Med*. 2010;23(S3):24–26.

CODES

ICD9
770.6 Transitory tachypnea of newborn

ICD10
P22.1 Transient tachypnea of newborn

FAQ
- Q: How long does the rapid breathing last?
- A: Most babies are better in 1 day, but TTN may persist for 2–3 days.
- Q: Are chest x-rays required?
- A: No. If the baby is eating well and having no other medical issues, observation is sufficient.

T

TRANSPOSITION OF THE GREAT ARTERIES

Bradley S. Marino

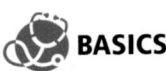 BASICS

DESCRIPTION

Abnormal anatomic relationship between the great arteries and the ventricles in which the aorta arises from the anatomic right ventricle and the pulmonary artery arises from the anatomic left ventricle

Incidence

Incidence is 20–30 per 100,000 live births, with a 60–70% male predilection.

Prevalence

Transposition of the great arteries represents up to 7% of all cases of congenital heart disease.

PATHOPHYSIOLOGY

- Systemic and pulmonary circulations are separated and function in parallel.
- Desaturated systemic venous blood is ejected from the right heart to the aorta, whereas the oxygenated pulmonary venous blood is ejected from the left ventricle into the lungs.
- Survival depends on defects that permit mixing between the two circulations (patent ductus arteriosus [PDA], patent foramen ovale [PFO], ventricular septal defect [VSD]).

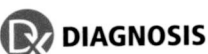 DIAGNOSIS

HISTORY

- Infants are of normal birth weight, or sometimes large for gestational age.
- Cyanosis
- Tachypnea often without retractions
- Poor feeding

PHYSICAL EXAM

- General:
  - Moderate to severe cyanosis
- Cardiovascular:
  - Heart sounds: Single loud S2, but no heart murmur is heard in infants with intact ventricular septum; soft systolic murmur in those infants with a VSD, and a systolic ejection murmur of valvar or subvalvar aortic or pulmonic stenosis may be heard.
- Respiratory:
  - Generally dyspnea and tachypnea present without retractions in a neonate without a VSD; with a large VSD and congestive heart failure (CHF), retractions may be present.
- Abdomen:
  - Hepatomegaly may occur with a large VSD and CHF.

DIAGNOSTIC TESTS & INTERPRETATION

Lab

Arterial blood gas:

- Hypoxemia (pO_2 often in low 30s) unchanged in 100% FiO_2. Infants with inadequate mixing have pO_2 <25 torr with metabolic acidosis.

Imaging

- Chest radiograph:
  - Mild cardiomegaly with an egg-shaped heart with narrow superior mediastinum (so-called egg on a string) and increased pulmonary vascular markings.
- EKG:
  - Initially normal, progressing to right ventricular hypertrophy and right axis deviation
- Echocardiogram:
  - 2D ECHO and color-flow Doppler studies usually provide all anatomic and functional information required for management of infants with D-transposition of the great arteries (D-TGA). The study should focus on the alignment of the great arteries and other associated anomalies, specifically defects that promote intercirculatory mixing, the presence of left or right ventricular outflow tract obstruction, and the coronary anatomy.

Pathological Findings

- In D-TGA, the aorta originates anteriorly from the right ventricle and carries desaturated blood to the body, and the pulmonary artery originates posteriorly from the left ventricle and carries oxygenated blood to the lungs. There is fibrous continuity between the pulmonary and mitral valves; subaortic conus (infundibulum) is present. In the normal heart, the aorta arises posteriorly from the left ventricle, there is fibrous continuity between the aortic and mitral valves, and subpulmonary conus is present.
- TGA types:
  - The most common type of TGA, known as D-TGA has transposed great arteries with cardiac segments (S,D,D): Situs solitus of the atria and viscera (S), dextroventricular segment situs (D), aortic valve annulus to the right of the pulmonary artery (D).
  - L-TGA or "corrected transposition," has transposed great arteries with cardiac segments (S,L,L): Situs solitus of the atria and viscera (S), levoventricular segment situs (L), and the aortic valve annulus is to the left of the pulmonary artery (L).

- Associated abnormalities include: PDA and PFO with intact ventricular septum (50%); VSD (40%), posterior malalignment VSD with left ventricular outflow tract obstruction (e.g., subpulmonic stenosis, pulmonary stenosis, pulmonary atresia; 10%), anterior malalignment VSD with right ventricular outflow tract obstruction (e.g., subaortic stenosis, aortic stenosis, coarctation of the aorta or interruption of the aortic arch; 10%); coronary branching abnormalities (33%); leftward juxtaposition of the atrial appendages (5%); and straddling of the atrioventricular valve,

DIFFERENTIAL DIAGNOSIS

The differential diagnosis for the neonate with TGA is that for the cyanotic neonate.

- Cardiac:
  - Lesions with ductal-dependent pulmonary blood flow:
    - Tricuspid atresia with normally related great arteries
    - Tetralogy of Fallot
    - Tetralogy of Fallot with pulmonic atresia
    - Critical pulmonic stenosis
    - Pulmonary atresia with intact ventricular septum
    - Ebstein anomaly
    - Heterotaxy (most forms)
  - Ductal-independent mixing lesions:
    - Total anomalous pulmonary venous connection without obstruction
    - Truncus arteriosus
  - Lesions with ductal-dependent systemic blood flow:
    - Hypoplastic left heart syndrome
    - Interrupted aortic arch
    - Critical coarctation of the aorta
    - Critical aortic stenosis
- Pulmonary:
  - Primary lung disease
  - Airway obstruction
  - Extrinsic compression of the lungs
- Neurologic:
  - CNS dysfunction
  - Respiratory neuromuscular dysfunction
- Hematologic:
  - Methemoglobinemia
  - Polycythemia

TREATMENT

MEDICATION (DRUGS)

- Correction of metabolic acidosis, hypoglycemia, and hypocalcemia improves myocardial function.
- Prostaglandin E1 (PGE1) is used for severe cyanosis to promote left (aorta) to right (pulmonary artery) shunting at the ductus arteriosus, thereby increasing pulmonary blood flow, distention of the left atrium and improved mixing at the atrial level. Side effects of PGE1 include apnea, fever, and hypotension.

SURGERY/OTHER PROCEDURES

- Interventional catheterization:
  - Balloon atrial septostomy (Rashkind procedure) is used in the severely hypoxemic infant with an intact or restrictive atrial septum to promote intercirculatory mixing at the atrial level and stabilize the neonate before definitive or palliative surgery.
- Definitive surgery for D-TGA includes procedures that redirect the pulmonary and systemic venous return at the atrial, ventricular, and great artery levels.
  - Atrial inversion: Atrial inversion procedures involve baffling the pulmonary venous blood flow to the tricuspid valve (systemic circulation), and the systemic venous blood flow to the mitral valve (pulmonary circulation). The 2 atrial inversion operations include the Mustard procedure, in which prosthetic or pericardial baffles are used to redirect the blood, and the Senning procedure, in which the baffles are composed of an atrial septal flap and the right atrial free wall. The Senning or Mustard procedures may be used in the following infants:
    - Infants with D-TGA with intact ventricular septum who have not had surgical repair within the first month of life.
    - Neonates with D-TGA with intact ventricular septum and severe pulmonic stenosis. Most centers would perform a Rastelli procedure for this anatomic variant (see susbsequent list items).
    - Neonates with D-TGA with "unswitchable coronaries" (<1% of cases).
  - Ventricular inversion:
    - D-TGA with a VSD and severe pulmonic stenosis: The Rastelli operation may be used to redirect blood flow at the ventricular level. In this operation, the proximal main pulmonary artery is divided and oversewn, and the left ventricular blood flow is baffled to the aorta by creating an intraventricular tunnel between the VSD and the aortic valve. A conduit is placed from the right ventricle to the pulmonary artery to redirect the right ventricular blood flow.

- Arterial switch:
  - D-TGA with intact ventricular septum and "switchable" coronaries: The arterial switch operation (ASO) is performed in which the great arteries are transected above their respective semilunar valves and switched with reimplantation of the coronary arteries into the neo-aortic root (native pulmonary valve root).
  - D-TGA with anterior malalignment VSD with severe aortic stenosis: ASO with VSD patch closure and transannular patch of the right ventricular outflow tract.

ONGOING CARE

PROGNOSIS

- Without treatment, mortality is 30% within the first week of life, 50% within the first month, 70% within the first 6 months, and 90% within the first year.
- In most centers, the mortality rate after ASO for D-TGA with intact ventricular septum or D-TGA with a VSD is <3%. Factors that have been shown to increase the mortality risk include an intramural course of the left coronary artery, retropulmonary course of the left coronary artery, complex arch abnormalities, right ventricular hypoplasia, multiple VSDs, and straddling atrioventricular valves.

COMPLICATIONS

- Complications of intra-atrial surgeries include obstruction of pulmonary venous return (<2% of cases), obstruction of systemic venous return (5% of cases), residual intra-atrial baffle shunt (20% of cases), tricuspid regurgitation (5–10%), absence of sinus rhythm (>50% of cases), supraventricular arrhythmias (50%), and moderately to severely depressed right ventricular function (20%). Follow-up observation is recommended every 12 months to detect arrhythmias, tricuspid regurgitation, or depressed right ventricular function that generally occur years after surgery. Arrhythmias include sinus node dysfunction (e.g., marked sinus bradycardia, ectopic atrial rhythm, junctional rhythm, or junctional bradycardia) and supraventricular tachycardia, especially atrial flutter.
- Complications after the Rastelli operation include left ventricular outflow tract obstruction, conduit obstruction, and complete heart block. Follow-up observation is recommended every 12 months to monitor for conduit obstruction, left ventricular outflow tract obstruction, and heart block.
- The most common complication after the ASO is neo-aortic root dilation with or without neo-aortic insufficiency. Other rarer complications include supravalvar pulmonary stenosis at the anastomotic site (5% of cases), supravalvar aortic stenosis at the anastomotic site (5% of cases), and coronary artery obstruction, that may lead to ischemia and infarction. These complications are uncommon and usually hemodynamically insignificant. Mortality varies depending on the period of time being assessed:
  - Early mortality is usually related to kinking or obstruction of the coronary arteries during transfer to the neo-aorta, an "unprepared" left ventricle, or hemorrhage from the multiple suture lines.
  - Late mortality (i.e., 1–2%) usually results from myocardial ischemia, pulmonary vascular obstructive disease, or during reoperation for supravalvar stenosis.

- Follow-up observation is recommended every 12 months to monitor for neo-aortic root dilation, neo-aortic valve insufficiency, supravalvar aortic or pulmonic stenosis, and coronary artery ischemia.

ADDITIONAL READING

- Bellinger DC, Wypij D, duDuplessis AJ, et al. Neurodevelopmental status at eight years in children with dextro-transposition of the great arteries: The Boston Circulatory Arrest Trial. *J Thorac Cardiovasc Surg.* 2003;126:1385–1396.
- Culbert EL, Ashburn DA, Cullen-Dean G, et al. Congenital Heart Surgeons Society. Quality of life of children after repair of transposition of the great arteries. *Circulation.* 2003;108:857–862.
- Formigari R, Toscano A, Giardini A, et al. Prevalence and predictors of neoaortic regurgitation after arterial switch operation for transposition of the great arteries. *J Thorac Cardiovasc Surg.* 2003; 126:1753–1759.
- Langley SM, Winlaw DS, Stumper O, et al. Midterm results after restoration of the morphologically left ventricle to the systemic circulation in patients with congenitally corrected transposition of the great arteries. *J Thorac Cardiovasc Surg.* 2003;125: 1229–1241.
- Marino BS, Wernovsky G, McElhinney D, et al. Neo-aortic valvar function after the arterial switch. *Cardiol Young.* 2006;16:481–489.
- Mavroudis C, Backer CL. Physiologic versus anatomic repair of congenitally corrected transposition of the great arteries. *Semin Thorac Cardiovasc Surg.* 2003;6:16–26.
- Pasquali SK, Hasselblad V, Li JS, et al. Coronary artery pattern and outcome of arterial switch operation for transposition of the great arteries: A meta-analysis. *Circulation.* 2002;106:2575–2580.
- Warnes CA, Transposition of the great arteries. *Circulation.* 2006;114:2699–2709.
- Williams WG, McCrindle BW, Ashburn DA, et al. Congenital Heart Surgeon's Society. Outcomes of 829 neonates with complete transposition of the great arteries 12–17 years after repair. *Eur J Cardiothorac Surg.* 2003;24:1–9.

CODES

ICD9
745.10 Transposition of great vessels (complete)

ICD10
Q20.3 Discordant ventriculoarterial connection

TRANSVERSE MYELITIS
Yang Mao-Draayer

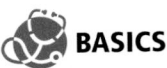

BASICS

DESCRIPTION
Inflammation in the spinal cord causing acute or subacute loss of motor, sensory, and autonomic function, often preceded by mid-back pain; may be postinfectious, postvaccination, or associated with multiple sclerosis (MS). While acute transverse myelitis (ATM) implies an inflammatory disease of the spinal cord, acute transverse myelopathy is a broader term that refers to any process that acutely impairs spinal cord function. Presumed pathophysiology of ATM is autoimmune-mediated inflammation and demyelination of the spinal cord. Postinfectious etiology largely predominates in children.

EPIDEMIOLOGY
Incidence
1–4/million per year, affecting all ages, with bimodal peaks between the ages of 10 and 19 years and between 30 and 39 years. Boys and girls are affected equally.

COMMONLY ASSOCIATED CONDITIONS
- ATM is most commonly associated with infection.
- It may be part of demyelinating disorders: May either occur as 1st episode of MS or in that disease setting; may also occur with demyelination of optic nerves (i.e., optic neuritis), also called Devic disease or neuromyelitis optica (NMO); may occur in monophasic demyelinating disease—acute disseminated encephalomyelitis (ADEM)—multiple demyelinating lesions in the brain as well as in the spinal cord.
- ATM may be associated with systemic inflammatory diseases (e.g., systemic lupus erythematosus, primary antiphospholipid syndrome, juvenile rheumatoid arthritis, sarcoidosis, connective tissue disease, vasculitis); may present with acute or recurrent transverse myelitis.
- ATM is rarely seen in association with metabolic causes of myelopathy (e.g., vitamin B_{12} deficiency).
- ATM does not usually occur in association with inherited demyelinating diseases (e.g., adrenomyeloneuropathy/leukodystrophy, Pelizaeus-Merzbacher, globoid cell leukodystrophy, and metachromatic leukodystrophy); these usually present with chronic myelopathy.

DIAGNOSIS

HISTORY
- Most prominent is neurologic dysfunction consistent with a spinal cord dysfunction at a specific level. Bilateral, but not necessarily symmetric, symptoms are usually present.
- ATM may be suggested by history of back pain, sensory level, and urinary/fecal incontinence or retention. The patient often has lower extremity weakness or inability to bear weight, possibly with decreased spontaneous use of hands.
- Details of the temporal course of the symptoms are important, because sudden onset of weakness raises the possibility of acute structural or vascular causes of myelopathy. In ATM, onset of spinal cord dysfunction usually progress in 4 hours to 21 days; the patient's signs usually plateau and evolve toward spasticity/hyperreflexia.
- ATM is often preceded by respiratory illness, vaccination, or systemic illness. One should determine if there is a prior history of infection or systemic inflammatory disease.
- Other important findings in history include vascular/ischemia, neoplasia, MS, radiation exposure, trauma, or immunodeficiency to rule out other causes of acute myelopathy.

PHYSICAL EXAM
- Extreme irritability: Extent of weakness may be assessed by spontaneous activity and how vigorously the child resists examination.
- Fever, hypertension, tachycardia, meningeal signs may be present; in such cases, CNS infection needs to be ruled out; point tenderness over the spine may suggest trauma or infection.
- Neurologic: Check visual acuity and color vision; funduscopic examination for optic nerve head pallor (optic neuritis).
- Increased tone: Spastic weakness is usually symmetric, legs more than arms.
- Reflexes are usually brisk, with positive Babinski sign.
- Sensory ataxia, a sensory level (a partial level is commonly seen) that may spare joint position, and vibration may be present.
- Urgent complication: Sphincter dysfunction, urinary retention or incontinence; check for loss of anal wink, bladder dilatation, and large post-void residual urine (>100 mL).

DIAGNOSTIC TESTS & INTERPRETATION
Diagnostic Procedures/Other
- A diagnosis of ATM requires evidence of inflammation of the spinal cord. MRI and CSF analysis are the 2 most important tests and are mandatory in suspected ATM. Enhancing spinal cord lesion or pleocytosis or increased IgG index is required for the diagnosis. If both tests are negative, repeat tests in 2–7 days is recommended.

- The 1st priority in acute myelopathy is to rule out structural causes—compressive myelopathy. Gadolinium-enhanced MRI of spine (above the level that could explain weakness or sensory deficit) excludes structural causes of myelopathy and can indicate transverse myelitis.
- The 2nd priority is to define the presence/absence of spinal cord inflammation and to rule out other CNS infections. Lumbar puncture is usually done after imaging, often showing normal or slightly increased protein levels and mild pleocytosis with lymphocyte predominance. Elevation of IgG index and presence of oligoclonal bands are indicative of ATM, MS, or other systemic inflammatory disease. CSF Gram stain; bacterial, viral, and fungal culture; VDRL, Lyme antibodies; and PCR of specific viruses should all be negative in ATM.
- The 3rd priority is to determine the extent of demyelination. Gadolinium-enhanced MRI of the brain and the orbit and evoked potential studies (e.g., visual evoked potential, somatosensory evoked potential) may identify other sites.
- Investigation for underlying systemic inflammatory/metabolic disorder includes ESR and ANA; for granulomatous disease or infection, incudes PPD/anergy panel, serum angiotensin-converting enzyme (ACE; elevated in sarcoidosis), RPR, Lyme titer; B_{12} and very-long-chain fatty acid (VLCFA).
- Viruses associated with ATM include the herpes viruses (EBV, VZV, HSV); CMV; mumps; rubella; influenza; hepatitis A, B, and C; and HIV. Positive IgM or >4-fold increase in IgG levels on 2 successive tests to a specific infectious agent suggests diagnosis of parainfectious ATM.

DIFFERENTIAL DIAGNOSIS
- Presentation of ATM in toddlers may resemble osteomyelitis, arthritis, toxic synovitis, or even a sudden abdominal problem: Extreme irritability, unwillingness to bear weight.
- Extremity weakness seen in ATM may resemble an acute neuromuscular disorder (e.g., Guillain-Barré syndrome or polymyositis), in which case the definitive myelopathic signs (e.g., spastic tone, hyperreflexia, upturned toes, sensory level) are not present. Guillain-Barré syndrome is frequently confused with ATM, particularly when the latter does not show typical upper motor neuron findings; normal MRI (except possible nerve root enhancement in GBS) and the albuminocytologic dissociation (high-protein, low cell count) in CSF from patients with Guillain-Barré syndrome help distinguish the 2 conditions.

- Other causes of myelopathy that require different treatment must be excluded—for example, urgent, surgically remediable cause of myelopathy (e.g., epidural abscess, tumor, arteriovenous malformation); emergency basis radiation, and/or high-dose IV corticosteroid therapy for neoplastic cord compression.
- ATM may be the presenting feature of MS, especially in patients with partial ATM and abnormal initial brain MRI; in such cases, MS treatments and follow-up MRIs should be considered.
- NMO (or Devic disease) is a rare (even rarer in children than adults) and aggressive demyelinating disease. When children present with recurrent transverse myelitis with an elongated (>3 vertebral segments) intramedullary spinal cord lesion, serum NMO antibody testing should be obtained to facilitate the diagnosis and treatment.
- Compressive myelopathies: Vertebral osteomyelitis/discitis; intrinsic or extrinsic tumor; spine trauma; epidural abscess
- Infectious causes of myelopathy:
  - Poliomyelitis: Concern about underlying immunodeficiency
  - Lyme disease: In children with possible exposure, serology is nonspecific but sensitive unless antibiotics are given early in the course, which ablates immune response
  - Syphilis: Usually chronic, tertiary form (tabes dorsalis), although meningovascular myelitis may cause acute myelopathy.
- Vascular causes: Cord ischemia (postcardiac surgery), cord arteriovenous malformation

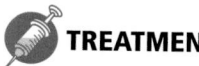 **TREATMENT**

ADDITIONAL TREATMENT
General Measures
- IV methylprednisolone may be useful in ATM or other acute demyelinating diseases based on observational studies. IV immunoglobulin or plasmapheresis may be a safe and effective therapeutic alternative in patients who do not respond to or are intolerant of IV methylprednisolone.
- Cyclophosphamide has been reported to be useful in myelitis associated with systemic inflammatory diseases.
- Symptomatic management: Anticipate urinary retention to prevent perforated bladder. Bowel/bladder regimen, catheterization, prophylactic antibiotics, and stool softeners are often used.

- Unlike acute polyneuropathy (i.e., Guillain-Barré syndrome), ATM rarely causes respiratory insufficiency unless patients have cervical lesions. In such cases, an intensive care setting to anticipate respiratory failure or autonomic instability, mechanical ventilation, and cautious use of antihypertensive agents may be necessary.
- Physical and occupational therapy (PT/OT) may help promote functional recovery and prevent contractures.

 ONGOING CARE

PROGNOSIS
- 1/3 of individuals with ATM recover completely, with the symptoms mostly resolved (gradually) in 3–6 months; 1/3 are left with moderate disability, and 1/3 have severe disability. Residual neurologic deficits include fixed weakness and sensory or autonomic deficits. Sphincter dysfunction improves more slowly than do other deficits. Treatment is largely symptomatic, and long-term PT/OT may be beneficial.
- Prognostic factors: Older age, increased deep tendon reflexes, and presence of the Babinski sign may indicate a better course. Rapid progression, back pain, and spinal shock predict poor recovery.
- ATM may be the presenting feature of MS, especially in patients with partial ATM and abnormal initial brain MRI; in such cases, follow-up MRIs and MS therapy should be considered.

ADDITIONAL READING

- Alper G, Petropoulou KA, Fitz CR, et al. Idiopathic acute transverse myelitis in children: An analysis and discussion of MRI findings. *Mult Scler.* 2011;17: 74–80.
- Dale RC, Brilot F, Banwell B. Pediatric central nervous system inflammatory demyelination: Acute disseminated encephalomyelitis, clinically isolated syndromes, neuromyelitis optica, and multiple sclerosis. *Curr Opin Neurol.* 2009;22:223–240.
- Defresne P, Hollenberg H, Husson B, et al. Acute transverse myelitis in children: Clinical course and prognostic factors. *J Child Neurol.* 2003;18: 401–406.

- Defresne P, Meyer L, Tardieu M, et al. Efficacy of high dose steroid therapy in children with severe acute transverse myelitis. *J Neurol Neurosurg Psychiatry.* 2001;71:272–274.
- Miyazawa R, Ikeuchi Y, Tomomasa T, et al. Determinants of prognosis of acute transverse myelitis in children. *Pediatr Int.* 2003;45:512–516.
- Transverse Myelitis Consortium Working Group. Proposed diagnostic criteria and nosology of acute transverse myelitis. *Neurology.* 2002;59:499–505.

 CODES

ICD9
341.20 Acute (transverse) myelitis NOS

ICD10
G37.3 Acute transverse myelitis in demyelinating disease of central nervous system

FAQ

- Q: What is the usual clinical course of ATM?
- A: The course of ATM in children proceeds through 3 stages: (a) Initial motor loss precedes sphincter dysfunction in most patients; there is often a sensory loss below certain levels, usually over 2–3 days; (b) plateau phase, where the mean duration of plateau is 1 week; and (c) recovery phase.
- Q: What causes the pain and irritability commonly seen in children with ATM?
- A: Pain in ATM may be as a result of (a) neuropathic pain from nerve root inflammation, (b) nociceptive pain from dural inflammation, (c) muscle spasm from motor dyscontrol, (d) bladder distention from dysautonomia, (e) psychologic distress from loss of motor control, or (f) dysesthesia from demyelination of spinothalamic tract.
- Q: When should MS be considered?
- A: MS should be considered when the history indicates other neurologic symptoms, such as internuclear ophthalmoplegia, optic neuritis, focal weakness, and numbness that lasts at least 24 hours to days that have now resolved completely, other lesions on brain/spine MRI at the time of presentation, or subsequent new MRI lesions.

T

TRICHINOSIS

Carolyn A. Paris
Jennifer R. Reid
George Anthony Woodward

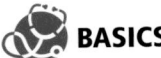 **BASICS**

DESCRIPTION
- Infection caused by ingestion of undercooked meat containing nematode (roundworm) larval cysts of the *Trichinella* genus
- Most common cause of infection worldwide

EPIDEMIOLOGY
- Worldwide distribution with an estimated 10,000 cases per year, and mortality rate of 0.2%, in main 55 countries reporting
- Historically, most US infections are due to *Trichinella spiralis* in commercial pork.
- Currently, more US infections are associated with wild game meat (especially bear) or through spillover to domestic animals.
- Occasional grouped outbreaks (e.g., families and communities with common exposure)
- Consider in patients with a history of travel, consumed foreign meat or wild game (e.g., bear, cougar, hyena, lion, panther, fox), horse, dog (China), seal, or walrus meat.
- Carried by rodents, domesticated animals (e.g., dogs, cats), raccoons, opossums, skunks
- Disease not transmissible person to person

Incidence
Between 2002–2007 in the United States, average of 11 cases annually:
- Decreasing number of cases are attributed to decline in prevalence of *Trichinella* in commercial swine (1.41% in 1900, 0.125% in 1966, and 0.013% in 1995), federal regulation preventing uncooked meat consumption by commercial swine, and increased public awareness regarding properly frozen and cooked meat.

Prevalence
~4% of cadavers in 1970 study with evidence of previous infection (additional estimates range from 10–20% prevalence)

RISK FACTORS
- Consumption of inadequately cooked meat, even in small quantities
- *Trichinella* species consumed
- Compromised immune status of host

GENERAL PREVENTION
- Consume only fully cooked meat, especially pork and wild game; meat should reach >160°F internally, no pink
  - Freezing kills *T. spiralis* in pork (<6 in. thick) at −20°F for 6 days, −10°F for 10 days, and −5°F for 20 days.
  - Freezing may not kill other *Trichinella* species, particularly in wild game.
- Freezing, curing, smoking, salting, and drying meat (including jerky) are not reliable sterilization methods.
- Routinely clean meat processing equipment.
- Irradiation may not kill *Trichinella* but should prevent ability to replicate.

- Avoid feeding swine uncooked meat scraps.
- Actively control rodents.
- Thoroughly cook all meat; internal temperature should reach >160°F.

PATHOPHYSIOLOGY
- *Trichinella* are obligate intracellular parasites capable of infecting only warm-blooded animals.
- At least 8 *Trichinella* species identified: *T. spiralis*, *T. britovi*, *T. pseudospiralis*, *T. papuae*, *T. nativa*, *T. nelsoni*, *T. murrelli*, and *T. zimbawensis*; *T. spiralis* most common worldwide.
- Life cycle of all species comprises 2 generations in the same host (broad range species—mammal, birds and reptiles), but only humans become clinically affected.
- Larvae in undercooked meat eaten by the patient are released after cyst wall digestion by gastric enzymes, pass to the small intestine, invade mucosa, then develop into adult worms.
- Incubation period 1–2 weeks
- Fertilized females release larvae (~500) over 2–3 weeks. Adult worms are expelled in feces; they do not multiply in a human host.
- Newborn larvae travel the bloodstream to seed skeletal muscles. There they grow 10-fold, coil, and encyst. Muscle fibers enlarge and become edematous; may have granulomatous reactions in nonskeletal muscle, but larvae are found only in skeletal muscle.
- Cysts (hyaline capsules) may calcify over several months to years.

ETIOLOGY
Consumption of undercooked infected meat; see Description

COMMONLY ASSOCIATED CONDITIONS
- Rheumatic syndromes: Polyarteritis nodosa–like systemic necrotizing vasculitis, symmetrical polyarteritis, glomerulonephritis.
- Immunocompromised hosts are at risk for more serious or prolonged infection

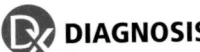 **DIAGNOSIS**

Requires combination of epidemiologic, clinical, and laboratory findings

HISTORY
- Ingestion of inadequately cooked meat (commercial pork, noncommercial pork, game animals, foreign meat)
- Others with similar symptoms and same dietary exposure

- Signs and symptoms:
  - Clinical severity varies, asymptomatic (subclinical) most common, fulminant to fatal rare; depends on *Trichinella* species and inoculum size
  - Children often have fewer and milder symptoms than adults.
  - Death can occur due to myocarditis, encephalitis, or pneumonia.
  - Many signs and symptoms (i.e., periorbital edema, muscle edema, eosinophilia due to allergic reaction to parasite antigens)
  - Nonspecific signs and symptoms may mimic other illnesses.
  - Enteral phase (24 hours to 7 days after infection): Symptoms due to intestinal ulceration from mucosal invasion by adult worms
    - Diarrhea, abdominal pain, nausea, vomiting, anorexia
    - May persist for weeks
  - Parenteral phase (1–8 weeks after infection): Symptoms due to systemic invasion:
    - General: Fever (begins at 2 weeks, peaks after 4 weeks, night spikes to 40–41°C), weakness, malaise, myalgias
    - Ocular: Periorbital edema, subconjunctival hemorrhage, conjunctivitis, disturbed vision, ocular pain, chemosis
    - Muscular: Myalgias, myositis (usually in extraocular muscles, then masseters, tongue, neck, limb flexors, lumbar muscles, intercostals, and diaphragm) with dyspnea, cough, hoarseness
    - Neurologic: Headache, focal paralysis, delirium, psychosis
    - Skin: Urticarial rash, subungual hemorrhages
    - Parenteral phase symptoms typically peak 2–3 weeks after infection.
    - Malaise and weakness may persist for weeks.
    - Cardiac: Myocarditis, arrhythmias secondary to myocarditis
  - Convalescent phase (begins 2nd month, may last months to years): Myalgias, weakness

PHYSICAL EXAM
Fever, periorbital edema, muscular tenderness, generalized edema, urticaria: See "Signs and symptoms" in the History section.

DIAGNOSTIC TESTS & INTERPRETATION
Lab
- Complete blood chemistry and differential: Eosinophilia (up to 70%, peaks 10–21 days post innoculation but prior to clinical symptoms), leukocytosis (moderate)
- Elevation of muscle enzymes (LDH, CPK, aldolase)
- Specific anti-*Trichinella* antibody detection
- Serologic tests are available through the US Centers for Disease Control and Prevention or state and some private and state labs.
- Detection of *Trichinella*-specific DNA by polymerase chain reaction (availability limited)

- *Trichinella* serology:
  – 2 tests required to ensure accurate diagnosis: 1st to detect antigen (ELISA) and the 2nd to detect antibodies to parasite surface antigens (FA)
  – Bentonite flocculation (1:5 or 4-fold increase), latex flocculation test, enzyme-linked immunosorbent assay, or immunofluorescence

Imaging
- X-ray: May show enlarged heart or calcified cysts in muscle (6–24 months post infection)
- Cardiac: Myocarditis may show ECG changes (premature contractions, prolonged PR interval, small QRS with intraventricular block, and flattening or inversion of T waves)
- Neurologic: Small CNS lesions, ring calcifications; IV enhancement on CT scan
- Electromyography: Results resemble those of polymyositis and inflammatory myopathies.

Diagnostic Procedures/Other
- Skeletal muscle biopsy (especially deltoid or gastrocnemius muscle from the patient at least 17 days after infection):
  – Inflammatory cells surround encysted larvae in necrotic muscle fibers.
  – Granulomatous reaction present in nonskeletal muscle but not encysted larvae.
  – Usually unnecessary, negative result possible in infected patient due to sampling error
- Can test suspected meat if available

DIFFERENTIAL DIAGNOSIS
- Infection: Viral syndromes, parasitic, spirochete, gastroenteritis, influenza, sinusitis, typhoid fever, measles, scarlet fever, meningitis, rheumatic fever, encephalitis, encephalomyelitis, poliomyelitis, tetanus, schistosomiasis, hookworm, Strongyloides, or helminthic infection
- Miscellaneous: Fever of unknown origin, dermatomyositis, myocarditis, inflammatory bowel disease, angioneurotic edema, rheumatoid arthritis, glomerulonephritis, polyneuritis, eosinophilic leukemia, polyarteritis nodosa, nonabsorption syndromes

 ## TREATMENT

MEDICATION (DRUGS)
First Line
- Systemic corticosteroids for severe symptoms (not recommended as monotherapy, may prolong adult worm survival in intestines) *plus*
- Albendazole (Albenza)
  – 15 mg/kg/day divided b.i.d for 15 days
  – Max dose 800 mg/day
  – Teratogenic/embryotoxic in rats
  – Approved <2 years
- Mebendazole and albendazole are most efficacious during the enteral phase (active against intestinal worms, little effect on muscle-embedded larvae).

Second Line
Pyrantel pamoate (Antiminth):
- Used during pregnancy; not approved <2 years
- Effective only against adult worms, not encysted larvae

ADDITIONAL TREATMENT
General Measures
- Most patients recover without specific therapy.
- Symptomatic treatment: Acetaminophen or NSAIDs, bed rest

ISSUES FOR REFERRAL
Cardiac, neurologic, pulmonary complications

IN-PATIENT CONSIDERATIONS
Admission Criteria
Cardiac, neurologic, or pulmonary complications indicate more severe disease.

Discharge Criteria
Resolution of cardiac symptoms

 ## ONGOING CARE

FOLLOW-UP RECOMMENDATIONS
- Expect improvement over several weeks.
- At 3–4 weeks, retreatment may be indicated if symptoms persist or there are ova in the feces.

Patient Monitoring
Cardiopulmonary monitoring

DIET
- Avoid further exposures.
- Breast-feeding may continue; the single case report of cessation of milk production was associated with parenteral mebendazole.

PATIENT EDUCATION
If concern for trichinosis exposure or symptoms, seek medical care early. Treatment is most efficacious the 1st week after exposure.

PROGNOSIS
- Mild to moderate illness usually resolves spontaneously with minimal sequelae. Muscle swelling and weakness may persist.
- Poorer prognosis (can be fulminant and fatal) with cardiac, CNS, or pulmonary involvement.
- Children usually are less symptomatic, have fewer complications, and recover more quickly.

COMPLICATIONS
- Cardiac: Myocarditis (may result in death 4–8 weeks after infection), secondary arrhythmias, hypotension, pericardial effusion
- Neurologic: Meningoencephalitis, CNS granulomas, headaches
- Pulmonary: Pneumonia, pneumonitis, pleural effusion, pulmonary embolism or infarct
- Renal: Glomerulonephritis
- Hepatic: Fatty change
- Muscular: Prolonged myalgias
- Ocular: Retinal hemorrhages
- Complications rarely are permanent.

ADDITIONAL READING
- American Academy of Pediatrics. Trichinellosis. In: *Red Book: 2009 report of the Committee on Infectious Diseases*. 28th ed. Elk Grove Village, IL: Author; 2009:673–674.
- Bruschi F, Murrell KD. New aspects of human trichinellosis: The impact of new *Trichinella* species. *Postgrad Med J*. 2002;78:15–22.
- Centers for Disease Control and Prevention. Trichinellosis surveillance—United States, 1997–2001. *MMWR Surveill Summ*. 2003; 52(SS06):1–8.
- Ozdemir D, Ozkan H, Akkoc N, et al. Acute trichinellosis in children compared with adults. *Pediatr Infect Dis J*. 2005;24:897–900.
- Gottstein B, Pozio E, Nockler K. Epidemiology, diagnosis, treatment, and control of trichinellosis. *Clin Microbiol Rev*. 2009;22(1):127–145.

 ## CODES

ICD9
124 Trichinosis

ICD10
B75 Trichinellosis

CLINICAL PEARLS
Additional names: Trichinelliasis, trichinellosis

FAQ
- Q: How can I prevent infection?
- A: Be sure meat is fully cooked (internal temperature ≥160°F [71°C], not pink) or frozen (−20°F for 6 days, −10°F for 10 days, or −5°F for 20 days). *Trichinella* larvae in game may be relatively resistant to freezing. Frozen bear meat has yielded infective larvae after >2 years of freezing.
- Q: Is trichinosis contagious from person to person?
- A: No, except through infected breast milk.
- Q: Do special precautions need to be taken when treating a patient with presumed trichinosis?
- A: Only thorough hand washing. No isolation required.
- Q: What should we recommend for a patient who has eaten contaminated meat?
- A: Treatment with mebendazole or thiabendazole should be considered.
- Q: What are the classic hallmarks of trichinosis?
- A: Diarrhea, abdominal pain, periorbital edema, myositis, fever, and eosinophilia, especially when combined with history of ingestion of potentially poorly cooked meat.

TUBERCULOSIS

Andrew P. Steenhoff
Barbara M. Watson (5th edition)

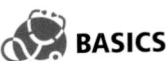 **BASICS**

DESCRIPTION

- Pediatric tuberculosis (TB) is the disease state caused by *Mycobacterium tuberculosis*, an acid-fast bacillus (AFB). Pediatric TB should be regarded as a spectrum of exposure through infection to disease because progression from an infected person (exposure) to infection and subsequently disease can occur much faster (within 3–6 months) in children <2 years of age (occurring within the incubation of the disease stated below).
- Progression through this spectrum depends on age; such disease progression being 40–50% for children up to 2 years old, ~20% for 2–4 year olds, and 10–15% for those ≥5 years old, the 5–10-year-old children being the most protected age group. Adolescence is another vulnerable age group.

EPIDEMIOLOGY

- The most common route of infection is via the respiratory tract. TB is spread from a person with disease by droplet nuclei that are inhaled by other people. A child becomes infected with TB after close and prolonged contact with an adult or adolescent who has active untreated infectious disease, usually pulmonary TB, in a poorly ventilated space. However, there are people who develop TB without knowledge of an infectious contact.
- Congenital infection occurs, although rarely, in the setting of an untreated mother in the last trimester of pregnancy.
- Infection with the tubercle bacillus needs to be differentiated from disease (i.e., TB).
- The interval between onset of infection and disease is 10–12 weeks.
- The greatest chance of disease occurring (i.e., of developing a positive result in tests using purified protein derivative [PPD], now renamed tuberculin skin test [TST]) is within the 1st 2 years after infection. However, for infants and children <5 years, progression through the spectrum of pediatric TB (exposure–infection–disease) is age dependent (see Description).
- Postpubertal adolescents and immunosuppressed people, including people with diabetes, with chronic renal failure, the malnourished, and those taking steroids for any reason have higher risks for progression of infection to disease.

GENERAL PREVENTION

- Prevention of disease by using isoniazid (isonicotinic acid hydrazide-INH), 10 mg/kg/day PO for 9 months, or if compliance is not anticipated, 2 times a week as direct observed therapy at 20 mg/kg, with a maximum dose of 900 mg usually administered by a school nurse, child care worker, or the local TB control program, ideally without breaks in treatment, although the patient has 12 months to complete the course. If a break occurs near the end of treatment, it need not be restarted, because such treatment is ~90% effective against development of active TB for 20 years in nonimmunosuppressed children. This recommendation prevents disease in the treated patient and, as a public health measure, interrupts transmission to contacts of that infected person with 90% efficacy.

- Other drugs for latent TB include 4 months of rifampicin if a child cannot tolerate INH, 4 months of INH and rifampin in case of granuloma or fibrosis consistent with latent tuberculosis infection (LTBI), and finally 6 months of INH by direct observed therapy is the last resort (for a total of 72 doses).
- Bacille Calmette-Guérin (BCG) vaccine is recommended only for infants and children who test negative to PPD and who are continually exposed to contagious adults or to adults with TB that is resistant to both INH and rifampin, and who cannot be kept away from the contagious adult.

COMMONLY ASSOCIATED CONDITIONS

- HIV infection: Factor in the increase in TB, because 1 in 240 US residents is infected with HIV, and the bacillus grows stronger and evades detection (chest radiographs may appear normal).
- Lymphoma
- Diabetes
- Chronic renal failure
- Malnutrition
- Immunosuppression, including chronic daily steroid use, high-dose steroid use or tumor necrosis factor-α (TNF-α) agonists, cancer chemotherapy
- Social issues: Incarcerated adolescents, infants and children in homeless shelters

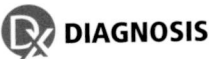 **DIAGNOSIS**

HISTORY

- Exposure: Family member with TB or positive skin test
- Migrant farm workers
- Immigration from a TB-endemic geographic area (e.g., Haiti, Southeast Asia, Africa, South and Central America, Russia, and elsewhere in Eastern Europe, where greater concern about drug-resistant strains ought to be exercised); visit by individuals from those countries; or visited the above countries
- Higher incidence in Native Americans
- Contact with adults who have active TB
- HIV-positive people
- Immunosuppressed state
- Incarcerated adolescents and their relatives who visit
- Homeless people
- Poor people in urban areas
- Exposure to milk from untested herds
- Malnutrition
- Long-term steroid usage

PHYSICAL EXAM

- Cervical and/or axillary adenopathy
- May reflect underlying disease or state (e.g., HIV, malnutrition, long-term steroid use)
- Pulmonary rales or clear chest
- Enlarged liver or spleen
- Site specific findings (e.g., gibbus [vertebral TB]) or focal neurologic signs (TB meningitis)

- Signs and symptoms:
  - Failure to thrive
  - Cervical or axillary lymphadenopathy without any other cause or that is prolonged
  - Cough >2 weeks
  - Weight loss
  - Change in sensorium
  - Fever in infants and adolescents, rarely in children 5–10 years of age
  - Decreased energy levels/playfulness >2 weeks

DIAGNOSTIC TESTS & INTERPRETATION
Lab

- Culture sputum, 3 gastric washings (early morning) performed with tube down over night, pleural fluid, CSF, urine
- Culture may take 2–3 weeks by the radiometric method.
- Positive culture results are found in <50% of children.

Imaging

Chest radiographs may show hilar adenopathy with or without atelectasis. However, any infiltrate, pleural effusion in a child with a positive TST result, and a risk factor for TB should be considered a TB suspect until proven otherwise. Infiltrates from bacterial or viral pathogens generally clear within 6–8 weeks; TB infiltrates tend not to clear so rapidly.

Diagnostic Procedures/Other

- Skin testing: TST
  - The Mantoux test comprises 5 tuberculin units with PPD administered intradermally. Details may be found at http://www.cdc.gov/tb.
  - The US Centers for Disease Control and Prevention does not recommend routine skin testing in low-risk groups in communities with low prevalence of TB.
  - Children at high risk should be tested annually:
    ○ Those in contact with adults from regions of the world with high TB prevalence
    ○ Children who spend time in homeless shelters
  - Those in contact with adults with TB, HIV, and other disease-producing immunosuppressed states: A skin test result may become positive 3–6 weeks after exposure; however, most commonly, it does not turn positive for 3 months—hence the rationale for treating an exposed child with INH and retesting with a PPD in 3 months.
  - A positive TST is a SENTINEL public health event indicating TB transmission in a community even if all other tests and examinations are negative.
  - A promising new molecular diagnostic test, Xpert MTB/RIF, is both simple and accurate. FDA approval is awaited.

DIFFERENTIAL DIAGNOSIS

- Malignancy
- Cervical or axillary adenopathy
- Pulmonary infiltrate: Other chronic organisms, disorders, and conditions (e.g., *Nocardia*, histoplasmosis). Infiltrates owing to bacterial or viral pathogens resolve faster than TB; thus, re-evaluation of a suspect in 8–12 weeks clarifies this differential.
- Hilar adenopathy: In TB it is usually unilateral, but Epstein-Barr virus, adenovirus, pertussis, and malignancy may possibly mimic symptoms.
- Miliary disease: Pulmonary effects, hepatosplenomegaly with or without CNS involvement
- GI disease: Most common differential diagnosis is Crohn disease.
- Meningitis: Fungal meningitis, partially treated bacterial meningitis (rarely)

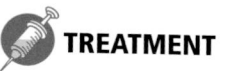 TREATMENT

MEDICATION (DRUGS)

- Initial treatment in areas with multidrug-resistant TB >4%: Until sensitivities are known, a 4-drug regimen should be started: INH, 10–15 mg/kg/day; rifampin, 10–20 mg/kg/day; pyrazinamide (PZA), 15–30 mg/kg/day; and either ethambutol, 15–20 mg/kg/day, or streptomycin, 20 mg/kg/day (depending on whether diagnosis is meningitis or miliary TB, for which a bactericide is desired); however, many cases in children of foreign-born parents are increasingly streptomycin resistant, making ethambutol a better choice.
- If the organism is sensitive to therapy, treatment with the initial 4 primary drugs should continue for the 1st 2 months; by then, all sputum specimens should have a negative result on culture, followed by 4 months of INH and rifampin. When this regimen is adhered to, prognosis and a complete cure are achieved in 97–98% of patients.
- If a cavity is seen in chest radiograph or sputum specimens continue to test positive, or the TB is miliary, disseminated, or meningeal, the duration of treatment needs to be longer (9–12 months).

ADDITIONAL TREATMENT
General Measures

- Hospitalization (if the patient has disease):
  - In cases of extensive disease (e.g., miliary TB or meningitis), and when an adult source case is not known, aggressive attempts should be made to obtain an organism from gastric aspirates, sputum induction, bronchoalveolar lavage, CSF, pleural or joint aspirate, bone aspirate, liver or tissue biopsy, and, in some cases, blood cultures.
- Isolation policies:
  - Unless the clinician can verify that the parent or any adult visitors are not themselves contagious, many infection control units require isolation of the child because the family members' state of contagion remains unknown at admission.
  - Nonpulmonary TB (e.g., GI TB, meningitis, bone TB, and TB with joint involvement) also does not require isolation.
  - Children >8 years of age and adolescents should be isolated until they have completed 10 days of therapy. Occasionally, immunocompromised children <8 years old also have cavitary disease and hence they too should be isolated.

 ONGOING CARE

FOLLOW-UP RECOMMENDATIONS
Patient Monitoring
Follow-up and contact tracing are key to making TB preventable.

PROGNOSIS
- Mortality for untreated TB is 40% over 4 years.
- For miliary TB and meningeal TB, prognosis depends on the stage of presentation as already discussed.
- For outbreaks of multidrug-resistant TB, death rates range from 70–90% within 4 months of diagnosis.

COMPLICATIONS
- Missed diagnosis: Failure to consider TB in a child who is failing to thrive and whose TST is negative
- TB meningitis: Outcome depends on the stage at which anti-TB medication starts:
  - If pharmacotherapy is started at stage I, complete recovery occurs in 94%, with neurologic sequelae in 6%.
  - If delayed until stage II, complete recovery occurs in 51%, with neurologic sequelae in 40% and death in 7%.
  - If delayed until stage III, complete recovery occurs in 18%, with neurologic sequelae in 61% and death in 20%.
- Miliary TB
- Bone TB: Most commonly spinal manifestation
- Renal TB: Presents as a fever of undetermined origin (FUO), with or without urinary symptoms
- Congenital TB manifests with hepatosplenomegaly; may have CSF abnormalities and abnormalities on CSF testing and chest radiograph: Patients too young for TST to be useful
- Drug toxicity: Pediatric patients are much more tolerant of anti-TB medications than adults; thus, regular monitoring of liver function test results is not routinely required, although clinical monitoring for symptoms such as abdominal pain and loss of appetite on a monthly basis remains the cornerstone for identifying any toxicity.
- Hepatitis with INH, rifampin, and PZA; neurologic and hematologic complications with INH; skin rashes predominantly with rifampin and INH, but reports have occurred with all anti-TB medications; ototoxicity with streptomycin; but ocular toxicity with ethambutol in the pediatric age group has not been documented, and therefore it is a safe drug to use. Management of common side effects and drug interactions may be found in the 2006 American Thoracic Society/US Centers for Disease Control and Prevention/Infectious Disease Society of America (see Additional Reading).

ADDITIONAL READING

- American Thoracic Society/US Centers for Disease Control and Prevention/Infectious Disease Society of America. Treatment of tuberculosis recommendations. *Am J Respir Crit Care Med*. 2006;147: 935–952.
- Boehme CC, Nabeta P, Hillemann D, et al. Rapid molecular detection of tuberculosis and rifampin resistance. *N Engl J Med*. 2010;363:1005–1015.
- Heymann SJ, Brewer TF, Wilson ME, et al. Pediatric tuberculosis: What needs to be done to decrease morbidity and mortality. *Pediatrics*. 2000;106:E1.
- MMWR trends in TB 2004. Global incidence of multidrug-resistant tuberculosis. *MMWR Recomm Rep*. 2004;53(10):1–24.
- National Tuberculosis Controllers Association; Centers for Disease Control and Prevention (CDC). Guidelines for the investigation of contacts of persons with infectious tuberculosis: Recommendations from the National Tuberculosis Controllers Association and CDC. *MMWR Recomm Rep*. 2005;54(RR-15):49–55.
- Newton SM, Brent AJ, Anderson S, et al. Paediatric tuberculosis. *Lancet Infect Dis*. 2008;8(8):498–510.
- Targeted tuberculin testing and treatment of latent tuberculosis infection. American Thoracic Society. *MMWR Recomm Rep*. 2000;49(RR-6):1–51.

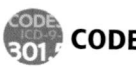 CODES

ICD9
- 011.90 Pulmonary tuberculosis, unspecified, unspecified
- 771.2 Other congenital infections specific to the perinatal period

ICD10
- A15.9 Respiratory tuberculosis unspecified
- P37.0 Congenital tuberculosis

FAQ

- Q: Should all children in close proximity to inner-city areas with a prevalence of TB be screened annually with PPD?
- A: The AAP and CDC encourage targeted screening based on risk factors indicated above. The targeted screening questionnaire should be administered at every visit until age 2 years, then annually thereafter. See tools at http://www.cdc.gov/tb.
- Q: Can we use the whole blood assay "QuantiFERON-TB Gold" to differentiate children who were born in other countries and had BCG instead of the TST (parents are requesting the test)?
- A: The test is not licensed for pediatric use and hence cannot be interpreted. A large study in navy recruits in 2006 demonstrated in foreign-born individuals with a TST >20 that the QuantiFERON-TB Gold Test was equivalent.

T

TUBEROUS SCLEROSIS COMPLEX

Garrick A. Applebee

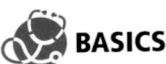 **BASICS**

DESCRIPTION
- Tuberous sclerosis complex (TSC) is a neurocutaneous syndrome characterized by a spectrum of signs and symptoms that present over a patient's lifetime, including neurologic disorders, multisystem tumor growth, and dermatologic manifestations.
- First described by Bourneville in 1880, the classic diagnostic triad of adenoma sebaceum, mental retardation, and seizures has been revised to include other manifestations because many patients with tuberous sclerosis do not exhibit this triad.

EPIDEMIOLOGY
Incidence
Current estimates suggest an incidence of 1 in 5,000 to 1 in 15,000 births. ~60–70% of cases reflect sporadic mutation; 30–40% of cases are familial.

RISK FACTORS
Genetics
- 2 clearly identified loci for familial and sporadic cases based on linkage analyses are 9q34 and 16p13, corresponding to TSC1 and TSC2 genes, respectively. TSC1 encodes the protein hamartin and TSC2 encodes the protein tuberin. Together, hamartin and tuberin join to form a regulatory complex of mTOR (the serine kinase mammalian target of rapamycin). Permanent activation of mTOR through mutations in the genes coding for these proteins causes dysregulation of cellular growth, differentiation, and migration, leading to the clinical symptoms and multisystem cellular overgrowth seen in TSC.
- >1,000 mutations in these genes are known to exist, leading to highly variable phenotypes in this disorder.
- TSC2 mutations: More common in sporadic cases, associated with more severe phenotypes
- 15–20% of cases meeting clinical criteria have no identifiable gene mutations.

ETIOLOGY
Tuberous sclerosis either is inherited in an autosomal-dominant pattern or results from a spontaneous/sporadic mutation.

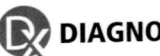 **DIAGNOSIS**

HISTORY
- Primary symptoms include seizures, mental defects, and skin lesions.
- All types of seizures are seen in TSC. Seizures may begin at any time and are present in 70–80% of patients. In infancy, infantile spasms are a common presenting seizure; 1/3 of patients develop infantile spasms.
- Mental retardation and neurobehavioral abnormalities (e.g., autism spectrum disorders, present in 25% of patients) may manifest as developmental delay, but some patients are without cognitive defect.
- Skin lesions may appear in infancy or during early childhood.
- It is important to take a full family history, reviewing involved systems.
- Inquire about history of seizures, mental retardation, skin lesions, and cardiac or renal disease/cancers.
- Screening for symptoms of hydrocephalus (headache, vomiting) is important: 10% of patients develop CSF obstruction from subependymal giant cell tumors.
- Women are primarily affected by pulmonary lymphangiomyomatosis, which may manifest as dyspnea or pneumothorax in early adulthood.

PHYSICAL EXAM
- Maintain a high level of suspicion for tuberous sclerosis in any patient presenting with:
  - Infantile spasms or childhood seizures
  - Autism
  - Intellectual impairment/developmental delay
  - Peculiar skin lesions
  - Ash leaf and café au lait spots are small (often <5 mm) but may be found anywhere on skin and are often present at birth. Examination with a Wood's lamp may help to identify hypopigmented lesions (e.g., ash leaf spots).
- Facial angiofibromas are typically found around the nose and cheeks and look like acne; they develop in later childhood to adolescence. They neither itch nor suppurate.
- Ungual fibromas appear around the nail bed.
- Shagreen patches are brownish leathery skin patches near the sacrum.

- Funduscopic examination may reveal whitish-yellow areas in epipapillary and peripapillary regions around the optic nerve head. They rarely impair vision. Papilledema may be seen with hydrocephalus.
- Signs of heart failure or tachyarrhythmia may be seen in infants with cardiac tumors.
- Flank pain, nausea, vomiting, and hematuria may suggest renal involvement.
- Procedures: Dilated funduscopic examination may also aid in full visualization of the optic nerve head.
- Definite diagnosis requires 2 major or 1 major plus 2 minor features:
  - Major criteria: Facial angiofibroma, ungual fibroma, shagreen patch, hypomelanotic papule (ash leaf spot), cortical tuber, subependymal giant cell tumor, retinal hamartoma, cardiac rhabdomyoma, renal angiomyolipoma, lymphangiomyomatosis
  - Minor criteria: Pitting in tooth enamel, hamartomatous rectal polyps, bone cysts, cerebral white matter radial migration lines, gingival fibromas, retinal achromic patch, "confetti" skin lesions (grouped lightly pigmented spots), multiple renal cysts
- As with other dominant, multisystem conditions, the findings in TSC have variable penetrance, and clinical manifestations may appear at different developmental points.
- Although seizures and mental retardation are common in TSC, they vary, are nonspecific, and so are not considered in the diagnostic criteria.

DIAGNOSTIC TESTS & INTERPRETATION
Lab
- Blood and CSF lab test results are typically normal unless renal function is significantly compromised by renal cysts or renal angiomyolipomas.
- ECG may reveal cardiac dysrhythmias, present in 47% of persons with cardiac rhabdomyomas.
- In patients with mental retardation or seizures, EEG helps to evaluate cerebral activity.
- In infants with suggestive history, an EEG may help diagnose infantile spasms, which are associated electrographically with a highly disorganized pattern of large-amplitude, asynchronous, sharp waves termed *hypsarrhythmia*.

- Later in childhood, patients with tuberous sclerosis may develop Lennox-Gastaut syndrome, which consists of mental retardation, seizures, and a characteristic EEG pattern of slow (i.e., 2.5 Hz) spike-wave complexes.

Imaging

- Subependymal or other cerebral calcifications on CT, often found in the course of emergent evaluation of new seizures, suggest TSC—consider MRI.
- Guidelines suggest MRI of the brain with gadolinium administration yearly or in alternate years until age 21 years and every 2–3 years thereafter. Imaging will identify tubers, subependymal nodules, hydrocephalus, and giant cell tumors. These appear hyperintense on T-weighted images and may enhance with gadolinium.
- Echocardiogram can detect cardiac rhabdomyomas in infants with tuberous sclerosis; prenatal ultrasound commonly identifies these tumors.
- CT of the lungs is indicated in women with TSC to screen for lymphangiomyomatosis.
- Renal ultrasound (every 1–2 years) or CT will demonstrate renal lesions.

Pathological Findings

Findings reflect the primary tissue in which lesions are identified:

- Brain:
  - 3 characteristic lesions are cortical tubers, subependymal nodules, and subependymal giant cell tumors.
  - In tubers, the cerebral cortical architecture is disrupted, and these regions may undergo calcification, which can be visible on skull radiographs or brain CT.
  - Subependymal nodules consist of large abnormal astrocytes emanating from the lateral ventricular surface.
  - Subependymal giant cell tumors are low-grade benign astrocytic neoplasms.
- Skin:
  - Facial angiofibromas may be mistaken for acne and are highly suggestive of tuberous sclerosis; they appear as pinkish-yellow plaques on the malar regions and nasolabial folds.
  - Ash leaf spots are hypopigmented hypomelanotic macules occurring anywhere on the body.

  - Ungual fibromas are fleshy growths along the lateral borders of the nail bed.
  - Shagreen patches are areas of shaggy leathery skin typically in the lumbosacral area.
- Retina:
  - Whitish-yellow angiomyolipomas or hamartomas occur near the optic nerve head or the retinal periphery and may calcify.
- Heart:
  - Rhabdomyomas in the ventricular wall occur in infancy and contain abundant nodules of large eosinophilic cells; this is the most common type of cardiac tumor of infancy and early childhood and may also occur in the absence of TSC.
- Kidney:
  - Renal cysts, polycystic kidneys, angiomyolipomas, and, more rarely, renal carcinomas
- Other organ systems:
  - Less commonly affected are the lungs, GI tract, spleen, vascular bed, and lymphatic system.

DIFFERENTIAL DIAGNOSIS

Neurocutaneous syndromes in which skin lesions, mental retardation, and seizures are characteristic features should be considered:

- Neurofibromatosis
- Sturge-Weber syndrome
- von Hippel–Lindau disease
- Neurocutaneous melanosis
- Albright syndrome
- Incontinentia pigmenti
- Linear sebaceous nevus

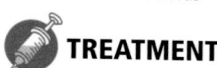 **TREATMENT**

MEDICATION (DRUGS)

- Rapamycin is an immunosuppressant agent that inhibits mTOR, thereby inhibiting the cellular proliferation seen in tuberous sclerosis patients. Its use in targeting a number of tuberous sclerosis complications is in development.
- Anticonvulsant therapy as needed. Infantile spasms may be treated with adrenocorticotropic hormone or vigabatrin (not available in the US)
- Medical management of heart failure or cardiac dysrhythmias is indicated in tuberous sclerosis patients with cardiac rhabdomyomas.

 ONGOING CARE

PROGNOSIS

Cognitive disability unfortunately will not improve unless the cognitive impairment results from uncontrolled seizures. Seizure control is medically refractory in up to 40% of cases, and some children require epilepsy surgery to remove cortical tubers or subependymal nodules. Cardiac tumors may also require surgical intervention. Renal angiomyolipomas can be embolized angiographically or surgically corrected. Subependymal giant cell astrocytomas that cause hydrocephalus may require resection.

ADDITIONAL READING

- Crino PB, Nathanson KL, Henske EP. The tuberous sclerosis complex. *New Engl J Med.* 2006; 355(13):1345–1356.
- Curatolo P, Bombardieri R, Cerminara C. Current management for epilepsy in tuberous sclerosis complex. *Curr Opin Neurol.* 2006;19:119–123.
- Au KS, Ward CH, Northrup H. Tuberous sclerosis complex: Disease modifiers and treatments. *Curr Opin Pediatr.* 2008;20(6):628–633.
- Franz DN. Tuberous sclerosis complex: Neurological, renal and pulmonary manifestations. *Neuropediatrics.* 2010;41(5):199–208.
- Crino PB. The pathophysiology of tuberous sclerosis complex. *Epilepsia.* 2010;51(Suppl 1):27–29.

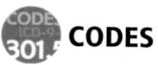 **CODES**

ICD9
759.5 Tuberous sclerosis

ICD10
Q85.1 Tuberous sclerosis

FAQ

- Q: Can tuberous sclerosis be transmitted in subsequent pregnancies?
- A: An affected patient with the tuberous sclerosis gene mutation has a 50% chance of transmitting the mutation to his or her children.
- Q: Is genetic testing available?
- A: Molecular genetic testing for mutations at the TSC1 and TSC2 loci are available but are not required for diagnosis because not all clinical cases of TSC have identifiable mutations.
- Q: Will my child need brain surgery?
- A: In the event of refractory seizures, removal of cortical tubers may help seizure control. Surgery may also be indicated in cases of obstructive hydrocephalus. If a brain tumor is detected by MRI, neurosurgical evaluation is indicated.

TULAREMIA

Brian T. Fisher
Louis M. Bell Jr. (5th edition)

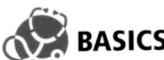 **BASICS**

DESCRIPTION

Tularemia is an infection caused by *Francisella tularensis*, a small, fastidious, nonmotile, gram-negative coccobacillus that requires cysteine-enriched agar for growth; 4 subspecies have been described:

- *Tularensis* (type A): Found primarily in North America; causes the most severe cases of tularemia in humans
- *Holarctica* (type B): Most widespread subspecies found in North America, Europe, and Asia; less virulent than *tularensis*
- *Novicida*: Found primarily in North America, but recent case report from Australia; does not require cysteine for growth; low virulence with occasional human infection
- *Mediasiatica*: Recovered from ticks and animals in Central Asia; not associated with disease in immunocompetent humans
- An additional species, *Francisella philomiragia*, has also been reported. This is a rare cause of human disease and is possibly associated with salt water exposure.
- Tularemia typically presents with fever, myalgias, and headache 3–6 days after initial exposure. The extent of the illness depends on infecting dose, subspecies, and route of entry.
- 4 clinical forms are typically described:
  - Ulceroglandular tularemia constitutes 75% of all cases. A papule, which ruptures and ulcerates, occurs at the site of entry. Regional lymphadenopathy and sometimes pharyngitis accompanies systemic symptoms of fever, myalgias, and headache. Bacteria may disseminate to end organ sites such as the spleen, liver, lungs, kidneys, and intestines:
    ○ Glandular tularemia is identical to the ulceroglandular form but without an identified primary skin lesion.
    ○ Oculoglandular tularemia occurs when the organism gains access via the conjunctival sac, usually from the patient rubbing the eyes with contaminated fingers. Yellow nodules and ulcers may appear on the palpebral conjunctiva associated with enlarged preauricular nodes.
  - Typhoidal tularemia presents with fever of unknown origin, without localizing lymphadenopathy or skin findings. Shock, pleuropulmonary findings, odynophagia, diarrhea, and bowel necrosis are often associated.

- Oropharyngeal tularemia occurs after the ingestion of contaminated food or water. An ulcerative or membranous tonsillitis accompanies a painful sore throat. Lower GI tract involvement with vomiting, diarrhea, and abdominal pain may be associated.
- Pneumonic tularemia occurs after inhalation of the organism. It can also be present in association with ulceroglandular and typhoidal tularemia. Pulmonary tularemia is the most fulminant and lethal form. Symptoms include fever, dry cough, and pleuritic chest pain. Tularemia in this form is a feared potential biological weapon because an exposure to only 1–10 colony-forming units can result in infection.

ALERT

- *F. tularensis* is currently listed as a class A bioterrorism agent because of its potential ease for dissemination and infection as well as potential for high case fatality rates.
- In the past, resistant forms of *F. tularensis* have been engineered, but the actual use of this organism as a bioterrorism agent has not been documented.
- The diagnosis of inhalation tularemia should raise the suspicion of bioterrorism.

EPIDEMIOLOGY

- *F. tularensis* is found primarily in the northern hemisphere from the 30–70° latitudes. A case of tularemia caused by subspecies *novicida* has been reported from Australia.
- Wild mammals (e.g., rabbits, hares, squirrels, beavers, deer, and rodents) may be infected, as well as invertebrates (e.g., ticks, deerflies, horseflies, and mosquitoes).
- Humans acquire tularemia after a bite by an infected arthropod or through contact with tissues or body fluids of an infected animal. The subspecies *holarctica* has been shown to persist in various water sources, and water-borne transmission to humans has been reported.
- Inhalational exposure can happen in the laboratory setting or after the organism is aerosolized during meat preparation.
- Most commonly reported during the summer months in children between 5 and 9 years of age and those >75 years old

RISK FACTORS

- Most frequently infected groups include hunters, trappers, farmers, and veterinarians.
- Activities involving wild animals or exposure to various arthropod vectors.
- Infection has been linked to landscapers using lawn mowers and brush cutters.
- Laboratory personnel working with samples known to be or potentially infected with Francisella.

GENERAL PREVENTION

- Isolation of the hospitalized patient:
  - Standard precautions are recommended for protection against secretions. Human-to-human transmission has not been reported.
- Control measures:
  - Protective clothing and insect repellent should be used to minimize insect bites.
  - Inspection for ticks and their immediate removal should be routine after outdoor activity in endemic areas.
  - Rubber gloves should be worn while handling or cooking wild animals (e.g., rabbits, lemmings) possibly contaminated with Francisella.
  - Laboratory workers should wear rubber gloves and masks in a biosafety level 3 environment when working with specimens potentially containing Francisella.

PATHOPHYSIOLOGY

- Entry into the human is via skin, mucous membranes, or inhalational.
- A primary lesion develops at the site of exposure.
- Local tender lymph node swelling ensues.
- After skin inoculation or inhalation, the organism can spread via the bloodstream to various organs.

ETIOLOGY

Human infection can result from various modes of entry:

- Skin contact with infected animals
- Vector-borne infection described after the bite of a tick, mosquito, horsefly, or deerfly
- Inhalation of aerosolized organism seen in laboratory workers, crop harvesting, disturbance of contaminated hay, and grass cutting.
- Ingestion of contaminated food products or water

DIAGNOSIS

HISTORY

- In the right clinical setting, a history that elicits any occupational exposure or recreational activity previously noted as risk factors should raise suspicion for tularemia.
- History of a recent tick, mosquito, or fly bite may be recalled among affected patients.
- A history of a papule that became ulcerated is classic for the ulceroglandular form.
- Fever >101°F for 2–3 weeks is common, with associated weight loss.

PHYSICAL EXAM

- A papule or ulcer may be seen at the inoculation site.
- Skin lesions should be sought, especially when lymphadenopathy is present.
- Lymph node swelling is typically tender with overlying erythema.
- After a 3–6-day incubation period, symptoms may include fever, myalgias, and headache.
- Hepatosplenomegaly, purulent conjunctivitis, adenopathy, an ulcerative skin lesion, and tonsillitis are other localized findings.

DIAGNOSTIC TESTS & INTERPRETATION
Lab

- Serum tube agglutination titers of 1:160 or greater are generally considered positive.
- A 4-fold rise in titers over a 2-week period is necessary to define a current infection.
- Cultures of blood, skin, ulcers, lymph nodes, gastric washings, and respiratory secretions require special media containing cysteine.
- Laboratory personnel should be made aware of the infection risk from specimens. Growth of the organism requires a biosafety level 3 laboratory.
- Polymerase chain reaction (PCR) tests are available in some laboratories. They are more sensitive than culture and can be performed on tissue samples. Current PCR techniques do not differentiate subspecies, but such techniques are under development.
- Fluorescent in situ hybridization techniques have been utilized in the research setting to differentiate subspecies and may be clinically useful in the future.

DIFFERENTIAL DIAGNOSIS

Depending on the form of tularemia, the infection can mimic other illnesses such as streptococcal or staphylococcal infection, mononucleosis, cutaneous anthrax, pasteurellosis, Q fever, legionellosis, typhoid fever, or mycobacterial disease. In general, tularemia should be considered in the following differential diagnoses:

- Fever of unknown origin
- Fever with purulent conjunctivitis
- Fever with hepatosplenomegaly
- Fever with skin ulcer

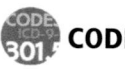 **TREATMENT**

MEDICATION (DRUGS)

- IV antibiotic therapy with streptomycin or gentamicin is considered 1st-line therapy.
- 2nd-line therapeutic options include ciprofloxacin, doxycycline, or chloramphenicol. Relapses have been associated with the latter two.
- Duration of treatment is typically 7–10 days. In severe disease, some experts recommend gentamicin in combination with ciprofloxacin.
- Vaccine:
  - A live attenuated vaccine has been in existence since the 1940s.
  - It is moderately effective against severe forms of tularemia.
  - Currently in the US, the vaccine is reserved for at-risk personnel.
  - Significant research into various vaccine techniques continues to evolve given concerns of *F. tularemia* as an agent of bioterrorism.

IN-PATIENT CONSIDERATIONS
Initial Stabilization

- If respiratory compromise is present, oxygen supplementation and/or assisted ventilation must be rapidly addressed.
- Recognition and prompt aggressive treatment of shock should be a major priority.

 ONGOING CARE

PROGNOSIS

When recognized and treated with appropriate antibiotics, the course is generally <1 month. Mortality is low, except in cases of fulminant disease or are otherwise immunocompromised. The subspecies *tularensis* is thought to be more virulent than the others. Both typhoidal and pneumonic tularemia are associated with the highest risk for mortality.

COMPLICATIONS

- Lymph node suppuration, meningitis, endocarditis, hepatitis, and renal failure have all been associated with tularemia.
- Infection with *F. tularensis* may be complicated by necrotic and granulomatous lesions in the liver and spleen as well as parenchymal degeneration.
- A sepsis syndrome with shock, fever, myalgias, and severe headache can be seen. Recognition and prompt aggressive treatment of shock should be a major priority.
- Skin manifestations, including vesiculopapular rash, erythema nodosum, and erythema multiforme have been associated with tularemia.

ADDITIONAL READING

- Barry EM, Cole LE, Santiago AE. Vaccines against tularemia. *Hum Vacc.* 2009;5:832–838.
- Cross JT, Schutze GE, Jacobs RF. Treatment of tularemia with gentamicin in pediatric patients. *Pediatr Infect Dis J.* 1995;14:152–151.
- Dennis DT, Inglesby TV, Henderson DA, et al. Tularemia as a biological weapon: Medical and public health management. *JAMA.* 2001;285: 2763–2773.
- Eliasson H, Broman T, Forsman M, et al. Tularemia: Current epidemiology and disease management. *Infect Dis Clin N Am.* 2006;20:289–311.
- Nigrovic LE, Wingerter SL. Tularemia. *Infect Dis Clin North Am.* 2008;22:489–504.
- Tarnvik A, Chu MC. New approaches to diagnosis and therapy of tularemia. *Ann N Y Acad Sci.* 2007;1105:378–404.

CODES

ICD9
- 021.0 Ulceroglandular tularemia
- 021.8 Other specified tularemia
- 021.9 Unspecified tularemia

ICD10
- A21.0 Ulceroglandular tularemia
- A21.8 Other forms of tularemia
- A21.9 Tularemia, unspecified

T

ULCERATIVE COLITIS

Judith Kelsen
Jonathan Markowitz

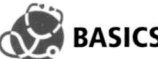 **BASICS**

DESCRIPTION
Ulcerative colitis (UC) is a disease characterized by remitting and relapsing inflammation of the large intestine. UC and Crohn disease (CD) are the disorders that represent the idiopathic inflammatory bowel diseases (IBDs). The hallmark symptoms of UC are abdominal cramping, diarrhea, and bloody stools. There are multiple patterns of presentation in children. UC routinely affects the rectum, with contiguous involvement extending proximally that can include the entire large intestine.

EPIDEMIOLOGY
- Yearly incidence is 2/100,000 in 10–19-year-olds
- 20–30% of patients with UC present before the age of 20 years.
- Incidence peaks between 15 and 30 years of age.
- Total prevalence is 50–75 per 100,000.

RISK FACTORS
Genetics
- HLA association: Bw52, DR2 (Japan); A2, Bw35, Bw40 (Ashkenazi Jews); A7, A11 (the Netherlands)
- Genome-wide association studies (GWAS) utilizing high-density SNP array technology has identified multiple loci associated with CD and UC.
- Recent study identified 5 new IBD susceptibility loci that are associated with early-onset disease.
- Higher concordance in monozygotic than in dizygotic twins
- Family history in ~15–20% of patients
- There is an increased incidence of family history in patients diagnosed prior to 20 years of age.

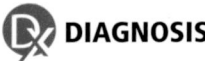 **DIAGNOSIS**

Patients with UC typically present with chronic symptoms of rectal bleeding, diarrhea, and abdominal pain that often occurs at the time of defecation. Rectal bleeding occurs in ~83–95% of patients with UC. Colonoscopy with histology is a gold standard in diagnosis of UC.

HISTORY
A detailed history is important in making the diagnosis:
- Rectal bleeding (90%)
- Abdominal pain (90%)
- Diarrhea (50%)
- Weight loss (10%)
- Growth failure
- Recent travel (enteric infections)
- Antibiotic use (*Clostridium difficile*)
- Family history of IBD
- Appendectomy is protective against developing UC.

PHYSICAL EXAM
- Fever
- Evidence of weight loss or poor growth
- Signs of anemia
- Uveitis
- Mouth sores
- Arthritis
- Abdominal tenderness or distention
- Perianal/Rectal examination (UC should not be associated with perianal disease.)

DIAGNOSTIC TESTS & INTERPRETATION
Lab
- CBC; anemia, iron deficiency
- Iron studies (iron deficiency)
- ESR, CRP; disease activity
- Electrolytes (hydration), CMP. Serum albumin may be low, hypoalbuminemia may be present in fulminant colitis.
- Hepatic function panel (hepatobiliary disease)
- Perinuclear antineutrophil cytoplasmic antibody (pANCA; positive in 80% of UC patients, 20% of CD patients)
- Stool for blood, white cells (colitis)
- Fecal calprotectin and fecal lactoferrin (FL): may be elevated during times of active inflammation.
- Stool cultures, *C. difficile* toxin A and B (infection)

Imaging
- Plain abdominal radiograph: This is important in diagnosing perforation, ileus, obstruction, and toxic megacolon. In toxic megacolon, the colon is dilated, and there are multiple air–fluid levels indicative of ileus. Serial x-rays are mandatory.
- Barium enema can demonstrate strictures and mucosal disease.
- An upper GI with small bowel follow-through (UGI/SBFT) can demonstrate the entire small bowel to exclude small intestinal disease indicative of CD.
- New imaging modalities, such as MR enterography, CT enterography, and ultrasound are currently being performed in place of UGI. MRI and US have the advantage of avoiding radiation exposure.
- MRI may have a role in differentiating transmural and mucosal inflammation and is also useful for demonstrating perianal fistulas that would indicate CD rather than UC.
- Ultrasound may be useful for evaluating associated hepatobiliary disease.
- Radionuclide imaging can differentiate between CD (small and large bowel involvement) and UC (only large bowel involvement).

Diagnostic Procedures/Other
- Colonoscopy (with biopsies) is a gold standard and is necessary to confirm the diagnosis of UC. It is critical to visualize the entire colon, including terminal ileum, to differentiate CD from UC.
- Upper endoscopy may increase chances of detecting CD.
- Endoscopic retrograde cholangiopancreatography (ERCP) is useful in diagnosing primary sclerosing cholangitis (3% of UC patients).

- Video capsule endoscopy (VCE) is more sensitive than UGI/SBFT for diagnosing small bowel disease indicative of CD rather than UC.
- Pitfalls:
  - The combination of positive pANCA and negative anti-*Saccharomyces cerevisiae* antibody (ASCA) has a reported sensitivity of 60–70% and a specificity of 95–97% for UC in adults. The sensitivity and specificity are poorer in pediatric patients.
  - Inflammation of the small intestine demonstrated by colonoscopy, VCE, UGI/SBFT, or radionuclide imaging is suggestive of CD, not UC.
  - Perianal disease (perianal skin tags, perianal fistulas, perianal abscess) is indicative of CD, not UC.
  - Infectious colitis (especially *C. difficile*) can mimic the findings of UC. *C. difficile* infection must be evaluated with assays for both toxin A and toxin B, or up to 40% of infections can be missed.
  - Toxic megacolon is a surgical emergency. The patient has a dilated colon with breakdown of its barrier to toxins entering the systemic circulation. Signs and symptoms include peritonitis, mental status changes, and fluid and electrolyte imbalance. Plain abdominal radiograph shows a segment or total colonic dilatation. Risk factors include 1st attack, pancolitis, concurrent use of opiates or anticholinergics, and recent barium enema or colonoscopy.

Pathological Findings
- Chronic or chronic active colitis, with inflammation limited to the mucosa
- Colitis: Crypt architectural distortion, cryptitis (aggregation of inflammatory cells in the crypt epithelium), crypt abscess
- Site of colon affected:
  - Rectum (virtually 100%)
  - Left side (50–60%)
  - Pancolitis (10%)
- Small intestine should not be involved, but occasionally the terminal ileum can show some inflammation on radiologic or histologic examination. This is thought to be from refluxed colonic contents (backwash ileitis).
- Skip lesions are not seen in UC.
- Chronic gastritis may be present in patients with UC.

DIFFERENTIAL DIAGNOSIS
- CD
- Infectious colitis: *Salmonella*, *Shigella*, *Campylobacter*, *Yersinia*, *Escherichia coli* (enterohemorrhagic), *Aeromonas*, amebiasis, *C. difficile*, cytomegalovirus
- STDs (herpes simplex, lymphogranuloma inguinale, chlamydia)
- Trauma due to anal sex or sexual abuse
- Congenital Hirschsprung enterocolitis
- Bleeding juvenile polyps
- Milk protein allergy
- Eosinophilic colitis
- Autoimmune enteropathy
- Irritable bowel syndrome (IBS)
- Appendicitis
- Hemolytic-uremic syndrome
- Henoch-Schönlein purpura

TREATMENT

MEDICATION (DRUGS)

- Mild disease can be treated with oral mesalamine, topical corticosteroid enema or foam, or mesalamine enema/suppositories.
- Moderate disease: Mesalamine, a short course of oral corticosteroid, low-residue diet
- Probiotics; may have important role in pouchitis
- Immunomodulators such as azathioprine and 6-mercaptopurine may help to maintain disease remission and minimize the need for recurrent courses of steroid. Methotrexate has fewer published data in UC but also may have efficacy.
- Infliximab: Monoclonal antibody against tumor necrosis factor (TNF)-α. It has become clinically important in the treatment of moderate to severe UC or steroid-resistant UC.
- Fulminant disease: Hospitalization, if concern for toxic megacolon—complete bowel rest with total parenteral nutrition, broad-spectrum antibiotics (IV ampicillin, gentamicin, and metronidazole), IV corticosteroids, serial abdominal radiographs, frequent examinations, stool chart (frequency, amount of blood, and volume of stool output); early surgical consult
- If treatment of acute symptoms with IV steroids fails (after 3–5 days), therapy with infliximab (usually given as a 5-mg/kg infusion) can be started. A 2nd dose is usually given ~2 weeks after the initial infusion.
- Pediatric Ulcerative Colitis Activity Index (PUCAI): Obtained on day 3–5; may identify patients with severe UC who will require escalation of therapy with infliximab or cyclosporine. Prevents unnecessary prolonged exposure to corticosteroids.
- IV cyclosporine infusion is an alternative to infliximab for treating fulminant colitis. Must be used with an immunomodulator and is nephrotoxic. Should be used by experienced clinicians. It is no longer 1st-line therapy due to adverse effects.
- Patients with fulminant disease who fail therapy with infliximab or cyclosporine should be referred for colectomy. Those with chronically active disease unresponsive to medication should also consider colectomy.
- Therapy of toxic megacolon is aimed at preventing perforation with decompression of the bowel. Management includes complete bowel rest, discontinuation of anticholinergics and narcotics, avoidance of endoscopy or barium enema, and broad-spectrum antibiotics; frequent examinations are required. Close communication with surgical colleagues is crucial.
- Methylprednisolone (IV): 1–2 mg/kg/day (equivalent to prednisone 60 mg maximum)
- Prednisone (PO): 1–2 mg/kg/day oral (up to maximum 60 mg/day)
- Mesalamine (PO): 40–60 mg/kg/day (maximum 4.8 g/day)
- Mesalamine (enema): 4 g at bedtime
- Mesalamine (suppository): 500 mg b.i.d.

- Hydrocortisone enema: 100 mg once a day to b.i.d.
- Hydrocortisone foam: 80 mg once a day to b.i.d.
- 6-mercaptopurine (6-MP) (PO): 1.0–1.5 mg/kg to start (keep absolute neutrophil count [ANC] >500)
- Azathioprine (PO): 2.0 mg/kg (keep ANC >500)
- Infliximab (IV): 2–3 mg/kg weeks 0, 2, 6, then every 8 weeks
- Cyclosporine (IV): 4 mg/kg/day for 2 weeks (therapeutic levels vary depending on the technique used in the laboratory)
- Cyclosporine (PO): 6–8 mg/kg/day for 6–8 months

SURGERY/OTHER PROCEDURES

- Urgently required for perforation, significant and persistent bleeding, toxic megacolon, and failure of medical treatment for fulminant colitis
- Can be electively performed for chronic incapacitating disease, growth failure, dysplastic changes in the colon, or long-standing disease (usually after 10 years)
- Because UC is limited to the colon, colectomy is considered a curative procedure.
- Ileoanal anastomosis and pouch construction is surgery of choice for most pediatric patients and usually is performed in 3 stages.

 ONGOING CARE

FOLLOW-UP RECOMMENDATIONS

Outpatient follow-up with a pediatric gastroenterologist should be arranged. Important parameters to follow as an outpatient include abdominal symptoms, stool frequency/consistency, height/weight, hemoglobin, WBC count (for patients on immunosuppressives), ESR, albumin, bilirubin and liver enzymes, fecal occult blood testing, and colonoscopic cancer screening (patients with long-standing disease). The PUCAI, a validated index for monitoring severe disease in pediatric patients.

COMPLICATIONS

- Bleeding
- Anemia
- Toxic megacolon
- Extraintestinal manifestations include hepatobiliary disease (3–5%), uveitis (up to 4%), arthritis affecting large joints (10%), spondylitis (6%), erythema nodosum (>5%), pyoderma gangrenosum (>1%), renal calculi (5%)
- Malignancy risk is 8% 10–25 years after colitis is diagnosed and it increases ~10% for every subsequent decade.
- Colonic stricture

ADDITIONAL READING

- Bousvaros A, Antonioli DA, Colletti RB, et al. Differentiating ulcerative colitis from Crohn disease in children and young adults: Report of a working group of the North American Society for Pediatric Gastroenterology, Hepatology, and Nutrition and the Crohn's and Colitis Foundation of America. *J Pediatr Gastroenterol Nutr*. 2007;44:653–674.
- Hyams JS, Lerer T, Griffiths A, et al. Outcome following infliximab therapy in children with ulcerative colitis. *Am J Gastroenterol*. 2010;105: 1430–1436.

- Loftus EV Jr. Epidemiology and risk factors for colorectal dysplasia and cancer in ulcerative colitis. *Gastroenterol Clin North Am*. 2006;35:517–531.
- Mallon P, McKay D, Kirk S, et al. Probiotics for induction of remission in ulcerative colitis. *Cochrane Database Syst Rev*. 2007;CD005573.
- Shikhare G, Kugathasan S. Inflammatory bowel disease in children: Current trends. *J Gastroenterol*. 2010;45:673–682.

CODES

ICD9
- 555.9 Regional enteritis of unspecified site
- 556.8 Other ulcerative colitis
- 556.9 Ulcerative colitis, unspecified

ICD10
- K51.90 Ulcerative colitis, unspecified, without complications
- K51.911 Ulcerative colitis, unspecified with rectal bleeding
- K51.912 Ulcerative colitis, unspecified with intestinal obstruction

FAQ

- Q: Will my child have this disease forever?
- A: Some people will have only the initial attack and then be symptom free, but usually an individual will have episodes of recurrences and remissions. Surgical removal of the colon represents a curative procedure, although some patients may develop inflammation in the pouch created out of the remaining bowel (pouchitis).
- Q: What is the cause of UC?
- A: Both genetic and environmental factors are important in the development of UC.
- Q: Where can I learn more about UC?
- A: The North American Society for Pediatric Gastroenterology, Hepatology and Nutrition provides a Web site for children with IBD and their families (www.gastrokids.org). The Crohn's and Colitis Foundation of America (www.CCFA.org) is a nonprofit organization dedicated to the care and education of people with CD and UC.
- Q: What new therapies will be used in the near future?
- A: Biologic agents, a broad category of therapies that uses our recently improved knowledge of the immune system, represent a new way of treating IBD, with several new treatments likely to be released within the next few years.

U

UPPER GASTROINTESTINAL BLEEDING

Maria R. Mascarenhas
Judith Kelsen

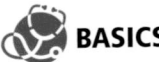

BASICS

DEFINITION
Vomiting of blood, whether bright red or dark, constitutes upper GI bleeding or hematemesis. This usually indicates bleeding from the GI tract proximal to the ligament of Treitz. The clinician must differentiate upper GI bleeding from hemoptysis (coughing up blood), nose bleeds, and bleeding from the mouth and pharynx. Sometimes, upper GI bleeding can present with melena or the passage of tarry stools.

GENERAL PREVENTION
- Avoid drugs that are likely to cause bleeding or gastritis, especially in a susceptible patient.
- In patients with chronic GI conditions, optimize therapy and monitoring.
- Correct coagulopathy
- Prophylactic sclerotherapy or banding is helpful for patients with known variceal bleeding.

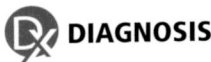

DIAGNOSIS

DIFFERENTIAL DIAGNOSIS
- 95% of the causes of upper GI bleeding are due to mucosal abnormalities or esophageal varices.
- Mucosal lesions are more likely to be associated with antecedent occult bleeding.
- In ~80–95% of patients, bleeding stops spontaneously.
- **Neonatal period**
  - Swallowed maternal blood
  - Necrotizing enterocolitis
  - Duodenal web, antral web
  - Hemorrhagic disease of the newborn
  - Esophagitis
  - Gastritis
  - Stress ulcer
  - Foreign body irritation
  - Vascular malformation
  - GI malformation
- **Infancy**
  - Esophagitis/gastritis
  - Stress ulcer
  - Mallory–Weiss tear
  - Pyloric stenosis
  - Vascular malformation
  - Duplication cysts
  - Metabolic disease
- **Preschool age**
  - Esophageal varices
  - Esophagitis/gastritis/ulcer
  - Foreign body/bezoar
  - Mallory–Weiss tear
  - Vascular malformation
  - Meckel diverticulum
- **School age**
  - Esophageal varices
  - Infection
  - Esophagitis/gastritis/ulcer
  - Mallory–Weiss tear
  - Inflammatory bowel disease
  - Drugs: NSAIDS, alpha-adrenergic antagonists
  - *Helicobacter pylori*
- All ages: Liver failure—coagulopathy, HSP

APPROACH TO THE PATIENT
Determine the cause of the bleeding and begin treatment. Place nasogastric (NG) tube and lavage contents of stomach to determine if bleeding is active and extent of bleeding.
- **Phase 1:** Determine whether the emesis contains blood; red food coloring, fruit-flavored drinks and juices, vegetables, and some medicines may resemble blood. A pH-buffered Gastroccult test identifies blood in the vomitus or gastric aspirate.
- **Phase 2:** Assess severity of bleeding. Is there a change in vital signs, hematocrit, BP, capillary filling, pulse?
- **Phase 3:** Determine the site of bleeding and begin treatment. Examine airway for bleeding: Epistaxis may contaminate emesis to make it resemble upper GI bleeding. Usually diagnosis requires imaging or endoscopy.

Hints for Screening Problems
- Bright red blood signifies active bleeding.
- Darker blood or coffee grounds blood usually means that the blood has had some time to become denatured by gastric acid.
- The rate of bleeding determines the clinical presentation. The more rapid the rate, the larger the volume of bleeding, leading to a greater drop in hemoglobin and change in pulse and BP. Slower bleeding usually presents with anemia and heme-positive stools.
- Any significant blood loss will lead to pallor, tachycardia, orthostasis, poor capillary refill, CNS changes (e.g., restlessness, confusion), and hypotension.
  - Hypotension is a late sign and may not be present even with significant blood loss because vasoconstriction maintains BP until decompensation occurs.
- Initial hemoglobin values may be unreliable because a delay in hemodilution may falsely produce near normal values.
- Absence of blood in the emesis or in NG lavage fluid does not rule out the upper GI tract as the site of bleeding, because a competent pylorus may mask bleeding from a duodenal site.
  - In some cases of massive upper GI bleeding, the patient may not vomit blood but may pass large, black, tarry, or sticky stools (e.g., melena).

HISTORY
- **Question:** Amount of blood (i.e., drops vs. 1 teaspoon vs. 1 tablespoon)?
- *Significance:* Indicates severity of bleeding
- **Question:** Presence of blood in emesis?
- *Significance:* Indicates bleeding from upper GI tract or swallowed blood. Vomitus may not have blood at all, but patient may have recently ingested foods that might resemble.
- **Question:** Source of bleeding?
- *Significance:* Hematemesis from the esophagus, stomach, or duodenum vs. hemoptysis vs. swallowed blood from the nose, mouth, or pharynx

- **Question:** Blood coughed?
- *Significance:* Indicative of hemoptysis
- **Question:** Bleeding from the nose?
- *Significance:* Swallowed and then vomited—did not originate in the upper GI tract
- **Question:** Prolonged retching before hematemesis?
- *Significance:* Suggests a Mallory–Weiss tear
- **Question:** Recent stress (e.g., burns, head trauma, surgery)?
- *Significance:* Suggests an ulcer or gastritis
- **Question:** Toxic ingestion?
- *Significance:* May result in an ulcerated esophagus, which can bleed. Ingestion of certain medications such as aspirin (as well as other anti-inflammatory drugs) and steroid therapy can lead to gastritis and ulcers. Ingestion of such drugs in combination with ethanol can lead to gastritis.
- **Question:** Abdominal pain and vomiting blood?
- *Significance:* Suggests esophagitis, gastritis, and peptic ulcers
- **Question:** Cracked nipples in a breastfeeding mother?
- *Significance:* May lead to the infant swallowing maternal blood and subsequent hematemesis
- **Question:** Gastroesophageal reflux?
- *Significance:* Suggests esophagitis
- **Question:** Past history of GI disease?
- *Significance:* Gastroesophageal reflux, peptic ulcer disease, or previous GI surgery may suggest symptoms are due to recurrence of disease.
- **Question:** Jaundice, hepatitis, or liver disease?
- *Significance:* Suggests portal hypertension and variceal bleeding
- **Question:** Neonatal history of umbilical vein catheterization or infection?
- *Significance:* Portal vein thrombosis (e.g., sepsis, shock, exchange transfusion, omphalitis, IV catheters) suggests portal hypertension and bleeding varices due to cavernous transformation of the portal vein.
- **Question:** Familial history of bleeding diathesis?
- *Significance:* Von Willebrand disease, hemophilia

PHYSICAL EXAM
- **Finding:** Any skin petechiae, ecchymosis, or hemangiomas?
- *Significance:* Evidence of chronic liver disease (e.g., spider angioma, palmar erythema, jaundice)
- **Finding:** Head, ears, eyes, nose, and throat—nasopharyngeal source of bleeding?
- *Significance:* Swallowed blood
- **Finding:** Freckles on buccal mucosa?
- *Significance:* Osler–Weber–Rendu syndrome, Peutz–Jeghers syndrome
- **Finding:** Oral thrush?
- *Significance:* Candidal esophagitis

- **Finding:** Oral mucosal lesions?
- *Significance:* Corrosive ingestions
- **Finding:** Abdomen?
- Significance:
  – Hepatosplenomegaly
  – Ascites
  – Portal hypertension
- **Finding:** Isolated splenomegaly?
- *Significance:* Cavernous transformation of the portal vein; portal hypertension
- **Finding:** Rectal examination—heme-positive stool may or may not be present?
- *Significance:* If positive, confirms the presence of upper GI bleeding.

DIAGNOSTIC TESTS & INTERPRETATION
Initial hemoglobin may not be accurate, and hemoglobin should be measured serially.

- **Test:** Gastroccult
- *Significance:* If possible, check the red substance for blood. In neonates, may need to check for fetal hemoglobin with the Apt test—a test to identify fetal hemoglobin.
- **Test:** CBC
- *Significance:* If leukopenia, anemia, or thrombocytopenia is present, consider chronic liver disease and portal hypertension. If anemia is present with normal erythrocyte indices, there is truly an acute cause for bleeding. If erythrocyte indices indicate iron-deficiency anemia, consider varices or a mucosal lesion (i.e., chronic blood loss).
- **Test:** Coagulation profile
- *Significance:* If PT or PTT is abnormal, consider liver disease or disseminated intravascular coagulation (DIC) with sepsis. If DIC screen is negative, consider liver disease. Make sure, however, that blood sample was not contaminated with heparin.
- **Test:** Bleeding time
- *Significance:* Abnormal in patients with previous history (or family history) of bleeding disorders
- **Test:** Liver function test results
- *Significance:* Abnormal in chronic liver disease
- **Test:** Upper endoscopy
- *Significance:* Diagnosis can be made in 75–90% of patients.
- **Test:** Capsule endoscopy
- *Significance:* May play a role in locating small bowel lesions
  – Sclerotherapy/banding, injection of ulcers, heated probes
  – Thermo-regulation, argon plasma coagulation

Imaging
- Barium tests:
  – Not as useful as esophagogastroduodenoscopy (EGD), but can identify a large ulcer. Air-contrast upper GI series is better than regular upper GI test.
- Bleeding scan:
  – Useful in the patient with significant bleeding in whom endoscopy undiagnostic. There are 2 types of scans: Technetium sulfur colloid and tagged erythrocyte. The former detects rapid bleeding, but can miss small bleeds, especially if patient is not bleeding during the scan. The latter can detect small bleeds, especially if intermittent.
  – Meckel scan: Can detect Meckel diverticulum as source of bleed
- Angiography:
  – Useful in detecting vascular causes of upper GI bleeding; can also be therapeutic (i.e., injection of coils into a vascular malformation may occlude it). Invasiveness and need for specialized training of clinicians are limitations.

 TREATMENT

ADDITIONAL TREATMENT
General Measures
Disease-specific therapy:
- Peptic ulcer disease:
  – Proton pump inhibitors
  – H2 blockers
  – Sucralfate
  – Prokinetic agents
  – *H. pylori* eradication
- Esophageal varices:
  – Vasopressin or somatostatin infusion
  – Sclerotherapy or banding
  – Sengstaken-Blakemore tube
  – Portosystemic shunts

Initial management of the emergency depends on diagnosis and clinical condition of the patient:
- Stabilize the patient with IV fluids and blood products if necessary
- Order laboratory tests: Complete blood chemistry, PT or PTT, EGD screen, liver function tests, blood type, and cross-match
- Insert an NG tube and lavage with saline to determine site as well as rate of ongoing bleeding. No need for cold saline.
- Monitor patient's vital signs and hemoglobin as necessary
- Make appropriate diagnosis and institute appropriate therapy (i.e., EGD, bleeding scans)

ISSUES FOR REFERRAL
Immediate referral if bleeding is profuse, if patient is hemodynamically unstable, or if bleeding will not stop. Refer any patient with evidence of chronic iron-deficiency anemia and heme-positive stools.

SURGERY/OTHER PROCEDURES
- Esophageal varices:
  – Sclerotherapy or banding
  – Sengstaken-Blakemore tube
  – Portosystemic shunts
- If bleeding stops quickly, workup is less emergent.

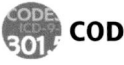 **ONGOING CARE**

- Monitor hemoglobin in the hospital until patient's condition is stable.
- Once patient is discharged, monitor patient's hemoglobin weekly as well as Hemoccult cards until stable.
- More specific follow-up depends on the underlying condition.

ADDITIONAL READING

- Chawla S, Seth D, Mahajan P, et al. Upper gastrointestinal bleeding in children. *Clin Pediatr (Phila)*. 2007;46(1):16–21.
- Fox VL. Gastrointestinal bleeding in infancy and childhood. *Gastroenterol Clin North Am*. 2000; 29:37–66.
- Jensen MK. Capsule endoscopy performed across the pediatric age range: Indications, incomplete studies, and utility in management of inflammatory bowel disease. *Gastrointest Endosc*. 2010;72(1):95–102.
- Kato S, Sherman P. What is new related to Helicobacter pylori infection in children and teenager? *Arch Pediatric Adolsc Med*. 2005;159(5): 415–421.
- Molleston JP. Variceal bleeding in children. *J Pediatr Gastroenterol Nutr*. 2003;37:538–545.
- Uppal K, Tubbs RS, Matusz P, et al. Meckel's diverticulum: A review. *Clin Anat*. 2011;24(4): 416–422.

CODES

ICD9
578.9 Hemorrhage, gastrointestinal (tract)
ICD10
K92.2 Gastrointestinal hemorrhage, unspecified

FAQ

- Q: When do you refer a patient?
- A: Any bleeding—immediate referral if bleed is large, the patient is hemodynamically unstable, and bleeding will not stop. Patients with evidence of chronic iron-deficiency anemia and heme-positive stools.
- Q: What makes upper GI bleeding an emergency?
- A: Any persistent bleed with change in vital signs; significant drop in hemoglobin

U

URETEROPELVIC JUNCTION OBSTRUCTION

J. Christopher Austin
Michael C. Carr

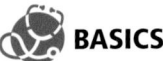 BASICS

DESCRIPTION
Ureteropelvic junction (UPJ) obstruction is a partial blockage of the kidney at the point where the renal pelvis transitions into the proximal ureter.

EPIDEMIOLOGY
- 45% of all cases of significant prenatal hydronephrosis are due to UPJ obstruction.
- Occurs more commonly in males (M/F 2:1)
- Left-sided lesion more common (66%)
- Bilateral in 10–40%
- 50% of patients have an additional genitourinary malformation (most common are vesicoureteral reflux, contralateral UPJ obstruction, multicystic dysplastic kidney, and renal agenesis).
- Of patients with VATER association, 21% have UPJ obstruction and thus should be screened with renal ultrasound. (VATER stands for vertebral defects, anal atresia, tracheoesophageal fistula with esophageal atresia, and radial and renal anomalies.)

PATHOPHYSIOLOGY
- The obstruction can cause varying degrees of hydronephrosis.
- Mild forms of UPJ obstruction result in dilation of the renal pelvis without loss of function.
- More severe forms result in dilation of the renal pelvis and calyces with loss of renal parenchyma and decreased function.
- In the most severe cases, the kidney may have cystic dysplasia and very poor function. Congenital hydronephrosis owing to an intrinsic narrowing is nearly always asymptomatic.
- When the obstruction is intermittent owing to a crossing vessel, the renal pelvis becomes distended (most commonly owing to the transient increase in urine output), which drapes it over the vessel and kinks the ureter, resulting in an acute obstruction. The acute distention of the renal pelvis results in pain (renal colic).

ETIOLOGY
- Intrinsic: A congenital narrowing of the UPJ, which is most commonly owing to abnormal musculature and fibrosis of this area, resulting in an adynamic segment
- Extrinsic: Kinking at the UPJ, which is most commonly owing to the renal pelvis draping over a lower pole crossing vessel. This type of obstruction can be intermittent.

DIAGNOSIS

HISTORY
- Antenatal:
  - If unilateral, timing and severity of hydronephrosis and status of the contralateral kidney are factors.
  - When bilateral or affecting a solitary kidney, renal insufficiency is a concern.
  - The presence of oligohydramnios, increased renal echogenicity, and cystic changes are indicators of poor renal function and dysplasia.
- Postnatal:
  - Feeding intolerance/respiratory distress (very rarely caused by UPJ obstruction)
- Older children:
  - History of episodic abdominal (may not lateralize well), flank, or back pain
  - Length of episodes (usually 30 minutes to several hours); associated nausea and vomiting
  - Relation of episodes to fluid intake; history of urinary tract infections or gross hematuria

PHYSICAL EXAM
- Newborn: Palpate kidneys. Affected kidney may feel enlarged but should not be tense. A tense mass can indicate a severe obstruction and should be imaged promptly.
- Older child: Careful abdominal exam for enlarged kidney and tenderness; costovertebral angle tenderness

DIAGNOSTIC TESTS & INTERPRETATION
Lab
- Newborn: If bilateral or a solitary kidney, serial assessments of renal function are necessary (serum electrolytes and creatinine) starting at 24–48 hours of age. With a normal contralateral kidney, no immediate laboratory testing is necessary.
- Older children: Urinalysis to detect hematuria or pyuria. Culture if infection suspected.

Imaging
Antenatally detected hydronephrosis: Infants with antenatally detected hydronephrosis typically are evaluated with 3 imaging studies—-renal/bladder ultrasound, voiding cystourethrogram (VCUG), and renal scan:

- Renal/Bladder ultrasound: In most cases, immediate imaging is not necessary. Because of a period of relative oliguria of a newborn in the 1st 24–48 hours of life, an ultrasound may underestimate the degree of hydronephrosis. This should not preclude evaluating an infant during this time as long as any normal study is followed up with a repeat study in 4–6 weeks. Evaluation should reveal the severity of dilation of the renal pelvis and calyces, changes in the amount and echogenicity of the parenchyma, and the presence of cortical cysts:
  - The evaluation of the full bladder is important for excluding dilated distal ureters, thickening of the bladder wall owing to outlet obstruction, and ureteroceles.
  - In cases of bilateral hydronephrosis, a solitary hydronephrotic kidney, or a tense kidney on physical examination, imaging should be promptly performed.
- VCUG: This study will detect the presence of vesicoureteral reflux as well as exclude the presence of posterior urethral valves and other abnormalities of the bladder:
  - The test can be delayed until after discharge from the nursery unless there is concern about posterior urethral valves, in which case it should be performed early.
- Renal scan: This study can quantify the differential renal function or the amount each kidney contributes to overall renal function (the normal differential is 50% ± 5% for each kidney):
  - The 2 most commonly used radionuclides are mercaptoacetyltriglycine (MAG-3) and diethylenetriamine penta-acetic acid (DTPA). In addition to the ability to detect diminished function, if there is poor drainage of the affected kidney, furosemide is given to wash out the radiotracer.
  - The time for washing out half of the accumulated radiotracer (T1/2) is often given in the report.
  - A prompt T1/2 (<10 minutes) is indicative of a nonobstructed kidney.
  - A slower T1/2 may be indicative of obstruction when it is >20 minutes. An intermediate T1/2 (10–20 minutes) is indeterminate for obstruction. Owing to effects of hydration, the amount of hydronephrosis, and variables in the timing of the diuretic administration, the T1/2 may be unreliable.

- Intravenous pyelogram (IVP): This study is most useful for evaluating the anatomy of the kidney and the ureters:
  - It can also be used for evaluating an older child with intermittent symptoms if it can be done during a symptomatic episode.
  - A normal study during a symptomatic episode of abdominal or flank pain excludes an intermittent UPJ obstruction as the cause of the child's pain.
  - If a normal study is obtained while the child is asymptomatic, an intermittent UPJ obstruction remains a possible cause.
- MRI: A new technique being studied that provides both anatomic and functional detail. Dynamic contrast-enhanced MRI requires sedation and placement of a bladder catheter. The images are obtained following infusion of gadolinium-DTPA. Lasix is given 15 minutes before the start of the study. This technique is being studied for use instead of ultrasound and renal scans in the hope that it will be a more precise tool in deciding whether or not the child requires surgical repair. The studies are currently preliminary, but this may be an important technique in the future.

DIFFERENTIAL DIAGNOSIS

- Vesicoureteral reflux: Higher grades of reflux will result in the dilation of the upper urinary tract.
- Distal ureteral obstruction: Obstruction at the level of the bladder owing to ureterovesical junction obstruction, ureterocele, or an ectopic ureter
- Bladder outlet obstruction: Dilation of the upper urinary tract secondary to obstruction of the lower urinary tract owing to posterior urethral valves, urethral atresia, or stricture
- Megacalycosis: Congenital dilation and increased numbers of calyces without significant renal pelvis dilation or obstruction
- Multicystic-dysplastic kidney: Can be difficult to differentiate severe hydronephrosis from cysts by ultrasound. Renal scan will demonstrate no function in multicystic-dysplastic kidneys.
- Triad syndrome: A triad of hypoplastic abdominal wall musculature, bilateral undescended testes, and dilation of the urinary tract (also known as "prune belly" syndrome or Eagle-Barrett syndrome)

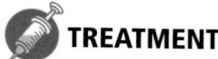 **TREATMENT**

ADDITIONAL TREATMENT
General Measures

- The decision to observe or surgically correct a UPJ obstruction depends on several factors. One must consider the age and overall health of the neonate, the amount of functional impairment of the kidney, whether it is a unilateral or bilateral process, the drainage pattern on renal scan, and whether or not it is symptomatic. There is no strict rule for who should be observed and who should undergo surgery. This decision should be made on an individual basis.

- Antibiotic prophylaxis: Newborns should be started on a once-a-day daily dose of amoxicillin or cephalexin at $\frac{1}{4}$ to $\frac{1}{2}$ the normal therapeutic dose. The antibiotic can be switched to trimethoprim, trimethoprim/sulfamethoxazole, or nitrofurantoin at 2 months of age. The duration that infants should be left on antibiotics is controversial among practicing pediatric urologists. Almost all agree that infants should be started on prophylactic antibiotics at birth. They should be continued at least until the infant undergoes a VCUG to exclude reflux. Several factors including age, sex, and degree of hydronephrosis are taken into account when deciding whether or not to stop the prophylaxis.
- Observation: Infants with the hydronephrosis thought to be owing to a narrowing at the UPJ are typically observed when there is preserved function (>40%) in the affected kidney and the contralateral kidney is normal. The pattern of drainage is taken into account, and if there is prompt drainage and normal differential function (50% ± 5%), these patients are followed with less frequent follow-up studies than those with less function or poor drainage. Most patients have follow-up imaging studies done at 3–6 month intervals during their 1st year of life, and they are gradually spaced out as time goes by if the hydronephrosis remains stable or improves.
- Older children with hydronephrosis owing to a UPJ obstruction are often detected during a symptomatic episode. If the UPJ obstruction is asymptomatic and the function of the kidney is preserved, the child may be observed as well.

SURGERY/OTHER PROCEDURES

- The gold standard for the repair of the UPJ obstruction has been a pyeloplasty:
  - During the procedure, the narrowed UPJ is most commonly excised and the ureter is reanastomosed to the renal pelvis.
  - This procedure is successful 95% of the time.
- Less invasive approaches include endoscopically incising the narrowing (endopyelotomy) or balloon dilation:
  - These approaches have been used in adults with rates of success in the 50–70% range but are considerably less invasive.
  - Endoscopic procedures have not been routinely offered as a 1st-line therapy for the treatment of UPJ obstructions because of their limited experience in children and the lower rates of success.

- Laparoscopic pyeloplasty is being performed in older children and adolescents and will likely be more common in the next several years. Robotically assisted procedures are now being done, further enhancing the minimally invasive approach. Both offer a similar rate of success to a traditional pyeloplasty with decreased perioperative morbidity because of the small incisions for the laparoscopic instruments.

ADDITIONAL READING

- Carr MC. Anomalies and surgery of the ureteropelvic junction in children. In: Walsh PC, Retik AB, Vaughan ED, et al., eds. *Campbell's Urology*. 8th ed. Philadelphia: WB Saunders; 2002.
- Perez-Brayfield MR, Kirsch AJ, Jones RA, et al. A prospective study comparing ultrasound, nuclear scintigraphy and dynamic contrast enhanced magnetic resonance imaging in the evaluation of hydronephrosis. *J Urol*. 2003;170:1330–1334.

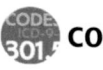 **CODES**

ICD9
- 593.4 Other ureteric obstruction
- 753.21 Congenital obstruction of ureteropelvic junction

ICD10
- N13.8 Other obstructive and reflux uropathy
- Q62.11 Congenital occlusion of ureteropelvic junction

FAQ

- Q: My unborn baby has hydronephrosis. My obstetrician told me that it is most likely a UPJ obstruction. Is my baby going to need surgery to correct this?
- A: Not necessarily; only ~1/3 of babies with significant hydronephrosis ultimately require surgical correction.
- Q: Will my child's kidney look normal after the surgery to fix it?
- A: Often the kidney has less dilation and an improved appearance, but not completely normal. Of greater importance is that there is no longer obstruction and the function is preserved or improved.

U

URETHRAL PROLAPSE

Stephen A. Zderic

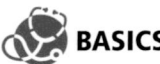 **BASICS**

DESCRIPTION
- Circular eversion of the distal urethral mucosa through the external urethral meatus
- Classification of urethral prolapse:
  - I: Minimal segmental inflammation
  - II: Circumferential prolapse with edema
  - III: Edematous mass protruding beyond the labia minora
  - IV: Severe hemorrhagic inflammation or necrosis and ulceration of the prolapse

EPIDEMIOLOGY
- Prepubertal girls <10 years of age
- Preponderance among African American females (90–100% of patients in reported series)
- Patients above average for height and weight

RISK FACTORS
Genetics
Predominance in African American females.

ETIOLOGY
Etiology unclear; proposed theories include:
- Poor adherence between smooth muscle layers of the urethra
- Estrogen deficiency
- Female circumcision

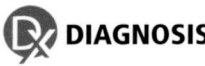 **DIAGNOSIS**

HISTORY
- 95% present with bleeding/bloody spotting on underwear.
- 21% have dysuria, frequency.
- Occasionally, a patient presents with urinary retention.
- Some are asymptomatic and detected only incidentally.

PHYSICAL EXAM
- Circular (doughnut-shaped) protrusion of urethral meatus with a reddish-purple mass surrounding the urethral meatus that is at the center
- Tissue appears inflamed and friable.
- To help distinguish between a urethral and vaginal mass, the vulva can be retracted downward and laterally.

DIAGNOSTIC TESTS & INTERPRETATION
Imaging
- If the appearance is atypical for urethral prolapse, ultrasound may be used to rule out bladder tumor (sarcoma botryoides) or prolapsed ureterocele.
- Urethral prolapse with typical presentation requires no imaging.

DIFFERENTIAL DIAGNOSIS
- Prolapsing ureterocele (or ectopic ureter, urethral polyp, bladder)
- Sarcoma botryoides
- Condyloma
- Hydrometrocolpos
- Periurethral abscess
- Trauma

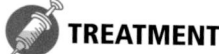 **TREATMENT**

ADDITIONAL TREATMENT
General Measures
- Do not try to manually reduce the prolapsed tissue.
- Conservative: Sitz baths followed by topical estrogen cream b.i.d.:
  – Some suggest topical antibiotics.
- Surgical: Most typical surgical approach is excision of prolapsed segment over a urethral Foley catheter, suturing the proximal urethral margin to the adjacent vestibule.

 ONGOING CARE

FOLLOW-UP RECOMMENDATIONS
Outpatient visit to assess success of estrogen cream or surgical repair

ADDITIONAL READING

- Anveden-Hertzenberg L, Gauderer MW, Elder JS. Urethral prolapse: An often misdiagnosed cause of vaginal bleeding in girls. *Ped Emerg Care*. 1995;11(4):212–214.
- Carlson NJ, Mercer LJ, Hajj SN. Urethral prolapse in the premenarchal female. *Int J Gynecol Obstet*. 1987;25(1):69–71.
- Hillyer S, Mooppan U, Kim H, et al. Diagnosis and treatment of urethral prolapse in children: Experience with 34 cases. *Urology*. 2009;73(5):1008–1011.

 CODES

ICD9
- 599.5 Prolapsed urethral mucosa
- 753.8 Other specified anomalies of bladder and urethra

ICD10
- N36.8 Other specified disorders of urethra
- Q64.71 Congenital prolapse of urethra

FAQ

- Q: What is the most common presenting complaint?
- A: Bleeding
- Q: What is the "first aid" for this problem?
- A: Avoid infection. You may use antibiotic cream. Keep tissue moist. Do not push the tissue back into the urethra.

U

URINARY TRACT INFECTION

Mercedes M. Blackstone

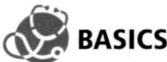 **BASICS**

DESCRIPTION
- Urinary tract infection (UTI) is significant growth of bacterial urinary tract pathogen(s):
  - For suprapubic aspirate, any growth is significant.
  - For urine obtained by catheterization, $\geq$50,000 CFU/mL, suspect if $\geq$10,000 CFU/mL.
  - For urine obtained by clean-catch technique, $\geq$100,000 CFU/mL
- Upper tract infection or pyelonephritis: Infection of the renal parenchyma; most febrile babies with a positive culture have upper tract infection.
- Lower tract infection or cystitis: Infection limited to the bladder, not involving the kidneys; occurs more in older children and adolescents; usually no fever

EPIDEMIOLOGY
Incidence
- Bimodal age distribution with peak incidence in infants <1 year (40 per 1,000)
- 2nd peak in adolescent females

Prevalence
- Overall prevalence of about 7% in febrile infants and young children; varies according to risk factors below
- Higher prevalence in white girls

RISK FACTORS
- Sex/Age: Boys are most at risk for UTI during 1st year of life; girls until school age and again in adolescence.
- Circumcision status: Uncircumcised males <1 year have 10 times the incidence of UTI compared with circumcised males.
- Race/Ethnicity: White children are 2–4 times more likely than blacks to have UTI:
  - May be due in part to differences in blood group antigens on the surfaces of uroepithelial cells, which affect bacterial adherence
- Abnormal urinary tract: Children with vesicoureteral reflux (VUR) and obstruction are at higher risk for UTI.
- Voiding dysfunction
  - Requiring frequent catheterization
  - Sexual activity
  - Clinical decision rule in febrile girls 2–24 months. Consider testing if $\geq$2 of following are present:
  - Temperature $\geq$39°C, fever for $\geq$2 days, white race, age <1 year, absence of another potential source of fever

GENERAL PREVENTION
- Teach correct wiping—front to back—to young children.
- Consider prophylactic antibiotics for select children with recurrent infection, VUR, urologic anomalies:
  - Existing evidence with 1-year follow-up does not support antibiotic prophylaxis for all patients with VUR.
- Attention to good voiding and stooling habits; treat constipation
- Consider single-dose postcoital antibiotics for adolescents with recurrent UTI.

PATHOPHYSIOLOGY
- Bacterial invasion of the urinary tract from ascending skin or gut flora
- Shorter urethra in females puts them at increased risk.
- Poor bladder emptying (neurogenic bladder, obstructive uropathies) facilitates movement of pathogens into the upper tract.
- In young infants, can be from hematogenous spread

ETIOLOGY
Urinary tract pathogens:
- *Escherichia coli* is responsible for about 80% of UTIs in children.
- Other fairly common microbes include *Klebsiella* species, *Enterococcus*, *Proteus mirabilis*.
- Less common: *Enterobacter cloacae*, group B hemolytic streptococci, *Citrobacter*, *Pseudomonas* species, *Staphylococcus aureus*, *Serratia* species, and *Staphylococcus saprophyticus* (teenage girls)

COMMONLY ASSOCIATED CONDITIONS
- ~5–10% of babies with febrile UTIs (pyelonephritis) are bacteremic, but the clinical course is likely unchanged.
- VUR or urinary anomalies

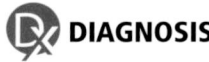 **DIAGNOSIS**

HISTORY
- Babies:
  - Symptoms are nonspecific, most often have fever alone
  - Can have vomiting, irritability, poor feeding, and lethargy
  - Rarely, failure to thrive or jaundice
- Older children:
  - Classic symptoms of the lower tract include urgency, frequency, dysuria, hesitancy, suprapubic discomfort, hematuria, and malodorous urine. Classic symptoms of the upper tract include chills, nausea, flank pain, and fever.
  - May have history of constipation
  - Can also present with secondary enuresis
- Special question:
  - Has the young child had a history of UTI, unexplained fevers, or urinary tract anomaly?

PHYSICAL EXAM
- Temperature and blood pressure should be documented
- Babies and toddlers: Often no physical findings or fever alone
  - Less common: Abdominal pain or distention, poor growth or weight gain, malodorous urine
  - Associated findings: May see evidence of foreign body, phimosis, labial adhesions, or midline abnormality of the lower back, which could indicate a neurogenic bladder
- Older children:
  - Lower tract: Suprapubic tenderness; may see evidence of constipation
  - Upper tract: Fever; costovertebral angle tenderness to percussion

DIAGNOSTIC TESTS & INTERPRETATION
Lab
- Urine culture collected sterilely is the gold standard for diagnosis:
  - Bladder catheterization in young children (or less commonly, suprapubic aspirate)
  - Midstream clean catch method for older cooperative children
  - A specimen should not be obtained by applying a bag to the perineum; contamination rates are too high.
- False positives:
  - Contaminated urine by perineum or stool organisms
- Cultures take 24–48 hours, so several rapid screening tests are available:
  - Conventional urinalysis: $\geq$5 WBC/HPF (uses centrifuged urine)
  - Enhanced urinalysis (combines microscopy on uncentrifuged urine with Gram stain): $\geq$10 WBC/mm^3 or positive Gram stain
    - High sensitivity and specificity; helpful in neonates
  - Urine dipstick alone equivalent to conventional microscopy:
    - Leukocyte esterase (LE) indicates presence of urinary leukocytes.
    - Nitrites are formed by nitrate-splitting bacteria (high rate of false negatives because urine has to sit in the bladder for $\geq$4 hours for nitrites to be detected).
    - Both suggest possible UTI; together they are highly specific.
- Serum testing is not routinely indicated in the patient with suspected UTI.
  - Blood culture: Not indicated in the well-appearing patient $\geq$2 months since bacteremia does not alter management
  - Inflammatory markers: White blood cell (WBC) count, C-reactive protein (CRP), erythrocyte sedimentation rate (ESR), and procalcitonin (PCT) may all be elevated in UTIs but are not particularly helpful in predicting diagnosis or distinguishing between upper and lower tract disease.
  - Serum creatinine: Not necessary for routine UTI but should be obtained in patients with recurrent disease or renal anomalies.

ALERT
Pitfalls:
- 10–25% of babies will have a negative urinalysis despite culture- or nuclear scan–documented UTI, so a culture should always be obtained in this population.
- Conversely, there are very high rates of asymptomatic bacteriuria in the pediatric population, so a mildly positive urinalysis should be weighed in the context of the pretest probability for UTI.
- Failure to culture by sterile means: Leads to a contaminated culture that is difficult to interpret
- Failure to screen a young child with another possible source of fever; children with otitis media, upper respiratory infections, and gastroenteritis can have a concurrent UTI.

Imaging
- There is controversy surrounding indications for imaging in routine UTIs.
- Ultrasound: Identifies hydronephrosis, congenital anomalies, and abscesses. Not good at detecting scars or VUR:
  - Recommended by AAP practice parameter for febrile children 2–24 months with UTI
  - If prenatal ultrasound beyond 32 weeks gestation was normal, may not be necessary.
- Voiding cystourethrogram (VCUG): Test of choice to detect and characterize VUR:
  - No longer routinely recommended by the AAP after first febrile UTI
  - Indicated for young children with recurrent febrile UTIs or an abnormal renal ultrasound
- In addition to the children covered by the AAP parameter, consider imaging for UTIs in all boys, children with recurrent infections, and children with voiding dysfunction or urinary abnormalities.
- Renal cortical scan: Detects acute pyelonephritis and renal scarring. Unclear utility in clinical setting; consider in febrile children if diagnosis is unclear.

DIFFERENTIAL DIAGNOSIS
- The differential diagnosis of isolated or prolonged fever is very broad.
- Infants: Gastroenteritis, occult bacteremia, occult pneumonia, meningitis, viral syndrome
- Older children and adolescents:
  - Common: Vaginal foreign body, vulvovaginitis/urethritis, epididymitis, gastroenteritis, sexually transmitted infection, pelvic inflammatory disease
  - Less common: Excessive drinking, urinary calculi, diabetes mellitus or insipidus, appendicitis, Kawasaki disease, tubo-ovarian abscess, ovarian torsion, group A streptococcal infection
  - Rare: Mass adjacent to bladder, spinal cord process (tumor, abscess), hypercalcemia

TREATMENT
MEDICATION (DRUGS)
First Line
- Empiric antibiotic therapy should be initiated in febrile children with suspected UTI in order to prevent scarring.
- *E. coli* is the most common pathogen associated with 1st UTI; it is typically sensitive to multiple antimicrobials.
- Gram staining, when available, can help guide empiric therapy.
- Empiric inpatient therapy: IV therapy with a 3rd-generation cephalosporin such as cefotaxime (120 mg/kg/day divided t.i.d.) or ceftriaxone (75 mg/kg/day) or the combination of ampicillin (100 mg/kg/day divided q.i.d.) and gentamicin (7.5 mg/kg/day divided t.i.d.):
  - High-risk patients who are immunocompromised, have indwelling catheters, or have recurrent UTIs should initially receive broad-spectrum antibiotics that cover the organisms involved in prior infections.

- Empiric outpatient therapy: Options include cefixime (8 mg/kg/day divided b.i.d.), cefdinir (14 mg/kg once daily), amoxicillin-clavulanate (45 mg/kg of amoxicillin component per day divided b.i.d.), amoxicillin (20–40 mg/kg/day divided b.i.d.), co-trimoxazole (6–12 mg TMP/kg/day divided b.i.d.), or cephalexin (50–100 mg/kg/day divided q.i.d.):
  - High rates of resistance to amoxicillin and co-trimoxazole in many communities make them poor initial choices in most cases.
- Antibiotic duration (IV/oral):
  - Children ≤2 years of age with a febrile UTI, recurrent UTI, or urinary tract abnormalities should receive a total of 7–14 days of antibiotic therapy.
  - Older children without fever or significant history who likely have an uncomplicated cystitis are eligible for a short course of antibiotics (5–7 days).
- Antibiotic prophylaxis after UTI:
  - Benefit somewhat unclear
  - AAP recommends the use of prophylactic antibiotics (co-trimoxazole 2 mg TMP/kg once daily or nitrofurantoin 1–2 mg/kg/day in 1–2 divided doses; maximum dose 100 mg/day) until imaging is completed.
  - Continued prophylaxis may be warranted for some patients with VUR; the duration is often determined in consultation with a urologist.

ONGOING CARE
FOLLOW-UP RECOMMENDATIONS
Patient Monitoring
- Consider a repeat urine culture after 2 days of therapy if the patient is not improving on an appropriate antibiotic regimen.
- Such patients should also receive imaging with ultrasound and consideration of VCUG or renal scan.
- Urinalysis and urine culture for subsequent febrile illnesses

PROGNOSIS
Prompt treatment of febrile UTIs reduces the risk for scarring and its sequelae. These children generally have a very good prognosis.

COMPLICATIONS
- Repeated febrile UTIs in young children may lead to renal scarring.
- Renal scarring in childhood carries a risk of hypertension, pre-eclampsia, and end-stage renal disease as an adult.

ADDITIONAL READING

- AAP, Committee on Quality Improvement, Subcommittee on Urinary Tract Infection. Practice parameter: The diagnosis, treatment, and evaluation of the initial urinary tract infection in febrile infants and young children. *Pediatrics.* 1999;103:843–852.
- AAP, Subcommittee on Urinary Tract Infection. Urinary tract infection: Clinical practice guideline for the diagnosis and management of the initial UTI in febrile infants and children 2 to 24 Months. *Pediatrics.* 2011;128:595–610.
- Gorelick MH, Shaw KN. Clinical decision rule to identify young febrile children at risk for UTI. *Arch Pediatr Adolesc Med.* 2000;154:386–390.
- McGillivray D, Mok E, Mulrooney E, et al. A head-to-head comparison: "Clean-void" bag versus catheter urinalysis in the diagnosis of urinary tract infection in young children. *J Pediatr.* 2005;147: 451–456.
- Montini G, Rigon L, Zucchetta P, et al. Prophylaxis after first febrile urinary tract infection in children? A multicenter, randomized, controlled noninferiority trial. *Pediatrics.* 2008;122(5):1064–1071.
- Schnadower D, Kuppermann N, Macias CG, et al; American Academy of Pediatrics Pediatric Emergency Medicine Collaborative Research Committee. Febrile infants with urinary tract infections at very low risk for adverse events and bacteremia. *Pediatrics.* 2010;126(6):1074–1083. Epub 2010 Nov 22.
- Shaikh N, Morone NE, Lopez J, et al. Does this child have a urinary tract infection? *JAMA.* 2007; 298(24):2895–2904.
- Shaikh N, Morone NE, Bost JE, et al. Prevalence of UTI in childhood: A meta-analysis. *Pediatr Infect Dis J.* 2008;27:302–308.

CODES

ICD9
- 590.80 Pyelonephritis, unspecified
- 595.9 Cystitis, unspecified
- 599.0 Urinary tract infection, site not specified

ICD10
- N11.9 Chronic tubulo-interstitial nephritis, unspecified
- N30.90 Cystitis, unspecified without hematuria
- N39.0 Urinary tract infection, site not specified

FAQ

- Q: Which children should have a radiologic evaluation after their 1st UTI?
- A: All boys, girls <3 years of age, and anyone with urologic abnormalities or recurrent UTIs. Imaging should be considered for febrile UTIs at any age.
- Q: Does a urine culture need to be done if the catheterized dipstick or urinalysis is negative?
- A: >10% of febrile infants with pyelonephritis will have a false-negative screening test (dipstick, urinalysis). A sterile urine culture should be done.

URTICARIA
Christopher P. Raab

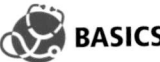 **BASICS**

DESCRIPTION
- Urticarial lesions are best described as raised, pruritic circumscribed erythematous papules.
- Single lesions may coalesce as they enlarge, forming generalized, raised, erythematous areas.
- They are transient, typically lasting several hours.
- Also known as "hives" or "nettle rash"
- Acute: <6 weeks duration
- Chronic: >6 weeks duration
- Other similar but nonurticarial entities:
  - Angioedema: Urticarial-like lesions that form in the deep dermal, subcutaneous, and submucosal layers
  - Anaphylaxis: Hypersensitivity reaction after exposure to an antigen, producing weakness, respiratory compromise secondary to airway edema, urticarial rash, pruritus, and hypotension; can lead to shock

EPIDEMIOLOGY
- Female:male ratio of 3:2
- No variation in race

Incidence
Lifetime incidence of 15–25%

GENERAL PREVENTION
When a trigger is identified, avoidance is the main preventive measure.

PATHOPHYSIOLOGY
- Immune mediated:
  - Antigen is cross-linked to IgE on a mast cell.
  - This causes mast cell activation leading to the release of vasoactive mediators, such as histamine, leukotrienes, prostaglandin D2, platelet-activating factor, and other vasoactive mediators.
  - These vasoactive mediators cause pruritus, vasodilatation, and capillary leak, which lead to the characteristic findings.
  - Common triggers include some medications such as penicillins, foods such as milk or eggs, and envenomations.
- Non–immune mediated:
  - Degranulation of mast cells secondary to other non-IgE reactions such as physical changes, chemicals, some medications such as beta-lactams and sulfa-containing drugs, and some foods
- Autoimmune mediated:
  - Degranulation of mast cells caused by cross-linking of IgE by IgG, or IgG binding to the high-affinity IgE (FcεRI) receptor on mast cells

ETIOLOGY
Acute Urticaria
- Viral infections are thought to make up ~80% of all cases of acute urticaria in children. Most commonly isolated causes include the following viruses:
  - Epstein-Barr
  - Coxsackie A and B
  - Hepatitis A, B, and C
- Parasitic infections
- Bacterial infections (especially group A strep)
- Medications: Most frequently reported include the following:
  - NSAIDs
  - Opiates
  - Vancomycin
- Radiocontrast
- Foods
- Transfusion of blood products
- Food additives and dyes
- Natural remedies including cranberry, feverfew, glucosamine, and ginger
- Insect venom including bees, wasps, hornets

Chronic Urticaria
- Idiopathic: Most have an unknown cause, but many feel that an association with an autoimmune mechanism is likely.
- Physical (~20–30%):
  - Dermatographism (9%): Stroking of skin causes linear urticaria at site of contact.
  - Cholinergic (5%): Diffuse erythema and elevated but pale urticarial lesions; intense pruritus. Associated with sweating reflex, so often associated with overheating or exertion. May be worsened in combination with other triggers in specific combinations.
  - Cold (3%): Urticarial lesions present at areas of skin exposed to low temperatures; has a familial and nonhereditary form.
  - Aquagenic: Urticarial lesions arise when the patient is exposed to water (e.g., bathtub, swimming pool).
  - Delayed pressure/vibratory: Deep or prolonged pressure on skin produces significant urticaria and often angioedema. Vibratory urticaria is a form of delayed pressure urticaria caused by repetitive vibration (e.g., use of a jackhammer).
- Mast cell disease:
  - Urticaria pigmentosa: Excessive number of mast cells in skin, bone marrow, lymph nodes, and other tissues. Flares are characterized by pruritus, flushing, tachycardia, nausea, and vomiting.
  - Systemic mastocytosis

- Systemic disease:
  - Rheumatologic:
    - Urticarial vasculitis: Erythematous wheals that resemble urticaria but histologically appear as leukocytoclastic vasculitis; often presents with systemic symptoms and lasts >24 hours
    - Muckle-Wells syndrome: Chronic recurrent urticaria, deafness, amyloidosis, and arthritis
  - Neoplasms
  - Infections: Parasites especially noted to cause chronic urticaria
  - Autoimmune: Antibodies to IgE or IgE receptor (FcεRI)

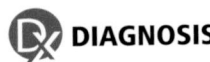 **DIAGNOSIS**

HISTORY
- Description of rash: Lesions may not be present at time of exam due to transient nature. Digital photos are often useful.
- Duration of symptoms, acute versus chronic:
  - If acute (<6 weeks), ask about:
    - Viral symptoms including rhinorrhea, cough, fever, congestion, malaise
    - Any medications (prescription or over the counter) or any herbal remedies
    - Any new foods or beverages
    - Any new exposures to perfumes, chemicals, or other skin products
  - If chronic (>6 weeks):
    - History of previous episodes including timing, exposures, any past history of urticaria or angioedema
    - Other symptoms or variations in presentation
    - Symptoms of systemic diseases, such as hyperthyroidism, systemic lupus erythematosus (SLE), rheumatoid arthritis, polymyositis, amyloidosis, infections, and lymphoma
    - Duration of lesions

PHYSICAL EXAM
- Appearance of rash: Has classic wheal and flare appearance
- Respiratory: Look for evidence of stridor, wheezing, or dyspnea. If present, be concerned for airway compromise or lower airway edema from an anaphylactic reaction.
- Facial or neck swelling: A concern for possible airway compromise
- A full physical exam should be performed to look for signs of systemic disease or malignancy, such as:
  - Upper respiratory tract infections
  - Thyromegaly
  - Lymphadenopathy or splenomegaly that suggests lymphoma
  - Joint examination for any evidence of connective tissue disease, rheumatoid arthritis, or SLE

DIAGNOSTIC TESTS & INTERPRETATION
Lab
- Testing is often fruitless unless indicated by history and physical examination.
- Skin testing may be performed if the causative agent is thought to be 1 of several food items.
- If symptoms are difficult to handle or persist >3 months, consider:
  – CBC with differential
  – ESR
  – Thyroid studies (thyroid-stimulating hormone [TSH], free T4, antithyroglobulin, and antiperoxisomal antibody)
- If symptoms are atypical, last >1 year, or are suggestive of urticarial vasculitis:
  – Complement studies
  – ANA titer
  – Liver function tests
  – Skin punch biopsy

DIFFERENTIAL DIAGNOSIS
- Viral exanthema
- Atopic dermatitis
- Contact dermatitis
- Insect bites
- Maculopapular drug rash
- Erythema multiforme
- Plant-induced eruptions
- Henoch-Schönlein purpura
- SLE

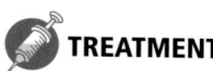 TREATMENT

Emergent treatment: If any difficulty breathing, stridor or wheezing, or other signs of anaphylaxis, give epinephrine 0.01 mL/kg of the 1:1,000 solution SC/IM.

MEDICATION (DRUGS)
- Acute urticaria:
  – Usually self-resolving but can treat with 2nd-generation nonsedating antihistamines
  – 1st-generation antihistamines: Diphenhydramine 1 mg/kg/dose or total 5 mg/kg/d divided PO q6h or hydroxyzine 2 mg/kg/day PO divided q6h for pruritus
- Chronic urticaria: See below.

First Line
Antihistamines/H1 antagonists:
- Less sedating, longer acting, and should be mainstay of therapy:
  – Cetirizine (Zyrtec): Dosing varies by age from 2.5–10 mg daily
  – Loratadine (Claritin): 5 mg daily
  – Fexofenadine (Allegra): Not indicated for those <6 years of age; >6 years of age can use 30 mg twice daily.
- 1st-generation antihistamines are effective but more sedating:
  – Diphenhydramine (Benadryl): 5 mg/kg/day divided q6h
  – Hydroxyzine (Atarax): 0.6 mg/kg/dose q6h
  – Cyproheptadine (Periactin): 2 mg up to 3 times a day: Primary treatment for cold urticaria

Second Line
Increase 2nd-generation H1 antagonist dose to maximum for age. In adult guidelines, increasing the dose up to 4-fold is more effective.

Third Line
- Addition of a second nonsedating 2nd-generation H1 antihistamine
- Leukotriene inhibitors: Minimal additive response noted in clinical studies
- Montelukast (Singulair): 5 mg daily
- Other:
  – Combined H1 and H2 antagonist
  – H2 antagonists: Added as 2nd agent because skin cells have both H1 and H2 receptors and a synergistic effect can be achieved by addition of an H2 blocker
  – Ranitidine (Zantac): 2–4 mg/kg/day divided twice daily; doxepin (Sinequan): A tricyclic antidepressant. >12 years of age 10–50 mg/day and can slowly titer up to 100 mg/day. Potent antihistamine but poorly tolerated due to sedation, hypotension, anticholinergic side effects, and massive weight gain
- Other immune-modifying agents used in chronic urticaria:
  – Other nonstandard therapies have been tried in small case studies: Cyclosporine, colchicines, dapsone, IV immunoglobulin (IVIG), plasmapheresis, methotrexate, cyclophosphamide, calcium channel blockers, ephedrine
  – Corticosteroids: Titer to lowest effective dose. Start with standard dose of 0.5–1 mg/kg/day of prednisone; often poorly tolerated secondary to substantial side effects including hypertension, immunosuppression, hyperglycemia, physical changes

 ONGOING CARE

FOLLOW-UP RECOMMENDATIONS
Patient Monitoring
- Watch for signs and symptoms of anaphylaxis; this is the major complication.
- Patients with chronic urticaria should follow up with their physician on a regular basis to monitor symptoms and response to therapies.

PROGNOSIS
Chronic urticaria:
- Resolution in 50% by 12 months
- Another 20% resolve by 5 years.
- 10–20% >20 years; many of those who continue to have symptoms are felt to have an autoimmune etiology.
- May have recurrences; physical urticaria subtypes are more likely to recur.

COMPLICATIONS
Anaphylaxis with resulting edema of the upper airway is the major life-threatening complication. The patient should seek immediate medical attention.

ADDITIONAL READING
- Dibbern D, Dreskin S. Urticaria and angioedema: An overview. *Immunol Allergy Clin North Am.* 2004; 24(2):141–162.
- Dibbern D. Urticaria: Selected highlights and recent advances. *Med Clin North Am.* 2006;90(1): 187–209.
- Powell RJ, Du Toit GL, Siddique N, et al. BSACI guidelines for the management of chronic urticaria and angio-oedema. *Clin Exp Allergy.* 2007;37: 631–650.
- Sheikh J. Advances in the treatment of chronic urticaria. *Immunol Allergy Clin North Am.* 2004;24(2):317–334.
- Bailey E, Shaker M. An update on childhood urticaria and angioedema. *Curr Opin Pediatr.* 2008;20(4):425–430.
- Zuberbier T, Asero R, Bindslev-Jensen C, et al. EAACI/GA2LEN/EDF/WAO guideline: Management of urticaria. *Allergy.* 2009;64(10):1427–1443.

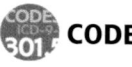 CODES

ICD9
- 708.0 Allergic urticaria
- 708.8 Other specified urticaria
- 708.9 Urticaria, unspecified

ICD10
- L50.0 Allergic urticaria
- L50.8 Other urticaria
- L50.9 Urticaria, unspecified

FAQ
- Q: When should I refer patients to a specialist, and to what specialty should I send them?
- A: Often, referral is made when a trigger cannot be identified, if it is felt to be a food or medication trigger, and/or the symptoms persist for >6 weeks. Refer to a dermatologist or allergist–immunologist experienced in the evaluation and workup of urticaria.
- Q: When should treatment with corticosteroids or other nonstandard therapies be used to treat chronic urticaria?
- A: Typically, these medications carry significant side effects and should be reserved for those patients in whom the urticaria is causing significant alterations in activities of daily living.
- Q: When does a patient need to be hospitalized or observed during an episode of urticaria?
- A: Concerning signs include extensive angioedema, respiratory symptoms such as stridor or wheezing, or nausea/vomiting. Symptoms of anaphylaxis should be treated with epinephrine and the patient observed for several hours to ensure that symptoms do not recur.

U

VACCINE ADVERSE EVENTS

Kristen Feemster

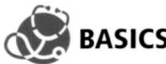 **BASICS**

ALERT

Adverse events after immunization may be a true vaccine-associated event or may be a coincidental event that would happen without immunization. Epidemiologic studies are important to establish causation.

DESCRIPTION

- A clinically significant event that occurs after administration of a vaccine and has been causally related to the vaccine
- All suspected adverse events should be reported; however, reporting does not imply causation.
- Contraindication to immunization = condition that increases risk of a serious adverse reaction
- Precaution for immunization = condition that might increase risk of an adverse event or may decrease effectiveness of vaccine to mount an immune response
  - Usually a temporary condition
  - Immunization indicated with a precaution if benefits outweigh risk

EPIDEMIOLOGY

- Adverse events monitored prelicensure to establish safety and postlicensure to identify rare adverse events that would not be detected in prelicensure studies. Reporting is guided by:
  - National Childhood Vaccine Injury Compensation Program:
    ○ Established by National Childhood Vaccine Injury Act of 1986 to establish a no-fault mechanism to manage claims of vaccine injury outside of the civil law system and provide compensation
    ○ Petitioners can file claims based on the Vaccine Injury Table (see "Patient Education") created by the program or can attempt to prove causation for an injury that is not listed.
    ○ Covers vaccines recommended for routine administration to children
    ○ Program also mandates reporting of adverse events by health care professionals and creation of vaccine information materials.
  - Vaccine Adverse Event Reporting System (VAERS)
    ○ Passive surveillance system to monitor all vaccines licensed in the US
    ○ All reports reviewed by FDA medical officers
    ○ Can detect possible unrecognized adverse events but limited ability to determine true causal relationships
    ○ Reporting to VAERS mandated by the National Childhood Vaccine Injury Compensation Program
  - Vaccine Safety Datalink
    ○ Active surveillance system formed by CDC in partnership with managed care organizations covering 9 million people
    ○ Can perform better observational studies to help determine causation

- Clinical Immunization Safety Assessment Network (CISA)
  ○ Network of 6 academic centers established by CDC in 2001 to develop research protocols to diagnose, evaluate, and manage adverse events
  ○ Develops evidence-based guidelines for immunizing people at risk for serious adverse events after vaccination

Incidence

- Difficult to measure incidence owing to current reporting systems for adverse events
- There are ~30,000 reports each year to VAERS.
  - 13% are considered serious adverse events.
- As of April 2011, there were almost 14,000 claims filed under the National Childhood Vaccine Injury Compensation Act since 1988 and about 2,500 families were compensated.

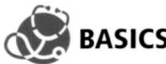 **DIAGNOSIS**

- Common mild adverse events after vaccination include:
  - Fever
  - Local erythema, swelling, and/or tenderness
  - Sleepiness and decreased appetite
  - Increased fussiness
  - Mild rash: Occurs in 1 of 25 people up to 1 month after varicella vaccination
- Moderate to serious adverse events to currently recommended vaccines are rare but include:
  - Syncope, particularly among adolescents
  - Febrile seizures (MMR, varicella, and DTaP vaccines)
  - Temporary joint pain or stiffness (MMR)
  - Temporary thrombocytopenia (MMR)
  - High fever
- To minimize the possibility of vaccine adverse events and to maximize the effectiveness of vaccination, the following contraindications and precautions should be followed.

Contraindications

General contraindications for vaccination include:

- History of an **anaphylactic** reaction to a vaccine component:
  - History of egg allergy no longer contraindication to influenza vaccination unless documented history of anaphylactic reaction
- Pregnancy with **live-virus vaccines** unless mother is at high risk for the vaccine-preventable condition
- Primary T-cell immunodeficiencies (i.e., severe combined immunodeficiency):
  - No live vaccines
  - Inactivated vaccines can be safely administered but may not generate an adequate immune response
- Primary B-cell immunodeficiencies:
  - If severe (i.e., X-linked agammaglobulinemia), no live bacterial vaccines, live-attenuated influenza vaccine (LAIV), or yellow fever vaccine
  - Less severe antibody deficiencies can receive live vaccines except for OPV.

- Phagocyte dysfunction:
  - No live bacterial vaccines
  - All live-virus and inactivated vaccines probably safe and effective
- Secondary immunosuppression (transplant, malignancy, autoimmune disease):
  - No live vaccines depending on degree of immunosuppression
  - Can achieve adequate response to vaccination within 3 months to 1 year after stopping immunosuppressive therapy
- HIV/AIDS:
  - Can give MMR and varicella vaccine unless severely immunocompromised
  - No OPV or LAIV
- High-dose corticosteroids >14 days:
  - No live virus vaccines until therapy discontinued for at least 1 month
- History of Guillain-Barré syndrome:
  - Contraindication for LAIV only
  - A precaution for receipt of MCV4 (conjugate meningococcal vaccine) ONLY if not at high risk for meningococcal disease
- Progressive neurologic disorder (infantile spasms, poorly controlled epilepsy):
  - Contraindication for **DTaP** only
  - Children with stable neurologic conditions can be vaccinated.
- Encephalopathy within 7 days of previous DTP, DTaP, or Tdap dose that is not attributable to another cause
- Hib conjugate vaccine should not be given to infants <6 weeks of age

Precautions

General **precautions** for receiving a vaccine include moderate to severe acute illness with or without fever. Vaccine-specific **precautions** include:

DTaP/DTP

- Fever ≥104°F or shocklike state within 48 hours of previous DTaP/DTP dose
- Persistent, inconsolable crying >3 hours within 48 hours of previous DTaP/DTP dose
- Seizure within 3 days of previous DTaP/DTP dose
- **Tdap:**
  - Progressive or unstable neurologic disorder
  - History of Arthus hypersensitivity reaction after previous tetanus toxoid–containing dose
    ○ Wait 10 years between doses of tetanus toxoid–containing vaccines.
- Any **tetanus toxoid–containing vaccine:**
  - Guillain-Barré within 6 weeks of a previous tetanus toxoid–containing vaccine dose
- **Hepatitis B:**
  - Infants <2,000 g in weight
- **Hepatitis A, IPV, and HPV vaccines:**
  - Pregnancy
- **Varicella:**
  - Receipt of antibody-containing blood product within past 11 months
  - Immunocompromised household contacts are not a contraindication or precaution but if rash develops 7–25 days after vaccination, should avoid direct contact with immunocompromised individual

- **MMR:**
  - Receipt of antibody-containing blood product within past 11 months
  - History of thrombocytopenic purpura
- **Rotavirus:**
  - Immunosuppression
  - Receipt of antibody-containing blood product within 6 weeks
  - Moderate to severe gastroenteritis
  - Previous history intussusceptions
- The following are NOT precautions or contraindications to the receipt of any vaccine:
  - Mild or recent illness
  - History of a mild to moderate local reaction to vaccine in the past
  - Concurrent antimicrobial therapy
  - Breastfeeding
  - History of other nonvaccine allergies
  - Stable neurologic conditions (e.g., cerebral palsy, developmental delay)

DIFFERENTIAL DIAGNOSIS
- Allergic reaction to an unrelated exposure
- Intercurrent illness

 ## ONGOING CARE

Approach to the Patient
- Before vaccination:
  - Discuss benefits and review potential adverse events so that families know what to expect.
  - Actively review Vaccine Information Sheets.
  - Solicit concerns so that they can be addressed.
- If a patient presents with a potential adverse event:
  - Take thorough history and perform exam to characterize symptoms and determine timing of symptom onset.
  - Evaluate for other potential causes of symptoms.
  - Determine likelihood of causality.
  - Report all adverse events to VAERS.
  - If the family would like to file a claim, refer to National Childhood Vaccine Injury Compensation Program.

MANAGEMENT
- **Addressing safety concerns:**
  - Despite increasing vaccine safety concerns, health care professionals are one of the most trusted sources of information regarding vaccines.
  - Actively review the required Vaccine Information Sheets with parents.
  - Emphasize benefits of vaccination and review potential consequences of not accepting vaccination.
  - Actively solicit concerns before vaccination.
  - If parents have specific concerns, refer to additional information sources such as the Vaccine Education Center at the Children's Hospital of Philadelphia or the "Parents Guide to Immunization" from the Centers for Disease Control and Prevention (see additional references in the "Patient Education" section)
  - Document vaccine discussions.

- **Reporting adverse events:**
  - VAERS is the primary reporting site for suspected adverse events. Health care providers, vaccine recipients, or parents of vaccine recipients and vaccine manufacturers can all report. However, health care providers are required to report:
    ○ Any adverse event listed by vaccine manufacturer as a contraindication for the receipt of additional doses of the vaccine
    ○ Any adverse event included on the VAERS table of reportable events that occurred within the specified time period
  - Health care providers, parents, and/or individuals who suspect a vaccine-related adverse event can report to VAERS.
- **Vaccine Injury Compensation Program:**
  - Covers all vaccines recommended for routine administration by the Advisory Commission of Immunization Practices
  - To qualify for compensation, must prove there was an injury listed in the Vaccine Injury Table that occurred within prescribed time period, prove that a vaccine caused an injury not listed on the table, or prove that a vaccine aggravated a preexisting condition
  - Effects of injury must last >6 months after vaccination and have resulted in hospitalization, surgery, or death.

Patient Education
- Vaccine Adverse Event Reporting System: http://vaers.hhs.gov
  - Table of reportable events: http://vaers.hhs.gov/resources/VAERS_Table_of_Reportable_Events_Following_Vaccination.pdf
- Vaccine Safety Datalink Project: www.cdc.gov/od/science/iso/vsd
- Clinical Immunization Safety Assessment Network: http://www.cdc.gov/vaccinesafety/cisa/
- National Childhood Vaccine Injury Compensation Program: http://www.hrsa.gov/vaccinecompensation/
  - Vaccine Injury Table: http://www.hrsa.gov/vaccinecompensation/table.htm
- The Brighton Collaboration: www.brightoncollaboration.org
  - International voluntary collaboration to develop standardized case definitions for adverse events
  - 25 published case definitions as of July 2011
- Vaccine Education Center at the Children's Hospital of Philadelphia: http://www.chop.edu/service/vaccine-education-center/home.html
  - Vaccine education information for health care providers, educators, and parents
- National Network for Immunization Information: www.immunizationinfo.org
  - Resources for communicating with families
- AAP Immunization Initiatives Web site: https://www2.aap.org/immunization/
  - Resources for parents and health care professionals
  - Refusal to vaccinate waivers

ADDITIONAL READING
- American Academy of Pediatrics. Active immunization. In: *Red book: Report of the Committee on Infectious Diseases*. Washington, DC: American Academy of Pediatrics; 2009:40–55.
- American Academy of Pediatrics. Immunization in special clinical circumstances. In: *Red book: Report of the Committee on Infectious Diseases*. Washington, DC: American Academy of Pediatrics; 2009:68–87.
- Atkinson WL, Kroger AL, Pickering LK. General immunization practices. In: Plotkin SA, Orenstein WA, Offit PA, eds. *Vaccine*. Philadelphia: Elsevier; 2008:84–109.
- Cook KM, Evans G. The National Vaccine Injury Compensation Program. *Pediatrics*. 2011;127: S74–S77.

 ## CODES

ICD9
- 995.20 Unspecified adverse effect of unspecified drug, medicinal and biological substance
- 999.9 Other and unspecified complications of medical care, not elsewhere classified

ICD10
- T50.905A Adverse effect of unspecified drugs, medicaments and biological substances, initial encounter
- T88.8XXA Other specified complications of surgical and medical care, not elsewhere classified, initial encounter

FAQ
- Q: Many parents request spacing vaccines. Is there evidence that giving multiple vaccines at a time is too much for a child's immune system?
- A: Recommended vaccines have a very small amount of antigen compared to natural infection and they activate a small proportion of immune system memory. Additionally, all vaccines given together have been tested when given at the same time to make sure they remain safe and effective.
- Q: What is the bottom line regarding autism and vaccines?
- A: Multiple studies including a recent Institute of Medicine report have not shown any causal relationship between thimerosal-containing vaccines and autism or MMR and autism. Additionally, the US court system through the Omnibus Autism Proceedings has recently ruled that there is insufficient evidence to show any causal relationship between thimerosal-containing vaccines or MMR and autism.

V

VAGINITIS

Marianne Ruby
Gary A. Emmett

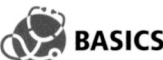 **BASICS**

DESCRIPTION

- Vaginitis is an inflammatory process of the vagina often caused by infection, but also caused by foreign bodies and other irritants.
- Vulvovaginitis is inflammation of the vulva and vagina; it is more common in prepubertal girls.
- Bacterial vaginosis is an overgrowth of vaginal flora, primarily anaerobic, associated with an elevation in vaginal pH, a malodorous discharge, and often a sensation of burning. This condition has been referred to as gardnerella, haemophilus, and nonspecific vaginitis.
- Vaginal discharge is a vaginal secretion that may or may not be associated with inflammation or infection.

ALERT
Any infection that raises suspicion of sexual abuse must be reported to the local authorities immediately.

EPIDEMIOLOGY

- Candidiasis may present cyclically with menses, possibly owing to changing estrogen levels.
- Gonorrhea is more likely to be symptomatic at the time of menses owing to easier access to the upper reproductive tract.
- Body mass index (BMI) at the extremes is associated with increased risk of vulvovaginitis.
- The epidemiology of bacterial vaginosis is not well known because it is not a reportable disease, and 50% of cases may be asymptomatic.

PATHOPHYSIOLOGY

- Physiologic leukorrhea is a normally occurring vaginal discharge that is clear or white, nonpruritic, nonirritating, and rarely malodorous:
  - The amount of discharge markedly varies from individual to individual and may be profuse.
  - In menstruating girls, as a result of varying estrogen levels, the volume of discharge varies with the menstrual cycle and is especially heavy at the time of ovulation.
- Candidiasis occurs more commonly when the glycogen level in the vaginal mucosa is increased, as in pregnancy and diabetes:
  - Use of antibiotics also increases the occurrence of candidiasis by eliminating competitive organisms.
- For bacterial vaginosis, the inciting cause is not known, but the etiologic cascade involves a decline in levels of lactobacillus, leading to an increased pH and increased overgrowth of normal bacterial flora. The change in the vaginal environment decreases the normal defenses against pathogens.
- The normal trauma of sexual intercourse may increase the likelihood of vaginitis by causing microscopic breakdown of the mucosal surface.
- During toileting, wiping from the anus toward the vagina may introduce bacteria not normal to the vagina and induce a vaginitis.

ETIOLOGY

- All ages:
  - Chemical irritants such as soaps, bubble baths, detergents, and fabric softeners
  - Allergic reactions
  - Foreign material, such as paper products, sand, soil, and small objects
  - *Candida albicans*, especially if exposed to antibiotics
  - Trauma from repeated rubbing, such as with masturbation
  - Sexual abuse
- Prepubertal females:
  - Diapers and nonbreathable clothing
  - Coliform bacteria from the child's toileting practices
  - β-Hemolytic group A streptococcus
  - Infestations, including pinworms and scabies
- Postpubertal females:
  - Noninflammatory, physiologic leukorrhea
  - Bacterial vaginosis
  - Trichomonas
  - *Chlamydia trachomatis*
  - Gonorrhea
  - Herpes simplex virus, types I and II
  - Human papilloma virus (HPV)
  - Chancroid
  - Lymphogranuloma venereum (LGV)
  - Behçet disease
  - Epstein-Barr virus

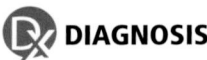 **DIAGNOSIS**

HISTORY

- Presence, color, odor, and duration of discharge
- Child is itchy or having a burning sensation or dysuria:
  - Itching and burning may be signs of vaginal inflammation.
  - Dysuria raises the suspicion for a urinary tract infection, but burning at the start of micturition (urination) may be seen with vulvovaginal inflammation.
- Conditions that make symptoms better or worse: Inflammation may be related to specific clothing, especially tight pants. Nighttime itching/discomfort may signal pinworm infestation.
- Treatment that has worked in the past may work again:
  - The success or failure of over-the-counter products may affect the treatment choices.
  - Over-the-counter treatment may affect culture results for candida.
- Any other recent health problems: Recent respiratory or gastrointestinal distress increases the risk for group A streptococcal infection.
- Any new medication, especially an antibiotic, introduced around the time of symptom onset:
  - Antibiotics increase the risk for candidal vaginitis.

- STIs should be considered if there is known sexual activity and should be considered even when sexual activity is denied.
- If appropriate, character and timing of the last menses: Gonorrhea is associated with increased symptoms at the time of menses. Some girls may have cyclic yeast infections associated with menses.
- Any new chemical exposures such as soaps, spermicides, or feminine hygiene products: Vaginitis often follows vaginal exposure to cleaning and other chemical agents.
- Any chronic illnesses such as diabetes, inflammatory bowel disease, or immunocompromised conditions: Vaginitis is much more common in these situations.
- Previously similar symptoms: Some people have a tendency toward repeated vaginal inflammation, especially candidiasis.

PHYSICAL EXAM

- Vital signs including height, weight, and temperature
- Calculate the BMI.
- Tanner pubertal development scores
- Examine the entire skin for other lesions or dermatoses.
- Abdominal examination to assess for abdominal pain and masses
- Evaluate external genitalia for tenderness, erythema, discharge, ulceration, edema, excoriation, traumatic injuries, warts (HPV), lymphadenopathy, and pigmentary changes.
- Evaluate vagina for findings above, if possible.

DIAGNOSTIC TESTS & INTERPRETATION
Lab
The following common gynecologic tests may help with differentiating normal physiologic leukorrhea from 3 common etiologies:

- Odor/"whiff" or "amine" test: Prepared with 10% KOH
- Wet mount of the vaginal discharge is mixed with saline for microscopic evaluation (see "Physical Exam").
- Nitrazine paper measures pH with lateral vaginal wall specimen.
- Chlamydial polymerase chain reaction (PCR) assay should be performed on all sexually active patients.
- Gonorrhea PCR or culture from cervical specimen
- Culture for fungi (yeast)
- Pap test starting at age 18 years with history of sexual activity

DIFFERENTIAL DIAGNOSIS
- Bacterial vaginosis
- Chlamydia
- Gonorrhea
- Trichomonas

- Candidiasis
- Herpes simplex virus infection
- HPV
- Physiologic leukorrhea
- Psoriasis
- Lichen sclerosis (hypotrophic dystrophy of the vulva)
- Congenital abnormalities, such as ectopic ureter
- Sexual abuse

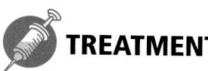

TREATMENT

MEDICATION (DRUGS)

- Topical steroids:
  - Lichen sclerosis requires very-high-potency topical steroids for amelioration. Apply to vulva twice daily for 2–4 weeks. Overuse may lead to thinning of the skin. Steroids can also promote the growth of yeast.
  - In moderate inflammation of the vulva caused by irritants, apply low-potency steroids lightly to vulva twice daily for 5–14 days, until symptoms have subsided for 2 days. Extreme overuse may also lead to skin thinning.
- Antifungal agents—including topical butoconazole, miconazole, and terconazole—applied as directed will relieve vaginal candidiasis; as an alternative, oral fluconazole 6 mg/kg in 1 dose to maximum dose of 150 mg may be effective.
- Antibiotics are used in many causes of vaginal infection:
  - Bacterial vaginosis is treated in older children with metronidazole 500 mg PO twice daily for 7 days or topically with metronidazole gel or clindamycin cream or suppository.
  - In infections with coliform bacteria, treat with amoxicillin at 40 mg/kg/d to maximum of 500 mg twice daily; β-hemolytic group A streptococcus will usually respond to the same dosage of amoxicillin.
  - In patients with penicillin allergy, trimethoprim/sulfa, azithromycin, or ciprofloxacin (in older children) is appropriate in either type of bacterial infection.
    - Chlamydia is treated with either azithromycin 1,000 mg PO in a single dose or doxycycline 100 mg PO twice daily for 7 days.
    - Uncomplicated gonorrhea is treated with ceftriaxone 250 mg IM once or azithromycin 1,000 mg PO or cefixime 400 mg PO once. Treat for chlamydia simultaneously unless the child is known not to have chlamydia.
    - Trichomonas responds to metronidazole 2 g in a single dose.
- Other anti-infective agents used in vaginitis include the following:
  - Herpes simplex virus is treated with famciclovir 250 mg 3 times daily for 7–10 days, with valacyclovir 1 g PO twice daily for 7–10 days, or with acyclovir 400 mg 3 times daily for 7–10 days. In recurring herpes simplex virus, prolonged use of these agents may be useful.
- In pinworms, mebendazole 100 mg is taken once by mouth. May be recommended for entire family, but is not used in pregnancy

ADDITIONAL TREATMENT

General Measures

- Removal of irritant/foreign body: In vaginitis caused by chemical irritants or foreign materials, the practitioner should attempt to identify and remove the cause. On occasion, especially in younger children, intravaginal foreign bodies may have to be removed under anesthesia.
- Promoting good hygiene: Girls should be educated in good toilet hygiene and proper front-to-back wiping.
- Sitz baths: Local treatment should include sitz baths (sitting in plain warm water) followed by air drying of the vulvar area, use of topical emollients (Vaseline or Aquaphor), and topical low-potency steroids (short course) to control inflammation and/or itching.
- Trauma from repeated rubbing or other causes is treated in the same manner.
- Congenital abnormalities, such as ectopic ureter, will respond to the above regimen but will eventually need definitive surgical treatment.

ONGOING CARE

FOLLOW-UP RECOMMENDATIONS

Patient Monitoring

- Follow-up appointment or phone call should be arranged 1 week following the initial diagnosis.
- To prevent recurrence in younger children, avoid irritants such as bubble bath, encourage proper wiping technique, and avoid unnecessary antibiotics.
- In sexually active adolescents, consistent use of condoms should be stressed to prevent the spread of STIs.

ALERT

- Antibiotic use may result in the development of candidiasis.
- Caution with over-the-telephone therapy of vaginal pruritus as candidiasis may be incorrect. If a patient using an antifungal is not better in 5 days, she must see the practitioner.

PROGNOSIS

When treated, patients with vaginitis, vulvovaginitis, and bacterial vaginosis generally do well.

COMPLICATIONS

- Pelvic inflammatory disease (PID)
- Scarring in the female reproductive tract
- Pelvic pain syndrome and infertility
- Untreated bacterial vaginosis has been associated with premature labor, premature rupture of membranes, and increased risk of acquiring STIs.

ADDITIONAL READING

- Brook I. Microbiology and management of polymicrobial female genital tract infections in adolescents. *J Pediatr Adolesc Gynecol.* 2002;15:217–226.
- Centers for Disease Control and Prevention (CDC). Sexually transmitted diseases treatment guidelines, 2010. *MMWR Recomm Rep.* 2010;59(RR-12):1–109.
- Eckert LO. Clinical practice: Acute vulvovaginitis. *N Engl J Med.* 2006;355:1244–1252.
- Freeto JP, Jay MS. "What's really going on down there?" A practical approach to the adolescent who has gynecologic complaints. *Pediatr Clin North Am.* 2006;53(3):529–545.
- Nyirjesy P. Vaginitis in the adolescent patient. *Pediatr Clin North Am.* 1999;46:733–745
- Schwebke JR. Gynecologic consequences of bacterial vaginosis. *Obstet Gynecol Clin North Am.* 2003;30:685–694.
- Syed T, Braverman P. Vaginitis in adolescents. *Adolesc Med Clin.* 2004;15(2):235–251
- Whaitir S, Kelly P. Genital gonorrhoea in children: Determining the source and mode of infection. *Arch Dis Child.* 2011;96:247–251. doi:10.1136/adc.2009

CODES

ICD9

- 041.9 Bacterial infection, unspecified, in conditions classified elsewhere and of unspecified site
- 616.10 Vaginitis and vulvovaginitis, unspecified

ICD10

- N76.0 Acute vaginitis
- N76.1 Subacute and chronic vaginitis

FAQ

- Q: Is the presence of gardnerella on vaginal culture sufficient to diagnose bacterial vaginosis?
- A: No. The diagnosis of bacterial vaginosis requires 3 of the following criteria: Elevated pH, fishy odor, clue cells on a wet mount, vaginal discharge, and/or a positive Gram stain.
- Q: Can vaginitis be confused with a urinary tract infection?
- A: Yes. Prominent vulvar and vestibular inflammation would strongly suggest a vulvovaginal source.
- Q: Can girls be asymptomatic for herpes simplex virus and HPV infections?
- A: Yes. Sexually active girls may carry these diseases without symptoms.

V

VASCULAR BRAIN LESIONS (CONGENITAL)

Sabrina E. Smith
Dennis J. Dlugos

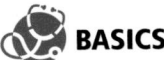 **BASICS**

DESCRIPTION

- Developmental venous anomalies (DVAs) are the most common vascular malformation of the brain, representing 60% of all central nervous system vascular malformations. Also known as venous angiomas, DVAs are made up of a cluster of venous radicles that drain into a collecting vein. They occur in 2.5–3% of the general population.
- DVAs are associated with cavernous malformations (see below) in 8–40% of cases, and 20% of patients with mucocutaenous venous malformations of the head and neck have DVAs. They are also associated with sinus pericranii, a communication between intracranial and extracranial venous drainage pathways in which blood may circulate bidirectionally.
- Cavernous malformations (CMs), also known as cavernous hemangiomas or cavernomas, are multilobulated, low-pressure and slow-flow vascular structures filled with blood, thrombus, or both. They do not contain elastin or smooth muscle. There is no intervening brain tissue except at the periphery of the lesion.
- Arteriovenous malformations (AVMs) are abnormal clusters of vessels that connect arteries and veins without a true capillary bed and have intervening gliotic brain tissue.
- Vein of Galen malformations (VOGMs) are a specific type of congenital arteriovenous malformation that involve the vein of Galen, which flows into the straight sinus after draining the internal cerebral veins and basal veins.
- Sturge–Weber syndrome (SWS), also known as encephalotrigeminal angiomatosis, is characterized by leptomeningeal angiomatosis, facial facial port wine stain (capillary malformation), and glaucoma. Some patients have all 3 findings, though others have just 1 or 2 features.

PATHOPHYSIOLOGY

- DVAs are an extreme variation of normal venous development. Typically, venous drainage in the brain occurs through a superficial system and a deep system. DVAs result when a deep venous territory drains toward the surface, or when a superficial territory drains to the deep venous system instead of draining in the expected direction. Intervening brain tissue is normal. The mechanism responsible for DVA formation is unknown.
- The pathogenesis of CMs is unknown, though the report of cases of new cavernoma development adjacent to a DVA suggests that DVAs may lead to CM formation. Most CMs occur sporadically, though familial syndromes exist. Several genes have been associated with familial CMs.

- The cause of AVM formation is unknown. A failure of normal capillary development with dysplastic vessels forming between primordial arteriovenous connections has been suggested.
- VOGMs are embryonic arteriovenous malformations consisting of choroidal arteries draining into the precursor of the vein of Galen. They develop between weeks 6 and 11 of fetal life.
- SWS occurs sporadically in 1/40,000–50,000 births, and no gene defect had been identified. The pathophysiology is thought to be venous dysplasia, in which the primordial venous plexus that is normally present at 5–8 weeks of gestation fails to regress. The location of this plexus around the cephalic end of the neural tube and under the ectoderm destined to form the facial skin accounts for the clinical features. Venous stasis occurs due to the absence of normal cortical venous structures, and hypoperfusion of brain tissue occurs. These findings are unilateral in the majority but can be bilateral in up to 20% of cases.

 DIAGNOSIS

HISTORY

- DVAs are usually benign and asymptomatic, coming to clinical attention as an incidental finding on a neuroimaging study.
- Headache, seizure, and intracerebral hemorrhage are common in patients with CMs and AVMs. Focal neurologic deficits may result from intracerebral hemorrhage or compression of underlying brain structures by the vascular malformation.
- 95% of newborns with VOGMs present in CHF. Others present with hydrocephalus, subarachnoid hemorrhage, intraventricular hemorrhage, or failure to thrive.
- Infants and older children usually present with hydrocephalus, headache, seizures, exercise-induced syncope, or subarachnoid hemorrhage.
- Facial port wine stain, seizures and glaucoma are common in SWS. Other neurologic symptoms include hemiparesis, developmental delay, mental retardation, and strokelike episodes presenting with hemiparesis and visual field defects.

PHYSICAL EXAM

- Physical exam is normal in children with DVAs and children with CMs or AVMs that have not ruptured. Focal neurologic deficits may persist following intracerebral hemorrhage associated with CMs or AVMs.

- In newborns with VOGMs, signs of congestive heart failure such as tachycardia, respiratory distress and hepatomegaly may occur. A continuous cranial bruit may be heard over the posterior skull, and bounding carotid pulses and peripheral pulses may be present. Scalp veins may be dilated.
- Older infants and children with VOGMs also may present with CHF, but more often demonstrate increased head circumference, focal neurologic signs, and failure to thrive. Proptosis may be noted.
- Children with SWS often have a facial port wine stain, most often in the V1 distribution. Glaucoma is also common. Hemiparesis or seizures may develop.

DIAGNOSTIC TESTS & INTERPRETATION

Routine blood studies are usually normal. Chest x-ray studies and electrocardiogram may reveal typical changes of high-output CHF in patients with VOGMs.

Imaging

- Neuroimaging studies are required for definitive diagnosis.
- DVAs can be visualized on contrast-enhanced CT or MRI. Diagnosis is made by visualization of the typical "caput medusa" appearance of the radially arranged veins draining into a collecting vein, seen as a linear or curvilinear focus of enhancement. They can also be visualized with conventional angiography, though this is not required unless a patient presents with an acute hemorrhage.
- MRI is better than CT at demonstrating CMs, which have a mulberry appearance. On MRI they are well-circumscribed lesions of mixed signal intensity on T1 and T2-weighted sequences. Contrast enhancement is variable. They are best seen on gradient-echo-T2-weighted images or susceptibility-weighted images, which are sensitive to hemosiderin or deoxyhemoglobin.
- AVMs can be seen with CT/CTA, MR/MRA and conventional angiography. Dynamic sequences are required to characterize the anatomy of feeding and draining vessels. Conventional angiography is the gold standard.
- VOGMs can be diagnosed on fetal ultrasound or MRI. In newborns cranial ultrasound shows a large, hypoechoic structure in the region of the vein of Galen. CT shows a high-density mass that enhances with contrast. MRI shows an area of decreased signal intensity or signal void because of high flow within the malformation. CT and MRI also show areas of cerebral ischemia or hemorrhage. Conventional angiography is required before intervention.
- In SWS, CT may show calcifications or atrophy. Gadolinium-enhanced MRI is the most sensitive study, showing leptomeningeal enhancement due to pial angiomatosis. Initial CT and MRI are often normal in the newborn period, so follow-up imaging is required.

DIFFERENTIAL DIAGNOSIS

- The differential diagnosis for headaches and seizures, common presenting symptoms of brain vascular malformations, is broad. CNS infection, vascular malformation and mass lesion can result in both. Other causes of seizure include dysplasia, remote brain injury, genetic and idiopathic. Other causes of headache include benign conditions such as migraine and tension headaches and structural abnormalities such as Chiari I malformations.
- VOGMs must be considered in any newborn with unexplained CHF (especially high-output failure), hydrocephalus, or intracranial hemorrhage. Other causes of high-output CHF in the newborn include anemia, hyperthyroidism, and other arteriovenous malformations.
- Intracranial hemorrhage may result from AVMs, CMs, aneurysms, bleeding diatheses, hypertension, or trauma in neonates and children. In older children, sickle cell disease, vasculopathies including moyamoya syndrome, and vasculitis can also lead to hemorrhage.

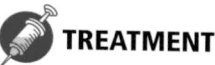 TREATMENT

ADDITIONAL TREATMENT
General Measures
- DVAs do not typically require treatment.
- Anticonvulsants should be used to treat seizures.
- Surgical resection is the only treatment option for CMs, though conservative management may be indicated if the risk of surgery outweighs the potential benefit.
- Treatment options for AVMs include resection via microsurgery, embolization, stereotactic radiosurgery and conservative management. Risk of hemorrhage ranges 0.9–34% per year, so decisions about treatment should be guided by symptoms at presentation and structural features of the AVM.
- Treatment of choice for VOGMs in all ages is endovascular embolization. Direct surgical intervention has unacceptable risks and is no longer recommended. Radiosurgery has been used in a small number of clinically stable older patients. Refractory CHF prompts intervention in neonates. Treatment in older infants and children is indicated to prevent cerebral ischemia (from arterial steal or from venous infarction) and to prevent hydrocephalus. Embolization can be completed in stages over a few months after CHF is controlled.
- Ventriculoperitoneal shunts may be required in patients who develop hydrocephalus following intracerebral hemorrhage related to CM or AVM, or in patients with VOGMs.

- Treatment in SWS is targeted to symptoms, using anticonvulsants for seizures and eye drops or ocular shunts for glaucoma. Low-dose aspirin is recommended at the time of diagnosis to prevent further brain injury due to impaired cerebral blood flow. Seizures can lead to ongoing brain injury by increasing metabolic demand in brain tissue that has abnormal perfusion at baseline, so aggressive seizure management is recommended. Some children with intractable epilepsy may be good candidates for epilepsy surgery.

 ONGOING CARE

- Generally, no specific follow-up is required for patients with DVAs.
- Follow-up with a neurologist is indicated for patients with CMs, AVMs, VOGMs, and SWS.
- Neurosurgical consultation is indicated for patients with CMs, AVMs, VOGMs.
- A follow-up CT or MRI is indicated to evaluate patients with new neurologic signs or symptoms.
- Ophthalmologic follow-up is indicated for patients with SWS and most patients with VOGMs, especially prior to treatment when hydrocephalus may develop.

PROGNOSIS
- Prognosis is excellent for patients with isolated DVAs.
- Prognosis for patients with CMs and AVMs depends on the size, location, presenting symptoms, and specific characteristics of the lesion. Patients who have experienced an intracerebral hemorrhage have worse prognosis than those who have not.
- For patients with VOGMs, earlier age of symptoms is associated with worse prognosis. Mortality in neonates with symptomatic lesions is 36%. In a recent meta-analysis of 337 patients treated with endovascular embolization between 2001 and 2010, 84% had a good or fair clinical outcome, and mortality was 16%.
- Prognosis in patients with SWS depends on the extent and location of involvement. Seizures occur in the majority (~85%) with low-normal intelligence or mental retardation in ~35%.

COMPLICATIONS
- Death can occur in patients with intracerebral hemorrhage due to CMs or AVMs.
- Mortality approaches 100% in untreated patients with VOGMs.
- In severe case of VOGMs, 80% of cardiac output may be delivered to the head because of the low vascular resistance within the malformation. Cardiac ischemia may occur because of decreased coronary artery blood flow.
- Intracerebral hemorrhage may occur as a result of CMs, AVMs, and VOGMs or as a complication of treatment.

- Longer-term complications from CMs, AVMs, and VOGMs include mental retardation, seizures, hydrocephalus, and chronic motor impairment.
- In patients with SWS, visual impairment can result if glaucoma is difficult to control. Persistent hemiparesis can develop.

PATIENT MONITORING
- Serial neuroimaging should be performed in patients with CMs, AVMs, and VOGMs to guide the timing of treatment and to assess for recurrence.
- Head circumference should be monitored in patients with VOGMs as a marker of hydrocephalus.

ADDITIONAL READING

- Geibprasert S, Pongpech S, Jiarakongmun P, Shroff MM, et al. Radiologic assessment of brain arteriovenous malformations: What clinicians need to know. *RadioGraphics*. 2010;30:483–501.
- Hartmann A, Mast H, Choi JH, Stapf C, et al. Treatment of arteriovenous malformations of the brain. *Curr Neurol Neurosci Rep*. 2007;7:28–34.
- Khullar D, Andeejani AMI, Bulsara KR. Evolution of treatment options for vein of Galen malformations: A review. *J Neurosurg Pedi*. 2010;6:444–451.
- Puttgen KB, Lin DDM. Neurocutaneous vascular syndromes. *Childs Nerv Syst*. 2010;26:1407–1415.
- Rammos SK, Maina R, Lanzino G. Developmental venous anomalies: Current concepts and implications for management. *Neurosurgery*. 2009;65:20–30.
- Ruiz DSM, Yilmaz H, Gailloud P. Cerebral developmental venous anomalies: Current concepts. *Ann Neurol*. 2009;66:271–283.

 CODES

ICD9
- 747.81 Anomalies of cerebrovascular system
- 759.6 Other hamartoses, not elsewhere classified

ICD10
- Q28.3 Other malformations of cerebral vessels
- Q85.8 Other phakomatoses, not elsewhere classified

FAQ

- Q: Can the AVM recur after treatment?
- A: Arteriovenous malformations have a propensity to recur. Imaging studies give a good indication of the likelihood of recurrence.
- Q: How does a vascular malformation cause seizures?
- A: Seizures can result from ischemia, hemorrhage, or acute hydrocephalus associated with the malformation.

VENTRICULAR SEPTAL DEFECT

Ronn E. Tanel
Stanford Ewing (5th edition)

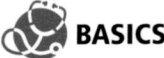 **BASICS**

DESCRIPTION

- A ventricular septal defect (VSD) is an opening in the ventricular septum, resulting in a communication between the left ventricle (LV) and the right ventricle (RV). The ventricular septum can be divided into 4 major areas:
  - Inlet/canal septum
  - Membranous/conoventricular septum
  - Muscular septum (largest)
  - Conal/infundibular/outlet septum (includes conal septal hypoplasia and malalignment types)
- There are several corresponding types of VSDs that have different natural histories and associated problems:
  - Inlet VSDs: Usually part of an atrioventricular (AV) canal defect, 5–7% of all VSDs
  - Membranous/conoventricular VSDs: 80% of all VSDs by classic teaching; fewer than muscular VSDs by echo data
  - Muscular VSDs: Usually single and small but can be multiple and of variable size; 5–20% of all VSDs by classic teaching, but 90% are inaudible
  - Conal septal hypoplasia VSDs: Usually large and unrestrictive; associated with aortic valve (AoV) cusp prolapse and aortic insufficiency
  - Anterior malalignment VSDs: Usually associated with RV outflow tract obstruction. Paradigms: Tetralogy of Fallot, double outlet RV
  - Posterior malalignment VSDs: Usually associated with LV outflow tract obstruction. Paradigms: Subaortic stenosis with coarctation or interrupted aortic arch
- There may also be multiple VSDs of different types in a single patient. Many complex forms of congenital heart disease include a VSD.

EPIDEMIOLOGY

Incidence
VSDs are the most common form of congenital heart disease, occurring in ~1.5–5.7 per 1,000 term births and ~ 4.5–7.0 per 1,000 preterm births, by classic teaching. Echo data show a high incidence of asymptomatic muscular VSDs, occurring in ~53 per 1,000 live births.

RISK FACTORS

Genetics
3% of children with VSDs have a parent with a VSD. VSD is the most common lesion in trisomies 21, 13, and 18, but >95% of children with VSDs have normal chromosomes. Congenital heart disease that includes a conal septal malalignment VSD (e.g., tetralogy of Fallot) or VSD with a conal truncal malformation (e.g., truncus arteriosus or interrupted aortic arch type B) have an 8–50% incidence of microdeletion of chromosome 22.

PATHOPHYSIOLOGY

- Both the size of the VSD and the ratio of pulmonary (PVR) to systemic vascular resistance (SVR) determine the direction and amount of shunting.
  - Small VSD: The VSD imposes high resistance to flow with a large LV-to-RV pressure gradient, usually resulting in normal RV pressures. The restrictive size results in a small left-to-right shunt. The VSD size is usually ≤1/4 the size of the AoV annulus. The workload of the ventricles is normal.
  - Moderate VSD: The VSD imposes modest resistance to flow, usually resulting in mildly elevated RV pressures. The amount of shunting can still be large and is determined by the PVR/SVR ratio. The VSD size is usually 1/3–2/3 the size of the AoV annulus. The workload of the ventricles is increased.
  - Large VSD: The VSD imposes no resistance to flow and is unrestrictive, resulting in systemic RV pressures and RV hypertension. The workload of the ventricles is markedly increased.
- The lower the PVR/SVR ratio, the greater the degree of left-to-right shunting. A large left-to-right shunt leads to pulmonary vascular congestion, tachypnea, tachycardia, and hepatomegaly, all signs of congestive heart failure (CHF). The amount of CHF correlates directly with shunt size, and usually peaks at 6–8 weeks of age, timed with the nadir of physiologic anemia. Lack of significant CHF in patients with a large VSD signifies elevated PVR and requires careful evaluation. Cardiac catheterization may be required in these patients to provide additional data.
- If a large VSD is left untreated, pulmonary vascular obstructive disease will eventually develop, leading to reversal of the shunt, cyanosis, and RV failure (Eisenmenger syndrome).

℞ DIAGNOSIS

HISTORY

- Small VSD: The child is usually asymptomatic, with normal growth and development. Most commonly, a murmur is detected at 1–6 weeks of age.
- Moderate VSD: The child is usually symptomatic with slow weight gain and sparing of longitudinal growth. There is often an increased incidence of respiratory infections. Sweating and fatigue with feeding may be present.
- Large VSD: The child is usually quite symptomatic, especially with a larger shunt, showing signs of CHF and marked failure to thrive.
- Children with Eisenmenger syndrome have cyanosis, fatigue, and symptoms of right heart failure.

PHYSICAL EXAM

- Small VSD:
  - The child usually appears healthy with normal growth.
  - The heart action is quiet but there is often an associated systolic thrill along the left sternal border with a membranous VSD, in contrast to a small muscular VSD.
  - Heart sounds are normal. A high-frequency, pansystolic murmur is present in membranous VSDs, whereas in muscular VSDs the murmur is not pansystolic.
  - The murmur is loudest over the region of the VSD.
- Moderate VSD:
  - The child usually appears in mild distress with tachycardia and tachypnea.
  - The heart action is increased and there is often still an associated thrill.
  - The P2 component of S2 may be normal or accentuated.
  - A medium frequency, pansystolic murmur is present over the location of the VSD.
  - A mid-diastolic rumble is present over the mitral listening area (apex), as a result of a significant shunt and indicates ≥2:1 pulmonary to systemic flow ratio. Hepatomegaly may be present.
- Large VSD:
  - The child usually appears ill with marked distress and marked tachycardia and tachypnea, proportional to the size of the left-to-right shunt.
  - The heart action is markedly increased without a thrill. The P2 component of S2 is loud and narrowly split as a result of pulmonary hypertension.
  - A soft, low-frequency pansystolic murmur is present over the VSD.
  - The loudness of the mid-diastolic rumble is proportional to the size of the left-to-right shunt.
  - CHF physical exam signs are proportional to the size of the left-to-right shunt, but are usually present to a significant degree.
- If significant aortic insufficiency develops, a high-frequency, early diastolic murmur is heard along the left sternal border.
- In newborns whose PVR has not yet fallen, the increased heart action remains the key to diagnosis as auscultation may be unimpressive.
- Likewise, in children with elevated PVR, the increased heart action remains the key to diagnosis. Auscultation shows a narrowly split S2 with a loud P2. The murmur loudness is dependent on VSD size and shunt, but often is soft or absent and unimpressive.

- Once Eisenmenger syndrome develops (secondary to pulmonary vascular obstructive changes), patients manifest cyanosis, clubbing, an increased RV impulse, a narrowly split S2 with a loud P2 component and a soft or absent VSD murmur. There may be a systolic murmur of tricuspid insufficiency at the left lower sternal border (LLSB), a high-frequency early diastolic murmur of pulmonary insufficiency, or an S3 at the LLSB. There is usually associated jugular venous distention and hepatomegaly, indicating high right-sided filling pressures.

DIAGNOSTIC TESTS & INTERPRETATION
Lab
- ECG:
  - Small VSD: Normal
  - Moderate VSD: Left ventricular hypertrophy (LVH)
  - Large VSD: Biventricular hypertrophy (BVH) and left atrial enlargement (LAE)
  - Eisenmenger syndrome: Right ventricular hypertrophy (RVH) and right atrial enlargement (RAE)
- Cardiac catheterization:
  - Generally reserved for patients with difficult VSD anatomy, associated lesions, or for the assessment of pulmonary vascular reactivity

Imaging
- Chest radiograph:
  - Small VSD: Normal
  - Moderate VSD: Hyperinflation, cardiomegaly, increased pulmonary vascular markings
  - Large VSD: Cardiomegaly, markedly increased pulmonary vascular markings, Kerley B lines
  - Eisenmenger syndrome: Normal heart size, prominent central pulmonary arteries, and decreased peripheral vascular markings
- Echocardiogram:
  - All children with a murmur consistent with a VSD should undergo echocardiogram to define the location, size, and number of VSDs and any associated defects. Color/spectral Doppler allows visualization of the shunt direction and the amount of restriction to the VSD, if any.

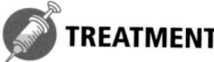 ## TREATMENT

ADDITIONAL TREATMENT
General Measures
- Small VSD: No intervention; observation and subacute bacterial endocarditis (SBE) prophylaxis for indicated procedures
- Moderate VSD: If signs of CHF develop, digoxin, diuretics, afterload reduction, and increased caloric intake are indicated.
- Large VSD: CHF often develops and requires aggressive therapy as noted above.
- Membranous and muscular VSDs often become smaller or close spontaneously. Generally, observation and/or medical therapy is indicated for a few months.

- Conoseptal hypoplasia and malalignment VSDs do not close spontaneously and therefore require surgical closure, often in infancy.
- After 1 year of life, a significant left-to-right shunt (Qp:Qs ≥2:1) or elevated pulmonary artery pressures are an indication for surgery.
- Children with elevated pulmonary artery pressures (≥1/2 systemic) should undergo repair before 2 years of age, even if CHF symptoms are controlled.
- Development of complications, including aortic insufficiency, subaortic membrane, and double-chamber RV, is usually an indication for surgical repair.
- Surgical correction may be contraindicated if the PVR is >8 Wood units/m^2.
- Recent series of surgical VSD closure report a mortality of 0.6–2.3%.
- Complete heart block occurs in <2% of patients postoperatively, but requires pacemaker therapy when it occurs.

 ## ONGOING CARE

PROGNOSIS
- Spontaneous closure: Usually by age 2 years; 90% of small muscular VSDs and 8–35% of small conoventricular VSDs
- Prognosis with surgical closure is excellent.
- The risk of Eisenmenger syndrome is considered minimal if large VSDs are surgically closed by 2 years of age.
- Caveat: Despite timely VSD surgical closure, a tiny percentage of patients still go on to develop Eisenmenger syndrome.

COMPLICATIONS
- All VSDs: Endocarditis—overall rate of 15 cases per 10,000 person-years of follow-up
- Moderate-to-large VSDs: LV volume overload, left atrial hypertension, CHF, poor growth, Eisenmenger syndrome
- Specific types:
  - Inlet VSDs: Often associated with cleft mitral valve with significant AV valve insufficiency
  - Membranous/conoventricular VSDs: Risk for development of aortic insufficiency, subaortic membrane, or double-chamber RV
  - Muscular VSDs: Isolated—near-zero risk for the development of subsequent lesions
  - Conal septal hypoplasia VSDs: Risk for development of aortic insufficiency
  - Malalignment VSDs: Usually associated with outflow tract obstruction and distal great artery hypoplasia/obstruction

PATIENT MONITORING
SBE prophylaxis is recommended for 6 months after complete closure (spontaneous or surgical) of a VSD.

ADDITIONAL READING
- Aquilar NE, Eugenio Lopez J. Ventricular septal defects. *Bol Asoc Med P R*. 2009;101:23–29.
- Hoffman JI, Kaplan S. The incidence of congenital heart disease. *J Am Coll Cardiol*. 2002;39: 1890–1900.
- Kidd L, Driscoll DJ, Gersony WM, et al. Second natural history study of congenital heart defects: Results of treatment of patients with ventricular septal defects. *Circulation*. 1993;87(Suppl 1): I38–I51.
- McDaniel NL. Ventricular and atrial septal defects. *Pediatr Rev*. 2001;22:265–270.
- Penny DJ, Vick GW. Ventricular septal defect. *Lancet*. 2011;377:1103–1112.

 ## CODES

ICD9
745.4 Ventricular septal defect

ICD10
Q21.0 Ventricular septal defect

FAQ
- Q: Should children with a murmur consistent with a VSD undergo echocardiogram?
- A: Yes, to define the location, size, and number of VSDs, and any associated lesions.
- Q: Should children with VSD have SBE prophylaxis?
- A: Based on the revised 2007 American Heart Association Guidelines, isolated VSD does not warrant SBE prophylaxis. However, SBE prophylaxis is recommended for 6 months following complete surgical or interventional catheterization closure (no residual defect) of a VSD.
- Q: Should asymptomatic children with a small VSD have activity restrictions?
- A: No, if there are no other problems

V

VENTRICULAR TACHYCARDIA

Arvind Hoskoppal
Jonathan R. Kaltman (5th edition)

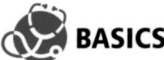

BASICS

DESCRIPTION

- Ventricular tachycardia (VT) is a series of 3 or more repetitive beats originating from the ventricle at a rate faster than the upper limit of normal for age. It usually is a wide complex rhythm, but can appear narrow in infants. VT may, but not always, have atrioventricular (AV) dissociation.
- Sustained ventricular tachycardia: Lasts >30 seconds
- Nonsustained ventricular tachycardia: Lasts from 3 beats–30 seconds
- May be monomorphic or polymorphic
- Torsades de pointes: Associated with congenital long QT syndrome, acquired long QT, and Brugada syndrome; the QRS complexes gradually change shape and axis throughout the tachycardia. VT may present at any age.
- Premature ventricular contractions (PVCs) have been reported in 0.8–2.2% of otherwise healthy children.

Genetics

- Long QT syndrome may be inherited in an autosomal-recessive or -dominant pattern. It is related to a variety of cardiac ion channel defects, and may be associated with hearing loss and/or a family history of sudden death.
- Brugada syndrome is related to a defect in the cardiac sodium channel (SCN 5A) and appears to be inherited in an autosomal-dominant pattern.

PATHOPHYSIOLOGY

VT may result from a reentrant mechanism, triggered mechanism, or abnormal automaticity.

ETIOLOGY

- Diverse and often overlapping
- Idiopathic
- Myocarditis or dilated cardiomyopathy
- Long QT syndrome (LQTS)
- RV dysplasia
- Brugada syndrome

- Congenital heart disease (e.g., tetralogy of Fallot, transposition of the great arteries, aortic stenosis, hypertrophic cardiomyopathy, myocardial tumors, Ebstein anomaly, and pulmonary vascular occlusive disease)
- Metabolic disturbances (hypoxia, acidosis, hypo/hyperkalemia, hypomagnesemia, hypothermia)
- Drug toxicity (e.g., digitalis toxicity, antiarrhythmic agents)
- Substance abuse (cocaine, methamphetamine)
- Myocardial ischemia (e.g., Kawasaki disease, congenital coronary anomalies)
- Trauma

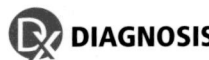

DIAGNOSIS

Based on electrocardiogram (ECG) or rhythm strip

HISTORY

- Varies widely, ranging from asymptomatic to sudden cardiac death
- Other symptoms include palpitations, presyncope or syncope, exercise intolerance, and dizziness.

PHYSICAL EXAM

- Can be normal; occasional heart rhythm irregularity secondary to frequent PVCs
- Acute, sustained VT may have signs of hemodynamic compromise, including lack of pulse
- Signs of underlying heart disease, if any are present

DIAGNOSTIC TESTS & INTERPRETATION

Lab

- Serum electrolytes, including magnesium and potassium levels, blood gas, and serum drug levels as appropriate
- Urine toxicology screen

- ECG:
  - ≥3 consecutive ventricular complexes faster than the upper limit of normal for age.
  - Bundle branch morphology (right or left) may indicate the site of origin of the VT. May have AV dissociation.
  - Typically, repolarization (T-wave) abnormalities are present.
  - The QTc interval should be measured in lead II during sinus rhythm.
  - Evaluate for Brugada syndrome in leads V1 and V2 (right bundle branch block, coved-type ST elevation, and T-wave inversion in the right precordial leads).
- Echocardiogram: Rule out congenital heart disease (CHD), pericardial and pleural effusions, tumors, and assess ventricular function.
- Ambulatory Holter monitor: Quantitative assessment of ventricular ectopy, and frequency of VT.
- Exercise stress test (>5 years old):
  - Benign PVCs are characteristically suppressed with exercise and return in the immediate recovery period.
  - Exacerbation or worsening of ventricular arrhythmias is concerning.
- Cardiac catheterization: Assessment of hemodynamics and possible coronary artery imaging
- Electrophysiologic study indications:
  - Confirm diagnosis and mechanism of a wide complex rhythm.
  - Evaluate suspected VT in the setting of structural or functional heart disease, syncope, or cardiac arrest.
  - Evaluate nonsustained VT in patients with CHD.
  - Determine appropriate medical therapy in a patient with inducible VT.
  - Evaluate syncope in the setting of palpitations (SVT versus VT).
  - Characterize VT with consideration for catheter ablation.
    - *Note*: Electrophysiologic studies are generally not helpful in individuals with LQTS.

DIFFERENTIAL DIAGNOSIS

Wide complex tachyarrhythmia:

- Should always suspect ventricular tachycardia until proven otherwise
- Supraventricular tachycardia (SVT) with aberrancy
- Antidromic tachycardia (antegrade conduction down an accessory pathway during an AV reciprocating tachycardia, e.g., Wolff–Parkinson–White syndrome)
- Atrial flutter or fibrillation with rapid antegrade conduction over an accessory pathway

 # TREATMENT

- **Acute:**
  - If the patient is hemodynamically compromised, prompt synchronized direct-current (1–2 joules/kg; adult, 100–400 joules) cardioversion is indicated.
  - Asynchronous cardioversion for ventricular fibrillation or pulseless ventricular tachycardia
  - Cardiopulmonary resuscitation as necessary
  - Lidocaine (1 mg/kg bolus over 1 minute, followed by an infusion at 20–50 mcg/kg/min, assuming normal liver and kidney function)
  - If torsades de pointes, $MgSO_4$ may be given.
  - Overdrive ventricular pacing may terminate the tachycardia; however, pacing may accelerate the VT or induce ventricular fibrillation.
  - IV amiodarone (side effect: hypotension, responds to volume)
- **Chronic:**
  - Medications:
    - Class IB (mexiletine and phenytoin). β-blockers (propranolol, atenolol, nadolol) are used in LQTS and may be effective in exercise-induced VT and postoperative CHD.
    - Class III agents (amiodarone and sotalol) should be avoided in patients with LQTS.
    - Class IC agents (flecainide) may be proarrhythmic and sudden death has been reported in patients with structural heart disease who were taking class IC agents.
  - Atrial pacing at rates slightly faster than VT rates may suppress tachycardia.
  - Catheter ablation using radiofrequency energy or cryoenergy
  - Automatic implantable cardioverter defibrillators

 # ONGOING CARE

PROGNOSIS

- Generally very good in patients with idiopathic VT and a structurally normal heart
- Suppression of ventricular ectopy with exercise has a favorable prognosis.
- In patients with heart disease (congenital or acquired) or LQTS, VT may increase the risk of presyncope, syncope, and possibly sudden death.

COMPLICATIONS

- Cardiovascular compromise (sudden death)
- Acquired cardiomyopathy (from long-standing VT and a lack of AV synchrony)

PATIENT MONITORING

- Depends on the underlying cause
- ECG, Holter monitor, and exercise stress test

ADDITIONAL READING

- Gilbert-Barness E, Barness LA. Pathogenesis of cardiac conduction disorders in children: Genetic and histopathologic aspects. *Am J Med Genet A.* 2006;140(19):1993–2006.
- Hebbar AK, Hueston WJ. Management of common arrhythmias: Part II. Ventricular arrhythmias and arrhythmias in special populations. *Am Fam Physician.* 2002;65(12):2491–2496.
- Kleinman ME, Chameides L, Schexnayder SM, et al. Part 14: Pediatric advanced life support: 2010 American Heart Association Guidelines for Cardiopulmonary Resuscitation and Emergency Cardiovascular Care. *Circulation* 2010;122: S876–S908.
- Sarrubbi B. The Wolff-Parkinson-White electrocardiogram pattern in athletes: How and when to evaluate the risk for dangerous arrhythmias, The opinion of the pediatric cardiologist. *J Cardiovasc Med (Hagerstown).* 2006; 7(4):271–278.
- Wren C. Cardiac arrhythmias in the fetus and newborn. *Semin Fetal Neonatal Med.* 2006; 11(3):182–190.
- Yabek SM. Ventricular arrhythmias in children with an apparently normal heart. *J Pediatr.* 1991; 119:1–11.

 # CODES

ICD9

- 426.82 Long QT syndrome
- 427.1 Paroxysmal ventricular tachycardia
- 746.89 Other specified congenital anomalies of heart

ICD10

- I45.81 Long QT syndrome
- I47.2 Ventricular tachycardia
- I49.8 Other specified cardiac arrhythmias

FAQ

- Q: Do frequent single PVCs require treatment?
- A: In an otherwise healthy child with a structurally normal heart, normal QT interval, and PVCs that suppress with exercise, no treatment is indicated.
- Q: Should siblings of patients with LQTS be evaluated?
- A: Yes, siblings and parents (even if asymptomatic) should have an ECG, Holter monitor, and exercise stress test for definitive evaluation of the QT interval. Commercial genetic testing is currently available to detect mutations in some of the most common genes that cause the Long QT syndrome. The test will positively identify ~75% of patients with the LQTS. Genetic testing may be considered in patients in whom there is a high suspicion of the LQTS.

V

VESICOURETERAL REFLUX

Hsi-Yang Wu
Howard M. Snyder

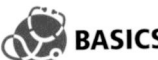 **BASICS**

DESCRIPTION
Vesicoureteral reflux (VUR) occurs when urine passes backward from the bladder to the ureters or kidneys.

EPIDEMIOLOGY
Prevalence
VUR occurs in ~1% of children. There are now clearly 2 different groups of patients:
- Those who were detected prenatally without any history of UTI:
  - ~20–30% of patients with prenatal hydronephrosis have VUR.
  - The ratio of males to females in this group is 3:1. This is believed to be caused by a period of high-pressure voiding in boys, which resolves by 18 months.
- Those who were detected after an acute UTI:
  - ~30–50% of children with UTI will have reflux, and they tend to be 2–3-year-old girls.
  - Since most children achieve urinary continence by this time, the cause of the UTI tends to be voiding immaturity and increased intravesical pressure.

RISK FACTORS
Genetics
- 30% of siblings will have low-grade reflux, but the great majority will have been asymptomatic, and renal scarring is rare.
- Parents with VUR have a 60% chance of having children with reflux:
  - Whether or not to screen siblings is controversial.
  - We elect to screen siblings with a history of recurrent febrile illnesses and girls who have not yet toilet trained.

PATHOPHYSIOLOGY
- VUR in combination with urinary tract infection can lead to pyelonephritis, renal scarring, and possibly end-stage renal disease. Primary VUR is classified into 5 grades by the International Reflux Study based on the voiding cystourethrogram (VCUG):
  - Grade I: Reflux into ureter
  - Grade II: Reflux into renal pelvis without dilation of calyces
  - Grade III: Blunting of calyces, mild dilation of ureter
  - Grade IV: Grossly dilated ureter, moderate calyceal dilation with maintained papillary impressions
  - Grade V: Grossly dilated ureter with loss of papillary impressions
- The grading scale is important because spontaneous resolution rates are significantly different between grades I–III and grades IV–V.

ETIOLOGY
- A combination of abnormal anatomy and abnormal voiding pressure:
  - Primary VUR results from either a short ureteral tunnel through the bladder wall or transient high-pressure voiding, which occurs normally in the 1st 18 months of life.
  - Patients with primary low-grade VUR can expect improvement and even resolution of the VUR with time as the ureteral tunnel grows or when bladder pressures decrease.
- Secondary VUR occurs when there is an associated lesion responsible for the abnormal anatomy or increased intravesical (bladder) pressure:
  - Patients with secondary reflux require treatment of their primary problem, and still may require surgery to treat their secondary reflux. Secondary reflux may occur in neurologically normal patients with dysfunctional voiding, ureteroceles, posterior ureteral valves, and prune belly syndrome, or in neurologically abnormal patients with spina bifida.
  - Although it may seem arbitrary, the distinction between primary and secondary reflux is important because the large prospective trials have been conducted on patients with primary reflux, and it is not appropriate to extend those findings to patients with secondary reflux.
  - Another important distinction is whether the diagnosis of VUR was made as a result of a prenatal diagnosis of hydronephrosis or whether the child presented with urinary tract infection.

℞ DIAGNOSIS

HISTORY
- Prenatal dilation of the urinary tract or UTI as presentation
- Family or sibling history of VUR
- Family history of UTI, suggestive of adherent uroepithelium
- Family history of renal failure
- Voiding history: Age at potty training
- Daytime or nighttime incontinence
- Frequency of urination
- Sensation of emptying the bladder completely
- Signs of dysfunctional voiding:
  - Urgency
  - Frequency
  - Damp underwear
  - Associated constipation: Frequency of bowel movements, suggestive of pelvic floor immaturity
- Evidence of holding urine during a bladder contraction:
  - Squatting, crossing legs
  - Compressing urethra with heel (Vincent's curtsy)

PHYSICAL EXAM
- Abdominal palpation (mainly to check for hard stool)
- Check for labial adhesions in girls
- Phimosis in boys
- Inspection and palpation of spine (possible neurogenic bladder)
- BP

DIAGNOSTIC TESTS & INTERPRETATION
Lab
A serum creatinine and urinalysis for proteinuria may be obtained if the renal ultrasound suggests significant renal scarring.

Imaging
- Renal/bladder ultrasound: This is usually obtained at the time of UTI, or if the patient had a prenatal diagnosis of hydronephrosis, at 1 week of life. The ultrasound is not as sensitive as dimercaptosuccinic acid (DMSA) scan for renal scarring. The lack of hydronephrosis does not mean that the patient does not have VUR. However, renal bladder ultrasound is a useful tool for following renal growth.
- VCUG: A contrast study is necessary for the 1st VCUG, to delineate the urethral anatomy in boys, and to accurately grade the reflux in both sexes:
  - An age-appropriate volume should be instilled in the bladder. The voiding portion of the study is important, since approximately 20% of VUR can be missed if voiding is not observed.
  - Follow-up VCUGs can be performed using radionuclide to decrease the radiation dose to the child.
- DMSA renal scan: The most accurate way to diagnose pyelonephritis and renal scarring:
  - Unfortunately, it is not possible to predict which patients will develop scarring after an acute episode.
  - If the diagnosis of upper tract infection versus cystitis is important, then the DMSA scan during an acute episode is useful.
  - The DMSA is not usually helpful with nonfebrile UTI in patients >6 months of age, since cystitis is rarely associated with high fevers.
  - Some advocate using DMSA to determine which patients require VCUG. This may allow for better segregation of high-risk patients.

DIFFERENTIAL DIAGNOSIS
In the prenatally detected group, hydronephrosis can also be due to ureteropelvic or ureterovesical junction obstruction. The important task is to differentiate primary from secondary VUR so that the parents can be appropriately counseled.

TREATMENT

ADDITIONAL TREATMENT
General Measures

- 4 prospective randomized controlled trials have concluded that medical management (prophylactic antibiotics) and surgery have essentially equal outcomes in regard to hypertension, growth, and renal scarring. Surgery was more effective at preventing pyelonephritis.
- The rate of renal scarring was equal in the medical and surgical arms of the International Reflux Study. However, the timing of renal scarring was different: In the medically treated arm, new renal scars continued to form during 5 years of follow-up, whereas in the surgical arm, the renal scars stopped within 10 months of surgery. Surgery was 95% successful in correcting reflux with a 4% complication rate. Surgery involves creation of a longer muscular backing for the ureter to create a flap-valve mechanism.
- Patients with low-grade reflux should be maintained on prophylactic antibiotics, since grades I to III have a significant rate of spontaneous resolution. Patients with high-grade reflux should be initially maintained on prophylactic antibiotics, but earlier consideration for surgical correction should be given owing to the lower rate of spontaneous resolution. Likewise, patients with reflux and renal scarring should be considered for earlier surgery since they have already shown a propensity toward UTI and renal damage.
- Antibiotic prophylaxis does not mean treatment-dose antibiotics. The antibiotics chosen are highly concentrated in the urine, and the use of high doses only selects out resistant organisms and leads to complications such as yeast infections. Amoxicillin at 10–15 mg/kg/d is used for the 1st 2 months of life, then trimethoprim/sulfamethoxazole (40 mg/200 mg/5 mL) at 0.25 mL/kg/d (equivalent to 2–3 mg/kg daily of trimethoprim) or nitrofurantoin at 1–2 mg/kg/d.
- Patients who are detected with VUR in infancy should probably have a contrast VCUG at 18 months to 2 years to determine the grade of reflux, since this can improve as voiding pressures normalize.
- In toilet-trained children, maintenance of a regular voiding pattern and regular bowel movements decreases the risk of febrile UTI and increases the chance of VUR resolution.
- Patients being managed on antibiotic prophylaxis undergo annual follow-up nuclear VCUG to document improvement or resolution of VUR. Grading is less precise with nuclear VCUG, but the radiation dose is lower. A renal ultrasound is also obtained to follow renal growth and check for gross renal scars.
- Indications for crossing over to surgery are:
  - Patient or parent wishes
  - Noncompliance with medical therapy
  - Breakthrough infections while on medical therapy (This is a relative indication. A careful review of voiding habits should be carried out to ensure that dysfunctional voiding is not responsible for the UTI. Lack of new renal scarring may suggest that continued medical management is appropriate.)
  - New renal scarring
  - Persistence of reflux after an appropriate period of antibiotic prophylaxis

- The use of injectable bulking agents has at best 80% success 1 year after 1 treatment, progressively decreasing as the grade of VUR increases. As additional experience is gained with injection therapy, success rates tend to increase. The minimally invasive nature of these treatments is balanced with a lower success rate. Deflux (dextranomer/hyaluronic acid) is the most commonly used injectable in the US and is widely used in treating grade I–III VUR. Deflux treatment in higher grades of VUR and the use of laparoscopic ureteral reimplantation are currently being explored in select patients.
- The use of continuous antibiotic prophylaxis has been questioned because while it decreases the risk of UTI, it has not been shown to decrease renal scarring compared to placebo. The NIH is currently sponsoring a multi-institutional trial to determine the benefits of continuous prophylaxis versus placebo treatment. The Swedish Reflux Trial showed a decreased rate of febrile UTI in girls with grades III–IV VUR who underwent injection therapy or prophylaxis, compared to those on surveillance. New renal scarring was less frequent in girls on prophylaxis compared to those on surveillance.
- The management of patients who continue to have VUR after several years of prophylactic antibiotics is controversial. Although most feel comfortable taking boys with VUR off antibiotics after age 6 because the risk of renal scarring is decreased and boys are at low risk for UTI, the adolescent girl is at increased risk for complications during pregnancy if she has a past history of UTI. The few studies on this subject seem to indicate that the patients with VUR and recurrent UTI are at risk for pregnancy-related complications whether or not the VUR has been surgically corrected, suggesting that the propensity toward UTI plays a more important factor.

ONGOING CARE

FOLLOW-UP RECOMMENDATIONS
Patient Monitoring
Patients with renal scarring should have annual BP checks and urinalysis for proteinuria.

PROGNOSIS

- In primary VUR, 80–90% of grades I and II reflux, 70% of grade III, 40% of grade IV, and 25% of grade V resolve over a 5-year period.
- The annual rate of spontaneous resolution is between 15% and 20% for grades I–III.
- Bilateral reflux is less likely to resolve than unilateral reflux.
- Patients age 5 years or older at presentation are less likely to resolve than those who present at <5 years of age.
- Ultimately the goal is prevention of renal scarring rather than resolution of the reflux, since low-pressure sterile reflux does not lead to renal scarring.
- The patient's propensity toward UTI must be considered as well as whether the reflux is resolving.

ADDITIONAL READING

- Brandstrom P, Neveus T, Sixt R, et al. The Swedish Reflux Trial: IV renal damage. *J Urol.* 2010;184(1): 292–297.
- Craig J, Simpson J, Williams G, et al. Antibiotic prophylaxis and recurrent urinary infection in children. *N Engl J Med.* 2009;361(18):1748–1759.
- Elder JS, Diaz M, Caldamone AA, et al. Endoscopic therapy for vesicoureteral reflux: A meta-analysis. I. Reflux resolution and urinary tract infection. *J Urol.* 2006;175:716–722.
- Keren R, Carpenter M, Greenfield S, et al. Is antibiotic prophylaxis in children with vesicoureteral reflux effective in preventing pyelonephritis and renal scars? A randomized, controlled trial. *Pediatrics.* 2008;122(6):1409–1410.
- Pennesi M, Travan L, Peratoner L, et al. Is antibiotic prophylaxis in children with vesicoureteral reflux effective in preventing pyelonephritis and renal scars? A randomized, controlled trial. *Pediatrics.* 2008;121(6):e1489–e1494.
- Peters C, Skoog S, Arant B, et al. Summary of the AUA guideline on management of primary vesicoureteral reflux in children. *J Urol.* 2010; 184(3):1134–1144.

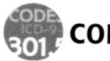

CODES

ICD9
- 593.70 Vesicoureteral reflux unspecified or without reflux nephropathy
- 753.8 Other specified anomalies of bladder and urethra

ICD10
- N13.70 Vesicoureteral-reflux, unspecified
- Q62.7 Congenital vesico-uretero-renal reflux

FAQ

- Q: How soon after a UTI should the VCUG be performed?
- A: Once the patient is clinically stable and afebrile and sterile urine has been documented, the VCUG can be performed.
- Q: Why not operate immediately to repair the reflux when it is diagnosed?
- A: Depending on the grade of reflux, many cases will resolve in time (see "Treatment").

V

VIRAL HEPATITIS

Jeremy King
Vani V. Gopalareddy

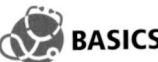 **BASICS**

DESCRIPTION

Viral hepatitis is defined as a systemic viral infection, in which the predominant manifestation is that of hepatic injury and dysfunction. It is primarily caused by hepatotropic viruses, which include hepatitis A to E; however, 10% of cases are caused by other viruses, such as Epstein-Barr virus (EBV), cytomegalovirus (CMV), herpes simplex virus (HSV), varicella-zoster virus (VZV), rubella, parvovirus, adenovirus, enteroviruses such as coxsackie B, and others. In the US, hepatitis B accounts for 40% of acute viral hepatitis cases, whereas hepatitis A and C account for 30% and 20%, respectively.

EPIDEMIOLOGY

Incidence

- Hepatitis A: 125,000–200,000 infections per year worldwide. ~22,000 US cases per year. 10% occur in daycare centers that care for children who are not toilet trained.
- Hepatitis B: 140,000–320,000 infections per year worldwide. ~40,000 US cases per year. Since the 1991 implementation of universal vaccination of infants, the incidence of acute hepatitis B virus (HBV) cases in US children has declined from 3.03 per 100,000 in 1990 to 0.34 in 2002.
- Hepatitis C: 20,000 infections per year in the US
- Hepatitis E: Common in poorly developed countries but rare in the US. Can cause chronic hepatitis in liver transplant patients

Prevalence

- Hepatitis B: US has a low prevalence with <1% of the population infected. Higher rates in certain subgroups such as immigrants from endemic areas, homosexuals, and parenteral drug users
- Hepatitis C: US has prevalence of 1.8%, representing ~3.9 million people (85% chronically infected)

RISK FACTORS

- Hepatitis A (transmission: Fecal–oral):
  - Daycare attendance, household exposure, travel to endemic areas
  - Maximum infectivity 2 weeks before jaundice
- Hepatitis B and C (transmission: Blood, body fluids, and sexual contact):
  - Recipients of blood or blood products
  - IV drug users
  - Multiple sexual partners
  - Homosexual males
  - Body piercing and tattoos
  - HIV-positive status
  - Infants born to a mother with hepatitis B or C
  - Household contacts with hepatitis B or C

GENERAL PREVENTION

- Good sanitation, hygiene, screening blood products, condom use, safe disposal of needles
- Hepatitis A:
  - Vaccine (Havrix, Vaqta): 0.5-mL dose IM and 2nd dose 6–12 months later
  - Current guidelines recommend that all children between the ages of 1 and 18 years should be vaccinated.
  - Use for travelers to endemic regions, daycare workers, and children with other liver diseases, and during outbreaks.
  - Avoid return to daycare center for 2 weeks after illness subsides.
  - Hepatitis A immunoglobulin for close contacts of infected individuals.
- Hepatitis B:
  - Screen all pregnant women.
  - Hepatitis B vaccine to all infants at birth; complete 3 vaccine series 0.5-mL dose IM during infancy
  - Vaccine and hepatitis B immunoglobulin to high-risk infants

PATHOPHYSIOLOGY

- Acute viral hepatitis tends to affect the liver parenchyma, whereas chronic viral hepatitis affects portal and periportal areas.
- In acute hepatitis, there is spotty necrosis, panlobular disarray, increased cellularity, pleomorphism of hepatocytes, and focal parenchymal necrosis.
- Chronic viral hepatitis is defined by continuing viral replication and inflammation of the liver for >6 months and affects the portal tracts predominantly but also extends into the parenchyma (interface hepatitis).
- Worsening injury leads to extensive fibrosis that occurs between portal tracts (portal bridging), nodular changes, and, finally, cirrhosis.

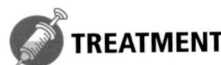 **DIAGNOSIS**

HISTORY

History should focus on risk factors for viral exposure, sick contacts, travel history, and high-risk behaviors. Family history of liver or autoimmune disease, medications, or drug and alcohol use should also be explored.

PHYSICAL EXAM

- Jaundice, hepatomegaly, or tenderness over the liver may or may not be present.
- Signs and symptoms:
  - Fever
  - Malaise and fatigue
  - Nausea and vomiting, anorexia
  - Jaundice: In hepatitis A, seen in 88% of adults but only 65% of children
  - Hepatomegaly
  - Right upper quadrant (RUQ) abdominal pain
  - Dark urine and pale stools
  - Arthralgias/arthritis
  - The vast majority of affected patients are minimally symptomatic or asymptomatic, especially with chronic infection.

DIAGNOSTIC TESTS & INTERPRETATION

Lab

- Liver function tests:
  - Marked elevation of aspartate aminotransferase/alanine aminotransferase (AST/ALT) during acute infection. May be normal to mildly elevated in chronically infected individuals
  - Bilirubin from mild to marked elevation
- In severe hepatitis, monitor PT/PTT, albumin, electrolytes, glucose, and CBC.
- Biochemical markers for each virus for diagnosis, management, and monitoring:
  - Antihepatitis A virus (HAV) IgM: Recent infection
  - Anti-HAV IgG: Past exposure or immunization acquired
  - Hepatitis B surface antigen (HBsAg): Current infection, acute or chronic
  - Hepatitis B surface antibody (HBsAb): Immunized or resolved infection
  - Hepatitis B "e" antigen (HBeAg): Significant infectivity, viral replication
  - Hepatitis B "e" antibody (HBeAb): End of severe infectivity (except in precore mutants). Endpoint for hepatitis B therapy
  - Hepatitis B virus core antigen (HBcore) IgM: Early phase of acute infection, not present in chronic HBV
  - HBcore total Ab: Exposed to HBV
  - HBV DNA: Quantification useful to assess viral load
  - HBV mutations: Useful to assess resistance to treatment with lamivudine
  - HDV Ab: Exposure to hepatitis D
  - HCV Ab: Exposure to HCV
  - HCV RNA: Quantitative, assess viral load; qualitative, assess presence/absence of virus
  - HCV genotype: Useful to determine duration of treatment and likelihood of response
  - HBV genotyping not clearly established to guide therapy or determine prognosis

Diagnostic Procedures/Other

Liver biopsy is often needed to determine type and extent of liver damage. It is usually indicated prior to initiation of antiviral therapy in children because risk of treatment may sometimes outweigh the benefit.

Pathological Findings

A wide array of histologic features is possible on liver biopsy, including inflammation, necrosis, and fibrosis, based on the severity and chronicity of disease.

DIFFERENTIAL DIAGNOSIS

- Many disorders give rise to elevated transaminases, and clues to a viral origin are based on the history, serology, and histologic findings.
- One often invokes the diagnosis of non-A, non-B, non-C hepatitis when the cause is almost certainly viral but no virus is isolated.
- Other possibilities include drug-induced, ischemic, alcoholic, or autoimmune hepatitis, as well as Wilson disease or α_1-antitrypsin deficiency.

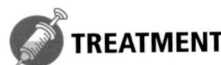 **TREATMENT**

MEDICATION (DRUGS)

- Hepatitis A:
  - No specific therapy is available.
  - Postexposure prophylaxis with pooled human serum globulin at dose of 0.02 mL/kg for household contacts, intimate exposure contacts, and children and staff in nursery or daycare centers with outbreaks

- Hepatitis B:
  - Postexposure prophylaxis with hepatitis B vaccine and hepatitis B immunoglobulin (HBIG) is indicated for neonates born to mothers who are hepatitis B carriers, after sexual contact with carriers, and after accidental exposure to infected blood products.
  - There is no treatment for acute hepatitis B, though lamivudine is reported to be effective in fulminant hepatitis due to HBV.
  - Chronic hepatitis B is treated with the antiviral agents interferon, adefovir, tenofovir, or entecavir when ALT is elevated.
  - The most successful treatment is still interferon with 33% success rate in meta-analysis of adult studies. Interferon-α: 10 MU/m^2 given 3 times a week for 6 months (not recommended for use in infants and very young children <2 years).
  - Response rates may be slightly lower for nucleoside analog reverse transcriptase inhibitors (nRTIs) like lamivudine, adefovir, and entecavir, although they have fewer side effects. Endpoint to stop treatment is not clear.
  - Lamivudine is no longer used owing to a high rate of resistance with prolonged treatment.
  - Adefovir dipivoxil (Hepsera) is approved for children >12 years at the dose of 10 mg/d and entecavir (Baraclude) for children >16 years at a dose of 0.5–1 mg daily.
  - Adefovir often works well in patients with lamivudine-resistant disease.
  - Tenofovir appears to have more potent antiviral activity than other nRTIs and rare resistance. It is not yet approved in children but trials in adolescents are under way.
  - The factor most predictive of treatment response in children with chronic hepatitis B is an elevated pretreatment ALT. Low viral DNA, young age, and female sex imply favorable response.
  - Each year, 5–10% of children spontaneously clear hepatitis Be antigen (HBeAg), at which point the disease usually becomes inactive, although a few will later reactivate.
  - Some pediatric studies suggest that antiviral therapy hastens but does not increase the rate of HbeAg seroconversion.
- Hepatitis C:
  - Antiviral therapy is indicated for children with progressive disease or advanced histologic features.
  - Pegylated interferon and ribavirin is the treatment of choice for chronic hepatitis C and was approved for children >3 years of age in 2008.
  - The combination dose is PEG-IFN (60 mcg/m^2 once weekly) + ribavirin (15 mg/d in 2 divided doses).
  - Treatment duration depends on genotype:
    - Genotypes 1 and 4: 1 year (type 1 most common in US)
    - Genotypes 2 and 3: 6–12 months (types more likely to respond to therapy)
  - Maintaining higher doses is possible by balancing side effects with erythropoietin and granulocyte-macrophage–colony-stimulating factor (GM-CSF) to counter hemolytic complications and leukopenia.
  - Several protease inhibitors have recently been approved for treatment of chronic HCV in adults in combination with PEG-IFN and ribavirin. Initial results are excellent, but these drugs are not yet approved for use in children.

ADDITIONAL TREATMENT
General Measures
- Severe cases need inpatient care; acute liver failure requires intensive care at a liver transplant center.
- Monitor and correct coagulation defects and fluid, electrolyte, and acid–base imbalances.
- Report acute cases to public health department.
- Patients with acute liver failure should be transferred to a pediatric transplant center.

ONGOING CARE
FOLLOW-UP RECOMMENDATIONS
- Serial measurement of serum AST/ALT, viral markers, α-fetoprotein, and ultrasound of the liver
- Liver biopsy pretreatment and for evaluation of disease progression

PROGNOSIS
- Hepatitis A:
  - Mild disease usual
  - Rarely results in relapsing, fulminant, or cholestatic disease
  - No chronic liver disease
  - Mortality <1%
  - Protective antibodies develop in response to infection and persist for life.
- Hepatitis B:
  - Fulminant hepatitis 1–2%
  - Mortality 0.5–2%
  - Chronic sequelae: Carrier state 10–95%, chronic hepatitis 5–10% (but 90% if vertically acquired), cirrhosis <5%, hepatocellular carcinoma (more common in HBV to viral integration into the genome)
- Hepatitis C:
  - Fulminant hepatitis 1%
  - Chronic sequelae: Carrier state 10–20%, chronic hepatitis 10–50%, cirrhosis 10–20%, hepatocellular carcinoma 5–10%
  - HCV is the most common indication for liver transplantation in adults.
  - In adult studies, sustained virologic response to therapy may decrease HCV-related hepatocellular carcinoma.

COMPLICATIONS
- Patients with advanced liver disease due to chronic hepatitis B or C are at risk of complications associated with cirrhosis and portal hypertension.
- Patients with chronic hepatitis B or with cirrhosis due to hepatitis C are at increased risk of hepatocellular carcinoma.
- Hepatitis B
  - Hepatitis D coinfection: Acute hepatitis B and D virus infection occur simultaneously:
    - Mortality rate of 1–10%
  - Hepatitis D superinfection: Acute hepatitis D occurs in a chronic carrier of hepatitis B:
    - Mortality rate of 5–20%
    - Acute liver failure occurs more frequently, chronic hepatitis 75%
    - Chronic HDV causes cirrhosis in 70–80% of patients and is a rapidly progressive disease compared with chronic hepatitis B alone. Cirrhosis has been noted to occur in as little as 2–10 years.

Pregnancy Considerations
Hepatitis E: Mortality of 20% caused by acute liver failure in pregnant women

ADDITIONAL READING

- Haber BA, Block JM, Jonas MM, et al. Recommendations for screening, monitoring and referral of pediatric chronic hepatitis B. *Pediatrics*. 2009;124(5):e1007–e1013.
- Hochman JA, Balistreri WF. Chronic viral hepatitis: Always be current! *Pediatr Rev*. 2003;24(12): 399–409.
- Laurer GM, Walker BD. Hepatitis C virus infection. *N Engl J Med*. 2001;345(1):41–52.
- Lok AS, McMahon BJ. Chronic hepatitis B. *Hepatology*. 2007;45(7):507–539.
- Mieli-Vergani G, Heller S, Jara P, et al. Autoimmune hepatitis. *J Pediatr Gastroenterol Nutr*. 2009; 49(2):158–164.
- Mohan N, Gonzalez-Peralta RP, Fujisawa T, et al. Chronic hepatitis C infection in children. *J Pediatr Gastroenterol Nutr*. 2010;50(2):123–131.
- Murray KF, Shah U, Mohan N, et al. Chronic hepatitis. *J Pediatr Gastroenterol Nutr*. 2010;47(2):225–233.
- Strader DB, Wright T, Thomas DL, et al. Diagnosis, management and treatment of hepatitis C. *Hepatology*. 2004;39(4):1147–1171.

CODES

ICD9
- 070.1 Viral hepatitis A without mention of hepatic coma
- 070.30 Viral hepatitis B without mention of hepatic coma, acute or unspecified, without mention of hepatitis delta
- 070.9 Unspecified viral hepatitis without mention of hepatic coma

ICD10
- B17.10 Acute hepatitis C without hepatic coma
- B19.9 Unspecified viral hepatitis without hepatic coma
- B19.10 Unspecified viral hepatitis B without hepatic coma

FAQ

- Q: Why do infants who acquire HBV at birth have a higher incidence of chronicity?
- A: The immaturity of the neonatal immune system contributes to the higher incidence of chronicity in this population. Furthermore, prenatal exposure to HBeAg may result in immune tolerance to the virus.
- Q: Should a mother with HCV positivity breastfeed?
- A: Transmission of HCV via breast milk is unlikely.

VOLVULUS

Joy L. Collins

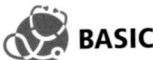 **BASICS**

DESCRIPTION

Volvulus is torsion of the gut upon itself or upon a narrow mesenteric pedicle. It may be acute and complete or chronic and intermittent. Segmental volvulus may occur in the small intestine or colon, but in children midgut volvulus is the most common form.

- Of patients with abnormal rotation, 50–80% will be symptomatic in infancy. Most patients will present by age 1 year with symptoms of acute bowel obstruction.
- Patients with a rotational anomaly may present with midgut volvulus without any preexisting symptoms.
- Malrotation with midgut volvulus is most common in neonates.

COMMONLY ASSOCIATED CONDITIONS

- Incomplete rotation of the intestine during fetal development is the most common form of malrotation.
- Incomplete malrotation results in a narrow mesenteric stalk for the midgut loop centered on the superior mesenteric artery and vein, and obstructing bands (Ladd bands) across the duodenum, predisposing to midgut volvulus.

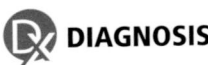 **DIAGNOSIS**

HISTORY

- Symptoms of acute or recurrent obstruction at birth or in the 1st year of life
- Recurrent bilious emesis (most important symptom) with or without acute abdomen
- ALERT: Some patients with midgut volvulus present with NONBILIOUS emesis.
- Feeding intolerance
- Chylous ascites and/or protein-losing enteropathy due to lymphatic congestion and bacterial overgrowth. These may present as history of abdominal distension, diarrhea, edema, or generalized/localized extremity swelling.
- In older children, recurrent abdominal pain and emesis. Older infants may have symptoms that mimic colic.
- Bloody stools or blood-tinged mucus per rectum

PHYSICAL EXAM

- Abdominal tenderness or fullness with or without distention
- Irritability, lethargy
- Brawny edema of abdominal wall
- Drawing up of legs
- Tachypnea and tachycardia

DIAGNOSTIC TESTS & INTERPRETATION

Lab

May see metabolic acidosis, thrombocytopenia

Imaging

- Abdominal radiograph may show dilated stomach and duodenum or may be normal.
- Abdominal ultrasound may show inversion of normal position of superior mesenteric artery (SMA) and vein (SMV; if SMV is located to left of SMA, suggestive of malrotation).
- Upper GI tract radiography may show abnormal position of the ligament of Treitz and, if volvulus is present, a corkscrew appearance of the midgut.
- The radiographic appearance, though, may be confusing because there are many patterns of duodenal malrotation reported. Abdominal radiograph may show double bubble sign of duodenal obstruction.

- In the absence of a corkscrew or Z-shaped duodenum, patterns that usually indicate volvulus or obstructing Ladd bands, colon position has greater prognostic implication, especially when the cecum is positioned in the right upper quadrant (RUQ) or left upper quadrant (LUQ).
- Barium enema shows an abnormal position of the cecum (but 10% of patients will have normal position of the cecum).
- In cases of colonic volvulus, contrast enema shows beak deformity at site of volvulus.

DIFFERENTIAL DIAGNOSIS

- Duodenal atresia
- Perforated viscus
- Necrotizing enterocolitis
- Meconium ileus or meconium plug syndrome
- Ileal atresia
- Hirschsprung enterocolitis
- Appendicitis
- Intussusception
- Pyelonephritis

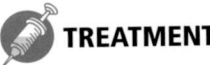 **TREATMENT**

ADDITIONAL TREATMENT

General Measures

- Emergent surgical exploration is indicated for volvulus
- Close monitoring of fluids and electrolytes to prevent shock, gastric suction, and intravenous antibiotics (as bowel resection may be required)
- Laparotomy with intestinal detorsion and resection of ischemic portions of the intestine

- Ladd procedure: Volvulus is untwisted in a counterclockwise direction, transduodenal bands are divided, mesenteric base is broadened, intestine is arranged in a position of nonrotation, and appendix is removed.
- If the entire midgut is ischemic, the volvulus may be untwisted, with re-exploration in 12–24 hours.
- Some surgeons feel that there is a role for laparoscopic approach to Ladd procedure in the stable patient.

 ONGOING CARE

FOLLOW-UP RECOMMENDATIONS
Patient Monitoring
- Prognosis depends on extent of involvement and degree of ischemia.
- Monitor closely for feeding intolerance postoperatively.
- Persistent symptoms after surgical repair suggest pseudo-obstructive motility disorder.
- Although rare, patients may have recurrent volvulus after a Ladd procedure.
- Pitfalls:
  – May take hours to days to become symptomatic
  – Symptoms may be mistaken for colic in infants or cyclic emesis in older children.
  – Delayed diagnosis may result in strangulation and infarction, leading to short gut syndrome.

COMPLICATIONS
- Intermittent or acute obstruction
- Strangulation resulting in ischemia and loss of midgut
- Protein-losing enteropathy can also result from strangulation.
- Short gut syndrome if significant length of intestine is lost or is poorly functional postoperatively

ADDITIONAL READING

- Hagendoorn J, Vieira-Travassos D, van der Zee D. Laparoscopic treatment of intestinal malrotation in neonates and infants: Retrospective study. *Surg Endosc.* 2011;25:217–220.
- Ismail A. Recurrent colonic volvulus in children. *J Pediatr Surg.* 1997;32:1739–1742.
- Jabra AA, Eng J, Zaleski CG, et al. CT of small-bowel obstruction in children: Sensitivity and specificity. *AJR Am J Roentgenol.* 2001;177:431–436.
- Malek MM, Burd RS. Surgical treatment of malrotation after infancy: A population based study. *J Pediatr Surg.* 2005;40(1):285–289.
- Murphy FL, Sparnon AL. Long-term complications following intestinal malrotation and the Ladd's procedure: A 15 year review. *Pediatr Surg Int.* 2006;22(4):326–329.
- Nehra D, Goldstein A. Intestinal malrotation: Varied clinical presentation from infancy through adulthood. *Surgery.* 2011;149(3):386–393.
- Rodriguez EJ, Gama MA, Ornstein SM, et al. Ascariasis causing small bowel volvulus. *Radiographics.* 2003;23:1291–1293.
- Salas S, Angel CA, Salas N, et al. Sigmoid volvulus in children and adolescents. *J Am Coll Surg.* 2000;190:717–723.

 CODES

ICD9
- 537.89 Other specified disorders of stomach and duodenum
- 560.2 Volvulus
- 751.4 Anomalies of intestinal fixation

ICD10
- K31.819 Angiodysplasia of stomach and duodenum without bleeding
- K56.2 Volvulus
- Q43.3 Congenital malformations of intestinal fixation

FAQ

- Q: In what age group is volvulus most common?
- A: Midgut volvulus is most common in the neonatal period.
- Q: How can the signs and symptoms of volvulus be distinguished from gastroesophageal reflux?
- A: Although both intermittent volvulus and gastroesophageal reflux (GER) may present with vomiting, the emesis in GER is not bilious. Bilious emesis, abdominal pain, and lethargy are signs of an abdominal obstruction, requiring further examination.
- Q: Should one think of intermittent volvulus in the differential diagnosis of children with presentation of protein-losing enteropathy?
- A: In children with unusual presentations of protein-losing enteropathy, especially with emesis as a contributing feature, exclude intermittent volvulus.
- Q: Have cases of gastric, small bowel, and colonic volvulus been reported?
- A: Yes, but rarely. Gastric volvulus patients do not manifest the full spectrum of signs and symptoms such as abdominal distension, vomiting, and abdominal pain. There are 2 main types of gastric volvulus: Organoaxial (longitudinal axis of rotation) and mesentericoaxial (transverse axis of rotation through greater and lesser stomach curves). In 2/3 of cases, there is an associated abnormality where the stomach is affixed to the esophagus.

  Small bowel volvulus has been reported in association with ascariasis.

  Colonic volvulus (usually sigmoid or cecum) is quite rare in children, and has been associated with Hirschsprung disease. Colonic volvulus also has been seen in mentally handicapped children, many times in association with aerophagia and chronic constipation. Colonic volvulus is a significant cause of death in the mentally handicapped population.

V

VOMITING

Matthew J. Ryan

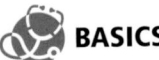

BASICS

DEFINITION

- Vomiting is the forceful expulsion of gastric contents through the mouth.
- Regurgitation is defined as small, effortless mouthfuls of food or stomach contents.
- Retching is contraction of the abdominal musculature against a closed glottis therefore there is no expulsion of stomach contents. This is also referred to as "dry heaves."

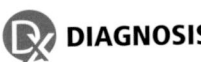

DIAGNOSIS

- Vomiting is a prominent feature of many disorders of infancy and childhood and is often the only presenting symptom of many diseases.
- Vomiting can be:
  - A defense mechanism to expel ingested toxins
  - An abnormality of or damage to the area postrema (a.k.a. the chemoreceptor trigger zone or vomiting center) located at the base of the fourth ventricle in the brain.
  - A result of intestinal obstruction or anatomic/mucosal abnormalities
  - The result of a generalized metabolic disease
- A full history should include medication and drug use, trauma, family history of migraines and, in adolescents, questions regarding feeding disorders (bulimia) and intercourse (pregnancy). Special attention should be directed to the timing of the emesis related to meals, position and time of day.

HISTORY

- Fever: Infectious causes of vomiting are common.
- Abdominal pain and frequent, forceful, or bilious emesis: Often associated with anatomic or obstructive intestinal disorder. Very commonly obstruction of a lumen (i.e., common bile duct stone or ureteropelvic junction (UPJ) obstruction) can present as vomiting.
- Age of patient: Pyloric stenosis and inborn errors of metabolism almost always present in infancy with vomiting, dehydration, and biochemical abnormalities.
- Mental retardation, pica, and patchy baldness: Indicate foreign body or hair ingestion and the development of a gastric bezoar.
- Nausea and epigastric pain related to meals: Often indicate gastritis, gastric emptying delay, or gallbladder disease

- Alleviated by meals: May signify gastroesophageal reflux or gastric ulcer
- Alternating vomiting and lethargy: May indicate intussusception
- Chronic headaches, fatigue, weakness, weight loss, and early morning vomiting: Neurologic causes of vomiting secondary to increased intracranial pressure
- Right- or left-sided abdominal pain: May indicate renal disease, inflammatory bowel disease
- Periodic chronic vomiting on a monthly basis may suggest a cyclic vomiting syndrome (CVS).

PHYSICAL EXAM

A careful and complete physical examination can often provide excellent clues as to the cause of vomiting in children:

- Visible bowel loops: Obstruction
- Palpation for bowel loops and tenderness, and auscultation for evidence of absent bowel sounds or borborygmi (rumbling bowel sounds): Intestinal obstruction
- Rectal examination: Testing the stool for occult blood
- Discoloration of skin and sclera: Jaundice (liver/gallbladder or metabolic disease)
- Orange tint of sclera or skin: Hypervitaminosis A
- Unusual odor: Metabolic disease
- Chronic vomiting: Evidence of neurologic dysfunction, including nystagmus, head tilt, papilledema, abnormal reflexes, and weakness
- Tense anterior fontanelle: May indicate meningitis, hydrocephalus, or vitamin A toxicity
- Enlarged parotid glands and hypersalivation: Bulimia and other feeding disorders
- Pelvic examination: Pregnancy, pelvic inflammatory disease, or ovarian disease

DIAGNOSTIC TESTS & INTERPRETATION

Lab

- CBC: Anemia and iron deficiency can occur with intestinal duplication and obstruction, gastritis/esophagitis, inflammatory bowel disease (IBD) and ulcer disease.
- Blood chemistry:
  - Electrolyte abnormalities are found in pyloric stenosis and metabolic abnormalities.
  - An elevated alanine aminotransferase, conjugated bilirubin, and gamma-glutamyl transferase (GGT) can indicate liver, gallbladder, or metabolic disease.
- Urinalysis: Pyelonephritis, nephrolithiasis
- Amylase/lipase: Pancreatitis
- BUN/creatinine: If elevated, renal disease
- Urine culture: UTI
- Stool studies: occult blood, infection

Imaging

- Plain abdominal radiographic study: Obstruction
- Abdominal ultrasound:
  - Liver, gallbladder, renal, pancreatic, ovarian, or uterine disease
  - In infants, abdominal ultrasound is the test of choice for pyloric stenosis.
  - Useful when considering abdominal abscess and appendicitis
- Contrast radiography: Intestinal anatomic abnormalities (malrotation, intussusception, volvulus)
- Gastroesophageal scintigraphy (gastric emptying study): Evaluate rate of gastric emptying
- Abdominal CT: Not generally indicated for evaluation of vomiting, although it is an effective tool when more anatomic abdominal detail is required (abscess, tumor). Also, a head CT is helpful in evaluation of neurologic causes of vomiting although brain MRI provides better imaging of the brain stem where the vomiting center is located.

Diagnostic Procedures/Surgery

- Endoscopy: Esophageal, gastric, and duodenal inflammation (esophagitis, gastritis, ulcer disease, celiac disease, eosinophilic enteritis) as well as for obtaining cultures for unusual infections (duodenal *Giardia*, *Helicobacter pylori*/cytomegalovirus gastritis)
- Gastroesophageal manometry to evaluate for primary or secondary motility disorders

DIFFERENTIAL DIAGNOSIS

- Disorders of GI tract:
  - Anatomic:
    - Esophageal: Stricture, web, ring, atresia
    - Stomach: Pyloric stenosis, web, duplication
    - Intestine: Duodenal atresia, malrotation, duplication
    - Colon: Hirschsprung disease, imperforate anus
  - Motility:
    - Achalasia
    - Gastroesophageal reflux
    - Intestinal pseudo-obstruction
  - Obstruction:
    - Foreign body/bezoar
    - Intussusception
    - Stricturing Crohn disease
    - Volvulus
    - Incarcerated hernia
  - Hepatobiliary disease
  - Eosinophilic enteritis
  - Appendicitis
  - Necrotizing enterocolitis
  - Peritonitis
  - Celiac disease
  - Peptic ulcer
  - Trauma:
    - Duodenal hematoma
    - Pancreatitis (pseudocyst)

- Neurologic:
  - Intracranial mass lesions:
    - Tumor
    - Cyst
    - Subdural hematoma
  - Cerebral edema
  - Hydrocephalus
  - Pseudotumor cerebri
  - Migraine (head, abdominal)
  - Seizures
  - Post concussion syndrome
- Renal:
  - Obstructive uropathy:
    - Ureteropelvic junction obstruction
    - Hydronephrosis
    - Nephrolithiasis
  - Renal insufficiency
  - Glomerulonephritis
  - Renal tubular acidosis
- Metabolic:
  - Inborn errors of metabolism:
    - Galactosemia
    - Fructose intolerance
    - Hereditary fructose intolerance
    - Amino acid or organic acid metabolism
    - Urea cycle defects
    - Fatty acid oxidation disorders
    - Lactic acidosis
- Infection:
  - Sepsis
  - Meningitis
  - UTI
  - Parasites
  - *Giardia*
  - *Ascaris*
  - *H. pylori*
  - Otitis media
  - Viral/Bacterial
  - Gastroenteritis
  - Viral hepatitis (A, B, C)
  - Pneumonia
  - *Bordetella pertussis*
- Endocrine:
  - Diabetes:
    - Diabetic ketoacidosis
    - Gastroparesis
  - Adrenal insufficiency
- Respiratory:
  - Sinusitis
  - Laryngitis
- Immunologic:
  - Food allergy
  - Anaphylaxis
  - Graft-versus-host disease
  - Chronic granulomatous disease

- Other:
  - Pregnancy
  - Rumination
  - Bulimia
  - Psychogenic
  - Motion sickness
  - Cyclic vomiting syndrome
  - Overfeeding
  - Pain
  - Medications:
    - Drugs (chemotherapy)
    - Vitamin toxicity
  - Vascular (superior mesenteric artery syndrome)
  - Porphyria
  - Familial dysautonomia

ALERT

Evidence of hematemesis, intestinal obstruction (bilious vomiting), dehydration, neurologic dysfunction, or an acute abdomen should be treated as a medical emergency, and hospitalization should be considered.

 TREATMENT

- Therapy should be directed toward the underlying etiology. Historically, antiemetic medications are contraindicated in cases of acute vomiting although some studies now suggest ondansetron may reduce frequency of admission.
- Oral rehydration therapy is typically the first line of treatment. IV fluids are appropriate if oral rehydration therapy fails or is contraindicated.
- Neurotransmitters involved in vomiting include dopamine, acetylcholine, histamine, endorphins, serotonin, and neurokinin. The mechanism of many antiemetic medications is blockade of these neurotransmitters.

ISSUES FOR REFERRAL
- Chronic vomiting (2–3 weeks)
- Weight loss
- Severe abdominal pain or irritability
- GI bleeding
- Evidence of intestinal obstruction
- Serum electrolyte abnormalities
- Abnormal neurologic examination
- Dehydration
- Signs of an acute abdomen
- Lethargy

ADDITIONAL READING

- Fedorowicz Z, Jagannath VA, Carter B. Antiemetics for reducing vomiting related to acute gastroenteritis in children and adolescents. *Cochrane Database Syst Rev.* 2011;(9):CD005506.
- Freedman SB, Adler M, Seshadri R, Powell EC. Oral ondansetron for gastroenteritis in a pediatric emergency department. *N Engl J Med.* 2006; 354(16):1698–1705.
- Li B. Cyclic vomiting syndrome: A brain-gut disorder. *Gastroenterol Clin.* 2003;32(3):997–1019.
- Li BUK, Sunku BK. Vomiting and nausea. In: Wyllie R, Hyams JS, eds. *Pediatric Gastrointestinal and Liver Disease*, 3rd ed. Philadelphia PA: Saunders; 2006.

 CODES

ICD9
- 536.2 Persistent vomiting
- 787.01 Nausea with vomiting
- 787.03 Vomiting alone

ICD10
- R11.10 Vomiting, unspecified
- R11.11 Vomiting without nausea
- R11.2 Nausea with vomiting, unspecified

FAQ

- Q: What are the most common causes of vomiting in an infant?
- A: Gastroesophageal Reflux and milk protein allergy although congenital pyloric stenosis, sepsis and malrotation must be ruled out.
- Q: What is the appropriate ER management for a patient presenting with hematemesis?
- A: Insertion of 2 large IVs with IV fluid rehydration are the initial steps to stabilize the patient. Oftentimes, NG lavage is both therapeutic and diagnostic to help determine the amount and briskness of the GI bleed.
- Q: Is bilious emesis always associated with small bowel obstruction?
- A: Repeated episodes of vomiting can cause duodenal contents to reflux into the stomach resulting in bile stained emesis without small bowel obstruction. Nevertheless, evaluation should include an abdominal film looking for air-fluid levels and bowel loop distension.

V

VON WILLEBRAND DISEASE

Char Witmer

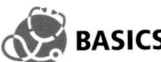 **BASICS**

DESCRIPTION
- An inherited bleeding disorder caused by either a quantitative deficiency or qualitative defect of the von Willebrand protein
- Characterized by mucocutaneous bleeding or bleeding after surgical procedures

EPIDEMIOLOGY
Prevalence
- The prevalence of von Willebrand disease in the general pediatric population is estimated to be ~1%.

RISK FACTORS
Genetics
- The gene for von Willebrand factor is found on chromosome 12.
- Type 1 (see "Pathophysiology") follows an autosomal dominant inheritance pattern with variable penetrance.
- Type 2 varies; it can be autosomal dominant or recessive.
- Type 3 follows an autosomal recessive inheritance pattern.

GENERAL PREVENTION
- Avoid contact sports.
- For patients with recurrent epistaxis, measures should be taken to avoid drying of the mucosa by applying petroleum jelly, humidifying the air, and reducing trauma to the nasal mucosa by keeping the fingernails short and discouraging nose picking.
- It may be advisable for patients to wear an emergency ID bracelet indicating that they have von Willebrand disease in the event they are involved in an accident that renders them unconscious.
- Avoid medications that negatively affect platelet function (i.e., ibuprofen, aspirin).
- Combination oral contraceptive pills are very effective for some patients with menorrhagia.
- Appropriate hemostatic therapy prior to dental extractions or surgical procedures to prevent bleeding

PATHOPHYSIOLOGY
- Von Willebrand factor is a large multimeric protein that allows platelets to adhere to sites of endothelial injury, initiating the primary step in hemostasis—formation of the platelet plug.
- Von Willebrand factor also serves as a carrier for factor VIII in the peripheral circulation, protecting it from degradation. Deficiency of von Willebrand factor results in a shorter factor VIII half-life, causing a lower level of circulating factor VIII.

- When the von Willebrand factor is either deficient or defective, primary hemostasis is compromised, resulting in a bleeding diathesis characterized by easy bruising, frequent epistaxis, menorrhagia, and prolonged bleeding following surgical or dental procedures.
- Von Willebrand disease is an inherited bleeding disorder; however, acquired forms of von Willebrand disease have been described in association with hypothyroidism, Wilms tumor, other neoplasms, cardiovascular disorders with increased shear stress, myeloproliferative disorders, uremia, and medications including ciprofloxacin, griseofulvin, and valproate therapy.
- Classification: There are three major categories of von Willebrand disease:
  - Type 1:
    ○ Mild to moderate quantitative deficiency of von Willebrand factor
    ○ The most common type, accounting for 70–80% of patients
    ○ Generally a mild bleeding disorder
  - Type 2:
    ○ Qualitative deficiency of von Willebrand factor
    ○ Diagnosed in 15–20% of patients
    ○ Tend to be more significant bleeding symptoms than in type 1
    ○ Type 2 von Willebrand disease is further classified into four subtypes.
    ○ Type 2A: Loss of the intermediate- and high-molecular-weight multimers. The loss is secondary to either abnormal assembly or secretion of multimers or increased proteolytic degradation. The multimer deficiency results in decreased platelet binding.
    ○ Type 2B: An abnormal von Willebrand factor that spontaneously binds to normal platelets, resulting in accelerated clearance of these platelets and loss of high-molecular-weight multimers. This can result in mild thrombocytopenia.
    ○ Type 2N: The abnormal von Willebrand factor does not bind factor VIII optimally. This decrease in binding results in a shorter plasma half-life of factor VIII, resulting in reduced plasma factor VIII levels. Type 2N can be confused with mild hemophilia.
    ○ Type 2M: The abnormal von Willebrand factor fails to bind normally to platelets. Normal multimers
  - Type 3:
    ○ Near-complete quantitative deficiency of von Willebrand factor, which also results in a secondary deficiency of factor VIII
    ○ Accounts for <5% of patients and results in a severe bleeding disorder

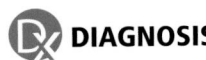 **DIAGNOSIS**

HISTORY
- A family history of von Willebrand disease or bleeding tendency is an important question in the evaluation for von Willebrand disease. However, be aware that variation in frequency and severity of bleeding symptoms can occur from person to person, even within an affected family.
- Mucosal bleeding is especially common in von Willebrand disease.
- Bruising is common, with increased quantity, increased size (>5 cm), and often in unusual locations with minimal trauma.
- Recurrent and/or prolonged epistaxis
- Menorrhagia occurs in 50–75% of women with von Willebrand disease.
- Excessive posttraumatic or postsurgical bleeding

PHYSICAL EXAM
- Bruises: Increased number, size, and/or unusual location
- May be entirely normal

DIAGNOSTIC TESTS & INTERPRETATION
Lab
- Screening tests for a bleeding disorder:
  - PT is normal in von Willebrand disease.
  - Activated partial thromboplastin time (aPTT) may be prolonged if there is a decrease in factor VIII levels but can be normal.
  - Platelet count is normal except in type 2B patients, who may have mild thrombocytopenia.
  - Bleeding time is usually prolonged, but may be normal in patients with mild type 1 von Willebrand disease (not recommended as a screening test).
  - Platelet function assay (PFA)-100 is usually prolonged, but may be normal in mild type 1 von Willebrand disease (not recommended as a screening test).
- Specific tests for von Willebrand disease include:
  - Von Willebrand factor antigen: Quantitation of von Willebrand factor by immunoassay
  - Von Willebrand factor activity (ristocetin cofactor): Assesses the function of von Willebrand factor using the antibiotic ristocetin, which induces platelet aggregation in the presence of von Willebrand factor
  - Factor VIII: Factor VIII clotting activity
  - Von Willebrand factor multimers: Multiple molecular forms of von Willebrand factor evaluated on agarose gel
    ○ Multimer analysis is important in delineating the type of von Willebrand disease. Do not send as part of the initial screening for von Willebrand disease.

DIFFERENTIAL DIAGNOSIS

- Primary hemostatic disorders:
  - Platelet function abnormalities, congenital thrombocytopenia
  - Mild inherited coagulation factor deficiencies
  - Hemophilia A (type 3 von Willebrand disease and type 2N are similar to mild and moderate factor VIII deficiency)
- Acquired and secondary hemostatic disorders:
  - Liver disease
  - Uremia
  - Acquired thrombocytopenia
  - Drugs that affect platelet function
  - Acquired factor inhibitors (extremely rare in children)
- Connective tissue disorders:
  - Ehlers-Danlos syndrome
  - Osteogenesis imperfecta
  - Scurvy
- Prolonged aPTT but no bleeding symptoms:
  - Inhibitor
  - Factor XII deficiency

ALERT

- The diagnosis of von Willebrand disease is not always straightforward:
- Because of normal physiologic variation in plasma levels of von Willebrand factor, repeated measurements over time may be necessary to establish the diagnosis.
- Conditions that may increase von Willebrand factor levels:
  - The newborn period
  - Surgery
  - Liver disease
  - Hyperthyroidism
  - High-stress states
  - Pregnancy
  - Inflammatory or infectious disease
  - Steroids
  - Oral contraceptives
  - Other estrogens

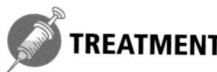

TREATMENT

General Measures

- There are several options for the management of bleeding in patients with von Willebrand disease. Superficial bleeding can usually be stopped by applying local pressure, ice, or topical thrombin, particularly in type 1.
- There are two main approaches to systemic therapy in von Willebrand disease: Increasing the release of endogenous von Willebrand factor or exogenous replacement of von Willebrand factor. The appropriate therapy depends on the type of von Willebrand disease and the clinical scenario.

MEDICATION (DRUGS)

- Desmopressin (DDAVP) is a synthetic analog of vasopressin that stimulates endothelial cell release of von Willebrand factor. It is effective in patients who have a functional von Willebrand factor, as in type 1 von Willebrand disease. It may be used for some patients with type 2 von Willebrand disease, but is ineffective in type 3:
  - Available in intravenous and intranasal formulations

- An infusion of 0.3 mcg/kg results in a 3–5-fold increase in von Willebrand factor and factor VIII; nasal administration is slightly less effective.
  - Side effects include facial flushing, light-headedness, or nausea.
  - Prior to use in a surgical setting, patients should have a trial to demonstrate an appropriate response (10% of patients do not respond).
  - May worsen thrombocytopenia in type 2B, not recommended
  - DDAVP may not be useful when prolonged hemostasis is required. After 24–48 hours, there is depletion of stored von Willebrand factor, causing it to be ineffective (tachyphylaxis).
  - It is important to remember that DDAVP will also cause fluid retention and, in some cases, hyponatremia. This can be avoided with fluid restriction following treatment.
- Humate-P or Alphanate:
  - Plasma-derived, intermediate-purity factor VIII concentrate products with adequate levels (especially large multimers) of von Willebrand factor
  - Therapy of choice for some patients with type 2 von Willebrand disease and all patients with type 3 von Willebrand disease
  - Useful in type 1 von Willebrand disease when prolonged hemostasis is necessary
- Aminocaproic acid or tranexamic acid:
  - Antifibrinolytics
  - Stabilize the fibrin clot by inhibiting the physiologic process of clot lysis
  - Best for oral mucosal bleeding
- Dose is 100 mg/kg given PO q6h

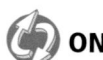 ONGOING CARE

PROGNOSIS

- Von Willebrand disease type 1 is often a very mild bleeding disorder and may go undetected.
- Most patients with von Willebrand disease have a normal life expectancy and, with proper education and treatment, minimal risk for permanent disability.
- Type 3 von Willebrand disease is a severe bleeding disorder, and life-threatening hemorrhage can occur.

COMPLICATIONS

- Significant perioperative bleeding can occur, especially with tonsillectomy, but the most common complications are recurrent epistaxis, prolonged bleeding with cuts and abrasions, and menorrhagia.
- Patients with type 3 von Willebrand disease have a more severe bleeding disorder and can have bleeding complications similar to those seen in hemophilia such as hemarthroses and intracranial hemorrhage.

ADDITIONAL READING

- Gill JC. Diagnosis and treatment of von Willebrand disease. *Hematol Oncol Clin North Am.* 2004;18: 1277–1299.
- Mannucci PM. Treatment of von Willebrand's disease. *N Engl J Med.* 2004;351:683–694.
- Mohri H. Acquired von Willebrand syndrome: Features and management. *Am J Hematol.* 2006;81:616–623.
- Pruthi RK. A practical approach to genetic testing for von Willebrand disease. *Mayo Clin Proc.* 2006;81: 679–691.
- Robertson J, Lillicrap D, James PD. Von Willebrand Disease. *Pediatr Clin North Am.* 2008;55(2): 377–392.

 CODES

ICD9
286.4 von Willebrand disease

ICD10
D68.0 Von Willebrand's disease

FAQ

- Q: What sports activities can a person with von Willebrand disease participate in safely?
- A: People with type 1 von Willebrand disease can participate in most activities, although it is usually advised to avoid situations in which significant trauma takes place, like contact sports such as football or boxing. Patients with type 3 should avoid activities with moderate trauma. For type 2 patients, the risk of bleeding varies.
- Q: Is life expectancy lower in people with von Willebrand disease?
- A: For most patients with von Willebrand disease, their life expectancy and quality of life will be normal.
- Q: Are there any medications contraindicated in a patient with von Willebrand disease?
- A: Aspirin should not be given, as it interferes with platelet function. Nonsteroidal anti-inflammatory agents cause a milder effect on platelets and should also be avoided when possible. Patients should use acetaminophen for fever or pain.

V

WARTS

Julia Belkowitz
Marney Gundlach (5th edition)

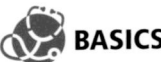 **BASICS**

DESCRIPTION

- Warts (verrucae) are benign epithelial tumors that can occur on any epithelial surface of the body and produce characteristic lesions at various anatomic sites.
- Types of warts:
  – Common warts (verruca vulgaris): Rough, minimally scaly papules and nodules on the fingers, hands, face, arms, and legs
  – Flat warts (verruca plana): Rough, flat-topped, minimally scaly papules on face, legs, and arms
  – Plantar warts (weight-bearing warts): Painful inward-growing papules and plaques on the bottom of the feet
  – Anogenital warts (condyloma acuminata): Skin-colored flat warts or moist, pink to brown, cauliflower-like lesions around the vagina and anal openings
  – Laryngeal warts (laryngeal papillomatosis): Transmitted vertically at delivery and present with stridor and progressive airway obstruction in children
- Transmission:
  – Humans are the only reservoir for human papillomavirus (HPV).
  – HPV can be transmitted by direct skin-to-skin or mucous membrane contact and by fomites.
  – Autoinoculation from common warts at another site should be considered as a possible mode of spread.
  – Clinical signs develop 1 month or more after inoculation.

EPIDEMIOLOGY

Prevalence
Affects 5–10% of children

GENERAL PREVENTION

- During contact sports, all lesions should be completely covered prior to participation. If the lesions are too extensive to completely cover, the athlete should not be allowed to participate.
- Quadrivalent HPV vaccination (protection against serotypes 6, 11, 16, 18) is recommended for girls ages 9–26 years for prevention of cervical cancer and genital warts and for boys 9–26 years to reduce likelihood of genital warts. Bivalent vaccine (protection against serotypes 16 and 18) is also available. Vaccinations are given in a 3-dose series.

PATHOPHYSIOLOGY

- The viruses have specific affinity for epidermal cells and cannot replicate in dermal connective tissue cells or other types of nonepithelial tissues.
- After implantation in the epidermis, the viruses enter the nuclei of lower and midepidermal cells. The viruses then take over the machinery of cell production. While replicating themselves, they induce a rapid proliferation of epithelial cells.
- The quantity of the virus, location of the warts, preexisting skin injury, and cell-mediated immunity all play a role in the transmission of the virus.

ETIOLOGY

- Warts are caused by HPV, which is a subgroup of papovaviruses, small double-stranded DNA viruses.
- There are >100 types of HPV:
  – Anogenital warts are often caused by types 6, 11 (most common), 16 and 18, and 31 and 45 (high risk).
  – Laryngeal papillomatosis is associated with types 6 and 11.

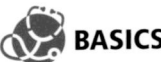 **DIAGNOSIS**

HISTORY

- Obtain wart exposure history from family members and caretakers.
- Determine the duration of the warts.
- Elicit any history of immunodeficiency.

PHYSICAL EXAM

- Common warts:
  – May be solitary or multiple and range in size from millimeters to centimeters
  – Linear patterns may be seen from autoinoculation.
  – Filiform or threadlike warts may be seen in the skin creases and on mucous membranes.
- Flat warts:
  – Small, rough, flat-topped, and minimally keratotic papules
  – Size ranges from 1–3 mm
- Plantar warts:
  – Painful, inward-growing, hyperkeratotic papules and plaques on the plantar surface of the feet
  – As a result of trauma from weight bearing, the surface of these lesions may have small black dots from thrombosed blood vessels.
- Anogenital warts:
  – May be skin-colored, flat warts or moist, pink to brown, cauliflower-like lesions in the skin creases, vulva, and scrotum, and in and around the vaginal and anal openings
  – In adolescent and adult males, the warts are localized to the penis (penile lesions are rarely seen in younger boys). The lesions are brown to slate-blue, pigmented macules and papules.
- Laryngeal warts:
  – Present with stridor and progressive airway obstruction in children

DIAGNOSTIC TESTS & INTERPRETATION
Tests are rarely needed.

Lab
Pap smears will show the presence of koilocytic cells in adolescent females with vulvar condyloma. HPV DNA testing is also available.

Diagnostic Procedures/Other
- Biopsy of flat warts shows koilocytic cells with an eccentric, shrunken nucleus surrounded by a perinuclear halo.
- Electron microscopy will show the distinctive viral particles.
- Antigen detection and molecular hybridization techniques have been used in adults to detect HPV in scrapings and biopsies of lesions.

DIFFERENTIAL DIAGNOSIS
- Common warts:
  – Molluscum contagiosum
  – Callus
- Flat warts:
  – Moles
  – Epidermal nevi
  – Tinea versicolor
  – Milia
  – Molluscum contagiosum
  – Granuloma annulare
  – Folliculitis
  – Lichen nitidus
  – Lichen planus
- Plantar warts:
  – Corns
  – Calluses
  – Foreign bodies
- Anogenital warts:
  – Irritant contact dermatitis
  – Molluscum contagiosum
  – Skin tags
  – Hemorrhoids
  – Condyloma lata of syphilis

ALERT
- Underlying immunodeficiency should be considered in any otherwise healthy child with extensive HPV infection. Hereditary severe combined immunodeficiency, acquired immunodeficiency syndrome, and selective T-cell immune defects should be considered.
- Treatment of genital warts in children and in those with immunodeficiency should be carried out in consultation with a dermatologist.
- Laryngeal papillomatosis should be treated by an otolaryngologist.

TREATMENT

When to expect improvement:

- Spontaneous resolution has been observed in common, flat, genital, and plantar warts. In healthy individuals, 75% of warts regress without treatment within 3 years without scarring.
- Any therapy and its side effects must be measured against the high rate of resolution without intervention.
- With the various treatment modalities, a response is generally seen within weeks to several months.
- Combination therapy is often required.

ADDITIONAL TREATMENT
General Measures
- Communication with families about expectations prior to therapy is important.
- Pain management using icepacks, EMLA, or other agents must be considered.
- For hyperkeratotic lesions, treatment response may be improved for many modalities if the lesion is first pared down with a scalpel or debrided with pumice or an emery board.

Additional Therapies
- Destructive techniques:
  - Salicylic acid:
    - Evidence for effectiveness of treatment
    - Can cause scarring
    - Should be considered 1st-line treatment, except in facial warts
  - Duct tape
    - Occlusion with duct tape for 6 days followed by debrided, and repeat treatment until resolution; inexpensive and associated with little discomfort
    - Causes local irritation and stimulates an immune response
    - Though early data seemed promising, more recent studies show no benefit over placebo.
  - Cryotherapy:
    - Involves using liquid nitrogen and deep-freezing the warts
    - Causes necrosis and blister formation
    - Is inexpensive, produces a rapid response, and does not require anesthesia; however, the treatment is painful and may lead to infection, scarring, and damage of normal skin
  - Cantharidin:
    - A topical applicant that triggers painless intraepidermal blisters
    - Should only be applied in the office setting
    - There is a high incidence of wart recurrence and postinflammatory pigment changes.
  - Electrocautery and CO_2 laser ablation:
    - Require local or general anesthesia
    - Can leave scars, and healing of the open wounds may take several months.
  - Phototherapies:
    - Yellow, pulsed, dye laser
    - Generates 585-nm light, which is absorbed by oxyhemoglobin in the skin and converted to heat energy
    - Pretreatment with salicylic acid may reduce the number of treatments required.
    - There is a small chance of scarring.
    - Treatment may be painful for young children.

- Photodynamic therapy:
  - Photosensitizing agent applied to wart; causes damage to cells
  - Benefits in recalcitrant warts demonstrated
- Immunotherapies
  - Cimetidine:
    - An H_2-blocker that causes nonspecific stimulation of T lymphocytes
    - This therapy has not been proven to be effective.
  - Intralesional therapies:
    - Direct injection of immune-stimulating antigen (e.g., *Candida* or mumps, etc.) treats both primary site and distant lesions.
    - Requires multiple treatments; needles can be painful and/or frightening to children.
    - Side effects include pruritus at site, fever, and myalgia.
  - Imiquimod:
    - The 1st member of a class of immune response modifiers
    - A 5% cream is applied to the warts and results in an increase in the production of cytokines, especially interferon-α.
    - The cream is approved for home treatment of adults with external anogenital warts.
    - Data have supported efficacy in children with warts.
  - Zinc
    - New use as immune modulator in warts
    - Oral administration in zinc-deficient patients shows resolution of lesions.
    - Inexpensive and painless, not yet well studied
- Antimitotic therapies:
  - Podophyllotoxin:
    - Applied to pared-down warts
    - Treatment takes several weeks to months.
    - May be painful and produce scarring
    - Especially useful in genital warts
    - Podophyllin resin not recommended owing to potential neurotoxicity
  - Retinoids
    - Topical home application of 0.05% tretinoin cream
    - Option for facial flat warts
    - Oral retinoids are not recommended.
- Chemotherapeutic agents such as 5-FU and bleomycin have been studied, but concerns about safety caution use.

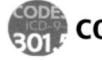 **ONGOING CARE**

FOLLOW-UP RECOMMENDATIONS
Patient Monitoring
Patients receiving treatment should be followed up at 3–4-week intervals to check the results and assess for any side effects.

PROGNOSIS
In healthy individuals, 75% of warts will spontaneously resolve without treatment within 3 years.

COMPLICATIONS
- Irritation and secondary infection of common warts may result in itching and pain.
- HPVs have also been associated with melanoma, keratoacanthoma, squamous cell carcinoma, leukoplakia, and oral carcinoma.
- Laryngeal warts can cause stridor and airway obstruction.

ADDITIONAL READING

- Boull C, Groth D. Update: Treatment of cutaneous viral warts in children. *Pediatr Dermatol*. 2011; 28:217–229.
- Herman BE, Corneli HM. A practical approach to warts in the emergency department. *Pediatr Emerg Care*. 2008;24(4):246–251.
- Sinclair KA, Woods CR, Sinal SH. Venereal warts in children. *Pediatr Rev*. 2011;32:115–121.
- Tyring S, Conant M, Marini M, et al. Imiquimod: An international update on therapeutic uses in dermatology. *Int J Dermatol*. 2002;41:810–816.

CODES

ICD9
- 078.10 Viral warts, unspecified
- 078.11 Condyloma acuminatum
- 078.19 Other specified viral warts

ICD10
- B07.0 Plantar wart
- B07.8 Other viral warts
- B07.9 Viral wart, unspecified

FAQ

- Q: How can one differentiate corns and/or calluses from warts?
- A: Using a no. 15 blade, pare down the surface of the wart. If the surface is smooth with normal markings without small black dots (thrombosed blood vessels) at the base, then they are not warts.
- Q: I am not sure if the lesions are warts. What else can I do in the office to confirm the diagnosis?
- A: Apply 3–5% acetic acid solution, and the lesions will turn white if they are warts. This, however, is not a specific test.
- Q: A child is seen for anogenital warts. What is the role of the physician?
- A: The child needs a complete medical examination. The anogenital area should be examined for any signs of sexual abuse. All skin lesions should be documented and possibly photographed. Serologic studies for syphilis and cultures for gonorrhea should be considered. Family members and caretakers should be asked about anogenital and common warts. Parents should be informed that anogenital warts could be caused by sexual abuse, particularly in children >3 years of age. Consultation with a child abuse expert should be considered.

W

WEIGHT LOSS
Mark F. Ditmar

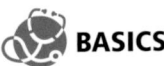

BASICS

DEFINITION
A documented decrease in weight from a previous measurement. Outside of the newborn period (weight loss in the first 2 weeks is common), acute illnesses resulting in fluid loss, and obese adolescents voluntarily on a designed weight reduction program, weight loss is an unusual and worrisome symptom, regardless of the percentage decline.

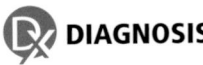

DIAGNOSIS

- Determine the acuity or chronicity and severity of weight loss, and the need for hospitalization
- Attempt to narrow the diagnostic possibilities by history and physical exam, particularly by assessing if the loss might be attributable to diminished intake, diminished absorption, or increased requirements.

DIFFERENTIAL DIAGNOSIS
- **Congenital/anatomic**
  - Congenital heart disease
  - Pyloric stenosis
  - GI malformation (duodenal atresia, annular pancreas, volvulus)
  - Short bowel syndrome
  - Lymphangiectasia
  - Superior mesenteric artery syndrome
  - Gastroesophageal reflux
  - Immunodeficiency disorders
  - Hirschsprung disease
- **Infectious**
  - Urinary tract infection (UTI)
  - Tuberculosis
  - Stomatitis
  - Osteomyelitis
  - HIV
  - Hepatitis
  - Parasitic disease
  - Abscess, intra-abdominal
  - Gastroenteritis
  - Pericarditis
  - Histoplasmosis
  - Acute severe febrile illness (pyelonephritis, pneumonia, septic arthritis)
- **Toxic, environmental, drugs**
  - Lead poisoning
  - Mercury poisoning
  - Vitamin A poisoning
  - Chronic methylphenidate, dextroamphetamine, or valproic acid use
  - Substance abuse, especially amphetamines and crack cocaine
- **Trauma**
  - Chronic subdural hematomas
- **Tumor**
  - Diencephalic syndrome
  - Leukemia
  - Lymphoma
  - Pheochromocytoma
  - Other neoplasms

- **Genetic/metabolic**
  - Diabetes mellitus
  - Diabetes insipidus
  - Hyperthyroidism
  - Cystic fibrosis
  - Shwachman syndrome
  - Addison disease
  - Hypercalcemia
  - Congenital adrenal hyperplasia
  - Lactose intolerance
  - Renal tubular acidosis
  - Chronic renal failure
  - Hypopituitarism
  - Inborn errors of metabolism
  - Storage diseases
  - Muscular dystrophy
  - Lipodystrophy
- **Allergic/inflammatory**
  - Inflammatory bowel disease
  - Juvenile idiopathic arthritis
  - Systemic lupus erythematosus
  - Sarcoidosis
  - Pancreatitis
  - Hepatitis
  - Celiac disease (gluten enteropathy)
- **Functional/miscellaneous**
  - Malnutrition
  - Child abuse
  - Postoperative
  - Dieting
  - Rumination syndrome
  - Depression/affective disorders
  - Anorexia nervosa
  - Inability to eat (new orthodontic appliances, loss of teeth, chronic mouth ulcerations)
  - Chronic congestive heart failure
  - Chronic pulmonary disease
  - Chronic renal disease
  - Iron deficiency
  - Zinc deficiency
  - Cerebral palsy
  - Postinfectious malabsorption
  - Factitious (e.g., scale error)

ALERT
Emergency care:
- Significant dehydration:
  - Abnormal vital signs with orthostasis, decreased urine output, decreased skin turgor, delayed capillary refill (>3 seconds)
  - Mandates cardiovascular support (IV hydration) and a more urgent diagnosis (e.g., inborn error of metabolism, obstructive GI disease, congenital adrenal hyperplasia, diabetic ketoacidosis)
- Abnormal mental status, significant lethargy may be seen in:
  - Severe dehydration
  - Hypoadrenalism
  - Hypoxic states
  - Toxic ingestions
  - Renal or respiratory failure
  - Increased intracranial pressure
  - Severe electrolyte abnormalities
- Increasing vomiting in the setting of known weight loss in infants:
  - High risk for dehydration, hypoglycemia, and electrolyte abnormalities

- Need to evaluate for treatable conditions (e.g., obstructive GI disease, inborn errors of metabolism, congenital adrenal hyperplasia, congenital heart disease) in which a delay is life-threatening
- Severe malnutrition (weight loss >20% of ideal body weight):
  - High risk for metabolic derangements, including dysrhythmias secondary to electrolyte abnormalities
- Aggressive evaluation is warranted.

HISTORY
Determine that weight loss is real and not due to scale error, different scales, different technique (e.g., clothed vs. unclothed).
- **Question:** Child's diet?
- *Significance*: A prospective 3-day dietary record can be useful for demonstrating insufficient caloric intake.
- **Question:** Age?
- *Significance*: The patient's age can very much indicate the most likely causes of weight loss to which questions about the history can be directed.
  - Patient <2 weeks old: Physiologic weight loss, underfeeding, inappropriate feeding, inborn errors of metabolism, congenital heart disease, gastroesophageal reflux
  - Patient <4 months old: Malnutrition, improper formula preparation, cystic fibrosis, gastroesophageal reflux, pyloric stenosis, congenital heart disease, congenital adrenal hyperplasia, inborn errors of metabolism
  - Patient 4 months to 8 years old: Chronic infection, cystic fibrosis, malabsorption, neglect/abuse, renal disease, liver disease, diabetes mellitus
  - Patient >8 years old: Eating disorder, chronic infection, neoplasm, renal disease, liver disease, substance abuse, diabetes mellitus, inflammatory bowel disease, collagen vascular disease
- **Question:** Cramping, bloating, or abnormally greasy, voluminous stools?
- *Significance*: Possible malabsorption
- **Question:** Vomiting, especially projectile?
- *Significance*: Suggestive of intestinal obstruction, gastroesophageal reflux, inborn errors of metabolism
- **Question:** Polyuria, polydipsia, and polyphagia?
- *Significance*: Possible diabetes mellitus
- **Question:** Headaches, especially early morning?
- *Significance*: Possible increased intracranial pressure, CNS malignancy
- **Question:** Maternal history of multiple miscarriages, neonatal deaths, or consanguinity?
- *Significance*: Possible inborn error of metabolism
- **Question:** History of severe infections, persistent candidal infections?

- *Significance*: Immunodeficiency, congenital or acquired
- **Question:** Fear of fatness, preoccupation with food, distorted body image, and/or amenorrhea?
- *Significance*: Possible eating disorder
- **Question:** Delayed puberty?
- *Significance*: Suggests chronic severe weight loss, pituitary abnormalities, anorexia nervosa
- **Question:** Foreign travel?
- *Significance*: Possible chronic infection (e.g., tuberculosis, parasitic disease)
- **Question:** Tiring during feeding or difficulty feeding due to cough and dyspnea?
- *Significance*: Suggests congestive heart failure in newborn/infant, hypothyroidism
- **Question:** Increased appetite with weight loss?
- *Significance*: Suggests hyperthyroidism, cystic fibrosis, pheochromocytoma
- **Question:** Altered mental status, seizures, unusual body/fluid odors?
- *Significance*: Inborn error of metabolism
- **Question:** Chronic sadness or irritability, insomnia or hypersomnia?
- *Significance*: Depression/affective disorder

PHYSICAL EXAM
- **Finding:** Clubbing?
- *Significance*: Suggests chronic cardiac, pulmonary, or intestinal disease
- **Finding:** Significant abdominal distension?
- *Significance*: Suggests celiac disease
- **Finding:** Hypothermia, bradycardia?
- *Significance*: Suggests anorexia nervosa, hypothyroidism
- **Finding:** Tachycardia, resting?
- *Significance*: Hyperthyroidism, pheochromocytoma, anemia, acute weight loss
- **Finding:** Orthostatic changes?
- *Significance*: Significant weight loss, possibly acute
- **Finding:** Hypotension, resting?
- *Significance*: Addison disease, anorexia nervosa, significant acute dehydration
- **Finding:** Visual field abnormalities?
- *Significance*: Suggests possible CNS malignancy
- **Finding:** Swollen joint?
- *Significance*: Juvenile idiopathic arthritis inflammatory bowel disease
- **Finding:** Muscle weakness?
- *Significance*: Connective tissue disorder, electrolyte abnormality, muscular dystrophy
- **Finding:** Enlarged liver and/or spleen?
- *Significance*: Suggests malignancy, chronic infection, storage disease, inborn error of metabolism

ALERT
- Be certain that the weight loss is real. In some studies, up to 25% of weight loss is an artifact as a result of measurement errors (e.g., excessive movement of scale, dressed vs. undressed patient).
- Newborns with weight loss, especially at the 2-week visit, may manifest passivity and paradoxical lack of interest in breastfeeding, although the reason for their problem is malnourishment due to inadequate intake (often from improper positioning or too infrequent feedings). They may not act "hungry." Observation of the feeding technique (by a practitioner with expertise or a lactation consultant) is vital.

DIAGNOSTIC TESTS & INTERPRETATION
- **Test:** CBC for evidence of:
- *Significance:*
  - Anemia—macrocytic associated with folate/B12 deficiency, microcytic with iron deficiency or chronic infection
  - Polycythemia—suggestive of chronic pulmonary or cardiac disease
  - Neutropenia—suggestive of hematologic malignancy, Shwachman syndrome, immunodeficiency
  - Lymphopenia—suggestive of immunodeficiency
  - Eosinophilia—suggestive of parasitic disease
  - Leukocytosis—suggestive of infection
  - Thrombocytosis—suggestive of chronic infection, malignancy
  - Lymphoblasts—suggestive of leukemia
- **Test:** Erythrocyte sedimentation rate
- *Significance*: May be elevated in inflammatory bowel disease, chronic infections, rheumatoid diseases
- **Test:** Serum electrolytes
- *Significance*: Abnormalities in dehydration, adrenal insufficiency (low sodium, high potassium), renal disease, anorexia nervosa
- **Test:** BUN, creatinine
- *Significance*: Abnormal in renal disease, dehydration
- **Test:** Stool for occult blood and pH, reducing substances (Clinitest)
- *Significance:*
  - Occult blood suggests inflammatory bowel disease.
  - Low pH and positive reducing substances suggest malabsorption.
- **Test:** Urinalysis
- *Significance:*
  - Hematuria and/or proteinuria suggest renal disease.
  - Glycosuria suggests diabetes mellitus.
  - Very low specific gravity suggests diabetes insipidus, chronic renal failure, and hypercalcemia.
  - Pyuria suggests UTI.
  - pH >6 suggests renal tubular acidosis (type I).
- **Test:** Urine culture
- *Significance*: Evaluation for UTI

- **Test:** Serum protein levels
- *Significance*: Very low levels imply impaired liver function, severe chronic weight loss, or protein malabsorption.
- **Test:** Tuberculosis skin test
- *Significance*: Possible chronic infection
- **Test:** Liver function tests
- *Significance*: Evaluation for hepatitis, chronic liver disease.

Depending on age and clinical findings, other tests to consider include: Thyroid function tests, sweat test, tests for malabsorption (e.g., lactose breath test, stool fat, stool for trypsin), tests for metabolic disease (e.g., plasma ammonia, lactate, serum/urine amino acids, urine organic acids), imaging studies (e.g., CT, MRI, bone scan), immunologic studies.

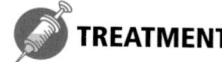

TREATMENT

ADDITIONAL TREATMENT
General Measures
Treatment is dependent on the etiology of the weight loss.

ISSUES FOR REFERRAL
Weight loss is a diagnostic exigency—a cause must be found or the loss self-resolved. If a diagnosis is not uncovered in the setting of continued weight loss, referral to a pediatric diagnostic center is indicated.

ADDITIONAL READING

- Kleinman RE, ed. *Pediatric nutrition handbook*, 6th ed. Elk Grove Village, IL: American Academy of Pediatrics, 2009.
- Macdonsal PD, Ross SRM, Frant L, et al. Neonatal weight loss in breast and formula fed infants. *Arch Dis Child Fetal Neonatal Ed*. 2003;88:F472–476.
- Schechter M. Weight loss/failure to thrive. *Pediatr Rev*. 2000;21:238–239.

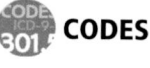

CODES

ICD9
783.21 Loss of weight

ICD10
R63.4 Abnormal weight loss

FAQ

- Q: How common is weight loss in the first 2 weeks of life?
- A: Formula-fed babies may lose up to 7% of birth weight and breastfed newborns up to 10% before regaining their birth weight by 2 weeks of age. An infant who has not regained his or her birth weight by 2 weeks requires evaluation and intervention.

W

WEST NILE VIRUS (AND OTHER ARBOVIRUS ENCEPHALITIS)

Jessica Newman
Jason Newland

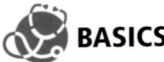 BASICS

DESCRIPTION
- Viruses transmitted by an arthropod vector that can cause CNS infections, undifferentiated febrile illness, acute polyarthropathy, and hemorrhagic fevers
- Most arboviral infections are asymptomatic.
- West Nile virus (WNV) is an arbovirus in the flavivirus family.
- WNV was 1st recognized in the US in 1999 during an outbreak of encephalitis in New York City.
- More than 150 arboviruses are known to cause human disease.
- Other arboviruses can produce similar syndromes or acute hemorrhagic fevers.

EPIDEMIOLOGY
- Arboviruses are spread by mosquitoes, ticks, and sand flies. The major vector for WNV in the US is the Culex mosquito. WNV has been spread through blood transfusions, transplanted organs, and rarely intrauterine.
- Arboviruses are maintained in nature through cycles of transmission among birds, horses, and small animals. Humans and domestic animals are infected incidentally as "dead-end" hosts.
- Disease among birds has been a hallmark of WNV in the US and has served as a sensitive surveillance indicator of WNV activity.
- Each North American arbovirus has specific geographic distributions and is associated with a different ratio of asymptomatic to clinical infections. These agents cause disease of variable severity and have distinct age-dependent effects. WNV has now been identified throughout the US and is also found in Europe, Africa, and Asia.

Incidence
- The peak incidence of arboviral encephalitis occurs during the late summer and early fall. Seasonality depends on the breeding and feeding seasons of the arthropod host.
- WNV is the leading cause of arboviral CNS disease. Encephalitis is most commonly seen in older adults, generally aged >60 years. Cases of WNV in children are unusual.
- Fewer than 10 and 20 cases, respectively, of Eastern equine encephalitis and Western equine encephalitis are reported nationally each year. Eastern equine encephalitis tends to produce a more fulminant illness than LaCrosse or Western equine encephalitis.

GENERAL PREVENTION
- Public health department efforts focus on surveillance of viral activity to predict and prevent outbreaks:
  - Active bird surveillance to detect the presence of WNV activity
  - Active mosquito surveillance to detect viral activity in mosquito populations
  - Passive surveillance by veterinarians and human health care professionals to detect neurologic illnesses consistent with encephalitis
  - Screening of blood and organ donors

- Personal precautions to avoid mosquito bites including use of repellents, protective clothing, and screens; avoiding peak feeding times (dawn and dusk); and installation of air conditioners
- Coordination of mosquito control programs in endemic infection areas
- Vaccines for prevention of most arbovirus infections are not available. A vaccine is available for Japanese encephalitis and yellow fever (YF) for travelers to endemic areas who are planning prolonged stays.
- Infection control measures:
  - Standard precautions are recommended for the hospitalized patient.
  - Respiratory precautions are recommended when vector mosquitoes are present.
  - Patients with dengue and YF can be viremic and should be protected against vector mosquitoes to avoid potential transmission

PATHOPHYSIOLOGY
- The incubation period for WNV and other arboviral encephalitis agents is 2–14 days (up to 21 days in immunocompromised hosts).
- The incubation period reflects the time necessary for viral replication, viremia, and subsequent invasion of the CNS.
- Virus replication begins locally at the site of the insect bite; transient viremia leads to spread of virus to liver, spleen, and lymph nodes. With continued viral replication and viremia, seeding of other organs including the CNS occurs.
- Virus can rarely be recovered from blood within the 1st week of onset of illness but not after neurologic symptoms have developed.

ETIOLOGY
- Arboviruses can be divided into 2 groups based on the predominant clinical syndrome.
- In the US, 7 arboviruses are important causes of encephalitis: WNV, California encephalitis virus (LaCrosse strain), Eastern equine encephalitis, Western equine encephalitis, St. Louis encephalitis, Powassan encephalitis virus, and Venezuelan equine encephalitis virus.
- Arboviruses such as yellow fever, dengue fever, and Colorado tick fever typically cause acute febrile diseases and hemorrhagic fevers and are not characterized by encephalitis.
- Clinical manifestations of WNV:
  - Asymptomatic: Most common
  - Self-limited febrile illness: 67% of symptomatic cases
  - Neuroinvasive disease: Aseptic meningitis, encephalitis, or flaccid paralysis—<1% cases

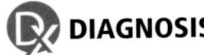 DIAGNOSIS

HISTORY
- The diagnosis of arboviral infections of the CNS is difficult.
- Characteristic epidemiology that suggests a specific etiology is an important part of the history.
- The season of disease, prevalent diseases within the community, and animal exposures may provide clues to the diagnosis:
  - Enteroviral infections are seen in the warmer months (summer and early fall) in temperate climates.
  - Mosquito propagation in damp climates or standing water during the summer months may increase the likelihood of arthropod-borne viruses.
  - History of an animal bite or bat exposure may suggest the possibility of rabies.
- WNV (symptomatic infection) is characterized by sudden onset of fever, headache, myalgias, muscle weakness, and GI symptoms (nausea, vomiting, or diarrhea).
- Neuroinvasive WNV can be characterized by neck stiffness and headache, mental status changes, movement disorders, or flaccid paralysis.

PHYSICAL EXAM
- Encephalitis caused by arboviruses is characterized by acute onset of fever and headache in almost all patients. Associated symptoms may include seizures, altered consciousness, disorientation, and behavioral disturbances. Neurologic signs are more commonly diffuse, but may be focal. These clinical findings can help to distinguish patients with meningitis, which is characterized by nuchal rigidity and fever usually without an altered sensorium.
- Other signs possibly observed in WNV infection:
  - A rash is seen in ~50% of patients and is described as nonpruritic, roseolar, or maculopapular on the chest, back, and arms, which lasts 1 week.
  - Diffuse lymphadenopathy is also common.
- Neurologic examination in WNV infection may reveal motor weakness or flaccid paralysis, increased deep tendon reflexes and extensor plantar responses, and tremor or abnormal movement of extremities

DIAGNOSTIC TESTS & INTERPRETATION
The diagnosis of arboviral encephalitis depends on the recognition of epidemiologic risk factors and typical signs and symptoms with the aid of laboratory and radiographic studies.

Lab
- Routine laboratory tests:
  - CBC typically reveals a mild leukocytosis.
  - Mild increase in ESR rate
  - Mild to moderate CSF pleocytosis, predominately mononuclear cells
  - Elevated CSF protein
  - Normal CSF glucose

- Serology:
  - IgM and IgG ELISA or IFA for WNV and other arboviruses are performed at state public health laboratories and the CDC.
  - The diagnosis of arbovirus encephalitis is made by 1 of the following:
    - Detection of virus-specific IgM antibodies in the CSF is confirmatory.
    - A 4-fold rise in serum antibody titers is confirmatory. Acute-phase titers should be collected 0–8 days after onset of symptoms. Convalescent phase titers should be collected 14–21 days after acute specimen. A single negative acute-phase specimen is inadequate for diagnosis, but a positive test can provide evidence of recent infection.
  - Isolation of the virus from tissue, blood, or CSF
  - Polymerase chain reaction (PCR) to detect viral RNA

Imaging
- Imaging studies such as MRI or CT can assist in ruling out other potential causes of encephalopathy or encephalitis.
- MRI has proved useful in differentiating postinfectious encephalomyelitis from acute viral encephalitis. The former is characterized by enhancement of multifocal white matter lesions.

Diagnostic Procedures/Other
EEG:
- Diffuse generalized slowing of brain waves
- Periodic high-voltage spike waves originating in the temporal lobe region and slow-wave complexes at 2–3-second intervals are suggestive of herpes simplex virus infection.

DIFFERENTIAL DIAGNOSIS
Infectious:
- Viral:
  - Herpes simplex virus
  - Enterovirus
  - HIV
  - HHV-6
  - Epstein-Barr virus
  - Cytomegalovirus
  - Lymphocytic choriomeningitis virus
  - Rabies
  - Mumps
  - Influenza
  - Adenovirus
- Nonviral:
  - Cat-scratch disease (*Bartonella henselae*)
  - *Mycoplasma pneumoniae*
  - Postinfectious encephalomyelitis: Generally follows a vague viral syndrome, usually upper respiratory tract, by days to weeks
  - Abscess/subdural empyema

- Meningitis:
  - Tuberculous
  - Cryptococcal or other fungal (histoplasmosis, coccidioidomycoses, blastomycoses)
  - Bacterial
  - Listeria
- Toxoplasmosis
- *Plasmodium falciparum* infection (malaria)
- Parasites (cysticercosis, echinococcus, amebiasis, trypanosomiasis)

Noninfectious: Tumor, carcinomatous meningitis, systemic lupus erythematosus, sarcoidosis, vasculitis, hemorrhage, toxic encephalopathy, metabolic disorders

TREATMENT

ADDITIONAL TREATMENT
General Measures
- No specific antiviral therapy is available.
- Supportive therapy including cardiorespiratory function, fluid and electrolyte balance, seizure control, and reduction of intracranial pressure is important.
- Consider IVIG and plasmapheresis for associated GBS.
- Recovery can be seen after prolonged periods of coma.

ONGOING CARE

FOLLOW-UP RECOMMENDATIONS
Patient Monitoring
- Neurobehavioral follow-up should be considered in children with severe or complicated disease.
- If WNV is diagnosed during pregnancy detailed fetal US should be considered 2–4 weeks after illness onset with evaluation for congenital anomalies and neurologic deficits.
- Infant serum should be tested for WNV IgM at birth and 6 months with IgG at 6 months.

PROGNOSIS
- Prognosis for recovery depends on the specific infecting agent and host factors such as age and underlying illness.
- Eastern equine and Japanese encephalitis have the worst prognoses, with mortality occurring in 30% of cases.

COMPLICATIONS
- Optic neuritis
- Seizures
- Coma
- Death
- Guillain-Barré syndrome
- Severe neurologic sequelae
- Myocarditis
- Pancreatitis
- Hepatitis

ADDITIONAL READING

- Asnis DS, Conetta R, Teixeira AA, et al. The West Nile virus outbreak of 1999 in New York: The Flushing Hospital experience. *Clin Infect Dis.* 2000;30:413–418.
- CDC. Guidelines for surveillance, prevention and control of West Nile virus infection—United States. *MMWR.* 2003;52:1160.
- Hayes EB. West Nile virus disease in children. *Pediatr Infect Dis J.* 2006 Nov;25(11):1065–1066.
- Lindsey NP, Hayes EB, Staples JE, et al. West Nile virus disease in children, United States 1999-2007. *Pediatrics.* 2009;123(6):e1084–e1089.
- Rizzo C, Esposito S, Azzari S, et al. West Nile virus infections in children: A disease pediatricians should think about. *Pediatr Infect Dis J.* 2011;301:65–66.
- Romero JR, Newland JG. Viral meningitis and encephalitis: Traditional and emerging viral agents. *Semin Pediatr Infect Dis.* 2003;14:72–82.

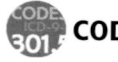 CODES

ICD9
- 062.2 Eastern equine encephalitis
- 064 Viral encephalitis transmitted by other and unspecified arthropods
- 066.40 West Nile Fever, unspecified

ICD10
- A83.2 Eastern equine encephalitis
- A85.2 Arthropod-borne viral encephalitis, unspecified
- A93.8 Other specified arthropod-borne viral fevers

FAQ
- Q: Should testing for arboviruses, including WNV, be performed on all patients with encephalitis?
- A: Diagnostic testing for arboviruses is not recommended for all patients with encephalitis. The prevalence of these diseases is low, and the diagnosis of more common causes of childhood encephalitis (e.g., herpes simplex virus) should be pursued initially. Patients with no other identifiable cause of encephalitis who have epidemiologic risk factors such as geographic location, season, and exposure history suggestive of arbovirus encephalitis should be evaluated. Testing of patients with aseptic meningitis or Guillain-Barré syndrome is low yield.

W

WHEEZING

Samuel Goldfarb
Lee Brooks

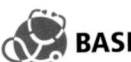 **BASICS**

DEFINITION

Wheezing is a continuous sound that is caused by turbulent airflow through an obstructed airway.

- Often described as musical in nature and with a variable pitch
- Wheezing is an expiratory sound; stridor is an inspiratory sound.
- Wheezing occurs from obstruction in the intrathoracic airway, whereas stridor is caused by an obstruction in the extrathoracic airway.
- If heard in both inspiration and expiration, there is a fixed obstruction or separate lesions in both the intrathoracic and extrathoracic airways.

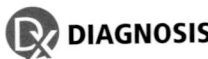 **DIAGNOSIS**

DIFFERENTIAL DIAGNOSIS

Extrathoracic (usually results in stridor rather than wheezing):

- **Nasal/nasopharynx**
  - Acute: Nasal turbinate edema or secretions, foreign body
  - Chronic: Adenoidal enlargement, nasal polyps, choanal stenosis, midface hypoplasia
- **Oropharynx**
  - Acute: Peritonsillar abscess, retropharyngeal abscess, palatine tonsillitis
  - Chronic: Adenotonsillar hypertrophy, macroglossia, micrognathia
- **Hypopharynx**
  - Acute: Acute nasal, nasopharyngeal, or oropharyngeal obstruction
  - Chronic: Hypopharyngeal hypotonia, glossoptosis, obesity, neoplasia
- **Larynx**
  - Acute: Laryngospasm, laryngotracheobronchitis (croup), epiglottitis, foreign body (large and irregular)
  - Chronic: Laryngomalacia, papillomatosis, hemangioma, granuloma, congenital cyst or web, laryngocele
- **Glottis**
  - Acute: Vocal cord paralysis or paresis, vocal cord inflammation or polyp, psychogenic wheezing
  - Chronic: Paradoxical vocal cord motion (vocal cord dysfunction), psychogenic wheezing, brainstem compression, injury to the vagus, glossopharyngeal or recurrent laryngeal nerves, papillomatosis
- **Subglottis/extrathoracic trachea**
  - Acute: Laryngotracheobronchitis (croup), bacterial, rachitic, recent endotracheal extubation
  - Chronic: Subglottic stenosis (congenital or after prolonged intubation), papillomatosis

Intrathoracic:

- **Trachea (extrinsic compression)**
  - Acute: Uncommon
  - Chronic:
    - Vascular: Vascular ring/sling, compression by an aberrant pulmonary artery
    - Cardiac: Left main bronchus compression, recurrent laryngeal nerve compression "cardiovocal syndrome"
    - Anterior mediastinum
    - Lymphoma, thymoma, teratoma
    - Middle mediastinum: Lymphoma, lymphadenopathy (tuberculosis, mycotic infection, sarcoidosis)
    - Posterior mediastinum: Neurogenic tumors, esophageal duplication or cyst, bronchogenic cyst
- **Trachea (intramural lesions)**
  - Acute: Uncommon
  - Chronic: Tracheomalacia
    - Congenital: Cartilaginous defect (Campbell–Williams syndrome), muscular defect (Mounier–Kuhn syndrome), s/p tracheoesophageal fistula repair, external compression/distortion, complete tracheal rings
    - Acquired: Chronic inflammation (recurrent infection, gastroesophageal reflux, recurrent aspiration), prolonged positive pressure ventilation, external compression
- **Trachea (intraluminal lesions)**
  - Acute: Foreign body (irregularly shaped and elongated), bacterial tracheitis (with chronic tracheostomy tube usage)
  - Chronic: Tracheal granulomas, hemangioma, papillomatosis, tracheal web
- **Bronchi/bronchioles**
  - Acute: Viral bronchiolitis, bronchopneumonia, foreign body (small, smooth shape), granuloma, neoplasia
  - Chronic: Asthma, bronchopulmonary dysplasia, bronchomalacia, carcinoid, adenoma

APPROACH TO THE PATIENT

- **Phase 1:** Determine the severity of the patient's general status and degree of respiratory distress and triage accordingly
- **Phase 2:** Construct a differential diagnosis
- **Phase 3:** Initiate appropriate therapies

HISTORY

- **Question:** Pattern of the wheezing?
- *Significance:*
  - A rapid onset suggests a foreign body or a postexposure exacerbation of asthma.
  - A slow onset suggests an infection.
  - Periods of recurrent wheezing suggest asthma.
  - Nocturnal and early morning wheezing or coughing are consistent with gastroesophageal reflux, sinusitis, and/or sensitivity to common bedroom allergens.
  - Wheezing in association with or soon after a meal can be seen in swallowing dysfunction, gastroesophageal reflux, or, less commonly, tracheoesophageal fistula.
  - Wheezing that worsens with crying is suggestive of tracheomalacia and/or bronchomalacia or a fixed intraluminal or extraluminal obstruction.

- **Question:** Wheezing correlated with exertion?
- *Significance:* Suggests asthma triggered by exercise
- **Question:** Multiple exacerbations with recurrent or chronic symptoms?
- *Significance:*
  - Recurrent cycles of exacerbations, with clearing in between, suggest a process such as asthma, cystic fibrosis, ciliary dyskinesia, and bronchopulmonary dysplasia.
  - Chronic or persistent wheezing is more common with fixed anatomic abnormalities.
- **Question:** Common triggers?
- *Significance:* Could be:
  - Smoke
  - Dust
  - Animal dander
  - Change in humidity or temperature
  - Change in seasons (pollens, grasses, molds)
  - Exercise
  - Infections (usually viral)
  - Inflammation of any sort
  - meals (aspiration, GERD, TEF)
- **Question:** Family history?
- *Significance:* A family history of wheezing, asthma, allergic rhinitis, or atopy suggests a diagnosis of asthma.
- **Question:** An episode of choking preceding the first onset of wheezing?
- *Significance:* Suggests foreign body aspiration

PHYSICAL EXAM

- **Finding:** Patient's degree of respiratory difficulty?
- *Significance:*
  - Tachypnea
  - Accessory muscle usage—use of intercostal and sternocleidomastoid muscles and abdominal musculature indicates increased expiratory effort to overcome airway obstruction.
  - Nasal flaring—with increasing respiratory difficulty, the nares will be dilated to decrease the resistance to air flow.
- **Finding:** Auscultate—assess airflow, adventitious sounds, and the inspiratory-to-expiratory ratio
- *Significance:*
  - Aeration: Decreased aeration is much worse prognostically than wheezing since it is directly related to the amount of aeration and ventilation. With decreased aeration, wheezing may not be audible.
  - Ratio of inspiration to exhalation: With increased intrathoracic airway obstruction, the time needed to exhale will become greater because of a greater decrease in airway caliber during exhalation. Normal ratio is 1:3.
- **Finding:** Presence of nasal crease, the "allergic salute" (i.e., rubbing the nose with the palm of the hand), atopic dermatitis, boggy nasal turbinates, clear postnasal drainage, allergic shiners, or Dennie lines?
- *Significance:* Suggestive of allergic rhinitis or atopic disease including asthma

- **Finding:** Patients with first-time, persistent, or atypical episodes of wheezing?
- *Significance:* "All that wheezes is not asthma": Although most episodes of wheezing will represent viral infections or asthma, clinicians need to be mindful of alternative diagnoses.
- **Finding:** The 3 *R*'s of asthma?
- *Significance:*
  - Recurrence: Symptoms that recur multiple times with full resolution in between episodes
  - Reactivity: Symptoms that can be triggered during exposures (temperature extremes, smoke, dust, humid or dry air, aromas, etc.)
  - Reversibility: Symptoms that resolve with bronchodilator therapy

DIAGNOSTIC TESTS & INTERPRETATION
- **Test:** Bronchodilator responsiveness
- *Significance:*
  - A postbronchodilator improvement in wheezing indicates a reversible process such as asthma.
  - A bronchodilator may worsen wheezing in disorders of airway wall rigidity such as bronchomalacia or tracheomalacia.
  - There may be no change following a bronchodilator in situations with foreign bodies, fixed airway obstruction due to significant inflammation (i.e., status asthmaticus) or airway remodeling.
- **Test:** Pulmonary function testing (spirometry)
- *Significance:*
  - Spirometry remains the standard and most helpful measure of pulmonary function.
  - Normative data have been described in children >6 years of age.
  - Methacholine challenge test is a provocative test to evaluate for asthma.
  - Exercise test with spirometry to evaluate for exercise-induced asthma
- **Test:** Pulse oximetry measurement of oxygen saturation (SpO$_2$)
- *Significance:* Pulse oximetry is an insensitive measure of mild-to-moderate respiratory difficulty during wheezing, but oxyhemoglobin saturation <92% may be seen in severe compromise.
- **Test:** Arterial blood gas
- *Significance:*
  - Arterial blood gases provide a direct measure of oxygenation (PaO$_2$) and ventilation (PaCO$_2$) and can also help to determine severity.
  - A normal or high normal PaCO$_2$ in a tachypneic patient (when it should be low) may be a sign of impending respiratory failure.

Lab
- **Test:** Microbiologic studies
- *Significance:*
  - Positive bacterial culture of sputum is helpful in directing or focusing antibiotic therapy. A Gram stain showing sheets of polymorphonuclear leukocytes and predominant organism is helpful to differentiate a potentially causative organism from the multitude of normal flora.
  - Positive respiratory virus screen or culture (often within 12 hours) can prevent needless antibiotic therapy and may be helpful in predicting future disease.

- **Test:** Tuberculosis skin test
- *Significance:* Mantoux purified protein derivative —tuberculosis
- **Test:** CBC including eosinophil count, quantitative immunoglobulins, IgE, complement, HIV testing, allergy skin testing

Imaging
Chest radiography (posteroanterior and lateral views): Should be strongly considered in all patients with new-onset wheezing or an asymmetric lung exam. Can show findings suggestive of airway obstruction (hyperinflation, hyperlucency, flattening of the diaphragms). Asymmetry in aeration on right and left lateral decubitus films suggests foreign body or other obstructing lesions on the side having the greatest air trapping.

TREATMENT
ADDITIONAL TREATMENT
General Measures
- A trial of bronchodilator therapy (e.g., albuterol) may be both therapeutic and diagnostic of the reversible airway obstruction characteristic of asthma.
- For acute asthma exacerbation—corticosteroids PO or IV
- Ipratropium bromide may be helpful in reducing airway secretions and reducing airway obstruction, but it is not FDA approved for treatment of asthma.
- Inhaled corticosteroids, antileukotriene agents, and less frequently methylxanthines (aminophylline and theophylline) are used as maintenance medications.
- Antibiotics should be used in patients with suspected pneumonia.
- In emergency setting epinephrine, terbutaline, and magnesium sulfate can be used along with supportive care such as supplemental oxygen.

ALERT
Factors that may indicate a respiratory emergency:
- Signs of mild-to-moderate respiratory difficulty: Tachypnea, intercostal and suprasternal retractions, nasal flaring, head bobbing and exaggerated shoulder movement during breathing, abdominal breathing and subcostal retractions, relative difficulty speaking in complete sentences, significant wheezing, prolonged exhalation, and low PaCO$_2$ in the face of tachypnea
- Signs of impending respiratory failure: Cyanosis, fatigue, inability to speak in >1- or 2-word phrases, altered mental status (e.g., confusion, agitation), decreased respiratory drive, inadequate ventilation (poor air flow), no audible wheezing, high normal or rising PaCO$_2$ in the face of tachypnea or respiratory distress
- Determine which patients require assisted ventilation (e.g., bag-mask ventilation, noninvasive [nasal] ventilation, or endotracheal intubation)
- Lack of response to aggressive bronchodilator therapy, without a history of asthma or recurrent wheeze, or biphasic adventitious sounds should immediately raise the suspicion of a fixed lesion.

ADDITIONAL READING
- Bel EH. Clinical phenotypes of asthma. *Curr Opin Pulm Med*. 2004;10:44–50.
- Covar RA, Spahn JD. Treating the wheezing infant. *Pediatr Clin North Am*. 2003;50:631–654.
- Grigg J. Asthma year in review 2006–7. *Pediatr Respir Rev*. 2008;9(2):134–138.
- McFadden ER. Acute severe asthma. *Am J Respir Crit Care Med*. 2003;168:740–759.

 CODES

ICD9
786.07 Wheezing

ICD10
R06.2 Wheezing

FAQ
- Q: What percent of recurrent wheezing resolves by school age?
- A: Roughly 40% of children with ≥1 episodes of wheezing before 3 years clear by 6 years of age.
- Q: Should chest radiographs be routinely obtained in children experiencing their first episodes of wheezing?
- A: For a child with new-onset asymmetric wheezing, a chest radiograph should be obtained. For a child with symmetric wheezing, chest radiography may not be helpful and should be ordered judiciously.

WILMS TUMOR

David T. Teachey

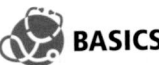 **BASICS**

DESCRIPTION
Wilms tumor is a malignant tumor of the kidney occurring in the pediatric age group. It is also called nephroblastoma.

EPIDEMIOLOGY
More common in girls than boys

Incidence
- 1 in 10,000 live births
- Increased incidence in children with neurofibromatosis

Prevalence
- Most common primary malignant renal tumor of childhood
- 5–6% of all childhood cancer

RISK FACTORS
Genetics
- 15–20% are presumed hereditary
- Familial cases are more often bilateral and occur at an earlier age.
- Associated with WAGR syndrome, Beckwith–Wiedemann syndrome, and Denys–Drash syndrome
- A tumor-suppressor gene related to Wilms tumor (*WT1*) has been localized to chromosome 11p13. Mutations in this gene occur in ~20% of Wilms tumors.
- Another tumor suppressor gene *WT2* (IGF2, H19, p57) has been localized on 11p15.

ETIOLOGY
- 20% of Wilms tumors have a mutation in the *WT1* tumor suppressor gene.
- Causes in the remaining 80% of patients are unknown.

COMMONLY ASSOCIATED CONDITIONS
- 12–15% of patients have other congenital anomalies
- May be associated with aniridia, hemihypertrophy, and cryptorchidism
- Associated syndromes: WAGR (Wilms tumor, aniridia, genitourinary [GU] abnormalities, mental retardation), Beckwith–Wiedemann syndrome (macroglossia, omphalocele, visceromegaly, hemihypertrophy), and Denys–Drash syndrome (ambiguous genitalia, progressive renal failure, and increased risk of Wilms tumor)

DIAGNOSIS

HISTORY
- Abdominal distention
- Abdominal pain (20–30% of cases)
- Hematuria (20–30% of cases)
- Fever, anorexia, vomiting
- Family history of Wilms tumor
- Rapid increase in abdominal size (suggestive of hemorrhage in the tumor)

PHYSICAL EXAM
- Asymptomatic abdominal mass extending from flank toward midline (most common presentation)
- Anemia (secondary to hemorrhage in the tumor)
- Fever
- Hypertension (owing to increased renin production in 25% of cases)
- Varicocele (indicates obstruction to spermatic vein owing to tumor thrombus in renal vein or inferior vena cava)
- Aniridia, hemihypertrophy, cryptorchidism, hypospadias
- Signs of Beckwith–Wiedemann and neurofibromatosis

DIAGNOSTIC TESTS & INTERPRETATION
Lab
- CBC
- Electrolytes
- Urine analysis: For microscopic hematuria
- Liver and kidney function tests
- Coagulation factors

Imaging
- Ultrasound of abdomen:
  - Diagnostic of mass of renal origin
  - Evaluate for extension of tumor into inferior vena cava.
- CT scan of abdomen, chest radiograph, and chest CT: To evaluate for metastatic disease
- Bone scan: Only if clear cell sarcoma, renal cell carcinoma, or rhabdoid tumor on pathology
- MRI of head: Only for clear cell sarcoma and rhabdoid tumors
- EKG and echocardiogram in patients that will receive anthracycline chemotherapy

Pathological Findings
- Gross pathology:
  - Often cystic with hemorrhages and necrosis
  - Usually no calcification (useful in differentiating from neuroblastoma, which is calcified on plain radiograph)
  - May extend into the inferior vena cava
- Histology:
  - Triphasic pattern blastemal, epithelial, and stromal cell
  - Blastemal cells aggregate into nodules like primitive glomeruli; the presence of diffuse anaplasia indicates a poor prognosis.
- Clinicopathologic staging:
  - Stage I: Tumor is restricted to one kidney and completely resected. The renal capsule is intact.
  - Stage II: Tumor extends beyond the kidney, but is completely excised.
  - Stage III: Residual nonhematogenous tumor is confined to the abdomen.
  - Stage IV: There is hematogenous spread to lungs, liver, bone, or brain.
  - Stage V: Bilateral disease

DIFFERENTIAL DIAGNOSIS
- Polycystic kidney
- Renal hematoma
- Renal abscess
- Neuroblastoma
- Other neoplasms of kidney: Clear-cell carcinoma, rhabdoid tumor

ALERT
Rarely, Wilms tumor may present with polycythemia. It can present as fever of unknown origin without any other signs or symptoms.

TREATMENT

SPECIAL THERAPY
Radiotherapy
- Not required for stage I and II patients unless anaplastic, clear cell, or rhabdoid
- Rradiotherapy to tumor bed with 1,080 cGy for stages III and IV. If gross tumor spillage or peritoneal seeding, treat whole abdomen
- Whole-lung radiation (1,200 cGy) for pulmonary metastasis

MEDICATION (DRUGS)
- Chemotherapy:
  - For stages I and II favorable histology: Vincristine and actinomycin D every 3 weeks for 6 months
  - For stages III and IV favorable histology, stage I–III focal anaplasia, and stage I diffuse anaplasia: Vincristine, actinomycin D, and doxorubicin for 6–15 months
  - Add cyclophosphamide and/or etoposide for higher-stage anaplastic tumors (stage IV focal or II–IV diffuse).
- Side effects of therapy:
  - Temporary loss of hair
  - Peripheral neuropathy
  - Impaired function of the remaining kidney over years following radiation
  - Cardiac toxicity with doxorubicin
  - Second malignant neoplasms in few cases

SURGERY/OTHER PROCEDURES
- Nephrectomy:
  - Preoperative chemotherapy in case of very large tumors with inferior vena cava extension
  - For bilateral disease, nephrectomy of more affected side and partial nephrectomy of the other side, followed by chemotherapy and radiation

 ONGOING CARE

PROGNOSIS
- Stages I and II: >90% cured
- Stage III: 85% cured
- Stage IV: 70% cured
- Favorable prognostic factors:
  - Tumor weight <250 g
  - Age at presentation <24 months
  - Stage I disease
  - Favorable histology
- Poor prognostic factors:
  - Diffuse anaplastic pathology
  - Clear cell sarcoma variant
  - Rhabdoid tumor variant
  - Lymph node involvement
  - Distant metastasis
  - Tumors with loss of heterozygosity (LOH) of chromosomes 1p and/or 16q

COMPLICATIONS
- Extension into inferior vena cava
- Metastasis to lungs and liver
- Cardiac toxicity secondary to doxorubicin
- Liver dysfunction secondary to actinomycin D and radiation therapy

FOLLOW-UP RECOMMENDATIONS
Patient Monitoring
- Every 3 months for 18 months, every 6 months for 1 year, and then yearly
- Chest radiograph, urinalysis, and abdominal ultrasound at regular intervals

ADDITIONAL READING
- Martinez CH, Dave S, Izawa J. Wilms' tumor. *Adv Exp Med Biol*. 2010;685:196–209.
- McLean TW, Buckley KS. Pediatric genitourinary tumors. *Curr Opin Oncol*. 2010;22:268–273.
- Davidoff AM. Wilms' tumor. *Curr Opin Pediatr*. 2009;21:357–364.
- Blakely ML, Ritchey ML. Controversies in the management of Wilms' tumor. *Semin Pediatr Surg*. 2001;10:127–131.
- Hohenstein P, Hastie ND. The many facets of the Wilms' tumor gene (WT1). *Hum Mol Genet*. 2006;15 Spec No2:R196–R201.

CODES

ICD9
189.0 Malignant neoplasm of kidney, except pelvis

ICD10
- C64.1 Malignant neoplasm of right kidney, except renal pelvis
- C64.2 Malignant neoplasm of left kidney, except renal pelvis
- C64.9 Malignant neoplasm of unsp kidney, except renal pelvis

FAQ
- Q: What should be done to protect the remaining kidney during sports?
- A: Children should wear a kidney guard to protect the unaffected kidney during contact sports.
- Q: Can a child grow and live normally with 1 kidney?
- A: Yes.

W

WILSON DISEASE

Waqar Waheed
Molly E. Rideout (5th edition)

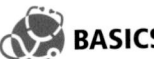 **BASICS**

DESCRIPTION
Wilson disease (WD), also known as hepatolenticular degeneration, is an autosomal recessive disorder of copper metabolism affecting the liver and brain.

EPIDEMIOLOGY
Children usually present with hepatic manifestations; adolescents and young adults may present with neurologic symptoms.

Incidence
- Incidence is 15–25 per million.
- Worldwide carrier rate is 1:100.

Prevalence
- Prevalence is 1:30,000.
- Most cases present between ages 5 and 35.
- Worldwide distribution

RISK FACTORS
Genetics
- Autosomal recessive inheritance with 1 of >200 known defects of the WD gene (ATP7B) on chromosome 13q14.3 membrane (ATPase)
- The affected protein facilitates biliary excretion of excess copper; incorporates copper into apo-ceruloplasmin for transport
- Heterozygotes are generally asymptomatic.
- Future siblings have 25% risk of disease.
- Direct mutational analysis is limited owing to the high number of mutations, except in isolated populations.

PATHOPHYSIOLOGY
- Loss of ATP7b function causes impaired biliary copper excretion (the only route for elimination of copper) and ceruloplasmin biosynthesis.
- Copper accumulates 1st in the liver, leading to cirrhosis.
- After liver is saturated, copper overflows and settles in the brain and other tissues.
- In the brain, copper collects primarily in the basal ganglia, leading to impaired motor control.
- Other tissues affected by copper accumulation are kidneys, heart, blood, and cornea.
- Failure to incorporate copper during ceruloplasmin biosynthesis produces an apoprotein that is rapidly degraded.

COMMONLY ASSOCIATED CONDITIONS
- Renal: Copper accumulation leads to Fanconi syndrome with tubular dysfunction, causing glycosuria, hypophosphatemia, and low uric acid.
- Hematologic: Hemolytic anemia, coagulopathy from liver failure
- Cardiac: Cardiomyopathy/dysrhythmias develop from copper deposits.

DIAGNOSIS

HISTORY
- Hepatic:
  - In children, symptoms of hepatic disease predominate, ranging in severity from asymptomatic hepatomegaly or elevated transaminases to chronic hepatitis to fulminant hepatic failure.
  - Average age for onset of hepatic symptoms ~10 years
  - Fulminant liver failure is associated with hemolysis and coagulopathy unresponsive to vitamin K
- Neurologic:
  - Neurologic symptoms are rare before age 10 years.
  - Neurologic signs in children: Behavior change, decline in school performance, poor hand–eye coordination, motor abnormalities—dystonia, tremors, dysphagia, dysarthria
- Psychiatric: Develop depression, anxiety, psychosis, and/or obsessive–compulsive disorder.
- Other: Nonspecific complaints are common—abdominal pain, nausea, anorexia, and fatigue.
- Signs and symptoms:
  - 45% of all patients present with liver disease, 35% with neurologic symptoms, 10% psychiatric
  - Remaining 10%: Hemolytic anemia, jaundice, cardiomyopathy, other
  - Consider WD in all cases of liver abnormality in which viral and autoimmune causes have been excluded.
  - WD accounts for 8–10% of all chronic active hepatitis in children.
  - Also consider WD in patients with unexplained neuropsychiatric symptoms.

PHYSICAL EXAM
- Ophthalmologic:
  - Kayser-Fleischer (KF) rings: Copper deposits on Descemet membrane of cornea (at limbus)
  - May require slit-lamp examination to see
  - 95% with neurologic signs have KF rings
  - 50–65% with hepatic presentation have KF rings
  - KF rings not pathognomonic for WD; may be seen in cholestatic liver disease
- Cardiovascular: Signs of cardiomyopathy, dysrhythmia, congestive heart failure
- Abdominal:
  - Hepatomegaly, ascites
  - Splenomegaly from portal hypertension
- Skin:
  - Jaundice due to hemolysis
  - Bleeding diathesis from liver disease
  - Edema
- Neurologic:
  - Movement disorders
  - Neurologic deficits

DIAGNOSTIC TESTS & INTERPRETATION
Lab
- Serum ceruloplasmin:
  - Low sensitivity and specificity
  - Level is usually low; however, up to 1/3 of patients have normal values.
  - An acute-phase reactant; during inflammation, infection, or trauma, level may increase to reference range.
  - Made mostly in the liver, it is the major carrier of copper in blood.
  - Very low (<50 mg/L): Strong evidence for WD
  - Low (<200 mg/L) plus symptoms and KF rings: Diagnostic of WD
  - Ceruloplasmin levels also low in renal or GI protein loss, Menkes disease, and end-stage liver disease
- Serum copper:
  - Low total serum copper (<80 mcg/dL) in WD
  - Level is decreased in proportion to decreased ceruloplasmin in circulation.
  - In acute fulminant liver failure, serum copper is increased owing to sudden release of stores (most is not bound to ceruloplasmin).
- Urinary copper excretion:
  - Reflects unbound copper in blood
  - Level is high in WD: >100 mcg/24 hours in symptomatic patient is diagnostic.
  - In equivocal cases, marked increase in urinary copper output after initiation of chelation therapy may help in diagnosis.
- Other:
  - Mild to moderate elevations of serum aminotransferase levels
  - Mutational analysis: useful for screening, if familial mutation is known

Imaging
- Abdominal ultrasound for liver size and pathology
- MRI of the brain with focus on basal ganglia should be obtained prior to initiation of therapy.
- "Face of the giant panda" sign that is characteristic of Wilson disease (red nuclei, substantia nigra, tegmentum)

Diagnostic Procedures/Other
- Liver biopsy is the definitive procedure for tissue diagnosis and hepatic disease staging.
- Biopsy should be obtained when diagnosis is not straightforward and in younger patients.
- Hepatic parenchymal copper concentration >250 mcg/g dry weight
- Hepatic copper level <50 mcg/g dry weight excludes WD.

DIFFERENTIAL DIAGNOSIS
- Liver disease:
  - Viral hepatitis
  - Autoimmune hepatitis/primary biliary cirrhosis
  - Menkes disease
  - Cholestatic disease from parenteral nutrition

- Neurologic disease:
  - Essential tremor
  - Sydenham or Huntington chorea
  - Hereditary dystonia
  - Other neurodegenerative diseases
- Psychiatric disease: Depression, psychoses
- KF rings: Seen in other causes cholestatic liver disease
- Low ceruloplasmin:
  - End-stage liver disease
  - Menkes disease
- Protein loss from GI or renal abnormalities

 TREATMENT

Early diagnosis is essential to limiting morbidity and mortality.

MEDICATION (DRUGS)
- **Penicillamine**
  - Mode of action (MOA):
    - Chelates copper and promotes renal excretion
    - Also induces metallothionein, interferes with collagen cross-linking, immunosuppressant
    - Improvement takes up to a year.
  - Dosages:
    - Initial dose: 1–1.5 g/d, b.i.d. or q.i.d., 1 or 2 hours after food
    - May start at a lower dose (250–500 mg/d) with gradual escalation over a few weeks.
    - Maintenance dose: 0.5–1 g/d
    - Fulminant liver failure if discontinued abruptly
  - Acute neurologic deterioration after initiation of therapy in up to 20%: Reduce dose to 250 mg/d
  - Side effects in 20–30%:
    - Pyridoxine deficiency, manifested by intercurrent infection or a growth spurt. B_6 supplementation 50 mg/wk
    - Skin complications due to interference with collagen and elastin formation
    - Hypersensitivity reactions (rash, fever, lymphadenopathy), bone marrow suppression, myasthenia gravis, optic neuritis, nephritis, lupuslike syndrome
    - Monitoring: CBC, liver function tests (LFTs), urinalysis, urine copper
- **Trientine**
  - Has become initial drug of choice
  - Used in combination with zinc
  - Chelates copper/promotes renal excretion
  - Dosages: Pediatric dose 20 mg/kg/d divided b.i.d.–t.i.d. to maximum of 750–1,000 mg/d
  - Maintenance therapy: 900–1,200 mg/d b.i.d. or t.i.d., empty stomach
  - Fewer side effects than penicillamine
  - Most improve with continued treatment.
  - Risk of sideroblastic anemia, hemorrhagic gastritis, nephritis, arthritis, worsened neurologic signs
  - Serum copper increases during treatment.
  - Also chelates iron, creating toxic complex; do not give supplemental Fe.
- **Zinc**
  - Routinely combined with trientine
  - Also used alone as maintenance therapy
  - Used successfully in asymptomatic or presymptomatic affected family members of individuals with Wilson disease

- MOA:
  - Interferes with absorption from GI tract by inducing metallothionein in enterocytes, which chelates metals. The copper is bound within the enterocyte and not absorbed into the portal circulation. It is shed in stool as enterocytes are normally shed.
  - Also induces copper binding metallothionein in the liver, thereby reducing the damaging effects of free copper
  - Dosage: 50 mg t.i.d., empty stomach
  - Side effects:
    - Few side effects: Gastric irritation, nausea (ameliorated by taking with meat [but no carbohydrates] or change the formulation to acetate, sulphate, or gluconate)
    - Take without food, except as above
    - After chelation for 4–6 months, with normal labs, usually OK to change to zinc for maintenance
    - May create a negative copper balance, removing all extra copper stores, resulting in improvement of hepatic and brain function, and loss of KF rings
    - Overtreatment may result in anemia or decreased wound healing from copper deficiency
    - No altered dose needed for surgery
    - Compliance with overall therapy monitored by urine zinc levels
- **Ammonium tetra-tiomolibdate**
  - Not FDA approved, limited data
  - Complex with copper in the intestinal tract, preventing absorption
  - Absorbed drugs form a complex with copper and albumin in blood. This complex is metabolized by liver and excreted in bile.
  - Particularly suited for treatment of neurologic manifestation in Wilson disease, as it is not associated with exacerbation on initiation of treatment.
  - S/E: Bone marrow suppression, ↑ aminotransferases
- **Antioxidants and experimental therapies**
  - Antioxidants (vitamin E/N-acetylcysteine) may protect against oxidative damage.

ADDITIONAL TREATMENT
General Measures
- Immunize for hepatitis A, B.
- Avoid excess alcohol.
- Well water or water via copper pipes needs to be tested: If >0.1 ppm Cu, find alternative source.

Additional Therapies
Patients with fulminant liver failure require liver transplant to survive.

SURGERY/OTHER PROCEDURES
- Orthotopic liver transplant required for fulminant liver failure or end-stage liver cirrhosis, which is resistant to chelation therapy.
- Uncertain indication for therapy-resistant neurologic symptoms. Several case reports suggest improved neurologic symptoms after transplantation.
- 5% with WD need liver transplants.

ONGOING CARE

FOLLOW-UP RECOMMENDATIONS
Patient Monitoring
- Patients require lifelong dietary copper restriction and chelation therapy.
- Continual monitoring for compliance and side effects of medications is crucial.
- Sudden discontinuation of therapy may precipitate fulminant hepatic failure.
- 1st-degree relatives >age 3 years should be screened with history, physical exam, LFTs, CBC, serum ceruloplasmin, 24-hour urine copper, and ophthalmologic examination for KF rings.
- Reproductive and genetic counseling for carriers should be offered. Prenatal testing

DIET
Low-copper diet for life: Avoid liver and other organ meats, shellfish, nuts, mushrooms, and chocolate.

PROGNOSIS
- If WD is recognized early and treated, most patients experience complete recovery.
- Progression to hepatocellular carcinoma is rare, unlike hemochromatosis.

ADDITIONAL READING

- Dina A, Jacob DA, Markowitz CE, et al. The "double panda sign" in Wilson's disease. *Neurology.* 2003;61:969.
- El-Youssef M. Wilson disease. *Mayo Clin Proc.* 2003;78:1126–1136.
- Gitlin J. Wilson disease. *Gastroenterology.* 2003;125:1868–1877.
- Huster D. Wilson's disease. *Best Pract Res Clin Gastroenterol.* 2010;24(5):531–539.
- Roberts E, Schilsky M. A practice guideline on Wilson disease: AASLD practice guidelines. *Hepatology.* 2003;37:1475–1492.
- www.wilsonsdisease.org

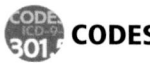 CODES

ICD9
275.1 Disorders of copper metabolism

ICD10
E83.01 Wilson's disease

FAQ

- Q: Are medications for WD safe during pregnancy?
- A: Women of reproductive age who are treated can have normal pregnancies. Doses of both trientine and penicillamine should be reduced during pregnancy, especially in the 3rd trimester, to promote wound healing in the case of a surgical delivery. Zinc doses can remain unchanged. Interruption of therapy is not recommended during pregnancy.

W

WISKOTT-ALDRICH SYNDROME

Elena Elizabeth Perez

BASICS

DESCRIPTION
- An X-linked primary immunodeficiency caused by a mutation in the WAS gene, and originally described as clinical triad of thrombocytopenia with small platelets, eczema, and recurrent infections with opportunistic and pyogenic organisms
- Also associated with IgA nephropathy, autoimmune disorders, and an increased incidence of B-cell lymphomas. Increased bleeding tendency secondary to thrombocytopenia likely results from impaired platelet production, increased turnover, and defective function.
- Disease variants also resulting from WAS gene mutations include X-linked thrombocytopenia (XLT) and X-linked neutropenia (XLN). Classic WAS is characterized by broad immunodeficiency, decreased number and function of T cells, disturbed marginal B-cell homeostasis, and skewed immunoglobulin isotypes, with defective antibody responses to vaccinations, impaired NK-cell cytotoxicity, and abnormal regulatory T-cell function as well as reduced phagocyte chemotaxis.

EPIDEMIOLOGY
- Presents in infancy with serious bleeding episodes secondary to thrombocytopenia (such as circumcision with increased bleeding, bloody diarrhea, ecchymoses)
- Recurrent infections usually start after 6 months of age:
  - Bacterial: Otitis media, sinusitis, meningitis, sepsis, and pneumonia
  - Viral infections: Herpes simplex virus, varicella with systemic complications
- Milder phenotypes may lack history of recurrent infections.
- Decline in T- and B-cell numbers with time
- Eczema is usually present by 1 year of age (may be resistant to therapy, sometimes requiring systemic antibiotics).

Incidence
- For WAS/XLT estimate is 10 in 1 million live births.
- Prevalence of XLT equal to WAS

RISK FACTORS
Genetics
- X-linked recessive disease
- Defective Wiskott-Aldrich syndrome protein gene located on X p11.22p–11.23
- ~60% of cases will have a positive family history for Wiskott-Aldrich syndrome.
- X-linked thrombocytopenia without the other findings is caused by mutations of the same gene.
- Genotype/phenotype correlation:
  - Lack of WASP expression: Increased infections, severe eczema, intestinal hemorrhage, death from intracranial bleeding, and malignancies
  - Survival rate significantly lower in WASP-negative patients

ETIOLOGY
- Mutations in the gene for the Wiskott-Aldrich syndrome protein (WAS)
- WAS protein (WASP) is involved in the reorganization of the actin cytoskeleton in hematopoietic cells:
  - Following activation of WASP, reorganization of actin cytoskeleton results in polarization of cells (e.g., polarized actin mesh in platelets for clotting and in macrophages for phagocytosis, and polarization of T or B cells to form immunologic synapses).
- WAS protein (WASp) is a cytoplasmic protein involved in cell mobility, immune regulation, cell signaling, cell-to-cell interactions, signaling, and cytotoxicity.
- Defects in WASp can lead to dysfunction in adaptive and innate immunity, immune surveillance, and platelet homeostasis and function as well as neutropenia.
- "Classic" WAS and XLT result from loss-of-function mutations.
- XLT can be misdiagnosed as idiopathic thrombocytopenic purpura (ITP) that does not carry increased risk of malignancy, so testing for WASp expression and WAS gene mutation is important in any male with thrombocytopenia and small platelets.
- XLN results from "activating" mutations in WAS that lead to increased actin polymerization; profound neutropenia, with or without associated lymphopenia; decreased T-cell proliferation in vitro; and increased risk of myelodysplastic changes in bone marrow.
- WASp is also important for regulatory T-cell function.

DIAGNOSIS

HISTORY
- Persistent or severe bleeding in infancy due to thrombocytopenia
- Recurrent infections, especially by bacteria with capsular polysaccharides (e.g., *Pneumococcus*)
- Eczema can be of variable severity:
  - "Acute on chronic"
  - 80% of cases associated with eczema
  - May result from imbalance of cytokines skewed toward Th2
- Older patients may report recurrent viral infections.
- Most common autoimmune features include autoimmune hemolytic anemia, cutaneous vasculitis, arthritis, and nephropathy.
- Less common autoimmune features include inflammatory bowel disease, idiopathic thrombocytopenic purpura, and neutropenia.
- Autoimmune features are poor prognostic indicators and can occur simultaneously.
- Maternal family history of Wiskott-Aldrich syndrome or X-linked thrombocytopenia

PHYSICAL EXAM
- Evaluation should focus on presence of infection.
- Dermatologic examination is significant for the extent of eczema and the presence of petechiae or ecchymoses.
- Splenomegaly

DIAGNOSTIC TESTS & INTERPRETATION
Lab
- CBC with differential
- Small platelets, decreased mean platelet volume, decreased platelet count
- Normal IgG, decreased IgM, increased IgA and IgE (reflecting immune dysregulation)
- Reduced or absent responses to polysaccharide antigens and isohemagglutinins to ABO antigens
- T- and B-lymphocyte enumeration and mitogen stimulation studies may progressively deteriorate with increasing age.

Diagnostic Procedures/Other
- WAS disease scoring system useful for defining clinical phenotypes associated with WAS mutations (XLN, XLT, vs. classic WAS)
- Sequencing of WAS gene
- Lymph node biopsy in suspected malignancy
- Bone marrow aspirate to evaluate thrombocytopenia

DIFFERENTIAL DIAGNOSIS
- Other causes of thrombocytopenia such as idiopathic thrombocytopenic purpura
- In 1 cohort, approximately 7% of patients diagnosed as having ITP actually had WAS as an underlying cause of thrombocytopenia.
- Severe atopic disease with dermatitis and secondary skin infections
- HIV infection
- Hyper-IgE syndrome
- Diagnosis should be considered in any boy who has congenital or early-onset thrombocytopenia with small platelets.
- Definitive diagnosis:
  - Male patient
  - Congenital thrombocytopenia ($<70,000/mm^3$)
  - Small platelets (mean platelet volume <0.5 fL)
  - Mutation in the Wiskott-Aldrich syndrome protein gene or absent Wiskott-Aldrich syndrome protein mRNA

TREATMENT

ADDITIONAL TREATMENT
General Measures
- Antibiotics for acute infections and prophylactically in postsplenectomy patients
- Splenectomy may be helpful for persistent severe thrombocytopenia in select patients. However, this may greatly increase the risk of overwhelming infections with encapsulated organisms.
- Splenectomy should be reserved for emergencies in classic WAS patients who are candidates for HCT, since it is a risk factor for death. Splenectomy in XLT with severe bleeding may increase platelet counts, but risk of severe infection requires lifelong antibiotic prophylaxis

- Thrombocytopenia precautions: No aspirin and avoidance of situations in which trauma (especially head trauma) is likely to occur, such as contact sports
- Platelet transfusions may be necessary for severe bleeding. Use irradiated blood products to avoid graft versus host disease, and cytomegalovirus-negative products in case of bone marrow transplantation.
- IV immunoglobulin replacement therapy is helpful in managing recurrent infections in some patients:
  – Hematopoietic stem cell transplantation is the treatment of choice for the classic WAS phenotype.
  – Allogeneic stem cell transplant from HLA genotypically identical sibling or 9/10 or 10/10 allele matched unrelated donor for any WAS patient with disease score 3–5 (see references) or with absent WASp expression
  – Outcomes are improving with 5-year survival rates >80% for matched sibling donors and similar for matched unrelated donor grafts <5 years of age. Transplant outcomes for patients >5 years of age with matched sibling or matched unrelated are also improving over time.
- Consider food allergy as exacerbating factor for eczema.
- First retroviral-based gene therapy trial in WAS recently completed in Germany with good immune reconstitution and increase in platelet counts in 9/10 patients. Lentiviral-based gene therapy trials are starting in the near future
- XLT patients have excellent long-term survival with supportive treatment, but HLA-matched sibling transplant can be considered owing to morbidity.

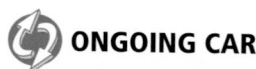 ## ONGOING CARE

FOLLOW-UP RECOMMENDATIONS
Patient Monitoring
- Signs and symptoms of malignancy should be evaluated expeditiously.
- As patients age, a progressive increase in infectious and autoimmune complications may occur.

COMPLICATIONS
- Progressive decline in immunologic function with an increase in infections. Humoral and cellular immune systems are affected.
- Increased frequency of autoimmune phenomena such as arthritis and vasculitis. The most common is hemolytic anemia. Vasculitis, Henoch-Schönlein purpura, inflammatory polyarthritis, and inflammatory bowel disease are also observed.
- ~100-fold increased risk of malignancy compared with the general pediatric population. Malignancy is more common in adolescents. Associated with Epstein-Barr virus
- Bleeding episodes can be life threatening.

- Immune reconstitution via stem cell transplant or gene therapy needed to prevent autoimmune disorders, lymphoma, and other malignancy
- Success of bone marrow transplant in last 10 years significantly improved.
- Splenectomy not recommended for classic WAS but may have role in XLT

ADDITIONAL READING

- Albert MH, Notarangelo LD, Ochs HD. Clinical spectrum, pathophysiology and treatment of the Wiskott-Aldrich syndrome. *Curr Opin Hematol*. 2011;18:42–48.
- Binder V, Albert M, Kabus M, et al. The genotype of the original Wiskott phenotype. *N Engl J Med*. 2006;355:1790–1793.
- Bosticardo M, Marangoni F, Aiuti A, et al. Recent advances in understanding the pathophysiology of Wiskott-Aldrich syndrome. *Blood*. 2009;113: 6288–6295.
- Bryant N, Watts R. Thrombocytopenic syndromes masquerading as childhood immune thrombocytopenic purpura. *Clin Pediatr*. 2011;50:255.
- Charrier S, Dupre L, Scaramuzza S, et al. Lentiviral vectors targeting WASP expression to hematopoietic cells, efficiently transduce and correct cells from WAS patients. *Gene Ther*. 2006;1–14.
- Imai K, Morio T, Zhu Y, et al. Clinical course of patients with WASP gene mutations. *Blood*. 2004;103(2):456–464.
- Jin Y, Mazza C, Christie J, et al. Mutations of the Wiskott-Aldrich syndrome protein (WASP): Hotspots, effect on transcription, and translation and phenotype/genotype correlation. *Blood*. 2004;104(13):4010–4019.
- Ochs HD. The Wiskott-Aldrich syndrome. *Clin Rev Allergy Immunol*. 2001;20:61–86.
- Schurman SH, Candotti F. Autoimmunity in Wiskott-Aldrich syndrome. *Curr Opin Rheum*. 2003;15:446–453.
- Shcherbina A, Candotti F, Rosen F, et al. High incidence of lymphomas in subgroups of Wiskott-Aldrich syndrome patients. *Br J Haematol*. 2003;121:529.

See Also (Topic, Algorithm, Electronic Media Element)
- Table 1

 ## CODES

ICD9
279.12 Wiskott-aldrich syndrome

ICD10
D82.0 Wiskott-Aldrich syndrome

FAQ

- Q: What is the life expectancy for patients with Wiskott-Aldrich syndrome?
- A: Before currently available therapies, most affected patients died in childhood. Currently, many patients live into their 3rd and 4th decades, even without bone marrow transplantation. Major causes of mortality are infections (44%), bleeding (23%), and malignancies (26%). Incidence of malignancy increases in 3rd decade of life. Successfully transplanted patients have a prolonged life expectancy. Patients with no gene expression have a poorer outcome.
- Q: Should patients with Wiskott-Aldrich syndrome receive live viral vaccines?
- A: These vaccines should be avoided because of the variable cellular immune defects associated with Wiskott-Aldrich syndrome. In general, patients receiving IV immunoglobulin do not require vaccinations.
- Q: What is the chance of a sibling having Wiskott-Aldrich syndrome?
- A: As with any X-linked disease, there is a 50% chance of another affected male child or asymptomatic carrier female. Genetic counseling should be offered to carrier females.
- Q: Can Wiskott-Aldrich syndrome be diagnosed prenatally?
- A: In families with affected males, fetal blood sampling can be performed in male fetuses to assess the size of the platelets. Small platelet size and family history of Wiskott-Aldrich syndrome suggest an affected infant.

W

YERSINIA ENTEROCOLITICA

Julia F. Shaklee
Louis M. Bell, Jr. (5th edition)
Eric J. Haas (5th edition)

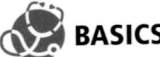

BASICS

DESCRIPTION
Yersinia enterocolitica is a gram-negative bacillus that produces an enteric infection characterized by fever, diarrhea, and abdominal pain that may mimic acute appendicitis.

EPIDEMIOLOGY
- *Y. enterocolitica* is an uncommon cause of infection in the US but affects infants and young children most frequently.
- Incidence is estimated at 9.4 per 100,000 for infants, 1.4 per 100,000 for young children, and 0.2 per 100,000 for other age groups.
- Transmission of *Y. enterocolitica* occurs through ingestion of contaminated food or water (particularly raw or undercooked pork or unpasteurized milk products) or contact with infected animals (swine are the principal reservoir). Fecal–oral and person-to-person transmission are also possible.
- Epidemics related to the improper handling of raw pork intestine (chitterlings) have been reported in the US, particularly during holiday festivities.
- Transmission through transfusion of contaminated blood products is also possible. In fact, the FDA has reported that contamination of the US blood supply by bacteria, although rare, is most frequently due to *Y. enterocolitica*.
- The incubation period is ~1–14 days (average 4–6).The average duration of organism excretion is ~2–3 weeks following diagnosis; however, asymptomatic carriage can persist even longer.
- Systemic disease or bacteremia occurs more commonly in young infants or those with predisposing conditions, including a clinical state of iron overload or deferoxamine therapy, immunosuppression, diabetes mellitus, malnutrition, and cirrhosis or other liver diseases.

GENERAL PREVENTION
- Infection control:
  - Enteric precautions are indicated for patients with enterocolitis until symptoms resolve.
- General measures:
  - Attempts to eliminate reservoirs and reduce frequency of ingesting contaminated foods and beverages are necessary.
  - Avoidance of undercooked meats, especially pork and unpasteurized milk, as well as preparation of meats near or during preparation of infant bottles for feeding is essential.

PATHOPHYSIOLOGY
- The portal of entry for *Y. enterocolitica* is the gastrointestinal tract.
- *Y. enterocolitica* adheres to epithelial cells and mucus, producing heat-stable enterotoxins, which play a role in the development of watery diarrhea.
- Another cytotoxin then directly injures the distal small and large bowel, producing stools characterized by blood and mucus.
- Release of these toxins leads to the development of an enterocolitis, most commonly in younger age groups.
- Mesenteric adenitis and/or terminal ileitis may lead to a pseudoappendicular syndrome, typically in the older child or young adult.
- Septicemia may lead to focal abscesses in a variety of organs, including the lung, liver, spleen, and kidney.

ETIOLOGY
- The genus *Yersinia* consists of 11 species, of which *Y. enterocolitica*, *Y. pseudotuberculosis*, and *Y. pestis* are the 3 most commonly encountered pathogens.
- *Y. enterocolitica* is a facultative, non–lactose-fermenting, urease-positive, gram-negative bacillus.
- Over 60 serotypes and 6 biotypes of *Y. enterocolitica* have been identified. Serotypes 0:3, 0:5.27, 0:8, and 0:9 and biotypes 2, 3, and 4 are most commonly isolated from patients. Serotype 0:3 is the most common type in the US.

DIAGNOSIS

Y. enterocolitica infection is uncommon in the US. Diagnosis is dependent upon elucidation of the pertinent exposure history as well as recognition of typical symptoms and laboratory testing.

HISTORY
- Enterocolitis is the most common manifestation of *Y. enterocolitica* infection in young children and is characterized by fever, abdominal pain, and diarrhea with blood or mucus.
  - 25% of patients have hematochezia.
  - Typical duration of illness is 1–3 weeks, but may be longer (up to several months).
  - The history taking should include exposure to unpasteurized milk products and raw pork or poultry, especially the preparation of pork chitterlings.

- A pseudoappendicitis syndrome due to mesenteric adenitis and/or terminal ileitis predominates in older children and adults and is associated with fever, right lower quadrant abdominal pain, and leukocytosis.
- *Yersinia* bacteremia is found most commonly in infants <1 year of age or those with predisposing conditions, particularly states of iron overload (e.g. sickle cell disease, thalassemia).
- Extraintestinal manifestations of *Y. enterocolitica* infection are uncommon and include pharyngitis, suppurative lymphadenitis, pyomyositis, osteomyelitis, abscess, UTI, pneumonia, endocarditis, meningitis, peritonitis, panophthalmitis, conjunctivitis, and septic arthritis.

PHYSICAL EXAM
Because of the wide range of clinical symptoms, including extraintestinal manifestations, the physical exam is nonspecific for this infection.

DIAGNOSTIC TESTS & INTERPRETATION
Lab
- *Y. enterocolitica* can be isolated from blood, sputum, CSF, urine, and bile; these specimens do not require selective culture media techniques. Stool samples should be plated on selective media such as cefsulodin-triclosan-novobiocin agar. If routine enteric media (MacConkey) are used, a cold enrichment technique will increase recovery of the organism. The laboratory should be notified that *Yersinia* is suspected if not routinely sought.
- Serologic methods (tube agglutination assay, ELISA) are available with a rise in titers noted 1 week after onset of symptoms and peak titers observed by the 2nd week of illness. These tests identify IgM, IgG, and IgA antibodies against *Y. enterocolitica*.
- Cross-reactivity between *Y. enterocolitica* and *Brucella abortus*, *Rickettsia* species, *Moraxella morganii*, *Salmonella* species, and thyroid tissue antigen make serodiagnosis of limited usefulness.

Imaging
Abdominal ultrasound can be used to distinguish pseudoappendicitis from acute appendicitis through demonstration of bowel wall edema in the terminal ileum and cecum.

DIFFERENTIAL DIAGNOSIS
- *Y. enterocolitica* should be considered in all patients with fever, abdominal pain, and stools with blood or mucus, as well as in patients with the extraintestinal manifestations described above.

- Pitfalls:
  – Not all bacterial colitis presents with bloody or mucus-appearing diarrhea. Therefore, suspicion should exist if the diarrhea is prolonged or environmental exposures pose a risk for developing infection.
  – The possibility of *Y. enterocolitica* bacteremia should be considered in blood transfusion–related illnesses, thalassemia, or prior history of liver disease.

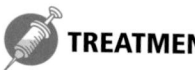 TREATMENT

ADDITIONAL TREATMENT
General Measures
- The benefit of treatment of uncomplicated enterocolitis, mesenteric adenitis, or pseudoappendicitis has not been established in immunocompetent hosts.
- Antimicrobial therapy has been shown to benefit patients with systemic infections, focal extraintestinal infections, and enterocolitis in an immunocompromised host.
- For most isolates, trimethoprim/sulfamethoxazole, chloramphenicol, aminoglycosides, tetracycline or doxycycline, fluoroquinolones, and 3rd-generation cephalosporins are effective treatment options.
- *Y. enterocolitica* is usually resistant to most penicillins and 1st-generation cephalosporins.

 ONGOING CARE

FOLLOW-UP RECOMMENDATIONS
- Symptoms of enterocolitis usually abate within 2 weeks of the onset of illness.
- Shedding of the organism in stool can last more than 6 weeks after diagnosis.
- For extraintestinal manifestations, the expected course is dependent upon the specific organ system involved.

PROGNOSIS
- The prognosis is usually quite good, as most infections are gastrointestinal.
- Systemic disease (i.e., septicemia with subsequent secondary spread) has higher morbidity and mortality. Mortality related to septicemia can be as high as 50%

COMPLICATIONS
- Postinfectious sequelae may occur 1–2 weeks after gastrointestinal symptoms and include erythema nodosum as well as reactive arthritis involving weight-bearing joints. These complications are seen most often in adults, particularly those with HLA-B27 antigen.
- Reiter syndrome, myocarditis, glomerulonephritis, erysipelas, chronic diarrhea persisting for months, and hemolytic anemia have also been reported.
- Intestinal perforation and ileocolic intussusception are possible.

ADDITIONAL READING

- Abdel-Haq NM, Asmar BI, Abuhammour WM, et al. Yersinia enterocolitica infection in children. *Pediatr Infect Dis J*. 2000;19:954–958.
- Dennis DT, Chow CC. Plague. *Pediatr Infect Dis J*. 2004;23:69–71.
- Natkin J, Beavis KG. Yersinia enterocolitica and Yersinia pseudotuberculosis. *Clin Lab Med*. 1999;19:523–536.

 CODES

ICD9
027.8 Other specified zoonotic bacterial diseases

ICD10
A04.6 Enteritis due to Yersinia enterocolitica

FAQ

- Q: How long is a child considered infectious with *Y. enterocolitica*?
- A: Although the typical course of enterocolitis is ~14 days, shedding of the organism in the stool can last 6 weeks or longer. Enteric precautions should be discussed with the child's parent or caregiver to ensure infection control.
- Q: If there is no history of stools with blood or mucus, can you exclude *Y. enterocolitica* as the likely infectious agent in a child with diarrhea?
- A: No. In fact, early in the course of illness, the diarrhea is more likely to be watery owing to the enterotoxins produced (see "Pathophysiology").
- Q: How is the diagnosis of *Y. enterocolitica* determined if you are unable to isolate the organism from a clinical specimen?
- A: When a diagnosis cannot be made during acute infection or in the clinical setting of postinfectious complications, a serologic titer of >1:128 is suggestive of previous infection of *Y. enterocolitica*. Keep in mind the possibility of cross-reactivity with *Brucella*, *Rickettsia*, *Morganella*, and *Salmonella* species as well as thyroid antigens.

Y

Appendix I
Syndromes Glossary

Megan Aylor, MD and Evan Fieldston, MD

4p syndrome (deletion 4p syndrome)—characterized by ocular hypertelorism, broad or beaked nose; microcephaly, low-set ears, pre-auricular dimples; hypotonia, severe mental deficiency, seizures; scoliosis.

5p syndrome—see "cri du chat syndrome."

13q syndrome (deletion 13q syndrome)—characterized by microcephaly, high nasal bridge, eye defect, thumb hypoplasia; typically involves malformations of the brain, heart, kidneys, and digits; usually lethal.

Aagenaes syndrome—autosomal-recessive; characterized by recurrent intrahepatic cholestasis, with lymphedema.

Aarskog syndrome—X-linked recessive; characterized by short stature, mild-to-moderate mental deficiency, musculoskeletal and genital anomalies; hypertelorism, small nose with anteverted nares, broad philtrum and nasal bridge, abnormal auricles and widow's peak, brachyclinodactyly, broad thumbs, broad feet with bulbous toes, simian crease, ptosis, syndactyly, "shawl" scrotum, cryptorchidism, inguinal hernia, hyperopic astigmatism, large corneas, ophthalmoplegia, strabismus, delayed puberty, mild pectus excavatum, prominent umbilicus; delayed bone age.

a beta lipoproteinemia—autosomal-recessive transmission of mutation in MTTP gene; characterized by inability to make beta-lipoproteins (i.e. LDL, VLDL, chylomicrons), preventing absorption of dietary fats and fat-soluble vitamins; early signs include failure to thrive, diarrhea, and acanthocytosis (star-shaped RBCs); childhood features include poor muscle control, ataxia, progressive pigmentary degeneration of the retina; by adulthood, there is significant cerebellar ataxia; absent or reduced lipoproteins and low carotene, vitamin A, and cholesterol levels.

acanthosis nigricans—skin disorder characterized by dark, thick, velvety skin in body folds and creases; can occur in healthy people or associated with medical problems, including obesity, glucose-resistance, diabetes, lymphoma, cancers of the GI or GU tracts, or those on hormones (i.e., growth hormone or oral contraceptives).

achondroplasia—autosomal-dominant, often new mutation; characterized by short limbs, short stature, megalocephaly, small foramen magnum (low risk of cord compression), caudal narrowing of spinal canal, low nasal bridge, prominent forehead, mild hypotonia, normal intelligence, relative glucose intolerance.

acrodermatitis enteropathica—autosomal-recessive; characterized by zinc deficiency due to abnormal absorption of zinc, manifest with vesicobullous and eczematous skin lesions in the perioral and perineal areas, cheeks, knees, and elbows; photophobia, conjunctivitis, and corneal dystrophy; chronic diarrhea; glossitis; nail dystrophy; growth retardation; superinfections and candidal infections; treatment requires lifelong zinc supplementation.

Adie syndrome—tonic pupil, usually characterized by mydriasis (dilated pupil) with little or no reaction to light, but may manifest as miotic, poorly reactive pupils; pupil may react to accommodation; associated with hyporeflexia.

agenesis of corpus callosum—cause unknown (suspected chromosomal, genetic, toxic, infectious, and mechanical etiologies depending on associated findings); complete or partial absence of the major tracts connecting the right and left hemispheres, usually associated with hydrocephalus, seizures, developmental delay, spasticity, and hypertelorism; can be isolated or found with Arnold-Chiari malformation, Dandy-Walker syndrome, Andermann syndrome, schizencephaly, holoprosencephaly, Aicardi syndrome, and midline facial defects; may also be seen in a variety of other syndromes, including Crouzon syndrome, fetal alcohol syndrome, Opitz syndrome, and Turner syndrome.

Aicardi syndrome—X-linked dominant, lethal in homozygous males; characterized by microcephaly, agenesis of corpus collosum, infantile spasms, chorioretinal lacunae, and costovertebral skeletal abnormalities.

Alagille syndrome (arteriohepatic dysplasia)—autosomal-dominant; characterized by paucity or absence of intrahepatic bile ducts with progressive destruction of bile ducts, cholestasis, peripheral pulmonic stenosis, peculiar facies (broad forehead, deep-set eyes that are widely spaced and underdeveloped, a small, pointed mandible), cardiac lesions, vertebral arch defects, and changes in the renal tubules and interstitium.

Albers-Schonberg disease (marble bone disease)—mostly autosomal-dominant, rarely autosomal-recessive; patients are prone to fractures and have mild anemia and craniofacial disproportion; radiologic changes include increased cortical bone density, longitudinal and transverse dense striations at the ends of the long bones, lucent and dense bands in the vertebrae, and thickening at the base of the skull.

Albright syndrome—see "McCune-Albright syndrome."

Alexander disease—caused by mutation in gene for glial fibrillary acidic protein (GFAP); 3 subtypes: Infantile, juvenile, adult; characterized by megaloencephaly in infants, dementia, spasticity and ataxia; may cause seizures in younger children; patients become mute, immobile, and dependent; hyaline eosinophilic inclusions occur in the footplates of astrocytes in subpial and subependymal regions; progressive disease with death with most patients dying within 10 years of onset; features similar to Canavan syndrome.

Alport syndrome—defective type IV collagen, most often X-linked, but with autosomal-dominant and -recessive forms; characterized by progressive nephritis to renal failure and neurosensory deafness; usually presents in infancy with hematuria, with proteinuria and hearing loss being later findings.

Andermann syndrome (Charlevoix disease)—autosomal-recessive; characterized by agenesis of the corpus collosum, mental deficiency, progressive neuropathy, and characteristic facies.

Andersen disease (glycogen storage disease, type IV)—caused by a defect of amylo(1,4 to 1,6) transglucosidase (brancher enzyme); characterized by hepatomegaly and failure to thrive in the 1st few months of life, progressing to liver cirrhosis and splenomegaly.

Angelman syndrome—maternal chromosome 15 interstitial deletion (genomic imprinting); "puppetlike" gait (ataxia and jerky arm movements), seizures, paroxysmal laughter, mental deficiency, absent or severely reduced speech, microcephaly; often blonde hair and blue eyes, characteristic facies with maxillary hypoplasia, large mouth, tongue protrusion and prognathia.

Apert syndrome (acrocephalosyndactyly)—autosomal-dominant; characterized by craniosynostosis, high and flat frontal bones, underdevelopment of the middle 3rd of the face, hypertelorism and proptosis; a narrow, high, arched palate; a short, beaked nose; syndactyly of the toes and digits; mental deficiency is common.

arthrogryposis multiplex congenita—congenital, usually nonhereditary fixed contracture of many if not all major joints; of heterogeneous cause, including neurologic, muscular, joint and tissue, and fetal crowding or in utero constraint on fetal movement.

Asperger syndrome—developmental disorder on the higher-functioning end of the autism spectrum; patients are often viewed as brilliant, eccentric, and physically awkward, fail to develop relationships with peers, have repetitive and stereotyped behaviors, usually with hand movements.

Ataxia-telangiectasia syndrome (Louis-Bar syndrome)—autosomal-recessive; characterized by progressive ataxia, degenerative central nervous system function, telangiectasia, lymphopenia, immune deficit (low to absent IgA and IgE), growth deficiency, and mental deficits.

Bart syndrome—autosomal-dominant dermolytic variant of epidermolysis bullosa; congenital aplasia of the skin; characterized by nail defects and recurrent blistering of the skin and mucous membranes.

Bartter syndrome—hypertrophy of the juxtaglomerular apparatus; characterized by hypokalemic alkalosis, hypochloremia, and hyperaldosteronism; patients have normal blood pressure but the renin level is elevated; may lead to mental retardation and small stature.

Beckwith-Wiedemann syndrome (exomphalos-macroglossia-gigantism syndrome)—usually sporadic; characterized by hypoglycemia, macrosomia, macroglossia, omphalocele, and visceromegaly; patients have unusual linear fissures in lobule of external ear, umbilical anomalies, and renal medullary dysplasia.

Behçet syndrome—unknown cause; vasculitis of large and small vessels; involves relapsing iridocyclitis and recurrent oral and genital ulcerations, white matter changes, aseptic meningitis, pulmonary aneurysm, arthritis, and arthralgias.

blind loop syndrome—stasis of small intestine, usually secondary to incomplete bowel obstruction or a problem of intestinal motility; can occur following GI surgery or from inflammatory bowel disease or scleroderma.

Bloch-Sulzberger syndrome (incontinentia pigmenti)—X-linked dominant; characterized by skin pigmentation disorder with malformation of eyes, teeth, bones, hair, nails, heart, and CNS; usually associated with mental deficiency and commonly with seizures.

Bloom syndrome—autosomal-recessive, more common in Ashkenazi Jews; chromosome instability leading to impaired growth, long, narrow face, pigmentation changes, dilated blood vessels in the skin, photosensitivity, and butterfly distribution of erythema and telangiectasia, mental deficiency, chronic lung problems, diabetes, male infertility, early menopause, and early development of cancer.

Blount disease (tibia vara)—unknown cause, possibly from effects of weight on growth plates; medial portion of tibia fails to develop normally causing angulation and irregularity of the medial aspect of the tibial metaphysis adjacent to the epiphysis; lower leg resembles bowleg, but is progressive and worsens over time; can involve one or both legs; more common in African American children, associated with obesity and early walking.

blue diaper syndrome—rare X-linked or autosomal-recessive disorder of defective tryptophan absorption; characterized by bluish stains on the diapers, digestive disturbances, irritability, fever, and visual difficulties.

Brill disease (Brill-Zinsser disease)—reactivation of dormant typhus, caused by epidemic form, *Rickettsia prowazekii*.

bronchiolitis obliterans—characterized by obstruction of bronchioles by granulation tissue; begins with necrotizing pneumonia secondary to viral infection (e.g., adenovirus, influenza, measles), tuberculosis (TB), or inhalation of fumes, talcum powder, or zinc.

Byler disease (Progressive Familial Intrahepatic Cholestasis)—autosomal-recessive; characterized by cholestasis, hepatomegaly, pruritus, splenomegaly, elevated bile acids, and gallstones.

Canavan syndrome—autosomal-recessive leukodystrophy; characterized by progressive neurological deficits, usually beginning in infancy, with macrocephaly, hypotonia, loss of milestones, seizures, swallowing difficulties, and sleep disturbance.

Caroli disease—autosomal-dominant; characterized by cystic dilatation of the intrahepatic bile ducts; characterized by recurrent bouts of cholangitis and biliary abscesses secondary to bile stasis and gallstones.

Caroli syndrome—autosomal-recessive; characterized by cystic dilatation of the intrahepatic bile ducts; more complex form of Caroli disease, leading to hepatic fibrosis; can be associated with polycystic kidney disease.

Cat-eye syndrome—duplication of segment of chromosome 22; characterized by coloboma of iris, down-slanting palpebral fissures, anal atresia, cardiac defects, renal agenesis; mild mental deficiency.

Charcot-Marie-Tooth disease (hereditary motor and sensory neuropathy (HMSN) or peroneal muscular atrophy)—various inheritance patterns; most common cause of chronic peripheral neuropathy; characterized by foot drop, high-arch foot; patients may have stocking-glove sensory loss.

CHARGE association—unknown etiology, likely insult in second month of gestation; characterized by coloboma, heart disease, choanal atresia, retarded growth and development and/or CNS anomalies, genital anomalies and/or hypogonadism, and ear anomalies and/or deafness.

Chédiak-Higashi syndrome—autosomal-recessive; characterized by partial oculocutaneous albinism, increased susceptibility to infection, lack of natural killer cells, and large, lysosomelike granules in many tissues; patients have splenomegaly, hypersplenism, hepatomegaly, lymphadenopathy, nystagmus, photophobia, and peripheral neuropathy.

Coats' disease (retinal telangiectasis)—telangiectasia of retinal vessels, with subretinal exudates; usually unilateral, but can be bilateral.

Cobb syndrome—noninherited very rare association of spinal angiomas or AVMs with congenital, cutaneous vascular malformations, such as port-wine stains or angiomas.

Cockayne syndrome—autosomal-recessive; characterized by dwarfism, microcephaly, mental retardation, birdlike facies, premature senility, and photosensitivity.

Congenital rubella syndrome—see "fetal rubella syndrome."

Cornelia de Lange syndrome (Brachmann-De Lange syndrome, de Lange syndrome)—unknown cause, most cases sporadic; characterized by prenatal growth retardation, microcephaly, hirsutism, synophris, anteverted nares, down-turned mouth, mental retardation, and congenital heart defects.

cri du chat syndrome (5p deletion syndrome)—usually sporadic; characterized by catlike cry in infancy, microcephaly, downward palpebral fissures, low birth weight, growth retardation, mental deficiency, hypotonia, round face, hypertelorism, epicanthal folds, and simian crease.

Crigler-Najjar syndrome, Type I (glucuronyl transferase deficiency)—autosomal-recessive; absence of hepatic uridine 5'-diphospho-glucuronosyltransferase activity leading to unconjugated hyperbilirubinemia on 1st day of life without evidence of hemolysis; requires phototherapy to prevent kernicterus.

Crigler-Najjar syndrome, Type II—autosomal-recessive; less severe unconjugated hyperbilirubinemia due to partial activity of uridine 5'-diphospho-glucuronosyltransferase; kernicterus is less common than in Type I.

Crouzon syndrome (craniofacial dysostosis)—autosomal-dominant with variable expression; characterized by exophthalmos due to shallow orbits, hypertelorism, craniosynostosis, and hypoplasia of maxilla; patients have oral cavity anomalies and premature closure of the external auditory meatus.

cyclic neutropenia—most often autosomal-dominant; lack of granulocyte macrophage colony-stimulating factor (GM-CSF); characterized by fever, mouth lesions, cervical adenitis, and gastroenteritis occurring every 3–6 weeks; neutrophil count may be zero.

De Sanctis-Cacchione syndrome—autosomal-recessive; characterized by xeroderma pigmentosum with mental retardation, dwarfism, and hypogonadism; skin is unable to repair itself after exposure to ultraviolet light; patients may have erythema, scaling bullae, crusting telangiectasia, keratoses, photophobia, corneal opacities, and tumors of the eyelids.

Diamond-Blackfan syndrome (congenital pure red cell aplasia)—failure of erythropoiesis; characterized by macrocytic anemia, pallor, weakness, elevated fetal hemoglobin, without hepatomegaly.

DiGeorge syndrome—microdeletion of 22q11.2 most often; characterized by thymic hypoplasia or aplasia with hypocalcemia; patients have tetany, seizures, abnormal facies, congenital heart disease, and increased incidence of infection.

Down syndrome—see "trisomy 21."

Dubin-Johnson syndrome—autosomal-recessive; characterized by elevated conjugated bilirubin, large amounts of coproporphyrin I in urine, and deposits of melaninlike pigment in hepatocellular lysosomes.

Dubowitz syndrome—autosomal-recessive; characterized by prenatal and postnatal growth retardation, mental retardation, hyperactivity, stubbornness and shyness, hypotonia, microcephaly, facial features that can resemble fetal alcohol syndrome, eczemalike skin disorder, and ocular abnormalities.

Eagle-Barrett syndrome (prune-belly syndrome)—characterized by deficiency of the abdominal musculature, dilatation and dysplasia of the urinary tract, cryptorchidism, dilatation of the posterior urethra, and a hypoplastic or absent prostate; associated with Trisomy 21, Trisomy 18, Tetralogy of Fallot, and ventricular septal defects.

ectodermal dysplasia—variable inheritance; characterized by poor development, or absence, of teeth, nails, hair, and sweat glands; hyperextensible skin, hypermobile joints, and easy bruisability.

Ehlers-Danlos syndrome—autosomal-dominant, variable expression (Type I); characterized by abnormal collagen leading to hyperextensible joints and skin, poor wound healing with parchment-thin scars, narrow maxilla, mitral valve prolapse, and aortic root dilatation. Types II-X have different modes of inheritance, severity of disease, and related findings.

Eisenmenger syndrome—combination of pulmonary hypertension and right-to-left cardiac shunting within the heart that is the progressive result of a structural heart defect that allows for left-to-right shunting and increased pulmonary blood flow; over time, pulmonary hypertension develops with reversal of the shunt direction; ventricular septal defects are the most common cause.

Fabry disease—X-linked deficiency of ceramide trihexosidase (alpha-galactosidase-A) leading to lipid storage disease; characterized by tingling and burning in the hands and feet; small, red maculopapular lesions on the buttocks, inguinal area, fingernails, and lips; and an inability to perspire; proteinuria, progressing to renal failure; increased risk of cardiovascular disease.

Farber syndrome—autosomal-recessive deficiency of acid ceramidase; characterized by subcutaneous nodules, arthritis, and laryngeal involvement with hoarseness.

fetal alcohol syndrome—characterized by prenatal and postnatal growth deficiency, microcephaly, hypoplastic maxillary bone; abnormal palpebral fissures; smooth philtrum with thin, smooth upper lip; epicanthal folds; cardiac septal defect; delayed development; and mental deficiency.

fetal hydantoin syndrome—characterized by prenatal and postnatal growth deficiency, wide anterior fontanel, midface hypoplasia, low nasal bridge, ocular hypertelorism, cupid bow upper lip, cleft lip and palate, mental deficiency, and cardiac defects.

fetal rubella syndrome—in utero rubella exposure (especially in the 1st trimester); characterized by mental deficiency, microcephaly, deafness, cataract, glaucoma, patent ductus arteriosus, cardiac septal defects, hepatosplenomegaly, anemia, and thrombocytopenia.

fetal valproate syndrome—midface hypoplasia, long philtrum, thin vermillion border, small mouth; aortic and ventricular abnormalities; long, thin fingers and toes; meningomyelocele.

fetal warfarin syndrome—Coumadin exposure, mostly in the 1st trimester, leading to nasal hypoplasia, mental deficiency, low birth weight, mild hypoplasia of nails and fingers, and stippled epiphyses on radiographs.

fibrodysplasia ossificans progressiva (FOP)—autosomal-dominant, single nucleotide defect, mostly fresh mutations; characterized by short hallux, ossification of muscles and subcutaneous tissues, and hearing loss; any trauma (e.g., surgery, biopsy, IM injections) can cause ectopic ossification.

Fragile X syndrome—X-linked in males and females, more easily recognized phenotype in males; characterized by mental deficiency, autism or autisticlike behaviors, macrocephaly, prognathism, dental crowding, large ears, blue eyes, mild connective tissue dysplasia, and macro-orchidism.

Friedreich ataxia—autosomal-recessive; progressive loss of large myelinated axons in peripheral nerves, with symptoms usually appearing in late childhood or adolescence; characterized by progressive cerebellar and spinal cord dysfunction; patients have high-arched foot, hammer toes, and cardiac failure.

fructose intolerance, hereditary—autosomal-recessive; involves deficiency of fructose-1-phosphate aldolase or fructose 1,6-diphosphatase; characterized by vomiting, diarrhea, hypoglycemic seizures, and jaundice.

Gardner syndrome—autosomal-dominant; variant of familial adenomatous polyposis; characterized by multiple GI polyps with malignant transformation, skin cysts, supernumerary teeth, and multiple osteoma.

Gaucher disease—autosomal-recessive deficiency of glucocerebrosidase, leading to accumulation and storage of glucocerebroside in the reticuloendothelial system; 3 types: (a) adult, or chronic, (b) acute neuropathic, or infantile, (c) subacute neuropathic, or juvenile; characterized by splenomegaly, hepatomegaly, delayed development, strabismus, swallowing difficulties, laryngeal spasm, opisthotonos, and bone pain.

Gianotti-Crosti syndrome (papular acrodermatitis of childhood)—infectious exanthem associated with nonicteric hepatitis; caused by a variety of viruses, often Hepatitis B and EBV; most common in children aged 3 months to 15 years, with 90% of cases in children 4 years and younger.

Gilbert syndrome—generally autosomal-recessive; reduced activity of glucuronyltransferase activity leading to mild unconjugated hyperbilirubinemia that worsens with stresses on the body, such as fasting.

Gilles de la Tourette syndrome—dominant trait with partial penetrance; characterized by multiple motor and vocal tics that begin before the age of 18; high rate of associated neurobehavioral difficulties, including obsessive-compulsive disorder, ADHD, anger control problems, and poor social skills.

Glanzmann thrombasthenia—autosomal-recessive; involves defective primary platelet aggregation (size and survival of platelets is normal).

Goldenhar syndrome—usually sporadic; characterized by oculo-auriculo-vertebral dysplasia and mandibular hypoplasia; patients have a hypoplastic zygomatic arch; malformed, displaced pinnae, and hearing loss.

Goltz syndrome—mostly sporadic and female, thought to be X-linked dominant; poikiloderma with focal dermal hypoplasia, syndactyly, polydactyly, spinal defects, colobomas, strabismus, nystagmus, and dental anomalies.

Gorlin syndrome—autosomal-dominant; characterized by basal cell carcinomas, macrocephaly, broad facies, and rib anomalies.

Gradenigo syndrome—complication of otitis media or mastoiditis; acquired palsy of the abducens nerve (CN VI) and pain in the trigeminal nerve distribution, with diplopia, ocular and facial pain, photophobia, and lacrimation.

Hand-Schuller-Christian disease—see "histiocytosis X."

Hartnup disease—autosomal-recessive defect in transport of monoamine monocarboxylic amino acids by intestinal mucosa and renal tubules; characterized by photosensitivity and a pellagralike skin rash; patients may have cerebellar ataxia.

histiocytosis X—formerly called eosinophilic granuloma, Langerhans cell histiocytosis,

Hand-Schuller-Christian disease, or Letterer-Siwe disease; abnormal increase in macrophages, monocytes, and dendritic cells; patients may have a few solitary bone lesions or seborrheic dermatitis of scalp, lymphadenopathy, hepatosplenomegaly, tooth loss, exophthalmos, or pulmonary infiltrates; skull x-rays notable for "punched out" lesions.

Holt-Oram syndrome—autosomal-dominant with variable expression; characterized by upper limb defects (including syndactyly, absent thumb, phocomelia), cardiac anomalies (including ostium secundum atrial septal defect, ventricular septal defect), and narrow shoulders.

homocystinuria syndrome—autosomal-recessive; deficient cystathioneine synthetase activity leading to mental deficiency, seizures, myopia, lens subluxation, malar flush, sparse fine hair, slim skeletal build, osteoporosis, vascular abnormalities, and thromboses.

Hunter syndrome (mucopolysaccharidosis II)—X-linked recessive; involves an accumulation of heparan sulfate and dermatan sulfate and enzyme deficiency of l-iduronate sulfatase; characterized by macrocephaly, coarse facial features, hypertrophy of internal organs, and mental deficiency.

Hurler syndrome (mucopolysaccharidosis IH)—autosomal-recessive; involves an accumulation of heparan sulfate and dermatan sulfate, and enzyme deficiency of α-l-iduronidase; characterized by coarse facial features, growth arrest, progressive mental deficiency, glaucoma, arthritis, and cardiac valvular disease.

Hutchinson-Gilford syndrome (progeria syndrome)—mostly sporadic; characterized by premature aging, severe growth failure, atherosclerosis, alopecia, and dystrophic nails.

Hyper-IgE (Job syndrome)—characterized by recurrent deep tissue and skin staphylococcal infections; patients have eosinophilia and IgE levels that are 10 times greater than normal.

incontinentia pigmenti—see "Bloch-Sulzberger syndrome."

Jeune thoracic dystrophy (asphyxiating thoracic dystrophy)—autosomal-recessive congenital dwarfism; characterized by small thorax, lung hypoplasia, respiratory distress, short limbs, and polydactyly; kidney lesions may progress to renal insufficiency or failure.

Job syndrome—see "Hyper-IgE."

Kabuki syndrome—sporadic; characterized by growth deficiency, mental deficiency, hypotonia, long palpebral fissures with eversion over the lateral portion of lower eyelid, ptosis, arching eyebrows, large protuberant ears, open mouth, cleft palate, extremity and rib deformities, joint hyperextensibility; cardiac anomalies.

Kallmann syndrome—genetic hypogonadism; characterized by isolated gonadotropin deficiency and anosmia.

Kartagener syndrome—autosomal-recessive; characterized by sinusitis, bronchiectasis, situs inversus, infertility and immotile cilia.

Kasabach-Merritt syndrome—characterized by giant hemangioma causing a consumptive coagulopathy, thrombocytopenia, and microangiopathic hemolytic anemia.

Kleine-Levin syndrome—characterized by unusual hunger, somnolence, and abnormal behavior.

Klinefelter syndrome—47 XXY karyotype; characterized by seminiferous tubule dysgenesis, testicular atrophy, eunuchoid habitus, gynecomastia, and behavior disorders.

Klippel-Feil syndrome—due to a defect in cervical spine development; characterized by a short neck, limited neck motion, and low occipital hairline. May also have associated genitourinary tract abnormalities.

Krabbe leukodystrophy—autosomal-recessive neurodegenerative disorder; characterized by lysosomal enzyme deficiency, leading to loss of myelin in white matter; patients develop hyperreexia, rigidity, swallowing difficulties, seizures, and blindness; usually presents by age 6 months, and most patients die by 2 years of age.

Larsen syndrome—usually autosomal-recessive; characterized by hyperlaxity, multiple congenital dislocations, and characteristic facies.

Laurence-Moon-Biedl syndrome—characterized by mental retardation, retinitis pigmentosa, hypogonadism, and spastic paraplegia.

Lawrence-Seip syndrome—association of acanthosis nigricans, generalized complete absence of subcutaneous fat, muscle hypertrophy, hyperlipemia, diabetes mellitus, and hepatosplenomegaly with cirrhosis.

Lennox-Gastaut syndrome (childhood epileptic encephalopathy)—characterized by intractable seizures of various types, mental retardation, and characteristic slow spike wave EEG pattern.

LEOPARD syndrome—autosomal-dominant with variable expression; characterized by lentigenes, EKG abnormalities, ocular hypertelorism, pulmonic stenosis, abnormalities of genitalia, retardation of growth, and deafness.

Lesch-Nyhan syndrome—X-linked disorder of purine metabolism; characterized by hyperuricemia as a result of diminished or absent hypoxanthine guanine phosphoribosyl transferase (HPRT) activity, choreoathetosis, compulsive self-mutilation, mental retardation, spastic cerebral palsy, and growth failure.

Letterer-Siwe disease—see "histiocytosis X."

Lowe syndrome (oculocerebrorenal syndrome)—X-linked disorder; characterized by congenital cataracts, hypotonia, mental retardation, rickets, and Fanconi syndrome.

Maffucci syndrome—characterized by multiple enchondroma of the bone and soft tissue hemangiomas; patients have short stature, skeletal deformities, scoliosis, and high risk of malignant transformation.

Marfan syndrome—mutation of fibrillin gene on chromosome 15; connective tissue disorder characterized by ectopia lentis, dilatation of the aorta, scoliosis, pneumothorax, pectus excavatum or carinatum, and long, thin extremities.

McCune-Albright syndrome—characterized by polyostotic fibrous dysplasia; multiple large café-au-lait macules with irregular edges, and endocrinopathies such as precocious puberty, hyperthyroidism, gigantism and Cushing syndrome; more commonly in girls.

MELAS syndrome—(Mitochondrial myopathy, Encephalopathy, Lactic Acidosis, and Strokelike episodes); causes seizures, hemiparesis, hemianopsia, or cortical blindness, sensorineural hearing loss, and short stature.

Menkes disease (kinky hair disease)—X-linked recessive progressive neurodegenerative disorder; characterized by short, friable, colorless scalp hair, failure to thrive, mental retardation, optic atrophy, hypopigmentation, hypothermia, growth failure, seizures, and progressive CNS failure.

Möbius syndrome—characterized by cranial nerve dysfunction causing bilateral facial weakness, feeding difficulties, and impairment of ocular abduction.

Morquio syndrome (mucopolysaccharidosis type IV)—characterized by skeletal dysplasia, short-trunk dwarfism, kyphoscoliosis, short neck, hypoplasia and corneal clouding and cardiac valve disease; patients have laxity of the odontoid processes, and are at risk for life-threatening atlantoaxial subluxation.

multiple hereditary exostosis—autosomal-dominant disorder characterized by presence of multiple osteochondromas (exostosis) occurring most commonly on the metaphysis of long bones, but may also occur on the ribs, scapula, vertebral bodies, and iliac crest; exostoses become calcified and cause skeletal deformities such as short stature, limb length discrepancy or deformity of the extremities.

nail-patella syndrome—autosomal-dominant; characterized by dystrophic and hypoplastic nails, hypoplastic patellae and iliac horns, and malformed radial heads; may lead to nephrotic syndrome and renal failure.

Niemann-Pick disease—autosomal-recessive disorder of lipid metabolism with 4 subtypes; characterized by failure to thrive, hepatomegaly, and rapidly progressive neurodegeneration; in its most severe form patients are normal at birth but by 6 months experience delayed development and loss of developmental milestones; 50% have a macular cherry red spot.

Noonan syndrome—autosomal-dominant; clinical features similar to Turner syndrome; characterized by cardiac disease (most commonly or pulmonary valve stenosis), hypertelorism, downward palpebral slant, epicanthal folds, webbed neck; short stature, and low set, posteriorly rotated ears; patients may also have cryptorchidism, and a bleeding diathesis.

Osler-Weber-Rendu syndrome (hereditary hemorrhagic telangiectasia)—autosomal-dominant vascular dysplasia; characterized by telangiectases of the skin, respiratory tract mucosa, lips, nails, and conjunctiva as well as arteriovenous malformations of the lung, liver, and brain.

Osteogenesis imperfecta, Type I—autosomal-dominant with variable expression; characterized by postnatal growth deficiency, fragile bone with frequent fractures, hyperextensibility, blue sclerae, yellowish or bluish gray teeth, and presenile deafness.

Osteogenesis imperfecta congenital (Type II)—mostly autosomal-dominant, but autosomal-recessive subtypes; characterized by short limbs, short broad bones, and defective ossification, deep blue sclerae; usually stillborn or die in infancy of respiratory failure.

Osteogenesis imperfecta, Type III—autosomal-dominant; more severe than Type I, with prenatal growth deficiency, multiple fractures present at birth, bluish sclera in infancy (normal in adulthood).

Osteogenesis imperfecta, Type IV—autosomal-dominant; normal or moderate short stature, significant bone deformities, normal sclera, femoral bowing in neonatal period that straightens with time.

Parinaud syndrome—characterized by weakness of upward gaze, nystagmus to convergence and accommodation, pupillary changes, and eyelid retraction; classically seen with pineal tumors.

Patau syndrome—see "trisomy 13."

Pelizaeus-Merzbacher disease—X-linked-recessive; characterized by abnormal myelin in the CNS, nystagmus, developmental delay, spasticity, and ataxia; patients may also have optic atrophy and seizures.

Peutz-Jeghers syndrome—autosomal-dominant; characterized by melanotic macules on the lips and mucous membranes, intestinal polyposis, and increased risk of malignancy.

Pickwickian syndrome—characterized by obesity and hypoventilation; patients may have sleep apnea, daytime somnolence and cyanosis.

Pierre Robin syndrome—characterized by severe micrognathia, glossoptosis, and cleft palate.

Poland syndrome—characterized by a unilateral absence or hypoplasia of the pectoralis muscle with ipsilateral breast hypoplasia and upper limb abnormalities.

Prader-Willi syndrome—autosomal-dominant disorder of chromosome 15 imprinting; characterized by hypotonia and initial failure to thrive, followed by marked obesity due to an insatiable appetite; other features include mental retardation, hypogonadism, small hands and feet, and short stature.

Progeria syndrome—see "Hutchinson-Gilford syndrome."

Prune-belly syndrome—see "Eagle-Barrett syndrome."

Rieger syndrome—sporadic autosomal-dominant; characterized by ocular abnormalities, hypodontia, and maxillary hypoplasia; less common features include renal, cardiac, neurologic, and umbilical abnormalities.

Riley-Day syndrome—autosomal-recessive familial dysautonomia occurring almost exclusively in persons of Ashkenazi Jewish decent; affects sensory and autonomic functions; characterized by poor feeding, aspiration, alacrima, excessive sweating with skin flushing, high threshold to pain, markedly decreased reflexes, smooth tongue and impaired taste, and erratic BP and temperature.

Rotor syndrome—autosomal-recessive; characterized by mild conjugated bilirubinemia and jaundice that may be exacerbated by infection, surgery, pregnancy, or drugs; usually asymptomatic with normal life expectancy; clinically, similar to Dubin-Johnson; however, patients with Rotor have normal appearing hepatocytes.

Rubinstein-Taybi syndrome—characterized by broad thumbs and toes, short stature, mental retardation, beaked nose, and congenital heart defects.

Russell-Silver syndrome—characterized by intrauterine growth retardation (IUGR), small triangular facies, 5th finger clinodactyly, hemihypertrophy, genitourinary malformations, and short stature.

Sandhoff disease (GM2-gangliosidosis type II)—autosomal-recessive progressive neurodegenerative disorder; characterized by deficient hexosaminidase activity leading to clinical manifestations nearly identical to Tay-Sachs disease, with macular cherry red spot, blindness, progressive loss of developmental milestones, and seizures, as well as hepatosplenomegaly, cardiac involvement, and mild skeletal abnormalities.

Sanfilippo syndrome, types A, B, C, and D (mucopolysaccharidosis types IIIA, B, C, and D)—autosomal recessive group of disorders caused by a deficiency in 1 of 4 distinct enzymes with clinically similar manifestations; characterized by accumulation of heparan sulfate, which leads to hyperactivity and destructive behavior and progresses to neurologic deterioration.

Scheie syndrome (mucopolysaccharidosis type IS)—autosomal recessive disease caused by an enzyme defect affecting α-L-iduronidase which leads to accumulation of heparan sulfate and dermatan sulfate; characterized by stiff joints, corneal clouding, aortic valve disease, and normal intellect.

scimitar syndrome—characterized by dextrocardia, hypoplasia of the right lung with systemic arterial supply, and anomalous right pulmonary vein draining in to the inferior vena cava, giving characteristic scimitar (curved swordlike) shape on chest radiograph.

Seckel syndrome—rare autosomal-recessive disorder; characterized by dwarfism, microcephaly, sharp facial features with underdeveloped chin, and mental retardation.

Shwachman-Diamond syndrome—autosomal-recessive; characterized by exocrine pancreatic dysfunction, bone marrow dysfunction with risk of malignant transformation, and skeletal abnormalities with moderate dwarfism.

Smith-Lemli-Opitz syndrome—autosomal-recessive disorder of cholesterol synthesis resulting in multiple malformations; characterized by growth retardation, microcephaly, ptosis, anteverted nares, micrognathia, syndactyly, hypospadius with cryptorchidism, and mental retardation.

Sotos syndrome (cerebral gigantism)—characterized by macrocephaly, large hands and feet, prominent mandible, rapid growth, mental retardation, and poor coordination.

Stickler syndrome—autosomal-dominant; characterized by progressive myopia, leading to retinal detachment and blindness; patients may also have Pierre Robin anomaly at birth and may develop sensorineural hearing loss and osteoarthritis during adolescence.

Sturge-Weber syndrome—characterized by a port-wine stain on the face at the 1st branch of the trigeminal nerve; patients have ipsilateral leptomeningeal angiomatosis with intracranial calcifications leading to seizures and mental retardation and may also have ocular complications, such as glaucoma.

Swyer-James syndrome—characterized by unilateral hyperlucent lung following bronchiolitis obliterans.

Tay-Sachs disease (GM2-gangliosidosis type I)—autosomal-recessive, most common among Ashkenazi Jews (carrier state 1 in 25); characterized by deficient hexosaminidase activity which leads to accumulation of GM2 gangliosides in the CNS; patients have loss of motor milestones, seizures, macular cherry-red spot, and progressive neurodegeneration leading to blindness, paralysis, and death within the 2nd or 3rd year of life.

Tourette syndrome—see "Gilles de la Tourette syndrome."

Treacher Collins syndrome—autosomal dominant with variable expression; characterized by mandibulofacial dysostosis; patients have hypoplastic zygomatic arches and mandibles, micrognathia, downward slanting palpebral fissures, coloboma of the lid, deformities of the external ear with associated conductive hearing deficits, and a cleft palate with or without cleft lip.

trisomy 13 (Patau syndrome)—characterized by midline defects including holoprosencephaly, aplasia cutis congenita, cleft lip, microphthalmia, postaxial polydactyly, clenched hands with overlapping fingers, and cardiovascular anomalies; majority abort spontaneously and most live born infants die within the 1st year of life.

trisomy 18 (Edwards syndrome)—characterized by a small face, prominent occiput, micrognathia, low-set ears, clenched hands with overriding fingers, a short sternum, and rocker bottom feet; patients are small for gestational age and have severe mental retardation,

cardiac and renal anomalies, and usually do not survive past the 1st year of life.

trisomy 21 (Down syndrome)—characterized by mental retardation and characteristic facies as well as congenital heart disease (particularly aterioventricular canal defects), GI disorders (Hirschprung disease, duodenal atresia), leukemia, hearing loss, and thyroid disease. One of the most common chromosomal abnormalities in liveborn children.

tuberous sclerosis—autosomal-dominant with highly variable expression; characterized by seizures, mental retardation, intracranial tubers and subependymal calcification, retinal hamartomas, cardiac rhabdomyomas, and renal hamartomas; pathognomonic skin lesions include hypopigmented macules (ash leaf spots), connective tissue nevi (shagreen patch), adenoma sebaceum, and subungual or periungual fibromas.

Turcot syndrome—characterized by adenomatous colonic polyposis associated with malignant brain tumors, especially medulloblastoma and glioblastoma.

Turner syndrome—classically, 45 XO karyotype, another 15% are mosaic and may have less marked features; characterized by gonadal dysplasia with sterility and primary amenorrhea, short stature, sparse pubic and axillary hair and underdeveloped breasts with wide spaced nipples; also low hairline, webbed neck, shield chest, congenital lymphedema of the extremities, cardiac disease (coarctation of the aorta), and increased carrying angle.

Usher syndrome—autosomal recessive; characterized by early retinitis pigmentosa, vestibular dysfunction, and sensorineural deafness.

vanishing testes syndrome—characterized by bilateral gonadal failure with normal external male genitalia, 46 XY karyotype, absent testes, and no male puberty.

VATER association—characterized by Vertebral defects, Anal atresia, Tracheoesophageal fistula with Esophageal atresia, and Radial and/or renal anomalies; may be expanded to VACTERL to include Congenital heart defects or other Limb defects.

Vogt-Koyanagi-Harada syndrome—disorder of melanocyte containing organs characterized by vitiligo, uveitis, dysacousis or tinnitus, aseptic meningitis, and premature graying of hair.

von Gierke disease (Glycogen Storage Disease Type I)—autosomal-recessive inherited defect in glucose-6-phosphatase; characterized by fasting hypoglycemia, growth retardation, hepatomegaly, lactic acidosis, hyperlipidemia, and hyperuricemia.

von Hippel–Landau disease—autosomal dominant with variable penetrance (chromosome 3); neurocutaneous syndrome predisposing to benign and malignant neoplasms, most commonly cerebellar, retinal or spinal hemangioblastoma; associated with pheochromocytoma, renal cell carcinoma, pancreatic tumors and cystic lesions of the kidneys, pancreas, liver, and epididymis.

Waardenburg syndrome—autosomal dominant; characterized by white forelock, heterochromic irides, lateral displacement of the inner canthi, broad nasal bridge, and sensorineural deafness.

Wegener granulomatosis—necrotizing granulomatous vasculitis involving (a) the airways, leading to rhinorrhea, chronic sinusitis, nasal ulceration; (b) the lungs, causing hemoptysis, dyspnea and cough; (c) the kidneys, manifested as hematuria and/or proteinuria due to glomerulonephritis; other symptoms include fever, malaise, weight loss, myalgias, arthralgias, ophthalmic involvement, neuropathies, and cutaneous nodules or ulcers.

Werner syndrome—autosomal recessive; characterized by short stature, gonadal atrophy, sclerodermalike skin changes, cataracts, subcutaneous calcification, premature arteriosclerosis, diabetes mellitus, and a wizened and prematurely aged facies.

Williams syndrome—deletion in subunit 7q11.23 (elastin allele); characterized by hypercalcemia in infants, supravalvular aortic stenosis, peripheral pulmonary artery stenosis, characteristic facies, mental retardation, growth delay, and stellate iris; affected children are often very talkative and musically inclined.

Wiskott-Aldrich syndrome—X-linked recessive; characterized by thrombocytopenia, severe eczema, and recurrent infections.

Wolff-Parkinson-White syndrome—accessory conduction pathway found in 25% of patients with supraventricular tachycardia; typical electrocardiographic findings include a short PR interval and slow upstroke of the QRS (delta wave); usually occurs in patients with a normal heart but also may occur in patients with Ebstein anomaly and cardiomyopathy; slightly increased risk for sudden death due to cardiac arrhythmia.

Wolman disease—autosomal-recessive lysosomal storage disease leading to fat deposition in visceral organs; fatal in infancy, this condition is characterized by intractable vomiting, failure to thrive, abdominal distention, steatorrhea, hepatosplenomegaly, and adrenal calcification.

Zellweger syndrome (cerebrohepatorenal syndrome)—autosomal-recessive disorder of peroxisome import characterized by hepatic cirrhosis, renal cysts, dysmorphic facies, seizures, mental retardation, hypotonia, glaucoma, and congenital stippled epiphyses.

Zollinger-Ellison syndrome—characterized by gastrin secreting islet cell tumors leading to gastric acid hypersecretion and production of duodenal and jejunal ulcers.

Appendix II
Cardiology Laboratory

Ilana Zeltser

BLOOD PRESSURE MEASUREMENT

Between 1% and 3% of the pediatric population has hypertension. Most cases of hypertension are early manifestations of essential hypertension. Approximately 10% of children have secondary hypertension, and 80% of these patients have underlying renal parenchymal or renal vascular disease. After renal disease, coarctation or hypoplasia of the aorta is the second most common cause of secondary hypertension.

Accurate determination of the blood pressure is an integral part of the physical examination. The blood pressure cuff must be the correct size; a small cuff will falsely overestimate the blood pressure. The blood pressure cuff should be 50% of the circumference and 2/3 the length of the extremity. Second, the patient should be sitting and calm. Finally, once the cuff is sufficiently inflated, the cuff should then be released slowly at a rate of 3 to 4 mmHg/sec. The 1st Korotkoff sound corresponds to the systolic pressure, although the 5th Korotkoff sound, the disappearance of sound, represents the diastolic pressure.

The report from the Second Task Force on Blood Pressure Control in Children published standard blood pressure measurements for children from birth to 18 years of age (Figure 1). These reference standards do not distinguish between racial or ethnic groups. In general, blood pressure increases with height, weight, age, and sexual maturation. Blood pressure is higher in males than in females during the 1st decade of life and tends to widen around the onset of puberty. Blood pressure follows a circadian rhythm, being highest late in the day and lowest at night while sleeping.

When cardiac disease is suspected, blood pressure measurements should be obtained in all 4 extremities. A difference of greater than 10 mmHg between upper and lower extremity blood pressures is pathologic and suggests the presence of aortic coarctation, aortic arch hypoplasia or interrupted aortic arch.

A. Girls

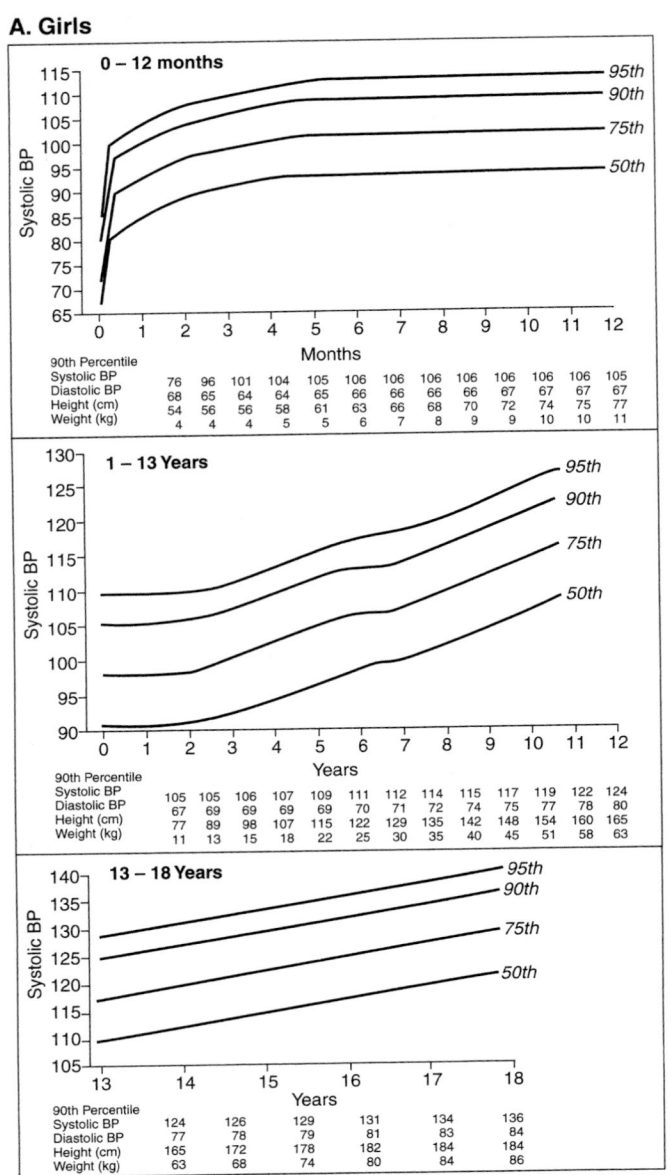

B. Boys

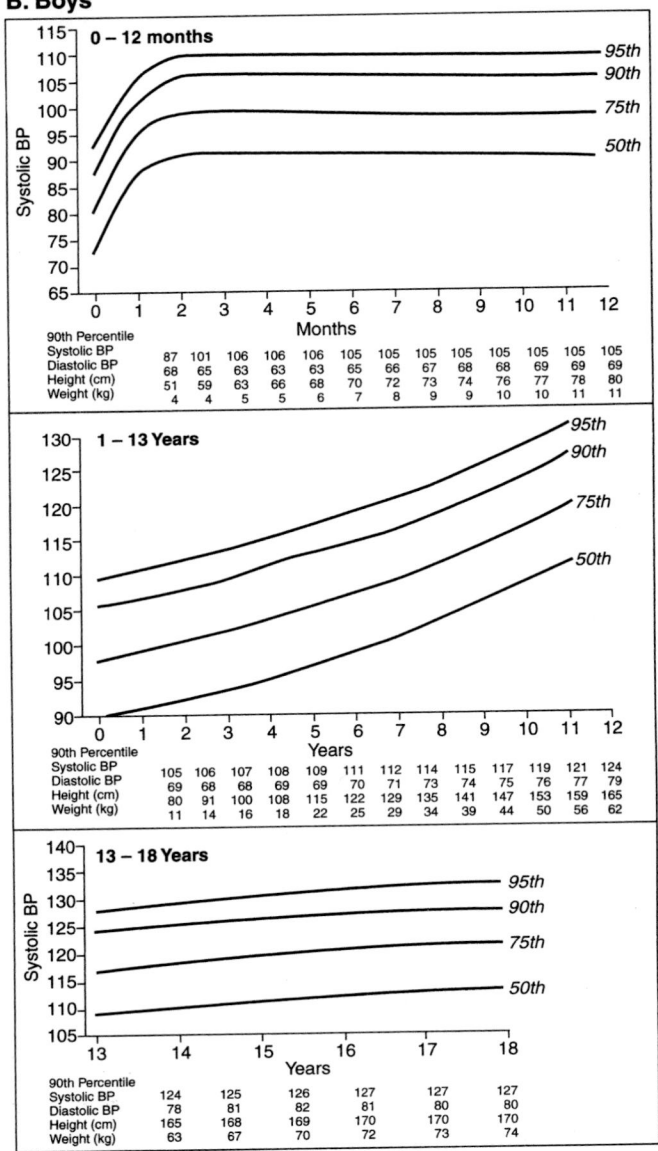

FIGURE 1. Standard blood pressure measurements in accordance with age and gender. A: Girls. B: Boys. BP, blood pressure. (From Horan MJ. Report of the Second Task Force on Blood Pressure Control in Children—1987. Pediatrics 1987;79:1–25, with permission).

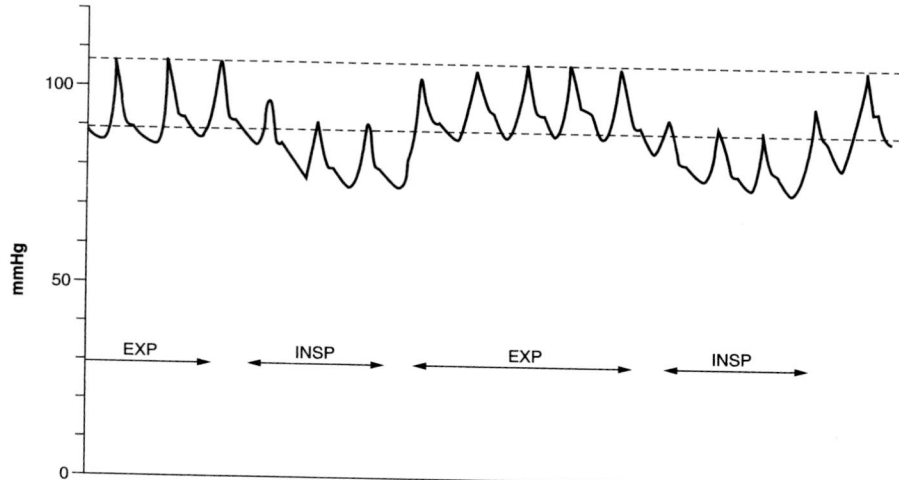

FIGURE 2. Pulsus paradoxus. EXP, expiration; INSP, inspiration. (Modified from Park MK. Pediatric cardiology for practitioners, 3rd ed. St. Louis: Mosby-Year Book 1996:15, with permission).

Pulse Pressure

The pulse pressure is the calculated difference between the systolic and diastolic pressures. A widened pulse pressure is present in: (a) high cardiac output states (anemia, fever, exercise, thyrotoxicosis), (b) diastolic run-off lesions (patent ductus arteriosus, aortic insufficiency, arteriovenous malformations), or (c) complete heart block. Narrow pulse pressure states may reflect: (a) low cardiac output states, (b) mitral or aortic valve stenosis, or (c) pericardial tamponade or constrictive pericarditis.

Hint: Normally, with inspiration, there is a small diminution of the systolic blood pressure compared to the diastolic pressure, resulting in a slight narrowing of the pulse pressure. Pulsus paradoxus exists when this response is exaggerated, and there is a greater than 10 mmHg drop in the systolic blood pressure

with inspiration, resulting in narrowing of the pulse pressure. Pulsus paradoxus indicates underlying cardiopulmonary disease and may be associated with cardiac tamponade, constrictive pericarditis, or severe respiratory compromise (e.g., status asthmaticus). See Figure 2 for a schematic illustration of pulsus paradoxus.

CYANOSIS

Central cyanosis can be detected when the absolute concentration of deoxygenated hemoglobin is at least 3 gm/dL in a child with a normal hemoglobin. The best indicator of cyanosis is the tongue, which is free of pigmentation and has a rich vascular supply. Whether or not cyanosis is manifest depends on (a) the hemoglobin and (b) factors that alter the affinity of

hemoglobin (temperature, serum pH, level of 2,3-diphosphoglycerate and the percentage of fetal versus adult hemoglobin). For example, a newborn with polycythemia (hemoglobin of 20 g/dL) and an arterial saturation of 80% will have 4 g/dL of deoxygenated hemoglobin and will appear cyanotic. In contrast, an anemic newborn (hemoglobin of 10 g/dL) with an arterial saturation of 80% will have only 2 g/dL of deoxygenated hemoglobin and will not appear cyanotic.

Hint: Central cyanosis should not be confused with acrocyanosis, a common physical finding in newborns as a result of peripheral vasoconstriction.

Hyperoxia Test

In infants with cyanosis and hypoxia, the differential diagnosis includes abnormalities of the cardiovascular, pulmonary, neurologic, and hematologic systems. In all neonates with hypoxemia, the hyperoxia test is a useful diagnostic tool to identify those neonates with a cardiovascular etiology. If a right radial arterial PaO_2 on 100% FiO_2 is less than 150 mmHg, severe congenital heart disease is likely. The infant is presumed to have ductal dependent congenital heart disease and the low PaO_2 is attributed to the obligatory mixing of oxygenated with deoxygenated blood within the circulatory system.

ELECTROCARDIOGRAPHY

The surface electrocardiogram (ECG) reflects the electrical activity in the heart and can provide information regarding the depolarization and repolarization of the heart muscle. The electrical signal represents the propagation of a wavefront through a cardiac chamber. Movement toward a recording electrode results in an upward deflection on the ECG, although movement away produces a negative deflection.

Correct ECG lead placement is of paramount importance in its accurate interpretation. The limb leads create a 360° frontal plane, although the precordial leads view the electrical activity in a horizontal plane (Figure 3). The standard ECG paper speed is 25 mm/sec with an amplitude of 1 mV/mm (Figure 4).

One should establish a systematic approach when interpreting ECGs. After noting the paper speed, standardization, and the patient's age, the signals can be analyzed. One should comment on the following: (a) rhythm, (b) rate, (c) axes of P, QRS, and T waves, (d) PR, QRS, and QT intervals, (e) waveform voltage, and (f) P, QRS, and T wave morphology (see Figure 4).

Rhythm

Sinus rhythm occurs when there is a P-wave prior to every QRS complex, and the axis of the P-wave is positive in leads I, II, and aVF.

Rate

Heart rate norms depend on the patient's age. In general, the heart decreases with increasing age (Table 1). When the ECG is at standard paper speed, 1 mm (1 small box) is equal to 0.04 seconds, and 5 mm (1 large box) is 0.2 seconds. Thus if there is one QRS complex every 0.2 seconds, then the heart rate is 300 beats/min. If the heart rate is inappropriately fast, then the rhythm may be sinus

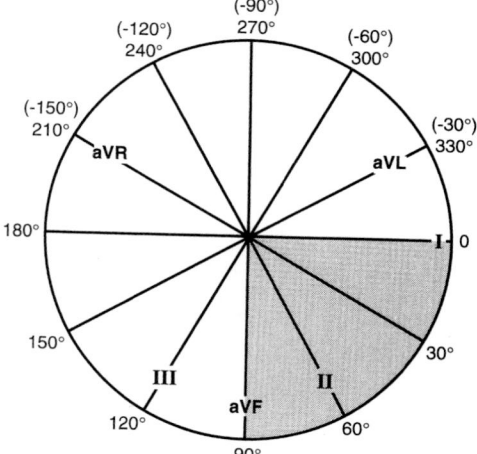

FIGURE 3. Hexaxial reference system (frontal axis). The shaded area represents the normal axis.

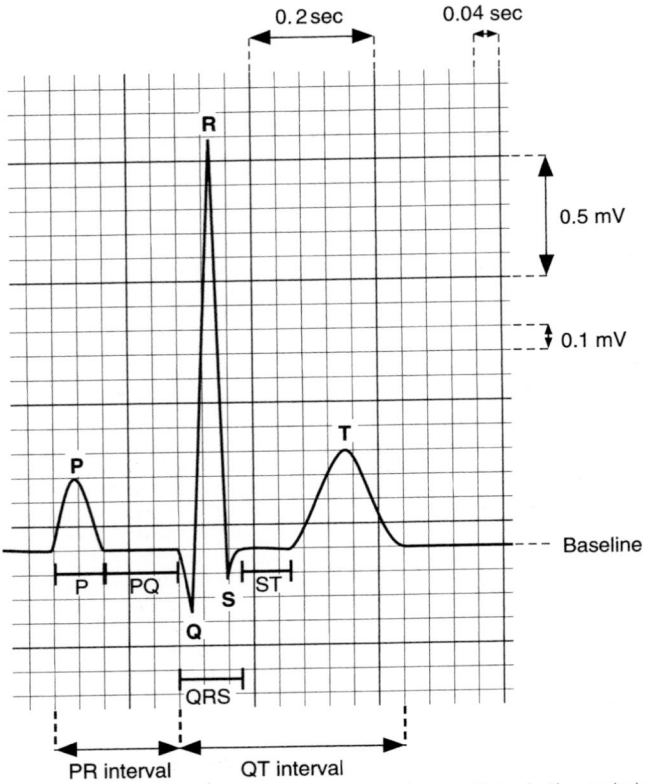

FIGURE 4. A normal electrocardiogram showing waveforms and intervals. The standard paper speed is 25 mm per second; therefore, a single 1-mm box equals 0.04 second, and a large (5-mm) box equals 0.20 second.

Axes

The limb leads are oriented in a hexaxial reference plane so that the angle between any two leads is 30°. With respect to the P-wave axis, the rhythm should be noted to be originating from the sinus node or an alternative pacemaker. The normal QRS axis changes with age. In the newborn period, the mean vector of depolarization is rightward, reflecting the dominance of the right ventricle in early infancy. As the left ventricular mass increases relative to the right side, the QRS axis shifts more leftward. Table 1 demonstrates expected ranges for the QRS axis with respect to age. When left axis deviation is present, there is frequently left ventricular hypertrophy or a left bundle branch block. Conversely, when right axis deviation is present, there is often right ventricular hypertrophy or a right bundle branch block. When the QRS axis is superior (northwest axis), an endocardial cushion defect or tricuspid atresia are possible.

The T-wave represents ventricular repolarization. Within the first 72 hours of life, the T-wave should invert in lead V1. As the left ventricle becomes progressively more dominant, the T-wave axis parallels the QRS axis. Thus, during adolescence, the T-wave becomes upright in lead V1 and the T wave axis becomes leftward. Finally, the QRS-T angle should be ≤90°. When there is an abnormally wide angle, the following are possible: (a) right or left ventricular hypertrophy associated with a strain pattern, (b) a ventricular conduction disturbance, or (c) myocardial dysfunction (see Figure 3).

Intervals

Measuring the intervals between deflections on the ECG evaluates the properties of the electrical conduction system. Refer to Table 1 for normal age-corrected values of intervals. The PR interval is measured from the onset of the P-wave to the beginning of the QRS complex and reflects the time for atrial depolarization and delay through the AV node. In general, with age, the heart rate is slower and the PR interval is longer. Abnormal prolongation of the PR interval, or 1st degree AV block, usually represents a delay in AV node conduction. This delay can be as a result of myocarditis, congenital heart disease, electrolyte abnormalities (hyperkalemia), hypoxia, ischemia, medications, or toxins (e.g., digitalis, quinidine). A short PR interval is present when there is either (a) an abnormal electrical connection between the atrium and ventricle, as seen in Wolff-Parkinson-White syndrome, Lown-Ganong-Levine syndrome, glycogen storage disease, or hypertrophic cardiomyopathy. Finally, a variable PR interval suggests either (a) a wandering atrial pacemaker or (b) Wenckebach phenomenon.

The QRS interval is measured from the onset of the Q-wave to the completion of the S-wave and represents ventricular depolarization. The QRS duration represents the intraventricular conduction time and is normally less than 0.09 seconds in children younger than 4 years and less than 0.1 seconds in children older than 4 years. When the QRS complex is wide, there is a delay or abnormal propagation of the electrical impulse through the ventricular myocardium. QRS widening is seen with a bundle branch block, preexcitation (e.g., Wolff-Parkinson-White syndrome), intraventricular block, ventricular arrhythmias and ventricular paced rhythms.

tachycardia or an arrhythmia. If sinus tachycardia is suspected, an underlying systemic process is usually responsible for stimulating the sinus node. Fever, anxiety, thyrotoxicosis, anemia and myocardial disease are among the more common causes of sinus tachycardia. Alternatively, if the heart rate is inappropriately slow, then the rhythm must be

differentiated between sinus bradycardia and an arrhythmia. Sinus bradycardia is common in trained athletes. Other etiologies of sinus bradycardia include increased intracranial pressure, hypothyroidism, malnutrition, anorexia, hypoxia, sinus node dysfunction, electrolyte abnormalities, and pharmaceuticals.

Table 1. Heart Rate, PR Interval, and QRS Duration

Age	Heart Rate (Beats/min)		PR Interval in Lead II (Seconds)		QRS Duration (Seconds)	
	Mean	Range	Mean	Range	Mean	Range
<1 day	126	95–155	0.106	0.082–0.138	0.05	0.025–0.069
1–7 days	135	100–180	0.107	0.079–0.130	0.05	0.025–0.068
8–30 days	160	120–190	0.100	0.075–0.128	0.053	0.026–0.075
1–3 months	147	95–200	0.098	0.075–0.126	0.052	0.027–0.069
3–6 months	139	114–170	0.105	0.078–0.137	0.053	0.028–0.075
6–12 months	130	95–170	0.105	0.077–0.138	0.055	0.03–0.070
1–3 years	121	95–150	0.113	0.090–0.140	0.056	0.032–0.070
3–5 years	98	70–130	0.119	0.092–0.150	0.058	0.03–0.069
5–8 years	86	65–120	0.124	0.094–0.155	0.059	0.035–0.075
8–12 years	86	65–120	0.129	0.093–0.165	0.062	0.038–0.079
12–16 years	86	65–120	0.135	0.098–0.169	0.065	0.040–0.081

Adapted with permission from Liebman J, Plonsey R, Gillette PC: *Pediatric Electrocardiography.* Baltimore, Williams & Wilkins, 1982, pp 96–97 and Cassels DE, Ziegler RF: *Electrocardiography in Infants and Children,* Philadelphia, WB Saunders, 1966, p 100.

Hint: Left bundle branch block is diagnosed when there is a monophasic R wave in lead I and no Q wave in lead V6. Right bundle branch block is diagnosed when there is a wide S wave in leads I and V6, right axis deviation, and an M-shaped (RSR' pattern) QRS complex in lead V1. Left anterior hemiblock can be diagnosed in the setting of left axis deviation associated with right bundle branch block.

Finally, the QT interval represents the time it takes for ventricular depolarization and repolarization. The QT interval is measured from the onset of the Q-wave to the termination of the T-wave. Given that the QT interval should shorten with increasing heart rates, the QT measurement should be adjusted for heart rate using the following formula: QTc = QT measured/square root of the R-R interval. The QTc interval is generally less than 0.45 seconds for infants younger than 6 months, and less than 0.44 seconds for children. The QTc is prolonged in Long QT syndrome wherein there are multiple genetic abnormalities of either the cardiac potassium or sodium channels. Other conditions that prolong the QTc interval include head injury, myocarditis, medications (such as, procainamide, amiodarone, quinidine) and electrolyte abnormalities (e.g., hypocalcemia, hypomagnesemia, hypokalemia).

Waveforms

Abnormal morphologic characteristics of the waveforms often indicate underlying pathology. When the P-wave amplitude is greater than 3 mm in lead II or lead V1, right atrial enlargement is present. If the P-wave has a duration greater than 0.1 seconds in lead II or is biphasic with a prominent negative component in lead V1, left atrial enlargement is present.

The amplitude of the QRS complex is evaluated in the precordial leads and depends on the child's age. The normal Q-wave represents septal depolarization and is seen in the inferolateral leads. The absence of Q-waves in leads V5 and V6, coupled with the presence of Q-waves in lead V1, is consistent with congenitally corrected transposition of the great arteries (L-TGA). Abnormally tall R-waves in lead V1 or deep S-waves in V5 and V6 represent right ventricular hypertrophy. Similarly, tall R-waves in leads V5 and V6 or deep S-waves in lead V1 represent left ventricular hypertrophy. Conversely, low-voltage QRS complexes suggest myocarditis, pericarditis, pericardial effusion, or hypothyroidism.

Finally, abnormalities of T-wave morphology can also suggest pathology. For example, tall, peaked T-waves can be seen with ventricular hypertrophy associated with strain, myocardial infarction, or hyperkalemia. Conversely, low-voltage, flat T-waves are associated with electrolyte abnormalities (hypokalemia, hypoglycemia), hypothyroidism, myocarditis, pericarditis, ischemia or medications (i.e., digitalis).

CHEST ROENTGENOGRAM

Despite the increasing use of alternative methods of noninvasive imaging, the plain chest roentgenogram continues to provide important information to the clinician when cardiac disease is suspected. The study is inexpensive, expedient, readily available, and minimally harmful, and therefore serves as a convenient tool in assessing patients. It can provide important information regarding cardiac size, pulmonary vascularity, and specific cardiac abnormalities. The normal cardiac silhouette in the anterior-posterior and lateral views is shown in Figure 5.

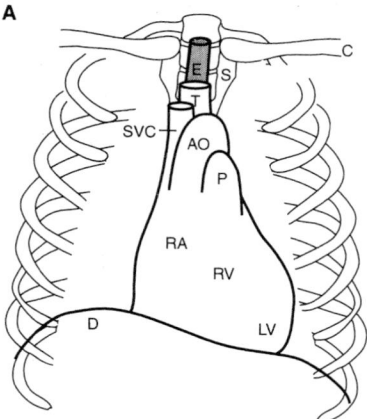

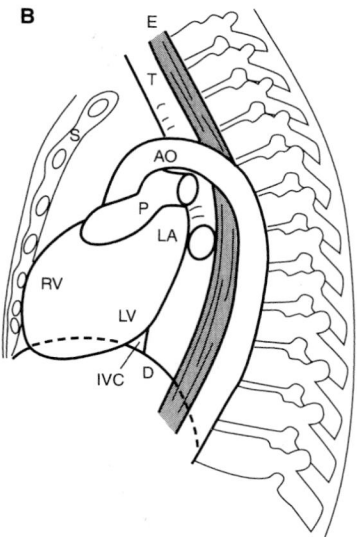

FIGURE 5. Normal cardiac silhouette. A: Anterior-posterior view. B: Lateral view. AO, aorta; C, clavicle; D, diaphragm; E, esophagus; IVC, inferior vena cava; LA, left atrium; LV, left ventricle; P, pulmonary outflow tract; RA, right atrium, RV, right ventricle; S, sternum; T, trachea; SVC, superior vena cava. (Modified from Sapire DW. Understanding and diagnosing pediatric heart disease. East Norwalk, CT: Appleton & Lange, 1991:64, with permission).

Heart Size

Cardiomegaly, or an enlarged heart, is associated with both congenital and acquired heart disease. Several factors influence the interpretation of cardiac size on a chest radiograph. First, given that the pericardium rests on the diaphragm, the apparent size of the heart will vary with the respiratory cycle and posture. For example, during exhalation or when a patient is in the supine position, the cardiac silhouette is horizontally stretched, and may appear larger. Conversely, during inspiration or in the standing position, the heart is most vertical and appears smaller. Second, the thymic shadow often blends with the cardiac silhouette making an accurate determination of heart size difficult.

A quantitative assessment of cardiac size should be made on the inspiratory film, when 9 to 10 ribs are visualized above the level of the diaphragm. The cardiothoracic ratio is then determined by comparing the transverse dimension of the heart relative to the

width of the thoracic cavity. The heart is considered enlarged if the cardiothoracic ratio exceeds 0.6 in the anterior-posterior dimension.

Individual cardiac chamber sizes can also be assessed on the standard plain film. For example, a large bulge appreciated to the right of the sternum suggests right atrial enlargement. Right ventricular hypertrophy is often demonstrated by an "up-tilting" of the apex of the heart from the diaphragm and an obliteration of the retrosternal space on the lateral projection. Left atrial enlargement is best seen in the lateral view as it displaces or compresses the esophagus. Left ventricular enlargement is best visualized in the anterior-posterior projection and appears as although the apex of the heart is "sagging."

Pulmonary Vascularity

When there is a suspicion of congenital heart disease, the appearance of the pulmonary vascular markings plays an important role in understanding the pathophysiology. In general, when a large left-to-right shunt is present (as in atrial septal defect, ventricular septal defect, patent ductus arteriosus) pulmonary arterial flow is increased and the vessels appear sharp and prominent. In the cyanotic neonate, when there is a paucity of pulmonary vascular markings, one must be suspicious of a right-sided obstructive lesion with a right-to-left shunt. In the case of pulmonary venous congestion, bronchial cuffing, and Kerley B lines, one must suspect pulmonary venous obstructive disease or congestive heart failure.

Specific Cardiac Lesions

Distinctive radiographic configurations have been associated with specific cardiac lesions. The "boot-shaped" heart seen in patients with tetralogy of Fallot reflects right ventricular hypertrophy and hypoplasia of the main pulmonary artery segment, causing a concavity of the upper left heart border. In patients with total anomalous pulmonary venous return without obstruction, a "snowman" or "figure-eight" pattern has been described. This radiographic finding represents right atrial and right ventricular enlargement secondary to the large left-to-right shunt and the presence of a large left-sided vertical vein. The chest roentgenogram of a patient with discrete aortic coarctation often shows a prominent indentation of the aorta resembling a "figure 3." The description of "an egg on a string" is used for the chest x-ray findings in patients with transposition of the great arteries, reflecting the narrowed mediastinum and right heart enlargement.

ECHOCARDIOGRAPHY

In pediatric patients, echocardiography is performed in a systematic manner and obtains subcostal, apical, parasternal, and suprasternal views (Figure 6).

M-Mode Echocardiography

A parasternal short-axis view using M-mode echocardiography reveals a cross section of the left ventricle and can be used to measure dimensions at different points in the cardiac cycle. Most commonly, it is used to obtain a shortening fraction (SF), calculated in the following manner:

$$SF = 100 \times [(LV \text{ end-diastolic dimension} - LV \text{ end-systolic dimension}) / LV \text{ end-diastolic dimension}]$$

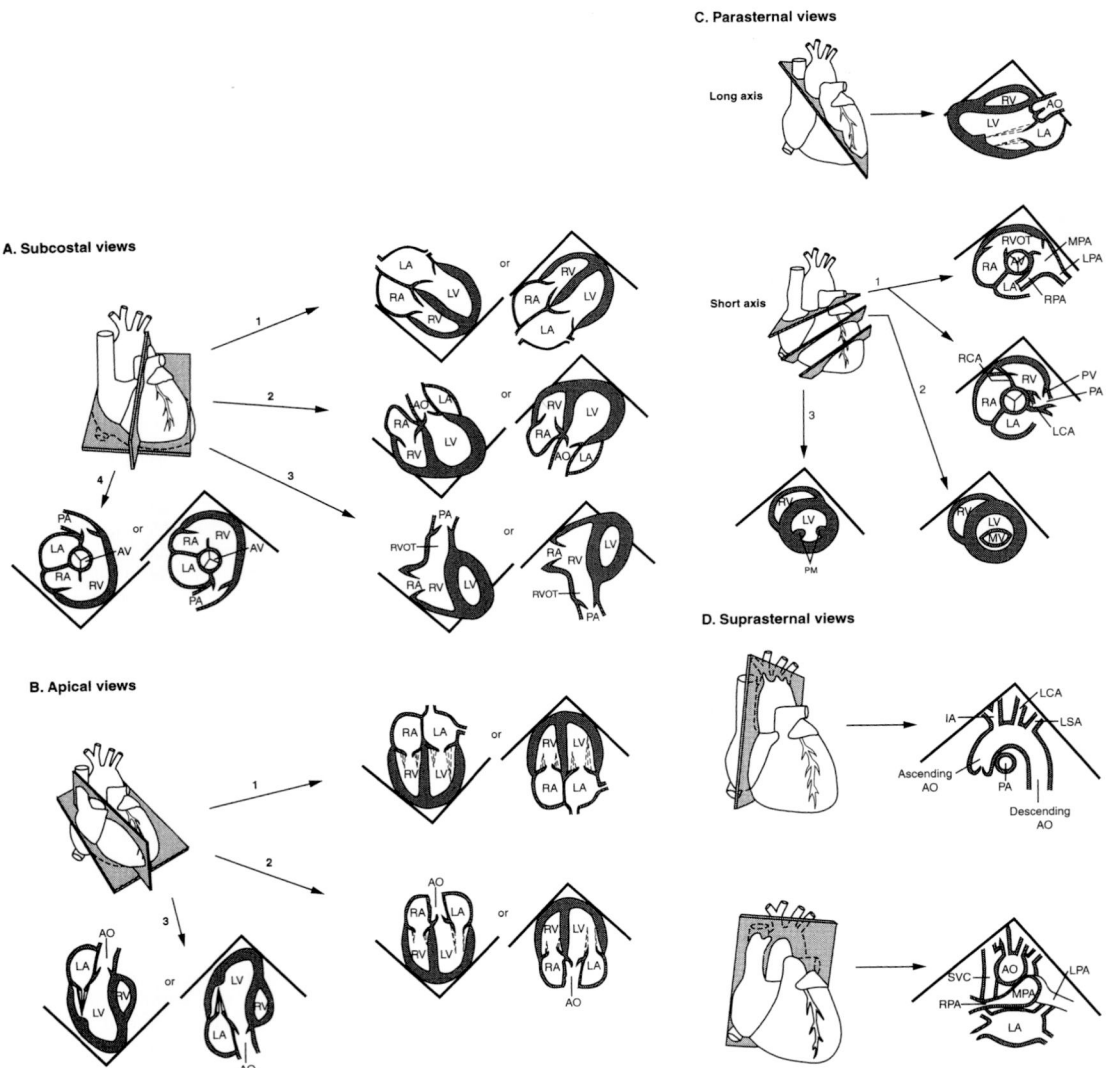

FIGURE 6. Echocardiographic series. The numbers represent different planes along a sweep of the echocardiographic beam. A: Subcostal views. B: Apical views. C: Parasternal views. D: Suprasternal views. AO, aorta; AV, aortic valve; IA, innominate artery; LA, left atrium; LCA, left coronary artery; LPA, left pulmonary artery; LSA, left subclavian artery; MPA, main pulmonary artery; MV, mitral valve; PA, pulmonary artery; PM, papillary muscle; PV, pulmonary valve; RA, right atrium; RCA, right coronary artery; RPA, right pulmonary artery; RV, right ventricle; RVOT, right ventricular outflow tract; SVC, superior vena cava. (Modified from Park MK. Pediatric cardiology for practitioners, 3rd ed. St. Louis: Mosby-Year Book, 1996:70–73, with permission).

The normal value for the SF is 28% to 38%, independent of age.

Doppler Echocardiography

Doppler echocardiography detects a frequency shift that reflects the direction and velocity of blood flow. Doppler echocardiography is used to detect valvular insufficiency or stenosis and abnormal flow patterns.

CARDIAC CATHETERIZATION

Cardiac catheterization allows sampling of oximetric and hemodynamic data. The normal pressures and oxygen saturations for children are shown in Figure 7. Cardiac catheterization, an invasive procedure, is often used in conjunction with angiography to confirm the diagnosis and physiology of acquired or congenital heart disease. The technique also has therapeutic applications, such as coil embolization of a patent ductus arteriosus, coil embolization of aortopulmonary collaterals, pulmonary artery angioplasty and stent placement, balloon valvuloplasty of semilunar valvular stenosis, and device closure of atrial and some ventricular septal defects.

Shunts

Data obtained from cardiac catheterization can be used to calculate the degree and direction of an intracardiac or extracardiac shunt. The calculation is based on the Fick principle, using oxygen as the indicator. The oxygen content equals the dissolved oxygen (which is usually negligible) plus the oxygen capacity [hemoglobin (g/dL) $\times$ 1.36 mL O_2/dL $\times$ 10] multiplied by the oxygen saturation (as a percentage).

Flow (Q) is equal to the oxygen consumption divided by the arteriovenous oxygen content difference:

$$Qp = VO_2/PV - PA$$
$$Qs = VO_2/AO - MV$$

in which
Qp = pulmonary flow
Qs = systemic flow
VO_2 = oxygen consumption per unit time
PV = pulmonary venous oxygen content
PA = pulmonary arterial oxygen content
MV = mixed venous oxygen content
AO = systemic arterial (aorta) oxygen content

A shunt is calculated with the effective pulmonary blood flow (Qp eff):

$$Qp\ eff = VO_2/PV - MV$$

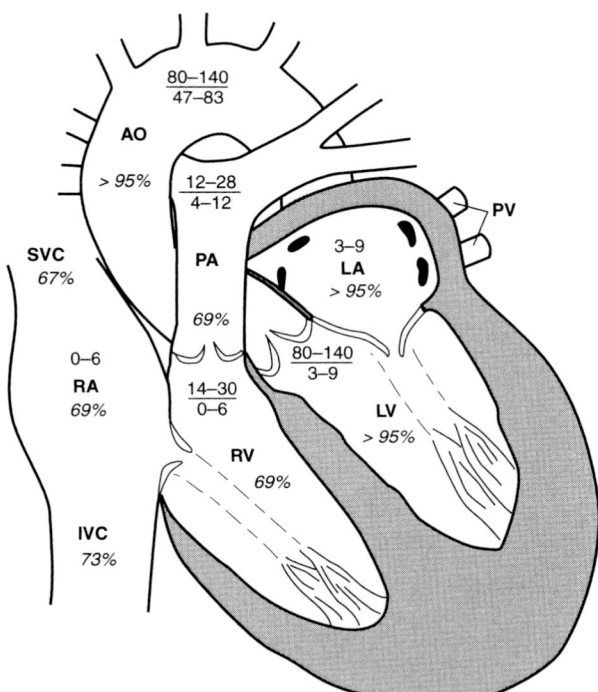

FIGURE 7. Normal pressures (systolic over diastolic, in mmHg), mean pressures, and oxygen saturations for children during cardiac catheterization. The data are based on information compiled from healthy patients between the ages of 2 months and 20 years. AO, aorta; IVC, inferior vena cava; LA, left atrium; LV, left ventricle; PA, pulmonary artery; PV, pulmonary vein; RA, right atrium; RV, right ventricle; SVC, superior vena cava.

A left-to-right shunt is the pulmonary flow less the effective pulmonary flow (Qp − Qp eff), and a right-to-left shunt is the systemic flow less the effective pulmonary flow (Qs − Qp eff).

Resistance

Systemic and pulmonary vascular resistance can also be calculated using the catheterization data. This calculation is based on Ohm's law (resistance equals the pressure change across the vascular bed divided by flow):

> Rs = AO − RA/Qs
> Rp = PA − LA/Qp
> in which
> Rs = systemic resistance
> Rp = pulmonary resistance
> AO = mean systemic (aorta) pressure
> RA = mean right atrial pressure
> PA = mean pulmonary artery pressure
> LA = mean left atrial pressure

A pulmonary resistance (Rp) of 2.5 Wood units or less is considered within the normal range; however, no vascular bed is static and variations in flow can affect the result obtained.

Appendix III
Surgical Glossary

Sanjeev K. Swami, MD

aortopexy—a procedure in which the aorta is approximated to the anterior thoracic wall; for the treatment of tracheomalacia.

Battle's sign—bruising over the mastoid process; seen in patients with a basilar skull fracture.

Bishop-Koop procedure—resection of a dilated loop of bowel proximal to meconium obstruction, with end-to-side anastomosis between the proximal bowel and obstructed loop, combined with end ileostomy; for the treatment of meconium ileus.

bladder augmentation—a procedure in which a portion of the intra-abdominal GI tract is used to increase the volume of the bladder.

Blalock-Taussig shunt—a procedure in which the subclavian artery is anastomosed to the pulmonary artery; provides pulmonary blood flow, for the temporary treatment of tetralogy of Fallot.

Boix-Ochoa procedure—restoration of the intra-abdominal esophageal length, repair of the esophageal hiatus, fixation of the esophagus to the hiatus, and restoration of the angle of His; for the treatment of incompetent lower esophageal sphincter.

Charcot triad—fever, jaundice, right upper quadrant pain; seen in patients with cholangitis.

Chordee correction—a procedure in which the corpus spongiosum is moved ventrally and the corpus cavernosa are approximated dorsally; for the treatment of chordee (abnormal penile curvature which can be associated with epispadias or hypospadias).

Clatworthy mesocaval shunt—division of the common iliac veins and side-to-end anastomosis of the inferior mesenteric vein to the left renal vein; for the treatment of portal hypertension.

Cohen procedure—trigonal reimplantation of the ureter; for the treatment of vesicoureteral reflux.

colonic conduit diversion—a procedure involving 2 stages: (1) a loop diversion using a colonic segment, and (2) an end-to-side anastomosis of the colonic segment to the GI tract.

colonic interposition—replacement of the esophagus with a colonic segment; for treatment of esophageal atresia or stricture when gastric mobilization is not feasible.

Dance sign—empty right lower quadrant, seen in patients with ileocecal intussusception.

diaphragmatic placation—surgical shortening of the diaphragm (abdominal, transthoracic, or bilateral); for the treatment of diaphragmatic eventration.

distal splenorenal shunt—see "Warren shunt."

Drapanas mesocaval shunt—prosthetic graft implantation from the inferior mesenteric vein to the inferior vena cava; for the treatment of portal hypertension.

Duckett transverse preputial island flap—technique in which a flap of foreskin is used to elongate the urethra; for the treatment of hypospadias.

Duhamel procedure—resection of the aganglionic colon above the dentate line with stable anastomosis to the rectal stump, normally performed in children 6–12 months of age; for the treatment of Hirschsprung disease (see "Martin modification").

end-to-side portocaval shunt—procedure in which the portal vein is divided and anastomosed to the inferior vena cava; for the treatment of portal hypertension.

esophagectomy—resection of the esophagus, with gastric pull-up and anastomosis with the cervical esophagus; for the treatment of esophageal atresia or stricture.

Fontan procedure—a procedure in which a graft is created to connect the pulmonary artery to the right atrium bypassing the right ventricle; for the treatment of hypoplastic left heart syndrome or other congenital heart diseases with single ventricle physiology.

Fredet-Ramstedt surgery—relaxation of the pyloric sphincter; for the treatment of pyloric stenosis.

gastroschisis—defect of the anterior abdominal wall lateral to the umbilicus (usually on the right), the viscera are not covered by a sac.

Glenn shunt—a shunt from the superior vena cava to the pulmonary artery, bypassing the right atrium and right ventricle; for the treatment of tricuspid atresia or stenosis.

Gridiron incision—see "McBurney incision."

Hegman procedure—surgical release of the tarsal, metatarsal, and intertarsal ligaments; for the treatment of metatarsus adductus.

Heller myotomy—myotomy of the anterior lower esophagus (always accompanied by a Thal fundoplication); for the treatment of achalasia.

ileal loop diversion—resection and implantation of ureters into an isolated ileal segment, with an ileal stoma and primary anastomosis of ileum to cecum.

ileal ureter—ileal interposition between the renal pelvis and bladder when the ureteral length is insufficient for anastomosis; for the treatment of urinary obstruction.

ileocecal conduit diversion—bilateral ureteral diversion and anastomosis to an isolated ileocecal segment and cecostomy with primary anastomosis of ileum to the right colon.

J-pouch—creation of an ileal reservoir in the distal ileum using a J-shaped conuration; used following colectomy.

Jateene procedure—arterial retransposition; for the treatment of transposition of the great vessels.

Kasai procedure—resection of atretic extrahepatic bile ducts and gallbladder with Roux-en-Y anastomosis of the jejunum to the remaining common hepatic duct; for the treatment of biliary atresia or other extrahepatic obstruction.

Kimura procedure (parasitized cecal patch)—a multistep operation in which (1) a side-to-side anastomosis is made with a portion of the distal ileum and the right colon, and (2) an ileoanal pull-through is performed; for the treatment of Hirschsprung disease.

King operation—resection of the knee with placement of a Kuntscher rod to the femur to the tibia, followed by a Syme amputation for the treatment of proximal focal femoral deficiency (PFFD).

Koch pouch diversion—a procedure involving bilateral ureteral diversion with anastomosis to a neobladder formed from an isolated ileal segment, combined with an ileal stoma and primary anastomosis of ileum to ileum.

Ladd's bands—fibrous bands found in the abdomen in patients with malrotation, often cause obstruction; resected during Ladd's procedure.

Ladd's procedure—restoration of intestinal anatomy from a malrotated state involving: counterclockwise reduction of midgut volvulus, splitting of Ladd's bands, division of peritoneal attachments to the cecum and ascending colon, and appendectomy; for the treatment of intestinal malrotation.

Lanz incision—an abdominal incision made in the left iliac fossa; for colostomy formation.

Left hepatectomy—resection of the left hepatic lobe (medial and lateral segments).

MAGPI procedure—distal advancement of the urethral meatus and granuloplasty; for the treatment of hypospadias.

Mainz pouch diversion—a procedure involving bilateral ureteral division with anastomosis to a neobladder formed from isolated cecum and terminal ileum; combined with an ileal stoma and primary anastomosis of the ileum to the right colon.

Martin modification (of Duhamel procedure)—right and transverse colectomy with ileoanal pull-through and side-to-side anastomosis of the remaining left colon to the ileum; procedure preserves some absorptive capacity of the large bowel; for the treatment of total colonic Hirschsprung disease.

McBurney (gridiron) incision—abdominal incision from the anterior superior iliac spine to the umbilicus; used for appendectomy.

Mikulicz procedure—a diverting enterostomy performed proximal to the meconium obstruction without resection; for the treatment of meconium ileus.

Mini-Pena procedure—anterior sagittal anorectoplasty; for the treatment of anterior rectoperianal tula (boys) or rectal-fourchette tula (girls).

Mitrofanoff technique—a modification of neobladder diversion procedures, in which vascularized appendix is used to create the stoma.

mustard technique—redirection of blood through an atrial septal defect (ASD) using a pericardial "baffle"; for the treatment of transposition of the great vessels; because of associated increased turbulence, this technique is not widely used today.

Mustardé procedure—correction, using simple mattress sutures, of a prominent ear with normal or absent antihelical folds.

Nissen fundoplication—a technique involving a 360° wrap of the gastric fundus around the gastroesophageal junction; for the treatment of incompetent lower esophageal sphincter; patient is rendered unable to vomit or belch.

Norwood procedure—a 3-stage palliative procedure including (1) atrial septectomy, transection, and ligation of the pulmonary artery, "neoaorta" formation using the proximal pulmonary artery, and creation of a synthetic aortopulmonary shunt (Blalock-Taussing shunt) or with a Sano Modification; (2) creation of a Glenn shunt; and (3) performance of a modified Fontan procedure; for the treatment of hypoplastic left heart syndrome.

onlay island flap—a technique in which a flap of foreskin is used to elongate the urethra; for the treatment of hypospadias.

omphalocele—defect of the anterior abdominal wall at the umbilicus, viscera covered by a sac.

orchiopexy—testicular pull-down and attachment; for the treatment of undescended testis. Also called "orchidopexy."

orthoplasty—surgical correction of excessive penile curvature.

parasitized cecal patch—see "Kimura procedure."

Pena procedure—posterior sagittal anorectoplasty performed in children 1–6 months of age; for the treatment of imperforate anus.

Pentalogy of Cantrell—diaphragmatic hernia, cardiac abnormalities, omphalocele, absence or malformation of the pericardium, and stern cleft.

Pfannenstiel incision—an abdominal incision used to gain access to the lower abdomen and bring pelvic organs within reach without dividing muscular tissue.

pharyngoplasty—elevation of the posterior pharyngeal wall following a primary cleft palate repair (to narrow the pharyngeal space); for the treatment of velopharyngeal incompetence.

Potts shunt—anastomosis of the descending aorta to the pulmonary artery for the permanent treatment of tetralogy of Fallot.

proximal splenorenal shunt—end-to-side anastomosis of the splenic vein to the left renal vein with splenectomy; for the treatment of portal hypertension.

pyeloplasty—resection of an atretic ureter with primary anastomosis to the renal pelvis; for the treatment of ureteropelvic junction obstruction.

pyloromyotomy—relaxation of the pyloric sphincter; for the treatment of pyloric stenosis.

Ramstedt operation—relaxation of the pyloric sphincter; for the treatment of pyloric stenosis.

Rashkind procedure—balloon atrial septostomy; for the treatment of transposition of the great vessels.

Rastelli repair—a technique involving the closure of a ventricular septal defect (VSD) with a patch and the creation of a conduit from the distal pulmonary artery to the right ventricle; for the treatment of transposition of the great vessels.

Ravitch procedure—a procedure involving (1) creation of osteotomies between the manubrium and costal cartilages, (2) a greenstick fracture of the manubrium, and (3) the temporary insertion (for 6 to 12 months) of a stabilizing bar; for the treatment of pectus excavatum or pectus carinatum.

right colon pouch—a procedure involving bilateral ureteral division with anastomosis to a neobladder (formed from an isolated segment of the right colon), combined with an ileal stoma and primary anastomosis of the ileum to the transverse colon.

right hepatectomy—resection of the right hepatic lobes (anterior and posterior segments).

rooftop (bilateral subcostal) incision—an abdominal incision used to access the liver and portal structures.

Roux-en-Y anastomosis—division of the jejunum distal to the ligament of Treitz with end-to-side anastomosis of the duodenum to the distal jejunum and anastomosis of the proximal jejunum (typically) to the bile duct.

Rovsing's sign—right lower quadrant pain with palpation of the left lower quadrant; seen in patients with appendicitis.

S-pouch—the creation of an ileal reservoir in the distal ileum using an S-shaped conuration following colectomy.

Sano modification—synthetic shunt connecting the right ventricle to the pulmonary arteries as part of a stage 1 Norwood procedure; provides pulmonary blood flow after ligation of proximal pulmonary arteries; for the treatment of hypoplastic left heart syndrome.

Santulli-Blanc enterostomy—a modification of the Bishop-Koop procedure that involves the resection of a distal dilated bowel segment with side-to-end anastomosis to the proximal enterostomy; for the treatment of meconium ileus.

Senning procedure (venous switch)—technique involving intraatrial redirection of venous return so that systemic caval return is shunted through the mitral valve to the left ventricle, and pulmonary return is brought through the tricuspid valve to the right ventricle; for the treatment of transposition of the great vessels.

side-to-side portocaval shunt—a procedure in which the portal vein is anastomosed to the inferior vena cava; for the treatment of portal hypertension.

side-to-side splenorenal shunt—side-to-side anastomosis of the splenic vein to the left renal vein; for the treatment of portal hypertension.

Sistrunk operation—complete excision of a thyroglossal duct cyst.

Soave procedure—a technique involving endorectal pull-through; for the correction of Hirschsprung disease.

Stamm gastrostomy—placement of an open gastrostomy tube; the opening is designed to close spontaneously on removal of the tube.

Sting procedure—subureteric Teflon injection; for the endoscopic correction of vesicoureteral reflux.

Sugiura procedure—a technique that involves lower esophageal transection and primary anastomosis, devascularization of the lower esophagus and stomach, and splenectomy; for the treatment of esophageal varices.

Swenson procedure—resection of the posterior rectal wall to the dentate line (aganglionic region); for the treatment of Hirschsprung disease; technically difficult and rarely performed.

Syme amputation—amputation of the foot, calculated to bring the end of the stump above the opposite knee at maturity; for the treatment of proximal focal femoral deficiency (PFFD).

Thal procedure—a procedure involving a 180° anterior wrap of the gastric fundus around the gastroesophageal junction, preserving the patient's ability to vomit and belch; for the treatment of incompetent lower esophageal sphincter.

Thiersch operation—a procedure in which a distal rectal segment that has prolapsed is approximated to the external sphincter muscle; for the treatment of rectal prolapse.

trisegmentectomy—resection of the right hepatic lobe and the quadrate lobe of the liver (right posterior segment, right anterior segment, and medial segment).

ureteropyelostomy—partial resection and side-to-side anastomosis of a partially duplicated ureter.

uretocalycostomy—a technique for the treatment of urinary obstruction involving division of the ureter (distal to the obstruction) and intrarenal anastomosis to the most dependent renal calyx; when the renal pelvis is insufficient for anastomosis, the lower pole of the kidney is resected.

vaginal switch operation—a procedure in which the vagina is separated from the urinary tract; for treatment of duplicated vagina.

Van Ness procedure—rotational 180° osteotomy of the femur in which the foot and ankle are brought to the level of the opposite knee; for prosthetic attachment for the treatment of femoral deficiency.

venous switch—see "Senning procedure."

ventricular-peritoneal shunt procedure—a procedure in which a Silastic catheter is positioned in a lateral ventricle and tunneled subcutaneously to drain into the peritoneal cavity; for the treatment of hydrocephalus. The shunt is occasionally positioned to drain into the central venous system, the pleura, or the right atrium.

Warren (distal splenorenal) shunt—a procedure in which the splenic vein is anastomosed to the left renal vein; for the treatment of portal hypertension.

Waterston aortopulmonary anastomosis—a procedure involving anastomosis of the ascending aorta and the right pulmonary artery; for the temporary treatment of tetralogy of Fallot.

Whipple procedure—resection of the pancreatic head, duodenum, and gallbladder with gastrojejunostomy, hepatojejunostomy, and pancreaticojejunostomy.

Appendix IV
Medications

Monica Darby, Shannon Manzi, and Susan McKamy

MEDICATIONS

Table 1. Medications

	Dosages	Dosage Forms
Acetaminophen (Feverall, Tylenol, Ofirmev)	***IV, PO or rectally:*** Premature infants, age <3 months: 10–12 mg/kg q8–12h. Infants, age <3 months: 10–15 mg/kg repeated q8h. Children: 10–15 mg/kg repeated q4–6h, up to 5 doses daily. (Do NOT exceed 75 mg/kg/day or 4 g/day). Adults: 325–650 mg q4–6h. Do not exceed 3 g/day.	Injection: 10 mg/mL Suspension: 160 mg/5 mL Suppositories: 120 mg, 325 mg, 650 mg Tablets: 160 mg, 325 mg, 500 mg Tablets, chewable: 80 mg Also available in combination with codeine; see codeine monograph.
Acetazolamide (Diamox)	***PO or IV:*** Children and adults: 8–30 mg/kg/day in 4 divided doses. Do not exceed 1 g/day. Lower doses are used for diuresis or correction of metabolic acidosis. The higher doses are used for the treatment of hydrocephalus or seizures. *Altitude sickness (adults):* 250 mg q8–12h beginning 24–48 hours before ascent and continuing for at least 48 hours after arrival.	Injection: 500 mg Tablets: 125, 250 mg Capsule, sustained release: 500 mg
Acetylcysteine (Mucomyst, Mucosil, Acetadote)	***Acetaminophen poisoning:*** *IV:* 150 mg/kg as an initial infusion over 1 hour followed by a second infusion of 50 mg/kg over 4 hours, followed by a third infusion of 100 mg/kg over 16 hours. Therapy may continue at a rate of 6.25 mg/kg/hr until acetaminophen level reaches 0 and AST/ALT levels decrease. *PO:* 140 mg/kg PO followed by 70 mg/kg for 17 doses administered q4h until acetaminophen levels are nontoxic. Usually administered as a 5% solution diluted in juice or soda. *Inhalation (administer 10% solution undiluted):* Infants: 2–4 mL of 10% soln repeated t.i.d. or q.i.d. Children and adolescents: 6–10 mL of 10% soln repeated t.i.d. or q.i.d.	Injection: 200 mg/mL in 30 mL vials Solution for inhalation: 10% or 20% in 10-mL and 30-mL vials
Acyclovir (Zovirax)	***PO:*** *Varicella zoster (chickenpox):* 80 mg/kg/day in 4 divided doses for 5 days. Do not exceed 800 mg/dose (3,200 mg/day). *Herpes simplex virus:* Children: 40–80 mg/kg/day in 3–4 divided doses. Adults: 200 mg q4h while awake (5 doses daily). Chronic suppressive therapy at a dose of 400 mg b.i.d. may be used for up to 1 year or longer. ***IV:*** *Neonatal HSV encephalitis:* Full term infants: 60 mg/kg/day in 3 divided doses for 10–14 days. *HSV encephalitis:* 1,500 mg/m^2/day in 3 divided doses for at least 10 days and up to 21 days. *Other HSV infections:* 750 mg/m^2/day in 3 divided doses for 7 days. *Varicella zoster infections:* 1,500 mg/m^2/day in 3 divided doses for 7 days. *Topically:* Apply ointment q3h up to 6 times daily for 7 days. Use a disposable finger cot or glove when applying the ointment to avoid transmission of the virus. Dosage may need to be adjusted in patients with renal dysfunction. Ensure adequate hydration.	Capsules: 200 mg Injection: 500-mg, 1-g vials Ointment: 5%, 15 g Suspension: 200 mg/5 mL
Adenosine (Adenocard)	***IV (given via rapid push followed by a saline flush):*** Neonates: 0.05 mg/kg initially followed by doses increasing in 0.05 mg/kg increments q2min to a maximum dose of 0.25 mg/kg. Children: 0.1 mg/kg initially, followed by increased doses (double dose to 0.2 mg/kg OR increase by 0.05 mg/kg increments) q2min to a maximum dose of 0.35 mg/kg or 12 mg/dose. Adults: 6 mg followed by 12 mg with a repeat dose of 12 mg, if needed.	Injection: 3 mg/mL (2-mL vial)

Table 1. Medications (continued)

	Dosages	Dosage Forms
Albumin, human (Albuminar, Albutein, Plasbumin)	***IV (as a 5% solution for hypovolemic patients or 25% for fluid- or sodium-restricted patients):*** Children: 0.5–1 g/kg infused over 2–4 hours. May repeat to a maximum of 6 g/kg/day. Adults: 25 g infused over 2–4 hours. Usually not to exceed 125 g/day.	Injection: 5% (50 mL, 250 mL, 500 mL); 25% (20 mL, 50 mL, 100 mL)
Albuterol (Proventil HFA, Ventolin HFA, Proair HFA)	***PO:*** Age 2–<6 years: 0.3–0.6 mg/kg/day in 3 divided doses to a maximum of 12 mg/day. Age ≥6–≤12 years: 6–8 mg/day in 3–4 divided doses to a maximum of 24 mg/day. Age >12 years: 6–16 mg/day in 3–4 divided doses to a maximum of 32 mg/day. ***Inhalation:*** *Metered-dose inhaler:* Age <12 years: 1–2 inhalations q.i.d. Age >12 years: 1–2 inhalations up to 6 times a day. Exacerbation: <10 kg: 2–4 puffs; 10–30 kg: 4–6 puffs; >30 kg: 6–8 puffs *Nebulization* of 0.5% solution: <10 kg = 0.25 mL, 10–30 kg: 0.5 mL; >30 kg: 1 mL usually repeated q4–6h, but may be administered more frequently (including continuously) in severely ill patients under controlled conditions.	Aerosol HFA: 90 mcg/actuation Solution for inhalation: 0.5%, 0.083% Syrup: 10 mg/5 mL Tablets: 2 mg, 4 mg Tablets, extended release: 4 mg, 8 mg
Allopurinol (Zyloprim)	***PO:*** *Neoplastic diseases:* Age <10 years: 10 mg/kg/day in 3 divided doses to a maximum of 300 mg/day. Age >10 years: 600–800 mg/day in 2 or 3 divided doses. ***IV:*** *Neoplastic diseases:* Age <10 years: 100 mg/m^2/dose q8h, max 600 mg/day Age >10 years: 200–400 mg/m^2/day divided in 1–3 doses, max 600 mg/day. Note: The metabolism of mercaptopurine and azathioprine is decreased by allopurinol. Decrease dose of mercaptopurine or azathioprine by 75%.	Tablets: 100 mg, 300 mg Injection: 3 mg/mL
Alprostadil (Prostin VR Pediatric)	***IV:*** A continuous infusion beginning at a dose of 0.05–0.1 mcg/kg/min. Dosage may be adjusted downward or gradually upward based on the patient's response. Usual dosage range is 0.01–0.4 mcg/kg/min.	Injection: 500 mcg/mL (1-mL vial)
Aluminum and magnesium hydroxides (Maalox, Mylanta)	***PO:*** Children: 5–15 mL 4–6 times daily or more frequently. Adults: 15–45 mL 4–6 times daily or more frequently.	Suspension: Aluminum hydroxide 200 mg, magnesium hydroxide 200 mg/5 mL with simethicone 20 mg/5 mL
Amikacin (Amikin)	***IV (dose should be based on ideal body weight):*** Neonates: Age 0–4 weeks, <1,200 g: 7.5 mg/kg/dose q18–24h. Age ≤7 days: 1,200–2,000 g: 7.5 mg/kg/dose q12–18h. >2,000 g: 10 mg/kg/dose q12h. Age >7 days: 1,200–2,000 g: 7.5 mg/kg/dose q8–12h. >2,000 g: 10 mg/kg/dose q8h or 30 mg/kg/dose q24h. Infants and children: 15–22.5 mg/kg/day in 3 divided doses daily. The dose for the treatment of nontuberculous mycobacterial infections is 15–30 mg/kg/day in 2 divided doses, to a maximum of 1.5 g/day as part of a multiple-drug regimen. Increase to 30 mg/kg/day for patients with cystic fibrosis. Adults: 15 mg/kg/day in 2–3 divided doses. Dosage adjustment is required in patients with renal dysfunction.	Injection: 50 mg/mL, 250 mg/mL

(continued)

Table 1. Medications (continued)

	Dosages	Dosage Forms
Aminocaproic acid (Amicar)	***IV:*** Children: 100 mg/kg over the first hour followed by an infusion of 33.3 mg/kg/hr or 100 mg/kg q6h. Maximum daily dose is 30 g. Older children and adults: 4–5 g over the first hour followed by an infusion of 1 g/hr for 8 hours or until control is achieved. ***PO:*** Doses are the same or alternatively, 100 mg/kg may be administered q4–6h to a maximum of 5 g/dose.	Injection: 250 mg/mL (20-mL vial) Solution: 1.25 g/5 mL (16-oz bottle) Tablet: 500 mg
Amiodarone (Cordarone)	***PO:*** Children (use BSA for children ≤1 year): Loading dose of 10–15 mg/kg/day or 600–800 mg/1.73 m^2/day in 1–2 divided doses for 4–14 days or until adequate control of arrhythmia is achieved or prominent adverse effects occur. Then reduce dosage to 5 mg/kg/day or 200–400 mg/1.73 m^2/day as a single dose for several weeks. A further dose reduction to 2.5 mg/kg/day should be attempted if the arrhythmia does not recur. Adults: Loading dose of 800–1,600 mg/day in 1–2 divided doses for 1–3 weeks, followed by dose of 600–800 mg/day in 1–2 divided doses for 1 month. Maintenance dose usually 400 mg/day, but may be lower for supraventricular arrhythmias. ***IV:*** Children (only limited information is available): Initial loading dose of 5 mg/kg over 1 hour followed by a continuous infusion of 5 mcg/kg/min has been used. The continuous infusion dosage may be increased to 10 mcg/kg/min and then to 15 mcg/kg/min until the desired effect is achieved. Due to the leaching of DEHP from IV administration sets, especially at the slow rates usually used in infants, bolus dosing q6h should be considered if IV therapy is expected to be long term. Adults: Loading dose of 150 mg administered over 10 minutes (15 mg/min) followed by 360 mg over 6 hours at a rate of 1 mg/min, followed by the maintenance dose of 540 mg over 18 hours at a rate of 0.5 mg/min. If necessary, maintenance infusion of 0.5 mg/min may be continued past the initial 24 hours. Additional bolus doses of 150 mg may be administered over 10 minutes for breakthrough arrhythmias. ***VT/VF dosing:*** Child: 5 mg/kg IV push Adult: 300 mg IV push	Injection: 50 mg/mL Tablets: 200 mg
Amitriptyline (Elavil, Endep)	***PO:*** *Chronic pain:* 0.1 mg/kg/day at bedtime initially, advancing to 0.5–2 mg/kg/day over a 2–3 week period. *Depression:* 1 mg/kg/day to start, advancing to a maximum of 5 mg/kg or 100 mg, whichever is less. Adolescents and adults: 25–50 mg at bedtime or in divided doses, increasing daily doses by 25 mg to a maximum of 100 mg/day for adolescents and 300 mg for adults. Dosage should be decreased to the lowest effective dose after symptom control has been reached.	Tablets: 10 mg, 25 mg, 50 mg, 75 mg, 100 mg, 150 mg
Amlodipine (Norvasc)	***PO:*** *Hypertension:* Children: 0.1 mg/kg/dose (max 10 mg) given once daily. Adults: 2.5–5 mg initial, max 10 mg/day. Doses may be titrated upward at 5–7 day.	Tablets: 2.5 mg, 5 mg, 10 mg
Amoxicillin (Amoxil, Trimox)	***PO:*** Children ≤20 kg: 20 mg/kg/day in 2 or 3 divided doses for UTIs. 40 mg/kg/day in 2 or 3 divided doses for otitis media, upper respiratory infection, or skin infections. Acute otitis media due to highly resistant strains of *S. pneumoniae* may require doses of 80–90 mg/kg/day in 2 or 3 divided doses. Children >20 kg and adults: 250–500 mg/dose t.i.d. or 500–875 mg b.i.d. Maximum daily dose is 3 g. *Endocarditis prophylaxis:* 50 mg/kg (up to 2 g) 1 hour before procedure. Dosage must be adjusted in patients with renal dysfunction.	Capsules: 250 mg, 500 mg Drops: 50 mg/mL Suspension: 125 mg/5 mL, 200 mg/5 mL, 250 mg/5 mL, 400 mg/5 mL Tablets, chewable: 125 mg, 200 mg, 250 mg, 400 mg Tablets: 500 mg, 875 mg

Table 1. Medications (continued)

	Dosages	Dosage Forms
Amoxicillin and clavulanic acid (Augmentin, Augmentin ES-600)	***PO (based on the amoxicillin component):*** 20–40 mg/kg/day in 3 divided doses to a maximum of 1.5 g/day, or 25–45 mg/kg/day in 2 divided doses to a maximum of 1.75 g/day using the b.i.d. formulation of the drug. Use the higher doses for respiratory tract infections and otitis media. Otitis media infections caused by multidrug-resistant *pneumococcus*: 80–90 mg/kg/day in 2 divided doses using the ES-600 suspension to avoid higher than recommended doses of clavulanic acid. Dosage must be adjusted in patients with renal dysfunction.	Suspension: Amoxicillin 125 mg and clavulanic acid 31.25 mg/ 5 mL; b.i.d. formulation—amoxicillin 200 mg and clavulanic acid 28.5 mg/5 mL; amoxicillin 250 mg and clavulanic acid 62.5 mg/5 mL; b.i.d. formulation—amoxicillin 400 mg and clavulanic acid 57 mg/5 mL; b.i.d. formulation—amoxicillin 600 mg and clavulanic acid 42.9 mg/5 mL Tablets: Amoxicillin 250 mg and clavulanic acid 125 mg; amoxicillin 500 mg and clavulanic acid 125 mg; b.i.d. formulation—amoxicillin 875 mg and clavulanic acid 125 mg Tablets, chewable: Amoxicillin 125 mg and clavulanic acid 31.25 mg; b.i.d. formulation—amoxicillin 200 mg and clavulanic acid 28.5 mg; amoxicillin 250 mg and clavulanic acid 62.5 mg; b.i.d. formulation—amoxicillin 400 mg and clavulanic acid 57 mg
Amphotericin B (Fungizone)	***IV (infusion over 2–8 hours):*** Begin with 0.25–0.5 mg/kg. Doses may be doubled on each subsequent day to a maximum of 1 mg/kg as the patient tolerates. Once therapy is established, alternate day doses at a maximum of 1.5 mg/kg/day may be used. Bladder irrigations of 50 mg daily in 1 L of sterile water instilled over 24 hours have been used to treat bladder infections. Do NOT confuse with liposomal amphotericin dosing.	Injection: 50-mg vial
Amphotericin B, cholesteryl (Amphotec)	***IV:*** Children and adults: 3–4 mg/kg/day as a single infusion. Doses of 6 mg/kg/day have been used to treat invasive *Candida* or *Cryptococcus* infections. Admix with 5% dextrose injection to a final concentration of ~0.6 mg/mL for administration over 3–4 hours. In patients who tolerate the longer infusion time well, the time can be shortened to 2 hours.	Injection: 50-mg vial, 100-mg vial
Amphotericin B, lipid complex (Abelcet)	***IV (infuse over 2 hours):*** Children and adults: 2.5–5 mg/kg/day in a single infusion. Admix with 5% dextrose to a final concentration of 1 mg/mL. A final concentration of 2 mg/mL may be used for pediatric patients or patients requiring fluid restriction.	Suspension for injection: 5 mg/mL
Amphotericin B Liposomal (AmBisome)	***IV (infuse over 2 hours):*** Children: 3–5 mg/kg/day Adults: 2–6 mg/kg/day Administer as an infusion at a concentration of 132 mg/mL over 2 hours. The infusion time may be decreased to 1 hour in patients who tolerate the 2 hr infusion.	Injection: 50-mg vial
Ampicillin (Principen)	***IV:*** *Meningitis:* Neonates, age <7 days: <2,000 g: 100 mg/kg/day in 2 divided doses. ≥2,000 g: 150 mg/kg/day in 3 divided doses. Neonates, age >7 days: <1,200 g: 100 mg/kg/day in 2 divided doses. 1,200–2,000 g: 150 mg/kg/day in 3 divided doses. >2,000 g: 200 mg/kg/day in 4 divided doses. Infants and children: 150–300 mg/kg/day in 4–6 divided doses to a maximum of 12 g/day. Adults: 150–200 mg/kg/day in 6–8 divided doses to a maximum total daily dose of 14 g. *Moderate infections:* Neonates, age <7 days: <2,000 g: 50 mg/kg/day in 2 divided doses. >2,000 g: 75 mg/kg/day in 3 divided doses.	Capsules: 250 mg, 500 mg Injection: 125-mg, 250-mg, 500-mg, 1-g, 2-g vials Suspension: 125 mg/5 mL, 250 mg/5 mL

(continued)

Table 1. Medications (continued)

	Dosages	Dosage Forms
Ampicillin (Principen) (*continued*)	Neonates, age <7 days: <1,200 g: 50 mg/kg/day in 2 divided doses. 1,200–2,000 g: 75 mg/kg/day in 3 divided doses. >2,000 g: 100 mg/kg/day in 4 divided doses. Infants, children, and adults: 50–100 mg/kg/day in 4–6 divided doses to a maximum total dose of 12 g/day. ***PO (mild to moderate infections):*** Children <20 kg: 50–75 mg/kg/day in 4 divided doses. Do not exceed adult doses for the same degree of infection. Children >20 kg and adults: 1–2 daily (250–500 mg/dose) in 4 divided doses. Dosage must be adjusted in patients with renal dysfunction.	
Ampicillin and sulbactam sodium (Unasyn)	***IV (dosed as ampicillin component):*** Infants and children: 100–200 mg/kg/day in 4 divided doses (max 8 g amp/day). Adults: 1.5–3 g (1–2 g ampicillin + 0.5–1 g sulbactam) given q6h. Maximum dose is 12 g/day (ampicillin + sulbactam). Dosage must be adjusted in patients with renal dysfunction.	Injection: 1.5 g (1 g ampicillin + 0.5 g sulbactam), 3 g (2 g ampicillin + 1 g sulbactam)
Ascorbic acid	***PO, IM, IV (IM preferred over IV):*** Children: Scurvy: 100–300 mg daily in 3–4 divided doses. Dietary supplementation: 35–100 mg daily. Adults: Scurvy: 200–500 mg daily in 2 divided doses. Dietary supplementation: 50–200 mg daily.	Injection: 250 mg/mL, 500 mg/mL Solution: 90 mg/mL Tablets: 100 mg, 250 mg, 500 mg, 1,000 mg
Aspirin (Anacin, Ascriptin, Bufferin, Easprin, Ecotrin)	***PO or rectally:*** *Analgesic, antipyretic:* Children: 10–15 mg/kg q4–6h. Adults: 325–1,000 mg q4–6h, up to 4 g/day. *Anti-inflammatory:* Children ≤25 kg: 60–90 mg/kg/day in 3–4 divided doses initially, with a usual range of 80–100 mg/kg/day. Monitor serum levels. Children >25 kg and adults: 2.4–3.6 g/day in 4 divided doses. Maximum total daily dose usually should not exceed 5.4 g. *Kawasaki syndrome:* 100 mg/kg/day in 4 divided doses until fever resolves; then 3–5 mg/kg once daily for 6–10 weeks after onset of the disease, or longer.	Suppositories: 300 mg, 325 mg, 600 mg, 650 mg Tablets: 325 mg, 500 mg, 650 mg Tablets, chewable: 81 mg Tablets, extended release: 165 mg, 325 mg, 500 mg, 650 mg, 975 mg Also available in buffered formulation, enteric-coated tablets, and chewing gum.
Atenolol (Tenormin)	***PO:*** Children: Initially 0.8–1 mg/kg/day in a single dose. Dosage may be increased to 1.5 mg/kg/day or a maximum of 2 mg/kg/day if necessary. Adults: Initially 25–50 mg/day, increasing to 50–100 mg/day as needed. The maximum dose for hypertension is 100 mg; for angina, 200 mg.	Tablets: 25 mg, 50 mg, 100 mg
Atomoxetine (Strattera)	***PO:*** Children ≤70 kg: 0.5 mg/kg/day initially to a maximum of 1.2 mg/kg/day. Doses may be given as a single daily dose or as 2 divided doses. Adolescents and adults >70 kg: 40 mg daily initially, increasing to a maximum daily dose of 100 mg.	Capsules: 10 mg, 18 mg, 25 mg, 40 mg, 60 mg, 80 mg, 100 mg
Atropine sulfate	***PO or IM:*** Preoperative: 0.02 mg/kg to a maximum dose of ~1 mg. *Bradycardia:* 0.02 mg/kg with a minimum dose of 0.1 mg and a maximum dose of 0.5 mg in children, 1 mg in adolescents, and 2 mg in adults. No longer in PALS algorithm, use only if suspicion of vagal stimulation. *Ophthalmic:* 1–2 drops of 0.5–1% solution in the eye.	Injection: 0.3 mg/mL, 0.4 mg/mL, 0.5 mg/mL, 0.8 mg/mL, 1 mg/mL Ointment, ophthalmic: 0.5%, 1% Solution, ophthalmic: 0.5%, 1%, 2%

Table 1. Medications (continued)

	Dosages	Dosage Forms
Azathioprine (Imuran)	**IV or PO:** *Transplant:* Initially 2–5 mg/kg/day as a single dose. Maintenance doses are usually 1–3 mg/kg/day. *Lupus:* 2–3 mg/kg/day as a single dose. *Rheumatoid arthritis:* 1 mg/kg/day as a single dose. Note: Metabolism of azathioprine is decreased by allopurinol; decrease dose of azathioprine by 75%.	Injection: 100-mg vial Tablets: 50 mg
Azelastine (Astelin)	**Intranasal metered dose spray:** Age 5–11 years: 1 spray in each nostril b.i.d. Age ≥12 years: 2 sprays in each nostril b.i.d.	Solution, nasal: 137 mcg/metered spray
Azithromycin (Zithromax)	**IV or PO:** *Otitis media* (age ≥6 months): 10 mg/kg (to a maximum of 500 mg) on the first day followed by 5 mg/kg/day (to a maximum of 250 mg) for 4 days. Alternatively, a dose of 30 mg/kg as a single dose (maximum 1,500 mg) or 10 mg/kg/day for 3 days (maximum 500 mg/day) may be used. *Pharyngitis/Tonsillitis:* Age ≥2 years: 12 mg/kg/day (to a maximum of 500 mg) for 5 days. Adults: 500 mg on the first day followed by 250 mg/day for 4 days. *Uncomplicated chlamydia infection:* 1 g as a single dose for patients >8 years of age weighing at least 45 kg. *Gonorrhea:* 2 g for patients weighing at least 45 kg. *Chancroid:* 20 mg/kg to a maximum dose of 1 g.	Tablets: 250, 500, 600 mg Suspension: 100 mg/5 mL, 200 mg/5 mL, 1-g packet Injection: 2 mg/mL
Aztreonam (Azactam)	**IV or IM:** Children over age 1 month: 60–100 mg/kg/day in 3–4 divided doses. Doses of up to 200 mg/kg/day have been used in cystic fibrosis patients. Maximum total daily dose is 8 g. Adults: 1–2 g q6–8h, depending on the severity of the infection. Dose adjustment is necessary in renal impairment.	Injection: 500-mg, 1-g, 2-g vials
Bacitracin; bacitracin and polymyxin B (Polysporin); bacitracin, neomycin, and polymyxin B (Neosporin)	**Ophthalmic:** Apply to eyes q3–4h. If both eyes involved, dispense separate tubes. **Topically:** Apply to affected area 1–3 times daily.	Ointment, topical (all 3): 15-g, 30-g tubes Ointment, ophthalmic (all 3): 3.5-g tube
Beclomethasone dipropionate (BeconaseAQ, QVAR)	**Intranasal aqueous formulation:** Age ≥6 years: 1–2 sprays in each nostril b.i.d. **Oral inhalation:** Age 6–12 years: 40 mcg b.i.d. Do not exceed 8 mcg b.i.d. Age >12 years: 40–80 mcg b.i.d. Do not exceed 320 mcg b.i.d.	Intranasal aerosol spray: 42 mcg/spray Oral inhalation aerosol: 40 mcg/spray, 80 mcg/spray
Betamethasone (Diprolene, Maxivate)	Apply a thin film to the skin 1–3 times daily. Avoid application to the face, groin, or axillae.	Dipropionate, augmented (Diprolene): 0.05% cream, lotion, gel, ointment Dipropionate: 0.05% cream, lotion, ointment Dipropionate with clotrimazole (antifungal) [Lotrisone] Valerate: 0.1% cream, lotion, ointment

(*continued*)

Table 1. Medications (continued)

	Dosages	Dosage Forms
Bisacodyl (Dulcolax)	**PO:** (*Higher doses for evacuation, lower for laxative*): Age 3–12 years: 5–10 mg as a single dose. Age >12 years: 5–15 mg as a single dose. Tablets are enteric coated and must not be chewed or crushed. **Rectally:** Age <2 years: 5 mg/day as a single dose. Age 2–11 years: 5–10 mg/day as a single dose. Age ≥12 years: 10 mg/day as a single dose.	Suppositories: 10 mg Tablets, enteric coated: 5 mg
Budesonide (Pulmicort, RhinocortAqua)	**Intranasal metered dose spray:** Age ≥6 years: 2 sprays in each nostril in the morning or as 2 divided doses. Dosage may be decreased to the lowest number of sprays that controls symptoms. **Oral inhalation powder:** Age 6–12 years: 1–2 puffs b.i.d. Age >12 years: 2–4 puffs b.i.d. **PO inhalation suspension for nebulization:** All patients: 0.5–2 mg daily as a single daily dose or in 2 divided doses.	Oral inhalation powder: 200 mcg/actuation Oral inhalation suspension: 0.25 mg/2 mL, 0.5 mg/2 mL Suspension, nasal: 32 mcg/actuation
Bumetanide (Bumex)	**PO or IV:** Neonates: 0.01–0.05 mg/kg/dose q24–48h. Infants and children: 0.015–0.1 mg/kg/dose q6–24h to a maximum of 10 mg/day. Adults: 0.5–1 mg/dose IV or 0.5–2 mg/dose PO once or twice daily to a maximum of 10 mg/day.	Injection: 0.25 mg/mL Tablets: 0.5 mg, 1 mg, 2 mg
Caffeine	**PO or IV:** *Loading dose:* 10 mg/kg caffeine base. If theophylline has been administered within the previous 3 days, a modified dose (50–75% of loading dose) may be given. *Maintenance:* 2.5 mg/kg caffeine base 24 hours after the loading dose. Dosage may be adjusted based on the patient's response and the results of serum level monitoring. Do not use caffeine and sodium benzoate injection in neonates.	Injection: 10 mg/mL base Solution: 10 mg/mL base
Calcitriol (Calcijex, Rocaltrol)	Individualize to maintain normal serum calcium levels. **PO:** *Hypocalcemia in premature infants:* 1 mcg/day for 5 days. *Renal failure:* Children: 0.25–2 mcg/day (hemodialysis) or 0.014–0.041 mcg/kg/day (no hemodialysis). Adults: 0.25–1 mcg/day. **IV:** *Hypocalcemia in premature infants:* 0.05 mcg/kg/day for 4 days. *Renal failure:* Children: 0.01–0.05 mcg/kg 3 times weekly (hemodialysis). Adults: 0.5–3 mcg 3 times weekly (hemodialysis).	Capsules: 0.25 mcg, 0.5 mcg Injection: 1 mcg/mL, 2 mcg/mL (1-mL ampules) Solution: 1 mcg/mL
Calcium salts	See dosage forms for calcium content of various salts. Dosage should be adjusted based on the desired response and serum calcium levels. **IV:** *Cardiac resuscitation:* **Calcium gluconate:** Children: 60–100 mg/kg/dose to a maximum of 3 g. Adults: 500 mg to 1 g/dose.	Calcium acetate = 25% Ca = 250 mg Ca per 1 g Ca acetate Calcium carbonate = 40% Ca = 400 mg Ca per 1 g Ca carbonate Calcium chloride = 27% Ca = 270 mg Ca per 1 g Ca chloride Calcium citrate = 21% Ca = 210 mg Ca per 1 g Ca citrate Calcium glubionate = 6.5% Ca = 65 mg Ca per 1 g Ca glubionate Calcium gluconate = 9% Ca = 90 mg Ca per 1 g Ca gluconate Calcium lactate = 13% Ca = 130 mg Ca per 1 g Ca lactate

Table 1. Medications (continued)

	Dosages	Dosage Forms
Calcium salts (*continued*)	Calcium **chloride:** Children: 20 mg/kg/dose to a maximum of 1 g. Adults: 2–4 mg/kg/dose to a maximum of 1 g. *Hypocalcemia (***gluconate*** salt):* Neonates: 200–800 mg/kg/day, usually as a continuous infusion. Infants and children: 200–500 mg/kg/day as a continuous infusion or in 4 divided doses. Adults: 2–15 g/day as a continuous infusion or in divided doses. *PO (carbonate, glubionate, or lactate salts):* Neonates: 20–80 mg elemental calcium/kg/day in 4–6 divided doses. Infants and children: 20–40 mg elemental calcium/kg/day in 4–6 divided doses. Adults: 400 mg to 1.2 g elemental calcium/day or more.	Injection: Chloride salt: 1 g (100 mg/mL) = 27 mg Ca/mL Gluconate salt: 1 g (100 mg/mL) = 9 mg Ca/mL Suspension: Carbonate salt: 1.25 g/5 mL = 500 mg Ca/5 mL Syrup: Glubionate salt: 1.8 g/5 mL = 115 mg Ca/5 mL Tablets: Acetate salt: 667 mg = 169 mg Ca (PhosLo) Carbonate salt: 650 mg = 260 mg Ca; 1.25 g = 500 mg Ca; 1.5 g = 600 mg Ca Citrate salt: 950 mg = 200 mg Ca (Citracal); 2376 mg = 500 mg Ca (Citracal Liquitab) Gluconate salt: 500 mg = 45 mg Ca; 650 mg = 58.5 mg Ca; 975 mg = 87.75 mg Ca; 1 g = 90 mg Ca Lactate salt: 325 mg = 42.25 mg Ca; 650 mg = 84.5 mg Ca
Calfactant (Infasurf)	*Intratracheally:* 3 mL/kg divided into 2–4 aliquots. Patients should be ventilated and repositioned between aliquots. May be repeated to a total of 3 doses at 12 hour intervals.	Suspension, intratracheal: 3 mL, 6 mL
Captopril (Capoten)	*PO:* Neonates: 0.01–0.05 mg/kg up to t.i.d., initially. Dose may be increased incrementally to a maximum of 0.5 mg/kg administered as frequently as q6h (2 mg/kg/day). Infants and children: 0.15–0.3 mg/kg up to t.i.d., initially. Dose may be increased incrementally to a maximum of 6 mg/kg/day in divided doses. Adolescents and adults: 12.5–25 mg q8–12h, initially. May be titrated upward to a maximum of 6 mg/kg/day or 450 mg.	Tablets: 12.5 mg, 25 mg, 50 mg, 100 mg
Carbamazepine (Carbatrol, Tegretol, Tegretol-XR)	*PO:* Initially 5–10 mg/kg/day in 2–4 divided doses, increasing slowly to a maximum of 35 mg/kg/day (1.6–2.4 g in adults). Suspension formulation should be administered in 3–4 daily doses; regular tablet formulations may be administered in 2–3 divided doses, extended release formulations may be administered in 2 divided doses.	Capsules, extended release: 200 mg, 300 mg. Suspension: 100 mg/5 mL Tablets, chewable: 100 mg Tablets: 200 mg Tablets, extended release: 100 mg, 200 mg, 400 mg
Carbamide peroxide (Debrox, Gly-Oxide)	*Ear:* Instill up to 5–10 drops in the ear and allow to remain for several minutes or longer. *PO:* Apply several drops to the affected area up to q.i.d.	Drops, oral: 10% (Cank-aid, Gly-Oxide, Orajel Brace-aid Rinse) Drops, otic: 6.5% (Auro Ear Drops, Debrox, Murine Ear Drops)
Cefaclor	*PO:* 20–40 mg/kg/day in 2–3 divided doses to a maximum of 2 g/24 hr.	Capsules: 250 mg, 500 mg Suspension: 125 mg/5 mL, 187 mg/5 mL, 250 mg/5 mL, 275 mg/5 mL
Cefadroxil	*PO:* Children: 30 mg/kg/day in 2 divided doses to a maximum of 2 g/day. Adults: 1–2 g/day in a single or 2 divided doses.	Capsules: 500 mg Suspension: 250 mg/5 mL, 500 mg/5 mL
Cefazolin (Ancef)	*IV or IM:* 50–150 mg/kg/day in 3 divided doses to a maximum of 6 g/day. Usual adult doses are 500 mg to 2 g/dose q8h. Dosing adjustment is necessary in renal impairment.	Injection: 500-mg, 1-g vials
Cefdinir (Omnicef)	*PO:* Age 6 months to 12 years: 14 mg/kg/day in 1 or 2 divided doses. Age >12 years or 43 kg: 600 mg daily in 1 or 2 divided doses.	Capsules: 300 mg Suspension: 125 mg/5 mL, 250 mg/5 mL

(continued)

Table 1. Medications (continued)

	Dosages	Dosage Forms
Cefixime (Suprax)	***PO:*** Children: 8–20 mg/kg/day in 1 or 2 divided doses to a maximum of 400 mg/day. Adults: 400 mg/day in 1 or 2 divided doses. *Otitis media:* Use suspension formula because higher serum levels are reached at the same dose when the suspension is administered.	Suspension: 100 mg/5 mL Tablets: 400 mg
Cefotaxime (Claforan)	***IV or IM:*** *Sepsis:* Infants and children: 100–150 mg/kg/day in 3–4 divided doses. Adults: 1–2 g q6–8h. *Meningitis:* Neonates, age <1 week: 50 mg/kg q12h. Neonates, age ≥1 week: 50 mg/kg q8h. Infants, age >4 weeks and children: 200 mg/kg/day in 4 divided doses. A dose of 300 mg/kg/day in 4 divided doses has been used for the treatment of pneumococcal meningitis. Maximum total daily dose is 12 g. Adults: 2 g q4–6h. Dosing adjustment is necessary in renal impairment.	Injection: 1-g, 2-g vials
Cefoxitin (Mefoxin)	***IV or IM:*** Neonates: 90–100 mg/kg/day in 3 divided doses. Children: 80–160 mg/kg/day depending on the severity of the infection in 4 divided doses. Adults: 1–2 g q6–8h to a maximum total daily dose of 12 g.	Injection: 1-g, 2-g vials
Cefpodoxime (Vantin)	***PO (with food to enhance absorption):*** Children: 10 mg/kg/day in 2 divided doses to a maximum of 800 mg/day. Adults: 200 mg/day in 2 divided doses for upper respiratory or uncomplicated UTI, 400 mg/day in 2 divided doses for lower respiratory tract infection (community-acquired pneumonia), 800 mg/day in 2 divided doses (skin, skin structure infection). Dosage adjustment is necessary in severe renal impairment.	Suspension: 50 mg/5 mL, 100 mg/5 mL Tablets: 100 mg, 200 mg
Cefprozil (Cefzil)	***PO:*** Children: *Otitis media:* 30 mg/kg/day in 2 divided doses to a maximum total daily dose of 1 g. *Pharyngitis, tonsillitis:* 15 mg/kg/day in 2 divided doses to a maximum total daily dose of 500 mg. Adults: *Lower respiratory tract:* 500 mg q12h. *Upper respiratory tract and skin:* 500 mg q24h. Dosage adjustment is necessary in renal impairment.	Suspension: 125 mg/5 mL, 250 mg/5 mL Tablets: 250 mg, 500 mg
Ceftazidime (Fortaz, Tazicef)	***IV or IM:*** Neonates: <2,000 g: 60 mg/kg/day in 2 divided doses. ≥2,000 g: 90 mg/kg/day in 3 divided doses. Infants and children: 90–150 mg/kg/day in 3 divided doses to a maximum total daily dose of 6 g. Adults: 3–6 g/day in 3 divided doses. Dosage adjustment is necessary in renal impairment.	Injection: 500 mg, 1 g, 2 g
Ceftriaxone (Rocephin)	***IV or IM:*** *PPNG (uncomplicated pharyngeal, urethral, endocervical, rectal):* <45 kg: 125 mg IM as a single dose. ≥45 kg: 250 mg IM as a single dose. *Infants born to a mother infected with PPNG:* 50 mg/kg IM to a maximum of 125 mg as a single dose.	Injection: 250-mg, 500-mg, 1-g, 2-g vials

Table 1. Medications (continued)

	Dosages	Dosage Forms
Ceftriaxone (Rocephin) (*continued*)	*Other serious infections (not including meningitis):* Children: 50–75 mg/kg/day in 2 divided doses. Do not exceed 2 g/day. Adults: Usually 1–2 g as a single daily dose or in 2 divided doses. *Otitis media:* 50 mg/kg as a single dose to a maximum dose of 1 g. *Meningitis:* Children: 100 mg/kg/day in 1–2 divided doses to a maximum total daily dose of 4 g.	
Cefuroxime (Ceftin, Zinacef)	**PO (administer with food to enhance absorption):** *Otitis media* (all ages): 30 mg/kg/day in 2 divided doses to a maximum total daily dose of 1 g. *Other infections* (all ages): 20 mg/kg/day in 2 divided doses to a maximum total daily dose of 500 mg. **IV:** Children: 50–100 mg/kg/day in 3–4 divided doses. A dose of 150 mg/kg/day in 3 divided doses is recommended for bone and joint infections. Do not exceed adult doses below. Adults: 2.25–4.5 g/day in 3 divided doses. Higher dose is necessary for severe infections and bone and joint infections. Dosage adjustment is necessary in renal impairment.	Injection: 750-mg, 1.5-g vials Suspension (axetil): 125 mg/5 mL, 250 mg/5 mL Tablets: 250 mg, 500 mg
Cephalexin (Keflex)	**PO:** Children: 50–100 mg/kg/day in 4 divided doses for otitis media and serious infections. Doses of 25–50 mg/kg/day in 2–4 divided doses may be used for less serious infections. Do not exceed adult doses. Adults: 1–4 g/day in 4 divided doses. Dosage must be adjusted in patients with renal dysfunction.	Capsules: 250 mg, 500 mg Suspension: 125 mg/5 mL, 250 mg/5 mL
Cetirizine (Zyrtec)	**PO:** Age 2–5 years: 2.5 mg/day. Dose may be increased to 5 mg/day as a single or 2 divided doses. Age ≥6 years: 5–10 mg/day as a single dose.	Syrup: 1 mg/mL Tablets: 5 mg, 10 mg
Charcoal (Actidose-Aqua, CharcoAid, Liqui-Char)	**PO:** Usually available as premixed solutions. Solutions containing sorbitol are not indicated for use in children. Do not administer with dairy due to decreased adsorptive capacity of the charcoal. Airway protection must be ensured. Single dose: Children: 1–2 g/kg up to 15–30 g as soon as possible after the ingestion, preferably after emesis. Adults: 30–100 g. Dose should be 5–10 times the amount of the ingested poison. Multiple dose (products without sorbitol): Infants: 1 g/kg q4–6h. Children and adults: 1–2 g/kg (up to 60 g) q2–6h.	Liquid: 25 g/120 mL, 50 g/240 mL
Chloral hydrate (Aquachloral)	**PO:** *Sedation before procedures:* 60–75 mg/kg 30 minutes to 1 hour before the procedure. May repeat with a half-dose (30–37.5 mg/kg) if the first dose is ineffective. Do not exceed 120 mg/kg or 2 g total.	Capsules: 500 mg Syrup: 500 mg/5 mL
Chloramphenicol (Chloromycetin)	**IV:** Infants and children: 50–100 mg/kg/day in 4 divided doses to a maximum total daily dose of 4 g. Adults: 50 mg/kg/day in 4 divided doses to a maximum total daily dose of 4 g. Serum levels must be monitored closely, especially in infants, and patients with renal or hepatic impairment.	Injection: 1-g vial

(continued)

Table 1. Medications (continued)

	Dosages	Dosage Forms
Chlorothiazide (Diuril)	**PO:** Infants <6 months: 20–40 mg/kg/day in 2 divided doses. Children: 20 mg/kg/day in 2 divided doses. Adults: 0.5–1 g/day in 1 or 2 divided doses. **IV:** Infants <6 months: 20–40 mg/kg/day in 2 divided doses, but doses of 2–8 mg/kg/day may be sufficient in some patients. Children: 4–20 mg/kg/day in 2 divided doses. Adults: 0.5–1 g/day.	Injection: 500 mg Suspension: 250 mg/5 mL Tablets: 250 mg, 500 mg
Chlorpromazine	**IV or PO:** *Nausea and vomiting or psychosis:* Age >6 months: 0.3–0.5 mg/kg IV q6–8h or 0.5–1 mg/kg PO q4–6h or 1 mg/kg rectally q6–8h as needed. Do not exceed adult doses. Adults: 25–50 mg IV q6–8h or 10–25 mg PO q4–6h or 50–100 mg rectally q6–8h. Doses may be increased in the treatment of psychoses; some adults may require as much as 800 mg/day until control is achieved. Dose should then be decreased to the usual maintenance levels of 200 mg/day for adults.	Injection: 25 mg/mL Tablets: 10 mg, 25 mg, 50 mg, 100 mg, 200 mg
Cholestyramine resin (Questran, Questran Light)	**PO:** Children: 240 mg/kg/day of the resin administered in 3 divided doses. Adults: 3–4 g t.i.d. or q.i.d. Doses should be administered mixed in liquids (4 g in 2–6 oz.) or with pulpy fruits (applesauce or pineapple). Many drugs bind with cholestyramine in the GI tract. Drugs should be administered 1 hour before or 4 hours after cholestyramine. Patients should also be cautioned to ingest plenty of fluids to avoid constipation and fecal impaction.	Powder: 4 g resin/9 g powder (Questran); 4 g resin/5 g powder (Questran Light, contains aspartame)
Cimetidine (Tagamet)	**PO or IV:** Initial dose: Children: 20–40 mg/kg/day in 4 divided doses daily. Adults: 300 mg q6h. PO, doses of 800 mg at bedtime or 400 mg b.i.d. may be used. A maximum total daily dose of 2.4 g should not be exceeded. Dosage must be adjusted in renal impairment.	Injection: 150 mg/mL Liquid: 300 mg/5 mL Tablets: 200 mg, 300 mg, 400 mg, 800 mg
Ciprofloxacin (Ciloxan, Cipro)	**PO (on an empty stomach):** Children: 20–30 mg/kg/day in 2 divided doses; up to 40 mg/kg/day may be used for patients with cystic fibrosis. Do not exceed 1.5 g/day. Adults: 500–1,500 mg/day in 2 divided doses. **IV (administer over 1 hour at a concentration of 1–2 mg/mL):** Children: 15–20 mg/kg/day in 2 divided doses; up to 30 mg/kg/day may be used in patients with cystic fibrosis. Do not exceed 800 mg/day. Adults: 400–800 mg/day in 2 divided doses. Dosage must be adjusted in patients with renal dysfunction. **Ophthalmic:** Administer 1–2 drops q2h while awake for 2 days and then q4h while awake for 5 days.	Injection: 10 mg/mL Ointment, ophthalmic: 0.3% base Solution, ophthalmic: 0.3% base Suspension: 250 mg/5 mL, 500 mg/5 mL Tablets: 250 mg, 500 mg, 750 mg
Citrate and citric acid (Polycitra, Tricitrates Solution)	**PO (dilute in water or juice):** Infants and children: 2–3 mEq/kg/day in 3–4 divided doses. Adults: 15–30 mL given q.i.d. Giving doses with meals decreases the saline laxative effect.	Equivalent to potassium 1 mEq, sodium 1 mEq, and bicarbonate 2 mEq per 1 mL

Table 1. Medications (continued)

	Dosages	Dosage Forms
Clarithromycin (Biaxin)	**PO:** Children: 15 mg/kg/day in 2 divided doses, not to exceed 1 g/day. Adults: 500 mg–1 g/day in 2 divided doses or 1 g daily as 2 extended release tablets	Suspension: 125 mg/5 mL, 250 mg/5 mL Tablets: 250 mg, 500 mg Tablets, extended release: 500 mg
Clindamycin (Cleocin)	**IV:** Neonates, age <7 days: ≤2,000 g: 10 mg/kg/day in 2 divided doses. >2,000 g: 15 mg/kg/day in 3 divided doses. Neonates, age >7 days: <1,200 g: 10 mg/kg/day in 2 divided doses. 1,200–2,000 g: 15 mg/kg/day in 3 divided doses. >2,000 g: 20 mg/kg/day in 3–4 divided doses. Infants and children: 25–40 mg/kg/day in 3–4 divided doses. Adults: 1.2–2.7 g/day in 2–4 divided doses. Maximum total daily dose should not exceed 4.8 g and should be used for life-threatening infections only. **PO:** Infants and children: 15–25 mg/kg/day in 3–4 divided doses for moderate to severe infections. Adults: 150–450 mg q6–8h to a maximum total daily dose of 1.8 g. **Topically:** Apply to the affected area b.i.d. Avoid the eyes, abraded skin, and mucous membranes.	Capsules: 150 mg Injection: 150 mg/mL Solution, oral: 75 mg/5 mL Solution, topical: 1%
Clonazepam (Klonopin)	**PO:** Age <10 years or weight <30 kg: Initially 0.01–0.03 mg/kg/day in 2–3 divided doses. Dose may be increased gradually (every third day) until seizures are controlled or adverse effects are seen. The usual maintenance dose range is 0.1–0.2 mg/kg/day. Adults, weight >30 kg: Initially 1.5 mg/day in 3 divided doses. Dose may be increased by 0.5–1 mg every third day to a maximum total daily dose of 20 mg. Usual maintenance dose is 0.05–0.2 mg/kg/day.	Tablets 0.5 mg, 1 mg, 2 mg Tablets, disintegrating: 0.125 mg, 0.25 mg, 0.5 mg, 1 mg, 2 mg
Clonidine (Catapres)	**PO:** *Hypertension:* 5–10 mcg/kg/day in 2–3 divided doses. In patients who experience sedation, the doses may be divided such that the patient receives a larger dose at bedtime and a smaller dose in the morning. Dose may be incrementally increased to 25 mcg/kg/day to a maximum dose of 0.9 mg/day, if necessary. *Attention deficit/hyperactivity disorder:* 5 mcg/kg/day in 4 divided doses has been used in some patients who have failed conventional therapy. Maximum dose is 0.3–0.4 mg/day. **TOP:** Once oral dose has been titrated to appropriate dose, may transition to patch at equivalent dose. Change every 7 days **Injectable:** Generally used as a component in epidural solutions at 0.5–2 mcg/kg/hr.	Tablet: 0.1 mg, 0.2 mg, 0.3 mg Patch: 0.1 mg/day, 0.2 mg/day, 0.3 mg/day Injection: 100, 500 mcg/mL
Clorazepate dipotassium (Tranxene)	**PO:** Age 9–12 years: Initially 3.75–7.5 mg b.i.d. Dose may be increased by 3.75 mg at weekly intervals to a maximum total daily dose of 60 mg. Age >12 years: Up to 7.5 mg up to t.i.d. May be increased by 7.5 mg at weekly intervals to a maximum total daily dose of 90 mg.	Tablets: 3.75 mg, 7.5 mg, 11.25 mg, 15 mg, 22.5 mg
Clotrimazole (Lotrimin, Mycelex)	**Vaginal cream:** 1 full applicator at bedtime for 7 days (1%) or 3 days (2%). **Vaginal suppository:** 1 suppository intravaginally at bedtime for 7 days or 2 at bedtime for 3 days or 500 mg as a single dose. **Topically:** Apply to affected areas b.i.d.	Cream, topical: 1% (30-g tube) Cream, vaginal: 1% (45-g), 2% (21 g) Solution, topical: 1% (10 mL, 30-mL Suppositories, vaginal: 100 mg, 200 mg

(continued)

Table 1. Medications (continued)

	Dosages	Dosage Forms
Codeine	**PO:** *Analgesic:* 0.5–1 mg/kg q4–6h as needed, to a maximum of 60 mg. Usual adult dose is 30 mg. *Antitussive:* 0.2–0.25 mg/kg q4–6h as needed, to a maximum of 30 mg.	Solution, oral (phosphate): 15 mg/5 mL Tablets (sulfate): 15 mg, 30 mg, 60 mg Also available in various combinations with acetaminophen: Elixir, oral: 12 mg codeine with 120 mg acetaminophen Tablets: 7.5 mg codeine with acetaminophen 300 mg (Tylenol w/Codeine No. 1), 15 mg codeine with acetaminophen 300 mg (Ace taminophon w/Codeine No. 2), 300 mg codeine with acetaminophen 300 mg (Tylenol w/Codeine No. 3), 60 mg codeine with acetaminophen 300 mg (Tylenol w/Codeine No. 4)
Cosyntropin (Cortrosyn)	**IV:** Age <2 years: 0.125 mg. Age >2 years: 0.25 mg.	Injection: 0.25 mg
Co-trimoxazole (trimethoprim and sulfamethoxazole; Bactrim, Septra)	**PO or IV (based on trimethoprim):** Age >2 months: *Treatment doses:* *Mild-to-moderate infections (urinary tract or otitis media):* 8 mg trimethoprim/kg/day in 2 divided doses. Maximum dose is 320 mg trimethoprim/day. *Pneumocystis carinii pneumonitis:* 20 mg trimethoprim/kg/day in 4 divided doses. *Prophylaxis doses:* *UTI:* 2 mg trimethoprim/kg/day as a single dose. *Pneumocystis carinii:* 150 mg/m²/day in 1 or 2 divided doses daily on 3 consecutive or alternating days per week. Dosage adjustment is necessary in patients with renal impairment. IV doses must be administered over 60–90 minutes and should be well diluted (1 mL injection in 25 mL infusate). Dosage must be adjusted in patients with renal dysfunction.	Injection: 16 mg trimethoprim and 80 mg sulfamethoxazole per 1 mL Suspension: 8 mg trimethoprim and 40 mg sulfamethoxazole per 1 mL Tablets: 80 mg trimethoprim and 400 mg sulfamethoxazole Tablets, double strength: 160 mg trimethoprim and 800 mg sulfamethoxazole
Cromolyn sodium (Crolom, Intal, Nasalcrom, Opticrom)	Children: *Metered-dose inhaler:* 2 inhalations q.i.d. *Nebulizer solution:* 20 mg nebulized q.i.d. *Intranasal spray:* 1 spray in each nostril 3–4 times daily. *Ophthalmic:* 1–2 drops in each eye 4–6 times daily.	Inhalation, metered dose: 800 mcg/spray Solution, nasal: 5.2 mg/spray Solution, nebulizer: 20 mg/2 mL Solution, ophthalmic: 4%
Crotamiton (Eurax)	**Topically:** Apply a thin layer to all skin surfaces from the neck to the toes and soles of the feet. Be sure to apply to all surfaces, including skin folds. Avoid the face and mucous membranes, including the urethral meatus. A second coat is applied 24 hours later. A cleansing bath should follow 48 hours after the second application. Treatment may be repeated after 7–10 days if the mites reappear. It is safe for use in infants and young children. If signs of irritation or hypersensitivity appear, remove the product immediately by bathing. Contaminated clothing and bed linens should be washed to avoid reinfestations.	Cream: 10% Lotion: 10%
Cyclosporine (Neoral, Sandimmune, Gengraf)	NOTE: The products are *not* bioequivalent. Clinical condition and serum levels must be monitored carefully when a patient's therapy is changed from one to the other, especially for patients receiving large doses (>10 mg/kg/day) of Sandimmune who are changed to Neoral or Gengraf therapy as significant drug toxicity may result. **PO (transplant):** *Sandimmune:* Initially 10–18 mg/kg/day (dose dependent on organ being transplanted) in 2 divided doses, tapering over several weeks with frequent monitoring to a maintenance dose usually in the range of 5–10 mg/kg/day. *Neoral or Gengraf:* Initially ~10 mg/kg/day in 2 divided doses, tapering over several weeks based on clinical condition and serum levels. **PO (other conditions):** Initially 2.5 mg/kg/day in 2 divided doses, max 4 mg/kg/day *Conversion from Sandimmune to Neoral or Gengraf:* Consult with pharmacist	Capsules (Neoral, Gengraf): 25 mg, 100 mg Capsules (Sandimmune): 25 mg, 100 mg Injection (Sandimmune): 50 mg/mL Solution, oral (Neoral, Gengraf and Sandimmune): 100 mg/mL

Table 1. Medications (continued)

	Dosages	Dosage Forms
Cyclosporine (Neoral, Sandimmune, Gengraf) (continued)	**IV (Sandimmune only):** IV dose is ~30% of the oral dose. Initial 5–6 mg/kg/day in 1 or 2 divided doses. Each dose should be administered over at least 2 hours.	
Dantrolene sodium (Dantrium)	**PO:** *Spasticity:* Age >5 years: 0.5 mg/kg given b.i.d. initially, but frequency may be increased gradually to t.i.d. or q.i.d. The maximum dose is 100 mg q.i.d. Adults: 25 mg daily initially, with increases in frequency and dose to a maximum of 400 mg/day in 4 divided doses. *Malignant hyperthermia prophylaxis:* 4–8 mg/kg/day in 3–4 divided doses daily for 1–2 days prior to surgery. **IV:** *Malignant hyperthermia prophylaxis:* 2.5 mg/kg administered over 1 hour ~1.25 hours before surgery. Repeat doses may be necessary. *Malignant hyperthermia crisis:* 1 mg/kg given rapidly. Repeat doses may be necessary, but it is usually not necessary to exceed 2.5 mg/kg. Maximum dose should not exceed 10 mg/kg.	Capsules: 25 mg, 50 mg, 100 mg Injection: 20 mg
Deferoxamine (Desferal)	**IV:** Children: *Acute iron intoxication:* 15 mg/kg/hr IV continuous infusion; maximum 6 g/24 hr. *Chronic iron overload:* 20–25 mg/kg/day IM or 500 mg-2 g IV with each unit of blood transfused, or 20–40 mg/kg/day SC over 8–12 hours up to 1–2 g/day.	Injection: 500-mg vial
Desmopressin acetate (DDAVP)	**Intranasally:** *Nocturnal enuresis in patients over age 6:* 20 mcg at bedtime with 1/2 of dose in each nostril. Dose may be increased or decreased depending on the patient's response. Usual range is 10–40 mcg/day. *Diabetes insipidus in patients ≥7 years of age:* Initially 5 mcg/day as a single dose or in 2 divided doses. Dosage should be titrated to the patient's response. The usual range is 5–40 mcg/day. **PO:** *Diabetes insipidus:* Children: Initially, 0.05 mg/dose with careful monitoring to prevent hyponatremia or water intoxication. Age >12 years: Initially, 0.05 mg b.i.d. Dosage may then be adjusted to maintain normal diurnal water turnover. The usual total daily dosage is in the range of 0.1–1.2 mg and may be administered in 2–3 divided doses. *Nocturnal enuresis in children >12 years:* 0.2–0.4 mg/day at bedtime. **IV:** *To increase factor VIII level:* 0.3 mcg/kg over 30 minutes. *Diabetes insipidus:* Adult doses are 2–4 mcg/day in 2 divided doses or ~1/10 of the intranasal dose necessary to control the patient's symptoms, if that is known.	Injection: 4 mcg/mL Solution, nasal: 100 mcg/mL/2.5 mL bottle with calibrated intranasal tube Spray, intranasal: 10 mcg/actuation metered dose Tablets: 0.1 mg, 0.2 mg
Dexamethasone (Decadron, Maxidex)	**IV, IM or PO:** *Bacterial meningitis:* 0.6 mg/kg/day in 4 divided doses for the first 4 days of antibiotic therapy. It must be started at the same time or before the first dose of antibiotic. *Cerebral edema:* 1–1.5 mg/kg/day in 4 divided doses to a maximum total daily dose of 16 mg. *Antiemetic therapy (chemotherapy-induced emesis):* 20 mg/m^2/day in 4 divided doses.	Elixir: 0.5 mg/5 mL Injection: 4 mg/mL, 10 mg/mL Solution, ophthalmic: 0.05%, 0.1% Solution, oral: 1 mg/mL Tablets: 0.5 mg, 0.75 mg, 1 mg, 1.5 mg, 2 mg, 4 mg, 6 mg

(continued)

Table 1. Medications (continued)

	Dosages	Dosage Forms
Dexamethasone (Decadron, Maxidex) (*continued*)	*Airway edema or extubation:* 0.5–2 mg/kg/day in 4 divided doses beginning 24 hours before and continuing for at least 24 hours after extubation. Maximum dose of 16 mg/day. *Croup:* 0.6 mg/kg PO/IM/IV x 1 dose, max 12 mg. Doses should be tapered when discontinuing long-term therapy. *Ophthalmic:* Instill drops or apply ointment t.i.d. or q.i.d.	
Dextroamphetamine sulfate (Dexedrine) **Dextroamphetamine mixed salts (Adderall)**	**PO:** Age 3–5 years: 2.5 mg/day given in the morning. Dosage may be increased 2.5 mg/day until a response is realized or side effects appear. Usual range is 0.1–0.5 mg/kg/day to a maximum of 40 mg. Age ≥6 years: 5 mg/day in the morning or at noon. Dosage may be increased in 5-mg increments at weekly intervals. Usual range is 0.1–0.5 mg/kg/day to a maximum of 40 mg.	Dextroamphetamine: Capsules, sustained release: 5 mg, 10 mg, 15 mg Tablets: 5 mg, 10 mg Dextroamphetamine mixed salts: Capsules, extended release (expressed in mg of salts): 5 mg, 10 mg, 15 mg, 20 mg, 25 mg, 30 mg Tablet (expressed in mg of salts): 5 mg, 7.5 mg, 10 mg, 12.5 mg, 15 mg, 20 mg, 30 mg
Diazepam (Diastat Rectal, Valium)	**IV:** *Status epilepticus:* 0.05–0.3 mg/kg (usual dose 0.2 mg/kg/dose) administered over 2–3 minutes and repeated q15–30min to a total maximum dose of 0.75 mg/kg or 30 mg, whichever is less. May be repeated in 2–4 hours, if necessary. *Sedation:* 0.04–0.2 mg/kg q2–4h to a maximum of 0.6 mg/kg within an 8-hour period. **PO for sedation or muscle relaxant:** 0.12–0.8 mg/kg/day in 3–4 divided doses to an adult dose of 6–40 mg/day. **Rectally (round dose off to closest dose available from manufacturer):** Age 2–5 years: 0.5 mg/kg. Age 6–11 years: 0.3 mg/kg Age ≥12 years: 0.2 mg/kg. Dose may be repeated q4–12h as necessary.	Gel, rectal (in rectal delivery system): 2.5 mg, 5 mg, 10 mg, 20 mg Injection: 5 mg/mL Solution, oral: 5 mg/5 mL Solution, concentrated oral: 5 mg/mL Tablets: 2 mg, 5 mg, 10 mg
Diazoxide (Proglycem)	**PO:** (*Hypoglycemia due to hyperinsulinism*): Newborns and infants: Initially 8 mg/kg/day in 2 or 3 divided doses. May be increased incrementally if response is inadequate to a maximum of 15 mg/kg/day. Children and adults: 3 mg/kg/day in 2 or 3 divided doses initially. May be increased to a maximum of 8 mg/kg/day.	Capsules: 50 mg Suspension, oral: 50 mg/mL
Dicloxacillin (Dycill, Dynapen, Pathocil)	**PO:** Children <40 kg: 25–50 mg/kg/day in 4 divided doses. Doses of 50–100 mg/kg/day in 4 divided doses have been used for osteomyelitis. Children ≥40 kg and adults: 125–500 mg/dose q6h.	Capsules: 250 mg, 500 mg
Digoxin (Lanoxicaps, Lanoxin) (See Table 3)	**IV or PO:** Should be based on lean body weight. Total digitalizing dose (TDD) is administered as follows: 1/2 TDD initially, then 1/4 TDD 8–12 hours later, then 1/4 TDD 8–12 hours after that. Maintenance doses are administered in 2 divided doses beginning 12 hours after the last digitalizing dose. Patients should be under continuous cardiographic monitoring during digitalization. IM doses are the same as oral doses, but that route of administration should be avoided.[†] Dosage must be adjusted in patients with renal dysfunction.	Capsules, liquid filled (Lanoxicaps): 0.1 mg, 0.2 mg (90–100% bioavailable) Injection: 0.1 mg/mL, 0.25 mg/mL (100% bioavailable IV) Solution: 0.05 mg/mL (75–87% bioavailable) Tablets: 0.125 mg, 0.25 mg (60–80% bioavailable)
Dihydroergotamine (D.H.E.)	**IV:** Age 6–9 years: 100–150 mcg/dose repeated q6h to a maximum of 8 doses. Age 10–12 years age: 200 mcg/dose repeated q6h to a maximum of 8 doses. Adolescents, age ≤16 years: 250–500 mcg/dose repeated q6h to a maximum of 8 doses. Adults: 500 mcg repeated hourly to a maximum of 2 mg (6 mg/wk) Total dose for entire course must not exceed 6 mg. Do not use erogtamines if patient has received MAOi in past 14 days.	Injection: 1 mg/mL

Table 1. Medications (continued)

	Dosages	Dosage Forms
Dimercaprol [BAL (British anti-lewisite)]	**Deep IM:** Lead toxicity (in conjunction with calcium EDTA): 4 mg/kg 6 times a day for 3–5 days.	Injection: 100 mg/mL (3-mL ampul)
Diphenhydramine	**IV, PO, IM:** Children: 5 mg/kg/day in 3 or 4 divided doses to a maximum of 300 mg/day. Adults: 10–50 mg repeated as often as q4h, not to exceed 400 mg/day. The drug may cause paradoxical excitement in children.	Capsules, tablets: 25 mg, 50 mg Elixir, solution, syrup: 12.5 mg/5 mL Injection: 10 mg/mL, 50 mg/mL
Dobutamine hydrochloride (Dobutrex)	**Continuous IV infusion:** 2–15 mcg/kg/min to a maximum of 40 mcg/kg/min. Start at the lower end of the range and titrate upward based on the patient's response.	Injection: 12.5 mg/mL
Docusate sodium (dioctyl sodium sulfosuccinate; Colace, D-S-S)	**PO:** (In 1–4 divided doses with a glass of water): Age <3 years: 10–40 mg/day. Age 3–6 years: 20–60 mg/day. Age >6–12 years: 40–150 mg/day. Age >12 years: 50–500 mg. Do not administer with mineral oil as absorption of the mineral oil may be increased.	Capsules: 50 mg, 100 mg, 240 mg, 250 mg Liquid: 150 mg/15 mL Syrup: 60 mg/15 mL Also available in combination with stimulant laxatives, including senna and casanthranol.
Dopamine hydrochloride (Dopastat, Intropin)	**Continuous IV infusion:** 2–20 mcg/kg/min, start higher at 5–10 mcg/kg/min in septic shock. Usual a maximum of 20 mcg/kg/min (50 mcg/kg/min has been documented but rarely offers additional support over 20 mcg/kg/min). Consider addition of second agent at 20 mcg/kg/min.	Injection in 5% dextrose: 0.8 mg/mL, 1.6 mg/mL, 3.2 mg/mL (premixed infusions) Injection: 40 mg/mL, 80 mg/mL, 160 mg/mL
Dornase alfa (Pulmozyme)	**Inhalation via approved compressor:** Age >5 years: 2.5 mg/day. Patients with cystic fibrosis may require 2.5 mg inh BID.	Solution, inhalation: 2.5 mg/2.5 mL
Doxycycline (Doxy-100, Vibramycin)	**PO or IV:** Age <8 years: Should not be used unless there is no alternative. Age ≥8 years: 2–5 mg/kg/day to a maximum of 200 mg/day in 1 or 2 divided doses. Adults: 100–200 mg/day in 1 or 2 divided doses. Inpatient treatment of PID 100 mg IV b.i.d. with cefoxitin 2 g IV q6h for at least 4 days or 2 days after patient improves, whichever is longer. Doxycycline should be continued PO to complete 10–14 days of therapy.	Capsules or tablets: 50 mg, 100 mg; Liquid: 5 mg/mL; Injection: 100 mg, 200 mg
Edetate calcium disodium (Calcium Disodium Versenate, Calcium EDTA)	**IV infusion:** Asymptomatic lead toxicity: Initial: Up to 1 g/m^2/24 hr or 50 mg/kg/24 hr in a continuous IV drip if possible or in 2–4 divided doses for 5 days. Subsequent courses: Up to 50 mg/kg/24 hr in a continuous IV drip if possible or in 2–4 divided doses for 3–5 days. Symptomatic lead toxicity or lead encephalopathy: Initial: 50 mg/kg/day or 1–1.5 g/m^2/24 hr in a continuous IV drip if possible or in 4 divided doses for 5–7 days; give with dimercaprol (BAL).	Injection: 200 mg/mL For intravenous infusion, dilute to a maximum concentration of 5 mg/mL with D$_5$W or normal saline. Infusions should be administered either continuously or over 1–2 hours if intermittent doses are used. Rapid infusion may increase intracranial pressure.
Edrophonium (Enlon, Reversol)	**IV:** Infants: Initially 0.1 mg; if no response, follow with an additional 0.4 mg for a maximum total dose of 0.5 mg. Children: Initial: 0.04 mg/kg followed by 0.16 mg/kg if no response; maximum total dose is 10 mg. Adults: 0.2 mg/kg up to 10 mg. Administer 2 mg initially, then titrate dose. Titration of therapy: 0.04 mg/kg 1 time; if strength improves, an increase in neostigmine or pyridostigmine dose is indicated.	Injection: 10 mg/mL May precipitate cholinergic crisis.

(continued)

Table 1. Medications (continued)

	Dosages	Dosage Forms
Enalapril, enalaprilat (Vasotec)	**PO:** Initially 0.1 mg/kg/day in 1 or 2 divided doses to the usual adult dose of 2.5–5 mg/kg/day. Dosage may be increased as required to a maximum of 0.5 mg/kg/day or 40 mg. **IV:** 5–10 mcg/kg (up to 0.625–1.25 mg) may be administered q8–24h as necessary for control of hypertension. Dosage must be decreased in patients with compromised renal function and also should be decreased in patients who are hyponatremic or volume depleted, in severe congestive heart failure, or in those who are receiving diuretics.	Injection: 1.25 mg/mL Tablets: 2.5 mg, 5 mg, 10 mg, 20 mg
Enoxaparin (Lovenox)	**SC:** *Prophylaxis:* Age <2 months: 0.75 mg/kg/dose q12h Age ≥2 months: 0.5 mg/kg/dose q12h. Adults >45 kg: 30 mg q12h. *Treatment of DVT or PE:* Age <2 months: 1.5 mg/kg/dose q12h. Age ≥2 months: 1 mg/kg/dose q12h. Adults >45 kg: 1 mg/kg/dose q12h. Doses should be adjusted based on antifactor Xa levels. Consult pharmacist for dosing in obese patients.	Injection: 100 mg/mL
Epinephrine (Adrenalin)	**IV:** *Asystole, or pulseless arrest:* Neonates: 0.01–0.03 mg/kg (0.1–0.3 mL/kg of a 1:10,000 solution) q3–5min as necessary. Infants to adults: An initial dose of 0.01 mg/kg; subsequent doses of 0.1 mg/kg may be repeated q3–5min as necessary. A continuous infusion may be started at a dose of 0.1–1 mcg/kg/min and titrated to effect. **IM:** *Anaphylaxis or respiratory failure:* 0.01 mg/kg IM of the 1:1,000 solution. 10–30 kg: 0.15 mg IM, >30 kg: 0.3 mg IM. **Nebulization:** 0.25–0.5 mL of a 2.25% racemic epinephrine solution diluted in 2.5–3 mL of normal saline for inhalation.	Injection: 1:10,000 (0.1 mg/mL), 1:1,000 (1 mg/mL) Injection pre-filled automatic syringe: EpiPen delivers 0.3 mg IM, EpiPen Jr. delivers 0.15 mg IM Solution, racemic for inhalation: 2.25%
Epoetin alfa (erythropoietin; Epogen, EPO, Procrit, r-HuEPO)	**IV or SC:** Initially 50–100 Unit/kg administered 1–3 times weekly until the hematocrit reaches 30–33%. Dosage should be lowered if the hematocrit exceeds that range or increases by >4 points in a 2-week period. It may be increased if the hematocrit does not reach the target range or fails to increase by 5–6 points in an 8-week period. The usual maintenance dose is 25 Unit/kg 3 times weekly. Hematocrit and serum iron levels should be monitored frequently. BP should also be monitored frequently.	Injection: 2,000 Unit/mL, 3,000 Unit/mL, 4,000 Unit/mL, 10,000 Unit/mL, 20,000 Unit/mL, 40,000 Unit/mL
Ergocalciferol (vitamin D₂, activated ergosterol; Calciferol, Drisdol)	**PO:** Healthy infants and children: 400 Units/day. Infants and children with malabsorption syndromes: 1,000 Units/day. Children with liver disease: 4,000–8,000 Units/day. Children with vitamin D–dependent rickets: 3,000–5,000 Units/day. Nutritional rickets with normal absorption: 1,000–5,000 Units/day; with malabsorption: 10,000–25,000 Units/day. **IM:** Should be retained for patients with rickets due to severe vitamin D deficiency. The dose for vitamin D–resistant rickets ranges from 50,000–500,000 Units/day, for hypoparathyroidism from 50,000–200,000 Units/day, and for familial hypophosphatemia from 10,000–80,000 Units/day. The range between therapeutic and toxic doses is narrow. Patients must be closely monitored. 1 mcg = 40 Units.	Capsules: 50,000 Units (1.25 mg) Injection (in sesame oil): 500,000 Units/mL (12.5 mg/mL) Solution, oral: 8,000 Units/mL (200 mcg/mL)

Table 1. Medications (continued)

	Dosages	Dosage Forms
Erythromycin (Ery-Tab, Eryc, Erythrocin, E.E.S.)	**PO:** Infants and children: Base, ethylsuccinate or stearate: 30–50 mg/kg/day in 3 or 4 divided doses do not exceed 2 g/day. Adults: Base: 250–500 mg q6–12h. Ethylsuccinate: 400–800 mg q6–12h. *Endocarditis prophylaxis* (penicillin-allergic patients): 20 mg/kg to a maximum of 1 g 2 hours before the procedure and 10 mg/kg to a maximum of 500 mg 6 hours later. *Bowel preparation* (erythromycin base, only): 20 mg/kg to a maximum of 1 g administered at 1:00, 2:00, and 11:00 P.M. on the day before surgery, usually combined with neomycin and mechanical cleansing of the bowel. **IV:** 15–50 mg/kg/day to a maximum of 4 g/day administered in 4 divided doses. **Ophthalmic ointment:** *Prophylaxis of neonates:* Apply a 0.5–1 cm ribbon of the ointment to each conjunctival sac. **Topically for acne:** Apply to the affected areas b.i.d. The skin should be washed, rinsed well, and dried before applying the erythromycin. Keep away from the eyes, nose, and mouth.	Base: Capsules, enteric-coated pellets: 250 mg Ointment, ophthalmic: 0.5% Gel, topical: 2% Solution, topical: 1.5%, 2% Tablets, enteric coated: 250 mg, 333 mg, 500 mg Tablets, film coated: 250 mg, 500 mg Ethylsuccinate: Suspension: 200 mg/5 mL, 400 mg/5 mL Tablets: 400 mg Stearate: Tablets: 250 mg, 500 mg
Erythromycin and sulfisoxazole	**PO (based on the erythromycin content):** Age ≤2 months: 40–50 mg/kg/day in 3 or 4 divided doses to a maximum of 2 g/day.	Suspension: 200 mg erythromycin and 600 mg sulfisoxazole per 5 mL
Etanercept (Enbrel)	**SC:** *The treatment of rheumatoid arthritis:* 0.4 mg/kg to a maximum dose of 25 mg given twice weekly 72–96 hours apart. Alternatively, 0.8 mg/kg to a maximum dose of 50 mg as a weekly dose may be used.	Injection, powder for reconstitution: 25 mg
Ethacrynic acid (Edecrin)	**PO:** 1 mg/kg administered 1–2 times daily. Do not exceed the usual adult dose of 50–200 mg/day. **IV:** 0.4–1 mg/kg up to 50 mg administered 1 or 2 times daily. Serum electrolytes must be closely monitored during ethacrynic acid therapy.	Injection: 50 mg Tablets: 25 mg
Ethambutol (Myambutol)	**PO:** (*Patient should be old enough to cooperate with an eye exam to detect optic neuritis*): Children: 15–20 mg/kg/day in a single dose. Adolescents and adults: 15–25 mg/kg/day in a single dose. Do not exceed 1.6 g/day.	Tablets: 100 mg, 400 mg
Ethosuximide (Zarontin)	**PO:** Age <6 years: 15 mg/kg/day in 2 divided doses to a maximum of 250 mg/dose. Age ≥6 years: 250 mg b.i.d. Dose may be increased by 250 mg/day q4–7 days to a maximum of 1.5 g/day or 40 mg/kg/day.	Capsules: 250 mg Syrup: 250 mg/5 mL
Famotidine (Pepcid)	**PO, IV:** Age >3 months to 1 year: 1 mg/kg/day in 2 divided doses may be used for GERD. Children and adults: 1 mg/kg/day in 2 divided doses up to 80 mg/day may be used for GERD. A dose of 0.5 mg/kg up to 40 mg may be used for peptic ulcer or esophagitis.	Injection: 10 mg/mL Powder for oral suspension: 40 mg/5 mL Tablets: 10 mg, 20 mg, 40 mg

(continued)

Table 1. Medications (continued)

	Dosages	Dosage Forms
Fentanyl citrate (Sublimaze)	**IV:** *(Slowly over a period of 3–5 minutes to avoid chest wall rigidity and to titrate to effect):* Children: 1–2 mcg/kg may be repeated at 30–60-minute intervals. For continuous therapy, after a bolus dose, a dose of 1 mcg/kg/hr initially may be increased or decreased as necessary to response. Older children and adults: 0.5–1 mcg/kg (25–50 mcg) may be repeated at 30–60-minute intervals. **Intranasal:** 1–2 mcg/kg intranasal x 1 dose if no IV access The doses listed are analgesic/sedation doses. Doses used for general anesthesia may be higher. **Transdermal:** Children >2 yrs who are receiving at least 60 mg in morphine equivalents/day may be transitioned to fentanyl patch. Consult pharmacist for conversion.	Injection: 50 mcg/mL Transdermal: 12.5 mcg/day, 25 mcg/day, 50 mcg/day, 75 mcg/day, 100 mcg/day
Ferrous sulfate (Feosol, Fer-In-Sol)	**PO (doses are expressed as elemental iron):** *Iron deficiency anemia:* Children: 3–6 mg/kg/day depending on the severity of the deficiency. Higher doses should be administered in 3 divided doses; moderate doses may be administered in 2 divided doses to avoid GI upset. For prophylaxis, 1–2 mg/kg/day in a single dose may be used. Adults: 120–240 mg iron daily in 2–4 divided doses. For prophylaxis, 60 mg iron daily as a single dose. Administration between meals increases absorption, but may result in more GI upset. Do not administer with antacids, eggs, or milk because they may decrease absorption of the iron. Many concentrations available, use caution. Ferrous sulfate contains 20% iron	Drops: 75 mg/0.6 mL (15 mg elemental Fe/0.6 mL) OR 75 mg/mL (15 mg elemental Fe/mL) Elixir: 220 mg/5 mL (44 mg elemental Fe/5 mL) Liquid 300 mg/5 mL (60 mg elemental Fe/5 mL) Suspension: 75 mg/1.5 mL (15 mg elemental Fe/1.5 mL) Tablets: 325 mg (65 mg elemental Fe); Tablet, slow release: 160 mg (50 mg elemental Fe), 140 mg (45 elemental Fe)
Fexofenadine (Allegra)	**PO:** Age 2–11 years: 30 mg b.i.d. Age >12 years: 60 mg b.i.d. or 180 mg daily.	Liquid: 6 mg/mL, Tablet: 30 mg, 60 mg, 180 mg, Tablet, orally disintegrating: 30 mg
Fluconazole (Diflucan)	**PO or IV:** *Oropharyngeal or esophageal candidiasis:* 6 mg/kg (up to 200 mg) on the first day; then 3 mg/kg/day (up to 100 mg). *Systemic candidiasis or cryptococcal meningitis:* 12 mg/kg (up to 400 mg) on the first day; then 6 mg/kg/day (up to 200 mg). *Prevention of candidiasis in bone marrow transplant:* 12 mg/kg/day (up to 400 mg) beginning several days before anticipated onset of neutropenia and continued until 7 days after neutrophil count is >1,000/mm³. *Vaginal candidiasis:* 150 mg as a single dose. Dosage should be adjusted in patients with renal dysfunction.	Injection: 2 mg/mL (ready to administer) Suspension: 10 mg/mL, 40 mg/mL Tablets: 50 mg, 100 mg, 150 mg, 200 mg
Flucytosine (Ancobon)	**PO:** Neonates: 50–100 mg/kg/day in 1–2 divided doses. Children and adults: 50–150 mg/kg/day in 4 divided doses. Dosage must be adjusted in renal impairment.	Capsules: 250 mg, 500 mg
Fludrocortisone (Florinef)	**PO:** Infants and children: 0.05–0.1 mg/day. Adults: 0.05–0.2 mg/day.	Tablets: 0.1 mg
Flumazenil (Mazicon, Romazicon)	**IV:** Children: 0.01 mg/kg (to a maximum of 0.2 mg) initially, followed by 0.005 mg/kg (to a maximum of 0.2 mg) every minute until a total cumulative dose of 1 mg has been reached. Adults: *Reversal of sedation:* 0.2 mg over 15 seconds; may repeat 0.2-mg dose q60sec to a maximum of 1 mg. May repeat doses q20min to a maximum of 3 mg in 1 hour. *Benzodiazepine overdose:* 0.2 mg over 30 seconds, then 0.3 mg over 30 seconds if desired level of consciousness is not reached. Additional 0.5-mg doses may be given every minute until a cumulative dose of 3 mg has been reached. If a partial response is noted, further 0.5-mg doses may be given until a cumulative dose of 5 mg is reached. Resedation may occur in patients who received long-acting benzodiazepines. Do not use in patients with seizure disorders dependent upon benzodiazepines for seizure control.	Injection: 0.1 mg/mL

Table 1. Medications (continued)

	Dosages	Dosage Forms
Flunisolide (AeroBid, Nasarel)	**Intranasal spray:** Age 6–14 years: 1 spray in each nostril t.i.d. or 2 sprays in each nostril b.i.d. initially. Maintenance dose is usually 1 spray in each nostril daily. Age >14 years: 2 sprays in each nostril b.i.d. or t.i.d. initially. After symptoms are controlled, dosage should be decreased to the lowest dose that will prevent symptoms from recurring. That may be as little as 1 spray in each nostril once daily for perennial rhinitis. The maximum dose is 4 sprays to each nostril daily. **Oral inhalation:** Age 6–15 years: 2 inhalations b.i.d. Adults: 2 inhalations b.i.d. initially, increasing to a maximum of 8 inhalations daily. Improvement in symptoms may take from several days to several weeks to occur, but therapy should not be continued for >3 weeks in the absence of efficacy. Dosage should be decreased to the lowest effective dose when symptoms abate.	Oral inhalation: 250 mcg/spray Spray, intranasal: 29 mcg/metered spray
Fluocinolone acetonide (Synalar)	**Topically:** Apply a thin layer to the affected area b.i.d. to q.i.d. Use the lowest effective potency product. Absorption is greater if the product is covered by anything that is occlusive (plastic pants, tight diapers).	Cream: 0.01%, 0.025% Ointment: 0.025% Shampoo: 0.01% Solution: 0.01%
Fluoride (Fluoritab, Karidium, Luride, Pediaflor)	**PO:** Dosage should be based on the fluoride content of the water supply. Long-term supplementation in areas with fluoridated water may result in dental fluorosis and osseous changes. Fluoride content of drinking water <0.3 ppm: Age 0–6 months: Do not supplement. Age >6 months–3 years: 0.25 mg/day. Age >3–6 years: 0.5 mg/day. Age >6–16 years: 1 mg/day. Fluoride content of drinking water 0.3–0.6 ppm: Age 0–3 years: Do not supplement. Age 3–6 years: 0.25 mg/day. Age >6–16 years: 0.5 mg/day. Fluoride content of drinking water >0.6 ppm: Do not supplement. *Dental gel:* Usually applied by a dentist. *Rinses:* Over-the-counter rinses may be used for patients over age 6 on a daily basis and contain 0.01–0.02% fluoride.	Most multivitamin combinations are available in formulations containing appropriate amounts of fluoride (Poly-Vi-Flor drops or chewable tablets, Tri-Vi-Flo drops, Vi-Daylin/F drops and chewable tablets). Products containing only fluoride: Drops: 0.25 mg/drop Solution: 0.5 mg/mL, 0.2 mg/mL (may be used PO or as a rinse) Tablets, chewable: 0.25 mg, 0.5 mg, 1 mg
Fluticasone (Flonase, Flovent)	**Intranasal metered dose spray:** Age ≥4 years: 1 spray in each nostril daily. Dosage may be increased to 2 sprays in each nostril daily if necessary. Adults: 2 sprays in each nostril daily. **Oral aerosol inhalation:** Age ≥4 years: 88 mcg b.i.d. for patients not previously treated with corticosteroids to a maximum of 440 mcg b.i.d. in patients who were previously treated with inhaled corticosteroids.	Spray oral inhalation: 44 mcg/actuation, 110 mcg/actuation, 220 mcg/actuation Suspension, nasal: 50 mcg/actuation
Fluticasone and Salmeterol (Advair)	**Oral powder inhalation:** Age 4–11 years: 1 inhalation daily of the fluticasone 100 mcg/salmeterol 50 mcg product. Age ≥12 years: 1 inhalation b.i.d. using the product that most closely matches the patient's previous steroid dosage. Use the lowest dose product for steroid naïve patients.	Powder for oral inhalation: 100 mcg fluticasone/50 mcg salmeterol/puff, 250 mcg fluticasone/50 mcg salmeterol/puff, 500 mcg fluticasone/50 mcg salmeterol/puff.
Folic acid	**PO, IV or IM:** Age <1 year: 0.1 mg/day. Age ≥1 year: 1 mg/day initially, then 0.1–0.4 mg/day.	Injection: 5 mg/mL Tablets: 0.4 mg, 0.8 mg, 1 mg

(continued)

Table 1. Medications (continued)

	Dosages	Dosage Forms
Fomepizole (Antizol, 4-MP, 4-methylpyrazole)	**IV:** *(Diluted to <25 mg/mL):* Children and Adults: 15 mg/kg loading dose, then 10 mg/kg/dose q12h for 4 doses, then 15 mg/kg/dose q12h until level is <20 mg/dL. Doses should be given q6h in children and q4h in adults during hemodialysis.	Injection: 1 gm/mL
Fosphenytoin See phenytoin Furosemide (Lasix)	**PO, IV, or IM:** Premature neonates (oral absorption may be poor): 1–2 mg/kg q12–24h. Oral doses up to 4 mg/kg may be used. Infants and children: 1–2 mg/kg q6–12h but not to exceed 6 mg/kg/day. May use as a continuous infusion 0.05–0.3 mg/kg/hr. Titrate to effect. Adults: 20–80 mg/day in divided doses to a maximum of 600 mg/day. Serum electrolyte levels should be monitored closely.	Injection: 10 mg/mL Solution: 10 mg/mL, 40 mg/5 mL Tablets: 20 mg, 40 mg, 80 mg
Gabapentin (Neurontin)	**PO:** Age 3–12 years: 10–15 mg/kg/day in 3 divided doses. The maintenance dose for patients 3–4 years of age is usually about 40 mg/kg/day and for patients 5 years and older is 25–35 mg/kg/day. Age >12 years: Initially, 300 mg on day 1, followed by rapid titration to 300 mg t.i.d. The usual maintenance dosage range is 900–1,800 mg/day in 3 divided doses to a maximum daily dose of 3,600 mg. It is not necessary to monitor gabapentin levels or the levels of other antiepileptic drugs the patient may be taking because there are no significant drug interactions. Withdrawal of gabapentin therapy should be accomplished over a period of at least 1 week. Dosage must be adjusted in patients with renal dysfunction.	Capsules: 100 mg, 300 mg, 400 mg Solution: 250 mg/5 mL Tablet: 100 mg, 300 mg, 400 mg, 600 mg, 800 mg
Ganciclovir (Cytovene, DHPG)	**IV:** *(As an infusion over 1 hour):* *Induction:* 10 mg/kg/day in 2 divided doses for 2–3 weeks. *Maintenance:* 5 mg/kg/day as a single dose for 7 days a week to 6 mg/kg/day for 5 days a week. **PO:** *Maintenance therapy only:* In adults, a dose of 1,000 mg t.i.d. with food is used. Valganciclovir is preferred in children when oral dosing required. Dosage must be adjusted in patients with renal dysfunction.	Capsules: 250 mg, 500 mg Injection: 500-mg vial
Gentamicin (Garamycin)	**IV or IM:** *(In obese patients it should be based on ideal, rather than actual, body weight):* Age <7 days: <1,000 g: 2.5 mg/kg q24h. 1,000–1,500 g: 2.5 mg/kg q18h. >1,500 g: 2.5 mg/kg q12 h. Age >7 days: 1,200–2,000 g: 2.5 mg/kg q12h. >2,000 g: 2.5 mg/kg q8h. ECMO patients: 2.5 mg/kg q18h. Age <10 years: 2.5 mg/kg q8h OR 7.5 mg/kg s24h. Age >10 years: 5–6 mg/kg/day administered in 3 divided doses. OR as a once daily dose. Note that many different dosing regimens exist. Follow institutional guidelines. If using for synergistic effect, use lower dose of 1–2 mg/kg IV q8h. Dosage must be adjusted in patients with renal dysfunction. **Ophthalmic solution:** 1–2 drops in the affected eye q2–4h. More frequent application (up to every hour) may be used initially in severe infections. **Ophthalmic ointment:** Apply a ribbon of ointment to the eye b.i.d. or t.i.d.	Injection: 10 mg/mL, 40 mg/mL Ointment, ophthalmic: 0.3% Solution, ophthalmic: 0.3%

Table 1. Medications (continued)

	Dosages	Dosage Forms
Glucagon	**IV, IM, or SC:** *Hypoglycemia* (dose may be repeated in 20 minutes if necessary): Neonates, Infants and Children <20 kg: 0.015–0.03 mg/kg/dose, to a maximum of 1 mg. Children >20 kg and Adults: 0.5–1 mg/dose.	Injection: 1 mg-vial
Glycopyrrolate (Robinul)	**IM:** *Preoperatively:* Age <2 years: 4.4–8.8 mcg/kg 30–60 minutes before the procedure. Age ≥2 years: 4.4 mcg/kg 30–60 minutes before the procedure. **PO:** *To control secretions* (glycopyrrolate is poorly absorbed from the GI tract): 50–100 mcg/kg administered t.i.d. or q.i.d. *Reversal of neuromuscular blockade:* 0.2 mg for each 1 mg neostigmine or 5 mg pyridostigmine administered.	Injection: 0.2 mg/mL Liquid: 1 mg/5 mL Tablets: 1 mg, 2 mg
Gonadorelin HCl [Factrel, LHRH (luteinizing hormone-release hormone), GnRH (gonadotropin-releasing hormone)]	**IV:** 2–5 mcg/kg to a maximum of 100 mcg.	Injection: 100 mcg
Griseofulvin (Microsize products: Grifulvin V, Grisactin; Ultramicrosize products: Fulvicin P/G, Grisactin Ultra, Gris-PEG)	Absorption of griseofulvin from the GI tract is somewhat dependent on the size of the particles of griseofulvin. The ultramicrosize is absorbed ~1.5 times as well as the microsize. Absorption is also increased by administering the dose with a fatty meal. Duration of therapy is dependent on the site of infection and ranges from 2–4 weeks for tinea corporis, to 4–8 weeks for tinea capitis and tinea pedis, to 3–6 months for tinea unguium. Children: Microsize: 15–20 mg/kg/day in 1 or 2 divided doses. Ultramicrosize: 10–13 mg/kg/day in 1 or 2 divided doses. Older children and adults: Microsize: 500 mg to 1 g/day in a single or 2 divided doses. Use higher dose for tinea pedis or tinea unguium. Ultramicrosize: 660–750 mg/day in a single or 2 divided doses. During long-term therapy, renal, hepatic, and hematopoietic function should be monitored. Patients should also be cautioned to avoid sunlight because photosensitivity reactions have occurred.	Microsize: Suspension: 125 mg/5 mL Tablets: 500 mg Ultramicrosize: Tablets: 125 mg, 250 mg, 330 mg
Haloperidol (Haldol)	**PO:** Age 3–12 years: *Agitation or hyperkinesia:* 0.01–0.03 mg/kg/day once daily. *Tourette disorder:* 0.05–0.075 mg/kg/day in 2 or 3 divided doses. *Psychotic disorders:* 0.05–0.15 mg/kg/day in 2 or 3 divided doses. **IM:** 1–3 mg q4–8h; maximum, 0.1 mg/kg/day. May use up to 5 mg/dose if >12 years and an imminent danger to themselves or others. Dose should be individually adjusted to patient. Not recommended for children under age 3. Do NOT interchange the decanoate salt (depot injection) with the lactate (immediate release) salt.	Injection: 5 mg/mL Injection, depot: 50 mg/mL Solution, concentrated oral: 2 mg/mL Tablets: 0.5 mg, 1 mg, 2 mg, 5 mg, 10 mg, 20 mg

(continued)

Table 1. Medications (continued)

	Dosages	Dosage Forms
Heparin sodium	**IV:** *Anticoagulation:* Children and adults: Continuous infusion: 50 Units/kg then 15–25 Units/kg/hr. Dose may be increased by 2–4 Units/kg/hr q6–8h based on the results of the APTT. Intermittent infusion: 50–100 Units/kg q4h. This method is less desirable than continuous infusion. *Line flushing:* *Central catheters:* May be flushed as infrequently as once daily with 2–3 mL of solution containing 10 Units/mL for patients under age 1 or 100 Units/mL for patients age 1 or older. *Peripheral catheters, locks:* Usually flushed q6–8h with 10 Units/mL concentration with a volume determined by the length of the catheter, but usually ~1 mL. Lines should be flushed before and after medication or blood administration or if blood is seen in the catheter. Preservative free heparin solutions should be used for all line flushes in children under age 2 months.	Injection: 1,000 Unit, 5,000 Unit, 10,000 Unit, 20,000 Unit, 40,000 Unit/mL Injection, preservative-free: 1,000 Unit, 5,000 Unit, 10,000 Unit/mL Solution, lock flush: 10 Unit/mL, 100 Unit/mL (available preserved and preservative-free)
Hydralazine (Apresoline)	**PO:** Children: 0.75–1 mg/kg/day in 2–4 divided doses, but not to exceed 25 mg/dose initially. May be increased slowly over 3 or 4 weeks to a maximum of 7.5 mg/kg/day (or 200 mg). Adults: Initially 10 mg q.i.d. May be increased by 10–25 mg/dose q2–5d to a maximum of 300 mg/day. **IV (ratio of PO to IV dosing is ~4:1):** Children: Initially 0.1–0.2 mg/kg (to a maximum of 20 mg) q4–6h. May be increased to a maximum of 1.7–3.5 mg/kg/day. Adults: Initially 10–20 mg q4–6h. May be increased to 40 mg/dose. Dose must be adjusted in renal impairment.	Injection: 20 mg/mL Tablets: 10 mg, 25 mg, 50 mg, 100 mg
Hydrochlorothiazide (Esidrix, HydroDIURIL, Oretic)	**PO:** *(Chlorothiazide, which is available as a suspension, is usually a better choice for children requiring low doses):* Age >6 months: 2 mg/kg/day in 2 divided doses. Adults: 25–100 mg/day in 1 or 2 doses.	Tablets: 25 mg, 50 mg
Hydrocortisone (Cortef, Cortenema, Cortifoam, Solu-Cortef)	**PO:** *Congenital adrenal hyperplasia:* Initially 30–36 mg/m²/day divided as 1/3 in the morning and 2/3 in the evening or 1/4 in the morning, 1/4 midday, and 1/2 in the evening. *Physiologic replacement:* 0.5–0.75 mg/kg/day. *Anti-inflammatory:* 2.5–10 mg/kg/day in 3 or 4 divided doses. **IV:** *Adrenal insufficiency:* Infants and young children: 1–2 mg/kg bolus, then 25–150 mg/day in 3 or 4 divided doses. Older children: 1–2 mg/kg bolus, then 150–250 mg/day in 3 or 4 divided doses. Adults: 15–240 mg/day in 1 or 2 divided doses. *Anti-inflammatory:* Infants and children: 1–5 mg/kg/day in 2–4 divided doses. Adults: 15–240 mg q12h. *Stress coverage (all patients):* 100 mg/m² as a single dose followed by 100 mg/m²/day in 6 divided doses. *Shock (succinate salt):* Children: 50 mg/kg then in 4 hours or q24h as needed. Adults: 500 mg to 2 g q2–6h.	Cream, topical: 0.5%, 1%, 2.5% Enema: 100 mg/60 mL (Cortenema) Foam, intrarectal: 90 mg/full applicator (Cortifoam), rectal/anal 1% (Proctofoam-HC) Injection (sodium phosphate): 50 mg/mL Injection (sodium succinate): 100-mg, 250-mg, 500-mg, 1-g vials Ointment, topical: 0.5%, 1%, 2.5% Suspension (cypionate): 10 mg/5 mL Tablets: 5 mg, 10 mg, 20 mg

Table 1. Medications (continued)

	Dosages	Dosage Forms
Hydrocortisone (Cortef, Cortenema, Cortifoam, Solu-Cortef) (continued)	*Rectal retention enemas:* 1 enema nightly for 21 days. May be continued for a longer period if effective or discontinued if no effect is seen. *Intrarectal foam:* 1 full applicator rectally nightly or b.i.d. for 2 or 3 weeks. Absorption of hydrocortisone may be greater from the foam formulation than the enema. Discontinue if not effective after 3 weeks. **Topically (low-potency corticosteroid in most formulations):** Apply a thin layer to the affected area t.i.d. or q.i.d.	
HYDROmorphone (Dilaudid)	***IV:*** Young children: 0.015–0.03 mg/kg q3–4h. Older children and adults: 1–4 mg q3–4h. Use lowest effective dose in opiate-naïve patients. ***PO:*** Young children: 0.04–0.07 mg/kg q3–4h. Older children and adults: 1–6 mg q3–4h depending on size and pain severity. *To convert a patient from oral to IV therapy:* Start with a ratio of 5:1. Ratios of up to 2:1 may be required in some patients on long-term chronic therapy. *To convert a patient from IV to oral therapy:* In a patient who is receiving a stable dose, use an IV to oral ratio of 1:3. Equianalgesic doses: Oral: 7.5 mg HYDROmorphone = 30 mg morphine. Parenteral: 1.5 mg HYDROmorphone = 10 mg morphine. Use caution when prescribing HYDROmorphone—interchanges with morphine have resulted in severe overdoses.	Injection: 1 mg/mL, 2 mg/mL, 4 mg/mL, 10 mg/mL Solution, oral: 1 mg/mL Suppositories, rectal: 3 mg Tablets: 2 mg, 4 mg, 8 mg
Hydroxychloroquine (Plaquenil)	***PO:*** SLE or JRA: 3–5 mg/kg/day in 1 or 2 divided doses to a maximum dose of 6.5 mg/kg/day.	Tablets: 200 mg
Hydroxyzine (Atarax, Vistaril)	***IM, IV or PO:*** Children: 2 mg/kg/day in 3 or 4 doses. Adults: 100–400 mg/day in 3 or 4 doses. Use lower doses for pruritus and higher doses for sedation. *Parenterally:* The use of hydroxyzine parenterally (IM, IV, SC) has been associated with severe adverse effects at the site of the injection. The reactions are characterized by local discomfort, sterile abscess, erythema, and tissue necrosis. Phlebitis and hemolysis have been reported after IV administration. The manufacturers recommend administration by deep IM injection into a well-developed large muscle. SC infiltration of the drug from an IM injection or extravasation of an IV injection must be avoided.	Capsule (pamoate): 25 mg, 50 mg, 100 mg Injection for IM use: 25 mg/mL, 50 mg/mL Solution, oral: 10 mg/5 mL Suspension, oral (pamoate): 25 mg/5 mL Tablets: 10 mg, 25 mg, 50 mg, 100 mg
Ibuprofen (Advil, Motrin, Nuprin)	***IV or PO:*** *Antipyretic:* 10 mg/kg/dose PO q6–8h, max 800 mg/dose. *Juvenile rheumatoid arthritis:* 30–70 mg/kg/day in 4 divided doses to a maximum of 2,400 mg/day. *Adult anti-inflammatory dose:* 400–800 mg q6–8h to a maximum of 3,200 mg/day.	Drops, concentrated: 40 mg/mL Suspension: 100 mg/5 mL Tablets: 200, 400, 600, 800 mg Tablet, chewable: 100 mg Capsules: 200 mg Injection:
Imipenem and cilastatin (Primaxin)	***IV infusion over 1 hour (expressed as mg of imipenem):*** Children: 50–100 mg/kg/day in 4 divided doses to a maximum of 4 g/day. Adults: 2–4 g/day in 3 or 4 divided doses. Dosage must be adjusted in patients with renal dysfunction.	Injection: Imipenem 250 mg and cilastatin 50 mg, imipenem 500 mg and cilastatin 500 mg

(continued)

Table 1. Medications (continued)

	Dosages	Dosage Forms
Imipramine (Tofranil)	**PO:** *Enuresis* in children under age 6: Initially 25 mg 1 hour before bedtime nightly. Dose may be increased to 50 mg in children age 6–12 or 75 mg in children over age 12 if the initial dose is ineffective. *Depression:* Children: 1.5 mg kg/day in 1–4 divided doses initially. May be increased in increments of about 1 mg/kg/day to a maximum of 5 mg/kg/day. Adolescents: 25–50 mg/day increased gradually to a maximum of 100 mg/day in a single or divided doses. Adults: 75–100 mg/day increased gradually to a maximum of 300 mg/day in a single or divided doses. Dosage should be decreased to the minimum effective dose after symptom control has been achieved. Administration of the total daily dose at bedtime may decrease the daytime sedative effects.	Tablets: 10 mg, 25 mg, 50 mg
Immune globulin, intramuscular	**IM:** *Measles prophylaxis:* 0.25 mL/kg within 6 days of exposure. In immunocompromised patients, use 0.5 mL/kg (15 mL maximum). *Hepatitis A pre-exposure prophylaxis:* Risk of exposure within 3 months: 0.02 mL/kg. Risk of exposure >3 months: 0.06 mL/kg. *Hepatitis A postexposure:* 0.02 mL/kg given within 2 weeks of exposure.	Injection, IM: 165 $\pm$ 15 mg (of protein) per mL (2 mL and 10 mL)
Immune globulin, intravenous (Gammagard S/D, Gammar-P IV, Gamunex, Iveegam, Octagam, Polygam S/D)	**IV as a slow infusion:** The rate of infusion varies from product to product but should always be initiated at a very slow rate and may be increased q30min to the manufacturer's maximum recommended rate or less as the patient tolerates. Infusion-related reactions usually abate if the rate of infusion is decreased. Anaphylactic hypersensitivity reactions may occur and are more likely in patients with IgA deficiency. *Immunodeficiency syndromes:* 100–400 mg/kg q2–4wks. *Idiopathic thrombocytopenic purpura:* Either 400 mg/kg/day for 2–5 consecutive days or 1 g/kg/day for 1 or 2 consecutive days may be used for induction. Maintenance doses are usually 400 mg/kg/dose q4–6wk but may be increased to 800–1,000 mg/kg if the lower dose is insufficient and are based on platelet counts and clinical response. *Kawasaki disease:* Usually 2 g/kg as a single dose. Alternatively, 400 mg/kg/day for 4 days may be used.	Gammagard S/D: Powder with diluent to make 5% solution Gammar-P IV: Powder with diluent to make 5% solution Gamunex solution 10% Iveegam: Powder with diluent to make 5% solution Octagam solution: 10% Polygam S/D: Powder with diluent to make 5% solution
Indomethacin IV (Indocin IV)	**IV push:** Further dilution of the reconstituted injection may result in precipitation of insoluble indomethacin. An initial 0.2 mg/kg/dose is followed by 2 doses based on the patient's postnatal age (PNA) *at the time of the first dose:* PNA <48 hours: 0.1 mg/kg at 12–24-hour intervals. PNA 2–7 days: 0.2 mg/kg at 12–24-hour intervals. PNA >7 days: 0.25 mg/kg at 12–24-hour intervals. The patient's renal and hepatic function should be monitored. Oral use in children is generally not recommended. Dosage must be adjusted in patients with renal dysfunction.	Injection (sodium trihydrate): 1 mg
Infliximab (Remicade)	**IV infusion:** Age ≥8 years: 5 mg/kg administered over 2 hours q2wk for 3 doses, then q4–8wk thereafter. Dosage may be increased to 10 mg/kg/dose if necessary. Infusion reactions common, administer per institutional protocol.	Injection: 100 mg

Table 1. Medications (continued)

	Dosages	Dosage Forms
Insulin	***IV:*** *Treatment of diabetic ketoacidosis:* start a continuous infusion of 0.1 units/kg/hr (usual range 0.05–0.2 units/kg/hr) to maintain steady, but slow, decrease of serum glucose levels of 50–100 mg/dl/hr. Only regular insulin should be used by this route. Euglycemia in ICU 0.01 unit/kg/hr ***SC:*** *Maintenance:* Most patients require 0.5–1 units/kg/day in 2–4 divided doses depending on how well controlled the patient's glucose levels have been. Patients should be warned not to change insulins without prior approval of their physicians. If regular insulin is to be mixed with other types of insulin, the regular insulin should always be measured first. Extemporaneously prepared doses of mixed insulins should be used as soon as possible after mixing to minimize the amount of the regular insulin that will be bound by excess protamine or zinc in the other insulin. The activity of regular insulin has a time to onset of 1/2–1 hour, peaks at 2–3 hours, and has a duration of 5–7 hours. The activity of isophane (NPH) insulin has a time to onset of ~1–2 hours, peaks at 4–12 hours, and has a duration of 18–24 hours.	All insulins below are 100 Units/mL *Rapid acting:* Aspart (NovoLog), Lispro (Humalog), Glulisine (Apidra) *Short acting:* Regular insulin *Intermediate acting:* Detemir, Isophane (NPH) *Long acting:* Glargine (Lantus) *Fixed combinations:* regular insulin 30 Units/mL with isophane insulin 70 Units/mL; regular insulin 50 Units/mL with isophane insulin 50 Units/mL; aspart insulin 30 Units/mL with aspart protamine insulin 70 Units/mL; lispro 25 Units/mL with lispro protamine 75 Units/mL
Ipratropium bromide (Atrovent)	***Nebulization: non acute:*** (*Evidence lacking for added benefit for maintenance therapy with beta2-agonists*): Children: 250–500 mcg q6h ***Metered inhaler: non-acute:*** (*Evidence lacking for added benefit for maintenance therapy with beta2-agonists*): Children and Adults: 1–3 actuations per dose every 6 hrs, not to exceed 12 inhalations per day. ***Nebulization (acute):*** Infants: 125–250 mcg t.i.d. Children <12 years (acute asthma in emergency department): 250–500 mcg every 20 minutes for 3 doses, then as needed (not shown to have further benefit in inpatient management per NIH guidelines). Children >12 years and Adults (acute asthma in emergency department) 500 mcg every 30 minutes for 3 doses, then as needed *Metered inhaler:* Children (acute): 4–8 puffs as needed Children >12 years and Adults: 8 puffs as needed	Aerosol HFA, metered dose: 17 mcg/actuation Solution for nebulization: 0.02%, 2.5 mL
Isoniazid (isonicotinic acid hydrazide, isonicotinyl hydrazide; INH)	***PO or IM:*** *Treatment:* Children: 10–20 mg/kg/day in 1 or 2 divided doses (up to 300 mg/day). Adults: 5 mg/kg/day up to 300 mg; 10 mg/kg should be used for disseminated disease. *Prophylaxis:* Children: 10 mg/kg/day in a single dose up to 300 mg/day. Adults: 300 mg/day. Liver function should be monitored during therapy because hepatitis may occur at any time. Patients whose diets are low in milk or meat should receive pyridoxine supplements at a dose of about 10–50 mg/day (1–2 mg/kg/day).	Solution, oral: 50 mg/5 mL Tablets: 100 mg, 300 mg
Isoproterenol (Isuprel)	***Continuous IV infusion:*** 0.05–3 mcg/kg/min up to 2–20 mcg/min.	Injection: 1:5,000 (0.2 mg/mL, 1 mg/5 mL)
Lansoprazole (Prilosec)	***PO or IV:*** Infants and children: Usual range is 0.4–2 mg/kg/day as a single dose. Adults: 15–30 mg daily. Higher doses may be used for pathological hypersecretory conditions.	Capsules: 15 mg, 30 mg Granules for oral suspension: 15 mg packet, 30 mg packet Tablets, PO disintegrating: 15 mg, 30 mg
Levalbuterol (Xopenex)	***Nebulized product for Inhalation (acute asthma exacerbation):*** Children: 0.075 mg/kg (minimum dose: 1.25 mg) every 20 minutes x 3 doses then 0.075–0.15 mg/kg (maximum dose 5 mg) every 1–4 hours as needed Adults: 1.25–5 mg every 30 minutes x 3 doses, then every 1–4 hours as needed	Solution for inhalation 0.63 mg/3 mL and 1.25 mg/3 mL Solution for inhalation (needs dilution): 0.63 mg/0.5 mL, 1.25 mg/0.5 mL Inhaler (HFA): 45 mcg/actuation

(continued)

Table 1. Medications (continued)

	Dosages	Dosage Forms
Levalbuterol (Xopenex) (*continued*)	***Nebulized product for Inhalation (non-acute):*** 0 to <5 years: 0.31–1.25 mg/dose every 4–6 hrs as needed Age 6–11 years: 0.31 mg/dose t.i.d. to a maximum dose of 0.63 mg t.i.d. Age >11 years: 0.63 mg t.i.d. to q.i.d. to a maximum of 1.25 mg t.i.d. with close monitoring for adverse effects. ***Inhaler (acute):*** Children: 4–8 puffs every 20 minutes ×3 doses, then every 1–4 hours as needed Adults: 4–8 puffs every 20 minutes for up to 4 hours, then every 1–4 hrs as needed Inhaler: ≥5 years and adults (non-acute): 2 inhalations every 4–6 hours as needed	
Levetiracetam (Keppra)	***PO or IV:*** *Status epilepticus:* 30 mg/kg over 5–15 min. Age 4–15 years: Initial dose: 10–20 mg/kg/day in 2 divided doses. May be increased to a maximum dose of 60 mg/kg/day. Age ≥16 years: 500 mg b.i.d. May be increased to a maximum daily dose of 1,500 mg b.i.d.	Injection: 100 mg/mL Solution 100 mg/mL Tablets: 250 mg, 500 mg, 750 mg, 1,000 mg
Levothyroxine sodium (Levothroid, Synthroid)	***PO:*** Age 0–6 months: 8–10 mcg/kg or 25–50 mcg/day. Age >6–<12 months: 6–8 mcg/kg or 50–75 mcg/day. Age 1–5 years: 5–6 mcg/kg or 75–100 mcg/day. Age 6–12 years: 4–5 mcg/kg or 100–150 mcg/day. Age >12 years: 2–3 mcg/kg or >150 mcg/day. ***IV:*** 1/2–3/4 of the oral dose for children or about half the oral dose for adults. The parenteral form of the drug is very unstable and should be used immediately after reconstitution without admixing with other solutions.	Injection: 100 mcg, 500 mcg Tablets: 25 mcg, 50 mcg, 75 mcg, 88 mcg, 100 mcg, 112 mcg, 125 mcg, 137 mcg, 150 mcg, 175 mcg, 200 mcg, 300 mcg
Lidocaine hydrochloride (Xylocaine)	***IV:*** *Cardiac arrhythmias:* 1 mg/kg loading dose followed by a continuous infusion of 20–50 mcg/kg/min. The loading dose may be repeated twice at 10–15-minute intervals, if necessary. 2 mg/kg RST/ETT ***Infiltration for local anesthesia:*** Dose depends on procedure, degree, and duration of anesthesia required and the vascularity of the site. Maximum recommended dose is 4.5 mg/kg (or 300 mg). Doses should not be repeated sooner than 2 hours. ***Topical:*** Apply to affected area as needed. Maximum dose should not exceed 3 mg/kg or be repeated within 2 hours. Patients treated with oral lidocaine viscous should be cautioned about the hazards of biting the numbed areas and swallowing difficulties.	Injection: 0.5%, 1%, 1.5%, 2%, 4%; 0.5% with epinephrine 1:200,000; 1% with epinephrine 1:100,000 or 1:200,000; 1.5% with epinephrine 1:200,000; 2% with epinephrine 1:100,000 or 1:200,000 Jelly: 2% Liquid, viscous: 2% Ointment: 2.5%, 5% Solution, topical: 2%, 4%
Linezolid (Zyvox)	***IV or PO for VRE infections:*** Age ≤11 years: 30 mg/kg/day in 3 divided doses. Age ≥12 years: 600 mg/dose q12h.	Injection: 200 mg, 600 mg Suspension: 100 mg/5 mL Tablets: 600 mg
Loperamide (Imodium)	***PO:*** *Acute diarrhea* (dosage is for the initial 24 hours): Age 2–6 years (13–20 kg): 1 mg t.i.d. Age >6–8 years (20–30 kg): 2 mg b.i.d. Age >8–12 years (>30 kg): 2 mg t.i.d. Adults: 4 mg initially followed by 2 mg after each unformed stool to a maximum of 8 mg in 24 hours (16 mg/24 hr under a physician's care). For subsequent days, use a dose of 0.1 mg/kg for children after each loose stool, but do not exceed dosage guidelines for the first day.	Capsules: 2 mg Solution, oral: 1 mg/5 mL Tablets: 2 mg

Table 1. Medications (continued)

	Dosages	Dosage Forms
Loperamide (Imodium) (*continued*)	*Chronic diarrhea:* Children: 0.08–0.24 mg/kg/day in 2 or 3 doses daily to a maximum of 2 mg/dose. Adults: 4 mg followed by 2 mg after each unformed stool until symptoms are controlled, then decreased to the lowest dose that will control symptoms. Usual maintenance dose is 4–8 mg/day.	
Loratadine (Claritin)	*PO:* Age 2–5 years: 5 mg/day in a single dose. Children ≥ 6 years and Adults: 10 mg/day in a single dose.	Syrup: 1 mg/mL Tablets: 10 mg Tablets, rapidly disintegrating: 10 mg
Lorazepam (Ativan)	*IV:* *Status epilepticus:* Neonates: 0.05 mg/kg over 2–5 minutes. Dose may be repeated in 10–15 minutes. Infants and children: 0.1 mg/kg over 2–5 minutes to a maximum of 4 mg/dose. A second dose may be given. Adolescents: 0.05–0.1 mg/kg over 2–5 minutes to a maximum of 4 mg. Dose may be repeated in 10–15 minutes. Adults: 4 mg over 2–5 minutes. Dose may be repeated in 10–15 minutes. *Adjunct to antiemetic therapy:* 0.02–0.04 mg/kg up to q6h. Do not exceed a maximum of 2 mg/dose. *PO or IV:* *Anxiety and sedation:* Infants and children: 0.02–0.1 mg/kg/dose every 4–8 hours. Adults: 2–6 mg/day, usually PO, in 2 or 3 divided doses.	Injection: 2 mg/mL, 4 mg/mL Solution, oral: 2 mg/mL Tablets: 0.5 mg, 1 mg, 2 mg
Magnesium citrate (Citrate of Magnesia, Evac-Q-Mag)	*PO:* (*Chill for better palatability*): Age <6: 2–4 mL/kg. Age 6–12 years: 100–150 mL. Age >12 years: 150–300 mL.	Solution: 300 mL (carbonated; contains 3.85–4.71 mEq Mg/5 mL)
Magnesium gluconate (Almora, Magonate, Magtrate)	*PO:* (*Expressed in terms of mEq of magnesium*): Children: 0.5–0.75 mEq/kg/day in 3 or 4 divided doses. Adults: 2.2–4.4 mEq (500–1,000 mg per dose) administered b.i.d. or t.i.d.	Liquid: 1,000 mg/5 mL (54 mg Mg = 4.4 mEq Mg) Tablets: 500 mg (27 mg Mg = 2.2 mEq Mg)
Magnesium hydroxide (Milk of Magnesia)	*PO:* Age <2 years: 0.5 mL/kg/dose. Age 2–5 years: 5–15 mL/day. Age 6–12 years: 15–30 mL/day. Age >12 years: 30–60 mL/day.	Suspension: Contains ~13.7 mEq Mg/5 mL
Magnesium sulfate	*IV:* [*Expressed in terms of magnesium sulfate (and mEq Mg)*]: *Hypomagnesemia* (monitor serum magnesium levels closely): Neonates: 25–50 mg/kg (0.2–0.4 mEq/kg) q8–12h for 2–3 doses. Infants and children: 25–50 mg/kg (0.2–0.4 mEq/kg) q4–6h for 3 or 4 doses with a maximum single dose of 2,000 mg (16 mEq). Torsades de pointes VT: 25–50 mg/kg/dose up to a maximum of 2 gm/dose Asthma 40 mg/kg over 20 min	Injection: 500 mg/mL (4.06 mEq/mL magnesium Mg)

(continued)

Table 1. Medications (continued)

	Dosages	Dosage Forms
Magnesium sulfate (*continued*)	Adults: 1 g (8 mEq) q6h for 4 doses. Doses of 2–3 g (16–24 mEq) have been used for severe hypomagnesemia. *Maintenance dose:* 30–60 mg/kg/day (0.25–0.5 mEq/kg/day) in 3 or 4 divided doses. *Management of seizures or hypertension in children:* 25–50 mg/kg (0.2–0.4 mEq/kg) q4–6h as needed. Administer the drug slowly (over 1–2 hours) in a concentration not >100 mg/mL. BP should be monitored frequently during infusions because hypotension has been reported with rapid administration.	
Mannitol (Osmitrol)	*IV:* Initial dose of 0.5–1 g/kg followed by doses of 0.25–0.5 g/kg q4–6h. A test dose of 0.2 g/kg (to a maximum of 12.5 g) over 3–5 minutes should produce a urine flow of about 1 mL/kg/hr for 2 or 3 hours. It should be used for patients with marked oliguria or inadequate renal function.	Injection: 5%, 10%, 15%, 20%, 25%
Meperidine hydrochloride (Demerol)	*PO, IV or IM:* Oral doses are about half as effective as IV doses but are generally used for less severe pain; therefore, the doses listed are for all routes of administration, but that should be kept in mind if a patient is being switched from parenteral to oral therapy. Children: 1–1.5 mg/kg q3–4h. A single dose of 2 mg/kg (to a maximum of 100 mg) may be used preoperatively. Adults: 50–150 mg q3–4h. Dosage adjustment is necessary in renal impairment. Long-term or high-dose therapy may result in accumulation of normeperidine, an active metabolite that is a CNS stimulant, especially in patients with renal failure.	Injection: 25 mg/mL, 50 mg/mL, 75 mg/mL, 100 mg/mL Solution, oral: 50 mg/5 mL Tablets: 50 mg, 100 mg
Meropenem (Merrem IV)	*IV:* *Mild-to-moderate infections:* Age ≥3 months: 60 mg/kg/day in 3 divided doses to a maximum total daily dose of 3 g. *Meningitis or severe infections:* Age ≥3 months: 120 mg/kg/day in 3 divided doses to a maximum total daily dose of 6 g.	Injection: 500 mg, 1 g
Mesalamine (Asacol, Pentasa, Rowasa)	*PO:* Children: 50 mg/kg/day divided every 6–12 hours (capsule) or every 8–12 hours (tablet) Adults: 1 g (capsules) q.i.d. or 800 mg (tablets) t.i.d. *Rectally:* 4 g enema administered at bedtime daily. The enema should be retained overnight (8 hours) for best results. The oral forms of the drug are formulated with an enteric coating to slowly release the drug.	Capsules (Pentasa): 250 mg Suspension, rectal: 4 g/60 mL Tablets (Asacol): 400 mg
Methylene blue (Urolene Blue)	*IV:* *Methemoglobinemia:* 1–2 mg/kg injected slowly over a period of several minutes. The dose may be repeated in 1 hour, if necessary. *PO:* *Adults with chronic methemoglobinemia:* 100–300 mg/day.	Injection: 10 mg/mL Tablets: 65 mg

Table 1. Medications (continued)

	Dosages	Dosage Forms
Methylphenidate (Concerta, Metadate, Ritalin)	**PO:** Age >6 years: Initially 0.3 mg/kg/day (2.5–5 mg/dose) before breakfast and lunch. That may be increased to the usual dosage range of 0.5–1 mg/kg/day or a maximum of 2 mg/kg/day or 60 mg. The sustained-release form may be given as a single dose at breakfast.	Capsules, extended release: (Metadate CD) 10 mg, 20 mg, 30 mg, 40 mg, 50 mg 60 mg; (Ritalin LA) 10 mg, 20 mg, 30 mg, 40 mg Tablets: 5 mg, 10 mg, 20 mg Tablets, chewable: 2.5 mg, 5 mg, 10 mg Tablets, extended release: 20 mg Tablets, osmotic extended release (Concerta): 18 mg, 27 mg, 36 mg, 54 mg
Methylprednisolone (A-methaPred, Depo-Medrol, Medrol, Solu-Medrol)	**IV:** *Status asthmaticus:* Initial dose: 2 mg/kg, followed by 1 mg/kg q6h. *"Pulse" therapy for lupus nephritis multiple sclerosis (MS) in older children and adults:* 1 g/day for 3 days. A dose of 30 mg/kg every other day for 6 doses has been used for children. **PO:** Children: 0.5–2 mg/kg/day in 2–4 divided doses. Adults: 2–60 mg/day in 1–4 divided doses. *Intra-articular, intralesional doses (acetate):* Adults: 4–40 mg or up to 80 mg for large joints q1–5wk.	Injection (acetate; Depo-Medrol): 20 mg/mL, 40 mg/mL, 80 mg/mL Injection (sodium succinate): 40-mg, 125-mg, 500-mg, 1-g, 2-g vials Tablets: 2 mg, 4 mg, 8 mg, 16 mg, 32 mg
Metoclopramide (Reglan)	**PO or IV:** *Gastroesophageal reflux:* Infants and Children: Initially 0.2–0.8 mg/kg/day in 4 divided doses before meals. Adults: 10–15 mg 30 minutes before meals and at bedtime. **IV:** *Antiemetic in chemotherapy-induced nausea:* 0.5–2 mg/kg administered 30 minutes before the chemotherapy and q4–6h as necessary. Extrapyramidal reactions are common at this dose and may be treated with diphenhydramine IV (1 mg/kg up to 50 mg) q6h or it may be given as a premedication 30 minutes prior to metoclopramide doses.	Injection: 5 mg/mL Solution, oral: 5 mg/5 mL, 10 mg/5 mL Tablets: 5 mg, 10 mg
Metolazone (Zaroxolyn)	**PO:** Infants and children: 0.2–0.4 mg/kg/day in 1–2 divided doses. Adults: 2.5–5 mg/day for the treatment of hypertension. Edema due to cardiac or renal disease may require doses of 5–20 mg/day.	Tablets: 2.5 mg, 5 mg, 10 mg
Metronidazole (Flagyl, Protostat)	**PO or IV:** *Anaerobic bacterial infections* (IV initially, then PO): Infants other than neonates to adults: 30 mg/kg/day in 3–4 divided doses, not to exceed 4 g/day. *Amebiasis* (usually PO): Infants and children: 35–50 mg/kg/day in 3 divided doses. Adults: 500–750 mg q8h. *Other parasitic infections* (usually PO): Infants and children: 15–30 mg/kg/day in 3 divided doses. Adults: 250 mg q8h or a single 2-g dose. *Trichomoniasis (adults): 2-g single dose* *Pelvic inflammatory disease:* Adults: 500 mg q12h. *Antibiotic-associated pseudomembranous colitis:* Infants and children: 30 mg/kg/day in 3 divided doses Max dose: 2 gm per day. Adults: 500 mg t.i.d. Oral doses may be taken with food to minimize stomach upset.	Injection: Available 5 mg/mL ready to infuse solution or 500-mg vial Tablets: 250 mg, 500 mg

(continued)

Table 1. Medications (continued)

	Dosages	Dosage Forms
Midazolam (Versed)	**IV (titrate dose slowly to avoid excessive dosing):** *Conscious sedation:* Children: 0.05–0.1 mg/kg just before the procedure to a maximum dose of 2 mg. Dose may be repeated q3 or 4 minutes up to 4 times. Adults: 0.5–2 mg over 2 minutes. Titrate to effect by repeating doses q2–3 minutes to a usual dose of 2.5–5 mg. *Infusion for sedation during mechanical ventilation:* Administer a loading dose of 0.05–0.2 mg/kg followed by a continuous infusion of 0.05–0.1 mg/kg/hr and titrate to effect. **PO:** 0.5 mg/kg to a maximum dose of 15 mg. **Intranasally:** 0.2–0.3 mg/kg/dose. The intranasal route of administration ia not FDA approved.	Injection: 1 mg/mL, 5 mg/mL Solution: 2 mg/mL
Mineral oil	**PO (do not administer concomitantly with docusate):** Children: 5–20 mL/day. Adults: 15–45 mL/day. **Rectally (as a retention enema):** Children: 30–60 mL. Adults: 60–150 mL.	Enema: 133 mL Liquid
Montelukast (Singulair)	**PO:** Age 6–23 months: 4 mg once daily given as the granules. Age 2–6 years age: 4 mg once daily. Age >6–14 years: 5 mg once daily. Age >14 years: 10 mg once daily.	Granules: 4 mg packet Tablets, chewable: 4 mg, 5 mg Tablets: 10 mg
Morphine sulfate (Astramorph PF, Duramorph, MSIR, MS Contin, Roxanol)	**IV or IM:** Neonates and infants under age 6 months: These patients are particularly sensitive to the respiratory depressant effects of opiates; therefore, the doses recommended are lower: 0.03–0.05 mg/kg every 4 to 8 hours. Infusions have been used in neonatal patients at a dose of 0.01 mg/kg/hr. The dose may be increased if necessary but should not exceed 0.03 mg/kg/hr. Infants over 6 months and children: 0.025–0.1 mg/kg q3–6h. Doses of up to 2.5 mg/kg have been used in severe pain such as sickle cell or cancer pain. The usual maximum dose is 10 mg. Adults: 2.5–10 mg q2–6h. **Epidurally:** 0.5–5 mg in the lumbar region. Dose may be repeated q24h. Maximum dose is 10 mg/24 hr. Use preservative free formulations. **Intrathecally:** 1/10 of epidural dose or about 0.2–1 mg/dose. Repeat doses are not recommended. Use preservative free formulations. **PO:** Prompt-release preparations are administered every 3 or 4 hours; controlled-release preparations are administered q8–12h. Oral doses are ~1/3 as effective as IV doses. Infants over 6 months and children: 0.2–0.5 mg/kg every 3 or 4 hours (prompt release) or 0.3–0.6 mg/kg q8–12h (extended release). Adults: 10–30 mg q3–4h (prompt release) or 15–30 mg q8–12h (extended release).	Injection: 0.5 mg/mL, 1 mg/mL, 2 mg/mL, 3 mg/mL, 4 mg/mL, 5 mg/mL, 8 mg/mL, 10 mg/mL, 15 mg/mL Solution: 10 mg/5 mL, 20 mg/5 mL, 20 mg/mL Suppositories: 5 mg, 10 mg, 20 mg, 30 mg Tablets: 15 mg, 30 mg Tablets, controlled release: 15 mg, 30 mg, 60 mg, 100 mg

Table 1. Medications (continued)

	Dosages	Dosage Forms
Mupirocin (pseudomonic acid A; Bactroban)	**Topically:** *Impetigo:* Apply ointment to affected area t.i.d. for 5–10 days. *Lacerations, minor suture infections or abrasions:* Apply cream to the affected area t.i.d. for 10 days. *Intranasal Staphylococcus aureus infection:* Apply 1/2 of the contents of a unit-dose tube of intranasal cream into each nostril 2–4 times daily for 5–14 days.	Cream (as mupirocin calcium): 2% mupirocin Cream, intranasal (as mupirocin calcium): 2% Ointment: 2%
Nalbuphine (Nubain)	**Parenterally:** *Reversal of morphine infusion side effects:* 0.025–0.05 mg/kg repeated q6h as necessary. *Analgesia:* Children, age >10 months: 0.1–0.14 mg/kg q3–6h as necessary to a maximum dose of 10 mg. Adults: 10–20 mg q3–6h.	Injection: 10 mg/mL, 20 mg/mL
Naloxone (Narcan)	**IV (preferred), IM, or SC:** *Neonatal opiate depression:* 0.01 mg/kg q2–3min until the desired response is obtained. Additional doses may be necessary at 1–2-hour intervals. *Opiate overdosage:* 0.1 mg/kg to a dose of 2 mg administered q2–3min until 5 doses (up to 10 mg) have been given. If the depressive condition is not reversed, causes other than opiate ingestion should be considered. Additional doses may be necessary because the duration of effect of the opiate is generally longer than that of naloxone. The drug may also be administered via continuous infusion, especially if higher doses are necessary. *Postoperative narcotic reversal (partial reversal):* 0.005–0.01 mg/kg q2–3min until the desired degree of reversal is achieved.	Injection: 0.4 mg/mL, 1 mg/mL
Naproxen (Aleve, Naprosyn)	**PO:** 5–15 mg/kg q8–12h to a maximum daily dose of 1 g. Lower dose is used for analgesia, higher for inflammatory diseases.	Suspension: 125 mg/5 mL Tablets: 250 mg, 375 mg, 500 mg
Neomycin, polymyxin B, and hydrocortisone (Cortisporin)	**Ophthalmic:** 1–2 drops to the affected eye q4–6h; apply finger pressure to the lacrimal sac for 1 minute after instillation. **Otic (both a suspension and a solution formulation are available.** The solution form may sting when instilled, but allows the ear canal to be examined easily): Instill 3–4 drops into the affected ear t.i.d. or q.i.d.	Solution or suspension, otic: Neomycin 5 mg/mL, polymyxin B 10,000 U/mL, and hydrocortisone 1% Suspension, ophthalmic: Neomycin 0.35%, polymyxin B 10,000 U, and hydrocortisone 1%
Neomycin sulfate (Neo-Fradin, Neo-Rx)	**PO:** *Bowel preparation:* 25 mg/kg (up to 1 g) at 1 P.M., 2 P.M., and 11 P.M. on the day before surgery (with erythromycin, cleansing enemas). *Hepatic coma:* 50–100 mg/kg/day in 3 or 4 divided doses up to 12 g/day.	Solution, oral: 125 mg/5 mL Tablets: 500 mg
Neostigmine (Prostigmin)	**IM:** *Myasthenia gravis test:* 0.04 mg/kg single dose **IV:** *Reversal of nondepolarizing neuromuscular blockade after surgery in conjunction with atropine or glycopyrrolate:* Infants: 0.025–0.1 mg/kg/dose. Children: 0.025–0.08 mg/kg/dose. Adults: 0.5–2.5 mg, total dose not to exceed 5 mg.	Injection: 0.5 mg/mL, 1 mg/mL

(continued)

Table 1. Medications (continued)

	Dosages	Dosage Forms
Nitrofurantoin (Furadantin, Macrodantin)	***PO:*** *Active infection:* Children (Furadantin): 5–7 mg/kg/day in 4 divided doses to a maximum of 400 mg/day. Adults: 50–100 mg every 6 hours Children >12 years and Adults (Macrodantin): 100 mg every 12 hours *Chronic suppression therapy:* Children: 1–2 mg/kg/day in 1 or 2 divided doses. Adults: 50–100 mg at bedtime daily. Administer with food or milk to decrease rate of absorption because high peak levels are associated with increased GI upset.	Capsules (macrocrystals): 25 mg, 50 mg, 100 mg Suspension: 25 mg/5 mL
Nitroprusside sodium (Nipride, Nitropress)	***IV as a continuous infusion:*** 0.3–0.5 mcg/kg/min initially, then titrate to effect. Usual dose is 3 mcg/kg/min. The maximum dose is 10 mcg/kg/min. Cyanide toxicity may occur during prolonged therapy or in patients with hepatic dysfunction. Administration of sodium thiosulfate may decrease blood cyanide levels. Thiocyanate may accumulate in patients with renal impairment.	Injection: 50 mg vial Protect solutions from light. Do not use if highly colored (blue, green, or red).
Norepinephrine (Levarterenol, Levophed, Noradrenalin)	***IV as a continuous infusion:*** Initially 0.05–0.1 mcg/kg/min, titrated to response. Maximum dose: 1–2 mcg/kg/min.	Injection: 1 mg/mL
Nystatin (Mycostatin, Nilstat)	***PO:*** Neonates: 100,000 Units administered q.i.d. Infants: 200,000 Units administered q.i.d. Children and adults: 400,000–1 million Units administered q.i.d. ***Topically:*** Apply ointment or cream to the affected area t.i.d. or q.i.d.	Cream: 100,000 Units/g [also available with triamcinolone, a topical steroid (Mycolog)] Ointment: 100,000 Units/g [also available with triamcinolone, a topical steroid (Mycolog)] Suspension: 100,000 Units/mL Tablets: 500,000 Units (intestinal infections only)
Octreotide (somatostatin analog; Sandostatin)	***IV or SC:*** The SC route is generally preferred because absorption is not immediate and the activity is somewhat prolonged. The drug may also be administered as a continuous infusion at a initial rate of 1 mcg/kg/hr. Pediatric experience is limited, but initial IV or SC doses of 1–10 mcg/kg with total daily doses of 2–50 mcg/kg in 2–4 divided doses have been used based on clinical response. Usual adult doses are 50 mcg 1 or 2 times daily initially, then titrate dose to the patient's response.	Injection: 50 mcg/mL, 100 mcg/mL, 200 mcg/mL, 500 mcg/mL, 1,000 mcg/mL
Ofloxacin (Floxin Otic, Ocuflox)	***Ophthalmic infections:*** *Bacterial conjunctivitis:* 1–2 drops in the affected eye q2–4h while awake for 2 days, then q.i.d. for up to 5 more days. *Bacterial keratitis:* 1–2 drops in the affected eye q30min while awake and 4–6 hours after retiring for 2 days, then every hour while awake for up to 4–6 more days, then q.i.d. until cure is attained. ***Otic infections:*** *Otitis externa:* Age 6 months–13 years: 5 drops in the affected ear canal daily for 7 days. Age >13 years: 10 drops in the affected ear canal daily for 7 days. *Suppurative otitis media in patients with perforated tympanic membranes:* 10 drops in the affected ear b.i.d. for 14 days. The tragus of the ear should be pumped several times to make sure the solution is in the ear canal and the patient should remain in a position with the ear up for 5 minutes.	Solution, ophthalmic: 0.3% Solution, otic: 0.3%

Table 1. Medications (continued)

	Dosages	Dosage Forms
Ofloxacin (Floxin Otic, Ocuflox) (continued)	*Otitis media in patients with tympanostomy tubes:* 5 drops in the affected ear b.i.d. for 10 days. The tragus of the ear should be pumped as above and the patient should remain in a position with the ear up for 5 minutes.	
Olopatadine (Patanol)	**Ophthalmic:** Age ≥3 years: 1–2 drops in each eye b.i.d. at 6–8h intervals.	Solution, ophthalmic: 0.1%
Omeprazole (Prilosec)	**PO with food or a meal:** Children: While safety and efficacy in children has not been established, a dose of 0.6–0.7 mg/kg/day as a single dose in the morning has been used. If necessary, a second dose may be given 12 hours later. The usual range of doses used is 0.3–3.3 mg/kg/day. Adults: 20 mg daily. Higher doses may be used for pathologic hypersecretory conditions. The usual starting dose is 60 mg daily, but doses of up to 360 mg daily have been used. Doses >80 mg/day should be given in 2–3 divided doses.	Capsules: 10 mg, 20 mg, 40 mg. The capsules contain enteric coated spheres. If the patient is unable to swallow capsules, the spheres may be put into an acidic juice, such as apple juice, for administration. Do not crush the spheres. Pediatric compounded liquids have been made as 2 mg/ml using a base of sodium bicarbonate 8.4% injectable solution.
Oseltamivir (Tamiflu)	**PO (within 2 days of onset of symptoms and continue for 5 days):** Treatment Age <1 year: 3 mg/kg/dose b.i.d. (not FDA-approved under 1 year, but dosing available from CDC) Age 1–12 years: ≤15 kg: 30 mg/dose b.i.d. 15 kg–23 kg: 45 mg/dose b.i.d. 23 kg–≤40 kg: 60 mg b.i.d. Age ≥13 years or >40 kg: 75 mg b.i.d.	Capsules: 75 mg. Powder for suspension: 6 mg/mL
Oxacillin	**IV:** Neonates, age <7 days: <2,000 g: 50–100 mg/kg/day in 2 divided doses. ≥2,000 g: 75–150 mg/kg/day in 3 divided doses. Neonates, age >7 days: <1,200 g: 50 mg/kg/day in 2 divided doses. 1,200–2,000 g: 75–100 mg/kg/day in 3 divided doses. >2,000 g: 100 mg/kg/day in 4 divided doses. Infants and children (depends on severity and site of infection). *Mild-to-moderate infections:* 100–150 mg/kg/day in 4 divided doses. *Severe infections, including osteomyelitis:* 100–200 mg/kg/day in 4–6 divided doses. Total maximum dose is 12 g/day. Adults: *Mild-to-moderate infections:* 500–1,000 mg q6h. *Severe infections:* 1–2 g q4–6h.	Injection: 1 g, 2 g
Oxcarbazepine (Trileptal)	**PO:** Age 2–16 years: 8–10 mg/kg/day (to a maximum of 600 mg daily) initially, with increases over a 2 week period to a target maintenance dose of 900 mg daily for patients weighing 20–29 kg, 1,200 mg daily for patients weighing >29–39 kg and 1,800 mg daily for patients weighing >39 kg. Doses of 6–60 mg/kg/day have been used in clinical trials, with patients in the age range of 2–4 years potentially needing the higher dosing range, achieved over at least 2–4 weeks. Adults: 600 mg daily in 2 divided doses initially, increasing over 1 week to the usual maintenance dose of 1,200 mg daily in two divided doses. Maximum daily dose is 2,400 mg.	Suspension: 60 mg/mL Tablets: 150 mg, 300 mg, 600 mg
Oxybutynin (Ditropan)	**PO:** Age ≤5 years: 0.2 mg/kg/dose given 2–3 times daily. Children, age >5 years: 5 mg administered b.i.d. or t.i.d. Adults: 5 mg b.i.d. or t.i.d., to a maximum of q.i.d.	Solution, oral: 5 mg/5 mL Tablets: 5 mg

(continued)

Table 1. Medications (continued)

	Dosages	Dosage Forms
Oxycodone	**PO (oxycodone component for combination products):** Children: 0.05–0.15 mg/kg/dose q4–6h. Adults: 5 mg q6h initially; may be increased to 10 mg q4h if necessary. Higher doses may be necessary for severe pain, using a plain oxycodone product.	Capsule: 5 mg Solution: 1 mg/mL Solution (concentrate): 20 mg/mL Tablets: 5 mg, 15 mg, 30 mg Also available in fixed combinations with acetaminophen or aspirin in capsule, liquid and tablet dosage forms.
Palivizumab (Synagis)	**IM:** Age ≤2 years: 15 mg/kg/dose given every month during RSV season, which is November through March in most of North America. Follow American Academy of Pediatrics' dosing and candidate selection recommendations.	Injection, lyophilized powder: 50 mg and 100 mg
Pancrelipase (Creon, Zenpep, Pancreaze)	**PO:** Depends on the condition being treated and the dietary content of the patient. Dosage is usually determined by the fat content of the diet. The usual starting dose is 4,000–8,000 Units of lipase activity before or with each meal or snack for children age 1–7, 4,000–12,000 Units for children age >7–12 years, or 4,000–33,000 Units for adults. Further dosage adjustments may be made based on the patient's symptoms. Typical dose: 1,000–2,500 units/kg/dose (of lipase activity per meal). The newer, enteric-coated products are designed to release the enzymes at pH >6 and are therefore more resistant to destruction by gastric acids.	Capsules, delayed release, containing enteric-coated spheres, microspheres, or microtablets Expressed in lipase USP units: Zenpep 5,000 units, 10,000 units, 15,000 units, 20,000 units Pancreaze 4,200 units, 10,500 units, 16,800 units, 21,000 units Creon 6,000 units, 12,000 units, 24,000 units
Penicillamine (Cuprimine, Depen)	Do not exceed a dose of 30 mg/kg/day. *Rheumatoid arthritis:* Children: Initial: 3 mg/kg/day (≤250 mg/day) for 3 months, then 6 mg/kg/day (≤500 mg/day) in divided doses b.i.d. for 3 months. Maximum: 10 mg/kg/day in 3 or 4 divided doses. *Wilson's disease:* Children: 20 mg/kg/day in 2–3 divided doses to a maximum of 1 g daily. Round dose off to the nearest 250 mg. Administer with pyridoxine supplementation	Capsules: 250 mg Tablets: 250 mg
Penicillin G, aqueous (potassium or sodium salt)	**IV:** Neonates, age <7 days: <2,000 g: 25,000 Units/kg/dose q12h. For meningitis, use 50,000 Units/kg/dose q12h. >2,000 g: 25,000 Units/kg/dose q8h. For meningitis, 50,000 Units/kg/dose q8h. Neonates, age >7 days: <1,200 g: 25,000 units/kg/dose q12h. For meningitis: 50,000 units/kg/dose q12h 1,200 g to <2,000 g: 25,000 Units/kg q8h. For meningitis, 50,000 Units/kg/dose q8h. >2,000 g: 25,000 Units/kg/dose q6h. For meningitis, 50,000 Units/kg/dose q6h. Infants and children: 100,000–250,000 Units/kg/day in 6 divided doses. Up to 400,000 Units/kg/day may be used for severe infections to a maximum of 24 million Units/day. Adults: 2–4 million Units/dose every 4–6 hours. The potassium salt contains 1.7 mEq of potassium and 0.3 mEq of sodium per 1 million Unit. The sodium salt contains 2 mEq of sodium per 1 million Unit. The potassium salt must be administered slowly at high doses due to the effect of the potassium.	Injection, potassium salt: 1 million Unit, 5 million Unit, 10 million Unit Injection, sodium salt: 5 million Unit
Penicillin G procaine, benzathine	**Deep IM:** Results in low but prolonged serum levels. May be given as a single daily dose. A dose of penicillin G benzathine will result in low serum levels for up to 4 weeks.	Injection, benzathine: 600,000 Units/mL Injection, benzathine and procaine: Combined equal parts of each in 300,000 Units, 600,000 Units, 1.2 million Units, 2.4 million Units; 900/300 (900,000 Units benzathine, 300,000 Units procaine)

Table 1. Medications (continued)

	Dosages	Dosage Forms
Penicillin G procaine, benzathine (*continued*)	Newborns: Avoid use in these patients because sterile abscess and procaine toxicity are of greater concern. Neonates > 1,200 g: 50,000 Units/kg as a single dose for asymptomatic congenital syphilis. Infants, Children and adults: 600,000–1.2 million Units/day. Maximum dose is 2.4 million U.	Injection, procaine: 600,000 Units/mL
Penicillin V potassium	**PO:** Children: 25–50 mg/kg/day in 3–4 divided doses. Adults: 125–500 mg/dose q6h. **Prophylaxis against pneumococcal infections: Sickle Cell Disease or Asplenia up to age 5 years (assuming adequate vaccination by age 5)** Age 2 months–3 years: 125 mg b.i.d. Age >3 years: 250 mg b.i.d. Prophylaxis of rheumatic fever: 250 mg b.i.d.	Liquid, oral: 125 mg/5 mL, 250 mg/5 mL Tablets: 250 mg, 500 mg
Pentobarbital (Nembutal)	**PO, IM:** *Sedation before surgery:* Children: 2–6 mg/kg to a maximum of 100 mg. **IV:** *For sedation before procedures:* Dose should be administered slowly and incrementally to avoid oversedation. Patients must be closely observed. Dosing is very patient-specific. The rate of injection should not exceed 1 mg/kg/min (50 mg/min in adults). Allow at least 1 minute to reach full effect. Children: Initially 2 mg/kg to a maximum of 100 mg. Incremental doses of 1–2 mg/kg may be used to a maximum total dose of 200 mg. Adults: Initially 100 mg. Incremental doses of 100–200 mg may be given to a maximum dose of 500 mg for healthy adults. *Barbiturate coma:* 10–15 mg/kg administered over 1–2 hours, followed by a maintenance infusion of 1 mg/kg/hr. Dosage may be increased to 2–3 mg/kg/hr to maintain burst suppression on EEG. Hypothermia may necessitate a decrease in dosage.	Injection: 50 mg/mL
Permethrin (Elimite Cream, Nix Cream Rinse)	*Scabies:* Age >2 months: Apply cream from head to toe. Wash cream off after 8–14 hours. May be reapplied after 1 week if live mites appear. *Head lice:* Apply cream rinse to hair that has been thoroughly washed, rinsed and towel dried. Saturate hair and scalp with cream rinse. Also apply to the ears and hairline at the nape of the neck. Rinse off after 10 minutes and remove remaining nits with the comb provided. May be repeated after 1 week if necessary.	Cream, topical: 5% Cream rinse: 1%
Phenobarbital	**IV or PO:** *Loading doses (usually IV for status epilepticus):* Neonates: 20 mg/kg in a single or 2 divided doses. Infants, children, and adults: 15–18 mg/kg a single or 2 divided doses. Allow 15–30 minutes for the drug to distribute into the CNS and for the seizures to stop. *Maintenance doses:* Neonates: 5 mg/kg/day in 2 divided doses. Infants: 5–6 mg/kg/day in 2 divided doses. Age 1–5 years: 6 mg/kg/day in 2 divided doses. Age >5–12 years: 4 mg/kg/day in 1 or 2 divided doses. Age >12 years: 1–2 mg/kg/day in 1 or 2 divided doses.	Elixir: 20 mg/5 mL Injection (sodium): 65 mg/mL, 130 mg/mL Tablets: 15 mg, 30 mg, 32 mg, 60 mg, 65 mg 100 mg

(continued)

Table 1. Medications (continued)

	Dosages	Dosage Forms
Phenylephrine (Neo-Synephrine, Mydfrin ophthalmic)	***Intranasally (do not use for longer than 3–5 days):*** Age 1 to <6 years: 0.125% solution 2–3 drops q4h as needed. Age 6–12 years: 0.25% solution 2–3 drops or 1–2 sprays q4h as needed. Age >12 years: 0.5% solution 2–3 drops or 1–2 sprays q4h as needed. 1% solution may be used in adults with extreme congestion. ***Ophthalmic:*** Neonates: Avoid 2.5% and use 1% phenylephrine combination products such as cyclopentolate/phenylephrine combination Infants: 1 drop of 2.5% solution 15–30 minutes before procedure. Children and adults: 1 drop of 2.5% or 10% solution; may repeat in 15–30 minutes. ***IV for severe hypotension or shock:*** A bolus dose of 5–20 mcg/kg (2–5 mg in adults) may be repeated q10–15 minutes. For infusion, initial doses of 0.1–0.5 mcg/kg/min are titrated to effect.	Injection: 10 mg/mL Solution, nasal drops or spray: 0.25%, 0.5%, 1% Solution, ophthalmic: 2.5%, 10%
Phenytoin (Dilantin)/ Fosphenytoin (Cerebyx)	Care must be taken when changing from one dosage form of the drug to another because some contain phenytoin sodium and some contain the free acid form of the drug. The free acid form is used for the Infatabs and the suspension. Phenytoin sodium is used for the injection and capsules. Phenytoin sodium contains 92% phenytoin. Injection labeled as 50 mg/mL phenytoin sodium contains 46 mg of phenytoin and capsules labeled 100 mg contain 92 mg phenytoin. Fosphenytoin should be ordered in terms of phenytoin equivalents. The patient's serum levels should be monitored whenever the dosage form is changed. In addition, the different brands of phenytoin capsules have different dissolution characteristics. Dilantin capsules are considered extended and may be dosed in adults as a single daily dose. The serum level range usually associated with clinical effectiveness is 10–20 mcg/mL; that associated with mild-to-moderate toxicity may be as low as 25–30 mcg/mL. *Loading dose (IV or PO):* 15–20 mg/kg in a single or divided doses. *Maintenance dose (IV or PO):* 5 mg/kg/day in 2 or 3 divided doses initially and then adjusted to response and serum levels. Usual ranges based on age (divided into 2 or 3 doses daily). Neonates: 5–8 mg/kg/day. Age 6 months to 3 years: 8–10 mg/kg/day. Age 4–6 years: 7.5–9 mg/kg/day. Age 7–9 years: 7–8 mg/kg/day. Age 10–16 years: 6–7 mg/kg/day. Adults: 5–6 mg/kg/day may be given as a single dose if extended-capsule preparation is used (usual dose = 300 mg daily). Higher doses are required in infants and young children due to lower absorption of the drug from the GI tract. IV doses of phenytoin should be administered at a maximum rate of about 1 mg/kg/min (50 mg/min in adults) to avoid cardiovascular side effects. The injection is not compatible with many solutions or medications. The line must be flushed well with saline before administration to avoid precipitation of phenytoin in the line. Extravasation of the drug must also be avoided because it is very alkaline and may cause severe tissue necrosis. Thorough flushing of the vessel after phenytoin administration will also decrease the incidence of local tissue inflammation that may occur even in the absence of extravasation. Fosphenytoin injection should be diluted with either 5% dextrose or normal saline to a concentration of 1.5–25 mg of phenytoin equivalents (2.3–37.5 mg fosphenytoin) per mL of diluent and may be administered at a rate of 2–3 mg phenytoin equivalents/kg/min (100–150 mg phenytoin equivalents/min in adults).	Capsule, phenytoin sodium, extended: 30 mg, 100 mg Injection, (fosphenytoin): 75 mg/1 mL (equivalent to 50 mg phenytoin sodium) Injection, phenytoin sodium: 50 mg/mL Suspension, phenytoin: 125 mg/5 mL Tablet, chewable, phenytoin: 50 mg
Phosphate (potassium and/or sodium)	Should be guided by the patient's serum phosphorus and potassium or sodium levels. Severe deficits should be replaced by the IV route because the oral route may result in diarrhea and oral absorption is unreliable. In general, the deficit should be made up by incorporating it into the patient's maintenance fluids.	Injection (potassium phosphate): 3 mmol (94 mg) phosphorus and 4.4 mEq potassium per milliliter Packets or capsules (Neutra-Phos): 250 mg (8 mmol) phosphorus, 7 mEq potassium, and 7 mEq sodium Packets or capsules (Neutra-Phos K): 250 mg (8 mmol) phosphorus, 14.25 mEq potassium

Table 1. Medications (continued)

	Dosages	Dosage Forms
Phosphate (potassium and/or sodium) (*continued*)	**IV maintenance:** Neonates: 0.5 mmol/kg up to 1–2 mmol/kg/day. Children: 0.5–1.5 mmol/kg/day Adults: 15–30 mmol/day Intermittent infusions should follow the guidelines outlined below for potassium infusions or sodium infusions because the 2 IV forms available are potassium phosphate (each 3 mmol of phosphate will also deliver 4.4 mEq of potassium) or sodium phosphate (each 3 mmol of phosphate will deliver 4 mEq of sodium). The guidelines below are meant for use in patients with severe hypophosphatemia (<1 mg/dL in adults; low values in children vary with age): Children: 0.08–0.3 mmol/kg with subsequent doses only after serum levels are checked and if the patient is symptomatic. Adults: 0.08 mmol/kg (uncomplicated hypophosphatemia) or 0.16 mmol/kg for prolonged deficits. Do not exceed 0.24 mmol/kg/dose (serum phosphorus ≥0.5 mg/dL) or 0.36 mmol/kg/dose (serum phosphorus <0.5 mg/dL). IV doses should be administered over a 6-hour period. Sodium phosphate doses should be diluted to be normal saline in component while potassium phosphate riders should be diluted according to presence of a peripheral line (<80 mEq/L potassium) or central line (diluted to <150 mEq/L potassium) **PO:** Should be taken with food to increase GI tolerance. Each packet or capsule should be mixed in 75 mL of water. Tablets should be taken with a full glass of water. IV formulations have also been administered as oral in small children or infants who cannot take oral capsules or packets. *Maintenance doses:* Children: 2–3 mmol/kg/day in 4 divided doses. Adults: 32–64 mmol/day (4–8 packets) in 4 divided doses. Do not administer at the same time as aluminum- and/or magnesium-containing antacids, sucralfate, or calcium because they may act to bind phosphorus.	Tablets (K-Phos Neutral): 250 mg (8 mmol) phosphorus, 1.1 mEq potassium, and 13 mEq sodium Tablets (Uro-KP-Neutral): 250 mg (8 mmol) phosphorus, 1.27 mEq potassium, and 10.9 mEq sodium
Phytonadione (vitamin K, Mephyton)	**IM or SC:** *Hemorrhagic disease of the newborn, prophylaxis:* 0.5–1 mg within 1 hour of birth and again 6–8 hours later, if needed. *Treatment:* 1–2 mg/day. *Treatment of deficiency caused by malabsorption or decreased synthesis or due to drugs* (administer IV cautiously and slowly): Children: 1–2 mg/day. Adults: 10 mg/day. *Treatment of oral anticoagulant overdose (highest doses used if bleeding or lack of need to continue anticoagulation):* Infants: 1–2 mg repeated q4–8h. Children and adults: 2.5–10 mg, may be repeated in 6–8 hours. **PO:** *Prevention of deficiency in malabsorption:* Children: 2.5–5 mg every other day or daily. Adults: 5–25 mg/day.	Injection: 1 mg/0.5 mL, 10 mg/mL Tablets: 5 mg
Piperacillin	**IV:** Neonates: 75 mg/kg/dose q8h. Infants and children: 200–300 mg/kg/day in 4–6 divided doses. Patients with cystic fibrosis may need doses of 350–500 mg/kg/day. Maximum dose is 24 g daily. Adults: 2–4 g/dose q4–6h to a maximum of 24 g daily.	Injection: 2 g, 3 g, 4 g

(continued)

Table 1. Medications (continued)

	Dosages	Dosage Forms
Piperacillin/Tazobactam (Zosyn)	**IV:** Neonates: 75 mg/kg/dose q8h (dosed on piperacillin component) Age 1<6 months: 150–300 mg/kg/day of piperacillin component in divided doses every 6–8 hours Age ≥6 months: 240–400 mg/kg/day (piperacillin component) in 4 divided doses daily to a maximum of 18 g of piperacillin. Adults: 2–4 g q6h to a maximum of 18 g of piperacillin.	Injection: 2 g piperacillin + 0.25 g tazobactam, 3 g piperacillin + 0.75 g tazobactam, 4 g piperacillin + 1 g tazobactam
Piroxicam (Feldene)	**PO:** Children: 0.2–0.3 mg/kg/day in a single daily dose to a maximum of 15 mg/day. Adults: 10–20 mg/day in a single dose.	Capsules: 10 mg, 20 mg
Polyethylene glycol electrolyte solution (Colyte, GoLYTELY, NuLytely)	**PO or NG after a 3–4-hour fast for bowel cleansing:** Children: 25–40 mL/kg/hr. Adults: 240 mL q10min. The patient should continue to drink the solution until the rectal effluent is clear. Rapid drinking of each portion is more effective than slow consumption. The first bowel movement should occur about an hour after starting. The solution is more palatable if chilled, but must not be poured over ice. Nothing, including other flavorings, should be added to the solution.	Powder for oral solution to make 4 L (GoLytely): PEG3350 236 g, sodium sulfate 22.74 g, sodium bicarbonate 6.74 g, sodium chloride 5.86 g, and potassium chloride 2.97 g Powder for oral solution to make 4L (Colyte): PEG3350 227.1 g, sodium sulfate 21.5 g, sodium bicarbonate 6.36 g, sodium chloride 5.53 g, and potassium chloride 2.82 g. Powder for oral solution to make 4L (Nulytely): PEG3350 420 g, sodium bicarbonate 5.72 g, sodium chloride 11.2 g, potassium chloride 1.48 g
Polyethylene glycol powder (GlycoLax, Miralax)	**PO:** Children 10–20 kg: 8.5 g mixed in 4 oz of water or juice daily. Alternative: 0.5–1.5 g/kg/day not to exceed 17 gm per dose. Children >20 kg and adults: 1 capful (17 gm) mixed in 8 oz of water or juice daily.	Powder (PEG3350): 255 g, 527 g
Potassium chloride	**PO:** Liquid doses must be well diluted before administration to avoid GI adverse effects. Capsules or tablets should be taken with a full glass of water. Capsules may be opened and emptied onto a soft food, but the beads should not be crushed or chewed. Total daily dose may be given in 1 or 2 divided doses if tolerated, or may be given in 3 or 4 divided doses to decrease GI upset. Dose is usually based on each patient's requirements and may depend on concurrent medications or medical conditions that result in potassium losses. The following may be used as general guidelines: *Normal daily requirement for either PO or IV replacement:* Newborn: 2–6 mEq/kg/day. Children: 2–3 mEq/kg/day. Adults: 40–80 mEq/day. *During diuretic therapy:* Children: 1–2 mEq/kg/day. Adults: 20–40 mEq/day. *For treatment of hypokalemia:* Children: 2–5 mEq/kg/day (individual doses should not exceed 1–2 mEq/kg/dose) Adults: 40–100 mEq/day. **IV:** Doses should be well diluted. Usually they are incorporated into the patient's daily fluid requirement. The maximum desirable concentration is 80 mEq/L. Greater concentrations up to 150 mEq/L in fluids should be used cautiously and only in patients with documented hypokalemia and if the patient has central intravenous access. Rates of infusion of potassium in fluids should not exceed 0.25 mEq/kg/hr in non-cardiac monitored areas.	Capsules, controlled release: 8 mEq (600 mg), 10 mEq (750 mg) Infusions diluted in D5W, NS or SWFI: 10 mEq, 20 mEq, 30 mEq, 40 mEq Injection, concentrated: 2 mEq/mL, 3 mEq/mL Liquids: 20 mEq/15 mL (10%), 40 mEq/15 mL (20%) Powders, effervescent packets: 20 mEq, 25 mEq Tablets, extended release: 8 mEq (600 mg), 10 mEq (750 mg), 20 mEq (1,500 mg) Other potassium salts are also available and may be desirable in patients who are acidotic. They include bicarbonate, citrate, acetate, and gluconate salts.

Table 1. Medications (continued)

	Dosages	Dosage Forms
Potassium chloride (continued)	In the case of a patient in whom a shorter infusion of potassium is necessary (potassium rider), the following guidelines may be used: Maximum concentration of the solution must not exceed 30 mEq/100 mL. The solutions should be infused using a pump to control the infusion rate. Infusion over 2–3 hours (0.3–0.5 mEq/kg/hr) is preferred. Rate of infusion of potassium should never exceed 1 mEq/kg/hr in children or 30 mEq/hr in adults. Administration of doses >0.3 mEq/kg/hr (riders) should be done only if the patient has an ECG monitor in place. Solutions should be mixed well to prevent layering of the potassium chloride, which may result in inadvertent rapid administration.	
Prednisolone **Prednisone**	**PO:** Depends on the condition being treated and the patient's response. The lowest dose possible should be used. Withdrawal of long-term therapy must be accomplished slowly by gradually tapering the dose. The guidelines below may be used for initial dosing. Children: *Anti-inflammatory or immunosuppressive:* 0.1–2 mg/kg/day in 1–4 divided doses. *Acute asthma:* 1 mg/kg/dose q6–12h depending on the severity of the attack. Every q6h dosing should be limited to 48 hours and then should be decreased to q12h. *Inflammatory bowel disease:* 1–3 mg/kg/day in 1–2 divided doses. *Nephrotic syndrome:* 2 mg/kg/day in 3 or 4 divided doses. *Organ transplants:* 1 mg/kg/day in 2 divided doses, tapering gradually to 0.15 mg/kg/day or lowest effective dose.	Liquid, as sodium phosphate: 5 mg/5 mL (Pediapred), 15 mg/5 mL (OraPred) Syrup (Prelone): 15 mg/5 mL Tablets: 5 mg Prednisone: Solution: 1 mg/mL, 5 mg/mL Syrup (Liquid Pred): 5 mg/5 mL Tablets: 1 mg, 2.5 mg, 5 mg, 10 mg, 20 mg, 50 mg
Primidone (Mysoline)	**PO:** Age <8 years: Initially 50–125 mg/day at bedtime or in 2 divided doses. Increase dose by 50–125 mg/day at weekly intervals to the normal range of 125–250 mg t.i.d. or 10–25 mg/kg/day. Age >8 years: Initially 125–250 mg/day at bedtime or in 2 divided doses. Increase dose by 125–250 mg/day at weekly intervals to the usual maintenance dose of 250 mg t.i.d. or q.i.d. Do not exceed 500 mg q.i.d. (2 g). Primidone is metabolized to phenobarbital and phenyl-ethylmalonamide (PEMA). Phenobarbital levels should be monitored in addition to primidone levels.	Tablets: 50 mg, 250 mg
Probenecid (Benemid)	*Prolong penicillin serum levels:* Age <2 years: Not recommended. Age 2–14 years: *Initial:* 25 mg/kg for 1 dose. *Maintenance:* 40 mg/kg/24 hr in 4 divided doses to a maximum of 2 g daily.	Tablets: 500 mg
Procainamide	**IV:** Children: Loading dose of 3–6 mg/kg to a maximum of 100 mg over 5 minutes. This may be repeated q5–10min to a maximum of 15 mg/kg (do not exceed 500 mg in 30 minutes). Follow with a maintenance infusion at a dose of 20–80 mcg/kg/min. Adults: Loading dose of 50–100 mg, repeated q5–10min to a maximum of 17 mg/kg or 1 g. Follow with a maintenance infusion at a usual dose of 1–4 mg/min (reduce dose in renal impairment).	Injection: 100 mg/mL, 500 mg/mL
Prochlorperazine (Compazine)	**PO or rectally as an antiemetic (avoid use in patients <2 years):** 0.4 mg/kg/day in 3 or 4 divided doses or alternatively by the patient's weight: 9–14 kg: 2.5 mg q12–24h as needed, to a maximum of 7.5 mg/day. >14–18 kg: 2.5 mg q8–12h as needed, to a maximum of 10 mg/day. >18–39 kg: 2.5 mg q8h or 5 mg q12h as needed, to a maximum of 15 mg/day. >40 kg: Rectally: 25 mg q12h. PO: 5–10 mg t.i.d. or q.i.d. **IM (avoid use in patients <2 years; IV is not recommended in children):** 0.1–0.15 mg/kg; may be repeated if necessary up to t.i.d. or q.i.d. Usual adult dose is 5–10 mg q4h to a maximum of 40 mg/day.	Injection: 5 mg/mL Suppositories: 25 mg Syrup: 5 mg/5 mL Tablets: 5 mg, 10 mg

(continued)

Table 1. Medications (continued)

	Dosages	Dosage Forms
Promethazine (Phenergan)	*Drug is contraindicated in children under age 2 due to risk of potentially fatal respiratory depression (Black Box Warning)* *Antihistamine* (usually PO): Children: 0.1 mg/kg q6h (not to exceed 12.5 mg/dose) during the day. A dose of 0.5 mg/kg (not to exceed 25 mg) may be used at bedtime. Adults: 12.5 mg q6h during the day with a 25-mg dose at bedtime. *Antiemetic* (PO, IM, or rectally; avoid IV use due to risk of serious tissue injury, including gangrene—Black box warning): Children: 0.25–1 mg/kg/dose (Not to exceed 25 mg) up to q4h. Adults: 12.5–25 mg q4h as needed. *Motion sickness* (PO): Children: 0.5 mg/kg 30 minutes to 1 hour before traveling; then q12h as needed. Adults: 25 mg 30 minutes to 1 hour before traveling; then q12h as needed. *Sedation* (all routes): Children: 0.5–1 mg/kg q6h as needed. Adults: 25–50 mg q6h as needed.	Injection: 25 mg/mL, 50 mg/mL Suppositories: 12.5 mg, 25 mg, 50 mg Syrup: 6.25 mg/5 mL Tablets: 12.5 mg, 25 mg, 50 mg
Propranolol (Inderal)	**PO:** *Arrhythmias:* Children: 0.5–1 mg/kg/day in 3 or 4 divided doses. Dosage may be titrated upward at 3–7-day intervals to the usual range of 2–4 mg/kg/day. If higher doses are necessary, up to 16 mg/kg/day (up to 640 mg) may be used. Adults: Usually 10–30 mg q6–8h. *Hypertension:* Children: 0.5–1 mg/kg/day in 2–4 divided doses, increasing at 3–7-day intervals to the usual range of 1–5 mg/kg/day. Adults: 40 mg b.i.d., increasing at 3–7-day intervals to a maximum dose of 640 mg/day (usual range 40–160 mg/day). *Migraine prophylaxis:* Children: 0.6–1.5 mg/kg/day in 3 divided doses. Adults: 80 mg/day in 3 or 4 divided doses. Dose may be increased to a maximum of 240 mg/day in divided doses or use a once daily sustained release capsule formulation. *Tetralogy spells:* Children: 1–2 mg/kg q6h. *Thyrotoxicosis:* Neonates: 2 mg/kg/day in 2–4 divided doses. Children: 1 mg/kg/day q.i.d. Adolescents and adults: 10–40 mg q6h. **IV:** Reserve for life-threatening arrhythmias. To be administered as an IV bolus *slowly over 10 minutes* under ECG monitoring. The IV dose is much smaller than the oral dose. Children: 0.01–0.1 mg/kg to a maximum of 1 mg for arrhythmias. For tetralogy spells, 0.15–0.25 mg/kg, which may be repeated once after 15 minutes. Adults: 1–3 mg. A second dose may be given, if necessary, after 2 minutes.	Capsules, sustained release: 60 mg, 80 mg, 120 mg, 160 mg Injection: 1 mg/mL Solution: 4 mg/mL, 8 mg/mL Tablets: 10 mg, 20 mg, 40 mg, 60 mg, 80 mg
Propylthiouracil	**PO:** Initially: Neonates: 5–10 mg/kg/day in 3 divided doses. Age <10 years: 5–7 mg/kg/day in 3 divided doses. Age ≥10 years: 150–300 mg/day in 3 divided doses. Adults: 300 mg/day in 3 divided doses. After control of symptoms has been achieved, the dose may be decreased to the lowest dose possible, usually 1/3–2/3 of the initial dose, administered in 3 doses daily.	Tablets: 50 mg

Table 1. Medications (continued)

	Dosages	Dosage Forms
Protamine sulfate	*IV:* 1 mg of protamine sulfate neutralizes 90 USP units of lung-derived Intravenous heparin or 115 USP Units of intestinal mucosa-derived intravenous heparin or 1 mg of LMWH. Because heparin disappears rapidly from the circulation, the dose of protamine decreases rapidly with time elapsed since the heparin infusion. The dose of protamine necessary after 30 minutes is half the dose above and that necessary after 2 hours is 1/4 the dose above. Because protamine itself is an anticoagulant, avoid overdosing. Protamine should be administered slowly, over a 1-minute period, and the dose should not exceed 50 mg.	Injection: 10 mg/mL
Psyllium (Fiberall, Hydrocil, Konsyl, Metamucil).	*PO (each dose should be accompanied by a full glass of water or other liquid):* Children: 1/2 the adult dose (1/2–1 packet or 1.7–3.4 g of psyllium) once daily to t.i.d. Adults: 1–2 packets or 3.4–6.8 g of psyllium once daily to t.i.d. Doses should be separated by 2 hours from other medications.	Powder: ~3.4 g/dose Powder, effervescent
Pyrantel pamoate	*PO (may be taken with juice or milk and without regard to the ingestion of food):* 11 mg/kg pyrantel base to a maximum of 1 g.	Suspension: 50 mg/mL pyrantel base
Ranitidine (Zantac)	*PO:* Children: 2–4 mg/kg/day in 2 divided doses initially. Dose may be higher, up to 10 mg/kg/day in GERD and hypersecretory conditions. Adults: 150 mg b.i.d. or 300 mg at bedtime. Dose may be higher or more frequently administered. Up to 600 mg/day has been used in hypersecretory conditions. *IV:* Neonates: 1–2 mg/kg/day in 2 divided doses (avoid use in <1,500 g neonates at risk for necrotizing enterocolitis unless compelling need) Children: 1–2 mg/kg/day in 3 or 4 divided doses. Do not exceed 6 mg/kg/day or 300 mg/day. Adults: 50 mg q8h. Do not exceed 400 mg/day. Dosage should be adjusted for renal dysfunction.	Capsule: 150 mg, 300 mg Injection: 25 mg/mL Syrup: 15 mg/mL Tablets: 75 mg, 150 mg, 300 mg Tablets, effervescent: 25 mg, 150 mg
Rifampin (Rifadin, Rimactane)	*PO (on an empty stomach):* *Tuberculosis:* Children: 10–20 mg/kg/day as a single daily dose to a maximum of 600 mg. Adults: 10 mg/kg/day as a single daily dose up to a maximum of 600 mg/day. *Meningococcal carriers:* Age <1 month: 10 mg/kg/day in 2 divided doses for 2 days. Infants and children: 20 mg/kg/day in 2 divided doses for 2 days, to a maximum dose of 1,200 mg/day. Adults: 600 mg/dose b.i.d. for 2 days. *Haemophilus influenzae type b prophylaxis:* Age <1 month: 10 mg/kg/day as a single dose for 4 days. Age >1 month and children: 20 mg/kg/day as a single dose for 4 days. Adults: 600 mg/day for 4 days. *Nasal carriers of Staphylococcus aureus:* Children: 15 mg/kg/day in 2 divided doses in combination with other antibiotics. Adults: 600 mg daily in combination with other antibiotics. *IV (over 30 minutes to 3 hours):* Same doses as for the oral route. Rifampin may cause a red-orange discoloration of the sweat, urine, tears, and other body fluids; soft contact lenses may be permanently stained.	Capsules: 150 mg, 300 mg Injection: 600 mg Suspension: Not commercially available, but may be made by mixing the powder from the capsules with simple syrup to form a 10 mg/mL suspension. Such suspensions are stable for 4 weeks at room temperature or refrigerated.

(continued)

Table 1. Medications (continued)

	Dosages	Dosage Forms
Salmeterol (Serevent Diskus)	*Salmeterol is a long acting drug and must not be used for acute exacerbations of asthma, is not a substitute for the use of steroids and should not be used without steroids for the treatment of chronic asthma.* **Powder (Diskus) for oral inhalation:** Age ≥4 years: 1 inhalation (50 mcg) b.i.d. ~12 hours apart is used for chronic asthma.	Inhalation, powder: 50 mcg/foil blister
Scopolamine (hyoscine; Isopto Hyoscine)	**IM, SC, or IV (anti-emetic):** Children: 0.006 mg/kg to a maximum dose of 0.3 mg. Adults: 0.3–0.65 mg. Transdermal patch (>12 years and adults; for motion sickness): Apply 1 patch behind the ear at least 4 hours prior to the exposure and then every 3 days as needed **Ophthalmic:** Children: 1 drop (up to q.i.d. for uveitis). Adults: 1–2 drops (up to q.i.d. for uveitis).	Injection: 0.4 mg/mL Solution, ophthalmic: 0.25% Transdermal patch, 1.5 mg
Silver sulfadiazine (Silvadene, SSD, Thermazene)	**Topically:** Applied to a thickness of 1/16-inch under sterile conditions (using a sterile glove) once or b.i.d. to a clean, debrided wound. Wound should always be covered with cream; reapply if it rubs off.	Cream: 10 mg/g
Sodium bicarbonate (NaHCO₃)	**IV:** *Cardiac arrest* (only after adequate ventilation has been established): 1 mEq/kg IV push initially; may repeat with a dose of 0.5 mEq/kg. Further doses should not be given until the patient's acid-base status has been determined. In infants, the concentration should not exceed 4.2% (0.5 mEq/mL). *Metabolic acidosis* (after measurement of blood gases and pH): Children: mEq HCO₃ = 0.3 × weight (kg) × base deficit (mEq/L) *OR* mEq HCO₃ = 0.5 × weight (kg) × [24-serum HCO₃ (mEq/L)]. Adults: mEq HCO₃ = 0.2 × weight (kg) × base deficit (mEq/L) *OR* mEq HCO₃ = 0.5 × weight (kg) × [24-serum HCO₃ (mEq/L)]. Doses should be administered slowly with frequent monitoring of acid-base balance. **PO:** *Urine alkalinization* (titrate dose to desired pH): Children: 1–10 mEq/kg/day in divided doses. Adults: 48 mEq initially followed by 12–24 mEq q4h. Doses up to 192 mEq/day have been used.	Injection: 4.2% (0.5 mEq/mL), 7.5% (0.9 mEq/mL), 8.4% (1 mEq/mL) Tablets: 325 mg, 650 mg
Sodium polystyrene sulfonate (Kayexalate)	**PO:** Children: Base the dose on the exchange rate of 1 mEq K⁺/g of resin in smaller children. Alternatively, a dose of 1 g/kg q6h may be used. Adults: 15 g administered once daily to q.i.d. **Rectally as a retention enema:** Children: 1 g/kg q2–6h. Adults: 30–50 g q6h. Enemas should be retained for as long as possible to increase ion exchange. Evacuation of the enema should be followed by a non-sodium-containing cleansing enema. Sorbitol is frequently used for making solutions because it helps to prevent constipation. Administer cautiously to patients who may be at risk of serum sodium level increases. It is not totally selective for potassium; small amounts of calcium and magnesium may also be lost.	Powder for oral or rectal use Suspension: 15 g/60 mL (with sorbitol) for oral or rectal use

Table 1. Medications (continued)

	Dosages	Dosage Forms
Sodium sulfacetamide (Bleph-10, Blephamide)	***Topically to the eye:*** Solutions: Apply 1–2 drops in the affected eye up to every 2 or 3 hours while awake. Ointment: Apply to the eye once daily to q.i.d. Drops will cause burning or stinging sensation. Ointment will cause blurred vision.	Ointment, ophthalmic: 10% Ointment, ophthalmic: 10% with prednisolone 0.2% Suspension, ophthalmic: 10%, 15%, 30% Solution, ophthalmic: 10% with prednisolone 0.25% Suspension, ophthalmic: 10% with prednisolone 0.2%
Spironolactone (Aldactone)	***PO:*** *Edema* (response may not be evident for up to 5 days): Children: 1–3 mg/kg/day in 1 or 2 divided doses. Adults: 100 mg/day with a range of 25–200 mg/day. *Primary aldosteronism:* Children: 125–375 mg/m^2/day in divided doses. Adults: 400 mg/day in 1 or 2 divided doses.	Tablets: 25 mg, 50 mg, 100 mg (A stable suspension may be made by crushing tablets and suspending the powder in simple syrup or cherry syrup.)
Streptomycin	***IM:*** Children: 20–40 mg/kg/24 hr in 1 to 2 divided doses. Adults: 1–2 g in 1 or 2 doses daily (doses >1 gm should be divided). Maximum dose 2 g/24 hr.	Injection: 1 g
Sucralfate (Carafate)	Sucralfate is not absorbed from the GI tract. It may bind with other drugs administered at the same time, lowering their effectiveness; therefore, it should be administered at least 2 hours before or after other drugs. ***PO:*** Children: Dosage has not been established, but 40–80 mg/kg/day in 4 divided doses has been used. Adults: 1 g q.i.d. The dose for stomatitis or mucositis is about 250 mg–500 mg of suspension swished around the mouth and then spit out or swallowed, repeated q.i.d.	Suspension: 1 g/10 mL Tablets: 1 g
Sulfasalazine (Azulfidine)	***PO:*** Age >2 years: Initially 40–60 mg/kg/day in 3–6 divided doses (not to exceed 4 g/day) then decreasing to a maintenance dose of 20–40 mg/kg/day in 4 divided doses to a maximum dose of 2 g/day. Adults: Initially 3–4 g/day in equally divided doses. Although doses as high as 12 g/day have been used, they are generally accompanied by an increased incidence of adverse effects. Maintenance doses are usually 2 g/day in 4 divided doses. The drug may cause a yellow discoloration of urine and skin.	Tablets: 500 mg Tablets, enteric coated: 500 mg
Sumatriptan (Imitrex)	***SC:*** Age ≥6 years and ≤30 kg: 0.06 mg/kg or 3 mg. Children >30 kg and adults: 6 mg. A second dose may be given at least 1 hour after the first dose if necessary. Do not exceed 2 doses in 24 hours. ***PO:*** Older adolescents and adults: 25 mg, 50 mg or 100 mg taken with fluids. A second dose may be taken after 2 hours. Daily dose should not exceed 200 mg.	Injection: 4 mg/0.5 mL, 6 mg/0.5 mL Tablet: 25 mg, 50 mg, 100 mg
Tacrolimus (FK-506, Prograf)	Patients are usually treated concurrently with an adrenal corticosteroid. ***PO:*** Children: 0.15–0.3 mg/kg/day in 2 divided doses. Adults: 0.1–0.2 mg/kg/day in 2 divided doses. Doses may be decreased to a lower maintenance dose.	

(continued)

Table 1. Medications (continued)

	Dosages	Dosage Forms
Tacrolimus (FK-506, Prograf) (continued)	**IV (as a continuous infusion):** Children: 0.01–0.06 mg/kg/day. Adults: 0.01–0.05 mg/kg/day. Conversion to oral therapy should take place as soon as the patient is able to tolerate oral medication.	Capsules: 1 mg, 5 mg Injection: 5 mg/mL
Terbinafine (Lamisil AF)	**Topically:** Age ≥12 years: Apply to affected area and surrounding skin for at least 1 week, but not more than 4 weeks.	Cream: 1% Solution (topical spray): 1%
Terbutaline (Brethine)	**PO:** Age <12 years: Initially 0.05 mg/kg/dose t.i.d., increased gradually as required to a maximum of 0.15 mg/kg/dose t.i.d. or total of 5 mg/24 hr. Age >12 years: Initially 2.5 mg t.i.d. Maintenance: Usually 2.5–5 mg or 0.075 mg/kg/dose t.i.d. **Parenteral, SC:** Age <12 years: 0.01 mg/kg to a maximum of 0.3 mg q15–20min for 3 doses. Age >12 years: 0.25 mg, repeated in 15–30 minutes if needed once only; a total dose of 0.5 mg should not be exceeded within a 4-hour period. Continuous infusion for status asthmaticus: Option to load IV with 10 mcg/kg (maximum 500 mcg) over 5 minutes, then start infusion of 0.2 mcg/kg/min to 4 mcg/kg/min.	Injection: 1 mg/mL (1-mL ampul) Tablets: 2.5 mg, 5 mg
Tetracycline	**PO (should be given on an empty stomach):** Age >8 years: 25–50 mg/kg/day in 4 divided doses not to exceed 3 g/day. Adults: 1–2 g/day in 2–4 divided doses.	Capsules: 250 mg, 500 mg Tablets: 250 mg, 500 mg
Theophylline	**IV or PO for apnea in infants:** Premature neonates with postconceptional age <40 weeks: 2 mg/kg/day in 2 divided doses. Term neonates, age <4 weeks: 5 mg/kg loading dose followed by 2–6 mg/kg/day in 2 or 3 divided doses. Term neonates, age >4 weeks: 5–7.5 mg/kg loading dose followed by 3–6 mg/kg/day in 3 divided doses. **Acute bronchospasm (all dosing should be based on lean body weight):** Loading dose: 1 mg/kg will increase serum theophylline concentration by 2 mcg/mL. Patients who have received no theophylline in the previous 24 hours may be given 5–7.5 mg/kg. Patients who have received theophylline within the previous 24 hours should have a serum concentration checked before receiving a partial loading dose. Serum theophylline level should be monitored 30 minutes after the end of a bolus infusion. Loading dose should be administered IV over 30 minutes or PO using an immediate-release product. For patients requiring a continuous IV infusion of theophylline, it should be started at the completion of the bolus dose at the following rate for children: Age 6 months to 1 year: 0.5 mg/kg/hr. Age >1–9 years: 0.9 mg/kg/hr. Age >9–12 years and adolescent smokers: 0.8 mg/kg/hr. Age >12–16 years (nonsmokers): 0.7 mg/kg/hr. Theophylline levels should be monitored 12–24 hours after beginning the infusion and daily while therapy continues. **Oral therapy for chronic bronchospasm:** Age 6 months to 1 year: 12–18 mg/kg/day. Age >1–9 years: 20–24 mg/kg/day. Age >9–12 years and adolescent smokers: 16 mg/kg/day. Age >12–16 years(nonsmokers): 13 mg/kg/day. Age >16 years(nonsmokers): 10 mg/kg/day (not to exceed 900 mg/day). Dose reduction should be made with liver dysfunction or cardiac dysfunction.	*Immediate release:* Elixir: 80 mg/15 ml Injection in D₅W: 0.4 mg/mL, 0.8 mg/mL, 1.6 mg/mL, 3.2 mg/mL, 4 mg/mL *Controlled release:* Capsules and tablets of various strengths and release properties: Frequency of dosing must be based on the characteristics of the product chosen. Immediate-release products must be administered q6h. Extended-release products may be administered every 8–12h or even q24h in adolescents using products designed for daily administration. Serum levels should be monitored frequently during early therapy to maintain serum levels between 10–20 mcg/mL. After a stable dose is achieved, monitoring should be done at least q6–12 months.

Table 1. Medications (continued)

	Dosages	Dosage Forms
Ticarcillin and clavulanate potassium (Timentin)	***IV (may be expressed in terms of ticarcillin content alone or in terms of the fixed ratio (30:1) of the commercially available combination product):*** Neonates <1,200 g or <7 days and 1,200–2,000 g: 150 mg/kg/day of ticarcillin component divided q12h Neonates 1,200–2,000 g and ≥7 days: 225 mg/kg/day of ticarcillin component divided q8h Neonates ≥2 kg: 225–300 mg/kg/day of ticarcillin component divided q8h Infants ≥3 months and children <60 kg: 200–300 mg/kg/day of ticarcillin (207–310 mg of ticarcillin/clavulanic acid) in 4–6 divided doses. ≥60 kg: 3 g ticarcillin + 0.1 g clavulanic acid (3.1 g of combination) q4–6h to a maximum of 24 g of ticarcillin daily. Dosage must be adjusted in patients with renal or hepatic dysfunction.	Injection: 3 g ticarcillin + 0.1 g clavulanic acid labeled as a combined total potency of 3.1 g (pharmacy bulk package containing 30 g ticarcillin + 1 g clavulanic acid)
Tobramycin (TobraDex, Tobrex)	***IV (assumes normal renal function):*** *Neonates <2 kg and <7 days: 2.5–3 mg/kg/dose q24–q36h* *Neonates: >2 kg and <7 days: 2.5 mg/kg/dose q12–q24h* *Neonates: <2 kg and >7 days: 3 mg/kg/dose q24h* *Neonates: >2 kg and >7 days: 5 mg/kg/day in 2 divided doses* ***Traditional dosing:*** Term Infants ≥3 months and children <5 years: 7.5 mg/kg/day in 3 divided doses. Children 5–10 years: 6 mg/kg/day in 3 divided doses. Older children and adults: 5 mg/kg/day in 3 divided doses. Patients with cystic fibrosis usually require higher doses (10 mg/kg/day in 3 divided doses). Dosage may be increased based on the results of serum level monitoring. Dosage must be adjusted in patients with renal dysfunction. ***Ophthalmic:*** Ointment: Apply a 1-cm ribbon of ointment to the eye b.i.d. or t.i.d. Solution: Apply 1–2 drops into the eye up to q30–60min in severe infections or q3–4h for moderate infections.	Injection: 10 mg/mL, 40 mg/mL Ointment, ophthalmic: 0.3% Ointment, ophthalmic: 0.3% with dexamethasone 0.1% Solution, ophthalmic: 0.3% Solution, ophthalmic: 0.3% with dexamethasone 0.1%
Tolmetin (Tolectin)	***PO for rheumatoid arthritis:*** Age >2 years: initially 20 mg/kg/day in 3 or 4 divided doses, adjusted to the patient's response. Usual maintenance dosage range is 15–30 mg/kg/day. Adults: 600 mg-1.8 g/day in 3 divided doses.	Capsules: 400 mg Tablets: 200 mg, 600 mg
Topiramate (Topamax)	***PO:*** Age 2–16 years: Initially, 1–3 mg/kg/day (or 25 mg) given daily at bedtime for 1 week. Gradually increase dose by 1–3 mg/kg/day and increase frequency to b.i.d. to the usual maintenance dosage range of 5–9 mg/kg/day. Age >16 years: Initially, 50 mg daily in 2 divided doses, then increase at weekly intervals by 50 mg/day to a usual adult dose range of 200–400 mg daily in 2 divided doses.	Capsule, sprinkle: 15 mg, 25 mg Tablet: 25 mg, 50 mg, 100 mg, 200 mg. Tablets should not be crushed since the drug has a very bitter taste. Broken tablets should be used immediately as the drug is not stable.
Trazodone (Desyrel)	***PO:*** Age 6–18 years: 1.5–2 mg/kg/day in 2 divided doses, increasing gradually to a maximum dose of 6 mg/kg/day in 3 divided doses. Adolescents: 25–50 mg/d, increased gradually to a maximum of 150 mg/day in divided doses. Adults: 150 mg/day in 3 divided doses increased gradually to a maximum of 600 mg/day.	Tablets: 50 mg, 100 mg, 150 mg, 300 mg

(continued)

Table 1. Medications (continued)

	Dosages	Dosage Forms
Tretinoin (Avita, Retin-A Micro, retinoic acid; Retin-A)	***Topically:*** Apply to the affected area once daily after cleaning, generally at bedtime. Avoid application to areas not being treated. Use should be discontinued if severe reddening, swelling, or peeling occurs. After healing, therapy may be restarted with the same or a different formulation administered less frequently.	Cream: 0.025%, 0.05%, 0.1% Gel: 0.01%, 0.025% Microsphere gel: 0.04%, 0.1% Solution: 0.05%
Trientine (Syprine)	***PO for copper chelation:*** Age 6 to 12 years: 500–750 mg daily in 2–4 divided doses to a maximum of 1.5 g daily. Adults: 750–1,250 mg daily in 2–4 divided doses to a maxiumum of 2 g daily. Capsules should be swallowed whole, on an empty stomach.	Capsule: 250 mg
Trifluridine (Viroptic)	***Topically to the eye:*** Apply 1 drop q2h while awake until re-epithelialization has occurred. Maximum daily dose of 9 drops should not be exceeded. After re-epithelialization has occurred, dosage should be reduced to 1 drop q4h for an additional 7 days to prevent recurrence, but the total length of therapy should not exceed 21 days.	Solution, ophthalmic: 1%
Trimethoprim (Primsol, Proloprim)	***PO:*** *UTI:* Age <12 years: 4 mg/kg/day in 2 divided doses for 10 days. Age ≥12 years: 100 mg b.i.d, or 200 mg once daily for 10 days. *Pneumocystis carinii pneumonia treatment (given with dapsone):* 15–20 mg/kg/day in 4 divided doses.	Solution: 50 mg/5 mL Tablet: 100 mg
Tropicamide (Mydriacyl, Ocu-Tropic, Tropicacyl)	***Topically to the eye:*** 1–2 drops into the eye(s) 15–20 minutes before exam. 0.5% solution is usually sufficient for exam. If cycloplegia for refraction is necessary, 1% solution must be used and repeated in 5 minutes. Exam must take place within 30 minutes because its effect is short.	Solution, ophthalmic: 0.5%, 1%
Ursodiol (Actigall, Urso 250, Urso Forte, Ursodeoxycholic acid)	***PO:*** *Cystic fibrosis*: 30 mg/kg/day in 2 divided doses. TPN Cholestasis (infants and young children): 30 mg/kg/day in 3 divided doses *Gallstones or cholestasis:* 8–10 mg/kg/day in 2–3 divided doses primarily in older children or adults.	Capsule: 300 mg Tablet: 250 mg, 500 mg
Valproic acid, valproate sodium, and divalproex sodium (Depacon, Depakene, Depakote, Depakote ER)	***PO (expressed in terms of valproic acid):*** Initially 15 mg/kg/day increasing by 5–10 mg/kg/day at weekly intervals until seizures are controlled or side effects occur. Usual maximum total daily dose is 60 mg/kg/day in 2–3 divided doses. Frequency of administration in part depends on dosage form, but dosage is usually divided. To prevent adverse GI effects, capsules (valproic acid) and solution are usually administered in 2 or 3 divided doses. Divalproex usually may be administered in 2 divided doses or as a single daily dose if the extended release tablet is used. The usual therapeutic serum concentration range is 50–100 mcg/mL. The oral solution has been administered rectally in patients who are NPO by diluting it 1:1 with tap water and administering it as a retention enema.	Capsules, sprinkles (divalproex sodium): 125 mg valproic acid Capsules (valproic acid): 250 mg Injection: 100 mg/mL Solution (valproate sodium): 250 mg valproic acid/5 mL Tablets (divalproex sodium): 125 mg, 250 mg, 500 mg valproic acid Tablets, extended release (divalproex sodium): 250 mg, 500 mg

Table 1. Medications (continued)

	Dosages	Dosage Forms
Valproic acid, valproate sodium, and divalproex sodium (Depacon, Depakene, Depakote, Depakote ER) *(continued)*	***IV (over 1 hour):*** For patients who are not on valproic acid therapy, use the dosing and frequency of administration guidelines outlined above for oral dosing but monitor trough levels since q6h dosing frequency may be needed. For patients already on valproic acid therapy, use the patient's total oral daily dose and divide with a frequency of dosing of every 6 hours for the IV route. The use of the injectable form for periods of more than 14 days has not been studied. Loading dose in refractory status epilepticus: 20–40 mg/kg.	
Vancomycin (Vancocin)	***IV (over at least 1 hour): If normal renal function for age:*** Neonates, age <7 days: <1,000 g: 10–15 mg/kg q24h. 1,000–2,000 g: 10–15 mg/kg q18h. >2,000 g: 10–15 mg/kg q12h. Neonates, age 7–30 days: <1,000 g: 10–15 mg/kg q18h. 1,000–2,000 g: 10–15 mg/kg q12h. >2,000 g: 10–15 mg/kg q8h. Infants >2 kg, age 31–60 days: 10–15 mg/kg q6–q8h. Age >2 months and >2 kg to Older Children: 40–60 mg/kg/day in 4 divided doses to a maximum dose of 4 g/day. Dose will depend on indication and desired trough level. Serum concentrations should be measured frequently while on therapy. Adults: 0.5 g q6h or 1 g q12h. Dosage adjustment is necessary in renal impairment. Doses of 60 mg/kg/day or more are usually required in children with staphylococcal or streptococcal CNS infections. ***Intrathecal:*** Neonates: 5–10 mg/day. Children: 5–20 mg/day. Adults: 20 mg/day. ***PO (not absorbed; do not use for systemic infections):*** Children: 40 mg/kg/day in 4 divided doses to a maximum daily dose of 2 g. The injectable form may be used PO. Adults: 0.5–2 g/day in 3 or 4 divided doses.	Capsules: 125 mg, 250 mg Injection: 500 mg, 1 g (5-g, 10-g pharmacy bulk packages)
Verapamil (Calan, Calan SR, Covera-HS, Isoptin SR, Verelan, Verelan PM)	***IV (push over 2–3 minutes):*** Age <1 year: 0.1–0.2 mg/kg (usually 0.75–2 mg). Age 1–16 years: 0.1–0.3 mg/kg to a maximum of 5 mg. May be repeated once in 30 minutes if not effective (maximum dose for second dose is 10 mg). Age >16 years: 0.075–0.15 mg/kg (5–10 mg) with a repeat dose in 30 minutes if necessary. ***PO (not well established in children and sustained or extended release products are not usually appropriate):*** Age 1–5 years: 4–8 mg/kg/day in 3 divided doses or ~40–80 mg q8h. Age >5 years: 80 mg q6–8h. Adults: 240–480 mg/day in 3 or 4 divided doses (1–2 doses daily using extended-release products for the treatment of hypertension).	Capsules, extended release: 120 mg, 180 mg, 240 mg Injection: 2.5 mg/mL Tablets: 40 mg, 80 mg, 120 mg Tablets, extended release: 120 mg, 180 mg, 240 mg
Vitamin E [alpha tocopherol, alpha tocopheryl acetate, tocopherol polyethylene glycol succinate (TPGS), Aquasol E]	***PO (water miscible or water soluble TPGS products are recommended, especially for patients with malabsorption):*** *Deficiency:* Infants: 25–50 units/day. *Children with malabsorption:* Consider use of a dose that is 2–5 times the RDA requirement for age or 1 mg/kg/day to raise and maintain plasma tocopherol levels. Patients with cystic fibrosis, thalassemia, or sickle-cell disease may require larger daily doses (400–800 U/day). Adults: 60–75 units/day.	Capsules: 100 U, 200 U, 400 U, 600 U, 1,000 U Capsules, water miscible: 100 U, 200 U, 400 U Solution, water miscible: 50 U/mL Solution (TPGS): 400 U/15 mL

(continued)

Table 1. Medications (continued)

	Dosages	Dosage Forms
Warfarin sodium (Coumadin)	**PO:** Infants and children: Loading dose 0.2 mg/kg (maximum 10 mg) if normal baseline INR. Usual maintenance dose is 0.1 mg/kg/day with a range of 0.05–0.34 mg/kg/day adjusted to achieve the desired PT/INR. Adults: 5–15 mg/day initially for 2–5 days until desired PT is reached. Usual maintenance dosage range is 2–10 mg/day.	Tablets: 1 mg, 2 mg, 2.5 mg, 3 mg, 4 mg, 5 mg, 6 mg, 7.5 mg, 10 mg
Voriconazole (VFEND)	**PO:** Age <12 years: Not established. However, in patients <25 kg, some centers have used 3–5 mg/kg/dose every 12 hours. Age ≥12 years or patients ≥40 kg: 100–300 mg q12h. **IV:** Age 2 years to <12 years: 5–8 mg/kg/dose q12h. Age ≥12 years: 6 mg/kg/dose q12h for 2 doses, followed by a maintenance dose of 4 mg/kg q12h. Consider serum trough concentration monitoring in select patients (e.g., in invasive aspergillosis)	Injection: 200 mg Suspension: 200 mg/5 ml Tablets: 50 mg, 200 m
Zafirlukast (Accolate)	**PO on an empty stomach:** Age 5–11 years: 10 mg b.i.d. Age ≥12 years: 20 mg b.i.d.	Tablet: 10 mg, 20 mg
Zanamivir (Relenza)	**Oral inhalation (Treatment of Influenza):** Age ≥7 years: 2 inhalations (10 mg) b.i.d. for 5 days beginning within 2 days of the onset of symptoms.	Powder for inhalation with device: 5 mg/actuation
Zidovudine (Retrovir)	**PO:** Age ≥4 weeks to <18 years: 240 mg/m^2/dose q12h to a maximum of 300 mg q12h or 160 mg/m^2 dose every 8 hrs (maximum 200 mg q8h). Alternatively, dosing may be based on weight: 4–8 kg: 12 mg/kg/dose twice daily or 8 mg/kg/dose t.i.d. ≥9 to <30 kg: 9 mg/kg/dose twice daily or 6 mg/kg/dose t.i.d. Children ≥30 kg and Adults: 300 mg b.i.d. or 200 mg t.i.d. Dosage may be decreased in patients who develop anemia and/or granulocytopenia. **IV:** Infants ≥6 weeks and Children <12 years: Continuous infusion: 20 mg/m^2/hr Intermittent infusion: 120 mg/m^2 by infusion over 1 hour q6h. Children ≥12 years and Adults: 1 mg/kg q4h 6 times daily. *Maternal-fetal HIV transmission prevention:* Maternal (>14 weeks of pregnancy): 100 mg q4h while awake (500 mg/day) or 200 mg t.i.d. or 300 mg b.i.d. until the onset of labor. During labor and delivery, 2 mg/kg over 1 hour followed by a continuous IV infusion of 1 mg/kg/hr until the umbilical cord is clamped. Infant (Term): 4 mg/kg PO q12h starting within 12 hours of birth and continuing for 6 weeks. For infants unable to tolerate oral drugs, 6 mg/kg/day IV in 4 evenly divided doses may be used. Dosage adjustment is necessary for premature infants and in severe renal impairment.	Capsules: 100 mg Injection: 10 mg/mL Solution: 50 mg/5 mL Tablets: 300 mg
Zinc	Response may not occur for 6–8 weeks. **PO:** Infants and children: 0.5–1 mg/kg/day of elemental zinc in 1–3 divided doses. Adults: 25–50 mg elemental zinc t.i.d. *Acrodermatitis enteropathica:* 10–45 mg/day elemental zinc. Zinc sulfate 4.4 mg = 1 mg elemental zinc (220 mg = 50 mg).	Zinc sulfate (23% zinc): Capsules: 220 mg (50 mg zinc) Injection: 1 mg/mL, 5 mg/mL (zinc) Tablets: 66 mg (15 mg zinc), 110 mg (25 mg zinc), 220 mg (50 mg zinc) Tablets: 10 mg (1.4 mg zinc), 15 mg (2 mg zinc), 50 mg (7 mg zinc), 78 mg (11 mg zinc)

Table 2. Citric Acid and Citrate Dosage Forms (Content per 1 mL)

Product	Sodium Citrate	Potassium Citrate	Citric Acid	Bicarbonate Equivalent
Oracit solution	98 mg (1 mEq Na)...	. . .	128 mg	1 mEq
Polycitra K solution	220 mg (2 mEq K)		66.8 mg	2 mEq
Polycitra-LC solution	100 mg (1 mEq Na)	110 mg (1 mEq K)	66.8 mg	2 mEq

Table 3. Digoxin Dosing

Age	Total Digitalizing Dose (mcg/kg)		Daily Maintenance Dose (mcg/kg Divided in 2 Doses)	
	PO	IV	PO	IV
Preterm infant	20–30	15–25	5–7.5	4–6
Full-term infant	25–40	20–30	6–10	5–8
1 month to 2 years	35–60	30–50	10–15	7.5–12
2 years to adult	30–40	25–35	7.5–15	6–9
Maximum dose	0.75–1.5 mg	0.5–1 mg	0.125–0.5 mg	0.1–0.4 mg

IV, intravenously; PO, orally.

Appendix V
Normal Laboratory Values

Henry R. Drott

% Saturation	20%–40%
Absolute B_1 count	76–462/μL
Absolute lymphocytecount (ALC)	1,266–3,022/μL
Absolute T3	919–2,419/μL
Absolute T4	614–1,447/μL
Absolute T8	267–1,133/μL
Absolute T11	1,025–2, 587/μL
Acetaminophen	10–20 mcg/mL
Acid phosphatase total	2–10 U/L
Alanine aminotransferase (ALT)	5–45 U/L
Albumin	3.7–5.6 g/dL
Aldolase	<6 U/L
Alkaline phosphatase (AP)	130–560 U/L
Alpha$_1$-antitrypsin	210–500 mg/dL
Alpha-fetoprotein (AFP)	0.6–5.6 ng/mL
Amikacin	
Peak	20–30 mcg/mL
Trough	0–10 mcg/mL
Ammonia	9–33 μmol/L
Amylase	30–100 U/L
Anion gap	7–20 mmol/L
Antithrombin III	91%–128%
Apolipoprotein A-I	102–215 mg/dL
Apolipoprotein B	45–125 mg/dL
Aspartate aminotransferase	
Newborn	35–140 U/L
Child	10–60 U/L
B_1 (TotalBcells)	4%–21%
Bands	0%–4%
Bicarbonate	20–26 mEq/L
Bilirubin	
$\delta\gamma$	0.3–0.6 mg/dL
Neonatal	2.0–12.0 mg/dL
Total	0.6–1.4 mg/dL
Unconjugated	0.2–1.0 mg/dL
Blasts	0%
Caffeine	5–20 mcg/mL
Calcium	8.9–10.7 mg/dL
Ionized	1.12–1.30 mmol/L
Stool	0–640 mg/24 h
Carbon dioxide	20–26 mmol/L
Carboxyhemoglobin	0%–2%
CD3+ and CD8+	17.4%–34.2%
CD14+	0%–10%
CD45+ and CD14−	90%–100%
Ceruloplasmin	23–48 mg/dL
CH50	104–356 U/mL
Chloramphenicol	5–20 mcg/mL
Chloride	96–106 mmol/L
Sweat	0–40 mmol/L
Cholesterol	111–220 mg/dL
High-density lipoprotein (HDL)	35–82 mg/dL
Low-density lipoprotein (LDL)	59–137 mg/dL
Complement	
C3	
Newborn	67–161 mg/dL
Child	90–187 mg/dL
C4	16–45 mg/dL
Copper	67–147 mcg/dL
Cortisol	
AM	10–25 mcg/dL
PM	2–10 mcg/dL
C-reactive protein (CRP), quantitative	0–1.2 mg/dL
Creatine kinase	
<age 1 year	60–305 U/L
>age 1 year	60–365 U/L
Creatinine	0.6–1.2 mg/dL
Cryoglobulin	
C3	0.0–0.028 mg/dL
IgA	0.0–0.026 mg/dL
IgG	0.0–0.157 mg/dL
IgM	0.0–0.224 mg/dL
Cyclosporin A	150–400 mcg/L
Digoxin	0.5–2.0 ng/mL
DNA binding	0–149 IU/mL
D-Xylose, posttest	36–63 mg/dL
	(25-g dose)
Erythrocyte sedimentation rate (ESR)	0–20 mm/h
Ethosuximide	25–100 mcg/mL
Factor II assay	27%–108%
Factor V assay	50%–200%
Factor VII assay	50%–200%
Factor VIII assay	50%–200%
Factor IX assay	
Newborn	14.5%–58.0%
Child	50%–200%
Factor X assay	50%–200%
Factor XI assay	50%–200%
Ferritin	23–70 ng/mL
Fibrin split products	0–10 mcg/mL
Fibrinogen	180–431 mg/dL
G-6-PD assay, quantitative	4.6–13.5 U/gHb
γ-Glutamyltransferase (GGT)	14–26 U/L
Gentamicin	
Peak	4–10 mcg/mL
Trough	0–2 mcg/mL
Glucose	75–110 mg/dL
CSF	32–82 mg/dL
Whole blood	60–115 mg/dL
Ham test	
Acidified	0%–1%
Unacidified	0%–1%
Haptoglobin	13–163 mg/dL
Hematocrit	36%–46%
Spun	36%–41%
Hemoglobin	13.5–17.0 g/dL
A_1C	3.8%–5.9%
Total	
Newborn	10–18 g/dL
Child	12–16.0 g/dL
HbA$_2$, quantitative	1.8%–3.6%
HbF, quantitative	0%–1.9%
Immunoglobulin A	
Newborn	0–5 mg/dL
Infant	27–169 mg/dL
Child	70–486 mg/dL

Immunoglobulin E	
Newborn	0–15 IU/mL
Child	0–200 IU/mL
Immunoglobulin G	
CSF	0.5–6 mg/dL
Child	635–1,775 mg/dL
Immunoglobulin M	
Child	71–237 mg/dL
Iron	50–180 mcg/dL
Urine	0–2.0 mg/24h
Iron-binding capacity	250–420 mcg/dL
Lactate	
CSF	0–3.3 mmol/L
Plasma	0.6–2.0 mmol/L
Lactate dehydrogenase (LDH)	340–670 U/L
Latex IgE	0–20 U
Lead, blood	0–10.0 mcg/dL
Lipase	25–110 U/L
Lyme antibodies (IgG/IgM)	0.00–0.79
Magnesium	1.5–2.5 mg/dL
Mean corpuscular hemoglobin (MCH)	26.0–34.0 pg
Mean corpuscular volume (MCV)	80.0–100.0 μm^3
Mean platelet volume	7.4–10.4 fl
Methemoglobin	0.0%–1.9%
Netilmicin	
Peak	5–10 mcg/mL
Trough	0–2 mcg/mL
Osmolality	
Urine	
Newborn	50–645 mOsm/kg
Child	50–1,500 mOsm/kg
Whole blood	275–296 mOsm/kg
Partial thromboplastin time	25.0–38.0 seconds
Peroxide hemolysis	0%–20%
Phenobarbital	15–40 mcg/mL
Phenytoin	10–20 mcg/mL
Phosphorus	2.7–4.7 mg/dL
Platelet aggregation, 10 mcgm	>60.1%
Platelet count	150–400 $10^3/\mu L$
Potassium	3.8–5.4 mmol/L
Prealbumin	22.0–45.0 mg/dL
Primidone	5–12 mcg/mL
Procainamide	4–10 mcg/mL
Prolactin	2.7–15.2 ng/mL
Protein, 24-hour total	0–150 mg/24h
Protein C	
Immunologic	50%–122%
Functional	59%–116%
Protein S, free	40%–111%

Protein, total	6.3–8.6 g/dL
Prothrombin time	10–12 seconds
Protoporphyrin, free RBC	30–80 $\mu mol/mol$ Hb
Pyruvate kinase assay	1.8–2.3 IU/mLRBC
RBC distribution width	11.5%–14.5%
Reptilase	18–22 seconds
Reticulocyte count	0.5%–1.5%
Ristocetin cofactor	48%–220%
Salicylate	<35 mg/dL
Sodium	136–145 mmol/L
Sucrose hemolysis	0%–5%
T3 (total T cells)	69%–86%
T4 (helper T cells)	39%–57%
T4–T8 ratio	0.7–2.5
T8 (suppressor T cells)	18%–45%
T11 (SRBC receptor)	75%–93%
Theophylline	10–20 mcg/mL
Thrombin time	11.3–16.3 seconds
Thyroid-stimulating hormone (thyrotropin)	0.5–5.0 $\mu IU/mL$
Thyroxine	
Newborn	3.0–14.4 mcg/dL
Infant	4.6–13.4 mcg/dL
Child	4.5–10.3 mcg/dL
Thyroxine-binding globulin	1.8–4.2 mg/dL
Tobramycin	
Peak	4–10 mcg/mL
Trough	0–2 mcg/mL
Total cell count	100
Total eosinophil count	100–300 mm^3
Total protein	
CSF	
Newborn	40–120 mg/dL
Child	15–40 mg/dL
Urine	0–20 mg/dL
Triglycerides	34–165 mg/dL
Triiodothyronine	0.9–2.25 ng/mL
Trypsin, stool	80–740 mcg/g
Urea nitrogen	2–19 mg/dL
Uric acid	2.1–5.0 mg/dL
Urine pH	4.8–7.8
Urine specific gravity; TS meter	1.003–1.1035
Valproic acid	50–100 mcg/mL
Vancomycin	
Peak	20–30 mcg/mL
Trough	0–12 mcg/mL
White blood cell count	
Newborn	9–30 $10^3/\mu L$
Child	4.5–11.0 $10^3/\mu L$
Zinc	68–94 mcg/dL

Appendix VI

Tables

Charles Schwartz

Table 1. Scoring System: Draw-a-Person Test

One Point Assigned per Feature:

Head present
Neck present
Neck, two dimensions
Eyes present
Eye detail: Brows or lashes
Nose present
Nose, two dimensions
   (not round ball)
Mouth present
Lips, two dimensions
Both nose and lips in two
   dimensions
Both chin and forehead shown
Bridge of nose (straight to eyes;
   narrower than base)
Hair I (any scribble)
Hair II (more detail)
Ears present

Fingers present
Correct number of fingers shown
Opposition of thumb shown
   (must include fingers)
Hands present
Arms present
Arms at side or engaged in activity
Feet: any indication
Attachment of arms to legs I
   (to trunk or anywhere)
Attachment of arms and legs II
   (at correct point on trunk)
Trunk present
Trunk in proportion, 2 dimensions
   (if greater than breadth)
Clothing I (anything)
Clothing II (two articles of clothing)

Mental Age (yr)	Points Scored by Boys	Points Scored by Girls
3	4	5
4	7	7
5	11	11
6	13	14
7	16	17
8	18	20

Table 2. Receptive Language Development (continued)

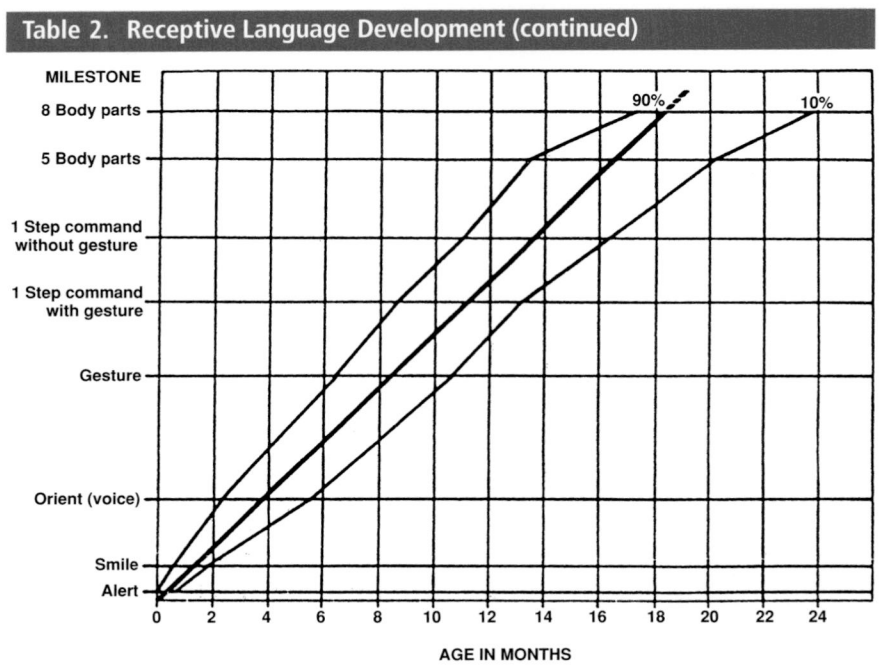

Table 3. Expressive Language Development (continued)

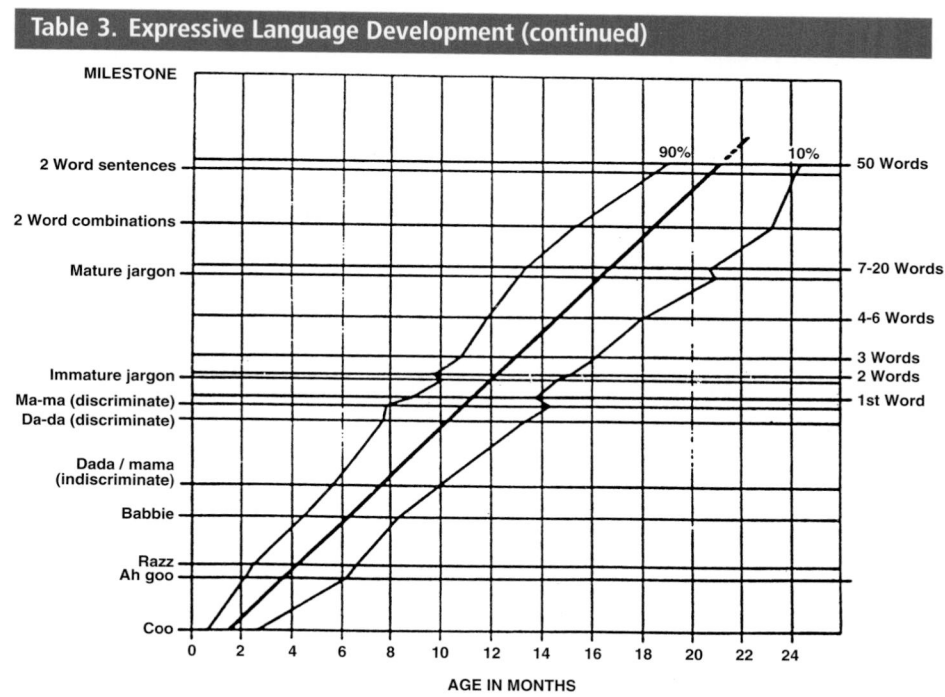

Table 4. Developmental Milestones from Birth to 5 Years

Age (Months)	Adaptive/Fine Motor	Language	Gross Motor	Personal–Social
1	Grasp reflex (hands fisted)	Facial response to sounds	Lifts head in prone position	Stares at face
2	Follows object with eyes past midline	Coos (vowel sounds)	Lifts head in prone position to 45°	Smiles in response to others
4	Hands open Brings objects to mouth	Laughs and squeals Turns toward voice	Sits: Head steady Rolls to supine	Smiles spontaneously
6	Palmar grasp of objects	Babbles (consonant sounds)	Sits independently Stands, hands held	Reaches for toys Recognizes strangers
9	Pincer grasp	Says "mama," "dada" nonspecifically, comprehends "no"	Pulls to stand	Feeds self Waves bye-bye
12	Helps turn pages of book	2–4 words Follows command with gesture	Stands independently Walks, one hand held	Points to indicate wants
15	Scribbles	4–6 words Follows command no gesture	Walks independently	Drinks from cup Imitates activities
18	Turns pages of book	10–20 words Points to 4 body parts	Walks up steps	Feeds self with spoon
24	Solves single-piece puzzles	Combines 2–3 words Uses "I" and "you"	Jumps Kicks ball	Removes coat Verbalizes wants
30	Imitates horizontal and vertical lines	Names all body parts	Rides tricycle using pedals	Pulls up pants Washes, dries hands
36	Copies circle Draws person with 3 parts	Gives full name, age, and sex Names 2 colors	Throws ball overhand Walks up stairs (alternating feet)	Toilet trained Puts on shirt, knows front from back
42	Copies cross	Understands "cold," "tired," "hungry"	Stands on one foot for 2–3 sec	Engages in associative play
48	Counts 4 objects Identifies some numbers and letters	Understands prepositions (under, on, behind, in front of) Asks "how" and "why"	Hops on one foot	Dresses with little assistance Shoes on correct feet
54	Copies square Draws person with 6 parts	Understands opposites	Broad-jumps 24 inches	Bosses and criticizes Shows off
60	Prints first name Counts 10 objects	Asks meaning of words	Skips (alternating feet)	Ties shoes

Table 2A. Causes of Failure to Thrive

Age at Onset	Diagnostic Considerations
Before birth (IUGR, prematurity)	Especially in "symmetric" IUGR, consider prenatal infections, congenital syndromes, teratogenic exposures (anticonvulsants, alcohol, etc.)
Neonatal	Incorrect formula preparation; failed breast-feeding; neglect; poor feeding interactions; metabolic, chromosomal, or anatomic abnormality (less common)
3–6 months	Underfeeding (possibly associated with poverty); improper formula preparation; milk protein intolerance; oral-motor dysfunction; celiac disease; HIV infection; cystic fibrosis; congenital heart disease; GE reflux
7–12 months	Autonomy struggles; overly fastidious parent; oral-motor dysfunction; delayed introduction of solids; intolerance of new foods
After 12 months	Coercive feeding; highly distractable child; distracting environment; acquired illness; new psychosocial stressor (divorce, job loss, new sibling, death in the family, etc.)

Reproduced from Frank DA, et al., with permission from the authors.

Table 3. Primitive Reflexes

Primitive Reflex	Age at Disappearance (Months)	Description
Palmar grasp	3–4	Pressing against the palmar surface of the infant's hand results in flexion of all fingers.
Rooting	3–4	Stroking the perioral skin at the corners of the mouth causes the mouth to open and turn to stimulated side.
Galant	2–3	Stroking along the paravertebral area causes lateral flexion of the trunk with the concavity toward the stimulated side.
Moro	4–6	Sudden movement of the head causes symmetric abduction and extension of the arms followed by gradual adduction and flexion of the arms over the body.
Asymmetric tonic neck	4–6	Turning the head to 1 side leads to extension of extremities on that side and flexion on the contralateral side. This puts the infant in the fencing position.
Tonic labyrinthine	2–3	In supine neck extension leads to shoulder retraction and trunk and lower extremity extension. This is reduced by neck flexion.
Positive support	2–3	Stimulation of the ball of the foot leads to co-contraction of opposing muscle groups, allowing weight to be borne.
Placing/Stepping	Variable	When the dorsal surface of one foot touches the underside of a table, the infant places the foot on the table top.

Table 4. Penile and Clitoral Length in the Newborn Infant

Gestational Age	Length (Mean ± SD) (cm)
Male Measure from pubic ramus to the tip of the glans with gentle traction applied.[a]	
30 wk	2.5 ± 0.4
34 wk	3.0 ± 0.4
Term	3.5 ± 0.4
Female Measure with labia majora separated and the prepuce skin retracted.[b]	
Term infants	4.0 ± 1.24
Preterm infants—The clitoris achieves full size by 24 wk gestation and may appear more prominent relative to the labia in premature infants.	

[a] Feldman KW, Smith DW. Fetal phallic growth and penile standards for newborn male infants. *J Pediatr.* 1975;86:395.

[b] Oberfield S, Mondok A, Shanrivar F, et al. Clitoral size in full-term infants. *Am J Perinatol.* 1989;6(4):453.

Table 5. Tanner Stages in the Female

Stage	Breast	Pubic Hair
1	Prepubertal, elevation of papilla only	Prepubertal
2	Enlargement of areola, elevation of breast and papilla ("breast bud")	Sparse, long, straight, slightly pigmented hair along labia
3	Further enlargement of breast and areola with no separation of contour	Hair is darker, curlier, and coarser with increased distribution on pubes
4	Areola and papilla form a second mount above the breast	Adult-type hair limited to pubes with no extension to medial thigh
5	Mature breast	Mature distribution of inverse triangle with spread to medial thighs

Table 6. Tanner Stages in the Male

Stage	Genital Development	Pubic Hair
1	Prepubertal	Prepubertal
2	Enlargement of testes (>4 mL volume) and scrotum with reddening of scrotal skin	Sparse, long, straight, slightly pigmented hair at base of penis
3	Growth of penis, primarily length, with further increase in size of testes and scrotum	Hair is darker and curlier with increased distribution on pubes
4	Further increase in length and breadth of penis with development of glans, increase in testes and scrotum	Adult-type hair limited to pubes with no extension to medial thigh
5	Adult size and shape	Mature distribution with spread to medial thighs and lower abdomen

Table 7. Normal Growth Rates

Age	Expected Growth Rate
1st year	25 cm (10 inches)/y
2nd year	12.5 cm (5 inches)/y
Childhood	6.25 cm (2.5 inches)/y
Adolescence, boys	15–38 cm (6–15 inches)
Adolescence, girls	15–25 cm (6–12 inches)

Table 8. Head Growth Velocity

Full-term		Preterm	
2 cm/mo	0–3 months	1 cm/wk	0–2 months
1 cm/mo	3–6 months	0.5 cm/wk	2–4 months
0.5 cm/mo	7–12 months	See full-term	>4 months

Table 9. Illustrations of the Primary and Permanent Dentition. *A* and *B,* The Numbers Represent the Average Age of Eruption for the Teeth, Indicated in Months for the Primary Teeth and Years for the Permanent Dentition. *C* and *D,* The Names of Specific Teeth in the Primary and Permanent Dentition are Shown

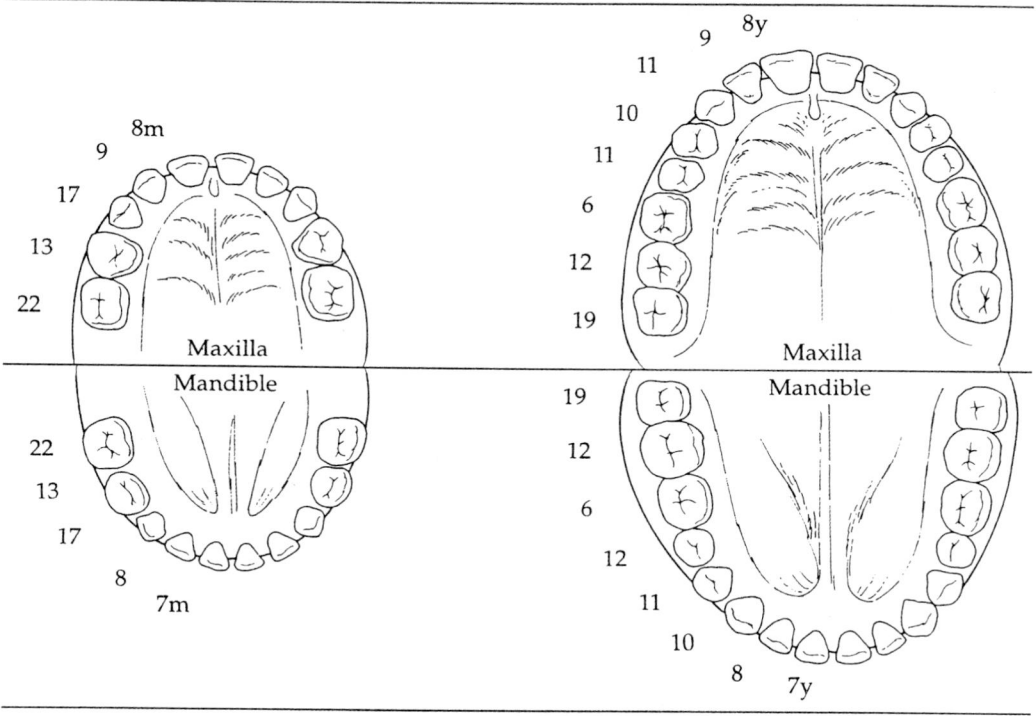

A. Primary Dentition

B. Permanent Dentition

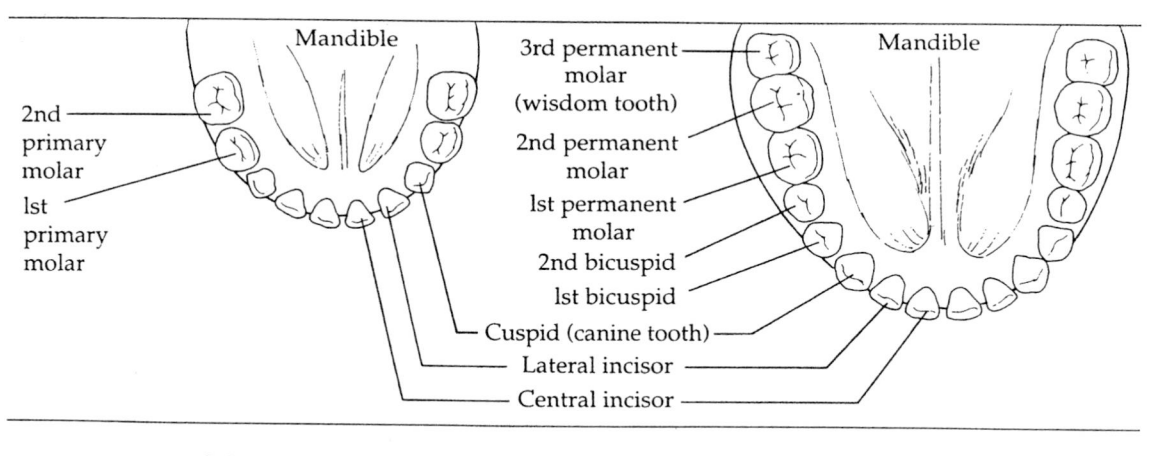

C. Primary Dentition

D. Permanent Dentition

Reproduced with permission from Nazif MM, Davis HW, McKibben DH, Roody MA. Arts of Pediatric Physical Diagnosis-3.

GROWTH CHART

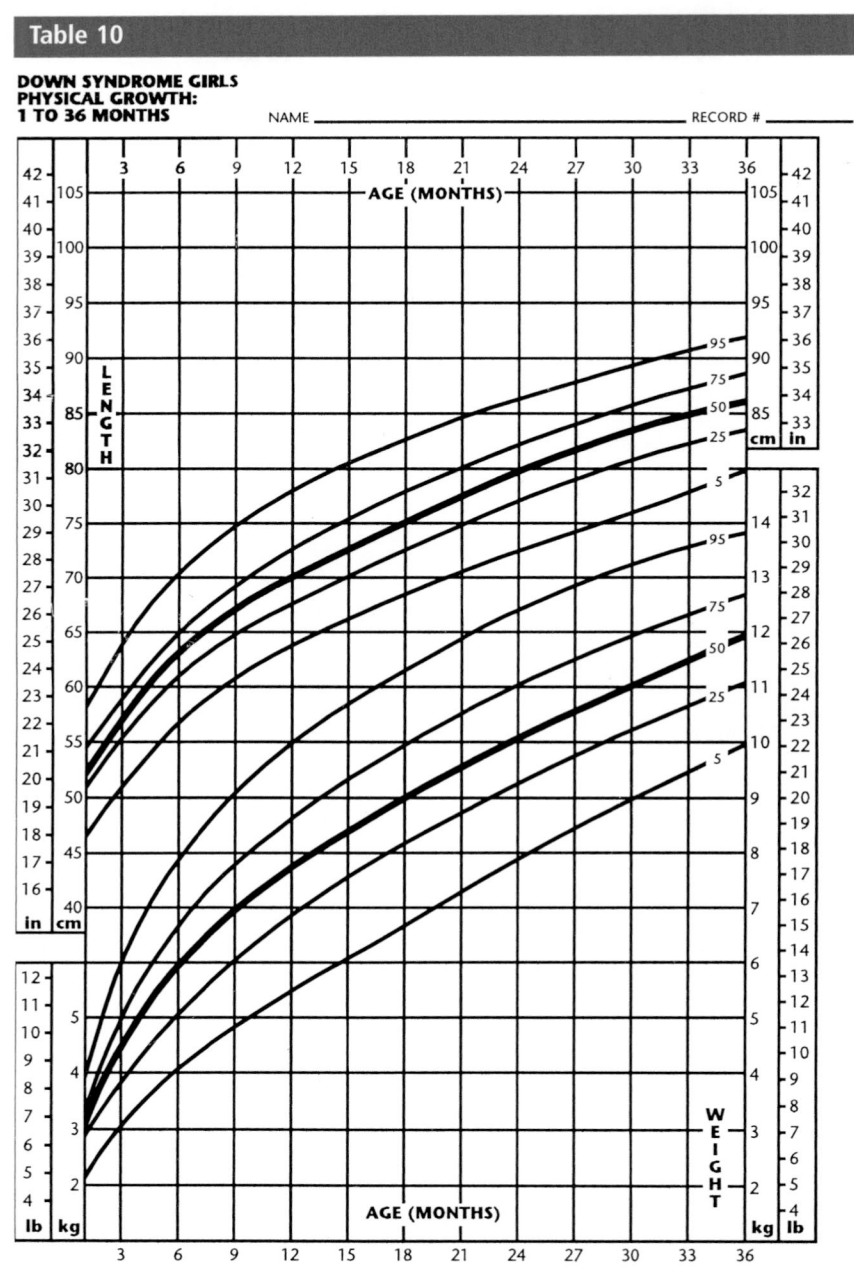

Table 10

DOWN SYNDROME GIRLS
PHYSICAL GROWTH:
1 TO 36 MONTHS

NAME _____ RECORD # _____

From Cronck C, Crocker AC, Pueschel SM, et al. Growth charts for children with Down syndrome: 1 month to 18 years of age. *Pediatrics*. 1988;81:102–110, with permission.

Table 10A

GIRLS WITH DOWN SYNDROME
PHYSICAL GROWTH:
2 TO 18 YEARS

NAME _____ RECORD # _____

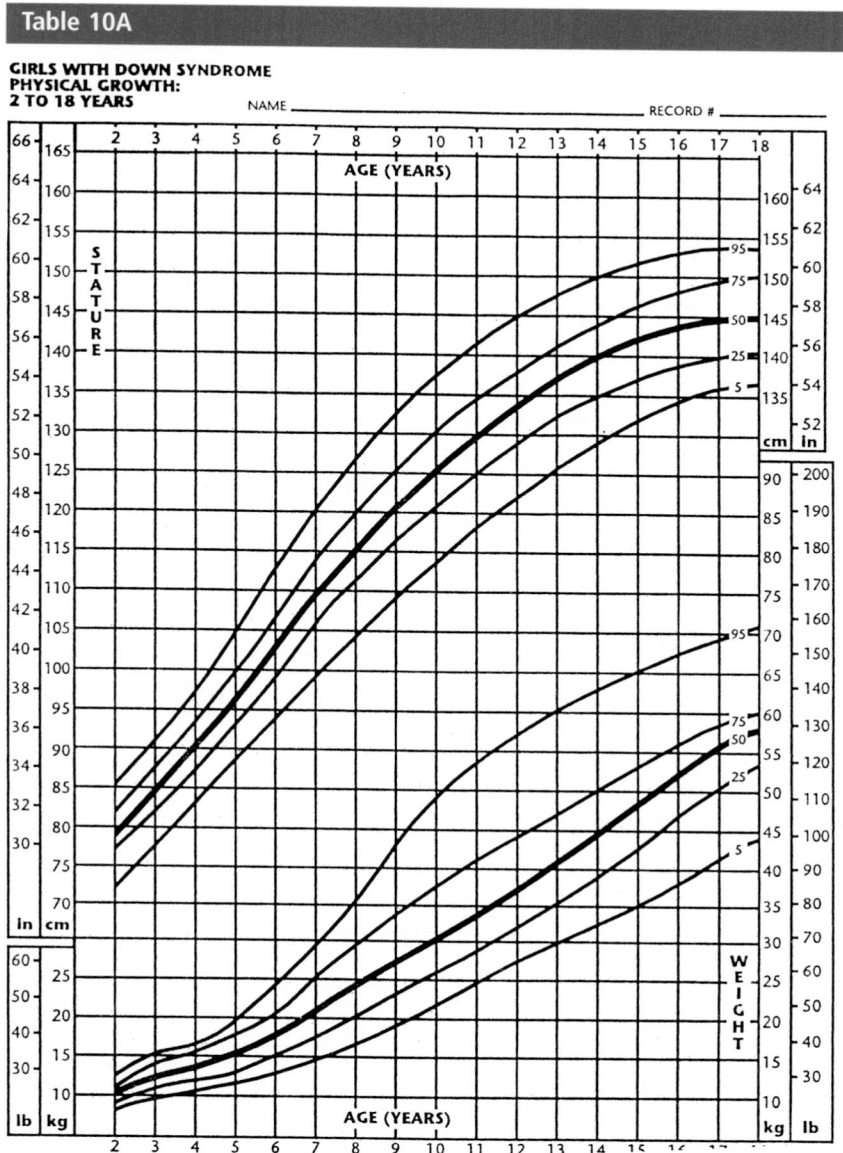

From Cronck C, Crocker AC, Pueschel SM, et al. Growth charts for children with Down syndrome: 1 month to 18 years of age. *Pediatrics.* 1988;81:102–110, with permission.

Table 11

**DOWN SYNDROME BOYS
PHYSICAL GROWTH:
1 TO 36 MONTHS**

NAME _____ RECORD # _____

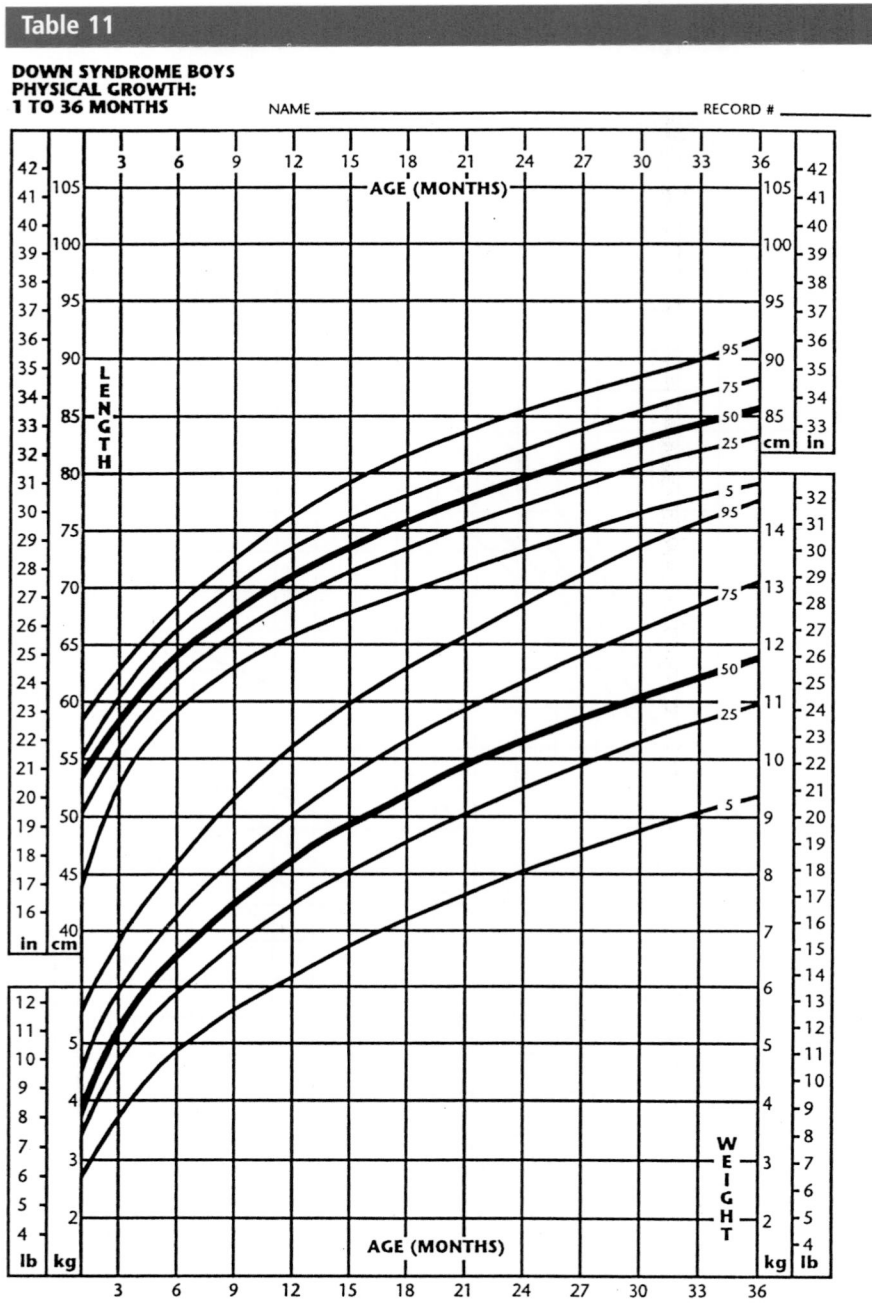

From Cronck C, Crocker AC, Pueschel SM, et al. Growth charts for children with Down syndrome: 1 month to 18 years of age. *Pediatrics*. 1988;81:102–110, with permission.

Table 11A

BOYS WITH DOWN SYNDROME
PHYSICAL GROWTH:
2 TO 18 YEARS

NAME _____ RECORD # _____

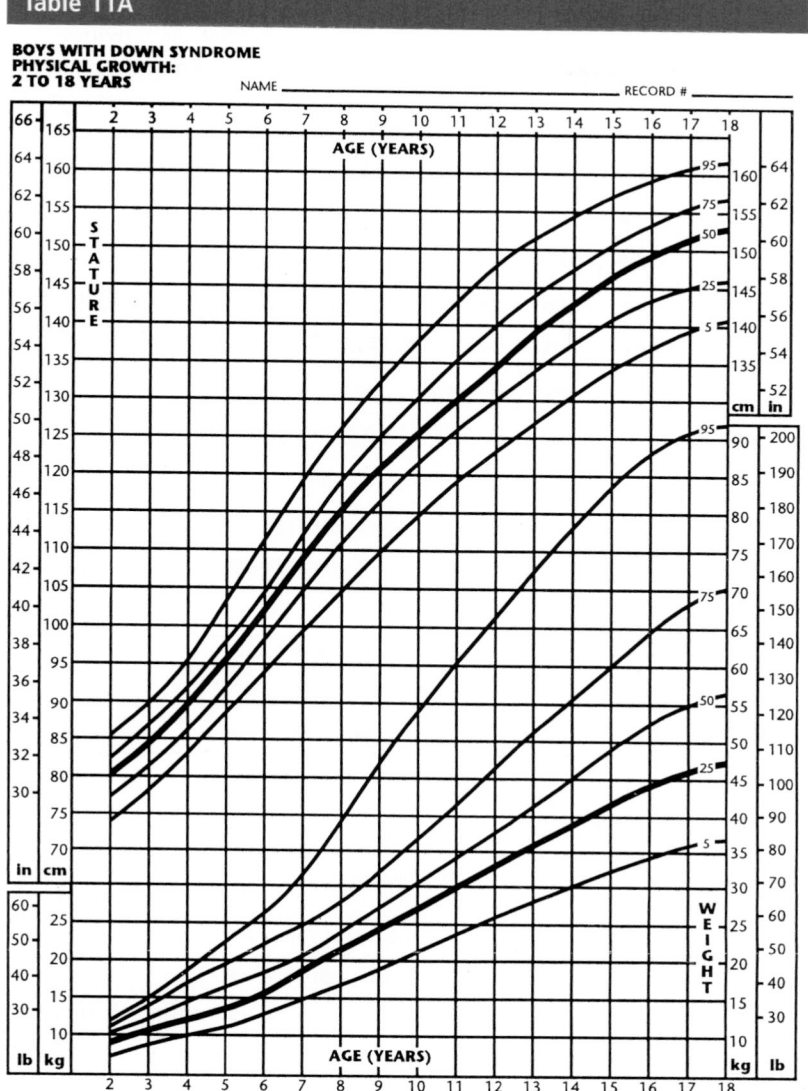

From Cronck C, Crocker AC, Pueschel SM, et al. Growth charts for children with Down syndrome: 1 month to 18 years of age. *Pediatrics*. 1988;81:102–110, with permission.

IMMUNIZATION

Table 12

DEPARTMENT OF HEALTH AND HUMAN SERVICES • CENTERS FOR DISEASE CONTROL AND PREVENTION

Recommended Immunization Schedule for Persons Aged 0–6 Years—UNITED STATES•2007

Vaccine ▼ Age ►	Birth	1 month	2 months	4 months	6 months	12 months	15 months	18 months	19–23 months	2–3 years	4–6 years
Hepatitis B[1]	HepB	HepB	see footnote†		HepB				HepB Series		
Rotavirus[2]			Rota	Rota	Rota						
Diphtheria, Tetanus, Pertussis[3]			DTaP	DTaP	DTaP		DTaP				DTaP
Haemophilus influenzae type b[4]			Hib	Hib	*Hib*[4]	Hib		Hib			
Pneumococcal[5]			PCV	PCV	PCV	PCV				PCV / PPV	
Inactivated Poliovirus			IPV	IPV		IPV					IPV
Influenza[6]						Influenza (Yearly)					
Measles, Mumps, Rubella[7]						MMR					MMR
Varicella[8]						Varicella					Varicella
Hepatitis A[9]						HepA (2 doses)				HepA Series	
Meningococcal[10]										MPSV4	

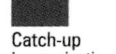

Range of recommended ages

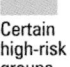

Catch-up immunization

Certain high-risk groups

This schedule indicates the recommended ages for routine administration of currently licensed childhood vaccines, as of December 1, 2006, for children aged 0–6 years. Additional information is available at http://www.cdc.gov/nip/recs/child-schedule.htm. Any dose not administered at the recommended age should be administered at any subsequent visit, when indicated and feasible. Additional vaccines may be licensed and recommended during the year. Licensed combination vaccines may be used whenever any components of the combination are indicated and other components of the vaccine are not contraindicated and if approved by the Food and Drug Administration for that dose of the series. Providers should consult the respective Advisory Committee on Immunization Practices statement for detailed recommendations. Clinically significant adverse events that follow immunization should be reported to the Vaccine Adverse Event Reporting System (VAERS). Guidance about how to obtain and complete a VAERS form is available at **http://www.vaers, hhs.gov** or by telephone, **800 822 7967.**

1. Hepatitis B vaccine (HepB). *(Minimum age: birth)*
At birth:
- Administer monovalent HepB to all newborns before hospital discharge.
- If mother is hepatitis surface antigen (HBsAg)-positive, administer HepB and 0.5 mL of hepatitis B immune globulin (HBIG) within 12 hours of birth.
- If mother's HBsAg status is unknown, administer HepB within 12 hours of birth. Determine the HBsAg status as soon as possible and if HBsAg-positive, administer HBIG (no later than age 1 week).
- If mother is HBsAg-negative, the birth dose can only be delayed with physician's order and mother's negative HBsAg laboratory report documented in the infant's medical record.

After the birth dose:
- The HepB series should be completed with either monovalent HepB or a combination vaccine containing HepB. The second dose should be administered at age 1–2 months. The final dose should be administered at age ≥24 weeks. Infants born to HBsAg-positive mothers should be tested for HBsAg and antibody to HBsAg after completion of ≥3 doses of a licensed HepB series, at age 9–18 months (generally at the next well-child visit).

4-month dose:
- It is permissible to administer 4 doses of HepB when combination vaccines are administered after the birth dose. If monovalent HepB is used for doses after the birth dose, a dose at age 4 months is not needed.

2. Rotavirus vaccine (Rota). *(Minimum age: 6 weeks)*
- Administer the first dose at age 6–12 weeks. Do not start the series later than age 12 weeks.
- Administer the final dose in the series by age 32 weeks. Do not administer a dose later than age 32 weeks.
- Data on safety and efficacy outside of these age ranges are insufficient.

3. Diphtheria and tetanus toxoids and acellular pertussis vaccine (DTaP). *(Minimum age: 6 weeks)*
- The fourth dose of DTaP may be administered as early as age 12 months, provided 6 months have elapsed since the third dose.
- Administer the final dose in the series at age 4–6 years.

4. *Haemophilus influenzae* type b conjugate vaccine (Hib). *(Minimum age: 6 weeks)*
- If PRP-OMP (PedvaxHIB® or ComVax® [Merck]) is administered at ages 2 and 4 months, a dose at age 6 months is not required.
- TriHiBit® (DTaP/Hib) combination products should not be used for primary immunization but can be used as boosters following any Hib vaccine in children aged ≥12 months.

5. Pneumococcal vaccine. *(Minimum age: 6 weeks for pneumococcal conjugate vaccine [PCV]; 2 years for pneumococcal polysaccharide vaccine [PPV])*
- Administer PCV at ages 24–59 months in certain high-risk groups. Administer PPV to children aged ≥2 years in certain high-risk groups. See *MMWR* 2000;49(No. RR-9):1–35.

6. Influenza vaccine. *(Minimum age: 6 months for trivalent inactivated influenza vaccine [TIV]; 5 years for live, attenuated influenza vaccine [LAIV])*
- All children aged 6–59 months and close contacts of all children aged 0–59 months are recommended to receive influenza vaccine.
- Influenza vaccine is recommended annually for children aged ≥59 months with certain risk factors, health-care workers, and other persons (including household members) in close contact with persons in groups at high risk. See *MMWR* 2006;55(No. RR-10):1–41.
- For healthy persons aged 5–49 years, LAIV may be used as an alternative to TIV.
- Children receiving TIV should receive 0.25 mL if aged 6–35 months or 0.5 mL if aged ≥3 years.
- Children aged <9 years who are receiving influenza vaccine for the first time should receive 2 doses (separated by ≥4 weeks for TIV and ≥6 weeks for LAIV).

7. Measles mumps and rubella vaccine (MMR). *(Minimum age: 12 months)*
- Administer the second dose of MMR at age 4–6 years. MMR may be administered before age 4–6 years, provided ≥4 weeks have elapsed since the first dose and both doses are administered at age ≥12 months.

8. Varicella vaccine. *(Minimum age: 12 months)*
- Administer the second dose of varicella vaccine at age 4–6 years. Varicella vaccine may be administered before age 4–6 years, provided that ≥3 months have elapsed since the first dose and both doses are administered at age ≥12 months. If second dose was administered ≥28 days following the first dose, the second dose does not need to be repeated.

9. Hepatitis A vaccine (HepA). *(Minimum age: 12 months)*
- HepA is recommended for all children aged 1 year (i.e., aged 12–23 months). The 2 doses in the series should be administered at least 6 months apart.
- Children not fully vaccinated by age 2 years can be vaccinated at subsequent visits.
- HepA is recommended for certain other groups of children, including in areas where vaccination programs target older children. See *MMWR* 2006;55(No. RR-7):1–23.

10. Meningococcal polysaccharide vaccine (MPSV4). *(Minimum age: 2 years)*
- Administer MPSV4 to children aged 2–10 years with terminal complement deficiencies or anatomic or functional asplenia and certain other high-risk groups. See *MMWR* 2005;54(No. RR-7):1–21.

The Recommended Immunization Schedules for Persons Aged 0–18 Years are approved by the Advisory Committee on Immunization Practices (http://www.cdc.gov/nip/acip), the American Academy of Pediatrics (http://www.aap.org), and the American Academy of Family Physicians (http://www.aafp.org).

SAFER•HEALTHIER•PEOPLE™

Table 12. (continued)

DEPARTMENT OF HEALTH AND HUMAN SERVICES • CENTERS FOR DISEASE CONTROL AND PREVENTION

Recommended Immunization Schedule for Persons Aged 7–18 Years—UNITED STATES • 2007

Vaccine ▼ Age ▶	7–10 years	11–12 YEARS	13–14 years	15 years	16–18 years
Tetanus, Diphtheria, Pertussis[1]	see footnote 1	Tdap	Tdap		
Human Papillomavirus[2]	see footnote 2	HPV (3 doses)	HPV Series		
Meningococcal[3]	MPSV4	MCV4		MCV4[3] / MCV4	
Pneumococcal[4]		PPV			
Influenza[5]		Influenza (Yearly)			
Hepatitis A[6]		HepA Series			
Hepatitis B[7]		HepB Series			
Inactivated Poliovirus[8]		IPV Series			
Measles, Mumps, Rubella[9]		MMR Series			
Varicella[10]		Varicella Series			

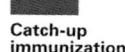

Range of recommended ages

Catch-up immunization

Certain high-risk groups

This schedule indicates the recommended ages for routine administration of currently licensed childhood vaccines, as of December 1, 2006, for children aged 7–18 years. Additional information is available at **http://www.cdc.gov/nip/recs/child-schedule.htm**. Any dose not administered at the recommended age should be administered at any subsequent visit, when indicated and feasible. Additional vaccines may be licensed and recommended during the year. Licensed combination vaccines may be used whenever any components of the combination are indicated and other components

of the vaccine are not contraindicated and if approved by the Food and Drug Administration for that dose of the series. Providers should consult the respective Advisory Committee on Immunization Practices statement for detailed recommendations. Clinically significant adverse events that follow immunization should be reported to the Vaccine Adverse Event Reporting System (VAERS). Guidance about how to obtain and complete a VAERS form is available at **http://www.vaers.hhs.gov** or by telephone, **800-822-7967**.

1. Tetanus and diphtheria toxoids and acellular pertussis vaccine (Tdap).
(Minimum age: 10 years for BOOSTRIX® and 11 years for ADACEL™)
- Administer at age 11–12 years for those who have completed the recommended childhood DTP/DTaP vaccination series and have not received a tetanus and diphtheria toxoids vaccine (Td) booster dose.
- Adolescents aged 13–18 years who missed the 11–12 year Td/Tdap booster dose should also receive a single dose of Tdap if they have completed the recommended childhood DTP/DTaP vaccination series.

2. Human papillomavirus vaccine (HPV). *(Minimum age: 9 years)*
- Administer the first dose of the HPV vaccine series to females at age 11–12 years.
- Administer the second dose 2 months after the first dose and the third dose 6 months after the first dose.
- Administer the HPV vaccine series to females at age 13–18 years if not previously vaccinated.

3. Meningococcal vaccine. *(Minimum age: 11 years for meningococcal conjugate vaccine [MCV4]; 2 years for meningococcal polysaccharide vaccine [MPSV4])*
- Administer MCV4 at age 11–12 years and to previously unvaccinated adolescents at high school entry (at approximately age 15 years).
- Administer MCV4 to previously unvaccinated college freshmen living in dormitories; MPSV4 is an acceptable alternative.
- Vaccination against invasive meningococcal disease is recommended for children and adolescents aged ≥2 years with terminal complement deficiencies or anatomic or functional asplenia and certain other high-risk groups. See *MMWR* 2005;54(No. RR-7):1–21. Use MPSV4 for children aged 2–10 years and MCV4 or MPSV4 for older children.

4. Pneumococcal polysaccharide vaccine (PPV). *(Minimum age: 2 years)*
- Administer for certain high-risk groups. See *MMWR* 1997;46(No. RR-8):1–24, and *MMWR* 2000;49(No. RR-9):1–35.

5. Influenza vaccine. *(Minimum age: 6 months for trivalent inactivated influenza vaccine [TIV]; 5 years for live, attenuated influenza vaccine [LAIV])*
- Influenza vaccine is recommended annually for persons with certain risk factors, health-care workers, and other persons (including household members) in close contact with persons in groups at high risk. See *MMWR* 2006;55 (No. RR-10):1–41.
- For healthy persons aged 5–49 years, LAIV may be used as an alternative to TIV.
- Children aged <9 years who are receiving influenza vaccine for the first time should receive 2 doses (separated by ≥4 weeks for TIV and ≥6 weeks for LAIV).

6. Hepatitis A vaccine (HepA). *(Minimum age: 12 months)*
- The 2 doses in the series should be administered at least 6 months apart.
- HepA is recommended for certain other groups of children, including in areas where vaccination programs target older children. See *MMWR* 2006;55 (No. RR-7):1–23.

7. Hepatitis B vaccine (HepB). *(Minimum age: birth)*
- Administer the 3-dose series to those who were not previously vaccinated.
- A 2-dose series of Recombivax H is licensed for children aged 11–15 years.

8. Inactivated poliovirus vaccine (IPV). *(Minimum age: 6 weeks)*
- For children who received an all-IPV or all-oral poliovirus (PV) series, a fourth dose is not necessary if the third dose was administered at age ≥4 years.
- If both PV and IPV were administered as part of a series, a total of 4 doses should be administered, regardless of the child s current age.

9. Measles, mumps, and rubella vaccine (MMR). *(Minimum age: 12 months)*
- If not previously vaccinated, administer 2 doses of MMR during any visit, with ≥4 weeks between the doses.

10. Varicella vaccine. *(Minimum age: 12 months)*
- Administer 2 doses of varicella vaccine to persons without evidence of immunity.
- Administer 2 doses of varicella vaccine to persons aged 13 years at least 3 months apart. Do not repeat the second dose, if administered ≥28 days after the first dose.
- Administer 2 doses of varicella vaccine to persons aged ≥13 years at least 4 weeks apart.

The Recommended Immunization Schedules for Persons Aged 0–18 Years are approved by the Advisory Committee on Immunization Practices (http://www.cdc.gov/nip/acip), the American Academy of Pediatrics (http://www.aap.org), and the American Academy of Family Physicians (http://www.aafp.org).

SAFER • HEALTHIER • PEOPLE™

Table 12. (continued)

Catch-up Immunization Schedule
for Persons Aged 4 Months–18 Years Who Start Late or Who Are More Than 1 Month Behind

UNITED STATES • 2007

The table below provides catch-up schedules and minimum intervals between doses for children whose vaccinations have been delayed. A vaccine series does not need to be restarted, regardless of the time that has elapsed between doses. Use the section appropriate for the child's age.

Vaccine	Minimum Age for Dose 1	Minimum Interval Between Doses			
		Dose 1 to Dose 2	Dose 2 to Dose 3	Dose 3 to Dose 4	Dose 4 to Dose 5
CATCH-UP SCHEDULE FOR PERSONS AGED 4 MONTHS–6 YEARS					
Hepatitis B[1]	Birth	4 weeks	**8 weeks** (and 16 weeks after first dose)		
Rotavirus[2]	6 wks	4 weeks	4 weeks		
Diphtheria, Tetanus, Pertussis[3]	6 wks	4 weeks	4 weeks	6 months	6 months[3]
Haemophilus influenzae type b[4]	6 wks	**4 weeks** if first dose administered at age <12 months **8 weeks (as final dose)** if first dose administered at age 12-14 months **No further doses needed** if first dose administered at age ≥15 months	**4 weeks[4]** if current age <12 months **8 weeks (as final dose)[4]** if current age ≥12 months and second dose administered at age <15 months **No further doses needed** if previous dose administered at age ≥15 months	**8 weeks (as final dose)** This dose only necessary for children aged 12 months–5 years who received 3 doses before age 12 months	
Pneumococcal[5]	6 wks	**4 weeks** if first dose administered at age <12 months and current age <24 months **8 weeks (as final dose)** if first dose administered at age ≥12 months or current age 24–59 months **No further doses needed** for healthy children if first dose administered at age ≥24 months	**4 weeks** if current age <12 months **8 weeks (as final dose)** if current age ≥12 months **No further doses needed** for healthy children if previous dose administered at age ≥24 months	**8 weeks (as final dose)** This dose only necessary for children aged 12 months–5 years who received 3 doses before age 12 months	
Inactivated Poliovirus[6]	6 wks	4 weeks	4 weeks	4 weeks[6]	
Measles, Mumps, Rubella[7]	12 mos	4 weeks			
Varicella[8]	12 mos	3 months			
Hepatitis A	12 mos	6 months			
CATCH-UP SCHEDULE FOR PERSONS AGED 7–18 YEARS					
Tetanus, Diphtheria/ Tetanus, Diphtheria, Pertussis[10]	7 yrs[10]	4 weeks	**8 weeks** if first dose administered at age <12 months **6 months** if first dose administered at age ≥12 months	**6 months** if first dose administered at age <12 months	
Human Papillomavirus[11]	9 yrs	4 weeks	12 weeks		
Hepatitis A	12 mos	6 months			
Hepatitis B[1]	Birth	4 weeks	**8 weeks** (and 16 weeks after first dose)		
Inactivated Poliovirus[6]	6 wks	4 weeks	4 weeks	4 weeks[6]	
Measles, Mumps, Rubella[7]	12 mos	4 weeks			
Varicella[8]	12 mos	**4 weeks** if first dose administered at age ≥13 years **3 months** if first dose administered at age <13 years			

1. **Hepatitis B vaccine (HepB).** *(Minimum age: birth)*
   - Administer the 3-dose series to those who were not previously vaccinated.
   - A 2-dose series of Recombivax HB® is licensed for children aged 11–15 years.
2. **Rotavirus vaccine (Rota).** *(Minimum age: 6 weeks)*
   - Do not start the series later than age 12 weeks.
   - Administer the final dose in the series by age 32 weeks. Do not administer a dose later than age 32 weeks.
   - Data on safety and efficacy outside of these age ranges are insufficient.
3. **Diphtheria and tetanus toxoids and acellular pertussis vaccine (DTaP).** *(Minimum age: 6 weeks)*
   - The fifth dose is not necessary if the fourth dose was administered at age ≥4 years.
   - DTaP is not indicated for persons aged ≥7 years.
4. ***Haemophilus influenzae* type b conjugate vaccine (Hib).** *(Minimum age: 6 weeks)*
   - Vaccine is not generally recommended for children aged ≥5 years.
   - If current age <12 months and the first 2 doses were PRP-P (PedvaxHIB® or Comvax® Merck), the third (and final) dose should be administered at age 12–15 months and at least 8 weeks after the second dose.
   - If first dose was administered at age 7–11 months, administer 2 doses separated by 4 weeks plus a booster at age 12–15 months.
5. **Pneumococcal conjugate vaccine (PCV).** *(Minimum age: 6 weeks)*
   - Vaccine is not generally recommended for children aged ≥5 years.
6. **Inactivated poliovirus vaccine (IPV).** *(Minimum age: 6 weeks)*
   - For children who received an all-IPV or all-oral poliovirus (OPV) series, a fourth dose is not necessary if third dose was administered at age ≥4 years.
   - If both OPV and IPV were administered as part of a series, a total of 4 doses should be administered, regardless of the child's current age.
7. **Measles, mumps, and rubella vaccine (MMR).** *(Minimum age: 12 months)*
   - The second dose of MMR is recommended routinely at age 4–6 years but may be administered earlier if desired.
   - If not previously vaccinated, administer 2 doses of MMR during any visit with ≥4 weeks between the doses.
8. **Varicella vaccine.** *(Minimum age: 12 months)*
   - The second dose of varicella vaccine is recommended routinely at age 4–6 years but may be administered earlier if desired.
   - Do not repeat the second dose in persons aged <13 years if administered ≥28 days after the first dose.
9. **Hepatitis A vaccine (HepA).** *(Minimum age: 12 months)*
   - HepA is recommended for certain groups of children, including in areas where vaccination programs target older children. See *MMWR* 2006 55(No. RR-7) 1–23.
10. **Tetanus and diphtheria toxoids vaccine (Td) and tetanus and diphtheria toxoids and acellular pertussis vaccine (Tdap).** *(Minimum ages: 7 years for Td, 10 years for BOOSTRIX®, and 11 years for ADACEL™)*
    - Tdap should be substituted for a single dose of Td in the primary catch-up series or as a booster if age appropriate; use Td for other doses.
    - A 5-year interval from the last Td dose is encouraged when Tdap is used as a booster dose. A booster (fourth) dose is needed if any of the previous doses were administered at age <12 months. Refer to ACIP recommendations for further information. See *MMWR* 2006 55(No. RR-3).
11. **Human papillomavirus vaccine (HPV).** *(Minimum age: 9 years)*
    - Administer the HPV vaccine series to females at age 13–18 years if not previously vaccinated.

Information about reporting reactions after immunization is available online at http://www.vaers.hhs.gov or by telephone via the 24-hour national toll-free information line 800-822-7967. Suspected cases of vaccine-preventable diseases should be reported to the state or local health department. Additional information, including precautions and contraindications for immunization, is available from the National Center for Immunization and Respiratory Diseases at http://www.cdc.gov/nip/default.htm or telephone, 800-CDC-INFO (800-232-4636).

DEPARTMENT OF HEALTH AND HUMAN SERVICES • CENTERS FOR DISEASE CONTROL AND PREVENTION • SAFER HEALTHIER PEOPLE

Table 13. Recommendations for Routine Immunization of HIV-Infected Children in the United States

Vaccine	Known Asymptomatic HIV Infection	Symptomatic HIV Infection
Hepatitis B	Yes	Yes
DTaP (or DTP)	Yes	Yes
IPV[a]	Yes	Yes
MMR	Yes	Yes[b]
Hib	Yes	Yes
Pneumococcal[c]	Yes	Yes
Influenza[d]	Yes	Yes
Varicella[e]	No	No

Adapted from the American Academy of Pediatrics. In Peter G, ed. *1997 Red Book: Report of the Committee on Infectious Diseases*, 24th ed. Elk Grove Village, IL: American Academy of Pediatrics, 1997.

DTP, diphtheria and tetanus toxoids and pertussis vaccine; DTaP, diphtheria and tetanus toxoids acellular pertussis vaccine; IPV, inactivated poliovirus vaccine; MMR, live-virus measles, mumps, and rubella; Hib, *Haemophilus influenzae* type b conjugate.

[a] Only inactivated polio vaccine (IPV) should be used for HIV-infected children, HIV-exposed infants whose status is indeterminate, and household contacts of HIV-infected patients.

[b] Severely immunocompromised HIV-infected children should not receive MMR vaccine.

[c] Pneumococcal vaccine should be administered at 2 years of age to all HIV-infected children. Children who are older than 2 years of age should receive pneumococcal vaccine at the time of diagnosis. Revaccination after 3 to 5 years is recommended in either circumstance.

[d] Influenza vaccine should be provided each fall and repeated annually for HIV-exposed infants 6 months of age and older, HIV-infected children and adolescents, and for household contacts of HIV-infected patients.

[e] Varicella vaccine is not currently indicated for HIV-exposed or HIV-infected patients, but studies are in progress to determine safety and possible indication.

Table 14. Guide to Tetanus Prophylaxis in Routine Wound Management

History of Absorbed Tetanus Toxoid (Doses)	Clean, Minor Wounds		All Other Wounds[a]	
	TD[b]	TIG[c]	TD[b]	TIG[c]
Unknown or <3	Yes	No	Yes	Yes
≥3[d]	No[e]	No	No[f]	No

Adapted from the American Academy of Pediatrics. In Peter G, ed. *1997 Red Book: Report of the Committee on Infectious Diseases*, 24th ed. Elk Grove Village, IL: American Academy of Pediatrics, 1997.

Td, adult-use tetanus and diphtheria toxoids; TIG, tetanus immune globulin (human).

[a] Such as, but not limited to, wounds contaminated with dirt, feces, soil, or saliva; puncture wounds; avulsions; and wounds resulting from missiles, crushing, burns, or frostbite.

[b] For children <7 years, diphtheria and tetanus toxoids and acellular pertussis (DTaP) or diphtheria-tetanus-pertussis (DTP) is recommended; if pertussis vaccine is contraindicated, diphtheria-tetanus toxoid (DT) is given. For persons ≥7 years of age, Td is recommended.

[c] Equine tetanus antitoxin should be used when TIG is not available.

[d] If only 3 doses of fluid toxoid have been received, a fourth dose of toxoid, preferably an adsorbed toxoid, should be given.

[e] Yes, if more than 10 years since the last dose.

[f] Yes, if more than 5 years since the last dose. (More frequent boosters are not needed and can accentuate side effects.)

Table 15. Suggested Intervals Between Immunoglobulin Administration and Measles Vaccination (MMR or Monovalent Measles Vaccine)

Indication for Immunoglobulin	Preparation	Route	Dose U or mL	Dose mg IgG/kg	Interval (Months)[a]
Tetanus	TIG	IM	250 U	10	3
Hepatitis A prophylaxis	IG				
Contact prophylaxis		IM	0.02 mL/kg	3.3	3
International travel		IM	0.06 mL/kg	10	3
Hepatitis B prophylaxis	HBIG	IM	0.06 mL/kg	10	3
Rabies prophylaxis	RIG	IM	20 IU/kg	22	4
Measles prophylaxis	IG				
Standard		IM	0.25 mL/kg	40	5
Immunocompromised host		IM	0.50 mL/kg	80	6
Varicella prophylaxis	VZIG	IM	125 U/10 kg (maximum, 625 U)	20–39	5
Blood transfusion					
Washed RBCs		IV	10 mL/kg	Negligible	0
RBCs, adenine-saline added		IV	10 mL/kg	10	3
Packed RBCs		IV	10 mL/kg	20–60	5
Whole blood		IV	10 mL/kg	80–100	6
Plasma or platelet products		IV	10 mL/kg	160	7
Replacement (or therapy) of immune deficiencies	IGIV	IV	...	300–400	8
ITP	IGIV	IV	...	400	8
RSV	IGIV	IV	...	750	9
ITP		IV	...	1,000	10
ITP or Kawasaki disease		IV	...	1,600–2,000	11

Adapted from the American Academy of Pediatrics. In: Peter G, ed. *1997 Red Book: Report of the Committee on Infectious Diseases*. 24th ed. Elk Grove Village, IL: American Academy of Pediatrics, 1997.

IG, immune globulin; IGIV, intravenous immune globulin; IM, intramuscular; ITP, immune (idiopathic) thrombocytopenic purpura; IV, intravenous; HBIG, hepatitis B immune globulin; MMR, measles-mumps-rubella vaccine; RBCs, red blood cells; RIG, rabies immune globulin; RSV-IGIV, respiratory syncytial virus intravenous immune globulin; TIG, tetanus immune globulin; VZIG, varicella-zoster immune globulin.

[a] These intervals should provide sufficient time for decreases in passive antibodies in all children to allow for an adequate response to the measles vaccine. Physicians should not assume that children are fully protected against measles during these intervals. Additional doses of IG or measles vaccine may be indicated after exposure to measles.

Table 16. Maternal Drug Use During Lactation

Avoid During Lactation		No Effects on Infant
Alcohol	Meperidine	Ampicillin
Chloramphenicol	Oral contraceptives	Caffeine
Cimetidine	Paregoric	Cephalosporins
Clindamycin	Phenobarbital	Erythromycin
Codeine	Propoxyphene	Furosemide
Diazepam	Radionuclide material	Haloperidol
Ergot	Sulfonamides	Hydralazine
Iodine	Tetracycline	
Isoniazid		
LSD		
Marijuana		

Adapted from Roberts RJ. *Drug therapy in infants*. Philadelphia: WB Saunders, 1984.

Table 17. Commercially Available Oral Rehydration Fluids (in mEq/L)

	Na$^+$	K$^+$	Cl$^-$	Base	Glucose
Pedialyte	45	20	35	30	2.5
Lytren	50	25	45	30	2.0
Rehydralyte	75	20	65	30	2.5
WHO formula	90	20	80	30	2.0

Table 18. Composition of Infant Formulas (per 100 mL)

Name (Manufacturer)	Kcal/oz	CHO (% of cal/type)	Fat (% of cal/type)	PRO (% of cal/type)	FE (mg)	VIT D (IU)	mg Ca/mg PO$_4$
Cow's Milk–based Standard Formulas							
Enfamil (Mead Johnson) with/without iron	20[a]	44%[a] Lactose	48% Palm olein, coconut oil, soy oil, sunflower oil	8% Cow's milk	1.22/0.34	41	52/36
Similac (Ross); with/without iron	20[a]	43% Lactose	48% Soy oil, coconut oil	9% Cow's milk	1.2/0.15	40	49/38
PM 60/75 (Ross)[b]	20	41% Lactose	50% Coconut oil, corn oil	9% Lactalbumin, casein	0.15	40	75/20
Gerber; with/without iron (Gerber)	20[c]	43% Lactose	49% Corn oil, coconut oil	9% Cow's milk	1.21/0.11	40	50/39
Good Start (Carnation)[b]	20[c]	44% Lactose, soy maltodextrin	46% Palm oil, safflower oil, coconut oil	10% Whey and whey protein	1.01	41	43/24
Soy-based Standard Formulas							
Isomil (Ross)	20	41% Corn syrup, sucrose	49% Coconut oil, soy oil	10% Soy protein isolate	1.2	40	70/50
Prosobee (Mead Johnson)	20	40% Corn syrup solids	48% Coconut oil, soy oil, palm oil	12% Soy protein isolate	1.3	42	63/49
Preterm Formulas							
Similac Special Care (Ross)	24[d]	42% Lactose (50%), polycose glucose polymers (50%)	47% MCT oil (50%), soy oil (30%), coconut oil (20%)	11% Nonfat milk whey (60%), casein (75%)	1.5/0.3	122	146/81
Enfamil Premature (Mead Johnson); with/without iron	24[d]	44% Lactose (50%), corn syrup solids	44% MCT oil (75%), soy oil (75%), coconut oil (20%)	12% Lactalbumin (60%), casein (75%)	1.5/0.2	219	134/75
Similac Neocare (Ross)[e]	22	41% Lactose (50%), glucose polymers (50%)	49% MCT oil (25%), LCT oil (75%)	10% Whey (50%), casein (50%)	1.3	59	78/46

(continued)

Table 18. Composition of Infant Formulas (per 50 mL) (continued)

Name (Manufacturer)	Kcal/oz	CHO (% of cal/type)	Fat (% of cal/type)	PRO (% of cal/type)	FE (mg)	VIT D (IU)	mg Ca/mg PO$_4$
Special Formulas[f]							
Nutramigen (Mead Johnson)	20	54% Modified corn starch, corn syrup solids	35% Corn oil, soy oil	11% Casein hydrolysate and amino acids	1.25	42	63/42
Pregestimil (Mead Johnson)	20	41% Corn syrup solids, modified cornstarch, dextrose	48% MCT oil (60%), corn oil, soy oil, safflower oil	11% Casein hydrolysate, amino acids	1.25	50	63/42
Portagen (Mead Johnson)	20	46% Corn syrup solids, sucrose	75% MCT oil (85%), corn oil, Lecithin	14% Sodium caseinate	1.25	52	63/47
Alimentum (Ross)[e]	20	41% Sucrose, modified tapioca starch	48% MCT oil (50%), safflower oil (75%), soy oil (10%)	11% Casein hydrolysate, amino acids	1.2	30	70/50
Lactofree (Mead Johnson)	20	42% Corn syrup solids	49% Palm olein, soy oil, coconut oil, sunflower oil	9% Cow's milk protein isolate	1.2	75	55/37
Neocate (Scientific Hospital Supplies, Inc.)	20	47% Corn syrup solids, dextrose, maltose, maltriose, oligosaccharides	41% Hybrid safflower oil, coconut oil, soy oil	12% Synthetic free amino acids	1.2	58	83/62

CHO, carbohydrate; CF, cystic fibrosis; FE, iron; LCT, long-chain triglyceride; MCT, medium-chain triglyceride; PRO, protein.
[a] Also available as 24 kcal/oz and 27 kcal/oz.
[b] Formula with a low renal solute load.
[c] Also available as 24 kcal/oz.
[d] Also available as 20 kcal/oz.
[e] Available only as ready-to-feed.

[f] Indications for Special Formulas

Name	Indications
Nutramigen	Cow's milk allergy, severe or multiple food allergies, severe or persistent diarrhea, galactosemia
Pregestimil	Malabsorption, intestinal resection, severe or persistent diarrhea, food allergies
Portagen	Steatorrhea secondary to CF, intestinal resections, pancreatic insufficiency, biliary atresia, lymphatic anomalies, celiac disease
Alimentum	Problems with digestion or absorption, severe or prolonged diarrhea, CF, steatorrhea, food allergies, intestinal resection
Lactofree	Lactose intolerance *without* cow's milk protein intolerance
Neocate	Cow's milk allergy, soy and protein hydrolysate intolerance, multiple food protein intolerance

SYNDROME AND OBESITY

Table 19. Uncommon Disorders Associated with Obesity

Alström-Hallgren syndrome. Autosomal-recessive trait, obesity, retinal degeneration with blindness in childhood, sensory nerve deafness, diabetes mellitis, small testes in males, and progressive nephropathy in adults.

Carpenter syndrome. Obesity; brachycephaly with craniosynostosis; peculiar facies with lateral displacement of inner canthi and apparent exophthalmos, flat nasal bridge, low-set ears, retrognathism, and high-arched palate; brachydactyly of hands with clinodactyly and partial syndactyly; preaxial polydactyly of feet with partial syndactyly; and mental retardation.

Cohen syndrome. Mild—childhood onset, truncal obesity, persistent hypotonia and muscle weakness, mild mental retardation, characteristic craniofacies with high nasal bridge, maxillary hypoplasia with mild downslant to palpebral fissures, high arched palate, short philtrum, small jaw, open mouth and prominent maxillary central incisors, mottled retina, myopia, strabismus, narrow hands and feet with shortening of metacarpals and metatarsals, simian crease, hyperextensible joints, lumbar lordosis, and mild scoliosis.

Cushing syndrome. Truncal obesity, hypertension, glucose intolerance, hirsutism, oligomenorrhea or amenorrhea, plethora, moon facies, buffalo hump, striae, ecchymoses, increased fatigability and weakness, and personality changes.

Growth hormone deficiency. Short stature, mild-to-moderate obesity.

Hyperinsulinemia. (From an insulin-secreting pancreatic tumor, hypersecretion by pancreatic beta cells or a hypothalamic lesion) Progressive obesity with hyperphagia, normal or excessive growth in stature, and signs and symptoms of hypoglycemia.

Hypothalamic dysfunction. (Due to tumor, trauma, or inflammation) Hyperinsulinemia and hyperphagia may be accompanied by headache, papilledema, impaired vision, amenorrhea or impotence, diabetes insipidus, hypothyroidism, adrenal insufficiency, somnolence, temperature dysregulation, seizures, and coma.

Hypothyroidism. Short stature; delayed sexual maturation; delayed union of epiphyses; lethargy; cold intolerance; hoarse voice; menorrhagia; decreased appetite; dry skin; aching muscles and delayed relaxation phase of deep tendon reflexes; progression to dull expressionless face; sparse hair; periorbital puffiness; large tongue; pale, cool, rough-feeling skin; and presence or absence of goiter.

Laurence-Moon-Biedl (Bardet-Biedl) syndrome. Autosomal-recessive trait, truncal obesity, retinal dystrophy/retinitis pigmentosa with progressively decreasing acuity, mental retardation, hypogenitalism, digital anomalies (polydactyly, syndactyly, or both), and nephropathy.

Polycystic ovary (Stein-Leventhal) syndrome. Irregular or absent menses, moderate hirsutism, weight gain shortly after menarche, increased ratio of luteinizing hormone to follicle-stimulating hormone, hyperandrogenemia, and increased levels of estrone with normal levels of estradiol. May occur in association with congenital adrenal hyperplasia, Cushing syndrome, hyperprolactinemia, or insulin resistance.

Prader-Willi syndrome. Obesity, hypotonia, and feeding problems in infancy; hyperphagia in childhood and adolescence; developmental delay; mental retardation; hypogonadism; short stature; small hands and feet; and strabismus.

Pseudohypoparathyroidism (type I). Short stature, round facies, short metatarsals and metacarpals, subcutaneous calcifications, moderate mental retardation, cataracts, coarse and dry skin, brittle hair and nails, hypocalcemia, and hyperphosphatemia.

Turner syndrome. Short stature, tendency to obesity, ovarian dysgenesis, broad chest with widely spaced nipples, prominent ears, narrow maxilla and small mandible, low posterior hairline, webbed posterior neck, elbow and knee anomalies, nail and skin anomalies, renal anomalies, and hearing impairment.

From Online Mendelian Inheritance in Man.

Table 20. 1989 Recommended Daily Dietary Allowance[a]

Age (Years) & Sex Group	Weight[b] (kg)	Weight[b] (lb)	Height[b] (cm)	Height[b] (In)	Fat-soluble Vitamins Vitamin A (mcg RE)[c]	Vitamin D (mcg)[d]	Vitamin E (mg TE)[e]	Vitamin K (mcg)	Water-soluble Vitamins Vitamin C (mg)	Thiamin (mg)	Riboflavin (mg)	Niacin (mg NE)[f]	Vitamin B$_6$ (mg)	Folate (mcg)	Vitamin B$_{12}$ (mcg)
Infants 0.0–0.5	6	13	60	24	375	7.5	3	5	30	0.3	0.4	5	0.3	25	0.3
0.5–1.0	9	20	71	28	375	10	4	10	35	0.4	0.5	6	0.6	35	0.5
Children 1–3	13	29	90	35	400	10	6	15	40	0.7	0.8	9	1.0	50	0.7
4–6	20	44	112	44	500	10	7	20	45	0.9	1.1	12	1.1	75	1.0
7–10	28	62	132	52	700	10	7	30	45	1.0	1.2	13	1.4	100	1.4
Males 11–14	45	99	157	62	1,000	10	10	45	50	1.3	1.5	17	1.7	150	2.0
15–18	66	145	176	69	1,000	10	10	65	60	1.5	1.8	20	2.0	200	2.0
Females 11–14	46	101	157	62	800	10	8	45	50	1.1	1.3	15	1.4	150	2.0
15–18	55	120	163	64	800	10	8	55	60	1.1	1.3	15	1.5	180	2.0

Adapted from the National Academy of Sciences-National Research Council.

[a] The allowances, expressed as average daily intakes over time, are intended to provide for individual variations among most normal persons as they live in the United States under usual environmental stresses. Diets should be based on a variety of common foods to provide other nutrients for which human requirements have been less well defined.
[b] The median weights and heights of those younger than 19 years were taken from Hammill PVV, et al. Physical growth: National Center for Health Statistics percentiles. *Am J Clin Nutr.* 1979;32:607–629. The use of these figures does not imply that the height-to-weight ratios are ideal.
[c] RE, retinol equivalent. 1 RE = 1 mcg retinol or 6 mcg beta-carotene.
[d] As cholecalciferol. 10 mcg cholecalciferol = 400 IU of vitamin D.
[e] TE, alpha-tocopherol equivalents. 1 TE = 1 mg d-alpha-tocopherol.
[f] NE, niacin equivalent. 1 NE = 1 mg of niacin or 60 mg of dietary tryptophan.

Table 21. Patient Teaching for Feeding Disorder

General Feeding Guidelines

The Importance of Role Modeling:

* Eat with your child. Young children eat better when adults are around!
* Eat a variety of fruits and vegetables.
* Use the food pyramid as a guide.

Establish a Consistent Mealtime Routine:

* Offer 3 meals and 2–3 snacks per day to help them develop a regular hunger-satiety schedule.
* Have children sit at the table for all meals; this will give them a signal that it is time to eat.
* Avoid asking children to eat, as this gives them the opportunity to refuse. Instead, use directives such as "Take a bite," or "It's time to pick up your spoon."
* Limit distractions during meals to help children focus on eating during mealtimes.
* Limit meal length to ~30 minutes.
* At the end of all meals, teach children to take "1 last bite" to signal the end of the meal. This can be a symbolic "last bite" where a spoon is gently touched to the child's lips.
* Once children have taken their "last bite," be sure to praise them to end the meal on a positive note.

Common Mealtime Concerns and Coping Strategies

Tantrums:

* Focus attention on children's appropriate mealtime behaviors.
* Cheer for children when they take a bite of food or show other appropriate mealtime behaviors. Be specific when praising them (e.g., "Great job taking your bite!" or "I like how you're picking up your spoon").
* Ignore refusal behaviors such as crying or throwing food off the table. Avoid responding or reacting to these behaviors. Instead, look away for ~20 seconds, and then remind them that it is time to take another bite. If the child throws food, wait until the end of the meal and have the child help pick up the food they have thrown.

Picky Eater:

* Children need to practice trying new food. It may take 10–15 trials of a new food before a child will learn to like the food.
* Have your child take "1 bite" of a new food at the end of 1 meal each day. Offer the same food every day for 1 week.
* Praise your child when he tastes new foods.

(continued)

Table 21. Patient Teaching for Feeding Disorder (continued)

Common Mealtime Concerns and Coping Strategies (*continued*)

The Grazer:

- Avoid allowing children to "graze" on small amounts of food and fluid throughout the day. These children do not feel hungry at mealtimes because they snack all day.
- Children who "graze" eat less (fewer calories) than children who have a consistent mealtime.
- Offer 3 meals and no more than 2–3 snacks each day.
- Remember that a snack can be a "mini meal" of nutrient dense foods and not necessarily "snack food."
- Restrict all snacks and drinks 30 minutes before and after meals. This way, children will not fill up on fluid just prior to or during the meal. By waiting 30 minutes until after the meal to offer fluid, children will not hold out for something to drink instead of eating.

The Short-Order Cook:

- "Short-order cook" caregivers may be preparing 4–5 meals hoping that their child will eat one of the choices.
- Offer the child a choice between 2 foods. Offer these choices at the start of the meal.
- If the child is too young or unable to choose, the caregiver may choose the food.
- When children refuse to eat, wait until the next meal or snack time to offer more food. This will teach children that they will not get a "better" food by refusing what has been offered.

INFECTIOUS DISEASES

Table 22. Risk Factors for Group B Streptococcal Infection

Maternal risk factors
Prolonged rupture of membranes (>18 hours)*
Premature rupture of membranes (<37 weeks' gestation)*
Preterm labor (<37 weeks' gestation)*
Fever >37.9°C (100.2°F)*
History of previous infant with GBS sepsis*
Clinical evidence of chorioamnionitis
GBS bacteriuria*
Multiple gestation
Diabetes

Fetal/Neonatal risk factors
Prematurity
Meconium passed in utero
Low 5-minute Apgar score (<6)
Male gender (sepsis four times more common in boys than in girls)

GBS, group B streptococci.
*Risk necessitating intrapartum antibiotic administration per 1996 Centers for Disease Control (CDC) guidelines.

Table 23. Signs and Symptoms of Sepsis in the Newborn

Respiratory distress	Tachypnea (respiratory rate >60/min), grunting, nasal flaring, retractions; sometimes present even without an oxygen requirement or abnormal chest x-ray
Temperature instability	Fever >37.9°C or hypothermia
Poor feeding	Lack of interest, abdominal distention, vomiting, diarrhea
Altered neurologic status	Lethargy, irritability, hypotonia, seizures (especially if meningitis is present)
Apnea	Especially in preterm infants
Poor perfusion	Mottled, grayish, capillary refill >3 s
Tachycardia	Often a late sign
Bulging fontanelle	Meningitis

Table 24. Neutrophil Indices

Neutrophil Indices	Normal Values
Absolute neutrophil count (ANC)[a]	>1,800/mm^3
Absolute band count (ABC)[b]	<2,000/mm^3
I:T ratio[c]	<0.2

[a] ANC = % total neutrophils × WBC count.
[b] ABC = % bands × WBC count.
[c] I:T = % immature (bands, metamyelocytes, myelocytes): % total (immature + segmented) neutrophils.

Table 25. Clinical Features Associated with Congenital Infection

Intrauterine growth retardation
Hydrops
Hepatosplenomegaly
Microcephaly, intracranial calcifications, hydrocephalus
Anemia, thrombocytopenia, petechiae
Jaundice (especially conjugated hyperbilirubinemia)
Pneumonitis
Cardiac malformations, myocarditis
Eye abnormalities (chorioretinitis, cataracts)
Bone abnormalities (osteochondritis, periostitis)

Table 26. Clinical Findings in Congenitally Infected Infants that Suggest a Specific Diagnosis

Infection	Suggestive Findings
Rubella	Cataracts, cloudy cornea, pigmented retina "Blueberry muffin" syndrome Vertical striation Malformation (PDA, pulmonary artery stenosis)
CMV	Microcephaly with periventricular calcifications Inguinal hernias in boys Petechiae with thrombocytopenia
Toxoplasmosis	Hydrocephalus with generalized calcifications Chorioretinitis
Syphilis	Osteochondritis and periostitis Eczematoid skin rash Mucocutaneous lesions (snuffles)
Herpes	Skin vesicles Keratoconjunctivitis Acute CNS findings

Modified with permission from Stagno S, Pass RF, Alford CA. Perinatal infections and maldevelopment. In: Bloom AD, James LS, eds. *The fetus and the newborn*, vol 17, Series 1. New York: Wiley-Liss, 1981.
CMV, cytomegalovirus; CNS, central nervous system; PDA, patent ductus arteriosus.

Table 27. Interpretation of Epstein-Barr Virus (EBV) Serology[a]

	IgG-VCA	IgM-VCA	EBV Nuclear Antigens	EBV Early Antigens
No evidence of infection	<10	<10	<2	<10
Acute infection	>10	≥10	<2	≥20
Convalescent infection	>10	Variable	>2	Variable
Remote past infection	≥10	<10	>2	≤20

[a] Values are expressed in reciprocal titers as measured by standard immunofluorescence methods.

Table 28. Croup (Laryngotracheobronchitis)—Severity Score for Croup Patients

Indicator of Severity of Illness	Score
Inspiratory stridor	
None	0
At rest, with stethoscope	1
At rest, without stethoscope	2
Retractions	
None	0
Mild	1
Moderate	2
Severe	3
Air entry	
Normal	0
Decreased	1
Severely decreased	2
Cyanosis	
None	0
With agitation	4
At rest	5
Level of consciousness	
Normal	0
Altered mental status	5
Mild Croup	0–3
Moderate to severe croup	>3

ABDOMINAL PAIN

Table 29. Classic Clinical Findings in Disorders Characterized by Abdominal Pain

Disorder	Typical Clinical Picture	Definitive Diagnostic Test
Peptic ulcer disease	Burning or sharp midepigastric pain that occurs 1–3 hours after meals and is exacerbated by spicy food and relieved by antacids; family history of peptic ulcer disease	Endoscopy
Pancreatitis	Episodic left upper quadrant pain that occurs 5–10 minutes after meals, radiates to the back, and is exacerbated by fatty foods	Pancreatic ultrasound or CT scan Serum amylase level ($\uparrow$)
Urinary tract infection	Suprapubic pain, burning on urination, urinary frequency, urinary urgency	Urine culture Urinalysis
Renal calculi	Severe periodic cramping pain that occurs in the flank and occasionally radiates to the groin; costovertebral angle tenderness; family history of renal calculi	Urinalysis Renal ultrasound
Periappendiceal abscess	Right lower quadrant pain; rebound and direct tenderness; anorexia and vomiting; fever	Barium enema Laparoscopy WBC count ($\uparrow$)
Gallbladder disease	Right upper quadrant pain that occurs 5–10 minutes after meals and is exacerbated by fatty foods; family history of gallstones	Gallbladder ultrasound
Menstrual pain	Cramping suprapubic pain that occurs during the menses	Trial with NSAIDs
Pelvic inflammatory disease (PID)	Suprapubic pain	Cervical culture
Functional abdominal pain (irritable bowel syndrome)	Cramping periumbilical pain that is exacerbated by eating and relieved by defecation	Trial with Metamucil
Lactose intolerance	Cramping periumbilical pain that increases following ingestion of dairy products and is accompanied by flatulence and bloating	Trial with a milk-free diet Breath hydrogen study for lactose deficiency
Inflammatory bowel disease	Right lower quadrant cramping and tenderness; anemia; guaiac-positive stool	Colonoscopy Barium enema Upper gastrointestinal series ESR ($\uparrow$), platelet count ($\uparrow$), WBC count ($\uparrow$)
Esophagitis	Epigastric and substernal pain that is relieved by antacids and exacerbated by lying down; history of iron deficiency; anemia; guaiac-positive stool	Endoscopy
Lead poisoning	Abdominal pain; history of pica; microcytic anemia; basophilic stippling	Serum lead level
Pancreatic pseudocyst	Left upper quadrant pain; recurrent vomiting; history of abdominal pain	Abdominal ultrasound
Sickle cell disease (SCD)	Periumbilical pain that responds to rest and rehydration	Sickle cell preparation Hemoglobin Electrophoresis
Abdominal epilepsy	Periodic severe abdominal pain that is often associated with seizures	Trial with anticonvulsants
Abdominal migraine	Severe abdominal pain; family history of migraine; recurrent headache, fever, and vomiting; unilateral or occipital headache; somatic complaints	Trial with antimigraine medications
Depression	Social withdrawal; decreased activity; irritability; poor attention span; difficulty sleeping	Trial with antidepressant medications
School avoidance	Nonspecific abdominal pain; severe anxiety reaction; pain that is more severe on weekdays and improves on weekends	

Modified with permission from Olson AD. Abdominal pain. In: Stockman JA, ed. *Difficult diagnosis in pediatrics*. Philadelphia: WB Saunders, 1990; p. 253.
ESR, erythrocyte sedimentation rate; NSAIDs, nonsteroidal antiinflammatory drugs; WBC, white blood cell; $\uparrow$, increased.

Table 30. Abdominal Masses Commonly Associated with Calcification

Neuroblastoma
Teratoma
   Ovarian
   Sacrococcygeal
Adrenal hematoma
Hepatic hemangioma
Meconium peritonitis

Table 31. Comparison of Functional Constipation and Hirschsprung Disease

	Functional Constipation	Hirschsprung Disease
Symptoms as a newborn	Rare	Almost always
Late onset (after 3 years)	Common	Rare
Difficult bowel training	Common	Rare
Stool size	Large	Small, ribbonlike
Urge to defecate	Rare	Common
Obstructive symptoms	Rare	Common
Enterocolitis	Rare	Sometimes
Failure to thrive	Rare	Common
Abdominal distention	Rare	Common
Stool in rectal ampulla	Common	None
Barium enema	Copious stool No transition zone	Delayed evacuation Transition zone
Rectal biopsy	Normal	No ganglion cells Increased anticholinesterase staining
Anorectal manometry	Distension of rectum causes relaxation of the internal sphincter	No sphincter relaxation

Table 32. Commonly Used Pediatric Medications that May Cause Cholestasis and Hepatotoxicity

Anticonvulsants
  Phenobarbital
  Diphenylhydantoin
  Carbamazepine
  Valproic acid
Antimicrobials
  Tetracycline
  Erythromycin (estolate preparations)
  Sulfonamides
  Ketoconazole
  Isoniazid
  Rifampin
  Griseofulvin

Immunosuppressants
  Cyclosporine
  Azathioprine
  Methotrexate
Steroids
  Corticosteroids
  Androgens
  Oral contraceptives
Miscellaneous drugs
  Acetaminophen
  Salicylates
  Chlorpromazine
  Cimetidine
  Iron preparations (with overdosage)

A large number of less commonly encountered agents, including antineoplastic agents, antidepressants, antipsychotics, and tranquilizers can also cause cholestasis and hepatotoxicity.

Table 33. Defects in Hepatic Bilirubin Conjugation

Disease	Defect	Genetics
Gilbert disease	Underactivity of the transferase, defective uptake of albumin-bound bilirubin from the plasma	Autosomal-recessive
Crigler-Najjar syndrome		
Type I	Complete absence of the transferase enzyme	Autosomal-recessive
Type II	Partial absence of the transferase enzyme (less severe than type I)	Autosomal-dominant

Table 34. Foods and Drugs Mimicking Blood in the Stool

False Hematochezia	False Melena	False Heme-positive Stools

Foods that contain
  Red dye
  Juice
  Candy
  Kool-Aid
  Jello
Tomatoes
Beets
Cranberries
	Spinach
	Blueberries
	Licorice
	Purple grapes
	Chocolate
	Grape juice
	Bismuth subsalicylate
	Iron supplements
		Red meat
		Cherries
		Tomato skin
		Iron supplements

Table 35. Clinical Signs of Dehydration in Children

Parameter	Mild	Moderate	Severe
Activity	Normal	Lethargic	Lethargic to comatose
Color	Pale	Gray	Mottled
Urine output	Decreased (<2–3 mL/kg/hr)	Oliguric (<1 mL/kg/hr)	Anuric
Fontanelle	Flat	Depressed	Sunken
Mucous membranes	Dry	Very dry	Cracked
Skin turgor	Slightly decreased	Markedly decreased	Tenting
Pulse	Normal to increased	Increased	Grossly tachycardic
Blood pressure	Normal	Normal	Decreased
Weight Loss	5%	10%	15%

Hypernatremic dehydration may be accompanied by moderate clinical signs. Reprinted with permission from Rogers MC: Shock. In: Rogers MC, Helfaer MA, eds. *Handbook of pediatric intensive care*, 2nd ed. Baltimore: Williams & Wilkins, 1994:140.

Table 36. Therapy for Hyperlipidemia

Type	Mechanism	Reduction in Cholesterol (%)	Effect on VLDL	Effect on HDL	Side Effect	Dose
Nonpharmacological therapy						
American Heart Association diet	Limits exogenous cholesterol	10–15	Decrease	Decrease		N/A
Exercise	Improves insulin resistance	Some decrease	Decrease	Increase		N/A
Weight Loss	Improves insulin resistance	Some decrease	Decrease	Mild increase		N/A
Pharmacological therapy						
Bile acid resins	Accelerate LDL disposal	20–30	Mild decrease	Mild increase	Epigastric distress, constipation, bloating, interferes with some drug absorption	Up to 24 g/day cholestyramine in divided doses
Nicotinic acid or niacin	Reduces VLDL and LDL synthesis increases HDL	25	50% decrease	30%–40% increase	Flushing, headache, tachycardia, gastrointestinal distress, activation of peptic ulcer disease and inflammatory bowel disease, hepatic dysfunction	Titrate up to 1 g 3 times/day
Probucol	Increases LDL disposal; reduces HDL/LDL	5–15		Decrease	Nausea, diarrhea, flatulence, eosinophilia, hepatic dysfunction, prolongation of QT interval	0.5 g 2 times/day
Gemfibrozil	Enhances VLDL breakdown; decreases VLDL production	Decrease	40%–50% decrease	20%–30% increase	Rarely myositis; should not be used in patients with renal disease, cholelithiasis, or liver dysfunction	600 mg 2 times/day
HMG CoA reductase inhibitor (lovastatin)	Inhibits cholesterol synthesis; increases LDL disposal	30–40			Elevated liver enzymes, myositis, cataracts in animals	20–40 mg 2 times/day

HDL, high-density lipoprotein; HMG CoA, 3-hydroxy-3-methylglutaryl coenzyme A; LDL, low-density lipoprotein; VLDL, very-low-density lipoprotein.

Table 36A. Expected Liver Span of Infants and Children

Age (yr)	Boys		Girls	
	Mean Estimated Liver Span	Standard Error of Mean	Mean Estimated Liver Span	Standard Error of Mean
6 mo	2.4	2.5	2.8	2.6
1	2.8	2.0	3.1	2.1
2	3.5	1.6	3.6	1.7
3	4.0	1.6	4.0	1.7
4	4.4	1.6	4.3	1.6
5	4.8	1.5	4.5	1.6
6	5.1	1.5	4.8	1.6
8	5.6	1.5	5.1	1.6
10	6.1	1.6	5.4	1.7
12	6.5	1.8	5.6	1.8
14	6.8	2.0	5.8	2.1
16	7.1	2.2	6.0	2.3
18	7.4	2.5	6.1	2.6
20	7.7	2.8	6.3	2.9

From Lawson EE, Grand RJ, Neff RK, et al. *Am J Dis Child* 1978;132:475, with permission.

Table 36B. Review of Liver Function Tests

I. LIVER FUNCTION TESTS

AP	AST	ALT	GGT	5 = NUC
Liver	Hepatocyte	Hepatocyte	Placenta	Biliary
Bone	Muscle	Muscle	Pancreas	
Intestine			Kidney	
Placenta			Bile	
Tumors			Ducts	
			Choroid	

II. "TRUE" LIVER FUNCTION TESTS
Prothrombin time
Albumin
Bile acids and salts
Factor II, V, VII, IX, X
   Vitamin k-dependent factors: II, VII, IX, X

III. LIVER FUNCTION TESTS
Clinical pearls for daily use:

	ALKALINE PHOSPHATASE	γ-GGT
Low	Zinc deficiency	Bile acid deficiency
	Wilson disease	
	Cystic fibrosis	
High	See other List	Cholestasis, ICP

IV. LIVER FUNCTION TESTS
Clinical pearls for daily use: Elevated transaminases and normal bilirubin, GGT, and alkaline phosphatase

Table 36C. Clinical Disease States and Age of Presentation of Hepatomegaly

Age	Clinical Disease States
Newborn (Birth–2 mo)	Intrauterine and intrapartum acquired infection (TORCH, syphilis, other)
	Erythroblastosis fetalis
	Neonatal hepatitis, α_1-antitrypsin, Alagille syndrome
	Biliary atresia
	Congestive heart failure
	Congenital paroxysmal atrial tachycardia
	Sepsis
Infant (2–12 mo)	Cystic fibrosis
	Metabolic disease: glycogen storage, α_1-antitrypsin deficiency, galactosemia, tyrosinemia, hereditary fructose intolerance, other
	Neonatal hepatitis, hepatitis B
	HIV infection (AIDS)
	Histiocytosis
	Malnutrition
	Tumors (intrinsic, metastatic)
	Cholelithiasis
	Choledochal cyst
Young child (1–6 yrs)	Viral hepatitis
	Drug-toxic hepatitis
	Parasitic
	Tumor
	Leukemia, lymphoma
Older child, adolescent (7–20 yrs)	Viral hepatitis
	Drug-toxic hepatitis
	Wilson disease
	Chronic active hepatitis
	Congenital hepatic fibrosis
	Focal nodular hyperplasia, adenoma
	α_1-Antitrypsin deficiency
	Reye syndrome
	Sickle cell anemia
	Cholelithiasis
	Juvenile rheumatoid arthritis, lupus erythematosus, sarcoidosis
	Leukemia, lymphoma
	Gonococcal perihepatitis
	Cystic fibrosis
	Diabetes

Adapted from Walker, WA, Mathia RK. *Pediatr Clin North Am* 1975;22:929.

Table 37. Assessment of Hypernatremia

Underlying Cause	ECF Volume	Urine Output	Urine Sodium	Specific Gravity
Sodium excess	Increased	Normal or increased	Increased	High
Water loss (DI)	Decreased	Increased	Decreased	High
Sodium and water loss (water > sodium)	Normal or decreased	Decreased	Increased	Low

DI, diabetes insipidus; ECF, extracellular fluid.

Table 38. Assessment of Hyponatremia

If Urine Output Decreased and UNq <20 mEq/L	If Urine Output Decreased and UNq >20 mEq/L	If Urine Output Normal or Increased and UNq >20 mEq/L	If Urine Output Normal or Increased and UNq >20 mEq/L
Effective intravascular volume, consider: CHF, nephrotic syndrome, dehydration, liver disease, third spacing conditions	Renal failure or increased ADH	Water intoxication	Renal NaCl wasting Nonoliguric renal failure, adrenal insufficiency Osmotic diuretic use or osmotic diuresis

Table 39. Conditions Associated with Increased ADH/ADH-Like Effect and Hyponatremia

Pain
Vomiting
CNS disorders: Including injuries, infection, tumors
Intrathoracic disorders: Including infections, mechanical ventilation
Drugs: Narcotics, barbiturates, carbamazepine, NSAIDs, cyclophosphamide, vincristine, others not commonly used in pediatrics

Table 40. Determination of Serum Osmolality

Reliable estimate under most circumstances:
Serum Osm = 2(Na mEq/L) + 10
Estimate when there is hyperglycemia or azotemia
Serum Osm = 2(Na) + glucose/18 + BUN/2.8

Table 41. Drugs Associated with Hyperkalemia

Potassium-sparing diuretics (e.g., spironolactone, triamterene, amiloride)
Potassium supplements (e.g., potassium chloride)
Potassium-containing penicillins
Stored blood
Cyclosporine
Nonsteroidal antiinflammatory drugs (NSAIDs)
Heparin
Angiotensin-converting enzyme (ACE) inhibitors
β-Adrenergic blockers
Chemotherapeutic agents

Table 42. Treatment of Hyperkalemia

Agent	Indication	Mechanism of Action	Dose	Side Effects/Potential Problems
10% calcium gluconate	ECG changes	Stabilizes membranes	1 mg/kg IV over 5–10 minutes	Hypercalcemia
Sodium bicarbonate	ECG changes or very high K^+ level	Shifts K^+ to intracellular compartment	1 mg/kg IV over 5–10 minutes	Sodium load
Glucose plus insulin	ECG changes or very high K^+ level	Shifts K^+ to intracellular compartment	0.25–0.5 gm/kg glucose plus 0.3 U insulin/gm glucose over 30–60 minutes	Hyper- or hypoglycemia
Kayexalate resin	To remove K^+ from body	K^+ binds to resin in gut	1 gm/kg PO or PR in 50%–70% sorbitol	Constipation
Furosemide	Symptomatic hyperkalemia	Enhances urinary K^+ excretion	1–2 mg/kg IV	May not be enough renal function to be effective
Hemo- or peritoneal dialysis	No renal function	Removes K^+ in dialysate	. . .	Risks associated with dialysis
Exchange transfusion	ECG changes or very high K^+ level	Donor blood has had most K^+ removed	Double volume	Risks associated with exchange transfusion

ECG, electrocardiogram; IV, intravenous; K^+, potassium; PO, orally; PR, parenterally.

Table 43. Drugs Associated with Hypokalemia

Drugs associated with increased renal loss
- Aminoglycoside toxicity
- Amphotericin B
- Cisplatin
- Penicillins in high doses
- Corticosteroids
- Diuretics (except for potassium-sparing ones)

Drugs associated with increased cellular uptake of potassium
- Terbutaline
- Epinephrine
- β-Adrenergic agents (e.g., albuterol)
- Theophylline toxicity
- Barium toxicity
- Insulin

Table 44. Oral Potassium Supplements

Preparation	Formulation	Potassium Supplied
Potassium phosphate	Tablet	1.1, 2.3, or 3.7 mEq
Potassium chloride	Extentabs	10 mEq
	Powder packet	20 mEq
	Effervescent tablets	20 mEq
	Liquid	20 mEq
Potassium citrate	Tablets, crystals, or syrup	1 mEq/mL (Polycitra) or 2 mEq/mL (Polycitra-K)
Potassium gluconate	Liquid	20 mEq/15 mL

Table 45. Commonly Used Calcium Preparations

Preparation	Elemental Calcium Content	Route
Calcium gluconate (10%)	1 mL = 9 mg = 0.45 mEq	IV
Calcium chloride (10%)	1 mL = 27 mg = 1.36 mEq	IV
Calcium glubionate (Neocalglucon)	1 mL = 23 mg = 1.12 mEq	PO

Table 46. Calcium Needs

Maintenance calcium (not precisely known)	20–50 mg/kg/d (elemental calcium)
Emergency calcium (for severe symptoms)	10–20 mg/kg (elemental calcium) slow IV with cardiac monitor

Table 47. Characteristics of Renal Tubular Acidosis

	Type 1	Type 2	Type 3
Renal function?	Normal	Normal	Normal or decreased
Failure to thrive?	Yes	Yes	Yes
Polyuria or polydipsia?	Yes	Yes	No
Potassium level?	Normal or low	Normal or low	Elevated
Bicarbonate leak?	Usually	Significant	Small
Urine maximally acid?	No (pH > 6)	Yes	Yes
Nephrocalcinosis or nephrolithiasis?	Yes	No	No
Fanconi syndrome?	No	Often	No
Osteomalacia or rickets?	Rarely	If Fanconi syndrome is present	No

Table 48. Toxins Removed by Hemodialysis

Toxin	Measured Level Suggestive of Need for Hemodialysis[a]
Acetaminophen	>100 mcg/mL in conjunction with antidote
Arsenic	Only with coexistent renal failure
Bromide	>150 mg/dL and severe symptoms
Chloral hydrate	250 mg/dL
Ethanol	600 mg/dL
Ethylene glycol	50 mg/dL
Isopropanol	400 mg/dL
Lithium	4 mEq/L in acute overdose
	As needed for severe symptoms in chronic overdose
Methanol	50 mq/dL
Salicylates	100–120 mg/dL in acute overdose
	60–800 mg/dL in chronic overdose

[a] The decision to perform hemodialysis should be based on physical findings as well as drug levels. A repeat measure should be obtained when the drug level is elevated to ensure that a laboratory error has not occurred. In addition, units of measure should be checked before instituting hemodialysis.

Table 49. Toxins Removed by Charcoal Hemoperfusion[a]

Toxin	Measured Level Suggestive of Need for Charcoal Hemoperfusion
Amitriptyline	Based on signs and symptoms
Chloral hydrate	250 mg/dL
Digitoxin	50 ng/mL with antidotal therapy
Digoxin	15 ng/mL with antidotal therapy
Ethchlorvinyl	150 mcg/mL
Glutethimide	40 mg/L
Methaqualone	40 mcg/mL
Notriptyline	Based on signs and symptoms
Pentobarbital	50 mg/L
Phenobarbital	100 mg/L
Theophylline	100 mcg/mL in acute overdose
	60 mcg/mL in chronic overdose

[a] The decision to perform hemoperfusion should be based on physical findings as well as drug levels. A repeat measure should be obtained when the drug level is elevated to ensure that a laboratory error has not occurred. In addition, units of measure should be checked before instituting hemodialysis.

Table 50. Normal Values for Fractional Excretion of Sodium (Fe$_{Na}$)

	Prerenal ARF	Intrinsic ARF
Adult or child	<1.0	>2.0
Infant (neonate)	<2.5	>2.5

ARF, acute renal failure.

Table 51. Causes of False-Positive Dipstick Reactions for Urinary Protein

Overlong immersion
Placing reagent strip directly in the urine stream
Alkaline urinary pH (pH >7.0)
Quaternary ammonium compounds and detergents
Pyuria
Bacteriuria
Mucoprotein

Table 52. Drugs that May Cause Hemolytic Anemia in Patients Who Have G6PD Deficiency

Acetanilid	Nitrofurantoin
Doxorubicin	Primaquine
Methylene blue	Pamaquine
Naphthalene	Sulfa drugs

Table 53. Clinical Aids in Distinguishing the Origin of Hematuria

Test For	Glomerular or Renal	Extrarenal
Urine color	Brown, tea or cola colored, cloudy, red	Red, pink
Clots	Usually absent	May be present
RBC casts	Frequently present	Never present
Red cell morphology	Dysmorphic or distorted	Normal RBC shape (eumorphic)
Urine stream	Bloody throughout entire stream	More bloody at initiation (suggesting distal urethral origin) or termination (suggesting trigonitis or cystitis)

Table 54. Characteristics of the Three Stages of Parapneumonic Pleural Effusions

	Exudative Stage	Fibrinolytic Stage	Organizing Stage (Empyema)
Appearance	Nonpurulent, not turbid	Nonpurulent, not turbid	Purulent, turbid
Fluid consistency	Free flowing	Loculated	Organized
Gram stain and culture results	Negative	Transitional	Positive (before antibiotic treatment)
Glucose	>100 mg/dL	<50 mg/dL	<50 mg/dL
Protein	<3 g/dL	>3 g/dL	>3 g/dL
pH	>7.30	<7.30	<7.30
WBCs	Few	PMNs	PMNs

PMNs, polymorphonuclear neutrophils; WBCs, white blood cells.

Table 55. Pleural Fluid Diagnostic Studies

Study	Transudate	Exudate
Biochemical		
Pleural LDH	<200 IU	≥200 IU
Pleural fluid/serum LDH ratio[a]	<0.6	≥0.6
Pleural fluid/serum protein ratio[a]	<0.5	≥0.5
Specific gravity	<1.016	≥1.016
Protein level	<3.0 g/dL	≥3.0 g/dL
Other studies		
Glucose	*Usually* >40 mg/dL	*Typically* <40 mg/dL
Amylase	May be elevated in some neoplasms, GI trauma, or surgery	
Rheumatoid factor, LE prep, ANA	Are occasionally helpful if collagen vascular disorders are within the differential	
Hematologic		
WBC count	Although high counts (>100/mm³) are suggestive of an exudate, the results are quite variable	
WBC differential	May actually provide more useful information	
Lymphocyte count	May be elevated in neoplasms, tuberculosis, and some fungal infections	
Segmented neutrophils	May be elevated in bacterial infections, connective tissue disease, pancreatitis, or pulmonary infarction	
Eosinophil count	May be elevated in bacterial infections, neoplasms, and connective tissue diseases	
RBC count	If >100,000/mm³, is suggestive of trauma, neoplasms, or pulmonary infarction	
Cytology and chromosomal studies	May show evidence of malignant cells or chromosomal abnormalities	
Microbiology		
Gram stain		
Fluid culture for aerobes and anaerobes		
Acid-fast stain (if tuberculosis is in the differential)		
Fungal culture		
Viral culture		
Counterimmune electrophoresis may aid in the detection of a bacterial infection)		

[a] These tests are more reliable in differentiating transudate from exudate than specific gravity or protein level.

Table 56. Normal Blood Gas Values from the Children's Hospital of Philadelphia Blood Gas Laboratory

Parameter	Age of Patient	Normal Value
pH	1 day	7.29–7.45
	3–24 months	7.34–7.46
	>7 years	7.37–7.41
Pco$_2$	1 day	27–40 mm Hg
	3–24 months	26–42 mm Hg
	>7 years	34–40 mm Hg
Po$_2$	1 day	37–97 mm Hg
	3–24 months	88–103 mm Hg
	>7 years	88–103 mm Hg
Base excess	1 day	>8–(−2)
	3–24 months	−7–0
	>7 years	−4–(+2)
HCO$_3$	1 day	19 mmol/L
	3–24 months	16/24 mmol/L
	>7 years	22–27 mmol/L
α_2 saturation	. . .	94%–99%
Venous pH	. . .	7.32–7.42
Venous CO$_2$		25–47 mm Hg
Venous O$_2$		25–47 mm Hg

CO$_2$, carbon dioxide; HCO$_3$, bicarbonate; O$_2$ = oxygen; Pco$_2$, carbon dioxide tension; Po$_2$, oxygen tension.

Table 57. Signs of Inhalation Injury

Pulmonary	CNS	Skin
Tachypnea	Confusion	Facial burns
Stridor	Dizziness	Singed nasal hairs
Hoarseness	Headache	Cyanosis
Rales	Hallucinations	Cherry red color
Wheezing	Restlessness	
Cough	Coma	
Retractions	Seizures	
Nasal flaring		
Carbonaceous sputum		

Table 58. Pulmonary Function Test

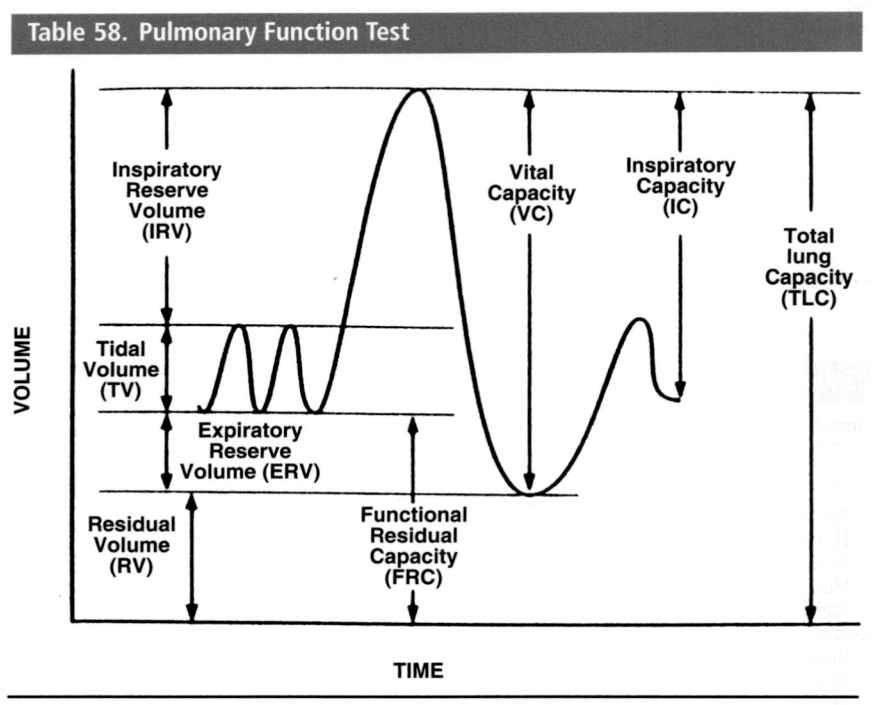

Table 59. Common Causes of Abnormally Wide Splitting of the Second Heart Sound (S₂)

Atrial septal defect (ASD)
Mild pulmonic stenosis
Complete right bundle branch block
Left ventricular paced beats
Massive pulmonary embolus

Table 60. Conditions Causing a Prominent Third Heart Sound (S₃)

Physiologic (infants and children)
Congestive heart failure (CHF)
Ventricular septal defect, with large pulmonary to systemic
　flow ratio
Mitral insufficiency
Tricuspid insufficiency
Hyperdynamic ventricle with high output (e.g., anemia, thyrotoxicosis,
　arteriovenous fistula)

Table 61. Conditions Causing a Prominent Fourth Heart Sound (S₄)

Left ventricular outflow tract obstruction (e.g., aortic stenosis)
Right ventricular outflow tract obstruction (e.g., pulmonic stenosis)
Hypertrophic cardiomyopathy
Heart block (atrium contracting against a closed valve)

Table 62. Drugs Associated with Rapid Heart Rates

Prescription drugs
　β-adrenergic agonists (e.g., albuterol)
　Methylxanthines (e.g., theophylline)
　Tricyclic antidepressants (e.g., imipramine)
　Nonsedating histamines (e.g., terfenadine)
Over-the-counter drugs
　Decongestants (e.g., pseudoephedrine)
　Diet aids (phenylpropanolamine)
　Inhaled bronchodilators (e.g., albuterol)
　Caffeine-containing products
Drugs of abuse
　Nicotine
　Cocaine
　Amphetamines
　Alcohol
　Marijuana
　LSD
　Phencyclidine
　Amyl nitrate

Table 63. Causes of Prolonged QT Interval

Congenital
　Hereditary
　　Jervell and Lange-Nielsen syndrome: Long QT interval, stress-induced
　　　syncope, congenital nerve deafness, autosomal-recessive
　　　inheritance
　　Romano-Ward syndrome: Long QT interval, stress-induced syncope,
　　　autosomal-dominant inheritance (usually incomplete
　　　penetrance)
　Sporadic
Acquired
　Electrolyte abnormalities
　　Hypocalcemia
　　Hypomagnesemia
　Metabolic disturbances
　　Malnutrition
　　Liquid protein diets
　Drugs
　　Phenothiazines (e.g., haloperidol)
　　Tricyclic antidepressants (e.g., imipramine)
　　Nonsedating antihistamines (e.g., terfenadine)
　　Class Ia antiarrhythmic agents (e.g., quinidine)
　　Class III antiarrhythmic agents (e.g., amiodarone)
　CNS trauma
　Cardiac abnormalities
　　Ischemia
　　Mitral valve prolapse
　　Myocarditis
　Intraventricular conduction abnormalities
　　Bundle branch blocks

Table 64. Structural Heart Disease Associated with Tachycardia

Defect	Type of Tachycardia
Congenital heart disease	
Mitral valve prolapse	SVT, VT
Aortic valve stenosis or regurgitation	VT
Ebstein anomaly of the tricuspid valve	SVT (WPW) commonly, VT less commonly
Tetralogy of Fallot	VT
Mustard/Senning repair of D-TGA	SVT (particularly atrial flutter)
Fontan repair of single ventricle	SVT (particularly atrial flutter)
Cardiomyopathy	
Hypertrophic cardiomyopathy	SVT, VT
Dilated cardiomyopathy	SVT, VT
Arrhythmogenic right ventricular dysplasia	VT (monomorphic, left bundle branch block)
Miscellaneous causes	
Cardiac tumor (atrial myxoma, rhabdomyosarcoma)	VT
Eisenmenger complex (pulmonary vascular disease and pulmonary hypertension)	SVT, VT (depending on tumor site)

D-TGA, D-transposition of the great arteries; SVT, supraventricular tachycardia; VT, ventricular tachycardia; WPW, Wolff-Parkinson-White syndrome.

Table 65. Poisons Causing Tachycardia

Tachycardia and hypertension
  Amphetamines
  Antihistamines
  Cocaine
  LSD/PCP
Tachycardia and hypotension
  β_2-Adrenergic agonists
    Albuterol
    Terbutaline
  Carbon monoxide
  Cyclic antidepressants
  Hydralazine
  Iron
  Phenothiazines
  Theophylline
  Any agent causing vomiting, diarrhea, or hemorrhage

LSD, lysergic acid diethylamide; PCP, phencyclidine hydrochloride.

Table 66. Poisons Causing Bradycardia

Bradycardia and hypertension
  α-Adrenergic agonists
    Phenylpropanolamine
    Ephedrine
  Clonidine
  Ergotamine
Bradycardia and hypotension
  α_1-Adrenergic antagonists
    Phentolamine
    Prazosin
  α_1-Adrenergic agonists
    Clonidine
    Tetrahydrozoline
  β-Adrenergic antagonists
    Propranolol
    Atenolol
    Metoprolol
  Calcium channel blockers
  Digitalis-containing drugs and plants
  Narcotics
  Organophosphate pesticides
  Sedative/Hypnotics

Table 67. Poisons Causing Cardiac Arrhythmias

Atrioventricular block
  Astemizole
  β-Adrenergic antagonists
  Calcium channel blockers
  Clonidine
  Cyclic antidepressants
  Digitalis-containing drugs and plants
Ventricular tachycardia
  Amphetamines
  Carbamazepine
  Chloral hydrate
  Chlorinated hydrocarbons
  Cocaine
  Cyclic antidepressants
  Digitalis-containing drugs or plants
  Phenothiazines (especially thioridazine)
  Theophylline
  Type Ia antiarrhythmic agents
    Quinidine
    Procainamide
  Type Ic antiarrhythmic agents
    Flecainide
    Encainide
Torsades de pointes (multifocal ventricular tachycardia)
  Amantadine
  Cyclic antidepressants
  Lithium
  Nonsedating antihistamines
    Astemizole
    Terfenadine
  Quinidine
  Phenothiazines
  Sotalol

Table 68. Revised Jones Criteria for Diagnosis of Acute Rheumatic Fever

Major Criteria	Minor Criteria
Carditis	Fever
Arthritis	Arthralgia
Rash (erythema marginatum)	Elevated ESR, CRP
Chorea (Sydenham)	Prolonged PR interval on ECG
Subcutaneous nodules	History of prior attack of rheumatic fever or rheumatic heart disease

Diagnosis is likely with the presence of two major and one minor criteria, or one major and two minor criteria. Supporting evidence of a preceding streptococcal infection includes a history of recent scarlet fever, a positive throat culture for group A *Streptococcus*, and an increased antistreptolysin O (ASO) titer (or titers for other streptococcal antibodies). Adapted from the Report of the Ad Hoc Committee of the American Heart Association Council on Rheumatic Fever and Congenital Heart Disease. *Circulation*. 1984;69:204A–208A. CRP, C-reactive protein; ECG, electrocardiogram; ESR, erythrocyte sedimentation rate.

Table 69. Range of Motion of Major Joints

	Flexion	Extension	Abduction	Adduction	Internal Rotation	External Rotation
Hip	120°	30°	50°	30°	35°	45°
Knee	135°	5°	0°	0°	10°	10°
Ankle	50°	20°	10°	20°	5° (eversion)	5° (inversion)
Shoulder	90°	45°	180°	45°	55°	45°
Elbow	135°	5°	0°	0°	90° (supination)	90° (pronation)
Wrist	80°	70°	20° (radial)	30° (lunar)	0°	0°

Table 70. Characteristics of Synovial Fluid

	Appearance	WBC/mm^2	% Neutrophils	% Glucose Synovial Blood
Normal	Clear	<2,000	<40	>50
Infectious	Turbid	>75,000	>75	<50
Inflammatory (JRA, SLE)	Clear/Turbid	5,000–75,000	50	≥50
Traumatic	Bloody/Clear	<5,000	<50	>50

Table 71. Relationship Between Short Stature, Bone Age, and Growth Velocity[a]

Bone age delayed—normal growth velocity	Constitutional short stature
Bone age normal—normal growth velocity	Genetic short stature
Bone age delayed—delayed growth velocity	Organic diseases

[a] Velocity = the rate of growth during a year.

Table 72. Clinical and Biochemical Features of Congenital Adrenal Hyperplasia (CAH)

Enzyme defect	Sexual Ambiguity		Additional Clinical Manifestations	Predominant Steroids
	Female	Male		
Desmolase	−	+	Salt wasting	...
3β-Hydroxysteroid dehydrogenase	+	+	Salt wasting	17-OH-pregnenolone, DHEA
21-Hydroxylase	+	−	Salt wasting	17-OH-progestone, androstenedione
11-Hydroxylase	+	−	Hypertension	11-Deoxycortisol
17-Hydroxylase	−	+	Hypertension	DOC, corticosterone

DHEA, dehydroepiandrosterone; DOE, deoxycorticosterone.

Table 73. Normal Serum Adrenal Steroid Levels in Newborn Infants

Steroid	Preterm Sick		Preterm Well	Full Term
	24–28 Weeks	31–35 Weeks	31–35 Weeks	
Cortisol (mcg/dL)	7.5 ± 4	6 ± 2.7	6.9 ± 3.8	6.2 ± 3.9
17-OH-Preg (ng/dL)	1794 ± 1818	1395 ± 694	942 ± 739	245 ± 291
17-OH-Pro (ng/dL)	651 ± 661	373 ± 317	169 ± 95	36 ± 13[a]
11-deoxycortisol (ng/dL)	662 ± 548	294 ± 239	111 ± 62	87 ± 42
DHEA (ng/dL)	1872 ± 4038	675 ± 502	920 ± 1227	286 ± 238
DHEAS (mcg/dL)	467 ± 312	459 ± 209	341 ± 93	162 ± 88
Androstenedione (ng/dL)	479 ± 1032	206 ± 86	215 ± 134	149 ± 67

Data based on information in Lee MM, Rajabopalan L, Berg G, et al. Serum adrenal steroid concentrations in premature infants. *J Clin Endocrinol Metab*. 1989;69:1133–1136, and in Wiener D, Smith J, Dahlem S, et al. Serum adrenal steroid levels in healthy term 3-day-old infants. *J Pediatr*. 1987;110(1):122–124.
17-OH-Preg, 17-OH-pregnenolone; 17-OH-Pro, 17-OH-progesterone; DHEA, dehydroepiandrosterone; DHEAS, dehydroepiandrosterone sulfate.
[a] 17-OH-Pro values in full-term sick newborns may be double or triple the baseline values. No data are available for other steroid hormones in sick full-term infants.

Table 74. Pharmacokinetics of Common Insulin Preparations

Insulin Preparation	Onset (Hours)	Peak (Hours)	Duration of Action (Hours)
Ultra-rapid-acting (Lispro)	0.25–0.50	1–2	2–3
Short-acting (Regular, Semilente)	0.5–1.0	2–4	4–6
Long-acting (NPH, Lente)	2–4	6–12	18–24
Very long-acting (Ultralente)	6–10	18–24	24–36

NPH, neutral protein Hagedorn insulin.

Table 75. Normal Thyroid Hormone Levels

T_4	Total	7.0–15.0 mcg/dL
	Free	0.8–2.3 ng/dL
T_3		100–250 ng/dL
TSH		0.5–5.0 mcg/dL

Table 76. Normal Ranges for Gonadotropin and Sex Steroid Levels: Females

	LH (mLU/mL)	FSH (mLU/mL)	Estradiol (ng/dL)	Testosterone (ng/dL)
0–1 year	0.02–7.0	0.24–14.2	0.5–5.0	<10
Prepubertal	0.02–0.3	1.0–4.2	<1.5	<3–10
Tanner 2	0.02–4.7	1.0–10.8	1.0–2.4	7.0–28
Tanner 3	0.10–12.0	1.5–12.8	0.7–6.0	15–35
Tanner 4	0.4–11.7	1.5–11.7	2.1–8.5	13–32
Tanner 5	0.4–11.7	1.0–9.2	3.4–17.0	20–38
Adult	. . .	. . .	. . .	10–55
Follicular phase	2.0–9.0	1.8–11.2	3.0–10.0	. . .
Midcycle	18.0–49	6.0–35.0	. . .	. . .
Luteal phase	2.0–11.0	1.8–11.2	7.0–30.0	. . .

FSH, follicle-stimulating hormone; LH, luteinizing hormone.

Table 77. Normal Ranges for Gonadotropin and Sex Steroid Levels: Males

	LH (mLU/mL)	FSH (mLU/mL)	Estradiol (ng/dL)	Testosterone (ng/dL)
0–1 year	0.02–7.0	0.16–4.1	1.0–3.2	<10
Prepubertal	0.02–0.3	0.26–3.0	<1.5	<3–10
Tanner 2	0.2–4.9	1.8–3.2	0.5–1.6	18–150
Tanner 3	0.2–5.0	1.2–5.8	0.5–2.5	100–320
Tanner 4	0.4–7.0	2.0–9.2	1.0–3.6	200–620
Tanner 5	0.4–7.0	2.6–11.0	1.0–3.6	350–970
Adult	1.5–9.0	2.0–9.2	0.8–3.5	350–1,030

FSH, follicle-stimulating hormone; LH, leuteinizing hormone.

Table 78. Classification of Total and LDL Cholesterol Levels in Children and Adolescents from Families with Hypercholesterolemia or Premature Cardiovascular Disease

Category	Total Cholesterol, mg/dL	LDL Cholesterol, mg/dL
Acceptable	<170	<110
Borderline	170–199	110–129
High	≥200	≥130

Table 79. Causes and Management of Rickets

Cause	Management
Calcium Deficiency	
Low intake	<6 months of age 400 mg/d
	6–12 months of age 600 mg/d
	1–10 years of age 800 mg/d
Extreme prematurity (birth weight <1,500 g)	Adjust intake to 200 mg/kg/d
Steatorrhea	25-OH-D_3 (5–7 mcg/kg/d) if serum levels are low and supplement dietary calcium between 25 and 100 mg/kg/d
Anticonvulsant (Phenobarbital or phenytoin)	**Calcium**
	<6 months of age 400 mg/d
	6–12 months of age 600 mg/d
	1–10 years of age 800 mg/d
	Vitamin D
	200 IU/d of ergocalciferol
Renal tubular acidosis	Base supplement: 3–10 mM/kg/d as $NaHCO_3$ or citrate
Vitamin D Deficiency	
Insufficient UV light exposure	200 IU/d of vitamin D of ergocalciferol
Breastfeed infants who are not supplemented with vitamin D	200 IU/d of vitamin D of ergocalciferol
Liver disease	4,000–8,000 IU/d ergocalciferol
Renal disorders	4,000–40,000 IU/d of Calcitriol
Nutritional rickets and osteomalacia	1,000–5,000 IU/day of ergocalciferol
Vitamin D–dependent rickets	3,000–5,000 IU/d of Calcitriol
Vitamin D–resistant rickets	40,000–80,000 IU/d of ergocalciferol with phosphate supplements, daily dosage is increased at 3–4 month intervals in 10,000–20,000 IU increments
Phosphorus Deficiency	
Diet (limited to premature infants)	Adjust formula or parenteral source to give 10 mg/kg/d
Antacid excess	Alternative gastric acid control
Excessive phosphaturia from tubular dysfunction	Supplemental P and calcitriol if low

Table 80. Classification of Rickets and Vitamin D Metabolite Levels

	Calcium	Phosphorus	Alkaline Phosphate	25 (OH)D
Deficient synthesis and supply No sunlight Poor diet Immaturity	N or ↓	↓	↑	↓
Malabsorption	N or ↓	↓	↑	↓
Liver disease	N or ↓	↓	↑	↓
Chronic renal failure	N or ↓	↑	↑	N
Vitamin D–dependent rickets (recessively inherited)	↓	↓	↑	N
Vitamin D–resistant rickets (sex-linked dominant)	N	↓	↑	N
Renal tubular disorders (defect of phosphate reabsorption)	N	↓	↑	N

N, normal; ↓, decreased; ↑, increased.

Table 81. Causes of Ataxia

Form of Ataxia	Major Causes	Other Causes
Acute ataxia	Ingestion Postinfectious cerebellitis	Migraine Neuroblastoma
Acute recurrent ataxia	Migraine Metabolic disease	. . .
Chronic ataxia	Congenital disorders with mental deficiency	. . .
Chronic progressive ataxia	Brain tumors Neuroectodermal tumors	Ataxia-telangiectasia Friedreich ataxia

Table 82. Glasgow Coma Scale

Eyes open			Best motor response	
Spontaneously	4		Obey commands	6
To speech	3		Localize pain	5
To pain	2		Withdrawal	4
None	1		Flexion to pain	3
Best verbal response			Extension to pain	2
Oriented	5		None	1
Confused	4			
Inappropriate	3			
Incomprehensible	2			
None	1			

Adapted from Fleisher G, Ludwig S, eds. *Textbook of pediatric emergency medicine*, 3rd ed. Baltimore: Williams & Wilkins, 1993:272.

Table 83. Glasgow Coma Scale (GCS) for Adults and Children and Modified Score for Infants

	Glasgow Coma Score (Adults/Older Children)		Modified Glasgow Coma Score (Infants)
Eye Opening	Spontaneous	4	Spontaneous
	To verbal stimuli	3	To speech
	To pain	2	To pain
	None	1	None
Best Verbal Response	Oriented	5	Coos and babbles
	Confused speech	4	Irritable, cries
	Inappropriate words	3	Cries to pain
	Nonspecific sounds	2	Moans to pain
	None	1	None
Best Motor Response	Follows commands	6	Normal spontaneous movements
	Localizes pain	5	Withdraws to touch
	Withdraws to pain	4	Withdraws to pain
	Flexes to pain	3	Abnormal flexion
	Extends to pain	2	Abnormal extension
	None	1	None

Table 84. Drugs that Can Cause Delirium or Coma

Drug	Physical Findings
Barbiturates	Small, reactive pupils; hypothermia; flaccidity; doll's eye reflex may be absent
Opiates	Pinpoint, reactive pupils; hypothermia; hypotension; hypoventilation; bradycardia
Psychedelics	Small, reactive pupils; hypertension; hyperventilation; dystonic posturing
Amphetamines	Dilated pupils, hyperthermia, hypertension, tachycardia, arrhythmia
Cocaine	Dilated pupils, hyperthermia, tachycardia
Atropine-scopolamine	Dilated pupils; hyperthermia; flushing; hot, dry skin; supraventricular tachycardia
Glutethimide	Midposition, irregular fixed pupils; hypothermia; flaccidity
Tricyclic antidepressants	Hyperthermia, hypotension, supraventricular tachycardia
Phenothiazines	Hypotension, arrhythmia, dystonia
Methaqualone	Same as with barbiturates; if severe tachycardia, dystonia

From Packer RJ, Berman PH. Coma. In: Fleisher GR, Ludwig S, eds. *Textbook of pediatric emergency medicine*, 3rd ed. Baltimore: Williams & Wilkins, 1993:126, with permission.

Table 85. Prognostic Indicators of Poor Neurologic Outcome in Near-Drowning Victims[a]

At the scene
    Submersion time >4–10 minutes
    Delay in beginning CPR
    Resuscitation >25 minutes
In the emergency department
    Necessity for CPR
    Fixed, dilated pupils
    pH <7.0
    GCS score <5
After initial resuscitation
    Persistent GCS score <5
    Persistent apnea

CPR, cardiopulmonary resuscitation; GCS, Glasgow Coma Scale.
[a] Applies to victims of warm water near-drownings only. Hypothermic victims of cold water near-drownings may have a better prognosis.

Table 86. Relationship of the Lesion to the Physical Findings

Lesion	Findings
Upper motor neuron involving corticospinal tract, thalamus, centrum, semiovale, motor cortex	Altered, normal or increased reflexes, bulk normal; strength normal or decreased
Cerebellum	Uncoordinated
Spinal (upper and lower motor)	Local pain, bowel and bladder dysfunction, if anterior horn cells involved, weakness and bulk, decreased absent reflexes, fasciculations
Peripheral	Loss of distal muscles, fasciculations less than spinal lesions; sensation is affected
Muscle	Weakness, muscle atrophy, decreased reflexes, pain, cramping, stiffness
Corticospinal tract	Increased tone, clasp knife character in flexion of arms and extension of legs
Extrapyramidal (basal ganglia)	Rigidity, normal reflexes, absent Babinski, voluntary movement is preserved, may have tremor, chorea, athetosis or dystonia

Table 87. Poisons Causing Coma

Coma with miosis
    Barbiturates and other sedative/hypnotics
    Bromide
    Chloral hydrate
    Clonidine
    Ethanol
    Narcotics
    Organophosphates
    PCP
    Phenothiazines
    Tetrahydrozoline
Coma with mydriasis
    Atropine/diphenoxylate
    Carbon monoxide
    Cyanide
    Cyclic antidepressants
    Glutethimide
    LSD

LSD, lysergic acid diethylamide; PCP, phencyclidine hydrochloride.

Table 88. Poisons Causing Seizures

Amoxapine
Amphetamines
Anticonvulsants
    Phenytoin
    Carbamazepine
Antihistamines and anticholinergic drugs or plants
Camphor
Carbon monoxide
Chlorinated hydrocarbons
Cocaine
Cyanide
Cyclic antidepressants
Isoniazid
Lead
Lidocaine
Meperidine
PCP
Phenothiazines
Phenylpropanolamine
Propoxyphene
Propranolol
Theophylline

PCP, phencyclidine hydrochloride.

Table 89. Differential Diagnosis of Metabolic Neurologic Dysfunction

Prominent Symptom	Diagnoses to Consider	Diagnostic Test	Metabolic Therapy
Myoclonic seizures	Ceroid	DNA, tissue EM	
	Lafora body disease	Muscle biopsy	
	Prion (GSS)	DNA	
	Mitochondrial	DNA, muscle biopsy	CoQ, other vitamins
	Aminoacidopathies	Blood biochemistry	Dietary
	Biotinidase deficiency	Blood biochemistry	Biotin supplement
	Organic acidurias	Blood biochemistry	Dietary, vitamins
Stroke	Homocystinuria	Blood/Urine test	B vitamins, betaine
	Mitochondrial	DNA, muscle biopsy	
Coma	Organic aciduria	Blood/Urine test	
	MSUD	Blood/Urine test	
	Hyperammonemias	Blood test	Dietary
Spasticity	Leukodystrophy	MRI, fibroblast analysis	Dietary
Visual loss	Leukodystrophy	MRI	
	Mitochondrial	DNA, muscle biopsy	
Psychosis	Leukodystrophy	MRI, blood biochemistry, DNA, fibroblast analysis	
	Porphyria	Blood/Urine Biochemistry	Avoid precipitants
	Wilson disease	Copper excretion, DNA	Penicillamine
	Homocystinuria	Blood biochemistry	(See above)
	Ceroid	DNA, tissue electron microscopy	
	Huntington disease	DNA	
Microcephaly	Ceroid	DNA, tissue EM	
	Rett syndrome	(Clinical features)	
	Krabbe disease	Blood biochemistry	
Macrocephaly	Storage disorders	DNA, blood biochemistry	
	Canavan disease	Urine biochemistry, DNA	
Neuropathy	Krabbe disease	MRI and blood biochemistry	
	Metachromatic leukodystrophy		
	Porphyria	Blood/Urine biochemistry	
	Mitochondrial	DNA, muscle biopsy	
	Friedreich ataxia	(Clinical features)	
	Abetalipoproteinemia		
	Disorders/deficiency of vitamin E	Blood biochemistry	Vitamin E
	Mitochondrial	Vitamin E level	Vitamin E
	Neuroaxonal dystrophy	DNA, muscle biopsy	
		MRI, nerve biopsy	
Myopathy	Fukuyama disease	MRI	
	Mitochondrial	DNA, muscle biopsy	
	Lactic acidoses	Blood biochemistry	
Ataxia	Ataxia telangiectasia	DNA	
	Leukodystrophies	MRI, blood biochemistry	
	Friedreich		
	Mitochondrial	(Clinical features)	
	Hartnup	DNA, muscle biopsy	
	Hyperammonemias	Blood biochemistry	
	Abetalipoproteinemia	Blood biochemistry	
	Sphingolipidoses	Blood biochemistry	
	Machado-Joseph, SCA-1 (hereditary ataxias)	Blood biochemistry, fibroblast analysis, DNA	

Table 90. Acquired Disorders Associated with Progressive Neurologic Dysfunction

Structural	Hormonal	Infectious	Environmental	Toxic	Immunologic
Hydrocephalus Brain tumor Vascular anomalies	Hypothyroidism Congenital adrenal hyperplasia (visuospatial deficits)	SSPE HIV Spirochetes	Malnutrition/Malabsorption syndromes Vitamin/Trace element deficiency (niacin, thiamine, folic acid, vitamin E, B$_{12}$, essential fatty acids) Physical abuse/neglect	Lead Organic chemicals Carbon monoxide Cocaine, hallucinogens, hypnotics Phenytoin (cerebellar degeneration)	Demyelination/Multiple sclerosis Opsoclonus/Myoclonus or cerebellar ataxia (neuroblastoma) Sydenham chorea Rasmussen encephalitis

Table 91. Epidural versus Acute Subdural Hematoma

	Epidural Hematoma	Subdural Hematoma
Common mechanism	Blunt direct trauma, frequently to parietal region	Acceleration-deceleration injury
Etiology	Arterial or venous	Venous (bridging veins below dura)
Incidence	Uncommon	Common
Peak age	Usually >2 years	Usually <1 year Peak at 6 months
Location	Unilateral Commonly parietal	75% bilateral Diffuse, over cerebral hemispheres
Skull fracture	Common	Uncommon
Associated seizures	Uncommon	Common
Retinal hemorrhages	Rare	Common
Decreased level of consciousness	Common	Almost always
Mortality	Rare	Uncommon
Morbidity in survivors	Low	High
Clinical findings	Dilated ipsilateral pupil, contralateral hemiparesis Period of lucidity prior to acute decompensation and rapid progression to herniation	Decreased level of consciousness Irritability, lethargy
Onset	Acute	Acute (within 24 hours), subacute (within 1 day–2 weeks), or chronic (after 2 weeks)
Findings on CT	Convex "lens-shaped" cerebral hemisphere	Concave, diffusely surrounding cerebral hemisphere

CT, computed tomography.

Table 92. Age-Related Prevalence of Principal Laparoscopic Findings in 121 Adolescent Females 11 to 17 Years Old with Acute Pelvic Pain (The Children's Hospital, Boston, 1980–1986)

Diagnosis	Number of Patients		
	Age 11–13	Age 14–15	Age 16–17
Ovarian cyst	12 (50%)	16 (35%)	19 (37%)
Acute pelvic inflammatory disease	4 (17%)	7 (16%)	10 (19%)
Adnexal torsion	0 (0%)	7 (16%)	2 (4%)
Endometriosis	0 (0%)	2 (4%)	4 (7%)
Ectopic pregnancy	0 (0%)	3 (7%)	1 (2%)
Appendicitis	3 (13%)	4 (9%)	6 (12%)
No pathology	5 (20%)	6 (13%)	10 (19%)
Total	24 (20%)	45 (37%)	52 (43%)

From Goldstein DP. Acute and chronic pelvic pain. *Pediatr Clin North Am*. 1989;36(3):576.

Table 93. Key Characteristics of Vaginal Discharges

	Presenting Symptoms	Discharge	Nonmenstrual pH	Amine/ Whiff Test	Vaginal Smear	Treatment
Nonspecific vaginitis	Foul-smelling discharge Itching	Scant to copious Brown to green in color	Variable	Negative	Leukocytes Bacteria and other debris	Improved perineal hygiene
Physiologic leukorrhea	None	Variable Scant to moderate Clear to white	<4.5	Negative	Normal epithelial cells Lactobacilli predominate	None
Bacterial vaginosis	Foul-smelling discharge	Gray-white	>4.7	Positive	Epithelial cells with bacteria ("clue cells") Gram-negative rods	Metronidazole Clindamycin
Candidiasis	Severe itching Vulvar inflammation	White, "curd-like"	<4.5	Negative	Fungal hyphae and buds	Topical or intravaginal imidazoles, triazoles Oral ketoconazole
Trichomonal vaginitis	Copious discharge Itching	Profuse Yellow to green	5.0–6.0	Occasionally present	Motile flagellated organisms	Metronidazole
Foreign body	Foul-smelling discharge	Foul-smelling Purulent Dark brown	Variable (usually >4.7)	Occasionally present	Leukocytes Epithelial cells with bacteria and debris	Remove foreign body Irrigate vagina
Contact vulvovaginitis	Vulvar inflammation Itching Edema	Scant White to yellow	Variable (usually <4.5)	Negative	Leukocytes Epithelial cells	Remove irritant Topical steroids

Table 94. Emergency Contraceptive Pills

Instructions for Use

Any of the birth control pills listed below can be used as ECPs. Use only the type of pill your health care provider prescribed for you. Use only one type of pill.

If You Are Taking	Number of Pills to Swallow as Soon as Possible (1st Dose)	Number of Pills to Swallow 12 Hours Later (2nd Dose)
Ovral	2 white pills	2 white pills
Lo/Ovral	4 white pills	4 white pills
Levlen	4 light-orange pills	4 light-orange pills
Nordette	4 light-orange pills	4 light-orange pills
Tri-Levlen	4 yellow pills	4 yellow pills
Triphasil	4 yellow pills	4 yellow pills
Alesse	5 pink pills	5 pink pills

- To reduce the chance of nausea, take an antinausea medicine (like Dramamine II or Benadryl) 1 hour **before** the first ECP dose; repeat according to labeled instructions. This may make you feel tired, so don't drive or drink any alcohol.
- Take the first ECP dose as soon as convenient **WITHIN 3 DAYS (72 HOURS)** after unprotected sex. Try to time the first dose so that the timing of the second dose will be convenient.
- Take the second ECP dose **12 hours after the first dose.**

IMPORTANT: Do not take any extra ECPs. More pills will probably not make the treatment work better. More pills will increase your risk of feeling sick to your stomach.

- Use condoms, spermicides, or a diaphragm if you have sex after taking ECPs until you get your period. Talk to your health care provider about other regular birth control methods you can use in the future.
- Your next period may be a few days early or late.

IMPORTANT: Do a home pregnancy test or see your health care provider if your period has not started **within 3 weeks** after ECP treatment. You may be pregnant.

Source: Program for Applied Technologies (PATH). *Emergency contraception: Resources for providers.* Seattle, 1997. This patient handout may be reproduced without permission of the publisher.

Table 95. Classification of Burns

Type of Burn	Affected Skin Layer	Appearance
First degree	Epidermis	Erythema, hypersensitivity
Second degree		
Superficial	Upper (papillary) dermis	Erythema, blistering, intact hairs, exquisite pain
Deep	Deep (reticular dermis)	Skin may be white or mottled and nonblanching, or blistered and moist; pain may or may not be present; hairs easily pulled
Third degree	Entire dermis	Dry, white or charred skin; leathery appearance, painless, no hair
Fourth degree	Subcutaneous tissue	Same as third degree; may have exposed muscle and bone

Table 96. "Rule of Nines"

Body Part	Percent of BSA		
	Infant	Child	Adolescent/Adult
Head	18%	13%	9%
Anterior trunk	18%	18%	18%
Posterior trunk	18%	18%	18%
Upper extremity (each)	9%	9%	9%
Lower extremity (each)	14%	16%	18%
Genitalia	1%	1%	1%

For small burns, a rough estimate of the affected BSA can be made by comparing the burn with the size of the child's palm (which represents approximately 1% of the BSA).
BSA, body surface area.

TOXICOLOGY

Table 97. Agents with Limited or Uncertain Binding to Activated Charcoal

Iron
Lithium
Heavy metals
  Arsenic
  Mercury
  Lead
  Thallium
Alcohols
  Methanol
  Ethanol
  Isopropanol
  Ethylene glycol
Hydrocarbons
  Kerosene
Gasoline
Mineral seal oil
Caustics[a]
  NaOH
  KOH
  HCL
  H_2SO_4
Low-molecular-weight
  compounds
Cyanide
Pesticides
  Organophosphates
  Carbamates

[a] Administration of activated charcoal may also impede further management.

Table 98. Agents Causing Hypoglycemia in Overdosed Children

Ethanol
Salicylates
Oral hypoglycemic agents
Propranolol
Insulin

Table 99. Poisons Not Detected on the Comprehensive Drug Screen[a]

β-Adrenergic antagonists
Calcium channel blockers
Carbon monoxide
Clonidine
Cyanide
Iron
LSD
Many benzodiazepines (alprazolam, midazolam, lorazepam)
Most plants and mushrooms

[a] Partial listing of some of the most common poisons.

Table 100. Poisons Causing Respiratory Depression or Apnea[a]

Antipsychotic agents
Carbamate pesticides
Chlorinated hydrocarbons
  Trichloroethylene
  1,1,1-trichloroethane
Clonidine
Coral snake envenomation
Cyclic antidepressants
Ethanol (especially when combined
  with sedative/hypnotics)
Exotic snake envenomation
  Cobras
  Sea snakes
  Mambas
Mojave rattlesnake envenomation
Narcotics
Nicotine
Organophosphate pesticides
Sedative/Hypnotics

[a] Partial list of representative poisons.

Table 101. Poisons Causing an Abnormal Anion Gap[a]

Increased anion gap with
  metabolic acidosis
  Carbon monoxide[b]
  Cyanide
  Ethanol[b]
  Ethylene glycol[b]
  Iron[b]
  Isoniazid
Methanol[b]
Salicylates[b]
Theophylline[b]
Decreased anion gap
  Bromide
  Lithium[b]
  Hypermagnesemia[b]
  Hypercalcemia[b]

[a] Partial list of representative poisons; anion gap = $Na^+ - (Cl^- + CO_2^-)$.
[b] Specific levels rapidly available.

Table 102. Common Poisons and Antidotes

Poison	Antidote	Administration
Acetaminophen	N-Acetylcysteine	Loading dose 140 mg/kg, then 17 doses at 70 mg/kg/dose. Dilute 20% solution to 5%–10% with juice or soda to improve palatability.
Anticholinergics	Physostigmine	
Benzodiazepines	Flumazenil	
β-Adrenergic antagonists	Glucagon	
Calcium channel blockers	Glucagon	
	Calcium gluconate 10%	0.3–0.6 mL/kg (8–16 mEq calcium/kg)
Carbon monoxide	Hyperbaric oxygen	
	Sodium thiosulfate 25%[a]	
Cyanide	Sodium nitrate 3%	Dose depends on hemoglobin (see cyanide antidote kit package insert). Do not exceed recommended dosage. Do not give to patients suffering from concomitant carbon monoxide exposure.
	Sodium thiosulfate 25%	Dose depends on hemoglobin (see cyanide antidote kit package insert).
Digitalis	Digitalis Fab fragments	Calculate dose based on level or dose ingested or 10 vials if acute overdose, 5 vials if chronic overdose.
Ethylene glycol	Ethanol	0.6 g/kg load over 1 hour followed by 100 mg/kg/hr infusion
	Pyridoxine	2 mg/kg and thiamine 0.5 mg/kg
Iron	Deferoxamine	5–15 mg/kg/hr IV infusion
Isoniazid	Pyridoxine	
Lead	Lead level 45–69 mcg/dL	
	Dimercaptosuccinic acid	10 mg/kg PO three times daily for 5 days, then twice daily for 14 days (may be useful at lower levels)
	or	
	Calcium NaEDTA	50–75 mg/kg/day divided, every 6 hours either IM or by slow IV infusion (IV use not FDA-approved)
	Lead level ≥70 mcg/dL	
	Calcium NaEDTA and	Administer as described above
	British anti-lewisite (BAL)	3–5 mg/kg IM every 4 hours for 5 days
Methanol	Folate	50–100 mg over 6 hours
	4-Methylpyrazole (investigational)	
Methemoglobinemia	Methylene blue 1%	1–2 mg/kg (0.1–0.2 mL/kg)
Narcotics	Naloxone	
Organophosphates	Atropine	0.1–0.5 mg/kg initial dose with additional doses as needed to counteract bronchorrhea
	Pralidoxime	25–50 mg/kg (up to 1 g); for severe cases, consider 10–15 mg/kg/hr infusion
Phenothiazines (dystonia)	Diphenhydramine	1–2 mg/kg IM or IV
	Benztropine	1–2 mg/kg IM or IV

IM, intramuscularly; IV, intravenously; FDA, Food and Drug Administration; NaEDTA, sodium ethylenediaminetetraacetic acid; PO, orally.
[a] Consider for possible cyanide inhalation if the patient suffers from smoke inhalation.

Table 103. Epidemiologic Aspects of Food Poisoning

Organism	Pathogenesis	Source	Prevention
Salmonella	Infection	Meats, poultry, eggs, dairy products	Proper cooking and food handling, pasteurization
Staphylococcus	Preformed enterotoxin	Meats, poultry, potato salad, cream-filled pastry, cheese, sausage	Careful food handling, rapid refrigeration
Clostridium prefringens	Enterotoxin	Meats, poultry	Avoid delay in serving foods, avoid cooling and rewarming foods
Clostridium botulinum	Preformed neurotoxin	Honey, home-canned foods, uncooked foods	Proper refrigeration (see text)
Vibrio parahaemolyticus	Infection enterotoxin	Sea fish, seawater, shellfish	Proper refrigeration
Bacillus cereus			
Diarrheal type	Sporulation enterotoxin	Many prepared foods	Proper refrigeration
Vomiting type	Preformed toxin	Cooked or fried rice, vegetables, meats, cereal, puddings	Proper refrigeration of cooked rice and other foods
Enterohemorrhagic E. coli 0157-H7	Cytotoxins	Milk, beef	Thorough cooking of beef, consumption of pasteurized milk products
Enterotoxigenic E. coli (traveler's diarrhea)	Enterotoxin	Food or water	Prognosis is not recommended for infants and young children

Table 104. Clinical Aspects of Food Poisoning

Organism	Incubation	Symptoms	Duration	Treatment
Bacillus cereus	Vomiting toxin 1–6 hr Diarrhea toxin 6–24 hr	Vomiting ± diarrhea; fever uncommon	8–24 hr	None
Brucella	Several days to months; usually >30 days	Weakness, fever, headache chills, arthralgia, weight loss; splenomegaly		Bactrim, tetracycline
Campylobacter	2–10 days; usually 2–5 days	Diarrhea (often bloody), abdominal pain, fever		Severe infection or immunocompromised; erythromycin, Cipro, or Norfloxacin
Clostridia botulinum	2 hr–8 days; usually 12–48 hr	Poor feeding, weak cry, constipation, diplopia, blurred vision, resp weakness; symmetric descending paralysis		Supportive, trivalent equine antitoxin to prevent further paralysis
Clostridia perfringens	6–24 hr	Diarrhea, abdominal cramps, vomiting and fever uncommon	<24 hr	None
Escherichia coli	→	→		Antibiotics in systemic infections
E. coli 0157:H7	1–10 days; usually 3–4 days	Diarrhea (often bloody), abdominal cramps, little or no fever. Can cause HUS.	5–10 days	Supportive
ETEC	6–48 hr	Diarrhea, abdominal cramps, nausea, fever, and vomiting; uncommon	5–10 days	Supportive
Listeria monocytogenes	2–6 wk	Meningitis, neonatal sepsis, fever	Variable	Ampicillin and gentamicin
Nontyphoidal Salmonella	6–48 hr	Diarrhea often with fever and abdominal cramps	<7 days	None unless <3 months or immunocompromised
Salmonella typi	3–60 days; usually 7–14 days	Fever, anorexia, malaise, headache, myalgias, ± diarrhea or constipation	3–4 wk	Chloramphenicol, ampicillin, amoxicillin, Bactrim, Cefotaxime, Ceftriaxone
Shigella	12 hr–6 days; usually 2–4 days	Diarrhea (often bloody), frequently fever, abdominal cramps	1 day–1 month	Bactrim, Cipro
Staphylococcus aureus	30 min–8 hr; usually 2–4 hr	Vomiting, diarrhea	<24 hr	None
Vibriosis	4–30 hr	Diarrhea, cramps, nausea, vomiting	Self limited	Usually none. Treatment for patients with liver disease or immunocompromised: Cefotaxime, gentamicin, Chloramphenicol, Tetracycline
Yersinia enterocolitica	1–10 days; usually 4–6 days	Diarrhea, abdominal pain (often severe), mesenteric adenitis, pseudo-appendicular syndrome	1–3 wks	Septicemia or enterocolitis in immunocompromised: Cefotaxime, aminoglycosides, tetracycline, Bactrim, chloramphenicol

Table 105. Nomogram for Estimating Severity of Acute Poisoning

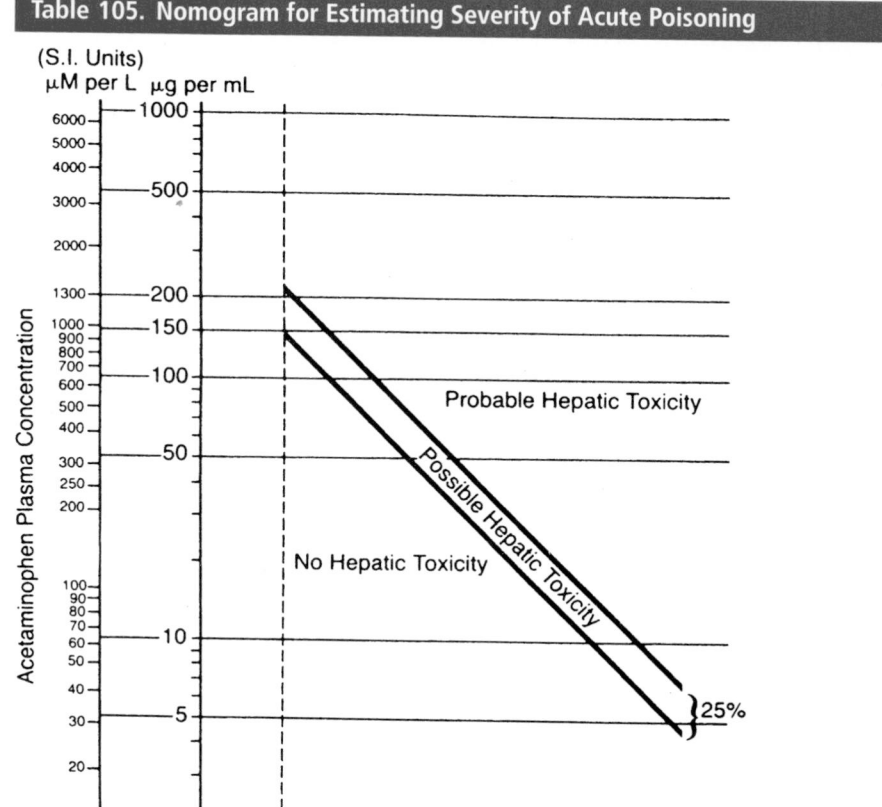

(S.I. Units)

μM per L   μg per mL

Acetaminophen Plasma Concentration

Probable Hepatic Toxicity

Possible Hepatic Toxicity

No Hepatic Toxicity

}25%

Hours After Ingestion

Table 106. Poisonous Plants

The following are a few common plants that are toxic:

Azalea	Laurel
Buttercup	Lily-of-the-valley
Calla lily	Mistletoe
Creeping Charlie—	Morning glory
ground ivy	Nightshade
Daffodil	Periwinkle
Delphinium	Philodendron
Elderberry	Poison ivy
Holly berries	Poison oak
Hyacinth bulbs	Rhododendron
Hydrangea	Sweet pea
Iris	Tomato vines
Ivy (Boston and	Tulip
English)	Wisteria
Jimson weed	Yew
Larkspur	

Table 107. Helpful Specific Drug Levels

Drug	Time to Peak Blood Level (Hours Postingestion)	Potential Intervention
Acetaminophen	4	N-Acetylcysteine administration
Carbamazepine	2–4[a],[b]	. . .
Carboxyhemoglobin	Immediate	Hyperbaric oxygen therapy
Digoxin	2–4	Fab (digoxin antibody) fragment
Ethanol	1/2–1[b]	. . .
Ethylene glycol	1/2–1	Ethanol infusion and hemodialysis
Iron	2–4	Deferoxamine administration
Isopropanol	1/2–1[b]	. . .
Lead	5 weeks[a]	Chelation and environmental abatement
Lithium	2–4	Hemodialysis
Methanol	1/2–1	Ethanol infusion and hemodialysis
Methemoglobinemia	Immediate	Methylene blue administration
Phenobarbital	2–4	Alkaline diuresis, multiple-dose activated charcoal
Phenytoin	1–2[a]	Multiple-dose activated charcoal
Salicylates	6–12[a]	Alkaline diuresis, multiple-dose activated charcoal, hemodialysis
Theophylline	1–36[a]	Multiple-dose activated charcoal, whole-bowel irrigation, charcoal hemoperfusion, hemodialysis

[a] Repeated measurement of levels is necessary because of significant variation in time to reach to peak level.
[b] The peak level is predictive of toxicity and clinical course. Adapted from Weisman RS, Howland MA, Verebey K. The toxicology laboratory. In: Goldfrank LR, Flomenbaum NE, Lewin NA, et al., eds. *Goldfrank's toxicologic emergencies,* 5th ed. East Norwalk, CT: Appleton & Lange, 1994:105.

Table 108. Regimens for the Treatment of Pelvic Inflammatory Disease (PID) in Adolescents

Outpatient regimens
  Regimen A
    Ofloxacin, 400 mg PO twice daily for 14 days
                    PLUS
    Metronidazole, 500 mg PO twice daily for 14 days
  Regimen B
    Ceftriaxone, 250 mg IM once
                    OR
    Cefoxitin (2 mg IM) plus probenecid (1 g PO) in a single dose concurrently once
                    OR
    Another parenteral third-generation cephalosporin (e.g., ceftizoxime or cefotaxime)
                    PLUS
    Doxycycline, 100 mg orally twice daily for 14 days
Inpatient regimens
  Parenteral regimen A
    Cefotetan, 2 g IV every 12 hours
                    OR
    Cefoxitin, 2 g IV every 6 hours
                    PLUS
    Doxycycline, 100 mg IV or PO every 12 hours
  Parenteral regimen B
    Clindamycin, 900 mg IV every 8 hours
                    PLUS
    Gentamicin loading dose IV or IM (2 mg/kg of body weight), followed by a maintenance dose (1.5 mg/kg) every 8 hours; single daily dosing may be substituted

The safety and effectiveness of fluoroquinolones (e.g., ciprofloxacin, ofloxacin, nurfloxacin, enoxacin) in patients younger than 18 years, pregnant women, and lactating women has not been established; therefore, fluoroquinolones are presently not recommended in these patients.
IM, intramuscularly; IV, intravenously; PO, orally.

Table 109. Uncomplicated Gonococcal Infection: Treatment in Children Beyond the Newborn Period and in Adolescents. Recommended Antimicrobial Regimens Include Therapy for Presumed Concomitant Infection with *Chlamydia trachomatis*[a]

Disease	Prepubertal Children Who Weigh <100 LB (45 kg)	Disease	Patients Who Weigh >100 LB (45 kg) and Are 9 Years or Older
Uncomplicated vulvovaginitis, urethritis, proctitis, or pharyngitis	Ceftriaxone, 125 mg IM,[b] in a single dose **OR** Spectinomycin[c] (max 2 g), IM, in a single dose **PLUS** Erythromycin,[e] 40 mg/kg/d in divided doses for 7 d	Uncomplicated endocervicitis, or urethritis	Ceftriaxone, 125 mg IM,[b] in a single dose **OR** Ciprofloxacin,[d] 500 mg orally, in a single dose **OR** Cefixime, 400 mg orally, in a single dose **OR** Oftoxacin,[d] 400 mg orally, in a single dose **OR** Spectinomycin,[c] 2 g IM, in a single dose **PLUS** Doxycycline, 100 mg orally, twice daily for 7 d[f] **OR** Azithromycin, 1 g orally, in a single dose

[a] Hospitalization should be considered, especially for patients who have been treated as outpatients and have failed to respond, and for those who are unlikely to adhere to treatment regimens.
[b] Some clinicians believe the discomfort of an IM injection can be reduced by using 1% lidocaine as a diluent.
[c] Spectinomycin is not recommended for treatment of pharyngeal infections; in persons who cannot take a cephalosporin, a quinolone, or spectinomycin, a 5-d oral regimen of trimethoprim-sulfamethoxazole may be given.
[d] Quinolones are contraindicated for persons younger than 18 years, pregnant women, and nursing women.
[e] Doxycycline can be given instead of erythromycin if the child is 9 years or older.
[f] Tetracycline, 500 mg, four times daily, can be substituted for doxycycline.
From American Academy of Pediatrics. In: Peter G, ed. *1994 Red book: Report of the Commitee on Infectious Diseases*, 23rd ed. Elk Grove Village, IL: American Academy of Pediatrics, 1994:199, with permission.

Table 110. Complicated Gonococcal Infection: Treatment for Children Beyond the Newborn Period and for Adolescents[a]

Disease	Prepubertal Children Who Weigh <100 LB (45 kg)	Disease	Patients Who Weigh >100 LB (45 kg) and Are 9 Years or Older
Ophthalmia, peritonitis, bacteremia, or arthritis	Ceftriaxone, 50 mg/kg/d (max 1 g/d) IV or IM,[c] once daily for 7 d	Gonococcal pharyngitis Pelvic inflammatory disease	Ceftriaxone, 125 mg IM,[c] in a single dose See Table 86

[a] In all cases, in addition to the recommended treatment for gonococcal infection, doxycycline (100 mg orally, twice daily for 7 d), tetracycline (500 mg, 4 times daily for 7 d), or azithromycin (1 g orally, in a single dose) is recommended on the presumption that the patient has concomitant infection with Chlamydia trachomatis, for children younger than 9 y and pregnant women, erythromycin is recommended.

[b] Hospitalization is required; follow-up cultures are necessary to ensure that treatment has been effective.

[c] Some clinicians believe the discomfort of IM injection can be reduced by using 1% lidocaine as a diluent.

[d] Such as the arthritis-dermatitis syndrome.

[e] Spectinomycin is not recommended for treatment of pharyngeal gonococcal infection. For patients who cannot take a cephalosporin, spectinomycin, or a quinolone, a 5-d oral regimen of trimethoprim-sulfamethoxazole may be given.

[f] Alternatively, parenteral therapy can be discontinued 24–48 h after improvement begins and a 7-d course is completed with an appropriate oral antimicrobial. Some experts advise a 10- to 14-d course of therapy.

From American Academy of Pediatrics. In: Peter G, ed. *1994 Red Book: Report of the Committee on Infectious Diseases,* 23rd ed. Elk Grove Village, IL: American Academy of Pediatrics, 1994:200, with permission.

Table 111. Late Effects of Chemotherapy and Radiation

Chemotherapy Agent	Possible Late Effects
Cyclophosphamide	Azoospermia, amenorrhea, hemorrhagic cystitis, secondary malignancies
Doxorubicin, daunomycin	Cardiomyopathy/Pericarditis, secondary leukemia
Methotrexate, actinomycin	Avascular necrosis, hepatitis or cirrhosis, learning disabilities with intrathecal use
Vincristine	Neuropathies
Steroids	Obesity, avascular necrosis, osteoporosis, cataracts
Cisplatin	Gynecomastia, nephritis, thrombotic thrombocytopenic purpura
Etoposide	Secondary leukemia
Radiation	
Cranium/Brain	Short stature or short trunk, obesity, learning disabilities, leukoencephalopathy, cranial neuropathies, alopecia, cataracts, hypothyroidism, second malignancies (brain, thyroid)
Head and neck	Nasolacrimal duct obstruction, chronic conjunctivitis, chronic otitis media, alopecia, cataracts, dental abnormalities, voice changes, facial deformities, neuropathies, esophagitis, second malignancies (thyroid, soft tissue sarcomas, bone tumors)
Mediastinum	Cardiomyopathy, hypothyroidism, second malignancies (thyroid, acute myeloid leukemia, breast cancer), pneumonitis/fibrosis, reduced cell-mediated immunity
Lungs	Pneumonitis or fibrosis
Spine	Short stature or short trunk, scoliosis, hypothyroidism, second malignancies (thyroid), delayed puberty
Bones	Atrophy or hypoplasia, avascular necrosis, osteoporosis, second malignancies (bone and soft-tissue sarcomas), osteochondromas
Total nodes	Reduced cell-mediated immunity, bone marrow dysfunction

Table 112. Red Eye: Common Causes by Location

Conjunctiva	Adnexa	Globe
Infectious conjunctivitis	Chalazion/Hordeolum	Corneal abrasion
Neonatal conjunctivitis	Dacryocystitis	Foreign body
Allergic conjunctivitis	Orbital cellulitis	
Periorbital cellulitis		

Table 113. Human Papilloma Viruses: Preferred Sites of Infectivity

Clinical Type	HPV Type
Verruca vulgaris (common warts)	1, 2, 4, 7, 26, 27, 29
Verruca plana (flat warts)	3, 10, 28, 41
Verruca plantaris (plantar warts)	1, 2, 4
Anogenital warts	1–6, 10, 11, 13, 16, 18, 31, 33, 35, 39, 41, 42
Laryngeal warts	6, 11, 13, 30, 40
Anogenital carcinoma	11, 16, 18, 31, 33, 42, 47
Bowenoid papulosis	16, 18, 30
Epidermodysplasia verruciformis	5, 8–10, 12, 14, 15, 17, 19–25, 16–38, 40

Table 114. Proper Child Safety Seat Use Chart: Buckle Everyone; Children Age 12 and Under Sit in Back!

	Infants	Toddler	Young Children
Weight	Birth to 1 year up to 20–22 lbs	Over 1 year and >20–40 lbs	>40–80 lbs
Type of seat	Infant only or rear-facing convertible	Convertible/forward-facing	Belt positioning booster seat
Seat position	Rear-facing only	Forward facing	Forward facing
Guidelines	Children to 1 year and at least 20 lbs in rear-facing seats Harness straps at or below shoulder level	Harness straps should be at or above shoulders Most seats require top slot for forward-facing	Belt positioning booster seats must be used with both lap and shoulder belts Make sure the lap belt fits low and tight across the lap/upper thigh area and the shoulder belt fits snug crossing the chest and shoulder to avoid abdominal injuries
Warning	All children age 12 and under should ride in the back seat	All children age 12 and under should ride in the back seat	All children age 12 and under should ride in the back seat

From National Highway Traffic Safety Administration, *www.nhtsa.dot.gov.*

Table 115. Pruritus

Causes of Pruritus in Children

Most Common	Less Common	Rare

Atopic dermatitis (eczema)
Contact dermatitis
Allergens: Plants (Rhus dermatitis: "Poison ivy"), cosmetics, dyes, systemic and topical medications (see "Differential Diagnosis")
Contact irritants (see table)
Cutaneous infections: Varicella-zoster virus (chicken pox), tinea infections, pinworm
Papular urticaria: Bites of fleas, mosquitos, etc.
Pediculosis (lice)
Mites: Scabies, chiggers
Seborrheic dermatitis
Xerosis (dry skin):
    Excess bathing
    Low humidity
	Anaphylaxis
	Cholestasis: Drug-induced (e.g., total parenteral nutrition, estrogens, phenothiazines, allopurinol)
	Extrahepatic biliary obstruction, biliary cirrhosis
	Cutaneous infections:
	    Cutaneous larva migrans "creeping eruption"
	    Hookworm, Cercariasis, Trichinosis
	Myiasis (maggots)
	Neurotic excoriations
	Chronic renal failure—with or without "uremic frost"
	Hepatic disease
	Hematopoietic neoplasms:
	    Hodgkin disease, leukemia, lymphoma
	Iron deficiency anemia
		Collagen-vascular disorders: Systemic lupus erythematosus, juvenile rheumatoid arthritis
		Congenital ectodermal disorders
		Systemic infections: HIV/AIDS, Parvovirus B19, Giardiasis, Ascariasis
		Endocrinologic disorders: Carcinoid syndrome, diabetes mellitus, hyper/hypothyroidism, hypoparathyroidism
		Neurologic syndromes: Cerebral abscess or tumor, multiple sclerosis
		Erythropoietic protoporphyria
		Psychosomatic disorders
		Solid organ neoplasms
		Polycythemia vera
		Mastocytosis

Note: Page numbers followed by f and t indicates figure and table respectively.

CCS0512